Optum

Coding Companion

AF824423

Cardiology/ Cardiothoracic/ Vascular Surgery

A comprehensive illustrated guide to coding and reimbursement

2025

optumcoding.com

Publisher's Notice

Coding Companion for Cardiology/Cardiothoracic/Vascular Surgery is designed to be an authoritative source of information about coding and reimbursement issues affecting cardiology, cardiovascular surgery, and vascular surgery procedures. Every effort has been made to verify accuracy and all information is believed reliable at the time of publication. Absolute accuracy cannot be guaranteed, however. This publication is made available with the understanding that the publisher is not engaged in rendering legal or other services that require a professional license.

American Medical Association Notice

Our Commitment to Accuracy

Optum is committed to producing accurate and reliable materials.

To report corrections, please email customerassistance@optum.com. You can also reach customer service by calling 1.800.464.3649, option 1.

Copyright

Made in the USA

ISBN 978-1-62254-920-7

Acknowledgments

Marianne Randall, CPC, *Senior Product Manager*
Stacy Perry, *Manager, Desktop Publishing*
Loraine Hewitt, *Subject Matter Expert*
Leanne Patterson, CPC, *Subject Matter Expert*
Tracy Betzler, *Senior Desktop Publishing Specialist*
Hope M. Dunn, *Senior Desktop Publishing Specialist*
Katie Russell, *Desktop Publishing Specialist*
Kimberli Turner, *Editor*

Subject Matter Experts

Leanne Patterson, CPC

Ms. Patterson has more than 20 years of experience in the health care profession. She has an extensive background in professional component coding, with proven expertise in assignment of E/M codes, general surgery coding, medical record documentation improvement, and HIPAA compliance. Her experience includes serving as Director of Compliance, conducting chart-to-claim audits, and physician education. She has been responsible for coding and denial management in large multi-specialty physician practices, and most recently has been part of a team developing content for products related to ICD-10-CM. Ms. Patterson is credentialed by and is a member of the AAPC.

Product Updates

Significant updates to this manual (CPT and HCPCS Level II codes and RVUs) will also be provided on our product updates page at Optumcoding.com, which can be accessed at the following: https://www.optumcoding.com/ProductUpdates/

Password: CAS25

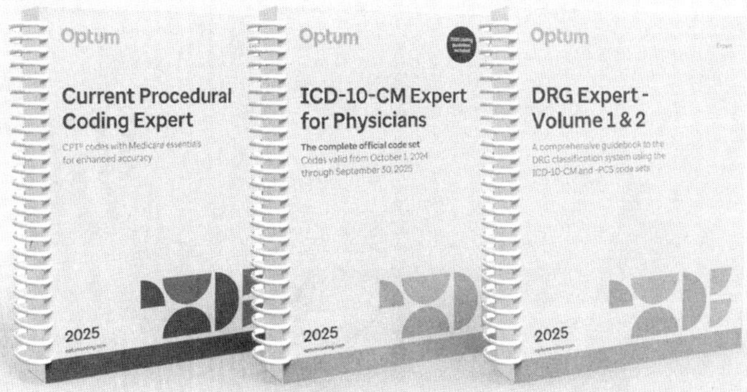

Ready to renew?

We make it easy

Optum offers many convenient ways to renew your coding resources so you always have the most up-to-date code sets when you need them.

Order online at **optumcoding.com** and see purchase history, track shipments, create a wish list or update your contact information.

Away from your computer? No problem. We also offer the following offline renewal options:

Phone: 1-800-464-3649, option 1

Fax: 1-801-982-4033 *(include purchase order)*

Mail: Optum, P.O. Box 88050, Chicago, IL 60680-9920
(include payment/purchase order)

Lock in your product price now and avoid rate increases later

Optum offers multi-year contracts for most book resources and online coding software. Call 1-800-464-3649, option 1, to learn how to lock in your rate.

Optum no longer accepts credit cards by fax or mail.

*Shipping charges and taxes still apply and cannot be used toward your account balance for eRewards coupons. Coupons expire 6 months after they are earned. Once a coupon expires, it will no longer be available for use. You must be signed in to your online account to have your purchases tracked for reward purposes. Offer valid online only – coupons cannot be earned with orders placed offline and coupons cannot be applied to orders placed offline. Customers who are already part of our Medallion or Reseller programs are not eligible for our eRewards program.

Optum

Contents

Getting Started with Coding Companion i
- CPT/HCPCS Codes i
- ICD-10-CM..........i
- Detailed Code Information i
- Appendix Codes and Descriptions..........i
- CCI Edits, RVUs, HCPCS, and Other Coding Updates i
- Index..........i
- General Guidelines i
- Sample Page and Key..........i

Evaluation and Management (E/M) Services Guidelines v

Cardiology/Cardiothoracic and Vascular Procedures and Services..........1
- E/M Services 1
- General (Musculoskeletal) 44
- Neck and Thorax..........46
- Larynx 63
- Trachea and Bronchi 68
- Lungs and Pleura 72
- Heart and Pericardium 142
- Arteries and Veins.......... 355
- Lymph Nodes.......... 651
- Mediastinum.......... 654
- Abdomen.......... 659
- Thyroid Gland 664
- Parathyroid.......... 665
- Nervous System 668
- Medicine 669
- HCPCS.......... 747
- Appendix 750

Correct Coding Initiative Update 30.3 811

Index 831

Getting Started with Coding Companion

Coding Companion for Cardiology/Cardiothoracic/Vascular Surgery is designed to be a guide to the specialty procedures classified in the CPT® book. It is structured to help coders understand procedures and translate physician narrative into correct CPT codes by combining many clinical resources into one, easy-to-use source book.

The book also allows coders to validate the intended code selection by providing an easy-to-understand explanation of the procedure and associated conditions or indications for performing the various procedures. As a result, data quality and reimbursement will be improved by providing code-specific clinical information and helpful tips regarding the coding of procedures.

CPT/HCPCS Codes

For ease of use, evaluation and management codes related to cardiology/cardiothoracic/vascular surgery are listed first in the *Coding Companion*. All other CPT codes in *Coding Companion* are listed in ascending numeric order. Included in the code set are all surgery, radiology, laboratory, and medicine codes pertinent to the specialty. Each CPT/HCPCS code is followed by its official CPT code description.

Resequencing of CPT Codes

The American Medical Association (AMA) employs a resequenced numbering methodology. According to the AMA, there are instances where a new code is needed within an existing grouping of codes, but an unused code number is not available to keep the range sequential. In the instance where the existing codes were not changed or had only minimal changes, the AMA assigned a code out of numeric sequence with the other related codes being grouped together. The resequenced codes and their descriptions have been placed with their related codes, out of numeric sequence.

CPT codes within the Optum *Coding Companion* series display in their resequenced order. **Resequenced codes are enclosed in brackets [ ] for easy identification.**

ICD-10-CM

The most current ICD-10-CM codes are provided, each listed with their full official description. Refer to the ICD-10-CM book for more ICD-10-CM coding information.

Detailed Code Information

One or more columns are dedicated to each procedure or service or to a series of similar procedures/services. Following the specific CPT code and its narrative, is a combination of features.

Appendix Codes and Descriptions

Some CPT/HCPCS codes are presented in a less comprehensive format in the appendix. The CPT/HCPCS codes appropriate to the specialty are included in the appendix with the official CPT/HCPCS code description, followed by an easy-to-understand explanation, relative value units, and Medicare edits. The Relative Value Unit/Medicare Edits table will not be included with any CPT/HCPCS code with a "0" (zero) value.

The codes in the appendix are presented in the following order:

- HCPCS
- E/M
- Surgery
- Radiology
- Pathology and Laboratory
- Medicine Services
- Category III

Category II codes are not published in this book. Refer to the CPT book for code descriptions.

CCI Edits, RVUs, HCPCS, and Other Coding Updates

The *Coding Companion* includes the list of codes from the official Centers for Medicare and Medicaid Services' National Correct Coding Policy Manual for Part B Medicare Contractors that are considered to be an integral part of the comprehensive code or mutually exclusive of it and should not be reported separately. The codes in the Correct Coding Initiative (CCI) section are from version 30.3, the most current version available at press time. CCI edits are updated quarterly and will be posted on the product updates page listed below. The website address is http://www.optumcoding.com/ProductUpdates/. The 2025 edition password is: **CAS25.** Log in frequently to ensure you receive the most current updates.

Index

A comprehensive index is provided for easy access to the codes. The index entries have several axes. A code can be looked up by its procedural name or by the diagnoses commonly associated with it. Codes are also indexed anatomically. For example:

32800 Repair lung hernia through chest wall

could be found in the index under the following main terms:

Hernia
Repair
Lung, 32800

or **Repair**
Lung
Hernia, 32800

General Guidelines

Providers

The AMA advises coders that while a particular service or procedure may be assigned to a specific section, it is not limited to use only by that specialty group (see paragraphs two and three under "Instructions for Use of the CPT Codebook" on page xv of the CPT Book). Additionally, the procedures and services listed throughout the book are for use by any qualified physician or other qualified health care professional or entity (e.g., hospitals, laboratories, or home health agencies). Keep in mind that there may be other policies or guidance that can affect who may report a specific service.

Supplies

Some payers may allow physicians to separately report drugs and other supplies when reporting the place of service as office or other nonfacility setting. Drugs and supplies are to be reported by the facility only when performed in a facility setting.

Professional and Technical Component

Radiology and some pathology codes often have a technical and a professional component. When physicians do not own their own equipment and send their patients to outside testing facilities, they should append modifier 26 to the procedural code to indicate they performed only the professional component.

Sample Page and Key

The following pages provide a sample page from the book displaying the format of *Coding Companion* with each element identified and explained.

33285-33286

1

33285 Insertion, subcutaneous cardiac rhythm monitor, including programming
33286 Removal, subcutaneous cardiac rhythm monitor

2

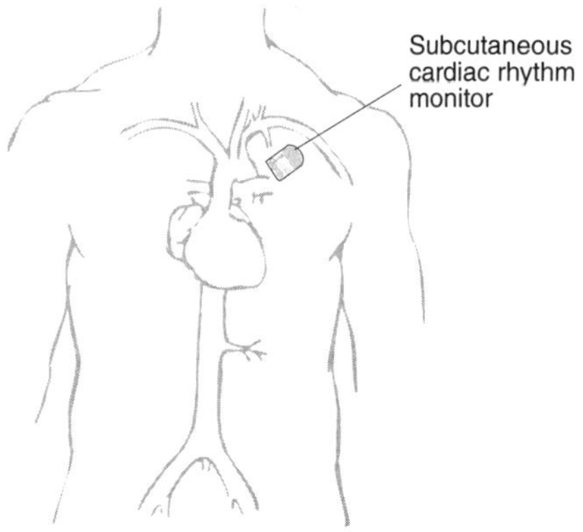

Explanation

3

The physician implants or removes an electronic device that is capable of recording heartrates and rhythms for over one year (subcutaneous cardiac rhythm monitor, cardiac event recorder, implantable loop recorder or ILR). In 33285, the physician uses a scalpel to make a small parasternal incision and dissects down to the level of subcutaneous tissue located over the left pectoral or mammary area. The monitor is implanted into the subcutaneous tissue. Electrodes that sense heart activity are located on the surface of the monitor, making it unnecessary to place transvenous leads. The device continuously and automatically monitors the heart's electrical activity when sensing the patient's rapid, irregular, or slow heartrate or can also be prompted by the patient in the course of experiencing symptoms. Programming of the device is included in this service. In 33286, the physician removes the monitor when sufficient information regarding the heart's activities has been obtained or when the batteries run out by incising down to the level of the recorder and removing it. In either surgery, the incision is closed with sutures. This type of recorder is capable of storing many separate events. When appropriate, a "programmer" is used by the physician to retrieve the information that can be displayed, stored, or printed.

Coding Tips

4

Code 33285 includes programming. For subsequent analysis and/or reprogramming, see 93285, 93291, and 93298.

ICD-10-CM Diagnostic Codes

5

G90.09	Other idiopathic peripheral autonomic neuropathy
I25.2	Old myocardial infarction
I44.0	Atrioventricular block, first degree
I44.1	Atrioventricular block, second degree
I44.2	Atrioventricular block, complete
I45.5	Other specified heart block
I45.6	Pre-excitation syndrome
I47.0	Re-entry ventricular arrhythmia
I47.11	Inappropriate sinus tachycardia, so stated
I47.21	Torsades de pointes
T82.518A	Breakdown (mechanical) of other cardiac and vascular devices and implants, initial encounter
T82.528A	Displacement of other cardiac and vascular devices and implants, initial encounter
T82.538A	Leakage of other cardiac and vascular devices and implants, initial encounter
T82.598A	Other mechanical complication of other cardiac and vascular devices and implants, initial encounter
T82.7XXA	Infection and inflammatory reaction due to other cardiac and vascular devices, implants and grafts, initial encounter
T82.827A	Fibrosis due to cardiac prosthetic devices, implants and grafts, initial encounter
T82.837A	Hemorrhage due to cardiac prosthetic devices, implants and grafts, initial encounter
T82.847A	Pain due to cardiac prosthetic devices, implants and grafts, initial encounter
T82.867A	Thrombosis due to cardiac prosthetic devices, implants and grafts, initial encounter
T82.897A	Other specified complication of cardiac prosthetic devices, implants and grafts, initial encounter
Z45.09	Encounter for adjustment and management of other cardiac device

Not all ICD-10-CM Codes are shown. Sample only.

Associated HCPCS Codes

6

C1764	Event recorder, cardiac (implantable)
E0616	Implantable cardiac event recorder with memory, activator, and programmer

AMA: 33285 2019,Oct; 2019,Apr **33286** 2019,Apr

Relative Value Units/Medicare Edits

7

Non-Facility RVU	Work	PE	MP	Total
33285	1.53	122.46	0.35	124.34
33286	1.5	2.03	0.34	3.87
Facility RVU	**Work**	**PE**	**MP**	**Total**
33285	1.53	0.69	0.35	2.57
33286	1.5	0.68	0.34	2.52

	FUD	Status	MUE	Modifiers				IOM Reference
33285	0	A	1(3)	51	N/A	N/A	N/A	None
33286	0	A	1(3)	51	N/A	N/A	N/A	

* with documentation

Terms To Know

8

event recorder. Portable, ambulatory heart monitor worn by the patient that makes electrocardiographic recordings of the length and frequency of aberrant cardiac rhythm to help diagnose heart conditions and to assess pacemaker functioning or programming.

implantable cardiovascular monitor. Implantable electronic device that stores cardiovascular physiologic data such as intracardiac pressure waveforms collected from internal sensors or data such as weight and blood pressure collected from external sensors. The information stored in these devices is used as an aid in managing patients with heart failure and other cardiac conditions that are non-rhythm related. The data may be transmitted via local telemetry or remotely to a surveillance technician or an internet-based file server.

1. CPT/HCPCS Codes and Descriptions

This edition of *Coding Companion* is updated with CPT and HCPCS codes for year 2025.

The following icons are used in *Coding Companion:*

- ● This CPT code is new for 2025.
- ▲ This CPT code description is revised for 2025.
- + This CPT code is an add-on code.

Add-on codes are not subject to bilateral or multiple procedure rules, reimbursement reduction, or appending modifier 50 or 51. Add-on codes describe additional intraservice work associated with the primary procedure performed by the same physician on the same date of service and are not reported as stand-alone procedures. Add-on codes for procedures performed on bilateral structures are reported by listing the add-on code twice.

- ★ This CPT code is identified by CPT as appropriate for audio-visual telemedicine services. Note: This icon is not appended to the synchronous audio-video visit codes 98000-98007.

The Centers for Medicare and Medicaid Services (CMS) have identified services that may be performed via telehealth. Payers may require telehealth/telemedicine to be reported with place of service 02 Telehealth Provided Other than the Patient's Home or 10 Telehealth Provided in Patient's Home and modifier 93 or 95 appended. If specialized equipment is used at the originating site, HCPCS Level II code Q3014 may be reported. Individual payers should be contacted for additional or different guidelines regarding telehealth/telemedicine services. Documentation should include the type of technology used for the treatment in addition to the patient evaluation, treatment, and consents.

According to CPT guidelines, the codes listed below may be used for reporting audio-only telemedicine services, when modifier 93 Synchronous Telemedicine Service Rendered Via Telephone or Other Real-Time Interactive Audio-Only Telecommunications System, is appended. These procedures involve electronic communication using interactive telecommunications equipment that at a minimum includes audio.

90785	90791	90792	90832	90833	90834	90836
90837	90838	90839	90840	90845	90846	90847
92507	92508	92521	92522	92523	92524	96041
96110	96116	96121	96156	96158	96159	96160
96161	96164	96165	96167	96168	96170	96171
97802	97803	97804	99406	99407	99408	99409
99497	99498					

2. Illustrations

The illustrations that accompany the *Coding Companion* series provide coders a better understanding of the medical procedures referenced by the codes and data. The graphics offer coders a visual link between the technical language of the operative report and the cryptic descriptions accompanying the codes. Although most pages will have an illustration, there will be some pages that do not.

3. Explanation

Every CPT code or series of similar codes is presented with its official CPT code description. However, sometimes these descriptions do not provide the coder with sufficient information to make a proper code selection. In *Coding Companion*, an easy-to-understand step-by-step clinical description of the procedure is provided. Technical language that might be used by the physician is included and defined. *Coding Companion* describes a common method of performing each procedure.

4. Coding Tips

Coding tips provide information on how the code should be used, provides related CPT codes, and offers help concerning common billing errors, modifier usage, and anesthesia. This information comes from consultants and subject matter experts at Optum and from the coding guidelines provided in the CPT book and by the Centers for Medicare and Medicaid Services (CMS).

5. ICD-10-CM Diagnostic Codes

ICD-10-CM diagnostic codes listed are common diagnoses or reasons the procedure may be necessary. This list in most cases is inclusive to the specialty. Some ICD-10-CM codes are further identified with the following icons:

- N Newborn: 0
- P Pediatric: 0-17
- M Maternity: 9-64
- A Adult: 15-124
- ☑ Laterality

Please note that in some instances the ICD-10-CM codes for only one side of the body (right) have been listed with the CPT code. The associated ICD-10-CM codes for the other side and/or bilateral may also be appropriate. Codes that refer to the right or left are identified with the ☑ icon to alert the user to check for laterality. In some cases, not every possible code is listed and the ICD-10-CM book should be referenced for other valid codes.

6. Associated HCPCS Codes

Medicare and some other payers require the use of HCPCS Level II codes and not CPT codes when reporting certain services. The HCPCS codes and their description are displayed in this field. If there is not a HCPCS code for this service, this field will not be displayed.

7. AMA References

The AMA references for *CPT Assistant* are listed by CPT code, with the most recent reference listed first. Generally only the last six years of references are listed.

8. Relative Value Units/Medicare Edits

Medicare edits are provided for most codes. These Medicare edits were current as of November 2024.

The 2025 Medicare edits were not available at the time this book went to press. Updated 2025 values will be posted at https://www.optumcoding.com/ProductUpdates/. The 2025 edition password is **CAS25**.

Relative Value Units

In a resource based relative value scale (RBRVS), services are ranked based on the relative costs of the resources required to provide those services as opposed to the average fee for the service, or average prevailing Medicare charge. The Medicare RBRVS defines three distinct components affecting the value of each service or procedure:

- Physician work component, reflecting the physician's time and skill
- Practice expense (PE) component, reflecting the physician's rent, staff, supplies, equipment, and other overhead
- Malpractice (MP) component, reflecting the relative risk or liability associated with the service
- Total RVUs are a sum of the work, PE, and MP RVUs

There are two groups of RVUs listed for each CPT code. The first RVU group is for facilities (Facility RVU), which includes provider services performed in hospitals, ambulatory surgical centers, or skilled nursing facilities. The second RVU group is for nonfacilities (Non-Facility RVU), which represents provider services performed in physician offices, patient's homes, or other nonhospital settings. The appendix includes RVU components for facility and non-facility. Because no values have been established by CMS for the Category III codes, no relative value unit/grids are identified. Refer to the RBRVS tool or guide for the RVUs when the technical (modifier TC) or professional (modifier 26) component of a procedure is provided.

Medicare Follow-Up Days (FUD)

Information on the Medicare global period is provided here. The global period is the time following a surgery during which routine care by the physician is considered postoperative and included in the surgical fee. Office visits or other routine care related to the original surgery cannot be separately reported if they occur during the global period.

Status

The Medicare status indicates if the service is separately payable by Medicare. The Medicare RBRVS includes:

A Active code—separate payment may be made

B Bundled code—payment is bundled into other service

C Carrier priced—individual carrier will price the code

I Not valid—Medicare uses another code for this service

N Non-covered—service is not covered by Medicare

R Restricted—special coverage instructions apply

T Paid as only service—These codes are paid only if there are no other services payable under the Physician Fee Schedule (PFS) billed on the same date by the same practitioner. If any other services payable under the PFS are billed on the same date by the same practitioner, these services are bundled into the service(s) for which payment is made.

X Statutory exclusion—no RVUs or payment

Medically Unlikely Edits

This column provides the maximum number of units allowed by Medicare. However, it is also important to note that not every code has a Medically Unlikely Edit (MUE) available. Medicare has assigned some MUE values that are not publicly available. If there is no information in the MUE column for a particular code, this doesn't mean that there is no MUE. It may simply mean that CMS has not released information on that MUE. Watch the remittance advice for possible details on MUE denials related to those codes. If there is not a published MUE, a dash will display in the field.

An additional component of the MUE edit is the MUE Adjudication Indicator (MAI). This edit is the result of an audit by the Office of the Inspector General (OIG) that identified inappropriate billing practices that bypassed the MUE edits. These included inappropriate reporting of bilateral services and split billing.

There are three MUE Adjudication Indicators.

- 1 Line Edit
- 2 Date of Service Edit: Policy
- 3 Date of Service Edit: Clinical

The MUE will be listed followed by the MAI value. For example code 33206 has a MUE value of 1 and a MAI value of 3. This will display in the MUE field as "1(3)."

Modifiers

Medicare identifies some modifiers that are required or appropriate to report with the CPT code. When the modifiers are not appropriate, it will be indicated with N/A. Four modifiers are included.

50 Bilateral Procedures

This modifier is used to identify when the same procedure is performed bilaterally. Medicare requires one line with modifier 50 and the reimbursement is 150 percent of the allowable. Other payers may require two lines and will reduce the second procedure.

51 Multiple Procedure

Medicare and other payers reduce the reimbursement of second and subsequent procedures performed at the same session to 50 percent of the allowable. For endoscopic procedures, the reimbursement is reduced by the value of the endoscopic base code.

62*Two Surgeons

Medicare identifies procedures that may be performed by co-surgeons. The reimbursement is split between both providers. Both surgeons must report the same code when using this modifier.

80*Assistant Surgeon

An assistant surgeon is allowed if modifier 80 is listed. Reimbursement is usually 20 percent of the allowable. For Medicare it is 16 percent to account for the patient's co-pay amount.

* with documentation

Modifiers 62 and 80 may require supporting documentation to justify the co- or assistant surgeon.

Medicare Official Regulatory Information

Medicare official regulatory information provides official regulatory guidelines. Also known as the CMS Online Manual System, the Internet-only Manuals (IOM) contain official CMS information pertaining to program issuances, instructions, policies, and procedures based on statutes, regulations, guidelines, models, and directives. Optum has provided the reference for the surgery codes. The full text of guidelines can be found online at https://www.cms.gov/medicare/regulations-guidance/manuals/internet-only-manuals-ioms.

9. Terms to Know

Some codes are accompanied by general information pertinent to the procedure, labeled "Terms to Know." This information is not critical to code selection, but is a useful supplement to coders hoping to expand their knowledge of the specialty.

Evaluation and Management (E/M) Services Guidelines

E/M Guidelines Overview

The E/M guidelines have sections that are common to all E/M categories and sections that are category specific. Most of the categories and many of the subcategories of service have special guidelines or instructions unique to that category or subcategory. Where these are indicated, eg, "Hospital Inpatient and Observation Care," special instructions are presented before the listing of the specific E/M services codes. It is important to review the instructions for each category or subcategory. These guidelines are to be used by the reporting physician or other qualified health care professional to select the appropriate level of service. These guidelines do not establish documentation requirements or standards of care. The main purpose of documentation is to support care of the patient by current and future health care team(s). These guidelines are for services that require a face-to-face encounter with the patient and/or family/caregiver. (For 99211 and 99281, the face-to-face services may be performed by clinical staff.)

▶In the **Evaluation and Management** section (98000-98016, 99202-99499), there are many code categories. Each category may have specific guidelines, or the codes may include specific details. These E/M guidelines are written for the following categories:

- Office or Other Outpatient Services
- Telemedicine Services
- Hospital Inpatient and Observation Care Services
- Consultations
- Emergency Department Services
- Nursing Facility Services
- Home or Residence Services
- Prolonged Service With or Without Direct Patient Contact on the Date of an Evaluation and Management Service◀

Classification of Evaluation and Management (E/M) Services

The E/M section is divided into broad categories, such as office visits, hospital inpatient or observation care visits, and consultations. Most of the categories are further divided into two or more subcategories of E/M services. For example, there are two subcategories of office visits (new patient and established patient) and there are two subcategories of hospital inpatient and observation care visits (initial and subsequent). The subcategories of E/M services are further classified into levels of E/M services that are identified by specific codes.

The basic format of codes with levels of E/M services based on medical decision making (MDM) or time is the same. First, a unique code number is listed. Second, the place and/or type of service is specified (eg, office or other outpatient visit). Third, the content of the service is defined. Fourth, time is specified. (A detailed discussion of time is provided in the Guidelines for Selecting Level of Service Based on Time.)

The place of service and service type are defined by the location where the face-to-face encounter with the patient and/or family/caregiver occurs. For example, service provided to a nursing facility resident brought to the office is reported with an office or other outpatient code.

New and Established Patients

Solely for the purposes of distinguishing between new and established patients, **professional services** are those face-to-face services rendered by physicians and other qualified health care professionals who may report evaluation and management services. A new patient is one who has not received any professional services from the physician or other qualified health care professional or another physician or other qualified health care professional of the **exact** same specialty **and subspecialty** who belongs to the same group practice, within the past three years.

An established patient is one who has received professional services from the physician or other qualified health care professional or another physician or other qualified health care professional of the **exact** same specialty **and subspecialty** who belongs to the same group practice, within the past three years. See Decision Tree for New vs Established Patients.

In the instance where a physician or other qualified health care professional is on call for or covering for another physician or other qualified health care professional, the patient's encounter will be classified as it would have been by the physician or other qualified health care professional who is not available. When advanced practice nurses and physician assistants are working with physicians, they are considered as working in the **exact** same specialty **and subspecialty** as the physician.

No distinction is made between new and established patients in the emergency department. E/M services in the emergency department category may be reported for any new or established patient who presents for treatment in the emergency department.

The Decision Tree for New vs Established Patients is provided to aid in determining whether to report the E/M service provided as a new or an established patient encounter.

Decision Tree for New vs Established Patients

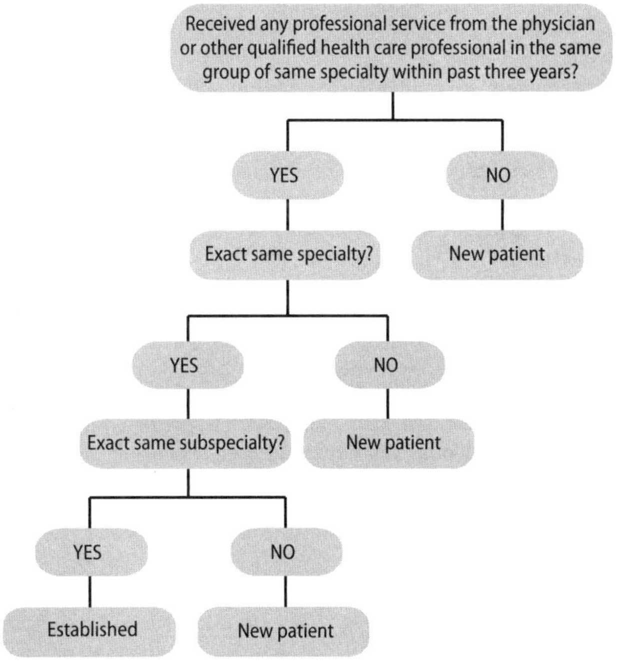

Initial and Subsequent Services

Some categories apply to both new and established patients (eg, hospital inpatient or observation care). These categories differentiate services by whether the service is the initial service or a subsequent service. For the purpose of distinguishing between initial or subsequent visits, professional services are those face-to-face services rendered by physicians and other qualified health care professionals who may report evaluation and management services. An initial service is when the patient has not received any professional services from the physician or

AMA CPT® Evaluation and Management (E/M) Services Guidelines reproduced with permission of the American Medical Association.

other qualified health care professional or another physician or other qualified health care professional of the exact same specialty and subspecialty who belongs to the same group practice, during the inpatient, observation, or nursing facility admission and stay.

A subsequent service is when the patient has received professional service(s) from the physician or other qualified health care professional or another physician or other qualified health care professional of the exact same specialty and subspecialty who belongs to the same group practice, during the admission and stay.

In the instance when a physician or other qualified health care professional is on call for or covering for another physician or other qualified health care professional, the patient's encounter will be classified as it would have been by the physician or other qualified health care professional who is not available. When advanced practice nurses and physician assistants are working with physicians, they are considered as working in the exact same specialty and subspecialty as the physician.

For reporting hospital inpatient or observation care services, a stay that includes a transition from observation to inpatient is a single stay. For reporting nursing facility services, a stay that includes transition(s) between skilled nursing facility and nursing facility level of care is the same stay.

Split or Shared Visits

Physician(s) and other qualified health care professional(s) (QHP[s]) may act as a team in providing care for the patient, working together during a single E/M service. The split or shared visits guidelines are applied to determine which professional may report the service. If the physician or other QHP performs a substantive portion of the encounter, the physician or other QHP may report the service. If code selection is based on total time on the date of the encounter, the service is reported by the professional who spent the majority of the face-to-face or non-face-to-face time performing the service. For the purpose of reporting E/M services within the context of team-based care, performance of a substantive part of the MDM requires that the physician(s) or other QHP(s) made or approved the management plan for the ***number and complexity of problems addressed at the encounter*** and takes responsibility for that plan with its inherent ***risk of complications and/or morbidity or mortality of patient management***. By doing so, a physician or other QHP has performed two of the three elements used in the selection of the code level based on MDM. If ***the amount and/or complexity of data to be reviewed and analyzed*** is used by the physician or other QHP to determine the reported code level, assessing an independent historian's narrative and the ordering or review of tests or documents do not have to be personally performed by the physician or other QHP, because the relevant items would be considered in formulating the management plan. Independent interpretation of tests and discussion of management plan or test interpretation must be personally performed by the physician or other QHP if these are used to determine the reported code level by the physician or other QHP.

Multiple Evaluation and Management Services on the Same Date

The following guidelines apply to services that a patient may receive for hospital inpatient care, observation care, or nursing facility care. For instructions regarding transitions to these settings from the office or outpatient, home or residence, or emergency department setting, see guidelines for **Hospital Inpatient and Observation Care Services or Nursing Facility Services**.

A patient may receive E/M services in more than one setting on a calendar date. A patient may also have more than one visit in the same setting on a calendar date. The guidelines for multiple E/M services on the same date address circumstances in which the patient has received multiple visits or services from the same physician or other QHP or another physician or other QHP of the exact same specialty and subspecialty who belongs to the same group practice.

Coding Tip

Instructions for Use of the CPT Codebook

When advanced practice nurses and physician assistants are working with physicians, they are considered as working in the exact same specialty and subspecialty as the physician. A "physician or other qualified health care professional" is an individual who is qualified by education, training, licensure/regulation (when applicable), and facility privileging (when applicable) who performs a professional service within his or her scope of practice and independently reports that professional service. These professionals are distinct from "clinical staff." A clinical staff member is a person who works under the supervision of a physician or other qualified health care professional, and who is allowed by law, regulation and facility policy to perform or assist in the performance of a specific professional service but does not individually report that professional service. Other policies may also affect who may report specific services.

CPT Coding Guidelines, Introduction, Instructions for Use of the CPT Codebook

Per day: The hospital inpatient and observation care services and the nursing facility services are "per day" services. When multiple visits occur over the course of a single calendar date in the same setting, a single service is reported. When using MDM for code level selection, use the aggregated MDM over the course of the calendar date. When using time for code level selection, sum the time over the course of the day using the guidelines for reporting time.

Multiple encounters in different settings or facilities: A patient may be seen and treated in different facilities (eg, a hospital-to-hospital transfer). When more than one primary E/M service is reported and time is used to select the code level for either service, only the time spent providing that individual service may be allocated to the code level selected for reporting that service. No time may be counted twice when reporting more than one E/M service. Prolonged services are also based on the same allocation and their relationship to the primary service. The designation of the facility may be defined by licensure or regulation. Transfer from a hospital bed to a nursing facility bed in a hospital with nursing facility beds is considered as two services in two facilities because there is a discharge from one type of designation to another. An intra-facility transfer for a different level of care (eg, from a routine unit to a critical care unit) does not constitute a new stay, nor does it constitute a transfer to a different facility.

Emergency department (ED) and services in other settings (same or different facilities): Time spent in an ED by a physician or other QHP who provides subsequent E/M services may be included in calculating total time on the date of the encounter when ED services are not reported and another E/M service is reported (eg, hospital inpatient and observation care services).

Discharge services and services in other facilities: Each service may be reported separately as long as any time spent on the discharge service is not counted towards the total time of a subsequent service in which code level selection for the subsequent service is based on time. This includes any hospital inpatient or observation care services (including admission and discharge services) time (99234, 99235, 99236) because these services may be selected based on MDM or time. When these services are reported with another E/M service on the same calendar date, time related to the hospital inpatient or observation care service (including admission and discharge services) may not be used for code selection of the subsequent service.

Discharge services and services in the same facility: If the patient is discharged and readmitted to the same facility on the same calendar date, report a subsequent care service instead of a discharge or initial service. For the purpose of E/M reporting, this is a single stay.

Discharge services and services in a different facility: If the patient is admitted to another facility, for the purpose of E/M reporting this is considered a different stay. Discharge and initial services may be reported as long as time spent on the discharge service is not counted towards the total time of the subsequent service reported when code level selection is based on time.

Critical care services (including neonatal intensive care services and pediatric and neonatal critical care): Reporting guidelines for intensive and critical care services that are performed on the same calendar date as another E/M service are described in the service specific section guidelines.

Transitions between office or other outpatient, home or residence, or emergency department and hospital inpatient or observation or nursing facility: See the guidelines for **Hospital Inpatient and Observation Care Services** or **Nursing Facility Services**. If the patient is seen in two settings and only one service is reported, the total time on the date of the encounter or the aggregated MDM is used for determining the level of the single reported service. If prolonged services are reported, use the prolonged services code that is appropriate for the primary service reported, regardless of where the patient was located when the prolonged services time threshold was met. The choice of the primary service is at the discretion of the reporting physician or other QHP.

Services Reported Separately

Any specifically identifiable procedure or service (ie, identified with a specific CPT code) performed on the date of E/M services may be reported separately.

The ordering and actual performance and/or interpretation of diagnostic tests/studies during a patient encounter are not included in determining the levels of E/M services when the professional interpretation of those tests/studies is reported separately by the physician or other qualified health care professional reporting the E/M service. Tests that do not require separate interpretation (eg, tests that are results only) and are analyzed as part of MDM do not count as an independent interpretation, but may be counted as ordered or reviewed for selecting an MDM level. The performance of diagnostic tests/studies for which specific CPT codes are available may be reported separately, in addition to the appropriate E/M code. The interpretation of the results of diagnostic tests/studies (ie, professional component) with preparation of a separate distinctly identifiable signed written report may also be reported separately, using the appropriate CPT code and, if required, with modifier 26 appended.

The physician or other qualified health care professional may need to indicate that on the day a procedure or service identified by a CPT code was performed, the patient's condition required a significant separately identifiable E/M service. The E/M service may be caused or prompted by the symptoms or condition for which the procedure and/or service was provided. This circumstance may be reported by adding modifier 25 to the appropriate level of E/M service. As such, different diagnoses are not required for reporting of the procedure and the E/M services on the same date.

History and/or Examination

E/M codes that have levels of services include a medically appropriate history and/or physical examination, when performed. The nature and extent of the history and/or physical examination are determined by the treating physician or other qualified health care professional reporting the service. The care team may collect information, and the patient or caregiver may supply information directly (eg, by electronic health record [EHR] portal or questionnaire) that is reviewed by the reporting physician or other qualified health care professional. The extent of history and physical examination is not an element in selection of the level of these E/M service codes.

Levels of E/M Services

Select the appropriate level of E/M services based on the following:

1. The level of the MDM as defined for each service, **or**
2. The total time for E/M services performed on the date of the encounter.

Within each category or subcategory of E/M service based on MDM or time, there are three to five levels of E/M services available for reporting purposes. Levels of E/M services are **not** interchangeable among the different categories or subcategories of service. For example, the first level of E/M services in the subcategory of office visit, new patient, does not have the same definition as the first level of E/M services in the subcategory of office visit, established patient. Each level of E/M services may be used by all physicians or other qualified health care professionals.

Guidelines for Selecting Level of Service Based on Medical Decision Making

Four types of MDM are recognized: straightforward, low, moderate, and high. The concept of the level of MDM does not apply to 99211, 99281.

MDM includes establishing diagnoses, assessing the status of a condition, and/or selecting a management option. MDM is defined by three elements. The elements are:

- ***The number and complexity of problem(s) that are addressed during the encounter.***
- ***The amount and/or complexity of data to be reviewed and analyzed.*** These data include medical records, tests, and/or other information that must be obtained, ordered, reviewed, and analyzed for the encounter. This includes information obtained from multiple sources or interprofessional communications that are not reported separately and interpretation of tests that are not reported separately. Ordering a test is included in the category of test result(s) and the review of the test result is part of the encounter and not a subsequent encounter. Ordering a test may include those considered but not selected after shared decision making. For example, a patient may request diagnostic imaging that is not necessary for their condition and discussion of the lack of benefit may be required. Alternatively, a test may normally be performed, but due to the risk for a specific patient it is not ordered. These considerations must be documented. Data are divided into three categories:
  - Tests, documents, orders, or independent historian(s). (Each unique test, order, or document is counted to meet a threshold number.)
  - Independent interpretation of tests (not separately reported).
  - Discussion of management or test interpretation with external physician or other qualified health care professional or appropriate source (not separately reported).
- ***The risk of complications and/or morbidity or mortality of patient management***. This includes decisions made at the encounter associated with diagnostic procedure(s) and treatment(s). This includes the possible management options selected and those considered but not selected after shared decision making with the patient and/or family. For example, a decision about hospitalization includes consideration of alternative levels of care. Examples may include a psychiatric patient with a sufficient degree of support in the outpatient setting or the decision to not hospitalize a patient with advanced dementia with an acute condition that would generally warrant inpatient care, but for whom the goal is palliative treatment.

Shared decision making involves eliciting patient and/or family preferences, patient and/or family education, and explaining risks and benefits of management options.

MDM may be impacted by role and management responsibility.

When the physician or other qualified health care professional is reporting a separate CPT code that includes interpretation and/or report, the interpretation and/or report is not counted toward the MDM

 ▶ ◀ = Contains new or revised text

when selecting a level of E/M services. When the physician or other qualified health care professional is reporting a separate service for discussion of management with a physician or another qualified health care professional, the discussion is not counted toward the MDM when selecting a level of E/M services.

The Levels of Medical Decision Making (MDM) table (Table 1) is a guide to assist in selecting the level of MDM for reporting an E/M services code. The table includes the four levels of MDM (ie, straightforward, low, moderate, high) and the three elements of MDM (ie, number and complexity of problems addressed at the encounter, amount and/or complexity of data reviewed and analyzed, and risk of complications and/or morbidity or mortality of patient management). To qualify for a particular level of MDM, two of the three elements for that level of MDM must be met or exceeded.

Examples in the table may be more or less applicable to specific settings of care. For example, the decision to hospitalize applies to the outpatient or nursing facility encounters, whereas the decision to escalate hospital level of care (eg, transfer to ICU) applies to the hospitalized or observation care patient. See also the introductory guidelines of each code family section.

The elements listed in Table 1, Levels of Medical Decision Making, are defined in the guidelines for number and complexity of problems addressed at the encounter, amount and/or complexity of data to be reviewed and analyzed, and risk of complications and/or morbidity or mortality of patient management.

Table 1: Levels of Medical Decision Making (MDM)

Elements of Medical Decision Making			
Level of MDM (Based on 2 out of 3 Elements of MDM)	**Number and Complexity of Problems Addressed at the Encounter**	**Amount and/or Complexity of Data to Be Reviewed and Analyzed** ***Each unique test, order, or document contributes to the combination of 2 or combination of 3 in Category 1 below.**	**Risk of Complications and/or Morbidity or Mortality of Patient Management**
Straightforward	**Minimal** • **1** self-limited or minor problem	**Minimal or none**	**Minimal risk of morbidity from additional diagnostic testing or treatment**
Low	**Low** • **2** or more self-limited or minor problems; **or** • **1** stable, chronic illness; **or** • **1** acute, uncomplicated illness or injury; **or** • **1** stable, acute illness; **or** • **1** acute, uncomplicated illness or injury requiring hospital inpatient or observation level of care	**Limited** *(Must meet the requirements of at least 1 out of 2 categories)* **Category 1: Tests and documents** • **Any combination of 2 from the following:** – Review of prior external note(s) from each unique source*; – Review of the result(s) of each unique test*; – Ordering of each unique test* **or** **Category 2: Assessment requiring an independent historian(s)** *(For the categories of independent interpretation of tests and discussion of management or test interpretation, see moderate or high)*	**Low risk of morbidity from additional diagnostic testing or treatment**
Moderate	**Moderate** • **1** or more chronic illnesses with exacerbation, progression, or side effects of treatment; **or** • **2** or more stable, chronic illnesses; **or** • **1** undiagnosed new problem with uncertain prognosis; **or** • **1** acute illness with systemic symptoms; **or** • **1** acute, complicated injury	**Moderate** *(Must meet the requirements of at least 1 out of 3 categories)* **Category 1: Tests, documents, or independent historian(s)** • **Any combination of 3 from the following:** – Review of prior external note(s) from each unique source*; – Review of the result(s) of each unique test*; – Ordering of each unique test*; – Assessment requiring an independent historian(s) **or** **Category 2: Independent interpretation of tests** • Independent interpretation of a test performed by another physician/other qualified health care professional (not separately reported); **or** **Category 3: Discussion of management or test interpretation** • Discussion of management or test interpretation with external physician/other qualified health care professional/appropriate source (not separately reported)	**Moderate risk of morbidity from additional diagnostic testing or treatment** *Examples only:* • Prescription drug management • Decision regarding minor surgery with identified patient or procedure risk factors • Decision regarding elective major surgery without identified patient or procedure risk factors • Diagnosis or treatment significantly limited by social determinants of health

Elements of Medical Decision Making			
Level of MDM (Based on 2 out of 3 Elements of MDM)	**Number and Complexity of Problems Addressed at the Encounter**	**Amount and/or Complexity of Data to Be Reviewed and Analyzed** ***Each unique test, order, or document contributes to the combination of 2 or combination of 3 in Category 1 below.**	**Risk of Complications and/or Morbidity or Mortality of Patient Management**
High	**High** • **1** or more chronic illnesses with severe exacerbation, progression, or side effects of treatment; **or** • **1** acute or chronic illness or injury that poses a threat to life or bodily function	**Extensive** *(Must meet the requirements of at least 2 out of 3 categories)* **Category 1: Tests, documents, or independent historian(s)** • **Any combination of 3 from the following:** – Review of prior external note(s) from each unique source*; – Review of the result(s) of each unique test*; – Ordering of each unique test*; – Assessment requiring an independent historian(s) **or** **Category 2: Independent interpretation of tests** • Independent interpretation of a test performed by another physician/other qualified health care professional (not separately reported); **or** **Category 3: Discussion of management or test interpretation** • Discussion of management or test interpretation with external physician/other qualified health care professional/appropriate source (not separately reported)	**High risk of morbidity from additional diagnostic testing or treatment** *Examples only:* • Drug therapy requiring intensive monitoring for toxicity • Decision regarding elective major surgery with identified patient or procedure risk factors • Decision regarding emergency major surgery • Decision regarding hospitalization or escalation of hospital-level care • Decision not to resuscitate or to de-escalate care because of poor prognosis • Decision regarding parenteral controlled substances

Number and Complexity of Problems Addressed at the Encounter

One element used in selecting the level of service is the number and complexity of the problems that are addressed at the encounter. Multiple new or established conditions may be addressed at the same time and may affect MDM. Symptoms may cluster around a specific diagnosis and each symptom is not necessarily a unique condition. Comorbidities and underlying diseases, in and of themselves, are not considered in selecting a level of E/M services **unless** they are addressed, and their presence increases the amount and/or complexity of data to be reviewed and analyzed or the risk of complications and/or morbidity or mortality of patient management. The final diagnosis for a condition does not, in and of itself, determine the complexity or risk, as extensive evaluation may be required to reach the conclusion that the signs or symptoms do not represent a highly morbid condition. Therefore, presenting symptoms that are likely to represent a highly morbid condition may "drive" MDM even when the ultimate diagnosis is not highly morbid. The evaluation and/or treatment should be consistent with the likely nature of the condition. Multiple problems of a lower severity may, in the aggregate, create higher risk due to interaction.

The term "risk" as used in the definition of this element relates to risk from the condition. While condition risk and management risk may often correlate, the risk from the condition is distinct from the risk of the management.

Problem: A problem is a disease, condition, illness, injury, symptom, sign, finding, complaint, or other matter addressed at the encounter, with or without a diagnosis being established at the time of the encounter.

Problem addressed: A problem is addressed or managed when it is evaluated or treated at the encounter by the physician or other qualified health care professional reporting the service. This includes consideration of further testing or treatment that may not be elected by virtue of risk/benefit analysis or patient/parent/guardian/surrogate choice. Notation in the patient's medical record that another professional is managing the problem without additional assessment or care coordination documented does not qualify as being addressed or managed by the physician or other qualified health care professional reporting the service. Referral without evaluation (by history, examination, or diagnostic study[ies]) or consideration of treatment does not qualify as being addressed or managed by the physician or other qualified health care professional reporting the service. For hospital inpatient and observation care services, the problem addressed is the problem status on the date of the encounter, which may be significantly different than on admission. It is the problem being managed or co-managed by the reporting physician or other qualified health care professional and may not be the cause of admission or continued stay.

Minimal problem: A problem that may not require the presence of the physician or other qualified health care professional, but the service is provided under the physician's or other qualified health care professional's supervision (see 99211, 99281).

Self-limited or minor problem: A problem that runs a definite and prescribed course, is transient in nature, and is not likely to permanently alter health status.

Stable, chronic illness: A problem with an expected duration of at least one year or until the death of the patient. For the purpose of defining chronicity, conditions are treated as chronic whether or not stage or severity changes (eg, uncontrolled diabetes and controlled diabetes are a single chronic condition). "Stable" for the purposes of categorizing MDM is defined by the specific treatment goals for an individual patient. A patient who is not at his or her treatment goal is not stable, even if the condition has not changed and there is no short-term threat to life or function. For example, a patient with persistently poorly controlled blood pressure for whom better control is a goal is not stable, even if the pressures are not changing and the patient is asymptomatic. The risk of morbidity **without** treatment is significant.

Acute, uncomplicated illness or injury: A recent or new short-term problem with low risk of morbidity for which treatment is considered. There is little to no risk of mortality with treatment, and full recovery without functional impairment is expected. A problem that is normally self-limited or minor but is not resolving consistent with a definite and prescribed course is an acute, uncomplicated illness.

Acute, uncomplicated illness or injury requiring hospital inpatient or observation level care: A recent or new short-term problem with low risk of morbidity for which treatment is required. There is little to no risk of mortality with treatment, and full recovery without functional impairment is expected. The treatment required is delivered in a hospital inpatient or observation level setting.

Stable, acute illness: A problem that is new or recent for which treatment has been initiated. The patient is improved and, while resolution may not be complete, is stable with respect to this condition.

Chronic illness with exacerbation, progression, or side effects of treatment: A chronic illness that is acutely worsening, poorly controlled, or progressing with an intent to control progression and requiring additional supportive care or requiring attention to treatment for side effects.

Undiagnosed new problem with uncertain prognosis: A problem in the differential diagnosis that represents a condition likely to result in a high risk of morbidity without treatment.

Acute illness with systemic symptoms: An illness that causes systemic symptoms and has a high risk of morbidity without treatment. For systemic general symptoms, such as fever, body aches, or fatigue in a minor illness that may be treated to alleviate symptoms, see the definitions for ***self-limited or minor problem*** or ***acute, uncomplicated illness or injury.*** Systemic symptoms may not be general but may be single system.

Acute, complicated injury: An injury which requires treatment that includes evaluation of body systems that are not directly part of the injured organ, the injury is extensive, or the treatment options are multiple and/or associated with risk of morbidity.

Chronic illness with severe exacerbation, progression, or side effects of treatment: The severe exacerbation or progression of a chronic illness or severe side effects of treatment that have significant risk of morbidity and may require escalation in level of care.

Acute or chronic illness or injury that poses a threat to life or bodily function: An acute illness with systemic symptoms, an acute complicated injury, or a chronic illness or injury with exacerbation and/or progression or side effects of treatment, that poses a threat to life or bodily function in the near term without treatment. Some symptoms may represent a condition that is significantly probable and poses a potential threat to life or bodily function. These may be included in this category when the evaluation and treatment are consistent with this degree of potential severity.

Amount and/or Complexity of Data to Be Reviewed and Analyzed

One element used in selecting the level of services is the amount and/or complexity of data to be reviewed or analyzed at an encounter.

Analyzed: The process of using the data as part of the MDM. The data element itself may not be subject to analysis (eg, glucose), but it is instead included in the thought processes for diagnosis, evaluation, or treatment. Tests ordered are presumed to be analyzed when the results are reported. Therefore, when they are ordered during an encounter, they are counted in that encounter. Tests that are ordered outside of an encounter may be counted in the encounter in which they are analyzed. In the case of a recurring order, each new result may be counted in the encounter in which it is analyzed. For example, an encounter that includes an order for monthly prothrombin times would count for one prothrombin time ordered and reviewed. Additional future results, if analyzed in a subsequent encounter, may be counted as a single test in that subsequent encounter. Any service for which the professional component is separately reported by the physician or other qualified health care professional reporting the E/M services is not counted as a data element ordered, reviewed, analyzed, or independently interpreted for the purposes of determining the level of MDM.

Test: Tests are imaging, laboratory, psychometric, or physiologic data. A clinical laboratory panel (eg, basic metabolic panel [80047]) is a single test. The differentiation between single or multiple tests is defined in accordance with the CPT code set. For the purpose of data reviewed and analyzed, pulse oximetry is not a test.

Unique: A unique test is defined by the CPT code set. When multiple results of the same unique test (eg, serial blood glucose values) are compared during an E/M service, count it as one unique test. Tests that have overlapping elements are not unique, even if they are identified with distinct CPT codes. For example, a CBC with differential would incorporate the set of hemoglobin, CBC without differential, and platelet count. A unique source is defined as a physician or other qualified health care professional in a distinct group or different specialty or subspecialty, or a unique entity. Review of all materials from any unique source counts as one element toward MDM.

Combination of data elements: A combination of different data elements, for example, a combination of notes reviewed, tests ordered, tests reviewed, or independent historian, allows these elements to be summed. It does not require each item type or category to be represented. A unique test ordered, plus a note reviewed and an independent historian would be a combination of three elements.

External: External records, communications and/or test results are from an external physician, other qualified health care professional, facility, or health care organization.

External physician or other qualified health care professional: An external physician or other qualified health care professional who is not in the same group practice or is of a different specialty or subspecialty. This includes licensed professionals who are practicing independently. The individual may also be a facility or organizational provider such as from a hospital, nursing facility, or home health care agency.

Discussion: Discussion requires an interactive exchange. The exchange must be direct and not through intermediaries (eg, clinical staff or trainees). Sending chart notes or written exchanges that are within progress notes does not qualify as an interactive exchange. The discussion does not need to be on the date of the encounter, but it is counted only once and only when it is used in the decision making of the encounter. It may be asynchronous (ie, does not need to be in person), but it must be initiated and completed within a short time period (eg, within a day or two).

Independent historian(s): An individual (eg, parent, guardian, surrogate, spouse, witness) who provides a history in addition to a history provided by the patient who is unable to provide a complete or reliable history (eg, due to developmental stage, dementia, or psychosis) or because a confirmatory history is judged to be necessary. In the case where there may be conflict or poor communication between multiple historians and more than one historian is needed, the independent historian requirement is met. It does not include translation services. The independent history does not need to be obtained in person but does need to be obtained directly from the historian providing the independent information.

Independent interpretation: The interpretation of a test for which there is a CPT code, and an interpretation or report is customary. This does not apply when the physician or other qualified health care professional who reports the E/M service is reporting or has previously reported the test. A form of interpretation should be documented but need not conform to the usual standards of a complete report for the test. A test that is ordered and independently interpreted may count both as a test ordered and interpreted.

Appropriate source: For the purpose of the **discussion of management** data element (see Table 1, Levels of Medical Decision Making), an appropriate source includes professionals who are not health care professionals but may be involved in the management of the patient (eg, lawyer, parole officer, case manager, teacher). It does not include discussion with family or informal caregivers. For the purpose of ***documents reviewed,*** documents from an appropriate source may be counted.

Risk of Complications and/or Morbidity or Mortality of Patient Management

One element used in selecting the level of service is the risk of complications and/or morbidity or mortality of patient management at an encounter. This is distinct from the risk of the condition itself.

Risk: The probability and/or consequences of an event. The assessment of the level of risk is affected by the nature of the event under consideration. For example, a low probability of death may be high risk, whereas a high chance of a minor, self-limited adverse effect of treatment may be low risk. Definitions of risk are based upon the usual behavior and thought processes of a physician or other qualified health care professional in the same specialty. Trained clinicians apply common language usage meanings to terms such as *high, medium, low,* or *minimal* risk and do not require quantification for these definitions (though quantification may be provided when evidence-based medicine has established probabilities). For the purpose of MDM, level of risk is based upon consequences of the problem(s) addressed at the encounter when appropriately treated. Risk also includes MDM related to the need to initiate or forego further testing, treatment, and/or hospitalization. The risk of patient management criteria applies to the patient management decisions made by the reporting physician or other qualified health care professional as part of the reported encounter.

Morbidity: A state of illness or functional impairment that is expected to be of substantial duration during which function is limited, quality of life is impaired, or there is organ damage that may not be transient despite treatment.

Social determinants of health: Economic and social conditions that influence the health of people and communities. Examples may include food or housing insecurity.

Surgery (minor or major, elective, emergency, procedure or patient risk):

Surgery—Minor or Major: The classification of surgery into minor or major is based on the common meaning of such terms when used by trained clinicians, similar to the use of the term "risk." These terms are not defined by a surgical package classification.

Surgery—Elective or Emergency: Elective procedures and emergent or urgent procedures describe the timing of a procedure when the timing is related to the patient's condition. An elective procedure is typically planned in advance (eg, scheduled for weeks later), while an emergent procedure is typically performed immediately or with minimal delay to allow for patient stabilization. Both elective and emergent procedures may be minor or major procedures.

Surgery—Risk Factors, Patient or Procedure: Risk factors are those that are relevant to the patient and procedure. Evidence-based risk calculators may be used, but are not required, in assessing patient and procedure risk.

Drug therapy requiring intensive monitoring for toxicity: A drug that requires intensive monitoring is a therapeutic agent that has the potential to cause serious morbidity or death. The monitoring is performed for assessment of these adverse effects and not primarily for assessment of therapeutic efficacy. The monitoring should be that which is generally accepted practice for the agent but may be patient-specific in some cases. Intensive monitoring may be long-term or short-term. Long-term intensive monitoring is not performed less than quarterly. The monitoring may be performed with a laboratory test, a physiologic test, or imaging. Monitoring by history or examination does not qualify. The monitoring affects the level of MDM in an encounter in which it is considered in the management of the patient. An example may be monitoring for cytopenia in the use of an antineoplastic agent between dose cycles. Examples of monitoring that do not qualify include monitoring glucose levels during insulin therapy, as the primary reason is the therapeutic effect (unless severe hypoglycemia is a current, significant concern); or annual electrolytes and renal function for a patient on a diuretic, as the frequency does not meet the threshold.

Parenteral controlled substances: The level of risk is based on the usual behavior and thought processes of a physician or other qualified health care professional in the same specialty and subspecialty and not simply based on the presence of an order for parenteral controlled substances.

Guidelines for Selecting Level of Service Based on Time

Certain categories of time-based E/M codes that do not have levels of services based on MDM (eg, Critical Care Services) in the E/M section use time differently. It is important to review the instructions for each category.

Time is **not** a descriptive component for the emergency department levels of E/M services because emergency department services are typically provided on a variable intensity basis, often involving multiple encounters with several patients over an extended period of time.

When time is used for reporting E/M services codes, the time defined in the service descriptors is used for selecting the appropriate level of services. The E/M services for which these guidelines apply require a face-to-face encounter with the physician or other qualified health care professional and the patient and/or family/caregiver. For office or other outpatient services, if the physician's or other qualified health care professional's time is spent in the supervision of clinical staff who perform the face-to-face services of the encounter, use 99211.

For coding purposes, time for these services is the total time on the date of the encounter. It includes both the face-to-face time with the patient and/or family/caregiver and non-face-to-face time personally spent by the physician and/or other qualified health care professional(s) on the day of the encounter (includes time in activities that require the physician or other qualified health care professional and does not include time in activities normally performed by clinical staff). It includes time regardless of the location of the physician or other qualified health care professional (eg, whether on or off the inpatient unit or in or out of the outpatient office). It does not include any time spent in the performance of other separately reported service(s).

Each service that may be reported using time for code level selection has a required time threshold. The concept of attaining a mid-point between levels does not apply. A full 15 minutes is required to report any unit of prolonged services codes 99417, 99418.

Physician(s) and other qualified health care professional(s) may each provide a portion of the face-to-face and non-face-to-face work related to the service. When time is being used to select the appropriate level of services for which time-based reporting is allowed, the time personally spent by the physician(s) and other qualified health care professional(s) assessing and managing the patient and/or counseling, educating, communicating results to the patient/family/caregiver on the date of the encounter is summed to define total time. Only distinct time should be summed (ie, when two or more individuals jointly meet with or discuss the patient, only the time of one individual should be counted).

When prolonged time occurs, the appropriate prolonged services code may be reported. The total time on the date of the encounter spent caring for the patient should be documented in the medical record when it is used as the basis for code selection.

Physician or other qualified health care professional time includes the following activities, when performed:

- preparing to see the patient (eg, review of tests)
- obtaining and/or reviewing separately obtained history
- performing a medically appropriate examination and/or evaluation
- counseling and educating the patient/family/caregiver
- ordering medications, tests, or procedures
- referring and communicating with other health care professionals (when not separately reported)

- documenting clinical information in the electronic or other health record
- independently interpreting results (not separately reported) and communicating results to the patient/family/caregiver
- care coordination (not separately reported)

Do not count time spent on the following:

- the performance of other services that are reported separately
- travel
- teaching that is general and not limited to discussion that is required for the management of a specific patient

For split or shared visits, see the split or shared visits guidelines.

Unlisted Service

An E/M service may be provided that is not listed in this section of the CPT codebook. When reporting such a service, the appropriate unlisted code may be used to indicate the service, identifying it by "Special Report," as discussed in the following paragraph. The "Unlisted Services" and accompanying codes for the E/M section are as follows:

99429 **Unlisted preventive** medicine service

99499 **Unlisted evaluation and management** service

Special Report

An unlisted service or one that is unusual, variable, or new may require a special report demonstrating the medical appropriateness of the service. Pertinent information should include an adequate definition or description of the nature, extent, and need for the procedure and the time, effort, and equipment necessary to provide the service. Additional items that may be included are complexity of symptoms, final diagnosis, pertinent physical findings, diagnostic and therapeutic procedures, concurrent problems, and follow-up care.

99202-99205

99202 Office or other outpatient visit for the evaluation and management of a new patient, which requires a medically appropriate history and/or examination and straightforward medical decision making. When using total time on the date of the encounter for code selection, 15 minutes must be met or exceeded.

99203 Office or other outpatient visit for the evaluation and management of a new patient, which requires a medically appropriate history and/or examination and low level of medical decision making. When using total time on the date of the encounter for code selection, 30 minutes must be met or exceeded.

99204 Office or other outpatient visit for the evaluation and management of a new patient, which requires a medically appropriate history and/or examination and moderate level of medical decision making. When using total time on the date of the encounter for code selection, 45 minutes must be met or exceeded.

99205 Office or other outpatient visit for the evaluation and management of a new patient, which requires a medically appropriate history and/or examination and high level of medical decision making. When using total time on the date of the encounter for code selection, 60 minutes must be met or exceeded.

Explanation

Providers report these codes for new patients being seen in the doctor's office, a multispecialty group clinic, or other outpatient environment. All require a medically appropriate history and/or examination. Code selection is based on the level of medical decision making (MDM) or total time personally spent by the physician and/or other qualified health care professional(s) on the date of the encounter. Factors to be considered in MDM include the number and complexity of problems addressed during the encounter, amount and complexity of data requiring review and analysis, and the risk of complications and/or morbidity or mortality associated with patient management. The most basic service is represented by 99202, which entails straightforward MDM. If time is used for code selection, a total time of 15 minutes must be met or exceeded on the day of the encounter. Report 99203 for a visit requiring a low level of MDM or meeting or exceeding 30 minutes of total time; 99204 for a visit requiring a moderate level of MDM or meeting or exceeding 45 minutes of total time; and 99205 for a visit requiring a high level of MDM or meeting or exceeding 60 minutes of total time.

Coding Tips

These codes are used to report office or other outpatient services for a new patient. A medically appropriate history and physical examination, as determined by the treating provider, should be documented. The level of history and physical examination are not considered when determining the level of service. Codes should be selected based upon the current CPT Medical Decision Making table. Alternatively, time alone may be used to select the appropriate level of service. Total time for reporting these services includes face-to-face and non-face-to-face time personally spent by the physician or other qualified health care professional on the date of the encounter. Medicare has identified these codes as telehealth/telemedicine services. CMS requires the use of a place of service (POS) indicator: POS 02 for telehealth services when the originating site is not the patient's home and POS 10 for telehealth services when the originating site is the patient's home. For prolonged services applicable to 99205, see 99417; for Medicare, see G2212. Medicare and commercial payers should be contacted regarding their coverage guidelines. For office or other outpatient services for an established patient, see 99211-99215.

ICD-10-CM Diagnostic Codes

The application of this code is too broad to adequately present ICD-10-CM diagnostic code links here. Refer to your ICD-10-CM book.

AMA: **99202** 2024,Sep; 2024,Jun; 2024,Jan; 2023,Dec; 2023,Nov; 2023,Oct; 2023,Sep; 2023,Aug; 2023,May; 2023,Apr; 2023,Mar; 2022,Dec; 2022,Nov; 2022,Oct; 2022,Sep; 2022,Aug; 2022,Jul; 2022,Jun; 2022,Apr; 2022,Feb; 2022,Jan; 2021,Nov; 2021,Oct; 2021,Sep; 2021,Aug; 2021,Jul; 2021,Jun; 2021,May; 2021,Apr; 2021,Mar; 2021,Feb; 2021,Jan; 2020,Dec; 2020,Nov; 2020,Oct; 2020,Sep; 2020,Jun; 2020,May; 2020,Mar; 2020,Feb; 2020,Jan; 2019,Oct; 2019,Jul; 2019,Jun; 2019,Feb; 2019,Jan; 2018,Oct; 2018,Sep; 2018,Apr; 2018,Mar **99203** 2024,Oct; 2024,Sep; 2024,Jun; 2024,Jan; 2023,Dec; 2023,Nov; 2023,Oct; 2023,Sep; 2023,Aug; 2023,May; 2023,Apr; 2023,Mar; 2022,Dec; 2022,Nov; 2022,Oct; 2022,Sep; 2022,Aug; 2022,Jul; 2022,Jun; 2022,Apr; 2022,Feb; 2022,Jan; 2021,Nov; 2021,Oct; 2021,Sep; 2021,Aug; 2021,Jul; 2021,Jun; 2021,May; 2021,Apr; 2021,Mar; 2021,Feb; 2021,Jan; 2020,Dec; 2020,Nov; 2020,Oct; 2020,Sep; 2020,Jun; 2020,May; 2020,Mar; 2020,Feb; 2020,Jan; 2019,Oct; 2019,Jul; 2019,Jun; 2019,Feb; 2019,Jan; 2018,Oct; 2018,Sep; 2018,Apr; 2018,Mar **99204** 2024,Oct; 2024,Sep; 2024,Jun; 2024,Jan; 2023,Dec; 2023,Nov; 2023,Oct; 2023,Sep; 2023,Aug; 2023,May; 2023,Apr; 2023,Mar; 2022,Dec; 2022,Nov; 2022,Oct; 2022,Sep; 2022,Aug; 2022,Jul; 2022,Jun; 2022,Apr; 2022,Feb; 2022,Jan; 2021,Nov; 2021,Oct; 2021,Sep; 2021,Aug; 2021,Jul; 2021,Jun; 2021,May; 2021,Apr; 2021,Mar; 2021,Feb; 2021,Jan; 2020,Dec; 2020,Nov; 2020,Oct; 2020,Sep; 2020,Jun; 2020,May; 2020,Mar; 2020,Feb; 2020,Jan; 2019,Oct; 2019,Jul; 2019,Jun; 2019,Feb; 2019,Jan; 2018,Oct; 2018,Sep; 2018,Apr; 2018,Mar **99205** 2024,Oct; 2024,Sep; 2024,Mar; 2024,Jan; 2023,Dec; 2023,Nov; 2023,Oct; 2023,Sep; 2023,Aug; 2023,May; 2023,Apr; 2023,Mar; 2022,Dec; 2022,Nov; 2022,Oct; 2022,Sep; 2022,Aug; 2022,Jul; 2022,Jun; 2022,Apr; 2022,Feb; 2022,Jan; 2021,Nov; 2021,Oct; 2021,Sep; 2021,Aug; 2021,Jul; 2021,Jun; 2021,May; 2021,Apr; 2021,Mar; 2021,Feb; 2021,Jan; 2020,Dec; 2020,Nov; 2020,Oct; 2020,Sep; 2020,Jun; 2020,May; 2020,Mar; 2020,Feb; 2020,Jan; 2019,Oct; 2019,Jul; 2019,Jun; 2019,Feb; 2019,Jan; 2018,Oct; 2018,Sep; 2018,Apr; 2018,Mar

Relative Value Units/Medicare Edits

Non-Facility RVU	Work	PE	MP	Total
99202	0.93	1.16	0.08	2.17
99203	1.6	1.59	0.16	3.35
99204	2.6	2.18	0.24	5.02
99205	3.5	2.79	0.33	6.62
Facility RVU	**Work**	**PE**	**MP**	**Total**
99202	0.93	0.4	0.08	1.41
99203	1.6	0.68	0.16	2.44
99204	2.6	1.13	0.24	3.97
99205	3.5	1.57	0.33	5.4

	FUD	Status	MUE	Modifiers				IOM Reference
99202	N/A	A	1(2)	N/A	N/A	N/A	80*	None
99203	N/A	A	1(2)	N/A	N/A	N/A	80*	
99204	N/A	A	1(2)	N/A	N/A	N/A	80*	
99205	N/A	A	1(2)	N/A	N/A	N/A	80*	

* with documentation

 ● New ▲ Revised + Add On ★ Telemedicine [Resequenced] ☑ Laterality

99211-99215

★**99211** Office or other outpatient visit for the evaluation and management of an established patient that may not require the presence of a physician or other qualified health care professional

99212 Office or other outpatient visit for the evaluation and management of an established patient, which requires a medically appropriate history and/or examination and straightforward medical decision making. When using total time on the date of the encounter for code selection, 10 minutes must be met or exceeded.

99213 Office or other outpatient visit for the evaluation and management of an established patient, which requires a medically appropriate history and/or examination and low level of medical decision making. When using total time on the date of the encounter for code selection, 20 minutes must be met or exceeded.

99214 Office or other outpatient visit for the evaluation and management of an established patient, which requires a medically appropriate history and/or examination and moderate level of medical decision making. When using total time on the date of the encounter for code selection, 30 minutes must be met or exceeded.

99215 Office or other outpatient visit for the evaluation and management of an established patient, which requires a medically appropriate history and/or examination and high level of medical decision making. When using total time on the date of the encounter for code selection, 40 minutes must be met or exceeded.

Explanation

Providers report these codes for established patients being seen in the doctor's office, a multispecialty group clinic, or other outpatient environment. All require a medically appropriate history and/or examination excluding the most basic service represented by 99211 that describes an encounter that may not require the presence of a physician or other qualified health care professional. For the remainder of codes within this range, code selection is based on the level of medical decision making (MDM) or total time personally spent by the physician and/or other qualified health care professional(s) on the date of the encounter. Factors to be considered in MDM include the number and complexity of problems addressed during the encounter, amount and complexity of data requiring review and analysis, and the risk of complications and/or morbidity or mortality associated with patient management. Report 99212 for a visit that entails straightforward MDM. If time is used for code selection, a total time of 10 minutes must be met or exceeded on the day of the encounter. Report 99213 for a visit requiring a low level of MDM or meeting or exceeding 20 minutes of total time; 99214 for a moderate level of MDM or meeting or exceeding 30 minutes of total time; and 99215 for a high level of MDM or meeting or exceeding 40 minutes of total time.

Coding Tips

These codes are used to report office or other outpatient services for an established patient. A medically appropriate history and physical examination, as determined by the treating provider, should be documented. The level of history and physical examination are not considered when determining the level of service. Codes should be selected based upon the current CPT Medical Decision Making table. Alternatively, time alone may be used to select the appropriate level of service. Total time for reporting these services includes face-to-face and non-face-to-face time personally spent by the physician or other qualified health care professional on the date of the encounter. Code 99211 does not require the presence of a physician or other qualified health care professional. Medicare has identified these codes as telehealth/telemedicine services. Code 99211, when performed as a telehealth service, may be reported by the performing provider by appending modifier 95 to the procedure code. CMS requires the use of a place of service (POS) indicator: POS 02 for telehealth services when the originating site is not the patient's home and POS 10 for telehealth services when the originating site is the patient's home. For prolonged services applicable to 99215, see 99417; for Medicare, see G2212. Medicare and commercial payers should be contacted regarding their coverage guidelines. For office or other outpatient services for a new patient, see 99202-99205.

ICD-10-CM Diagnostic Codes

The application of this code is too broad to adequately present ICD-10-CM diagnostic code links here. Refer to your ICD-10-CM book.

AMA: 99211 2024,Sep; 2024,Jun; 2024,Jan; 2023,Dec; 2023,Nov; 2023,Oct; 2023,Sep; 2023,Aug; 2023,Jul; 2023,May; 2023,Apr; 2023,Mar; 2022,Dec; 2022,Nov; 2022,Oct; 2022,Sep; 2022,Aug; 2022,Jul; 2022,Jun; 2022,Apr; 2022,Jan; 2021,Nov; 2021,Oct; 2021,Sep; 2021,Jun; 2021,May; 2021,Apr; 2021,Mar; 2021,Feb; 2021,Jan; 2020,Dec; 2020,Nov; 2020,Oct; 2020,Sep; 2020,Jun; 2020,May; 2020,Mar; 2020,Feb; 2020,Jan; 2019,Oct; 2019,Jul; 2019,Jun; 2019,Feb; 2019,Jan; 2018,Oct; 2018,Sep; 2018,Apr; 2018,Mar **99212** 2024,Sep; 2024,Jun; 2024,Jan; 2023,Dec; 2023,Nov; 2023,Sep; 2023,Aug; 2023,Jul; 2023,Jun; 2023,May; 2023,Apr; 2023,Mar; 2022,Dec; 2022,Nov; 2022,Oct; 2022,Sep; 2022,Aug; 2022,Jul; 2022,Jun; 2022,Apr; 2022,Feb; 2022,Jan; 2021,Nov; 2021,Oct; 2021,Sep; 2021,Aug; 2021,Jul; 2021,Jun; 2021,May; 2021,Apr; 2021,Mar; 2021,Feb; 2021,Jan; 2020,Dec; 2020,Nov; 2020,Oct; 2020,Sep; 2020,Jun; 2020,May; 2020,Mar; 2020,Feb; 2020,Jan; 2019,Oct; 2019,Jul; 2019,Jun; 2019,Feb; 2019,Jan; 2018,Oct; 2018,Sep; 2018,Apr; 2018,Mar **99213** 2024,Oct; 2024,Sep; 2024,Jun; 2024,Jan; 2023,Dec; 2023,Nov; 2023,Oct; 2023,Sep; 2023,Aug; 2023,Jul; 2023,Jun; 2023,May; 2023,Apr; 2023,Mar; 2022,Dec; 2022,Nov; 2022,Oct; 2022,Sep; 2022,Aug; 2022,Jul; 2022,Jun; 2022,Apr; 2022,Feb; 2022,Jan; 2021,Nov; 2021,Oct; 2021,Sep; 2021,Aug; 2021,Jul; 2021,Jun; 2021,May; 2021,Apr; 2021,Mar; 2021,Feb; 2021,Jan; 2020,Dec; 2020,Nov; 2020,Oct; 2020,Sep; 2020,Jun; 2020,May; 2020,Mar; 2020,Feb; 2020,Jan; 2019,Oct; 2019,Jul; 2019,Jun; 2019,Feb; 2019,Jan; 2018,Oct; 2018,Sep; 2018,Apr; 2018,Mar **99214** 2024,Oct; 2024,Sep; 2024,Jun; 2024,Jan; 2023,Dec; 2023,Nov; 2023,Sep; 2023,Aug; 2023,Jul; 2023,Jun; 2023,May; 2023,Apr; 2023,Mar; 2022,Dec; 2022,Nov; 2022,Oct; 2022,Sep; 2022,Aug; 2022,Jul; 2022,Jun; 2022,Apr; 2022,Feb; 2022,Jan; 2021,Nov; 2021,Oct; 2021,Sep; 2021,Aug; 2021,Jul; 2021,Jun; 2021,May; 2021,Apr; 2021,Mar; 2021,Feb; 2021,Jan; 2020,Dec; 2020,Nov; 2020,Oct; 2020,Sep; 2020,Jun; 2020,May; 2020,Mar; 2020,Feb; 2020,Jan; 2019,Oct; 2019,Jul; 2019,Jun; 2019,Feb; 2019,Jan; 2018,Oct; 2018,Sep; 2018,Apr; 2018,Mar **99215** 2024,Oct; 2024,Sep; 2024,Jun; 2024,Jan; 2023,Dec; 2023,Nov; 2023,Oct; 2023,Sep; 2023,Aug; 2023,Jul; 2023,Jun; 2023,May; 2023,Apr; 2023,Mar; 2022,Dec; 2022,Nov; 2022,Oct; 2022,Sep; 2022,Aug; 2022,Jul; 2022,Jun; 2022,Apr; 2022,Feb; 2022,Jan; 2021,Nov; 2021,Oct; 2021,Sep; 2021,Aug; 2021,Jul; 2021,Jun; 2021,May; 2021,Apr; 2021,Mar; 2021,Feb; 2021,Jan; 2020,Dec; 2020,Nov; 2020,Oct; 2020,Sep; 2020,Jun; 2020,May; 2020,Mar; 2020,Feb; 2020,Jan; 2019,Oct; 2019,Jul; 2019,Jun; 2019,Feb; 2019,Jan; 2018,Oct; 2018,Sep; 2018,Apr; 2018,Mar

Relative Value Units/Medicare Edits

Non-Facility RVU	Work	PE	MP	Total
99211	0.18	0.51	0.01	0.7
99212	0.7	0.94	0.06	1.7
99213	1.3	1.33	0.1	2.73
99214	1.92	1.79	0.14	3.85
99215	2.8	2.4	0.22	5.42
Facility RVU	**Work**	**PE**	**MP**	**Total**
99211	0.18	0.07	0.01	0.26
99212	0.7	0.29	0.06	1.05
99213	1.3	0.56	0.1	1.96
99214	1.92	0.83	0.14	2.89
99215	2.8	1.27	0.22	4.29

	FUD	Status	MUE	Modifiers				IOM Reference
99211	N/A	A	1(3)	N/A	N/A	N/A	80*	None
99212	N/A	A	2(3)	N/A	N/A	N/A	80*	
99213	N/A	A	2(3)	N/A	N/A	N/A	80*	
99214	N/A	A	2(3)	N/A	N/A	N/A	80*	
99215	N/A	A	1(3)	N/A	N/A	N/A	80*	

* with documentation

Terms To Know

established patient. Patient who has received professional services in a face-to-face setting within the last three years from the same physician/qualified health care professional or another physician/qualified health care professional of the exact same specialty and subspecialty who belongs to the same group practice. If the patient is seen by a physician/qualified health care professional who is covering for another physician/qualified health care professional, the patient will be considered the same as if seen by the physician/qualified health care professional who is unavailable.

outpatient. Person who has not been admitted as an inpatient but who is registered on the hospital or CAH records as an outpatient and receives services (rather than supplies alone) directly from the hospital or CAH. (Code of Federal Regulations, section 410.2.)

[98000, 98001, 98002, 98003]

- ● **98000** Synchronous audio-video visit for the evaluation and management of a new patient, which requires a medically appropriate history and/or examination and straightforward medical decision making. When using total time on the date of the encounter for code selection, 15 minutes must be met or exceeded.
- ● **98001** Synchronous audio-video visit for the evaluation and management of a new patient, which requires a medically appropriate history and/or examination and low medical decision making. When using total time on the date of the encounter for code selection, 30 minutes must be met or exceeded.
- ● **98002** Synchronous audio-video visit for the evaluation and management of a new patient, which requires a medically appropriate history and/or examination and moderate medical decision making. When using total time on the date of the encounter for code selection, 45 minutes must be met or exceeded.
- ● **98003** Synchronous audio-video visit for the evaluation and management of a new patient, which requires a medically appropriate history and/or examination and high medical decision making. When using total time on the date of the encounter for code selection, 60 minutes must be met or exceeded.

Explanation

Providers report these codes for new patients being seen via telehealth using synchronous audio-video as an alternative to an in-person visit. The provider and patient interact from different locations through real-time communication in which they can see and hear each other. All require a medically appropriate history and/or examination. Code selection is based on the level of medical decision making (MDM) or total time personally spent by the physician and/or other qualified health care professional(s) on the date of the encounter. Factors to be considered in MDM include the number and complexity of problems addressed during the encounter, amount and complexity of data requiring review and analysis, and the risk of complications and/or morbidity or mortality associated with patient management. The most basic service is represented by 98000, which entails straightforward MDM. If time is used for code selection, a total time of 15 minutes must be met or exceeded on the day of the encounter. Report 98001 for a visit requiring a low level of MDM or meeting or exceeding 30 minutes of total time; 98002 for a visit requiring a moderate level of MDM or meeting or exceeding 45 minutes of total time; and 98003 for a visit requiring a high level of MDM or meeting or exceeding 60 minutes of total time.

Coding Tips

These codes are used to report synchronous, real-time, audio-video interactive telecommunication services for a new patient. A medically appropriate history and physical examination, as determined by the treating provider, should be documented. Codes should be selected based upon the current CPT Medical Decision Making table. Alternatively, time alone may be used to select the appropriate level of service. Total time for reporting these services includes non-face-to-face time personally spent by the physician or other qualified health care professional on the date of the encounter. These services may be initiated by the patient, family, caregiver, physician, or other qualified health care professional (OQHP). Time spent establishing a connection or arranging the appointment should not be counted when reporting based on time. If the audio-video connection is lost during an encounter and only audio is restored, the service responsible for the bulk of the time should be reported. Do not report these codes on the same day as an in-person E/M visit; add the elements or time of each visit together and report only one E/M service. For prolonged services applicable to 98003, see 99417. Medicare does not recognize these services for payment. Refer to office and other outpatient E/M codes (99202-99215) and other services currently on the Medicare telehealth list to report audio-video and audio-only telecommunication services furnished via synchronous two-way communication technology. Medicare and commercial payers should be contacted regarding their coverage guidelines.

ICD-10-CM Diagnostic Codes

The application of this code is too broad to adequately present ICD-10-CM diagnostic code links here. Refer to your ICD-10-CM book.

Relative Value Units/Medicare Edits

Non-Facility RVU	Work	PE	MP	Total
98000				
98001				
98002				
98003				
Facility RVU	**Work**	**PE**	**MP**	**Total**
98000				
98001				
98002				
98003				

	FUD	Status	MUE	Modifiers				IOM Reference
98000	N/A		-	N/A	N/A	N/A	N/A	None
98001	N/A		-	N/A	N/A	N/A	N/A	
98002	N/A		-	N/A	N/A	N/A	N/A	
98003	N/A		-	N/A	N/A	N/A	N/A	

* with documentation

Terms To Know

new patient. Patient who is receiving face-to-face care from a physician or other qualified health care professional of the exact same specialty and subspecialty who belongs to the same group practice for the first time in three years. For OPPS hospitals, a patient who has not been registered as an inpatient or outpatient, including off-campus provider-based clinic or emergency department, within the past three years.

synchronous services. Services that entail real-time communication between the patient and/or family and a physician or other qualified health care professional (QHP) when both are located at different physical sites.

telemedicine. Medical information exchanged from site to site via electronic communication. Examples include patient evaluation and consultation, monitoring, education and other clinical services.

[98004, 98005, 98006, 98007]

- **98004** Synchronous audio-video visit for the evaluation and management of an established patient, which requires a medically appropriate history and/or examination and straightforward medical decision making. When using total time on the date of the encounter for code selection, 10 minutes must be met or exceeded.
- **98005** Synchronous audio-video visit for the evaluation and management of an established patient, which requires a medically appropriate history and/or examination and low medical decision making. When using total time on the date of the encounter for code selection, 20 minutes must be met or exceeded.
- **98006** Synchronous audio-video visit for the evaluation and management of an established patient, which requires a medically appropriate history and/or examination and moderate medical decision making. When using total time on the date of the encounter for code selection, 30 minutes must be met or exceeded.
- **98007** Synchronous audio-video visit for the evaluation and management of an established patient, which requires a medically appropriate history and/or examination and high medical decision making. When using total time on the date of the encounter for code selection, 40 minutes must be met or exceeded.

Explanation

Providers report these codes for established patients being seen via telehealth using synchronous audio-video as an alternative to an in-person visit. The provider and patient interact from different locations through real-time communication in which they can see and hear each other. All require a medically appropriate history and/or examination. Code selection is based on the level of medical decision making (MDM) or total time personally spent by the physician and/or other qualified health care professional(s) on the date of the encounter. Factors to be considered in MDM include the number and complexity of problems addressed during the encounter, amount and complexity of data requiring review and analysis, and the risk of complications and/or morbidity or mortality associated with patient management. The most basic service is represented by 98004, which entails straightforward MDM. If time is used for code selection, a total time of 10 minutes must be met or exceeded on the day of the encounter. Report 98005 for a visit requiring a low level of MDM or meeting or exceeding 20 minutes of total time; 98006 for a visit requiring a moderate level of MDM or meeting or exceeding 30 minutes of total time; and 98007 for a visit requiring a high level of MDM or meeting or exceeding 40 minutes of total time.

Coding Tips

These codes are used to report synchronous, real-time, audio-video interactive telecommunication services for an established patient. A medically appropriate history and physical examination, as determined by the treating provider, should be documented. Codes should be selected based upon the current CPT Medical Decision Making table. Alternatively, time alone may be used to select the appropriate level of service. Total time for reporting these services includes non-face-to-face time personally spent by the physician or other qualified health care professional on the date of the encounter. These services may be initiated by the patient, family, caregiver, physician, or other qualified health care professional (OQHP), and do not require a specific time interval from the last in-person visit or telemedicine visit. Time spent establishing a connection or arranging the appointment should not be counted when reporting based on time. If the audio-video connection is lost during an encounter and only audio is restored, the service responsible for the bulk of the time should be reported. These codes may be used to report regular follow-up in lieu of an in-person visit if the patient requires reassessment for a condition related to a treatment plan from a previous E/M visit. Do not report these codes for routine telecommunications or when communicating laboratory results related to a previous E/M service. Do not report these codes on the same day as an in-person E/M visit; add the elements or time of each visit together and report only one E/M service. For prolonged services applicable to 98007, see 99417. Medicare does not recognize these services for payment. Refer to office and other outpatient E/M codes (99202-99215) and other services currently on the Medicare telehealth list to report audio-video and audio-only telecommunication services furnished via synchronous two-way communication technology. Medicare and commercial payers should be contacted regarding their coverage guidelines.

ICD-10-CM Diagnostic Codes

The application of this code is too broad to adequately present ICD-10-CM diagnostic code links here. Refer to your ICD-10-CM book.

Relative Value Units/Medicare Edits

Non-Facility RVU	Work	PE	MP	Total
98004				
98005				
98006				
98007				
Facility RVU	**Work**	**PE**	**MP**	**Total**
98004				
98005				
98006				
98007				

	FUD	Status	MUE	Modifiers				IOM Reference
98004	N/A		-	N/A	N/A	N/A	N/A	None
98005	N/A		-	N/A	N/A	N/A	N/A	
98006	N/A		-	N/A	N/A	N/A	N/A	
98007	N/A		-	N/A	N/A	N/A	N/A	

* with documentation

Terms To Know

established patient. Patient who has received professional services in a face-to-face setting within the last three years from the same physician/qualified health care professional or another physician/qualified health care professional of the exact same specialty and subspecialty who belongs to the same group practice. If the patient is seen by a physician/qualified health care professional who is covering for another physician/qualified health care professional, the patient will be considered the same as if seen by the physician/qualified health care professional who is unavailable.

synchronous services. Services that entail real-time communication between the patient and/or family and a physician or other qualified health care professional (QHP) when both are located at different physical sites.

telemedicine. Medical information exchanged from site to site via electronic communication. Examples include patient evaluation and consultation, monitoring, education and other clinical services.

[98008, 98009, 98010, 98011]

- ● **98008** Synchronous audio-only visit for the evaluation and management of a new patient, which requires a medically appropriate history and/or examination, straightforward medical decision making, and more than 10 minutes of medical discussion. When using total time on the date of the encounter for code selection, 15 minutes must be met or exceeded.
- ● **98009** Synchronous audio-only visit for the evaluation and management of a new patient, which requires a medically appropriate history and/or examination, low medical decision making, and more than 10 minutes of medical discussion. When using total time on the date of the encounter for code selection, 30 minutes must be met or exceeded.
- ● **98010** Synchronous audio-only visit for the evaluation and management of a new patient, which requires a medically appropriate history and/or examination, moderate medical decision making, and more than 10 minutes of medical discussion. When using total time on the date of the encounter for code selection, 45 minutes must be met or exceeded.
- ● **98011** Synchronous audio-only visit for the evaluation and management of a new patient, which requires a medically appropriate history and/or examination, high medical decision making, and more than 10 minutes of medical discussion. When using total time on the date of the encounter for code selection, 60 minutes must be met or exceeded.

Explanation

Providers report these codes for new patients being seen via telehealth using synchronous audio as an alternative to an in-person visit. The provider and patient interact from different locations through real-time communication in which they can hear each other. The visit must include more than 10 minutes of medical discussion. Video communication is not required for these services. All require a medically appropriate history and/or examination. Code selection is based on the level of medical decision making (MDM) or total time personally spent by the physician and/or other qualified health care professional(s) on the date of the encounter. Factors to be considered in MDM include the number and complexity of problems addressed during the encounter, amount and complexity of data requiring review and analysis, and the risk of complications and/or morbidity or mortality associated with patient management. The most basic service is represented by 98008, which entails straightforward MDM. If time is used for code selection, a total time of 15 minutes must be met or exceeded on the day of the encounter. Report 98009 for a visit requiring a low level of MDM or meeting or exceeding 30 minutes of total time; 98010 for a visit requiring a moderate level of MDM or meeting or exceeding 45 minutes of total time; and 98011 for a visit requiring a high level of MDM or meeting or exceeding 60 minutes of total time.

Coding Tips

These codes are used to report synchronous, real-time, audio only interactive telecommunication services for a new patient. A medically appropriate history and physical examination, as determined by the treating provider, should be documented. Codes should be selected based upon the current CPT Medical Decision Making table. Alternatively, time alone may be used to select the appropriate level of service. Total time for reporting these services includes non-face-to-face time personally spent by the physician or other qualified health care professional on the date of the encounter. These services may be initiated by the patient, family, caregiver, physician, or other qualified health care professional (OQHP). Time spent establishing a connection or arranging the appointment should not be counted when reporting based on time. These services require more than 10 minutes of medical discussion, defined as synchronous (real-time) interactive verbal communication. Do not report these codes for routine telecommunications or when communicating laboratory results related to a previous E/M service. Do not report these codes on the same day as an in-person E/M visit; add the elements or time of each visit together and report only one E/M service. For prolonged services applicable to 98011, see 99417. Medicare does not recognize these services for payment. Refer to office and other outpatient E/M codes (99202-99215) and other services currently on the Medicare telehealth list to report audio-video and audio-only telecommunication services furnished via synchronous two-way communication technology. Medicare and commercial payers should be contacted regarding their coverage guidelines.

ICD-10-CM Diagnostic Codes

The application of this code is too broad to adequately present ICD-10-CM diagnostic code links here. Refer to your ICD-10-CM book.

Relative Value Units/Medicare Edits

Non-Facility RVU	Work	PE	MP	Total
98008				
98009				
98010				
98011				
Facility RVU	**Work**	**PE**	**MP**	**Total**
98008				
98009				
98010				
98011				

	FUD	Status	MUE	Modifiers				IOM Reference
98008	N/A		-	N/A	N/A	N/A	N/A	None
98009	N/A		-	N/A	N/A	N/A	N/A	
98010	N/A		-	N/A	N/A	N/A	N/A	
98011	N/A		-	N/A	N/A	N/A	N/A	

* with documentation

Terms To Know

synchronous services. Services that entail real-time communication between the patient and/or family and a physician or other qualified health care professional (QHP) when both are located at different physical sites.

telemedicine. Medical information exchanged from site to site via electronic communication. Examples include patient evaluation and consultation, monitoring, education and other clinical services.

[98012, 98013, 98014, 98015]

- ● **98012** Synchronous audio-only visit for the evaluation and management of an established patient, which requires a medically appropriate history and/or examination, straightforward medical decision making, and more than 10 minutes of medical discussion. When using total time on the date of the encounter for code selection, 10 minutes must be exceeded.
- ● **98013** Synchronous audio-only visit for the evaluation and management of an established patient, which requires a medically appropriate history and/or examination, low medical decision making, and more than 10 minutes of medical discussion. When using total time on the date of the encounter for code selection, 20 minutes must be met or exceeded.
- ● **98014** Synchronous audio-only visit for the evaluation and management of an established patient, which requires a medically appropriate history and/or examination, moderate medical decision making, and more than 10 minutes of medical discussion. When using total time on the date of the encounter for code selection, 30 minutes must be met or exceeded.
- ● **98015** Synchronous audio-only visit for the evaluation and management of an established patient, which requires a medically appropriate history and/or examination, high medical decision making, and more than 10 minutes of medical discussion. When using total time on the date of the encounter for code selection, 40 minutes must be met or exceeded.

Explanation

Providers report these codes for established patients being seen via telehealth using synchronous audio as an alternative to an in-person visit. The provider and patient interact from different locations through real-time communication in which they can hear each other. The visit must include more than 10 minutes of medical discussion. Video communication is not required for these services. All require a medically appropriate history and/or examination. Code selection is based on the level of medical decision making (MDM) or total time personally spent by the physician and/or other qualified health care professional(s) on the date of the encounter. Factors to be considered in MDM include the number and complexity of problems addressed during the encounter, amount and complexity of data requiring review and analysis, and the risk of complications and/or morbidity or mortality associated with patient management. The most basic service is represented by 98012, which entails straightforward MDM. If time is used for code selection, a total time of 10 minutes must be exceeded on the day of the encounter. Report 98013 for a visit requiring a low level of MDM or meeting or exceeding 20 minutes of total time; 98014 for a visit requiring a moderate level of MDM or meeting or exceeding 30 minutes of total time; and 98015 for a visit requiring a high level of MDM or meeting or exceeding 40 minutes of total time.

Coding Tips

These codes are used to report synchronous, real-time, audio only interactive telecommunication services for an established patient. A medically appropriate history and physical examination, as determined by the treating provider, should be documented. Codes should be selected based upon the current CPT Medical Decision Making table. Alternatively, time alone may be used to select the appropriate level of service. Total time for reporting these services includes non-face-to-face time personally spent by the physician or other qualified health care professional on the date of the encounter. These services may be initiated by the patient, family, caregiver, physician, or other qualified health care professional (OQHP), and do not require a specific time interval from the last in-person visit or telemedicine visit. These codes may be used to report regular follow-up in lieu of an in-person visit if the patient requires reassessment for a condition related to a treatment plan from a previous E/M visit. Time spent establishing a connection or arranging the appointment should not be counted when reporting based on time. These services require more than 10 minutes of medical discussion, defined as synchronous (real-time) interactive verbal communication. Do not report these codes for routine telecommunications or when communicating laboratory results related to a previous E/M service. Do not report on the same day as an in-person E/M visit, add the elements or time of each visit together and report only one E/M service. For prolonged services applicable to 98015, see 99417. Medicare does not recognize these services for payment. Refer to office and other outpatient E/M codes (99202-99215) and other services currently on the Medicare telehealth list to report audio-video and audio-only telecommunication services furnished via synchronous two-way communication technology. Medicare and commercial payers should be contacted regarding their coverage guidelines. When home and outpatient INR monitoring (93792-93793) is evaluated during a synchronous telemedicine service, do not report these codes separately. If providing care plan oversight (CPO) during the same call(s), do not report these codes in addition to 99374-99380. Do not report these codes during the same month as complex chronic care management services 99487 or 99489; or during the service time of transition care management services 99495 or 99496.

ICD-10-CM Diagnostic Codes

The application of this code is too broad to adequately present ICD-10-CM diagnostic code links here. Refer to your ICD-10-CM book.

Relative Value Units/Medicare Edits

Non-Facility RVU	Work	PE	MP	Total
98012				
98013				
98014				
98015				
Facility RVU	**Work**	**PE**	**MP**	**Total**
98012				
98013				
98014				
98015				

	FUD	Status	MUE	Modifiers				IOM Reference
98012	N/A		-	N/A	N/A	N/A	N/A	None
98013	N/A		-	N/A	N/A	N/A	N/A	
98014	N/A		-	N/A	N/A	N/A	N/A	
98015	N/A		-	N/A	N/A	N/A	N/A	

* with documentation

Terms To Know

synchronous services. Services that entail real-time communication between the patient and/or family and a physician or other qualified health care professional (QHP) when both are located at different physical sites.

telemedicine. Medical information exchanged from site to site via electronic communication. Examples include patient evaluation and consultation, monitoring, education and other clinical services.

[98016]

- ● **98016** Brief communication technology-based service (eg, virtual check-in) by a physician or other qualified health care professional who can report evaluation and management services, provided to an established patient, not originating from a related evaluation and management service provided within the previous 7 days nor leading to an evaluation and management service or procedure within the next 24 hours or soonest available appointment, 5-10 minutes of medical discussion.

Explanation

A brief, synchronous service using communication technology is performed by a physician or other qualified health care professional to determine if an office visit or other evaluation and management (E/M) service is needed for an established patient. This virtual check-in or triage service is initiated by the patient. This code requires at least five minutes of real-time medical discussion and should not be reported if the problem discussed is related to an E/M encounter that occurred within the previous seven days or when the problem leads to an E/M encounter or procedure within the following 24 hours or next available appointment opening.

Coding Tips

This code is used to report a brief, synchronous, real-time, audio only interactive telecommunication service for an established patient. This service is based on the time of the medical discussion only, MDM is not applicable. This telehealth service is patient initiated and used to determine if a more extensive E/M service may be required. If this service leads to another E/M service on the same date, and time is used for code level selection, add the time of each visit together and report only one E/M service. Do not report this code if less than five minutes of medical discussion is provided. Do not report 98016 in addition to 98000-98015.

ICD-10-CM Diagnostic Codes

The application of this code is too broad to adequately present ICD-10-CM diagnostic code links here. Refer to your ICD-10-CM book.

Relative Value Units/Medicare Edits

Non-Facility RVU	Work	PE	MP	Total
98016				
Facility RVU	**Work**	**PE**	**MP**	**Total**
98016				

	FUD	Status	MUE	Modifiers				IOM Reference
98016	N/A		-	N/A	N/A	N/A	N/A	None

* with documentation

Terms To Know

established patient. Patient who has received professional services in a face-to-face setting within the last three years from the same physician/qualified health care professional or another physician/qualified health care professional of the exact same specialty and subspecialty who belongs to the same group practice. If the patient is seen by a physician/qualified health care professional who is covering for another physician/qualified health care professional, the patient will be considered the same as if seen by the physician/qualified health care professional who is unavailable.

99221-99223

99221 Initial hospital inpatient or observation care, per day, for the evaluation and management of a patient, which requires a medically appropriate history and/or examination and straightforward or low level medical decision making. When using total time on the date of the encounter for code selection, 40 minutes must be met or exceeded.

99222 Initial hospital inpatient or observation care, per day, for the evaluation and management of a patient, which requires a medically appropriate history and/or examination and moderate level of medical decision making. When using total time on the date of the encounter for code selection, 55 minutes must be met or exceeded.

99223 Initial hospital inpatient or observation care, per day, for the evaluation and management of a patient, which requires a medically appropriate history and/or examination and high level of medical decision making. When using total time on the date of the encounter for code selection, 75 minutes must be met or exceeded.

Explanation

Initial hospital inpatient or observation service codes describe the first encounter with the patient by a physician or qualified clinician. CPT guidelines indicate these services may be reported for the first encounter by the provider of the same specialty/subspecialty of the same group practice. Transition from observation to inpatient status does not qualify as an initial hospital encounter. Codes are reported per day and do not differentiate between new or established patients. Under the initial inpatient or observation care category, there are three levels represented by 99221, 99222, and 99223. All services require a medically appropriate history and/or examination. Code selection is based on the level of medical decision making (MDM) or total time personally spent by the physician and/or other qualified health care professional(s) on the date of the encounter. Factors to be considered in MDM include the number and complexity of problems addressed during the encounter, amount and complexity of data requiring review and analysis, and the risk of complications and/or morbidity or mortality associated with patient management. Report 99221 for a visit that entails straightforward or low MDM. If time is used for code selection, a total time of 40 minutes must be met or exceeded on the day of encounter. Report 99222 for a visit requiring a moderate level of MDM or meeting or exceeding 55 minutes of total time. Report 99223 for a high level of MDM or meeting or exceeding 75 minutes of total time. Note that these codes include services provided to patients in a "partial hospital" setting.

Coding Tips

These codes are used to report initial hospital inpatient or observation services. A medically appropriate history and physical examination, as determined by the treating provider, should be documented. The level of history and physical examination are not considered when determining the level of service. Codes should be selected based upon the current CPT Medical Decision Making table. Alternatively, time alone may be used to select the appropriate level of service. Total time for reporting these services includes face-to-face and non-face-to-face time personally spent by the physician or other qualified health care professional on the date of the encounter. CPT guidelines indicate these services may be reported for the initial encounter by one provider of the same specialty/subspecialty of the same group practice. All other providers should report 99231-99233 or 99252-99255. Medicare and some payers may require the admitting/supervising provider to append modifier AI. Observation services do not need to be provided in a designated observation unit. Medicare has identified these codes as telehealth/telemedicine services. Telemedicine services may be reported by the performing provider by using the appropriate place of service (POS) indicator; POS 02 for telehealth when the originating site is not the patient's home. For prolonged services applicable to 99223, see 99418; for Medicare, see G0316. Medicare and commercial payers should be contacted regarding their coverage guidelines. For subsequent inpatient or observation care, see 99231-99233. For discharge from an inpatient or observation stay on a different date of service than the admission, see 99238-99239. For patients admitted to hospital inpatient or observation care for a minimum of eight hours and discharged on the same date, see 99234-99236. Services provided in another setting on the same date may be separately reported if appropriate with modifier 25 appended.

ICD-10-CM Diagnostic Codes

The application of this code is too broad to adequately present ICD-10-CM diagnostic code links here. Refer to your ICD-10-CM book.

AMA: **99221** 2024,Sep; 2024,Mar; 2023,Dec; 2023,Oct; 2023,Aug; 2023,May; 2023,Feb; 2023,Jan; 2022,Dec; 2022,Nov; 2022,Oct; 2022,Sep; 2022,Aug; 2022,Jul; 2022,May; 2022,Apr; 2021,Oct; 2021,Jan; 2020,Dec; 2020,Oct; 2020,Sep; 2020,Mar; 2019,Jul; 2018,Dec; 2018,Oct; 2018,Jun **99222** 2024,Sep; 2024,Mar; 2023,Dec; 2023,Oct; 2023,May; 2023,Feb; 2023,Jan; 2022,Dec; 2022,Nov; 2022,Oct; 2022,Sep; 2022,Aug; 2022,Jul; 2022,May; 2022,Apr; 2021,Oct; 2021,Jan; 2020,Dec; 2020,Oct; 2020,Sep; 2020,Mar; 2019,Jul; 2018,Dec; 2018,Oct; 2018,Jun **99223** 2024,Sep; 2024,Mar; 2023,Dec; 2023,Oct; 2023,Jul; 2023,May; 2023,Feb; 2023,Jan; 2022,Dec; 2022,Nov; 2022,Oct; 2022,Sep; 2022,Aug; 2022,Jul; 2022,May; 2022,Apr; 2021,Oct; 2021,Sep; 2021,Jan; 2020,Dec; 2020,Oct; 2020,Sep; 2020,Mar; 2019,Jul; 2018,Dec; 2018,Oct; 2018,Jun

Relative Value Units/Medicare Edits

Non-Facility RVU	Work	PE	MP	Total
99221	1.63	0.65	0.18	2.46
99222	2.6	1.05	0.23	3.88
99223	3.5	1.38	0.26	5.14
Facility RVU	**Work**	**PE**	**MP**	**Total**
99221	1.63	0.65	0.18	2.46
99222	2.6	1.05	0.23	3.88
99223	3.5	1.38	0.26	5.14

	FUD	Status	MUE	Modifiers				IOM Reference
99221	N/A	A	1(3)	N/A	N/A	N/A	80*	None
99222	N/A	A	1(3)	N/A	N/A	N/A	80*	
99223	N/A	A	1(3)	N/A	N/A	N/A	80*	

* with documentation

99231-99233

★**99231** Subsequent hospital inpatient or observation care, per day, for the evaluation and management of a patient, which requires a medically appropriate history and/or examination and straightforward or low level of medical decision making. When using total time on the date of the encounter for code selection, 25 minutes must be met or exceeded.

★**99232** Subsequent hospital inpatient or observation care, per day, for the evaluation and management of a patient, which requires a medically appropriate history and/or examination and moderate level of medical decision making. When using total time on the date of the encounter for code selection, 35 minutes must be met or exceeded.

★**99233** Subsequent hospital inpatient or observation care, per day, for the evaluation and management of a patient, which requires a medically appropriate history and/or examination and high level of medical decision making. When using total time on the date of the encounter for code selection, 50 minutes must be met or exceeded.

Explanation

Subsequent hospital inpatient or observation service codes describe visits that occur after the first encounter with a patient by a physician or qualified clinician. Codes are reported per day and do not differentiate between new or established patients. Under the subsequent inpatient or observation care category, there are three levels represented by 99231, 99232, and 99233. All services require a medically appropriate history and/or examination. Code selection is based on the level of medical decision making (MDM) or total time personally spent by the physician and/or other qualified health care professional(s) on the date of the encounter. Factors to be considered in MDM include the number and complexity of problems addressed during the encounter, amount and complexity of data requiring review and analysis, and the risk of complications and/or morbidity or mortality associated with patient management. Report 99231 for a visit that entails straightforward or low MDM. If time is used for code selection, a total time of 25 minutes must be met or exceeded on the day of encounter. Report 99232 for a visit requiring a moderate level of MDM or meeting or exceeding 35 minutes of total time. Report 99233 for a high level of MDM or meeting or exceeding 50 minutes of total time.

Coding Tips

These codes are used to report subsequent hospital inpatient or observation services. A medically appropriate history and physical examination, as determined by the treating provider, should be documented. The level of history and physical examination are not considered when determining the level of service. Codes should be selected based upon the current CPT Medical Decision Making table. Alternatively, time alone may be used to select the appropriate level of service. Total time for reporting these services includes face-to-face and non-face-to-face time personally spent by the physician or other qualified health care professional on the date of the encounter. Observation services do not need to be provided in a designated observation unit. Medicare and the CPT codebook have identified these codes as telehealth/telemedicine services. Telemedicine services may be reported by the performing provider by adding modifier 95 to the procedure code and/or using the appropriate place of service (POS) indicator; POS 02 for telehealth when the originating site is not the patient's home. For prolonged services applicable to 99233, see 99418; for Medicare, see G0316. Medicare and commercial payers should be contacted regarding their coverage guidelines. For initial inpatient or observation care, see 99221-99223. For discharge from an inpatient or observation stay on a different date of service than the admission, see 99238-99239. For patients admitted to hospital inpatient or observation care for a minimum of eight hours and discharged on the same date, see 99234-99236; for admission and discharge on the same date of less than eight hours, see 99221-99223.

ICD-10-CM Diagnostic Codes

The application of this code is too broad to adequately present ICD-10-CM diagnostic code links here. Refer to your ICD-10-CM book.

AMA: 99231 2024,Sep; 2023,Dec; 2023,Oct; 2023,May; 2023,Feb; 2023,Jan; 2022,Dec; 2022,Nov; 2022,Oct; 2022,Sep; 2022,Aug; 2022,Jul; 2022,Apr; 2021,Dec; 2021,Oct; 2021,Jun; 2021,Jan; 2020,Dec; 2020,Sep; 2020,Mar; 2019,Jul; 2018,Dec; 2018,Oct; 2018,Jun **99232** 2024,Sep; 2024,Jan; 2023,Dec; 2023,Oct; 2023,May; 2023,Feb; 2023,Jan; 2022,Dec; 2022,Nov; 2022,Oct; 2022,Sep; 2022,Aug; 2022,Jul; 2022,Apr; 2021,Dec; 2021,Oct; 2021,Jun; 2021,Jan; 2020,Dec; 2020,Sep; 2020,Mar; 2019,Jul; 2018,Dec; 2018,Oct; 2018,Jun **99233** 2024,Sep; 2023,Dec; 2023,Oct; 2023,Jul; 2023,May; 2023,Feb; 2023,Jan; 2022,Dec; 2022,Nov; 2022,Oct; 2022,Sep; 2022,Aug; 2022,Jul; 2022,Apr; 2021,Dec; 2021,Oct; 2021,Jun; 2021,Jan; 2020,Dec; 2020,Sep; 2020,Mar; 2019,Jul; 2018,Dec; 2018,Oct; 2018,Jun

Relative Value Units/Medicare Edits

Non-Facility RVU	Work	PE	MP	Total
99231	1.0	0.38	0.09	1.47
99232	1.59	0.63	0.12	2.34
99233	2.4	0.94	0.18	3.52
Facility RVU	**Work**	**PE**	**MP**	**Total**
99231	1.0	0.38	0.09	1.47
99232	1.59	0.63	0.12	2.34
99233	2.4	0.94	0.18	3.52

	FUD	Status	MUE	Modifiers				IOM Reference
99231	N/A	A	1(3)	N/A	N/A	N/A	80*	None
99232	N/A	A	1(3)	N/A	N/A	N/A	80*	
99233	N/A	A	1(3)	N/A	N/A	N/A	80*	

* with documentation

99234-99236

99234 Hospital inpatient or observation care, for the evaluation and management of a patient including admission and discharge on the same date, which requires a medically appropriate history and/or examination and straightforward or low level of medical decision making. When using total time on the date of the encounter for code selection, 45 minutes must be met or exceeded.

99235 Hospital inpatient or observation care, for the evaluation and management of a patient including admission and discharge on the same date, which requires a medically appropriate history and/or examination and moderate level of medical decision making. When using total time on the date of the encounter for code selection, 70 minutes must be met or exceeded.

99236 Hospital inpatient or observation care, for the evaluation and management of a patient including admission and discharge on the same date, which requires a medically appropriate history and/or examination and high level of medical decision making. When using total time on the date of the encounter for code selection, 85 minutes must be met or exceeded.

Explanation

Hospital inpatient or observation care services in cases where the patient is admitted and discharged on the same date of service by the supervising or qualified clinician are reported with 99234-99236. Two or more encounters are required on the same date: an admission encounter and a discharge encounter. These codes also require a minimum hospital stay of eight hours. Codes do not differentiate between new or established patients. Under this care category, there are three levels represented by 99234, 99235, and 99236. All services require a medically appropriate history and/or examination. Code selection is based on the level of medical decision making (MDM) or total time personally spent by the physician and/or other qualified health care professional(s) on the date of the encounter. Factors to be considered in MDM include the number and complexity of problems addressed during the encounter, amount and complexity of data requiring review and analysis, and the risk of complications and/or morbidity or mortality associated with patient management. Report 99234 for a visit that entails straightforward or low MDM. If time is used for code selection, a total time of 45 minutes must be met or exceeded on the day of the encounter. Report 99235 for a visit requiring a moderate level of MDM or meeting or exceeding 70 minutes of total time. Report 99236 for a high level of MDM or meeting or exceeding 85 minutes of total time.

Coding Tips

These codes are used to report hospital inpatient or observation services for the patient admitted and discharged on the same date of service. A medically appropriate history and physical examination, as determined by the treating provider, should be documented. The level of history and physical examination are not considered when determining the level of service. Codes should be selected based upon the current CPT Medical Decision Making table. Alternatively, time alone may be used to select the appropriate level of service. Total time for reporting these services includes face-to-face and non-face-to-face time personally spent by the physician or other qualified health care professional on the date of the encounter. Two or more encounters are required with one assessment as the initial and the other as the discharge. Medicare has identified these codes as telehealth/telemedicine services. Telemedicine services may be reported by the performing provider by using the appropriate place of service (POS) indicator; POS 02 for telehealth when the originating site is not the patient's home. For prolonged services applicable to 99236, see 99418; for Medicare, see G0316. Medicare and commercial payers should be contacted regarding their coverage guidelines. For patients admitted to hospital inpatient or observation care for less than eight hours on the same date of service, see 99221-99223. For initial hospital inpatient or observation care, see 99221-99223; subsequent inpatient or observation care, see 99231-99233. For discharge from an inpatient or observation stay on a different date of service than the admission, see 99238-99239.

ICD-10-CM Diagnostic Codes

The application of this code is too broad to adequately present ICD-10-CM diagnostic code links here. Refer to your ICD-10-CM book.

AMA: **99234** 2024,Sep; 2023,Dec; 2023,Jan; 2022,Dec; 2022,Nov; 2022,Sep; 2022,Aug; 2022,Jul; 2022,May; 2022,Apr; 2021,Oct; 2021,Jan; 2020,Dec; 2020,Sep; 2020,Mar; 2019,Jul; 2018,Dec; 2018,Oct; 2018,Apr **99235** 2024,Sep; 2023,Dec; 2023,Jan; 2022,Dec; 2022,Nov; 2022,Sep; 2022,Aug; 2022,Jul; 2022,May; 2022,Apr; 2021,Oct; 2021,Jan; 2020,Dec; 2020,Sep; 2020,Mar; 2019,Jul; 2018,Dec; 2018,Oct; 2018,Apr **99236** 2024,Sep; 2023,Dec; 2023,Jan; 2022,Dec; 2022,Nov; 2022,Sep; 2022,Aug; 2022,Jul; 2022,May; 2022,Apr; 2021,Oct; 2021,Jan; 2020,Dec; 2020,Sep; 2020,Mar; 2019,Jul; 2018,Dec; 2018,Oct; 2018,Apr

Relative Value Units/Medicare Edits

Non-Facility RVU	Work	PE	MP	Total
99234	2.0	0.73	0.17	2.9
99235	3.24	1.25	0.24	4.73
99236	4.3	1.56	0.32	6.18
Facility RVU	**Work**	**PE**	**MP**	**Total**
99234	2.0	0.73	0.17	2.9
99235	3.24	1.25	0.24	4.73
99236	4.3	1.56	0.32	6.18

	FUD	Status	MUE	Modifiers				IOM Reference
99234	N/A	A	1(3)	N/A	N/A	N/A	80*	None
99235	N/A	A	1(3)	N/A	N/A	N/A	80*	
99236	N/A	A	1(3)	N/A	N/A	N/A	80*	

* with documentation

99238-99239

99238 Hospital inpatient or observation discharge day management; 30 minutes or less on the date of the encounter

99239 more than 30 minutes on the date of the encounter

Explanation

Hospital discharge services are time-based codes that, when reported, describe the amount of time spent by the qualified clinician that is responsible for discharge services for inpatient or observation care. These discharge day management codes include all final steps involved in the discharge of a patient from the hospital on a date that differs from the date of admission, including the last patient exam, discussing the hospital stay, instructions for ongoing care as it relates to all pertinent caregivers, as well as preparing the medical discharge records, prescriptions, and/or referrals as applicable. Time reported should be for the total duration of time spent by the provider even when the time spent on that date is not continuous. For a hospital discharge duration of 30 minutes or less, report 99238; for a duration of greater than 30 minutes, report 99239.

Coding Tips

These codes are used to report all discharge day services for the hospital inpatient or observation patient, including examination, discharge and follow-up care instructions, and preparation of all medical records. These are time-based codes and time spent with the patient must be documented in the medical record. Medicare has identified these codes as telehealth/telemedicine services. Telemedicine services may be reported by the performing provider by using the appropriate place of service (POS) indicator; POS 02 for telehealth when the originating site is not the patient's home. Medicare and commercial payers should be contacted regarding their coverage guidelines. For patients admitted to hospital inpatient or observation care for a minimum of eight hours and discharged on the same date, see 99234-99236; for admission and discharge on the same date of less than eight hours, see 99221-99223. For services performed by other providers on the date of discharge including instructions to the patient or family/caregiver and post-discharge coordination services, see codes 99231-99233.

ICD-10-CM Diagnostic Codes

The application of this code is too broad to adequately present ICD-10-CM diagnostic code links here. Refer to your ICD-10-CM book.

AMA: 99238 2023,Dec; 2023,Jul; 2023,Jan; 2022,Dec; 2022,Aug; 2022,Jul; 2021,Jan; 2019,Jul; 2018,Dec **99239** 2023,Dec; 2023,Jan; 2022,Dec; 2022,Aug; 2022,Jul; 2021,Jan; 2019,Jul; 2018,Dec

Relative Value Units/Medicare Edits

Non-Facility RVU	Work	PE	MP	Total
99238	1.5	0.8	0.11	2.41
99239	2.15	1.1	0.15	3.4
Facility RVU	**Work**	**PE**	**MP**	**Total**
99238	1.5	0.8	0.11	2.41
99239	2.15	1.1	0.15	3.4

	FUD	Status	MUE	Modifiers				IOM Reference
99238	N/A	A	1(3)	N/A	N/A	N/A	80*	None
99239	N/A	A	1(3)	N/A	N/A	N/A	80*	

* with documentation

99242-99245

★99242 Office or other outpatient consultation for a new or established patient, which requires a medically appropriate history and/or examination and straightforward medical decision making. When using total time on the date of the encounter for code selection, 20 minutes must be met or exceeded.

★99243 Office or other outpatient consultation for a new or established patient, which requires a medically appropriate history and/or examination and low level of medical decision making. When using total time on the date of the encounter for code selection, 30 minutes must be met or exceeded.

★99244 Office or other outpatient consultation for a new or established patient, which requires a medically appropriate history and/or examination and moderate level of medical decision making. When using total time on the date of the encounter for code selection, 40 minutes must be met or exceeded.

★99245 Office or other outpatient consultation for a new or established patient, which requires a medically appropriate history and/or examination and high level of medical decision making. When using total time on the date of the encounter for code selection, 55 minutes must be met or exceeded.

Explanation

Office or other outpatient consultation service codes describe encounters where another qualified clinician's advice or opinion regarding diagnosis and treatment is rendered at the request of the primary treating provider. Consultations may also be requested by another appropriate source (e.g., a third-party payer may request a second opinion). The request for a consultation must be documented in the medical record, as well as a written report of the consultation findings. During a consultation, diagnostic or therapeutic services may be initiated at the same encounter or at a follow-up visit. Office or other outpatient sites include the physician's office, a home or residence, or the emergency department. Consultation codes do not differentiate between new or established patients. All services require a medically appropriate history and/or examination. Code selection is based on the level of medical decision making (MDM) or total time personally spent by the physician and/or other qualified health care professional(s) on the date of the encounter. Factors to be considered in MDM include the number and complexity of problems addressed during the encounter, amount and complexity of data requiring review and analysis, and the risk of complications and/or morbidity or mortality associated with patient management. Report 99242 for a visit that entails straightforward MDM. If time is used for code selection, a total time of 20 minutes must be met or exceeded on the day of the encounter. Report 99243 for a visit requiring a low level of MDM or meeting or exceeding 30 minutes of total time; 99244 for a moderate level of MDM or meeting or exceeding 40 minutes of total time; and 99245 for a high level of MDM or meeting or exceeding 55 minutes of total time.

Coding Tips

These codes are used to report consultations in the office or outpatient setting including home, residence, or emergency department. A medically appropriate history and physical examination, as determined by the treating provider, should be documented. The level of history and physical examination are not considered when determining the level of service. Codes should be selected based upon the current CPT Medical Decision Making table. Alternatively, time alone may be used to select the appropriate level of service. Total time for reporting these services includes face-to-face and non-face-to-face time personally spent by the physician or other qualified health care professional on the date of the encounter. Managing the patient's entire care or for the care of a specific condition or problem is considered a transfer of care and not

 ● New ▲ Revised + Add On ★ Telemedicine [Resequenced] ☑ Laterality

a consultation service. For a transfer of care service, report codes for new or established office or other outpatient services or codes for home or residence services. Consultation codes are not covered by Medicare and some payers and are reported using new or established outpatient E/M codes. Consultation services should not be reported when the care and management of a problem or condition is assumed prior to the initial examination of the patient. In these situations, the appropriate initial or subsequent evaluation and management service should be reported. Subsequent care is reported using the appropriate codes for established patients in the specific site of service. The CPT codebook has identified these codes as telehealth/telemedicine services. Telemedicine services may be reported by the performing provider by adding modifier 95 to the procedure code and using the appropriate place of service (POS) indicator. For prolonged services applicable to 99245, see 99417. Commercial payers should be contacted regarding their coverage guidelines. For office or other outpatient services for a new patient, see 99202-99205; for an established patient, see 99211-99215. For inpatient consultation services, see 99252-99255.

ICD-10-CM Diagnostic Codes

The application of this code is too broad to adequately present ICD-10-CM diagnostic code links here. Refer to your ICD-10-CM book.

AMA: **99242** 2024,Sep; 2023,Dec; 2023,Oct; 2023,Mar; 2023,Feb; 2022,Dec; 2022,Nov; 2022,Oct; 2022,Sep; 2022,Aug; 2022,Jul; 2022,May; 2022,Apr; 2022,Feb; 2021,Oct; 2021,Mar; 2021,Jan; 2020,Dec; 2020,Nov; 2020,Oct; 2020,Sep; 2020,Mar; 2019,Jul; 2018,Apr; 2018,Mar **99243** 2024,Sep; 2023,Dec; 2023,Oct; 2023,Mar; 2023,Feb; 2022,Dec; 2022,Nov; 2022,Oct; 2022,Sep; 2022,Aug; 2022,Jul; 2022,May; 2022,Apr; 2022,Feb; 2021,Oct; 2021,Mar; 2021,Jan; 2020,Dec; 2020,Nov; 2020,Oct; 2020,Sep; 2020,Mar; 2019,Jul; 2018,Apr; 2018,Mar **99244** 2024,Sep; 2023,Dec; 2023,Oct; 2023,Mar; 2023,Feb; 2022,Dec; 2022,Nov; 2022,Oct; 2022,Sep; 2022,Aug; 2022,Jul; 2022,May; 2022,Apr; 2022,Feb; 2021,Oct; 2021,Mar; 2021,Jan; 2020,Dec; 2020,Nov; 2020,Oct; 2020,Sep; 2020,Mar; 2019,Jul; 2018,Apr; 2018,Mar **99245** 2024,Sep; 2023,Dec; 2023,Oct; 2023,Mar; 2023,Feb; 2022,Dec; 2022,Nov; 2022,Oct; 2022,Sep; 2022,Aug; 2022,Jul; 2022,May; 2022,Apr; 2022,Feb; 2021,Oct; 2021,Mar; 2021,Jan; 2020,Dec; 2020,Nov; 2020,Oct; 2020,Sep; 2020,Mar; 2019,Jul; 2018,Apr; 2018,Mar

Relative Value Units/Medicare Edits

Non-Facility RVU	Work	PE	MP	Total
99242	1.08	1.1	0.07	2.25
99243	1.8	1.46	0.11	3.37
99244	2.69	1.96	0.16	4.81
99245	3.75	2.3	0.23	6.28
Facility RVU	**Work**	**PE**	**MP**	**Total**
99242	1.08	0.51	0.07	1.66
99243	1.8	0.71	0.11	2.62
99244	2.69	1.14	0.16	3.99
99245	3.75	1.38	0.23	5.36

	FUD	Status	MUE	Modifiers				IOM Reference
99242	N/A	I	0(3)	N/A	N/A	N/A	N/A	None
99243	N/A	I	0(3)	N/A	N/A	N/A	N/A	
99244	N/A	I	0(3)	N/A	N/A	N/A	N/A	
99245	N/A	I	0(3)	N/A	N/A	N/A	N/A	

* with documentation

99252-99255

★99252 Inpatient or observation consultation for a new or established patient, which requires a medically appropriate history and/or examination and straightforward medical decision making. When using total time on the date of the encounter for code selection, 35 minutes must be met or exceeded.

★99253 Inpatient or observation consultation for a new or established patient, which requires a medically appropriate history and/or examination and low level of medical decision making. When using total time on the date of the encounter for code selection, 45 minutes must be met or exceeded.

★99254 Inpatient or observation consultation for a new or established patient, which requires a medically appropriate history and/or examination and moderate level of medical decision making. When using total time on the date of the encounter for code selection, 60 minutes must be met or exceeded.

★99255 Inpatient or observation consultation for a new or established patient, which requires a medically appropriate history and/or examination and high level of medical decision making. When using total time on the date of the encounter for code selection, 80 minutes must be met or exceeded.

Explanation

Inpatient or observation consultation service codes describe encounters with patients admitted to the hospital in inpatient or observation status, those residing in nursing facilities, or to patients in a partial hospital setting where another qualified clinician's advice or opinion regarding diagnosis and treatment is rendered at the request of the primary treating provider. The request for a consultation must be documented in the patient's medical record, as well as a written report of the findings of the consultation to the primary treating physician. During the course of a consultation, diagnostic or therapeutic services may be initiated at the same encounter or at a follow-up visit. Consultation codes do not differentiate between new or established patients. Only one inpatient or observation consultation services code should be reported per admission. Subsequent consultation services during the same hospital stay are reported with subsequent inpatient or observation hospital care codes or subsequent nursing facility care codes. All services require a medically appropriate history and/or examination. Code selection is based on the level of medical decision making (MDM) or total time personally spent by the physician and/or other qualified health care professional(s) on the date of the encounter. Factors to be considered in MDM include the number and complexity of problems addressed during the encounter, amount and complexity of data requiring review and analysis, and the risk of complications and/or morbidity or mortality associated with patient management. Report 99252 for a visit that entails straightforward MDM. If time is used for code selection, a total time of 35 minutes must be met or exceeded on the day of the encounter. Report 99253 for a visit requiring a low level of MDM or meeting or exceeding 45 minutes of total time; 99254 for a moderate level of MDM or meeting or exceeding 60 minutes of total time; and 99255 for a high level of MDM or meeting or exceeding 80 minutes of total time.

Coding Tips

These codes are used to report consultations in the inpatient or observation setting. A medically appropriate history and physical examination, as determined by the treating provider, should be documented. The level of history and physical examination are not considered when determining the level of service. Codes should be selected based upon the current CPT Medical Decision Making table. Alternatively, time alone may be used to select the appropriate level of service. Total time for reporting these services includes face-to-face and non-face-to-face time personally spent by the physician or other qualified health care professional on the date of the encounter. For observation services, the patient is not required to be physically located in a designated observation area within a hospital; however, if such an area is utilized, these codes should be reported. CPT guidelines indicate these services may be reported for the first encounter by the provider of the same specialty/subspecialty of the same group practice. Managing the patient's entire care or for the care of a specific condition or problem is considered a transfer of care and not a consultation service. For a transfer of care service, report codes for hospital inpatient or observation services or nursing facility services. Consultation codes are not covered by Medicare and some payers and are reported using new or established inpatient E/M codes. Consultation services should not be reported when the care and management of a problem or condition is assumed prior to the initial examination of the patient. In these situations, the appropriate initial or subsequent evaluation and management service should be reported. Do not report an inpatient and outpatient consultation when both are related to the same inpatient admission. The CPT codebook has identified these codes as telehealth/telemedicine services. Telemedicine services may be reported by the performing provider by adding modifier 95 to the procedure code and using the appropriate place of service (POS) indicator. For prolonged services applicable to 99255, see 99418. Commercial payers should be contacted regarding their coverage guidelines. For initial hospital care services, see 99221-99223; for subsequent hospital care services, see 99231-99233. For office or other outpatient consultation services, see 99242-99245.

ICD-10-CM Diagnostic Codes

The application of this code is too broad to adequately present ICD-10-CM diagnostic code links here. Refer to your ICD-10-CM book.

AMA: **99252** 2024,Sep; 2024,Mar; 2023,Dec; 2023,Oct; 2023,Jul; 2023,May; 2023,Mar; 2022,Dec; 2022,Nov; 2022,Oct; 2022,Sep; 2022,Aug; 2022,Jul; 2022,May; 2022,Apr; 2022,Feb; 2021,Oct; 2021,Jan; 2020,Dec; 2020,Sep; 2020,Mar; 2019,Jul **99253** 2024,Sep; 2024,Mar; 2023,Dec; 2023,Oct; 2023,Jul; 2023,May; 2023,Mar; 2022,Dec; 2022,Nov; 2022,Oct; 2022,Sep; 2022,Aug; 2022,Jul; 2022,May; 2022,Apr; 2022,Feb; 2021,Oct; 2021,Sep; 2021,Jan; 2020,Dec; 2020,Sep; 2020,Mar; 2019,Jul **99254** 2024,Sep; 2024,Mar; 2023,Dec; 2023,Oct; 2023,Jul; 2023,May; 2023,Mar; 2022,Dec; 2022,Nov; 2022,Oct; 2022,Sep; 2022,Aug; 2022,Jul; 2022,May; 2022,Apr; 2022,Feb; 2021,Oct; 2021,Jan; 2020,Dec; 2020,Sep; 2020,Mar; 2019,Jul **99255** 2024,Sep; 2024,Mar; 2023,Dec; 2023,Oct; 2023,Jul; 2023,May; 2023,Mar; 2022,Dec; 2022,Nov; 2022,Oct; 2022,Sep; 2022,Aug; 2022,Jul; 2022,May; 2022,Apr; 2022,Feb; 2021,Oct; 2021,Jan; 2020,Dec; 2020,Sep; 2020,Mar; 2019,Jul

Relative Value Units/Medicare Edits

Non-Facility RVU	Work	PE	MP	Total
99252	1.5	0.52	0.09	2.11
99253	2.0	0.84	0.12	2.96
99254	2.72	1.23	0.16	4.11
99255	3.86	1.44	0.23	5.53
Facility RVU	**Work**	**PE**	**MP**	**Total**
99252	1.5	0.52	0.09	2.11
99253	2.0	0.84	0.12	2.96
99254	2.72	1.23	0.16	4.11
99255	3.86	1.44	0.23	5.53

	FUD	Status	MUE	Modifiers				IOM Reference
99252	N/A	I	0(3)	N/A	N/A	N/A	N/A	None
99253	N/A	I	0(3)	N/A	N/A	N/A	N/A	
99254	N/A	I	0(3)	N/A	N/A	N/A	N/A	
99255	N/A	I	0(3)	N/A	N/A	N/A	N/A	

* with documentation

Terms To Know

consultation. Advice or opinion regarding diagnosis and treatment or determination to accept transfer of care of a patient that is rendered by a medical professional at the request of the primary care provider. Consultations may also be requested by another appropriate source. A request for consultation must be documented in the medical record, as well as a written report of the findings of the consultation. Since January 1, 2010, Medicare no longer recognizes CPT consultation codes; however, telehealth consultation services reported with HCPCS Level II codes are a paid service under the Medicare Physician Fee Schedule (MPFS).

99281-99285

99281 Emergency department visit for the evaluation and management of a patient that may not require the presence of a physician or other qualified health care professional

99282 Emergency department visit for the evaluation and management of a patient, which requires a medically appropriate history and/or examination and straightforward medical decision making

99283 Emergency department visit for the evaluation and management of a patient, which requires a medically appropriate history and/or examination and low level of medical decision making

99284 Emergency department visit for the evaluation and management of a patient, which requires a medically appropriate history and/or examination and moderate level of medical decision making

99285 Emergency department visit for the evaluation and management of a patient, which requires a medically appropriate history and/or examination and high level of medical decision making

Explanation

Emergency department service codes describe E/M services provided to patients in the emergency department (ED). ED codes are typically reported per day and do not differentiate between new or established patients. Other procedures or services performed in conjunction with the emergency room encounter may be reported separately. Under the emergency department services category, there are five levels represented by 99281-99285. For the lowest level of care, 99281, services can be performed by clinical staff and must be face-to-face. The presence of a physician or qualified clinician is not required, but services are performed under their supervision. There are no time or MDM requirements for 99281. The remaining levels, 99282-99285, require a medically appropriate history and/or examination. Code selection is based on the level of medical decision making (MDM). Factors to be considered in MDM include the number and complexity of problems addressed during the encounter, amount and complexity of data requiring review and analysis, and the risk of complications and/or morbidity or mortality associated with patient management. Time is not listed as a component in the code descriptors for emergency department services as these types of services are provided based on the varying intensity of the patient's condition and may involve emergency providers caring for several patients over an extended period involving multiple encounters, making it difficult for the clinician to accurately detail the amount of time spent face-to-face with the patient. Report 99282 for a visit that entails straightforward MDM; 99283 for a visit requiring a low level of MDM; 99284 for a moderate level of MDM; and 99285 for a high level of MDM.

Coding Tips

These codes are used to report emergency department services for a new or established patient. A medically appropriate history and physical examination, as determined by the treating provider, should be documented. The level of history and physical examination are not considered when determining the level of service. Codes should be selected based upon the current CPT Medical Decision Making table. Time is not a factor when selecting this E/M service. An emergency department is typically described as an organized hospital-based facility available 24 hours a day, providing unscheduled episodic services to patients in need of urgent medical attention. If a provider evaluates a patient in the ED as a convenience for the provider rather than a necessity for emergency care, report codes for office or other outpatient services. Medicare has identified these codes as telehealth/telemedicine services. Telemedicine services may be reported by the performing provider by using the appropriate place of service (POS) indicator; POS 02 for telehealth when the originating site is not the patient's home. Medicare and commercial payers should be contacted regarding their coverage guidelines. For critical care services provided in the emergency department, see 99291-99292. For observation care services provided to a patient located in the emergency department, see 99221-99223. For patients admitted to hospital inpatient or observation care for a minimum of eight hours and discharged on the same date, see 99234-99236. Report place of service code 23 for services provided in the hospital emergency room.

ICD-10-CM Diagnostic Codes

The application of this code is too broad to adequately present ICD-10-CM diagnostic code links here. Refer to your ICD-10-CM book.

AMA: 99281 2023,Aug; 2023,Jul; 2023,May; 2023,Mar; 2022,Dec; 2022,Nov; 2022,Oct; 2022,Sep; 2022,Aug; 2022,Jul; 2022,May; 2021,Sep; 2021,May; 2021,Mar; 2021,Jan; 2020,Dec; 2020,Oct; 2020,Jul; 2019,Jul **99282** 2024,Apr; 2023,Aug; 2023,Jul; 2023,Mar; 2022,Dec; 2022,Nov; 2022,Oct; 2022,Sep; 2022,Aug; 2022,Jul; 2022,May; 2021,Sep; 2021,May; 2021,Mar; 2021,Jan; 2020,Dec; 2020,Oct; 2020,Jul; 2019,Jul **99283** 2024,Apr; 2023,Aug; 2023,Jul; 2023,Mar; 2022,Dec; 2022,Nov; 2022,Oct; 2022,Sep; 2022,Aug; 2022,Jul; 2022,May; 2021,Sep; 2021,May; 2021,Mar; 2021,Jan; 2020,Dec; 2020,Oct; 2020,Jul; 2019,Jul **99284** 2024,Apr; 2023,Aug; 2023,Jul; 2023,Mar; 2022,Dec; 2022,Nov; 2022,Oct; 2022,Sep; 2022,Aug; 2022,Jul; 2022,May; 2021,Sep; 2021,May; 2021,Mar; 2021,Jan; 2020,Dec; 2020,Oct; 2020,Jul; 2019,Jul **99285** 2024,Apr; 2023,Aug; 2023,Jul; 2023,Mar; 2022,Dec; 2022,Nov; 2022,Oct; 2022,Sep; 2022,Aug; 2022,Jul; 2022,May; 2021,Sep; 2021,May; 2021,Mar; 2021,Jan; 2020,Dec; 2020,Oct; 2020,Jul; 2020,Jan; 2019,Jul

Relative Value Units/Medicare Edits

Non-Facility RVU	Work	PE	MP	Total
99281	0.25	0.06	0.03	0.34
99282	0.93	0.21	0.1	1.24
99283	1.6	0.34	0.17	2.11
99284	2.74	0.56	0.29	3.59
99285	4.0	0.78	0.42	5.2
Facility RVU	**Work**	**PE**	**MP**	**Total**
99281	0.25	0.06	0.03	0.34
99282	0.93	0.21	0.1	1.24
99283	1.6	0.34	0.17	2.11
99284	2.74	0.56	0.29	3.59
99285	4.0	0.78	0.42	5.2

	FUD	Status	MUE	Modifiers				IOM Reference
99281	N/A	A	1(3)	N/A	N/A	N/A	80*	None
99282	N/A	A	1(3)	N/A	N/A	N/A	80*	
99283	N/A	A	1(3)	N/A	N/A	N/A	80*	
99284	N/A	A	1(3)	N/A	N/A	N/A	80*	
99285	N/A	A	1(3)	N/A	N/A	N/A	80*	

* with documentation

99288

99288 Physician or other qualified health care professional direction of emergency medical systems (EMS) emergency care, advanced life support

Explanation

This code is used to report qualified clinician direction of emergency medical systems (EMS) emergency care or advanced life support in the emergency department (ED). This can involve the clinician communicating via a two-way voice system with emergency medical technicians in an ambulance or with other rescue personnel who are outside of the hospital emergency department. Clinician direction of the performance of medically necessary procedures includes, but is not limited to, telemetry of cardiac rhythm; cardiac and/or pulmonary resuscitation; endotracheal or esophageal obturator airway intubation; administration of intravenous (IV) fluids and/or intramuscular (IM), intra-tracheal, or subcutaneous drugs; and/or electrical conversion of cardiac arrhythmia.

Coding Tips

This code is used by a facility-based practitioner (emergency department, critical care unit) who is directing remote emergency care or advanced life support in the urgent care of the patient. Time is not a factor when selecting this E/M service. This service may be reported in addition to other E/M services on the same date when documented in the patient record.

ICD-10-CM Diagnostic Codes

The application of this code is too broad to adequately present ICD-10-CM diagnostic code links here. Refer to your ICD-10-CM book.

AMA: **99288** 2022,Nov; 2022,Aug; 2022,Jul; 2022,May; 2021,Jan; 2019,Jul

Relative Value Units/Medicare Edits

Non-Facility RVU	Work	PE	MP	Total
99288	0.0	0.0	0.0	0.0
Facility RVU	**Work**	**PE**	**MP**	**Total**
99288	0.0	0.0	0.0	0.0

	FUD	Status	MUE	Modifiers				IOM Reference
99288	N/A	B	0(3)	N/A	N/A	N/A	N/A	None

* with documentation

Terms To Know

emergency department. Organized hospital-based facility for the provision of unscheduled episodic services to patients who present for immediate medical attention. The facility must be available 24 hours a day.

qualified health care professional. Educated, licensed or certified, and regulated professional operating under a specified scope of practice to provide patient services that are separate and distinct from other clinical staff.

99291-99292

99291 Critical care, evaluation and management of the critically ill or critically injured patient; first 30-74 minutes

\+ **99292** each additional 30 minutes (List separately in addition to code for primary service)

Explanation

Critical care services are reported by a physician or other qualified health care provider for critically ill or injured patients. Critical illnesses or injuries are defined as those with impairment to one or more vital organ systems with an increased risk of rapid or imminent health deterioration. Critical care services require direct patient/provider involvement with highly complex decision making in order to evaluate, control, and support vital systems functions to treat one or more vital organ system failures and/or to avoid further decline of the patient's condition. Vital organ system failure includes, but is not limited to, failure of the central nervous, circulatory, or respiratory systems; kidneys; liver; shock; and other metabolic processes. Generally, critical care services necessitate the interpretation of many physiologic parameters and/or other applications of advanced technology as available in a critical care unit, pediatric intensive care unit, respiratory care unit, in an emergency facility, patient room or other hospital department; however, in emergent situations, critical care may be provided where these elements are not available. Critical care may be provided so long as the patient's condition continues to warrant the level of care according to the criteria described. Care provided to patients residing in a critical care unit but not fitting the criteria for critical care is reported using other E/M codes, as appropriate. These codes are time based codes, meaning the total time spent must be documented and includes direct patient care bedside or time spent on the patient's floor or unit (reviewing laboratory results or imaging studies and discussing the patient's care with medical staff, time spent with family members, caregivers, or other surrogate decision makers to gather information on the patient's medical history, reviewing the patient's condition or prognosis, and discussing various treatment options or limitations of treatment), as long as the clinician is immediately available and not providing services to any other patient during the same time period. Time spent outside of the patient's unit or floor, including telephone calls, caregiver discussions, or time spent in actions that do not directly contribute to the patient's care rendered in the critical unit are not reported as critical care. Report these codes for attendance of the patient during transport for patients 24 months of age or older to or from a facility. Code 99291 represents the first 30 to 74 minutes of critical care and is reported once per day. Additional time beyond the first 74 minutes is reported in 30 minute increments with 99292.

Coding Tips

These codes are used to report critical care services. These are time-based services and the total time spent providing critical care must be documented in the medical record. All time spent providing critical care on the same date of service is added together and does not need to be contiguous. Time is reported for practitioner time spent in care of the critically ill or injured patient at the patient's bedside and on the floor/unit. Time spent off the patient unit, even if related to patient care, is not counted. Do not report critical care for patients who may be in the critical care unit but are not currently critically ill. The following services are considered inclusive to the critical care codes when reported by the clinician: interpretation of cardiac output measurements, chest x-rays, pulse oximetry, blood gases, collection and interpretation of physiologic data, computer data such as ECGs, gastric intubation, vascular access, and ventilation management. Code 99291 is reported once per day. Code 99292 is reported in addition to code 99291. Medicare and some other payers may allow 99292 to be reported alone when critical care is reported by another physician of the same group and specialty the same date as another provider reporting 99291. Medicare has identified these codes as telehealth/telemedicine services. Telemedicine services may be reported by the performing provider by using the appropriate place of service (POS) indicator; POS 02 for telehealth when the originating site is not the patient's home. Medicare and commercial payers should be contacted regarding their coverage guidelines. For care of the critically ill neonate, see 99468-99469; for patients 29 days through 24 months, see 99471-99472; and for patients 2 through 5 years, see 99475-99476.

ICD-10-CM Diagnostic Codes

The application of this code is too broad to adequately present ICD-10-CM diagnostic code links here. Refer to your ICD-10-CM book.

AMA: **99291** 2023,Mar; 2023,Feb; 2022,Dec; 2022,Nov; 2022,Sep; 2022,Aug; 2022,Jul; 2022,May; 2022,Mar; 2022,Jan; 2021,Sep; 2021,Jun; 2021,Jan; 2020,Feb; 2020,Jan; 2019,Dec; 2019,Aug; 2019,Jul; 2018,Dec; 2018,Jun **99292** 2023,Feb; 2022,Dec; 2022,Nov; 2022,Sep; 2022,Aug; 2022,Jul; 2022,May; 2022,Mar; 2022,Jan; 2021,Jan; 2020,Feb; 2019,Dec; 2019,Aug; 2019,Jul; 2018,Dec; 2018,Jun

Relative Value Units/Medicare Edits

Non-Facility RVU	Work	PE	MP	Total
99291	4.5	3.26	0.42	8.18
99292	2.25	1.1	0.23	3.58
Facility RVU	**Work**	**PE**	**MP**	**Total**
99291	4.5	1.39	0.42	6.31
99292	2.25	0.7	0.23	3.18

	FUD	Status	MUE	Modifiers				IOM Reference
99291	N/A	A	1(2)	N/A	N/A	N/A	80*	None
99292	N/A	A	8(3)	N/A	N/A	N/A	80*	

* with documentation

99304-99306

99304 Initial nursing facility care, per day, for the evaluation and management of a patient, which requires a medically appropriate history and/or examination and straightforward or low level of medical decision making. When using total time on the date of the encounter for code selection, 25 minutes must be met or exceeded.

99305 Initial nursing facility care, per day, for the evaluation and management of a patient, which requires a medically appropriate history and/or examination and moderate level of medical decision making. When using total time on the date of the encounter for code selection, 35 minutes must be met or exceeded.

99306 Initial nursing facility care, per day, for the evaluation and management of a patient, which requires a medically appropriate history and/or examination and high level of medical decision making. When using total time on the date of the encounter for code selection, 50 minutes must be met or exceeded.

Explanation

Initial nursing facility service codes describe the first encounter with a patient by a physician or qualified clinician in nursing facilities and skilled nursing facilities, or for services in a psychiatric residential treatment center and intermediate care facility for patients with intellectual disabilities. Initial nursing facility codes may be reported once per admission, per physician or qualified clinician, per stay. Initial nursing facility codes do not differentiate between new or established patients. Under the initial nursing facility care category, there are three levels represented by 99304, 99305, and 99306. All services require a medically appropriate history and/or examination. Code selection is based on the level of medical decision making (MDM) or total time personally spent by the physician and/or other qualified health care professional(s) on the date of the encounter. Factors to be considered in MDM include the number and complexity of problems addressed during the encounter, amount and complexity of data requiring review and analysis, and the risk of complications and/or morbidity or mortality associated with patient management. Report 99304 for a visit that entails straightforward or low MDM. If time is used for code selection, a total time of 25 minutes must be met or exceeded on the day of the encounter. Report 99305 for a visit requiring a moderate level of MDM or meeting or exceeding 35 minutes of total time. Report 99306 for a high level of MDM or meeting or exceeding 50 minutes of total time. For high MDM, an additional component is recognized for initial nursing facility codes for the number and complexity of problems addressed: multiple morbidities requiring intensive management, for the patient who is at risk of worsening status or hospital admission and requiring frequent evaluations with possible changes to medications and/or treatment.

Coding Tips

These codes are used to report the initial encounter in the nursing/skilled nursing facility setting, psychiatric residential treatment center, or care facility for individuals with intellectual disabilities. A medically appropriate history and physical examination, as determined by the treating provider, should be documented. The level of history and physical examination are not considered when determining the level of service. Codes should be selected based upon the current CPT Medical Decision Making table. Alternatively, time alone may be used to select the appropriate level of service. Total time for reporting these services includes face-to-face and non-face-to-face time personally spent by the physician or other qualified health care professional on the date of the encounter. CPT guidelines indicate these services are reported by the principal/admitting provider; initial services performed as consultations may be reported using 99304-99306 or inpatient observation consultation codes 99252-99255. Medicare and some payers may allow providers of different specialties to report initial nursing facility services and require the principal/admitting provider to append modifier AI. When the patient is admitted to the nursing facility during the course of another encounter from a different site of service, such as the physician's office or the emergency department, the services in the initial site can be reported separately. Transitions from the skilled nursing facility level to the nursing facility level do not qualify as a new stay. Hospital inpatient or observation discharge services may be reported separately when performed on the same date of service. Medicare has identified these codes as telehealth/telemedicine services. Telemedicine services may be reported by the performing provider by using the appropriate place of service (POS) indicator; POS 02 for telehealth when the originating site is not the patient's home. For prolonged services applicable to 99306, see 99418; for Medicare, see G0317. Medicare and commercial payers should be contacted regarding their coverage guidelines. For care plan oversight services provided to nursing facility residents, see 99379-99380. For subsequent nursing facility care services, see 99307-99310. For nursing facility discharge services, see 99315-99316.

ICD-10-CM Diagnostic Codes

The application of this code is too broad to adequately present ICD-10-CM diagnostic code links here. Refer to your ICD-10-CM book.

AMA: **99304** 2024,Sep; 2023,Dec; 2023,Jan; 2022,Dec; 2022,Nov; 2022,Oct; 2022,Aug; 2022,Jul; 2022,May; 2022,Apr; 2021,Jan; 2020,Dec; 2020,Nov; 2020,Sep; 2020,Mar; 2019,Jul **99305** 2024,Sep; 2023,Dec; 2023,Jan; 2022,Dec; 2022,Nov; 2022,Oct; 2022,Aug; 2022,Jul; 2022,May; 2022,Apr; 2021,Jan; 2020,Dec; 2020,Nov; 2020,Sep; 2020,Mar; 2019,Jul **99306** 2024,Sep; 2023,Dec; 2023,Jan; 2022,Dec; 2022,Nov; 2022,Oct; 2022,Aug; 2022,Jul; 2022,May; 2022,Apr; 2021,Jan; 2020,Dec; 2020,Nov; 2020,Sep; 2020,Mar; 2019,Jul

Relative Value Units/Medicare Edits

Non-Facility RVU	Work	PE	MP	Total
99304	1.5	0.78	0.11	2.39
99305	2.5	1.3	0.17	3.97
99306	3.5	1.69	0.23	5.42
Facility RVU	**Work**	**PE**	**MP**	**Total**
99304	1.5	0.78	0.11	2.39
99305	2.5	1.3	0.17	3.97
99306	3.5	1.69	0.23	5.42

	FUD	Status	MUE	Modifiers				IOM Reference
99304	N/A	A	1(2)	N/A	N/A	N/A	80*	None
99305	N/A	A	1(2)	N/A	N/A	N/A	80*	
99306	N/A	A	1(2)	N/A	N/A	N/A	80*	

* with documentation

99307-99310

★**99307** Subsequent nursing facility care, per day, for the evaluation and management of a patient, which requires a medically appropriate history and/or examination and straightforward medical decision making. When using total time on the date of the encounter for code selection, 10 minutes must be met or exceeded.

★**99308** Subsequent nursing facility care, per day, for the evaluation and management of a patient, which requires a medically appropriate history and/or examination and low level of medical decision making. When using total time on the date of the encounter for code selection, 20 minutes must be met or exceeded.

★**99309** Subsequent nursing facility care, per day, for the evaluation and management of a patient, which requires a medically appropriate history and/or examination and moderate level of medical decision making. When using total time on the date of the encounter for code selection, 30 minutes must be met or exceeded.

★**99310** Subsequent nursing facility care, per day, for the evaluation and management of a patient, which requires a medically appropriate history and/or examination and high level of medical decision making. When using total time on the date of the encounter for code selection, 45 minutes must be met or exceeded.

Explanation

Subsequent nursing facility care service codes describe visits that occur after the first encounter of the patient's nursing facility admission by the supervising qualified clinician. Codes are reported per day and do not differentiate between new or established patients. All services require a medically appropriate history and/or examination. Code selection is based on the level of medical decision making (MDM) or total time personally spent by the physician and/or other qualified health care professional(s) on the date of the encounter. Factors to be considered in MDM include the number and complexity of problems addressed during the encounter, amount and complexity of data requiring review and analysis, and the risk of complications and/or morbidity or mortality associated with patient management. Report 99307 for a visit that entails straightforward MDM. If time is used for code selection, a total time of 10 minutes must be met or exceeded on the day of the encounter. Report 99308 for a visit requiring a low level of MDM or meeting or exceeding 20 minutes of total time; 99309 for a moderate level of MDM or meeting or exceeding 30 minutes of total time; and 99310 for a high level of MDM or meeting or exceeding 45 minutes of total time.

Coding Tips

These codes are used to report the subsequent encounters in the nursing/skilled nursing facility setting, psychiatric residential treatment center, or care facility for individuals with intellectual disabilities. A medically appropriate history and physical examination, as determined by the treating provider, should be documented. The level of history and physical examination are not considered when determining the level of service. Codes should be selected based upon the current CPT Medical Decision Making table. Alternatively, time alone may be used to select the appropriate level of service. Total time for reporting these services includes face-to-face and non-face-to-face time personally spent by the physician or other qualified health care professional on the date of the encounter. Subsequent nursing facility services include review of the medical record, including all diagnostic studies, as well as changes noted in the patient's condition and response to treatment since the last evaluation. Medicare and the CPT codebook have identified these codes as telehealth/telemedicine services. Telemedicine services may be reported by the performing provider by adding modifier 95 to the procedure code and/or using the appropriate place of service (POS) indicator; POS 02 for telehealth when the originating site is not the patient's home. For prolonged services applicable to 99310, see 99418; for Medicare, see G0317. Medicare and commercial payers should be contacted regarding their coverage guidelines. For care plan oversight services provided to nursing facility residents, see 99379-99380. For initial nursing facility care services, see 99304-99306; for nursing facility discharge services, see 99315-99316. Report place of service (POS) code 31 for the skilled nursing facility; report POS code 32 for the nursing facility; report POS code 54 for intermediate care facility; and report POS code 56 for the psychiatric residential treatment center.

ICD-10-CM Diagnostic Codes

The application of this code is too broad to adequately present ICD-10-CM diagnostic code links here. Refer to your ICD-10-CM book.

AMA: 99307 2024,Sep; 2023,Dec; 2022,Dec; 2022,Nov; 2022,Oct; 2022,Aug; 2022,Jul; 2022,May; 2022,Apr; 2021,Jan; 2020,Dec; 2020,Nov; 2020,Sep; 2020,Mar; 2019,Jul **99308** 2024,Sep; 2023,Dec; 2022,Dec; 2022,Nov; 2022,Oct; 2022,Aug; 2022,Jul; 2022,May; 2022,Apr; 2021,Jan; 2020,Dec; 2020,Nov; 2020,Sep; 2020,Mar; 2019,Jul **99309** 2024,Sep; 2023,Dec; 2022,Dec; 2022,Nov; 2022,Oct; 2022,Aug; 2022,Jul; 2022,May; 2022,Apr; 2021,Jan; 2020,Dec; 2020,Nov; 2020,Sep; 2020,Mar; 2019,Jul **99310** 2024,Sep; 2023,Dec; 2022,Dec; 2022,Nov; 2022,Oct; 2022,Aug; 2022,Jul; 2022,May; 2022,Apr; 2021,Jan; 2020,Dec; 2020,Nov; 2020,Sep; 2020,Mar; 2019,Jul

Relative Value Units/Medicare Edits

Non-Facility RVU	Work	PE	MP	Total
99307	0.7	0.45	0.05	1.2
99308	1.3	0.83	0.09	2.22
99309	1.92	1.16	0.13	3.21
99310	2.8	1.58	0.2	4.58
Facility RVU	**Work**	**PE**	**MP**	**Total**
99307	0.7	0.45	0.05	1.2
99308	1.3	0.83	0.09	2.22
99309	1.92	1.16	0.13	3.21
99310	2.8	1.58	0.2	4.58

	FUD	Status	MUE	Modifiers				IOM Reference
99307	N/A	A	1(2)	N/A	N/A	N/A	80*	None
99308	N/A	A	1(2)	N/A	N/A	N/A	80*	
99309	N/A	A	1(2)	N/A	N/A	N/A	80*	
99310	N/A	A	1(2)	N/A	N/A	N/A	80*	

* with documentation

Terms To Know

medical decision making. Consideration of the differential diagnoses, the amount and/or complexity of data reviewed and considered (medical records, test results, correspondence from previous treating physicians, etc.), current diagnostic studies ordered, and treatment or management options and risk (complications of the patient's condition, the potential for complications, continued morbidity, risk of mortality, any comorbidities associated with the patient's disease process).

99315-99316

99315 Nursing facility discharge management; 30 minutes or less total time on the date of the encounter

99316 more than 30 minutes total time on the date of the encounter

Explanation

Nursing facility discharge services are time-based codes that describe the amount of time spent by the clinician during all final steps involved in the discharge of a patient from the nursing facility, including the last patient exam, discussing the nursing facility stay, instructions for ongoing care as it relates to all pertinent caregivers, and preparing the medical discharge records, prescriptions, and/or referrals as applicable. A face-to-face service with the patient or family/caregiver is required and may occur on a date that is prior to the date that the patient leaves the facility. Time reported should be for the total duration of time spent by the provider on the date of the encounter, even when the time spent on that date is not continuous. For a nursing facility discharge duration of 30 minutes or less, report 99315; for a duration of greater than 30 minutes, report 99316. These codes are reported following initial and subsequent nursing facility care codes 99304-99306 and 99307-99310.

Coding Tips

These codes are used to report all discharge services for the nursing facility resident on the date of the face-to-face encounter. This code includes patient examination, follow-up care instructions to appropriate caregivers, prescriptions, referrals, and preparation of all medical records. These are time-based codes and floor unit time spent caring for the patient must be documented in the medical record. All time spent providing discharge services on the same date of service is added together and does not need to be contiguous. Medicare has identified these codes as telehealth/telemedicine services. Telemedicine services may be reported by the performing provider by using the appropriate place of service (POS) indicator: POS 02 for telehealth services when the originating site is not the patient's home. Medicare and commercial payers should be contacted regarding their coverage guidelines. For initial nursing facility care services, see 99304-99306; for subsequent nursing facility care services, see 99307-99310. Report place of service (POS) code 31 for the skilled nursing facility; report POS code 32 for the nursing facility; report POS code 54 for intermediate care facility; and report POS code 56 for the psychiatric residential treatment center.

ICD-10-CM Diagnostic Codes

The application of this code is too broad to adequately present ICD-10-CM diagnostic code links here. Refer to your ICD-10-CM book.

AMA: 99315 2023,Dec; 2022,Dec; 2022,Nov; 2022,Oct; 2022,Aug; 2022,Jul; 2022,May; 2022,Apr; 2021,Jan; 2020,Nov; 2020,Mar; 2019,Jul **99316** 2023,Dec; 2022,Dec; 2022,Nov; 2022,Oct; 2022,Aug; 2022,Jul; 2022,May; 2022,Apr; 2021,Jan; 2020,Nov; 2020,Mar; 2019,Jul

Relative Value Units/Medicare Edits

Non-Facility RVU	Work	PE	MP	Total
99315	1.5	0.83	0.1	2.43
99316	2.5	1.23	0.17	3.9
Facility RVU	**Work**	**PE**	**MP**	**Total**
99315	1.5	0.83	0.1	2.43
99316	2.5	1.23	0.17	3.9

	FUD	Status	MUE	Modifiers				IOM Reference
99315	N/A	A	1(2)	N/A	N/A	N/A	80*	None
99316	N/A	A	1(2)	N/A	N/A	N/A	80*	

* with documentation

Terms To Know

discharge plan. Treatment plan by the provider for continued patient care after discharge that may include home care, the services of case managers or other health care providers, or transfer to another facility.

nursing facility. Services provided to inpatients of a skilled nursing facility, intermediate care facility, long-term care facility, or psychiatric residential treatment center that provides convalescent, rehabilitative, or long-term care of patients.

99341-99345

99341 Home or residence visit for the evaluation and management of a new patient, which requires a medically appropriate history and/or examination and straightforward medical decision making. When using total time on the date of the encounter for code selection, 15 minutes must be met or exceeded.

99342 Home or residence visit for the evaluation and management of a new patient, which requires a medically appropriate history and/or examination and low level of medical decision making. When using total time on the date of the encounter for code selection, 30 minutes must be met or exceeded.

99344 Home or residence visit for the evaluation and management of a new patient, which requires a medically appropriate history and/or examination and moderate level of medical decision making. When using total time on the date of the encounter for code selection, 60 minutes must be met or exceeded.

99345 Home or residence visit for the evaluation and management of a new patient, which requires a medically appropriate history and/or examination and high level of medical decision making. When using total time on the date of the encounter for code selection, 75 minutes must be met or exceeded.

Explanation

Home or residence services codes are reported by providers for E/M services rendered to new patients in a home or residence, including a private residence or temporary lodging. Short-term accommodations such as a hotel, campground, hostel, or cruise ship are included, along with an assisted living facility, group home, custodial care facility, and residential substance abuse treatment facility. All services require a medically appropriate history and/or examination. Code selection is based on the level of medical decision making (MDM) or total time personally spent by the physician and/or other qualified health care professional(s) on the date of the encounter. Travel time is not included when selecting a level based on total time. Factors to be considered in MDM include the number and complexity of problems addressed during the encounter, amount and complexity of data requiring review and analysis, and the risk of complications and/or morbidity or mortality associated with patient management. Report 99341 for a visit that entails straightforward MDM. If time is used for code selection, a total time of 15 minutes must be met or exceeded on the day of the encounter. Report 99342 for a visit requiring a low level of MDM or meeting or exceeding 30 minutes of total time; 99344 for a moderate level of MDM or meeting or exceeding 60 minutes of time; and 99345 for a high level of MDM or meeting or exceeding 75 minutes of total time.

Coding Tips

These codes are used to report the new patient evaluation and management services provided in a private residence, temporary lodging, or short-term accommodation such as hotel, campground, hostel, or cruise ship, are also included along with an assisted living facility, group home, custodial care facility, and residential substance abuse treatment facility for a new patient. A medically appropriate history and physical examination, as determined by the treating provider, should be documented. The level of history and physical examination are not considered when determining the level of service. Codes should be selected based upon the current CPT Medical Decision Making table. Alternatively, time alone may be used to select the appropriate level of service. Total time for reporting these services includes face-to-face and non-face-to-face time personally spent by the physician or other qualified health care professional on the date of the encounter. Note that E/M services provided in a group home that is licensed as an intermediate care facility for individuals with intellectual disabilities should be reported with codes for initial hospital inpatient and observation care or initial nursing facility care. For commercial payers, consider assigning the appropriate consultation code, see 99242-99245. Medicare has identified these codes as telehealth/telemedicine services. Telemedicine services may be reported by the performing provider by using the appropriate place of service (POS) indicator; POS 02 for telehealth when the originating site is not the patient's home and POS 10 for telehealth services when the originating site is the patient's home. For prolonged services applicable to 99345, see 99417; for Medicare, see G0318. Medicare and commercial payers should be contacted regarding their coverage guidelines. For care plan oversight provided in the home under the care of a hospice agency, see 99377-99378; provided under the care of a home health agency, see 99374-99375. Report place of service (POS) code 12 for services rendered in a private residence.

ICD-10-CM Diagnostic Codes

The application of this code is too broad to adequately present ICD-10-CM diagnostic code links here. Refer to your ICD-10-CM book.

AMA: **99341** 2024,Sep; 2023,Dec; 2023,Aug; 2023,Mar; 2022,Dec; 2022,Nov; 2022,Oct; 2022,Jul; 2022,May; 2022,Apr; 2021,Jan; 2020,Dec; 2020,Nov; 2020,Sep; 2020,Mar; 2019,Jul; 2018,Apr **99342** 2024,Sep; 2023,Dec; 2023,Aug; 2023,Mar; 2022,Dec; 2022,Nov; 2022,Oct; 2022,Jul; 2022,May; 2022,Apr; 2021,Jan; 2020,Dec; 2020,Nov; 2020,Sep; 2020,Mar; 2019,Jul; 2018,Apr **99344** 2024,Sep; 2023,Dec; 2023,Aug; 2023,Mar; 2022,Dec; 2022,Nov; 2022,Oct; 2022,Jul; 2022,May; 2022,Apr; 2021,Jan; 2020,Dec; 2020,Nov; 2020,Sep; 2020,Mar; 2019,Jul; 2018,Apr **99345** 2024,Sep; 2023,Dec; 2023,Aug; 2023,Mar; 2022,Dec; 2022,Nov; 2022,Oct; 2022,Jul; 2022,May; 2022,Apr; 2021,Jan; 2020,Dec; 2020,Nov; 2020,Sep; 2020,Mar; 2019,Jul; 2018,Apr

Relative Value Units/Medicare Edits

Non-Facility RVU	Work	PE	MP	Total
99341	1.0	0.42	0.05	1.47
99342	1.65	0.6	0.08	2.33
99344	2.87	1.2	0.16	4.23
99345	3.88	1.88	0.25	6.01
Facility RVU	**Work**	**PE**	**MP**	**Total**
99341	1.0	0.42	0.05	1.47
99342	1.65	0.6	0.08	2.33
99344	2.87	1.2	0.16	4.23
99345	3.88	1.88	0.25	6.01

	FUD	Status	MUE	Modifiers				IOM Reference
99341	N/A	A	1(2)	N/A	N/A	N/A	80*	None
99342	N/A	A	1(2)	N/A	N/A	N/A	80*	
99344	N/A	A	1(2)	N/A	N/A	N/A	80*	
99345	N/A	A	1(2)	N/A	N/A	N/A	80*	

* with documentation

Terms To Know

new patient. Patient who is receiving face-to-face care from a physician or other qualified health care professional of the exact same specialty and subspecialty who belongs to the same group practice for the first time in three years. For OPPS hospitals, a patient who has not been registered as an inpatient or outpatient, including off-campus provider-based clinic or emergency department, within the past three years.

99347-99350

99347 Home or residence visit for the evaluation and management of an established patient, which requires a medically appropriate history and/or examination and straightforward medical decision making. When using total time on the date of the encounter for code selection, 20 minutes must be met or exceeded.

99348 Home or residence visit for the evaluation and management of an established patient, which requires a medically appropriate history and/or examination and low level of medical decision making. When using total time on the date of the encounter for code selection, 30 minutes must be met or exceeded.

99349 Home or residence visit for the evaluation and management of an established patient, which requires a medically appropriate history and/or examination and moderate level of medical decision making. When using total time on the date of the encounter for code selection, 40 minutes must be met or exceeded.

99350 Home or residence visit for the evaluation and management of an established patient, which requires a medically appropriate history and/or examination and high level of medical decision making. When using total time on the date of the encounter for code selection, 60 minutes must be met or exceeded.

Explanation

Home or residence services codes are reported by providers for E/M services rendered to established patients in a home or residence, including a private residence or temporary lodging. Short-term accommodations such as a hotel, campground, hostel, or cruise ship are included, along with an assisted living facility, group home, custodial care facility, and residential substance abuse treatment facility. All services require a medically appropriate history and/or examination. Code selection is based on the level of medical decision making (MDM) or total time personally spent by the physician and/or other qualified health care professional(s) on the date of the encounter. Travel time is not included when selecting a level based on total time. Factors to be considered in MDM include the number and complexity of problems addressed during the encounter, amount and complexity of data requiring review and analysis, and the risk of complications and/or morbidity or mortality associated with patient management. Report 99347 for a visit that entails straightforward MDM. If time is used for code selection, a total time of 20 minutes must be met or exceeded on the day of the encounter. Report 99348 for a visit requiring a low level of MDM or meeting or exceeding 30 minutes of total time; 99349 for a moderate level of MDM or meeting or exceeding 40 minutes of time; and 99350 for a high level of MDM or meeting or exceeding 60 minutes of total time.

Coding Tips

These codes are used to report the established patient evaluation and management services provided in a private residence, temporary lodging, or short-term accommodation such as hotel, campground, hostel, or cruise ship, are also included along with an assisted living facility, group home, custodial care facility, and residential substance abuse treatment facility for an established patient. A medically appropriate history and physical examination, as determined by the treating provider, should be documented. The level of history and physical examination are not considered when determining the level of service. Codes should be selected based upon the current CPT Medical Decision Making table. Alternatively, time alone may be used to select the appropriate level of service. Total time for reporting these services includes face-to-face and non-face-to-face time personally spent by the physician or other qualified health care professional on the date of the encounter. Note that E/M services provided in a group home that is licensed as an intermediate care facility for individuals with intellectual disabilities should be reported with codes for initial hospital inpatient and observation care or initial nursing facility care. For commercial payers, consider assigning the appropriate consultation code, see 99242-99245. Medicare has identified these codes as telehealth/telemedicine services. Telemedicine services may be reported by the performing provider by using the appropriate place of service (POS) indicator; POS 02 for telehealth when the originating site is not the patient's home and POS 10 for telehealth services when the originating site is the patient's home. For prolonged services applicable to 99350, see 99417; for Medicare, see G0318. Medicare and commercial payers should be contacted regarding their coverage guidelines. For care plan oversight provided in the home under the care of a hospice agency, see 99377-99378; provided under the care of a home health agency, see 99374-99375. Report place of service (POS) code 12 for services rendered in a private residence.

ICD-10-CM Diagnostic Codes

The application of this code is too broad to adequately present ICD-10-CM diagnostic code links here. Refer to your ICD-10-CM book.

AMA: **99347** 2024,Sep; 2023,Dec; 2023,Aug; 2023,Mar; 2022,Dec; 2022,Nov; 2022,Oct; 2022,Jul; 2022,May; 2022,Apr; 2021,Jan; 2020,Dec; 2020,Nov; 2020,Sep; 2020,Mar; 2019,Jul; 2018,Apr **99348** 2024,Sep; 2023,Dec; 2023,Aug; 2023,Mar; 2022,Dec; 2022,Nov; 2022,Oct; 2022,Jul; 2022,May; 2022,Apr; 2021,Jan; 2020,Dec; 2020,Nov; 2020,Sep; 2020,Mar; 2019,Jul; 2018,Apr **99349** 2024,Sep; 2024,Jun; 2023,Dec; 2023,Aug; 2023,Mar; 2022,Dec; 2022,Nov; 2022,Oct; 2022,Jul; 2022,May; 2022,Apr; 2021,Jan; 2020,Dec; 2020,Nov; 2020,Sep; 2020,Mar; 2019,Jul; 2018,Apr **99350** 2024,Sep; 2023,Dec; 2023,Aug; 2023,Mar; 2022,Dec; 2022,Nov; 2022,Oct; 2022,Jul; 2022,May; 2022,Apr; 2021,Jan; 2020,Dec; 2020,Nov; 2020,Sep; 2020,Mar; 2019,Jul; 2018,Apr

Relative Value Units/Medicare Edits

Non-Facility RVU	Work	PE	MP	Total
99347	0.9	0.4	0.05	1.35
99348	1.5	0.7	0.08	2.28
99349	2.44	1.19	0.16	3.79
99350	3.6	1.68	0.24	5.52
Facility RVU	**Work**	**PE**	**MP**	**Total**
99347	0.9	0.4	0.05	1.35
99348	1.5	0.7	0.08	2.28
99349	2.44	1.19	0.16	3.79
99350	3.6	1.68	0.24	5.52

	FUD	Status	MUE	Modifiers				IOM Reference
99347	N/A	A	1(3)	N/A	N/A	N/A	80*	None
99348	N/A	A	1(3)	N/A	N/A	N/A	80*	
99349	N/A	A	1(3)	N/A	N/A	N/A	80*	
99350	N/A	A	1(3)	N/A	N/A	N/A	80*	

* with documentation

99358-99359

99358 Prolonged evaluation and management service before and/or after direct patient care; first hour

\+ **99359** each additional 30 minutes (List separately in addition to code for prolonged service)

Explanation

Prolonged time without direct contact with the patient that is performed by the physician or other qualified clinician on a different day than a related E/M service can be reported with 99358 and 99359. For example, the provider may review records for a patient who received a face-to-face E/M service on a previous date or will receive care on a future date. The reported E/M service does not have to be selected based on time to report these prolonged timed services. Time reported for prolonged care should be for the total duration of time spent by the provider even when the time spent on that date is not continuous. Report 99358 for the first hour of prolonged care without direct patient care that is performed on a different date than the face-to-face E/M service and 99359 for each additional 30 minutes.

Coding Tips

These codes are used to report prolonged services on another date before and/or after face-to-face patient care beyond the usual service. These are time-based codes and time spent with the patient must be documented in the medical record. Time spent on other separately reported services excluding the E/M service should not be counted toward the prolonged service time. Do not include time spent for care plan oversight services, chronic care management, principal care management, home and outpatient international normalized ratio (INR) monitoring, medical team conferences, interprofessional telephone/internet/electronic health record consultations, or online digital E/M services. Codes 99358-99359 may be reported on a different date of service than the primary service and do not require the primary service to have an established time. Prolonged service of less than 30 minutes should not be reported separately. Report 99358 only once per day for the initial hour of prolonged service care; for each additional 30-minute block of time beyond the initial hour, see 99359. Do not report 99358-99359 on the same date of service as 99202-99205, 99212-99215, 99221-99223, 99231-99236, 99242-99245, 99252-99255, 99281-99285, 99304-99310, 99341-99345, 99347-99350, 99417-99418, 99483, G2212, or G0316-G0318. Report 99359 in addition to 99358. For prolonged services provided: by a physician or other qualified health care professional with or without direct patient contact in the office or other outpatient setting (i.e., 99205 or 99215), see 99417, for Medicare, see G2212; in an inpatient or observation setting, see 99418, for Medicare, see G0316; in a nursing facility, see 99418, for Medicare, see G0317; in a home or residence, see 99417, for Medicare, see G0318. For prolonged services provided by clinical staff, see 99415-99416.

ICD-10-CM Diagnostic Codes

The application of this code is too broad to adequately present ICD-10-CM diagnostic code links here. Refer to your ICD-10-CM book.

AMA: **99358** 2024,Oct; 2023,Nov; 2023,Mar; 2022,Dec; 2022,Nov; 2022,Aug; 2022,Jul; 2022,Jun; 2022,May; 2022,Jan; 2021,Sep; 2021,Jan; 2020,Sep; 2020,Feb; 2019,Jul; 2019,Jun; 2019,Jan; 2018,Oct **99359** 2024,Oct; 2023,Nov; 2023,Mar; 2022,Dec; 2022,Nov; 2022,Aug; 2022,Jul; 2022,May; 2022,Jan; 2021,Sep; 2021,Jan; 2020,Sep; 2019,Jul; 2019,Jun; 2019,Jan; 2018,Oct

Relative Value Units/Medicare Edits

Non-Facility RVU	Work	PE	MP	Total
99358	1.8	0.74	0.11	2.65
99359	0.75	0.33	0.05	1.13
Facility RVU	**Work**	**PE**	**MP**	**Total**
99358	1.8	0.7	0.11	2.61
99359	0.75	0.29	0.05	1.09

	FUD	Status	MUE	Modifiers				IOM Reference
99358	N/A	I	1(2)	N/A	N/A	N/A	80*	None
99359	N/A	I	2(3)	N/A	N/A	N/A	80*	

* with documentation

Terms To Know

other qualified health care professional. Individual who is qualified by education, training, licensure/regulation, and facility privileging to perform a professional service within his or her scope of practice and independently (or as incident-to) report the professional service without requiring physician supervision. Payers may state exemptions in writing or state and local regulations may not follow this definition for performance of some services. Always refer to any relevant plan policies and federal and/or state laws to determine who may perform and report services.

prolonged physician services. Extended pre- or post-service care provided to a patient whose condition requires services beyond the usual.

[99415, 99416]

\+ **99415** Prolonged clinical staff service (the service beyond the highest time in the range of total time of the service) during an evaluation and management service in the office or outpatient setting, direct patient contact with physician supervision; first hour (List separately in addition to code for outpatient Evaluation and Management service)

\+ **99416** Prolonged clinical staff service (the service beyond the highest time in the range of total time of the service) during an evaluation and management service in the office or outpatient setting, direct patient contact with physician supervision; each additional 30 minutes (List separately in addition to code for prolonged service)

Explanation

Prolonged clinical staff services describe special situations in which the physician's staff provide assistance to a patient beyond the usual time associated with circumstances requiring observation of the patient, such as in cases where the patient was administered a new medication or inhaled drug requiring monitoring to ensure patient safety in the office or outpatient setting. Such cases do not necessitate the clinician being face-to-face with the patient throughout the entire time; observation and monitoring of the patient can be performed by a member of the clinician's staff under the provider's supervision. Report these codes in conjunction with the designated E/M service code, along with any other service provided at the same encounter. Codes in this category should report the total amount of face-to-face time spent with the patient and/or family or caregiver by the clinical staff on the same date of service even if the time is not continuous; time spent rendering other separately reportable services other than the E/M service does not count toward the prolonged services time. Report the first hour of prolonged services on a given date with 99415; for each additional 30 minutes of prolonged services, report 99416.

Coding Tips

These codes are used to report prolonged face-to-face services beyond the highest total time indicated in the code description provided by the clinical staff in the office or outpatient setting. These are time-based codes and time spent with the patient must be documented in the medical record. Time spent on other separately reported services excluding the E/M service should not be counted toward the prolonged service time. These codes are reported in addition to the other E/M service provided on the same date of service. A provider must be available to provide direct supervision of the clinical staff. Report 99415 only once per day for the initial hour of prolonged service care; for each additional 30-minute block of time beyond the initial hour, see 99416. Prolonged service of less than 30 minutes should not be reported separately. For prolonged services with or without direct patient contact provided by the physician or other qualified health care provider in the office or other outpatient setting, see 99417, for Medicare, see G2212; in the inpatient or observation setting, see 99418, for Medicare, see G0316. Do not report 99415-99416 with 99417. Report 99415 in addition to 99202-99205 and 99212-99215. Report 99416 in addition to 99415.

ICD-10-CM Diagnostic Codes

The application of this code is too broad to adequately present ICD-10-CM diagnostic code links here. Refer to your ICD-10-CM book.

AMA: 99415 2024,Mar; 2022,Nov; 2022,Jul; 2022,May; 2021,Jan; 2020,Nov; 2020,Sep; 2020,Feb; 2019,Jul **99416** 2024,Mar; 2022,Nov; 2022,Jul; 2022,May; 2021,Jan; 2020,Nov; 2020,Sep; 2020,Feb; 2019,Jul

Relative Value Units/Medicare Edits

Non-Facility RVU	Work	PE	MP	Total
99415	0.0	0.6	0.02	0.62
99416	0.0	0.28	0.01	0.29
Facility RVU	**Work**	**PE**	**MP**	**Total**
99415	0.0	0.6	0.02	0.62
99416	0.0	0.28	0.01	0.29

	FUD	Status	MUE	Modifiers				IOM Reference
99415	N/A	A	1(2)	N/A	N/A	N/A	80*	None
99416	N/A	A	3(3)	N/A	N/A	N/A	80*	

* with documentation

Terms To Know

add-on code. CPT code representing a procedure performed in addition to the primary procedure and designated with a + symbol in the CPT book. Add-on codes are never reported as a stand-alone service but are reported secondarily in addition to the primary procedure.

clinical staff. Someone who works for, or under, the direction of a physician or qualified health care professional and does not bill services separately. The person may be licensed or regulated to help the physician perform specific duties.

[99417, 99418]

+ ★**99417** Prolonged outpatient evaluation and management service(s) time with or without direct patient contact beyond the required time of the primary service when the primary service level has been selected using total time, each 15 minutes of total time (List separately in addition to the code of the outpatient Evaluation and Management service)

+ ★**99418** Prolonged inpatient or observation evaluation and management service(s) time with or without direct patient contact beyond the required time of the primary service when the primary service level has been selected using total time, each 15 minutes of total time (List separately in addition to the code of the inpatient and observation Evaluation and Management service)

Explanation

Prolonged time (with and without direct patient contact combined) that is provided by the physician or other qualified health care professional on the date of an evaluation and management service can be reported with 99417 (outpatient) or 99418 (inpatient or observation). These codes are assigned only when the code for the primary E/M service has been selected based solely on total time, and only after exceeding the required time to report the highest-level of service by at least 15 minutes. For example, when reporting an E/M service for an established patient (99215), code 99417 would not be reported until at least 15 minutes of time beyond 40 minutes has been accumulated (55 minutes) on the day of the encounter. Time spent on procedures that can be reported separately are not included in the prolonged time.

Coding Tips

These codes are used to report prolonged service time by the physician or other qualified health care professional provided on the same date as the highest level of service of the associated E/M service. The prolonged time may be with or without direct patient contact. This service is reported only when time was the criteria used to select the code for the primary E/M service and the time exceeds the minimum time required to report these levels of service by at least 15 minutes. Code 99417 may be reported once for each additional 15 minutes spent providing prolonged services. The CPT codebook has identified these codes as telehealth/telemedicine services. Telemedicine services may be reported by the performing provider by adding modifier 95 to the procedure code and using the appropriate place of service (POS) indicator. Time spent on procedures that can be reported separately are not included in the prolonged time. Report 99417 for prolonged time for an outpatient evaluation and management service for the combination of time with and without direct patient contact that goes beyond the required time of codes 98003, 98007, 98011, 98015, 99205, 99215, 99245, 99345, 99350, or 99483. Report 99418 for prolonged time for an inpatient or observation evaluation and management service for the combination of time with and without direct patient contact that goes beyond the required time of codes 99223, 99233, 99236, 99255, 99306, or 99310. Each code can be reported for each 15 minutes of prolonged time. Prolonged services provided on a date other than the date of the face-to-face encounter may be reported with 99358-99359. Prolonged services provided by clinical staff are reported with 99415-99416. Do not report 99417-99418 with 90833, 90836, 90838, or 99358-99359; do not report 99417 with 99415-99416 or G0318; do not report 99418 with G0316 or G0317.

ICD-10-CM Diagnostic Codes

This/these CPT code(s) are add-on code(s). See the primary procedure code that this code is performed with for your ICD-10-CM code selections.

AMA: 99417 2024,Oct; 2023,Mar; 2022,Dec; 2022,Nov; 2022,Aug; 2022,Jul; 2022,May; 2021,Jan; 2020,Nov; 2020,Sep **99418** 2023,Mar; 2023,Jan; 2022,Nov; 2022,Oct

Relative Value Units/Medicare Edits

Non-Facility RVU	Work	PE	MP	Total
99417	0.61	0.27	0.04	0.92
99418	0.81	0.31	0.05	1.17
Facility RVU	**Work**	**PE**	**MP**	**Total**
99417	0.61	0.24	0.04	0.89
99418	0.81	0.31	0.05	1.17

	FUD	Status	MUE	Modifiers				IOM Reference
99417	N/A	I	6(3)	N/A	N/A	N/A	N/A	None
99418	N/A	I	4(3)	N/A	N/A	N/A	N/A	

* with documentation

Terms To Know

inpatient. Time period in which a patient is housed in a hospital or facility offering medical, surgical, and/or psychiatric services, usually without interruption.

outpatient. Person who has not been admitted as an inpatient but who is registered on the hospital or CAH records as an outpatient and receives services (rather than supplies alone) directly from the hospital or CAH. (Code of Federal Regulations, section 410.2.)

prolonged physician services. Extended pre- or post-service care provided to a patient whose condition requires services beyond the usual.

99360

99360 Standby service, requiring prolonged attendance, each 30 minutes (eg, operative standby, standby for frozen section, for cesarean/high risk delivery, for monitoring EEG)

Explanation

Standby services are those requested of a qualified clinician that involves prolonged attendance without face-to-face contact with the patient (e.g., operative or cesarean/high-risk delivery standby, EEG monitoring, or standby to obtain a frozen section specimen). The clinician on standby is not permitted to provide care or services to other patients during the standby period. This code should not be used to report time spent proctoring another individual nor should it be used if the standby period ends with the standby clinician performing a procedure that is subject to the surgical package. This code encompasses the total duration of time spent on standby on a given date; standby services of less than 30 minutes total duration are not reported separately. A second and subsequent period of standby, after the initial 30 minutes, may be reported contingent that each unit of standby service equates to a full 30 minutes.

Coding Tips

This code is used to report standby services requested by another clinician for prolonged attendance without face-to-face patient contact. This is a time-based code representing the total duration of time spent providing standby services and must be documented in the medical record. Standby services of less than 30 minutes should not be reported separately. Report each additional 30 minutes of time beyond the initial time only when a full 30-minute period is provided. Report this code in addition to 99460 or 99465, if applicable. Do not report 99360 with 99464.

ICD-10-CM Diagnostic Codes

The application of this code is too broad to adequately present ICD-10-CM diagnostic code links here. Refer to your ICD-10-CM book.

AMA: 99360 2022,Nov; 2022,Jul; 2021,Jan; 2019,Jul

Relative Value Units/Medicare Edits

Non-Facility RVU	Work	PE	MP	Total
99360	1.2	0.47	0.07	1.74
Facility RVU	**Work**	**PE**	**MP**	**Total**
99360	1.2	0.47	0.07	1.74

	FUD	Status	MUE	Modifiers				IOM Reference
99360	N/A	X	1(3)	N/A	N/A	N/A	N/A	None

* with documentation

99366-99368

99366 Medical team conference with interdisciplinary team of health care professionals, face-to-face with patient and/or family, 30 minutes or more, participation by nonphysician qualified health care professional

99367 Medical team conference with interdisciplinary team of health care professionals, patient and/or family not present, 30 minutes or more; participation by physician

99368 participation by nonphysician qualified health care professional

Explanation

A medical team conference is defined as a service where at least three qualified health care professionals from different specialties or disciplines, each of whom provides direct care to the patient, actively engage in the evolution, revision, coordination, and implementation of health care services needed by the patient. The conferences may or may not involve the presence of the patient, family members, community agencies, surrogate decision makers/legal guardians, and/or caregivers. Medical team clinicians should report the time spent in a team conference with the patient and/or family present with the appropriate E/M code, using time as a key controlling factor for selecting a code when counseling and/or coordination of care dominates the service. The individual clinician must be directly involved with rendering face-to-face services outside of the conference visit with other clinicians or agencies. All medical professionals participating on the medical team must document their own individual participation in the team conference, in addition to their contributed information and follow-up treatment recommendations. However, only one individual from the same specialty may report a code from this category at the same encounter. No individuals may report a code from range 99366-99368 if participation in the medical team conference is a part of a facility or organizational service contractually provided by the facility or organization. Team conferences commence upon review of the individual patient case and conclude once the review has come to a conclusion. Record keeping and report generation time is not reportable. The clinician must report all time for which he or she was present. Reportable time is not limited to the time that the clinician is communicating with other team members, the patient, and/or the patient's family. Note that time spent in medical team conferences should not be used toward determining other E/M services such as care plan oversight services, home, domiciliary, or rest home care plan oversight, prolonged services, psychotherapy, or any other E/M service. Nonphysician qualified health care professionals may report 99366, medical team conference, direct (face-to-face) contact with patient and/or family, when the patient is present for any or all of the medical conference with a duration of at least 30 minutes. This includes such providers as speech-language pathologists, physical therapists, occupational therapists, social workers, and dieticians. Medical conferences of less than 30 minutes duration are not reported. Codes 99367-99368 describe team conferences without direct, face-to-face patient and/or family contact.

Coding Tips

These codes are used to report medical team conferences, with direct patient and/or family contact (99366) or without direct patient and/or family contact (99367-99368). For medical team participation by a nonphysician health care professional with direct patient and/or family contact, see 99366; without direct patient or family contact, see 99368. For medical team participation by the physician without direct patient and/or family contact, see 99367. Time required for record keeping and generating reports is not counted. The time for the team conference starts when review of an individual patient begins and ends when the review is completed. The health care professional who reports the service should be present for all time reported. Do not count time used for other services such as prolonged services (99358-99359), E/M services, psychotherapy, or care plan oversight (99374-99380). Medical team meetings of less than 30 minutes should not be reported separately. For physician participation with face-to-face patient contact, report the appropriate E/M code. Do not report codes 99367-99368 in the same month as 99437, 99439, 99487, or 99489-99491.

ICD-10-CM Diagnostic Codes

The application of this code is too broad to adequately present ICD-10-CM diagnostic code links here. Refer to your ICD-10-CM book.

AMA: **99366** 2023,Nov; 2022,Nov; 2022,Jul; 2022,Jan; 2021,Jan; 2019,Jul; 2018,Apr **99367** 2023,Nov; 2022,Nov; 2022,Jul; 2022,Jan; 2021,Jan; 2019,Dec; 2019,Jul; 2018,Apr **99368** 2023,Nov; 2022,Nov; 2022,Jul; 2022,Jan; 2021,Jan; 2019,Jul; 2018,Apr

Relative Value Units/Medicare Edits

Non-Facility RVU	Work	PE	MP	Total
99366	0.82	0.35	0.05	1.22
99367	1.1	0.43	0.07	1.6
99368	0.72	0.28	0.04	1.04
Facility RVU	**Work**	**PE**	**MP**	**Total**
99366	0.82	0.32	0.05	1.19
99367	1.1	0.43	0.07	1.6
99368	0.72	0.28	0.04	1.04

	FUD	Status	MUE	Modifiers				IOM Reference
99366	N/A	B	0(3)	N/A	N/A	N/A	N/A	None
99367	N/A	B	0(3)	N/A	N/A	N/A	N/A	
99368	N/A	B	0(3)	N/A	N/A	N/A	N/A	

* with documentation

Terms To Know

interdisciplinary care. Two or more health care professions working in a collaborative manner for the benefit of the patient.

other qualified health care professional. Individual who is qualified by education, training, licensure/regulation, and facility privileging to perform a professional service within his or her scope of practice and independently (or as incident-to) report the professional service without requiring physician supervision. Payers may state exemptions in writing or state and local regulations may not follow this definition for performance of some services. Always refer to any relevant plan policies and federal and/or state laws to determine who may perform and report services.

99374-99380

99374 Supervision of a patient under care of home health agency (patient not present) in home, domiciliary or equivalent environment (eg, Alzheimer's facility) requiring complex and multidisciplinary care modalities involving regular development and/or revision of care plans by that individual, review of subsequent reports of patient status, review of related laboratory and other studies, communication (including telephone calls) for purposes of assessment or care decisions with health care professional(s), family member(s), surrogate decision maker(s) (eg, legal guardian) and/or key caregiver(s) involved in patient's care, integration of new information into the medical treatment plan and/or adjustment of medical therapy, within a calendar month; 15-29 minutes

99375 30 minutes or more

99377 Supervision of a hospice patient (patient not present) requiring complex and multidisciplinary care modalities involving regular development and/or revision of care plans by that individual, review of subsequent reports of patient status, review of related laboratory and other studies, communication (including telephone calls) for purposes of assessment or care decisions with health care professional(s), family member(s), surrogate decision maker(s) (eg, legal guardian) and/or key caregiver(s) involved in patient's care, integration of new information into the medical treatment plan and/or adjustment of medical therapy, within a calendar month; 15-29 minutes

99378 30 minutes or more

99379 Supervision of a nursing facility patient (patient not present) requiring complex and multidisciplinary care modalities involving regular development and/or revision of care plans by that individual, review of subsequent reports of patient status, review of related laboratory and other studies, communication (including telephone calls) for purposes of assessment or care decisions with health care professional(s), family member(s), surrogate decision maker(s) (eg, legal guardian) and/or key caregiver(s) involved in patient's care, integration of new information into the medical treatment plan and/or adjustment of medical therapy, within a calendar month; 15-29 minutes

99380 30 minutes or more

Explanation

Care plan oversight (CPO) services are reported for the primary supervising health care provider's time in reviewing and adjusting treatment plans. These services may include review of multiple modalities; patient status relevant laboratory tests; communication with other health care team members, family members, and/or patient advocates; and developing a new course of action or any adjustments to the current plan. Codes are reported within one calendar month and are classified according to the place of service. The initial service for each location is approximately 15 to 29 minutes in duration; each additional 30 minutes is reported separately. Report 99374-99375 for patients in a home health setting; 99377-99378 for hospice patients; and 99379-99380 for patients residing in a nursing facility. Note that only one clinician is eligible to report CPO services for a specific time period in order to demonstrate the singular or lead role the clinician has with a particular patient.

Coding Tips

Codes 99374-99380 are used to report care plan oversight (CPO) services of the physicians' supervision of patients in nursing facilities, under the care of home health agencies, or hospice benefits that require complex or multidisciplinary care modalities requiring ongoing provider involvement in the plan of care. These are time-based codes and time spent involved in care plan activities must be documented in the medical record. Total time for care plan oversight provided within a 30-day period determines code selection. Only one clinician is eligible to report CPO services for a specific time period in order to demonstrate the singular or lead role the clinician has with a particular patient. CPO services should not be reported until after the end of the month in which the services are performed. Coverage of these services varies by payer. Check with the payer for specific coverage guidelines. These codes may be reported separately from other E/M services provided in these settings. Do not report 99374-99378 with complex chronic care coordination services 99487-99489 for the same month. Do not report these codes for time reported with 98012-98016, 98966-98968, or 99421-99423.

ICD-10-CM Diagnostic Codes

The application of this code is too broad to adequately present ICD-10-CM diagnostic code links here. Refer to your ICD-10-CM book.

AMA: **99374** 2023,Nov; 2022,Nov; 2022,Jul; 2022,Jan; 2021,Jan; 2020,Mar; 2019,Jul; 2019,Jan **99375** 2023,Nov; 2022,Nov; 2022,Jul; 2022,Jan; 2021,Jan; 2020,Mar; 2019,Jul; 2019,Jan **99377** 2023,Nov; 2022,Nov; 2022,Jul; 2022,Jan; 2021,Jan; 2020,Mar; 2019,Jul; 2019,Jan **99378** 2023,Nov; 2022,Nov; 2022,Jul; 2022,Jan; 2021,Jan; 2020,Mar; 2019,Jul; 2019,Jan **99379** 2023,Nov; 2022,Nov; 2022,Jul; 2022,Jan; 2021,Jan; 2020,Mar; 2019,Jul; 2019,Jan **99380** 2023,Nov; 2022,Nov; 2022,Jul; 2022,Jan; 2021,Jan; 2020,Mar; 2019,Jul; 2019,Jan

Relative Value Units/Medicare Edits

Non-Facility RVU	Work	PE	MP	Total
99374	1.1	0.87	0.07	2.04
99375	1.73	1.2	0.1	3.03
99377	1.1	0.87	0.07	2.04
99378	1.73	1.2	0.1	3.03
99379	1.1	0.87	0.07	2.04
99380	1.73	1.2	0.1	3.03
Facility RVU	**Work**	**PE**	**MP**	**Total**
99374	1.1	0.43	0.07	1.6
99375	1.73	0.67	0.1	2.5
99377	1.1	0.43	0.07	1.6
99378	1.73	0.67	0.1	2.5
99379	1.1	0.43	0.07	1.6
99380	1.73	0.67	0.1	2.5

	FUD	Status	MUE	Modifiers				IOM Reference
99374	N/A	B	0(3)	N/A	N/A	N/A	N/A	None
99375	N/A	I	0(3)	N/A	N/A	N/A	N/A	
99377	N/A	B	0(3)	N/A	N/A	N/A	N/A	
99378	N/A	I	0(3)	N/A	N/A	N/A	N/A	
99379	N/A	B	0(3)	N/A	N/A	N/A	N/A	
99380	N/A	B	0(3)	N/A	N/A	N/A	N/A	

* with documentation

Terms To Know

care plan oversight services. Physician's ongoing review and revision of a patient's care plan involving complex or multidisciplinary care modalities.

domiciliary. Facility, such as an assisted living, group home, custodial care, or an intermediate care facility, that provides room and board on a long-term basis and may include personal assistance services.

99381-99387

99381 Initial comprehensive preventive medicine evaluation and management of an individual including an age and gender appropriate history, examination, counseling/anticipatory guidance/risk factor reduction interventions, and the ordering of laboratory/diagnostic procedures, new patient; infant (age younger than 1 year)
99382 early childhood (age 1 through 4 years)
99383 late childhood (age 5 through 11 years)
99384 adolescent (age 12 through 17 years)
99385 18-39 years
99386 40-64 years
99387 65 years and older

Explanation

Initial preventive medicine services are typically well-patient examinations for new patients with code selection dependent upon the patient's age. These services include applicable patient history and examination, guidance/recommendation regarding personal risk factors, and any laboratory and/or diagnostic procedures ordered. Clinicians are not required to report minor or self-limiting problems or complaints noted during the course of the preventive examination when those problems do not require any additional work or necessitate performing the key components of a problem oriented E/M service. Report 99381 for infants younger than 1 year of age; 99382 for children 1 to 4 years of age; 99383 for children 5 to 11 years of age; 99384 for adolescents12 to 17 years of age; 99385 for adult patients 18 to 39 years of age; 99386 for patients 40 to 64 years of age; and 99387 for patients 65 years of age and older.

Coding Tips

These codes are used to report preventive medicine services for a new patient. Time is not a factor when selecting these E/M services. Code selection is determined based on whether the patient is new or established and the age of the patient. When documentation supports that a significant, separately identifiable problem-oriented evaluation and management (E/M) service is rendered, the appropriate code for the E/M service may be reported separately. Append modifier 25 to the service code selected to indicate that a separately identifiable E/M service was provided on the same date of service as the preventive medicine service. Immunizations and vaccines including counseling when provided, and ancillary services, including laboratory, radiology, or screening tests, performed at the time of the preventive service may be reported separately. Preventive medicine services are not covered by Medicare. For preventive services provided to an established patient, see 99391-99397.

ICD-10-CM Diagnostic Codes

The application of this code is too broad to adequately present ICD-10-CM diagnostic code links here. Refer to your ICD-10-CM book.

AMA: 99381 2024,Sep; 2022,Dec; 2022,Nov; 2022,Jul; 2021,Nov; 2021,Feb; 2021,Jan; 2019,Jul **99382** 2024,Sep; 2022,Dec; 2022,Nov; 2022,Jul; 2021,Nov; 2021,Feb; 2021,Jan; 2019,Jul **99383** 2024,Sep; 2022,Dec; 2022,Nov; 2022,Jul; 2021,Nov; 2021,Feb; 2021,Jan; 2019,Jul **99384** 2024,Sep; 2022,Dec; 2022,Nov; 2022,Jul; 2021,Nov; 2021,Feb; 2021,Jan; 2019,Jul **99385** 2024,Sep; 2022,Dec; 2022,Nov; 2022,Jul; 2021,Nov; 2021,Feb; 2021,Jan; 2019,Jul **99386** 2024,Sep; 2022,Dec; 2022,Nov; 2022,Jul; 2021,Nov; 2021,Feb; 2021,Jan; 2019,Jul **99387** 2024,Sep; 2022,Dec; 2022,Nov; 2022,Jul; 2021,Nov; 2021,Feb; 2021,Jan; 2019,Jul

Relative Value Units/Medicare Edits

Non-Facility RVU	Work	PE	MP	Total
99381	1.5	1.68	0.09	3.27
99382	1.6	1.72	0.1	3.42
99383	1.7	1.75	0.1	3.55
99384	2.0	1.86	0.12	3.98
99385	1.92	1.83	0.12	3.87
99386	2.33	1.99	0.14	4.46
99387	2.5	2.19	0.15	4.84
Facility RVU	**Work**	**PE**	**MP**	**Total**
99381	1.5	0.58	0.09	2.17
99382	1.6	0.62	0.1	2.32
99383	1.7	0.66	0.1	2.46
99384	2.0	0.78	0.12	2.9
99385	1.92	0.74	0.12	2.78
99386	2.33	0.9	0.14	3.37
99387	2.5	0.97	0.15	3.62

	FUD	Status	MUE	Modifiers				IOM Reference
99381	N/A	N	0(3)	N/A	N/A	N/A	N/A	None
99382	N/A	N	0(3)	N/A	N/A	N/A	N/A	
99383	N/A	N	0(3)	N/A	N/A	N/A	N/A	
99384	N/A	N	0(3)	N/A	N/A	N/A	N/A	
99385	N/A	N	0(3)	N/A	N/A	N/A	N/A	
99386	N/A	N	0(3)	N/A	N/A	N/A	N/A	
99387	N/A	N	0(3)	N/A	N/A	N/A	N/A	

* with documentation

Terms To Know

preventive medicine service. Evaluation and management service provided as a periodic health screening and/or prophylactic service that does not typically include management of new or existing diagnoses or problems.

99391-99397

99391 Periodic comprehensive preventive medicine reevaluation and management of an individual including an age and gender appropriate history, examination, counseling/anticipatory guidance/risk factor reduction interventions, and the ordering of laboratory/diagnostic procedures, established patient; infant (age younger than 1 year)
99392 early childhood (age 1 through 4 years)
99393 late childhood (age 5 through 11 years)
99394 adolescent (age 12 through 17 years)
99395 18-39 years
99396 40-64 years
99397 65 years and older

Explanation

Periodic comprehensive preventive medicine services are typically well-patient examinations for established patients presenting for reevaluations and/or management of overall health condition with code selection dependent upon the patient's age. These services include applicable patient history and examination, guidance/recommendation regarding personal risk factors, and any laboratory and/or diagnostic procedures ordered. Clinicians are not required to report minor or self-limiting problems or complaints noted during the course of the preventive examination when those problems do not require any additional work or necessitate performing the key components of a problem oriented E/M service. Report 99391 for infants younger than 1 year of age; 99392 for children 1 to 4 years of age; 99393 for children 5 to 11 years of age; 99394 for adolescents12 to 17 years of age; 99395 for adult patients 18 to 39 years of age; 99396 for patients 40 to 64 years of age; and 99397 for patients 65 years of age and older.

Coding Tips

These codes are used to report preventive medicine services for an established patient. Time is not a factor when selecting these E/M services. Code selection is determined based on whether the patient is new or established and the age of the patient. When documentation supports that a significant, separately identifiable problem-oriented evaluation and management (E/M) service is rendered, the appropriate code for the E/M service may be reported separately. Append modifier 25 to the service code selected to indicate that a separately identifiable E/M service was provided on the same date of service as the preventive medicine service. Immunizations and vaccines including counseling when provided, and ancillary services, including laboratory, radiology, or screening tests, performed at the time of the preventive service may be reported separately. Preventive medicine services are not covered by Medicare. For preventive services provided to a new patient, see 99381-99387.

ICD-10-CM Diagnostic Codes

The application of this code is too broad to adequately present ICD-10-CM diagnostic code links here. Refer to your ICD-10-CM book.

AMA: 99391 2022,Dec; 2022,Nov; 2022,Jul; 2021,Nov; 2021,Feb; 2021,Jan; 2019,Jul **99392** 2023,Mar; 2022,Dec; 2022,Nov; 2022,Jul; 2021,Nov; 2021,Feb; 2021,Jan; 2019,Jul **99393** 2024,Sep; 2022,Dec; 2022,Nov; 2022,Jul; 2021,Nov; 2021,Feb; 2021,Jan; 2019,Jul **99394** 2024,Sep; 2023,Jul; 2022,Dec; 2022,Nov; 2022,Jul; 2021,Nov; 2021,Feb; 2021,Jan; 2019,Jul **99395** 2024,Sep; 2022,Dec; 2022,Nov; 2022,Jul; 2021,Nov; 2021,Feb; 2021,Jan; 2019,Jul **99396** 2024,Sep; 2022,Dec; 2022,Nov; 2022,Jul; 2021,Nov; 2021,Feb; 2021,Jan; 2019,Jul **99397** 2024,Sep; 2022,Dec; 2022,Nov; 2022,Jul; 2021,Nov; 2021,Feb; 2021,Jan; 2019,Jul

Relative Value Units/Medicare Edits

Non-Facility RVU	Work	PE	MP	Total
99391	1.37	1.49	0.08	2.94
99392	1.5	1.54	0.09	3.13
99393	1.5	1.53	0.09	3.12
99394	1.7	1.61	0.1	3.41
99395	1.75	1.63	0.11	3.49
99396	1.9	1.69	0.12	3.71
99397	2.0	1.87	0.12	3.99
Facility RVU	**Work**	**PE**	**MP**	**Total**
99391	1.37	0.53	0.08	1.98
99392	1.5	0.58	0.09	2.17
99393	1.5	0.58	0.09	2.17
99394	1.7	0.66	0.1	2.46
99395	1.75	0.68	0.11	2.54
99396	1.9	0.74	0.12	2.76
99397	2.0	0.78	0.12	2.9

	FUD	Status	MUE	Modifiers				IOM Reference
99391	N/A	N	0(3)	N/A	N/A	N/A	N/A	None
99392	N/A	N	0(3)	N/A	N/A	N/A	N/A	
99393	N/A	N	0(3)	N/A	N/A	N/A	N/A	
99394	N/A	N	0(3)	N/A	N/A	N/A	N/A	
99395	N/A	N	0(3)	N/A	N/A	N/A	N/A	
99396	N/A	N	0(3)	N/A	N/A	N/A	N/A	
99397	N/A	N	0(3)	N/A	N/A	N/A	N/A	

* with documentation

Terms To Know

preventive medicine service. Evaluation and management service provided as a periodic health screening and/or prophylactic service that does not typically include management of new or existing diagnoses or problems.

99401-99404

99401 Preventive medicine counseling and/or risk factor reduction intervention(s) provided to an individual (separate procedure); approximately 15 minutes

99402 approximately 30 minutes

99403 approximately 45 minutes

99404 approximately 60 minutes

Explanation

Preventive medicine individual counseling services are face-to-face services performed by a qualified clinician in order to foster healthy living and/or avert illness/injury. Risk factor counseling may be utilized in the absence of illness. These services may include counseling/evaluation of family issues, appropriate diet and exercise, high-risk behavior, avoidance of injury, dental issues, and discussion of available laboratory and/or diagnostic results. Report 99401 for encounters lasting 15 minutes; 99402 for 30 minutes; 99403 for 45 minutes; and 99404 for a duration of 60 minutes.

Coding Tips

These codes are used to report counseling services provided to patients to support healthy living and reduce risk of illness or injury. These services are provided face-to-face by the physician or other qualified health care provider. These are time-based codes and time spent with the patient must be documented in the medical record. These separate procedures by definition are usually a component of a more complex service and are not identified separately. When performed alone or with other unrelated procedures/services they may be reported. When documentation supports that a significant, separately identifiable problem-oriented evaluation and management (E/M) service is rendered, the appropriate code for the E/M service may be reported separately. Append modifier 25 to the service code selected to indicate that a separately identifiable E/M service was provided on the same date of service as the counseling service. Do not report 96156-96159 or 96164-96171 with 99401-99404 on the same date of service. For preventive medicine counseling provided in a group setting, see 99411-99412. For behavior change intervention services, see 99406-99409.

ICD-10-CM Diagnostic Codes

The application of this code is too broad to adequately present ICD-10-CM diagnostic code links here. Refer to your ICD-10-CM book.

AMA: **99401** 2022,Nov; 2022,Oct; 2022,Jul; 2022,Apr; 2022,Jan; 2021,Jan; 2020,Aug; 2019,Jul **99402** 2022,Nov; 2022,Oct; 2022,Jul; 2022,Apr; 2022,Jan; 2021,Jan; 2020,Aug; 2019,Jul **99403** 2022,Nov; 2022,Oct; 2022,Jul; 2022,Apr; 2022,Jan; 2021,Jan; 2020,Aug; 2019,Jul **99404** 2022,Nov; 2022,Oct; 2022,Jul; 2022,Apr; 2022,Jan; 2021,Jan; 2020,Aug; 2019,Jul

Relative Value Units/Medicare Edits

Non-Facility RVU	Work	PE	MP	Total
99401	0.48	0.64	0.03	1.15
99402	0.98	0.83	0.06	1.87
99403	1.46	1.02	0.09	2.57
99404	1.95	1.21	0.12	3.28
Facility RVU	**Work**	**PE**	**MP**	**Total**
99401	0.48	0.19	0.03	0.7
99402	0.98	0.38	0.06	1.42
99403	1.46	0.57	0.09	2.12
99404	1.95	0.76	0.12	2.83

	FUD	Status	MUE	Modifiers				IOM Reference
99401	N/A	N	0(3)	N/A	N/A	N/A	N/A	None
99402	N/A	N	0(3)	N/A	N/A	N/A	N/A	
99403	N/A	N	0(3)	N/A	N/A	N/A	N/A	
99404	N/A	N	0(3)	N/A	N/A	N/A	N/A	

* with documentation

Terms To Know

counseling. Discussion with a patient and/or family concerning one or more of the following areas: diagnostic results, impressions, recommended diagnostic studies, prognosis, risks, benefits of management (treatment) options, instructions for management (treatment) and/or follow-up, importance of compliance with chosen management (treatment) options, risk factor reduction, and patient and family education.

preventive medicine service. Evaluation and management service provided as a periodic health screening and/or prophylactic service that does not typically include management of new or existing diagnoses or problems.

99406-99409

★**99406** Smoking and tobacco use cessation counseling visit; intermediate, greater than 3 minutes up to 10 minutes
★**99407** intensive, greater than 10 minutes
★**99408** Alcohol and/or substance (other than tobacco) abuse structured screening (eg, AUDIT, DAST), and brief intervention (SBI) services; 15 to 30 minutes
★**99409** greater than 30 minutes

Explanation

Individual behavior change intervention services are counseling and/or intervention services directed at high-risk behaviors such as tobacco, alcohol, and substance abuse. These services can be reported as treatment of the condition or in relation to the condition that has the potential of causing illness or injury. Additionally, the encounter uses validated instruments to determine the patient's opinion related to behavior change and providing input on a plan to change behavior with appropriate actions and motivation. Report 99406 for smoking and tobacco cessation counseling requiring three to 10 minutes of time and 99407 for counseling requiring more than ten minutes. Report 99408 for alcohol and/or substance abuse screening utilizing such instruments as AUDIT, DAST, and intervention services requiring 15 to 30 minutes; for more than 30 minutes, report 99409.

Coding Tips

These codes are used to report interventional counseling services provided to patients to promote behavioral change when the behavior is considered an illness itself or to change the behavior before it results in an illness. These are time-based codes and time spent with the patient must be documented in the medical record. When documentation supports that a significant, separately identifiable problem-oriented evaluation and management (E/M) service is rendered, the appropriate code for the E/M service may be reported separately. Append modifier 25 to the service code selected to indicate that a separately identifiable E/M service was provided on the same date of service as the counseling service. Codes 99408 and 99409 should only be reported for the initial screening and brief intervention. Do not report 99407 with 99406. Do not report 99409 with 99408. Do not report 99408 or 99409 with 96160-96161. Do not report 96156-96159 or 96164-96171 with 99406-99409 on the same date of service. The CPT codebook has identified these codes as telehealth/telemedicine services that may also be audio only services. Medicare has identified 99406 and 99407 as telehealth/telemedicine services that may also be audio only services. Telemedicine services may be reported by the performing provider by adding modifier 93 or 95 to these procedure code and using the appropriate place of service (POS) indicator; POS 02 for telehealth when the originating site is not the patient's home and POS 10 for telehealth services when the originating site is the patient's home. Modifier 33 may be appended when these services are performed as a preventive service as identified by the U.S. Preventive Services Task Force (USPSTF). Medicare and commercial payers should be contacted regarding their coverage guidelines. For preventive medicine counseling provided to an individual, see 99401-99404. For preventive medicine counseling provided in a group setting, see 99411-99412.

ICD-10-CM Diagnostic Codes

The application of this code is too broad to adequately present ICD-10-CM diagnostic code links here. Refer to your ICD-10-CM book.

AMA: **99406** 2024,Sep; 2024,Apr; 2022,Nov; 2022,Oct; 2022,Aug; 2022,Jul; 2021,Jan; 2020,Sep; 2020,Aug; 2019,Jul **99407** 2024,Sep; 2022,Nov; 2022,Oct; 2022,Aug; 2022,Jul; 2021,Jan; 2020,Aug; 2019,Jul **99408** 2024,Sep; 2022,Nov; 2022,Oct; 2022,Aug; 2022,Jul; 2021,Jan; 2020,Aug; 2019,Jul **99409** 2024,Sep; 2022,Nov; 2022,Oct; 2022,Aug; 2022,Jul; 2021,Jan; 2020,Aug; 2019,Jul

Relative Value Units/Medicare Edits

Non-Facility RVU	Work	PE	MP	Total
99406	0.24	0.18	0.02	0.44
99407	0.5	0.28	0.04	0.82
99408	0.65	0.33	0.04	1.02
99409	1.3	0.59	0.08	1.97
Facility RVU	**Work**	**PE**	**MP**	**Total**
99406	0.24	0.09	0.02	0.35
99407	0.5	0.2	0.04	0.74
99408	0.65	0.25	0.04	0.94
99409	1.3	0.5	0.08	1.88

	FUD	Status	MUE	Modifiers				IOM Reference
99406	N/A	A	1(2)	N/A	N/A	N/A	80*	None
99407	N/A	A	1(2)	N/A	N/A	N/A	80*	
99408	N/A	N	0(3)	N/A	N/A	N/A	N/A	
99409	N/A	N	0(3)	N/A	N/A	N/A	N/A	

* with documentation

Terms To Know

AUDIT. Alcohol use disorder identification test.

DAST. Drug abuse screening test.

 N Newborn: 0 P Pediatric: 0-17 M Maternity: 9-64 A Adult: 15-124 AMA: CPT Assist

99411-99412

99411 Preventive medicine counseling and/or risk factor reduction intervention(s) provided to individuals in a group setting (separate procedure); approximately 30 minutes

99412 approximately 60 minutes

Explanation

Preventive medicine group counseling services are face-to-face services performed by a qualified clinician in order to foster healthy living and/or avert illness/injury. Risk factor counseling may be utilized in the absence of illness in a group setting. These services may include counseling/evaluation of family issues, appropriate diet and exercise, high-risk behavior, avoidance of injury, dental issues, and discussion of available laboratory and/or diagnostic results. Report 99411 for encounters of 30 minutes duration and 99412 for encounters lasting 60 minutes.

Coding Tips

These codes are used to report counseling services provided to patients to support healthy living and reduce risk of illness or injury. These services are provided face-to-face by the physician or other qualified health care provider. These are time-based codes and time spent with the patient must be documented in the medical record. These separate procedures are usually a component of a more complex service and are not identified separately. When performed alone or with other unrelated procedures/services they may be reported. When documentation supports that a significant, separately identifiable problem-oriented evaluation and management (E/M) service is rendered, the appropriate code for the E/M service may be reported separately. Append modifier 25 to the service code selected to indicate that a separately identifiable E/M service was provided on the same date of service as the counseling service. Do not report 96156-96159 or 96164-96171 with 99411-99412 on the same date of service. For group counseling of patients with symptoms or established illness, see 99078. For preventive medicine counseling provided to an individual, see 99401-99404. For behavior change intervention services, see 99406-99409.

ICD-10-CM Diagnostic Codes

The application of this code is too broad to adequately present ICD-10-CM diagnostic code links here. Refer to your ICD-10-CM book.

AMA: **99411** 2022,Nov; 2022,Oct; 2022,Jul; 2021,Jan; 2020,Aug; 2019,Jul **99412** 2022,Nov; 2022,Oct; 2022,Jul; 2021,Jan; 2020,Aug; 2019,Jul

Relative Value Units/Medicare Edits

Non-Facility RVU	Work	PE	MP	Total
99411	0.15	0.44	0.01	0.6
99412	0.25	0.48	0.02	0.75
Facility RVU	**Work**	**PE**	**MP**	**Total**
99411	0.15	0.06	0.01	0.22
99412	0.25	0.1	0.02	0.37

	FUD	Status	MUE	Modifiers				IOM Reference
99411	N/A	N	0(3)	N/A	N/A	N/A	N/A	None
99412	N/A	N	0(3)	N/A	N/A	N/A	N/A	

* with documentation

[99421, 99422, 99423]

99421 Online digital evaluation and management service, for an established patient, for up to 7 days, cumulative time during the 7 days; 5-10 minutes

99422 Online digital evaluation and management service, for an established patient, for up to 7 days, cumulative time during the 7 days; 11-20 minutes

99423 Online digital evaluation and management service, for an established patient, for up to 7 days, cumulative time during the 7 days; 21 or more minutes

Explanation

Online medical evaluation services are non-face-to-face encounters originating from the established patient to the physician or other qualified health care professional for evaluation or management of a problem. The patient initiates the digital communication through a Health Insurance Portability and Accountability Act (HIPAA) compliant platform. The service includes all asynchronous (not in real-time) communication with the patient, review of the initial patient query and medical records, personal interaction with clinical staff by the provider related to the patient query, and development of a plan including ordering any necessary prescriptions or tests. The service may include more than one provider responding to the same patient and is only reportable once during seven days for the same encounter. These codes are not reported if the online patient request is related to an E/M service that occurred within the previous seven days or within the global period following a procedure. Report 99421 if the cumulative time during the seven-day period is five to 10 minutes; 99422 for 11 to 20 minutes; and 99423 for 21 or more minutes.

Coding Tips

These codes are used to report non-face-to-face patient services initiated by an established patient via an on-line inquiry. Providers must provide a timely response to the inquiry and the encounter must be stored permanently to report this service. These services are reported once in a seven-day period and are reported for the cumulative time devoted to the service over the seven days. Cumulative time of less than five minutes should not be reported. A new/unrelated problem initiated within seven days of a previous E/M visit that addresses a different problem may be reported separately. Medicare and other payers may not reimburse separately for these services. Check with the specific payer to determine coverage. For nonphysician on-line medical services, see 98970, 98971, and 98972. Do not report these services when performed concurrently with other billable services, such as 99202-99205, 99212-99215, 99242-99245, or when using the following for the same communication: 99091, 99374-99380, 99424-99427, 99437, 99487-99489, 99491, and 99495-99496. Do not report these services for INR monitoring when reporting 93792 or 93793.

ICD-10-CM Diagnostic Codes

The application of this code is too broad to adequately present ICD-10-CM diagnostic code links here. Refer to your ICD-10-CM book.

AMA: **99421** 2023,Nov; 2022,Nov; 2022,Jul; 2022,Jan; 2021,Sep; 2021,Jan; 2020,Mar; 2020,Jan **99422** 2023,Nov; 2022,Nov; 2022,Jul; 2022,Jan; 2021,Sep; 2021,Jan; 2020,Mar; 2020,Jan **99423** 2023,Nov; 2022,Nov; 2022,Jul; 2022,Jan; 2021,Sep; 2021,Jan; 2020,Mar; 2020,Jan

Relative Value Units/Medicare Edits

Non-Facility RVU	Work	PE	MP	Total
99421	0.25	0.18	0.02	0.45
99422	0.5	0.34	0.04	0.88
99423	0.8	0.54	0.06	1.4
Facility RVU	**Work**	**PE**	**MP**	**Total**
99421	0.25	0.11	0.02	0.38
99422	0.5	0.21	0.04	0.75
99423	0.8	0.34	0.06	1.2

	FUD	Status	MUE	Modifiers				IOM Reference
99421	N/A	A	1(2)	N/A	N/A	N/A	80*	None
99422	N/A	A	1(2)	N/A	N/A	N/A	80*	
99423	N/A	A	1(2)	N/A	N/A	N/A	80*	

* with documentation

Terms To Know

established patient. Patient who has received professional services in a face-to-face setting within the last three years from the same physician/qualified health care professional or another physician/qualified health care professional of the exact same specialty and subspecialty who belongs to the same group practice. If the patient is seen by a physician/qualified health care professional who is covering for another physician/qualified health care professional, the patient will be considered the same as if seen by the physician/qualified health care professional who is unavailable.

other qualified health care professional. Individual who is qualified by education, training, licensure/regulation, and facility privileging to perform a professional service within his or her scope of practice and independently (or as incident-to) report the professional service without requiring physician supervision. Payers may state exemptions in writing or state and local regulations may not follow this definition for performance of some services. Always refer to any relevant plan policies and federal and/or state laws to determine who may perform and report services.

99446-99449 [99451, 99452]

99446 Interprofessional telephone/Internet/electronic health record assessment and management service provided by a consultative physician or other qualified health care professional, including a verbal and written report to the patient's treating/requesting physician or other qualified health care professional; 5-10 minutes of medical consultative discussion and review

99447 11-20 minutes of medical consultative discussion and review

99448 21-30 minutes of medical consultative discussion and review

99449 31 minutes or more of medical consultative discussion and review

99451 Interprofessional telephone/Internet/electronic health record assessment and management service provided by a consultative physician or other qualified health care professional, including a written report to the patient's treating/requesting physician or other qualified health care professional, 5 minutes or more of medical consultative time

99452 Interprofessional telephone/Internet/electronic health record referral service(s) provided by a treating/requesting physician or other qualified health care professional, 30 minutes

Explanation

Interprofessional telephone/internet/electronic health record consultation services are utilized when the attending qualified clinician requests the input of a physician or qualified clinician with specific knowledge of the condition. This specialist may assist in diagnosis or treatment of the patient without seeing the patient and often occurs when the situation is urgent and/or complex in nature. The patient may be a new or established patient with a new problem or exacerbation of a current problem in the eyes of the consultant; however, the consultant may not have seen the patient within the previous 14 days. This code may not be reported for transfer of care or to schedule a face-to-face with the consultant within the next 14 days or next available appointment opening. This discussion includes appropriate review of medical records, laboratory and radiology results, medication review/tolerance, and pathology results. The consult should account for more than 50 percent of the time in discussion; if more than one discussion is necessary, the time is cumulative with the code reported one time. The patient's medical record should contain a request for consult with an explanation as to the medical necessity of the request and the consultant should provide a verbal and written report to the requesting/treating clinician. These codes are not reportable if the discussion requires less than five minutes of time. Report 99446 for encounters of five to 10 minutes duration; 99447 for 11 to 20 minutes; 99448 for 21 to 30 minutes; and 99449 for encounters of more than 30 minutes duration. Report 99451 for encounters of five or more minutes that include a written report only from the consultant. The attending qualified clinician can report 99452 when 16 to 30 minutes of the clinician's time is spent preparing for or communicating with the consultant; 99452 can only be reported once during a 14-day period.

Coding Tips

These codes are used to report a consultative assessment and management service requested by the patient's treating clinician for guidance from the specialist in treating the patient. These are time-based codes and time spent in medical consultation must be documented in the medical record. These codes do not differentiate between a new or established patient. Do not report these codes for the sole purpose of arranging a transfer of care or other face-to-face services. Report 99446-99449 for time spent in telephone/internet/electronic health record assessment and review with a verbal and written report of findings. Report 99451 for a written report of findings without a verbal report. Report 99452 for 16 to 30 minutes spent by the provider in a service day, preparing for or communicating with the consultant. Do not report 99452 on the same date as an E/M service; time and work of the referral service should be included in the total time or MDM component of the E/M service. Do not report consultations of less than five minutes. For telephone services conducted by the physician or OQHP directly with the patient, see 98008-98016. For on-line digital medical evaluation and management services provided by the physician directly with the patient, see 99421-99423. For nonphysician telephone services, see 98966-98968.

ICD-10-CM Diagnostic Codes

The application of this code is too broad to adequately present ICD-10-CM diagnostic code links here. Refer to your ICD-10-CM book.

AMA: **99446** 2023,Mar; 2022,Jul; 2021,Sep; 2021,Jan; 2019,Jul; 2019,Jun; 2019,Jan **99447** 2023,Mar; 2022,Jul; 2021,Sep; 2021,Jan; 2019,Jul; 2019,Jun; 2019,Jan **99448** 2023,Mar; 2022,Jul; 2021,Sep; 2021,Jan; 2019,Jul; 2019,Jun; 2019,Jan **99449** 2023,Mar; 2022,Jul; 2021,Sep; 2021,Jan; 2019,Jul; 2019,Jun; 2019,Jan **99451** 2023,Mar; 2022,Jul; 2021,Sep; 2021,Jan; 2019,Jul; 2019,Jun; 2019,Jan **99452** 2024,Oct; 2023,Mar; 2022,Jul; 2021,Sep; 2021,Jan; 2020,Sep; 2020,Jun; 2019,Jul; 2019,Jun; 2019,Jan

Relative Value Units/Medicare Edits

Non-Facility RVU	Work	PE	MP	Total
99446	0.35	0.15	0.03	0.53
99447	0.7	0.31	0.07	1.08
99448	1.05	0.46	0.09	1.6
99449	1.4	0.62	0.11	2.13
99451	0.7	0.29	0.05	1.04
99452	0.7	0.27	0.04	1.01
Facility RVU	**Work**	**PE**	**MP**	**Total**
99446	0.35	0.15	0.03	0.53
99447	0.7	0.31	0.07	1.08
99448	1.05	0.46	0.09	1.6
99449	1.4	0.62	0.11	2.13
99451	0.7	0.29	0.05	1.04
99452	0.7	0.27	0.04	1.01

	FUD	Status	MUE	Modifiers				IOM Reference
99446	N/A	A	1(2)	N/A	N/A	N/A	80*	None
99447	N/A	A	1(2)	N/A	N/A	N/A	80*	
99448	N/A	A	1(2)	N/A	N/A	N/A	80*	
99449	N/A	A	1(2)	N/A	N/A	N/A	80*	
99451	N/A	A	1(2)	N/A	N/A	N/A	80*	
99452	N/A	A	1(2)	N/A	N/A	N/A	80*	

* with documentation

[99453, 99454]

99453 Remote monitoring of physiologic parameter(s) (eg, weight, blood pressure, pulse oximetry, respiratory flow rate), initial; set-up and patient education on use of equipment

99454 Remote monitoring of physiologic parameter(s) (eg, weight, blood pressure, pulse oximetry, respiratory flow rate), initial; device(s) supply with daily recording(s) or programmed alert(s) transmission, each 30 days

Explanation

A physician or other qualified health care professional orders an FDA-defined remote patient monitoring (RPM) device that is used by a patient for the purposes of collecting, monitoring, and reporting health-related data to the provider, including, but not limited to, weight, blood pressure, or pulse oximetry. This technology allows for the gathering of health data from the patient in one location and the electronic transmission of that data to a provider in a different location for review and subsequent recommendations, particularly in patients with ongoing and/or chronic disease processes. Code 99453 reports the work involved with orienting the patient to the RPM process, the initial device set-up, and patient instruction and training for each episode of care. An episode of care is described as starting at the time the RPM device service begins and is complete when the established treatment goal has been reached. Code 99454 reports the supply of the actual device including the daily recordings and program alert transmissions for a 30-day period. These codes should not be reported for monitoring if the duration is less than 16 days.

Coding Tips

These codes are used to report the remote physiological monitoring services of a medically approved device ordered by the physician or other qualified health care professional. Code 99453 is used to report initial patient education with set up and instruction. Code 99454 is used to report each 30 days of device recording and transmission. For self-measured blood pressure monitoring, see 99473-99474. For remote therapeutic monitoring, see 98975-98978.

ICD-10-CM Diagnostic Codes

The application of this code is too broad to adequately present ICD-10-CM diagnostic code links here. Refer to your ICD-10-CM book.

AMA: **99453** 2024,Feb; 2023,Feb; 2022,Oct; 2022,Jul; 2022,Apr; 2022,Feb; 2021,Sep; 2021,Feb; 2021,Jan; 2020,Nov; 2020,Apr; 2019,Jul; 2019,Mar; 2019,Jan **99454** 2024,Feb; 2023,Feb; 2022,Oct; 2022,Jul; 2022,Apr; 2022,Feb; 2021,Sep; 2021,Jan; 2020,Nov; 2020,Apr; 2019,Oct; 2019,Jul; 2019,Mar; 2019,Jan

Relative Value Units/Medicare Edits

Non-Facility RVU	Work	PE	MP	Total
99453	0.0	0.58	0.02	0.6
99454	0.0	1.41	0.01	1.42
Facility RVU	**Work**	**PE**	**MP**	**Total**
99453	0.0	0.58	0.02	0.6
99454	0.0	1.41	0.01	1.42

	FUD	Status	MUE	Modifiers				IOM Reference
99453	N/A	A	1(2)	N/A	N/A	N/A	80*	None
99454	N/A	A	1(2)	N/A	N/A	N/A	80*	

* with documentation

[99091]

99091 Collection and interpretation of physiologic data (eg, ECG, blood pressure, glucose monitoring) digitally stored and/or transmitted by the patient and/or caregiver to the physician or other qualified health care professional, qualified by education, training, licensure/regulation (when applicable) requiring a minimum of 30 minutes of time, each 30 days

Explanation

A physician or other qualified health care professional collects and interprets physiologic data. The data (e.g., blood pressure) is stored digitally and may be transmitted by the patient and/or the caregiver to the provider. The report should contain the time it took the provider to acquire the physiologic data, review and interpret the data, and modify any care plan due to the additional data acquisition. A minimum of 30 minutes every 30 days must be spent in the collection and interpretation of data to report this service.

Coding Tips

This code is used to report the collection and interpretation of physiological data. The data is stored or transmitted from a patient-based device and reviewed by a qualified provider. Do not use 99091 to report transfer and interpretation of data from hospital or laboratory computers. Report 99091 once per 30 days when at least 30 minutes of provider time is spent. Do not report 99091 in the same calendar month when reporting 99374-99380, 99424-99427, 99437, 99457, 99487 or 99491. Do not report 99091 when a more specific code is available (see 93227, 93272, 95250, etc.).

ICD-10-CM Diagnostic Codes

The application of this code is too broad to adequately present ICD-10-CM diagnostic code links here. Refer to your ICD-10-CM book.

AMA: 99091 2023,Nov; 2022,Apr; 2022,Feb; 2022,Jan; 2021,May; 2020,Nov; 2020,Apr; 2020,Mar; 2020,Feb; 2019,Oct; 2019,Jun; 2019,Mar; 2019,Jan; 2018,Dec; 2018,Jun; 2018,Mar; 2018,Feb

Relative Value Units/Medicare Edits

Non-Facility RVU	Work	PE	MP	Total
99091	1.1	0.43	0.08	1.61
Facility RVU	**Work**	**PE**	**MP**	**Total**
99091	1.1	0.43	0.08	1.61

	FUD	Status	MUE	Modifiers				IOM Reference
99091	N/A	A	1(2)	N/A	N/A	N/A	80*	None

* with documentation

[99473, 99474]

99473 Self-measured blood pressure using a device validated for clinical accuracy; patient education/training and device calibration

99474 Self-measured blood pressure using a device validated for clinical accuracy; separate self-measurements of two readings one minute apart, twice daily over a 30-day period (minimum of 12 readings), collection of data reported by the patient and/or caregiver to the physician or other qualified health care professional, with report of average systolic and diastolic pressures and subsequent communication of a treatment plan to the patient

Explanation

Self-measured blood pressure monitoring (SMBP) has been shown to be an effective approach to lowering blood pressure (BP), improving control in patients with hypertension, and increasing patient compliance with antihypertensive therapy. Also known as out-of-office BP measurement or home BP monitoring, the practice involves the use of devices that have been validated for clinical accuracy. Devices that measure blood pressure over the upper arm remain the most accurate choice compared to other available options, and remain the standard for proper BP measurement over finger, wrist, mobile health, and wearable devices. Report 99473 for patient education/training and device calibration. Report 99474 for separate self-measurements of two readings, one minute apart, twice daily over a 30-day period with a minimum of 12 readings. This includes collection of data reported by the patient and/or caregiver to the physician or other qualified health care professional, with a report of average systolic and diastolic pressures and subsequent communication of a treatment plan to the patient.

Coding Tips

These codes are used to report patient measured blood pressure using a medically validated device. Code 99473 is used to report initial patient education and device calibration. Code 99474 is used to report each 30 days of collected data reported by the patient and an appropriate treatment plan provided to the patient. Code 99473 may only be reported once per device and code 99474 may only be reported once per calendar month. These codes should not be reported in the same calendar month as 93784, 93786, 93788, 93790, 99091, 99424-99427, 99437, 99439, 99453, 99454, 99457, 99487, or 99489-99491.

ICD-10-CM Diagnostic Codes

The application of this code is too broad to adequately present ICD-10-CM diagnostic code links here. Refer to your ICD-10-CM book.

AMA: 99473 2023,Nov; 2023,Feb; 2022,Sep; 2022,Jul; 2022,Feb; 2021,Jan; 2020,Apr; 2020,Feb; 2020,Jan **99474** 2023,Nov; 2023,Feb; 2022,Sep; 2022,Jul; 2022,Feb; 2021,Jan; 2020,Apr; 2020,Feb; 2020,Jan

Relative Value Units/Medicare Edits

Non-Facility RVU	Work	PE	MP	Total
99473	0.0	0.42	0.01	0.43
99474	0.18	0.31	0.01	0.5
Facility RVU	**Work**	**PE**	**MP**	**Total**
99473	0.0	0.42	0.01	0.43
99474	0.18	0.07	0.01	0.26

	FUD	Status	MUE	Modifiers				IOM Reference
99473	N/A	A	1(2)	N/A	N/A	N/A	80*	None
99474	N/A	A	1(2)	N/A	N/A	N/A	80*	

* with documentation

Terms To Know

diastolic. Pertaining to the time in between ventricular contractions (systole), when ventricular filling occurs.

other qualified health care professional. Individual who is qualified by education, training, licensure/regulation, and facility privileging to perform a professional service within his or her scope of practice and independently (or as incident-to) report the professional service without requiring physician supervision. Payers may state exemptions in writing or state and local regulations may not follow this definition for performance of some services. Always refer to any relevant plan policies and federal and/or state laws to determine who may perform and report services.

systolic. Pressure in the arteries when the heart contracts (systole).

treatment plan. Plan of care established by the provider outlining specific deficits and planned treatment that may be submitted to the case manager when seeking certification for a plan member.

[99457, 99458]

99457 Remote physiologic monitoring treatment management services, clinical staff/physician/other qualified health care professional time in a calendar month requiring interactive communication with the patient/caregiver during the month; first 20 minutes

\+ **99458** Remote physiologic monitoring treatment management services, clinical staff/physician/other qualified health care professional time in a calendar month requiring interactive communication with the patient/caregiver during the month; each additional 20 minutes (List separately in addition to code for primary procedure)

Explanation

The provider or clinical staff utilizes the results obtained from an FDA-defined remote patient physiologic monitoring (RPM) device to oversee the patient's treatment plan. The device is ordered by a physician or other qualified health care provider and used by the patient for the purposes of collecting, monitoring, and reporting health-related data, including, but not limited to, weight, blood pressure, or pulse oximetry. This technology allows for the gathering of health data from the patient in one location and the electronic transmission of that data to a provider in a different location for review and subsequent recommendations, particularly in patients with ongoing and/or chronic disease processes. Report these codes to identify time spent managing care when the patient or the practice does not meet requirements for reporting a more specific service. These codes may be reported simultaneously with chronic care management, principal care management, transitional care management, and behavioral health integration services. Time involved in performing this service should remain separate and distinct from other services and does not count toward the required time for both services in a single month. Live and interactive communication with the patient and/or caregiver is required; data may be patient-reported or device-generated. Report 99457 for the first 20 minutes of clinician time per calendar month and 99458 for each additional 20 minutes.

Coding Tips

These codes are used to report treatment management of a patient currently monitored remotely for physiological parameters. Report 99457 once per calendar month when at least 20 minutes of live interactive communication is provided, regardless of the number of modalities performed. Report 99458 for each additional 20 minutes minimum of monitoring during the same month. Use 99457-99458 only when another more specific code is not available. Codes 99457 and 99458 may be reported with 99424-99427, 99437, 99439, 99487, 99489, 99490, 99491, 99495, 99496, 99484, and 99492-99494, but may not be performed concurrently. Do not report 99457 or 99458 with 99202-99205, 99211-99215, 99221-99223, 99231-99233, 99252-99255, or 99341-99350. Do not report 99457 with 93264 or 99091, or in the same month as 99473-99474.

ICD-10-CM Diagnostic Codes

The application of this code is too broad to adequately present ICD-10-CM diagnostic code links here. Refer to your ICD-10-CM book.

AMA: **99457** 2023,Feb; 2022,Oct; 2022,Jul; 2022,Apr; 2022,Feb; 2022,Jan; 2021,Sep; 2021,Jan; 2020,Apr; 2020,Feb; 2019,Jul; 2019,Jun; 2019,Mar; 2019,Jan **99458** 2022,Oct; 2022,Jul; 2022,Apr; 2022,Feb; 2022,Jan; 2021,Sep; 2021,Jan; 2020,Feb

Relative Value Units/Medicare Edits

Non-Facility RVU	Work	PE	MP	Total
99457	0.61	0.82	0.04	1.47
99458	0.61	0.53	0.04	1.18
Facility RVU	**Work**	**PE**	**MP**	**Total**
99457	0.61	0.24	0.04	0.89
99458	0.61	0.24	0.04	0.89

	FUD	Status	MUE	Modifiers				IOM Reference
99457	N/A	A	1(2)	N/A	N/A	N/A	80*	None
99458	N/A	A	3(3)	N/A	N/A	N/A	80*	

* with documentation

Terms To Know

monitoring. Recording of events; keep track, regulate, or control patient activities and record findings.

other qualified health care professional. Individual who is qualified by education, training, licensure/regulation, and facility privileging to perform a professional service within his or her scope of practice and independently (or as incident-to) report the professional service without requiring physician supervision. Payers may state exemptions in writing or state and local regulations may not follow this definition for performance of some services. Always refer to any relevant plan policies and federal and/or state laws to determine who may perform and report services.

treatment plan. Plan of care established by the provider outlining specific deficits and planned treatment that may be submitted to the case manager when seeking certification for a plan member.

99464-99465

99464 Attendance at delivery (when requested by the delivering physician or other qualified health care professional) and initial stabilization of newborn

99465 Delivery/birthing room resuscitation, provision of positive pressure ventilation and/or chest compressions in the presence of acute inadequate ventilation and/or cardiac output

Explanation

Delivery/birthing room attendance and resuscitation services are reported when special newborn circumstances require additional attendance and/or care. Report 99464 when attendance during delivery is requested by the delivering health care professional with newborn stabilization. Report 99465 for delivery/birthing room resuscitation, including any positive pressure ventilation and/or chest compression when required due to unsatisfactory ventilation or cardiac output.

Coding Tips

These codes are used to report stabilization or resuscitation services provided to a newborn in the delivery or birthing center. Additional services performed as a necessary part of the resuscitation service, including intubation and vascular lines, may be reported in addition to 99465. These additional services should only be reported when necessary for resuscitation not as a convenience prior to admission to a neonatal intensive care unit. These codes may be reported in addition to 99221-99223, 99291, 99460, 99468, and 99477. Do not report 99465 with 99464.

ICD-10-CM Diagnostic Codes

The application of this code is too broad to adequately present ICD-10-CM diagnostic code links here. Refer to your ICD-10-CM book.

AMA: **99464** 2022,Jul; 2021,Jan; 2019,Jul; 2018,Jun **99465** 2023,Nov; 2022,Jul; 2021,Jan; 2019,Jul; 2018,Jun

Relative Value Units/Medicare Edits

Non-Facility RVU	Work	PE	MP	Total
99464	1.5	0.55	0.1	2.15
99465	2.93	1.08	0.2	4.21
Facility RVU	**Work**	**PE**	**MP**	**Total**
99464	1.5	0.55	0.1	2.15
99465	2.93	1.08	0.2	4.21

	FUD	Status	MUE	Modifiers				IOM Reference
99464	N/A	A	1(2)	N/A	N/A	N/A	80*	None
99465	N/A	A	1(2)	N/A	N/A	N/A	80*	

* with documentation

99468-99472, 99475-99476

99468 Initial inpatient neonatal critical care, per day, for the evaluation and management of a critically ill neonate, 28 days of age or younger

99469 Subsequent inpatient neonatal critical care, per day, for the evaluation and management of a critically ill neonate, 28 days of age or younger

99471 Initial inpatient pediatric critical care, per day, for the evaluation and management of a critically ill infant or young child, 29 days through 24 months of age

99472 Subsequent inpatient pediatric critical care, per day, for the evaluation and management of a critically ill infant or young child, 29 days through 24 months of age

99475 Initial inpatient pediatric critical care, per day, for the evaluation and management of a critically ill infant or young child, 2 through 5 years of age

99476 Subsequent inpatient pediatric critical care, per day, for the evaluation and management of a critically ill infant or young child, 2 through 5 years of age

Explanation

Inpatient neonatal and pediatric critical care services are reported for neonates (28 days of age or younger) and pediatric patients (29 days through less than 6 years of age) beginning with the date of admission to the critical care unit and for all following days that the patient remains in the unit. Codes are only reportable once daily, per patient, by a single provider within the admission range of the specific facility. Several services are included in the care of these patients and are not separately reportable by the provider, such as monitoring vital signs, any required vascular access, ventilation oversight, blood gas, pulse oximetry measurement, evaluation of car seat, blood transfusion, oral/nasogastric tube insertion, suprapubic bladder aspiration and/or bladder catheter placement, and lumbar puncture. Facilities, however, may report these services separately. Report 99468 for initial inpatient neonates; 99469 for subsequent inpatient neonates; 99471 for initial inpatient pediatric patients aged 29 days to 24 months; 99472 for subsequent inpatient pediatric patients aged 29 days to 24 months; 99475 for initial inpatient pediatric patients 2 to 5 years of age; and 99476 for subsequent inpatient pediatric patients 2 to 5 years of age.

Coding Tips

These codes are used to report inpatient neonatal and pediatric critical care services. Code selection is determined based on whether the service is an initial or subsequent encounter and the age of the patient. These codes are reported on a per day basis. Report an initial critical care code for the first day of service and a subsequent critical care code for the following day(s) of service for the same patient admission. These codes may only be reported by one physician and only once per day, per patient. The following services are considered inclusive to the critical care codes when reported by the physician: interpretation of cardiac output measurements, chest x-rays, gastric intubation, temporary transcutaneous pacing, airway management, ventilation management, pulse oximetry, blood gases, collection and interpretation of physiologic data, computer data such as ECGs, blood transfusion, nasogastric tube placement, bladder aspiration, catheterization, lumbar puncture, vascular access, and car seat evaluation. Codes 99468, 99471, and 99475 for initial critical care services should only be reported once per hospital stay. Medicare has identified these codes as telehealth/telemedicine services. Telemedicine services may be reported by the performing provider by using the appropriate place of service (POS) indicator; POS 02 for telehealth when the originating site is not the patient's home. Medicare and commercial payers should be contacted regarding their coverage guidelines. For initiation of selective head or total body hypothermia, see 99184. For neonatal and pediatric patients that receive critical care services in the outpatient setting, see 99291-99292. For critical care provided to patients 6 years of age or older, see 99291-99292. For neonatal patients that are not critically ill but require intensive monitoring or other intensive care, see 99477-99480. Report services for patients who improve and do not require critical or intensive care services with codes 99231-99233. When the patient status changes the transferring provider may only report one services for that date, 99221-99233, 99291-99292, 99460-99462, or 99477-99480 as appropriate.

ICD-10-CM Diagnostic Codes

The application of this code is too broad to adequately present ICD-10-CM diagnostic code links here. Refer to your ICD-10-CM book.

AMA: **99468** 2023,May; 2023,Feb; 2022,Dec; 2022,Sep; 2022,Jul; 2021,Jan; 2019,Jul; 2018,Dec; 2018,Jun **99469** 2023,May; 2023,Feb; 2022,Dec; 2022,Sep; 2022,Jul; 2021,Jan; 2019,Jul; 2018,Dec; 2018,Jun **99471** 2023,Feb; 2023,Jan; 2022,Dec; 2022,Sep; 2022,Jul; 2021,Jan; 2019,Jul; 2018,Dec; 2018,Jun **99472** 2023,Feb; 2023,Jan; 2022,Dec; 2022,Sep; 2022,Jul; 2021,Jan; 2019,Jul; 2018,Dec; 2018,Jun **99475** 2023,Feb; 2023,Jan; 2022,Dec; 2022,Sep; 2022,Jul; 2021,Jan; 2019,Jul; 2018,Dec; 2018,Jun **99476** 2023,Feb; 2023,Jan; 2022,Dec; 2022,Sep; 2022,Jul; 2021,Jan; 2019,Jul; 2018,Dec; 2018,Jun

Relative Value Units/Medicare Edits

Non-Facility RVU	Work	PE	MP	Total
99468	18.46	6.76	1.26	26.48
99469	7.99	2.92	0.54	11.45
99471	15.98	5.85	1.11	22.94
99472	7.99	3.12	0.64	11.75
99475	11.25	4.34	0.94	16.53
99476	6.75	2.64	0.56	9.95
Facility RVU	**Work**	**PE**	**MP**	**Total**
99468	18.46	6.76	1.26	26.48
99469	7.99	2.92	0.54	11.45
99471	15.98	5.85	1.11	22.94
99472	7.99	3.12	0.64	11.75
99475	11.25	4.34	0.94	16.53
99476	6.75	2.64	0.56	9.95

	FUD	Status	MUE	Modifiers				IOM Reference
99468	N/A	A	1(2)	N/A	N/A	N/A	80*	None
99469	N/A	A	1(2)	N/A	N/A	N/A	80*	
99471	N/A	A	1(2)	N/A	N/A	N/A	80*	
99472	N/A	A	1(2)	N/A	N/A	N/A	80*	
99475	N/A	A	1(2)	N/A	N/A	N/A	80*	
99476	N/A	A	1(2)	N/A	N/A	N/A	80*	

* with documentation

[99437, 99439, 99490, 99491]

99490 Chronic care management services with the following required elements: multiple (two or more) chronic conditions expected to last at least 12 months, or until the death of the patient, chronic conditions that place the patient at significant risk of death, acute exacerbation/decompensation, or functional decline, comprehensive care plan established, implemented, revised, or monitored; first 20 minutes of clinical staff time directed by a physician or other qualified health care professional, per calendar month.

+ **99439** Chronic care management services with the following required elements: multiple (two or more) chronic conditions expected to last at least 12 months, or until the death of the patient, chronic conditions that place the patient at significant risk of death, acute exacerbation/decompensation, or functional decline, comprehensive care plan established, implemented, revised, or monitored; each additional 20 minutes of clinical staff time directed by a physician or other qualified health care professional, per calendar month (List separately in addition to code for primary procedure)

99491 Chronic care management services with the following required elements: multiple (two or more) chronic conditions expected to last at least 12 months, or until the death of the patient, chronic conditions that place the patient at significant risk of death, acute exacerbation/decompensation, or functional decline, comprehensive care plan established, implemented, revised, or monitored; first 30 minutes provided personally by a physician or other qualified health care professional, per calendar month.

+ **99437** Chronic care management services with the following required elements: multiple (two or more) chronic conditions expected to last at least 12 months, or until the death of the patient, chronic conditions that place the patient at significant risk of death, acute exacerbation/decompensation, or functional decline, comprehensive care plan established, implemented, revised, or monitored; each additional 30 minutes by a physician or other qualified health care professional, per calendar month (List separately in addition to code for primary procedure)

Explanation

Care management services are defined as those management and support services that are 1) rendered by clinical staff while under the direction of a clinician who may be a physician or other qualified health care professional (QHP) or 2) provided personally by a physician or other QHP to a patient who resides in a personal residence or in an assisted living facility, domiciliary, or rest home. Some components of care management services include the establishment, implementation, monitoring, or revision of the patient's individual care plan; coordination of the care provided by other agencies and professionals; and education afforded to the patient or their caregiver regarding the patient's care plan, condition, and prognosis. Intended to improve coordination of care and patient engagement while reducing hospitalizations and disjointed care, care management services also take into account the patient's other medical conditions, psychosocial needs, and normal activities of daily living (ADL). Chronic care management services are represented by resequenced codes 99490, 99439, 99491, and 99437. Typically, patients receiving this care have a minimum of two and possibly more chronic ongoing or episodic health conditions that are anticipated to last at least one year (or until the patient expires) and that put the patient at increased risk of death, exacerbation, or functional decline. Chronic care management services include the establishment, implementation, revision, or monitoring of a comprehensive care plan. Code 99490 should be reported once per calendar month for the first 20 minutes of clinical staff time when directed by a physician or other QHP; for each additional 20 minutes, report 99439. Code 99439 should not be reported more than twice per calendar month. Code 99491 is also reported once per calendar month and represents the first 30 minutes provided personally by the physician or other QHP involved with care management activities; report 99437 for each additional 30 minutes.

Coding Tips

These codes are used to report care management services provided by the clinical staff under the direction of a qualified health care professional or directly by a physician or other qualified health care professional to a patient residing at home or in an assisted living facility, domiciliary, or rest home. These are time-based codes and total time spent performing care management services during the calendar month should be documented in the patient record. Do not report these codes if all elements listed in the code description are not performed. If the physician provides face-to-face E/M visits in the same calendar month, these visits may be reported separately. Do not count clinical staff time for a particular day if the physician reports an E/M service on that day. Code 99490 and 99491 may only be reported once per calendar month by the provider that assumes the care management role for the patient. Do not report 99490 if less than 20 minutes of chronic care management is provided in the calendar month. Code 99439 should be reported in addition to 99490 for each additional 20 minutes of clinical staff time provided. Report 99491 when more than 30 minutes of chronic care management is provided by the physician or other qualified health care provider in the same calendar month. Code 99437 should be reported in addition to 99491 for each additional 30 minutes of physician time provided. Do not report 99439 or 99490 with 99437 or 99491 during the same calendar month; do not report any of these codes with 99487 or 99489. Do not report these codes with 90951-90970 for ESRD services or in the postoperative period of a reported surgery. Do not report these codes with 99374-99380, 99424-99427, 99437, 99487, 99489, 99491, or 99605-99607 in the same calendar month. Do not report these codes for service time reported with 93792-93793, 98012-98016, 98960-98962, 98966-98968, 98970-98972, 99071, 99078, 99080, 99091, 99358-99359, 99366-99368, 99421-99423, or 99605-99607; or 99437 and 99491 with 99495 or 99496.

ICD-10-CM Diagnostic Codes

The application of this code is too broad to adequately present ICD-10-CM diagnostic code links here. Refer to your ICD-10-CM book.

AMA: 99437 2023,Nov; 2022,Aug; 2022,Jul; 2022,Apr; 2022,Jan **99439** 2023,Nov; 2022,Jul; 2022,Jan; 2021,Jan **99490** 2023,Nov; 2022,Jul; 2022,Jan; 2021,Jan; 2020,Apr; 2020,Feb; 2019,Jan; 2018,Oct; 2018,Jul; 2018,Apr; 2018,Mar; 2018,Feb **99491** 2023,Nov; 2022,Dec; 2022,Aug; 2022,Jul; 2022,Jan; 2021,Jan; 2020,Apr; 2018,Oct

Relative Value Units/Medicare Edits

Non-Facility RVU	Work	PE	MP	Total
99490	1.0	0.81	0.07	1.88
99439	0.7	0.69	0.05	1.44
99491	1.5	0.94	0.1	2.54
99437	1.0	0.72	0.07	1.79
Facility RVU	**Work**	**PE**	**MP**	**Total**
99490	1.0	0.42	0.07	1.49
99439	0.7	0.29	0.05	1.04
99491	1.5	0.64	0.1	2.24
99437	1.0	0.43	0.07	1.5

	FUD	Status	MUE	Modifiers				IOM Reference
99490	N/A	A	1(2)	N/A	N/A	N/A	80*	None
99439	N/A	A	2(2)	N/A	N/A	N/A	80*	
99491	N/A	A	1(2)	N/A	N/A	N/A	80*	
99437	N/A	A	2(3)	N/A	N/A	N/A	80*	

* with documentation

Terms To Know

coordination of care. Care provided concurrently with counseling that includes treatment instructions to the patient or caregiver; special accommodations for home, work, school, vacation, or other locations; coordination with other providers and agencies; and living arrangements.

qualified health care professional. Educated, licensed or certified, and regulated professional operating under a specified scope of practice to provide patient services that are separate and distinct from other clinical staff.

99487-99489

99487 Complex chronic care management services with the following required elements: multiple (two or more) chronic conditions expected to last at least 12 months, or until the death of the patient, chronic conditions that place the patient at significant risk of death, acute exacerbation/decompensation, or functional decline, comprehensive care plan established, implemented, revised, or monitored, moderate or high complexity medical decision making; first 60 minutes of clinical staff time directed by a physician or other qualified health care professional, per calendar month.

\+ **99489** each additional 30 minutes of clinical staff time directed by a physician or other qualified health care professional, per calendar month (List separately in addition to code for primary procedure)

Explanation

Care management services are defined as those management and support services that are 1) rendered by clinical staff while under the direction of a clinician who may be a physician or other qualified health care professional (QHP) or 2) provided personally by a physician or other QHP to a patient who resides in a personal residence or in an assisted living facility, domiciliary, or rest home. Some components of care management services include the establishment, implementation, monitoring, or revision of the patient's individual care plan; coordination of the care provided by other agencies and professionals; and education afforded to the patient or their caregiver regarding the patient's care plan, condition, and prognosis. Intended to improve coordination of care and patient engagement while reducing hospitalizations and disjointed care, care management services also consider the patient's other medical conditions, psychosocial needs, and normal activities of daily living (ADL). Complex chronic care management services (99487, 99489) are provided to patients who typically have a minimum of two and possibly more chronic ongoing or episodic health conditions that are anticipated to last at least one year (or until the patient expires) and that put the patient at increased risk of death, exacerbation, or functional decline. Included is the establishment, implementation, revision, or monitoring of a comprehensive care plan that requires moderate or high complexity medical decision making. Code 99487 is reported once per calendar month for the first 60 minutes of clinical staff time when directed by a physician or other QHP; for each additional 30 minutes, report 99489. Code 99489 should not be reported more than twice per calendar month.

Coding Tips

These codes are used to report care management services provided by the clinical staff under the direction of a qualified health care professional to a patient residing at home or in an assisted living facility, domiciliary, or rest home. These are time-based codes and total time spent performing care management services during the calendar month should be documented in the patient record. Do not report these codes if all elements listed in the code description are not performed. If the physician provides face-to-face E/M visits in the same calendar month, these visits may be reported separately. Do not count clinical staff time for a particular day if the physician reports an E/M service on that day. Code 99487 may only be reported once per calendar month by the provider that assumes the care management role for the patient. Code 99489 should only be reported in addition to 99487. Do not report 99487 if less than 60 minutes of complex chronic care management is provided in a calendar month. Do not report 99489 if less than 30 minutes of additional time beyond the first 60 minutes of complex chronic care is provided. Do not report these codes in addition to 90951-90970 for ESRD services or in the postoperative period of a reported surgery. Do not report these codes in addition to 99374-99380, 99424-99427, 99437, 99439, or 99490-99491 in the same calendar month. Do not report 99487 or 99489 for service time reported with 93792-93793, 98012-98016, 98960-98962, 98966-98968, 98970-98972, 99071, 99078, 99080, 99091, 99358-99359, 99366-99368, 99421-99423, or 99605-99607.

ICD-10-CM Diagnostic Codes

The application of this code is too broad to adequately present ICD-10-CM diagnostic code links here. Refer to your ICD-10-CM book.

AMA: **99487** 2024,Jul; 2023,Nov; 2022,Jul; 2022,Jan; 2021,Jan; 2020,Apr; 2020,Mar; 2020,Feb; 2019,Jan; 2018,Oct; 2018,Jul; 2018,Apr; 2018,Mar; 2018,Feb **99489** 2023,Nov; 2022,Jul; 2022,Jan; 2021,Jan; 2020,Apr; 2020,Mar; 2020,Feb; 2019,Jan; 2018,Oct; 2018,Jul; 2018,Apr; 2018,Mar; 2018,Feb

Relative Value Units/Medicare Edits

Non-Facility RVU	Work	PE	MP	Total
99487	1.81	2.1	0.12	4.03
99489	1.0	1.1	0.07	2.17
Facility RVU	**Work**	**PE**	**MP**	**Total**
99487	1.81	0.75	0.12	2.68
99489	1.0	0.42	0.07	1.49

	FUD	Status	MUE	Modifiers				IOM Reference
99487	N/A	A	1(2)	N/A	N/A	N/A	80*	None
99489	N/A	A	10(3)	N/A	N/A	N/A	80*	

* with documentation

[99424, 99425, 99426, 99427]

99424 Principal care management services, for a single high-risk disease, with the following required elements: one complex chronic condition expected to last at least 3 months, and that places the patient at significant risk of hospitalization, acute exacerbation/decompensation, functional decline, or death, the condition requires development, monitoring, or revision of disease-specific care plan, the condition requires frequent adjustments in the medication regimen and/or the management of the condition is unusually complex due to comorbidities, ongoing communication and care coordination between relevant practitioners furnishing care; first 30 minutes provided personally by a physician or other qualified health care professional, per calendar month.

\+ **99425** Principal care management services, for a single high-risk disease, with the following required elements: one complex chronic condition expected to last at least 3 months, and that places the patient at significant risk of hospitalization, acute exacerbation/decompensation, functional decline, or death, the condition requires development, monitoring, or revision of disease-specific care plan, the condition requires frequent adjustments in the medication regimen and/or the management of the condition is unusually complex due to comorbidities, ongoing communication and care coordination between relevant practitioners furnishing care; each additional 30 minutes provided personally by a physician or other qualified health care professional, per calendar month (List separately in addition to code for primary procedure)

99426 Principal care management services, for a single high-risk disease, with the following required elements: one complex chronic condition expected to last at least 3 months, and that places the patient at significant risk of hospitalization, acute exacerbation/decompensation, functional decline, or death, the condition requires development, monitoring, or revision of disease-specific care plan, the condition requires frequent adjustments in the medication regimen and/or the management of the condition is unusually complex due to comorbidities, ongoing communication and care coordination between relevant practitioners furnishing care; first 30 minutes of clinical staff time directed by physician or other qualified health care professional, per calendar month.

\+ **99427** Principal care management services, for a single high-risk disease, with the following required elements: one complex chronic condition expected to last at least 3 months, and that places the patient at significant risk of hospitalization, acute exacerbation/decompensation, functional decline, or death, the condition requires development, monitoring, or revision of disease-specific care plan, the condition requires frequent adjustments in the medication regimen and/or the management of the condition is unusually complex due to comorbidities, ongoing communication and care coordination between relevant practitioners furnishing care; each additional 30 minutes of clinical staff time directed by a physician or other qualified health care professional, per calendar month (List separately in addition to code for primary procedure)

Explanation

Principal care management services are provided to patients for a single high-risk disease. There is one complex condition that is chronic and expected to last a minimum of three months that puts the patient at substantial risk of exacerbation, functional decline, hospitalization, or death. The disease-specific care plan related to this condition requires on-going development, monitoring, or revising. Frequent adjustments to the medication regimen are required, or patient comorbidities increase the complexity of the condition's management. Communication and care coordination between those furnishing care is required on an ongoing basis. Report 99424 once per calendar month for the first 30 minutes of care provided personally by a physician or other qualified health care professional (QHP); report 99425 for each additional 30 minutes. Report 99426 once per calendar month for the first 30 minutes of clinical staff time when directed by a physician or other QHP; for each additional 20 minutes, report 99427.

Coding Tips

These codes are used to report care management services provided by the clinical staff under the direction of a qualified health care professional or directly by a physician or other qualified health care professional to a patient residing at home or in an assisted living facility, domiciliary, or rest home. These are time-based codes and total time spent performing care management services during the calendar month should be documented in the patient record. Do not report these codes if all elements listed in the code description are not performed. If the physician provides face-to-face E/M visits in the same calendar month, these visits may be reported separately. Do not count clinical staff time for a particular day if the physician reports an E/M service on that day. Do not report 99424 if less than 30 minutes of principal care management is provided in the calendar month. Code 99425 should be reported in addition to 99424 for each additional 30 minutes of physician time provided. Report 99426 when more than 30 minutes of principal care management is provided by the clinical staff in the same calendar month. Code 99427 should be reported in addition to 99426 for each additional 30 minutes of clinical staff time. Do not report these codes with 90951-90970 for ESRD services or in the postoperative period of a reported surgery. Do not report these codes with 99374-99380, 99426-99427, 99437, 99439, 99473-99474, 99487, 99489, or 99490-99491 in the same calendar month. Do not report these codes for service time reported with 93792-93793, 98012-98016, 98960-98962, 98966-98968, 98970-98972, 99071, 99078, 99080, 99091, 99358-99359, 99366-99368, 99421-99423, or 99605-99607.

ICD-10-CM Diagnostic Codes

The application of this code is too broad to adequately present ICD-10-CM diagnostic code links here. Refer to your ICD-10-CM book.

AMA: 99424 2023,Nov; 2022,Dec; 2022,Nov; 2022,Aug; 2022,Jul; 2022,Apr; 2022,Jan **99425** 2023,Nov; 2022,Dec; 2022,Nov; 2022,Aug; 2022,Jul; 2022,Apr; 2022,Jan **99426** 2023,Nov; 2022,Nov; 2022,Jul; 2022,Apr; 2022,Jan **99427** 2023,Nov; 2022,Nov; 2022,Jul; 2022,Apr; 2022,Jan

Relative Value Units/Medicare Edits

Non-Facility RVU	Work	PE	MP	Total
99424	1.45	0.92	0.11	2.48
99425	1.0	0.73	0.07	1.8
99426	1.0	0.78	0.08	1.86
99427	0.71	0.66	0.05	1.42
Facility RVU	**Work**	**PE**	**MP**	**Total**
99424	1.45	0.65	0.11	2.21
99425	1.0	0.45	0.07	1.52
99426	1.0	0.39	0.08	1.47
99427	0.71	0.27	0.05	1.03

	FUD	Status	MUE	Modifiers				IOM Reference
99424	N/A	A	1(2)	N/A	N/A	N/A	80*	None
99425	N/A	A	2(3)	N/A	N/A	N/A	80*	
99426	N/A	A	1(2)	N/A	N/A	N/A	80*	
99427	N/A	A	2(3)	N/A	N/A	N/A	80*	

* with documentation

Terms To Know

comorbid condition. Condition present that is not the primary reason for treating the patient, but one that affects the patient's care.

qualified health care professional. Educated, licensed or certified, and regulated professional operating under a specified scope of practice to provide patient services that are separate and distinct from other clinical staff.

99495-99496

★**99495** Transitional care management services with the following required elements: Communication (direct contact, telephone, electronic) with the patient and/or caregiver within 2 business days of discharge, At least moderate level of medical decision making during the service period, Face-to-face visit, within 14 calendar days of discharge

★**99496** Transitional care management services with the following required elements: Communication (direct contact, telephone, electronic) with the patient and/or caregiver within 2 business days of discharge, High level of medical decision making during the service period, Face-to-face visit, within 7 calendar days of discharge

Explanation

Transitional care management services are reported for patients requiring moderate to high level of medical decision making who are transitioning from an inpatient or observation facility, partial hospital, or a nursing facility to a home or community type setting, including a private residence or temporary lodging. Short-term accommodations such as a hotel, campground, hostel, or cruise ship are included, along with an assisted living facility, custodial care facility, residential substance abuse treatment facility, or a group home that is not licensed as an intermediate care facility for individuals with intellectual disabilities. The start date is the day of discharge and lasts through the following 29 days. These services include one face-to-face encounter in addition to other services performed within the specific timeframe by a physician or qualified clinician or by licensed clinical staff under qualified clinician direction. Initial communication (direct contact, which may include telephonic or electronic means) must occur within two business days of discharge with review of the patient's medication regimen by the date of the initial face-to-face encounter. The date of the first face-to-face encounter and medical decision making drives the code selection. Subsequent evaluation and management services by the same provider may be reported separately. Only one provider may report transitional care management services during the 30 days following discharge. Report 99495 when MDM is of at least a moderate level during the service period, in addition to the face-to-face encounter within 14 days of hospital discharge. Report 99496 when MDM is a high level during the service period and the face-to-face encounter is within seven days of hospital discharge. Note that MDM for transitional care management is determined by the decision making over the entire service period.

Coding Tips

These codes are used to report services provided to a new or established patient whose medical or psychological issues necessitate a moderate or high level of medical decision making while transitioning from an inpatient facility, partial hospital, observation status, or skilled nursing facility to an assisted living facility, home, domiciliary, or rest home. Transitional care management (TCM) services require a face-to-face visit, initial patient contact, and medication reconciliation all within a specific timeframe. Do not report these codes if all elements listed in the code description are not performed. These codes may only be reported one time within 30 days of discharge and by only one provider. Code 99495 requires the face-to-face visit within 14 calendar days of discharge. Code 99496 requires one face-to-face visit within seven calendar days of discharge. If the physician or other qualified health care professional provides more than one face-to-face E/M visit within the 30 days, these visits may be reported separately. Medicare and the CPT codebook have identified these codes as telehealth/telemedicine services. Telemedicine services may be reported by the performing provider by adding modifier 95 to the procedure code and/or using the appropriate place of service (POS) indicator; POS 02 for telehealth when the originating site is not the patient's home and POS 10 for telehealth services when the originating site is the patient's home. Medicare and commercial payers should be contacted regarding their coverage guidelines.

ICD-10-CM Diagnostic Codes

The application of this code is too broad to adequately present ICD-10-CM diagnostic code links here. Refer to your ICD-10-CM book.

AMA: 99495 2024,Sep; 2022,Dec; 2022,Jul; 2022,Jan; 2021,Jan; 2020,Mar; 2020,Feb; 2020,Jan; 2019,Jan; 2018,Jul; 2018,Apr; 2018,Mar; 2018,Feb **99496** 2024,Sep; 2022,Dec; 2022,Jul; 2022,Jan; 2021,Jan; 2020,Mar; 2020,Feb; 2020,Jan; 2019,Jan; 2018,Jul; 2018,Apr; 2018,Mar; 2018,Feb

Relative Value Units/Medicare Edits

Non-Facility RVU	Work	PE	MP	Total
99495	2.78	3.25	0.18	6.21
99496	3.79	4.37	0.24	8.4
Facility RVU	**Work**	**PE**	**MP**	**Total**
99495	2.78	1.2	0.18	4.16
99496	3.79	1.62	0.24	5.65

	FUD	Status	MUE	Modifiers				IOM Reference
99495	N/A	A	1(2)	N/A	N/A	N/A	80*	None
99496	N/A	A	1(2)	N/A	N/A	N/A	80*	

* with documentation

Terms To Know

medical decision making. Consideration of the differential diagnoses, the amount and/or complexity of data reviewed and considered (medical records, test results, correspondence from previous treating physicians, etc.), current diagnostic studies ordered, and treatment or management options and risk (complications of the patient's condition, the potential for complications, continued morbidity, risk of mortality, any comorbidities associated with the patient's disease process).

other qualified health care professional. Individual who is qualified by education, training, licensure/regulation, and facility privileging to perform a professional service within his or her scope of practice and independently (or as incident-to) report the professional service without requiring physician supervision. Payers may state exemptions in writing or state and local regulations may not follow this definition for performance of some services. Always refer to any relevant plan policies and federal and/or state laws to determine who may perform and report services.

99497-99498

★99497 Advance care planning including the explanation and discussion of advance directives such as standard forms (with completion of such forms, when performed), by the physician or other qualified health care professional; first 30 minutes, face-to-face with the patient, family member(s), and/or surrogate

+ ★99498 each additional 30 minutes (List separately in addition to code for primary procedure)

Explanation

Advance care planning services are reported for the discussion and explanation of advanced directives by a qualified clinician. These services are time-based services that do not involve any active management of problems during the course of the face-to-face service between the provider and a patient, family member, or surrogate and may be reported on the same day as another E/M service. Report 99497 for the first 30 minutes of advance care planning and 99498 for each additional 30 minutes.

Coding Tips

These codes are used to report counseling and discussion of advance care directives face-to-face with the patient, family member, or surrogate. An advance directive document appointing an agent and/or recording of the wishes of the patient's medical treatment should be recorded in the medical record. These codes may be reported separately when performed on the same day as another E/M service. Use 99498 in addition to 99497. These codes may be reported in addition to the following E/M codes when performed on the same date of service: 99202-99215, 99221-99223, 99231-99236, 99238-99239, 99242-99245, 99252-99255, 99281-99285, 99304-99310, 99315-99316, 99341-99345, 99347-99350, 99381-99397, and 99495-99496. Do not report these codes when reporting 99291-99292, 99468-99469, 99471-99472, 99475-99480, or 99483 on the same date of service. Medicare and the CPT codebook have identified these codes as telehealth/telemedicine services that may also be audio only services. Telemedicine services may be reported by the performing provider by adding modifier 93 or 95 to these procedure code and using the appropriate place of service (POS) indicator; POS 02 for telehealth when the originating site is not the patient's home and POS 10 for telehealth services when the originating site is the patient's home. Medicare and commercial payers should be contacted regarding their coverage guidelines.

ICD-10-CM Diagnostic Codes

The application of this code is too broad to adequately present ICD-10-CM diagnostic code links here. Refer to your ICD-10-CM book.

AMA: 99497 2022,Dec; 2022,Aug; 2022,Jul; 2021,Jan; 2018,Apr **99498** 2022,Dec; 2022,Aug; 2022,Jul; 2021,Jan; 2018,Apr

Relative Value Units/Medicare Edits

Non-Facility RVU	Work	PE	MP	Total
99497	1.5	0.86	0.1	2.46
99498	1.4	0.63	0.1	2.13
Facility RVU	**Work**	**PE**	**MP**	**Total**
99497	1.5	0.64	0.1	2.24
99498	1.4	0.61	0.1	2.11

	FUD	Status	MUE	Modifiers				IOM Reference
99497	N/A	A	1(2)	N/A	N/A	N/A	80*	None
99498	N/A	A	3(3)	N/A	N/A	N/A	80*	

* with documentation

Terms To Know

advance directive. Legal documents, such as living wills and durable powers of attorney for health care decisions, stating medical preferences in the event the patient should become incapable of voicing his or her opinion.

20101

20101 Exploration of penetrating wound (separate procedure); chest

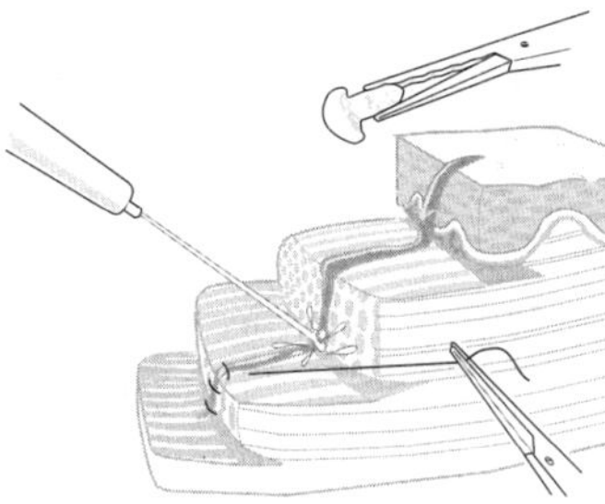

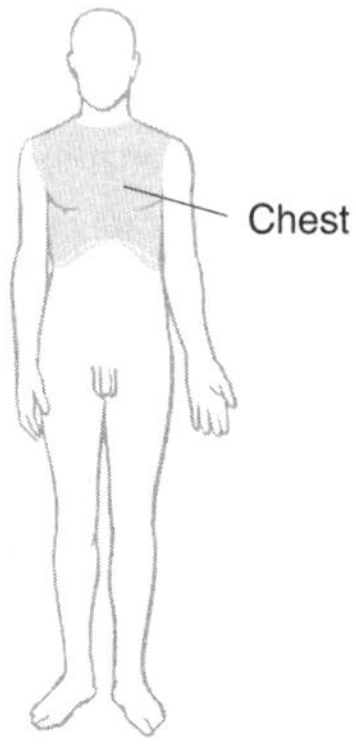

A penetrating wound of the chest is explored. The depth of the wound is assessed and the tissues debrided of fragments. Repairs and closures are made as needed

Explanation

The physician explores a penetrating wound of the chest in the operating room, such as a gunshot or stab wound, to help identify damaged structures. Nerve, organ, and blood vessel integrity is assessed. The wound may be enlarged to help assess the damage. Debridement, removal of foreign bodies, and ligation or coagulation of minor blood vessels in the subcutaneous tissues, fascia, and muscle are also included in this code. Damaged tissues are debrided and repaired when possible. The wound is closed (if clean) or packed open if contaminated by the penetrating body.

Coding Tips

This separate procedure by definition is usually a component of a more complex service and is not identified separately. When performed alone or with other unrelated procedures/services, it may be reported. If performed alone, list the code; if performed with other procedures/services, list the code and append modifier 59 or an X{EPSU} modifier. This code includes debridement, enlargement of the wound (to determine penetration), removal of foreign body, and minor blood vessel ligation or coagulation. If major repair is performed on a major structure or major blood vessel, requiring thoracotomy, then 20101 is not reported separately. For simple, intermediate, or complex repair that does not require enlargement of the wound, report the specific codes for repair instead of 20101. Surgical trays, A4550, are not separately reimbursed by Medicare; however, other third-party payers may cover them. Check with the specific payer to determine coverage.

ICD-10-CM Diagnostic Codes

S21.111A Laceration without foreign body of right front wall of thorax without penetration into thoracic cavity, initial encounter

S21.112A Laceration without foreign body of left front wall of thorax without penetration into thoracic cavity, initial encounter

S21.121A Laceration with foreign body of right front wall of thorax without penetration into thoracic cavity, initial encounter

S21.122A Laceration with foreign body of left front wall of thorax without penetration into thoracic cavity, initial encounter

S21.131A Puncture wound without foreign body of right front wall of thorax without penetration into thoracic cavity, initial encounter

S21.132A Puncture wound without foreign body of left front wall of thorax without penetration into thoracic cavity, initial encounter

S21.141A Puncture wound with foreign body of right front wall of thorax without penetration into thoracic cavity, initial encounter

S21.142A Puncture wound with foreign body of left front wall of thorax without penetration into thoracic cavity, initial encounter

S21.151A Open bite of right front wall of thorax without penetration into thoracic cavity, initial encounter

S21.152A Open bite of left front wall of thorax without penetration into thoracic cavity, initial encounter

S21.211A Laceration without foreign body of right back wall of thorax without penetration into thoracic cavity, initial encounter

S21.212A Laceration without foreign body of left back wall of thorax without penetration into thoracic cavity, initial encounter

S21.221A Laceration with foreign body of right back wall of thorax without penetration into thoracic cavity, initial encounter

S21.222A Laceration with foreign body of left back wall of thorax without penetration into thoracic cavity, initial encounter

S21.231A Puncture wound without foreign body of right back wall of thorax without penetration into thoracic cavity, initial encounter

S21.232A Puncture wound without foreign body of left back wall of thorax without penetration into thoracic cavity, initial encounter

S21.241A Puncture wound with foreign body of right back wall of thorax without penetration into thoracic cavity, initial encounter

S21.242A Puncture wound with foreign body of left back wall of thorax without penetration into thoracic cavity, initial encounter

S21.251A Open bite of right back wall of thorax without penetration into thoracic cavity, initial encounter

S21.252A Open bite of left back wall of thorax without penetration into thoracic cavity, initial encounter

S29.021A Laceration of muscle and tendon of front wall of thorax, initial encounter

S29.022A Laceration of muscle and tendon of back wall of thorax, initial encounter

S29.091A Other injury of muscle and tendon of front wall of thorax, initial encounter

S29.092A Other injury of muscle and tendon of back wall of thorax, initial encounter

S29.8XXA Other specified injuries of thorax, initial encounter

Relative Value Units/Medicare Edits

Non-Facility RVU	Work	PE	MP	Total
20101	3.23	13.19	0.83	17.25
Facility RVU	**Work**	**PE**	**MP**	**Total**
20101	3.23	2.24	0.83	6.3

	FUD	Status	MUE	Modifiers				IOM Reference
20101	10	A	2(3)	51	N/A	N/A	N/A	None

* with documentation

20985

\+ **20985** Computer-assisted surgical navigational procedure for musculoskeletal procedures, image-less (List separately in addition to code for primary procedure)

Explanation

Imageless computer-assisted surgery (CAS) is an adjunct process used in conjunction with certain orthopaedic procedures. Using such tools as markers, reference frames, intraoperative sensing, and computer workstations, imageless computer-assisted navigational procedures increase visualization of the surgical field and aid in precise navigation with minimally invasive approaches. Imageless navigation uses angles and measurements (kinematics) for anatomy determination. Through direct imageless applications, landmarks are established on a universal limb model. This application requires touch-pointing the anatomic landmarks, which are then registered in the computer for use in accurate navigation and measurement in relation to any bone or instrument movement as the surgery is performed. This application provides a way to establish coordinates as an aid for precisely locating anatomical structures in open or percutaneous procedures without the use of preoperative or intraoperative images. Code 20985 is reported in addition to the procedure code when the physician uses an imageless system to help determine coordinates.

Coding Tips

Do not report 20985 with 61781–61783. For computer-assisted navigational procedures with image guidance based on images that are acquired preoperatively and intraoperatively, see 0054T and 0055T.

ICD-10-CM Diagnostic Codes

This/these CPT code(s) are add-on code(s). See the primary procedure code that this code is performed with for your ICD-10-CM code selections.

Relative Value Units/Medicare Edits

Non-Facility RVU	Work	PE	MP	Total
20985	2.5	1.29	0.51	4.3
Facility RVU	**Work**	**PE**	**MP**	**Total**
20985	2.5	1.29	0.51	4.3

	FUD	Status	MUE	Modifiers				IOM Reference
20985	N/A	A	2(3)	N/A	N/A	N/A	80*	None

* with documentation

Terms To Know

CT. Computed tomography.

fluoroscopy. Radiology technique that allows visual examination of part of the body or a function of an organ using a device that projects an x-ray image on a fluorescent screen.

ultrasound. Imaging using ultra-high sound frequency bounced off body structures.

21501-21502

21501 Incision and drainage, deep abscess or hematoma, soft tissues of neck or thorax;

21502 with partial rib ostectomy

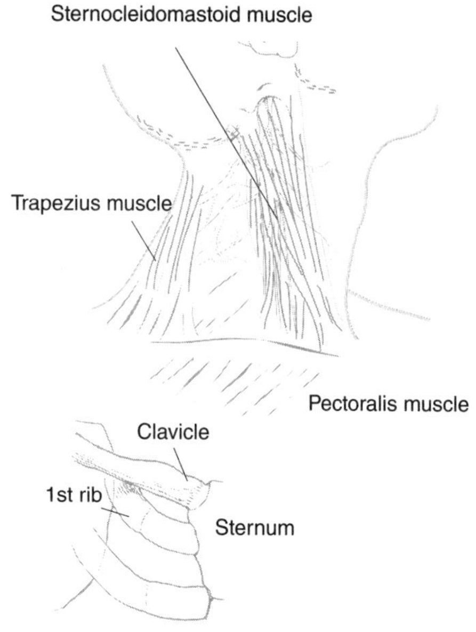

A deep abscess or hematoma of the soft tissues of the neck or thorax is incised and drained

Explanation

The physician performs surgery to remove or drain an abscess or hematoma from the deep soft tissues of the neck or thorax. With proper anesthesia administered, the physician makes an incision overlying the site of the abscess or hematoma of the neck or thorax. Dissection is carried down through the deep subcutaneous tissues and may be continued into the fascia or muscle to expose the abscess or hematoma. The incision may be extended if the mass is larger than expected. The abscess or hematoma is incised and the contents are drained. The area is irrigated and the incision is repaired in layers with sutures, staples, and/or Steri-strips; closed with drains in place; or simply left open to further facilitate drainage of infection. Report 21502 if a partial rib ostectomy is performed during this procedure.

Coding Tips

If significant additional time and effort are documented, append modifier 22 and submit a cover letter and operative report. For a biopsy of the soft tissue of the neck or thorax, see 21550. For subfascial incision and drainage, see 22010–22015.

ICD-10-CM Diagnostic Codes

L03.221	Cellulitis of neck
L03.312	Cellulitis of back [any part except buttock]
L03.313	Cellulitis of chest wall
S10.83XA	Contusion of other specified part of neck, initial encounter
S20.211A	Contusion of right front wall of thorax, initial encounter
S20.212A	Contusion of left front wall of thorax, initial encounter
S20.213A	Contusion of bilateral front wall of thorax, initial encounter
S20.214A	Contusion of middle front wall of thorax, initial encounter
S20.221A	Contusion of right back wall of thorax, initial encounter
S20.222A	Contusion of left back wall of thorax, initial encounter
S20.223A	Contusion of bilateral back wall of thorax, initial encounter
S20.224A	Contusion of middle back wall of thorax, initial encounter
T81.41XA	Infection following a procedure, superficial incisional surgical site, initial encounter
T81.42XA	Infection following a procedure, deep incisional surgical site, initial encounter

AMA: 21501 2023,Apr; 2021,Sep **21502** 2023,Apr; 2021,Sep

Relative Value Units/Medicare Edits

Non-Facility RVU	Work	PE	MP	Total
21501	3.98	9.96	0.82	14.76
21502	7.55	5.91	1.85	15.31
Facility RVU	**Work**	**PE**	**MP**	**Total**
21501	3.98	5.45	0.82	10.25
21502	7.55	5.91	1.85	15.31

	FUD	Status	MUE	Modifiers				IOM Reference
21501	90	A	3(3)	51	N/A	N/A	N/A	None
21502	90	A	1(3)	51	N/A	N/A	80	

* with documentation

Terms To Know

abscess. Circumscribed collection of pus resulting from bacteria, frequently associated with swelling and other signs of inflammation.

cellulitis. Infection of the skin and subcutaneous tissues, most often caused by *Staphylococcus* or *Streptococcus* bacteria secondary to a cutaneous lesion. Progression of the inflammation may lead to abscess and tissue death, or even systemic infection-like bacteremia.

contusion. Superficial injury (bruising) produced by impact without a break in the skin.

drain. Device that creates a channel to allow fluid from a cavity, wound, or infected area to exit the body.

hematoma. Tumor-like collection of blood in some part of the body caused by a break in a blood vessel wall, usually as a result of trauma.

incision and drainage. Cutting open body tissue for the removal of tissue fluids or infected discharge from a wound or cavity.

infected postoperative seroma. Infection within a pocket of serum following surgery.

ostectomy. Excision of bone.

secondary. Second in order of occurrence or importance, or appearing during the course of another disease or condition.

soft tissue. Nonepithelial tissues outside of the skeleton that includes subcutaneous adipose tissue, fibrous tissue, fascia, muscles, blood and lymph vessels, and peripheral nervous system tissue.

21510

21510 Incision, deep, with opening of bone cortex (eg, for osteomyelitis or bone abscess), thorax

A deep, surgical incision extends to the bone and into the bone cortex

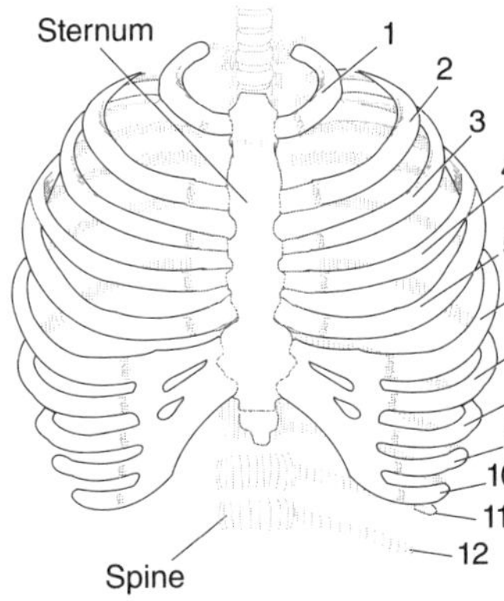

Explanation

The physician incises the bone cortex of infected bone in the thorax to treat an abscess or osteomyelitis. The physician makes an incision over the affected area. Dissection is carried down through the soft tissues to expose the bone. The periosteum is split and reflected from the bone overlying the infected area. A curette may be used to scrape away the abscess or infected portion down to healthy bony tissue or drill holes may be made through the cortex into the medullary canal in a window outline around the infected or abscessed bone. The area is drained and debrided of infected bony and soft tissue. The physician irrigates the area with antibiotic solution, the periosteum is closed over the bone, and the soft tissues are sutured closed; or the wound is packed and left open, allowing the area to drain. Secondary closure is performed approximately three weeks later. Dressings are changed daily.

Coding Tips

If significant additional time and effort are documented, append modifier 22 and submit a cover letter and operative report. When 21510 is performed with another separately identifiable procedure, the highest dollar value code is listed as the primary procedure, and subsequent procedures are appended with modifier 51.

ICD-10-CM Diagnostic Codes

L03.313	Cellulitis of chest wall
M46.23	Osteomyelitis of vertebra, cervicothoracic region
M46.24	Osteomyelitis of vertebra, thoracic region
M46.25	Osteomyelitis of vertebra, thoracolumbar region
M86.08	Acute hematogenous osteomyelitis, other sites
M86.18	Other acute osteomyelitis, other site
M86.28	Subacute osteomyelitis, other site
M86.38	Chronic multifocal osteomyelitis, other site
M86.48	Chronic osteomyelitis with draining sinus, other site
M86.58	Other chronic hematogenous osteomyelitis, other site
M86.68	Other chronic osteomyelitis, other site
M86.8X8	Other osteomyelitis, other site
T81.41XA	Infection following a procedure, superficial incisional surgical site, initial encounter
T81.42XA	Infection following a procedure, deep incisional surgical site, initial encounter
T81.43XA	Infection following a procedure, organ and space surgical site, initial encounter
T81.44XA	Sepsis following a procedure, initial encounter
T81.49XA	Infection following a procedure, other surgical site, initial encounter

AMA: 21510 2023,Apr; 2021,Sep

Relative Value Units/Medicare Edits

Non-Facility RVU	Work	PE	MP	Total
21510	6.2	5.95	1.53	13.68
Facility RVU	**Work**	**PE**	**MP**	**Total**
21510	6.2	5.95	1.53	13.68

	FUD	Status	MUE	Modifiers				IOM Reference
21510	90	A	1(3)	51	N/A	N/A	80*	None

* with documentation

Terms To Know

abscess. Circumscribed collection of pus resulting from bacteria, frequently associated with swelling and other signs of inflammation.

cellulitis. Infection of the skin and subcutaneous tissues, most often caused by *Staphylococcus* or *Streptococcus* bacteria secondary to a cutaneous lesion. Progression of the inflammation may lead to abscess and tissue death, or even systemic infection-like bacteremia.

debride. To remove all foreign objects and devitalized or infected tissue from a burn or wound to prevent infection and promote healing.

dissect. Cut apart or separate tissue for surgical purposes or for visual or microscopic study.

infected postoperative seroma. Infection within a pocket of serum following surgery.

osteomyelitis. Inflammation of bone that may remain localized or spread to the marrow, cortex, or periosteum, in response to an infecting organism, usually bacterial and pyogenic.

osteotomy. Surgical cutting of a bone.

periosteum. Double-layered connective membrane on the outer surface of bone.

secondary. Second in order of occurrence or importance, or appearing during the course of another disease or condition.

sequestrectomy. Surgical excision of a nonviable piece of bone that has become walled off, or sequestered, away from living bone during necrosis.

● New ▲ Revised + Add On ★ Telemedicine [Resequenced] ☑ Laterality

21550

21550 Biopsy, soft tissue of neck or thorax

Explanation

The physician performs a biopsy of the soft tissues of the neck or thorax. With proper anesthesia administered, the physician identifies the mass through palpation and x-ray (reported separately), if needed. An incision is made over the site and dissection is taken down to the subcutaneous fat or further into the fascia or muscle to reach the lesion. A portion of the tissue mass is excised and submitted for pathology. The area is irrigated and the incision is closed with layered sutures.

Coding Tips

Note that 21550 is for incisional biopsy. A biopsy is not reported separately when followed by an excisional removal during the same operative session. When 21550 is performed with another separately identifiable procedure, the highest dollar value code is listed as the primary procedure, and subsequent procedures are appended with modifier 51. If a needle biopsy of soft tissue is needed, see 20206. Surgical trays, A4550, are not separately reimbursed by Medicare; however, other third-party payers may cover them. Check with the specific payer to determine coverage.

ICD-10-CM Diagnostic Codes

C49.0	Malignant neoplasm of connective and soft tissue of head, face and neck
C49.3	Malignant neoplasm of connective and soft tissue of thorax
C76.0	Malignant neoplasm of head, face and neck
C76.1	Malignant neoplasm of thorax
C79.89	Secondary malignant neoplasm of other specified sites
D09.8	Carcinoma in situ of other specified sites
D21.0	Benign neoplasm of connective and other soft tissue of head, face and neck
D21.3	Benign neoplasm of connective and other soft tissue of thorax
L03.221	Cellulitis of neck
L03.313	Cellulitis of chest wall
R22.1	Localized swelling, mass and lump, neck
R22.2	Localized swelling, mass and lump, trunk

AMA: 21550 2023,Jan

Relative Value Units/Medicare Edits

Non-Facility RVU	Work	PE	MP	Total
21550	2.11	5.62	0.31	8.04
Facility RVU	**Work**	**PE**	**MP**	**Total**
21550	2.11	2.28	0.31	4.7

	FUD	Status	MUE	Modifiers				IOM Reference
21550	10	A	2(3)	51	N/A	N/A	N/A	None

* with documentation

Terms To Know

biopsy. Tissue or fluid removed for diagnostic purposes through analysis of the cells in the biopsy material.

soft tissue. Nonepithelial tissues outside of the skeleton.

21555-21556 [21552, 21554]

21555 Excision, tumor, soft tissue of neck or anterior thorax, subcutaneous; less than 3 cm

21552 Excision, tumor, soft tissue of neck or anterior thorax, subcutaneous; 3 cm or greater

21556 Excision, tumor, soft tissue of neck or anterior thorax, subfascial (eg, intramuscular); less than 5 cm

21554 Excision, tumor, soft tissue of neck or anterior thorax, subfascial (eg, intramuscular); 5 cm or greater

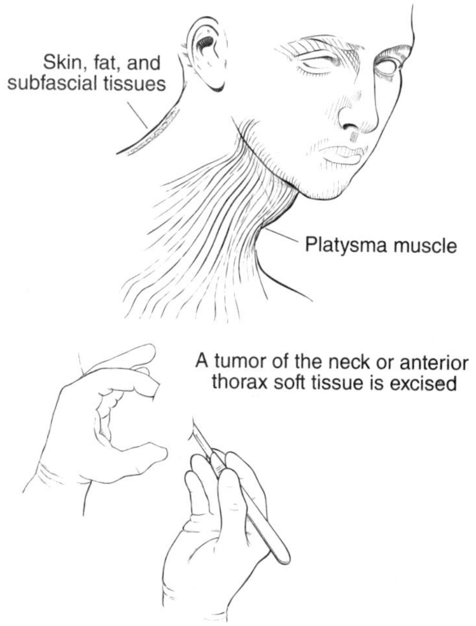

Explanation

The physician removes a tumor from the soft tissue of the neck or anterior thorax (chest) that is located in the subcutaneous tissue in 21552 or 21555 and in the deep soft tissue, below the fascial plane or within the muscle, in 21554 or 21556. With the proper anesthesia administered, the physician makes an incision in the skin overlying the mass and dissects down to the tumor. The extent of the tumor is identified and a dissection is undertaken all the way around the tumor. A portion of neighboring soft tissue may also be removed to ensure adequate removal of all tumor tissue. A drain may be inserted and the incision is repaired with layers of sutures, staples, or Steri-strips. Report 21555 for excision of subcutaneous tumors whose resected area is less than 3 cm and 21552 for excision of subcutaneous tumors 3 cm or greater. Report 21556 for excision of subfascial or intramuscular tumors whose resected area is less than 5 cm and 21554 for excision of subfascial or intramuscular tumors 5 cm or greater.

Coding Tips

If significant additional time and effort are documented, append modifier 22 and submit a cover letter and operative report. When 21555 is performed with another separately identifiable procedure, the highest dollar value code is listed as the primary procedure, and subsequent procedures are appended with modifier 51. A biopsy is not identified separately when followed by an excisional removal during the same operative session. Report any free grafts or flaps separately. For excision of a chest wall tumor involving ribs, see 21601–21603. Surgical trays, A4550, are not separately reimbursed by

Medicare; however, other third-party payers may cover them. Check with the specific payer to determine coverage.

ICD-10-CM Diagnostic Codes

C49.0	Malignant neoplasm of connective and soft tissue of head, face and neck
C49.3	Malignant neoplasm of connective and soft tissue of thorax
C76.0	Malignant neoplasm of head, face and neck
C76.1	Malignant neoplasm of thorax
D17.1	Benign lipomatous neoplasm of skin and subcutaneous tissue of trunk
D17.39	Benign lipomatous neoplasm of skin and subcutaneous tissue of other sites
D21.0	Benign neoplasm of connective and other soft tissue of head, face and neck
D21.3	Benign neoplasm of connective and other soft tissue of thorax
D48.110	Desmoid tumor of head and neck

AMA: **21552** 2022,Oct **21554** 2022,Oct **21555** 2022,Oct; 2018,Sep **21556** 2022,Oct; 2018,Sep

Relative Value Units/Medicare Edits

Non-Facility RVU	Work	PE	MP	Total
21555	3.96	8.35	0.81	13.12
21552	6.49	5.56	1.51	13.56
21556	7.66	6.88	1.5	16.04
21554	11.13	8.58	2.39	22.1
Facility RVU	**Work**	**PE**	**MP**	**Total**
21555	3.96	4.57	0.81	9.34
21552	6.49	5.56	1.51	13.56
21556	7.66	6.88	1.5	16.04
21554	11.13	8.58	2.39	22.1

	FUD	Status	MUE	Modifiers				IOM Reference
21555	90	A	2(3)	51	N/A	N/A	N/A	None
21552	90	A	2(3)	51	N/A	N/A	80	
21556	90	A	2(3)	51	N/A	N/A	N/A	
21554	90	A	2(3)	51	N/A	N/A	80	

* with documentation

Terms To Know

fascia. Fibrous sheet or band of tissue that envelops organs, muscles, and groupings of muscles.

flap. Mass of flesh and skin partially excised from its location but retaining its blood supply that is moved to another site to repair adjacent or distant defects.

free graft. Unattached piece of skin and tissue moved to another part of the body and sutured into place to repair a defect.

Merkel cell carcinoma. Rare form of skin cancer that typically presents on the face, head, or neck as a flesh-colored or bluish-red lesion. This neoplasm is fast growing and can metastasize quickly to other areas of the body. Risk factors include older patients with weakened immune systems and/or long-term exposure to the sun.

21557-21558

21557 Radical resection of tumor (eg, sarcoma), soft tissue of neck or anterior thorax; less than 5 cm

21558 5 cm or greater

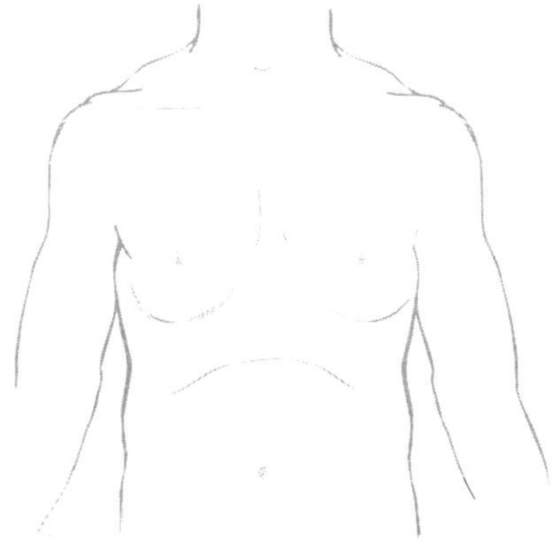

Radical resection of soft tissue tumor of the neck or anterior thorax

Explanation

The physician performs a radical resection of a malignant soft tissue tumor (i.e., sarcoma) from the neck or anterior thorax, not involving bone. An incision is made over the tumor and dissection exposes it. The tumor and any adjacent tissue that may be affected by the spread of the neoplasm are excised. Large resections may be needed. The type and stage of the lesion determines the extent of the tumor margin resection area. Muscle or fascia may need to be repaired and drains may be placed. The surgical wound may be closed using simple or intermediate repair or separately reportable complex closure, adjacent tissue transfer, or graft. Report 21557 for excision of tumors whose resected area is less than 5 cm and 21558 for excision of tumors 5 cm or greater.

Coding Tips

An excisional biopsy is not reported separately when a therapeutic excision is performed during the same surgical session. Report any free grafts or flaps separately. Surgical trays, A4550, are not separately reimbursed by Medicare; however, other third-party payers may cover them. Check with the specific payer to determine coverage. For radical resection of cutaneous tumors, see 11600–11620.

ICD-10-CM Diagnostic Codes

C49.0	Malignant neoplasm of connective and soft tissue of head, face and neck
C49.3	Malignant neoplasm of connective and soft tissue of thorax
C76.0	Malignant neoplasm of head, face and neck
C76.1	Malignant neoplasm of thorax

AMA: **21557** 2022,Oct; 2020,Apr; 2018,Sep **21558** 2022,Oct; 2020,Apr; 2018,Sep

Neck and Thorax

Relative Value Units/Medicare Edits

Non-Facility RVU	Work	PE	MP	Total
21557	14.75	10.96	3.17	28.88
21558	21.58	14.03	4.64	40.25
Facility RVU	**Work**	**PE**	**MP**	**Total**
21557	14.75	10.96	3.17	28.88
21558	21.58	14.03	4.64	40.25

	FUD	Status	MUE	Modifiers				IOM Reference
21557	90	A	1(3)	51	N/A	62*	80	None
21558	90	A	1(3)	51	N/A	62*	80	

* with documentation

Terms To Know

anterior. Situated in the front area or toward the belly surface of the body.

complex. Composite or collection of related things, such as symptoms, anatomical parts, or surgical procedures.

fascia. Fibrous sheet or band of tissue that envelops organs, muscles, and groupings of muscles.

flap. Mass of flesh and skin partially excised from its location but retaining its blood supply that is moved to another site to repair adjacent or distant defects.

graft. Tissue implant from another part of the body or another person.

intermediate repair. *1)* Surgical closure of a wound requiring closure of one or more of the deeper subcutaneous tissue and non-muscle fascia layers in addition to the skin. *2)* Contaminated wounds with single layer closure that need extensive cleaning or foreign body removal. *3)* Wounds with limited undermining less than the width of the wound.

malignant. Any condition tending to progress toward death, specifically an invasive tumor with a loss of cellular differentiation that has the ability to spread or metastasize to other body areas.

radical. Extensive surgery.

resection. Surgical removal of a part or all of an organ or body part.

soft tissue. Nonepithelial tissues outside of the skeleton.

21600

21600 Excision of rib, partial

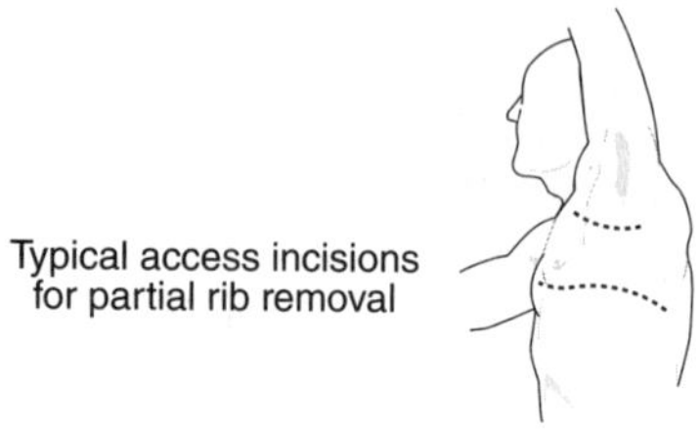

A portion of a single rib is surgically removed

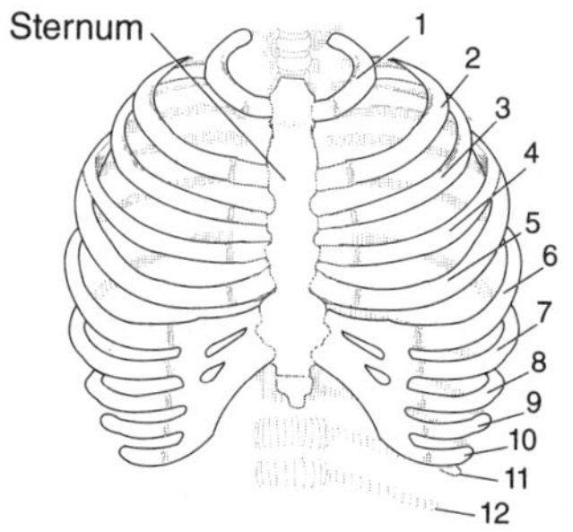

The ribs are the framework of the thoracic cage. Ten pairs connect anteriorly to the sternum and two pairs (11 and 12) float. Ribs numbered 7 to 10 fuse to form the costal margin before attaching to the sternum

Explanation

The physician removes part of one rib. With the patient under anesthesia, the physician makes an incision in the skin of the chest overlying the rib. The tissues are dissected deep to the rib itself. The rib is identified. The physician removes the desired part of the rib using a saw and other instruments. The remaining pieces of the rib and the wound itself are irrigated and debrided. The incision is sutured in layers.

Coding Tips

If this procedure is a component of a more complex service, it is not reported separately. When 21600 is performed with another separately identifiable procedure, the highest dollar value code is listed as the primary procedure, and subsequent procedures are appended with modifier 51. For an excision of the first and/or cervical rib, see 21615–21616. For resection of the cervical rib with division of scalenus anticus, see 21705. For an excision of a chest wall tumor involving the ribs, see 21601–21603. For radical chest wall or rib cage debridement due to an injury that includes bone, skin, and subcutaneous tissue, see 11044 and 11047.

ICD-10-CM Diagnostic Codes

C41.3	Malignant neoplasm of ribs, sternum and clavicle
D16.7	Benign neoplasm of ribs, sternum and clavicle
M86.38	Chronic multifocal osteomyelitis, other site
M86.48	Chronic osteomyelitis with draining sinus, other site
M86.58	Other chronic hematogenous osteomyelitis, other site
M86.68	Other chronic osteomyelitis, other site
Q76.6	Other congenital malformations of ribs
Q76.8	Other congenital malformations of bony thorax

Relative Value Units/Medicare Edits

Non-Facility RVU	Work	PE	MP	Total
21600	7.26	8.24	1.68	17.18
Facility RVU	**Work**	**PE**	**MP**	**Total**
21600	7.26	8.24	1.68	17.18

	FUD	Status	MUE	Modifiers				IOM Reference
21600	90	A	5(3)	51	N/A	62*	80	None

* with documentation

Terms To Know

benign. Mild or nonmalignant in nature.

debride. To remove all foreign objects and devitalized or infected tissue from a burn or wound to prevent infection and promote healing.

dissect. Cut apart or separate tissue for surgical purposes or for visual or microscopic study.

excision. Surgical removal of an organ or tissue.

infection. Presence of microorganisms in body tissues that may result in cellular damage.

irrigation. To wash out or cleanse a body cavity, wound, or tissue with water or other fluid.

malignant. Any condition tending to progress toward death, specifically an invasive tumor with a loss of cellular differentiation that has the ability to spread or metastasize to other body areas.

ostectomy. Excision of bone.

osteomyelitis. Inflammation of bone that may remain localized or spread to the marrow, cortex, or periosteum, in response to an infecting organism, usually bacterial and pyogenic.

primary. Principal or first in the order of occurrence or importance.

secondary. Second in order of occurrence or importance, or appearing during the course of another disease or condition.

21601-21603

21601 Excision of chest wall tumor including rib(s)

21602 Excision of chest wall tumor involving rib(s), with plastic reconstruction; without mediastinal lymphadenectomy

21603 Excision of chest wall tumor involving rib(s), with plastic reconstruction; with mediastinal lymphadenectomy

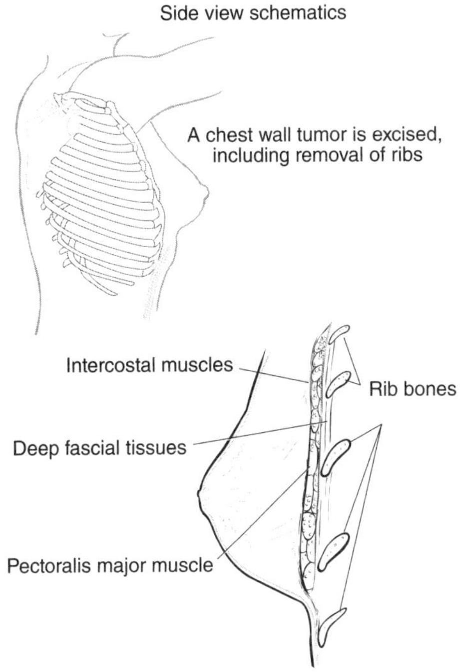

Explanation

The physician excises a chest wall tumor, including ribs. An incision in the skin of the chest overlying the site of the tumor is made. The tumor and surrounding tissue are excised. The tissue removed includes at least one adjacent rib above or below the tumor site and any associated intercostal muscles. It may also include rib cage resection and/or an en bloc resection of muscles, including the pectoralis minor or major, the serratus anterior, or the latissimus dorsi. The physician ligates or cauterizes bleeding vessels. A chest tube may be placed to re-expand the lung. The incision is repaired with layered closure and a pressure dressing is applied to the wound. In 21602, the physician excises a chest wall tumor, involving ribs, with plastic reconstruction. The tumor and surrounding tissue are excised and includes at least one adjacent rib above and below the tumor site and all intervening intercostal muscles. It may also include an en bloc resection of muscles, including the pectoralis minor or major, the serratus anterior, or the latissimus dorsi. In 21603, lymphatic tissue lying within the mediastinum is also removed. The physician ligates or cauterizes bleeding vessels. A chest tube may be placed to re-expand the lung. Plastic reconstruction is done and may involve rib grafts and/or a myocutaneous flap. A pressure dressing is applied to the wound.

Coding Tips

For a tumor of the neck or thorax not involving the ribs, see 21555–21557. An excisional biopsy is not reported separately when a therapeutic excision is performed during the same surgical session. Do not report 21601–21603 with 32100, 32503, 32504, 32551, 32554, or 32555.

ICD-10-CM Diagnostic Codes

C41.3	Malignant neoplasm of ribs, sternum and clavicle
C49.3	Malignant neoplasm of connective and soft tissue of thorax

Neck and Thorax

C76.1	Malignant neoplasm of thorax
C79.51	Secondary malignant neoplasm of bone
C79.89	Secondary malignant neoplasm of other specified sites
D09.8	Carcinoma in situ of other specified sites
D16.7	Benign neoplasm of ribs, sternum and clavicle
D21.3	Benign neoplasm of connective and other soft tissue of thorax
D36.0	Benign neoplasm of lymph nodes
D36.7	Benign neoplasm of other specified sites
D48.0	Neoplasm of uncertain behavior of bone and articular cartilage
D48.111	Desmoid tumor of chest wall
D48.7	Neoplasm of uncertain behavior of other specified sites
R22.2	Localized swelling, mass and lump, trunk

AMA: **21601** 2019,Dec **21602** 2019,Dec **21603** 2019,Dec

Relative Value Units/Medicare Edits

Non-Facility RVU	Work	PE	MP	Total
21601	17.78	12.21	4.47	34.46
21602	22.19	18.31	5.39	45.89
21603	25.17	18.92	6.21	50.3
Facility RVU	**Work**	**PE**	**MP**	**Total**
21601	17.78	12.21	4.47	34.46
21602	22.19	18.31	5.39	45.89
21603	25.17	18.92	6.21	50.3

	FUD	Status	MUE	Modifiers				IOM Reference
21601	90	A	2(3)	51	N/A	62*	80	None
21602	90	A	1(3)	51	N/A	62*	80	
21603	90	A	1(3)	51	N/A	62*	80	

* with documentation

Terms To Know

cautery. Destruction or burning of tissue by means of a hot instrument, an electric current, or a caustic chemical, such as silver nitrate.

en bloc removal. Take out as a whole or all in one mass.

lymphadenectomy. Dissection of lymph nodes free from the vessels and removal for examination by frozen section in a separate procedure to detect early-stage metastases.

mediastinum. Collection of organs and tissues that separate the pleural sacs. Located between the sternum and spine above the diaphragm, it contains the heart and great vessels, trachea and bronchi, esophagus, thymus, lymph nodes, and nerves.

21610

21610 Costotransversectomy (separate procedure)

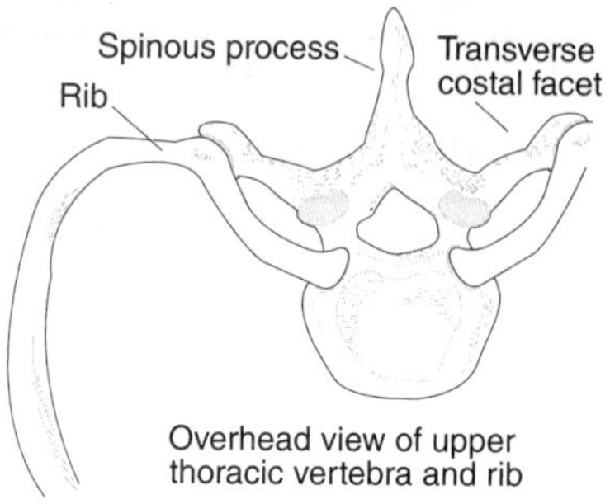

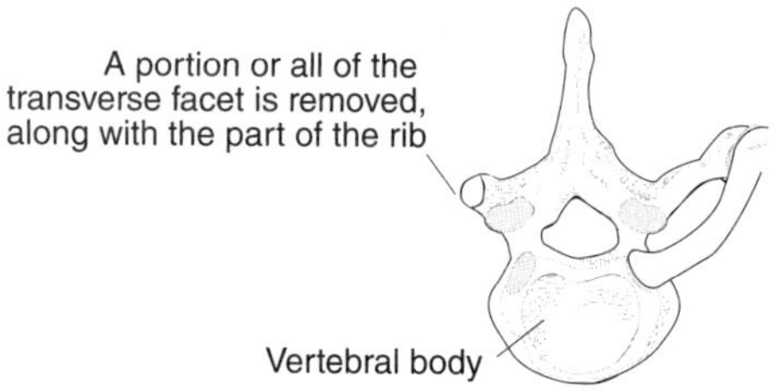

Explanation

The physician resects the costovertebral joint. The physician makes a posterior incision overlying the joint. The tissues are dissected from the joint and the transverse process is cut from the vertebral body. The physician removes all or a portion of the adjacent rib. The incision is closed in sutured layers.

Coding Tips

This separate procedure by definition is usually a component of a more complex service and is not identified separately. When performed alone or with other unrelated procedures/services, it may be reported. If performed alone, list the code; if performed with other procedures/services, list the code and append modifier 59 or an X{EPSU} modifier. This procedure involves partial or complete excision of the affected rib at the costovertebral joint.

ICD-10-CM Diagnostic Codes

A18.01	Tuberculosis of spine
C41.2	Malignant neoplasm of vertebral column
C41.3	Malignant neoplasm of ribs, sternum and clavicle
C79.51	Secondary malignant neoplasm of bone
C7B.03	Secondary carcinoid tumors of bone
D16.6	Benign neoplasm of vertebral column
D16.7	Benign neoplasm of ribs, sternum and clavicle
M86.38	Chronic multifocal osteomyelitis, other site
M86.48	Chronic osteomyelitis with draining sinus, other site
M86.58	Other chronic hematogenous osteomyelitis, other site
M86.68	Other chronic osteomyelitis, other site
M86.8X8	Other osteomyelitis, other site
Q76.6	Other congenital malformations of ribs
Q76.8	Other congenital malformations of bony thorax

Relative Value Units/Medicare Edits

Non-Facility RVU	Work	PE	MP	Total
21610	15.91	14.34	6.62	36.87
Facility RVU	**Work**	**PE**	**MP**	**Total**
21610	15.91	14.34	6.62	36.87

	FUD	Status	MUE	Modifiers				IOM Reference
21610	90	A	1(3)	51	N/A	N/A	80	None

* with documentation

Terms To Know

anomaly. Irregularity in the structure or position of an organ or tissue.

benign. Mild or nonmalignant in nature.

congenital. Present at birth, occurring through heredity or an influence during gestation up to the moment of birth.

dissect. Cut apart or separate tissue for surgical purposes or for visual or microscopic study.

facet. Smooth surface area where the transverse and articular processes of certain vertebrae articulate with another vertebra.

incision. Act of cutting into tissue or an organ.

malignant. Any condition tending to progress toward death, specifically an invasive tumor with a loss of cellular differentiation that has the ability to spread or metastasize to other body areas.

neoplasm. New abnormal growth, tumor.

ostectomy. Excision of bone.

osteoarthrosis. Most common form of a noninflammatory degenerative joint disease with degenerating articular cartilage, bone enlargement, and synovial membrane changes.

osteomyelitis. Inflammation of bone that may remain localized or spread to the marrow, cortex, or periosteum, in response to an infecting organism, usually bacterial and pyogenic.

resect. Cutting out or removing a portion or all of a bone, organ, or other structure.

transverse. Crosswise at right angles to the long axis of a structure or part.

vertebral body. Disc-shaped portion of a vertebra that is anteriorly located and bears weight.

21615-21616

21615 Excision first and/or cervical rib;
21616 with sympathectomy

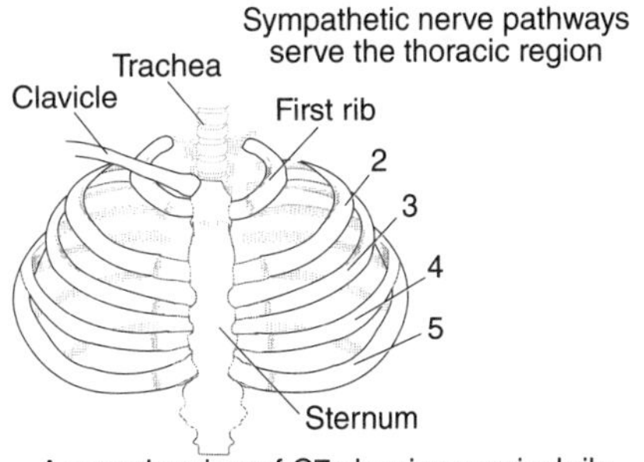

A superior view of C7 showing cervical rib; attachment anteriorly may be to the first rib, or its costal cartilage (Type II), or even the sternum (Type IV); no anterior attachment is also found (Type I)

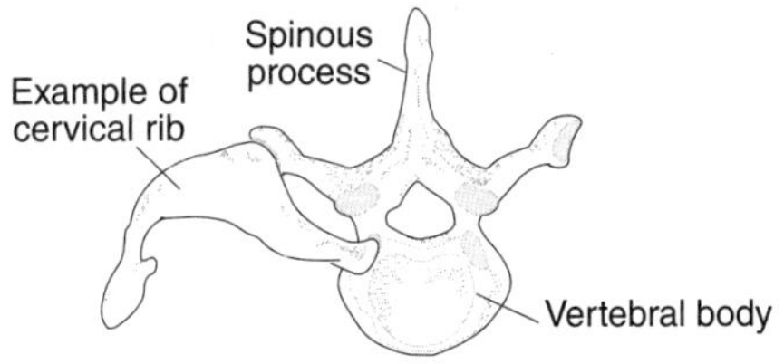

A cervical rib is present on the seventh vertebra in about 1 percent of the population

Explanation

The physician performs surgery to remove the first rib and/or an extraneous cervical rib. With the patient under anesthesia, an incision is made in the skin just above the clavicle on the affected side and carried deep to the rib. The rib is identified and the attached soft tissues are dissected from the bone. The physician excises the rib using a saw and other surgical instruments. The rib is freed from its articulation and removed. The wound is irrigated and closed in layers. A dressing is applied. Report 21616 if a sympathetic nerve pathway is cut during the procedure.

Coding Tips

These are unilateral procedures. If performed bilaterally, some payers require that the service be reported twice with modifier 50 appended to the second code, while others require identification of the service only once with modifier 50 appended. Check with individual payers. Modifier 50 identifies a procedure performed identically on the opposite side of the body (mirror image). For a partial rib excision, see 21600. For resection of a cervical rib with division scalenus anticus, see 21705.

ICD-10-CM Diagnostic Codes

G54.0	Brachial plexus disorders
I74.2	Embolism and thrombosis of arteries of the upper extremities
M54.12	Radiculopathy, cervical region
M95.4	Acquired deformity of chest and rib
Q76.5	Cervical rib

Relative Value Units/Medicare Edits

Non-Facility RVU	Work	PE	MP	Total
21615	10.45	5.62	2.59	18.66
21616	12.69	5.47	3.16	21.32
Facility RVU	**Work**	**PE**	**MP**	**Total**
21615	10.45	5.62	2.59	18.66
21616	12.69	5.47	3.16	21.32

	FUD	Status	MUE	Modifiers				IOM Reference
21615	90	A	1(2)	51	50	62*	80	None
21616	90	A	1(2)	51	50	N/A	80	

* with documentation

Terms To Know

cervicalgia. Pain localized to the cervical region, generally referring to the posterior or lateral regions of the neck.

debride. To remove all foreign objects and devitalized or infected tissue from a burn or wound to prevent infection and promote healing.

dissect. Cut apart or separate tissue for surgical purposes or for visual or microscopic study.

embolism. Obstruction of a blood vessel resulting from a clot or foreign substance.

excision. Surgical removal of an organ or tissue.

irrigate. Washing out, lavage.

lesion. Area of damaged tissue that has lost continuity or function, due to disease or trauma. Lesions may be located on internal structures such as the brain, nerves, or kidneys, or visible on the skin.

neuritis. Inflammation of a nerve or group of nerves, often manifested by loss of function and reflexes, pain, and numbness or tingling.

ostectomy. Excision of bone.

radiculitis. Pain along an inflamed nerve, with inflammation of the root of the associated spinal nerve.

Raynaud's phenomenon. Vascular disorder resulting in bilateral decreased circulation of the fingers and toes causing a pale or bluish appearance, numbness, tingling, and pain brought on by cold or emotions and relieved with heat.

resection. Surgical removal of a part or all of an organ or body part.

sympathectomy. Surgical interruption or transection of a sympathetic nervous system pathway.

thrombosis. Condition arising from the presence or formation of blood clots within a blood vessel that may cause vascular obstruction and insufficient oxygenation.

21620

21620 Ostectomy of sternum, partial

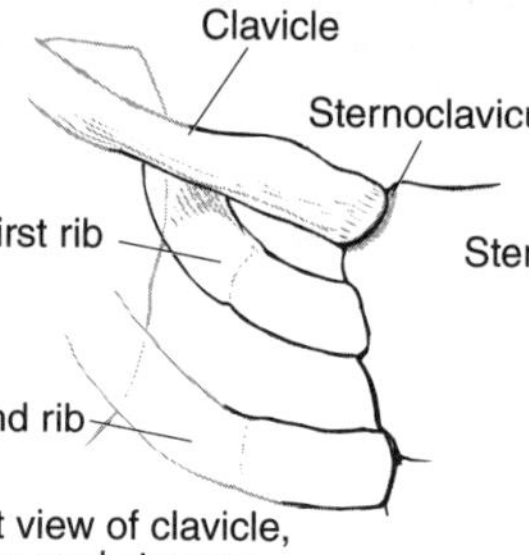

Front view of clavicle, ribs, and sternum

The sternum is the flat, elongated bone that makes up the anterior structure of the thoracic cage. It has three parts: the manubrium (uppermost), the body, and the xiphoid process (lowermost)

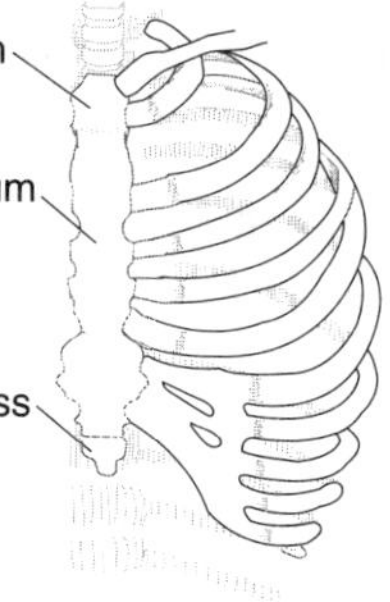

Explanation

The physician removes a portion of the sternum from the chest. With the patient under anesthesia, the physician makes an incision in the skin overlying the sternum. This is carried deep through the subcutaneous tissues to the bone. The sternum is identified and the attached soft tissues are carefully dissected from the bone. The physician marks the portion of the sternum to be removed. The bone is cut in the appropriate places using a saw and other surgical instruments. The remaining portion of the bone is irrigated and smoothed as needed. The wound is closed in layers and a dressing is applied.

Coding Tips

When this procedure is performed to access the chest cavity for open heart surgery, it is incidental to that procedure and is not reported separately. If significant additional time and effort are documented, append modifier 22 and submit a cover letter and operative report. When 21620 is performed with another separately identifiable procedure, the highest dollar value code is listed as the primary procedure, and subsequent procedures are appended with modifier 51.

ICD-10-CM Diagnostic Codes

C41.3	Malignant neoplasm of ribs, sternum and clavicle
D16.7	Benign neoplasm of ribs, sternum and clavicle
Q76.7	Congenital malformation of sternum

Relative Value Units/Medicare Edits

Non-Facility RVU	Work	PE	MP	Total
21620	7.28	6.16	1.72	15.16
Facility RVU	**Work**	**PE**	**MP**	**Total**
21620	7.28	6.16	1.72	15.16

	FUD	Status	MUE	Modifiers				IOM Reference
21620	90	A	1(2)	51	N/A	62*	80	None

* with documentation

Terms To Know

aseptic necrosis. Death of bone tissue resulting from a disruption in the vascular supply, caused by a noninfectious disease process, such as a fracture or the administration of immunosuppressive drugs.

benign. Mild or nonmalignant in nature.

chronic. Persistent, continuing, or recurring.

debridement. Removal of dead or contaminated tissue and foreign matter from a wound.

incision. Act of cutting into tissue or an organ.

irrigate. Washing out, lavage.

malignant. Any condition tending to progress toward death, specifically an invasive tumor with a loss of cellular differentiation that has the ability to spread or metastasize to other body areas.

ostectomy. Excision of bone.

osteomyelitis. Inflammation of bone that may remain localized or spread to the marrow, cortex, or periosteum, in response to an infecting organism, usually bacterial and pyogenic.

secondary. Second in order of occurrence or importance, or appearing during the course of another disease or condition.

soft tissue. Nonepithelial tissues outside of the skeleton that includes subcutaneous adipose tissue, fibrous tissue, fascia, muscles, blood and lymph vessels, and peripheral nervous system tissue.

21627

21627 Sternal debridement

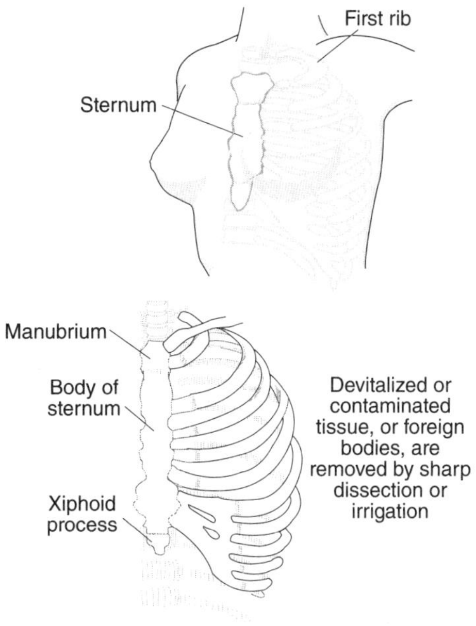

There are three parts of the sternum: the manubrium (uppermost), the body, and the xiphoid process

Explanation

The physician performs a debridement of the sternum. With the patient under anesthesia, the physician makes an incision in the skin overlying the sternum. The incision is carried deep to the bone. The sternum is debrided as warranted using any of a variety of hand or powered surgical instruments. Irrigation is used so that debridement can be completed as extensively as indicated. The wound may be loosely packed and a dressing applied or it may be closed in layers and a dressing applied.

Coding Tips

This procedure is usually performed to treat postoperative infection following open thoracic surgery. It may also be performed following open injury complicated by infection. For closure of sternotomy separation with or without debridement, see 21750.

ICD-10-CM Diagnostic Codes

C41.3	Malignant neoplasm of ribs, sternum and clavicle
D16.7	Benign neoplasm of ribs, sternum and clavicle
S21.121A	Laceration with foreign body of right front wall of thorax without penetration into thoracic cavity, initial encounter
S21.122A	Laceration with foreign body of left front wall of thorax without penetration into thoracic cavity, initial encounter
S21.141A	Puncture wound with foreign body of right front wall of thorax without penetration into thoracic cavity, initial encounter
S21.142A	Puncture wound with foreign body of left front wall of thorax without penetration into thoracic cavity, initial encounter
S21.321A	Laceration with foreign body of right front wall of thorax with penetration into thoracic cavity, initial encounter
S21.322A	Laceration with foreign body of left front wall of thorax with penetration into thoracic cavity, initial encounter
S21.341A	Puncture wound with foreign body of right front wall of thorax with penetration into thoracic cavity, initial encounter

S21.342A Puncture wound with foreign body of left front wall of thorax with penetration into thoracic cavity, initial encounter

S21.351A Open bite of right front wall of thorax with penetration into thoracic cavity, initial encounter

S21.352A Open bite of left front wall of thorax with penetration into thoracic cavity, initial encounter

T81.41XA Infection following a procedure, superficial incisional surgical site, initial encounter

T81.42XA Infection following a procedure, deep incisional surgical site, initial encounter

T81.43XA Infection following a procedure, organ and space surgical site, initial encounter

T81.44XA Sepsis following a procedure, initial encounter

T81.49XA Infection following a procedure, other surgical site, initial encounter

AMA: 21627 2023,Apr; 2021,Sep

Relative Value Units/Medicare Edits

Non-Facility RVU	Work	PE	MP	Total
21627	7.3	7.55	1.69	16.54
Facility RVU	**Work**	**PE**	**MP**	**Total**
21627	7.3	7.55	1.69	16.54

	FUD	Status	MUE	Modifiers				IOM Reference
21627	90	A	1(2)	51	N/A	N/A	80	None

* with documentation

Terms To Know

aseptic necrosis. Death of bone tissue resulting from a disruption in the vascular supply, caused by a noninfectious disease process, such as a fracture or the administration of immunosuppressive drugs.

chronic. Persistent, continuing, or recurring.

debridement. Removal of dead or contaminated tissue and foreign matter from a wound.

infected postoperative seroma. Infection within a pocket of serum following surgery.

irrigation. To wash out or cleanse a body cavity, wound, or tissue with water or other fluid.

lesion. Area of damaged tissue that has lost continuity or function, due to disease or trauma.

malignant. Any condition tending to progress toward death, specifically an invasive tumor with a loss of cellular differentiation that has the ability to spread or metastasize to other body areas.

secondary. Second in order of occurrence or importance, or appearing during the course of another disease or condition.

soft tissue. Nonepithelial tissues outside of the skeleton that includes subcutaneous adipose tissue, fibrous tissue, fascia, muscles, blood and lymph vessels, and peripheral nervous system tissue.

21630

▲ **21630** Radical resection of sternum

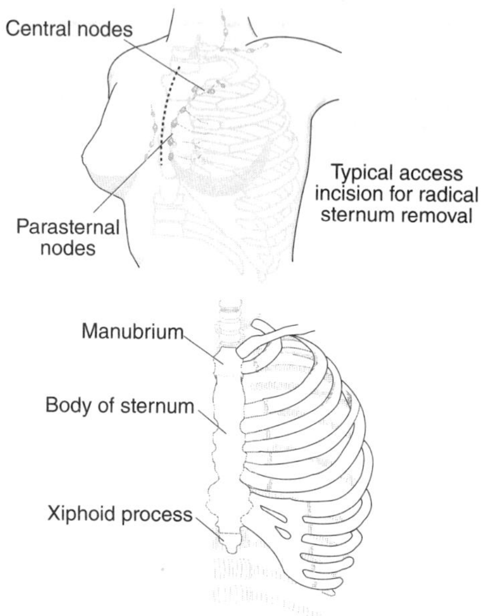

The sternum is the flat, elongated bone that makes up the anterior structure of the thoracic cage

Explanation

The physician removes most or all of the sternum from the chest. With the patient under anesthesia, the physician makes a long incision overlying the sternum and anterior chest. This is carried deep to the bone. Dissection is performed around the sternum. Ribs are disarticulated as needed and thorough debridement is accomplished. Using saws and other surgical instruments, the physician removes the bone. Internal fixation devices (reported separately) are often needed to support the ribs and chest wall. The wound is irrigated and closed in layers.

Coding Tips

Debridement, irrigation, and closure are not reported separately. If significant additional time and effort are documented, append modifier 22 and submit a cover letter and operative report. When 21630 is performed with another separately identifiable procedure, the highest dollar value code is listed as the primary procedure, and subsequent procedures are appended with modifier 51. If internal fixation devices are necessary, report separately; see 21825.

ICD-10-CM Diagnostic Codes

C41.3 Malignant neoplasm of ribs, sternum and clavicle

C77.1 Secondary and unspecified malignant neoplasm of intrathoracic lymph nodes

C78.1 Secondary malignant neoplasm of mediastinum

C79.51 Secondary malignant neoplasm of bone

T81.42XA Infection following a procedure, deep incisional surgical site, initial encounter

AMA: 21630 2023,Apr; 2021,Sep

Relative Value Units/Medicare Edits

Non-Facility RVU	Work	PE	MP	Total
21630	19.18	16.7	3.55	39.43
Facility RVU	**Work**	**PE**	**MP**	**Total**
21630	19.18	16.7	3.55	39.43

	FUD	Status	MUE	Modifiers				IOM Reference
21630	90	A	1(2)	51	N/A	62*	80	None

* with documentation

Terms To Know

aseptic necrosis. Death of bone tissue resulting from a disruption in the vascular supply, caused by a noninfectious disease process, such as a fracture or the administration of immunosuppressive drugs.

lymphadenectomy. Dissection of lymph nodes free from the vessels and removal for examination by frozen section in a separate procedure to detect early-stage metastases.

malignant. Any condition tending to progress toward death, specifically an invasive tumor with a loss of cellular differentiation that has the ability to spread or metastasize to other body areas.

neoplasm. New abnormal growth, tumor.

resection. Surgical removal of a part or all of an organ or body part.

21700-21705

21700 Division of scalenus anticus; without resection of cervical rib

21705 with resection of cervical rib

Numerous structures cross or attach to the first rib, including the anterior scalenus

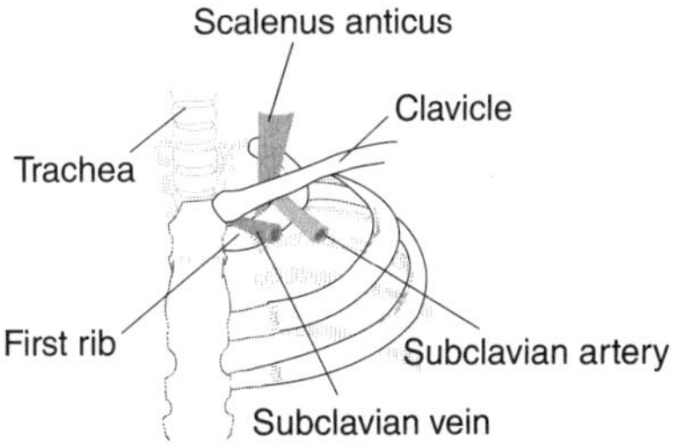

Superior view of C7 showing cervical rib, which usually occurs bilaterally

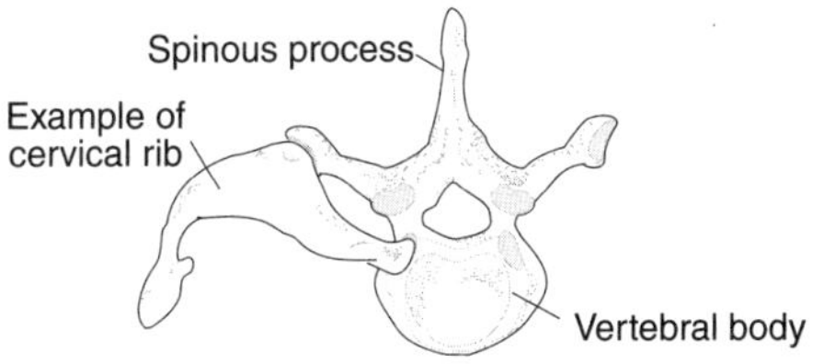

Explanation

The physician performs a surgical procedure where the scalenus anticus muscle is divided, usually for the purpose of treating thoracic outlet syndrome. With the patient under anesthesia, the physician makes an incision overlying the scalene muscle. This incision is carried deep to the muscle. The muscle is exposed and identified. A discission of the muscle is performed in line of the fibers. This relieves the pressure on the neurovascular structures. The wound is thoroughly irrigated and closed in layers. Report 21700 if the procedure does not include resection of the cervical rib. Report 21705 if resection of the cervical rib is performed during the procedure.

Coding Tips

When 21700 or 21705 is performed with another separately identifiable procedure, the highest dollar value code is listed as the primary procedure, and subsequent procedures are appended with modifier 51. For resection of the cervical rib without division of scalenus anticus, see 21615–21616.

ICD-10-CM Diagnostic Codes

G54.0 Brachial plexus disorders

Q76.5 Cervical rib

Relative Value Units/Medicare Edits

Non-Facility RVU	Work	PE	MP	Total
21700	6.31	2.75	1.57	10.63
21705	9.92	3.47	2.46	15.85
Facility RVU	**Work**	**PE**	**MP**	**Total**
21700	6.31	2.75	1.57	10.63
21705	9.92	3.47	2.46	15.85

	FUD	Status	MUE	Modifiers				IOM Reference
21700	90	A	1(2)	51	50	N/A	80	None
21705	90	A	1(2)	51	50	N/A	80	

* with documentation

21740

21740 Reconstructive repair of pectus excavatum or carinatum; open

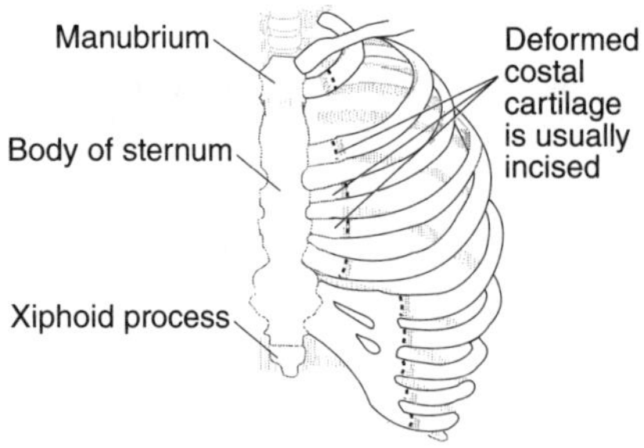

In some instances a convex sternum (left) is everted and reattached

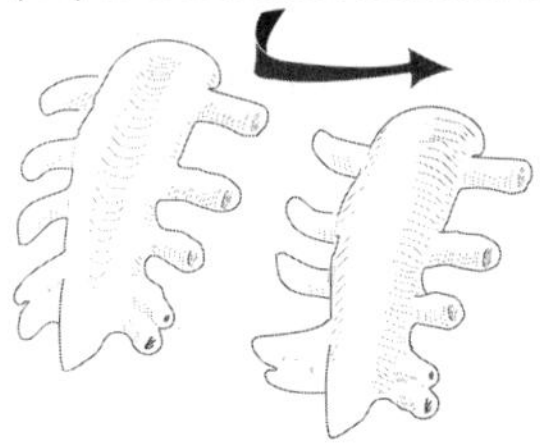

Explanation

The physician performs surgery on the anterior chest to correct pectus excavatum (a depression in the chest wall) or pectus carinatum (a forward projection of the chest wall). With the patient under anesthesia, the physician makes an incision overlying the anterior sternum. This is carried deep to the bone. The costal cartilages are exposed and deformed rib ends are freed from their sternal attachments. The sternum is mobilized and restored to its normal position. Internal fixation devices are employed to hold the sternum in corrected alignment. The physician irrigates the wound and closes it in layers with sutures.

Coding Tips

If significant additional time and effort are documented, append modifier 22 and submit a cover letter and operative report. Internal fixation devices are not reported separately. Report radiological services separately. For minimally invasive approach, see 21742 and 21743.

ICD-10-CM Diagnostic Codes

Q67.6	Pectus excavatum
Q67.7	Pectus carinatum

Relative Value Units/Medicare Edits

Non-Facility RVU	Work	PE	MP	Total
21740	17.57	8.68	4.34	30.59
Facility RVU	**Work**	**PE**	**MP**	**Total**
21740	17.57	8.68	4.34	30.59

	FUD	Status	MUE	Modifiers				IOM Reference
21740	90	A	1(2)	51	N/A	62*	80	None

* with documentation

21742-21743

21742 Reconstructive repair of pectus excavatum or carinatum; minimally invasive approach (Nuss procedure), without thoracoscopy

21743 minimally invasive approach (Nuss procedure), with thoracoscopy

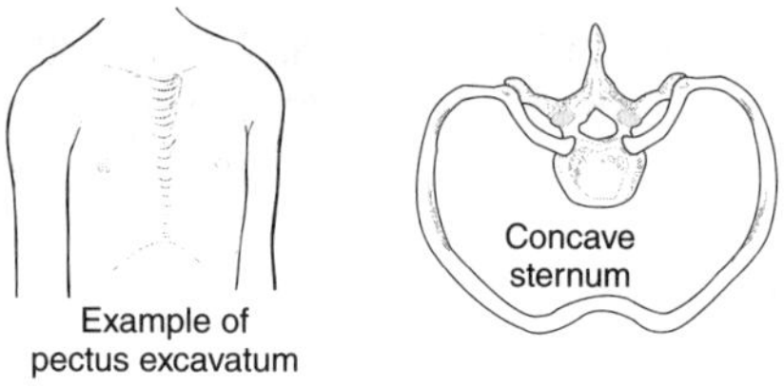

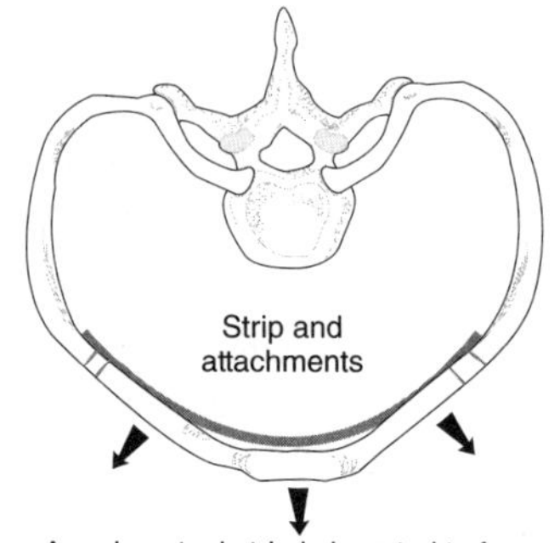

A spring steel strip is inserted to force the sternum into normal anatomic shape

Explanation

The physician performs a Nuss procedure, also known as minimally invasive repair of pectus excavatum (MIRPE), without thoracoscopy in 21742 and with thoracoscopy in 21743. Pectus excavatum is a depression of the sternum and chest, giving a sunken appearance. The chest is first marked at strategic points and the length of a curved steel bar, called the Lorenz pectus bar, to be inserted into the sternum is measured and shaped to fit the individual's chest. Midaxillary line incisions are made on the right and left side aligned with the deepest depression point. A skin tunnel is raised from the incisions and another small lateral incision is made for insertion of a thoracoscope. The skin incisions are elevated and a long introducer instrument is inserted through the right intercostal space at the top of the pectus ridge and slowly advanced across the anterior mediastinal space with videoscopic guidance. The sternum is forcefully lifted as the introducer is passed to the other side. Once behind the sternum, the tip is pushed through the intercostal space at the top of the pectus ridge on the left side and brought out through that skin incision. Umbilical tape is pulled through the tunnel and used to guide the prepared bar. The bar is inserted with the convex curve facing posteriorly and rotated with a flipping instrument until the convex curve faces anteriorly. The bar can be pulled back out and bent in a more ideal curvature for correction as many times as needed. Usually only one bar is placed. With the bar in position, a stabilizing bar is sutured around the pectus bar and to the muscle. Sutures are placed in the lateral chest wall musculature as well as one other fixation point to the side of the sternum around one rib and the pectus bar. Wounds are closed and the patient is extubated while deeply anesthetized and kept well sedated for a few days with pain management therapy.

Coding Tips

If significant additional time and effort are documented, append modifier 22 and submit a cover letter and operative report. Internal fixation devices are not reported separately. Radiological services are not reported separately. For reconstructive repair of the pectus excavatum or carinatum, invasive approach, see 21740.

ICD-10-CM Diagnostic Codes

Q67.6	Pectus excavatum
Q67.7	Pectus carinatum

AMA: 21742 2019,Nov **21743** 2019,Nov

Relative Value Units/Medicare Edits

Non-Facility RVU	Work	PE	MP	Total
21742	0.0	0.0	0.0	0.0
21743	0.0	0.0	0.0	0.0
Facility RVU	**Work**	**PE**	**MP**	**Total**
21742	0.0	0.0	0.0	0.0
21743	0.0	0.0	0.0	0.0

	FUD	Status	MUE	Modifiers				IOM Reference
21742	90	C	1(2)	51	N/A	62*	80	None
21743	90	C	1(2)	51	N/A	62*	80	

* with documentation

Terms To Know

alignment. Establishment of a straight line or harmonious relationship between structures.

anterior. Situated in the front area or toward the belly surface of the body; an anatomical reference point used to show the position and relationship of one body structure to another.

congenital. Present at birth, occurring through heredity or an influence during gestation up to the moment of birth.

incision. Act of cutting into tissue or an organ.

invasive. Insertion of an instrument, device, or foreign matter into the body or requiring puncture or incision of the skin.

lateral. On/to the side.

pectus carinatum. Congenital abnormality of the anterior chest wall with protrusion of the sternum, rounding the appearance of the chest.

pectus excavatum. Congenital abnormality of the anterior chest wall with depression of the sternum, sinking the appearance of the chest.

posterior. Located in the back part or caudal end of the body.

reconstruction. Recreating, restoring, or rebuilding a body part or organ.

21750

21750 Closure of median sternotomy separation with or without debridement (separate procedure)

The sternotomy edges may be debrided

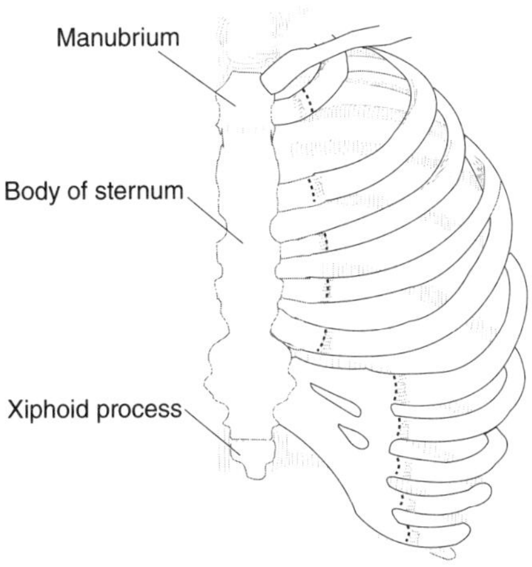

Internal fixation may be required

Explanation

The physician performs surgery on the sternum bone to put the bone back together following previous surgical separation. With the patient under anesthesia, the physician makes an incision overlying the sternum. The incision is carried deep to the bone and the separated pieces are identified. The physician may debride soft tissue or bone. The bony fragments are manipulated back together and held in place. The physician uses wire or other internal fixation devices to maintain the bone in appropriate position. The wound is irrigated and closed in layers.

Coding Tips

This separate procedure by definition is usually a component of a more complex service and is not identified separately. When performed alone or with other unrelated procedures/services, it may be reported. If performed alone, list the code; if performed with other procedures/services, list the code and append modifier 59 or an X{EPSU} modifier. Sternal debridement is included in this procedure and should not be reported separately. For sternal debridement only, see 21627. When 21750 is performed with another separately identifiable procedure, the highest dollar value code is listed as the primary procedure, and subsequent procedures are appended with modifier 51.

ICD-10-CM Diagnostic Codes

I97.88	Other intraoperative complications of the circulatory system, not elsewhere classified
I97.89	Other postprocedural complications and disorders of the circulatory system, not elsewhere classified
J95.89	Other postprocedural complications and disorders of respiratory system, not elsewhere classified
T81.328A	Disruption or dehiscence of closure of other specified internal operation (surgical) wound, initial encounter
T81.42XA	Infection following a procedure, deep incisional surgical site, initial encounter

T81.43XA	Infection following a procedure, organ and space surgical site, initial encounter
T81.44XA	Sepsis following a procedure, initial encounter
T81.49XA	Infection following a procedure, other surgical site, initial encounter
T81.89XA	Other complications of procedures, not elsewhere classified, initial encounter

Relative Value Units/Medicare Edits

Non-Facility RVU	Work	PE	MP	Total
21750	11.4	6.08	2.71	20.19
Facility RVU	**Work**	**PE**	**MP**	**Total**
21750	11.4	6.08	2.71	20.19

	FUD	Status	MUE	Modifiers				IOM Reference
21750	90	A	1(2)	51	N/A	62*	80	None

* with documentation

Terms To Know

debridement. Removal of dead or contaminated tissue and foreign matter from a wound.

infection. Presence of microorganisms in body tissues that may result in cellular damage.

irrigate. Washing out, lavage.

lesion. Area of damaged tissue that has lost continuity or function, due to disease or trauma. Lesions may be located on internal structures such as the brain, nerves, or kidneys, or visible on the skin.

malunion. Fracture that has united in a faulty position due to inadequate reduction of the original fracture, insufficient holding of a previously well-reduced fracture, contracture of the soft tissues, or comminuted or osteoporotic bone causing a slow disintegration of the fracture.

manipulation. Skillful treatment by hand to reduce fractures and dislocations or provide therapy through forceful passive movement of a joint beyond its active limit of motion.

median sternotomy. Standard incision for open chest cardiac surgeries, from above the bellybutton to just under the chin, down the center of the chest through the sternum into the thoracic cavity.

nonunion. Failure of two ends of a fracture to mend or completely heal.

soft tissue. Nonepithelial tissues outside of the skeleton that includes subcutaneous adipose tissue, fibrous tissue, fascia, muscles, blood and lymph vessels, and peripheral nervous system tissue.

21811-21813

21811 Open treatment of rib fracture(s) with internal fixation, includes thoracoscopic visualization when performed, unilateral; 1-3 ribs

21812 4-6 ribs

21813 7 or more ribs

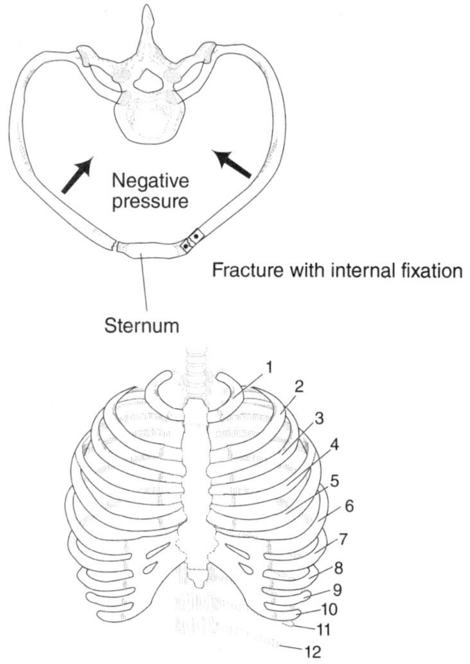

Explanation

The physician performs surgery on one or more unilateral rib fractures requiring internal fixation. With the patient under anesthesia, the physician makes an incision overlying the fractured rib. This is carried deep to the bone. The fracture is found, the pieces are identified, and dead tissue is debrided as needed. The physician manipulates and aligns the fracture fragments into an acceptable position and stabilizes the fragments using devices such as pins, rods, screws, or wires. The wound is irrigated and closed in layers. Report 21811 for treatment of one to three ribs; 21812 for four to six ribs; and 21813 for seven or more ribs. This includes thoracoscopic visualization when utilized.

Coding Tips

These codes are unilateral procedures. If performed bilaterally, some payers require that the service be reported twice with modifier 50 appended to the second code while others require identification of the service only once with modifier 50 appended. Check with individual payers. Modifier 50 identifies a procedure performed identically on the opposite side of the body (mirror image).

ICD-10-CM Diagnostic Codes

M96.A2	Fracture of one rib associated with chest compression and cardiopulmonary resuscitation
M96.A3	Multiple fractures of ribs associated with chest compression and cardiopulmonary resuscitation
S22.31XA	Fracture of one rib, right side, initial encounter for closed fracture ☑
S22.31XB	Fracture of one rib, right side, initial encounter for open fracture ☑
S22.31XG	Fracture of one rib, right side, subsequent encounter for fracture with delayed healing ☑

S22.31XK Fracture of one rib, right side, subsequent encounter for fracture with nonunion ☑

S22.41XA Multiple fractures of ribs, right side, initial encounter for closed fracture ☑

S22.41XB Multiple fractures of ribs, right side, initial encounter for open fracture ☑

S22.41XG Multiple fractures of ribs, right side, subsequent encounter for fracture with delayed healing ☑

S22.41XK Multiple fractures of ribs, right side, subsequent encounter for fracture with nonunion ☑

AMA: **21811** 2022,May **21812** 2022,May **21813** 2022,May

Relative Value Units/Medicare Edits

Non-Facility RVU	Work	PE	MP	Total
21811	10.79	4.29	2.58	17.66
21812	13.0	5.22	3.09	21.31
21813	17.61	7.07	4.52	29.2
Facility RVU	**Work**	**PE**	**MP**	**Total**
21811	10.79	4.29	2.58	17.66
21812	13.0	5.22	3.09	21.31
21813	17.61	7.07	4.52	29.2

	FUD	Status	MUE	Modifiers				IOM Reference
21811	0	A	1(2)	51	50	N/A	80	None
21812	0	A	1(2)	51	50	N/A	80	
21813	0	A	1(2)	51	50	N/A	80	

* with documentation

Terms To Know

debride. To remove all foreign objects and devitalized or infected tissue from a burn or wound to prevent infection and promote healing.

manipulate. Treatment by hand.

manubrium. Sternum.

21820

21820 Closed treatment of sternum fracture

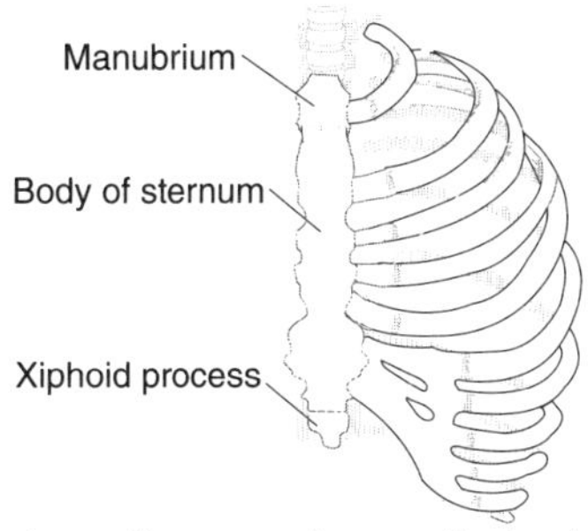

Fractures often occur at or near the juncture of the manubrium and the body of the sternum

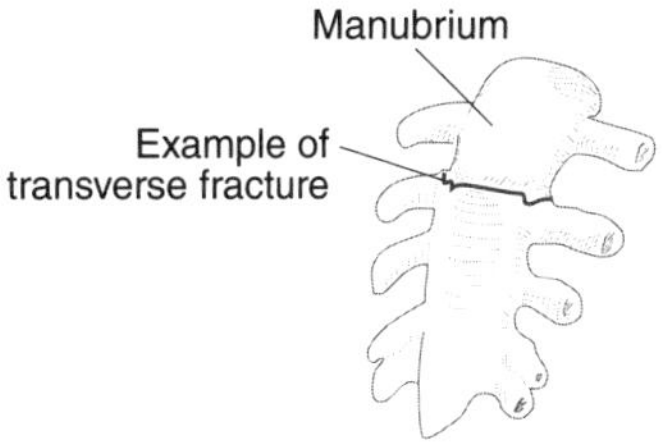

Explanation

Separately reportable x-rays are used to identify if a fracture of the sternum is present. If the fracture is non-displaced and stable, closed treatment is initiated. Braces or splints are not used. The patient's activity is modified while the fracture heals.

Coding Tips

Closed treatment may be reported even for nondisplaced sternum fractures requiring no splinting or bracing. When 21820 is performed with another separately identifiable procedure, the highest dollar value code is listed as the primary procedure, and subsequent procedures are appended with modifier 51. For open treatment, see 21825.

ICD-10-CM Diagnostic Codes

M96.A1 Fracture of sternum associated with chest compression and cardiopulmonary resuscitation

S22.21XA Fracture of manubrium, initial encounter for closed fracture

S22.22XA Fracture of body of sternum, initial encounter for closed fracture

S22.23XA Sternal manubrial dissociation, initial encounter for closed fracture

S22.24XA Fracture of xiphoid process, initial encounter for closed fracture

AMA: **21820** 2022,May

Relative Value Units/Medicare Edits

Non-Facility RVU	Work	PE	MP	Total
21820	1.36	3.02	0.29	4.67
Facility RVU	**Work**	**PE**	**MP**	**Total**
21820	1.36	2.96	0.29	4.61

	FUD	Status	MUE	Modifiers				IOM Reference
21820	90	A	1(2)	51	N/A	N/A	N/A	None

* with documentation

21825

21825 Open treatment of sternum fracture with or without skeletal fixation

Explanation

The physician performs an open surgical reduction of a sternum fracture. The patient is positioned supine on the operating table. A longitudinal incision is made along the midportion of the sternum. Dissection exposes the fractured sternum. The surgeon reduces the fracture. If fixation is needed to keep the fracture stable, the physician drills holes on either side of the fracture. Wire is passed through the holes and around the fracture and the wire ends are twisted together to immobilize the fracture. The incision is repaired in layers with sutures, staples, or Steri-strips.

Coding Tips

Any wiring or internal fixation is not reported separately. Report open treatment of rib fractures separately, see 21811–21813. When 21825 is performed with another separately identifiable procedure, the highest dollar value code is listed as the primary procedure, and subsequent procedures are appended with modifier 51. For closed treatment of a sternum fracture, see 21820. For sternoclavicular dislocation, see 23520–23532.

ICD-10-CM Diagnostic Codes

M96.A1	Fracture of sternum associated with chest compression and cardiopulmonary resuscitation
S22.21XA	Fracture of manubrium, initial encounter for closed fracture
S22.21XB	Fracture of manubrium, initial encounter for open fracture
S22.22XA	Fracture of body of sternum, initial encounter for closed fracture
S22.22XB	Fracture of body of sternum, initial encounter for open fracture
S22.23XA	Sternal manubrial dissociation, initial encounter for closed fracture
S22.23XB	Sternal manubrial dissociation, initial encounter for open fracture
S22.24XA	Fracture of xiphoid process, initial encounter for closed fracture
S22.24XB	Fracture of xiphoid process, initial encounter for open fracture

AMA: 21825 2022,May

Relative Value Units/Medicare Edits

Non-Facility RVU	Work	PE	MP	Total
21825	7.76	7.1	1.82	16.68
Facility RVU	**Work**	**PE**	**MP**	**Total**
21825	7.76	7.1	1.82	16.68

	FUD	Status	MUE	Modifiers				IOM Reference
21825	90	A	1(2)	51	N/A	62*	80	None

* with documentation

Terms To Know

fixation. Act or condition of being attached, secured, fastened, or held in position.

internal skeletal fixation. Repair involving wires, pins, screws, and/or plates placed through or within the fractured area to stabilize and immobilize the injury.

sternum. Long and flat bone in the center of the chest. It attaches to the ribs to help protect the heart and lungs from injury.

31500

31500 Intubation, endotracheal, emergency procedure

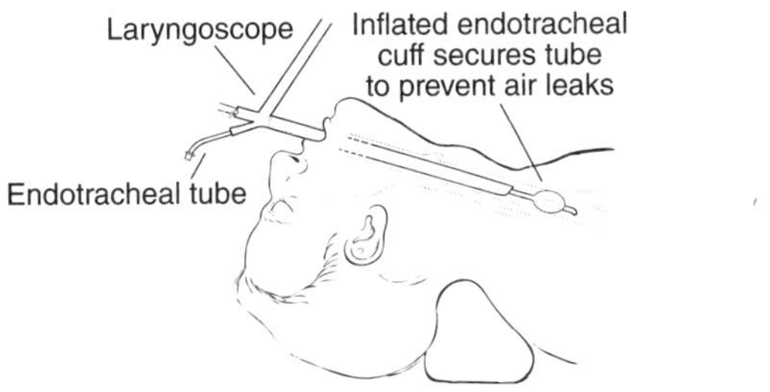

An emergency endotracheal intubation is performed

Explanation

The physician places an endotracheal tube to provide air passage in emergency situations. The patient is ventilated with a mask and bag and positioned by extending the neck anteriorly and the head posteriorly. The physician places the laryngoscope into the patient's mouth and advances the blade toward the epiglottis until the vocal cords are visible. An endotracheal tube is inserted between the vocal cords and advanced to the proper position. The cuff of the endotracheal tube is inflated.

Coding Tips

Emergency endotracheal intubation may be reported separately when performed in connection with critical care; see 99291 or 99292 and notes for definitions of critical care and other procedures that may be reported. Anesthesia services are included in code 31500 and should not be reported separately. Code 31500 is included in bundled pediatric and neonatal critical care service codes 99468–99472, 99475, and 99476 and intensive care service codes 99477–99480.

ICD-10-CM Diagnostic Codes

I26.01	Septic pulmonary embolism with acute cor pulmonale
I26.02	Saddle embolus of pulmonary artery with acute cor pulmonale
I26.93	Single subsegmental thrombotic pulmonary embolism without acute cor pulmonale
I26.94	Multiple subsegmental thrombotic pulmonary emboli without acute cor pulmonale
I27.82	Chronic pulmonary embolism
I50.21	Acute systolic (congestive) heart failure
I50.22	Chronic systolic (congestive) heart failure
I50.23	Acute on chronic systolic (congestive) heart failure
I50.811	Acute right heart failure
I50.812	Chronic right heart failure
I50.813	Acute on chronic right heart failure
I50.814	Right heart failure due to left heart failure
I97.110	Postprocedural cardiac insufficiency following cardiac surgery
I97.111	Postprocedural cardiac insufficiency following other surgery
I97.120	Postprocedural cardiac arrest following cardiac surgery
I97.121	Postprocedural cardiac arrest following other surgery
J44.0	Chronic obstructive pulmonary disease with (acute) lower respiratory infection
J44.1	Chronic obstructive pulmonary disease with (acute) exacerbation
J4A.0	Restrictive allograft syndrome
J81.0	Acute pulmonary edema
J82.81	Chronic eosinophilic pneumonia
J82.82	Acute eosinophilic pneumonia
J84.170	Interstitial lung disease with progressive fibrotic phenotype in diseases classified elsewhere
J84.178	Other interstitial pulmonary diseases with fibrosis in diseases classified elsewhere
J95.821	Acute postprocedural respiratory failure
J95.822	Acute and chronic postprocedural respiratory failure
J95.84	Transfusion-related acute lung injury (TRALI)
J95.87	Transfusion-associated dyspnea (TAD)
J96.01	Acute respiratory failure with hypoxia
J96.02	Acute respiratory failure with hypercapnia
J96.21	Acute and chronic respiratory failure with hypoxia
J96.22	Acute and chronic respiratory failure with hypercapnia

AMA: 31500 2021,Jul; 2018,Jun

Relative Value Units/Medicare Edits

Non-Facility RVU	Work	PE	MP	Total
31500	3.0	0.74	0.43	4.17
Facility RVU	**Work**	**PE**	**MP**	**Total**
31500	3.0	0.74	0.43	4.17

	FUD	Status	MUE	Modifiers				IOM Reference
31500	0	A	2(3)	N/A	N/A	N/A	N/A	None

* with documentation

Terms To Know

epiglottis. Lid-like cartilaginous tissue that covers the entrance to the larynx and blocks food from entering the trachea.

intubation. Insertion of a tube into a hollow organ, canal, or cavity within the body.

larynx. Musculocartilaginous structure between the trachea and the pharynx that functions as the valve preventing food and other particles from entering the respiratory tract, as well as the voice mechanism.

31515

31515 Laryngoscopy direct, with or without tracheoscopy; for aspiration

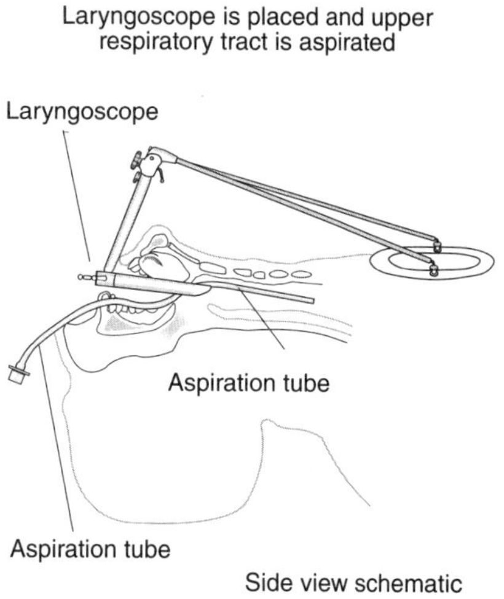

Explanation

The physician uses an aspirator to remove excess saliva or semi-solid foreign material from the larynx. After applying topical anesthesia to the oral cavity and pharynx, the physician inserts the laryngoscope through the patient's mouth. An aspirator is fed through the laryngoscope and the larynx is cleared of saliva and semi-solid foreign material. If a tracheoscopy is performed, a bronchoscope is inserted through the laryngoscope for microscopic visualization of the trachea and bronchi. No other procedure is performed.

Coding Tips

Laryngoscopy code selection is dependent on two variables. Laryngoscopy procedures may be either direct or indirect, and they may be performed with either a rigid or flexible scope. A direct laryngoscopy allows the physician to see the larynx through a scope in the throat. In contrast, when an indirect laryngoscopy is performed, the physician uses mirrors to visualize the larynx. Code 31515 refers to direct visualization with a rigid laryngoscope. Report the appropriate endoscopy for each anatomic site examined. Surgical endoscopy includes a diagnostic endoscopy; however, diagnostic endoscopy can be identified separately when performed at the same surgical session as an open procedure.

ICD-10-CM Diagnostic Codes

J04.0 Acute laryngitis
J05.0 Acute obstructive laryngitis [croup]
J38.3 Other diseases of vocal cords
J38.7 Other diseases of larynx
J39.0 Retropharyngeal and parapharyngeal abscess
J39.8 Other specified diseases of upper respiratory tract
J69.0 Pneumonitis due to inhalation of food and vomit
J69.1 Pneumonitis due to inhalation of oils and essences
J69.8 Pneumonitis due to inhalation of other solids and liquids
J95.01 Hemorrhage from tracheostomy stoma
J95.02 Infection of tracheostomy stoma
J95.09 Other tracheostomy complication
J95.859 Other complication of respirator [ventilator]
J95.88 Other intraoperative complications of respiratory system, not elsewhere classified
J95.89 Other postprocedural complications and disorders of respiratory system, not elsewhere classified
O89.01 Aspiration pneumonitis due to anesthesia during the puerperium [M]
P24.01 Meconium aspiration with respiratory symptoms [N]
P24.11 Neonatal aspiration of (clear) amniotic fluid and mucus with respiratory symptoms [N]
P24.21 Neonatal aspiration of blood with respiratory symptoms [N]
P24.31 Neonatal aspiration of milk and regurgitated food with respiratory symptoms [N]
P24.81 Other neonatal aspiration with respiratory symptoms [N]
R04.1 Hemorrhage from throat
R04.2 Hemoptysis
R04.81 Acute idiopathic pulmonary hemorrhage in infants [P]
R04.89 Hemorrhage from other sites in respiratory passages
R09.3 Abnormal sputum
T81.41XA Infection following a procedure, superficial incisional surgical site, initial encounter
T81.42XA Infection following a procedure, deep incisional surgical site, initial encounter
T81.43XA Infection following a procedure, organ and space surgical site, initial encounter
T81.44XA Sepsis following a procedure, initial encounter
T81.49XA Infection following a procedure, other surgical site, initial encounter

AMA: 31515 2020,Dec; 2019,Sep

Relative Value Units/Medicare Edits

Non-Facility RVU	Work	PE	MP	Total
31515	1.8	4.36	0.24	6.4
Facility RVU	**Work**	**PE**	**MP**	**Total**
31515	1.8	1.28	0.24	3.32

	FUD	Status	MUE	Modifiers				IOM Reference
31515	0	A	1(3)	51	N/A	N/A	N/A	None

* with documentation

Terms To Know

direct laryngoscopy. Endoscopic instrument, such as a flexible or rigid fiberoptic scope, inserted into the larynx for direct viewing capabilities of the voice box and vocal cords.

larynx. Musculocartilaginous structure between the trachea and the pharynx that functions as the valve preventing food and other particles from entering the respiratory tract, as well as the voice mechanism. Also called the voicebox, the larynx is composed of three single cartilages: cricoid, epiglottis, and thyroid; and three paired cartilages: arytenoid, corniculate, and cuneiform.

trachea. Tube descending from the larynx and branching into the right and left main bronchi.

 [N] Newborn: 0 [P] Pediatric: 0-17 [M] Maternity: 9-64 [A] Adult: 15-124 AMA: CPT Assist

31520-31526

31520 Laryngoscopy direct, with or without tracheoscopy; diagnostic, newborn
31525 diagnostic, except newborn
31526 diagnostic, with operating microscope or telescope

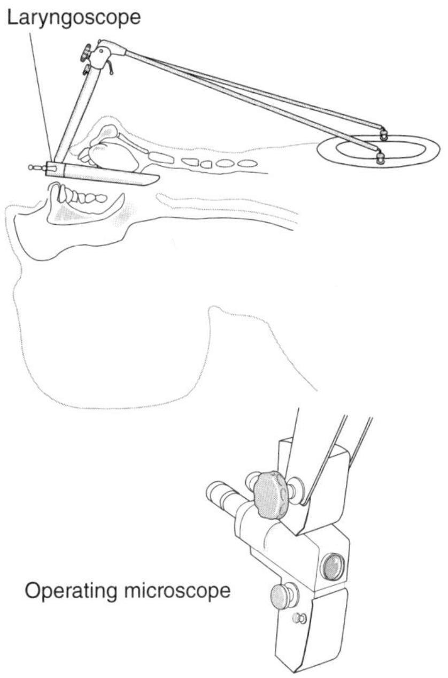

Explanation

The physician places a rigid laryngoscope to examine the patient's larynx. The physician administers a topical anesthetic to the oral cavity, pharynx, and larynx and inserts the laryngoscope through the patient's mouth. The interior of the larynx of a newborn is examined in 31520 and of a patient other than a newborn in 31525. In 31526, the physician uses an operating microscope or a telescope to examine the interior of the larynx. For all procedures, if a tracheoscopy is performed, a bronchoscope is inserted through the laryngoscope for microscopic visualization of the trachea and bronchi. No other procedure is performed at this time.

Coding Tips

Laryngoscopy code selection is dependent on two variables. Laryngoscopy procedures may be direct or indirect, and they may be performed with a rigid or flexible scope. A direct laryngoscopy allows the physician to see the larynx through a scope in the throat. In contrast, when an indirect laryngoscopy is performed, the physician uses mirrors to visualize the larynx. Report the appropriate endoscopy for each anatomic site examined. Surgical endoscopy includes a diagnostic endoscopy; however, diagnostic endoscopy can be identified separately when performed at the same surgical session as an open procedure. Do not append modifier 63 to 31520 as the description or nature of the procedure includes infants up to 4 kg. Use of an operating microscope is included in 31526. Do not report 69990 separately.

ICD-10-CM Diagnostic Codes

C15.3 Malignant neoplasm of upper third of esophagus
C33 Malignant neoplasm of trachea
D02.1 Carcinoma in situ of trachea
J04.11 Acute tracheitis with obstruction
J04.2 Acute laryngotracheitis
J37.1 Chronic laryngotracheitis
J39.0 Retropharyngeal and parapharyngeal abscess
P24.01 Meconium aspiration with respiratory symptoms N
P24.11 Neonatal aspiration of (clear) amniotic fluid and mucus with respiratory symptoms N
P24.21 Neonatal aspiration of blood with respiratory symptoms N
P26.0 Tracheobronchial hemorrhage originating in the perinatal period N
P28.31 Primary central sleep apnea of newborn
P28.32 Primary obstructive sleep apnea of newborn
P28.33 Primary mixed sleep apnea of newborn
P28.41 Central neonatal apnea of newborn
P28.42 Obstructive apnea of newborn
P28.43 Mixed neonatal apnea of newborn
Q31.5 Congenital laryngomalacia
Q32.0 Congenital tracheomalacia
R04.1 Hemorrhage from throat
R04.2 Hemoptysis
R05.1 Acute cough
R05.2 Subacute cough
R05.3 Chronic cough
R05.8 Other specified cough
R06.03 Acute respiratory distress
R47.02 Dysphasia
R47.1 Dysarthria and anarthria
R47.81 Slurred speech
R49.0 Dysphonia
R49.1 Aphonia
S11.022A Laceration with foreign body of trachea, initial encounter
S11.024A Puncture wound with foreign body of trachea, initial encounter
T27.0XXA Burn of larynx and trachea, initial encounter
T27.1XXA Burn involving larynx and trachea with lung, initial encounter
Z03.822 Encounter for observation for suspected aspirated (inhaled) foreign body ruled out

AMA: 31520 2020,Dec; 2019,Sep **31525** 2020,Dec; 2019,Sep **31526** 2020,Dec; 2019,Sep

Relative Value Units/Medicare Edits

Non-Facility RVU	Work	PE	MP	Total
31520	2.56	1.74	0.38	4.68
31525	2.63	4.52	0.39	7.54
31526	2.57	1.74	0.38	4.69
Facility RVU	**Work**	**PE**	**MP**	**Total**
31520	2.56	1.74	0.38	4.68
31525	2.63	1.77	0.39	4.79
31526	2.57	1.74	0.38	4.69

	FUD	Status	MUE	Modifiers				IOM Reference
31520	0	A	1(3)	51	N/A	N/A	80*	None
31525	0	A	1(3)	51	N/A	N/A	N/A	
31526	0	A	1(3)	51	N/A	N/A	N/A	

* with documentation

31527-31529

31527 Laryngoscopy direct, with or without tracheoscopy; with insertion of obturator
31528 with dilation, initial
31529 with dilation, subsequent

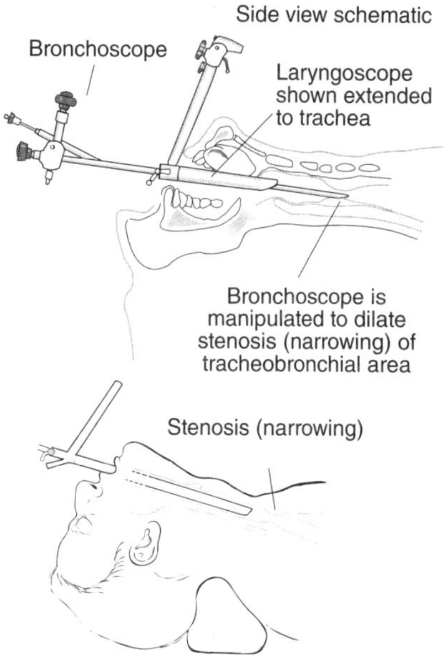

Explanation

In 31527, the physician administers a topical anesthetic to the oral cavity, pharynx, and larynx and inserts the laryngoscope through the patient's mouth. The interior of the larynx is examined. An obturator is an object that is used to close an opening. A wire is threaded through a cannulated needle that has been placed into the larynx. The end of the wire is grasped with forceps and drawn out through the laryngoscope. The wire is drawn through the obturator and threaded through another needle in the supraglottic space. The external ends of the wire are knotted over a stent. In 31528-31529, the physician dilates a tracheobronchial stenosis. A topical or general anesthetic is administered, and the laryngoscope inserted into the patient's mouth. The interior of the larynx is examined. The physician manipulates the laryngoscope to dilate areas of the tracheobronchial stenosis. Use 31528 for initial dilations (i.e., when it is the first dilation of a new area or for a new clinical condition, it has been three years or longer since the last dilation, previous dilations were performed by a physician from a different group practice, or it is the first lifetime dilation for the patient) and 31529 to report subsequent dilations. If a tracheoscopy is performed, a bronchoscope is inserted through the laryngoscope for visualization of the trachea and bronchi.

Coding Tips

Laryngoscopy code selection is dependent on two variables. Laryngoscopy procedures may be either direct or indirect, and they may be performed with either a rigid or flexible scope. Codes 31527–31529 refer to direct visualization with a rigid laryngoscope. Report the appropriate endoscopy for each anatomic site examined. Surgical endoscopy includes a diagnostic endoscopy; however, diagnostic endoscopy can be identified separately when performed at the same surgical session as an open procedure.

ICD-10-CM Diagnostic Codes

D38.1	Neoplasm of uncertain behavior of trachea, bronchus and lung
J37.1	Chronic laryngotracheitis
Q32.0	Congenital tracheomalacia
Q32.1	Other congenital malformations of trachea
S10.0XXA	Contusion of throat, initial encounter
S17.0XXA	Crushing injury of larynx and trachea, initial encounter
T17.320A	Food in larynx causing asphyxiation, initial encounter
T17.328A	Food in larynx causing other injury, initial encounter
T17.390A	Other foreign object in larynx causing asphyxiation, initial encounter
T17.398A	Other foreign object in larynx causing other injury, initial encounter
T27.0XXA	Burn of larynx and trachea, initial encounter
T27.1XXA	Burn involving larynx and trachea with lung, initial encounter
T27.4XXA	Corrosion of larynx and trachea, initial encounter
T27.5XXA	Corrosion involving larynx and trachea with lung, initial encounter

AMA: 31527 2020,Dec; 2019,Sep **31528** 2023,Nov; 2021,May; 2020,Dec; 2019,Sep **31529** 2023,Nov; 2020,Dec; 2019,Sep

Relative Value Units/Medicare Edits

Non-Facility RVU	Work	PE	MP	Total
31527	3.27	2.07	0.47	5.81
31528	2.37	1.59	0.35	4.31
31529	2.68	1.74	0.39	4.81
Facility RVU	**Work**	**PE**	**MP**	**Total**
31527	3.27	2.07	0.47	5.81
31528	2.37	1.59	0.35	4.31
31529	2.68	1.74	0.39	4.81

	FUD	Status	MUE	Modifiers				IOM Reference
31527	0	A	1(2)	51	N/A	N/A	80*	None
31528	0	A	1(2)	51	N/A	N/A	80*	
31529	0	A	1(3)	51	N/A	N/A	80*	

* with documentation

Terms To Know

dilation. Artificial increase in the diameter of an opening or lumen made by medication or by instrumentation.

direct laryngoscopy. Endoscopic instrument, such as a flexible or rigid fiberoptic scope, inserted into the larynx for direct viewing capabilities of the voice box and vocal cords.

larynx. Musculocartilaginous structure between the trachea and the pharynx that functions as the valve preventing food and other particles from entering the respiratory tract, as well as the voice mechanism. Also called the voicebox, the larynx is composed of three single cartilages: cricoid, epiglottis, and thyroid; and three paired cartilages: arytenoid, corniculate, and cuneiform.

obturator. Prosthesis used to close an acquired or congenital opening in the palate that aids in speech and chewing.

stenosis. Narrowing or constriction of a passage.

trachea. Tube descending from the larynx and branching into the right and left main bronchi.

31592

31592 Cricotracheal resection

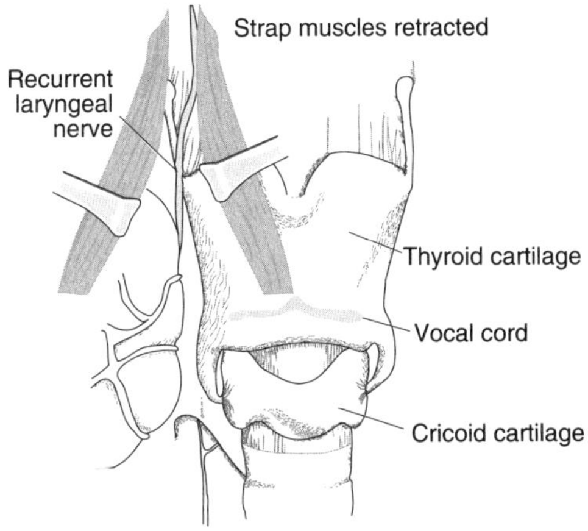

Cricotracheal resection is performed

Explanation

The physician removes a narrowed portion of the trachea usually below the larynx. A horizontal skin incision is made across the base of the neck or, in some cases, a sternotomy may be necessary. The prior tracheotomy stoma is removed when applicable. Flaps are lifted from the level of the hyoid bone to the suprasternal notch. The cricoid cartilage is split vertically and examined to be certain one intact ring between the area of resection and stoma is available in order for appropriate anastomosis between the trachea and larynx. Sutures are placed on both sides of the trachea just under the lowest level of the resection. Portions of the cricoid cartilage are removed from the anterior and lateral positions, avoiding the cricoarytenoid joint. The area of stenosis is removed with focus on avoiding the underlying esophagus. Upon removal of the narrowed portion, the ends are tied with absorbable sutures within the tracheal wall. Skin incisions are closed with sutures or staples. Sutures join the skin on the lower chin to the chest to prevent backward movement of the head or a neck brace may be utilized to keep sutures intact. This procedure may be performed as a single or double stage procedure depending on the exact location of the stenosis. In a single stage (SSCTR) procedure, a previously placed tracheotomy tube is removed and an endotracheal tube inserted. In a double stage (DSCTR) procedure, a stent may be inserted above the tracheotomy tube or a T-tube may be utilized instead of the tracheotomy tube. This allows the airway to remain open and is removed four to six weeks postop.

Coding Tips

Harvesting of the graft and rotational or advancement flaps performed through the same incision are not reported separately. For tracheostomy, see 31600–31610. For excision of a tracheal stenosis and anastomosis, see 31780 and 31781.

ICD-10-CM Diagnostic Codes

J38.01	Paralysis of vocal cords and larynx, unilateral
J38.02	Paralysis of vocal cords and larynx, bilateral
J38.3	Other diseases of vocal cords
J38.6	Stenosis of larynx

Relative Value Units/Medicare Edits

Non-Facility RVU	Work	PE	MP	Total
31592	25.0	23.44	3.64	52.08
Facility RVU	**Work**	**PE**	**MP**	**Total**
31592	25.0	23.44	3.64	52.08

	FUD	Status	MUE	Modifiers				IOM Reference
31592	90	A	1(2)	51	N/A	62*	80*	None

* with documentation

Terms To Know

larynx. Musculocartilaginous structure between the trachea and the pharynx that functions as the valve preventing food and other particles from entering the respiratory tract, as well as the voice mechanism.

stenosis. Narrowing or constriction of a passage.

sternotomy. Incision into the sternum, the bone that forms the front of the chest cavity and connects with the ribs.

trachea. Tube descending from the larynx and branching into the right and left main bronchi.

tracheotomy. Formation of a tracheal opening on the neck surface with tube insertion to allow for respiration in cases of obstruction or decreased patency. A tracheotomy may be planned or performed on an emergency basis for temporary or long-term use.

31600-31610

31600 Tracheostomy, planned (separate procedure);
31601 younger than 2 years
31603 Tracheostomy, emergency procedure; transtracheal
31605 cricothyroid membrane
31610 Tracheostomy, fenestration procedure with skin flaps

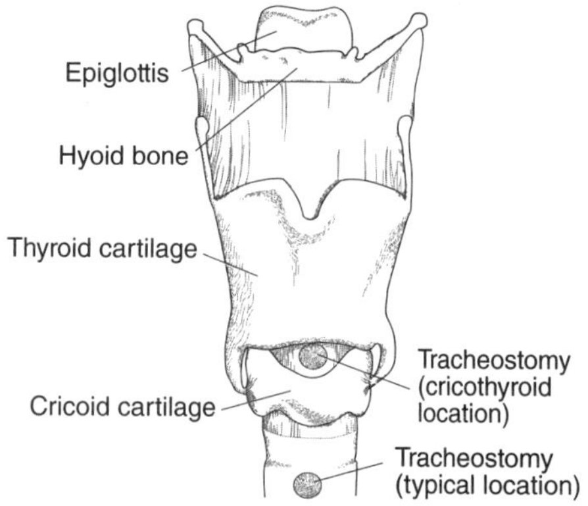

A tracheostomy is often performed just below the first tracheal ring and provides the patient with a controllable airway

Explanation

The physician creates a tracheostomy. The physician makes a horizontal neck incision and dissects the muscles to expose the trachea. The thyroid isthmus is cut if necessary. The trachea is incised and an airway is inserted. After bleeding is controlled, a stoma is created by suturing the skin to the tissue layers. In 31600, the tracheostomy is a planned procedure. In 31601, it is a planned procedure performed on patients younger than 2 years of age. In 31603, it is performed under emergency conditions by puncturing the trachea and inserting a cannula. In 31605, it is performed under emergency conditions by puncturing the cricothyroid membrane located just above the cricoid and inserting a cannula. This is not a true tracheostomy and is usually converted to a tracheostomy once the situation is no longer emergent. In 31610, skin flaps are used to create a more permanent stoma.

Coding Tips

Note that 31600 and 31601, separate procedures by definition, are usually a component of a more complex service and are not identified separately. When performed alone or with other unrelated procedures/services, they may be reported. If performed alone, list the code; if performed with other procedures/services, list the code and append modifier 59 or an X{EPSU} modifier. For a Bjork flap created in addition to the tracheostomy, use 31600, 31601, or 31603 as applicable. Creation of a Bjork flap does not justify reporting 31610. For endotracheal intubation, see 31500. For tracheal aspiration under direct vision, see 31515.

ICD-10-CM Diagnostic Codes

J43.0	Unilateral pulmonary emphysema [MacLeod's syndrome]
J43.1	Panlobular emphysema
J43.2	Centrilobular emphysema
J43.8	Other emphysema
J80	Acute respiratory distress syndrome
J95.821	Acute postprocedural respiratory failure
J95.822	Acute and chronic postprocedural respiratory failure
J95.87	Transfusion-associated dyspnea (TAD)
J96.01	Acute respiratory failure with hypoxia
J96.02	Acute respiratory failure with hypercapnia
J96.11	Chronic respiratory failure with hypoxia
J96.12	Chronic respiratory failure with hypercapnia
J96.21	Acute and chronic respiratory failure with hypoxia
J96.22	Acute and chronic respiratory failure with hypercapnia
P22.0	Respiratory distress syndrome of newborn N
P27.0	Wilson-Mikity syndrome
P27.1	Bronchopulmonary dysplasia originating in the perinatal period
P28.2	Cyanotic attacks of newborn N
P28.5	Respiratory failure of newborn N
Q31.1	Congenital subglottic stenosis
Q32.0	Congenital tracheomalacia
Q32.1	Other congenital malformations of trachea
Q32.2	Congenital bronchomalacia
Q32.3	Congenital stenosis of bronchus
R06.03	Acute respiratory distress
S17.0XXA	Crushing injury of larynx and trachea, initial encounter
T27.0XXA	Burn of larynx and trachea, initial encounter
T27.4XXA	Corrosion of larynx and trachea, initial encounter

AMA: 31600 2023,Jul; 2020,Dec; 2019,Sep **31601** 2020,Dec **31603** 2020,Dec **31610** 2020,Dec

Relative Value Units/Medicare Edits

Non-Facility RVU	Work	PE	MP	Total
31600	5.56	2.43	1.08	9.07
31601	8.0	4.23	1.18	13.41
31603	6.0	2.39	1.12	9.51
31605	6.45	2.08	1.26	9.79
31610	12.0	14.97	1.84	28.81
Facility RVU	**Work**	**PE**	**MP**	**Total**
31600	5.56	2.43	1.08	9.07
31601	8.0	4.23	1.18	13.41
31603	6.0	2.39	1.12	9.51
31605	6.45	2.08	1.26	9.79
31610	12.0	14.97	1.84	28.81

	FUD	Status	MUE	Modifiers				IOM Reference
31600	0	A	1(2)	51	N/A	N/A	N/A	None
31601	0	A	1(2)	51	N/A	62*	80	
31603	0	A	1(2)	51	N/A	N/A	N/A	
31605	0	A	1(2)	51	N/A	N/A	N/A	
31610	90	A	1(2)	51	N/A	N/A	N/A	

* with documentation

Terms To Know

respiratory distress syndrome. Premature neonates with respiratory distress and associated with reduced amounts of lung surfactant. Frequently fatal.

trachea. Tube descending from the larynx and branching into the right and left main bronchi.

tracheostomy. Formation of a tracheal opening on the neck surface with tube insertion to allow for respiration in cases of obstruction or decreased patency. A tracheostomy may be planned or performed on an emergency basis for temporary or long-term use.

31612

31612 Tracheal puncture, percutaneous with transtracheal aspiration and/or injection

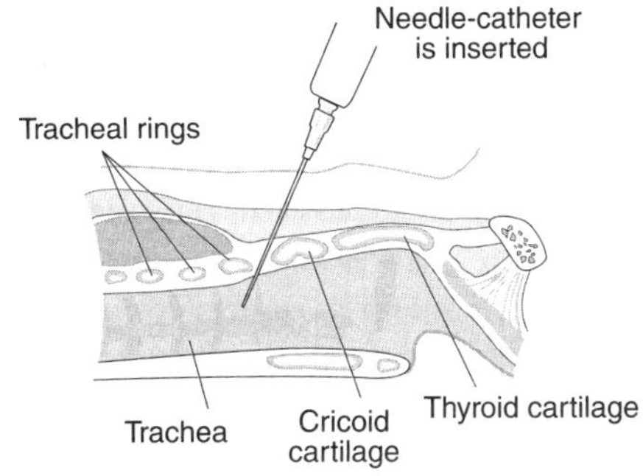

Midsagittal view showing needle placement

Explanation

The physician punctures the trachea with a needle to aspirate secretions or inject a therapeutic agent. The physician palpates the site and inserts a hollow point needle. Secretions are aspirated or a therapeutic agent is injected. The needle is removed.

Coding Tips

For tracheal aspiration under direct vision, see 31515. For catheter aspiration of tracheobronchial tree, see 31725.

ICD-10-CM Diagnostic Codes

A48.1	Legionnaires' disease
J44.0	Chronic obstructive pulmonary disease with (acute) lower respiratory infection
J44.1	Chronic obstructive pulmonary disease with (acute) exacerbation
J44.81	Bronchiolitis obliterans and bronchiolitis obliterans syndrome
J45.20	Mild intermittent asthma, uncomplicated
J45.21	Mild intermittent asthma with (acute) exacerbation
J45.22	Mild intermittent asthma with status asthmaticus
J45.31	Mild persistent asthma with (acute) exacerbation
J45.32	Mild persistent asthma with status asthmaticus
J45.41	Moderate persistent asthma with (acute) exacerbation
J45.42	Moderate persistent asthma with status asthmaticus
J45.51	Severe persistent asthma with (acute) exacerbation
J45.52	Severe persistent asthma with status asthmaticus
J4A.0	Restrictive allograft syndrome
J68.0	Bronchitis and pneumonitis due to chemicals, gases, fumes and vapors
J69.0	Pneumonitis due to inhalation of food and vomit
J69.8	Pneumonitis due to inhalation of other solids and liquids
O74.0	Aspiration pneumonitis due to anesthesia during labor and delivery M
O74.1	Other pulmonary complications of anesthesia during labor and delivery M
O89.01	Aspiration pneumonitis due to anesthesia during the puerperium M
O89.09	Other pulmonary complications of anesthesia during the puerperium M
P24.01	Meconium aspiration with respiratory symptoms N
P24.11	Neonatal aspiration of (clear) amniotic fluid and mucus with respiratory symptoms N
P24.21	Neonatal aspiration of blood with respiratory symptoms N
P24.31	Neonatal aspiration of milk and regurgitated food with respiratory symptoms N
P24.81	Other neonatal aspiration with respiratory symptoms N

Relative Value Units/Medicare Edits

Non-Facility RVU	Work	PE	MP	Total
31612	0.91	1.75	0.14	2.8
Facility RVU	**Work**	**PE**	**MP**	**Total**
31612	0.91	0.38	0.14	1.43

	FUD	Status	MUE	Modifiers				IOM Reference
31612	0	A	1(3)	51	N/A	N/A	80*	None

* with documentation

Terms To Know

anomaly. Irregularity in the structure or position of an organ or tissue.

aspirate. To withdraw fluid or air from a body cavity by suction.

congenital. Present at birth, occurring through heredity or an influence during gestation up to the moment of birth.

meconium aspiration syndrome. Newborn respiratory complications resulting from the passage and subsequent aspiration of meconium (fetal intestinal waste material) prior to or during delivery.

trachea. Tube descending from the larynx and branching into the right and left main bronchi.

31615

31615 Tracheobronchoscopy through established tracheostomy incision

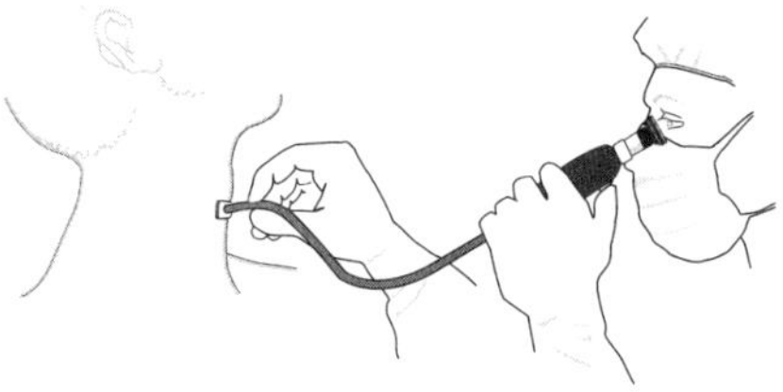

Examination using flexible fiberoptic bronchoscope

Explanation

The physician views the airway using a bronchoscope placed through an existing tracheostomy. The physician examines the conducting airways. The bronchoscope is removed.

Coding Tips

When medically necessary, report moderate (conscious) sedation provided by the performing physician with 99151-99153. When provided by another physician, report 99155-99157. This procedure is similar to a diagnostic bronchoscopy, 31622, except that in 31615 the endoscope is passed through an existing tracheostomy instead of through the oral or nasal cavity. Report the appropriate endoscopy for each anatomic site examined. Surgical endoscopy includes a diagnostic endoscopy; however, diagnostic endoscopy can be identified separately when performed at the same surgical session as an open procedure. For tracheobronchoscopy with bronchial alveolar lavage, report 31624 with modifier 52 appended. For tracheoscopy, see 31515–31574. Surgical trays, A4550, are not separately reimbursed by Medicare; however, other third-party payers may cover them. Check with the specific payer to determine coverage.

ICD-10-CM Diagnostic Codes

B25.0	Cytomegaloviral pneumonitis
B44.0	Invasive pulmonary aspergillosis
B59	Pneumocystosis
C33	Malignant neoplasm of trachea
C34.01	Malignant neoplasm of right main bronchus ☑
C34.11	Malignant neoplasm of upper lobe, right bronchus or lung ☑
C34.2	Malignant neoplasm of middle lobe, bronchus or lung
C34.81	Malignant neoplasm of overlapping sites of right bronchus and lung ☑
C78.01	Secondary malignant neoplasm of right lung ☑
C78.39	Secondary malignant neoplasm of other respiratory organs
C7A.090	Malignant carcinoid tumor of the bronchus and lung
D02.1	Carcinoma in situ of trachea
D02.21	Carcinoma in situ of right bronchus and lung ☑
D14.2	Benign neoplasm of trachea
D14.31	Benign neoplasm of right bronchus and lung ☑
D38.1	Neoplasm of uncertain behavior of trachea, bronchus and lung
D3A.090	Benign carcinoid tumor of the bronchus and lung
D86.0	Sarcoidosis of lung
D86.1	Sarcoidosis of lymph nodes
J44.0	Chronic obstructive pulmonary disease with (acute) lower respiratory infection
J44.1	Chronic obstructive pulmonary disease with (acute) exacerbation
J44.81	Bronchiolitis obliterans and bronchiolitis obliterans syndrome
J47.0	Bronchiectasis with acute lower respiratory infection
J47.1	Bronchiectasis with (acute) exacerbation
J47.9	Bronchiectasis, uncomplicated
J4A.0	Restrictive allograft syndrome
J67.7	Air conditioner and humidifier lung
J67.8	Hypersensitivity pneumonitis due to other organic dusts
J68.0	Bronchitis and pneumonitis due to chemicals, gases, fumes and vapors
J68.4	Chronic respiratory conditions due to chemicals, gases, fumes and vapors
J69.0	Pneumonitis due to inhalation of food and vomit
J69.1	Pneumonitis due to inhalation of oils and essences
J69.8	Pneumonitis due to inhalation of other solids and liquids
J70.2	Acute drug-induced interstitial lung disorders
J70.3	Chronic drug-induced interstitial lung disorders
J70.5	Respiratory conditions due to smoke inhalation
J95.851	Ventilator associated pneumonia
J96.01	Acute respiratory failure with hypoxia
J96.02	Acute respiratory failure with hypercapnia
J96.11	Chronic respiratory failure with hypoxia
J96.12	Chronic respiratory failure with hypercapnia
J96.21	Acute and chronic respiratory failure with hypoxia
J96.22	Acute and chronic respiratory failure with hypercapnia
Q32.0	Congenital tracheomalacia
Q32.1	Other congenital malformations of trachea
Q32.2	Congenital bronchomalacia
T17.510A	Gastric contents in bronchus causing asphyxiation, initial encounter
T17.518A	Gastric contents in bronchus causing other injury, initial encounter
T17.520A	Food in bronchus causing asphyxiation, initial encounter
T17.810A	Gastric contents in other parts of respiratory tract causing asphyxiation, initial encounter
T17.818A	Gastric contents in other parts of respiratory tract causing other injury, initial encounter
T17.820A	Food in other parts of respiratory tract causing asphyxiation, initial encounter
T17.828A	Food in other parts of respiratory tract causing other injury, initial encounter

AMA: 31615 2021,Aug; 2020,Dec

Relative Value Units/Medicare Edits

Non-Facility RVU	Work	PE	MP	Total
31615	1.84	3.09	0.25	5.18
Facility RVU	**Work**	**PE**	**MP**	**Total**
31615	1.84	1.37	0.25	3.46

	FUD	Status	MUE	Modifiers				IOM Reference
31615	0	A	1(3)	51	N/A	N/A	N/A	None

* with documentation

31760

31760 Tracheoplasty; intrathoracic

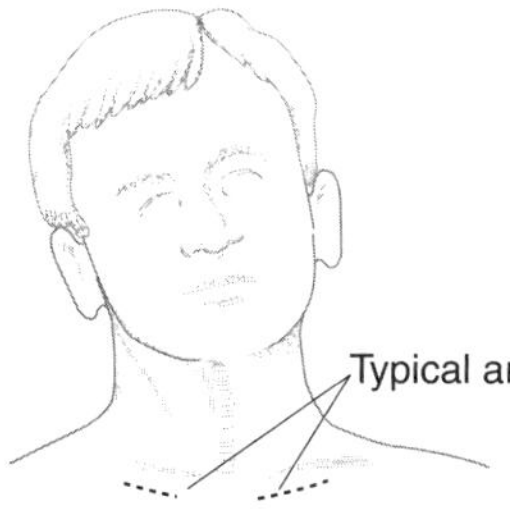

Any of a wide variety of surgical repairs may be made to the tracheopharyngeal area using an intrathoracic surgical approach

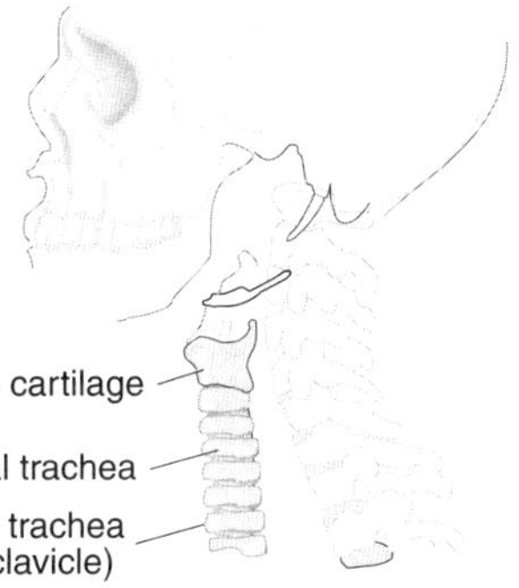

Explanation

The physician makes an incision in the thorax and approaches the trachea by opening the rib cage. An airway is inserted and the trachea is incised. Surgical repair of the trachea is undertaken. End-to-end anastomosis of the trachea may be performed. For satisfactory reconstruction, it may be necessary for the physician to surgically repair the trachea using splints constructed from rib or costal cartilage to patch the length of the trachea. Once repair is achieved, the airway is removed and the incisions are closed.

Coding Tips

When 31760 is performed with another separately identifiable procedure, the highest dollar value code is listed as the primary procedure, and subsequent procedures are appended with modifier 51. Report any free grafts or flaps separately.

ICD-10-CM Diagnostic Codes

C33	Malignant neoplasm of trachea
C78.39	Secondary malignant neoplasm of other respiratory organs
D02.1	Carcinoma in situ of trachea
D14.2	Benign neoplasm of trachea
D38.1	Neoplasm of uncertain behavior of trachea, bronchus and lung
Q32.0	Congenital tracheomalacia
Q32.1	Other congenital malformations of trachea
Q39.1	Atresia of esophagus with tracheo-esophageal fistula
Q39.2	Congenital tracheo-esophageal fistula without atresia
S11.021A	Laceration without foreign body of trachea, initial encounter
S11.022A	Laceration with foreign body of trachea, initial encounter
S11.023A	Puncture wound without foreign body of trachea, initial encounter
S11.024A	Puncture wound with foreign body of trachea, initial encounter
S11.025A	Open bite of trachea, initial encounter
S17.0XXA	Crushing injury of larynx and trachea, initial encounter
T27.0XXA	Burn of larynx and trachea, initial encounter
T27.1XXA	Burn involving larynx and trachea with lung, initial encounter
T27.4XXA	Corrosion of larynx and trachea, initial encounter
T27.5XXA	Corrosion involving larynx and trachea with lung, initial encounter
Z85.12	Personal history of malignant neoplasm of trachea

Relative Value Units/Medicare Edits

Non-Facility RVU	Work	PE	MP	Total
31760	23.48	11.49	5.8	40.77
Facility RVU	**Work**	**PE**	**MP**	**Total**
31760	23.48	11.49	5.8	40.77

	FUD	Status	MUE	Modifiers				IOM Reference
31760	90	A	1(2)	51	N/A	62*	80	None

* with documentation

Terms To Know

anastomosis. Surgically created connection between ducts, blood vessels, or bowel segments to allow flow from one to the other.

cartilage. Variety of fibrous connective tissue that is inherently nonvascular. Usually found in the joints, it aids in movement and provides a cushion to absorb jolts and shocks.

free graft. Unattached piece of skin and tissue moved to another part of the body and sutured into place to repair a defect.

malignant. Any condition tending to progress toward death, specifically an invasive tumor with a loss of cellular differentiation that has the ability to spread or metastasize to other body areas.

reconstruction. Recreating, restoring, or rebuilding a body part or organ.

tracheoesophageal fistula. Abnormal opening between the trachea and the esophagus. There are three types of tracheoesophageal fistulas; congenital, formed from a previous tracheostomy, and fistula not caused by previous surgery.

32035-32036

32035 Thoracostomy; with rib resection for empyema
32036 with open flap drainage for empyema

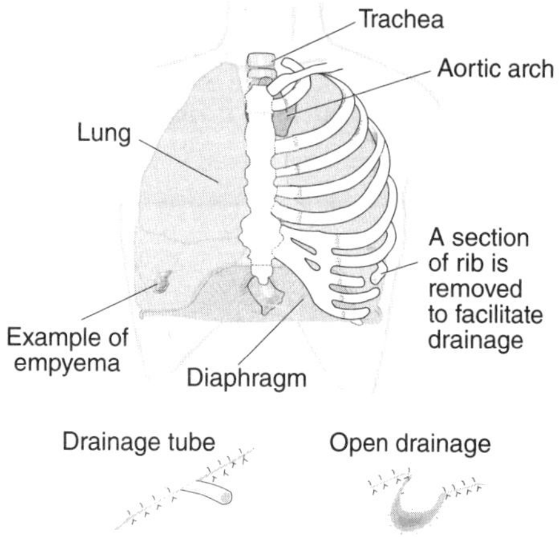

Explanation

The physician removes the purulent fluid of an empyema by creating a drainage wound in the chest. Using a scalpel, an incision is made through the skin of the chest and the incision is deepened to expose a portion of a rib. In 32035, to enter the chest cavity, a short segment of the exposed rib is removed using rib cutters. The resulting defect in the chest wall allows for the continuous release of pus from the empyema (abscess in the chest cavity). In 32036, to create a drainage site, a short segment of the rib is removed using rib cutters. The resulting defect in the chest wall allows for the continuous release of pus from the empyema. To ensure that the drainage wound stays open, a flap is created in the skin and subcutaneous tissues.

Coding Tips

Open flap drainage (32036) requires a subsequent procedure for closure once the empyema has resolved. For closure of the chest wall following open flap drainage for empyema, see 32810. For tube thoracostomy for empyema, see 32551. Wound exploration resulting from penetrating trauma without thoracotomy is reported with 20101.

ICD-10-CM Diagnostic Codes

J86.0 Pyothorax with fistula
J86.9 Pyothorax without fistula

Relative Value Units/Medicare Edits

Non-Facility RVU	Work	PE	MP	Total
32035	11.29	7.85	2.78	21.92
32036	12.3	8.35	2.96	23.61
Facility RVU	**Work**	**PE**	**MP**	**Total**
32035	11.29	7.85	2.78	21.92
32036	12.3	8.35	2.96	23.61

	FUD	Status	MUE	Modifiers				IOM Reference
32035	90	A	1(2)	51	50	62*	80	None
32036	90	A	1(3)	51	50	62*	80	

* with documentation

32096-32098

32096 Thoracotomy, with diagnostic biopsy(ies) of lung infiltrate(s) (eg, wedge, incisional), unilateral
32097 Thoracotomy, with diagnostic biopsy(ies) of lung nodule(s) or mass(es) (eg, wedge, incisional), unilateral
32098 Thoracotomy, with biopsy(ies) of pleura

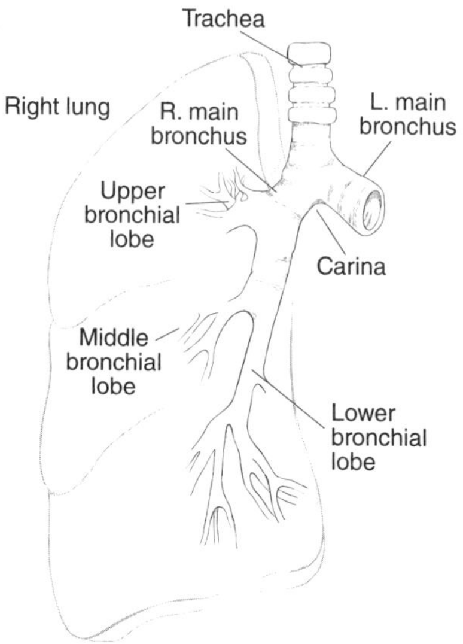

Explanation

The physician removes a sample of tissue from the lung or the pleura. Using a scalpel, the skin between two ribs is incised and the tissues separated to expose the inside of the chest cavity. A representative sample of tissue is removed from the lung or pleura using a biopsy needle or by cutting with a scalpel or scissors. The surgical wound is closed by suturing. Report 32096 when the biopsy is performed to sample unilateral lung infiltrates. Report 32097 when the biopsy is of a unilateral lung nodule or mass. Report 32098 when the tissue biopsied is the pleura.

Coding Tips

Note that 32096 and 32097 are unilateral procedures. If performed bilaterally, some payers require that the service be reported twice with modifier 50 appended to the second code while others require identification of the service only once with modifier 50 appended. Check with individual payers. Modifier 50 identifies a procedure performed identically on the opposite side of the body (mirror image). Codes 32096 and 32097 should only be reported once per lung. Do not report 32096 or 32097 with 32440, 32442, 32445, or 32488. A diagnostic wedge biopsy is characterized by removing tissue without concern for resection margins. A therapeutic wedge resection involves close attention to resection margins and complete resection. For wound exploration as a result of penetrating trauma not by thoracotomy, see 20101.

ICD-10-CM Diagnostic Codes

A15.6 Tuberculous pleurisy
B59 Pneumocystosis
C34.01 Malignant neoplasm of right main bronchus ☑
C34.02 Malignant neoplasm of left main bronchus ☑
C34.11 Malignant neoplasm of upper lobe, right bronchus or lung ☑
C34.12 Malignant neoplasm of upper lobe, left bronchus or lung ☑
C34.2 Malignant neoplasm of middle lobe, bronchus or lung
C34.31 Malignant neoplasm of lower lobe, right bronchus or lung ☑

C34.32	Malignant neoplasm of lower lobe, left bronchus or lung ☑
C34.81	Malignant neoplasm of overlapping sites of right bronchus and lung ☑
C34.82	Malignant neoplasm of overlapping sites of left bronchus and lung ☑
C38.4	Malignant neoplasm of pleura
C38.8	Malignant neoplasm of overlapping sites of heart, mediastinum and pleura
C45.0	Mesothelioma of pleura
C46.51	Kaposi's sarcoma of right lung ☑
C46.52	Kaposi's sarcoma of left lung ☑
C78.01	Secondary malignant neoplasm of right lung ☑
C78.02	Secondary malignant neoplasm of left lung ☑
C78.2	Secondary malignant neoplasm of pleura
C7A.090	Malignant carcinoid tumor of the bronchus and lung
D02.21	Carcinoma in situ of right bronchus and lung ☑
D02.22	Carcinoma in situ of left bronchus and lung ☑
D14.31	Benign neoplasm of right bronchus and lung ☑
D14.32	Benign neoplasm of left bronchus and lung ☑
D19.0	Benign neoplasm of mesothelial tissue of pleura
D38.1	Neoplasm of uncertain behavior of trachea, bronchus and lung
D38.2	Neoplasm of uncertain behavior of pleura
D3A.090	Benign carcinoid tumor of the bronchus and lung
D86.0	Sarcoidosis of lung
J60	Coalworker's pneumoconiosis A
J61	Pneumoconiosis due to asbestos and other mineral fibers A
J62.0	Pneumoconiosis due to talc dust
J62.8	Pneumoconiosis due to other dust containing silica
J63.0	Aluminosis (of lung)
J63.1	Bauxite fibrosis (of lung)
J63.2	Berylliosis
J63.3	Graphite fibrosis (of lung)
J63.4	Siderosis
J63.5	Stannosis
J63.6	Pneumoconiosis due to other specified inorganic dusts
J66.0	Byssinosis
J66.1	Flax-dressers' disease
J66.2	Cannabinosis
J66.8	Airway disease due to other specific organic dusts
J67.8	Hypersensitivity pneumonitis due to other organic dusts
J67.9	Hypersensitivity pneumonitis due to unspecified organic dust
J68.0	Bronchitis and pneumonitis due to chemicals, gases, fumes and vapors
J68.4	Chronic respiratory conditions due to chemicals, gases, fumes and vapors
J70.2	Acute drug-induced interstitial lung disorders
J82.81	Chronic eosinophilic pneumonia
J82.82	Acute eosinophilic pneumonia
J82.83	Eosinophilic asthma
J84.112	Idiopathic pulmonary fibrosis
J84.113	Idiopathic non-specific interstitial pneumonitis
J84.115	Respiratory bronchiolitis interstitial lung disease
J84.117	Desquamative interstitial pneumonia
J84.170	Interstitial lung disease with progressive fibrotic phenotype in diseases classified elsewhere
J84.178	Other interstitial pulmonary diseases with fibrosis in diseases classified elsewhere
J84.2	Lymphoid interstitial pneumonia
J84.82	Adult pulmonary Langerhans cell histiocytosis A
J84.848	Other interstitial lung diseases of childhood
J84.89	Other specified interstitial pulmonary diseases
J85.0	Gangrene and necrosis of lung
J86.0	Pyothorax with fistula
J86.9	Pyothorax without fistula
J91.0	Malignant pleural effusion
J92.0	Pleural plaque with presence of asbestos
M32.13	Lung involvement in systemic lupus erythematosus
M33.01	Juvenile dermatomyositis with respiratory involvement
M33.11	Other dermatomyositis with respiratory involvement
M33.21	Polymyositis with respiratory involvement
M35.02	Sjögren syndrome with lung involvement

AMA: **32096** 2021,Apr **32097** 2021,Apr

Relative Value Units/Medicare Edits

Non-Facility RVU	Work	PE	MP	Total
32096	13.75	6.64	3.33	23.72
32097	13.75	6.68	3.33	23.76
32098	12.91	6.47	3.09	22.47
Facility RVU	**Work**	**PE**	**MP**	**Total**
32096	13.75	6.64	3.33	23.72
32097	13.75	6.68	3.33	23.76
32098	12.91	6.47	3.09	22.47

	FUD	Status	MUE	Modifiers				IOM Reference
32096	90	A	1(3)	51	N/A	62*	80	None
32097	90	A	1(3)	51	N/A	62*	80	
32098	90	A	1(2)	51	N/A	62*	80	

* with documentation

Terms To Know

effusion. Escape of fluid from within a body cavity.

hemoptysis. Coughing up or spitting out blood or blood-streaked sputum.

pleura. One of the two membranes that surround the lungs. The visceral pleura encases the lung and the parietal pleura lines the inner chest walls.

pleurisy. Inflammation of the serous membrane that lines the lungs and the thoracic cavity. Pleurisy may cause effusion within the cavity or have exudate in the pleural space or on the membrane surface.

thoracotomy. Surgical procedure for opening the chest wall in order to access the lungs, esophagus, trachea, aorta, heart, and diaphragm.

32100

32100 Thoracotomy; with exploration

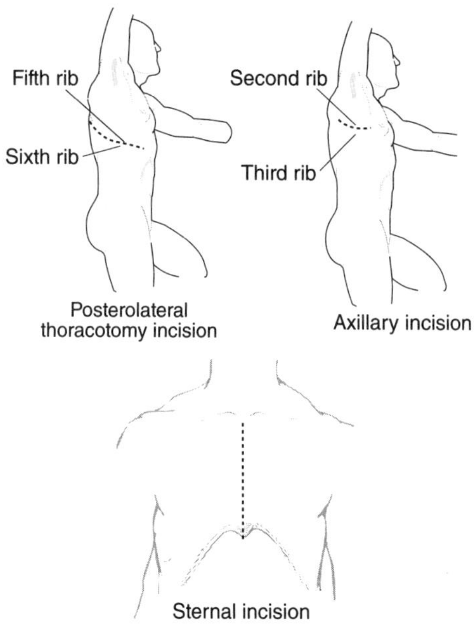

Any of a number of access incisions may be used

Explanation

The physician opens the chest cavity widely to directly visualize and assess the organs and structures in the chest. Using a scalpel, the surgeon makes a long incision around the side of the chest between two of the ribs. The incision is carried through all of the tissue layers into the chest cavity. Rib spreaders are inserted into the wound and the ribs are spread apart exposing the lung, heart, and other structures. Alternately, the chest cavity can be opened and the operation performed through a vertical incision in the center of the chest through the sternum. The skin incision is carried down to the sternum bone and a saw is used to split the sternum. With the sternum split in half, the chest is entered by spreading the sternum apart with a set of rib spreaders. The chest cavity is explored and the anatomy visualized using a gloved hand and large gauze sponges. The surgical instruments are removed. A chest tube(s) may be used to provide drainage for the chest cavity. When the procedure is complete, if applicable, the sternotomy is repaired using wires to bring the two halves of the sternum together, and the operative wound is closed by sutures or staples.

Coding Tips

Report 32100 for a major thoracotomy when the chest cavity is opened to fully explore any lesions. For a thoracotomy with a biopsy, see 32096, 32097, and 32098. For exploration of a chest wound not requiring thoracotomy, see 20101. Do not report 32100 with 21601-21603, 32503, 32504, 33955-33957, 33963, or 33964.

ICD-10-CM Diagnostic Codes

C34.01 Malignant neoplasm of right main bronchus ☑
C34.11 Malignant neoplasm of upper lobe, right bronchus or lung ☑
C34.2 Malignant neoplasm of middle lobe, bronchus or lung
C34.31 Malignant neoplasm of lower lobe, right bronchus or lung ☑
C34.81 Malignant neoplasm of overlapping sites of right bronchus and lung ☑
C46.51 Kaposi's sarcoma of right lung ☑
D14.31 Benign neoplasm of right bronchus and lung ☑
D3A.090 Benign carcinoid tumor of the bronchus and lung
S26.01XA Contusion of heart with hemopericardium, initial encounter
S26.020A Mild laceration of heart with hemopericardium, initial encounter
S26.021A Moderate laceration of heart with hemopericardium, initial encounter
S26.022A Major laceration of heart with hemopericardium, initial encounter
S26.11XA Contusion of heart without hemopericardium, initial encounter
S26.12XA Laceration of heart without hemopericardium, initial encounter
S27.0XXA Traumatic pneumothorax, initial encounter
S27.1XXA Traumatic hemothorax, initial encounter
S27.2XXA Traumatic hemopneumothorax, initial encounter
S27.311A Primary blast injury of lung, unilateral, initial encounter
S27.312A Primary blast injury of lung, bilateral, initial encounter ☑
S27.321A Contusion of lung, unilateral, initial encounter
S27.322A Contusion of lung, bilateral, initial encounter ☑
S27.331A Laceration of lung, unilateral, initial encounter
S27.332A Laceration of lung, bilateral, initial encounter ☑
S27.411A Primary blast injury of bronchus, unilateral, initial encounter
S27.412A Primary blast injury of bronchus, bilateral, initial encounter ☑
S27.421A Contusion of bronchus, unilateral, initial encounter
S27.422A Contusion of bronchus, bilateral, initial encounter ☑
S27.431A Laceration of bronchus, unilateral, initial encounter
S27.432A Laceration of bronchus, bilateral, initial encounter ☑
S27.51XA Primary blast injury of thoracic trachea, initial encounter
S27.52XA Contusion of thoracic trachea, initial encounter
S27.53XA Laceration of thoracic trachea, initial encounter
S27.63XA Laceration of pleura, initial encounter
S27.802A Contusion of diaphragm, initial encounter
S27.803A Laceration of diaphragm, initial encounter
S27.812A Contusion of esophagus (thoracic part), initial encounter
S27.813A Laceration of esophagus (thoracic part), initial encounter
S28.0XXA Crushed chest, initial encounter

AMA: 32100 2019,Dec

Relative Value Units/Medicare Edits

Non-Facility RVU	Work	PE	MP	Total
32100	13.75	7.05	3.27	24.07
Facility RVU	**Work**	**PE**	**MP**	**Total**
32100	13.75	7.05	3.27	24.07

	FUD	Status	MUE	Modifiers				IOM Reference
32100	90	A	1(3)	51	N/A	62*	80	None

* with documentation

32110

32110 Thoracotomy; with control of traumatic hemorrhage and/or repair of lung tear

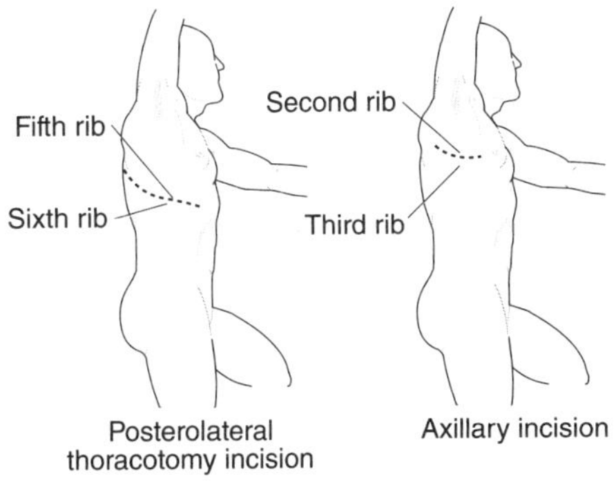

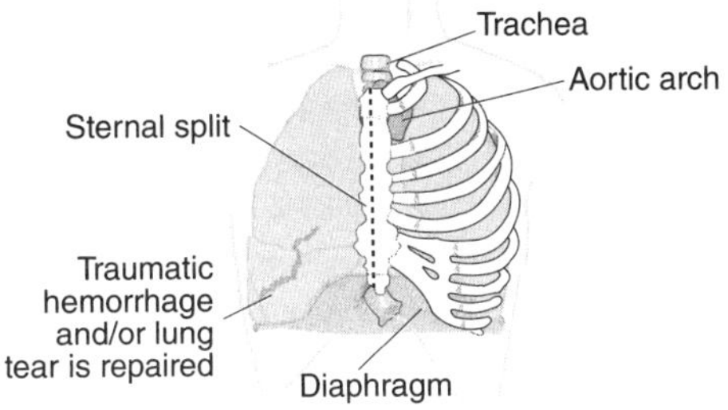

Explanation

The physician opens the chest cavity widely to directly visualize and assess the organs and structures in the chest. Using a scalpel, the surgeon makes a long incision around the side of the chest between two of the ribs. The incision is carried through all of the tissue layers into the chest cavity. Rib spreaders are inserted into the wound and the ribs are spread apart exposing the lung, heart, and other structures. Alternately, the chest cavity can be opened and the operation performed through a vertical incision in the center of the chest through the sternum. The skin incision is carried down to the sternum bone and a saw is used to split the sternum. With the sternum split in half, the chest is entered by spreading the sternum apart with a set of rib spreaders. The chest cavity is explored and the anatomy visualized using a gloved hand and large gauze sponges. The site of the hemorrhage or lung tear is identified and repaired. The surgical instruments are removed. A chest tube(s) may be used to provide drainage for the chest cavity. When the procedure is complete, if applicable, the sternotomy is repaired using wires to bring the two halves of the sternum together, and the operative wound is closed by sutures or staples.

Coding Tips

When 32110 is performed with another separately identifiable procedure, the highest dollar value code is listed as the primary procedure, and subsequent procedures are appended with modifier 51. If traumatic hemorrhage is controlled through a thoracoscope, not open thoracotomy, see 32654.

ICD-10-CM Diagnostic Codes

S21.311A Laceration without foreign body of right front wall of thorax with penetration into thoracic cavity, initial encounter

S21.321A Laceration with foreign body of right front wall of thorax with penetration into thoracic cavity, initial encounter

S21.331A Puncture wound without foreign body of right front wall of thorax with penetration into thoracic cavity, initial encounter

S21.341A Puncture wound with foreign body of right front wall of thorax with penetration into thoracic cavity, initial encounter

S21.351A Open bite of right front wall of thorax with penetration into thoracic cavity, initial encounter

S21.411A Laceration without foreign body of right back wall of thorax with penetration into thoracic cavity, initial encounter

S21.421A Laceration with foreign body of right back wall of thorax with penetration into thoracic cavity, initial encounter

S21.431A Puncture wound without foreign body of right back wall of thorax with penetration into thoracic cavity, initial encounter

S21.441A Puncture wound with foreign body of right back wall of thorax with penetration into thoracic cavity, initial encounter

S21.451A Open bite of right back wall of thorax with penetration into thoracic cavity, initial encounter

S25.411A Minor laceration of right pulmonary blood vessels, initial encounter ☑

S25.421A Major laceration of right pulmonary blood vessels, initial encounter ☑

S25.811A Laceration of other blood vessels of thorax, right side, initial encounter ☑

S27.0XXA Traumatic pneumothorax, initial encounter

S27.1XXA Traumatic hemothorax, initial encounter

S27.2XXA Traumatic hemopneumothorax, initial encounter

S27.311A Primary blast injury of lung, unilateral, initial encounter

S27.312A Primary blast injury of lung, bilateral, initial encounter ☑

S27.321A Contusion of lung, unilateral, initial encounter

S27.322A Contusion of lung, bilateral, initial encounter ☑

S27.331A Laceration of lung, unilateral, initial encounter

S27.332A Laceration of lung, bilateral, initial encounter ☑

S27.391A Other injuries of lung, unilateral, initial encounter

S27.392A Other injuries of lung, bilateral, initial encounter ☑

S28.0XXA Crushed chest, initial encounter

Relative Value Units/Medicare Edits

Non-Facility RVU	Work	PE	MP	Total
32110	25.28	12.49	6.04	43.81
Facility RVU	**Work**	**PE**	**MP**	**Total**
32110	25.28	12.49	6.04	43.81

	FUD	Status	MUE	Modifiers				IOM Reference
32110	90	A	1(3)	51	N/A	62*	80	None

* with documentation

Terms To Know

spontaneous tension pneumothorax. Air leaking from the lung and trapped in the lung lining.

thoracotomy. Surgical procedure for opening the chest wall in order to access the lungs, esophagus, trachea, aorta, heart, and diaphragm.

 ● New ▲ Revised + Add On ★ Telemedicine [Resequenced] ☑ Laterality

32120

32120 Thoracotomy; for postoperative complications

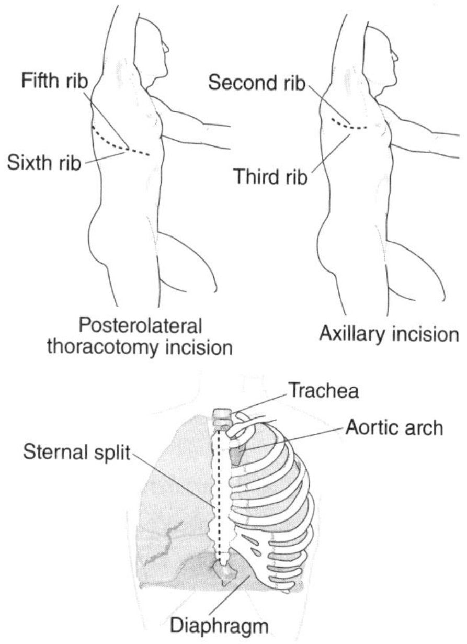

Explanation

The physician performs a thoracotomy to identify any thoracic postoperative complications. The physician opens the chest cavity widely to directly visualize and assess the organs and structures in the chest. Using a scalpel, the surgeon makes a long incision around the side of the chest between two of the ribs. The incision is carried through all of the tissue layers into the chest cavity. Rib spreaders are inserted into the wound and the ribs are spread apart exposing the lung, heart, and other structures. Alternately, the chest cavity can be opened and the operation performed through a vertical incision in the center of the chest through the sternum. The skin incision is carried down to the sternum bone and a saw is used to split the sternum. With the sternum split in half, the chest is entered by spreading the sternum apart with a set of rib spreaders. The chest cavity is explored and the anatomy visualized using a gloved hand and large gauze sponges. The surgical instruments are removed. A chest tube(s) may be used to provide drainage for the chest cavity. When the procedure is complete, if applicable, the sternotomy is repaired using wires to bring the two halves of the sternum together, and the operative wound is closed by sutures or staples.

Coding Tips

When 32120 is performed with another separately identifiable procedure, the highest dollar value code is listed as the primary procedure, and subsequent procedures are appended with modifier 51.

ICD-10-CM Diagnostic Codes

J95.811	Postprocedural pneumothorax
J95.812	Postprocedural air leak
J95.830	Postprocedural hemorrhage of a respiratory system organ or structure following a respiratory system procedure
J95.831	Postprocedural hemorrhage of a respiratory system organ or structure following other procedure
J95.860	Postprocedural hematoma of a respiratory system organ or structure following a respiratory system procedure
J95.861	Postprocedural hematoma of a respiratory system organ or structure following other procedure
J95.862	Postprocedural seroma of a respiratory system organ or structure following a respiratory system procedure
J95.863	Postprocedural seroma of a respiratory system organ or structure following other procedure
J95.89	Other postprocedural complications and disorders of respiratory system, not elsewhere classified
T81.41XA	Infection following a procedure, superficial incisional surgical site, initial encounter
T81.42XA	Infection following a procedure, deep incisional surgical site, initial encounter
T81.43XA	Infection following a procedure, organ and space surgical site, initial encounter
T81.44XA	Sepsis following a procedure, initial encounter
T81.49XA	Infection following a procedure, other surgical site, initial encounter
T81.510A	Adhesions due to foreign body accidentally left in body following surgical operation, initial encounter
T81.520A	Obstruction due to foreign body accidentally left in body following surgical operation, initial encounter
T81.530A	Perforation due to foreign body accidentally left in body following surgical operation, initial encounter
T81.538A	Perforation due to foreign body accidentally left in body following other procedure, initial encounter

Relative Value Units/Medicare Edits

Non-Facility RVU	Work	PE	MP	Total
32120	14.39	8.06	3.49	25.94
Facility RVU	**Work**	**PE**	**MP**	**Total**
32120	14.39	8.06	3.49	25.94

	FUD	Status	MUE	Modifiers				IOM Reference
32120	90	A	1(3)	51	N/A	62*	80	None

* with documentation

Terms To Know

empyema. Accumulation of pus within the respiratory or pleural cavity.

fistula. Abnormal tube-like passage between two body cavities or organs or from an organ to the outside surface.

thoracotomy. Surgical procedure for opening the chest wall in order to access the lungs, esophagus, trachea, aorta, heart, and diaphragm.

 N Newborn: 0 P Pediatric: 0-17 M Maternity: 9-64 A Adult: 15-124 AMA: CPT Assist

32124

32124 Thoracotomy; with open intrapleural pneumonolysis

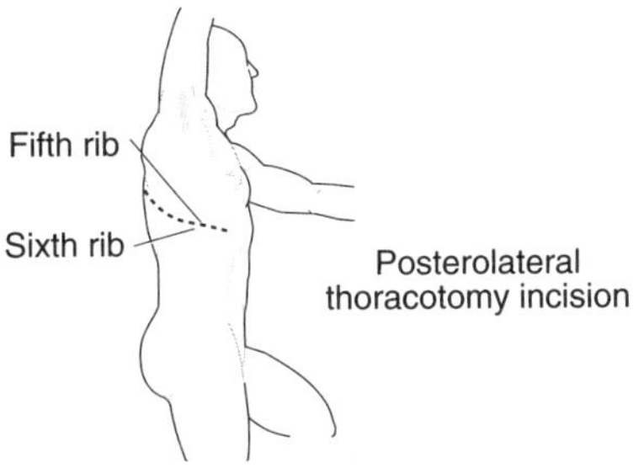

Adhesions between lung tissue and the inside surface of the chest cavity are released

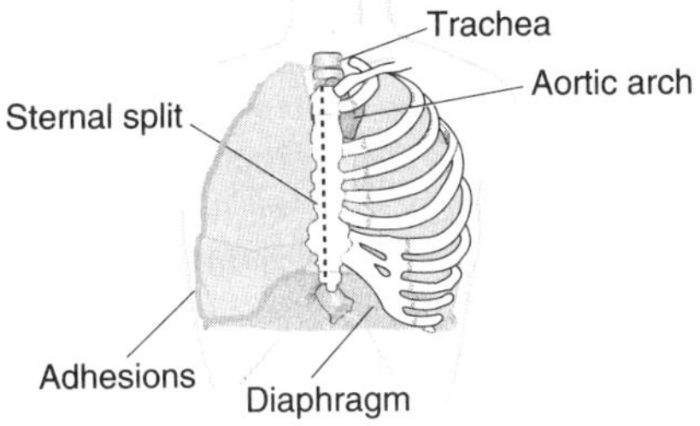

Explanation

The physician opens the chest cavity widely to directly visualize and separate the surface of the lung, which has become adherent to the inside surface of the chest cavity. Using a scalpel, the surgeon makes a long incision around the side of the chest between two of the ribs. The incision is carried through all of the tissue layers into the chest cavity. Rib spreaders are inserted into the wound and the ribs are spread apart exposing the lung. Alternately, the chest cavity can be opened and the operation performed through a vertical incision in the center of the chest through the sternum. The skin incision is carried down to the sternum bone and a saw is used to split the sternum. With the sternum split in half, the chest is entered by spreading the sternum apart with a set of rib spreaders. Using a gloved hand and a large moist gauze sponge, the surgeon manually divides the tissues attaching the lung to the wall of the chest cavity. When the procedure is complete, the instruments and gauze sponges are removed. A chest tube(s) may be used to provide drainage for the chest cavity. If applicable, the sternotomy is repaired using wires to bring the two halves of the sternum together, and the operative wound is closed by sutures or staples.

Coding Tips

If total decortication, including intrapleural pneumonolysis, is performed via thoracoscopy, see 32652.

ICD-10-CM Diagnostic Codes

A15.0	Tuberculosis of lung
A15.6	Tuberculous pleurisy
B90.9	Sequelae of respiratory and unspecified tuberculosis

Relative Value Units/Medicare Edits

Non-Facility RVU	Work	PE	MP	Total
32124	15.45	8.31	3.63	27.39
Facility RVU	**Work**	**PE**	**MP**	**Total**
32124	15.45	8.31	3.63	27.39

	FUD	Status	MUE	Modifiers				IOM Reference
32124	90	A	1(3)	51	N/A	62*	80	None

* with documentation

Terms To Know

adhesion. Abnormal fibrous connection between two structures, soft tissue or bony structures, that may occur as the result of surgery, infection, or trauma.

complication. Condition arising after the beginning of observation and treatment that modifies the course of the patient's illness or the medical care required, or an undesired result or misadventure in medical care.

decortication of lung. Removal of a constricting membrane or layer of pleural tissue from a portion of the lung surface to allow for lung expansion.

effusion. Escape of fluid from within a body cavity.

empyema. Accumulation of pus within the respiratory or pleural cavity.

fistula. Abnormal tube-like passage between two body cavities or organs or from an organ to the outside surface.

iatrogenic. Adversely induced in the patient; caused by medical treatment.

incision. Act of cutting into tissue or an organ.

late effect. Abnormality, dysfunction, or other residual condition produced after the acute phase of an illness, injury, or disease is over. There is no time limit on when late effects can appear.

pleurisy. Inflammation of the serous membrane that lines the lungs and the thoracic cavity. Pleurisy may cause effusion within the cavity or have exudate in the pleural space or on the membrane surface.

thoracotomy. Surgical procedure for opening the chest wall in order to access the lungs, esophagus, trachea, aorta, heart, and diaphragm.

32140

32140 Thoracotomy; with cyst(s) removal, includes pleural procedure when performed

Explanation

The physician opens the chest cavity widely to remove one or more lung cysts. Using a scalpel, the surgeon makes a long incision around the side of the chest between two of the ribs. The incision is carried through all of the tissue layers into the chest cavity. Rib spreaders are inserted into the wound and the ribs are spread apart exposing the lung. Alternately, the chest cavity can be opened and the operation performed through a vertical incision in the center of the chest through the sternum. The skin incision is carried down to the sternum bone and a saw is used to split the sternum. With the sternum split in half, the chest is entered by spreading the sternum apart with a set of rib spreaders. Space is made in the chest by packing the uninvolved lung away from the operative field by using large moist gauze sponges. In order to perform the procedure, the pleural surface may require an operative procedure such as pneumonolysis (separation of the surface of the lung that has become adherent to the inside surface of the chest cavity). The lung cyst is located and removed by sharp and blunt dissection of the tissues. When the procedure is complete, the instruments and gauze sponges are removed. A chest tube(s) may be used to provide drainage for the chest cavity. If applicable, the sternotomy is repaired using wires to bring the two halves of the sternum together, and the operative wound is closed by sutures or staples.

Coding Tips

For surgical thoracoscopy with excision of a pericardial cyst, tumor, or mass, see 32661; with excision of a mediastinal cyst, tumor, or mass, see 32662.

ICD-10-CM Diagnostic Codes

B67.1	Echinococcus granulosus infection of lung
J98.4	Other disorders of lung
Q33.0	Congenital cystic lung

Relative Value Units/Medicare Edits

Non-Facility RVU	Work	PE	MP	Total
32140	16.66	8.64	4.11	29.41
Facility RVU	**Work**	**PE**	**MP**	**Total**
32140	16.66	8.64	4.11	29.41

	FUD	Status	MUE	Modifiers				IOM Reference
32140	90	A	1(3)	51	N/A	62*	80	None

* with documentation

Terms To Know

cyst. Elevated encapsulated mass containing fluid, semisolid, or solid material with a membranous lining.

excision. Surgical removal of an organ or tissue.

lesion. Area of damaged tissue that has lost continuity or function, due to disease or trauma.

thoracotomy. Surgical procedure for opening the chest wall in order to access the lungs, esophagus, trachea, aorta, heart, and diaphragm.

32141

32141 Thoracotomy; with resection-plication of bullae, includes any pleural procedure when performed

Explanation

The physician opens the chest cavity widely to remove one or more lung bullae (large non-functional air sacs). Using a scalpel, the surgeon makes a long incision around the side of the chest between two of the ribs. The incision is carried through all of the tissue layers into the chest cavity. Rib spreaders are inserted into the wound and the ribs are spread apart exposing the lung. Alternately, the chest cavity can be opened and the operation performed through a vertical incision in the center of the chest through the sternum. The skin incision is carried down to the sternum bone and a saw is used to split the sternum. With the sternum split in half, the chest is entered by spreading the sternum apart with a set of rib spreaders. Space is made in the chest by packing the uninvolved lung away from the operative field using large moist gauze sponges. In order to perform the procedure, the pleural surface may require an operative procedure such as pneumonolysis (separation of the surface of the lung that has become adherent to the inside surface of the chest cavity). The lung bullae is located and removed by sharp and blunt dissection of the tissues and often by folding and suturing of the tissues (plication). When the procedure is complete, the instruments and gauze sponges are removed. A chest tube(s) may be used to provide drainage for the chest cavity. If applicable, the sternotomy is repaired using wires to bring the two halves of the sternum together, and the operative wound is closed by sutures or staples.

Coding Tips

To report thoracoscopy with excision or plication of bullae, including any pleural procedure, see 32655. For excision/plication of emphysematous lungs for lung volume reduction, see 32491.

ICD-10-CM Diagnostic Codes

J43.0	Unilateral pulmonary emphysema [MacLeod's syndrome]
J43.1	Panlobular emphysema
J43.2	Centrilobular emphysema
J43.8	Other emphysema
J43.9	Emphysema, unspecified

Relative Value Units/Medicare Edits

Non-Facility RVU	Work	PE	MP	Total
32141	27.18	11.21	6.53	44.92
Facility RVU	**Work**	**PE**	**MP**	**Total**
32141	27.18	11.21	6.53	44.92

	FUD	Status	MUE	Modifiers				IOM Reference
32141	90	A	1(3)	51	N/A	62*	80	None

* with documentation

Terms To Know

pleura. One of the two membranes that surround the lungs. The visceral pleura encases the lung and the parietal pleura lines the inner chest walls.

plication. Surgical technique involving folding, tucking, or pleating to reduce the size of a hollow structure or organ.

thoracotomy. Surgical procedure for opening the chest wall in order to access the lungs, esophagus, trachea, aorta, heart, and diaphragm.

32150-32151

32150 Thoracotomy; with removal of intrapleural foreign body or fibrin deposit
32151 with removal of intrapulmonary foreign body

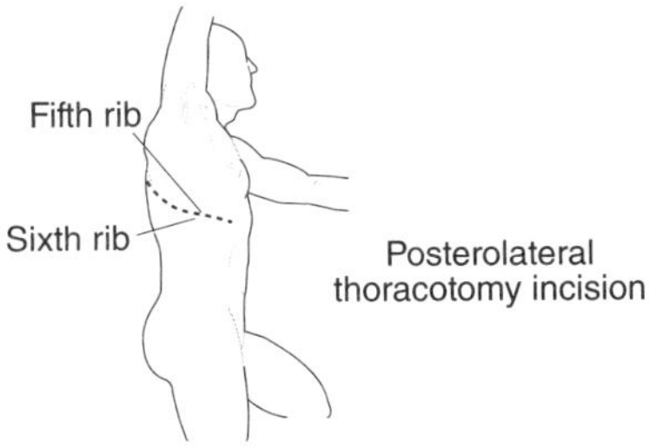

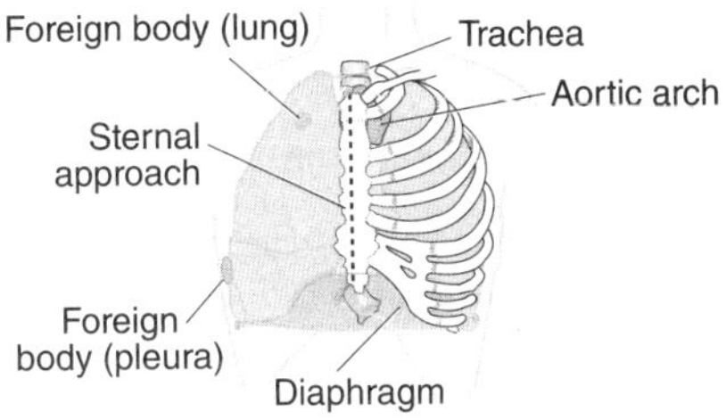

Explanation

The physician opens the chest cavity widely to remove a foreign body or fibrin deposit (thick insoluble protein deposit formed after the clotting of blood). Using a scalpel, the surgeon makes a long incision around the side of the chest between two of the ribs. The incision is carried through all of the tissue layers into the chest cavity. Rib spreaders are inserted into the wound and the ribs are spread apart exposing the lung. Alternately, the chest cavity can be opened and the operation performed through a vertical incision in the center of the chest through the sternum. The skin incision is carried down to the sternum bone and a saw is used to split the sternum. With the sternum split in half, the chest is entered by spreading the sternum apart with a set of rib spreaders. Space is made in the chest by packing the uninvolved lung away from the operative field using large moist gauze sponges. The foreign body or fibrin deposit is located and removed by sharp and blunt dissection. When the procedure is complete, the instruments and gauze sponges are removed. A chest tube(s) may be used to provide drainage for the chest cavity. If applicable, the sternotomy is repaired using wires to bring the two halves of the sternum together, and the operative wound is closed by sutures or staples. Report 32150 for removal of an intrapleural foreign body or fibrin deposits and 32151 for removal of an intrapulmonary foreign body.

Coding Tips

If removal of an intrapleural foreign body or a fibrin deposit is achieved by thoracoscopy, see 32653.

ICD-10-CM Diagnostic Codes

J92.0	Pleural plaque with presence of asbestos
J92.9	Pleural plaque without asbestos
J94.2	Hemothorax
S21.321A	Laceration with foreign body of right front wall of thorax with penetration into thoracic cavity, initial encounter
S21.322A	Laceration with foreign body of left front wall of thorax with penetration into thoracic cavity, initial encounter
S21.341A	Puncture wound with foreign body of right front wall of thorax with penetration into thoracic cavity, initial encounter
S21.342A	Puncture wound with foreign body of left front wall of thorax with penetration into thoracic cavity, initial encounter
S21.421A	Laceration with foreign body of right back wall of thorax with penetration into thoracic cavity, initial encounter
S21.422A	Laceration with foreign body of left back wall of thorax with penetration into thoracic cavity, initial encounter
S21.441A	Puncture wound with foreign body of right back wall of thorax with penetration into thoracic cavity, initial encounter
S21.442A	Puncture wound with foreign body of left back wall of thorax with penetration into thoracic cavity, initial encounter
S27.1XXA	Traumatic hemothorax, initial encounter
S27.2XXA	Traumatic hemopneumothorax, initial encounter
S27.311A	Primary blast injury of lung, unilateral, initial encounter
S27.312A	Primary blast injury of lung, bilateral, initial encounter ☑
S27.321A	Contusion of lung, unilateral, initial encounter
S27.322A	Contusion of lung, bilateral, initial encounter ☑
S27.331A	Laceration of lung, unilateral, initial encounter
S27.332A	Laceration of lung, bilateral, initial encounter ☑
S27.63XA	Laceration of pleura, initial encounter
S27.893A	Laceration of other specified intrathoracic organs, initial encounter
T81.510A	Adhesions due to foreign body accidentally left in body following surgical operation, initial encounter
T81.520A	Obstruction due to foreign body accidentally left in body following surgical operation, initial encounter
T81.530A	Perforation due to foreign body accidentally left in body following surgical operation, initial encounter
T81.590A	Other complications of foreign body accidentally left in body following surgical operation, initial encounter

Relative Value Units/Medicare Edits

Non-Facility RVU	Work	PE	MP	Total
32150	16.82	9.34	4.06	30.22
32151	16.94	8.72	4.18	29.84
Facility RVU	**Work**	**PE**	**MP**	**Total**
32150	16.82	9.34	4.06	30.22
32151	16.94	8.72	4.18	29.84

	FUD	Status	MUE	Modifiers				IOM Reference
32150	90	A	1(3)	51	N/A	62*	80	None
32151	90	A	1(3)	51	N/A	62*	80	

* with documentation

Terms To Know

blunt dissection. Surgical technique used to expose an underlying area by separating along natural cleavage lines of tissue, without cutting.

effusion. Escape of fluid from within a body cavity.

fibrin. Main fibrous composition of blood clots.

pleura. One of the two membranes that surround the lungs. The visceral pleura encases the lung and the parietal pleura lines the inner chest walls.

thoracotomy. Surgical procedure for opening the chest wall in order to access the lungs, esophagus, trachea, aorta, heart, and diaphragm.

● New ▲ Revised + Add On ★ Telemedicine [Resequenced] ☑ Laterality

32160

32160 Thoracotomy; with cardiac massage

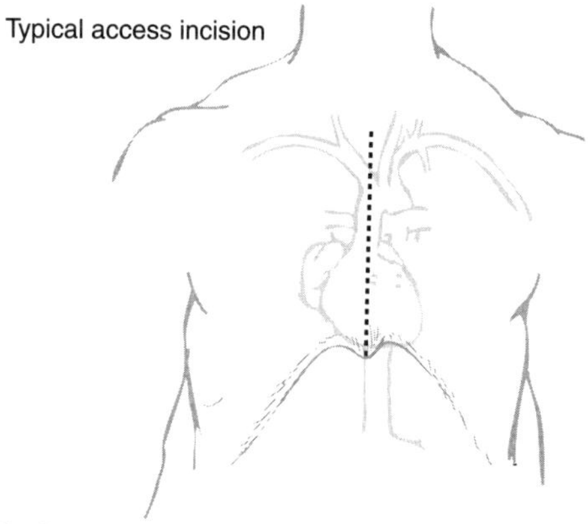

The heart is accessed through a major thoracotomy and direct cardiac massage is initiated

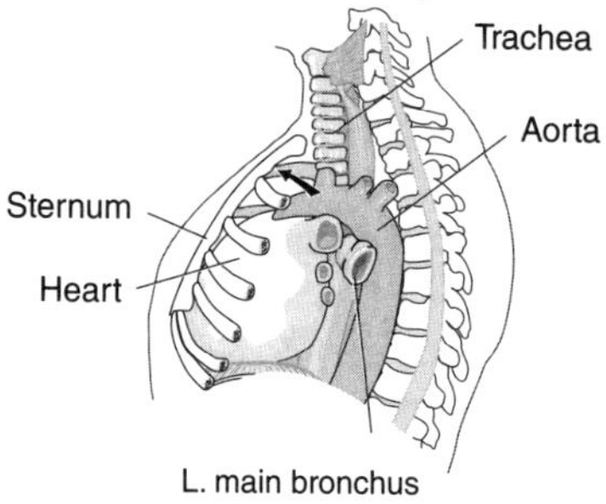

Explanation

The physician opens the chest cavity widely to perform manual cardiac massage in the case of cardiac arrest. Using a scalpel, the surgeon makes a long incision around the side of the chest between two of the ribs. The incision is carried through all of the tissue layers into the chest cavity. Rib spreaders are inserted into the wound and the ribs are spread apart exposing the lung. Alternately, the chest cavity can be opened and the operation performed through a vertical incision in the center of the chest through the sternum. The skin incision is carried down to the sternum bone and a saw is used to split the sternum. With the sternum split in half, the chest is entered by spreading the sternum apart with a set of rib spreaders. Space is made in the chest by packing the uninvolved lung away from the operative field using large moist gauze sponges. The heart is exposed and squeezed rhythmically to mimic cardiac contractions, thus pumping blood through the body. The heart may be directly contra-shocked to produce spontaneous heartbeats. When the procedure is complete, the instruments and gauze sponges are removed. A chest tube(s) may be used to provide drainage for the chest cavity. If applicable, the sternotomy is repaired using wires to bring the two halves of the sternum together, and the operative wound is closed by sutures or staples.

Coding Tips

For closed cardiopulmonary resuscitation, see 92950. For other resections of the lung, see 32480–32504.

ICD-10-CM Diagnostic Codes

I46.2	Cardiac arrest due to underlying cardiac condition
I46.8	Cardiac arrest due to other underlying condition
I46.9	Cardiac arrest, cause unspecified
I97.120	Postprocedural cardiac arrest following cardiac surgery
I97.121	Postprocedural cardiac arrest following other surgery
I97.710	Intraoperative cardiac arrest during cardiac surgery
I97.711	Intraoperative cardiac arrest during other surgery

Relative Value Units/Medicare Edits

Non-Facility RVU	Work	PE	MP	Total
32160	13.1	7.59	3.04	23.73
Facility RVU	**Work**	**PE**	**MP**	**Total**
32160	13.1	7.59	3.04	23.73

	FUD	Status	MUE	Modifiers				IOM Reference
32160	90	A	1(3)	51	N/A	62*	80	None

* with documentation

Terms To Know

cardiac arrest. Sudden, unexpected cessation of cardiac action, including absence of heart sounds and/or blood pressure.

incision. Act of cutting into tissue or an organ.

massage. Systematic and patterned stroking, kneading, and therapeutic friction applied to soft tissue by hand.

resuscitation. Restoration to life or consciousness of one apparently dead, it includes such measures as artificial respiration and cardiac massage or electrical shock.

sternotomy. Incision into the sternum, the bone that forms the front of the chest cavity and connects with the ribs.

suture. Numerous stitching techniques employed in wound closure.

thoracotomy. Surgical procedure for opening the chest wall in order to access the lungs, esophagus, trachea, aorta, heart, and diaphragm.

32200

32200 Pneumonostomy, with open drainage of abscess or cyst

Explanation

The physician treats an abscess or cyst in the lung by draining the pus or fluid directly through the chest wall. Using a scalpel, the skin between two ribs is incised and the tissues separated to expose the inside of the chest cavity. The lung is cut with scissors or a scalpel down to the abscess or the cyst. The abscess or cyst is opened and the fluid is allowed to drain through the wound created in the lung and the chest wall. A rubber drainage tube may be left in place to maintain or facilitate drainage. The incision is not sutured closed. The outside incision is dressed with bulky gauze dressing to absorb the drainage.

Coding Tips

A pneumonostomy is performed for abscess or cyst within the lung. For empyema, an accumulation of pus in the pleural space, see 32035–32036. For drainage of an abscess in the thoracic cavity by tube thoracostomy, see 32551. For a percutaneous image-guided drainage of an abscess or cyst of the lungs by catheter placement, see 49405.

ICD-10-CM Diagnostic Codes

B67.1	Echinococcus granulosus infection of lung
J85.0	Gangrene and necrosis of lung
J85.1	Abscess of lung with pneumonia
J85.2	Abscess of lung without pneumonia
J86.0	Pyothorax with fistula
J86.9	Pyothorax without fistula
J98.4	Other disorders of lung
Q33.0	Congenital cystic lung

Relative Value Units/Medicare Edits

Non-Facility RVU	Work	PE	MP	Total
32200	18.68	10.61	4.6	33.89
Facility RVU	**Work**	**PE**	**MP**	**Total**
32200	18.68	10.61	4.6	33.89

	FUD	Status	MUE	Modifiers				IOM Reference
32200	90	A	2(3)	51	N/A	62*	80	None

* with documentation

Terms To Know

abscess. Circumscribed collection of pus resulting from bacteria, frequently associated with swelling and other signs of inflammation.

emphysematous bleb. Formation of blisters or vesicles greater than 1.0 mm within an emphysematous lung, containing serum or blood.

empyema. Accumulation of pus within the respiratory or pleural cavity.

mediastinum. Collection of organs and tissues that separate the pleural sacs. Located between the sternum and spine above the diaphragm, it contains the heart and great vessels, trachea and bronchi, esophagus, thymus, lymph nodes, and nerves.

pneumonotomy. Surgical incision into a lung.

thoracostomy. Creation of an opening in the chest wall for drainage.

32215

32215 Pleural scarification for repeat pneumothorax

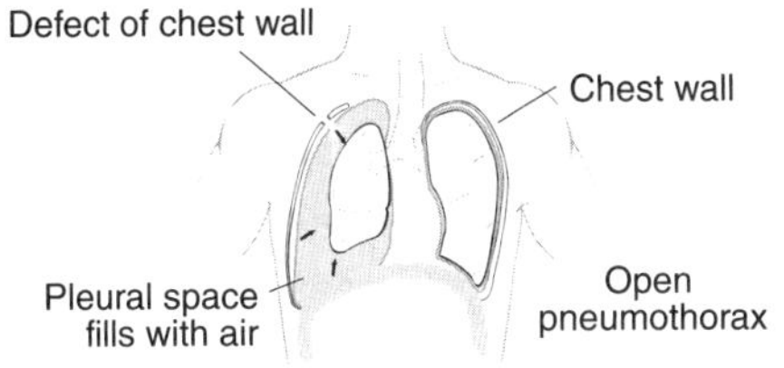

Pneumothorax is the presence of air in the pleural space. The lung may collapse, as shown, and a life-threatening situation arise

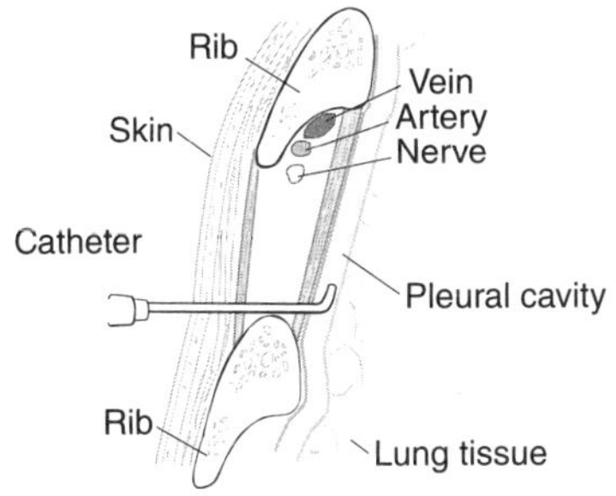

Injecting an abrasive chemical solution into the pleural space causes it to scar and adhere to the cavity walls. The pleural space is effectively eliminated, preventing pneumothorax

Explanation

The physician treats repeat pneumothorax by producing adhesions between the surface of the lung and the inside surface of the chest cavity. To create the adhesions, a chemical solution is injected into the chest cavity and allowed to circulate over the surface of the lung and the inside surface of the chest cavity. The physician injects the solution by passing a tube into the chest cavity. The physician passes a trocar over the top of a rib and punctures through the chest tissues between the ribs and enters the pleural cavity. With the end of the trocar in the chest cavity, the physician advances the plastic tube into the chest cavity. The sharp instrument is removed leaving one end of the plastic catheter in place within the chest cavity. A syringe is attached to the outside end of the catheter and fluid is injected into the chest cavity. The fluid selected is designed to cause the formation of adhesive scar tissue between the surface of the lung and the inside surface of the chest cavity. Once the lung adheres to the chest wall it can no longer collapse and allow the formation of a pneumothorax.

Coding Tips

To report chemical pleurodesis for recurrent or persistent pneumothorax, see 32560.

ICD-10-CM Diagnostic Codes

J93.0	Spontaneous tension pneumothorax
J93.11	Primary spontaneous pneumothorax
J93.12	Secondary spontaneous pneumothorax
J93.81	Chronic pneumothorax
J93.83	Other pneumothorax
J95.811	Postprocedural pneumothorax
J95.812	Postprocedural air leak
P25.1	Pneumothorax originating in the perinatal period N

Relative Value Units/Medicare Edits

Non-Facility RVU	Work	PE	MP	Total
32215	13.05	7.62	3.22	23.89
Facility RVU	**Work**	**PE**	**MP**	**Total**
32215	13.05	7.62	3.22	23.89

	FUD	Status	MUE	Modifiers				IOM Reference
32215	90	A	1(2)	51	50	62*	80	None

* with documentation

Terms To Know

adhesion. Abnormal fibrous connection between two structures, soft tissue or bony structures, that may occur as the result of surgery, infection, or trauma.

catheter. Flexible tube inserted into an area of the body for introducing or withdrawing fluid.

iatrogenic pneumothorax. Air trapped in the lining of the lung following surgery.

pleura. One of the two membranes that surround the lungs. The visceral pleura encases the lung and the parietal pleura lines the inner chest walls.

scarification. Process of making scratches or small cuts in the skin or tissue.

spontaneous tension pneumothorax. Air leaking from the lung and trapped in the lung lining.

trocar. Cannula or a sharp pointed instrument used to puncture and aspirate fluid from cavities.

32220-32225

32220 Decortication, pulmonary (separate procedure); total
32225 partial

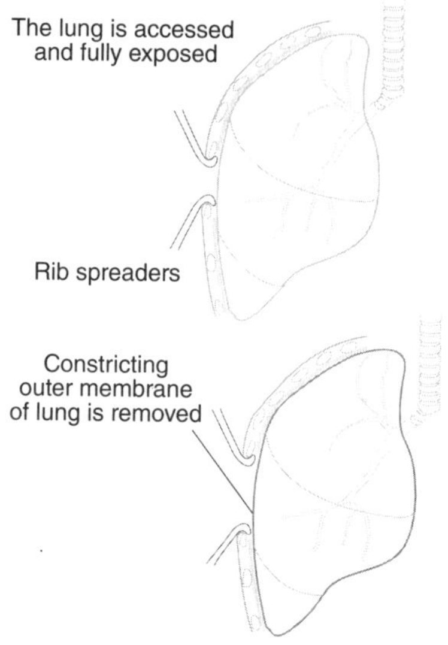

Explanation

The physician removes a constricting membrane or layer of tissue from the surface of the lung (decortication) in order to permit the lung to fully expand. The physician opens the chest cavity widely. Using a scalpel, the surgeon makes a long incision around the side of the chest between two of the ribs. The incision is carried through all the tissue layers into the chest cavity. Rib spreaders are inserted into the wound and the ribs are spread apart exposing the lung. The constricting membrane is stripped off the surface of the lung. In 32225, only a portion of the lung surface is removed. The chest wall incision is sutured closed in layers. A chest tube(s) may be used to provide drainage for the chest cavity. Alternately, the chest cavity can be opened by a vertical incision in the front of the chest through the sternum. The skin incision is carried down to the sternum bone and a saw is used to split the sternum. With the sternum split in half, the chest is entered by spreading the sternum apart with a set of rib spreaders. When the procedure is complete, the wound is closed by using wires to bring the two halves of the sternum together and the skin is closed by suturing.

Coding Tips

These separate procedures by definition are usually a component of a more complex service and are not identified separately. When performed alone or with other unrelated procedures/services, they may be reported. If performed alone, list the code; if performed with other procedures/services, list the code and append modifier 59 or an X{EPSU} modifier. If the procedure is attempted thoracoscopically, but requires major thoracotomy for completion, report 32220 or 32225 for the open portion of the procedure and report a diagnostic thoracoscopy, 32601, as a secondary procedure. For decortication and parietal pleurectomy, see 32320. For surgical thoracoscopy with partial pulmonary decortication, see 32651; with total decortication, including intrapleural pneumonolysis, see 32652.

ICD-10-CM Diagnostic Codes

A15.0	Tuberculosis of lung
A15.6	Tuberculous pleurisy
C38.4	Malignant neoplasm of pleura
C45.0	Mesothelioma of pleura

C78.2	Secondary malignant neoplasm of pleura
J86.0	Pyothorax with fistula
J86.9	Pyothorax without fistula
J91.0	Malignant pleural effusion
J94.1	Fibrothorax
J94.2	Hemothorax
N80.B2	Endometriosis of lung
N80.B6	Endometriosis of cardiothoracic space
S27.1XXA	Traumatic hemothorax, initial encounter
S27.2XXA	Traumatic hemopneumothorax, initial encounter

Relative Value Units/Medicare Edits

Non-Facility RVU	Work	PE	MP	Total
32220	26.65	14.29	6.48	47.42
32225	16.75	8.73	4.04	29.52
Facility RVU	**Work**	**PE**	**MP**	**Total**
32220	26.65	14.29	6.48	47.42
32225	16.75	8.73	4.04	29.52

	FUD	Status	MUE	Modifiers				IOM Reference
32220	90	A	1(2)	51	50	62*	80	None
32225	90	A	1(2)	51	50	62*	80	

* with documentation

Terms To Know

abscess. Circumscribed collection of pus resulting from bacteria, frequently associated with swelling and other signs of inflammation.

fibrosis. Formation of fibrous tissue as part of the restorative process.

incision. Act of cutting into tissue or an organ.

malignant. Any condition tending to progress toward death, specifically an invasive tumor with a loss of cellular differentiation that has the ability to spread or metastasize to other body areas.

neoplasm. New abnormal growth, tumor.

secondary. Second in order of occurrence or importance, or appearing during the course of another disease or condition.

32310

32310 Pleurectomy, parietal (separate procedure)

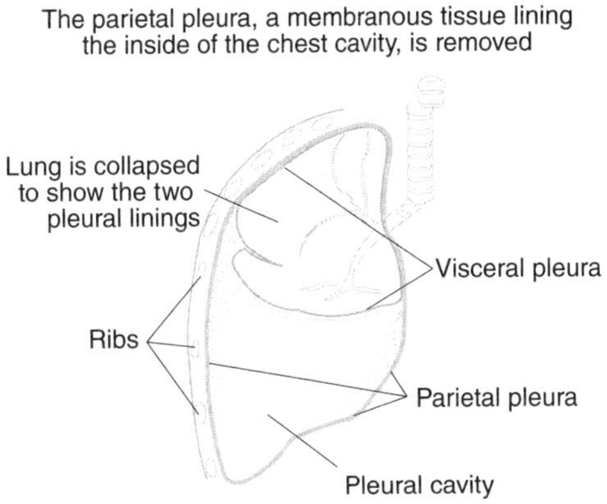

Explanation

The physician removes the membranous tissue lining the inside surface of the chest cavity (the parietal pleura). The physician opens the chest cavity widely to gain access to the inside surface of the chest. Using a scalpel, the surgeon makes a long incision around the side of the chest between two of the ribs. The incision is carried through all the tissue layers into the chest cavity. Rib spreaders are inserted into the wound and the ribs are spread apart exposing the lung. The parietal pleura is stripped from the inside surface of the chest. The chest wall incision is sutured closed in layers. A chest tube(s) may be used to provide drainage for the chest cavity. Alternately, the chest cavity can be opened and the operation performed through a vertical incision in the center of the chest through the sternum. The skin incision is carried down to the sternum bone and a saw is used to split the sternum. With the sternum split in half, the chest is entered by spreading the sternum apart with a set of rib spreaders. When the procedure is complete, the wound is closed by using wires to bring the two halves of the sternum together and the skin is closed over the sternum by suturing.

Coding Tips

This separate procedure by definition is usually a component of a more complex service and is not identified separately. When performed alone or with other unrelated procedures/services, it may be reported. If performed alone, list the code; if performed with other procedures/services, list the code and append modifier 59 or an X{EPSU} modifier. If the procedure is attempted thoracoscopically, but requires major thoracotomy for completion, report 32310 for the open portion of the procedure and report a diagnostic thoracoscopy, 32601, as a secondary procedure. For surgical thoracoscopy with parietal pleurectomy, see 32656.

ICD-10-CM Diagnostic Codes

A15.0	Tuberculosis of lung
C38.4	Malignant neoplasm of pleura
C45.0	Mesothelioma of pleura
C78.2	Secondary malignant neoplasm of pleura
J86.0	Pyothorax with fistula
J86.9	Pyothorax without fistula
J91.0	Malignant pleural effusion
J93.0	Spontaneous tension pneumothorax
J93.11	Primary spontaneous pneumothorax
J93.12	Secondary spontaneous pneumothorax
J93.81	Chronic pneumothorax

Lungs and Pleura

● New ▲ Revised + Add On ★ Telemedicine [Resequenced] ☑ Laterality

J93.82	Other air leak
J93.83	Other pneumothorax
J94.1	Fibrothorax
J94.2	Hemothorax
J94.8	Other specified pleural conditions
J95.811	Postprocedural pneumothorax
J95.812	Postprocedural air leak
N80.B1	Endometriosis of pleura
P25.1	Pneumothorax originating in the perinatal period N
S27.2XXA	Traumatic hemopneumothorax, initial encounter

Relative Value Units/Medicare Edits

Non-Facility RVU	Work	PE	MP	Total
32310	15.28	8.24	3.77	27.29
Facility RVU	**Work**	**PE**	**MP**	**Total**
32310	15.28	8.24	3.77	27.29

	FUD	Status	MUE	Modifiers				IOM Reference
32310	90	A	1(3)	51	N/A	62*	80	None

* with documentation

Terms To Know

diaphragm. Muscular wall separating the thorax and its structures from the abdomen.

pleura. One of the two membranes that surround the lungs. The visceral pleura encases the lung and the parietal pleura lines the inner chest walls.

pneumothorax. Collapsed lung due to air or gas trapped in the pleural space formed by the membrane that encloses the lungs and lines the thoracic cavity.

Lungs and Pleura

32320

32320 Decortication and parietal pleurectomy

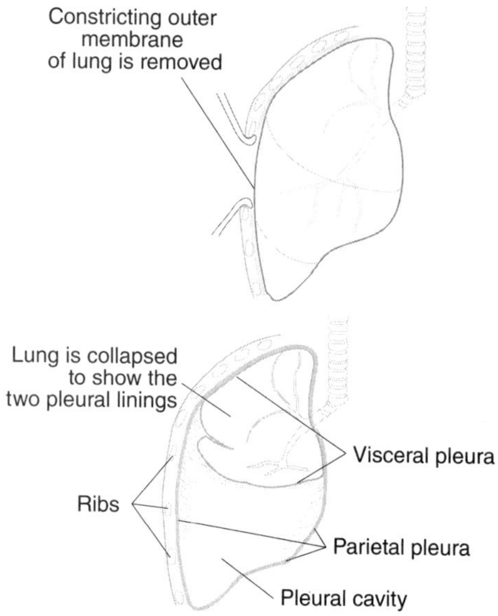

Explanation

The physician removes a constricting membrane or layer of tissue from a portion of the surface of the lung (decortication) in order to permit the lung to fully expand and also removes the membranous tissue lining the inside surface of the chest cavity (the parietal pleura). The physician opens the chest cavity widely. Using a scalpel, the surgeon makes a long incision around the side of the chest between two of the ribs. The incision is carried through all the tissue layers into the chest cavity. Rib spreaders are inserted into the wound and the ribs are spread apart exposing the lung. The constricting membrane is stripped off the surface of the lung. The parietal pleura is stripped from the inside surface of the chest. The chest wall incision is sutured closed in layers. A chest tube(s) may be used to provide drainage for the chest cavity. Alternately, the chest cavity can be opened and the operation performed through a vertical incision in the center of the chest through the sternum. The skin incision is carried down to the sternum bone and a saw is used to split the sternum. With the sternum split in half, the chest is entered by spreading the sternum apart with a set of rib spreaders. When the procedure is complete, the wound is closed by using wires to bring the two halves of the sternum together and the skin is closed over the sternum by suturing.

Coding Tips

For partial decortication only, see 32225. For total decortication only, see 32220. For parietal pleurectomy only, see 32310. For surgical thoracoscopy with partial pulmonary decortication, see 32651. For surgical thoracoscopy with parietal pleurectomy, see 32656.

ICD-10-CM Diagnostic Codes

A15.0	Tuberculosis of lung
A15.6	Tuberculous pleurisy
C38.4	Malignant neoplasm of pleura
C45.0	Mesothelioma of pleura
C78.2	Secondary malignant neoplasm of pleura
J86.0	Pyothorax with fistula
J86.9	Pyothorax without fistula
J91.0	Malignant pleural effusion

N Newborn: 0 P Pediatric: 0-17 M Maternity: 9-64 A Adult: 15-124 AMA: CPT Assist

J93.0	Spontaneous tension pneumothorax
J93.11	Primary spontaneous pneumothorax
J93.12	Secondary spontaneous pneumothorax
J93.81	Chronic pneumothorax
J93.82	Other air leak
J93.83	Other pneumothorax
J94.1	Fibrothorax
J94.2	Hemothorax
J94.8	Other specified pleural conditions
J95.811	Postprocedural pneumothorax
J95.812	Postprocedural air leak
N80.B1	Endometriosis of pleura
P25.1	Pneumothorax originating in the perinatal period N
S27.2XXA	Traumatic hemopneumothorax, initial encounter

Relative Value Units/Medicare Edits

Non-Facility RVU	Work	PE	MP	Total
32320	27.25	13.7	6.61	47.56
Facility RVU	**Work**	**PE**	**MP**	**Total**
32320	27.25	13.7	6.61	47.56

	FUD	Status	MUE	Modifiers				IOM Reference
32320	90	A	1(3)	51	N/A	62*	80	None

* with documentation

Terms To Know

decortication of lung. Removal of a constricting membrane or layer of pleural tissue from a portion of the lung surface to allow for lung expansion.

pleura. One of the two membranes that surround the lungs. The visceral pleura encases the lung and the parietal pleura lines the inner chest walls.

pleural effusion. Collection of lymph and other fluid within the pleural space.

pneumothorax. Collapsed lung due to air or gas trapped in the pleural space formed by the membrane that encloses the lungs and lines the thoracic cavity.

32400

32400 Biopsy, pleura, percutaneous needle

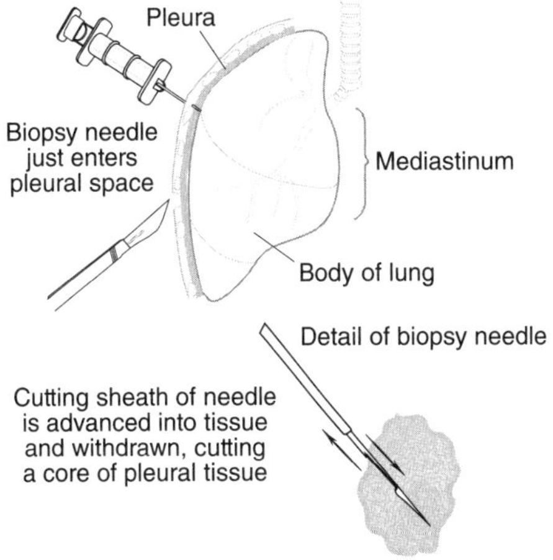

Explanation

The physician obtains a sample of the lining of the lung and/or the lining of the inside of the chest cavity by needle biopsy. Using a pleural biopsy needle, the physician passes the needle over the top of a rib, punctures through the chest tissues between two ribs, enters the pleural cavity and slightly punctures the surface of the lung. With the end of the needle in the chest cavity, the physician withdraws a piece of tissue. The needle is withdrawn and the puncture site covered with a bandage. The procedure is often done under radiological guidance to assure more precise placement of the needle.

Coding Tips

For fine needle aspiration, see 10004-10012 and 10021. For percutaneous biopsy, lung or mediastinum, see 32408. For a diagnostic thoracoscopy with biopsy of the lungs and pleural space, see 32607, 32608, and/or 32609. For open biopsy of the pleura, see 32098. If imaging guidance is performed, see 76942, 77002, 77012, or 77021.

ICD-10-CM Diagnostic Codes

A15.6	Tuberculous pleurisy
C38.4	Malignant neoplasm of pleura
C38.8	Malignant neoplasm of overlapping sites of heart, mediastinum and pleura
C45.0	Mesothelioma of pleura
C78.2	Secondary malignant neoplasm of pleura
D19.0	Benign neoplasm of mesothelial tissue of pleura
D38.2	Neoplasm of uncertain behavior of pleura
J86.0	Pyothorax with fistula
J86.9	Pyothorax without fistula
J90	Pleural effusion, not elsewhere classified
J91.0	Malignant pleural effusion
J91.8	Pleural effusion in other conditions classified elsewhere
J92.0	Pleural plaque with presence of asbestos
J92.9	Pleural plaque without asbestos
J94.0	Chylous effusion
J94.1	Fibrothorax
J94.2	Hemothorax
J94.8	Other specified pleural conditions

M32.13	Lung involvement in systemic lupus erythematosus
N80.B1	Endometriosis of pleura
Q34.0	Anomaly of pleura

AMA: **32400** 2023,Jan; 2019,Apr

Relative Value Units/Medicare Edits

Non-Facility RVU	Work	PE	MP	Total
32400	1.76	3.1	0.18	5.04
Facility RVU	**Work**	**PE**	**MP**	**Total**
32400	1.76	0.52	0.18	2.46

	FUD	Status	MUE	Modifiers				IOM Reference
32400	0	A	2(3)	51	N/A	N/A	N/A	None

* with documentation

Terms To Know

effusion. Escape of fluid from within a body cavity.

percutaneous approach. Method used to gain access to a body organ or specific area by puncture or minor incision through the skin or mucous membrane and/or any other body layers necessary to reach the procedure site.

pleura. One of the two membranes that surround the lungs. The visceral pleura encases the lung and the parietal pleura lines the inner chest walls.

32408

32408 Core needle biopsy, lung or mediastinum, percutaneous, including imaging guidance, when performed

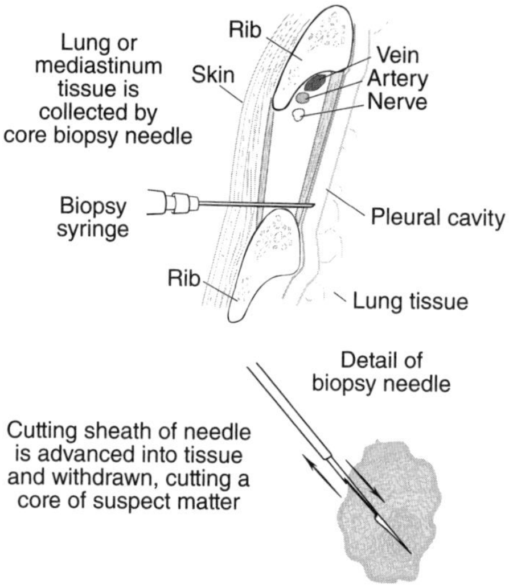

Explanation

The physician obtains a sample of the lung or the mediastinum (the tissues in the center of the chest between the two lung cavities) by puncturing through the space between two of the ribs with a needle. The procedure is often done under radiological guidance, which is included in this code when performed, to assure more precise placement of the needle. Using a core biopsy needle, the physician passes the needle over the top of a rib, punctures through the chest tissues, enters the pleural cavity, and punctures the area of concern in the lung or the mediastinum. With the end of the needle in the chest cavity, the physician withdraws a piece of tissue. The needle is withdrawn and the puncture site covered with a bandage.

Coding Tips

This code is reported only once per lesion sampled in a single session. Imaging guidance (76942, 77002, 77012, 77021) is included in this procedure and is not reported separately. If multiple lesions are biopsied, report 32408 for each site taken on separate lesions and append modifier 59 to additional codes. For open biopsy of the lung, see 32096 and 32097. For biopsy of the mediastinum, open, see 39000 and 39010. For thoracoscopic (VATS) biopsy of the lung, pleura, pericardium, or mediastinal space, see 32604, 32606, 32607, 32608, and 32609. For fine needle aspiration, see 10004-10012 and 10021.

ICD-10-CM Diagnostic Codes

A15.0	Tuberculosis of lung
C34.11	Malignant neoplasm of upper lobe, right bronchus or lung ☑
C34.12	Malignant neoplasm of upper lobe, left bronchus or lung ☑
C34.2	Malignant neoplasm of middle lobe, bronchus or lung
C34.31	Malignant neoplasm of lower lobe, right bronchus or lung ☑
C34.32	Malignant neoplasm of lower lobe, left bronchus or lung ☑
C34.81	Malignant neoplasm of overlapping sites of right bronchus and lung ☑
C34.82	Malignant neoplasm of overlapping sites of left bronchus and lung ☑
C37	Malignant neoplasm of thymus
C38.1	Malignant neoplasm of anterior mediastinum
C38.2	Malignant neoplasm of posterior mediastinum

C38.8 Malignant neoplasm of overlapping sites of heart, mediastinum and pleura
C46.51 Kaposi's sarcoma of right lung ☑
C46.52 Kaposi's sarcoma of left lung ☑
C78.01 Secondary malignant neoplasm of right lung ☑
C78.02 Secondary malignant neoplasm of left lung ☑
C78.1 Secondary malignant neoplasm of mediastinum
C7A.090 Malignant carcinoid tumor of the bronchus and lung
C7A.091 Malignant carcinoid tumor of the thymus
C81.02 Nodular lymphocyte predominant Hodgkin lymphoma, intrathoracic lymph nodes
C81.12 Nodular sclerosis Hodgkin lymphoma, intrathoracic lymph nodes
C81.22 Mixed cellularity Hodgkin lymphoma, intrathoracic lymph nodes
C81.32 Lymphocyte depleted Hodgkin lymphoma, intrathoracic lymph nodes
C81.42 Lymphocyte-rich Hodgkin lymphoma, intrathoracic lymph nodes
C81.72 Other Hodgkin lymphoma, intrathoracic lymph nodes
C82.02 Follicular lymphoma grade I, intrathoracic lymph nodes
C82.12 Follicular lymphoma grade II, intrathoracic lymph nodes
C82.32 Follicular lymphoma grade IIIa, intrathoracic lymph nodes
C82.52 Diffuse follicle center lymphoma, intrathoracic lymph nodes
C83.02 Small cell B-cell lymphoma, intrathoracic lymph nodes
C83.12 Mantle cell lymphoma, intrathoracic lymph nodes
C83.32 Diffuse large B-cell lymphoma, intrathoracic lymph nodes
C83.52 Lymphoblastic (diffuse) lymphoma, intrathoracic lymph nodes
C83.72 Burkitt lymphoma, intrathoracic lymph nodes
D02.21 Carcinoma in situ of right bronchus and lung ☑
D02.22 Carcinoma in situ of left bronchus and lung ☑
D09.3 Carcinoma in situ of thyroid and other endocrine glands
D14.31 Benign neoplasm of right bronchus and lung ☑
D14.32 Benign neoplasm of left bronchus and lung ☑
D15.2 Benign neoplasm of mediastinum
D17.4 Benign lipomatous neoplasm of intrathoracic organs
D38.1 Neoplasm of uncertain behavior of trachea, bronchus and lung
D38.3 Neoplasm of uncertain behavior of mediastinum
D38.4 Neoplasm of uncertain behavior of thymus
D3A.090 Benign carcinoid tumor of the bronchus and lung
Z11.1 Encounter for screening for respiratory tuberculosis

AMA: 32408 2023,Jan; 2021,Sep; 2021,Apr

Relative Value Units/Medicare Edits

Non-Facility RVU	Work	PE	MP	Total
32408	3.18	21.68	0.32	25.18
Facility RVU	**Work**	**PE**	**MP**	**Total**
32408	3.18	0.96	0.32	4.46

	FUD	Status	MUE	Modifiers				IOM Reference
32408	0	A	2(3)	51	N/A	N/A	N/A	None

* with documentation

32440

32440 Removal of lung, pneumonectomy;

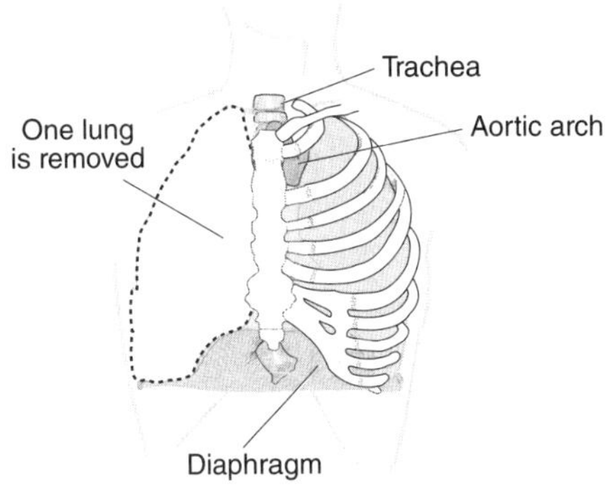

Bronchus and blood vessels are ligated at the root of the lung

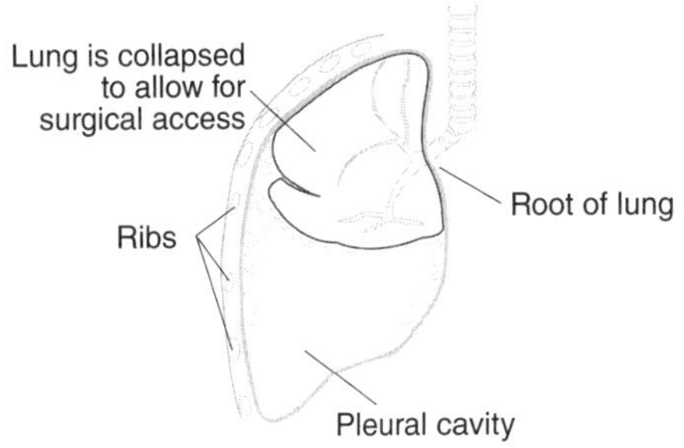

Explanation

The physician removes one lung in its entirety. The physician opens the chest cavity widely to gain access to the lung to be removed. Using a scalpel, the surgeon makes a long incision around the side of the chest between two of the ribs. The incision is carried through all of the tissue layers into the chest cavity. Rib spreaders are inserted into the wound and the ribs are spread apart exposing the lung, heart, and other structures. Alternately, the chest cavity can be opened and the operation performed through a vertical incision in the center of the chest through the sternum. The skin incision is carried down to the sternum bone and a saw is used to split the sternum. With the sternum split in half, the chest is entered by spreading the sternum apart with a set of rib spreaders. The root of the lung is found by pushing aside the deflated lung with a gloved hand and large moist gauze sponges. Within the root of the lung, the blood vessels and bronchial tubes are clamped, tied off, and cut. The lung is removed through the wide chest incision. The instruments and gauze sponges are removed. A chest tube(s) may be used to provide drainage for the chest cavity. When the procedure is complete, if applicable, the sternotomy is repaired using wires to bring the two halves of the sternum together, and the operative wound is closed by sutures or staples.

Coding Tips

For total pneumonectomy, extrapleural, see 32445. For single lobectomy, see 32480; bilobectomy, see 32482; for removal of partial lobe by segmentectomy, see 32484. For lung transplantation, see 32850–32856. For heart-lung transplant, including recipient cardiectomy-pneumonectomy, see 33935.

ICD-10-CM Diagnostic Codes

C34.01 Malignant neoplasm of right main bronchus ☑
C34.02 Malignant neoplasm of left main bronchus ☑
C34.11 Malignant neoplasm of upper lobe, right bronchus or lung ☑
C34.12 Malignant neoplasm of upper lobe, left bronchus or lung ☑
C34.2 Malignant neoplasm of middle lobe, bronchus or lung

C34.31	Malignant neoplasm of lower lobe, right bronchus or lung ☑
C34.32	Malignant neoplasm of lower lobe, left bronchus or lung ☑
C34.81	Malignant neoplasm of overlapping sites of right bronchus and lung ☑
C34.82	Malignant neoplasm of overlapping sites of left bronchus and lung ☑
C46.51	Kaposi's sarcoma of right lung ☑
C46.52	Kaposi's sarcoma of left lung ☑
C78.01	Secondary malignant neoplasm of right lung ☑
C78.02	Secondary malignant neoplasm of left lung ☑
C7A.090	Malignant carcinoid tumor of the bronchus and lung
D02.21	Carcinoma in situ of right bronchus and lung ☑
D02.22	Carcinoma in situ of left bronchus and lung ☑
D38.1	Neoplasm of uncertain behavior of trachea, bronchus and lung
J85.0	Gangrene and necrosis of lung

Relative Value Units/Medicare Edits

Non-Facility RVU	Work	PE	MP	Total
32440	27.28	12.42	6.7	46.4
Facility RVU	**Work**	**PE**	**MP**	**Total**
32440	27.28	12.42	6.7	46.4

	FUD	Status	MUE	Modifiers				IOM Reference
32440	90	A	1(2)	51	N/A	62*	80	None

* with documentation

Terms To Know

ligate. To tie off a blood vessel or duct with a suture or a soft, thin wire (ligature wire).

sternotomy. Incision into the sternum, the bone that forms the front of the chest cavity and connects with the ribs.

32442

32442 Removal of lung, pneumonectomy; with resection of segment of trachea followed by broncho-tracheal anastomosis (sleeve pneumonectomy)

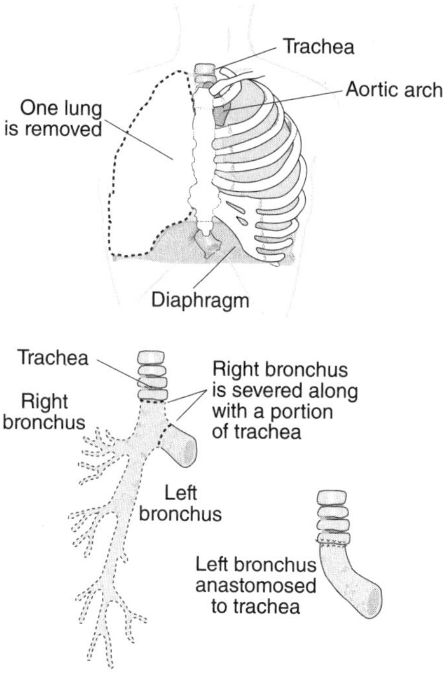

A total pneumonectomy is performed along with resection of a segment of the trachea followed by anastomosis

Explanation

The physician removes one lung in its entirety. The physician opens the chest cavity widely to gain access to the lung to be removed. Using a scalpel, the surgeon makes a long incision around the side of the chest between two of the ribs. The incision is carried through all of the tissue layers into the chest cavity. Rib spreaders are inserted into the wound and the ribs are spread apart exposing the lung, heart, and other structures. Alternately, the chest cavity can be opened and the operation performed through a vertical incision in the center of the chest through the sternum. The skin incision is carried down to the sternum bone and a saw is used to split the sternum. With the sternum split in half, the chest is entered by spreading the sternum apart with a set of rib spreaders. The root of the lung is found by pushing aside the deflated lung with a gloved hand and large moist gauze sponges. Within the root of the lung, the blood vessels and bronchial tubes are clamped, tied off, and cut. The lung and a segment of the trachea are removed through the wide chest incision. The trachea is sutured to the main bronchial tube of the remaining lung in the other half of the chest. The instruments and gauze sponges are removed. A chest tube(s) may be used to provide drainage for the chest cavity. When the procedure is complete, if applicable, the sternotomy is repaired using wires to bring the two halves of the sternum together, and the operative wound is closed by sutures or staples.

Coding Tips

For removal of lung, other than total pneumonectomy with circumferential resection of segment of bronchus followed by broncho-bronchial anastomosis (sleeve lobectomy), see 32486.

ICD-10-CM Diagnostic Codes

C33	Malignant neoplasm of trachea

C34.01	Malignant neoplasm of right main bronchus ☑
C34.02	Malignant neoplasm of left main bronchus ☑
C34.11	Malignant neoplasm of upper lobe, right bronchus or lung ☑
C34.12	Malignant neoplasm of upper lobe, left bronchus or lung ☑
C34.2	Malignant neoplasm of middle lobe, bronchus or lung
C34.31	Malignant neoplasm of lower lobe, right bronchus or lung ☑
C34.32	Malignant neoplasm of lower lobe, left bronchus or lung ☑
C34.81	Malignant neoplasm of overlapping sites of right bronchus and lung ☑
C34.82	Malignant neoplasm of overlapping sites of left bronchus and lung ☑
C46.51	Kaposi's sarcoma of right lung ☑
C46.52	Kaposi's sarcoma of left lung ☑
C78.01	Secondary malignant neoplasm of right lung ☑
C78.02	Secondary malignant neoplasm of left lung ☑
C7A.090	Malignant carcinoid tumor of the bronchus and lung
D02.21	Carcinoma in situ of right bronchus and lung ☑
D02.22	Carcinoma in situ of left bronchus and lung ☑
D38.1	Neoplasm of uncertain behavior of trachea, bronchus and lung
D3A.090	Benign carcinoid tumor of the bronchus and lung

Relative Value Units/Medicare Edits

Non-Facility RVU	Work	PE	MP	Total
32442	56.47	19.37	13.99	89.83
Facility RVU	**Work**	**PE**	**MP**	**Total**
32442	56.47	19.37	13.99	89.83

	FUD	Status	MUE	Modifiers				IOM Reference
32442	90	A	1(2)	51	N/A	62*	80	None

* with documentation

Terms To Know

carcinoma in situ. Malignancy that arises from the cells of the vessel, gland, or organ of origin that remains confined to that site or has not invaded neighboring tissue.

Kaposi's sarcoma. Malignant neoplasm caused by vascular proliferation of cutaneous tumors characterized by channels lined with endothelial tissue containing vascular spaced.

resection. Surgical removal of a part or all of an organ or body part.

32445

32445 Removal of lung, pneumonectomy; extrapleural

Explanation

The physician removes one lung in its entirety and the pleural membranes covering the lung and the inside surface of the chest cavity (the parietal pleura). The physician opens the chest cavity widely to gain access to the lung to be removed. Using a scalpel, the surgeon makes a long incision around the side of the chest between two of the ribs. The incision is carried through all of the tissue layers down to the membrane lining the chest cavity. Rib spreaders are inserted into the wound and the ribs are spread apart, taking care to preserve the integrity of the chest lining. Holding a gauze sponge, the surgeon strips away the lining inside the chest all the way around to the root of the lung. This creates a sac of the parietal pleura that contains the lung. Within the root of the lung, the blood vessels and bronchial tubes are clamped, tied off, and cut. The lung and the pleural tissues of the inside of the chest wall are removed through the wide chest incision. After the removal of the instruments and gauze sponges, the chest incision is sutured closed in layers. A chest tube(s) may be used to provide drainage for the chest cavity.

Coding Tips

If extrapleural pneumonectomy with empyectomy is performed, report 32540 in addition to 32445. For chest wall tumor resection performed with lung resection, see 21601-21603. For a single lobectomy, see 32480; bilobectomy, see 32482. For removal of a partial lobe by segmentectomy, see 32484. For lung transplantation, see 32850–32856. For a heart-lung transplant, including recipient cardiectomy-pneumonectomy, see 33935.

ICD-10-CM Diagnostic Codes

C45.0	Mesothelioma of pleura

Relative Value Units/Medicare Edits

Non-Facility RVU	Work	PE	MP	Total
32445	63.84	24.37	15.81	104.02
Facility RVU	**Work**	**PE**	**MP**	**Total**
32445	63.84	24.37	15.81	104.02

	FUD	Status	MUE	Modifiers				IOM Reference
32445	90	A	1(2)	51	N/A	62*	80	None

* with documentation

Terms To Know

carcinoma in situ. Malignancy that arises from the cells of the vessel, gland, or organ of origin that remains confined to that site or has not invaded neighboring tissue.

empyectomy. Removal of an accumulation of pus.

Kaposi's sarcoma. Malignant neoplasm caused by vascular proliferation of cutaneous tumors characterized by channels lined with endothelial tissue containing vascular spaced.

lobectomy. Excision of a lobe of an organ such as the liver, thyroid, lung, or brain.

pulmonary congestion. Excessive retention of interstitial fluid in the lungs and pulmonary vessels.

32480-32482

32480 Removal of lung, other than pneumonectomy; single lobe (lobectomy)

32482 2 lobes (bilobectomy)

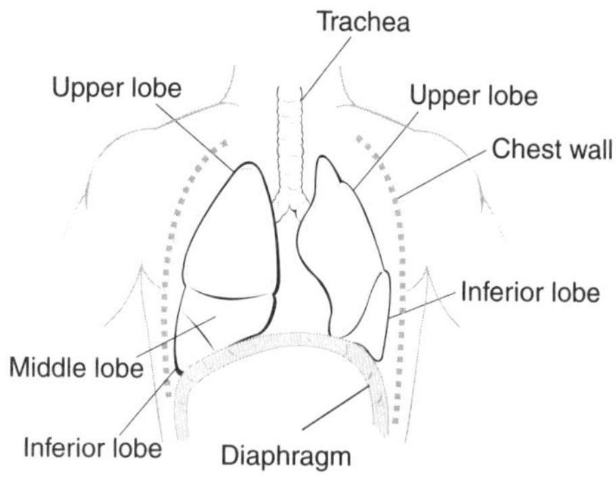

Explanation

The physician opens the chest cavity widely to gain access to the lung to be removed. Using a scalpel, the surgeon makes a long incision around the side of the chest between two of the ribs. The incision is carried through all of the tissue layers into the chest cavity. Rib spreaders are inserted into the wound and the ribs are spread apart exposing the lung. Alternately, the chest cavity can be opened and the operation performed through a vertical incision in the center of the chest through the sternum. The skin incision is carried down to the sternum bone and a saw is used to split the sternum. With the sternum split in half, the chest is entered by spreading the sternum apart with a set of rib spreaders. The lobe(s) to be removed is identified and isolated in the operative field by pushing aside the deflated lung with a gloved hand and large moist gauze sponges. Within the lobe(s) of the lung, the main blood vessels and bronchial tubes are clamped, tied off, and cut. The lobe(s) is removed through the wide chest incision. The instruments and gauze sponges are removed. A chest tube(s) may be used to provide drainage for the chest cavity. When the procedure is complete, if applicable, the sternotomy is repaired using wires to bring the two halves of the sternum together, and the operative wound is closed by sutures or staples. Report 32480 when one lobe is removed and 32482 when two lobes are removed.

Coding Tips

Diagnostic lung biopsies with intraoperative pathology that determines the need for resection or other definitive procedures should be reported using only the most complex service performed. If lung resection is performed with chest wall tumor resection, report the appropriate chest wall tumor resection code (21601–21603) in addition to 32480 or 32482. When concurrent decortication is performed with a lobectomy or segmentectomy, report 32320 in addition to 32480 or 32482. If bronchoplasty is performed at the time of a lobectomy, report 32501 in addition to 32480 or 32482. For removal of a single segment, see 32484; with circumferential resection of bronchus and reanastomosis, see 32486; for completion pneumonectomy, see 32488. For total pneumonectomy, see 32440. For surgical thoracoscopy, with total or segmental lobectomy, see 32663.

ICD-10-CM Diagnostic Codes

A15.0 Tuberculosis of lung
B44.0 Invasive pulmonary aspergillosis
B44.1 Other pulmonary aspergillosis
C34.01 Malignant neoplasm of right main bronchus ☑
C34.02 Malignant neoplasm of left main bronchus ☑
C34.11 Malignant neoplasm of upper lobe, right bronchus or lung ☑
C34.12 Malignant neoplasm of upper lobe, left bronchus or lung ☑
C34.2 Malignant neoplasm of middle lobe, bronchus or lung
C34.31 Malignant neoplasm of lower lobe, right bronchus or lung ☑
C34.32 Malignant neoplasm of lower lobe, left bronchus or lung ☑
C34.81 Malignant neoplasm of overlapping sites of right bronchus and lung ☑
C34.82 Malignant neoplasm of overlapping sites of left bronchus and lung ☑
C46.51 Kaposi's sarcoma of right lung ☑
C46.52 Kaposi's sarcoma of left lung ☑
C78.01 Secondary malignant neoplasm of right lung ☑
C78.02 Secondary malignant neoplasm of left lung ☑
C79.89 Secondary malignant neoplasm of other specified sites
C7A.090 Malignant carcinoid tumor of the bronchus and lung
D02.21 Carcinoma in situ of right bronchus and lung ☑
D02.22 Carcinoma in situ of left bronchus and lung ☑
D14.31 Benign neoplasm of right bronchus and lung ☑
D14.32 Benign neoplasm of left bronchus and lung ☑
D38.1 Neoplasm of uncertain behavior of trachea, bronchus and lung
D3A.090 Benign carcinoid tumor of the bronchus and lung
J43.0 Unilateral pulmonary emphysema [MacLeod's syndrome]
J43.1 Panlobular emphysema
J43.2 Centrilobular emphysema
J43.8 Other emphysema
J47.0 Bronchiectasis with acute lower respiratory infection
J47.1 Bronchiectasis with (acute) exacerbation
J85.0 Gangrene and necrosis of lung
J85.1 Abscess of lung with pneumonia
J85.2 Abscess of lung without pneumonia
J98.4 Other disorders of lung
Q33.2 Sequestration of lung

Relative Value Units/Medicare Edits

Non-Facility RVU	Work	PE	MP	Total
32480	25.82	11.65	6.27	43.74
32482	27.44	12.62	6.69	46.75
Facility RVU	**Work**	**PE**	**MP**	**Total**
32480	25.82	11.65	6.27	43.74
32482	27.44	12.62	6.69	46.75

	FUD	Status	MUE	Modifiers				IOM Reference
32480	90	A	1(2)	51	N/A	62*	80	None
32482	90	A	1(2)	51	N/A	62*	80	

* with documentation

Terms To Know

bronchiectasis. Dilation of the bronchi with mucous production and persistent cough due to infection or chronic conditions that causes diminished lung capacity and frequent infections of the lung.

32484

32484 Removal of lung, other than pneumonectomy; single segment (segmentectomy)

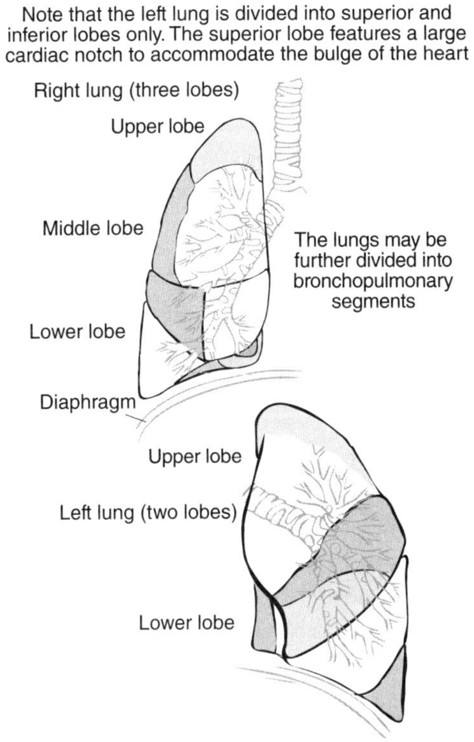

Explanation

The physician removes a segment of a lobe of one lung. The physician opens the chest cavity widely to gain access to the lung to be removed. Using a scalpel, the surgeon makes a long incision around the side of the chest between two of the ribs. The incision is carried through all of the tissue layers into the chest cavity. Rib spreaders are inserted into the wound and the ribs are spread apart exposing the lung. Alternately, the chest cavity can be opened and the operation performed through a vertical incision in the center of the chest through the sternum. The skin incision is carried down to the sternum bone and a saw is used to split the sternum. With the sternum split in half, the chest is entered by spreading the sternum apart with a set of rib spreaders. The segment to be removed is identified and isolated in the operative field by pushing aside the deflated lung with a gloved hand and large moist gauze sponges. Within the segment of the lung, the main blood vessels and bronchial tubes are clamped, tied off, and cut. The segment is removed through the wide chest incision. The instruments and gauze sponges are removed. A chest tube(s) may be used to provide drainage for the chest cavity. When the procedure is complete, if applicable, the sternotomy is repaired using wires to bring the two halves of the sternum together, and the operative wound is closed by sutures or staples.

Coding Tips

Diagnostic lung biopsies with intraoperative pathology that determines the need for resection or other definitive procedures should be reported using only the most complex service performed. If lung resection is performed with chest wall tumor resection, report the appropriate chest wall tumor resection code (21601–21603) in addition to 32484. When concurrent decortication is performed with lobectomy or segmentectomy, report 32320 in addition to 32484. If bronchoplasty is performed at the time of a segmentectomy, report 32501 in addition to 32484. For removal of a single lobe, see 32480; two lobes, see 32482; with circumferential resection of bronchus and reanastomosis, see 32486; for completion pneumonectomy, see 32488. For total pneumonectomy, see 32440. For surgical thoracoscopy, with total or segmental lobectomy, see 32663.

ICD-10-CM Diagnostic Codes

A15.0	Tuberculosis of lung
B44.0	Invasive pulmonary aspergillosis
B44.1	Other pulmonary aspergillosis
C34.01	Malignant neoplasm of right main bronchus ☑
C34.11	Malignant neoplasm of upper lobe, right bronchus or lung ☑
C34.2	Malignant neoplasm of middle lobe, bronchus or lung
C34.31	Malignant neoplasm of lower lobe, right bronchus or lung ☑
C34.81	Malignant neoplasm of overlapping sites of right bronchus and lung ☑
C46.51	Kaposi's sarcoma of right lung ☑
C78.01	Secondary malignant neoplasm of right lung ☑
C7A.090	Malignant carcinoid tumor of the bronchus and lung
D02.21	Carcinoma in situ of right bronchus and lung ☑
D14.31	Benign neoplasm of right bronchus and lung ☑
D38.1	Neoplasm of uncertain behavior of trachea, bronchus and lung
D3A.090	Benign carcinoid tumor of the bronchus and lung
J43.0	Unilateral pulmonary emphysema [MacLeod's syndrome]
J43.1	Panlobular emphysema
J43.2	Centrilobular emphysema
J43.8	Other emphysema
J47.0	Bronchiectasis with acute lower respiratory infection
J47.1	Bronchiectasis with (acute) exacerbation
J85.0	Gangrene and necrosis of lung
J85.1	Abscess of lung with pneumonia
J85.2	Abscess of lung without pneumonia
J98.4	Other disorders of lung
Q33.2	Sequestration of lung

Relative Value Units/Medicare Edits

Non-Facility RVU	Work	PE	MP	Total
32484	25.38	10.78	6.18	42.34
Facility RVU	**Work**	**PE**	**MP**	**Total**
32484	25.38	10.78	6.18	42.34

	FUD	Status	MUE	Modifiers				IOM Reference
32484	90	A	2(3)	51	N/A	62*	80	None

* with documentation

Terms To Know

emphysema. Pathological condition in which there is destructive enlargement of the air sacs in the lungs resulting in damage and lack of elasticity to the alveolar walls, commonly seen in long-term smokers.

pneumonectomy. Surgical removal of a lung or lung tissue.

segmentectomy. Removal of a segment of a gland or an organ.

32486

32486 Removal of lung, other than pneumonectomy; with circumferential resection of segment of bronchus followed by broncho-bronchial anastomosis (sleeve lobectomy)

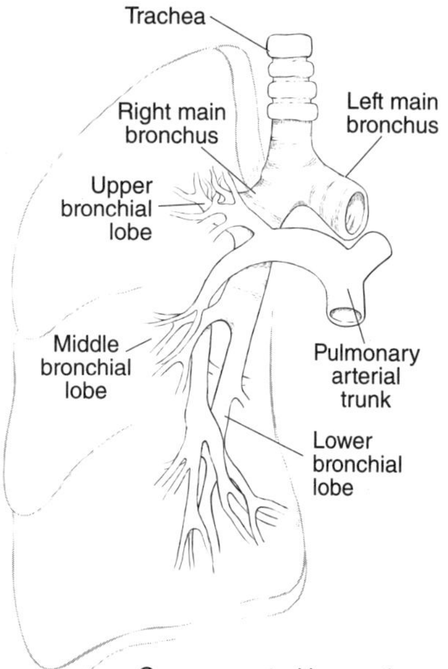

One segment with resection of bronchus and anastomosis

Explanation

The physician removes a portion (lobectomy, bilobectomy, or segmentectomy) of one lung and repairs a bronchial tube that has been partially resected. The physician opens the chest cavity widely to gain access to the lung to be removed. Using a scalpel, the surgeon makes a long incision around the side of the chest between two of the ribs. The incision is carried through all of the tissue layers into the chest cavity. Rib spreaders are inserted into the wound and the ribs are spread apart exposing the lung. Alternately, the chest cavity can be opened and the operation performed through a vertical incision in the center of the chest through the sternum. The skin incision is carried down to the sternum bone and a saw is used to split the sternum. With the sternum split in half, the chest is entered by spreading the sternum apart with a set of rib spreaders. The portion of lung to be removed is identified and isolated in the operative field by pushing aside the deflated lung with a gloved hand and large moist gauze sponges. Within the lung, main blood vessels and bronchial tubes are clamped, tied off, and cut. The resected part of the lung is removed through the wide chest incision. The segment of diseased or damaged bronchial tube is removed. The healthy end of the smaller bronchial tube in the remaining lobe is sutured to the main bronchial tube in the root of the lung. The instruments and gauze sponges are removed. A chest tube(s) may be used to provide drainage for the chest cavity. When the procedure is complete, if applicable, the sternotomy is repaired using wires to bring the two halves of the sternum together, and the operative wound is closed by sutures or staples.

Coding Tips

Diagnostic lung biopsies with intraoperative pathology that determines the need for resection or another definitive procedure should be reported using only the most complex service performed. When a diagnostic wedge resection is performed and followed by a more complex procedure on the same anatomic location, report add-on codes 32507 or 32668 with the more complex procedure. When a therapeutic wedge resection is performed on a different lobe than a more complex lung resection, append modifier 59 or an X{EPSU} modifier. If a lung resection is performed with chest wall tumor resection, report the appropriate chest wall tumor resection code (21601–21603) in addition to 32486. When concurrent decortication is performed with a lobectomy or segmentectomy, report 32320 in addition to 32486. If bronchoplasty is performed at the time of a lobectomy, bilobectomy, or segmentectomy, report 32501 in addition to the applicable procedure: 32480–32484. For removal of a single lobe, see 32480; two lobes, see 32482; single segment, see 32484; for completion pneumonectomy, see 32488. For total pneumonectomy, see 32440. For surgical thoracoscopy, with total or segmental lobectomy, see 32663.

ICD-10-CM Diagnostic Codes

A15.0	Tuberculosis of lung
B44.0	Invasive pulmonary aspergillosis
B44.1	Other pulmonary aspergillosis
C34.01	Malignant neoplasm of right main bronchus ☑
C34.11	Malignant neoplasm of upper lobe, right bronchus or lung ☑
C34.2	Malignant neoplasm of middle lobe, bronchus or lung
C34.31	Malignant neoplasm of lower lobe, right bronchus or lung ☑
C34.81	Malignant neoplasm of overlapping sites of right bronchus and lung ☑
C46.51	Kaposi's sarcoma of right lung ☑
C78.01	Secondary malignant neoplasm of right lung ☑
C79.89	Secondary malignant neoplasm of other specified sites
C7A.090	Malignant carcinoid tumor of the bronchus and lung
D02.21	Carcinoma in situ of right bronchus and lung ☑
D14.31	Benign neoplasm of right bronchus and lung ☑
D38.1	Neoplasm of uncertain behavior of trachea, bronchus and lung
D3A.090	Benign carcinoid tumor of the bronchus and lung
J43.0	Unilateral pulmonary emphysema [MacLeod's syndrome]
J43.1	Panlobular emphysema
J43.2	Centrilobular emphysema
J43.8	Other emphysema
J47.0	Bronchiectasis with acute lower respiratory infection
J47.1	Bronchiectasis with (acute) exacerbation
J85.0	Gangrene and necrosis of lung
J85.1	Abscess of lung with pneumonia
J85.2	Abscess of lung without pneumonia
J98.4	Other disorders of lung
Q33.2	Sequestration of lung

Relative Value Units/Medicare Edits

Non-Facility RVU	Work	PE	MP	Total
32486	42.88	15.42	10.64	68.94
Facility RVU	**Work**	**PE**	**MP**	**Total**
32486	42.88	15.42	10.64	68.94

	FUD	Status	MUE	Modifiers				IOM Reference
32486	90	A	1(3)	51	N/A	62*	80	None

* with documentation

32488

32488 Removal of lung, other than pneumonectomy; with all remaining lung following previous removal of a portion of lung (completion pneumonectomy)

Note that the left lung is divided into superior and inferior lobes only. The superior lobe features a large cardiac notch to accommodate the bulge of the heart

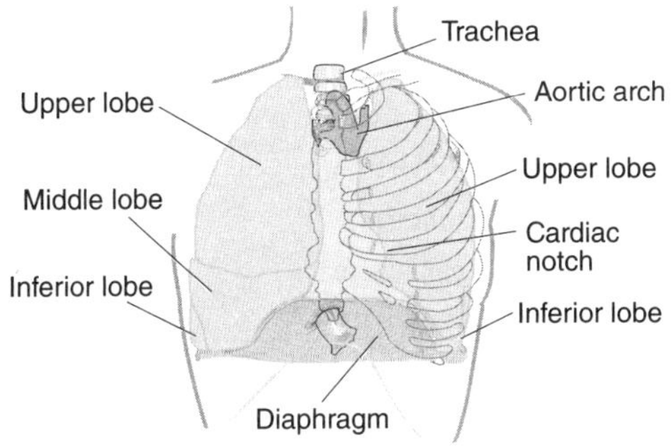

Explanation

The physician removes the remaining portion(s) of a lung from a prior partial lung removal. The physician opens the chest cavity widely to gain access to the lung to be removed. Using a scalpel, the surgeon makes a long incision around the side of the chest between two of the ribs. The incision is carried through all of the tissue layers into the chest cavity. Rib spreaders are inserted into the wound and the ribs are spread apart exposing the lung. Alternately, the chest cavity can be opened and the operation performed through a vertical incision in the center of the chest through the sternum. The skin incision is carried down to the sternum bone and a saw is used to split the sternum. With the sternum split in half, the chest is entered by spreading the sternum apart with a set of rib spreaders. The remaining portion of lung is isolated in the operative field by pushing aside the deflated lung with a gloved hand and large moist gauze sponges. Within the root of the lung, the blood vessels and bronchial tubes are clamped, tied off, and cut. The lung is removed through the wide chest incision. The instruments and gauze sponges are removed. A chest tube(s) may be used to provide drainage for the chest cavity. When the procedure is complete, if applicable, the sternotomy is repaired using wires to bring the two halves of the sternum together, and the operative wound is closed by sutures or staples.

Coding Tips

If a lung resection is performed with chest wall tumor resection, report the appropriate chest wall tumor resection code (21601–21603) in addition to 32488. When concurrent decortication is performed with a lobectomy or segmentectomy, report 32320 in addition to 32488. For removal of a single lobe, see 32480; two lobes, see 32482; single segment, see 32484; with circumferential resection of bronchus and reanastomosis, see 32486. For a total pneumonectomy, see 32440. For a surgical thoracoscopy, with a total or segmental lobectomy, see 32663. For lobectomy or segmentectomy with concomitant decortication, see 32320 in addition to the code for lung removal.

ICD-10-CM Diagnostic Codes

A15.0	Tuberculosis of lung
B44.0	Invasive pulmonary aspergillosis
B44.1	Other pulmonary aspergillosis
C34.01	Malignant neoplasm of right main bronchus ☑
C34.02	Malignant neoplasm of left main bronchus ☑
C34.11	Malignant neoplasm of upper lobe, right bronchus or lung ☑
C34.12	Malignant neoplasm of upper lobe, left bronchus or lung ☑
C34.2	Malignant neoplasm of middle lobe, bronchus or lung
C34.31	Malignant neoplasm of lower lobe, right bronchus or lung ☑
C34.32	Malignant neoplasm of lower lobe, left bronchus or lung ☑
C34.81	Malignant neoplasm of overlapping sites of right bronchus and lung ☑
C34.82	Malignant neoplasm of overlapping sites of left bronchus and lung ☑
C46.51	Kaposi's sarcoma of right lung ☑
C46.52	Kaposi's sarcoma of left lung ☑
C78.01	Secondary malignant neoplasm of right lung ☑
C78.02	Secondary malignant neoplasm of left lung ☑
C79.89	Secondary malignant neoplasm of other specified sites
C7A.090	Malignant carcinoid tumor of the bronchus and lung
D02.21	Carcinoma in situ of right bronchus and lung ☑
D02.22	Carcinoma in situ of left bronchus and lung ☑
D14.31	Benign neoplasm of right bronchus and lung ☑
D14.32	Benign neoplasm of left bronchus and lung ☑
D38.1	Neoplasm of uncertain behavior of trachea, bronchus and lung
D3A.090	Benign carcinoid tumor of the bronchus and lung
J43.0	Unilateral pulmonary emphysema [MacLeod's syndrome]
J43.1	Panlobular emphysema
J43.2	Centrilobular emphysema
J43.8	Other emphysema
J47.0	Bronchiectasis with acute lower respiratory infection
J47.1	Bronchiectasis with (acute) exacerbation
J85.0	Gangrene and necrosis of lung
J85.1	Abscess of lung with pneumonia
J85.2	Abscess of lung without pneumonia
J98.4	Other disorders of lung
Q33.2	Sequestration of lung

Relative Value Units/Medicare Edits

Non-Facility RVU	Work	PE	MP	Total
32488	42.99	16.88	10.65	70.52
Facility RVU	**Work**	**PE**	**MP**	**Total**
32488	42.99	16.88	10.65	70.52

	FUD	Status	MUE	Modifiers				IOM Reference
32488	90	A	1(2)	51	N/A	62*	80	None

* with documentation

Terms To Know

aspergillosis. Infection by Aspergillus species, mainly A. Fumigatus, A. flavus group, or A. terreus group.

bronchiectasis. Dilation of the bronchi with mucous production and persistent cough due to infection or chronic conditions that causes diminished lung capacity and frequent infections of the lung.

32491

32491 Removal of lung, other than pneumonectomy; with resection-plication of emphysematous lung(s) (bullous or non-bullous) for lung volume reduction, sternal split or transthoracic approach, includes any pleural procedure, when performed

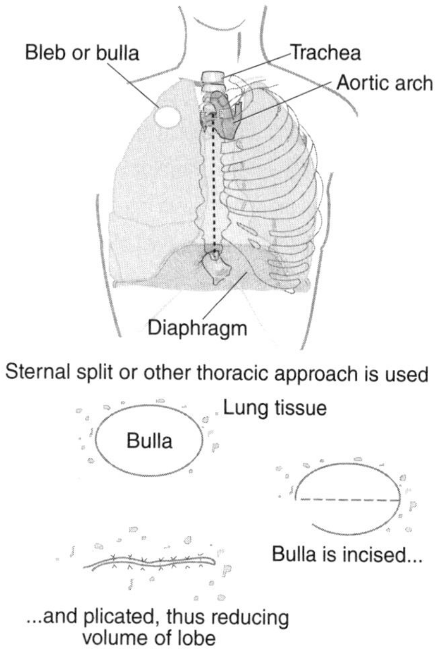

Emphysematous lungs may develop open areas of damaged tissue called blebs or bullae. Removal or plication of a bleb reduces lung volume

Explanation

The physician removes part of an emphysematous lung. Using a scalpel, the surgeon makes a long incision around the side of the chest between two of the ribs. The incision is carried through all of the tissue layers into the chest cavity. Rib spreaders are inserted into the wound and the ribs are spread apart exposing the lung. Alternately, the chest cavity can be opened and the operation performed through a vertical incision in the center of the chest through the sternum. The skin incision is carried down to the sternum bone and a saw is used to split the sternum. With the sternum split in half, the chest is entered by spreading the sternum apart with a set of rib spreaders. Space is made in the chest by packing the uninvolved lung away from the operative field using large moist gauze sponges. In order to perform the procedure, the pleural surface may require an operative procedure such as pneumonolysis (separation of the surface of the lung that has become adherent to the inside surface of the chest cavity). The lung tissue to be removed is identified and isolated in the operative field by pushing aside the deflated lung with a gloved hand and large moist gauze sponges. The lung tissue may be further isolated using a row of staples. The emphysematous lung tissue is removed by sharp and blunt dissection and often by folding and suturing of the tissues (plication). When the procedure is complete, the instruments and gauze sponges are removed. A chest tube(s) may be used to provide drainage for the chest cavity. If applicable, the sternotomy is repaired using wires to bring the two halves of the sternum together, and the operative wound is closed by sutures or staples.

Coding Tips

Diagnostic lung biopsies with intraoperative pathology that determines the need for resection, or another definitive procedure, should be reported using only the most complex service performed. When a diagnostic wedge resection is performed and followed by a more complex procedure on the same anatomic location, report add-on codes 32507 or 32668 with the more complex procedure. When a therapeutic wedge resection is performed on a different lobe than a more complex lung resection, append modifier 59 or an X{EPSU} modifier. For a thoracotomy with excision or plication of bullae, with or without any pleural procedure, see 32141. For a surgical thoracoscopy with excision-plication of bullae, including any pleural procedure, see 32655. For open wedge resection of the lung, see 32505, 32506, or 32507. When lung resection is performed with chest wall tumor resection, use 21601-21603 to report the appropriate chest wall tumor resection, in addition to lung resection codes 32480, 32482, 32484, 32486, 32488, 32505, 32506, and 32507.

ICD-10-CM Diagnostic Codes

J43.0	Unilateral pulmonary emphysema [MacLeod's syndrome]
J43.1	Panlobular emphysema
J43.2	Centrilobular emphysema
J43.8	Other emphysema
J43.9	Emphysema, unspecified
J98.2	Interstitial emphysema
J98.3	Compensatory emphysema
T79.7XXA	Traumatic subcutaneous emphysema, initial encounter

Relative Value Units/Medicare Edits

Non-Facility RVU	Work	PE	MP	Total
32491	25.24	12.16	6.23	43.63
Facility RVU	**Work**	**PE**	**MP**	**Total**
32491	25.24	12.16	6.23	43.63

	FUD	Status	MUE	Modifiers				IOM Reference
32491	90	R	1(2)	51	50	62*	80	None

* with documentation

Terms To Know

emphysema. Pathological condition in which there is destructive enlargement of the air sacs in the lungs resulting in damage and lack of elasticity to the alveolar walls, commonly seen in long-term smokers.

emphysematous bleb. Formation of blisters or vesicles greater than 1.0 mm within an emphysematous lung, containing serum or blood.

excision. Surgical removal of an organ or tissue.

plication. Surgical technique involving folding, tucking, or pleating to reduce the size of a hollow structure or organ.

thoracotomy. Surgical procedure for opening the chest wall in order to access the lungs, esophagus, trachea, aorta, heart, and diaphragm.

32501

\+ **32501** Resection and repair of portion of bronchus (bronchoplasty) when performed at time of lobectomy or segmentectomy (List separately in addition to code for primary procedure)

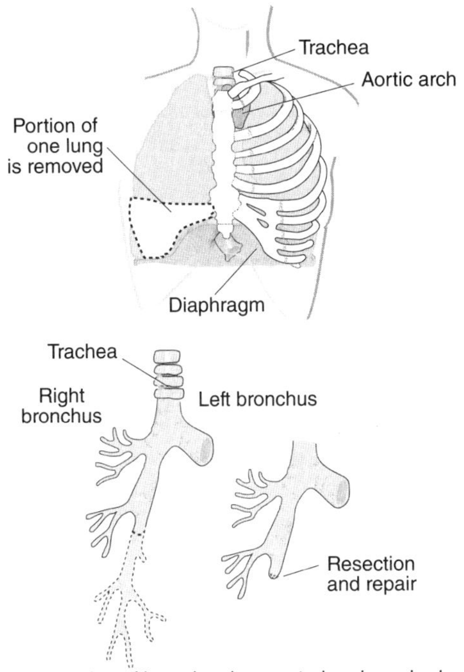

A portion of bronchus is resected and repaired

Explanation

During lobectomy or segmentectomy, the physician repairs part of a bronchus. After removing the lobes or lobe segments (see codes 32480, 32482, 32484 for procedure description), the segment of diseased or damaged bronchial tube is repaired and sutured to the main bronchial tube in the root of the lung. The remaining instruments and gauze sponges are removed from the chest cavity. The chest incision is sutured closed in layers (sternal wires are used if the chest was entered through a midline sternal incision). A chest tube(s) may be used to provide drainage for the chest cavity. List this code separately in addition to the primary procedure.

Coding Tips

Use 32501 in addition to 32480, 32482, and 32484. Also report 32501 when plastic closure is required to preserve function of a lung following the removal of a portion of that lung. It is not to be used in the instance of closure of the proximal end of a bronchus resection. For removal of lung, other than total pneumonectomy, with circumferential resection of segment of bronchus followed by broncho-bronchial anastomosis (sleeve lobectomy), see 32486.

ICD-10-CM Diagnostic Codes

This/these CPT code(s) are add-on code(s). See the primary procedure code that this code is performed with for your ICD-10-CM code selections. Diagnostic code(s) would be the same as the actual procedure performed.

Relative Value Units/Medicare Edits

Non-Facility RVU	Work	PE	MP	Total
32501	4.68	1.29	1.17	7.14
Facility RVU	**Work**	**PE**	**MP**	**Total**
32501	4.68	1.29	1.17	7.14

	FUD	Status	MUE	Modifiers				IOM Reference
32501	N/A	A	1(3)	N/A	N/A	62*	80	None

* with documentation

Terms To Know

bronchoplasty. Reconstruction or plastic repair of the bronchus.

excision. Surgical removal of an organ or tissue.

incision. Act of cutting into tissue or an organ.

lobectomy. Excision of a lobe of an organ such as the liver, thyroid, lung, or brain.

pneumonectomy. Surgical removal of a lung or lung tissue.

resection. Surgical removal of a part or all of an organ or body part.

segmentectomy. Removal of a segment of a gland or an organ.

sternotomy. Incision into the sternum, the bone that forms the front of the chest cavity and connects with the ribs.

trachea. Tube descending from the larynx and branching into the right and left main bronchi.

32503-32504

32503 Resection of apical lung tumor (eg, Pancoast tumor), including chest wall resection, rib(s) resection(s), neurovascular dissection, when performed; without chest wall reconstruction(s)

32504 with chest wall reconstruction

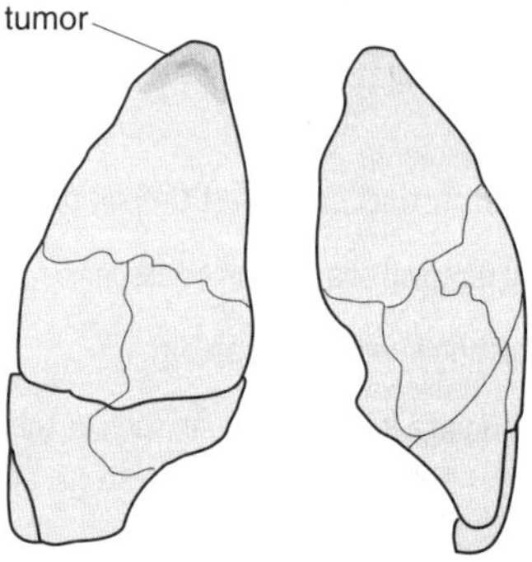

Explanation

The physician removes a tumor from the apex of the lung, such as a Pancoast tumor, as well as a portion of the chest wall. The patient may be intubated with a double lumen endotracheal tube to verify correct positioning and to evaluate endobronchial disease. The chest cavity is entered using an anterior or posterior incision. The posterior incision is made along the outline of the scapula, entering the pleural space at the third or fourth intercostal space. In some cases, an anterior transcervical approach is used. The necessary extended en bloc resection of the chest wall includes posterior portions of the first three ribs, part of the upper thoracic vertebrae (including the transverse process), the intercostal nerves, the lower trunk of the brachial plexus, the stellate ganglion, a section of the dorsal sympathetic ganglion, and the portion of the involved lung. For tumors that are situated peripherally, the apical segment of the upper lobe of the lung is separated from the remaining superior lobe. The apex of the lung is left attached to the chest wall. The first through third, fourth, or fifth ribs are sectioned anteriorly. The subclavian artery is sharply dissected from the surrounding structures. A subperiosteal dissection is performed around the first rib, which is transected, and the subclavian vessels are mobilized superiorly. If preoperative magnetic resonance imaging demonstrated vessel involvement, an initial anterior approach is performed to dissect or graft the vessels. The ribs are disarticulated and the tumor, along with the involved chest wall, is gradually mobilized. Next, the segmental vessels are identified, doubly ligated, and transected. The parietal pleura are bluntly dissected along the anterior border of the spinal column. The tumor and the involved chest wall that has remained attached to the inferior trunk of the brachial plexus is excised, using caution to spare the T1 nerve root as it crosses beneath the angle of the first rib to join the C8 nerve root. If a tumor has invaded the vertebral bodies, the subclavian artery, or the C8 to T1 nerve routes, a multidisciplinary approach may be necessary. At the completion of the procedure, two large chest tubes are placed: one at the apex of the chest to drain any residual air and the other to drain fluids. Report 32504 when chest wall reconstruction is performed.

Coding Tips

When a diagnostic wedge resection is performed and followed by a more complex procedure on the same anatomic location, report add-on codes 32507 or 32668 with the more complex procedure. When a therapeutic wedge resection is performed on a different lobe than a more complex lung resection, append modifier 59 or an X{EPSU} modifier. Do not report 32503 or 32504 with 21601-21603, 32100, 32551, 32554, or 32555.

ICD-10-CM Diagnostic Codes

C34.10 Malignant neoplasm of upper lobe, unspecified bronchus or lung

C34.11 Malignant neoplasm of upper lobe, right bronchus or lung ☑

C34.12 Malignant neoplasm of upper lobe, left bronchus or lung ☑

AMA: 32503 2019,Dec **32504** 2019,Dec

Relative Value Units/Medicare Edits

Non-Facility RVU	Work	PE	MP	Total
32503	31.74	13.42	7.84	53.0
32504	36.54	14.75	9.06	60.35
Facility RVU	**Work**	**PE**	**MP**	**Total**
32503	31.74	13.42	7.84	53.0
32504	36.54	14.75	9.06	60.35

	FUD	Status	MUE	Modifiers				IOM Reference
32503	90	A	1(2)	51	N/A	62*	80	None
32504	90	A	1(2)	51	N/A	62*	80	

* with documentation

Terms To Know

apex. Highest point of a root end of a tooth, or the end of any organ.

en bloc removal. Take out as a whole or all in one mass.

ligate. To tie off a blood vessel or duct with a suture or a soft, thin wire (ligature wire).

Pancoast syndrome. Neoplasm of upper lobe of the lung.

pleura. One of the two membranes that surround the lungs. The visceral pleura encases the lung and the parietal pleura lines the inner chest walls.

transection. Transverse dissection; to cut across a long axis; cross section.

32505-32507

32505 Thoracotomy; with therapeutic wedge resection (eg, mass, nodule), initial

\+ **32506** with therapeutic wedge resection (eg, mass or nodule), each additional resection, ipsilateral (List separately in addition to code for primary procedure)

\+ **32507** with diagnostic wedge resection followed by anatomic lung resection (List separately in addition to code for primary procedure)

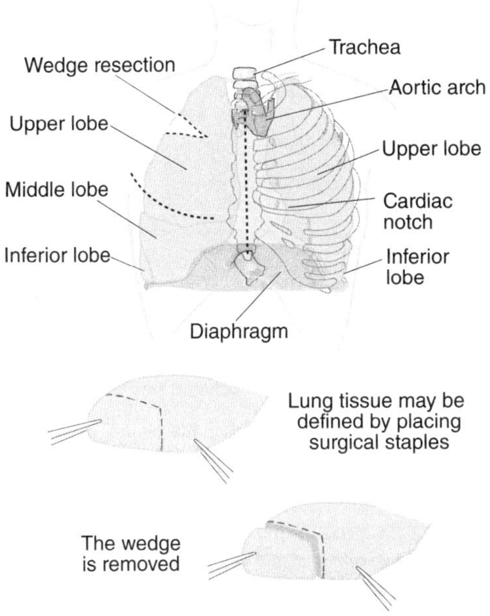

A wedge resection, single or multiple, is taken from a lung

Explanation

The physician removes a wedge-shaped portion(s) of a lobe(s) on one or both lungs. The physician opens the chest cavity widely to gain access to the lung to be removed. Using a scalpel, the surgeon makes a long incision around the side of the chest between two of the ribs. The incision is carried through all of the tissue layers into the chest cavity. Rib spreaders are inserted into the wound and the ribs are spread apart exposing the lung. Alternately, the chest cavity can be opened and the operation performed through a vertical incision in the center of the chest through the sternum. The skin incision is carried down to the sternum bone and a saw is used to split the sternum. With the sternum split in half, the chest is entered by spreading the sternum apart with a set of rib spreaders. The area to be removed is identified and isolated in the operative field by pushing aside the deflated lung with a gloved hand and large moist gauze sponges. The healthy portions of the lung surrounding the area(s) to be removed are clamped and the unhealthy portion is removed by cutting the lung tissue isolated by the clamps. Sutures or surgical clips are used to repair the cut portion of the remaining lung tissue. The instruments and gauze sponges are removed. A chest tube(s) may be used to provide drainage for the chest cavity. When the procedure is complete, if applicable, the sternotomy is repaired using wires to bring the two halves of the sternum together and the operative wound is closed by sutures or staples. Report 32505 for the initial therapeutic wedge resection and 32506 for each additional wedge resection on the same side. Report 32507 when the wedge resection is followed by a lung resection.

Coding Tips

Report 32506 in addition to 32505. Report 32507 in addition to 32440, 32442, 32445, 32480, 32482, 32484, 32486, 32488, 32503, and 32504. Therapeutic wedge resection codes (32505, 32506, 32666, or 32667) should not be reported in addition to the more complex lung procedures (lobectomy) unless wedge resection is performed on a different lobe or lung. When a diagnostic wedge resection is performed and followed by a more complex procedure on the same anatomic location, report 32507 or 32668 with the more complex procedure. When a therapeutic wedge resection is performed on a different lobe than a more complex lung resection, append modifier 59 or X{EPSU}. If lung resection and chest wall tumor resection are performed at the same operative session, report the appropriate chest wall tumor resection code (21601-21603) in addition to lung resection codes 32480, 32482, 32484, 32486, 32488, and 32505-32507. If the procedure is attempted thoracoscopically, but requires major thoracotomy for completion, report 32505-32507 for the open portion of the procedure and report a diagnostic thoracoscopy, 32601, as a secondary procedure. Do not report 32505 with 32440, 32442, 32445, or 32488. For surgical thoracoscopy with wedge resection of lung, see 32666-32668.

ICD-10-CM Diagnostic Codes

A15.0	Tuberculosis of lung
B44.0	Invasive pulmonary aspergillosis
B44.1	Other pulmonary aspergillosis
C34.11	Malignant neoplasm of upper lobe, right bronchus or lung ☑
C34.12	Malignant neoplasm of upper lobe, left bronchus or lung ☑
C34.2	Malignant neoplasm of middle lobe, bronchus or lung
C34.31	Malignant neoplasm of lower lobe, right bronchus or lung ☑
C34.32	Malignant neoplasm of lower lobe, left bronchus or lung ☑
C34.81	Malignant neoplasm of overlapping sites of right bronchus and lung ☑
C34.82	Malignant neoplasm of overlapping sites of left bronchus and lung ☑
C46.51	Kaposi's sarcoma of right lung ☑
C46.52	Kaposi's sarcoma of left lung ☑
C78.01	Secondary malignant neoplasm of right lung ☑
C78.02	Secondary malignant neoplasm of left lung ☑
C7A.090	Malignant carcinoid tumor of the bronchus and lung
D02.21	Carcinoma in situ of right bronchus and lung ☑
D02.22	Carcinoma in situ of left bronchus and lung ☑
D14.31	Benign neoplasm of right bronchus and lung ☑
D14.32	Benign neoplasm of left bronchus and lung ☑
D38.1	Neoplasm of uncertain behavior of trachea, bronchus and lung
D3A.090	Benign carcinoid tumor of the bronchus and lung
D86.0	Sarcoidosis of lung
J43.0	Unilateral pulmonary emphysema [MacLeod's syndrome]
J43.1	Panlobular emphysema
J43.2	Centrilobular emphysema
J47.0	Bronchiectasis with acute lower respiratory infection
J47.1	Bronchiectasis with (acute) exacerbation
J85.0	Gangrene and necrosis of lung
J85.1	Abscess of lung with pneumonia
J85.2	Abscess of lung without pneumonia
J98.4	Other disorders of lung
Q33.2	Sequestration of lung

Relative Value Units/Medicare Edits

Non-Facility RVU	Work	PE	MP	Total
32505	15.75	8.03	3.83	27.61
32506	3.0	0.85	0.73	4.58
32507	3.0	0.84	0.73	4.57
Facility RVU	**Work**	**PE**	**MP**	**Total**
32505	15.75	8.03	3.83	27.61
32506	3.0	0.85	0.73	4.58
32507	3.0	0.84	0.73	4.57

	FUD	Status	MUE	Modifiers				IOM Reference
32505	90	A	1(2)	51	N/A	62*	80	None
32506	N/A	A	3(3)	N/A	N/A	62*	80	
32507	N/A	A	2(3)	N/A	N/A	62*	80	

* with documentation

Terms To Know

resection. Surgical removal of a part or all of an organ or body part.

sternotomy. Incision into the sternum, the bone that forms the front of the chest cavity and connects with the ribs.

therapeutic procedure. Manner of effecting change through the application of clinical skills and/or services that attempt to improve function.

thoracotomy. Surgical procedure for opening the chest wall in order to access the lungs, esophagus, trachea, aorta, heart, and diaphragm.

wedge excision. Surgical removal of a section of tissue that is thick at one edge and tapers to a thin edge.

32540

32540 Extrapleural enucleation of empyema (empyemectomy)

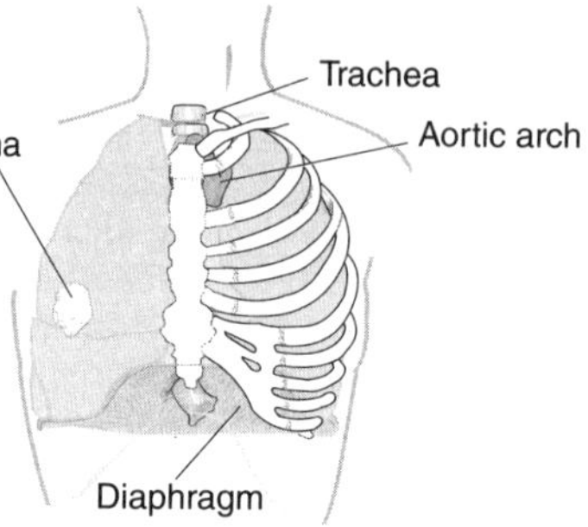

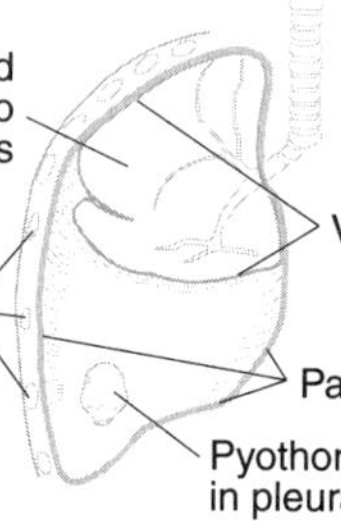

An empyema is a pocket of pus within a body cavity and may also be referred to as a pyothorax, or pus in the pleural cavity

Explanation

The physician removes an empyema (an abscess in the chest cavity between the lung and the chest wall) in its entirety, including the pleural membranes surrounding the abscess. The physician opens the chest cavity to gain access to the abscess. Using a scalpel, the surgeon makes an incision around the side of the chest between two of the ribs. The incision is carried through all the tissue layers down to the membrane lining the chest cavity. Rib spreaders are inserted into the wound and the ribs are spread apart exposing the tissues, taking care to preserve the integrity of the chest lining. Holding a gauze sponge, the surgeon strips away the lining adherent to the chest wall and the abscess and carries this all the way around the abscess. This creates a sac that contains the abscess. The intact mass is shelled out through the chest incision. After the removal of the instruments and gauze sponges, the chest incision is sutured closed in layers leaving a drainage tube or the wound is partially closed to allow drainage.

Coding Tips

When performed at the time of a lung excision, report 32540 with the appropriate lung removal code, 32440–32491. For tube thoracotomy with or without water seal for abscess, hemothorax, or empyema (separate procedure), see 32551. For thoracostomy, with rib resection for empyema, see 32035; with open flap drainage for empyema, see 32036. For pneumonostomy with open drainage of abscess or cyst, see 32200.

ICD-10-CM Diagnostic Codes

A15.6	Tuberculous pleurisy
J86.0	Pyothorax with fistula
J86.9	Pyothorax without fistula

Relative Value Units/Medicare Edits

Non-Facility RVU	Work	PE	MP	Total
32540	30.35	13.21	7.52	51.08
Facility RVU	**Work**	**PE**	**MP**	**Total**
32540	30.35	13.21	7.52	51.08

	FUD	Status	MUE	Modifiers				IOM Reference
32540	90	A	1(3)	51	N/A	62*	80	None

* with documentation

Terms To Know

abscess. Circumscribed collection of pus resulting from bacteria, frequently associated with swelling and other signs of inflammation.

empyema. Accumulation of pus within the respiratory or pleural cavity.

fistula. Abnormal tube-like passage between two body cavities or organs or from an organ to the outside surface.

lesion. Area of damaged tissue that has lost continuity or function, due to disease or trauma. Lesions may be located on internal structures such as the brain, nerves, or kidneys, or visible on the skin.

resection. Surgical removal of a part or all of an organ or body part.

thoracostomy. Creation of an opening in the chest wall for drainage.

thoracotomy. Surgical procedure for opening the chest wall in order to access the lungs, esophagus, trachea, aorta, heart, and diaphragm.

32550

32550 Insertion of indwelling tunneled pleural catheter with cuff

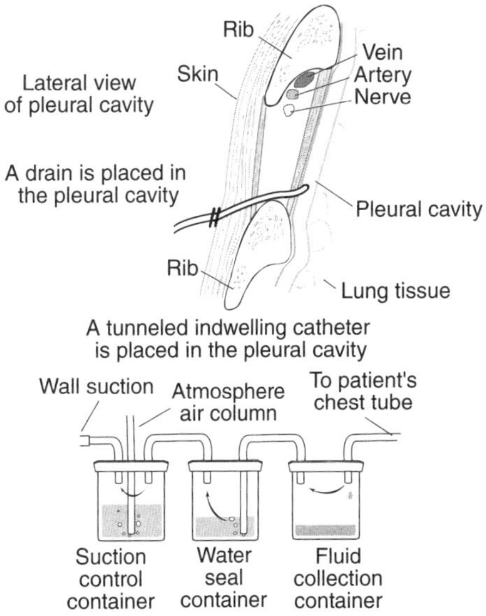

Explanation

The physician inserts a tunneled, indwelling pleural catheter to aid quality of life and long-term management of malignant effusion. The catheter allows drainage on an outpatient or home basis and consists of flexible rubber tubing with a safety drainage valve to provide access to the pleural cavity and prevent air and fluid entering. A polyester cuff secures the catheter in place and helps prevent infection. Using separately reportable imaging guidance, the physician inserts the catheter percutaneously through a small incision in the anterior axillary area. The pleural catheter is threaded over a guidewire to access the pleural cavity, tunneled under the skin along the chest wall, and brought out that side in the lower chest. After placement, the patient may drain pleural fluid at home periodically into vacuum bottles by connecting the matching drainage line access tip to the valve.

Coding Tips

When medically necessary, report moderate (conscious) sedation provided by the performing physician with 99151-99153. When provided by another physician, report 99155-99157. Supplies used when providing this procedure may be reported with the appropriate HCPCS Level II codes. Check with the specific payer to determine coverage. If performed on the same side of the chest, do not report 32550 with 32554–32557. If imaging guidance is performed, see 75989.

ICD-10-CM Diagnostic Codes

A15.6	Tuberculous pleurisy
A15.7	Primary respiratory tuberculosis
J90	Pleural effusion, not elsewhere classified
J91.0	Malignant pleural effusion
J91.8	Pleural effusion in other conditions classified elsewhere
J94.0	Chylous effusion
M32.13	Lung involvement in systemic lupus erythematosus

Relative Value Units/Medicare Edits

Non-Facility RVU	Work	PE	MP	Total
32550	3.92	18.58	0.54	23.04
Facility RVU	**Work**	**PE**	**MP**	**Total**
32550	3.92	1.54	0.54	6.0

	FUD	Status	MUE	Modifiers				IOM Reference
32550	0	A	2(3)	N/A	N/A	N/A	N/A	None

* with documentation

Terms To Know

malignant neoplasm. Any cancerous tumor or lesion exhibiting uncontrolled tissue growth that can progressively invade other parts of the body with its disease-generating cells.

pleura. One of the two membranes that surround the lungs. The visceral pleura encases the lung and the parietal pleura lines the inner chest walls.

32551

32551 Tube thoracostomy, includes connection to drainage system (eg, water seal), when performed, open (separate procedure)

The conventional three-bottle water seal system evacuates the pleural space without backpressure. The negative pressure works to reinflate the lung and seal any leakage

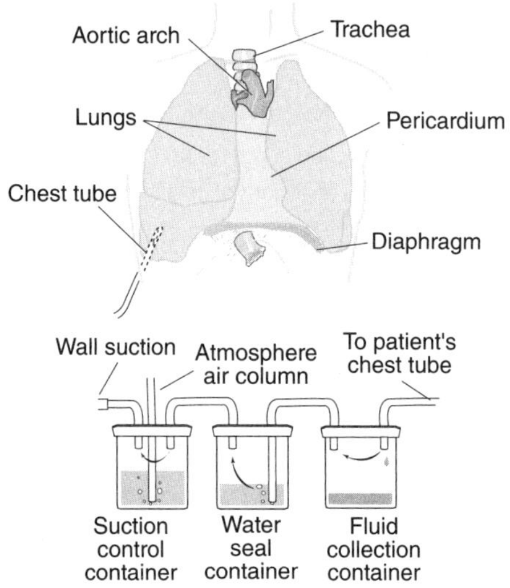

Explanation

The physician removes fluid and/or air from the chest cavity by puncturing through the space between the ribs. To enter the chest cavity, the physician passes a trocar over the top of a rib, punctures through the chest tissues between the ribs, and enters the pleural cavity. Separately reportable imaging guidance may be used. With the end of the trocar in the chest cavity, the physician advances the plastic tube into the chest cavity. The sharp trocar is removed leaving one end of the plastic catheter in place within the chest cavity. A large syringe is attached to the outside end of the catheter and the fluid (blood or pus) is removed from the chest cavity by pulling back on the plunger of the syringe. The outside end of the tube may be connected to a drainage system, such as a water seal, to prevent air from being sucked into the chest cavity and to allow continuous or intermittent removal of air or fluid.

Coding Tips

When medically necessary, report moderate (conscious) sedation provided by the performing physician with 99151-99153. When provided by another physician, report 99155-99157. Do not report 32551 with 33020 or 33025 if a pleural drain is placed on the same side. For pleural drainage, percutaneous, with insertion of an indwelling catheter, see 32556–32557. Do not report 32551 with 43287 or 43288. For radiological supervision and interpretation, see 75989.

ICD-10-CM Diagnostic Codes

J86.0	Pyothorax with fistula
J86.9	Pyothorax without fistula
J90	Pleural effusion, not elsewhere classified
J91.0	Malignant pleural effusion
J91.8	Pleural effusion in other conditions classified elsewhere
J93.0	Spontaneous tension pneumothorax
J93.11	Primary spontaneous pneumothorax
J93.12	Secondary spontaneous pneumothorax
J93.81	Chronic pneumothorax

J93.82 Other air leak
J93.83 Other pneumothorax
J94.0 Chylous effusion
J94.2 Hemothorax
J94.8 Other specified pleural conditions
J95.811 Postprocedural pneumothorax
P26.0 Tracheobronchial hemorrhage originating in the perinatal period N
P26.1 Massive pulmonary hemorrhage originating in the perinatal period N
P26.8 Other pulmonary hemorrhages originating in the perinatal period N
S27.0XXA Traumatic pneumothorax, initial encounter
S27.1XXA Traumatic hemothorax, initial encounter
S27.2XXA Traumatic hemopneumothorax, initial encounter

AMA: 32551 2023,Mar; 2021,Nov; 2019,Dec; 2018,Jul

Relative Value Units/Medicare Edits

Non-Facility RVU	Work	PE	MP	Total
32551	3.04	1.02	0.53	4.59
Facility RVU	**Work**	**PE**	**MP**	**Total**
32551	3.04	1.02	0.53	4.59

	FUD	Status	MUE	Modifiers				IOM Reference
32551	0	A	2(3)	51	50	N/A	N/A	None

* with documentation

Terms To Know

hemothorax. Blood collecting in the pleural cavity.

pneumothorax. Collapsed lung due to air or gas trapped in the pleural space formed by the membrane that encloses the lungs and lines the thoracic cavity.

thoracostomy. Creation of an opening in the chest wall for drainage.

trocar. Cannula or a sharp pointed instrument used to puncture and aspirate fluid from cavities.

32552

32552 Removal of indwelling tunneled pleural catheter with cuff

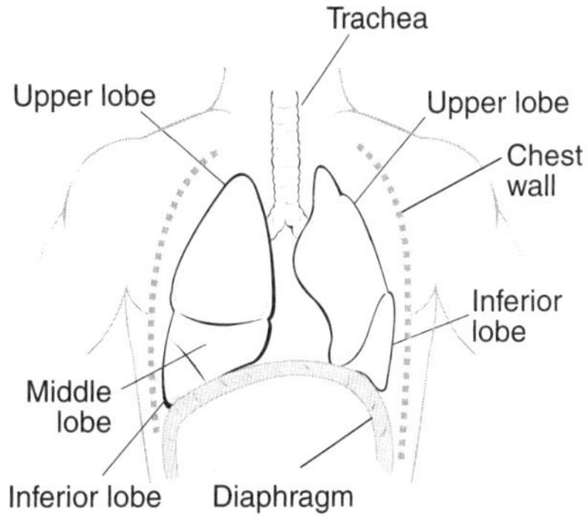

Explanation

The physician removes a previously placed, indwelling tunneled pleural catheter with cuff. Following administration of local anesthesia along the subcutaneous catheter tunnel, blunt dissection is used to release the cuff and the catheter is meticulously withdrawn. Conscious sedation may be required.

Coding Tips

For insertion of an indwelling tunneled pleural catheter with cuff, see 32550. For insertion of a chest tube, see 32551.

ICD-10-CM Diagnostic Codes

T85.79XA Infection and inflammatory reaction due to other internal prosthetic devices, implants and grafts, initial encounter
Z48.03 Encounter for change or removal of drains

Relative Value Units/Medicare Edits

Non-Facility RVU	Work	PE	MP	Total
32552	2.53	2.56	0.37	5.46
Facility RVU	**Work**	**PE**	**MP**	**Total**
32552	2.53	1.76	0.37	4.66

	FUD	Status	MUE	Modifiers				IOM Reference
32552	10	A	2(2)	51	N/A	N/A	80*	None

* with documentation

Terms To Know

tunneled catheter. Catheter inserted into a central vein via a chest incision and maneuvered under the skin to a distal outlet location enabling secure placement with decreased risk of infection and can stay in place for extended periods of time. This procedure is commonly performed in an operating room.

32553

32553 Placement of interstitial device(s) for radiation therapy guidance (eg, fiducial markers, dosimeter), percutaneous, intra-thoracic, single or multiple

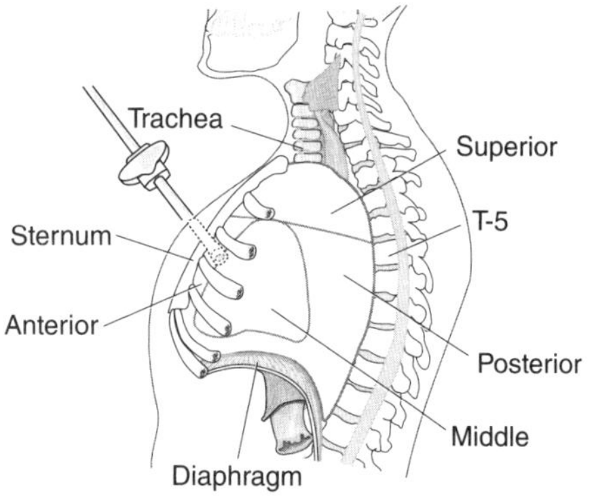

Percutaneous placement of interstitial device into the thorax

Explanation

The physician places one or more interstitial devices such as gold seeds (fiducial markers) for radiation therapy guidance or a dosimeter to gauge the amount of radiation received. Implanted percutaneously in and/or around an intrathoracic soft tissue tumor, these act as radiographic landmarks to define the position of the target lesion. Under CT or other image guidance, the physician injects a small capsule or seed into the intrathoracic tissue using a needle injection device. Allowing for precision in targeting radiation and/or for measuring the radiation doses received, an injected fiducial marker is visible by ultrasound and fluoroscopy and permits accurate triangulation of the tissue to be treated. An injected capsule dosimeter relays radiation dose information so that the clinical team can monitor for any deviation between the radiation plan and the actual radiation received.

Coding Tips

Report the device separately. When medically necessary, report moderate (conscious) sedation provided by the performing physician with 99151-99153. When provided by another physician, report 99155-99157. For radiology services, see 76942, 77002, 77012, and 77021. When percutaneous placement of interstitial devices related to intra-abdominal, intrapelvic, and/or retroperitoneal radiation therapy guidance is required, see 49411.

ICD-10-CM Diagnostic Codes

C33	Malignant neoplasm of trachea
C34.01	Malignant neoplasm of right main bronchus ☑
C34.02	Malignant neoplasm of left main bronchus ☑
C34.11	Malignant neoplasm of upper lobe, right bronchus or lung ☑
C34.12	Malignant neoplasm of upper lobe, left bronchus or lung ☑
C34.2	Malignant neoplasm of middle lobe, bronchus or lung
C34.31	Malignant neoplasm of lower lobe, right bronchus or lung ☑
C34.32	Malignant neoplasm of lower lobe, left bronchus or lung ☑
C34.81	Malignant neoplasm of overlapping sites of right bronchus and lung ☑
C34.82	Malignant neoplasm of overlapping sites of left bronchus and lung ☑
C38.4	Malignant neoplasm of pleura
C45.0	Mesothelioma of pleura
C46.51	Kaposi's sarcoma of right lung ☑
C46.52	Kaposi's sarcoma of left lung ☑
C76.1	Malignant neoplasm of thorax
C78.01	Secondary malignant neoplasm of right lung ☑
C78.02	Secondary malignant neoplasm of left lung ☑
C78.2	Secondary malignant neoplasm of pleura
C79.89	Secondary malignant neoplasm of other specified sites
C7A.090	Malignant carcinoid tumor of the bronchus and lung
D02.21	Carcinoma in situ of right bronchus and lung ☑
D02.22	Carcinoma in situ of left bronchus and lung ☑
D09.3	Carcinoma in situ of thyroid and other endocrine glands
D09.8	Carcinoma in situ of other specified sites
D14.31	Benign neoplasm of right bronchus and lung ☑
D14.32	Benign neoplasm of left bronchus and lung ☑
D19.0	Benign neoplasm of mesothelial tissue of pleura
D38.1	Neoplasm of uncertain behavior of trachea, bronchus and lung
D38.2	Neoplasm of uncertain behavior of pleura
D3A.090	Benign carcinoid tumor of the bronchus and lung

AMA: 32553 2023,Jan

Relative Value Units/Medicare Edits

Non-Facility RVU	Work	PE	MP	Total
32553	3.55	11.13	0.36	15.04
Facility RVU	**Work**	**PE**	**MP**	**Total**
32553	3.55	1.22	0.36	5.13

	FUD	Status	MUE	Modifiers				IOM Reference
32553	0	A	1(2)	51	N/A	N/A	80	None

* with documentation

Terms To Know

in situ. Located in the natural position or contained within the origin site, not spread into neighboring tissue.

Kaposi's sarcoma. Malignant neoplasm caused by vascular proliferation of cutaneous tumors characterized by channels lined with endothelial tissue containing vascular spaced.

ultrasound. Imaging using ultra-high sound frequency bounced off body structures.

32554-32555

32554 Thoracentesis, needle or catheter, aspiration of the pleural space; without imaging guidance
32555 with imaging guidance

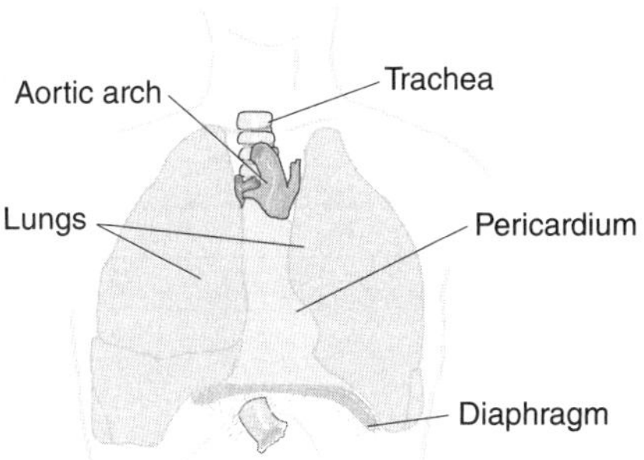

The pleural space is aspirated

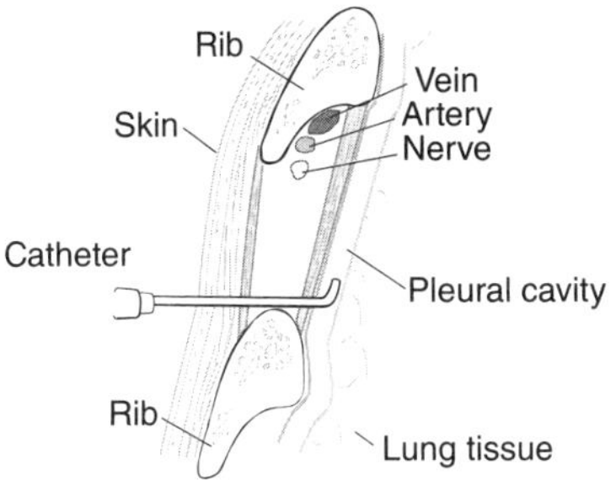

Explanation

The physician removes fluid and/or air from the chest cavity by puncturing through the space between the ribs with a hollow needle (cannula) and entering the chest cavity. The fluid (blood or pus) is removed from the chest cavity by pulling back on the plunger of the syringe attached to the cannula. Report 32554 if the procedure is performed without imaging guidance. Report 32555 when imaging guidance is used during the procedure.

Coding Tips

Do not report 32554 or 32555 with 32550, 32551, 76942, 77002, 77012, 77021, or 75989. For percutaneous insertion of a pleural catheter, see 32556 and 33557.

ICD-10-CM Diagnostic Codes

A15.6	Tuberculous pleurisy
J86.0	Pyothorax with fistula
J86.9	Pyothorax without fistula
J90	Pleural effusion, not elsewhere classified
J91.0	Malignant pleural effusion
J91.8	Pleural effusion in other conditions classified elsewhere
J93.0	Spontaneous tension pneumothorax
J93.11	Primary spontaneous pneumothorax
J94.0	Chylous effusion
J94.2	Hemothorax
J94.8	Other specified pleural conditions
J95.4	Chemical pneumonitis due to anesthesia
M32.13	Lung involvement in systemic lupus erythematosus
M35.02	Sjögren syndrome with lung involvement
N80.B1	Endometriosis of pleura

AMA: **32554** 2023,Jan; 2019,Dec **32555** 2023,Jan; 2019,Dec

Relative Value Units/Medicare Edits

Non-Facility RVU	Work	PE	MP	Total
32554	1.82	4.98	0.21	7.01
32555	2.27	6.86	0.22	9.35
Facility RVU	**Work**	**PE**	**MP**	**Total**
32554	1.82	0.58	0.21	2.61
32555	2.27	0.71	0.22	3.2

	FUD	Status	MUE	Modifiers				IOM Reference
32554	0	A	2(3)	51	50	N/A	N/A	None
32555	0	A	2(3)	51	50	N/A	N/A	

* with documentation

Terms To Know

aspirate. To withdraw fluid or air from a body cavity by suction.

cannula. Tube inserted into a blood vessel, duct, or body cavity to facilitate passage.

effusion. Escape of fluid from within a body cavity.

percutaneous. Through the skin.

pleura. One of the two membranes that surround the lungs. The visceral pleura encases the lung and the parietal pleura lines the inner chest walls.

Lungs and Pleura

● New ▲ Revised + Add On ★ Telemedicine [Resequenced] ☑ Laterality

32556-32557

32556 Pleural drainage, percutaneous, with insertion of indwelling catheter; without imaging guidance
32557 with imaging guidance

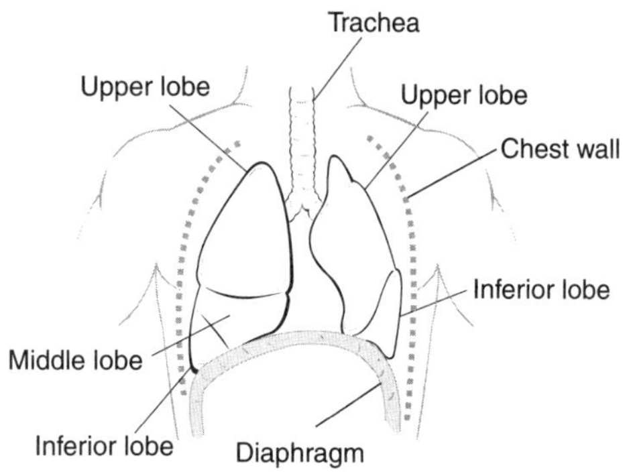

Explanation

The physician removes fluid and/or air from the chest cavity. The patient is positioned dependent upon the location of the fluid (blood or pus) on preprocedural imaging. The chest cavity is accessed by puncturing through the space between the ribs with a needle. Once the fluid is accessed via the needle(s), a guidewire is inserted to the most distal point of the fluid in the pleural cavity. A catheter (i.e., pigtail catheter) is inserted the length of the guidewire and the chest cavity is drained. In some instances, the catheter is connected to a water seal system. Report 32556 if the procedure is performed without imaging guidance. Report 32557 when imaging guidance is used during the procedure.

Coding Tips

Do not report 32556 or 32557 with 32550, 32551, 76942, 77002, 77012, 77021, or 75989. For an open procedure, see 32551. For needle or catheter aspiration of the pleural space via thoracentesis, see 32554 and 32555. For insertion of an indwelling tunneled pleural catheter with a cuff, see 32550.

ICD-10-CM Diagnostic Codes

A15.6	Tuberculous pleurisy
J86.0	Pyothorax with fistula
J86.9	Pyothorax without fistula
J90	Pleural effusion, not elsewhere classified
J91.0	Malignant pleural effusion
J91.8	Pleural effusion in other conditions classified elsewhere
J94.0	Chylous effusion
J94.2	Hemothorax
M32.13	Lung involvement in systemic lupus erythematosus
N80.B1	Endometriosis of pleura
S27.0XXA	Traumatic pneumothorax, initial encounter
S27.1XXA	Traumatic hemothorax, initial encounter

AMA: 32556 2023,Jan **32557** 2023,Jan

Relative Value Units/Medicare Edits

Non-Facility RVU	Work	PE	MP	Total
32556	2.5	19.23	0.37	22.1
32557	3.12	16.17	0.31	19.6
Facility RVU	**Work**	**PE**	**MP**	**Total**
32556	2.5	0.79	0.37	3.66
32557	3.12	0.94	0.31	4.37

	FUD	Status	MUE	Modifiers				IOM Reference
32556	0	A	2(3)	51	50	N/A	N/A	None
32557	0	A	2(3)	51	50	N/A	N/A	

* with documentation

Terms To Know

fistula. Abnormal tube-like passage between two body cavities or organs or from an organ to the outside surface.

pleural effusion. Collection of lymph and other fluid within the pleural space.

pyothorax. Collection of pus in the pleural space that is commonly caused by an infection that spreads from the lung, such as bacterial pneumonia or a lung abscess.

32560

32560 Instillation, via chest tube/catheter, agent for pleurodesis (eg, talc for recurrent or persistent pneumothorax)

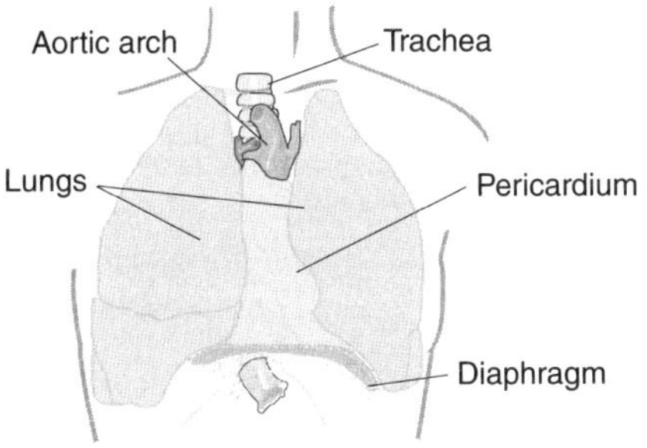

Pleurodesis is the insertion of a caustic chemical into the pleural space, inducing inflammation to eliminate repeated effusion and/or pneumothorax

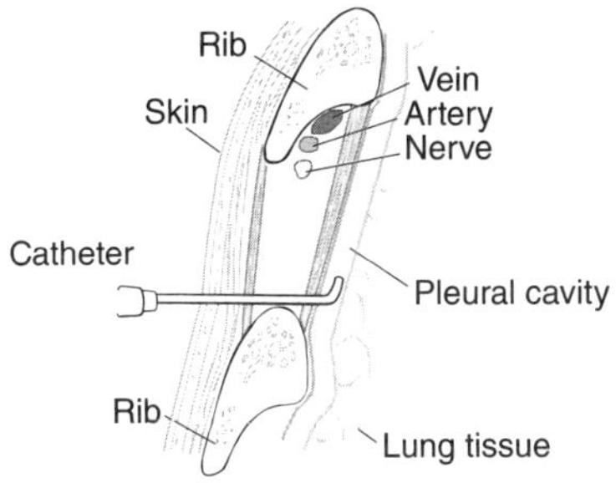

Explanation

The physician instills an agent for pleurodesis, such as talc for recurrent or persistent pneumothorax, into the chest cavity via a chest tube or catheter by puncturing through the space between the ribs. The physician passes a trocar over the top of a rib, punctures through the chest tissues, and enters the pleural cavity. With the end of the trocar, the physician advances the plastic tube into the chest cavity within the pleural space, specifically between the layers of the visceral and parietal pleura. The sharp instrument is removed leaving one end of the plastic catheter in place. A syringe is attached to the outside end of the catheter and the agent is injected into the pleural space. The agent selected is designed to eradicate the pleural space preventing reoccurrence of pleural effusion.

Coding Tips

For thoracentesis with aspiration of the pleural space, see 32554 and 32555. For treatment of pneumothorax with thoracentesis, with insertion of an indwelling catheter, see 32556 and 32557. For pleural scarification by other methods, see 32215. For insertion of a chest tube, see 32551. For thoracoscopy with pleurodesis, see 32650.

ICD-10-CM Diagnostic Codes

J86.0	Pyothorax with fistula
J86.9	Pyothorax without fistula
J90	Pleural effusion, not elsewhere classified
J91.0	Malignant pleural effusion
J91.8	Pleural effusion in other conditions classified elsewhere
J93.0	Spontaneous tension pneumothorax
J93.11	Primary spontaneous pneumothorax
J93.12	Secondary spontaneous pneumothorax
J93.81	Chronic pneumothorax
J93.82	Other air leak
J93.83	Other pneumothorax
J94.0	Chylous effusion
J94.8	Other specified pleural conditions
J95.811	Postprocedural pneumothorax
J95.812	Postprocedural air leak
L60.5	Yellow nail syndrome
M32.13	Lung involvement in systemic lupus erythematosus

Relative Value Units/Medicare Edits

Non-Facility RVU	Work	PE	MP	Total
32560	1.54	5.78	0.24	7.56
Facility RVU	**Work**	**PE**	**MP**	**Total**
32560	1.54	0.46	0.24	2.24

	FUD	Status	MUE	Modifiers				IOM Reference
32560	0	A	1(3)	51	N/A	N/A	N/A	None

* with documentation

Terms To Know

dyspnea. Difficult or labored breathing.

effusion. Escape of fluid from within a body cavity.

emphysematous bleb. Formation of blisters or vesicles greater than 1.0 mm within an emphysematous lung, containing serum or blood.

fistula. Abnormal tube-like passage between two body cavities or organs or from an organ to the outside surface.

pleurisy. Inflammation of the serous membrane that lines the lungs and the thoracic cavity. Pleurisy may cause effusion within the cavity or have exudate in the pleural space or on the membrane surface.

pleurisy. Inflammation of the serous membrane that lines the lungs and the thoracic cavity. Pleurisy may cause effusion within the cavity or have exudate in the pleural space or on the membrane surface.

spontaneous tension pneumothorax. Air leaking from the lung and trapped in the lung lining.

thoracentesis. Surgical puncture of the chest cavity with a specialized needle or hollow tubing to aspirate fluid from within the pleural space for diagnostic or therapeutic reasons.

trocar. Cannula or a sharp pointed instrument used to puncture and aspirate fluid from cavities.

32561-32562

32561 Instillation(s), via chest tube/catheter, agent for fibrinolysis (eg, fibrinolytic agent for break up of multiloculated effusion); initial day
32562 subsequent day

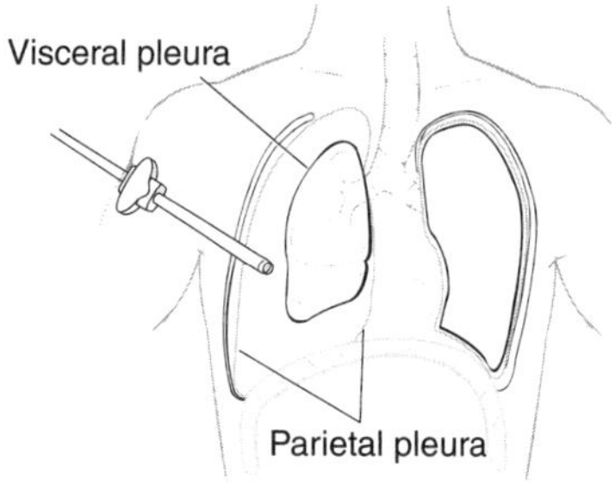

Explanation

The physician instills a fibrinolytic agent (one that breaks up fibrinous adhesions) into the chest cavity via a chest tube or catheter by puncturing through the space between the ribs. To enter the chest cavity, the physician passes a trocar over the top of a rib, punctures through the chest tissues, and enters the pleural cavity. With the end of the trocar in the chest cavity, the physician advances the plastic tube into the chest cavity. The sharp instrument is removed, leaving one end of the plastic catheter in place within the chest cavity. A syringe is attached to the outside end of the catheter and a fibrinolytic agent, such as a saline mixture with Streptokinase or urokinase, is injected into the chest cavity. The agent selected is designed to break up multiloculated pleural effusions and facilitate adequate drainage. Report 32561 for the first day of instillation and 32562 for each subsequent day.

Coding Tips

These codes should be reported only once per day even if multiple instillations are performed. For insertion of a chest tube, see 32551.

ICD-10-CM Diagnostic Codes

A15.6	Tuberculous pleurisy
J90	Pleural effusion, not elsewhere classified
J91.0	Malignant pleural effusion
J91.8	Pleural effusion in other conditions classified elsewhere
J94.0	Chylous effusion
J94.2	Hemothorax
J94.8	Other specified pleural conditions
M32.13	Lung involvement in systemic lupus erythematosus

Relative Value Units/Medicare Edits

Non-Facility RVU	Work	PE	MP	Total
32561	1.39	1.29	0.16	2.84
32562	1.24	1.16	0.14	2.54
Facility RVU	**Work**	**PE**	**MP**	**Total**
32561	1.39	0.43	0.16	1.98
32562	1.24	0.39	0.14	1.77

	FUD	Status	MUE	Modifiers				IOM Reference
32561	0	A	1(2)	51	N/A	N/A	80	None
32562	0	A	1(2)	51	N/A	N/A	80	

* with documentation

32601

32601 Thoracoscopy, diagnostic (separate procedure); lungs, pericardial sac, mediastinal or pleural space, without biopsy

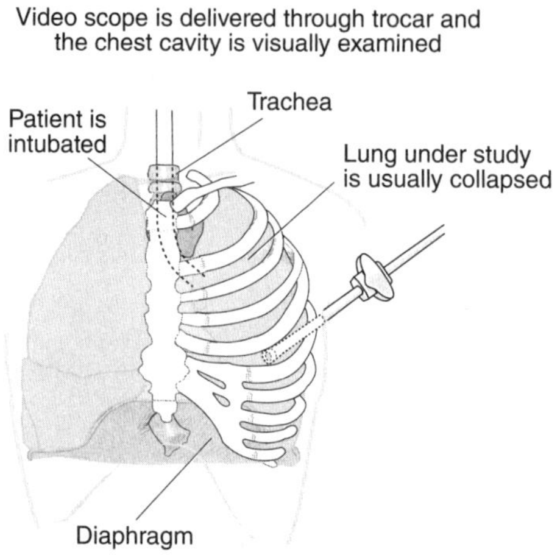

Explanation

The physician examines the inside of the chest cavity through a rigid or flexible fiberoptic endoscope. The procedure can be done under local or general anesthesia. The surgeon makes a small incision between two ribs and by blunt dissection and the use of a trocar enters the thoracic cavity. The endoscope is passed through the trocar and into the chest cavity. The lung is usually partially collapsed by instilling air into the chest through the trocar, or if general anesthesia is used, the lung may be collapsed through a double lumen endotracheal tube inserted through the mouth into the trachea. The contents of the chest cavity are examined by direct visualization and/or the use of a video camera. Still photographs may be taken as part of the procedure. At the conclusion of the procedure, the endoscope and the trocar are removed. A chest tube for drainage and re-expansion of the lung is usually inserted through the wound used for the thoracoscopy.

Coding Tips

This separate procedure by definition is usually a component of a more complex service and not identified separately. When performed alone or with other unrelated procedures/services, it may be reported. If performed alone, list the code; if performed with other procedures/services, list the code and append modifier 59 or an X{EPSU} modifier. Report the appropriate endoscopy for each anatomic site examined. Surgical thoracoscopy (video-assisted thoracic surgery or VATS) always includes diagnostic thoracoscopy. For thoracoscopic biopsies of lung infiltrates, lung nodules, or masses, or for pleural biopsies, see 32607–32609. For a thoracotomy to biopsy lung or pleura, see 32096, 32097, or 32098.

ICD-10-CM Diagnostic Codes

A18.84	Tuberculosis of heart
A39.53	Meningococcal pericarditis
A54.83	Gonococcal heart infection
B33.23	Viral pericarditis
C34.01	Malignant neoplasm of right main bronchus ☑
C34.02	Malignant neoplasm of left main bronchus ☑
C34.2	Malignant neoplasm of middle lobe, bronchus or lung
C34.31	Malignant neoplasm of lower lobe, right bronchus or lung ☑
C34.32	Malignant neoplasm of lower lobe, left bronchus or lung ☑
C38.0	Malignant neoplasm of heart

C38.1 Malignant neoplasm of anterior mediastinum
C38.2 Malignant neoplasm of posterior mediastinum
C38.4 Malignant neoplasm of pleura
C45.0 Mesothelioma of pleura
C46.51 Kaposi's sarcoma of right lung ☑
C76.1 Malignant neoplasm of thorax
C78.01 Secondary malignant neoplasm of right lung ☑
C78.1 Secondary malignant neoplasm of mediastinum
C78.2 Secondary malignant neoplasm of pleura
C81.02 Nodular lymphocyte predominant Hodgkin lymphoma, intrathoracic lymph nodes
C81.12 Nodular sclerosis Hodgkin lymphoma, intrathoracic lymph nodes
C81.22 Mixed cellularity Hodgkin lymphoma, intrathoracic lymph nodes
C81.32 Lymphocyte depleted Hodgkin lymphoma, intrathoracic lymph nodes
C81.42 Lymphocyte-rich Hodgkin lymphoma, intrathoracic lymph nodes
C82.02 Follicular lymphoma grade I, intrathoracic lymph nodes
C82.12 Follicular lymphoma grade II, intrathoracic lymph nodes
C82.32 Follicular lymphoma grade IIIa, intrathoracic lymph nodes
C82.52 Diffuse follicle center lymphoma, intrathoracic lymph nodes
C82.62 Cutaneous follicle center lymphoma, intrathoracic lymph nodes
C83.02 Small cell B-cell lymphoma, intrathoracic lymph nodes
C83.12 Mantle cell lymphoma, intrathoracic lymph nodes
C83.32 Diffuse large B-cell lymphoma, intrathoracic lymph nodes
C83.52 Lymphoblastic (diffuse) lymphoma, intrathoracic lymph nodes
C83.72 Burkitt lymphoma, intrathoracic lymph nodes
C84.02 Mycosis fungoides, intrathoracic lymph nodes
C84.12 Sezary disease, intrathoracic lymph nodes
C85.22 Mediastinal (thymic) large B-cell lymphoma, intrathoracic lymph nodes
I01.0 Acute rheumatic pericarditis
I09.2 Chronic rheumatic pericarditis
I30.0 Acute nonspecific idiopathic pericarditis
I30.1 Infective pericarditis
I31.0 Chronic adhesive pericarditis
I31.1 Chronic constrictive pericarditis
I31.31 Malignant pericardial effusion in diseases classified elsewhere
I31.39 Other pericardial effusion (noninflammatory)
J85.0 Gangrene and necrosis of lung
J85.1 Abscess of lung with pneumonia
J85.3 Abscess of mediastinum
J86.0 Pyothorax with fistula
J90 Pleural effusion, not elsewhere classified
J91.0 Malignant pleural effusion
J91.8 Pleural effusion in other conditions classified elsewhere
J93.0 Spontaneous tension pneumothorax
J93.11 Primary spontaneous pneumothorax
J93.12 Secondary spontaneous pneumothorax
J93.81 Chronic pneumothorax
J94.0 Chylous effusion
J94.1 Fibrothorax
J94.2 Hemothorax
M32.12 Pericarditis in systemic lupus erythematosus
M32.13 Lung involvement in systemic lupus erythematosus

AMA: 32601 2024,Jan

Relative Value Units/Medicare Edits

Non-Facility RVU	Work	PE	MP	Total
32601	5.5	2.27	1.32	9.09
Facility RVU	**Work**	**PE**	**MP**	**Total**
32601	5.5	2.27	1.32	9.09

	FUD	Status	MUE	Modifiers				IOM Reference
32601	0	A	1(3)	51	N/A	N/A	80*	None

* with documentation

Terms To Know

blunt dissection. Surgical technique used to expose an underlying area by separating along natural cleavage lines of tissue, without cutting.

cannula. Tube inserted into a blood vessel, duct, or body cavity to facilitate passage.

pleura. One of the two membranes that surround the lungs. The visceral pleura encases the lung and the parietal pleura lines the inner chest walls.

trocar. Cannula or a sharp pointed instrument used to puncture and aspirate fluid from cavities.

VATS. Video-assisted thoracic surgery. Less invasive technique than open thoracic surgery for various procedures on the heart and lungs. The surgeon typically gains access to the chest cavity using trocars (slender tube-like instruments), through which an endoscope and the surgical instruments are passed. The patient's internal organs can then be viewed intraoperatively on a monitor.

32604

32604 Thoracoscopy, diagnostic (separate procedure); pericardial sac, with biopsy

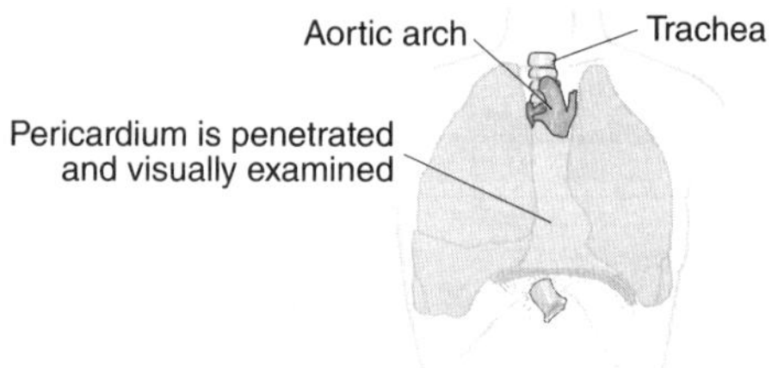

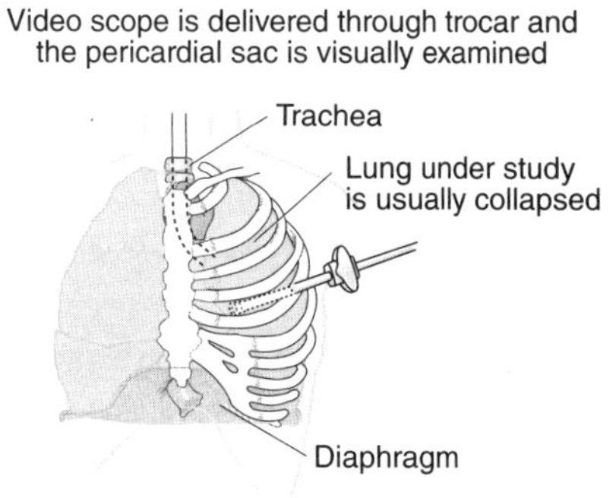

Explanation

The physician examines the pericardial sac using a rigid or flexible fiberoptic endoscope. The procedure can be done under local or general anesthesia. The physician makes a small incision between two ribs and by blunt dissection and the use of a trocar enters the thoracic cavity. The endoscope is passed through the trocar and into the chest cavity. The lung is usually partially collapsed by instilling air into the chest through the trocar or, if general anesthesia is used, the lung may be collapsed through a double lumen endotracheal tube inserted through the mouth into the trachea. The endoscope is advanced to and into the pericardial sac as the physician views the structures and the anatomy of the area through the scope. The contents of the pericardial sac are examined by direct visualization and/or the use of a video camera. Still photographs may be taken as part of the procedure. The pericardial tissue selected for biopsy is identified and the biopsy is taken using a device inserted through the endoscope. At the conclusion of the procedure, the endoscope and the trocar are withdrawn. A chest tube for drainage and re-expansion of the lung is usually inserted through the wound used for the thoracoscopy.

Coding Tips

This separate procedure by definition is usually a component of a more complex service and is not identified separately. When performed alone or with other unrelated procedures/services, it may be reported. If performed alone, list the code; if performed with other procedures/services, list the code and append modifier 59 or X{EPSU}. Report the appropriate endoscopy for each anatomic site examined. Surgical thoracoscopy (video-assisted thoracic surgery or VATS) always includes diagnostic thoracoscopy. For diagnostic thoracoscopy of the pericardial sac without biopsy, see 32601. To report pericardial biopsy, open, see 39010.

ICD-10-CM Diagnostic Codes

A18.84	Tuberculosis of heart
A39.53	Meningococcal pericarditis
A52.06	Other syphilitic heart involvement
A54.83	Gonococcal heart infection
A69.29	Other conditions associated with Lyme disease
B33.23	Viral pericarditis
C38.0	Malignant neoplasm of heart
C45.2	Mesothelioma of pericardium
I01.0	Acute rheumatic pericarditis
I09.2	Chronic rheumatic pericarditis
I30.0	Acute nonspecific idiopathic pericarditis
I30.1	Infective pericarditis
I30.8	Other forms of acute pericarditis
I31.0	Chronic adhesive pericarditis
I31.1	Chronic constrictive pericarditis
I31.2	Hemopericardium, not elsewhere classified
I31.31	Malignant pericardial effusion in diseases classified elsewhere
I31.39	Other pericardial effusion (noninflammatory)
I31.8	Other specified diseases of pericardium
I32	Pericarditis in diseases classified elsewhere
M32.12	Pericarditis in systemic lupus erythematosus

AMA: 32604 2021,Apr

Relative Value Units/Medicare Edits

Non-Facility RVU	Work	PE	MP	Total
32604	8.77	3.17	2.17	14.11
Facility RVU	**Work**	**PE**	**MP**	**Total**
32604	8.77	3.17	2.17	14.11

	FUD	Status	MUE	Modifiers				IOM Reference
32604	0	A	1(3)	51	N/A	N/A	80*	None

* with documentation

Terms To Know

biopsy. Tissue or fluid removed for diagnostic purposes through analysis of the cells in the biopsy material.

diagnostic procedures. Procedure performed on a patient to obtain information to assess the medical condition of the patient or to identify a disease and to determine the nature and severity of an illness or injury.

pericarditis. Inflammation affecting the pericardium, the fibroserous membrane that surrounds the heart.

32606

32606 Thoracoscopy, diagnostic (separate procedure); mediastinal space, with biopsy

Video scope is delivered through trocar and the mediastinal space is visually examined

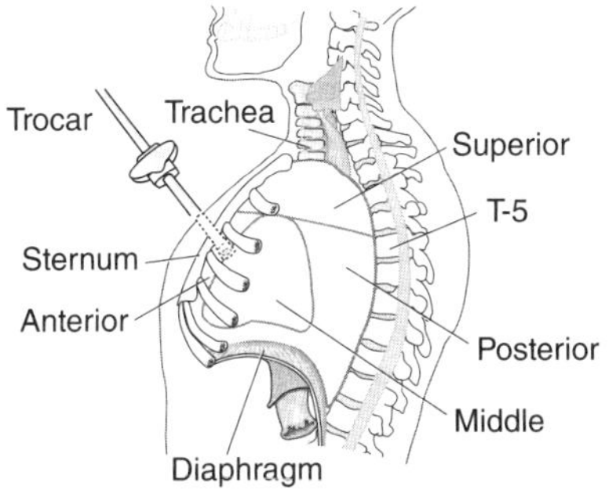

The mediastinal space is the general region between the left and right lungs

Explanation

The physician examines the inside of the mediastinal space through a rigid or flexible fiberoptic endoscope. The procedure can be done under local or general anesthesia. The physician makes a small incision between two ribs and by blunt dissection and the use of a trocar enters the thoracic cavity. The endoscope is passed through the trocar and into the chest cavity. The lung is usually partially collapsed by instilling air into the chest through the trocar or, if general anesthesia is used, the lung may be collapsed through a special double lumen endotracheal tube inserted through the mouth into the trachea. As the physician views the structures and the anatomy of the area through the endoscope, the endoscope is advanced into the mediastinum (area inside the center of the chest cavity between the lungs). The contents of the mediastinal space are examined by direct visualization and/or by the use of a video camera. Still photographs may be taken as part of the procedure. The tissue selected for biopsy is identified and a biopsy taken using a device inserted through the endoscope. At the conclusion of the procedure, the endoscope and the trocar are withdrawn. A chest tube for drainage and re-expansion of the lung is usually inserted through the wound used for the thoracoscopy.

Coding Tips

This separate procedure by definition is usually a component of a more complex service and is not identified separately. When performed alone or with other unrelated procedures/services, it may be reported. If performed alone, list the code; if performed with other procedures/services, list the code and append modifier 59 or an X{EPSU} modifier. Report the appropriate endoscopy for each anatomic site examined. Surgical thoracoscopy (video-assisted thoracic surgery or VATS) always includes diagnostic thoracoscopy. For diagnostic thoracoscopy in the mediastinal space, see 32601. For biopsy of the lung or mediastinum by percutaneous needle, see 32408. For mediastinoscopy, with or without biopsy, see 39401.

ICD-10-CM Diagnostic Codes

C33 Malignant neoplasm of trachea
C34.01 Malignant neoplasm of right main bronchus ☑
C34.02 Malignant neoplasm of left main bronchus ☑
C38.0 Malignant neoplasm of heart
C38.1 Malignant neoplasm of anterior mediastinum
C38.2 Malignant neoplasm of posterior mediastinum
C38.8 Malignant neoplasm of overlapping sites of heart, mediastinum and pleura
C78.1 Secondary malignant neoplasm of mediastinum
C7A.090 Malignant carcinoid tumor of the bronchus and lung
C81.02 Nodular lymphocyte predominant Hodgkin lymphoma, intrathoracic lymph nodes
C81.12 Nodular sclerosis Hodgkin lymphoma, intrathoracic lymph nodes
C81.22 Mixed cellularity Hodgkin lymphoma, intrathoracic lymph nodes
C81.32 Lymphocyte depleted Hodgkin lymphoma, intrathoracic lymph nodes
C81.42 Lymphocyte-rich Hodgkin lymphoma, intrathoracic lymph nodes
C81.72 Other Hodgkin lymphoma, intrathoracic lymph nodes
C82.02 Follicular lymphoma grade I, intrathoracic lymph nodes
C82.12 Follicular lymphoma grade II, intrathoracic lymph nodes
C82.32 Follicular lymphoma grade IIIa, intrathoracic lymph nodes
C82.52 Diffuse follicle center lymphoma, intrathoracic lymph nodes
C82.62 Cutaneous follicle center lymphoma, intrathoracic lymph nodes
C82.82 Other types of follicular lymphoma, intrathoracic lymph nodes
C83.02 Small cell B-cell lymphoma, intrathoracic lymph nodes
C83.12 Mantle cell lymphoma, intrathoracic lymph nodes
C83.32 Diffuse large B-cell lymphoma, intrathoracic lymph nodes
C83.52 Lymphoblastic (diffuse) lymphoma, intrathoracic lymph nodes
C83.72 Burkitt lymphoma, intrathoracic lymph nodes
C84.02 Mycosis fungoides, intrathoracic lymph nodes
C84.12 Sezary disease, intrathoracic lymph nodes
C84.Z2 Other mature T/NK-cell lymphomas, intrathoracic lymph nodes
C85.22 Mediastinal (thymic) large B-cell lymphoma, intrathoracic lymph nodes
C85.82 Other specified types of non-Hodgkin lymphoma, intrathoracic lymph nodes
D14.31 Benign neoplasm of right bronchus and lung ☑
D14.32 Benign neoplasm of left bronchus and lung ☑
D15.0 Benign neoplasm of thymus
D15.2 Benign neoplasm of mediastinum
D38.3 Neoplasm of uncertain behavior of mediastinum
D38.4 Neoplasm of uncertain behavior of thymus
D3A.090 Benign carcinoid tumor of the bronchus and lung

AMA: 32606 2021,Apr

Relative Value Units/Medicare Edits

Non-Facility RVU	Work	PE	MP	Total
32606	8.39	3.14	2.06	13.59
Facility RVU	**Work**	**PE**	**MP**	**Total**
32606	8.39	3.14	2.06	13.59

	FUD	Status	MUE	Modifiers				IOM Reference
32606	0	A	1(3)	51	N/A	N/A	80*	None

* with documentation

32607

32607 Thoracoscopy; with diagnostic biopsy(ies) of lung infiltrate(s) (eg, wedge, incisional), unilateral

Video scope is delivered through trocar and the chest cavity is visually examined

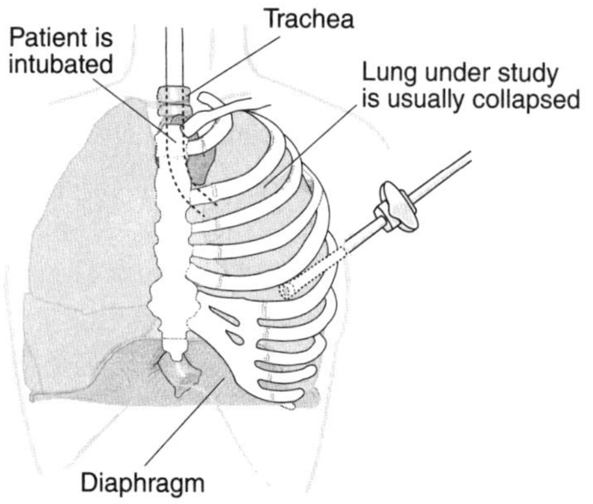

Lung infiltrates are biopsied

Explanation

The physician biopsies lung infiltrates through a rigid or flexible fiberoptic endoscope. This procedure can be done under local or general anesthesia. The surgeon makes a small incision between two ribs and by blunt dissection and the use of a trocar enters the thoracic cavity. The endoscope is passed through the trocar and into the chest cavity. One lung is usually partially collapsed by instilling air into the chest through the trocar or, if general anesthesia is used, the lung may be collapsed through a double lumen endotracheal tube inserted through the mouth into the trachea. The contents of the chest cavity are examined by direct visualization and/or the use of a video camera. Still photographs may be taken as part of the procedure. The lung infiltrates selected for biopsy are identified and the biopsy is taken using a device inserted through the endoscope. At the conclusion of the procedure, the endoscope and the trocar are removed. A chest tube for drainage and re-expansion of the lung is usually inserted through the wound used for the thoracoscopy.

Coding Tips

This is a unilateral procedure. If performed bilaterally, some payers require that the service be reported twice with modifier 50 appended to the second code while others require identification of the service only once with modifier 50 appended. Check with the individual payers. Modifier 50 identifies a procedure performed identically on the opposite side of the body (mirror image). This code should only be reported once per lung. Do not report 32607 with 32440, 32442, 32445, 32488, or 32671.

ICD-10-CM Diagnostic Codes

C34.11	Malignant neoplasm of upper lobe, right bronchus or lung ☑
C34.2	Malignant neoplasm of middle lobe, bronchus or lung
C34.31	Malignant neoplasm of lower lobe, right bronchus or lung ☑
C34.81	Malignant neoplasm of overlapping sites of right bronchus and lung ☑
C78.01	Secondary malignant neoplasm of right lung ☑
D02.21	Carcinoma in situ of right bronchus and lung ☑
D14.31	Benign neoplasm of right bronchus and lung ☑
D38.1	Neoplasm of uncertain behavior of trachea, bronchus and lung
D86.0	Sarcoidosis of lung
J60	Coalworker's pneumoconiosis [A]
J61	Pneumoconiosis due to asbestos and other mineral fibers [A]
J62.0	Pneumoconiosis due to talc dust
J62.8	Pneumoconiosis due to other dust containing silica
J63.0	Aluminosis (of lung)
J63.1	Bauxite fibrosis (of lung)
J63.2	Berylliosis
J63.3	Graphite fibrosis (of lung)
J63.4	Siderosis
J63.5	Stannosis
J63.6	Pneumoconiosis due to other specified inorganic dusts
J66.0	Byssinosis
J66.1	Flax-dressers' disease
J66.2	Cannabinosis
J66.8	Airway disease due to other specific organic dusts
J67.8	Hypersensitivity pneumonitis due to other organic dusts
J68.0	Bronchitis and pneumonitis due to chemicals, gases, fumes and vapors
J68.4	Chronic respiratory conditions due to chemicals, gases, fumes and vapors
J70.2	Acute drug-induced interstitial lung disorders
J82.81	Chronic eosinophilic pneumonia
J82.82	Acute eosinophilic pneumonia
J84.112	Idiopathic pulmonary fibrosis
J84.113	Idiopathic non-specific interstitial pneumonitis
J84.115	Respiratory bronchiolitis interstitial lung disease
J84.117	Desquamative interstitial pneumonia
J84.170	Interstitial lung disease with progressive fibrotic phenotype in diseases classified elsewhere
J84.178	Other interstitial pulmonary diseases with fibrosis in diseases classified elsewhere
J84.2	Lymphoid interstitial pneumonia
J84.82	Adult pulmonary Langerhans cell histiocytosis [A]
M32.13	Lung involvement in systemic lupus erythematosus
M33.01	Juvenile dermatomyositis with respiratory involvement
M33.11	Other dermatomyositis with respiratory involvement
M33.21	Polymyositis with respiratory involvement
M35.02	Sjögren syndrome with lung involvement
N80.B2	Endometriosis of lung

AMA: 32607 2021,Apr

Relative Value Units/Medicare Edits

Non-Facility RVU	Work	PE	MP	Total
32607	5.5	2.25	1.32	9.07
Facility RVU	**Work**	**PE**	**MP**	**Total**
32607	5.5	2.25	1.32	9.07

	FUD	Status	MUE	Modifiers				IOM Reference
32607	0	A	1(3)	51	N/A	N/A	80*	None

* with documentation

32608

32608 Thoracoscopy; with diagnostic biopsy(ies) of lung nodule(s) or mass(es) (eg, wedge, incisional), unilateral

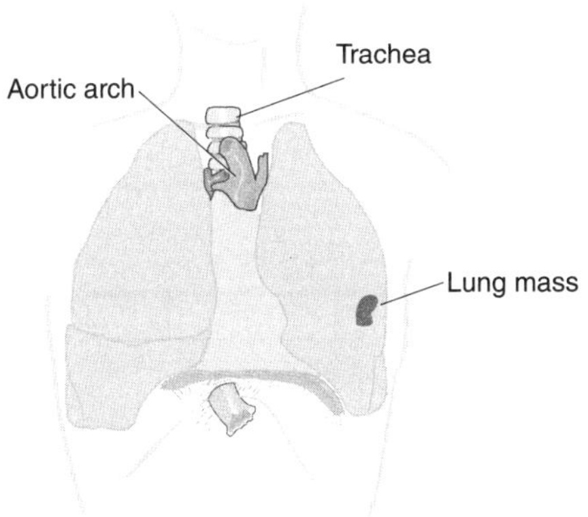

Video scope is delivered through trocar, and the pericardial sac is visually examined and nodules or masses are biopsied

Explanation

The physician biopsies a lung nodule or mass through a rigid or flexible fiberoptic endoscope. This procedure can be done under local or general anesthesia. The surgeon makes a small incision between two ribs and by blunt dissection and the use of a trocar enters the thoracic cavity. The endoscope is passed through the trocar and into the chest cavity. One lung is usually partially collapsed by instilling air into the chest through the trocar or, if general anesthesia is used, the lung may be collapsed through a double lumen endotracheal tube inserted through the mouth into the trachea. The contents of the chest cavity are examined by direct visualization and/or the use of a video camera. Still photographs may be taken as part of the procedure. The lung nodule(s) or mass(es) selected for biopsy is identified and the biopsy is taken using a device inserted through the endoscope. At the conclusion of the procedure, the endoscope and the trocar are removed. A chest tube for drainage and re-expansion of the lung is usually inserted through the wound used for the thoracoscopy.

Coding Tips

This is a unilateral procedure. If performed bilaterally, some payers require that the service be reported twice with modifier 50 appended to the second code while others require identification of the service only once with modifier 50 appended. Check with individual payers. Modifier 50 identifies a procedure performed identically on the opposite side of the body (mirror image). This code may only be reported once per lung. Do not report 32608 with 32440, 32442, 32445, 32488, or 32671.

ICD-10-CM Diagnostic Codes

B67.1	Echinococcus granulosus infection of lung
C34.11	Malignant neoplasm of upper lobe, right bronchus or lung ☑
C34.12	Malignant neoplasm of upper lobe, left bronchus or lung ☑
C34.2	Malignant neoplasm of middle lobe, bronchus or lung
C34.31	Malignant neoplasm of lower lobe, right bronchus or lung ☑
C34.32	Malignant neoplasm of lower lobe, left bronchus or lung ☑
C34.81	Malignant neoplasm of overlapping sites of right bronchus and lung ☑
C34.82	Malignant neoplasm of overlapping sites of left bronchus and lung ☑
C46.51	Kaposi's sarcoma of right lung ☑
C46.52	Kaposi's sarcoma of left lung ☑
C78.01	Secondary malignant neoplasm of right lung ☑
C78.02	Secondary malignant neoplasm of left lung ☑
D02.21	Carcinoma in situ of right bronchus and lung ☑
D02.22	Carcinoma in situ of left bronchus and lung ☑
D14.31	Benign neoplasm of right bronchus and lung ☑
D14.32	Benign neoplasm of left bronchus and lung ☑
D38.1	Neoplasm of uncertain behavior of trachea, bronchus and lung
D86.0	Sarcoidosis of lung
J85.0	Gangrene and necrosis of lung
R91.1	Solitary pulmonary nodule

AMA: **32608** 2021,Apr

Relative Value Units/Medicare Edits

Non-Facility RVU	Work	PE	MP	Total
32608	6.84	2.63	1.68	11.15
Facility RVU	**Work**	**PE**	**MP**	**Total**
32608	6.84	2.63	1.68	11.15

	FUD	Status	MUE	Modifiers				IOM Reference
32608	0	A	1(3)	51	N/A	N/A	80*	None

* with documentation

Terms To Know

dissection. Separating by cutting tissue or body structures apart.

endoscopy. Visual inspection of the body using a fiberoptic scope.

general anesthesia. State of unconsciousness produced by an anesthetic agent or agents, inducing amnesia by blocking the awareness center in the brain, and rendering the patient unable to control protective reflexes, such as breathing.

32609

32609 Thoracoscopy; with biopsy(ies) of pleura

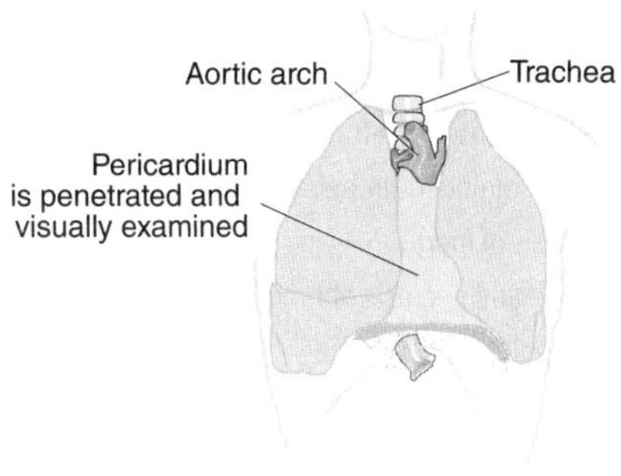

Video scope is delivered through trocar and the pericardial sac is visually examined and biopsies obtained

Explanation

The physician biopsies the pleura through a rigid or flexible fiberoptic endoscope. This procedure can be done under local or general anesthesia. The surgeon makes a small incision between two ribs and by blunt dissection and the use of a trocar enters the thoracic cavity. The endoscope is passed through the trocar and into the chest cavity. One lung is usually partially collapsed by instilling air into the chest through the trocar or, if general anesthesia is used, the lung may be collapsed through a double lumen endotracheal tube inserted through the mouth into the trachea. The contents of the chest cavity are examined by direct visualization and/or the use of a video camera. Still photographs may be taken as part of the procedure. The area of the pleura selected for biopsy is identified and the biopsy is taken using a device inserted through the endoscope. At the conclusion of the procedure, the endoscope and the trocar are removed. A chest tube for drainage and re-expansion of the lung is usually inserted through the wound used for the thoracoscopy.

Coding Tips

Surgical thoracoscopy (video-assisted thoracic surgery or VATS) always includes diagnostic thoracoscopy.

ICD-10-CM Diagnostic Codes

A15.6	Tuberculous pleurisy
C38.4	Malignant neoplasm of pleura
C38.8	Malignant neoplasm of overlapping sites of heart, mediastinum and pleura
C45.0	Mesothelioma of pleura
C78.2	Secondary malignant neoplasm of pleura
D19.0	Benign neoplasm of mesothelial tissue of pleura
D38.2	Neoplasm of uncertain behavior of pleura
J86.0	Pyothorax with fistula
J86.9	Pyothorax without fistula
J90	Pleural effusion, not elsewhere classified
J91.0	Malignant pleural effusion
J91.8	Pleural effusion in other conditions classified elsewhere
J92.0	Pleural plaque with presence of asbestos
J92.9	Pleural plaque without asbestos
J94.0	Chylous effusion
J94.1	Fibrothorax
J94.2	Hemothorax
J94.8	Other specified pleural conditions
M32.13	Lung involvement in systemic lupus erythematosus
N80.B1	Endometriosis of pleura
Q34.0	Anomaly of pleura

AMA: **32609** 2021,Apr

Relative Value Units/Medicare Edits

Non-Facility RVU	Work	PE	MP	Total
32609	4.58	1.98	0.99	7.55
Facility RVU	**Work**	**PE**	**MP**	**Total**
32609	4.58	1.98	0.99	7.55

	FUD	Status	MUE	Modifiers				IOM Reference
32609	0	A	1(3)	51	N/A	N/A	80*	None

* with documentation

Terms To Know

dissection. Separating by cutting tissue or body structures apart.

hemoptysis. Coughing up or spitting out blood or blood-streaked sputum.

pleura. One of the two membranes that surround the lungs. The visceral pleura encases the lung and the parietal pleura lines the inner chest walls.

pleural effusion. Collection of lymph and other fluid within the pleural space.

pleurisy. Inflammation of the serous membrane that lines the lungs and the thoracic cavity. Pleurisy may cause effusion within the cavity or have exudate in the pleural space or on the membrane surface.

trachea. Tube descending from the larynx and branching into the right and left main bronchi.

trocar. Cannula or a sharp pointed instrument used to puncture and aspirate fluid from cavities.

32650

32650 Thoracoscopy, surgical; with pleurodesis (eg, mechanical or chemical)

Pleurodesis is performed

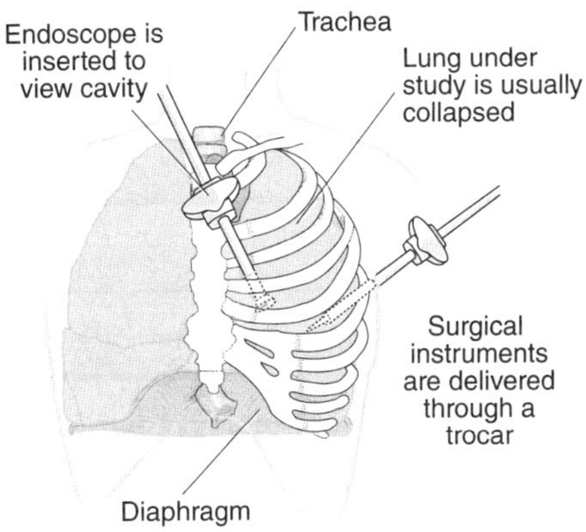

Explanation

The physician examines the inside of the chest cavity through a rigid or flexible fiberoptic endoscope and induces adhesion of the surface of the lung to the inside surface of the chest cavity. The procedure can be done under local or general anesthesia. The physician makes a small incision between two ribs and by blunt dissection and the use of a trocar enters the thoracic cavity. The endoscope is passed through the trocar and into the chest cavity. The lung is usually partially collapsed by instilling air into the chest through the trocar or, if general anesthesia is used, the lung may be collapsed through a double lumen endotracheal tube inserted through the mouth into the trachea. The contents of the chest cavity are examined by direct visualization and/or by the use of a video camera. Still photographs may be taken as part of the procedure. A second trocar and instruments may be inserted into the chest cavity through a second wound in the chest. Adhesion may be induced in one of two ways: by abrading the surfaces of the lung and the inside of the chest cavity or by the instillation of chemicals into the chest cavity that bath the surfaces of the lung and the inside of the chest cavity. Most commonly, a chemical solution is instilled into the chest through the endoscope or second puncture site. At the conclusion of the procedure, the endoscope and the trocar are removed. A chest tube for drainage and re-expansion of the lung is usually inserted through the wound used for the thoracoscopy.

Coding Tips

Surgical thoracoscopy always includes diagnostic thoracoscopy. For percutaneous chemical pleurodesis, see 32560. For pleural scarification for repeat pneumothorax, see 32215.

ICD-10-CM Diagnostic Codes

J86.0	Pyothorax with fistula
J86.9	Pyothorax without fistula
J90	Pleural effusion, not elsewhere classified
J91.0	Malignant pleural effusion
J91.8	Pleural effusion in other conditions classified elsewhere
J93.0	Spontaneous tension pneumothorax
J93.11	Primary spontaneous pneumothorax
J93.12	Secondary spontaneous pneumothorax
J93.81	Chronic pneumothorax
J93.82	Other air leak
J93.83	Other pneumothorax
J94.0	Chylous effusion
J94.8	Other specified pleural conditions
J95.811	Postprocedural pneumothorax
J95.812	Postprocedural air leak
M32.13	Lung involvement in systemic lupus erythematosus
N80.B1	Endometriosis of pleura

Relative Value Units/Medicare Edits

Non-Facility RVU	Work	PE	MP	Total
32650	10.83	6.48	2.58	19.89
Facility RVU	**Work**	**PE**	**MP**	**Total**
32650	10.83	6.48	2.58	19.89

	FUD	Status	MUE	Modifiers				IOM Reference
32650	90	A	1(2)	51	50	62*	80	None

* with documentation

Terms To Know

emphysematous bleb. Formation of blisters or vesicles greater than 1.0 mm within an emphysematous lung, containing serum or blood.

pleurodesis. Injection of a sclerosing agent into the pleural space for creating adhesions between the parietal and the visceral pleura to treat a collapsed lung caused by air trapped in the pleural cavity, or severe cases of pleural effusion.

32651-32652

32651 Thoracoscopy, surgical; with partial pulmonary decortication
32652 with total pulmonary decortication, including intrapleural pneumonolysis

Portion of constricting outer membrane of lung is removed

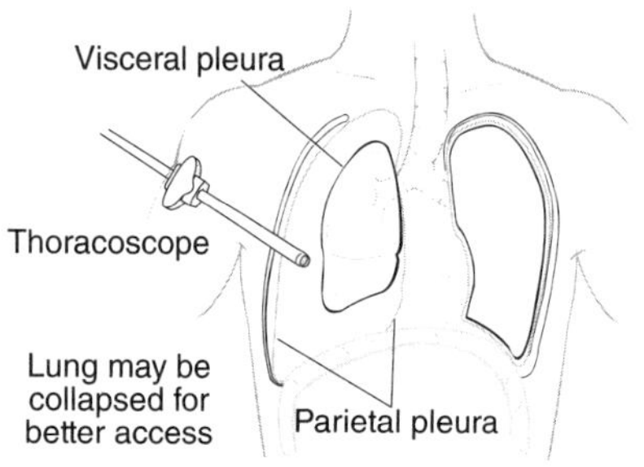

Adhesions between lung tissue and the inside surface of the chest cavity may be released

Explanation

The physician examines the inside of the chest cavity through a rigid or flexible fiberoptic endoscope and removes a portion of the tissue covering the surface of the lung. The procedure can be done under local or general anesthesia. The physician makes a small incision between two ribs and by blunt dissection and the use of a trocar enters the thoracic cavity. The endoscope is passed through the trocar and into the chest cavity. The lung is usually partially collapsed by instilling air into the chest through the trocar or, if general anesthesia is used, the lung may be collapsed through a double lumen endotracheal tube inserted through the mouth into the trachea. The contents of the chest cavity are examined by direct visualization and/or by the use of a video camera. Still photographs may be taken as part of the procedure. A second and/or third trocar and instruments may be inserted into the chest cavity through a second and/or third wound in the chest. Under direct visualization through the endoscope, the physician strips away the membranous tissues covering a portion of the lung (or all of the lung ins 32652) using instruments inserted into the chest through the secondary sites. Code 32652 includes intrapleural pneumonolysis in which the physician divides the tissues attaching the lung to the wall of the chest cavity. At the conclusion of the procedure, the endoscope and the trocar are removed. A chest tube for drainage and re-expansion of the lung is usually inserted through the wound used for the thoracoscopy.

Coding Tips

Surgical thoracoscopy always includes diagnostic thoracoscopy. For a major thoracotomy with open intrapleural pneumonolysis, see 32124. For total pulmonary decortication (separate procedure), see 32220; partial, see 32225. For decortication and parietal pleurectomy, see 32320.

ICD-10-CM Diagnostic Codes

A15.6	Tuberculous pleurisy
C38.4	Malignant neoplasm of pleura
C38.8	Malignant neoplasm of overlapping sites of heart, mediastinum and pleura
C45.0	Mesothelioma of pleura
C78.2	Secondary malignant neoplasm of pleura
D19.0	Benign neoplasm of mesothelial tissue of pleura
J86.0	Pyothorax with fistula
J86.9	Pyothorax without fistula
J92.0	Pleural plaque with presence of asbestos
J92.9	Pleural plaque without asbestos
J94.1	Fibrothorax

Relative Value Units/Medicare Edits

Non-Facility RVU	Work	PE	MP	Total
32651	18.78	9.08	4.57	32.43
32652	29.13	12.86	7.14	49.13
Facility RVU	**Work**	**PE**	**MP**	**Total**
32651	18.78	9.08	4.57	32.43
32652	29.13	12.86	7.14	49.13

	FUD	Status	MUE	Modifiers				IOM Reference
32651	90	A	1(2)	51	50	62*	80	None
32652	90	A	1(2)	51	50	62*	80	

* with documentation

Terms To Know

decortication. Removal of the cortical substance, the encapsulating or encasing material, of an organ, such as the kidneys or lungs.

effusion. Escape of fluid from within a body cavity.

pneumothorax. Collapsed lung due to air or gas trapped in the pleural space formed by the membrane that encloses the lungs and lines the thoracic cavity.

32653

32653 Thoracoscopy, surgical; with removal of intrapleural foreign body or fibrin deposit

Fibrin is an insoluble protein residue associated with clotting of blood

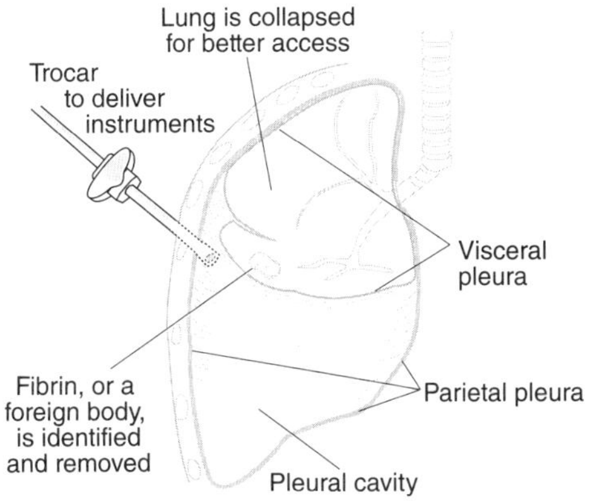

Surgical thoracoscopy is performed

Explanation

The physician examines the inside of the chest cavity through either a rigid or flexible fiberoptic endoscope and removes a foreign body or a fibrin deposit (the thick tissue much like remains of a blood clot). The procedure can be done under local or general anesthesia. The surgeon makes a small incision between two ribs and, by blunt dissection and the use of a trocar, enters the thoracic cavity. The endoscope is passed through the trocar and into the chest cavity. The lung is usually partially collapsed by instilling air into the chest through the trocar or, if general anesthesia is used, the lung may be collapsed through a special double lumen endotracheal tube inserted through the mouth into the trachea. The contents of the chest cavity are examined by direct visualization and/or by the use of a video camera. Still photographs may be taken as part of the procedure. A second and/or third trocar and instruments may be inserted into the chest cavity through a second and/or third wound in the chest. The foreign body or fibrin deposit is located and removed using instruments through the scope or the secondary sites. At the conclusion of the procedure, the endoscope and the trocar are removed. A chest tube for drainage and re-expansion of the lung is usually inserted through the wound used for the thoracoscopy.

Coding Tips

Surgical thoracoscopy always includes diagnostic thoracoscopy. For a thoracotomy with removal of an intrapleural foreign body or a fibrin deposit, see 32150.

ICD-10-CM Diagnostic Codes

J94.2	Hemothorax
S21.321A	Laceration with foreign body of right front wall of thorax with penetration into thoracic cavity, initial encounter
S21.322A	Laceration with foreign body of left front wall of thorax with penetration into thoracic cavity, initial encounter
S21.341A	Puncture wound with foreign body of right front wall of thorax with penetration into thoracic cavity, initial encounter
S21.342A	Puncture wound with foreign body of left front wall of thorax with penetration into thoracic cavity, initial encounter
S21.421A	Laceration with foreign body of right back wall of thorax with penetration into thoracic cavity, initial encounter
S21.422A	Laceration with foreign body of left back wall of thorax with penetration into thoracic cavity, initial encounter
S21.441A	Puncture wound with foreign body of right back wall of thorax with penetration into thoracic cavity, initial encounter
S21.442A	Puncture wound with foreign body of left back wall of thorax with penetration into thoracic cavity, initial encounter
S27.1XXA	Traumatic hemothorax, initial encounter
S27.2XXA	Traumatic hemopneumothorax, initial encounter
S27.311A	Primary blast injury of lung, unilateral, initial encounter
S27.312A	Primary blast injury of lung, bilateral, initial encounter ☑
S27.321A	Contusion of lung, unilateral, initial encounter
S27.322A	Contusion of lung, bilateral, initial encounter ☑
S27.331A	Laceration of lung, unilateral, initial encounter
S27.332A	Laceration of lung, bilateral, initial encounter ☑
S27.63XA	Laceration of pleura, initial encounter
S27.893A	Laceration of other specified intrathoracic organs, initial encounter
T81.510A	Adhesions due to foreign body accidentally left in body following surgical operation, initial encounter
T81.518A	Adhesions due to foreign body accidentally left in body following other procedure, initial encounter
T81.520A	Obstruction due to foreign body accidentally left in body following surgical operation, initial encounter
T81.528A	Obstruction due to foreign body accidentally left in body following other procedure, initial encounter
T81.530A	Perforation due to foreign body accidentally left in body following surgical operation, initial encounter
T81.538A	Perforation due to foreign body accidentally left in body following other procedure, initial encounter
T81.590A	Other complications of foreign body accidentally left in body following surgical operation, initial encounter
T81.598A	Other complications of foreign body accidentally left in body following other procedure, initial encounter

Relative Value Units/Medicare Edits

Non-Facility RVU	Work	PE	MP	Total
32653	18.17	8.93	4.24	31.34
Facility RVU	**Work**	**PE**	**MP**	**Total**
32653	18.17	8.93	4.24	31.34

	FUD	Status	MUE	Modifiers				IOM Reference
32653	90	A	1(3)	51	N/A	62*	80	None

* with documentation

32654

32654 Thoracoscopy, surgical; with control of traumatic hemorrhage

Hemorrhage is usually controlled by identifying the site and clipping or cauterizing damaged vessels

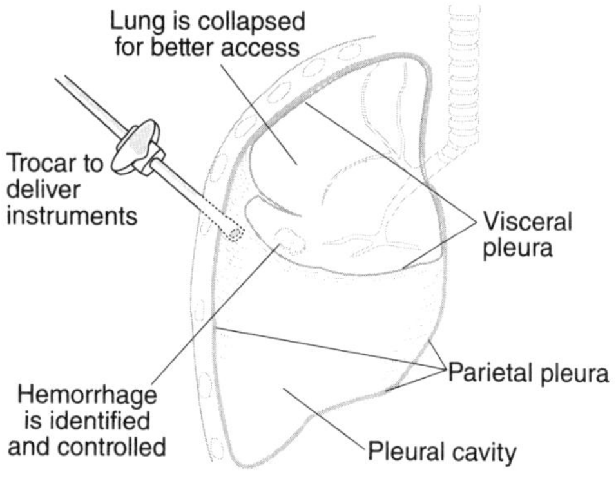

Surgical thoracoscopy is performed

Explanation

The physician examines the inside of the chest cavity through either a rigid or flexible fiberoptic endoscope and controls bleeding from a wound to the chest. The procedure can be done under local or general anesthesia. The physician makes a small incision between two ribs and, by blunt dissection and the use of a trocar, enters the thoracic cavity. The endoscope is passed through the trocar and into the chest cavity. The lung is usually partially collapsed by instilling air into the chest through the trocar or, if general anesthesia is used, the lung may be collapsed through a special double lumen endotracheal tube inserted through the mouth into the trachea. The contents of the chest cavity are examined by direct visualization and/or by the use of a video camera. Still photographs may be taken as part of the procedure. A second and/or third trocar and instruments may be inserted into the chest cavity through a second and/or third wound in the chest. Under direct visualization through the endoscope, the physician manipulates the instruments inserted through the secondary sites and localizes the site of the bleeding. The hemorrhage is controlled by clipping or cauterizing the damaged blood vessel. At the conclusion of the procedure, the endoscope and the trocar(s) are removed. A chest tube for drainage and re-expansion of the lung is usually inserted through the wound used for the thoracoscopy.

Coding Tips

Surgical thoracoscopy always includes diagnostic thoracoscopy. Code 32654 should not be billed with thoracoscopic intervention codes. It is intended to be used only when bleeding occurs spontaneously or as the result of trauma, not when it results from another surgical intervention. For a major thoracotomy with control of a traumatic hemorrhage and/or repair of a lung tear, see 32110.

ICD-10-CM Diagnostic Codes

S21.311A Laceration without foreign body of right front wall of thorax with penetration into thoracic cavity, initial encounter
S21.321A Laceration with foreign body of right front wall of thorax with penetration into thoracic cavity, initial encounter
S21.331A Puncture wound without foreign body of right front wall of thorax with penetration into thoracic cavity, initial encounter
S21.341A Puncture wound with foreign body of right front wall of thorax with penetration into thoracic cavity, initial encounter
S21.351A Open bite of right front wall of thorax with penetration into thoracic cavity, initial encounter
S21.411A Laceration without foreign body of right back wall of thorax with penetration into thoracic cavity, initial encounter
S21.421A Laceration with foreign body of right back wall of thorax with penetration into thoracic cavity, initial encounter
S21.431A Puncture wound without foreign body of right back wall of thorax with penetration into thoracic cavity, initial encounter
S21.441A Puncture wound with foreign body of right back wall of thorax with penetration into thoracic cavity, initial encounter
S21.451A Open bite of right back wall of thorax with penetration into thoracic cavity, initial encounter
S25.491A Other specified injury of right pulmonary blood vessels, initial encounter ☑
S25.811A Laceration of other blood vessels of thorax, right side, initial encounter ☑
S25.891A Other specified injury of other blood vessels of thorax, right side, initial encounter ☑
S27.0XXA Traumatic pneumothorax, initial encounter
S27.1XXA Traumatic hemothorax, initial encounter
S27.2XXA Traumatic hemopneumothorax, initial encounter
S27.311A Primary blast injury of lung, unilateral, initial encounter
S27.312A Primary blast injury of lung, bilateral, initial encounter ☑
S27.321A Contusion of lung, unilateral, initial encounter
S27.322A Contusion of lung, bilateral, initial encounter ☑
S27.331A Laceration of lung, unilateral, initial encounter
S27.332A Laceration of lung, bilateral, initial encounter ☑
S27.391A Other injuries of lung, unilateral, initial encounter
S27.392A Other injuries of lung, bilateral, initial encounter ☑
S28.0XXA Crushed chest, initial encounter

Relative Value Units/Medicare Edits

Non-Facility RVU	Work	PE	MP	Total
32654	20.52	9.76	4.73	35.01
Facility RVU	**Work**	**PE**	**MP**	**Total**
32654	20.52	9.76	4.73	35.01

	FUD	Status	MUE	Modifiers				IOM Reference
32654	90	A	1(3)	51	50	62*	80	None

* with documentation

Terms To Know

cauterize. Heat or chemicals used to burn or cut.

dissection. Separating by cutting tissue or body structures apart.

hemoptysis. Coughing up or spitting out blood or blood-streaked sputum.

hemorrhage. Internal or external bleeding with loss of significant amounts of blood.

32655-32656

32655 Thoracoscopy, surgical; with resection-plication of bullae, includes any pleural procedure when performed

32656 with parietal pleurectomy

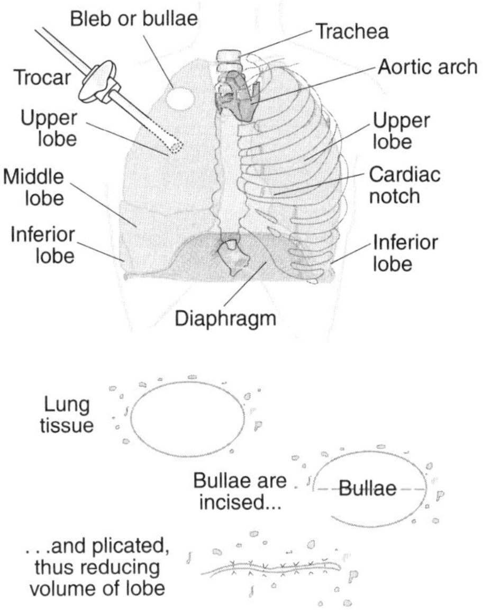

Emphysematous lungs may develop open areas of damaged tissue called blebs or bullae

Explanation

The physician examines the inside of the chest cavity through a rigid or flexible fiberoptic endoscope and removes one or more lung bullae (large nonfunctional air sacs) in 32655 and removes the inside lining of the chest cavity (the parietal pleura) in 32656. The physician makes a small incision between two ribs and by blunt dissection and the use of a trocar enters the thoracic cavity. The endoscope is passed through the trocar and into the chest cavity. The lung is usually partially collapsed by instilling air into the chest through the trocar or the lung may be collapsed through a double lumen endotracheal tube inserted through the mouth into the trachea. The contents of the chest cavity are examined by direct visualization and/or by the use of a video camera. Still photographs may be taken as part of the procedure. A second and/or third trocar and instruments may be inserted into the chest cavity through a second and/or third wound in the chest. Under direct visualization through the endoscope, the physician manipulates the instruments inserted through the secondary sites and localizes the items to be removed. In 32655, the bulla(e) is removed by sharp and blunt dissection of the tissues, which often requires folding and suturing of the tissues (plication). In order to perform the procedure, the pleural surface may require an operative procedure such as pneumonolysis (separation of the surface of the lung that has become adherent to the inside surface of the chest cavity). In 32656, the physician manipulates the instruments inserted through the secondary sites and strips away the parietal pleura from the inside surface of the chest. At the conclusion of the procedure, the endoscope and the trocar(s) are removed. A chest tube for drainage and re-expansion of the lung is usually inserted through the wound used for the thoracoscopy.

Coding Tips

When a diagnostic wedge resection is performed and followed by a more complex procedure on the same anatomic location, report add-on codes 32507 or 32668 with the more complex procedure. When a therapeutic wedge resection is performed on a different lobe than a more complex lung resection, append modifier 59 or an X{EPSU} modifier. Surgical thoracoscopy always includes diagnostic thoracoscopy. For thoracoscopic lung volume reduction, see 32672. For thoracoscopic wedge resection, see 32666, 32667, or 32668. For a major thoracotomy with excision-plication of bullae, with or without any pleural procedure, see 32141. For open parietal pleurectomy (separate procedure), see 32310. For open decortication and parietal pleurectomy, see 32320.

ICD-10-CM Diagnostic Codes

A15.0	Tuberculosis of lung
C38.4	Malignant neoplasm of pleura
C45.0	Mesothelioma of pleura
C78.2	Secondary malignant neoplasm of pleura
J43.0	Unilateral pulmonary emphysema [MacLeod's syndrome]
J43.1	Panlobular emphysema
J43.2	Centrilobular emphysema
J43.8	Other emphysema
J86.0	Pyothorax with fistula
J86.9	Pyothorax without fistula
J91.0	Malignant pleural effusion
J93.0	Spontaneous tension pneumothorax
J93.11	Primary spontaneous pneumothorax
J93.12	Secondary spontaneous pneumothorax
J93.81	Chronic pneumothorax
J94.1	Fibrothorax
J94.2	Hemothorax
J95.811	Postprocedural pneumothorax
J95.812	Postprocedural air leak
N80.B1	Endometriosis of pleura
P25.1	Pneumothorax originating in the perinatal period N
S27.0XXA	Traumatic pneumothorax, initial encounter
S27.2XXA	Traumatic hemopneumothorax, initial encounter

AMA: 32655 2024,Feb **32656** 2024,Feb

Relative Value Units/Medicare Edits

Non-Facility RVU	Work	PE	MP	Total
32655	16.17	8.25	3.95	28.37
32656	13.26	7.37	3.23	23.86
Facility RVU	**Work**	**PE**	**MP**	**Total**
32655	16.17	8.25	3.95	28.37
32656	13.26	7.37	3.23	23.86

	FUD	Status	MUE	Modifiers				IOM Reference
32655	90	A	1(3)	51	50	62*	80	None
32656	90	A	1(2)	51	50	62*	80	

* with documentation

Lungs and Pleura

32658

32658 Thoracoscopy, surgical; with removal of clot or foreign body from pericardial sac

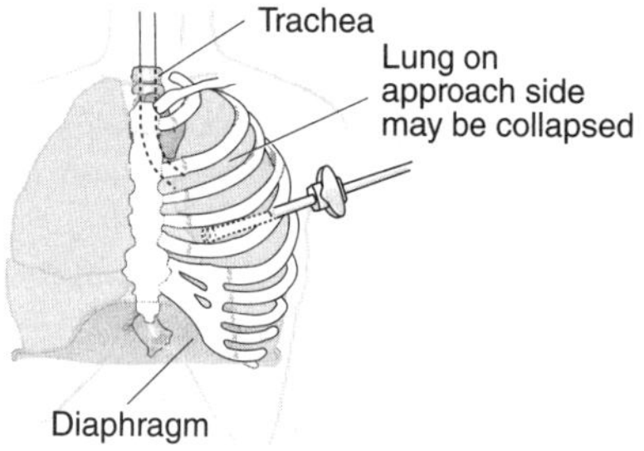

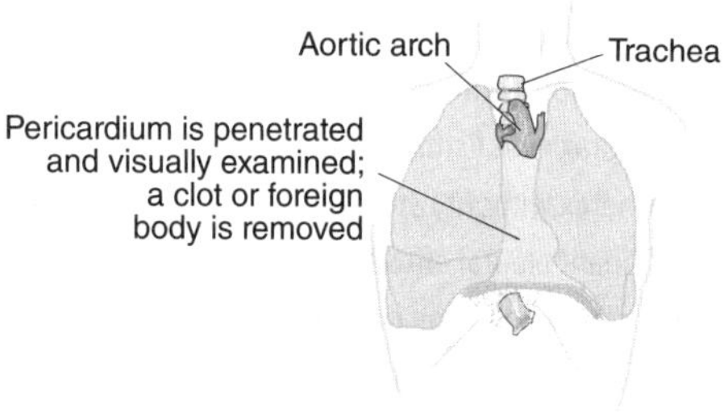

Explanation

The physician examines the inside of the pericardial sac through either a rigid or flexible fiberoptic endoscope and removes a blood clot or foreign body. The procedure can be done under local or general anesthesia. The physician makes a small incision between two ribs and, by blunt dissection and the use of a trocar, enters the thoracic cavity. The endoscope is passed through the trocar and into the chest cavity. The lung is usually partially collapsed by instilling air into the chest through the trocar or, if general anesthesia is used, the lung may be collapsed through a special double lumen endotracheal tube inserted through the mouth into the trachea. The endoscope is advanced to and into the pericardial sac as the physician views the structures and the anatomy of the area through the scope. The contents of the pericardial sac are examined by direct visualization and/or by the use of a video camera. Still photographs may be taken as part of the procedure. The clot and/or foreign body is identified and removed using a device through the endoscope or using a second instrument introduced into the area through a second insertion site in the chest. At the conclusion of the procedure, the endoscope and the trocar are withdrawn. A chest tube for drainage and re-expansion of the lung is usually inserted through the wound used for the thoracoscopy.

Coding Tips

Surgical thoracoscopy always includes diagnostic thoracoscopy. For an open pericardiotomy for the removal of a clot or foreign body (primary procedure), see 33020.

ICD-10-CM Diagnostic Codes

I23.0	Hemopericardium as current complication following acute myocardial infarction A
I31.2	Hemopericardium, not elsewhere classified
I31.4	Cardiac tamponade
S26.01XA	Contusion of heart with hemopericardium, initial encounter
S26.020A	Mild laceration of heart with hemopericardium, initial encounter
S26.021A	Moderate laceration of heart with hemopericardium, initial encounter
S26.022A	Major laceration of heart with hemopericardium, initial encounter
S26.09XA	Other injury of heart with hemopericardium, initial encounter

Relative Value Units/Medicare Edits

Non-Facility RVU	Work	PE	MP	Total
32658	11.71	6.66	2.88	21.25
Facility RVU	**Work**	**PE**	**MP**	**Total**
32658	11.71	6.66	2.88	21.25

	FUD	Status	MUE	Modifiers				IOM Reference
32658	90	A	1(3)	51	N/A	62*	80	None

* with documentation

Terms To Know

contusion. Superficial injury (bruising) produced by impact without a break in the skin.

dissection. Separating by cutting tissue or body structures apart.

foreign body. Any object or substance found in an organ and tissue that does not belong under normal circumstances.

infection. Presence of microorganisms in body tissues that may result in cellular damage.

trocar. Cannula or a sharp pointed instrument used to puncture and aspirate fluid from cavities.

N Newborn: 0 P Pediatric: 0-17 M Maternity: 9-64 A Adult: 15-124 AMA: CPT Assist

32659-32661

32659 Thoracoscopy, surgical; with creation of pericardial window or partial resection of pericardial sac for drainage

32661 with excision of pericardial cyst, tumor, or mass

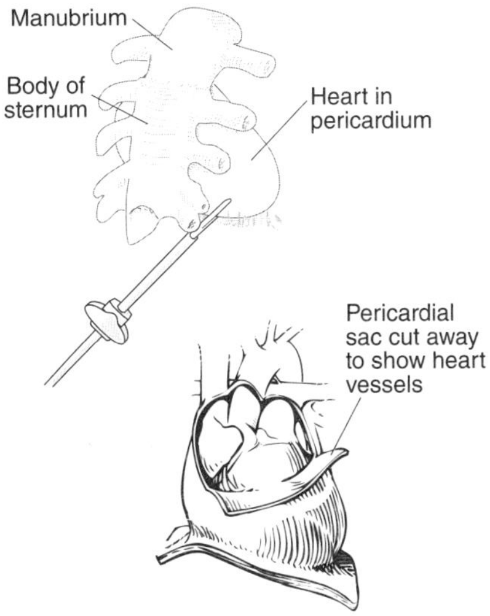

The pericardial sac is accessed through the use of a variety of endoscopic techniques

Explanation

The physician operates on the pericardial sac (the sac surrounding the heart) through a rigid or flexible fiberoptic endoscope and creates a hole in the pericardial sac for drainage. The procedure can be done under local or general anesthesia. The physician makes a small incision between two ribs and by blunt dissection and the use of a trocar enters the thoracic cavity. The endoscope is passed through the trocar and into the chest cavity. The lung is usually partially collapsed by instilling air into the chest through the trocar or, if general anesthesia is used, the lung may be collapsed through a double lumen endotracheal tube inserted through the mouth into the trachea. The endoscope is advanced to and into the pericardial sac as the physician views the structures and the anatomy of the area through the scope. The contents of the pericardial sac are examined by direct visualization and/or by the use of a video camera. Still photographs may be taken as part of the procedure. Using an instrument introduced through the endoscope or through a second wound in the chest, the physician creates an opening in the pericardial sac to allow constant drainage from the sac. The drainage opening is made by the creation of a window (a flap) in the pericardium or by resecting (cutting away) a portion of the pericardium. At the conclusion of the procedure, the endoscope and the trocar are withdrawn. A chest tube for drainage and re-expansion of the lung is usually inserted through the wound used for the thoracoscopy. In 32661, a cyst, tumor, or mass lesion inside the pericardial sac is also excised.

Coding Tips

Surgical thoracoscopy always includes diagnostic thoracoscopy. For an open creation of a pericardial window or partial resection for drainage, see 33025. For open pericardiectomy, see 33030–33031. For open excision of a pericardial cyst or tumor, see 33050.

ICD-10-CM Diagnostic Codes

A18.84	Tuberculosis of heart
A39.53	Meningococcal pericarditis
A52.06	Other syphilitic heart involvement
A54.83	Gonococcal heart infection
A69.29	Other conditions associated with Lyme disease
B33.23	Viral pericarditis
C38.0	Malignant neoplasm of heart
C45.2	Mesothelioma of pericardium
I01.0	Acute rheumatic pericarditis
I09.2	Chronic rheumatic pericarditis
I23.0	Hemopericardium as current complication following acute myocardial infarction A
I30.0	Acute nonspecific idiopathic pericarditis
I30.1	Infective pericarditis
I30.8	Other forms of acute pericarditis
I31.2	Hemopericardium, not elsewhere classified
I31.31	Malignant pericardial effusion in diseases classified elsewhere
I31.39	Other pericardial effusion (noninflammatory)
I31.4	Cardiac tamponade
I32	Pericarditis in diseases classified elsewhere
M32.12	Pericarditis in systemic lupus erythematosus
N80.B4	Endometriosis of the pericardial space
S26.01XA	Contusion of heart with hemopericardium, initial encounter
S26.020A	Mild laceration of heart with hemopericardium, initial encounter
S26.021A	Moderate laceration of heart with hemopericardium, initial encounter
S26.022A	Major laceration of heart with hemopericardium, initial encounter
S26.09XA	Other injury of heart with hemopericardium, initial encounter

Relative Value Units/Medicare Edits

Non-Facility RVU	Work	PE	MP	Total
32659	11.94	7.0	2.9	21.84
32661	13.33	7.09	3.3	23.72
Facility RVU	**Work**	**PE**	**MP**	**Total**
32659	11.94	7.0	2.9	21.84
32661	13.33	7.09	3.3	23.72

	FUD	Status	MUE	Modifiers				IOM Reference
32659	90	A	1(2)	51	N/A	62*	80	None
32661	90	A	1(3)	51	N/A	62*	80	

* with documentation

32662

32662 Thoracoscopy, surgical; with excision of mediastinal cyst, tumor, or mass

A cyst, tumor, or mass within the mediastinal space is removed in a thoracoscopic surgical procedure

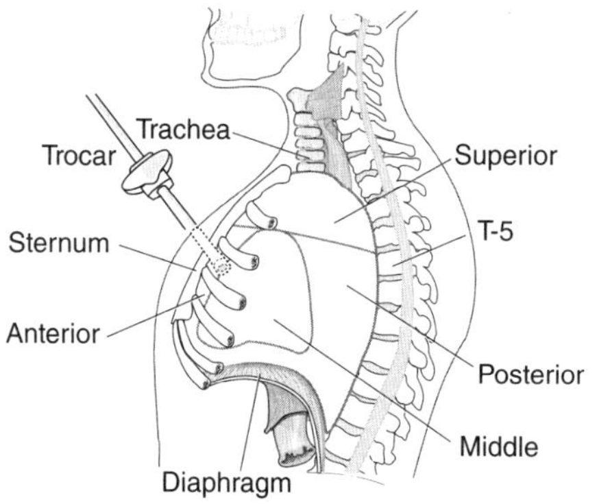

Explanation

The physician removes a cyst, tumor, or mass from the mediastinum through either a rigid or flexible fiberoptic endoscope. The procedure can be done under local or general anesthesia. The physician makes a small incision between two ribs and by blunt dissection and the use of a trocar enters the thoracic cavity. The endoscope is passed through the trocar and into the chest cavity. The lung is usually partially collapsed by instilling air into the chest through the trocar or, if general anesthesia is used, the lung may be collapsed through a special double lumen endotracheal tube inserted through the mouth into the trachea. As the physician views the structures and the anatomy of the area through the endoscope, the endoscope is advanced to and into the mediastinum (area inside the center of the chest cavity between the lungs). The contents of the mediastinal space are examined by direct visualization and/or by the use of a video camera. Still photographs may be taken as part of the procedure. The cyst, tumor, or mass is identified and removed using instruments guided through the endoscope or by using instruments introduced into the area through a second and/or third insertion site in the chest. At the conclusion of the procedure, the endoscope and the trocar are withdrawn. A chest tube for drainage and re-expansion of the lung is usually inserted through the wound used for the thoracoscopy.

Coding Tips

Surgical thoracoscopy always includes diagnostic thoracoscopy. For open excision of a mediastinal cyst, see 39200. For open excision of a mediastinal tumor, see 39220.

ICD-10-CM Diagnostic Codes

C33 Malignant neoplasm of trachea
C34.01 Malignant neoplasm of right main bronchus ☑
C34.02 Malignant neoplasm of left main bronchus ☑
C38.0 Malignant neoplasm of heart
C38.1 Malignant neoplasm of anterior mediastinum
C38.2 Malignant neoplasm of posterior mediastinum
C38.8 Malignant neoplasm of overlapping sites of heart, mediastinum and pleura
C78.1 Secondary malignant neoplasm of mediastinum
C7A.090 Malignant carcinoid tumor of the bronchus and lung
C81.02 Nodular lymphocyte predominant Hodgkin lymphoma, intrathoracic lymph nodes
C81.12 Nodular sclerosis Hodgkin lymphoma, intrathoracic lymph nodes
C81.22 Mixed cellularity Hodgkin lymphoma, intrathoracic lymph nodes
C81.32 Lymphocyte depleted Hodgkin lymphoma, intrathoracic lymph nodes
C81.42 Lymphocyte-rich Hodgkin lymphoma, intrathoracic lymph nodes
C81.72 Other Hodgkin lymphoma, intrathoracic lymph nodes
C82.02 Follicular lymphoma grade I, intrathoracic lymph nodes
C82.12 Follicular lymphoma grade II, intrathoracic lymph nodes
C82.32 Follicular lymphoma grade IIIa, intrathoracic lymph nodes
C82.52 Diffuse follicle center lymphoma, intrathoracic lymph nodes
C82.62 Cutaneous follicle center lymphoma, intrathoracic lymph nodes
C82.82 Other types of follicular lymphoma, intrathoracic lymph nodes
C83.02 Small cell B-cell lymphoma, intrathoracic lymph nodes
C83.12 Mantle cell lymphoma, intrathoracic lymph nodes
C83.32 Diffuse large B-cell lymphoma, intrathoracic lymph nodes
C83.52 Lymphoblastic (diffuse) lymphoma, intrathoracic lymph nodes
C83.72 Burkitt lymphoma, intrathoracic lymph nodes
C84.02 Mycosis fungoides, intrathoracic lymph nodes
C84.12 Sezary disease, intrathoracic lymph nodes
C84.Z2 Other mature T/NK-cell lymphomas, intrathoracic lymph nodes
C85.22 Mediastinal (thymic) large B-cell lymphoma, intrathoracic lymph nodes
C85.82 Other specified types of non-Hodgkin lymphoma, intrathoracic lymph nodes
D14.31 Benign neoplasm of right bronchus and lung ☑
D14.32 Benign neoplasm of left bronchus and lung ☑
D15.0 Benign neoplasm of thymus
D15.2 Benign neoplasm of mediastinum
D38.3 Neoplasm of uncertain behavior of mediastinum
D38.4 Neoplasm of uncertain behavior of thymus
D3A.090 Benign carcinoid tumor of the bronchus and lung

Relative Value Units/Medicare Edits

Non-Facility RVU	Work	PE	MP	Total
32662	14.99	7.85	3.69	26.53
Facility RVU	**Work**	**PE**	**MP**	**Total**
32662	14.99	7.85	3.69	26.53

	FUD	Status	MUE	Modifiers				IOM Reference
32662	90	A	1(3)	51	N/A	62*	80	None

* with documentation

Lungs and Pleura

32663

32663 Thoracoscopy, surgical; with lobectomy (single lobe)

Lung segments are defined by bronchopulmonary branches and the tissues they serve. The schematic below shows just some of the main segments within the larger lobes

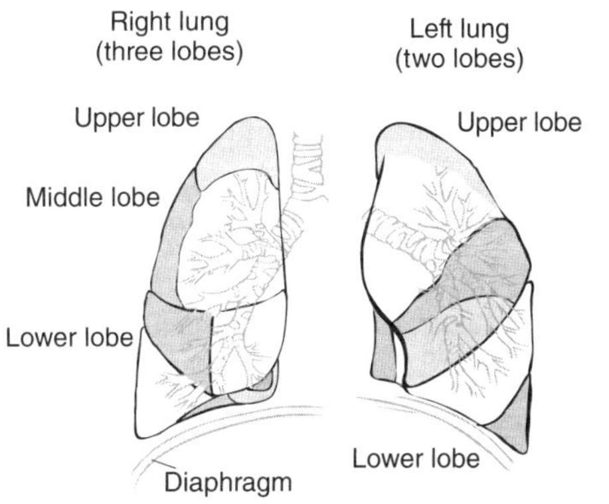

The major lobes of the lung differ from right to left. The right lung has three lobes and the left two, due to the space given over to the heart and pericardium

Explanation

The physician removes an entire lobe of one lung through a rigid or flexible fiberoptic endoscope. The physician makes a small incision between two ribs and by blunt dissection and the use of a trocar enters the thoracic cavity. The endoscope is passed through the trocar and into the chest cavity. The lung is usually partially collapsed by instilling air into the chest through the trocar or the lung may be collapsed through a double lumen endotracheal tube inserted through the mouth into the trachea. The contents of the chest cavity are examined by direct visualization and/or by the use of a video camera. Still photographs may be taken as part of the procedure. Additional instruments may be inserted into the chest cavity through a second and/or third wound in the chest. Under direct visualization through the endoscope, the physician manipulates the instruments inserted through the secondary sites and clamps the blood vessels and bronchial tubes going to the lobe of the lung to be removed. With the clamps in place, the lobe is removed by dividing the vessel and bronchial tubes isolated by the clamps. Any cut portions of the remaining lung tissue are repaired by suturing or clipping with surgical clips. At the conclusion of the procedure, the endoscope and the trocar(s) are removed. A chest tube for drainage and re-expansion of the lung is usually inserted through the wound used for the thoracoscopy.

Coding Tips

Surgical thoracoscopy always includes diagnostic thoracoscopy. For a thoracoscopic segmentectomy, see 32669. For open lung resections, see 32480-32488.

ICD-10-CM Diagnostic Codes

A15.0 Tuberculosis of lung
B44.0 Invasive pulmonary aspergillosis
B44.1 Other pulmonary aspergillosis
C34.01 Malignant neoplasm of right main bronchus ☑
C34.02 Malignant neoplasm of left main bronchus ☑
C34.11 Malignant neoplasm of upper lobe, right bronchus or lung ☑
C34.12 Malignant neoplasm of upper lobe, left bronchus or lung ☑
C34.2 Malignant neoplasm of middle lobe, bronchus or lung
C34.31 Malignant neoplasm of lower lobe, right bronchus or lung ☑
C34.32 Malignant neoplasm of lower lobe, left bronchus or lung ☑
C34.81 Malignant neoplasm of overlapping sites of right bronchus and lung ☑
C34.82 Malignant neoplasm of overlapping sites of left bronchus and lung ☑
C46.51 Kaposi's sarcoma of right lung ☑
C46.52 Kaposi's sarcoma of left lung ☑
C78.01 Secondary malignant neoplasm of right lung ☑
C78.02 Secondary malignant neoplasm of left lung ☑
C79.89 Secondary malignant neoplasm of other specified sites
C7A.090 Malignant carcinoid tumor of the bronchus and lung
D02.21 Carcinoma in situ of right bronchus and lung ☑
D02.22 Carcinoma in situ of left bronchus and lung ☑
D14.31 Benign neoplasm of right bronchus and lung ☑
D14.32 Benign neoplasm of left bronchus and lung ☑
D38.1 Neoplasm of uncertain behavior of trachea, bronchus and lung
D3A.090 Benign carcinoid tumor of the bronchus and lung
J43.0 Unilateral pulmonary emphysema [MacLeod's syndrome]
J43.1 Panlobular emphysema
J43.2 Centrilobular emphysema
J43.8 Other emphysema
J47.0 Bronchiectasis with acute lower respiratory infection
J47.1 Bronchiectasis with (acute) exacerbation
J85.0 Gangrene and necrosis of lung
J85.1 Abscess of lung with pneumonia
J85.2 Abscess of lung without pneumonia
J98.4 Other disorders of lung
Q33.2 Sequestration of lung

Relative Value Units/Medicare Edits

Non-Facility RVU	Work	PE	MP	Total
32663	24.64	10.6	6.05	41.29
Facility RVU	**Work**	**PE**	**MP**	**Total**
32663	24.64	10.6	6.05	41.29

	FUD	Status	MUE	Modifiers				IOM Reference
32663	90	A	1(3)	51	N/A	62*	80	None

* with documentation

Terms To Know

bronchiectasis. Dilation of the bronchi with mucous production and persistent cough due to infection or chronic conditions that causes diminished lung capacity and frequent infections of the lung.

32664

32664 Thoracoscopy, surgical; with thoracic sympathectomy

A thoracic sympathectomy is performed using thoracoscopic technique

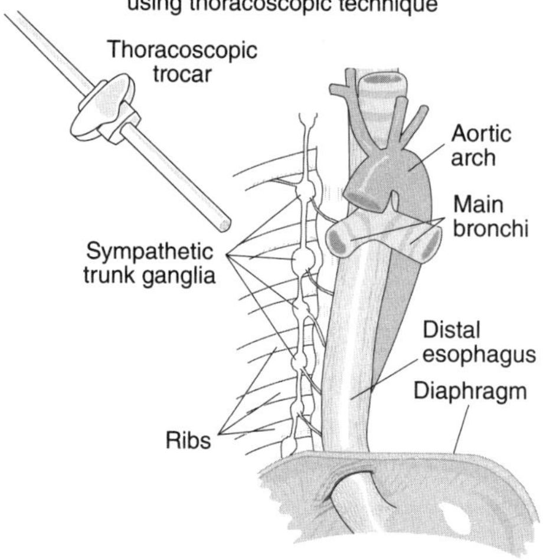

Schematic showing sympathetic nerve trunk in relation to select thoracic structures. The sympathetic trunk ganglia lie on the juncture of the rib and spine and there are usually about 10 on each side

Explanation

The physician performs a sympathectomy inside of the chest cavity through a rigid or flexible fiberoptic endoscope. The procedure can be done under local or general anesthesia. The physician makes a small incision between two ribs and by blunt dissection and the use of a trocar enters the thoracic cavity. The endoscope is passed through the trocar and into the chest cavity. The lung is usually partially collapsed by instilling air into the chest through the trocar or, if general anesthesia is used, the lung may be collapsed through a double lumen endotracheal tube inserted through the mouth into the trachea. The contents of the chest cavity are examined by direct visualization and/or by the use of a video camera. Still photographs may be taken as part of the procedure. A second and/or third trocar and instruments may be inserted into the chest cavity through a second and/or third wound in the chest. Under direct visualization through the endoscope, the physician manipulates the instruments inserted through the secondary sites and localizes and isolates a portion of the sympathetic nerves as they course deeply through the chest. The sympathectomy is accomplished by clipping and/or cutting the nerves. At the conclusion of the procedure, the endoscope and the trocar(s) are removed. A chest tube for drainage and re-expansion of the lung is usually inserted through the wound used for the thoracoscopy.

Coding Tips

Surgical thoracoscopy always includes a diagnostic thoracoscopy. For open cervicothoracic sympathectomy, see 64804. For thoracolumbar sympathectomy, see 64809. For exploratory thoracoscopy with or without biopsy, see 32601–32609.

ICD-10-CM Diagnostic Codes

G90.511	Complex regional pain syndrome I of right upper limb ☑
G90.512	Complex regional pain syndrome I of left upper limb ☑
G90.513	Complex regional pain syndrome I of upper limb, bilateral ☑
G90.521	Complex regional pain syndrome I of right lower limb ☑
G90.522	Complex regional pain syndrome I of left lower limb ☑
G90.523	Complex regional pain syndrome I of lower limb, bilateral ☑
G90.59	Complex regional pain syndrome I of other specified site
I73.00	Raynaud's syndrome without gangrene
I73.01	Raynaud's syndrome with gangrene
L74.510	Primary focal hyperhidrosis, axilla
L74.511	Primary focal hyperhidrosis, face
L74.512	Primary focal hyperhidrosis, palms
L74.513	Primary focal hyperhidrosis, soles
L74.52	Secondary focal hyperhidrosis

AMA: **32664** 2024,Apr

Relative Value Units/Medicare Edits

Non-Facility RVU	Work	PE	MP	Total
32664	14.28	7.36	3.53	25.17
Facility RVU	**Work**	**PE**	**MP**	**Total**
32664	14.28	7.36	3.53	25.17

	FUD	Status	MUE	Modifiers				IOM Reference
32664	90	A	1(2)	51	50	62*	80	None

* with documentation

Terms To Know

dissection. Separating by cutting tissue or body structures apart.

endoscopy. Visual inspection of the body using a fiberoptic scope.

ganglion. Fluid-filled, benign cyst appearing on a tendon sheath or aponeurosis, frequently connecting to an underlying joint.

hyperhidrosis. Condition of excessive perspiration beyond what the body requires for normal temperature control.

instillation. Administering a liquid slowly over time, drop by drop.

manipulation. Skillful treatment by hand to reduce fractures and dislocations or provide therapy through forceful passive movement of a joint beyond its active limit of motion.

sympathectomy. Surgical interruption or transection of a sympathetic nervous system pathway.

sympathetic nerves. Self-regulating nerves that are part of the autonomic nervous system and that innervate the involuntary motor systems that prepare the body for intense activity.

trocar. Cannula or a sharp pointed instrument used to puncture and aspirate fluid from cavities.

32665

32665 Thoracoscopy, surgical; with esophagomyotomy (Heller type)

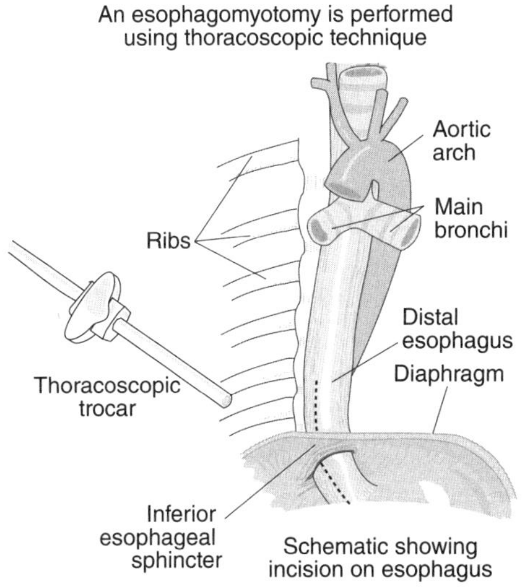

The failure of the distal esophagus to relax during swallowing is called achalasia and this procedure is a treatment for the condition. Heller procedure involves incising just the outer muscle layers of the esophagus

Explanation

The physician repairs a diseased and malfunctioning esophagus by operating through a series of several ports through the chest wall, guided under direct visualization through an endoscope introduced into the chest cavity. The physician makes a small incision between two ribs and by blunt dissection and the use of a trocar enters the thoracic cavity. The endoscope is passed through the trocar and into the chest cavity. The lung is usually partially collapsed by instilling air into the chest through the trocar or the lung may be collapsed through a double lumen endotracheal tube inserted through the mouth into the trachea. The contents of the chest cavity are examined by direct visualization and/or by the use of a video camera. Still photographs may be taken as part of the procedure. Several other trocars and instruments are inserted into the chest cavity through a series of similar puncture wounds placed at various locations in the chest. A second fiberoptic endoscope is passed through the mouth and guided into the esophagus just above the stomach to assist in the procedure. Under direct visualization through the chest endoscope, the physician manipulates the instruments inserted through the secondary chest sites and operates on the esophagus just above its junction with the stomach. The esophagus is presented to the physician by flexing the tip of the scope inside the esophagus. The outer longitudinal muscle of the esophagus is identified, and cut in a longitudinal fashion and the incision is carried down through the circular muscle layer of the esophagus. The length of the incision is carried onto the surface of the stomach about one centimeter. The depth of the incision in the esophageal wall is down to but not through the mucosal tissues lining the inside of the esophagus. Care is taken not to enter the inside of the esophagus. The incision relaxes the esophagus just above the stomach and allows food to more easily enter the stomach in those patients who have difficulty swallowing due to disease in this area of the esophagus. At the conclusion of the procedure, the endoscope and the trocar(s) are removed. A chest tube for drainage and re-expansion of the lung is usually inserted through the wound used for the thoracoscopy.

Coding Tips

Surgical thoracoscopy always includes a diagnostic thoracoscopy. For open esophagomyotomy (Heller type), thoracic approach, see 43331. For exploratory thoracoscopy with or without biopsy, see 32601–32609. Do not report 32665 with 43497.

ICD-10-CM Diagnostic Codes

K22.0	Achalasia of cardia
K22.2	Esophageal obstruction
K22.4	Dyskinesia of esophagus
K22.5	Diverticulum of esophagus, acquired
Q39.0	Atresia of esophagus without fistula
Q39.1	Atresia of esophagus with tracheo-esophageal fistula
Q39.3	Congenital stenosis and stricture of esophagus
Q39.4	Esophageal web
Q39.6	Congenital diverticulum of esophagus

Relative Value Units/Medicare Edits

Non-Facility RVU	Work	PE	MP	Total
32665	21.53	9.56	5.31	36.4
Facility RVU	**Work**	**PE**	**MP**	**Total**
32665	21.53	9.56	5.31	36.4

	FUD	Status	MUE	Modifiers				IOM Reference
32665	90	A	1(2)	51	N/A	62*	80	None

* with documentation

Terms To Know

achalasia. Failure of the smooth muscles within the gastrointestinal tract to relax at points of junction; most commonly referring to the esophagogastric sphincter's failure to relax when swallowing.

blunt dissection. Surgical technique used to expose an underlying area by separating along natural cleavage lines of tissue, without cutting.

dyskinesia of esophagus. Difficult or impaired voluntary muscle movement of the esophagus.

fistula. Abnormal tube-like passage between two body cavities or organs or from an organ to the outside surface.

instillation. Administering a liquid slowly over time, drop by drop.

stenosis. Narrowing or constriction of a passage.

trocar. Cannula or a sharp pointed instrument used to puncture and aspirate fluid from cavities.

32666-32667

32666 Thoracoscopy, surgical; with therapeutic wedge resection (eg, mass, nodule), initial unilateral

\+ **32667** with therapeutic wedge resection (eg, mass or nodule), each additional resection, ipsilateral (List separately in addition to code for primary procedure)

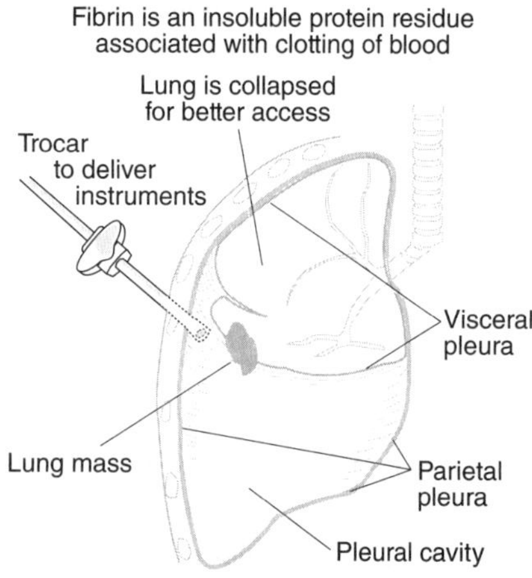

Surgical thoracoscopy is performed. The pleural cavity is visualized and a mass or nodule is removed via wedge resection

Explanation

The physician performs a wedge resection of a lung mass or nodule through a rigid or flexible fiberoptic endoscope. The physician makes a small incision between two ribs and by blunt dissection and the use of a trocar enters the thoracic cavity. The endoscope is passed through the trocar and into the chest cavity. The lung is usually partially collapsed by instilling air into the chest through the trocar or the lung may be collapsed through a double lumen endotracheal tube inserted through the mouth into the trachea. The contents of the chest cavity are examined by direct visualization and/or by the use of a video camera. Still photographs may be taken as part of the procedure. Additional instruments may be inserted into the chest cavity through a second and/or third wound in the chest. Under direct visualization through the endoscope, the physician manipulates the instruments inserted through the secondary sites and clamps the blood vessels and bronchial tubes going to the sections of lung to be removed. With the clamps in place, the tissue is removed. Any cut portions of the lung tissue are repaired by suturing or clipping with surgical clips. At the conclusion of the procedure, the endoscope and the trocar(s) are removed. A chest tube for drainage and re-expansion of the lung is usually inserted through the wound used for the thoracoscopy. Report 32666 for the initial therapeutic wedge resection and 32667 for each additional resection on the same side.

Coding Tips

Note that 32666 is a unilateral procedure. If performed bilaterally, some payers require that the service be reported twice with modifier 50 appended to the second code while others require identification of the service only once with modifier 50 appended. Check with individual payers. Modifier 50 identifies a procedure performed identically on the opposite side of the body (mirror image). When a diagnostic wedge resection is performed and followed by a more complex procedure on the same anatomic location, report 32507 or 32668 with the more complex procedure. When a therapeutic wedge resection is performed on a different lobe than a more complex lung resection, append modifier 59 or an X{EPSU} modifier. Do not report these codes with 32440, 32442, 32445, 32488, or 32671.

ICD-10-CM Diagnostic Codes

A15.0	Tuberculosis of lung
B44.0	Invasive pulmonary aspergillosis
B44.1	Other pulmonary aspergillosis
C34.11	Malignant neoplasm of upper lobe, right bronchus or lung ☑
C34.12	Malignant neoplasm of upper lobe, left bronchus or lung ☑
C34.2	Malignant neoplasm of middle lobe, bronchus or lung
C34.31	Malignant neoplasm of lower lobe, right bronchus or lung ☑
C34.32	Malignant neoplasm of lower lobe, left bronchus or lung ☑
C34.81	Malignant neoplasm of overlapping sites of right bronchus and lung ☑
C34.82	Malignant neoplasm of overlapping sites of left bronchus and lung ☑
C46.51	Kaposi's sarcoma of right lung ☑
C46.52	Kaposi's sarcoma of left lung ☑
C78.01	Secondary malignant neoplasm of right lung ☑
C78.02	Secondary malignant neoplasm of left lung ☑
C7A.090	Malignant carcinoid tumor of the bronchus and lung
D02.21	Carcinoma in situ of right bronchus and lung ☑
D02.22	Carcinoma in situ of left bronchus and lung ☑
D14.31	Benign neoplasm of right bronchus and lung ☑
D14.32	Benign neoplasm of left bronchus and lung ☑
D38.1	Neoplasm of uncertain behavior of trachea, bronchus and lung
D3A.090	Benign carcinoid tumor of the bronchus and lung
D86.0	Sarcoidosis of lung
J43.0	Unilateral pulmonary emphysema [MacLeod's syndrome]
J43.1	Panlobular emphysema
J43.2	Centrilobular emphysema
J43.8	Other emphysema
J47.0	Bronchiectasis with acute lower respiratory infection
J47.1	Bronchiectasis with (acute) exacerbation
J85.0	Gangrene and necrosis of lung
J85.1	Abscess of lung with pneumonia
J85.2	Abscess of lung without pneumonia
J98.4	Other disorders of lung
Q33.2	Sequestration of lung

Relative Value Units/Medicare Edits

Non-Facility RVU	Work	PE	MP	Total
32666	14.5	7.76	3.56	25.82
32667	3.0	0.85	0.74	4.59
Facility RVU	**Work**	**PE**	**MP**	**Total**
32666	14.5	7.76	3.56	25.82
32667	3.0	0.85	0.74	4.59

	FUD	Status	MUE	Modifiers				IOM Reference
32666	90	A	1(3)	51	50	62*	80	None
32667	N/A	A	3(3)	N/A	N/A	62*	80	

* with documentation

32668

\+ **32668** Thoracoscopy, surgical; with diagnostic wedge resection followed by anatomic lung resection (List separately in addition to code for primary procedure)

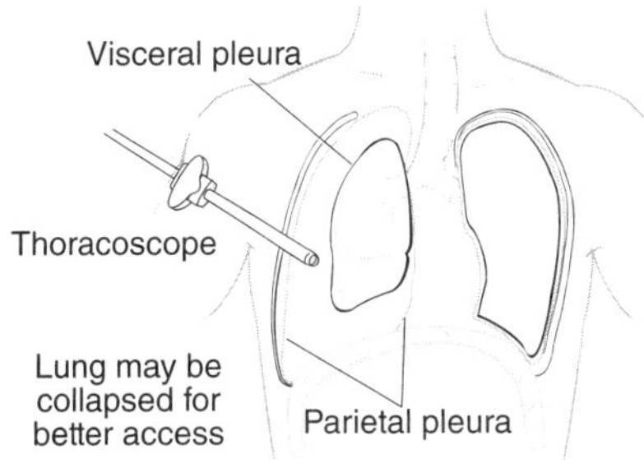

Explanation

The physician performs a wedge resection followed by a lung resection through a rigid or flexible fiberoptic endoscope. The physician makes a small incision between two ribs and by blunt dissection and the use of a trocar enters the thoracic cavity. The endoscope is passed through the trocar and into the chest cavity. The lung is usually partially collapsed by instilling air into the chest through the trocar or the lung may be collapsed through a double lumen endotracheal tube inserted through the mouth into the trachea. The contents of the chest cavity are examined by direct visualization and/or by the use of a video camera. Still photographs may be taken as part of the procedure. Additional instruments may be inserted into the chest cavity through a second and/or third wound in the chest. Under direct visualization through the endoscope, the physician manipulates the instruments inserted through the secondary sites and clamps the blood vessels and bronchial tubes going to the sections of lung to be removed. With the clamps in place, the tissue is removed. Any cut portions of the lung tissue are repaired by suturing or clipping with surgical clips. At the conclusion of the procedure, the endoscope and the trocar(s) are removed. A chest tube for drainage and re-expansion of the lung is usually inserted through the wound used for the thoracoscopy.

Coding Tips

Report 32668 in addition to 32440, 32442, 32445, 32480, 32482, 32484, 32486, 32488, 32503, 32504, 32663, 32669, 32670, or 32671. When a diagnostic wedge resection is performed and followed by a more complex procedure on the same anatomic location, report 32507 or 32668 with the more complex procedure. When a therapeutic wedge resection is performed on a different lobe than a more complex lung resection, append modifier 59 or an X{EPSU} modifier.

ICD-10-CM Diagnostic Codes

This/these CPT code(s) are add-on code(s). See the primary procedure code that this code is performed with for your ICD-10-CM code selections. Diagnostic code(s) would be the same as the actual procedure performed.

Relative Value Units/Medicare Edits

Non-Facility RVU	Work	PE	MP	Total
32668	3.0	0.85	0.74	4.59
Facility RVU	**Work**	**PE**	**MP**	**Total**
32668	3.0	0.85	0.74	4.59

	FUD	Status	MUE	Modifiers				IOM Reference
32668	N/A	A	2(3)	N/A	N/A	62*	80	None

* with documentation

32669-32671

32669 Thoracoscopy, surgical; with removal of a single lung segment (segmentectomy)

32670 with removal of two lobes (bilobectomy)

32671 with removal of lung (pneumonectomy)

Lung segments are defined by bronchopulmonary branches and the tissues they serve. The schematic below shows just some of the main segments within the larger lobes

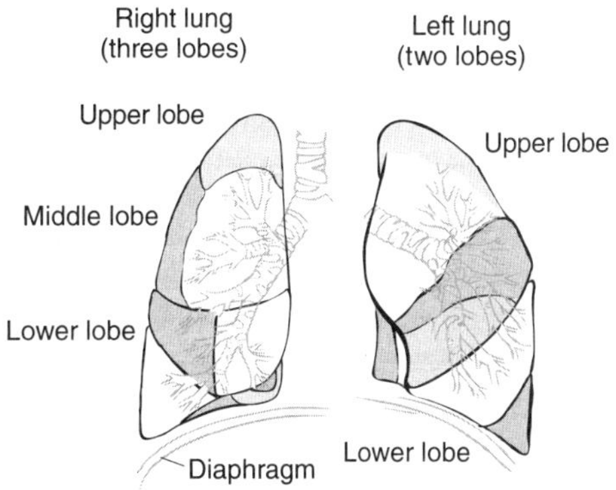

The major lobes of the lung differ from right to left. The right lung has three lobes and the left two, due to the space given over to the heart and pericardium

Explanation

The physician removes a segment of the lung or an entire lung through a rigid or flexible fiberoptic endoscope. The physician makes a small incision between two ribs and by blunt dissection and the use of a trocar enters the thoracic cavity. The endoscope is passed through the trocar and into the chest cavity. The lung is usually partially collapsed by instilling air into the chest through the trocar or the lung may be collapsed through a double lumen endotracheal tube inserted through the mouth into the trachea. The contents of the chest cavity are examined by direct visualization and/or by the use of a video camera. Still photographs may be taken as part of the procedure. Additional instruments may be inserted into the chest cavity through a second and/or third wound in the chest. Under direct visualization through the endoscope, the physician manipulates the instruments inserted through the secondary sites and clamps the blood vessels and bronchial tubes going to the sections of lung to be removed. With the clamps in place, the tissue is removed. Any cut portions of the lung tissue are repaired by suturing or clipping with surgical clips. At the conclusion of the procedure, the endoscope and the trocar(s) are removed. A chest tube for drainage and re-expansion of the lung is usually inserted through the wound used for the thoracoscopy. Report 32669 when the physician removes a single lung segment, 32670 when the physician removes two lobes of a lung, and 32671 when an entire lung is removed.

Coding Tips

Surgical thoracoscopy always includes a diagnostic thoracoscopy. Diagnostic lung biopsies with an intraoperative pathology that determines the need for resection or another definitive procedure should be reported using only the most complex service performed.

ICD-10-CM Diagnostic Codes

A15.0 Tuberculosis of lung

B44.0 Invasive pulmonary aspergillosis

B44.1 Other pulmonary aspergillosis

C34.01 Malignant neoplasm of right main bronchus ☑

C34.02	Malignant neoplasm of left main bronchus ☑
C34.11	Malignant neoplasm of upper lobe, right bronchus or lung ☑
C34.12	Malignant neoplasm of upper lobe, left bronchus or lung ☑
C34.2	Malignant neoplasm of middle lobe, bronchus or lung
C34.31	Malignant neoplasm of lower lobe, right bronchus or lung ☑
C34.32	Malignant neoplasm of lower lobe, left bronchus or lung ☑
C34.81	Malignant neoplasm of overlapping sites of right bronchus and lung ☑
C34.82	Malignant neoplasm of overlapping sites of left bronchus and lung ☑
C46.51	Kaposi's sarcoma of right lung ☑
C46.52	Kaposi's sarcoma of left lung ☑
C78.01	Secondary malignant neoplasm of right lung ☑
C78.02	Secondary malignant neoplasm of left lung ☑
C7A.090	Malignant carcinoid tumor of the bronchus and lung
D02.21	Carcinoma in situ of right bronchus and lung ☑
D02.22	Carcinoma in situ of left bronchus and lung ☑
D14.31	Benign neoplasm of right bronchus and lung ☑
D14.32	Benign neoplasm of left bronchus and lung ☑
D38.1	Neoplasm of uncertain behavior of trachea, bronchus and lung
D3A.090	Benign carcinoid tumor of the bronchus and lung
D86.0	Sarcoidosis of lung
J85.0	Gangrene and necrosis of lung
J85.1	Abscess of lung with pneumonia
J85.2	Abscess of lung without pneumonia
J98.4	Other disorders of lung
Q33.2	Sequestration of lung

Relative Value Units/Medicare Edits

Non-Facility RVU	Work	PE	MP	Total
32669	23.53	10.33	5.79	39.65
32670	28.52	11.77	6.92	47.21
32671	31.92	12.44	7.89	52.25
Facility RVU	**Work**	**PE**	**MP**	**Total**
32669	23.53	10.33	5.79	39.65
32670	28.52	11.77	6.92	47.21
32671	31.92	12.44	7.89	52.25

	FUD	Status	MUE	Modifiers				IOM Reference
32669	90	A	2(3)	51	N/A	62*	80	None
32670	90	A	1(2)	51	N/A	62*	80	
32671	90	A	1(2)	51	N/A	62*	80	

* with documentation

32672

32672 Thoracoscopy, surgical; with resection-plication for emphysematous lung (bullous or non-bullous) for lung volume reduction (LVRS), unilateral includes any pleural procedure, when performed

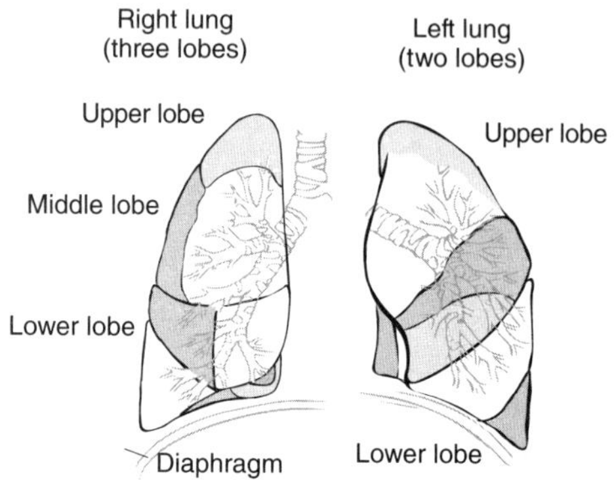

Explanation

The physician removes part of an emphysematous lung. A small incision is made between two ribs and by blunt dissection and the use of a trocar the thoracic cavity is entered. The endoscope is passed through the trocar and into the chest cavity. The lung is usually partially collapsed by instilling air into the chest through the trocar or the lung may be collapsed through a double lumen endotracheal tube inserted through the mouth into the trachea. The contents of the chest cavity are examined by direct visualization and/or by the use of a video camera. Still photographs may be taken as part of the procedure. Additional instruments may be inserted into the chest cavity through a second and/or third wound in the chest. Under direct visualization through the endoscope, the physician manipulates the instruments inserted through the secondary sites and clamps the blood vessels and bronchial tubes going to the section(s) of lung to be removed. With the clamps in place, the emphysematous lung tissue is removed by sharp and blunt dissection and often by folding and suturing of the tissues (plication). Any cut portions of the lung tissue are repaired by suturing or clipping with surgical clips. At the conclusion of the procedure, the endoscope and the trocar(s) are removed. A chest tube for drainage and re-expansion of the lung is usually inserted through the wound used for the thoracoscopy.

Coding Tips

Surgical thoracoscopy always includes a diagnostic thoracoscopy. For an open resection-plication of emphysematous lung(s), see 32491.

ICD-10-CM Diagnostic Codes

J43.0	Unilateral pulmonary emphysema [MacLeod's syndrome]
J43.1	Panlobular emphysema
J43.2	Centrilobular emphysema
J43.8	Other emphysema
J43.9	Emphysema, unspecified

Relative Value Units/Medicare Edits

Non-Facility RVU	Work	PE	MP	Total
32672	27.0	11.15	6.65	44.8
Facility RVU	**Work**	**PE**	**MP**	**Total**
32672	27.0	11.15	6.65	44.8

	FUD	Status	MUE	Modifiers				IOM Reference
32672	90	A	1(3)	51	N/A	62*	80	None

* with documentation

Terms To Know

emphysema. Pathological condition in which there is destructive enlargement of the air sacs in the lungs resulting in damage and lack of elasticity to the alveolar walls, commonly seen in long-term smokers.

emphysematous bleb. Formation of blisters or vesicles greater than 1.0 mm within an emphysematous lung, containing serum or blood.

LVRS. Lung volume reduction surgery. Treatment for patients with severe or end-stage emphysema. LVRS allows the remaining compressed lung to expand and thus improve respiratory function.

plication. Surgical technique involving folding, tucking, or pleating to reduce the size of a hollow structure or organ.

resection. Surgical removal of a part or all of an organ or body part.

trocar. Cannula or a sharp pointed instrument used to puncture and aspirate fluid from cavities.

32673

32673 Thoracoscopy, surgical; with resection of thymus, unilateral or bilateral

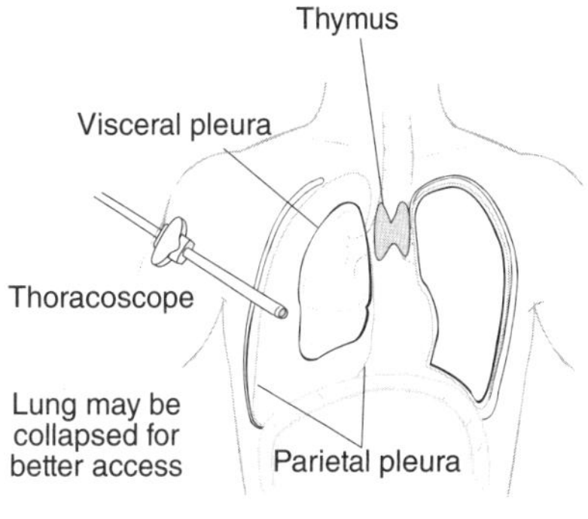

Thymus is resected

Explanation

The physician removes one or both lobes of the thymus gland via thoracoscopic approach. A small incision is made between two ribs and by blunt dissection and the use of a trocar the thoracic cavity is entered. The endoscope is passed through the trocar and into the chest cavity. Additional instruments may be inserted into the chest cavity through a second and/or third wound in the chest. Under direct visualization through the endoscope, the physician manipulates the instruments inserted through the secondary sites and the superior lobe of the thymus is separated from the inferior aspect of the thyroid. The blood supply to the thymus is divided and the thymus is dissected free from the pericardium and removed. A chest tube for drainage is usually inserted through the wound used for the thoracoscopy.

Coding Tips

Surgical thoracoscopy always includes a diagnostic thoracoscopy. For exploratory thoracoscopy with or without biopsy, see 32601–32609. For an open thymectomy, see 60520, 60521, or 60522. For open excision of a mediastinal cyst, see 39200. For open excision of a mediastinal tumor, see 39220.

ICD-10-CM Diagnostic Codes

C37	Malignant neoplasm of thymus
C7A.091	Malignant carcinoid tumor of the thymus
D15.0	Benign neoplasm of thymus
D38.4	Neoplasm of uncertain behavior of thymus
D3A.091	Benign carcinoid tumor of the thymus

Relative Value Units/Medicare Edits

Non-Facility RVU	Work	PE	MP	Total
32673	21.13	9.62	5.19	35.94
Facility RVU	**Work**	**PE**	**MP**	**Total**
32673	21.13	9.62	5.19	35.94

	FUD	Status	MUE	Modifiers				IOM Reference
32673	90	A	1(2)	51	N/A	62*	80	None

* with documentation

Lungs and Pleura

● New ▲ Revised + Add On ★ Telemedicine [Resequenced] ☑ Laterality

32674

\+ **32674** Thoracoscopy, surgical; with mediastinal and regional lymphadenectomy (List separately in addition to code for primary procedure)

Lymph nodes within the mediastinal space are removed in a thoracoscopic surgical procedure

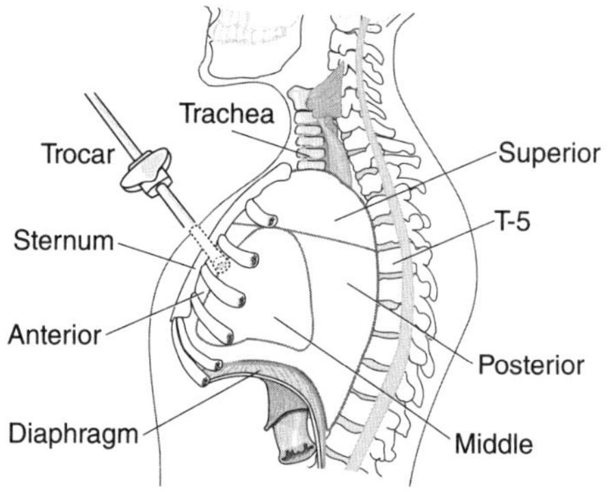

The mediastinal space is the general region between the left and right lungs

Explanation

A regional and mediastinal lymphadenectomy is performed via a thoracoscopic approach. A small incision is made between two ribs and by blunt dissection and the use of a trocar the thoracic cavity is entered. The endoscope is passed through the trocar and into the chest cavity. Additional instruments may be inserted into the chest cavity through a second and/or third wound in the chest. Under direct visualization through the endoscope, the physician manipulates the instruments inserted through the secondary sites and removes the lymph nodes near the lungs, around the heart, and behind the trachea. The area is irrigated, and the operative incision is closed with sutures. A chest tube for drainage is usually inserted through the wound used for the thoracoscopy.

Coding Tips

Surgical thoracoscopy always includes a diagnostic thoracoscopy. Report 32674 in addition to 21601, 31760, 31766, 31786, 32096-32200, 32220-32320, 32440-32491, 32503-32505, 32601-32663, 32666, 32669-32673, 32815, 33025, 33030, 33050-33130, 39200-39220, 39560-39561, 43101, 43112, 43117-43118, 43122-43123, 43287, 43288, 43351, 60270, and 60505. For mediastinal and regional lymphadenectomy by thoracotomy, see 38746.

ICD-10-CM Diagnostic Codes

This/these CPT code(s) are add-on code(s). See the primary procedure code that this code is performed with for your ICD-10-CM code selections. Diagnostic code(s) would be the same as the actual procedure performed.

Relative Value Units/Medicare Edits

Non-Facility RVU	Work	PE	MP	Total
32674	4.12	1.16	1.03	6.31
Facility RVU	**Work**	**PE**	**MP**	**Total**
32674	4.12	1.16	1.03	6.31

	FUD	Status	MUE	Modifiers				IOM Reference
32674	N/A	A	1(2)	N/A	N/A	62*	80	None

* with documentation

32800

32800 Repair lung hernia through chest wall

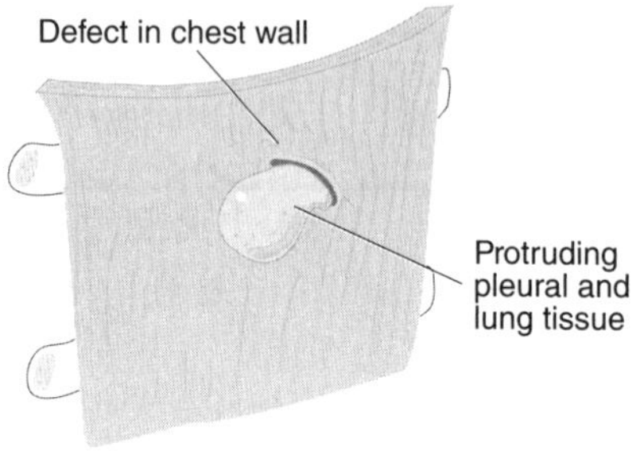

A hernia is a protrusion, usually through a wall containment, and the defect may be congenital

Explanation

The physician repairs a hernia of the chest wall that allows the bulging of the lung through a defect in the chest wall. The physician makes an incision through the skin overlying the defect and carries the incision down to the inside lining of the chest cavity. The defect is repaired by the folding and suturing of tissues or the rotation of muscle and/or thick fibrous tissue flaps over the area and suturing of the flap over the defect. Alternately, the defect can be covered by a synthetic mesh material which is sutured in place. The incision is then closed in layers of sutures.

Coding Tips

Lung hernias may be congenital or acquired and result from a defect in the chest wall causing the lung to protrude through the defect.

ICD-10-CM Diagnostic Codes

J98.4	Other disorders of lung
S21.311A	Laceration without foreign body of right front wall of thorax with penetration into thoracic cavity, initial encounter
S21.312A	Laceration without foreign body of left front wall of thorax with penetration into thoracic cavity, initial encounter
S21.321A	Laceration with foreign body of right front wall of thorax with penetration into thoracic cavity, initial encounter
S21.322A	Laceration with foreign body of left front wall of thorax with penetration into thoracic cavity, initial encounter
S21.331A	Puncture wound without foreign body of right front wall of thorax with penetration into thoracic cavity, initial encounter
S21.332A	Puncture wound without foreign body of left front wall of thorax with penetration into thoracic cavity, initial encounter
S21.341A	Puncture wound with foreign body of right front wall of thorax with penetration into thoracic cavity, initial encounter
S21.342A	Puncture wound with foreign body of left front wall of thorax with penetration into thoracic cavity, initial encounter
S21.351A	Open bite of right front wall of thorax with penetration into thoracic cavity, initial encounter
S21.352A	Open bite of left front wall of thorax with penetration into thoracic cavity, initial encounter
S21.411A	Laceration without foreign body of right back wall of thorax with penetration into thoracic cavity, initial encounter
S21.412A	Laceration without foreign body of left back wall of thorax with penetration into thoracic cavity, initial encounter

S21.421A	Laceration with foreign body of right back wall of thorax with penetration into thoracic cavity, initial encounter
S21.422A	Laceration with foreign body of left back wall of thorax with penetration into thoracic cavity, initial encounter
S21.431A	Puncture wound without foreign body of right back wall of thorax with penetration into thoracic cavity, initial encounter
S21.432A	Puncture wound without foreign body of left back wall of thorax with penetration into thoracic cavity, initial encounter
S21.441A	Puncture wound with foreign body of right back wall of thorax with penetration into thoracic cavity, initial encounter
S21.442A	Puncture wound with foreign body of left back wall of thorax with penetration into thoracic cavity, initial encounter
S21.451A	Open bite of right back wall of thorax with penetration into thoracic cavity, initial encounter
S21.452A	Open bite of left back wall of thorax with penetration into thoracic cavity, initial encounter
S27.893A	Laceration of other specified intrathoracic organs, initial encounter
T81.530A	Perforation due to foreign body accidentally left in body following surgical operation, initial encounter
T81.590A	Other complications of foreign body accidentally left in body following surgical operation, initial encounter

Relative Value Units/Medicare Edits

Non-Facility RVU	Work	PE	MP	Total
32800	15.71	8.38	3.88	27.97
Facility RVU	**Work**	**PE**	**MP**	**Total**
32800	15.71	8.38	3.88	27.97

	FUD	Status	MUE	Modifiers				IOM Reference
32800	90	A	1(3)	51	N/A	62*	80	None

* with documentation

Terms To Know

acquired. Produced by outside influences and not by genetics or birth defect.

anomaly. Irregularity in the structure or position of an organ or tissue.

congenital. Present at birth, occurring through heredity or an influence during gestation up to the moment of birth.

hernia. Protrusion of a body structure through tissue.

incision. Act of cutting into tissue or an organ.

suture. Numerous stitching techniques employed in wound closure.

32810

32810 Closure of chest wall following open flap drainage for empyema (Clagett type procedure)

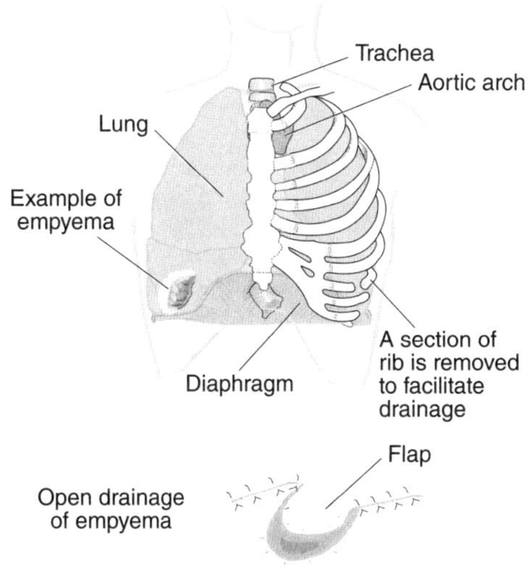

Closure of skin flap is performed

Explanation

The physician treats a draining empyema (accumulation of pus in the chest cavity) by resecting a rib, irrigating the empyema space with an antibiotic solution intermittently over an extended period of time, and closing of the empyema space in six to eight weeks. This code reports the closure portion only.

Coding Tips

Treatment of empyema, an accumulation of pus in the pleural cavity, by open flap drainage requires a second procedure for closure of the flap. This procedure reports the closure portion only. Modifier 58 should be appended to indicate that this is a staged or related procedure performed by the same physician. For thoracostomy with initial creation of an open flap drainage for empyema, see 32036.

ICD-10-CM Diagnostic Codes

A15.6	Tuberculous pleurisy
J86.0	Pyothorax with fistula
J86.9	Pyothorax without fistula

Relative Value Units/Medicare Edits

Non-Facility RVU	Work	PE	MP	Total
32810	14.95	8.15	3.7	26.8
Facility RVU	**Work**	**PE**	**MP**	**Total**
32810	14.95	8.15	3.7	26.8

	FUD	Status	MUE	Modifiers				IOM Reference
32810	90	A	1(3)	51	N/A	N/A	80	None

* with documentation

32815

32815 Open closure of major bronchial fistula

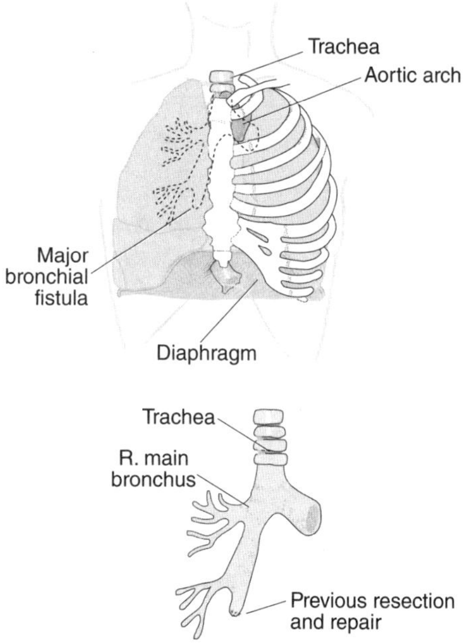

In some instances, the site of a previous bronchial surgery develops into a fistula between the stub and surrounding tissues or pleura

Explanation

The physician repairs a major bronchial fistula (an abnormal passageway between the remaining end of a bronchial tube and the chest that occurs sometimes after the removal of a lung or portion of a lung). The physician enters the chest cavity through a vertical incision made in the middle of the front of the chest. The incision is carried down to the sternum which is split in order to enter the chest cavity at the root of the lung near the center of the chest. The fistula exposure often requires the resection of one or two of the upper ribs. The end of the bronchial tube is located and the stump of the bronchial tube is reamputated and the inside lining of the bronchial tube is treated with silver nitrate to destroy the mucus forming cells lining the bronchus. The stump is sutured or stapled. The chest defect created is repaired and the sternum closed using wire sutures and the skin closed in layers of sutures. A chest tube may be inserted into the chest cavity for drainage.

Coding Tips

For thoracoplasty, Schede type or extrapleural, all stages, with closure of bronchopleural fistula, see 32906.

ICD-10-CM Diagnostic Codes

J86.0 Pyothorax with fistula

Relative Value Units/Medicare Edits

Non-Facility RVU	Work	PE	MP	Total
32815	50.03	20.32	12.28	82.63
Facility RVU	**Work**	**PE**	**MP**	**Total**
32815	50.03	20.32	12.28	82.63

	FUD	Status	MUE	Modifiers				IOM Reference
32815	90	A	1(3)	51	N/A	62*	80	None

* with documentation

32820

32820 Major reconstruction, chest wall (posttraumatic)

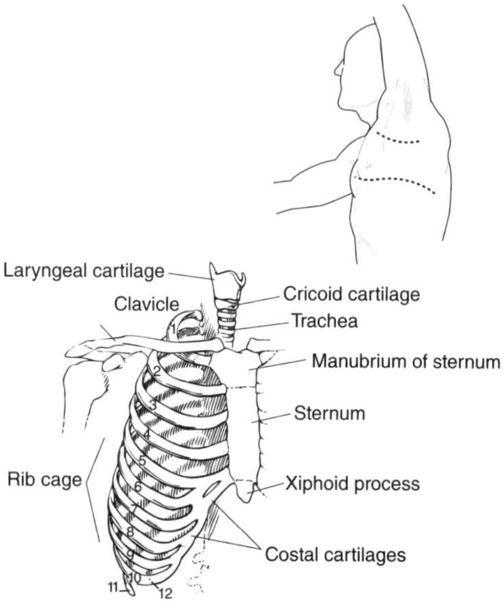

The ribs are the framework of the thoracic cage. Ten pairs connect anteriorly to the sternum and two pairs (11 and 12) float. Ribs numbered 7 to 10 fuse to form the costal margin before attaching to the sternum

Explanation

The physician repairs and reconstructs the chest wall following a major disfiguring injury to the chest (e.g. a shotgun blast). The purpose of the repair is to restore structure and coverage of the chest wall as well as fill any vacant spaces within the chest to prevent infection. The chest wall consists of three layers: the soft tissue layer, including the skin, subcutaneous tissue and muscle; the skeletal layer, consisting of the ribs, cartilage and sometimes the sternum; and the pleural space (parietal cavity). During the procedure, the parietal cavity is checked for air leaks and repaired if necessary. Any empty pleural space may be filled with muscle flap, omentum, or prosthetic material. Bone grafts, muscle or omental flaps or methyl methacrylate reinforced mesh is used to reconstruct the ribs and/or sternum damaged in the trauma. Repair of the soft tissue layer using skin flaps is included in the reconstruction. Skin autograft or substitutes required to close the defect may be reported separately.

Coding Tips

Report 32820 only for reconstruction following trauma. Reconstruction following excision or resection of chest wall tumors should be reported with 21602–21603. For an excision of a chest wall tumor involving the ribs, with plastic reconstruction, without mediastinal lymphadenectomy, see 21602; with mediastinal lymphadenectomy, see 21603. For removal of lung, see 32480–32491.

ICD-10-CM Diagnostic Codes

S21.151A Open bite of right front wall of thorax without penetration into thoracic cavity, initial encounter

S21.152A Open bite of left front wall of thorax without penetration into thoracic cavity, initial encounter

S21.211A Laceration without foreign body of right back wall of thorax without penetration into thoracic cavity, initial encounter

S21.212A Laceration without foreign body of left back wall of thorax without penetration into thoracic cavity, initial encounter

S21.221A Laceration with foreign body of right back wall of thorax without penetration into thoracic cavity, initial encounter

S21.222A Laceration with foreign body of left back wall of thorax without penetration into thoracic cavity, initial encounter

S21.231A Puncture wound without foreign body of right back wall of thorax without penetration into thoracic cavity, initial encounter

S21.232A Puncture wound without foreign body of left back wall of thorax without penetration into thoracic cavity, initial encounter

S21.241A Puncture wound with foreign body of right back wall of thorax without penetration into thoracic cavity, initial encounter

S21.242A Puncture wound with foreign body of left back wall of thorax without penetration into thoracic cavity, initial encounter

S21.251A Open bite of right back wall of thorax without penetration into thoracic cavity, initial encounter

S21.252A Open bite of left back wall of thorax without penetration into thoracic cavity, initial encounter

S21.311A Laceration without foreign body of right front wall of thorax with penetration into thoracic cavity, initial encounter

S21.312A Laceration without foreign body of left front wall of thorax with penetration into thoracic cavity, initial encounter

S21.321A Laceration with foreign body of right front wall of thorax with penetration into thoracic cavity, initial encounter

S21.322A Laceration with foreign body of left front wall of thorax with penetration into thoracic cavity, initial encounter

S21.331A Puncture wound without foreign body of right front wall of thorax with penetration into thoracic cavity, initial encounter

S21.332A Puncture wound without foreign body of left front wall of thorax with penetration into thoracic cavity, initial encounter

S21.341A Puncture wound with foreign body of right front wall of thorax with penetration into thoracic cavity, initial encounter

S21.342A Puncture wound with foreign body of left front wall of thorax with penetration into thoracic cavity, initial encounter

S21.351A Open bite of right front wall of thorax with penetration into thoracic cavity, initial encounter

S21.352A Open bite of left front wall of thorax with penetration into thoracic cavity, initial encounter

S21.411A Laceration without foreign body of right back wall of thorax with penetration into thoracic cavity, initial encounter

S21.412A Laceration without foreign body of left back wall of thorax with penetration into thoracic cavity, initial encounter

S21.421A Laceration with foreign body of right back wall of thorax with penetration into thoracic cavity, initial encounter

S21.422A Laceration with foreign body of left back wall of thorax with penetration into thoracic cavity, initial encounter

S21.431A Puncture wound without foreign body of right back wall of thorax with penetration into thoracic cavity, initial encounter

S21.432A Puncture wound without foreign body of left back wall of thorax with penetration into thoracic cavity, initial encounter

S21.441A Puncture wound with foreign body of right back wall of thorax with penetration into thoracic cavity, initial encounter

S21.442A Puncture wound with foreign body of left back wall of thorax with penetration into thoracic cavity, initial encounter

S21.451A Open bite of right back wall of thorax with penetration into thoracic cavity, initial encounter

S21.452A Open bite of left back wall of thorax with penetration into thoracic cavity, initial encounter

S22.21XB Fracture of manubrium, initial encounter for open fracture

S22.22XB Fracture of body of sternum, initial encounter for open fracture

S22.23XB Sternal manubrial dissociation, initial encounter for open fracture

S22.24XB Fracture of xiphoid process, initial encounter for open fracture

S22.41XB Multiple fractures of ribs, right side, initial encounter for open fracture ☑

S22.5XXA Flail chest, initial encounter for closed fracture

S22.5XXB Flail chest, initial encounter for open fracture

S27.0XXA Traumatic pneumothorax, initial encounter

S27.1XXA Traumatic hemothorax, initial encounter

S27.2XXA Traumatic hemopneumothorax, initial encounter

S27.893A Laceration of other specified intrathoracic organs, initial encounter

S28.0XXA Crushed chest, initial encounter

S29.091A Other injury of muscle and tendon of front wall of thorax, initial encounter

S29.092A Other injury of muscle and tendon of back wall of thorax, initial encounter

S29.8XXA Other specified injuries of thorax, initial encounter

T21.21XA Burn of second degree of chest wall, initial encounter

T21.31XA Burn of third degree of chest wall, initial encounter

T21.61XA Corrosion of second degree of chest wall, initial encounter

T21.71XA Corrosion of third degree of chest wall, initial encounter

T81.31XA Disruption of external operation (surgical) wound, not elsewhere classified, initial encounter

T81.328A Disruption or dehiscence of closure of other specified internal operation (surgical) wound, initial encounter

AMA: 32820 2023,Mar

Relative Value Units/Medicare Edits

Non-Facility RVU	Work	PE	MP	Total
32820	22.51	11.45	5.56	39.52
Facility RVU	**Work**	**PE**	**MP**	**Total**
32820	22.51	11.45	5.56	39.52

	FUD	Status	MUE	Modifiers				IOM Reference
32820	90	A	1(2)	51	N/A	62*	80	None

* with documentation

Terms To Know

autograft. Any tissue harvested from one anatomical site of a person and grafted to another anatomical site of the same person. Most commonly, blood vessels, skin, tendons, fascia, and bone are used as autografts.

flap. Mass of flesh and skin partially excised from its location but retaining its blood supply that is moved to another site to repair adjacent or distant defects.

omentum. Fold of peritoneal tissue suspended between the stomach and neighboring visceral organs of the abdominal cavity.

32850

32850 Donor pneumonectomy(s) (including cold preservation), from cadaver donor

Explanation

The physician performs a donor pneumonectomy(ies) for transplant from a cadaver donor. In cases where the donor has been declared brain dead, adequate functioning of the heart, lungs, and circulatory system are maintained prior to removal of the organ. During surgical removal of the lung(s), the donor may be placed on a cardiopulmonary bypass machine to maintain perfusion to the organs. The physician makes a long, mid-line vertical incision through all the layers of the skin down to the sternum bone. The sternum is split and the chest cavity entered. Each lung is removed in one block by dividing the trachea and the major arteries and veins that carry blood to and from the heart. The lung(s) is preserved for transplantation into the recipient. The organ(s) remains under refrigeration, specially packed in a sealable container with some preserving solution and kept on ice in a suitable carrier.

Coding Tips

Lung transplantation involves three distinct components. Code 32850 reports only the cadaver pneumonectomy. Backbench work (32855–32856), which involves preparation of the cadaver donor lung allograft prior to transplant, is reported separately. Transplant of the cadaver lung including recipient pneumonectomy and care of the recipient (32851–32854) is also reported separately. Any additional repair or resection procedures on the donor lung are also reported separately, see 32491, 32505–32507, 35216, and 35276. Donor pneumonectomy and any backbench work, repair, or resection procedures on the donor lung are usually the financial responsibility of the recipient.

ICD-10-CM Diagnostic Codes

Z52.89 Donor of other specified organs or tissues

Relative Value Units/Medicare Edits

Non-Facility RVU	Work	PE	MP	Total
32850	0.0	0.0	0.0	0.0
Facility RVU	**Work**	**PE**	**MP**	**Total**
32850	0.0	0.0	0.0	0.0

	FUD	Status	MUE	Modifiers				IOM Reference
32850	N/A	X	1(2)	N/A	N/A	N/A	N/A	None

* with documentation

Terms To Know

allograft. Graft from one individual to another of the same species.

cardiectomy. Surgical removal of the heart, may be for transplant or replacement with mechanical heart.

cardiopulmonary bypass. Venous blood is diverted to a heart-lung machine, which mechanically pumps and oxygenates the blood temporarily so the heart can be bypassed while an open procedure on the heart or coronary arteries is performed. During bypass, the lungs are deflated and immobile.

donor. Person from whom tissues or organs are removed for transplantation.

incision. Act of cutting into tissue or an organ.

pneumonectomy. Surgical removal of a lung or lung tissue.

32851-32852

32851 Lung transplant, single; without cardiopulmonary bypass
32852 with cardiopulmonary bypass

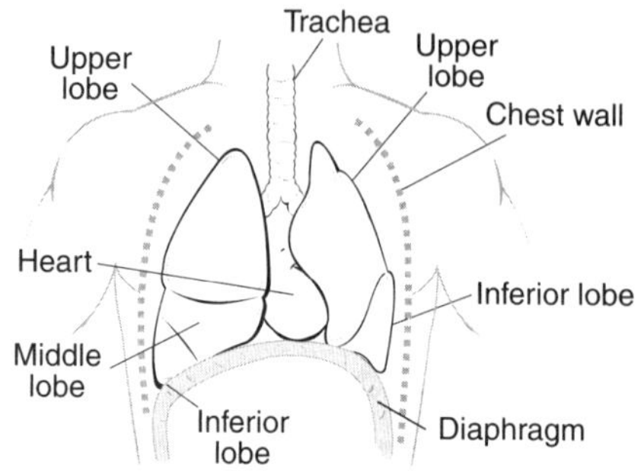

One lung is transplanted with or without cardiopulmonary bypass

Explanation

The physician performs a single lung transplantation of the recipient patient. A long, mid-line vertical incision is made through all the layers of the skin down to the sternum bone. The sternum is split, and the chest cavity entered. In 32851, the patient's oxygenation and circulation are maintained by the patient's own heart and other lung during the procedure, while in 32852, the patient is placed on a cardiopulmonary bypass machine to maintain circulation to the organs. The patient's original lung is deflated and the root of the lung isolated and the major arteries and veins that carry blood to and from the heart are identified and divided. The main bronchial tube to that lung is severed and the lung removed. The donor lung is placed in the chest cavity and its bronchial tube and arteries and veins sutured to the patients where the former lung was attached. Circulation and functioning of the donor lung are assured and the chest is closed. The sternum is closed using wire sutures and the skin closed in layers of sutures. A chest tube(s) is inserted into the chest cavity for drainage.

Coding Tips

Lung transplantation involves three distinct components. Codes 32851–32852 report only the transplant of the cadaver lung including recipient pneumonectomy and care of the recipient. Cadaver pneumonectomy (32850) is reported separately. Backbench work (32855–32856), which involves preparation of the cadaver donor lung allograft prior to transplant, is reported separately. Any additional repair or resection procedures on the donor lung are also reported separately, see 32491, 32505–32507, 35216, and 35276. Donor pneumonectomy and any backbench work, repair, or resection procedures on the donor lung are usually the financial responsibility of the recipient. For transplant of bilateral lungs, see 32853-32854.

ICD-10-CM Diagnostic Codes

D86.0 Sarcoidosis of lung
D86.2 Sarcoidosis of lung with sarcoidosis of lymph nodes
E84.0 Cystic fibrosis with pulmonary manifestations
E88.01 Alpha-1-antitrypsin deficiency
I27.0 Primary pulmonary hypertension
I27.21 Secondary pulmonary arterial hypertension
I27.22 Pulmonary hypertension due to left heart disease
I27.23 Pulmonary hypertension due to lung diseases and hypoxia
I27.24 Chronic thromboembolic pulmonary hypertension
I27.29 Other secondary pulmonary hypertension

I27.81 Cor pulmonale (chronic)
I27.82 Chronic pulmonary embolism
I27.83 Eisenmenger's syndrome
I27.89 Other specified pulmonary heart diseases
J44.1 Chronic obstructive pulmonary disease with (acute) exacerbation
J60 Coalworker's pneumoconiosis A
J61 Pneumoconiosis due to asbestos and other mineral fibers A
J62.0 Pneumoconiosis due to talc dust
J62.8 Pneumoconiosis due to other dust containing silica
J63.0 Aluminosis (of lung)
J63.1 Bauxite fibrosis (of lung)
J63.2 Berylliosis
J63.3 Graphite fibrosis (of lung)
J63.4 Siderosis
J63.5 Stannosis
J63.6 Pneumoconiosis due to other specified inorganic dusts
J68.4 Chronic respiratory conditions due to chemicals, gases, fumes and vapors
J68.8 Other respiratory conditions due to chemicals, gases, fumes and vapors
J70.1 Chronic and other pulmonary manifestations due to radiation
J84.01 Alveolar proteinosis
J84.112 Idiopathic pulmonary fibrosis
J84.113 Idiopathic non-specific interstitial pneumonitis
J84.114 Acute interstitial pneumonitis
J84.115 Respiratory bronchiolitis interstitial lung disease
J84.117 Desquamative interstitial pneumonia
J84.170 Interstitial lung disease with progressive fibrotic phenotype in diseases classified elsewhere
J84.178 Other interstitial pulmonary diseases with fibrosis in diseases classified elsewhere
J84.2 Lymphoid interstitial pneumonia
J84.81 Lymphangioleiomyomatosis
J84.82 Adult pulmonary Langerhans cell histiocytosis A
J84.83 Surfactant mutations of the lung
J84.843 Alveolar capillary dysplasia with vein misalignment
J84.89 Other specified interstitial pulmonary diseases
P26.1 Massive pulmonary hemorrhage originating in the perinatal period N
P26.8 Other pulmonary hemorrhages originating in the perinatal period N
P27.1 Bronchopulmonary dysplasia originating in the perinatal period
P29.30 Pulmonary hypertension of newborn
P29.38 Other persistent fetal circulation

Relative Value Units/Medicare Edits

Non-Facility RVU	Work	PE	MP	Total
32851	59.64	22.12	14.64	96.4
32852	65.5	23.06	15.17	103.73
Facility RVU	**Work**	**PE**	**MP**	**Total**
32851	59.64	22.12	14.64	96.4
32852	65.5	23.06	15.17	103.73

	FUD	Status	MUE	Modifiers				IOM Reference
32851	90	A	1(2)	51	N/A	62*	80	None
32852	90	A	1(2)	51	N/A	62*	80	

* with documentation

Terms To Know

agenesis. Absence of an organ due to developmental failure in the prenatal period.

asbestosis. Lung disease caused by long-term inhalation of asbestos particles. Asbestos exposure has been linked to lung cancer, most commonly mesothelioma.

dysplasia. Abnormality or alteration in the size, shape, and organization of cells from their normal pattern of development.

fibrosis. Formation of fibrous tissue as part of the restorative process.

hypoplasia. Condition in which there is underdevelopment of an organ or tissue.

meconium. First stool passed by a fetus, sometimes while still in the uterus. In this event, the meconium combines with the maternal amniotic fluid. Complications may occur if meconium is aspirated by the fetus while in utero or at the time of birth.

32853-32854

32853 Lung transplant, double (bilateral sequential or en bloc); without cardiopulmonary bypass

32854 with cardiopulmonary bypass

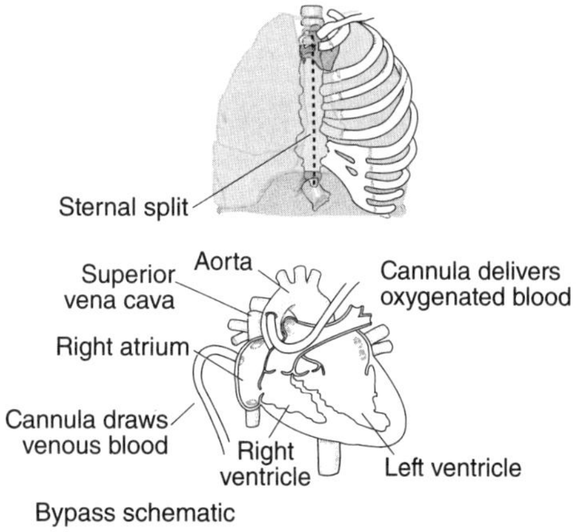

Cardiopulmonary bypass, also known as extracorporeal circulation, is a blood oxygenation technique used in many types of open heart surgeries

Explanation

The physician performs a double lung transplantation of the recipient patient, either in a bilateral sequential fashion or performed en bloc. A long, midline vertical incision is made through all the layers of the skin down to the sternum bone. The sternum is split, and the chest cavity entered. The patient's original lungs are deflated, the root of the lung isolated, and the major arteries and veins that carry blood to and from the heart are identified and divided. The tracheal tube to the lungs is severed and the lungs are removed. The donor lungs are placed in the chest cavity as a single unit or one at a time. The tracheal tube and arteries and veins are sutured to the site where the former lungs were attached. Circulation and functioning of the donor lungs are assured and the chest is closed. The sternum is closed using wire sutures and the skin closed in layers. Chest tubes are inserted into the chest cavities for drainage. The transplantation procedure in 32853 is accomplished without cardiopulmonary bypass, while in 32854 the patient is placed on a cardiopulmonary bypass machine to maintain circulation to the organs.

Coding Tips

Lung transplantation involves three distinct components. Codes 32853–32854 report only the transplant of the cadaver lung including recipient pneumonectomy and care of the recipient. Cadaver pneumonectomy (32850) is reported separately. Backbench work (32855–32856), which involves preparation of the cadaver donor lung allograft prior to transplant, is reported separately. Any additional repair or resection procedures on the donor lung are also reported separately, see 32491, 32505–32507, 35216, and 35276. Donor pneumonectomy and any backbench work, repair, or resection procedures on the donor lung are usually the financial responsibility of the recipient. For transplant of a unilateral lung, see 32851-32852.

ICD-10-CM Diagnostic Codes

D86.0	Sarcoidosis of lung
D86.2	Sarcoidosis of lung with sarcoidosis of lymph nodes
E84.0	Cystic fibrosis with pulmonary manifestations
E88.01	Alpha-1-antitrypsin deficiency
I27.0	Primary pulmonary hypertension
I27.21	Secondary pulmonary arterial hypertension
I27.22	Pulmonary hypertension due to left heart disease
I27.23	Pulmonary hypertension due to lung diseases and hypoxia
I27.24	Chronic thromboembolic pulmonary hypertension
I27.29	Other secondary pulmonary hypertension
I27.81	Cor pulmonale (chronic)
I27.82	Chronic pulmonary embolism
I27.83	Eisenmenger's syndrome
I27.89	Other specified pulmonary heart diseases
J44.1	Chronic obstructive pulmonary disease with (acute) exacerbation
J60	Coalworker's pneumoconiosis A
J61	Pneumoconiosis due to asbestos and other mineral fibers A
J62.0	Pneumoconiosis due to talc dust
J62.8	Pneumoconiosis due to other dust containing silica
J63.0	Aluminosis (of lung)
J63.1	Bauxite fibrosis (of lung)
J63.2	Berylliosis
J63.3	Graphite fibrosis (of lung)
J63.4	Siderosis
J63.5	Stannosis
J63.6	Pneumoconiosis due to other specified inorganic dusts
J68.4	Chronic respiratory conditions due to chemicals, gases, fumes and vapors
J68.8	Other respiratory conditions due to chemicals, gases, fumes and vapors
J70.1	Chronic and other pulmonary manifestations due to radiation
J84.01	Alveolar proteinosis
J84.112	Idiopathic pulmonary fibrosis
J84.113	Idiopathic non-specific interstitial pneumonitis
J84.114	Acute interstitial pneumonitis
J84.115	Respiratory bronchiolitis interstitial lung disease
J84.117	Desquamative interstitial pneumonia
J84.170	Interstitial lung disease with progressive fibrotic phenotype in diseases classified elsewhere
J84.178	Other interstitial pulmonary diseases with fibrosis in diseases classified elsewhere
J84.2	Lymphoid interstitial pneumonia
J84.81	Lymphangioleiomyomatosis
J84.82	Adult pulmonary Langerhans cell histiocytosis A
J84.83	Surfactant mutations of the lung
J84.843	Alveolar capillary dysplasia with vein misalignment
J84.89	Other specified interstitial pulmonary diseases
P26.1	Massive pulmonary hemorrhage originating in the perinatal period N
P26.8	Other pulmonary hemorrhages originating in the perinatal period N
P27.1	Bronchopulmonary dysplasia originating in the perinatal period
P29.30	Pulmonary hypertension of newborn
P29.38	Other persistent fetal circulation

Relative Value Units/Medicare Edits

Non-Facility RVU	Work	PE	MP	Total
32853	84.48	29.45	20.73	134.66
32854	90.0	30.57	21.99	142.56
Facility RVU	**Work**	**PE**	**MP**	**Total**
32853	84.48	29.45	20.73	134.66
32854	90.0	30.57	21.99	142.56

	FUD	Status	MUE	Modifiers				IOM Reference
32853	90	A	1(2)	51	N/A	62*	80	None
32854	90	A	1(2)	51	N/A	62*	80	

* with documentation

Terms To Know

cardiopulmonary bypass. Venous blood is diverted to a heart-lung machine, which mechanically pumps and oxygenates the blood temporarily so the heart can be bypassed while an open procedure on the heart or coronary arteries is performed. During bypass, the lungs are deflated and immobile.

dysplasia. Abnormality or alteration in the size, shape, and organization of cells from their normal pattern of development.

fibrosis. Formation of fibrous tissue as part of the restorative process.

hypoplasia. Condition in which there is underdevelopment of an organ or tissue.

32855-32856

32855 Backbench standard preparation of cadaver donor lung allograft prior to transplantation, including dissection of allograft from surrounding soft tissues to prepare pulmonary venous/atrial cuff, pulmonary artery, and bronchus; unilateral

32856 bilateral

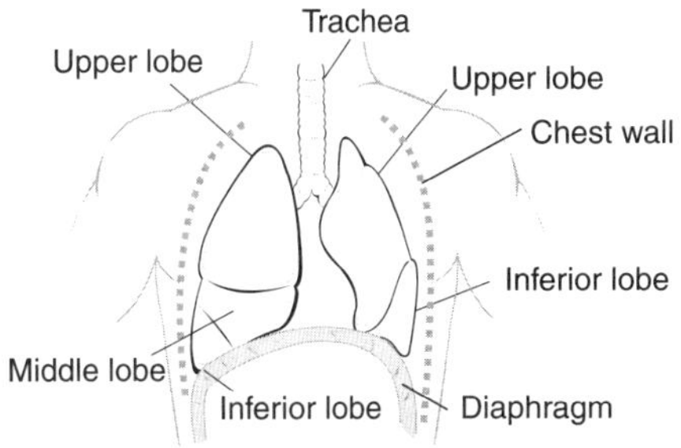

Backbench preparation is performed on one or both lungs from a cadaver in preparation for transplant

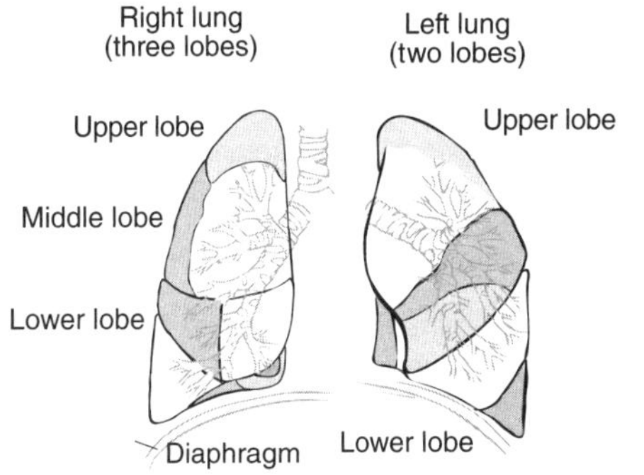

Explanation

The physician performs a standard backbench preparation of one or both lungs following procurement from a cadaver donor. Backbench or back table preparation refers to procedures performed on the donor organs following procurement to prepare the donor organs for transplant. Both lungs are removed or the heart and lungs are removed en bloc. If the heart and lungs are removed en bloc, back table separation of the heart and lungs is performed. The lungs are inspected following procurement to identify any injury or abnormality not noted prior to procurement. The physician prepares the lungs by dissecting free any residual soft tissue. Attention is focused on the pulmonary venous/atrial cuff, pulmonary artery, and bronchus. The pulmonary venous/atrial cuff is inspected and any residual tissue removed. The pulmonary artery, which was divided at its bifurcation, is inspected and any residual tissue removed. The aorta, which was divided distal to the innominate artery, is inspected and residual tissue removed. When all residual soft tissue has been removed and the vessels prepared, the lung(s) is ready for transplant. Report 32855 for backbench preparation of one lung (unilateral). Report 32856 for backbench preparation of both lungs (bilateral).

Coding Tips

Lung transplantation involves three distinct components. Codes 32855–32856 report only the backbench work, which involves preparation of the cadaver donor lung allograft prior to transplant. Cadaver pneumonectomy (32850) is reported separately. Transplant of the cadaver lung including recipient pneumonectomy and care of the recipient (32851–32854) is also reported separately. Any additional repair or resection procedures on the donor lung are also reported separately, see 32491, 32505–32507, 35216, and 35276. Donor pneumonectomy and any backbench work, repair, or resection procedures on the donor lung are usually the financial responsibility of the recipient.

ICD-10-CM Diagnostic Codes

The application of this code is too broad to adequately present ICD-10-CM diagnostic code links here. Refer to your ICD-10-CM book.

Relative Value Units/Medicare Edits

Non-Facility RVU	Work	PE	MP	Total
32855	0.0	0.0	0.0	0.0
32856	0.0	0.0	0.0	0.0
Facility RVU	**Work**	**PE**	**MP**	**Total**
32855	0.0	0.0	0.0	0.0
32856	0.0	0.0	0.0	0.0

	FUD	Status	MUE	Modifiers				IOM Reference
32855	N/A	C	1(2)	51	N/A	62*	80	None
32856	N/A	C	1(2)	51	N/A	62*	80	

* with documentation

Terms To Know

abscess. Circumscribed collection of pus resulting from bacteria, frequently associated with swelling and other signs of inflammation.

allograft. Graft from one individual to another of the same species.

asbestosis. Lung disease caused by long-term inhalation of asbestos particles. Asbestos exposure has been linked to lung cancer, most commonly mesothelioma.

backbench preparation. Procedures performed on a donor organ following procurement to prepare the organ for transplant into the recipient. Excess fat and other tissue may be removed, the organ may be perfused, and vital arteries may be sized, repaired, or modified to fit the patient. These procedures are done on a back table in the operating room before transplantation can begin.

cadaver. Dead body.

empyema. Accumulation of pus within the respiratory or pleural cavity.

32900

32900 Resection of ribs, extrapleural, all stages

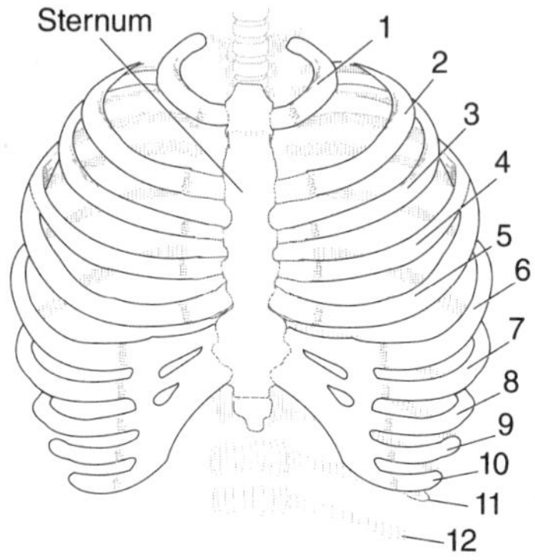

A rib, or a portion of a single rib, is surgically removed without entry into the thoracic cavity

Explanation

The physician resects a rib(s) without entering the chest cavity. The surgeon make an incision in the skin overlying the rib to be removed and carries that incision through the tissues down to the rib. The tissues are dissected away from the rib taking care not to puncture through the pleural membrane on the inside surface of the rib. This avoids the egress of air into the chest cavity. With the tissue removed from the surface of the rib, the rib is cut at two places and the intervening section removed. The resulting defect may be covered by the use of muscle flaps grafted to the area. The remaining tissues and skin are closed by suturing in layers.

Coding Tips

Report this procedure only when performed for the purpose of surgical collapse of the thoracic cavity. For radical resection of the chest wall and rib cage for tumor, see 21601. For partial excision of a rib, see 21600. For excision of the first and/or cervical rib, see 21615. For excision of the first and/or cervical rib with sympathectomy, see 21616. For division of scalenus anticus with resection of the cervical rib, see 21705.

ICD-10-CM Diagnostic Codes

C41.3	Malignant neoplasm of ribs, sternum and clavicle
D16.7	Benign neoplasm of ribs, sternum and clavicle
M41.124	Adolescent idiopathic scoliosis, thoracic region
M41.125	Adolescent idiopathic scoliosis, thoracolumbar region
M41.24	Other idiopathic scoliosis, thoracic region
M41.25	Other idiopathic scoliosis, thoracolumbar region
M41.34	Thoracogenic scoliosis, thoracic region
M41.35	Thoracogenic scoliosis, thoracolumbar region
M41.44	Neuromuscular scoliosis, thoracic region
M41.45	Neuromuscular scoliosis, thoracolumbar region
M41.54	Other secondary scoliosis, thoracic region
M41.55	Other secondary scoliosis, thoracolumbar region
M41.84	Other forms of scoliosis, thoracic region
M41.85	Other forms of scoliosis, thoracolumbar region
M86.38	Chronic multifocal osteomyelitis, other site
M86.48	Chronic osteomyelitis with draining sinus, other site
M86.58	Other chronic hematogenous osteomyelitis, other site
M86.68	Other chronic osteomyelitis, other site

M95.4	Acquired deformity of chest and rib
M99.82	Other biomechanical lesions of thoracic region
M99.88	Other biomechanical lesions of rib cage
Q67.6	Pectus excavatum
Q76.6	Other congenital malformations of ribs

Relative Value Units/Medicare Edits

Non-Facility RVU	Work	PE	MP	Total
32900	23.81	10.58	5.89	40.28
Facility RVU	**Work**	**PE**	**MP**	**Total**
32900	23.81	10.58	5.89	40.28

	FUD	Status	MUE	Modifiers				IOM Reference
32900	90	A	1(2)	51	N/A	62*	80	None

* with documentation

Terms To Know

benign. Mild or nonmalignant in nature.

deformity. Irregularity or malformation of the body.

dissection. Separating by cutting tissue or body structures apart.

excision. Surgical removal of an organ or tissue.

graft. Tissue implant from another part of the body or another person.

incision. Act of cutting into tissue or an organ.

malignant. Any condition tending to progress toward death, specifically an invasive tumor with a loss of cellular differentiation that has the ability to spread or metastasize to other body areas.

neoplasm. New abnormal growth, tumor.

ostectomy. Excision of bone.

pectus excavatum. Congenital abnormality of the anterior chest wall with depression of the sternum, sinking the appearance of the chest.

resection. Surgical removal of a part or all of an organ or body part.

sympathectomy. Surgical interruption or transection of a sympathetic nervous system pathway.

32905-32906

32905 Thoracoplasty, Schede type or extrapleural (all stages);
32906 with closure of bronchopleural fistula

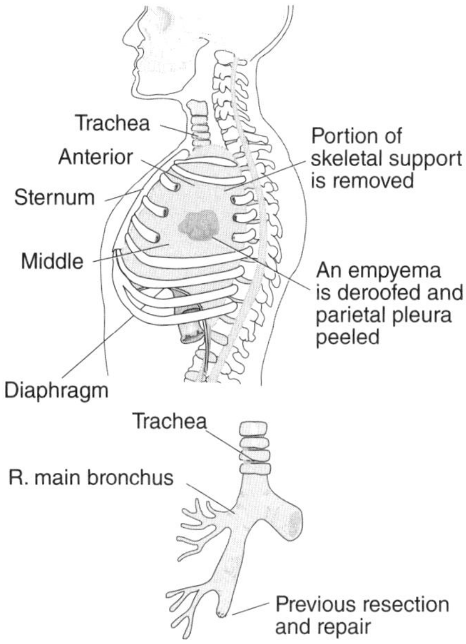

In some instances, the site of a previous bronchial surgery has developed a fistula between the stub and pleura

Explanation

The physician performs a thoracoplasty, which is the removal of the skeletal support of a portion of the chest (32905), and also closes a bronchopleural fistula (32906) to treat chronic thoracic empyema (accumulation of pus in the chest cavity) when there is insufficient lung tissue to fill the chest space. The procedure is carried out primarily on the upper chest. An incision is made through the skin down to the ribs. The Schede operation consists of the extensive unroofing of an empyema space by resecting the overlying ribs and portions of membrane lining the chest cavity (parietal pleural peel). In 32906, the bronchopleural fistula (an abnormal passageway between the remaining end of a bronchial tube that occurs sometimes after the removal of a lung or portion of a lung) is identified and resected, then closed by suturing. Closure of the fistula sometimes requires the use of muscle flap grafts taken from outside the chest cavity. The muscles in the area are partially closed over gauze packing and the skin partially closed by suturing in layers. As the packing is withdrawn in stages a few days later, it is hoped that freshly granulation tissue fills in the space formerly occupied by the empyema. The original Schede type operation is rarely performed but several modifications are currently done.

Coding Tips

For open closure of a major bronchial fistula, see 32815. For resection of the first rib for thoracic outlet syndrome, see 21615–21616.

ICD-10-CM Diagnostic Codes

A15.6	Tuberculous pleurisy
J86.0	Pyothorax with fistula
J86.9	Pyothorax without fistula

Relative Value Units/Medicare Edits

Non-Facility RVU	Work	PE	MP	Total
32905	23.29	10.44	5.75	39.48
32906	29.3	12.09	7.26	48.65
Facility RVU	**Work**	**PE**	**MP**	**Total**
32905	23.29	10.44	5.75	39.48
32906	29.3	12.09	7.26	48.65

	FUD	Status	MUE	Modifiers				IOM Reference
32905	90	A	1(2)	51	N/A	62*	80	None
32906	90	A	1(2)	51	N/A	62*	80	

* with documentation

Terms To Know

closure. Repairing an incision or wound by suture or other means.

empyema. Accumulation of pus within the respiratory or pleural cavity.

fistula. Abnormal tube-like passage between two body cavities or organs or from an organ to the outside surface.

graft. Tissue implant from another part of the body or another person.

granulation tissue. Loose collection of fibroblasts, inflammatory cells, and new vessels in an edematous fleshy projection that forms at the base of open wounds over which new skin forms, unless excessive granulation tissue, or proud flesh, rises above the wound surface.

incision. Act of cutting into tissue or an organ.

open fracture. Exposed break in a bone, always considered compound due to its high risk of infection from the open wound leading to the fracture. Broken bone ends may protrude through the skin and contaminants or foreign bodies are often embedded in the tissues.

resection. Surgical removal of a part or all of an organ or body part.

spontaneous tension pneumothorax. Air leaking from the lung and trapped in the lung lining.

32940

32940 Pneumonolysis, extraperiosteal, including filling or packing procedures

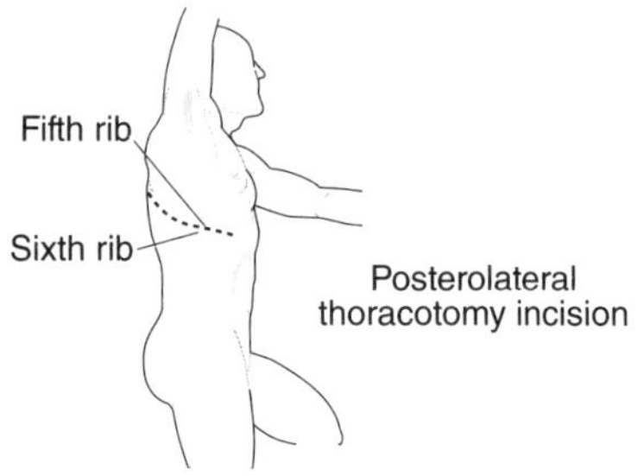

Adhesions between lung tissue and the inside surface of the chest cavity are released in an open surgical procedure

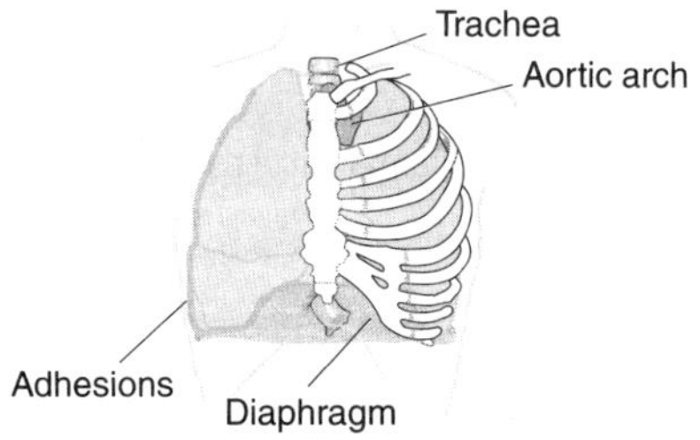

Following lysis, the pleural space may require packing or filling to prevent scar tissue development

Explanation

The physician opens the chest cavity and separates the surface of the lung which has become adherent to the inside surface of the chest cavity. Using a scalpel, the surgeon makes an incision around the side of the chest between two of the ribs. The incision is carried through all the tissue layers down to the tissue lining the chest cavity. Rib spreaders are inserted into the wound and the ribs are spread apart exposing the membrane lining the chest cavity (the parietal pleura). The surgeon separates the tissue between the periosteal membrane adherent to the inside surface of the lung and the parietal pleural membrane. This allows the movement of the lung within the chest cavity. The area or space created is packed or filled and the incision is closed in layers of sutures.

Coding Tips

Pneumolysis procedures are defined by site. Code 32940 reports extraperiosteal lysis of adhesions. For major thoracotomy with open intrapleural pneumonolysis, see 32124. For surgical thoracoscopy with total pulmonary decortication, including intrapleural pneumonolysis, see 32652.

ICD-10-CM Diagnostic Codes

A15.0	Tuberculosis of lung
A15.6	Tuberculous pleurisy
B90.9	Sequelae of respiratory and unspecified tuberculosis

Relative Value Units/Medicare Edits

Non-Facility RVU	Work	PE	MP	Total
32940	21.34	9.9	5.26	36.5
Facility RVU	**Work**	**PE**	**MP**	**Total**
32940	21.34	9.9	5.26	36.5

	FUD	Status	MUE	Modifiers				IOM Reference
32940	90	A	1(3)	51	N/A	62*	80	None

* with documentation

Terms To Know

adhesion. Abnormal fibrous connection between two structures, soft tissue or bony structures, that may occur as the result of surgery, infection, or trauma.

decortication. Removal of the cortical substance, the encapsulating or encasing material, of an organ, such as the kidneys or lungs.

emphysema. Pathological condition in which there is destructive enlargement of the air sacs in the lungs resulting in damage and lack of elasticity to the alveolar walls, commonly seen in long-term smokers.

empyema. Accumulation of pus within the respiratory or pleural cavity.

incision. Act of cutting into tissue or an organ.

late effect. Abnormality, dysfunction, or other residual condition produced after the acute phase of an illness, injury, or disease is over. There is no time limit on when late effects can appear.

lysis. Destruction, breakdown, dissolution, or decomposition of cells or substances by a specific catalyzing agent.

pleurisy. Inflammation of the serous membrane that lines the lungs and the thoracic cavity. Pleurisy may cause effusion within the cavity or have exudate in the pleural space or on the membrane surface.

pneumolysis. Breakdown of tissue attaching the lungs to the wall of the chest cavity, causing lung collapse.

thoracotomy. Surgical procedure for opening the chest wall in order to access the lungs, esophagus, trachea, aorta, heart, and diaphragm.

32960

32960 Pneumothorax, therapeutic, intrapleural injection of air

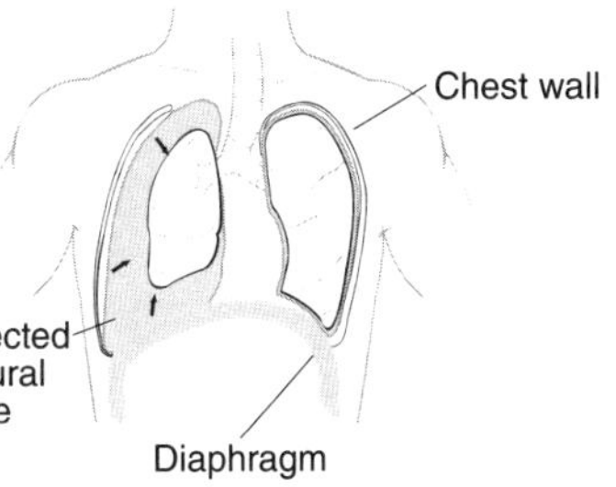

A pleural cavity is normally negatively pressurized and the introduction of atmospheric air causes the lung to begin to collapse

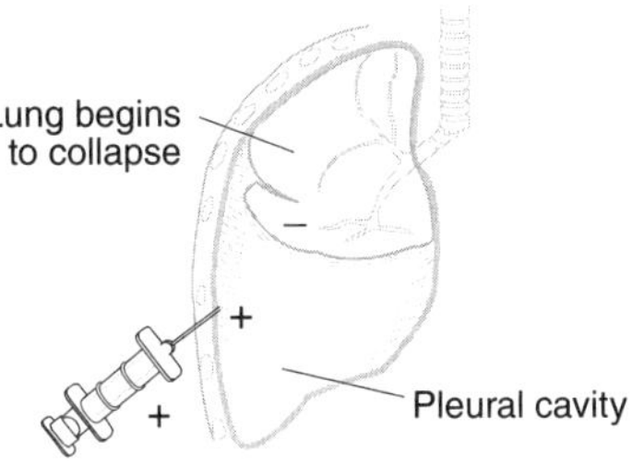

Air is injected into the thoracic cavity for therapeutic purposes

Explanation

The physician partially collapses a lung by injecting air into the chest cavity by puncturing through the space between the ribs. Using a needle attached to a syringe the physician passes the needle over the top of a rib and punctures through the chest tissues and enters the pleural cavity. With the end of the needle in the chest cavity, the physician injects air into the chest cavity to create a partial collapse of one lung, most commonly used to treat tuberculosis. A small plastic tube may be passed through the chest and left in place for repeated injections of air.

Coding Tips

This procedure reports the surgical creation of a pneumothorax used to treat pulmonary effusion, tuberculosis, and other conditions. Do not confuse with procedures performed to correct a spontaneous or traumatic pneumothorax. For thoracentesis for aspiration of the pleural space, see 32554 and 32555. For chemical pleurodesis for recurrent or persistent pneumothorax, see 32560.

ICD-10-CM Diagnostic Codes

A15.0	Tuberculosis of lung
A15.6	Tuberculous pleurisy
A15.7	Primary respiratory tuberculosis

Relative Value Units/Medicare Edits

Non-Facility RVU	Work	PE	MP	Total
32960	1.84	1.8	0.15	3.79
Facility RVU	**Work**	**PE**	**MP**	**Total**
32960	1.84	0.68	0.15	2.67

	FUD	Status	MUE	Modifiers				IOM Reference
32960	0	A	1(2)	51	N/A	N/A	N/A	None

* with documentation

32997

32997 Total lung lavage (unilateral)

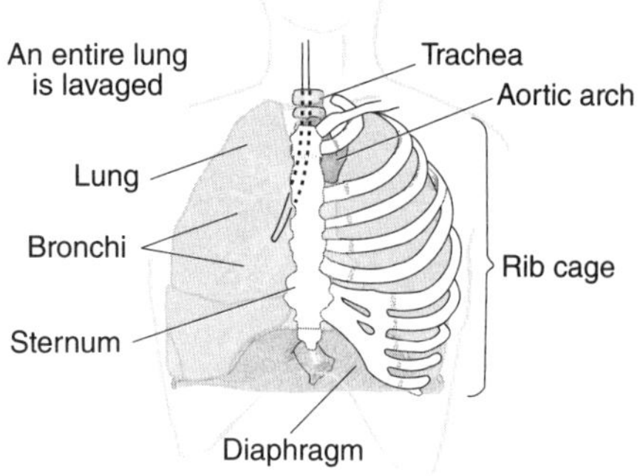

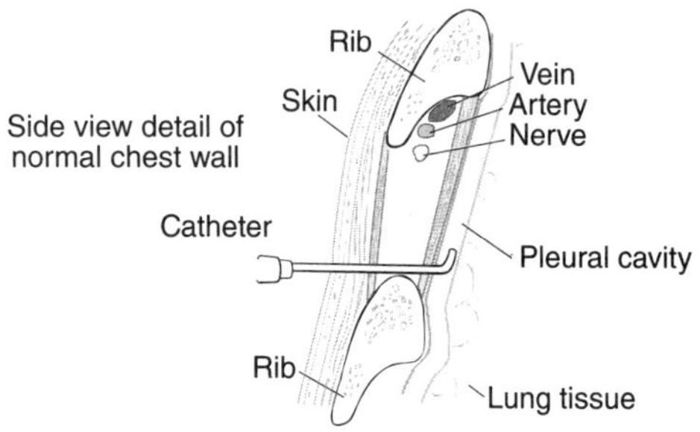

Explanation

The physician performs total lavage on one lung. The physician views the airway using a fiberoptic or rigid bronchoscopy. Under appropriate anesthesia, the bronchoscope is introduced through the nasal or oral cavity and advanced to the lungs. Saline is introduced through the bronchoscope and the lung tissue is washed or bathed. The saline is removed by suction and the solution containing the cells that have been obtained in the procedure may be sent to pathology to diagnose certain diseases, such as cancer. This procedure may also be performed to treat specific diseases or injuries.

Coding Tips

This is a unilateral procedure. If performed bilaterally, some payers require that the service be reported twice with modifier 50 appended to the second code, while others require identification of the service only once with modifier 50 appended. Check with individual payers. Modifier 50 identifies a procedure performed identically on the opposite side of the body (mirror image). For bronchial alveolar lavage performed endoscopically, see 31624.

ICD-10-CM Diagnostic Codes

E84.0	Cystic fibrosis with pulmonary manifestations
J44.0	Chronic obstructive pulmonary disease with (acute) lower respiratory infection
J44.1	Chronic obstructive pulmonary disease with (acute) exacerbation
J45.22	Mild intermittent asthma with status asthmaticus
J45.32	Mild persistent asthma with status asthmaticus
J45.42	Moderate persistent asthma with status asthmaticus
J45.52	Severe persistent asthma with status asthmaticus
J68.0	Bronchitis and pneumonitis due to chemicals, gases, fumes and vapors
J69.0	Pneumonitis due to inhalation of food and vomit
J69.1	Pneumonitis due to inhalation of oils and essences
J69.8	Pneumonitis due to inhalation of other solids and liquids
J84.01	Alveolar proteinosis

Relative Value Units/Medicare Edits

Non-Facility RVU	Work	PE	MP	Total
32997	7.31	2.0	0.57	9.88
Facility RVU	**Work**	**PE**	**MP**	**Total**
32997	7.31	2.0	0.57	9.88

	FUD	Status	MUE	Modifiers				IOM Reference
32997	0	A	1(2)	51	50	N/A	N/A	None

* with documentation

Terms To Know

abscess. Circumscribed collection of pus resulting from bacteria, frequently associated with swelling and other signs of inflammation.

catheter. Flexible tube inserted into an area of the body for introducing or withdrawing fluid.

empyema. Accumulation of pus within the respiratory or pleural cavity.

fistula. Abnormal tube-like passage between two body cavities or organs or from an organ to the outside surface.

instillation. Administering a liquid slowly over time, drop by drop.

intubation. Insertion of a tube into a hollow organ, canal, or cavity within the body.

lavage. Washing.

32998 [32994]

32998 Ablation therapy for reduction or eradication of 1 or more pulmonary tumor(s) including pleura or chest wall when involved by tumor extension, percutaneous, including imaging guidance when performed, unilateral; radiofrequency

32994 Ablation therapy for reduction or eradication of 1 or more pulmonary tumor(s) including pleura or chest wall when involved by tumor extension, percutaneous, including imaging guidance when performed, unilateral; cryoablation

In a percutaneous approach, radiofrequency is used to destroy or reduce a pulmonary tumor

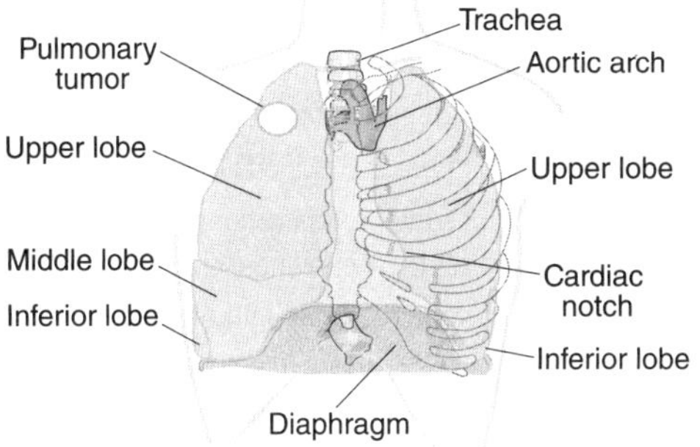

Explanation

In 32998, the physician uses the heat created from high-frequency radio waves to destroy one or more tumors in the lung, pleura, or chest wall. A small incision is made in the skin of the chest and the lesion is accessed by inserting an ablation probe connected to a radiofrequency generator between the ribs. Under imaging guidance, the ablation probe is advanced into the lesion of the lung, pleura, or chest wall. Treatment with the heat probe usually takes several minutes and may include repositioning the probe within the lesion so that overlapping ablations treat the entire tumor. The incision is closed with sutures. This process may be repeated for multiple lesions within the same lung. Report 32994 when the procedure is performed using cryoablation. Imaging guidance is included in these procedures, when performed.

Coding Tips

These are unilateral procedures. If performed bilaterally, some payers require that the service be reported twice with modifier 50 appended to the second code, while others require identification of the service only once with modifier 50 appended. Check with individual payers. Modifier 50 identifies a procedure performed identically on the opposite side of the body (mirror image).

ICD-10-CM Diagnostic Codes

C34.11 Malignant neoplasm of upper lobe, right bronchus or lung ☑
C34.12 Malignant neoplasm of upper lobe, left bronchus or lung ☑
C34.2 Malignant neoplasm of middle lobe, bronchus or lung
C34.31 Malignant neoplasm of lower lobe, right bronchus or lung ☑
C34.32 Malignant neoplasm of lower lobe, left bronchus or lung ☑
C34.81 Malignant neoplasm of overlapping sites of right bronchus and lung ☑
C34.82 Malignant neoplasm of overlapping sites of left bronchus and lung ☑
C38.4 Malignant neoplasm of pleura
C38.8 Malignant neoplasm of overlapping sites of heart, mediastinum and pleura
C45.0 Mesothelioma of pleura
C49.3 Malignant neoplasm of connective and soft tissue of thorax
C78.01 Secondary malignant neoplasm of right lung ☑
C78.02 Secondary malignant neoplasm of left lung ☑
C78.2 Secondary malignant neoplasm of pleura
C7A.090 Malignant carcinoid tumor of the bronchus and lung
D02.21 Carcinoma in situ of right bronchus and lung ☑
D02.22 Carcinoma in situ of left bronchus and lung ☑
D14.31 Benign neoplasm of right bronchus and lung ☑
D14.32 Benign neoplasm of left bronchus and lung ☑
D19.0 Benign neoplasm of mesothelial tissue of pleura
D38.1 Neoplasm of uncertain behavior of trachea, bronchus and lung
D38.2 Neoplasm of uncertain behavior of pleura
D3A.090 Benign carcinoid tumor of the bronchus and lung
D48.111 Desmoid tumor of chest wall
D48.112 Desmoid tumor, intrathoracic
J91.0 Malignant pleural effusion

Relative Value Units/Medicare Edits

Non-Facility RVU	Work	PE	MP	Total
32998	9.03	80.9	0.97	90.9
32994	9.03	132.36	0.97	142.36
Facility RVU	**Work**	**PE**	**MP**	**Total**
32998	9.03	2.79	0.97	12.79
32994	9.03	2.77	0.97	12.77

	FUD	Status	MUE	Modifiers				IOM Reference
32998	0	A	1(2)	51	50	N/A	80	None
32994	0	A	1(2)	51	50	N/A	80	

* with documentation

Terms To Know

ablation. Removal or destruction of a body part or tissue or its function. Ablation may be performed by surgical means, hormones, drugs, radiofrequency, heat, chemical application, or other methods.

mediastinum. Collection of organs and tissues that separate the pleural sacs. Located between the sternum and spine above the diaphragm, it contains the heart and great vessels, trachea and bronchi, esophagus, thymus, lymph nodes, and nerves.

pleura. One of the two membranes that surround the lungs. The visceral pleura encases the lung and the parietal pleura lines the inner chest walls.

33016

33016 Pericardiocentesis, including imaging guidance, when performed

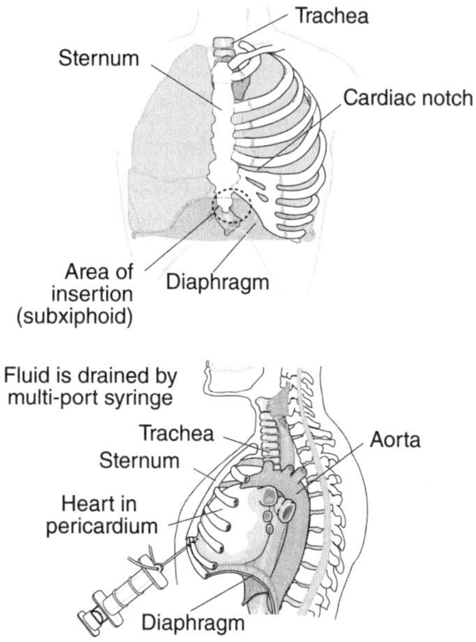

A centesis syringe is inserted into the pericardial sac and excess fluid is aspirated

Explanation

The physician drains fluid from the pericardial space. The physician may perform this procedure using anatomic landmarks or under fluoroscopic or echocardiographic (ultrasound) guidance, which is not separately reportable. The physician places a long needle below the sternum and directs it into the pericardial space. When pericardial fluid is aspirated, the physician may advance a guidewire through the needle into the pericardial space and exchange the needle over the guidewire for a drainage catheter. The physician removes as much pericardial fluid as is required, removes the needle or catheter, and dresses the wound.

Coding Tips

When medically necessary, report moderate (conscious) sedation provided by the performing physician with 99151–99153. When provided by another physician, report 99155–99157. Imaging guidance is included in this procedure and is not reported separately. If a catheter is used and removed at the end of the procedure, the removal is not reported separately. Do not report 33016 with 76942, 77002, 77012, or 77021. Do not report 33016 with 93303–93325 when echocardiography is performed solely for pericardiocentesis guidance. For pericardial drainage, see 33017–33019.

ICD-10-CM Diagnostic Codes

A18.84	Tuberculosis of heart
A39.53	Meningococcal pericarditis
A43.8	Other forms of nocardiosis
A52.06	Other syphilitic heart involvement
A54.83	Gonococcal heart infection
B33.23	Viral pericarditis
C38.0	Malignant neoplasm of heart
C45.2	Mesothelioma of pericardium
C79.89	Secondary malignant neoplasm of other specified sites
D15.1	Benign neoplasm of heart
D48.7	Neoplasm of uncertain behavior of other specified sites
I01.0	Acute rheumatic pericarditis
I09.2	Chronic rheumatic pericarditis
I23.0	Hemopericardium as current complication following acute myocardial infarction A
I24.1	Dressler's syndrome
I30.0	Acute nonspecific idiopathic pericarditis
I30.1	Infective pericarditis
I30.8	Other forms of acute pericarditis
I31.0	Chronic adhesive pericarditis
I31.1	Chronic constrictive pericarditis
I31.2	Hemopericardium, not elsewhere classified
I31.31	Malignant pericardial effusion in diseases classified elsewhere
I31.39	Other pericardial effusion (noninflammatory)
I31.4	Cardiac tamponade
I31.8	Other specified diseases of pericardium
I32	Pericarditis in diseases classified elsewhere
I97.89	Other postprocedural complications and disorders of the circulatory system, not elsewhere classified
M32.12	Pericarditis in systemic lupus erythematosus
P29.89	Other cardiovascular disorders originating in the perinatal period N
P54.8	Other specified neonatal hemorrhages N
S26.01XA	Contusion of heart with hemopericardium, initial encounter
S26.09XA	Other injury of heart with hemopericardium, initial encounter
T86.298	Other complications of heart transplant
T86.39	Other complications of heart-lung transplant

AMA: 33016 2022,Aug; 2020,Jan

Relative Value Units/Medicare Edits

Non-Facility RVU	Work	PE	MP	Total
33016	4.4	1.5	0.97	6.87
Facility RVU	**Work**	**PE**	**MP**	**Total**
33016	4.4	1.5	0.97	6.87

	FUD	Status	MUE	Modifiers				IOM Reference
33016	0	A	1(3)	51	N/A	N/A	N/A	None

* with documentation

Terms To Know

percutaneous. Through the skin.

pericardiocentesis. Puncture of a cavity for the purpose of removing fluid from the pericardial sac.

33017-33018

33017 Pericardial drainage with insertion of indwelling catheter, percutaneous, including fluoroscopy and/or ultrasound guidance, when performed; 6 years and older without congenital cardiac anomaly

33018 birth through 5 years of age or any age with congenital cardiac anomaly

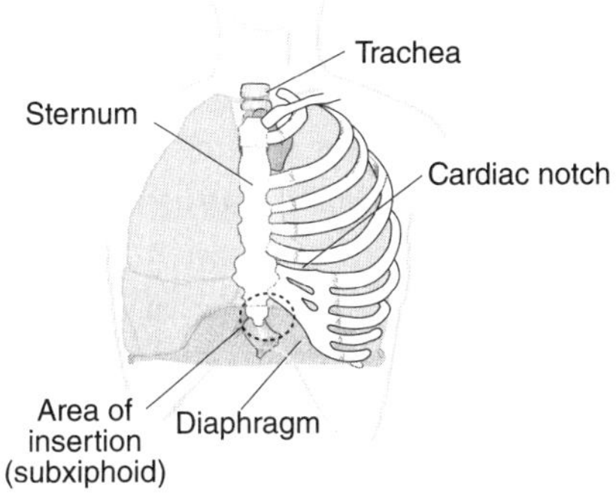

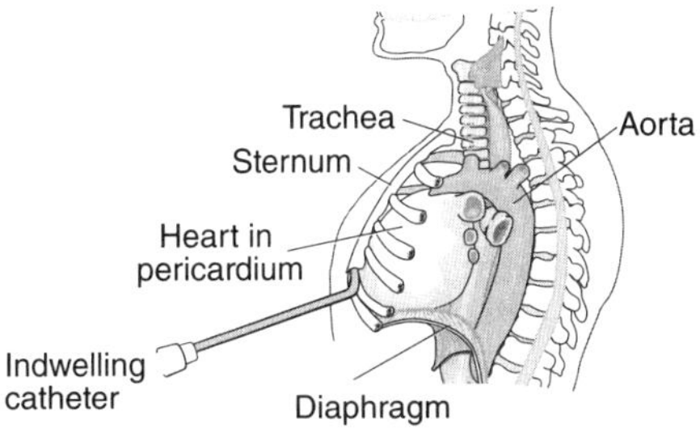

Indwelling catheter is inserted percutaneously for drainage of pericardium

Explanation

The physician drains fluid from the pericardial space. The physician may perform these procedures using anatomic landmarks or under fluoroscopic or echocardiographic (ultrasound) guidance, which is included in these codes and not reported separately. The physician places a long needle percutaneously below the sternum and directs it into the pericardial space. When pericardial fluid flows back through the needle, the physician passes a guidewire through the needle into the pericardial space. The physician exchanges the needle over the wire for an indwelling drainage catheter. The physician attaches the catheter to a drainage bag, sutures the indwelling catheter into place on the chest wall, and dresses the wound. Report 33017 when the procedure is performed on ages 6 years and older without a congenital cardiac anomaly. Report 33018 when the procedure is performed on newborns to 5 years of age with a congenital cardiac anomaly, such as dextrocardia, heterotaxy, mesocardia, or a single ventricle anomaly, or for any age within the first 90-day postop period following surgical repair of a congenital cardiac anomaly.

Coding Tips

When medically necessary, report moderate (conscious) sedation provided by the performing physician with 99151–99153. When provided by another physician, report 99155–99157. Imaging guidance is included in these procedures and is not reported separately. Do not report 33017 or 33018 with 75989, 76942, 77002, 77012, or 77021. Do not report 33017 or 33018 with 93303–93325 when echocardiography is performed solely for pericardiocentesis guidance. Do not report these codes when a catheter is placed to aspirate fluid and then removed at the end of the procedure. For pericardiocentesis, see 33016.

ICD-10-CM Diagnostic Codes

A18.84	Tuberculosis of heart
A39.53	Meningococcal pericarditis
A52.06	Other syphilitic heart involvement
A54.83	Gonococcal heart infection
B33.23	Viral pericarditis
C38.0	Malignant neoplasm of heart
C45.2	Mesothelioma of pericardium
C79.89	Secondary malignant neoplasm of other specified sites
D15.1	Benign neoplasm of heart
I01.0	Acute rheumatic pericarditis
I09.2	Chronic rheumatic pericarditis
I23.0	Hemopericardium as current complication following acute myocardial infarction A
I24.1	Dressler's syndrome
I30.0	Acute nonspecific idiopathic pericarditis
I30.1	Infective pericarditis
I31.0	Chronic adhesive pericarditis
I31.1	Chronic constrictive pericarditis
I31.2	Hemopericardium, not elsewhere classified
I31.31	Malignant pericardial effusion in diseases classified elsewhere
I31.39	Other pericardial effusion (noninflammatory)
I31.4	Cardiac tamponade
I32	Pericarditis in diseases classified elsewhere
M32.12	Pericarditis in systemic lupus erythematosus
Q20.4	Double inlet ventricle
Q20.6	Isomerism of atrial appendages
Q24.0	Dextrocardia
Q89.3	Situs inversus
S26.01XA	Contusion of heart with hemopericardium, initial encounter
T86.298	Other complications of heart transplant
T86.39	Other complications of heart-lung transplant

AMA: **33017** 2022,Aug; 2020,Mar; 2020,Jan **33018** 2020,Mar; 2020,Jan

Relative Value Units/Medicare Edits

Non-Facility RVU	Work	PE	MP	Total
33017	4.62	1.59	1.04	7.25
33018	5.4	1.83	1.24	8.47
Facility RVU	**Work**	**PE**	**MP**	**Total**
33017	4.62	1.59	1.04	7.25
33018	5.4	1.83	1.24	8.47

	FUD	Status	MUE	Modifiers				IOM Reference
33017	0	A	1(3)	51	N/A	N/A	N/A	None
33018	0	A	1(3)	51	N/A	N/A	N/A	

* with documentation

33019

33019 Pericardial drainage with insertion of indwelling catheter, percutaneous, including CT guidance

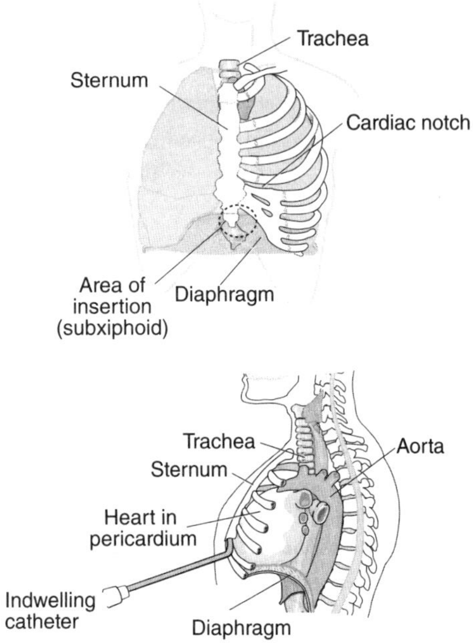

Indwelling catheter is inserted percutaneously for drainage of pericardium

Explanation

The physician drains fluid from the pericardial space. The physician performs this procedure under CT guidance, which is included in this code and not reported separately. The physician places a long needle percutaneously below the sternum and directs it into the pericardial space. When pericardial fluid flows back through the needle, the physician passes a guidewire through the needle into the pericardial space. The physician exchanges the needle over the wire for an indwelling drainage catheter. The physician attaches the catheter to a drainage bag, sutures the indwelling catheter into place on the chest wall, and dresses the wound.

Coding Tips

When medically necessary, report moderate (conscious) sedation provided by the performing physician with 99151–99153. When provided by another physician, report 99155–99157. Imaging (CT) guidance is included in this procedure and is not reported separately. Do not report 33019 with 75989, 76942, 77002, 77012, or 77021. Do not report 33019 when a catheter is placed to aspirate fluid and then removed at the end of the procedure. For pericardial drainage with insertion of an indwelling catheter, percutaneous, using fluoroscopy and/or ultrasound guidance, see 33017–33018.

ICD-10-CM Diagnostic Codes

A18.84	Tuberculosis of heart
A39.53	Meningococcal pericarditis
A43.8	Other forms of nocardiosis
A52.06	Other syphilitic heart involvement
A54.83	Gonococcal heart infection
B33.23	Viral pericarditis
C38.0	Malignant neoplasm of heart
C45.2	Mesothelioma of pericardium
C79.89	Secondary malignant neoplasm of other specified sites
D15.1	Benign neoplasm of heart
D48.7	Neoplasm of uncertain behavior of other specified sites
I01.0	Acute rheumatic pericarditis
I09.2	Chronic rheumatic pericarditis
I23.0	Hemopericardium as current complication following acute myocardial infarction A
I24.1	Dressler's syndrome
I30.0	Acute nonspecific idiopathic pericarditis
I30.1	Infective pericarditis
I30.8	Other forms of acute pericarditis
I31.0	Chronic adhesive pericarditis
I31.1	Chronic constrictive pericarditis
I31.2	Hemopericardium, not elsewhere classified
I31.31	Malignant pericardial effusion in diseases classified elsewhere
I31.39	Other pericardial effusion (noninflammatory)
I31.4	Cardiac tamponade
I31.8	Other specified diseases of pericardium
I32	Pericarditis in diseases classified elsewhere
I97.89	Other postprocedural complications and disorders of the circulatory system, not elsewhere classified
M32.12	Pericarditis in systemic lupus erythematosus
P29.89	Other cardiovascular disorders originating in the perinatal period N
P54.8	Other specified neonatal hemorrhages N
S26.01XA	Contusion of heart with hemopericardium, initial encounter
S26.09XA	Other injury of heart with hemopericardium, initial encounter
T86.298	Other complications of heart transplant
T86.39	Other complications of heart-lung transplant

AMA: 33019 2020,Jan

Relative Value Units/Medicare Edits

Non-Facility RVU	Work	PE	MP	Total
33019	4.29	1.34	0.52	6.15
Facility RVU	**Work**	**PE**	**MP**	**Total**
33019	4.29	1.34	0.52	6.15

	FUD	Status	MUE	Modifiers				IOM Reference
33019	0	A	1(3)	51	N/A	N/A	N/A	None

* with documentation

33020

33020 Pericardiotomy for removal of clot or foreign body (primary procedure)

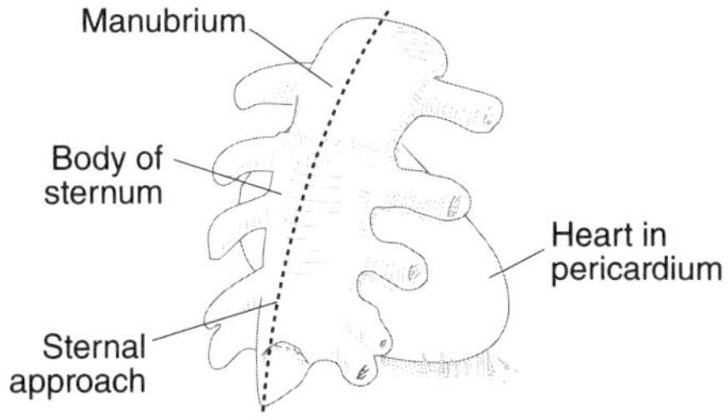

The pericardium is accessed, typically via the sternum, and a clot or foreign body is removed

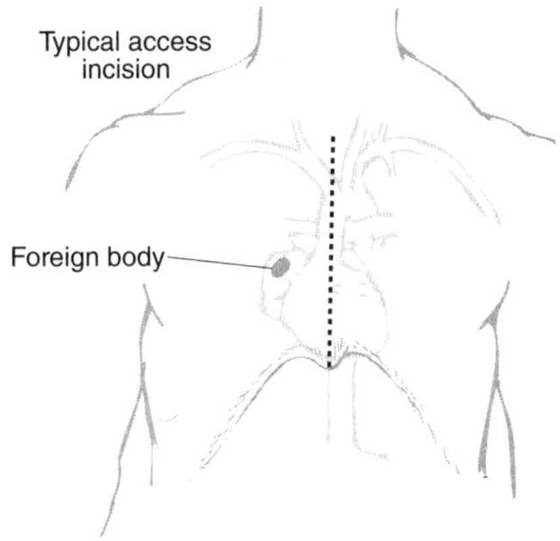

Explanation

The physician removes a clot or foreign body from the pericardial space. The physician performs a midline sternotomy, incising skin, fascia, and the sternum. The pericardium is incised and the clot or foreign body is removed. The pericardium is repaired loosely, leaving gaps for blood and fluid to drain into the pleural space. The sternum is reanastomosed with sternal wires and the skin is sutured in layers. In a less invasive approach for smaller clots or foreign matter, a needle is inserted through the skin under the sternum until it reaches the pericardial sac guided by fluoroscopy or echocardiography. A catheter is inserted to retrieve foreign matter or a catheter with a balloon attachment may also be used. The inflation of the balloon creates an opening within the desired location. The balloon catheter is removed and replaced with another catheter used to retrieve the foreign matter or clot.

Coding Tips

If this procedure is attempted thoracoscopically, but requires thoracotomy for completion, report 33020 for the open portion of the procedure and report a diagnostic thoracoscopy, 32601, as a secondary procedure. Do not report 33020 with 32551 if a pleural drain is placed on the same side. For thoracoscopic removal of a pericardial blood clot or foreign body, see 32658.

ICD-10-CM Diagnostic Codes

I30.0	Acute nonspecific idiopathic pericarditis
I30.8	Other forms of acute pericarditis
I31.1	Chronic constrictive pericarditis
I31.2	Hemopericardium, not elsewhere classified
I31.31	Malignant pericardial effusion in diseases classified elsewhere
I31.39	Other pericardial effusion (noninflammatory)
S21.311A	Laceration without foreign body of right front wall of thorax with penetration into thoracic cavity, initial encounter
S21.321A	Laceration with foreign body of right front wall of thorax with penetration into thoracic cavity, initial encounter
S21.331A	Puncture wound without foreign body of right front wall of thorax with penetration into thoracic cavity, initial encounter
S21.341A	Puncture wound with foreign body of right front wall of thorax with penetration into thoracic cavity, initial encounter
S21.351A	Open bite of right front wall of thorax with penetration into thoracic cavity, initial encounter
S21.411A	Laceration without foreign body of right back wall of thorax with penetration into thoracic cavity, initial encounter
S21.421A	Laceration with foreign body of right back wall of thorax with penetration into thoracic cavity, initial encounter
S21.431A	Puncture wound without foreign body of right back wall of thorax with penetration into thoracic cavity, initial encounter
S21.441A	Puncture wound with foreign body of right back wall of thorax with penetration into thoracic cavity, initial encounter
S21.451A	Open bite of right back wall of thorax with penetration into thoracic cavity, initial encounter
S26.01XA	Contusion of heart with hemopericardium, initial encounter
S26.020A	Mild laceration of heart with hemopericardium, initial encounter
S26.021A	Moderate laceration of heart with hemopericardium, initial encounter
S26.022A	Major laceration of heart with hemopericardium, initial encounter
S26.09XA	Other injury of heart with hemopericardium, initial encounter
S26.11XA	Contusion of heart without hemopericardium, initial encounter
S26.12XA	Laceration of heart without hemopericardium, initial encounter
S26.19XA	Other injury of heart without hemopericardium, initial encounter
S28.0XXA	Crushed chest, initial encounter
S38.1XXA	Crushing injury of abdomen, lower back, and pelvis, initial encounter

AMA: 33020 2021,Nov

Relative Value Units/Medicare Edits

Non-Facility RVU	Work	PE	MP	Total
33020	14.31	6.7	3.36	24.37
Facility RVU	**Work**	**PE**	**MP**	**Total**
33020	14.31	6.7	3.36	24.37

	FUD	Status	MUE	Modifiers				IOM Reference
33020	90	A	1(3)	51	N/A	62*	80	None

* with documentation

33025

33025 Creation of pericardial window or partial resection for drainage

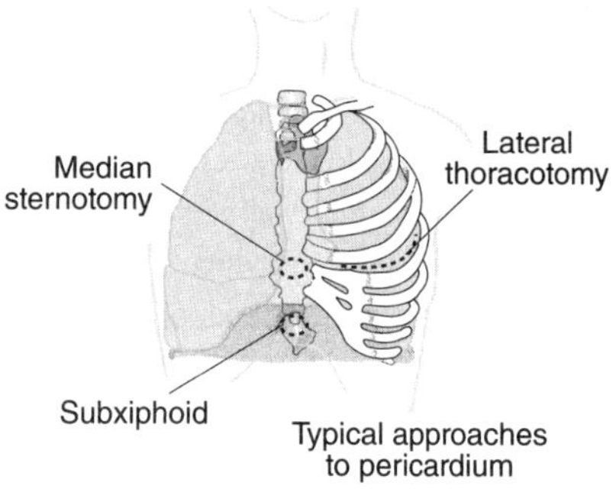

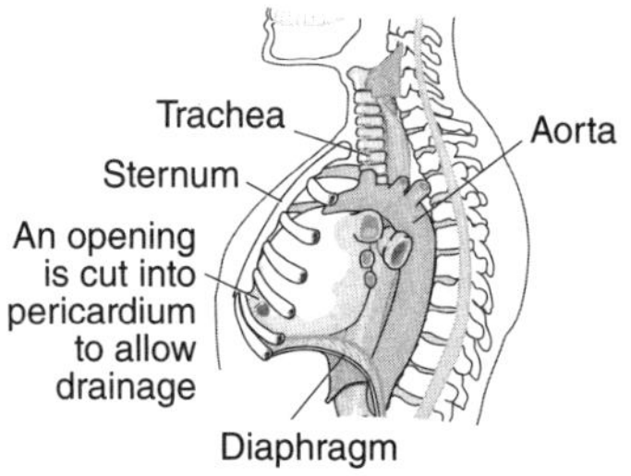

The pericardium is surgically accessed and constricting pericardial matter is removed from around the ventricle (partial) and sometimes from around the atria and cavae (total)

Explanation

The physician gains access to the pericardium in one of three ways: an incision into the subxiphoid space, the chest wall (thoracotomy), or thoracoscopically. The physician may make an incision in the pericardium or use electrocautery to open the pericardium large enough to allow drainage of pericardial fluid into the pleural space. This may require the use of a clamp or forceps to retract the surrounding tissues; however, if the pericardium is distended, a needle aspiration may be utilized under thoracoscopic guidance. The physician closes the sternal or chest wall incision and dresses the wound. The physician may leave chest tubes and/or a mediastinal drainage tube in place following the procedure.

Coding Tips

If this procedure is attempted thoracoscopically, but requires thoracotomy for completion, report 33025 for the open portion of the procedure and report a diagnostic thoracoscopy, 32601, as a secondary procedure. Thoracentesis and thoracostomy are included in this procedure and should not be reported separately. Do not report 33020 with 32551 if pleural drain is placed on the same side. For thoracoscopic creation of a pericardial window or partial resection of the pericardial sac for drainage, see 32659.

ICD-10-CM Diagnostic Codes

A18.84	Tuberculosis of heart
C38.0	Malignant neoplasm of heart
C45.2	Mesothelioma of pericardium
C79.89	Secondary malignant neoplasm of other specified sites
C7B.09	Secondary carcinoid tumors of other sites
C7B.8	Other secondary neuroendocrine tumors
D15.1	Benign neoplasm of heart
I01.0	Acute rheumatic pericarditis
I24.1	Dressler's syndrome
I30.0	Acute nonspecific idiopathic pericarditis
I30.1	Infective pericarditis
I30.8	Other forms of acute pericarditis
I31.0	Chronic adhesive pericarditis
I31.1	Chronic constrictive pericarditis
I31.2	Hemopericardium, not elsewhere classified
I31.31	Malignant pericardial effusion in diseases classified elsewhere
I31.39	Other pericardial effusion (noninflammatory)
I31.4	Cardiac tamponade
I31.8	Other specified diseases of pericardium
J98.51	Mediastinitis
M32.12	Pericarditis in systemic lupus erythematosus
T81.41XA	Infection following a procedure, superficial incisional surgical site, initial encounter
T81.42XA	Infection following a procedure, deep incisional surgical site, initial encounter
T81.43XA	Infection following a procedure, organ and space surgical site, initial encounter
T81.44XA	Sepsis following a procedure, initial encounter

AMA: **33025** 2021,Nov

Relative Value Units/Medicare Edits

Non-Facility RVU	Work	PE	MP	Total
33025	13.2	6.44	3.17	22.81
Facility RVU	**Work**	**PE**	**MP**	**Total**
33025	13.2	6.44	3.17	22.81

	FUD	Status	MUE	Modifiers				IOM Reference
33025	90	A	1(2)	51	N/A	62*	80	None

* with documentation

Terms To Know

acute. Sudden, severe.

chronic. Persistent, continuing, or recurring.

neoplasm. New abnormal growth, tumor.

pericarditis. Inflammation affecting the pericardium, the fibroserous membrane that surrounds the heart.

pericardium. Thin and slippery case in which the heart lies that is lined with fluid so that the heart is free to pulse and move as it beats.

resection. Surgical removal of a part or all of an organ or body part.

thoracentesis. Surgical puncture of the chest cavity with a specialized needle or hollow tubing to aspirate fluid from within the pleural space for diagnostic or therapeutic reasons.

thoracotomy. Surgical procedure for opening the chest wall in order to access the lungs, esophagus, trachea, aorta, heart, and diaphragm.

33030-33031

33030 Pericardiectomy, subtotal or complete; without cardiopulmonary bypass
33031 with cardiopulmonary bypass

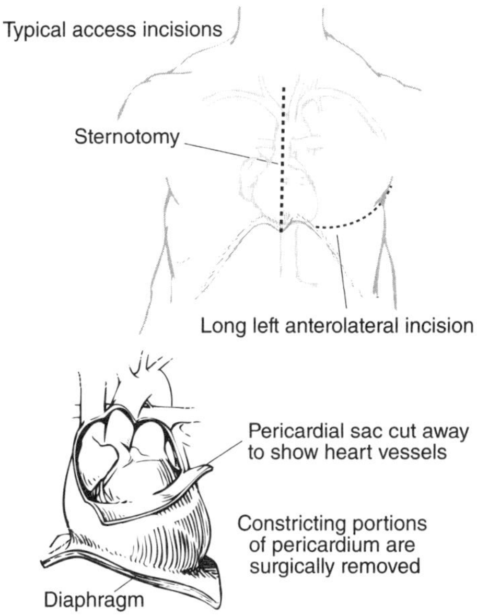

Constricting pericardial matter is removed from around the ventricle (partial) and sometimes also from around the atria and cavae (total)

Explanation

The physician gains access to the pericardium through an incision through the sternum (median sternotomy). The physician cuts away most or all of the pericardial tissue while the heart is still beating (without cardiopulmonary bypass), taking care to leave the phrenic nerves intact. The physician closes the sternal or chest wall incision and dresses the wound. The physician may leave chest tubes and/or a mediastinal drainage tube in place following the procedure. Report 33031 if the procedure is performed with cardiopulmonary bypass.

Coding Tips

If this procedure is attempted thoracoscopically, but requires thoracotomy for completion, report 33030 or 33031 for the open portion of the procedure and report a diagnostic thoracoscopy, 32601, as a secondary procedure. Thoracotomy, thoracentesis, and ECG monitoring are included and should not be reported separately.

ICD-10-CM Diagnostic Codes

A18.84	Tuberculosis of heart
C38.0	Malignant neoplasm of heart
C45.2	Mesothelioma of pericardium
C79.89	Secondary malignant neoplasm of other specified sites
C7B.09	Secondary carcinoid tumors of other sites
C7B.8	Other secondary neuroendocrine tumors
D15.1	Benign neoplasm of heart
D48.7	Neoplasm of uncertain behavior of other specified sites
I01.0	Acute rheumatic pericarditis
I24.1	Dressler's syndrome
I30.0	Acute nonspecific idiopathic pericarditis
I30.1	Infective pericarditis
I30.8	Other forms of acute pericarditis
I31.0	Chronic adhesive pericarditis
I31.1	Chronic constrictive pericarditis
I31.2	Hemopericardium, not elsewhere classified
I31.31	Malignant pericardial effusion in diseases classified elsewhere
I31.39	Other pericardial effusion (noninflammatory)
I31.8	Other specified diseases of pericardium
M32.12	Pericarditis in systemic lupus erythematosus
N80.B4	Endometriosis of the pericardial space
S26.01XA	Contusion of heart with hemopericardium, initial encounter
S26.020A	Mild laceration of heart with hemopericardium, initial encounter
S26.021A	Moderate laceration of heart with hemopericardium, initial encounter
S26.022A	Major laceration of heart with hemopericardium, initial encounter
T81.41XA	Infection following a procedure, superficial incisional surgical site, initial encounter
T81.42XA	Infection following a procedure, deep incisional surgical site, initial encounter
T81.43XA	Infection following a procedure, organ and space surgical site, initial encounter
T81.44XA	Sepsis following a procedure, initial encounter

Relative Value Units/Medicare Edits

Non-Facility RVU	Work	PE	MP	Total
33030	36.0	14.24	8.68	58.92
33031	45.0	16.89	10.86	72.75
Facility RVU	**Work**	**PE**	**MP**	**Total**
33030	36.0	14.24	8.68	58.92
33031	45.0	16.89	10.86	72.75

	FUD	Status	MUE	Modifiers				IOM Reference
33030	90	A	1(2)	51	N/A	62*	80	None
33031	90	A	1(2)	51	N/A	62*	80	

* with documentation

Terms To Know

cardiopulmonary bypass. Venous blood is diverted to a heart-lung machine, which mechanically pumps and oxygenates the blood temporarily so the heart can be bypassed while an open procedure on the heart or coronary arteries is performed. During bypass, the lungs are deflated and immobile.

late effect. Abnormality, dysfunction, or other residual condition produced after the acute phase of an illness, injury, or disease is over. There is no time limit on when late effects can appear.

thoracotomy. Surgical procedure for opening the chest wall in order to access the lungs, esophagus, trachea, aorta, heart, and diaphragm.

33050

33050 Resection of pericardial cyst or tumor

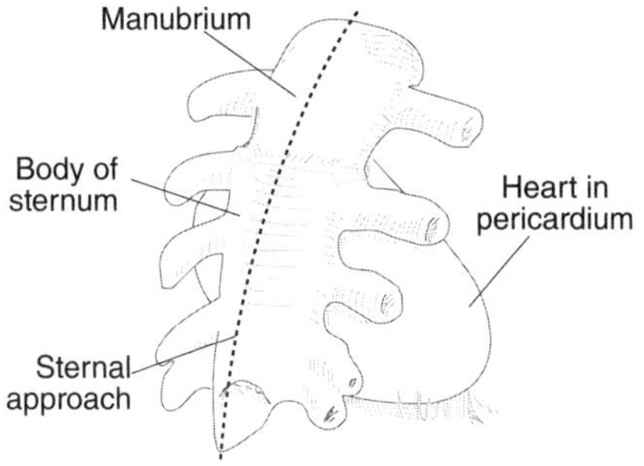

The pericardium is accessed, typically by a sternal split but other accesses may be employed. A pericardial cyst or tumor is removed

Explanation

The physician gains access to the pericardium through an incision through the sternum (median sternotomy) or the chest wall (lateral thoracotomy). If cardiopulmonary bypass is performed, the physician places cardiopulmonary bypass catheters (usually through incisions in the right atrial appendage and aorta or femoral artery). The physician stops the heart by infusing cardioplegia solution into the coronary circulation. The physician cuts away the pericardial cyst or tumor. The physician takes the patient off cardiopulmonary bypass, if used, closes the surgical incisions, and dresses the sternal or chest wall wound. The physician may leave chest tubes and/or a mediastinal drainage tube in place following the procedure.

Coding Tips

If significant additional time and effort are documented, append modifier 22 and submit a cover letter and operative report. For an open pericardial biopsy, see 39010. To report excision of a pericardial cyst, tumor, or mass thoracoscopically, see 32661. For resection of an external cardiac tumor, see 33130.

ICD-10-CM Diagnostic Codes

C38.0	Malignant neoplasm of heart
C45.2	Mesothelioma of pericardium
C79.89	Secondary malignant neoplasm of other specified sites
D15.1	Benign neoplasm of heart
D48.7	Neoplasm of uncertain behavior of other specified sites
I31.8	Other specified diseases of pericardium
Q24.8	Other specified congenital malformations of heart

Relative Value Units/Medicare Edits

Non-Facility RVU	Work	PE	MP	Total
33050	16.97	8.71	4.19	29.87
Facility RVU	**Work**	**PE**	**MP**	**Total**
33050	16.97	8.71	4.19	29.87

	FUD	Status	MUE	Modifiers				IOM Reference
33050	90	A	1(2)	51	N/A	62*	80	None

* with documentation

33120-33130

33120 Excision of intracardiac tumor, resection with cardiopulmonary bypass
33130 Resection of external cardiac tumor

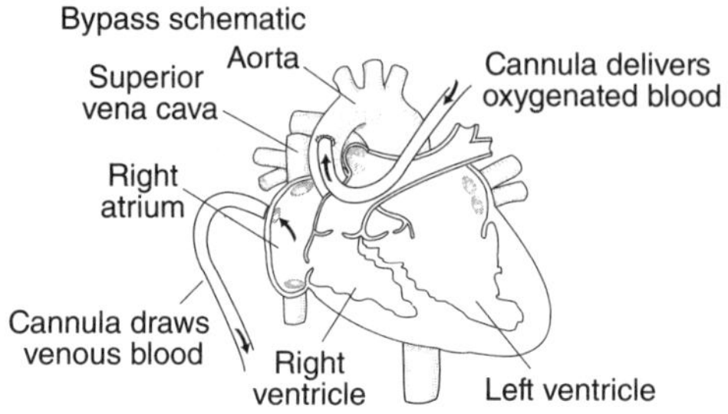

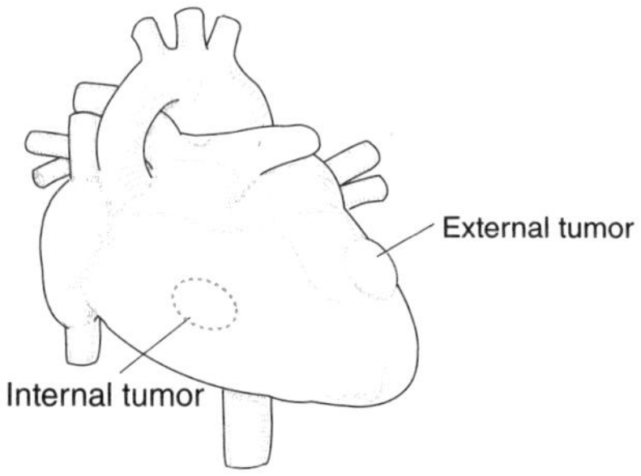

An external or internal cardiac tumor is removed

Explanation

Cardiopulmonary bypass is employed. Venous tubes are placed in both caval veins. The part of the heart that is opened depends on where the tumor is located. Every effort is made to avoid making an incision in any ventricular wall. After the heart is opened, the tumor is resected with a margin of normal heart tissue. Any problems created by this resection (damage to heart valves, holes in the walls between heart chambers or the outside of the heart, injury to coronary arteries) are repaired. All holes in the heart are closed. Cardiopulmonary bypass is stopped when heart function returns. In 33130, cardiopulmonary bypass is only required if a significant portion of the heart or major vessel must be removed with the tumor to get a margin of normal tissue around the tumor. The tumor and surrounding normal tissue are removed. Defects created in the heart, coronary arteries, or major vessels are repaired.

Coding Tips

Procedure codes for reporting tumor excision of the heart are classified by site. They may be pericardial, involving only the fibroserous sac surrounding the heart; external, involving the outer portion of the heart; or internal, requiring incision into the heart wall. If significant additional time and effort is documented, append modifier 22 and submit a cover letter and operative report. For excision of a pericardial tumor, see 33050. To report myocardial resection for ventricular aneurysm, see 33542.

ICD-10-CM Diagnostic Codes

C38.0	Malignant neoplasm of heart
C45.2	Mesothelioma of pericardium
C79.89	Secondary malignant neoplasm of other specified sites
C7B.09	Secondary carcinoid tumors of other sites
D15.1	Benign neoplasm of heart
D48.7	Neoplasm of uncertain behavior of other specified sites

Relative Value Units/Medicare Edits

Non-Facility RVU	Work	PE	MP	Total
33120	38.45	13.79	9.22	61.46
33130	24.17	10.42	5.59	40.18
Facility RVU	**Work**	**PE**	**MP**	**Total**
33120	38.45	13.79	9.22	61.46
33130	24.17	10.42	5.59	40.18

	FUD	Status	MUE	Modifiers				IOM Reference
33120	90	A	1(3)	51	N/A	62*	80	None
33130	90	A	1(3)	51	N/A	62*	80	

* with documentation

Terms To Know

absorbable sutures. Strands used for suture or repair of tissue prepared from collagen or a synthetic polymer and capable of being absorbed by tissue over time.

benign. Mild or nonmalignant in nature.

carcinoma in situ. Malignancy that arises from the cells of the vessel, gland, or organ of origin that remains confined to that site or has not invaded neighboring tissue.

lesion. Area of damaged tissue that has lost continuity or function, due to disease or trauma. Lesions may be located on internal structures such as the brain, nerves, or kidneys, or visible on the skin.

malignant. Any condition tending to progress toward death, specifically an invasive tumor with a loss of cellular differentiation that has the ability to spread or metastasize to other body areas.

neoplasm. New abnormal growth, tumor.

nonabsorbable sutures. Strands of natural or synthetic material that resist absorption into living tissue and are removed once healing is under way. Nonabsorbable sutures are commonly used to close skin wounds and repair tendons or collagenous tissue.

tumor. Pathological swelling or enlargement; a neoplastic growth of uncontrolled, abnormal multiplication of cells.

33140-33141

33140 Transmyocardial laser revascularization, by thoracotomy; (separate procedure)

\+ **33141** Transmyocardial laser revascularization, by thoracotomy; performed at the time of other open cardiac procedure(s) (List separately in addition to code for primary procedure)

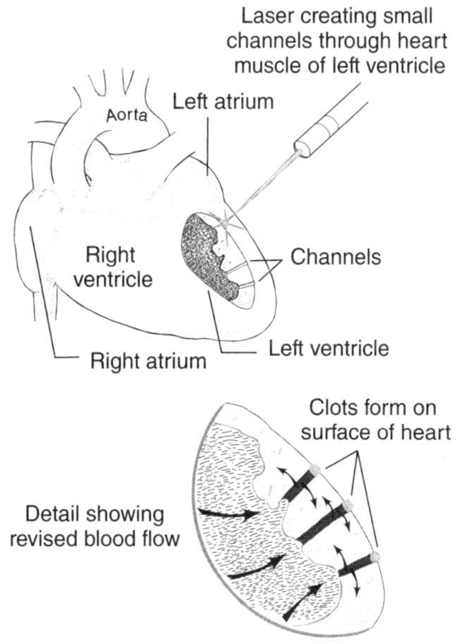

Small holes are burned by laser into the heart tissue to encourage revascularization of diseased muscle

Explanation

The physician performs transmyocardial laser revascularization to restore the flow of blood and oxygen to the heart. Varying approaches may be employed. The procedure is frequently performed on the beating heart, although cardiopulmonary bypass may be initiated. In the beating heart: Using a scalpel the physician makes a 10 centimeters to 15 centimeters incision on the left side of the chest between the ribs and exposes the surface of the heart. The area of ischemia (in still vital tissue) is identified. A laser is inserted through the chest opening and is fired (between heartbeats) through the filled left ventricle. Between 10 channels to 40 channels (small holes) are created to encourage new capillary growth in the area. As the channels are created pressure is applied to each to help close the openings. When the procedure is completed the laser is removed and the wound is closed with layered sutures. If cardiopulmonary bypass was initiated it is discontinued, the patient is rewarmed, and the heartbeat is restored. Report 33140 if the transmyocardial laser revascularization is performed alone. Report 33141 when it is performed at the time of another open cardiac procedure.

Coding Tips

Note that 33140, a separate procedure by definition, is usually a component of a more complex service and is not identified separately. When performed alone or with other unrelated procedures/services, it may be reported. If performed alone, list the code; if performed with other procedures/services, list the code and append modifier 59 or an X{EPSU} modifier. Report 33141 in addition to 33390–33391, 33404–33496, 33510–33536, and 33542.

ICD-10-CM Diagnostic Codes

I20.0	Unstable angina
I20.1	Angina pectoris with documented spasm
I20.2	Refractory angina pectoris

I20.81 Angina pectoris with coronary microvascular dysfunction
I21.01 ST elevation (STEMI) myocardial infarction involving left main coronary artery
I21.02 ST elevation (STEMI) myocardial infarction involving left anterior descending coronary artery
I21.09 ST elevation (STEMI) myocardial infarction involving other coronary artery of anterior wall
I21.11 ST elevation (STEMI) myocardial infarction involving right coronary artery
I21.19 ST elevation (STEMI) myocardial infarction involving other coronary artery of inferior wall
I21.21 ST elevation (STEMI) myocardial infarction involving left circumflex coronary artery
I21.29 ST elevation (STEMI) myocardial infarction involving other sites
I21.4 Non-ST elevation (NSTEMI) myocardial infarction
I21.A1 Myocardial infarction type 2
I21.B Myocardial infarction with coronary microvascular dysfunction
I22.0 Subsequent ST elevation (STEMI) myocardial infarction of anterior wall
I22.1 Subsequent ST elevation (STEMI) myocardial infarction of inferior wall
I22.2 Subsequent non-ST elevation (NSTEMI) myocardial infarction
I22.8 Subsequent ST elevation (STEMI) myocardial infarction of other sites
I24.0 Acute coronary thrombosis not resulting in myocardial infarction
I24.89 Other forms of acute ischemic heart disease
I25.110 Atherosclerotic heart disease of native coronary artery with unstable angina pectoris A
I25.111 Atherosclerotic heart disease of native coronary artery with angina pectoris with documented spasm A
I25.112 Atherosclerotic heart disease of native coronary artery with refractory angina pectoris A
I25.118 Atherosclerotic heart disease of native coronary artery with other forms of angina pectoris A
I25.3 Aneurysm of heart
I25.41 Coronary artery aneurysm
I25.42 Coronary artery dissection
I25.5 Ischemic cardiomyopathy
I25.6 Silent myocardial ischemia
I25.710 Atherosclerosis of autologous vein coronary artery bypass graft(s) with unstable angina pectoris A
I25.711 Atherosclerosis of autologous vein coronary artery bypass graft(s) with angina pectoris with documented spasm A
I25.712 Atherosclerosis of autologous vein coronary artery bypass graft(s) with refractory angina pectoris A
I25.720 Atherosclerosis of autologous artery coronary artery bypass graft(s) with unstable angina pectoris A
I25.721 Atherosclerosis of autologous artery coronary artery bypass graft(s) with angina pectoris with documented spasm A
I25.722 Atherosclerosis of autologous artery coronary artery bypass graft(s) with refractory angina pectoris A
I25.730 Atherosclerosis of nonautologous biological coronary artery bypass graft(s) with unstable angina pectoris A
I25.731 Atherosclerosis of nonautologous biological coronary artery bypass graft(s) with angina pectoris with documented spasm A
I25.732 Atherosclerosis of nonautologous biological coronary artery bypass graft(s) with refractory angina pectoris A
I25.750 Atherosclerosis of native coronary artery of transplanted heart with unstable angina
I25.751 Atherosclerosis of native coronary artery of transplanted heart with angina pectoris with documented spasm
I25.752 Atherosclerosis of native coronary artery of transplanted heart with refractory angina pectoris A
I25.760 Atherosclerosis of bypass graft of coronary artery of transplanted heart with unstable angina A
I25.761 Atherosclerosis of bypass graft of coronary artery of transplanted heart with angina pectoris with documented spasm A
I25.762 Atherosclerosis of bypass graft of coronary artery of transplanted heart with refractory angina pectoris A
I25.790 Atherosclerosis of other coronary artery bypass graft(s) with unstable angina pectoris A
I25.791 Atherosclerosis of other coronary artery bypass graft(s) with angina pectoris with documented spasm A
I25.792 Atherosclerosis of other coronary artery bypass graft(s) with refractory angina pectoris A
I25.810 Atherosclerosis of coronary artery bypass graft(s) without angina pectoris A
I25.811 Atherosclerosis of native coronary artery of transplanted heart without angina pectoris
I25.812 Atherosclerosis of bypass graft of coronary artery of transplanted heart without angina pectoris A
I25.82 Chronic total occlusion of coronary artery
I25.83 Coronary atherosclerosis due to lipid rich plaque A
I25.84 Coronary atherosclerosis due to calcified coronary lesion
I25.89 Other forms of chronic ischemic heart disease
Q24.5 Malformation of coronary vessels

Relative Value Units/Medicare Edits

Non-Facility RVU	Work	PE	MP	Total
33140	28.34	10.74	6.56	45.64
33141	2.54	0.7	0.62	3.86
Facility RVU	**Work**	**PE**	**MP**	**Total**
33140	28.34	10.74	6.56	45.64
33141	2.54	0.7	0.62	3.86

	FUD	Status	MUE	Modifiers				IOM Reference
33140	90	A	1(2)	51	N/A	N/A	80	None
33141	N/A	A	1(2)	N/A	N/A	62*	80	

* with documentation

Heart and Pericardium

33202

33202 Insertion of epicardial electrode(s); open incision (eg, thoracotomy, median sternotomy, subxiphoid approach)

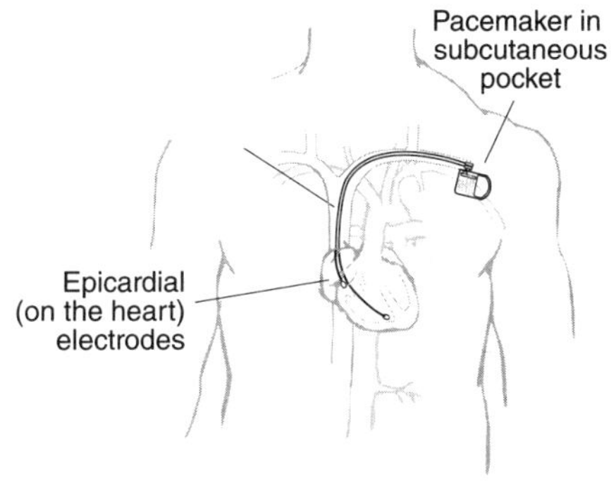

Epicardial electrodes are placed outside the heart in an open procedure

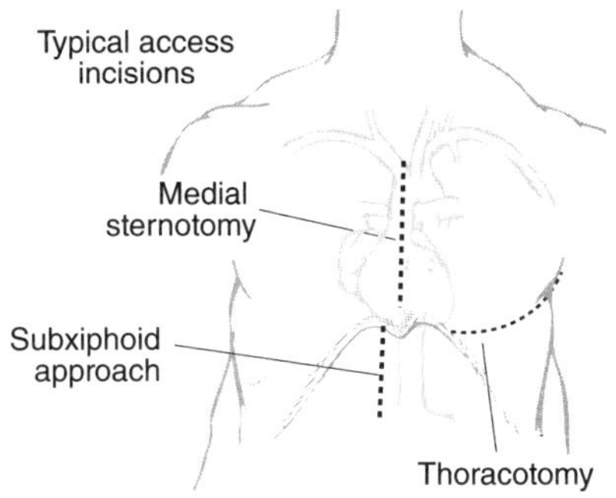

Explanation

The physician places one or more electrical leads on the outside of the heart (epicardial electrodes) by open chest incision. The incision can be in the middle of the chest (midline sternotomy), a vertical incision just below the ribcage (subxiphoid), or between the ribs on the left side of the body (thoracotomy). The chest cavity is opened. After the heart is exposed, electrodes are affixed to the appropriate areas of the heart muscle. The electrodes are tested and then tunneled under the coastal margin to the upper abdomen to a pulse generator or to the infraclavicular area if the generator is in that area. The physician closes the incision with layered sutures.

Coding Tips

Report 33202 when an epicardial lead is placed by the same physician during the same session with the insertion of a pulse generator when performed with 33212, 33213, 33221, 33230, 33231, or 33240. For endoscopic placement of epicardial electrodes by thoracoscopy or pericardioscopy, see 33203.

ICD-10-CM Diagnostic Codes

G90.01	Carotid sinus syncope
I44.0	Atrioventricular block, first degree
I44.1	Atrioventricular block, second degree
I44.2	Atrioventricular block, complete
I45.5	Other specified heart block
I45.6	Pre-excitation syndrome
I45.81	Long QT syndrome
I47.11	Inappropriate sinus tachycardia, so stated
I47.19	Other supraventricular tachycardia
I48.0	Paroxysmal atrial fibrillation
I48.11	Longstanding persistent atrial fibrillation
I48.19	Other persistent atrial fibrillation
I48.21	Permanent atrial fibrillation
I49.2	Junctional premature depolarization
I49.5	Sick sinus syndrome
I49.8	Other specified cardiac arrhythmias
Q24.6	Congenital heart block

AMA: 33202 2019,Mar; 2019,Jan

Relative Value Units/Medicare Edits

Non-Facility RVU	Work	PE	MP	Total
33202	13.2	6.44	3.17	22.81
Facility RVU	**Work**	**PE**	**MP**	**Total**
33202	13.2	6.44	3.17	22.81

	FUD	Status	MUE	Modifiers				IOM Reference
33202	90	A	1(2)	51	N/A	N/A	N/A	None

* with documentation

Terms To Know

atrioventricular block. Condition in which there is a disturbance of electrical conduction, such as a delay, intermittence, or absence in the transmission of an impulse from the atria to the ventricles and categorized according to degree of severity.

electrode. Electric terminal specialized for a particular electrochemical reaction that acts as a medium between a body surface and another instrument, commonly termed a lead.

epicardial electrode. Stimulation device that is attached to or inserted into the heart muscle and connected to a generator.

ventricular tachycardia. Excessively rapid ventricular rhythm of the heart, usually more than 150 beats per minute, with an origin beat generated in the ventricle, commonly from atrioventricular dissociation.

33203

33203 Insertion of epicardial electrode(s); endoscopic approach (eg, thoracoscopy, pericardioscopy)

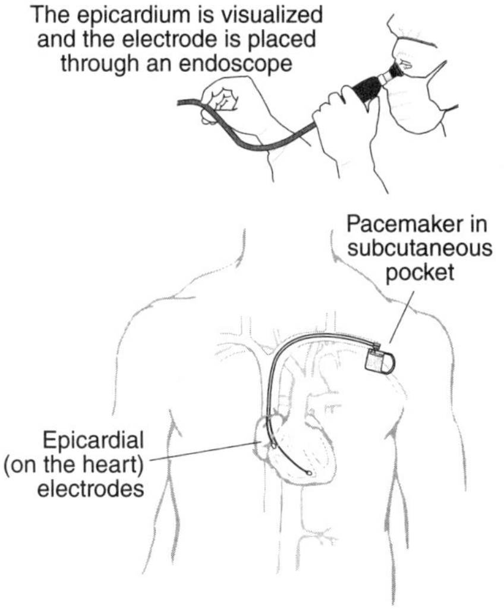

Explanation

The physician places electrical leads on the outside of the heart (epicardial electrodes) using an endoscopic approach. Three trocars are placed in the left anterior chest wall and the left lung is collapsed. A small incision is made in the chest (thoracostomy) and a 12 mm trocar is placed. The thoracoscope (endoscope) is inserted. Two additional trocars are placed under thoracoscopic visualization in the inframammary anterolateral region. Under thoracoscopic guidance, the pericardium is grasped and incised. The lateral trocar is removed and the incision enlarged to allow passage of the epicardial electrode placement device and the electrodes through the intercostal space. The electrodes are placed intrapericardially. The pericardium is approximated with a single stitch to hold the electrodes in place. The electrodes are tested and then tunneled under the costal margin to the upper abdomen to a pulse generator or over the ribs to the infraclavicular area if the generator is in that area. The thoracoscope is removed and a thoracostomy tube is placed at this site. The lung is expanded and the incisions closed with layered sutures.

Coding Tips

Report 33203 when an epicardial lead is placed by the same physician during the same session with the insertion of a pulse generator when performed with 33212, 33213, 33221, 33230, 33231, or 33240. For placement of epicardial electrodes by thoracotomy, see 33202.

ICD-10-CM Diagnostic Codes

G90.01	Carotid sinus syncope
I44.0	Atrioventricular block, first degree
I44.1	Atrioventricular block, second degree
I44.2	Atrioventricular block, complete
I45.5	Other specified heart block
I45.6	Pre-excitation syndrome
I45.81	Long QT syndrome
I47.11	Inappropriate sinus tachycardia, so stated
I48.0	Paroxysmal atrial fibrillation
I48.11	Longstanding persistent atrial fibrillation
I48.19	Other persistent atrial fibrillation
I48.21	Permanent atrial fibrillation
I49.2	Junctional premature depolarization
I49.5	Sick sinus syndrome
I49.8	Other specified cardiac arrhythmias
Q24.6	Congenital heart block

AMA: 33203 2019,Mar; 2019,Jan

Relative Value Units/Medicare Edits

Non-Facility RVU	Work	PE	MP	Total
33203	13.97	6.54	3.46	23.97
Facility RVU	**Work**	**PE**	**MP**	**Total**
33203	13.97	6.54	3.46	23.97

	FUD	Status	MUE	Modifiers				IOM Reference
33203	90	A	1(2)	51	N/A	N/A	N/A	None

* with documentation

Terms To Know

atrioventricular block. Condition in which there is a disturbance of electrical conduction, such as a delay, intermittence, or absence in the transmission of an impulse from the atria to the ventricles and categorized according to degree of severity.

ventricular tachycardia. Excessively rapid ventricular rhythm of the heart, usually more than 150 beats per minute, with an origin beat generated in the ventricle, commonly from atrioventricular dissociation.

33206-33208

33206 Insertion of new or replacement of permanent pacemaker with transvenous electrode(s); atrial
33207 ventricular
33208 atrial and ventricular

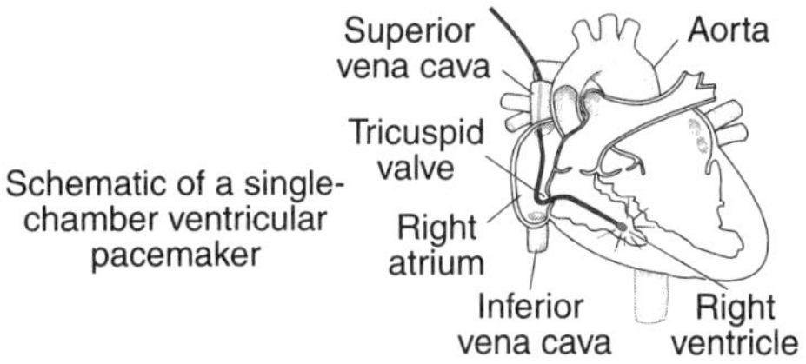

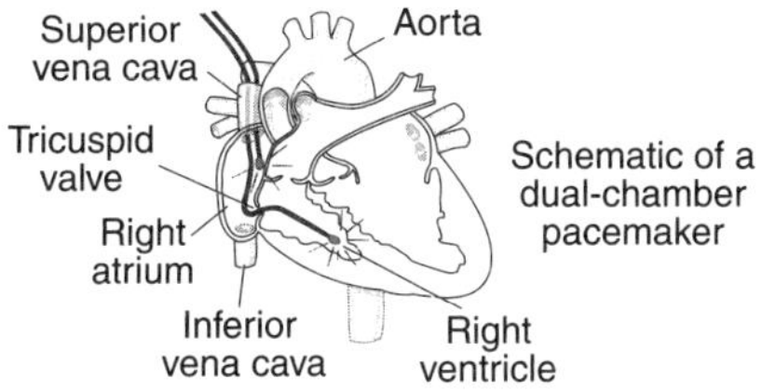

Explanation

The physician inserts or replaces a permanent pacemaker with transvenous electrodes. Under appropriate anesthesia, the physician gains access to the central caval veins typically via a percutaneous approach through the subclavian vein or employing a cut-down technique to the cephalic vein. Less commonly, the axillary, internal jugular, or femoral vein may be used. The vein is penetrated with a large needle and a wire is passed through it. A fluoroscope is used to guide the wire into the right atrium. A pocket for the pacemaker generator is created and the wire is tested. The wire is connected to the generator and the generator is closed in its pocket. Report 33206 if the guide and pacemaker wires are placed in the right atrium only; 33207 if the guide and pacemaker wires are placed in the right ventricle only; and 33208 if the elements of 33206 and 33207 are combined.

Coding Tips

When medically necessary, report moderate (conscious) sedation provided by the performing physician with 99151-99153. When provided by another physician, report 99155-99157. Codes 33206–33208 report a global service that includes subcutaneous placement of the pulse generator and transcutaneous placement of the electrode. These procedures include any repositioning or replacement, as well as fluoroscopic guidance. For removal and replacement of a pacemaker pulse generator and transvenous electrodes, report 33233 with 33234 or 33235 and 33206, 33207, or 33208. For removal and replacement of an implantable pacing cardioverter-defibrillator, see 33249. For removal and replacement of a subcutaneous implantable defibrillator, see 33270. Removal of subcutaneous leads may be reported separately with 33272. Do not report device evaluation codes (93260, 93261, 93279–93298) in addition to pulse generator and lead insertion/revision codes. Do not report 33206–33208 with 33227–33229. Do not report 33206, 33207, or 33208 with 33216 or 33217.

ICD-10-CM Diagnostic Codes

I44.0	Atrioventricular block, first degree
I44.1	Atrioventricular block, second degree
I44.2	Atrioventricular block, complete
I44.39	Other atrioventricular block
I44.4	Left anterior fascicular block
I44.5	Left posterior fascicular block
I44.69	Other fascicular block
I45.0	Right fascicular block
I45.19	Other right bundle-branch block
I45.2	Bifascicular block
I45.3	Trifascicular block
I45.4	Nonspecific intraventricular block
I45.5	Other specified heart block
I45.6	Pre-excitation syndrome
I45.81	Long QT syndrome
I47.11	Inappropriate sinus tachycardia, so stated
I47.19	Other supraventricular tachycardia
I48.0	Paroxysmal atrial fibrillation
I48.11	Longstanding persistent atrial fibrillation
I48.19	Other persistent atrial fibrillation
I48.21	Permanent atrial fibrillation
I49.2	Junctional premature depolarization
I49.5	Sick sinus syndrome
I49.8	Other specified cardiac arrhythmias
I50.21	Acute systolic (congestive) heart failure
I50.22	Chronic systolic (congestive) heart failure
I50.23	Acute on chronic systolic (congestive) heart failure
I50.31	Acute diastolic (congestive) heart failure
I50.32	Chronic diastolic (congestive) heart failure
I50.33	Acute on chronic diastolic (congestive) heart failure
I50.41	Acute combined systolic (congestive) and diastolic (congestive) heart failure
I50.42	Chronic combined systolic (congestive) and diastolic (congestive) heart failure
I50.43	Acute on chronic combined systolic (congestive) and diastolic (congestive) heart failure
I50.811	Acute right heart failure
I50.812	Chronic right heart failure
I50.813	Acute on chronic right heart failure
I50.814	Right heart failure due to left heart failure
I50.82	Biventricular heart failure
I50.83	High output heart failure
I50.84	End stage heart failure
I51.7	Cardiomegaly
I97.110	Postprocedural cardiac insufficiency following cardiac surgery
I97.111	Postprocedural cardiac insufficiency following other surgery
I97.120	Postprocedural cardiac arrest following cardiac surgery
I97.121	Postprocedural cardiac arrest following other surgery
I97.130	Postprocedural heart failure following cardiac surgery
I97.131	Postprocedural heart failure following other surgery
I97.190	Other postprocedural cardiac functional disturbances following cardiac surgery
I97.710	Intraoperative cardiac arrest during cardiac surgery
I97.711	Intraoperative cardiac arrest during other surgery
Q24.6	Congenital heart block
T82.110A	Breakdown (mechanical) of cardiac electrode, initial encounter
T82.111A	Breakdown (mechanical) of cardiac pulse generator (battery), initial encounter

T82.118A	Breakdown (mechanical) of other cardiac electronic device, initial encounter
T82.120A	Displacement of cardiac electrode, initial encounter
T82.121A	Displacement of cardiac pulse generator (battery), initial encounter
T82.128A	Displacement of other cardiac electronic device, initial encounter
T82.190A	Other mechanical complication of cardiac electrode, initial encounter
T82.191A	Other mechanical complication of cardiac pulse generator (battery), initial encounter
T82.817A	Embolism due to cardiac prosthetic devices, implants and grafts, initial encounter
T82.827A	Fibrosis due to cardiac prosthetic devices, implants and grafts, initial encounter
T82.837A	Hemorrhage due to cardiac prosthetic devices, implants and grafts, initial encounter
T82.847A	Pain due to cardiac prosthetic devices, implants and grafts, initial encounter
T82.857A	Stenosis of other cardiac prosthetic devices, implants and grafts, initial encounter
T82.867A	Thrombosis due to cardiac prosthetic devices, implants and grafts, initial encounter
Z45.018	Encounter for adjustment and management of other part of cardiac pacemaker

AMA: 33206 2019,Oct; 2019,Mar; 2019,Jan **33207** 2019,Oct; 2019,Mar; 2019,Jan **33208** 2019,Oct; 2019,Mar; 2019,Jan

Relative Value Units/Medicare Edits

Non-Facility RVU	Work	PE	MP	Total
33206	7.14	4.66	1.61	13.41
33207	7.8	4.52	1.77	14.09
33208	8.52	4.8	1.93	15.25
Facility RVU	**Work**	**PE**	**MP**	**Total**
33206	7.14	4.66	1.61	13.41
33207	7.8	4.52	1.77	14.09
33208	8.52	4.8	1.93	15.25

	FUD	Status	MUE	Modifiers				IOM Reference
33206	90	A	1(3)	51	N/A	62	N/A	None
33207	90	A	1(3)	51	N/A	62	N/A	
33208	90	A	1(3)	51	N/A	62	N/A	

* with documentation

33210-33211

33210 Insertion or replacement of temporary transvenous single chamber cardiac electrode or pacemaker catheter (separate procedure)

33211 Insertion or replacement of temporary transvenous dual chamber pacing electrodes (separate procedure)

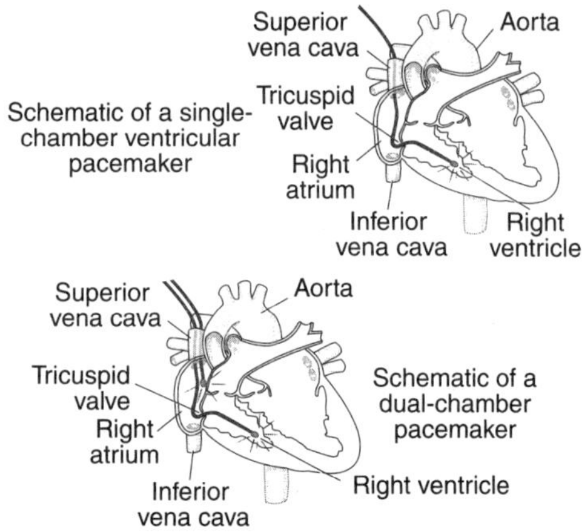

Explanation

Access to the central caval veins is obtained through the subclavian vein or jugular vein. The vein is penetrated with a large needle and a wire is passed through it. A fluoroscope is used to guide the wire into the right atrium. The wire is connected to a generator that is not implanted but temporarily placed outside the body. Report 33210 when a single chamber temporary transvenous electrode or pacemaker catheter is placed and 33211 when a dual chamber electrode(s) is inserted or replaced.

Coding Tips

When medically necessary, report moderate (conscious) sedation provided by the performing physician with 99151-99153. When provided by another physician, report 99155-99157. These separate procedures by definition are usually a component of a more complex service and are not identified separately. When performed alone or with other unrelated procedures/services they may be reported. If performed alone, list the code; if performed with other procedures/services, list the code and append 59 or an X{EPSU} modifier. Fluoroscopy is included in 33210 and 33211 and is not reported separately. Do not report device evaluation codes (93260, 93261, 93279–93298) in addition to pulse generator and lead insertion/revision codes.

ICD-10-CM Diagnostic Codes

I21.01	ST elevation (STEMI) myocardial infarction involving left main coronary artery
I21.02	ST elevation (STEMI) myocardial infarction involving left anterior descending coronary artery
I21.11	ST elevation (STEMI) myocardial infarction involving right coronary artery
I21.A1	Myocardial infarction type 2
I21.B	Myocardial infarction with coronary microvascular dysfunction
I22.0	Subsequent ST elevation (STEMI) myocardial infarction of anterior wall
I22.1	Subsequent ST elevation (STEMI) myocardial infarction of inferior wall
I44.0	Atrioventricular block, first degree
I44.1	Atrioventricular block, second degree
I44.2	Atrioventricular block, complete

I45.2 Bifascicular block
I45.3 Trifascicular block
I45.6 Pre-excitation syndrome
I45.81 Long QT syndrome
I46.2 Cardiac arrest due to underlying cardiac condition
I46.8 Cardiac arrest due to other underlying condition
I47.11 Inappropriate sinus tachycardia, so stated
I49.2 Junctional premature depolarization
I49.5 Sick sinus syndrome
I97.110 Postprocedural cardiac insufficiency following cardiac surgery
I97.111 Postprocedural cardiac insufficiency following other surgery
I97.120 Postprocedural cardiac arrest following cardiac surgery
I97.121 Postprocedural cardiac arrest following other surgery
I97.130 Postprocedural heart failure following cardiac surgery
I97.131 Postprocedural heart failure following other surgery
I97.710 Intraoperative cardiac arrest during cardiac surgery
I97.711 Intraoperative cardiac arrest during other surgery
Q24.6 Congenital heart block
T82.110A Breakdown (mechanical) of cardiac electrode, initial encounter
T82.120A Displacement of cardiac electrode, initial encounter
T82.817A Embolism due to cardiac prosthetic devices, implants and grafts, initial encounter
T82.827A Fibrosis due to cardiac prosthetic devices, implants and grafts, initial encounter
T82.837A Hemorrhage due to cardiac prosthetic devices, implants and grafts, initial encounter
T82.847A Pain due to cardiac prosthetic devices, implants and grafts, initial encounter
T82.867A Thrombosis due to cardiac prosthetic devices, implants and grafts, initial encounter

AMA: 33210 2023,Jun; 2022,Jul; 2021,Dec; 2019,Oct; 2019,Jan **33211** 2022,Jul; 2019,Oct; 2019,Jan

Relative Value Units/Medicare Edits

Non-Facility RVU	Work	PE	MP	Total
33210	3.05	1.04	0.63	4.72
33211	3.14	1.13	0.67	4.94
Facility RVU	**Work**	**PE**	**MP**	**Total**
33210	3.05	1.04	0.63	4.72
33211	3.14	1.13	0.67	4.94

	FUD	Status	MUE	Modifiers				IOM Reference
33210	0	A	1(3)	51	N/A	N/A	N/A	None
33211	0	A	1(3)	51	N/A	N/A	N/A	

* with documentation

33212-33214 [33221]

33212 Insertion of pacemaker pulse generator only; with existing single lead
33213 with existing dual leads
33221 Insertion of pacemaker pulse generator only; with existing multiple leads
33214 Upgrade of implanted pacemaker system, conversion of single chamber system to dual chamber system (includes removal of previously placed pulse generator, testing of existing lead, insertion of new lead, insertion of new pulse generator)

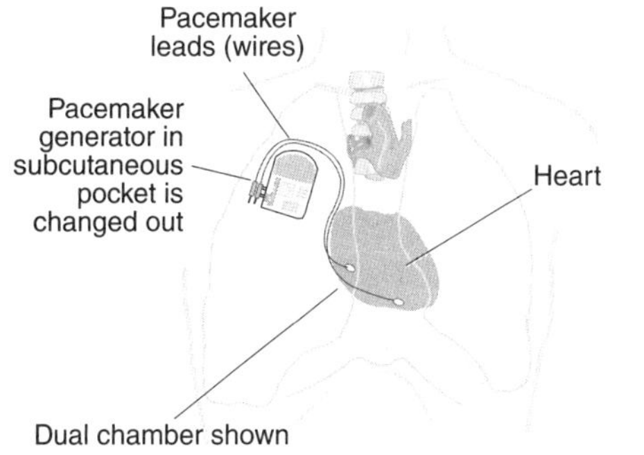

The generator consists of a battery, programmable circuitry, and is attached to the wire leads to the heart

Explanation

A single or dual chamber pacemaker pulse generator is inserted or replaced and connected to previously placed, existing leads. If this is an initial insertion, a pocket for the pacemaker generator is created subcutaneously in the subclavicular region or underneath the abdominal muscles just below the ribcage. The generator is inserted into the pocket. The pocket is closed. Report 33212 if a single chamber (atrial or ventricular) pacemaker pulse generator is inserted, 33213 if a dual chamber (atrial and ventricular) pacemaker pulse generator is inserted, or 33221 for the insertion of the generator with multiple existing leads. In 33214, a single chamber system is converted to a dual chamber system. The existing pacemaker generator pocket is opened and the single chamber generator removed. The dual chamber generator is placed into the existing pocket. The existing pacer wire is tested and connected to the generator. A second lead is placed and tested. The pocket is closed.

Coding Tips

When medically necessary, report moderate (conscious) sedation provided by the performing physician with 99151-99153. When provided by another physician, report 99155-99157. When documentation indicates the replacement of the pulse generator, see 33227–33229, but do not report these codes with 33214. Do not report 33212, 33213, or 33221 with 33233 for removal and replacement of the pacemaker pulse generator. Do not report these codes with 33216 or 33217. When epicardial lead placement is performed with insertion of the generator, see 33202 and/or 33203 in addition to 33212, 33213, and 33221. Revision of skin pocket is included and not reported separately. Fluoroscopy is included in 33212, 33214, and 33221 and is not reported separately. Do not report device evaluation codes (93260, 93261, 93279–93298) in addition to pulse generator and lead insertion/revision codes.

ICD-10-CM Diagnostic Codes

I44.0 Atrioventricular block, first degree
I44.1 Atrioventricular block, second degree
I44.2 Atrioventricular block, complete

I44.4	Left anterior fascicular block
I44.5	Left posterior fascicular block
I45.0	Right fascicular block
I45.2	Bifascicular block
I45.6	Pre-excitation syndrome
I45.81	Long QT syndrome
I47.11	Inappropriate sinus tachycardia, so stated
I47.19	Other supraventricular tachycardia
I48.0	Paroxysmal atrial fibrillation
I48.11	Longstanding persistent atrial fibrillation
I48.19	Other persistent atrial fibrillation
I48.21	Permanent atrial fibrillation
I49.2	Junctional premature depolarization
I49.5	Sick sinus syndrome
I50.21	Acute systolic (congestive) heart failure
I50.22	Chronic systolic (congestive) heart failure
I50.23	Acute on chronic systolic (congestive) heart failure
I50.31	Acute diastolic (congestive) heart failure
I50.32	Chronic diastolic (congestive) heart failure
I50.33	Acute on chronic diastolic (congestive) heart failure
I50.41	Acute combined systolic (congestive) and diastolic (congestive) heart failure
I50.42	Chronic combined systolic (congestive) and diastolic (congestive) heart failure
I50.43	Acute on chronic combined systolic (congestive) and diastolic (congestive) heart failure
I50.811	Acute right heart failure
I50.812	Chronic right heart failure
I50.813	Acute on chronic right heart failure
I50.814	Right heart failure due to left heart failure
I50.82	Biventricular heart failure
I50.83	High output heart failure
I50.84	End stage heart failure
Q24.6	Congenital heart block
T82.111A	Breakdown (mechanical) of cardiac pulse generator (battery), initial encounter
T82.121A	Displacement of cardiac pulse generator (battery), initial encounter

AMA: 33212 2019,Oct; 2019,Mar; 2019,Jan **33213** 2019,Oct; 2019,Mar; 2019,Jan **33214** 2019,Oct; 2019,Mar; 2019,Jan **33221** 2019,Oct; 2019,Mar; 2019,Jan

Relative Value Units/Medicare Edits

Non-Facility RVU	Work	PE	MP	Total
33212	5.01	3.39	1.15	9.55
33213	5.28	3.51	1.21	10.0
33221	5.55	3.76	1.25	10.56
33214	7.59	4.84	1.7	14.13
Facility RVU	**Work**	**PE**	**MP**	**Total**
33212	5.01	3.39	1.15	9.55
33213	5.28	3.51	1.21	10.0
33221	5.55	3.76	1.25	10.56
33214	7.59	4.84	1.7	14.13

	FUD	Status	MUE	Modifiers				IOM Reference
33212	90	A	1(3)	51	N/A	N/A	N/A	None
33213	90	A	1(3)	51	N/A	N/A	N/A	
33221	90	A	1(3)	51	N/A	N/A	N/A	
33214	90	A	1(3)	51	N/A	62	80*	

* with documentation

Terms To Know

fluoroscopy. Radiology technique that allows visual examination of part of the body or a function of an organ using a device that projects an x-ray image on a fluorescent screen.

pacemaker. Implantable cardiac device that controls the heart's rhythm and maintains regular beats by artificial electric discharges. This device consists of the pulse generator with a battery and the electrodes, or leads, which are placed in single or dual chambers of the heart, usually transvenously.

pulse generator. Circuit used to generate pulses. Pulse generators contain the battery, the electronic circuit, and the connector in a hermetically sealed encasement. Pulse generators may be temporary transcutaneous or placed in a subcutaneous pocket.

33215-33217

33215 Repositioning of previously implanted transvenous pacemaker or implantable defibrillator (right atrial or right ventricular) electrode
33216 Insertion of a single transvenous electrode, permanent pacemaker or implantable defibrillator
33217 Insertion of 2 transvenous electrodes, permanent pacemaker or implantable defibrillator

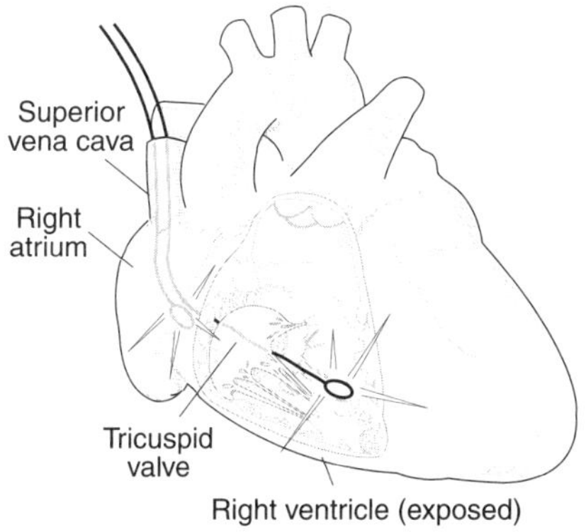

Schematic showing leads and electrodes to both right chambers

Explanation

In 33215, a previously placed transvenous right atrial or right ventricular electrode is repositioned. This is done when the system does not function due to improper placement of the electrode wire itself. The generator is removed and the wire is tested to ensure that the wire is not defective, but simply in the wrong place. It is reattached to the generator in its new position and tested again. In 33216, the physician inserts a single transvenous electrode and in 33217 two transvenous electrodes when there is a malfunction or complication with the electrode wire of a permanent pacemaker or implantable defibrillator. The generator is removed and the wire is tested. When the wire is found defective, another transvenous electrode is inserted. Access to the central caval veins is obtained through the subclavian vein or jugular vein. The vein is penetrated with a large needle and a wire is passed through it. Fluoroscopy is used to guide the wire into position. The wire is connected to the generator and the wound is closed. Various head and body positions are tested again to ensure adequate pacing.

Coding Tips

When medically necessary, report moderate (conscious) sedation provided by the performing physician with 99151-99153. When provided by another physician, report 99155-99157. These codes report insertion or repositioning of electrodes on permanent pacemakers or implantable defibrillators. Do not report 33216–33217 with 33206–33208, 33212–33214, 33221, 33227–33231, 33240, 33249, or 33262–33264. Revision of skin pocket is included and is not reported separately. Imaging guidance is included in these procedures and is not reported separately. For insertion and replacement of a cardiac venous system electrode, see 33224 and 33225. Do not report device evaluation codes (93260, 93261, 93279–93298) in addition to pulse generator and lead insertion/revision codes. Supplies used when providing these procedures may be reported with C1777. Check with the specific payer to determine coverage.

ICD-10-CM Diagnostic Codes

I11.0	Hypertensive heart disease with heart failure
I13.0	Hypertensive heart and chronic kidney disease with heart failure and stage 1 through stage 4 chronic kidney disease, or unspecified chronic kidney disease
I13.2	Hypertensive heart and chronic kidney disease with heart failure and with stage 5 chronic kidney disease, or end stage renal disease
I16.0	Hypertensive urgency
I16.1	Hypertensive emergency
I21.01	ST elevation (STEMI) myocardial infarction involving left main coronary artery
I21.02	ST elevation (STEMI) myocardial infarction involving left anterior descending coronary artery
I21.11	ST elevation (STEMI) myocardial infarction involving right coronary artery
I21.21	ST elevation (STEMI) myocardial infarction involving left circumflex coronary artery
I21.4	Non-ST elevation (NSTEMI) myocardial infarction
I21.A1	Myocardial infarction type 2
I21.B	Myocardial infarction with coronary microvascular dysfunction
I22.0	Subsequent ST elevation (STEMI) myocardial infarction of anterior wall
I22.1	Subsequent ST elevation (STEMI) myocardial infarction of inferior wall
I22.2	Subsequent non-ST elevation (NSTEMI) myocardial infarction
I25.2	Old myocardial infarction
I25.5	Ischemic cardiomyopathy
I25.6	Silent myocardial ischemia
I42.0	Dilated cardiomyopathy
I44.0	Atrioventricular block, first degree
I44.1	Atrioventricular block, second degree
I44.2	Atrioventricular block, complete
I44.4	Left anterior fascicular block
I44.5	Left posterior fascicular block
I45.0	Right fascicular block
I45.2	Bifascicular block
I45.4	Nonspecific intraventricular block
I45.6	Pre-excitation syndrome
I45.81	Long QT syndrome
I46.2	Cardiac arrest due to underlying cardiac condition
I46.8	Cardiac arrest due to other underlying condition
I47.0	Re-entry ventricular arrhythmia
I47.11	Inappropriate sinus tachycardia, so stated
I47.19	Other supraventricular tachycardia
I47.21	Torsades de pointes
I48.0	Paroxysmal atrial fibrillation
I48.11	Longstanding persistent atrial fibrillation
I48.21	Permanent atrial fibrillation
I48.3	Typical atrial flutter
I48.4	Atypical atrial flutter
I49.01	Ventricular fibrillation
I49.02	Ventricular flutter
I49.2	Junctional premature depolarization
I49.5	Sick sinus syndrome
I50.1	Left ventricular failure, unspecified
I50.21	Acute systolic (congestive) heart failure
I50.22	Chronic systolic (congestive) heart failure
I50.23	Acute on chronic systolic (congestive) heart failure

I50.31	Acute diastolic (congestive) heart failure
I50.32	Chronic diastolic (congestive) heart failure
I50.33	Acute on chronic diastolic (congestive) heart failure
I50.41	Acute combined systolic (congestive) and diastolic (congestive) heart failure
I50.42	Chronic combined systolic (congestive) and diastolic (congestive) heart failure
I50.43	Acute on chronic combined systolic (congestive) and diastolic (congestive) heart failure
I50.811	Acute right heart failure
I50.812	Chronic right heart failure
I50.813	Acute on chronic right heart failure
I50.814	Right heart failure due to left heart failure
I50.82	Biventricular heart failure
I50.83	High output heart failure
I50.84	End stage heart failure
Q24.6	Congenital heart block
T82.110A	Breakdown (mechanical) of cardiac electrode, initial encounter
T82.120A	Displacement of cardiac electrode, initial encounter
T82.817A	Embolism due to cardiac prosthetic devices, implants and grafts, initial encounter
T82.827A	Fibrosis due to cardiac prosthetic devices, implants and grafts, initial encounter
T82.837A	Hemorrhage due to cardiac prosthetic devices, implants and grafts, initial encounter
T82.847A	Pain due to cardiac prosthetic devices, implants and grafts, initial encounter
T82.867A	Thrombosis due to cardiac prosthetic devices, implants and grafts, initial encounter
Z95.0	Presence of cardiac pacemaker
Z95.810	Presence of automatic (implantable) cardiac defibrillator

AMA: 33215 2019,Oct; 2019,Mar; 2019,Jan **33216** 2019,Oct; 2019,Mar; 2019,Jan **33217** 2019,Oct; 2019,Mar; 2019,Jan

Relative Value Units/Medicare Edits

Non-Facility RVU	Work	PE	MP	Total
33215	4.92	3.12	1.13	9.17
33216	5.62	4.09	1.27	10.98
33217	5.59	4.04	1.27	10.9
Facility RVU	**Work**	**PE**	**MP**	**Total**
33215	4.92	3.12	1.13	9.17
33216	5.62	4.09	1.27	10.98
33217	5.59	4.04	1.27	10.9

	FUD	Status	MUE	Modifiers				IOM Reference
33215	90	A	2(3)	51	N/A	N/A	N/A	None
33216	90	A	1(3)	51	N/A	N/A	N/A	
33217	90	A	1(3)	51	N/A	N/A	N/A	

* with documentation

33218-33220

33218 Repair of single transvenous electrode, permanent pacemaker or implantable defibrillator

33220 Repair of 2 transvenous electrodes for permanent pacemaker or implantable defibrillator

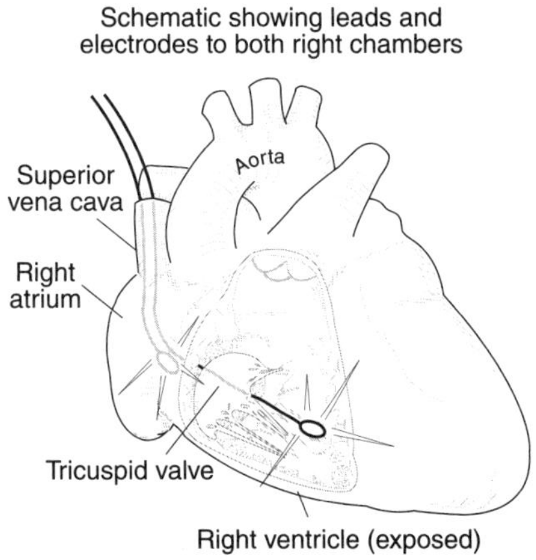

Explanation

A previously placed transvenous electrode is repaired. The permanent pacemaker or implantable defibrillator pocket is opened and the generator is removed. The electrode wire is tested. Repairs are performed on the electrode. The wire is tested again and reconnected to the generator. The generator is placed back in its pocket and the pocket is closed. Report 33218 if a single electrode is repaired and 33220 if two electrodes are repaired.

Coding Tips

When medically necessary, report moderate (conscious) sedation provided by the performing physician with 99151-99153. When provided by another physician, report 99155-99157. These codes report repair of electrodes on permanent pacemakers or implantable defibrillators. For repair of a single permanent pacemaker or implantable defibrillator electrode in addition to the replacement of the pulse generator, report 33218 with 33227–33229 or 33262–33264. For repair of two transvenous electrodes for permanent pacemaker or implantable defibrillator in addition to replacement of the pulse generator, report 33220 with 33228, 33229, 33263, or 33264.

ICD-10-CM Diagnostic Codes

T82.110A	Breakdown (mechanical) of cardiac electrode, initial encounter
T82.120A	Displacement of cardiac electrode, initial encounter
T82.190A	Other mechanical complication of cardiac electrode, initial encounter
T82.7XXA	Infection and inflammatory reaction due to other cardiac and vascular devices, implants and grafts, initial encounter
T82.817A	Embolism due to cardiac prosthetic devices, implants and grafts, initial encounter
T82.827A	Fibrosis due to cardiac prosthetic devices, implants and grafts, initial encounter
T82.837A	Hemorrhage due to cardiac prosthetic devices, implants and grafts, initial encounter
T82.847A	Pain due to cardiac prosthetic devices, implants and grafts, initial encounter
T82.857A	Stenosis of other cardiac prosthetic devices, implants and grafts, initial encounter

T82.867A Thrombosis due to cardiac prosthetic devices, implants and grafts, initial encounter

T82.897A Other specified complication of cardiac prosthetic devices, implants and grafts, initial encounter

Z45.09 Encounter for adjustment and management of other cardiac device

Z95.0 Presence of cardiac pacemaker

Z95.810 Presence of automatic (implantable) cardiac defibrillator

AMA: 33218 2019,Oct; 2019,Mar; 2019,Jan **33220** 2019,Oct; 2019,Mar; 2019,Jan

Relative Value Units/Medicare Edits

Non-Facility RVU	Work	PE	MP	Total
33218	5.82	4.38	1.32	11.52
33220	5.9	4.0	1.36	11.26
Facility RVU	**Work**	**PE**	**MP**	**Total**
33218	5.82	4.38	1.32	11.52
33220	5.9	4.0	1.36	11.26

	FUD	Status	MUE	Modifiers				IOM Reference
33218	90	A	1(3)	51	N/A	N/A	N/A	None
33220	90	A	1(3)	51	N/A	N/A	N/A	

* with documentation

Terms To Know

cardioverter-defibrillator. Device that uses both low energy cardioversion or defibrillating shocks and antitachycardia pacing to treat ventricular tachycardia or ventricular fibrillation.

complication. Condition arising after the beginning of observation and treatment that modifies the course of the patient's illness or the medical care required, or an undesired result or misadventure in medical care.

heartbeat. Contraction of the heart muscles in a rhythmic pattern, circulating about 70 ml of blood and taking less than a second to complete.

in situ. Located in the natural position or contained within the origin site, not spread into neighboring tissue.

pacemaker. Implantable cardiac device that controls the heart's rhythm and maintains regular beats by artificial electric discharges. This device consists of the pulse generator with a battery and the electrodes, or leads, which are placed in single or dual chambers of the heart, usually transvenously.

transvenous electrode. Electrode placed using a transvenous catheter and wedged into the endocardium of the right ventricle or atrium.

33222-33223

33222 Relocation of skin pocket for pacemaker

33223 Relocation of skin pocket for implantable defibrillator

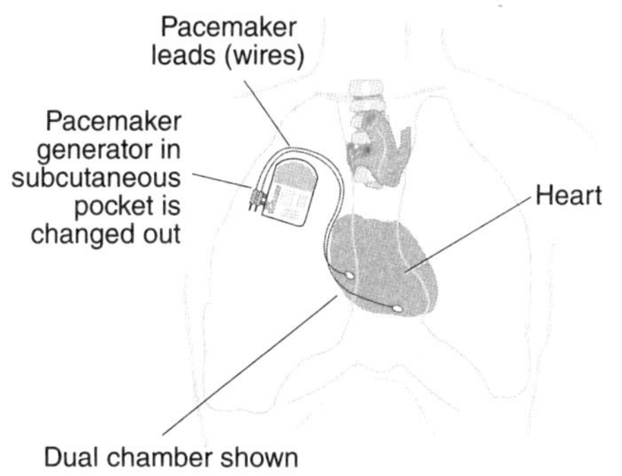

Explanation

The physician relocates a pacemaker or defibrillator pocket due to infection, erosion, or complications from the original generator placement. The pocket is opened and the generator is removed. A new pocket is formed in the subcutaneous tissue within the reach of the already present electrodes. The electrodes are brought through a new subcutaneous tunnel into the new pocket. The old pocket is closed. The existing or new generator is placed in the new pocket and the electrodes are connected. The pocket is closed. Report 33222 when a permanent pacemaker pocket is relocated and 33223 when an implantable defibrillator pocket is relocated.

Coding Tips

When medically necessary, report moderate (conscious) sedation provided by the performing physician with 99151-99153. When provided by another physician, report 99155-99157. Do not report 33222 or 33223 with 10140, 10180, 11042–11047, or 13100–13102.

ICD-10-CM Diagnostic Codes

M79.81 Nontraumatic hematoma of soft tissue

T81.41XA Infection following a procedure, superficial incisional surgical site, initial encounter

T81.42XA Infection following a procedure, deep incisional surgical site, initial encounter

T81.43XA Infection following a procedure, organ and space surgical site, initial encounter

T81.49XA Infection following a procedure, other surgical site, initial encounter

T81.83XA Persistent postprocedural fistula, initial encounter

T81.89XA Other complications of procedures, not elsewhere classified, initial encounter

T82.7XXA Infection and inflammatory reaction due to other cardiac and vascular devices, implants and grafts, initial encounter

T82.817A Embolism due to cardiac prosthetic devices, implants and grafts, initial encounter

T82.827A Fibrosis due to cardiac prosthetic devices, implants and grafts, initial encounter

T82.837A Hemorrhage due to cardiac prosthetic devices, implants and grafts, initial encounter

T82.847A Pain due to cardiac prosthetic devices, implants and grafts, initial encounter

T82.855A Stenosis of coronary artery stent, initial encounter

Heart and Pericardium

T82.857A	Stenosis of other cardiac prosthetic devices, implants and grafts, initial encounter
T82.867A	Thrombosis due to cardiac prosthetic devices, implants and grafts, initial encounter
T82.897A	Other specified complication of cardiac prosthetic devices, implants and grafts, initial encounter
Z45.018	Encounter for adjustment and management of other part of cardiac pacemaker
Z45.02	Encounter for adjustment and management of automatic implantable cardiac defibrillator

AMA: 33222 2019,Oct; 2019,Jan **33223** 2019,Oct; 2019,Jan

Relative Value Units/Medicare Edits

Non-Facility RVU	Work	PE	MP	Total
33222	4.85	4.21	1.12	10.18
33223	6.3	4.34	1.45	12.09
Facility RVU	**Work**	**PE**	**MP**	**Total**
33222	4.85	4.21	1.12	10.18
33223	6.3	4.34	1.45	12.09

	FUD	Status	MUE	Modifiers				IOM Reference
33222	90	A	1(3)	51	N/A	N/A	N/A	None
33223	90	A	1(3)	51	N/A	N/A	80*	

* with documentation

Terms To Know

cardioverter-defibrillator. Device that uses both low energy cardioversion or defibrillating shocks and antitachycardia pacing to treat ventricular tachycardia or ventricular fibrillation.

hematoma. Tumor-like collection of blood in some part of the body caused by a break in a blood vessel wall, usually as a result of trauma.

pacemaker. Implantable cardiac device that controls the heart's rhythm and maintains regular beats by artificial electric discharges. This device consists of the pulse generator with a battery and the electrodes, or leads, which are placed in single or dual chambers of the heart, usually transvenously.

seroma. Swelling caused by the collection of serum, or clear fluid, in the tissues.

33224

33224 Insertion of pacing electrode, cardiac venous system, for left ventricular pacing, with attachment to previously placed pacemaker or implantable defibrillator pulse generator (including revision of pocket, removal, insertion, and/or replacement of existing generator)

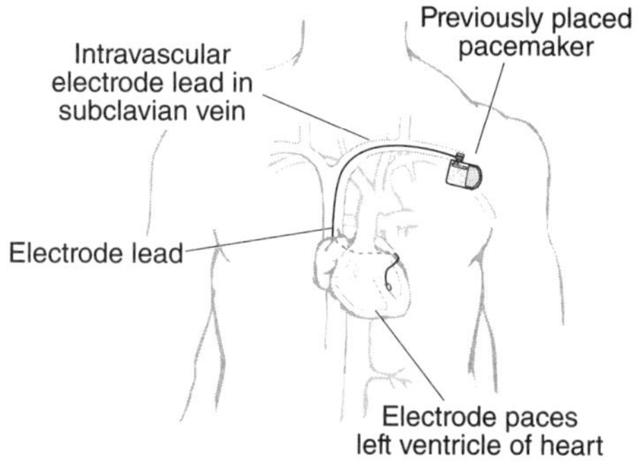

A pacing electrode is placed in the venous system and attached to a previously placed pacemaker or defibrillator generator

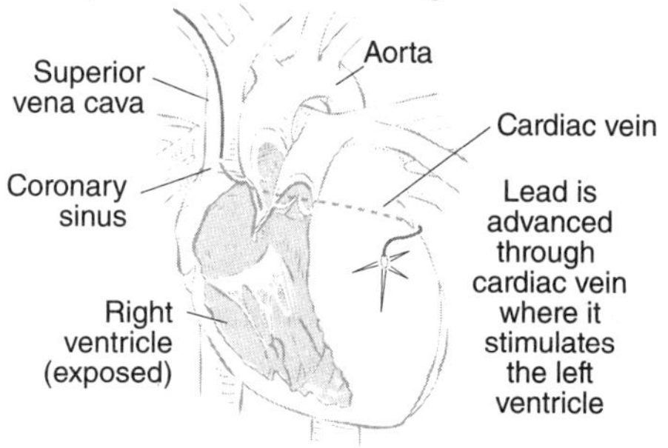

Explanation

If biventricular pacing is required, an additional electrode is placed in the left ventricle. With the pacemaker or implantable defibrillator already in place, the physician gains access transvenously through the subclavian or jugular vein. This procedure is done under local anesthesia. A fluoroscope may be used for guidance and a pacing electrode is inserted in the left ventricular chamber of the heart, usually in the coronary sinus tributary. The electrode is connected to the pulse generator and the pocket is closed. The generator pocket may be revised and/or the existing generator removed, inserted, or replaced. In rare cases, when transvenous approach cannot be used, the device is implanted in the pocket underneath the skin in the lower abdomen (epicardial approach). Implantation using this approach is done under general anesthesia.

Coding Tips

This code reports the insertion of an electrode on a previously placed permanent pacemaker or implantable defibrillator for left ventricular pacing. Fluoroscopy is included in 33224 and is not reported separately. For epicardial electrode placement at the time of insertion of a pacing electrode in the cardiac venous system, report 33202 or 33203 with 33224. For repositioning of an electrode for left ventricular pacing, see 33226. For insertion of a single chamber electrode, see 33216. For insertion of a dual chamber electrode, see 33217. To report body surface-activation mapping to optimize electrical synchrony, 0695T may be reported with 33224. Do not report device evaluation codes (93260, 93261, 93279–93298) in addition to pulse generator and lead insertion/revision codes. Supplies used when providing this procedure may be reported with HCPCS Level II code C1900. Check with the specific payer to determine coverage.

ICD-10-CM Diagnostic Codes

I11.0	Hypertensive heart disease with heart failure
I13.2	Hypertensive heart and chronic kidney disease with heart failure and with stage 5 chronic kidney disease, or end stage renal disease
I16.0	Hypertensive urgency
I16.1	Hypertensive emergency
I21.01	ST elevation (STEMI) myocardial infarction involving left main coronary artery
I21.02	ST elevation (STEMI) myocardial infarction involving left anterior descending coronary artery
I21.11	ST elevation (STEMI) myocardial infarction involving right coronary artery
I21.21	ST elevation (STEMI) myocardial infarction involving left circumflex coronary artery
I21.4	Non-ST elevation (NSTEMI) myocardial infarction
I21.A1	Myocardial infarction type 2
I21.B	Myocardial infarction with coronary microvascular dysfunction
I22.0	Subsequent ST elevation (STEMI) myocardial infarction of anterior wall
I22.1	Subsequent ST elevation (STEMI) myocardial infarction of inferior wall
I22.2	Subsequent non-ST elevation (NSTEMI) myocardial infarction
I25.2	Old myocardial infarction
I25.5	Ischemic cardiomyopathy
I25.6	Silent myocardial ischemia
I42.0	Dilated cardiomyopathy
I42.1	Obstructive hypertrophic cardiomyopathy
I42.2	Other hypertrophic cardiomyopathy
I42.3	Endomyocardial (eosinophilic) disease
I42.4	Endocardial fibroelastosis
I42.5	Other restrictive cardiomyopathy
I42.6	Alcoholic cardiomyopathy
I42.7	Cardiomyopathy due to drug and external agent
I43	Cardiomyopathy in diseases classified elsewhere
I44.0	Atrioventricular block, first degree
I44.1	Atrioventricular block, second degree
I44.2	Atrioventricular block, complete
I44.39	Other atrioventricular block
I44.4	Left anterior fascicular block
I44.5	Left posterior fascicular block
I45.0	Right fascicular block
I45.2	Bifascicular block
I45.3	Trifascicular block
I45.4	Nonspecific intraventricular block
I45.6	Pre-excitation syndrome
I45.81	Long QT syndrome
I46.2	Cardiac arrest due to underlying cardiac condition
I46.8	Cardiac arrest due to other underlying condition
I47.0	Re-entry ventricular arrhythmia
I47.11	Inappropriate sinus tachycardia, so stated
I47.19	Other supraventricular tachycardia
I47.21	Torsades de pointes
I47.29	Other ventricular tachycardia
I48.0	Paroxysmal atrial fibrillation
I48.11	Longstanding persistent atrial fibrillation
I48.19	Other persistent atrial fibrillation
I48.21	Permanent atrial fibrillation
I49.01	Ventricular fibrillation
I49.02	Ventricular flutter
I49.2	Junctional premature depolarization
I49.5	Sick sinus syndrome
I50.1	Left ventricular failure, unspecified
I50.21	Acute systolic (congestive) heart failure
I50.22	Chronic systolic (congestive) heart failure
I50.23	Acute on chronic systolic (congestive) heart failure
I50.31	Acute diastolic (congestive) heart failure
I50.32	Chronic diastolic (congestive) heart failure
I50.33	Acute on chronic diastolic (congestive) heart failure
I50.41	Acute combined systolic (congestive) and diastolic (congestive) heart failure
I50.42	Chronic combined systolic (congestive) and diastolic (congestive) heart failure
I50.43	Acute on chronic combined systolic (congestive) and diastolic (congestive) heart failure
I50.811	Acute right heart failure
I50.812	Chronic right heart failure
I50.813	Acute on chronic right heart failure
I50.814	Right heart failure due to left heart failure
I50.82	Biventricular heart failure
I50.83	High output heart failure
I50.84	End stage heart failure
I51.7	Cardiomegaly
Q24.6	Congenital heart block
Z95.0	Presence of cardiac pacemaker
Z95.810	Presence of automatic (implantable) cardiac defibrillator

AMA: **33224** 2019,Oct; 2019,Jan

Relative Value Units/Medicare Edits

Non-Facility RVU	Work	PE	MP	Total
33224	9.04	3.9	2.05	14.99
Facility RVU	**Work**	**PE**	**MP**	**Total**
33224	9.04	3.9	2.05	14.99

	FUD	Status	MUE	Modifiers				IOM Reference
33224	0	A	1(3)	51	N/A	N/A	N/A	None

* with documentation

Heart and Pericardium

33225

\+ **33225** Insertion of pacing electrode, cardiac venous system, for left ventricular pacing, at time of insertion of implantable defibrillator or pacemaker pulse generator (eg, for upgrade to dual chamber system) (List separately in addition to code for primary procedure)

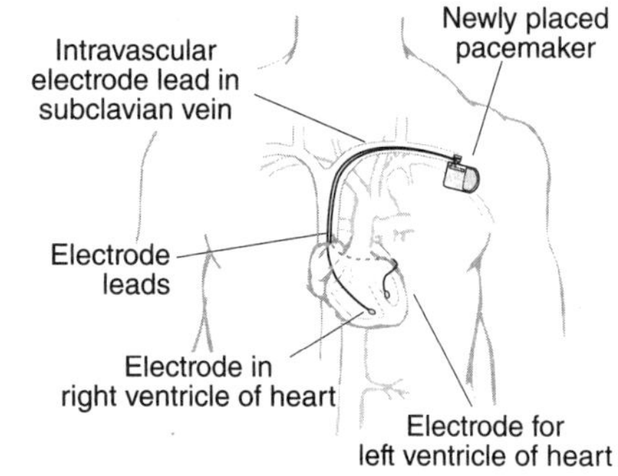

A pacing electrode is placed in the venous system at the time a pacemaker or defibrillator generator is inserted

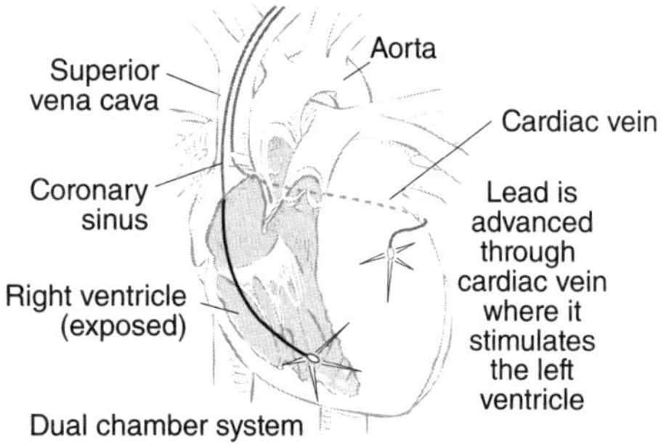

Explanation

If biventricular pacing is required, an additional electrode is placed in the left ventricle. During insertion of an implantable defibrillator or pacemaker pulse generator, the physician gains access transvenously through the subclavian or jugular vein. This procedure is done under local anesthesia. A fluoroscope may be used for guidance and a pacing electrode is inserted in the left ventricular chamber of the heart, usually in the coronary sinus tributary. The generator is upgraded to a dual chamber system. The electrode is connected to the pulse generator and the pocket is closed. In rare cases, when transvenous approach cannot be used, the device is implanted in the pocket underneath the skin in the lower abdomen (epicardial approach). Implantation using this approach is done under general anesthesia.

Coding Tips

Fluoroscopy is included in 33225 and is not reported separately. This code reports the insertion of an electrode at the time of insertion of an implantable defibrillator or pacemaker pulse generator for left ventricular pacing and includes an upgrade to a dual chamber system and pocket revision. Report 33225 in addition to 33206, 33207, 33208, 33212, 33213, 33214, 33216, 33217, 33221, 33223, 33228, 33229, 33230, 33231, 33233, 33234, 33235, 33240, 33249, 33263, and 33264. Use 33225 in addition to 33222 when a pacemaker generator pocket is relocated and 33223 when an implantable defibrillator pocket is relocated. For insertion of an electrode for a previously placed implantable defibrillator or pacemaker pulse generator, see 33224. For repositioning of an electrode for left ventricular pacing, see 33226. To report body surface-activation mapping to optimize electrical synchrony, 0695T may be reported with 33225. Do not report device evaluation codes (93260, 93261, 93279–93298) in addition to pulse generator and lead insertion/revision codes.

ICD-10-CM Diagnostic Codes

This/these CPT code(s) are add-on code(s). See the primary procedure code that this code is performed with for your ICD-10-CM code selections. Diagnostic code(s) would be the same as the actual procedure performed.

AMA: 33225 2019,Oct; 2019,Jan

Relative Value Units/Medicare Edits

Non-Facility RVU	Work	PE	MP	Total
33225	8.33	3.29	1.89	13.51
Facility RVU	**Work**	**PE**	**MP**	**Total**
33225	8.33	3.29	1.89	13.51

	FUD	Status	MUE	Modifiers				IOM Reference
33225	N/A	A	1(3)	N/A	N/A	N/A	N/A	None

* with documentation

Terms To Know

arrhythmia. Irregular heartbeat.

cardioverter-defibrillator. Device that uses both low energy cardioversion or defibrillating shocks and antitachycardia pacing to treat ventricular tachycardia or ventricular fibrillation.

electrode. Electric terminal specialized for a particular electrochemical reaction that acts as a medium between a body surface and another instrument, commonly termed a lead.

fluoroscopy. Radiology technique that allows visual examination of part of the body or a function of an organ using a device that projects an x-ray image on a fluorescent screen.

pacemaker. Implantable cardiac device that controls the heart's rhythm and maintains regular beats by artificial electric discharges. This device consists of the pulse generator with a battery and the electrodes, or leads, which are placed in single or dual chambers of the heart, usually transvenously.

transvenous electrode. Electrode placed using a transvenous catheter and wedged into the endocardium of the right ventricle or atrium.

33226

33226 Repositioning of previously implanted cardiac venous system (left ventricular) electrode (including removal, insertion and/or replacement of existing generator)

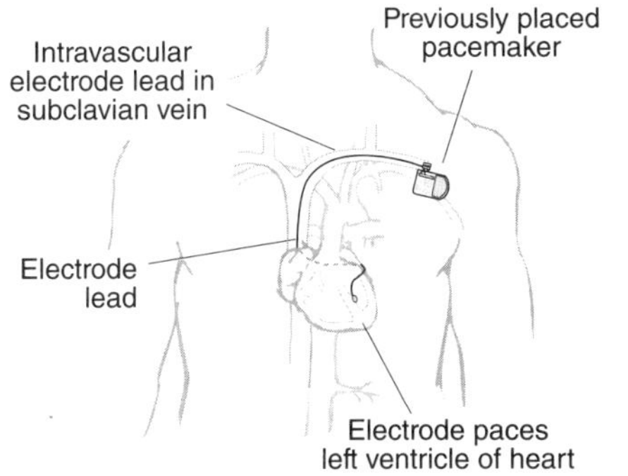

A pacing electrode in the venous system is repositioned

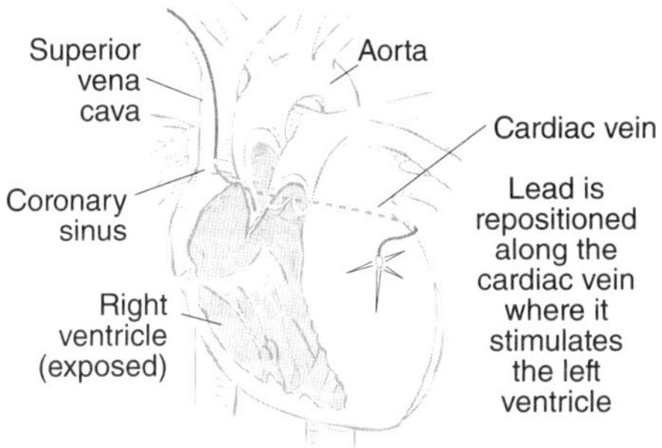

Explanation

The physician gains access transvenously through the subclavian or jugular vein. A fluoroscope may be used for guidance and the pacing electrode that is already in place in the ventricular chamber of the heart, usually in the coronary sinus tributary, is repositioned. The generator pocket may be revised and/or the existing generator removed, inserted, or replaced. The electrode is connected to the generator and the pocket is closed.

Coding Tips

This code reports the repositioning of an electrode in a previously placed pacing cardioverter-defibrillator or pacemaker pulse generator for left ventricular pacing. Fluoroscopy is included in 33226 and is not reported separately. For insertion of an electrode for a previously placed pacing cardioverter-defibrillator or pacemaker pulse generator, see 33224. For insertion of an electrode at the time of insertion of a pacing cardioverter-defibrillator or pacemaker pulse generator for left ventricular pacing, see 33225. To report body surface-activation mapping to optimize electrical synchrony, 0695T may be reported with 33226. For insertion of a single chamber electrode, see 33216. For insertion of a dual chamber electrode, see 33217.

ICD-10-CM Diagnostic Codes

T82.110A Breakdown (mechanical) of cardiac electrode, initial encounter

T82.120A Displacement of cardiac electrode, initial encounter

T82.190A Other mechanical complication of cardiac electrode, initial encounter

T82.7XXA Infection and inflammatory reaction due to other cardiac and vascular devices, implants and grafts, initial encounter

T82.817A Embolism due to cardiac prosthetic devices, implants and grafts, initial encounter

T82.827A Fibrosis due to cardiac prosthetic devices, implants and grafts, initial encounter

T82.837A Hemorrhage due to cardiac prosthetic devices, implants and grafts, initial encounter

T82.847A Pain due to cardiac prosthetic devices, implants and grafts, initial encounter

T82.857A Stenosis of other cardiac prosthetic devices, implants and grafts, initial encounter

T82.867A Thrombosis due to cardiac prosthetic devices, implants and grafts, initial encounter

T82.897A Other specified complication of cardiac prosthetic devices, implants and grafts, initial encounter

Z45.09 Encounter for adjustment and management of other cardiac device

Z95.0 Presence of cardiac pacemaker

Z95.810 Presence of automatic (implantable) cardiac defibrillator

AMA: **33226** 2019,Oct; 2019,Jan

Relative Value Units/Medicare Edits

Non-Facility RVU	Work	PE	MP	Total
33226	8.68	3.67	2.0	14.35
Facility RVU	**Work**	**PE**	**MP**	**Total**
33226	8.68	3.67	2.0	14.35

	FUD	Status	MUE	Modifiers				IOM Reference
33226	0	A	1(3)	51	N/A	N/A	N/A	None

* with documentation

Terms To Know

electrode. Electric terminal specialized for a particular electrochemical reaction that acts as a medium between a body surface and another instrument, commonly termed a lead.

fluoroscopy. Radiology technique that allows visual examination of part of the body or a function of an organ using a device that projects an x-ray image on a fluorescent screen.

pacemaker. Implantable cardiac device that controls the heart's rhythm and maintains regular beats by artificial electric discharges. This device consists of the pulse generator with a battery and the electrodes, or leads, which are placed in single or dual chambers of the heart, usually transvenously.

33233

33233 Removal of permanent pacemaker pulse generator only

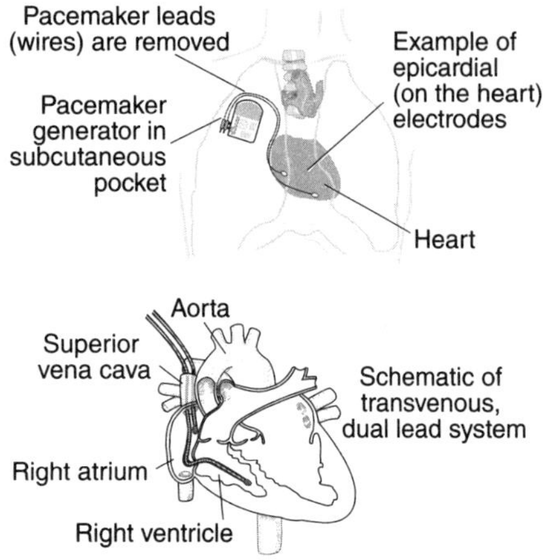

An implanted permanent pacemaker generator is removed

Explanation

In 33233, only the permanent pacemaker pulse generator is removed. The pacemaker generator pocket is opened. The generator is disconnected from the wire(s) and removed. The wire(s) is left in place in the pocket and the pocket is closed.

Coding Tips

When medically necessary, report moderate (conscious) sedation provided by the performing physician with 99151-99153. When provided by another physician, report 99155-99157. An inactive pacemaker does not always require removal. Procedure 33233 reports removal of the pacemaker generator only. For removal with replacement of the pulse generator during the same surgical session, see 33227–33229. For removal of transvenous pacemaker electrodes, see 33234–33235. For removal of a permanent epicardial pacemaker system and/or electrodes by thoracotomy, see 33236–33237. For removal of transvenous electrodes by thoracotomy, see 33238.

ICD-10-CM Diagnostic Codes

T82.111A Breakdown (mechanical) of cardiac pulse generator (battery), initial encounter

T82.121A Displacement of cardiac pulse generator (battery), initial encounter

T82.191A Other mechanical complication of cardiac pulse generator (battery), initial encounter

T82.7XXA Infection and inflammatory reaction due to other cardiac and vascular devices, implants and grafts, initial encounter

T82.817A Embolism due to cardiac prosthetic devices, implants and grafts, initial encounter

T82.827A Fibrosis due to cardiac prosthetic devices, implants and grafts, initial encounter

T82.837A Hemorrhage due to cardiac prosthetic devices, implants and grafts, initial encounter

T82.847A Pain due to cardiac prosthetic devices, implants and grafts, initial encounter

T82.857A Stenosis of other cardiac prosthetic devices, implants and grafts, initial encounter

T82.867A Thrombosis due to cardiac prosthetic devices, implants and grafts, initial encounter

Z45.018 Encounter for adjustment and management of other part of cardiac pacemaker

AMA: 33233 2019,Oct; 2019,Mar

Relative Value Units/Medicare Edits

Non-Facility RVU	Work	PE	MP	Total
33233	3.14	3.06	0.72	6.92
Facility RVU	**Work**	**PE**	**MP**	**Total**
33233	3.14	3.06	0.72	6.92

	FUD	Status	MUE	Modifiers				IOM Reference
33233	90	A	1(2)	51	N/A	N/A	N/A	None

* with documentation

Terms To Know

complication. Condition arising after the beginning of observation and treatment that modifies the course of the patient's illness or the medical care required, or an undesired result or misadventure in medical care.

epicardial electrode. Stimulation device that is attached to or inserted into the heart muscle and connected to a generator.

infection. Presence of microorganisms in body tissues that may result in cellular damage.

pacemaker. Implantable cardiac device that controls the heart's rhythm and maintains regular beats by artificial electric discharges. This device consists of the pulse generator with a battery and the electrodes, or leads, which are placed in single or dual chambers of the heart, usually transvenously.

revision. Reordering or rearrangement of tissue to suit a particular need or function.

thoracotomy. Surgical procedure for opening the chest wall in order to access the lungs, esophagus, trachea, aorta, heart, and diaphragm.

transvenous electrode. Electrode placed using a transvenous catheter and wedged into the endocardium of the right ventricle or atrium.

[33227, 33228, 33229]

33227 Removal of permanent pacemaker pulse generator with replacement of pacemaker pulse generator; single lead system

33228 Removal of permanent pacemaker pulse generator with replacement of pacemaker pulse generator; dual lead system

33229 Removal of permanent pacemaker pulse generator with replacement of pacemaker pulse generator; multiple lead system

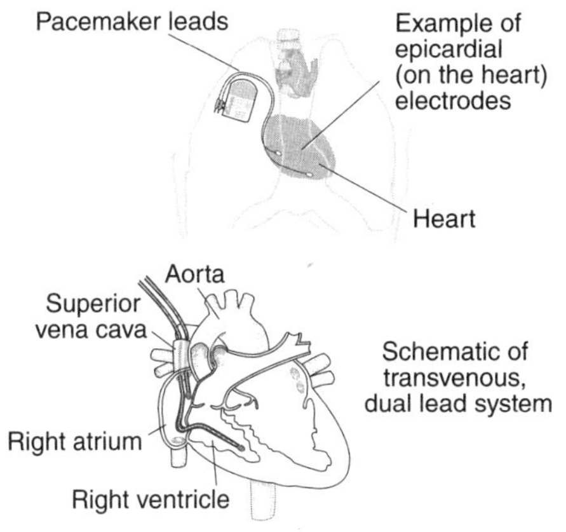

Explanation

A permanent pacemaker pulse generator is removed and replaced. The pacemaker generator pocket is opened. The existing generator is disconnected from the wire(s) and removed. The wire(s) is left in place in the pocket and a new permanent pacemaker pulse generator is inserted. The existing pacer wire(s) is tested and connected to the generator. The pocket is closed. Report 33227 for removal and replacement of a single lead system generator, 33228 for a dual lead system generator, and 33229 for a multiple lead system generator.

Coding Tips

When medically necessary, report moderate (conscious) sedation provided by the performing physician with 99151-99153. When provided by another physician, report 99155-99157. These codes are used when removal and replacement of the permanent pulse generator are performed during the same operative session. For removal and replacement of the pacemaker pulse generator, as well as the transvenous electrodes, see 33233 with 33234 or 33235 and 33206–33208. Do not report 33227–33229 with 33214, 33216, 33217, or 33233.

ICD-10-CM Diagnostic Codes

T82.111A	Breakdown (mechanical) of cardiac pulse generator (battery), initial encounter
T82.121A	Displacement of cardiac pulse generator (battery), initial encounter
T82.191A	Other mechanical complication of cardiac pulse generator (battery), initial encounter
T82.7XXA	Infection and inflammatory reaction due to other cardiac and vascular devices, implants and grafts, initial encounter
T82.817A	Embolism due to cardiac prosthetic devices, implants and grafts, initial encounter
T82.827A	Fibrosis due to cardiac prosthetic devices, implants and grafts, initial encounter
T82.837A	Hemorrhage due to cardiac prosthetic devices, implants and grafts, initial encounter
T82.847A	Pain due to cardiac prosthetic devices, implants and grafts, initial encounter
T82.857A	Stenosis of other cardiac prosthetic devices, implants and grafts, initial encounter
T82.867A	Thrombosis due to cardiac prosthetic devices, implants and grafts, initial encounter
T82.897A	Other specified complication of cardiac prosthetic devices, implants and grafts, initial encounter
Z45.018	Encounter for adjustment and management of other part of cardiac pacemaker
Z95.0	Presence of cardiac pacemaker

AMA: **33227** 2019,Oct; 2019,Mar **33228** 2019,Oct; 2019,Mar **33229** 2019,Oct; 2019,Mar

Relative Value Units/Medicare Edits

Non-Facility RVU	Work	PE	MP	Total
33227	5.25	3.57	1.21	10.03
33228	5.52	3.69	1.26	10.47
33229	5.79	3.9	1.32	11.01
Facility RVU	**Work**	**PE**	**MP**	**Total**
33227	5.25	3.57	1.21	10.03
33228	5.52	3.69	1.26	10.47
33229	5.79	3.9	1.32	11.01

	FUD	Status	MUE	Modifiers				IOM Reference
33227	90	A	1(3)	51	N/A	N/A	N/A	None
33228	90	A	1(3)	51	N/A	N/A	N/A	
33229	90	A	1(3)	51	N/A	N/A	N/A	

* with documentation

Terms To Know

dual chamber system. System that includes a pulse generator and one electrode inserted into the right atrium and one into the right ventricle.

multiple-lead device. Implantable cardiac device (pacemaker or implantable cardioverter-defibrillator [ICD]) in which pacing and sensing components are placed in three or more chambers of the heart.

pacemaker. Implantable cardiac device that controls the heart's rhythm and maintains regular beats by artificial electric discharges. This device consists of the pulse generator with a battery and the electrodes, or leads, which are placed in single or dual chambers of the heart, usually transvenously.

pulse generator. Circuit used to generate pulses. Pulse generators contain the battery, the electronic circuit, and the connector in a hermetically sealed encasement. Pulse generators may be temporary transcutaneous or placed in a subcutaneous pocket.

33234-33235

33234 Removal of transvenous pacemaker electrode(s); single lead system, atrial or ventricular

33235 dual lead system

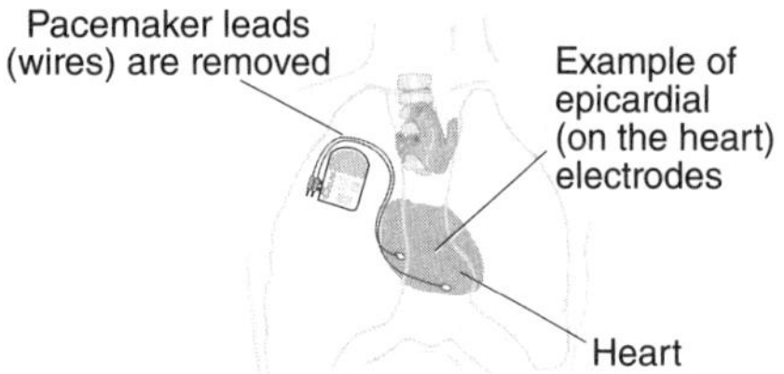

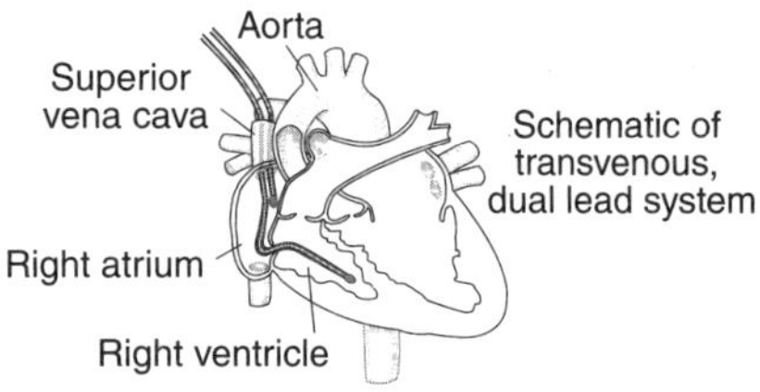

Explanation

In 33234 and 33235, only the transvenous electrode(s) are removed. In 33234, the generator pocket is opened and the wire is disconnected from the generator. The wire is dissected from the scar tissue that has formed around it. Once the wire is completely freed, it is twisted in a direction opposite to that used for insertion (counter clockwise). The wire is withdrawn. Bleeding from the tracts leading to the vein is controlled with sutures. A new wire may be placed, but is reported separately. Report 33235 for a dual lead system (removal of two wires).

Coding Tips

When medically necessary, report moderate (conscious) sedation provided by the performing physician with 99151-99153. When provided by another physician, report 99155-99157. Procedures 33234 and 33235 report removal of pacemaker leads without concurrent replacement. For removal with replacement of generator and leads during the same surgical session, see 33206–33208. For transvenous leads inserted when a pulse generator is in place, see 33216 and 33217. For removal of a permanent pacemaker pulse generator without replacement, see 33233. For removal of a pacemaker system and/or electrodes by thoracotomy, see 33236–33238. Unsuccessful transvenous extraction of electrodes converted to an open procedure should be reported using thoracotomy code 33238 for pacemaker electrodes or 33243 for cardioverter-defibrillator electrodes.

ICD-10-CM Diagnostic Codes

T82.110A	Breakdown (mechanical) of cardiac electrode, initial encounter
T82.120A	Displacement of cardiac electrode, initial encounter
T82.190A	Other mechanical complication of cardiac electrode, initial encounter
T82.7XXA	Infection and inflammatory reaction due to other cardiac and vascular devices, implants and grafts, initial encounter
T82.817A	Embolism due to cardiac prosthetic devices, implants and grafts, initial encounter
T82.827A	Fibrosis due to cardiac prosthetic devices, implants and grafts, initial encounter
T82.837A	Hemorrhage due to cardiac prosthetic devices, implants and grafts, initial encounter
T82.847A	Pain due to cardiac prosthetic devices, implants and grafts, initial encounter
T82.857A	Stenosis of other cardiac prosthetic devices, implants and grafts, initial encounter
T82.867A	Thrombosis due to cardiac prosthetic devices, implants and grafts, initial encounter
Z45.018	Encounter for adjustment and management of other part of cardiac pacemaker

AMA: 33234 2019,Oct; 2019,Mar **33235** 2019,Oct; 2019,Mar

Relative Value Units/Medicare Edits

Non-Facility RVU	Work	PE	MP	Total
33234	7.66	4.89	1.73	14.28
33235	9.9	6.61	2.26	18.77
Facility RVU	**Work**	**PE**	**MP**	**Total**
33234	7.66	4.89	1.73	14.28
33235	9.9	6.61	2.26	18.77

	FUD	Status	MUE	Modifiers				IOM Reference
33234	90	A	1(2)	51	N/A	N/A	N/A	None
33235	90	A	1(2)	51	N/A	N/A	N/A	

* with documentation

Terms To Know

complication. Condition arising after the beginning of observation and treatment that modifies the course of the patient's illness or the medical care required, or an undesired result or misadventure in medical care.

epicardial electrode. Stimulation device that is attached to or inserted into the heart muscle and connected to a generator.

infection. Presence of microorganisms in body tissues that may result in cellular damage.

pacemaker. Implantable cardiac device that controls the heart's rhythm and maintains regular beats by artificial electric discharges. This device consists of the pulse generator with a battery and the electrodes, or leads, which are placed in single or dual chambers of the heart, usually transvenously.

revision. Reordering or rearrangement of tissue to suit a particular need or function.

suture. Numerous stitching techniques employed in wound closure.

thoracotomy. Surgical procedure for opening the chest wall in order to access the lungs, esophagus, trachea, aorta, heart, and diaphragm.

transvenous electrode. Electrode placed using a transvenous catheter and wedged into the endocardium of the right ventricle or atrium.

33236-33237

33236 Removal of permanent epicardial pacemaker and electrodes by thoracotomy; single lead system, atrial or ventricular
33237 dual lead system

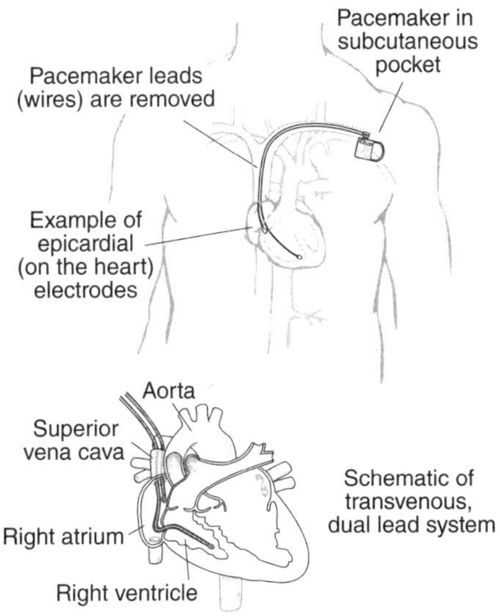

Pacemaker and electrodes are removed

Explanation

Code 33236 reports the removal of a single lead epicardial pacemaker system and electrodes. The old pacemaker pocket is opened and the generator is removed. The old wires are cut and the incision is closed. The old chest incision is opened. The wires are pulled into the chest and they are followed onto the heart surface. The electrodes are detached from the heart. The chest incision is closed. Report 33237 if a dual lead epicardial system is being removed.

Coding Tips

Procedures 33236 and 33237 report removal of the pacemaker system only. For removal of transvenous electrodes not requiring thoracotomy, see 33234–33235. For removal of transvenous electrodes by thoracotomy, see 33238. For insertion of epicardial electrodes, see 33202 and 33203.

ICD-10-CM Diagnostic Codes

T82.110A	Breakdown (mechanical) of cardiac electrode, initial encounter
T82.111A	Breakdown (mechanical) of cardiac pulse generator (battery), initial encounter
T82.120A	Displacement of cardiac electrode, initial encounter
T82.121A	Displacement of cardiac pulse generator (battery), initial encounter
T82.190A	Other mechanical complication of cardiac electrode, initial encounter
T82.191A	Other mechanical complication of cardiac pulse generator (battery), initial encounter
T82.7XXA	Infection and inflammatory reaction due to other cardiac and vascular devices, implants and grafts, initial encounter
T82.817A	Embolism due to cardiac prosthetic devices, implants and grafts, initial encounter
T82.827A	Fibrosis due to cardiac prosthetic devices, implants and grafts, initial encounter
T82.837A	Hemorrhage due to cardiac prosthetic devices, implants and grafts, initial encounter
T82.847A	Pain due to cardiac prosthetic devices, implants and grafts, initial encounter
T82.867A	Thrombosis due to cardiac prosthetic devices, implants and grafts, initial encounter

AMA: 33236 2019,Oct; 2019,Mar **33237** 2019,Oct; 2019,Mar

Relative Value Units/Medicare Edits

Non-Facility RVU	Work	PE	MP	Total
33236	12.73	7.55	2.92	23.2
33237	13.84	7.85	3.2	24.89
Facility RVU	**Work**	**PE**	**MP**	**Total**
33236	12.73	7.55	2.92	23.2
33237	13.84	7.85	3.2	24.89

	FUD	Status	MUE	Modifiers				IOM Reference
33236	90	A	1(2)	51	N/A	62	80*	None
33237	90	A	1(2)	51	N/A	62	80*	

* with documentation

Terms To Know

complication. Condition arising after the beginning of observation and treatment that modifies the course of the patient's illness or the medical care required, or an undesired result or misadventure in medical care.

dual chamber system. System that includes a pulse generator and one electrode inserted into the right atrium and one into the right ventricle.

epicardial electrode. Stimulation device that is attached to or inserted into the heart muscle and connected to a generator.

infection. Presence of microorganisms in body tissues that may result in cellular damage.

pacemaker. Implantable cardiac device that controls the heart's rhythm and maintains regular beats by artificial electric discharges. This device consists of the pulse generator with a battery and the electrodes, or leads, which are placed in single or dual chambers of the heart, usually transvenously.

pulse generator. Component of a pacemaker or an implantable cardioverter defibrillator that contains the battery and the electronics for producing the electrical discharge sent to the heart to control cardiac rhythm. Insertion or replacement of the pulse generator may be done alone, not in conjunction with insertion or replacement of the entire pacemaker system.

single-lead device. Implantable cardiac device (pacemaker or implantable cardioverter-defibrillator [ICD]) in which pacing and sensing components are placed in only one chamber of the heart.

thoracotomy. Surgical procedure for opening the chest wall in order to access the lungs, esophagus, trachea, aorta, heart, and diaphragm.

33238

33238 Removal of permanent transvenous electrode(s) by thoracotomy

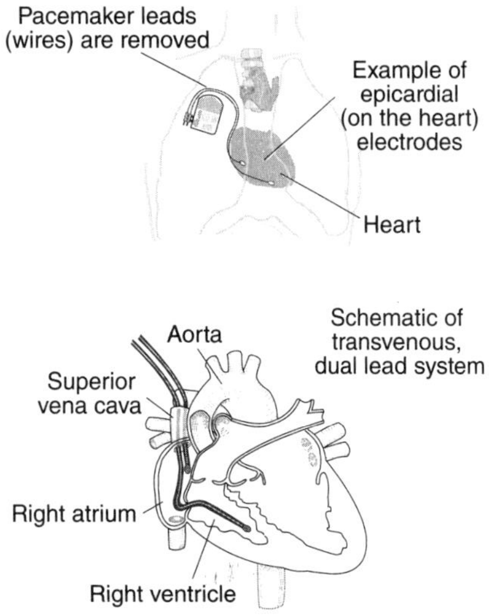

Removal of transvenous electrode(s)

Explanation

The physician removes a transvenous electrode(s) by thoracotomy. Prior to this procedure, the pacemaker pocket was opened, the generator removed, and the wires cut. The right chest is opened and the superior caval vein is dissected out. Tourniquets are placed around the vein above and below the planned site of opening. The tourniquets are tightened and a hole is made in the caval vein. The cut ends of the wires are pulled out through the hole in the caval vein. The ends of the wires that are still in the heart are twisted counterclockwise until they are free and are withdrawn through the caval vein. The hole in the caval vein is closed and the tourniquets released. The chest is closed.

Coding Tips

Procedure 33238 reports removal of pacemaker components only. For removal with replacement of generator and leads during the same surgical session, see 33206–33208. For transvenous leads inserted when a pulse generator is in place, see 33216 and 33217. Note that 33238 may require vein or heart repair with graft; report this separately. For removal of a permanent pacemaker pulse generator, see 33233. For removal of transvenous electrodes not requiring thoracotomy, see 33234–33235. For removal of an epicardial pacemaker system or electrodes by thoracotomy, see 33236–33237.

ICD-10-CM Diagnostic Codes

T82.110A Breakdown (mechanical) of cardiac electrode, initial encounter
T82.120A Displacement of cardiac electrode, initial encounter
T82.190A Other mechanical complication of cardiac electrode, initial encounter
T82.7XXA Infection and inflammatory reaction due to other cardiac and vascular devices, implants and grafts, initial encounter
T82.817A Embolism due to cardiac prosthetic devices, implants and grafts, initial encounter
T82.827A Fibrosis due to cardiac prosthetic devices, implants and grafts, initial encounter
T82.837A Hemorrhage due to cardiac prosthetic devices, implants and grafts, initial encounter
T82.847A Pain due to cardiac prosthetic devices, implants and grafts, initial encounter
T82.857A Stenosis of other cardiac prosthetic devices, implants and grafts, initial encounter
T82.867A Thrombosis due to cardiac prosthetic devices, implants and grafts, initial encounter

AMA: **33238** 2019,Oct

Relative Value Units/Medicare Edits

Non-Facility RVU	Work	PE	MP	Total
33238	15.4	9.15	3.61	28.16
Facility RVU	**Work**	**PE**	**MP**	**Total**
33238	15.4	9.15	3.61	28.16

	FUD	Status	MUE	Modifiers				IOM Reference
33238	90	A	1(2)	51	N/A	62	80*	None

* with documentation

Terms To Know

complication. Condition arising after the beginning of observation and treatment that modifies the course of the patient's illness or the medical care required, or an undesired result or misadventure in medical care.

epicardial electrode. Stimulation device that is attached to or inserted into the heart muscle and connected to a generator.

infection. Presence of microorganisms in body tissues that may result in cellular damage.

pacemaker. Implantable cardiac device that controls the heart's rhythm and maintains regular beats by artificial electric discharges. This device consists of the pulse generator with a battery and the electrodes, or leads, which are placed in single or dual chambers of the heart, usually transvenously.

thoracotomy. Surgical procedure for opening the chest wall in order to access the lungs, esophagus, trachea, aorta, heart, and diaphragm.

tourniquet. Device used to apply compressive force to a blood vessel in a limb and slow or prevent blood flow to and from the area.

transvenous electrode. Electrode placed using a transvenous catheter and wedged into the endocardium of the right ventricle or atrium.

33240 [33230, 33231]

33240 Insertion of implantable defibrillator pulse generator only; with existing single lead

33230 Insertion of implantable defibrillator pulse generator only; with existing dual leads

33231 Insertion of implantable defibrillator pulse generator only; with existing multiple leads

Schematic showing epicardial ICD leads and electrodes

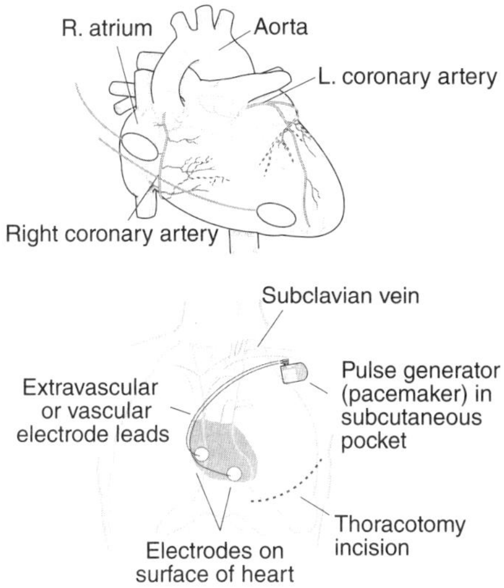

Explanation

This operation is done only when defibrillator electrodes are already in place. The previous pocket is opened or a new pocket is created for the implantable defibrillator pulse generator. The defibrillator pulse generators are implanted subcutaneously usually in an infraclavicular or abdominal pocket with the assistance of fluoroscopy. The electrodes are tested. The electrodes are connected to the defibrillator pulse generator and it is placed in the pocket. The pocket is closed with sutures, adhesive strips, or special glue. Report 33240 when there is an existing single lead (electrode); 33230 when there are existing dual leads (electrodes); and 33231 when there are existing multiple leads (electrodes).

Coding Tips

When medically necessary, report moderate (conscious) sedation provided by the performing physician with 99151-99153. When provided by another physician, report 99155-99157. These codes are appropriate for reporting "battery" change. Epicardial lead placement codes (33202, 33203) can be reported in addition to 33230, 33231, and 33240 when performed by the same physician during the same operative session. For repositioning of a previously implanted electrode, see 33215. For electrode repair, see 33218–33220. Fluoroscopy is included with these procedures and should not be reported separately. For pocket revision, see 33223. Do not report 33230–33231 or 33240 with 33216, 33217, or 33241. Do not report 33240 with 33271, 93260, or 93261. When pulse generator replacement is performed, see 33262–33264. Do not report device evaluation codes (93260, 93261, 93279–93298) in addition to pulse generator and lead insertion/revision codes. Defibrillator threshold testing (DFT) during transvenous implantable defibrillator insertion/replacement is reported separately with 93640 and/or 93641.

ICD-10-CM Diagnostic Codes

I11.0	Hypertensive heart disease with heart failure
I13.0	Hypertensive heart and chronic kidney disease with heart failure and stage 1 through stage 4 chronic kidney disease, or unspecified chronic kidney disease
I13.2	Hypertensive heart and chronic kidney disease with heart failure and with stage 5 chronic kidney disease, or end stage renal disease
I16.0	Hypertensive urgency
I16.1	Hypertensive emergency
I21.01	ST elevation (STEMI) myocardial infarction involving left main coronary artery
I21.02	ST elevation (STEMI) myocardial infarction involving left anterior descending coronary artery
I21.09	ST elevation (STEMI) myocardial infarction involving other coronary artery of anterior wall
I21.11	ST elevation (STEMI) myocardial infarction involving right coronary artery
I21.19	ST elevation (STEMI) myocardial infarction involving other coronary artery of inferior wall
I21.21	ST elevation (STEMI) myocardial infarction involving left circumflex coronary artery
I21.29	ST elevation (STEMI) myocardial infarction involving other sites
I21.4	Non-ST elevation (NSTEMI) myocardial infarction
I21.A1	Myocardial infarction type 2
I21.B	Myocardial infarction with coronary microvascular dysfunction
I22.0	Subsequent ST elevation (STEMI) myocardial infarction of anterior wall
I22.1	Subsequent ST elevation (STEMI) myocardial infarction of inferior wall
I22.2	Subsequent non-ST elevation (NSTEMI) myocardial infarction
I22.8	Subsequent ST elevation (STEMI) myocardial infarction of other sites
I25.2	Old myocardial infarction
I25.5	Ischemic cardiomyopathy
I25.6	Silent myocardial ischemia
I25.89	Other forms of chronic ischemic heart disease
I42.0	Dilated cardiomyopathy
I42.1	Obstructive hypertrophic cardiomyopathy
I42.2	Other hypertrophic cardiomyopathy
I42.5	Other restrictive cardiomyopathy
I42.8	Other cardiomyopathies
I44.0	Atrioventricular block, first degree
I44.1	Atrioventricular block, second degree
I44.2	Atrioventricular block, complete
I44.39	Other atrioventricular block
I44.4	Left anterior fascicular block
I44.5	Left posterior fascicular block
I44.69	Other fascicular block
I45.0	Right fascicular block
I45.19	Other right bundle-branch block
I45.2	Bifascicular block
I45.4	Nonspecific intraventricular block
I45.5	Other specified heart block

I45.6 Pre-excitation syndrome
I45.81 Long QT syndrome
I46.2 Cardiac arrest due to underlying cardiac condition
I46.8 Cardiac arrest due to other underlying condition
I47.0 Re-entry ventricular arrhythmia
I47.11 Inappropriate sinus tachycardia, so stated
I47.19 Other supraventricular tachycardia
I47.21 Torsades de pointes
I47.29 Other ventricular tachycardia
I48.0 Paroxysmal atrial fibrillation
I48.11 Longstanding persistent atrial fibrillation
I48.19 Other persistent atrial fibrillation
I48.21 Permanent atrial fibrillation
I49.01 Ventricular fibrillation
I49.02 Ventricular flutter
I49.2 Junctional premature depolarization
I49.5 Sick sinus syndrome
I49.8 Other specified cardiac arrhythmias
I50.1 Left ventricular failure, unspecified
I50.21 Acute systolic (congestive) heart failure
I50.22 Chronic systolic (congestive) heart failure
I50.23 Acute on chronic systolic (congestive) heart failure
I50.31 Acute diastolic (congestive) heart failure
I50.32 Chronic diastolic (congestive) heart failure
I50.33 Acute on chronic diastolic (congestive) heart failure
I50.41 Acute combined systolic (congestive) and diastolic (congestive) heart failure
I50.42 Chronic combined systolic (congestive) and diastolic (congestive) heart failure
I50.43 Acute on chronic combined systolic (congestive) and diastolic (congestive) heart failure
I50.811 Acute right heart failure
I50.812 Chronic right heart failure
I50.813 Acute on chronic right heart failure
I50.814 Right heart failure due to left heart failure
I50.82 Biventricular heart failure
I50.83 High output heart failure
I50.84 End stage heart failure
Q24.6 Congenital heart block
Q24.8 Other specified congenital malformations of heart
T82.110A Breakdown (mechanical) of cardiac electrode, initial encounter
T82.111A Breakdown (mechanical) of cardiac pulse generator (battery), initial encounter
T82.120A Displacement of cardiac electrode, initial encounter
T82.121A Displacement of cardiac pulse generator (battery), initial encounter
T82.190A Other mechanical complication of cardiac electrode, initial encounter
T82.191A Other mechanical complication of cardiac pulse generator (battery), initial encounter
T82.598A Other mechanical complication of other cardiac and vascular devices and implants, initial encounter
T82.7XXA Infection and inflammatory reaction due to other cardiac and vascular devices, implants and grafts, initial encounter
T82.817A Embolism due to cardiac prosthetic devices, implants and grafts, initial encounter
T82.827A Fibrosis due to cardiac prosthetic devices, implants and grafts, initial encounter
T82.837A Hemorrhage due to cardiac prosthetic devices, implants and grafts, initial encounter
T82.847A Pain due to cardiac prosthetic devices, implants and grafts, initial encounter
T82.855A Stenosis of coronary artery stent, initial encounter
T82.857A Stenosis of other cardiac prosthetic devices, implants and grafts, initial encounter
T82.867A Thrombosis due to cardiac prosthetic devices, implants and grafts, initial encounter
T82.897A Other specified complication of cardiac prosthetic devices, implants and grafts, initial encounter
Z45.02 Encounter for adjustment and management of automatic implantable cardiac defibrillator
Z95.810 Presence of automatic (implantable) cardiac defibrillator

AMA: 33230 2019,Oct; 2019,Jan **33231** 2019,Oct; 2019,Jan **33240** 2019,Oct; 2019,Jan

Relative Value Units/Medicare Edits

Non-Facility RVU	Work	PE	MP	Total
33240	5.8	3.75	1.33	10.88
33230	6.07	3.58	1.4	11.05
33231	6.34	4.07	1.43	11.84
Facility RVU	**Work**	**PE**	**MP**	**Total**
33240	5.8	3.75	1.33	10.88
33230	6.07	3.58	1.4	11.05
33231	6.34	4.07	1.43	11.84

	FUD	Status	MUE	Modifiers				IOM Reference
33240	90	A	1(3)	51	N/A	N/A	N/A	None
33230	90	A	1(3)	51	N/A	N/A	N/A	
33231	90	A	1(3)	51	N/A	N/A	N/A	

* with documentation

Terms To Know

defibrillation. Arrest of cardiac arrhythmias (atrial or ventricular) with restoration of normal rhythm, usually by applying brief electroshock to the heart.

dual-lead device. Implantable cardiac device (pacemaker or implantable cardioverter-defibrillator [ICD]) in which pacing and sensing components are placed in only two chambers of the heart.

pulse generator. Component of a pacemaker or an implantable cardioverter defibrillator that contains the battery and the electronics for producing the electrical discharge sent to the heart to control cardiac rhythm. Insertion or replacement of the pulse generator may be done alone, not in conjunction with insertion or replacement of the entire pacemaker system.

33241

33241 Removal of implantable defibrillator pulse generator only

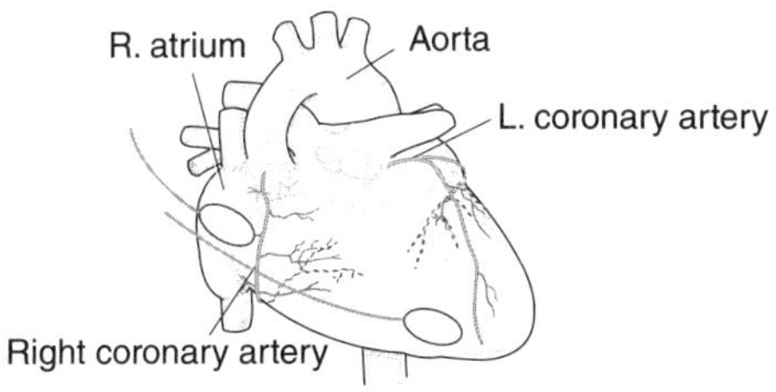

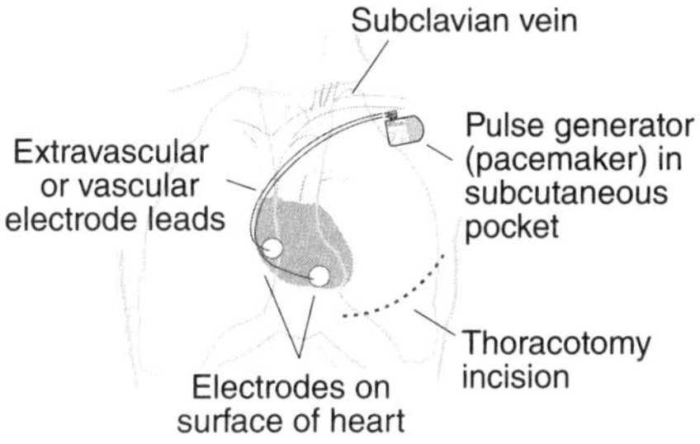

Pulse generator is removed

Explanation

The physician removes only the implantable defibrillator pulse generator. The pulse generator may be removed due to a complication or malfunction. The subcutaneous generator pocket is opened and the generator is removed. The electrodes are detached from the generator and the electrodes are placed in the pocket. The pocket is closed.

Coding Tips

When medically necessary, report moderate (conscious) sedation provided by the performing physician with 99151-99153. When provided by another physician, report 99155-99157. For removal and replacement of an implantable defibrillator pulse generator and electrodes, report 33243 or 33244 and 33249 for transvenous electrodes or 33270 and 33272 for subcutaneous electrodes with 33241. Do not report 33241 with 33230, 33231, or 33240, which includes removal and replacement of an implantable defibrillator pulse generator only. Do not report 33241 in addition to 93260 or 93261. For generator replacement only, see 33262–33264. Fluoroscopy is included and should not be reported separately.

ICD-10-CM Diagnostic Codes

T82.111A Breakdown (mechanical) of cardiac pulse generator (battery), initial encounter

T82.121A Displacement of cardiac pulse generator (battery), initial encounter

T82.191A Other mechanical complication of cardiac pulse generator (battery), initial encounter

T82.598A Other mechanical complication of other cardiac and vascular devices and implants, initial encounter

T82.7XXA Infection and inflammatory reaction due to other cardiac and vascular devices, implants and grafts, initial encounter

T82.817A Embolism due to cardiac prosthetic devices, implants and grafts, initial encounter

T82.827A Fibrosis due to cardiac prosthetic devices, implants and grafts, initial encounter

T82.837A Hemorrhage due to cardiac prosthetic devices, implants and grafts, initial encounter

T82.847A Pain due to cardiac prosthetic devices, implants and grafts, initial encounter

T82.857A Stenosis of other cardiac prosthetic devices, implants and grafts, initial encounter

T82.867A Thrombosis due to cardiac prosthetic devices, implants and grafts, initial encounter

T82.897A Other specified complication of cardiac prosthetic devices, implants and grafts, initial encounter

Z45.02 Encounter for adjustment and management of automatic implantable cardiac defibrillator

Z95.810 Presence of automatic (implantable) cardiac defibrillator

AMA: 33241 2019,Oct

Relative Value Units/Medicare Edits

Non-Facility RVU	Work	PE	MP	Total
33241	3.04	2.63	0.7	6.37
Facility RVU	**Work**	**PE**	**MP**	**Total**
33241	3.04	2.63	0.7	6.37

	FUD	Status	MUE	Modifiers				IOM Reference
33241	90	A	1(2)	51	N/A	N/A	N/A	None

* with documentation

Terms To Know

atrioventricular block. Condition in which there is a disturbance of electrical conduction, such as a delay, intermittence, or absence in the transmission of an impulse from the atria to the ventricles and categorized according to degree of severity.

cardioverter-defibrillator. Device that uses both low energy cardioversion or defibrillating shocks and antitachycardia pacing to treat ventricular tachycardia or ventricular fibrillation.

electrode. Electric terminal specialized for a particular electrochemical reaction that acts as a medium between a body surface and another instrument, commonly termed a lead.

myocardial infarction. Obstruction of circulation to the heart, resulting in necrosis.

pulse generator. Circuit used to generate pulses. Pulse generators contain the battery, the electronic circuit, and the connector in a hermetically sealed encasement. Pulse generators may be temporary transcutaneous or placed in a subcutaneous pocket.

ventricular tachycardia. Excessively rapid ventricular rhythm of the heart, usually more than 150 beats per minute, with an origin beat generated in the ventricle, commonly from atrioventricular dissociation.

[33262, 33263, 33264]

33262 Removal of implantable defibrillator pulse generator with replacement of implantable defibrillator pulse generator; single lead system

33263 Removal of implantable defibrillator pulse generator with replacement of implantable defibrillator pulse generator; dual lead system

33264 Removal of implantable defibrillator pulse generator with replacement of implantable defibrillator pulse generator; multiple lead system

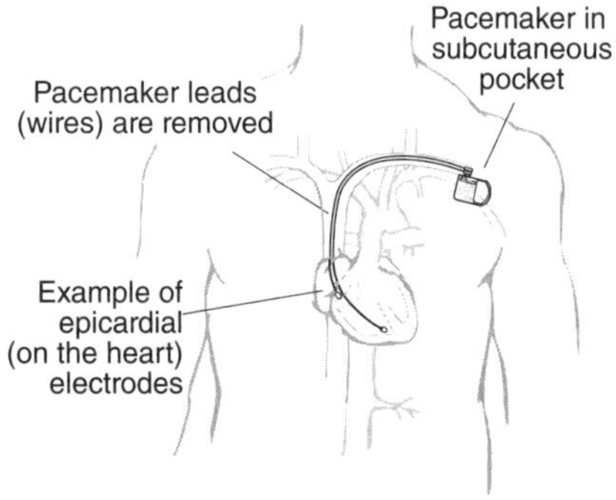

Explanation

An implantable defibrillator pulse generator is removed and replaced. The pulse generator may be removed due to a complication or malfunction. The generator pocket is opened. The existing generator is disconnected from the wire(s) and removed. The wire(s) is left in place in the pocket and a new pulse generator is inserted. The existing wire(s) is tested and connected to the new generator. The pocket is closed. Report 33262 for removal and replacement of a single lead system generator; 33263 for a dual lead system generator; and 33264 for a multiple lead system generator.

Coding Tips

When medically necessary, report moderate (conscious) sedation provided by the performing physician with 99151-99153. When provided by another physician, report 99155-99157. Do not report 33262–33264 with 33216, 33217, or 33241. Do not report 33262 with 33271, 93260, 93261, or 0614T. For removal of electrodes via thoracotomy and removal/replacement of a pulse generator, use 33243 in addition to 33241 or 33262–33264. For transvenous removal of electrodes and removal/replacement of a pulse generator, use 33244 in addition to 33241 or 33262–33264. For repair of an implantable defibrillator pulse generator and/or leads, see 33218 and 33220. For removal of electrodes with removal or replacement of an implantable defibrillator pulse generator, report 33272 in addition to 33241 or 33262. Revision of a skin pocket is included and is not reported separately.

ICD-10-CM Diagnostic Codes

I11.0	Hypertensive heart disease with heart failure
I13.0	Hypertensive heart and chronic kidney disease with heart failure and stage 1 through stage 4 chronic kidney disease, or unspecified chronic kidney disease
I13.2	Hypertensive heart and chronic kidney disease with heart failure and with stage 5 chronic kidney disease, or end stage renal disease
I16.0	Hypertensive urgency
I16.1	Hypertensive emergency
I21.01	ST elevation (STEMI) myocardial infarction involving left main coronary artery
I21.02	ST elevation (STEMI) myocardial infarction involving left anterior descending coronary artery
I21.11	ST elevation (STEMI) myocardial infarction involving right coronary artery
I21.21	ST elevation (STEMI) myocardial infarction involving left circumflex coronary artery
I21.4	Non-ST elevation (NSTEMI) myocardial infarction
I21.A1	Myocardial infarction type 2
I21.B	Myocardial infarction with coronary microvascular dysfunction
I22.0	Subsequent ST elevation (STEMI) myocardial infarction of anterior wall
I22.1	Subsequent ST elevation (STEMI) myocardial infarction of inferior wall
I22.2	Subsequent non-ST elevation (NSTEMI) myocardial infarction
I25.2	Old myocardial infarction
I25.5	Ischemic cardiomyopathy
I25.6	Silent myocardial ischemia
I42.0	Dilated cardiomyopathy
I44.0	Atrioventricular block, first degree
I44.1	Atrioventricular block, second degree
I44.2	Atrioventricular block, complete
I44.4	Left anterior fascicular block
I44.5	Left posterior fascicular block
I45.0	Right fascicular block
I45.2	Bifascicular block
I45.4	Nonspecific intraventricular block
I45.6	Pre-excitation syndrome
I45.81	Long QT syndrome
I46.2	Cardiac arrest due to underlying cardiac condition
I46.8	Cardiac arrest due to other underlying condition
I47.0	Re-entry ventricular arrhythmia
I47.11	Inappropriate sinus tachycardia, so stated
I47.21	Torsades de pointes
I48.0	Paroxysmal atrial fibrillation
I48.11	Longstanding persistent atrial fibrillation
I48.21	Permanent atrial fibrillation
I49.01	Ventricular fibrillation
I49.02	Ventricular flutter
I49.2	Junctional premature depolarization
I49.5	Sick sinus syndrome
I50.1	Left ventricular failure, unspecified
I50.21	Acute systolic (congestive) heart failure
I50.22	Chronic systolic (congestive) heart failure
I50.23	Acute on chronic systolic (congestive) heart failure
I50.31	Acute diastolic (congestive) heart failure
I50.32	Chronic diastolic (congestive) heart failure
I50.33	Acute on chronic diastolic (congestive) heart failure
I50.41	Acute combined systolic (congestive) and diastolic (congestive) heart failure
I50.42	Chronic combined systolic (congestive) and diastolic (congestive) heart failure
I50.43	Acute on chronic combined systolic (congestive) and diastolic (congestive) heart failure
I50.811	Acute right heart failure

N Newborn: 0 P Pediatric: 0-17 M Maternity: 9-64 A Adult: 15-124 AMA: CPT Assist

I50.812 Chronic right heart failure
I50.813 Acute on chronic right heart failure
I50.814 Right heart failure due to left heart failure
I50.82 Biventricular heart failure
I50.83 High output heart failure
I50.84 End stage heart failure
Q24.6 Congenital heart block
T82.111A Breakdown (mechanical) of cardiac pulse generator (battery), initial encounter
T82.121A Displacement of cardiac pulse generator (battery), initial encounter
T82.598A Other mechanical complication of other cardiac and vascular devices and implants, initial encounter
T82.817A Embolism due to cardiac prosthetic devices, implants and grafts, initial encounter
T82.827A Fibrosis due to cardiac prosthetic devices, implants and grafts, initial encounter
T82.837A Hemorrhage due to cardiac prosthetic devices, implants and grafts, initial encounter
T82.847A Pain due to cardiac prosthetic devices, implants and grafts, initial encounter
T82.855A Stenosis of coronary artery stent, initial encounter
T82.857A Stenosis of other cardiac prosthetic devices, implants and grafts, initial encounter
T82.867A Thrombosis due to cardiac prosthetic devices, implants and grafts, initial encounter
Z45.02 Encounter for adjustment and management of automatic implantable cardiac defibrillator
Z95.810 Presence of automatic (implantable) cardiac defibrillator

AMA: **33262** 2019,Oct **33263** 2019,Oct **33264** 2019,Oct

Relative Value Units/Medicare Edits

Non-Facility RVU	Work	PE	MP	Total
33262	5.81	3.86	1.32	10.99
33263	6.08	3.95	1.39	11.42
33264	6.35	4.1	1.46	11.91
Facility RVU	**Work**	**PE**	**MP**	**Total**
33262	5.81	3.86	1.32	10.99
33263	6.08	3.95	1.39	11.42
33264	6.35	4.1	1.46	11.91

	FUD	Status	MUE	Modifiers				IOM Reference
33262	90	A	1(3)	51	N/A	N/A	N/A	None
33263	90	A	1(3)	51	N/A	N/A	N/A	
33264	90	A	1(3)	51	N/A	N/A	N/A	

* with documentation

33243-33244

33243 Removal of single or dual chamber implantable defibrillator electrode(s); by thoracotomy
33244 by transvenous extraction

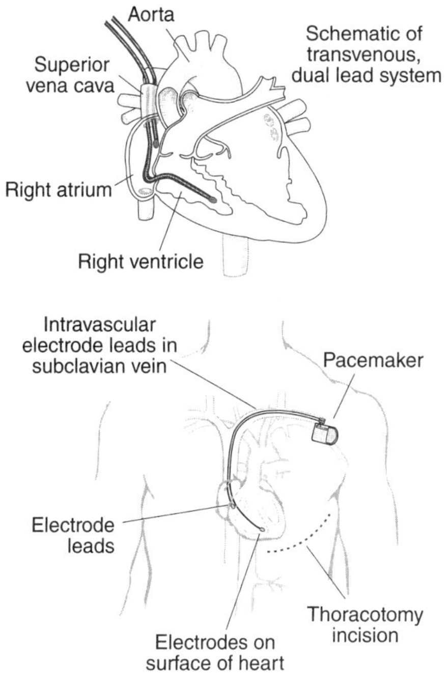

Defibrillator electrodes are removed

Explanation

In 33243, single or dual chamber implantable defibrillator electrodes are removed. Electrodes may be removed due to a complication or malfunction. The generator pocket is opened and the electrode wires are disconnected. The old chest incision is opened and the electrodes are dissected out and removed. The chest incision is closed. In 33244, electrodes only are removed by transvenous extraction, which is currently the most common technique for removing electrodes since most implantable defibrillator electrodes are now placed transvenously. Electrodes may be removed due to a complication or malfunction. The generator pocket is opened and the wire is disconnected from the generator. The wire is dissected from the scar tissue that has formed around it. Once the wire is completely freed, it is twisted in a direction opposite to that used for insertion (counterclockwise). The wire is withdrawn. Bleeding from the tracts leading to the vein is controlled with sutures. A new wire may be placed, but it is reported separately.

Coding Tips

When medically necessary, report moderate (conscious) sedation provided by the performing physician with 99151-99153. When provided by another physician, report 99155-99157. Removal of the pulse generator and electrodes requires reporting of multiple codes. For removal of an electrode by thoracotomy and removal of the pulse generator, report 33243 in addition to 33241. For removal of an electrode by transvenous extraction and removal of the pulse generator, report 33244 in addition to 33241. A transvenous extraction is normally attempted initially, but if it is unsuccessful a thoracotomy is performed. Removal and reinsertion of a new implantable defibrillator system also requires reporting of multiple codes. Report 33241 and 33243 or 33244 for the removal portion of the procedure. Report 33249 for insertion of the new system. For insertion or repositioning of implantable defibrillator electrodes without concurrent insertion of a pulse generator, see 33215–33217. For repair of implantable defibrillator electrodes, see 33218 or 33220.

Unsuccessful transvenous extraction of electrodes converted to an open procedure should be reported using thoracotomy code 33243.

ICD-10-CM Diagnostic Codes

T82.110A	Breakdown (mechanical) of cardiac electrode, initial encounter
T82.120A	Displacement of cardiac electrode, initial encounter
T82.190A	Other mechanical complication of cardiac electrode, initial encounter
T82.7XXA	Infection and inflammatory reaction due to other cardiac and vascular devices, implants and grafts, initial encounter
T82.817A	Embolism due to cardiac prosthetic devices, implants and grafts, initial encounter
T82.827A	Fibrosis due to cardiac prosthetic devices, implants and grafts, initial encounter
T82.837A	Hemorrhage due to cardiac prosthetic devices, implants and grafts, initial encounter
T82.847A	Pain due to cardiac prosthetic devices, implants and grafts, initial encounter
T82.857A	Stenosis of other cardiac prosthetic devices, implants and grafts, initial encounter
T82.867A	Thrombosis due to cardiac prosthetic devices, implants and grafts, initial encounter
T82.897A	Other specified complication of cardiac prosthetic devices, implants and grafts, initial encounter
Z45.02	Encounter for adjustment and management of automatic implantable cardiac defibrillator
Z95.810	Presence of automatic (implantable) cardiac defibrillator

AMA: **33243** 2019,Oct; 2019,Jan **33244** 2019,Oct; 2019,Jan

Relative Value Units/Medicare Edits

Non-Facility RVU	Work	PE	MP	Total
33243	23.57	11.41	5.67	40.65
33244	13.74	8.54	3.16	25.44
Facility RVU	**Work**	**PE**	**MP**	**Total**
33243	23.57	11.41	5.67	40.65
33244	13.74	8.54	3.16	25.44

	FUD	Status	MUE	Modifiers				IOM Reference
33243	90	A	1(2)	51	N/A	62*	80	None
33244	90	A	1(2)	51	N/A	62*	N/A	

* with documentation

Terms To Know

cardioverter-defibrillator. Device that uses both low energy cardioversion or defibrillating shocks and antitachycardia pacing to treat ventricular tachycardia or ventricular fibrillation.

33249

33249 Insertion or replacement of permanent implantable defibrillator system, with transvenous lead(s), single or dual chamber

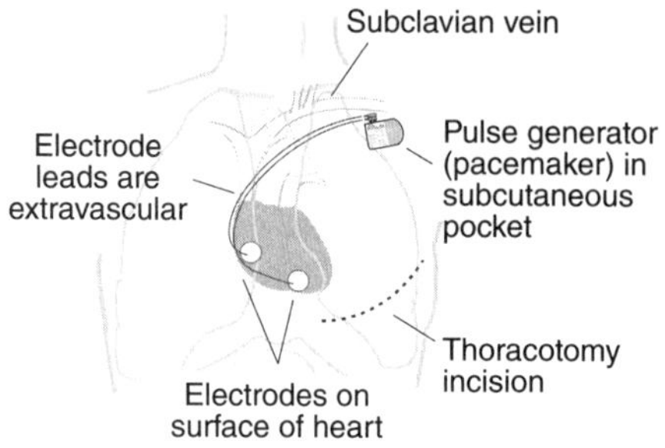

Single or dual chamber electrodes are inserted or repositioned by thoracotomy, with insertion of pulse generator

Explanation

The physician inserts or replaces a permanent implantable defibrillator system, including the pulse generator with transvenous electrode placement. Transvenous placement is currently the most common technique for placing implantable defibrillator electrodes. An implantable defibrillator is a device designed to administer an electric shock to control cardiac arrhythmias and restore a normal heartbeat. Local anesthesia is administered. An incision is made in the infraclavicular area. The subcutaneous tissue is opened and a pocket is created for the pulse generator. The electrode catheter is advanced through the superior vena cava into the heart and placed in the appropriate site in the right ventricle (single chamber system) or in the right ventricle and atrium (dual chamber system). Multiple leads may be required for both single and dual chamber systems. Once all leads are placed, they are tested and connected to the pulse generator that is placed in the previously prepared pocket. All incisions are closed. All radiological supervision and guidance is included.

Coding Tips

When medically necessary, report moderate (conscious) sedation provided by the performing physician with 99151-99153. When provided by another physician, report 99155-99157. For transvenous insertion of electrodes only, see 33216 and 33217; do not report these codes in addition to 33249. For repair of AICD transvenous electrodes, see 33218 or 33220. Removal with reinsertion of an implantable defibrillator system requires reporting of multiple codes. Report 33241 and 33243 or 33244 for the removal portion of the procedure and 33249 for the reinsertion. For insertion of epicardial electrodes by thoracotomy without concurrent pulse generator insertion, see 33202. For insertion of epicardial electrodes by endoscopy (thoracostomy or pericardioscopy) without concurrent pulse generator insertion, see 33203. Revision of a skin pocket is included and is not reported separately. Fluoroscopy is included in this procedure and is not reported separately. Do not report device evaluation codes (93260, 93261, 93279–93298) in addition to pulse generator and lead insertion/revision codes. Defibrillator threshold testing (DFT) during transvenous implantable defibrillator insertion/replacement is reported separately with 93640 or 93641.

ICD-10-CM Diagnostic Codes

I11.0	Hypertensive heart disease with heart failure
I13.0	Hypertensive heart and chronic kidney disease with heart failure and stage 1 through stage 4 chronic kidney disease, or unspecified chronic kidney disease

I13.2	Hypertensive heart and chronic kidney disease with heart failure and with stage 5 chronic kidney disease, or end stage renal disease
I16.0	Hypertensive urgency
I16.1	Hypertensive emergency
I21.01	ST elevation (STEMI) myocardial infarction involving left main coronary artery
I21.02	ST elevation (STEMI) myocardial infarction involving left anterior descending coronary artery
I21.11	ST elevation (STEMI) myocardial infarction involving right coronary artery
I21.21	ST elevation (STEMI) myocardial infarction involving left circumflex coronary artery
I21.4	Non-ST elevation (NSTEMI) myocardial infarction
I21.A1	Myocardial infarction type 2
I21.B	Myocardial infarction with coronary microvascular dysfunction
I22.0	Subsequent ST elevation (STEMI) myocardial infarction of anterior wall
I22.1	Subsequent ST elevation (STEMI) myocardial infarction of inferior wall
I22.2	Subsequent non-ST elevation (NSTEMI) myocardial infarction
I25.2	Old myocardial infarction
I25.5	Ischemic cardiomyopathy
I25.6	Silent myocardial ischemia
I42.0	Dilated cardiomyopathy
I42.1	Obstructive hypertrophic cardiomyopathy
I44.0	Atrioventricular block, first degree
I44.1	Atrioventricular block, second degree
I44.2	Atrioventricular block, complete
I44.4	Left anterior fascicular block
I44.5	Left posterior fascicular block
I45.0	Right fascicular block
I45.2	Bifascicular block
I45.6	Pre-excitation syndrome
I45.81	Long QT syndrome
I46.2	Cardiac arrest due to underlying cardiac condition
I46.8	Cardiac arrest due to other underlying condition
I47.0	Re-entry ventricular arrhythmia
I47.11	Inappropriate sinus tachycardia, so stated
I47.21	Torsades de pointes
I48.0	Paroxysmal atrial fibrillation
I48.21	Permanent atrial fibrillation
I49.01	Ventricular fibrillation
I49.02	Ventricular flutter
I49.2	Junctional premature depolarization
I49.5	Sick sinus syndrome
I50.21	Acute systolic (congestive) heart failure
I50.22	Chronic systolic (congestive) heart failure
I50.23	Acute on chronic systolic (congestive) heart failure
I50.31	Acute diastolic (congestive) heart failure
I50.32	Chronic diastolic (congestive) heart failure
I50.33	Acute on chronic diastolic (congestive) heart failure
I50.41	Acute combined systolic (congestive) and diastolic (congestive) heart failure
I50.42	Chronic combined systolic (congestive) and diastolic (congestive) heart failure
I50.43	Acute on chronic combined systolic (congestive) and diastolic (congestive) heart failure
I50.811	Acute right heart failure
I50.812	Chronic right heart failure
I50.813	Acute on chronic right heart failure
I50.814	Right heart failure due to left heart failure
I50.82	Biventricular heart failure
I50.83	High output heart failure
I50.84	End stage heart failure
T82.110A	Breakdown (mechanical) of cardiac electrode, initial encounter
T82.111A	Breakdown (mechanical) of cardiac pulse generator (battery), initial encounter
T82.120A	Displacement of cardiac electrode, initial encounter
T82.121A	Displacement of cardiac pulse generator (battery), initial encounter
T82.817A	Embolism due to cardiac prosthetic devices, implants and grafts, initial encounter
T82.827A	Fibrosis due to cardiac prosthetic devices, implants and grafts, initial encounter
T82.837A	Hemorrhage due to cardiac prosthetic devices, implants and grafts, initial encounter
T82.847A	Pain due to cardiac prosthetic devices, implants and grafts, initial encounter
T82.857A	Stenosis of other cardiac prosthetic devices, implants and grafts, initial encounter
T82.867A	Thrombosis due to cardiac prosthetic devices, implants and grafts, initial encounter
Z45.02	Encounter for adjustment and management of automatic implantable cardiac defibrillator
Z95.810	Presence of automatic (implantable) cardiac defibrillator

AMA: 33249 2019,Oct; 2019,Jan

Relative Value Units/Medicare Edits

Non-Facility RVU	Work	PE	MP	Total
33249	14.92	8.53	3.4	26.85
Facility RVU	**Work**	**PE**	**MP**	**Total**
33249	14.92	8.53	3.4	26.85

	FUD	Status	MUE	Modifiers				IOM Reference
33249	90	A	1(3)	51	N/A	62*	N/A	None

* with documentation

[33270, 33271]

33270 Insertion or replacement of permanent subcutaneous implantable defibrillator system, with subcutaneous electrode, including defibrillation threshold evaluation, induction of arrhythmia, evaluation of sensing for arrhythmia termination, and programming or reprogramming of sensing or therapeutic parameters, when performed

33271 Insertion of subcutaneous implantable defibrillator electrode

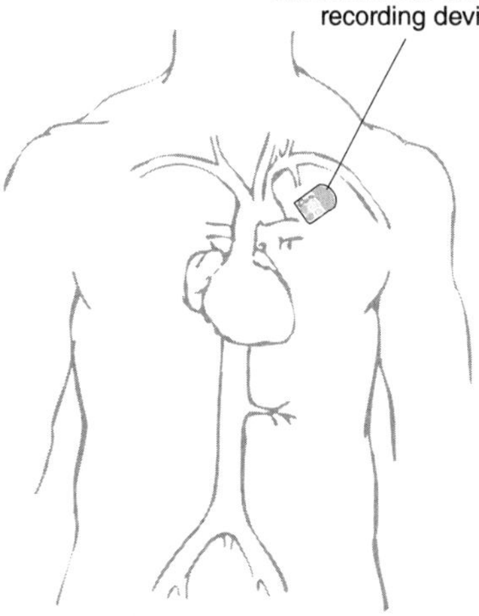

Explanation

In 33270, the physician performs initial insertion or replacement of a permanent subcutaneous implantable defibrillator (S-ICD) system, including the pulse generator and lead. The pulse generator is placed in a subcutaneous pocket on the left side of the chest next to the ribs. Two small incisions are made above the sternum and the lead wire is threaded through and sutured into place. The lead is connected to the pulse generator. The physician records cardiac electrical signals from the leads and paces the heart through the leads to determine pacing threshold. The physician uses the S-ICD pulse generator to pace the heart into an arrhythmia, such as ventricular tachycardia or fibrillation. The S-ICD detects and terminates the arrhythmia using pacing or by shocking the heart through the lead. The physician may reprogram the treatment parameters to optimize the device function to best treat the patient's arrhythmia. The incisions are closed. Report 33271 for insertion of the lead only.

Coding Tips

Do not report 33270 with 33271, 93260, 93261, or 93644. Do not report 33271 with 33240, 33262, 33270, 93260, or 93261. For removal and replacement of an implantable defibrillator generator and subcutaneous electrode, report 33270 and 33272 with 33241. For insertion or replacement of a cardiac venous system electrode, see 33224 and 33225. Revision of a skin pocket is included and is not reported separately. Radiological supervision and interpretation is included and is not reported separately. Device evaluation (93260–93261 and 93279–93298) is included and is not reported separately. For insertion or replacement with a substernal electrode, see 0571T. For insertion of a substernal defibrillator electrode, see 0572T.

ICD-10-CM Diagnostic Codes

I11.0	Hypertensive heart disease with heart failure
I13.0	Hypertensive heart and chronic kidney disease with heart failure and stage 1 through stage 4 chronic kidney disease, or unspecified chronic kidney disease
I13.2	Hypertensive heart and chronic kidney disease with heart failure and with stage 5 chronic kidney disease, or end stage renal disease
I16.0	Hypertensive urgency
I16.1	Hypertensive emergency
I21.01	ST elevation (STEMI) myocardial infarction involving left main coronary artery
I21.02	ST elevation (STEMI) myocardial infarction involving left anterior descending coronary artery
I21.11	ST elevation (STEMI) myocardial infarction involving right coronary artery
I21.21	ST elevation (STEMI) myocardial infarction involving left circumflex coronary artery
I21.4	Non-ST elevation (NSTEMI) myocardial infarction
I21.A1	Myocardial infarction type 2
I21.B	Myocardial infarction with coronary microvascular dysfunction
I22.0	Subsequent ST elevation (STEMI) myocardial infarction of anterior wall
I22.1	Subsequent ST elevation (STEMI) myocardial infarction of inferior wall
I22.2	Subsequent non-ST elevation (NSTEMI) myocardial infarction
I25.2	Old myocardial infarction
I25.5	Ischemic cardiomyopathy
I25.6	Silent myocardial ischemia
I42.0	Dilated cardiomyopathy
I42.1	Obstructive hypertrophic cardiomyopathy
I44.0	Atrioventricular block, first degree
I44.1	Atrioventricular block, second degree
I44.2	Atrioventricular block, complete
I44.4	Left anterior fascicular block
I44.5	Left posterior fascicular block
I45.0	Right fascicular block
I45.2	Bifascicular block
I45.4	Nonspecific intraventricular block
I45.6	Pre-excitation syndrome
I45.81	Long QT syndrome
I46.2	Cardiac arrest due to underlying cardiac condition
I46.8	Cardiac arrest due to other underlying condition
I47.0	Re-entry ventricular arrhythmia
I47.11	Inappropriate sinus tachycardia, so stated
I47.21	Torsades de pointes
I48.0	Paroxysmal atrial fibrillation
I48.11	Longstanding persistent atrial fibrillation
I48.21	Permanent atrial fibrillation
I49.01	Ventricular fibrillation
I49.02	Ventricular flutter
I49.2	Junctional premature depolarization
I49.5	Sick sinus syndrome
I50.21	Acute systolic (congestive) heart failure
I50.22	Chronic systolic (congestive) heart failure
I50.23	Acute on chronic systolic (congestive) heart failure
I50.31	Acute diastolic (congestive) heart failure
I50.32	Chronic diastolic (congestive) heart failure
I50.33	Acute on chronic diastolic (congestive) heart failure

I50.41 Acute combined systolic (congestive) and diastolic (congestive) heart failure
I50.42 Chronic combined systolic (congestive) and diastolic (congestive) heart failure
I50.43 Acute on chronic combined systolic (congestive) and diastolic (congestive) heart failure
I50.811 Acute right heart failure
I50.812 Chronic right heart failure
I50.813 Acute on chronic right heart failure
I50.814 Right heart failure due to left heart failure
I50.82 Biventricular heart failure
I50.83 High output heart failure
I50.84 End stage heart failure
T82.110A Breakdown (mechanical) of cardiac electrode, initial encounter
T82.111A Breakdown (mechanical) of cardiac pulse generator (battery), initial encounter
T82.817A Embolism due to cardiac prosthetic devices, implants and grafts, initial encounter
T82.827A Fibrosis due to cardiac prosthetic devices, implants and grafts, initial encounter
T82.837A Hemorrhage due to cardiac prosthetic devices, implants and grafts, initial encounter
T82.847A Pain due to cardiac prosthetic devices, implants and grafts, initial encounter
T82.867A Thrombosis due to cardiac prosthetic devices, implants and grafts, initial encounter
Z45.02 Encounter for adjustment and management of automatic implantable cardiac defibrillator
Z95.810 Presence of automatic (implantable) cardiac defibrillator

AMA: 33270 2019,Oct; 2019,Jan **33271** 2019,Oct; 2019,Jan

Relative Value Units/Medicare Edits

Non-Facility RVU	Work	PE	MP	Total
33270	9.1	5.34	2.06	16.5
33271	7.5	4.21	1.72	13.43
Facility RVU	**Work**	**PE**	**MP**	**Total**
33270	9.1	5.34	2.06	16.5
33271	7.5	4.21	1.72	13.43

	FUD	Status	MUE	Modifiers				IOM Reference
33270	90	A	1(3)	51	N/A	N/A	N/A	None
33271	90	A	1(3)	51	N/A	N/A	N/A	

* with documentation

Terms To Know

electrode. Electric terminal specialized for a particular electrochemical reaction that acts as a medium between a body surface and another instrument, commonly termed a lead.

subcutaneous pocket. Small space created under the skin in a suitable location for holding an implantable device, such as the pulse generator of a pacemaker or cardioverter defibrillator.

[33272]

33272 Removal of subcutaneous implantable defibrillator electrode

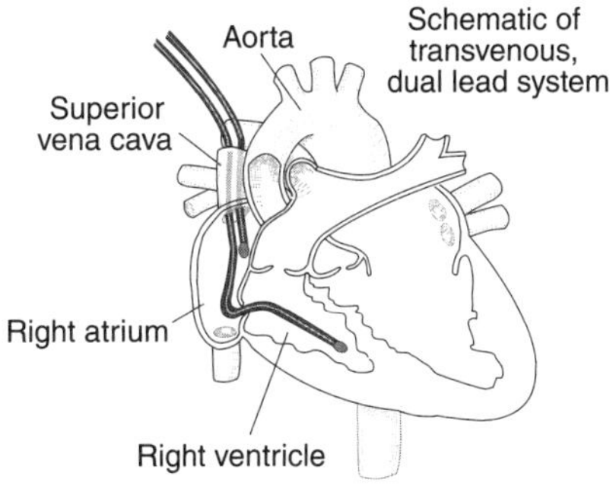

Explanation

The physician performs a procedure to remove the subcutaneous implantable defibrillator lead only. The lead may be removed due to a complication or malfunction. An incision is made in the area above the sternum where the lead is located. The lead is disconnected from the pulse generator, pulled through, and removed. The incision is repaired.

Coding Tips

Insertion or replacement of a pulse generator (33241) may be reported separately, when performed. Radiological supervision and interpretation is included and is not reported separately. Removal and replacement of the pulse generator and electrodes requires reporting of multiple codes: report 33272 in addition to 33241 or 33270. For repositioning of a previously implanted subcutaneous defibrillator electrode, see 33273. Do not report 33272 with 93260 or 93261. For removal of a substernal defibrillator electrode, see 0573T.

ICD-10-CM Diagnostic Codes

T82.110A Breakdown (mechanical) of cardiac electrode, initial encounter
T82.120A Displacement of cardiac electrode, initial encounter
T82.190A Other mechanical complication of cardiac electrode, initial encounter
T82.7XXA Infection and inflammatory reaction due to other cardiac and vascular devices, implants and grafts, initial encounter
T82.817A Embolism due to cardiac prosthetic devices, implants and grafts, initial encounter
T82.827A Fibrosis due to cardiac prosthetic devices, implants and grafts, initial encounter
T82.837A Hemorrhage due to cardiac prosthetic devices, implants and grafts, initial encounter
T82.847A Pain due to cardiac prosthetic devices, implants and grafts, initial encounter
T82.857A Stenosis of other cardiac prosthetic devices, implants and grafts, initial encounter
T82.867A Thrombosis due to cardiac prosthetic devices, implants and grafts, initial encounter
T82.897A Other specified complication of cardiac prosthetic devices, implants and grafts, initial encounter
Z45.02 Encounter for adjustment and management of automatic implantable cardiac defibrillator
Z95.810 Presence of automatic (implantable) cardiac defibrillator

AMA: **33272** 2019,Oct; 2019,Jan

Relative Value Units/Medicare Edits

Non-Facility RVU	Work	PE	MP	Total
33272	5.42	3.6	1.24	10.26
Facility RVU	**Work**	**PE**	**MP**	**Total**
33272	5.42	3.6	1.24	10.26

	FUD	Status	MUE	Modifiers				IOM Reference
33272	90	A	1(3)	51	N/A	N/A	N/A	None

* with documentation

Terms To Know

electrode. Electric terminal specialized for a particular electrochemical reaction that acts as a medium between a body surface and another instrument, commonly termed a lead.

pulse generator. Circuit used to generate pulses. Pulse generators contain the battery, the electronic circuit, and the connector in a hermetically sealed encasement. Pulse generators may be temporary transcutaneous or placed in a subcutaneous pocket.

subcutaneous. Below the skin.

supervision and interpretation. Radiology services that usually contain an invasive component and are reported by the radiologist for supervision of the procedure and the personnel involved with performing the examination, reading the film, and preparing the written report.

[33273]

33273 Repositioning of previously implanted subcutaneous implantable defibrillator electrode

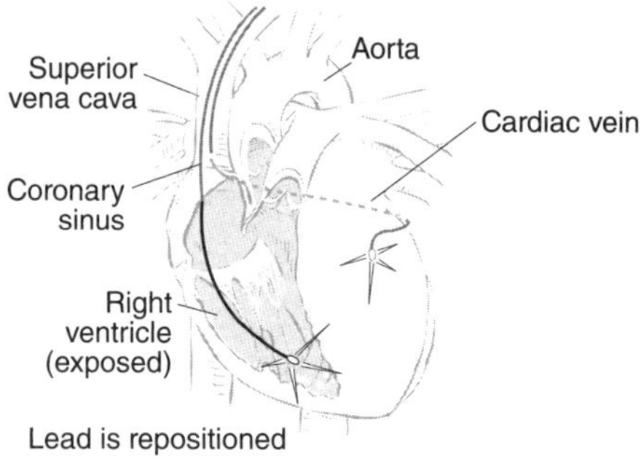

Explanation

A previously placed implanted subcutaneous defibrillator lead (electrode) is repositioned. This procedure is performed when the system does not function due to improper placement of the lead. An incision is made over the previous subcutaneous pocket on the left side of the chest next to the ribs. The lead is disconnected from the pulse generator. The generator is removed and the lead is tested for proper function. It is then reattached to the generator in the new position and retested. The incision is closed.

Coding Tips

Do not report 33273 with 93260 or 93261. Radiological supervision and interpretation is included and is not reported separately. For insertion or replacement of a previously placed subcutaneous defibrillator system, see 33270. For insertion of a subcutaneous implantable defibrillator electrode, see 33271. For removal of a subcutaneous implantable defibrillator electrode, see 33272. For repositioning of a substernal defibrillator electrode, see 0574T.

ICD-10-CM Diagnostic Codes

T82.120A	Displacement of cardiac electrode, initial encounter
T82.897A	Other specified complication of cardiac prosthetic devices, implants and grafts, initial encounter
Z45.02	Encounter for adjustment and management of automatic implantable cardiac defibrillator
Z95.810	Presence of automatic (implantable) cardiac defibrillator

AMA: **33273** 2019,Oct; 2019,Jan

Relative Value Units/Medicare Edits

Non-Facility RVU	Work	PE	MP	Total
33273	6.5	3.88	1.51	11.89
Facility RVU	**Work**	**PE**	**MP**	**Total**
33273	6.5	3.88	1.51	11.89

	FUD	Status	MUE	Modifiers				IOM Reference
33273	90	A	1(3)	51	N/A	N/A	N/A	None

* with documentation

[33274, 33275]

33274 Transcatheter insertion or replacement of permanent leadless pacemaker, right ventricular, including imaging guidance (eg, fluoroscopy, venous ultrasound, ventriculography, femoral venography) and device evaluation (eg, interrogation or programming), when performed

33275 Transcatheter removal of permanent leadless pacemaker, right ventricular, including imaging guidance (eg, fluoroscopy, venous ultrasound, ventriculography, femoral venography), when performed

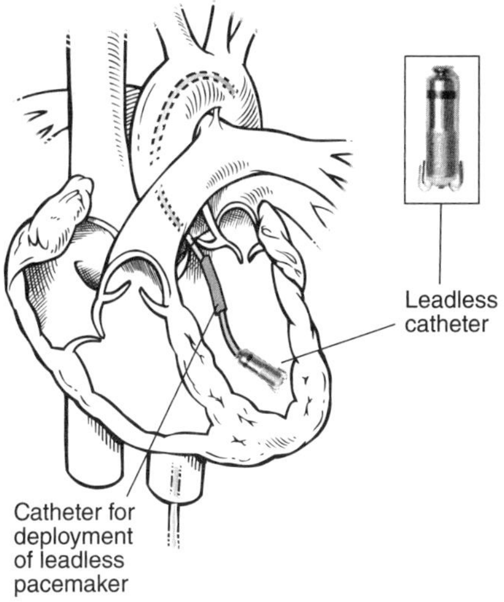

Explanation

The physician performs transcatheter insertion, replacement, or removal of a ventricular permanent leadless pacemaker. This pacemaker is a single-chamber unit without leads that is placed into the right ventricle. The size varies based on manufacturer, but is approximately 7 mm x 26 mm and weighs 2 grams. The less invasive and shorter implantation procedure of a leadless pacemaker reduces recovery time and eliminates complications related to the transvenous leads and the subcutaneous pulse generator used in traditional pacemaker implantation, specifically infections. The battery typically lasts seven to 15 years, and the pacing, amplitude, and impedance are all relative to the traditional pacemaker. The femoral vein is entered and the device is fed into the right ventricle using a special catheter. Once attached, a continued connection allows for measurements to be taken and to determine positioning. All imaging and device evaluations are included in the procedures and should not be reported separately. For insertion or replacement of the pacemaker, report 33274; for removal of the pacemaker, report 33275.

Coding Tips

Do not report these codes with 75820, 76000, 77002, 76937, or 93566. Do not report 33275 with 33274. Do not report 33274 or 33275 with 93451, 93453, 93456, 93457, 93460, 93461, 93593, 93594, or 93596–93598 unless complete right heart catheterization is performed for reasons distinct from the leadless pacemaker procedure. For subsequent leadless pacemaker device evaluation, see 93279, 93286, 93288, 93294, 93296, 0804T, or 0826T. For insertion, replacement, repositioning, or removal of pacemakers with leads, see 33202-33208, 33212-33221, 33227-33229, and 33233-33237. Do not report 33274 or 33275 with 0795T–0803T or 0823T–0825T. For a dual-chamber leadless pacemaker, see 0795T–0803T. For insertion or replacement of a right ventricle leadless pacemaker as part of a complete dual-chamber leadless pacemaker, see 0797T; removal, see 0800T.

ICD-10-CM Diagnostic Codes

I44.0	Atrioventricular block, first degree
I44.1	Atrioventricular block, second degree
I44.2	Atrioventricular block, complete
I44.39	Other atrioventricular block
I44.4	Left anterior fascicular block
I44.5	Left posterior fascicular block
I44.69	Other fascicular block
I45.0	Right fascicular block
I45.19	Other right bundle-branch block
I45.2	Bifascicular block
I45.3	Trifascicular block
I45.4	Nonspecific intraventricular block
I45.5	Other specified heart block
I45.6	Pre-excitation syndrome
I45.81	Long QT syndrome
I47.11	Inappropriate sinus tachycardia, so stated
I47.19	Other supraventricular tachycardia
I48.0	Paroxysmal atrial fibrillation
I48.21	Permanent atrial fibrillation
I49.2	Junctional premature depolarization
I49.5	Sick sinus syndrome
I49.8	Other specified cardiac arrhythmias
I50.1	Left ventricular failure, unspecified
I50.21	Acute systolic (congestive) heart failure
I50.22	Chronic systolic (congestive) heart failure
I50.23	Acute on chronic systolic (congestive) heart failure
I50.31	Acute diastolic (congestive) heart failure
I50.32	Chronic diastolic (congestive) heart failure
I50.33	Acute on chronic diastolic (congestive) heart failure
I50.41	Acute combined systolic (congestive) and diastolic (congestive) heart failure
I50.42	Chronic combined systolic (congestive) and diastolic (congestive) heart failure
I50.43	Acute on chronic combined systolic (congestive) and diastolic (congestive) heart failure
I50.810	Right heart failure, unspecified
I50.811	Acute right heart failure
I50.812	Chronic right heart failure
I50.813	Acute on chronic right heart failure
I50.814	Right heart failure due to left heart failure
I50.82	Biventricular heart failure
I50.83	High output heart failure
I50.84	End stage heart failure
I50.89	Other heart failure
I51.7	Cardiomegaly
Q24.6	Congenital heart block
T82.110A	Breakdown (mechanical) of cardiac electrode, initial encounter
T82.111A	Breakdown (mechanical) of cardiac pulse generator (battery), initial encounter
T82.120A	Displacement of cardiac electrode, initial encounter

T82.121A	Displacement of cardiac pulse generator (battery), initial encounter
T82.190A	Other mechanical complication of cardiac electrode, initial encounter
T82.191A	Other mechanical complication of cardiac pulse generator (battery), initial encounter
T82.7XXA	Infection and inflammatory reaction due to other cardiac and vascular devices, implants and grafts, initial encounter
T82.817A	Embolism due to cardiac prosthetic devices, implants and grafts, initial encounter
T82.827A	Fibrosis due to cardiac prosthetic devices, implants and grafts, initial encounter
T82.837A	Hemorrhage due to cardiac prosthetic devices, implants and grafts, initial encounter
T82.847A	Pain due to cardiac prosthetic devices, implants and grafts, initial encounter
T82.857A	Stenosis of other cardiac prosthetic devices, implants and grafts, initial encounter
T82.867A	Thrombosis due to cardiac prosthetic devices, implants and grafts, initial encounter
T82.897A	Other specified complication of cardiac prosthetic devices, implants and grafts, initial encounter
Z45.018	Encounter for adjustment and management of other part of cardiac pacemaker
Z95.0	Presence of cardiac pacemaker

AMA: 33274 2024,Mar; 2019,Mar; 2019,Jan **33275** 2024,Mar; 2019,Mar; 2019,Jan

Relative Value Units/Medicare Edits

Non-Facility RVU	Work	PE	MP	Total
33274	7.8	4.51	1.77	14.08
33275	8.59	4.3	1.99	14.88
Facility RVU	**Work**	**PE**	**MP**	**Total**
33274	7.8	4.51	1.77	14.08
33275	8.59	4.3	1.99	14.88

	FUD	Status	MUE	Modifiers				IOM Reference
33274	90	A	1(3)	51	N/A	62	N/A	None
33275	90	A	1(3)	51	N/A	N/A	N/A	

* with documentation

Terms To Know

catheterization. Use or insertion of a tubular device into a duct, blood vessel, hollow organ, or body cavity for injecting or withdrawing fluids for diagnostic or therapeutic purposes.

fluoroscopy. Radiology technique that allows visual examination of part of the body or a function of an organ using a device that projects an x-ray image on a fluorescent screen.

transcatheter. Procedure or treatment performed via a catheter.

venography. Radiographic study of the veins.

[33276, 33277]

33276 Insertion of phrenic nerve stimulator system (pulse generator and stimulating lead[s]), including vessel catheterization, all imaging guidance, and pulse generator initial analysis with diagnostic mode activation, when performed

\+ **33277** Insertion of phrenic nerve stimulator transvenous sensing lead (List separately in addition to code for primary procedure)

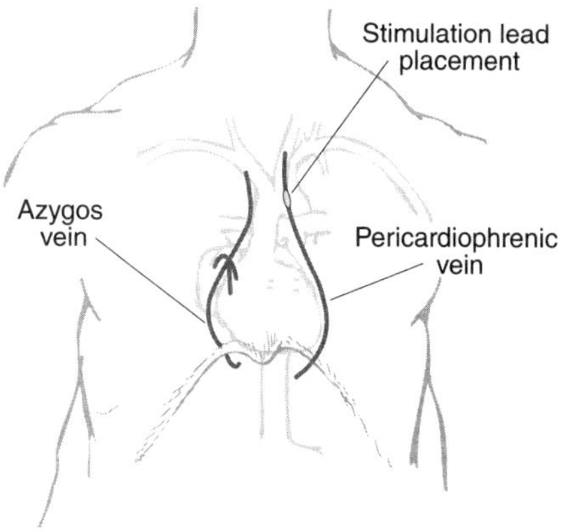

Phrenic nerve stimulator system is inserted

Explanation

The physician treats central sleep apnea with insertion of a phrenic nerve stimulator system, which consists of a pulse generator much like a pacemaker, a stimulation electrode, and, when appropriate, a sensing electrode. Respiration sensing is accomplished by the electrodes determining the patient's position at rest/activity to allow for programming of applicable delivery times. This unit assists stable breathing by preventing episodes of apnea followed by rapid breathing. With the patient under appropriate anesthesia (typically conscious sedation), the physician creates a subcutaneous or submuscular pocket in the pectoral region of the chest and inserts the implantable pulse generator (IPG). Using standard transvenous implantation techniques, venous access is obtained through the axillary, cephalic, or subclavian vein; access wires are then advanced into the inferior vena cava. The stimulating lead is inserted and placed in the left pericardiophrenic vein or the right brachiocephalic vein. The sensing electrode, if deemed necessary, is inserted into the azygos vein (on the back of the thorax, which flows into the superior vena cava). The electrodes are connected to the generator and tested prior to pocket closure. Report 33276 for insertion of the pulse generator and one or more stimulating leads; this includes the initial analysis with diagnostic mode activation if performed and all imaging guidance and vessel catheterization. In addition, report 33277 for insertion of the transvenous sensing lead if applicable.

Coding Tips

Vessel catheterization and imaging guidance is included in these procedures and not separately reported. Report 33277 with 33276 and 33287. For therapeutic activation of a phrenic nerve stimulation system, see 93150–93153. Do not report 33276 with 93150–93153. For insertion of a phrenic nerve sensing lead other than at initial insertion of a phrenic nerve stimulator, see 33999.

ICD-10-CM Diagnostic Codes

G12.21	Amyotrophic lateral sclerosis A
G47.31	Primary central sleep apnea
G47.35	Congenital central alveolar hypoventilation syndrome

Heart and Pericardium

G47.37	Central sleep apnea in conditions classified elsewhere
G82.51	Quadriplegia, C1-C4 complete
G82.52	Quadriplegia, C1-C4 incomplete
G82.53	Quadriplegia, C5-C7 complete
G82.54	Quadriplegia, C5-C7 incomplete
J96.01	Acute respiratory failure with hypoxia
J96.02	Acute respiratory failure with hypercapnia
J96.11	Chronic respiratory failure with hypoxia
J96.12	Chronic respiratory failure with hypercapnia
J96.21	Acute and chronic respiratory failure with hypoxia
J96.22	Acute and chronic respiratory failure with hypercapnia
J98.6	Disorders of diaphragm
Z99.11	Dependence on respirator [ventilator] status

AMA: 33276 2024,Apr **33277** 2024,Apr

Relative Value Units/Medicare Edits

Non-Facility RVU	Work	PE	MP	Total
33276	9.5	5.39	2.16	17.05
33277	5.43	2.24	1.25	8.92
Facility RVU	**Work**	**PE**	**MP**	**Total**
33276	9.5	5.39	2.16	17.05
33277	5.43	2.24	1.25	8.92

	FUD	Status	MUE	Modifiers				IOM Reference
33276	90	A	1(2)	51	N/A	N/A	N/A	None
33277	N/A	A	1(2)	N/A	N/A	N/A	N/A	

* with documentation

Terms To Know

phrenic nerves. Two nerves that arise mainly from the fourth cervical nerve, providing motor nerve function to a side of the diaphragm, and serve in the breathing function. The right nerve plays a role in liver function.

pulse generator. Circuit used to generate pulses. Pulse generators contain the battery, the electronic circuit, and the connector in a hermetically sealed encasement. Pulse generators may be temporary transcutaneous or placed in a subcutaneous pocket.

[33278, 33279, 33280]

33278 Removal of phrenic nerve stimulator, including vessel catheterization, all imaging guidance, and interrogation and programming, when performed; system, including pulse generator and lead(s)

33279 Removal of phrenic nerve stimulator, including vessel catheterization, all imaging guidance, and interrogation and programming, when performed; transvenous stimulation or sensing lead(s) only

33280 Removal of phrenic nerve stimulator, including vessel catheterization, all imaging guidance, and interrogation and programming, when performed; pulse generator only

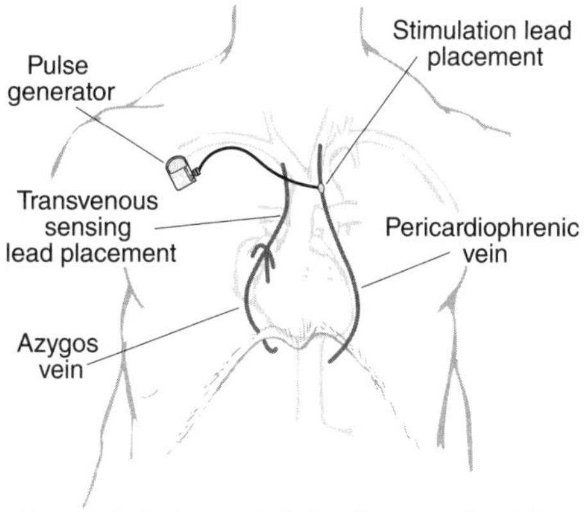

Removal of all or part of phrenic nerve stimulator

Explanation

The phrenic nerve stimulator system for treatment of central sleep apnea consists of a pulse generator much like a pacemaker, a stimulation electrode, and a sensing electrode. Respiration sensing is accomplished by the electrodes determining the patient's position at rest/activity to allow for programming of applicable delivery times. This unit assists stable breathing by preventing episodes of apnea followed by rapid breathing. In 33279, the physician removes one or more transvenous stimulation or sensing leads. The generator pocket is opened, and the generator disconnected from the appropriate lead (electrode). The lead is dissected from any scar tissue that has formed around it and withdrawn, bleeding is controlled, and the pocket is closed with sutures. In 33280, only the pulse generator is removed. The physician opens the generator pocket. The generator is disconnected from the electrodes and removed. The electrodes remain within the pocket and the pocket is closed. In 33278, the entire system, consisting of the pulse generator and the leads, is removed. These codes include interrogation and programming if performed and all imaging guidance and vessel catheterization.

Coding Tips

Vessel catheterization and imaging guidance are included in these procedures and are not reported separately. Report 33279 once for removal of one or more leads. Do not report 33278–33280 with 33276, 33277, 33281, 33287, or 33288. For removal and replacement of a phrenic nerve stimulator, see 33287 and 33288. For repositioning of a phrenic nerve stimulator transvenous leads, see 33281.

ICD-10-CM Diagnostic Codes

T85.113A	Breakdown (mechanical) of implanted electronic neurostimulator, generator, initial encounter
T85.191A	Other mechanical complication of implanted electronic neurostimulator of peripheral nerve electrode (lead), initial encounter

Heart and Pericardium

T85.193A Other mechanical complication of implanted electronic neurostimulator, generator, initial encounter
Z45.42 Encounter for adjustment and management of neurostimulator
Z96.82 Presence of neurostimulator

AMA: **33278** 2024,Apr **33279** 2024,Apr **33280** 2024,Apr

Relative Value Units/Medicare Edits

Non-Facility RVU	Work	PE	MP	Total
33278	9.55	5.21	2.21	16.97
33279	5.42	3.58	1.25	10.25
33280	3.04	2.82	0.31	6.17
Facility RVU	**Work**	**PE**	**MP**	**Total**
33278	9.55	5.21	2.21	16.97
33279	5.42	3.58	1.25	10.25
33280	3.04	2.82	0.31	6.17

	FUD	Status	MUE	Modifiers				IOM Reference
33278	90	A	1(2)	51	N/A	N/A	N/A	None
33279	90	A	1(2)	51	N/A	N/A	N/A	
33280	90	A	1(2)	51	N/A	N/A	N/A	

* with documentation

Terms To Know

catheterization. Use or insertion of a tubular device into a duct, blood vessel, hollow organ, or body cavity for injecting or withdrawing fluids for diagnostic or therapeutic purposes.

phrenic nerves. Two nerves that arise mainly from the fourth cervical nerve, providing motor nerve function to a side of the diaphragm, and serve in the breathing function. The right nerve plays a role in liver function.

pulse generator. Circuit used to generate pulses. Pulse generators contain the battery, the electronic circuit, and the connector in a hermetically sealed encasement. Pulse generators may be temporary transcutaneous or placed in a subcutaneous pocket.

subcutaneous pocket. Small space created under the skin in a suitable location for holding an implantable device, such as the pulse generator of a pacemaker or cardioverter defibrillator.

[33281]

33281 Repositioning of phrenic nerve stimulator transvenous lead(s)

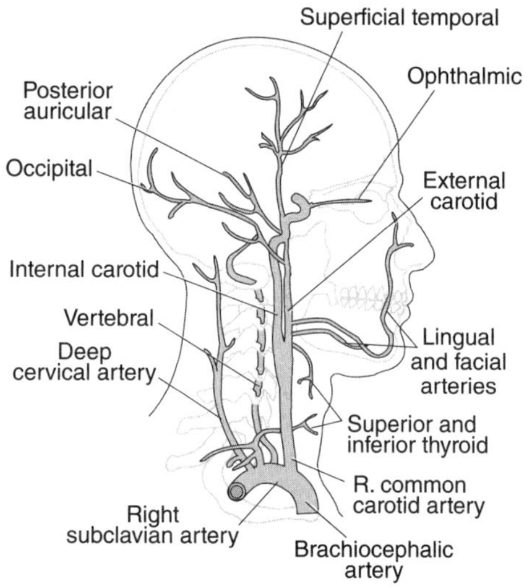

Repositioning of stimulator lead in right brachiocephalic vein

Explanation

One or more previously placed phrenic nerve stimulation and/or sensing transvenous leads are repositioned. This may be done when the system does not function due to improper placement of the electrode itself. The generator is removed, and the electrode is tested to ensure that it is not defective, but simply in the wrong place. It is reattached to the generator in its new position and tested again. This code includes all imaging guidance and vessel catheterization necessary to complete the procedure.

Coding Tips

Vessel catheterization and imaging guidance are included in this procedure and are not reported separately. Do not report 33281 with 33276 or 33277. Report 33281 once per patient per day.

ICD-10-CM Diagnostic Codes

T85.121A Displacement of implanted electronic neurostimulator of peripheral nerve electrode (lead), initial encounter
Z45.42 Encounter for adjustment and management of neurostimulator
Z96.82 Presence of neurostimulator

AMA: **33281** 2024,Apr

Relative Value Units/Medicare Edits

Non-Facility RVU	Work	PE	MP	Total
33281	6.0	3.71	1.38	11.09
Facility RVU	**Work**	**PE**	**MP**	**Total**
33281	6.0	3.71	1.38	11.09

	FUD	Status	MUE	Modifiers				IOM Reference
33281	90	A	1(2)	51	N/A	N/A	N/A	None

* with documentation

Heart and Pericardium

[33287, 33288]

33287 Removal and replacement of phrenic nerve stimulator, including vessel catheterization, all imaging guidance, and interrogation and programming, when performed; pulse generator

33288 Removal and replacement of phrenic nerve stimulator, including vessel catheterization, all imaging guidance, and interrogation and programming, when performed; transvenous stimulation or sensing lead(s)

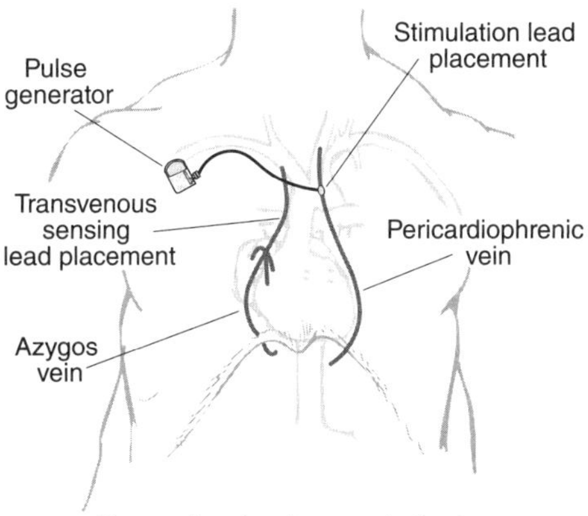

Removal and replacement of pulse generator or transvenous leads

Explanation

The physician removes and replaces an existing phrenic nerve stimulator pulse generator in 33287. The generator pocket is opened. The existing generator is disconnected from any attached electrodes (leads) and removed. The leads are left in place in the pocket and a new pulse generator is inserted. The existing leads are tested and connected to the generator and the pocket is closed. In 33288, the physician removes and replaces one or more transvenous stimulation or sensing leads. The generator pocket is opened, and the generator disconnected from the appropriate lead. The lead is dissected from any scar tissue that has formed around it and extracted. A replacement lead is advanced into the targeted location, connected to the pulse generator, and tested. These codes include interrogation and programming if performed and all imaging guidance and vessel catheterization.

Coding Tips

Vessel catheterization and imaging guidance are included in these procedures and are not reported separately. Do not report 33287 with 33276 or 33278. Report 33288 once for removal of one or more leads. Do not report 33288 with 33277, 33279, or 33281. For removal of a phrenic nerve stimulator without replacement, see 33278, 33279, and 33280.

ICD-10-CM Diagnostic Codes

T85.113A	Breakdown (mechanical) of implanted electronic neurostimulator, generator, initial encounter
T85.193A	Other mechanical complication of implanted electronic neurostimulator, generator, initial encounter
Z45.42	Encounter for adjustment and management of neurostimulator
Z96.82	Presence of neurostimulator

AMA: 33287 2024,Apr **33288** 2024,Apr

Relative Value Units/Medicare Edits

Non-Facility RVU	Work	PE	MP	Total
33287	6.05	4.0	1.39	11.44
33288	8.51	4.61	1.96	15.08
Facility RVU	**Work**	**PE**	**MP**	**Total**
33287	6.05	4.0	1.39	11.44
33288	8.51	4.61	1.96	15.08

	FUD	Status	MUE	Modifiers				IOM Reference
33287	90	A	1(2)	51	N/A	N/A	N/A	None
33288	90	A	1(2)	51	N/A	N/A	N/A	

* with documentation

Terms To Know

electrode. Electric terminal specialized for a particular electrochemical reaction that acts as a medium between a body surface and another instrument, commonly termed a lead.

phrenic nerves. Two nerves that arise mainly from the fourth cervical nerve, providing motor nerve function to a side of the diaphragm, and serve in the breathing function. The right nerve plays a role in liver function.

pulse generator. Circuit used to generate pulses. Pulse generators contain the battery, the electronic circuit, and the connector in a hermetically sealed encasement. Pulse generators may be temporary transcutaneous or placed in a subcutaneous pocket.

33250-33251

33250 Operative ablation of supraventricular arrhythmogenic focus or pathway (eg, Wolff-Parkinson-White, atrioventricular node re-entry), tract(s) and/or focus (foci); without cardiopulmonary bypass

33251 with cardiopulmonary bypass

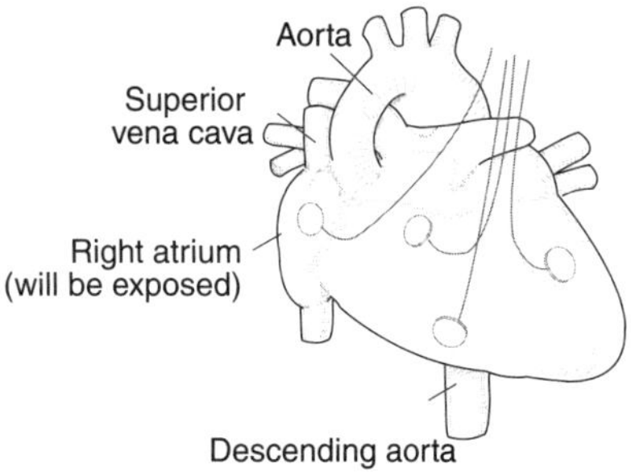

Mapping grid of electrodes is placed on the heart to determine the source of arrhythmia

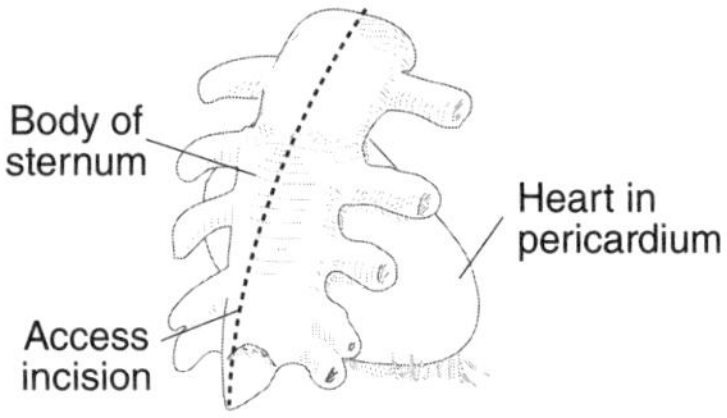

The source of a cardiac arrhythmia is determined in an open surgical procedure and supraventricular tissues are ablated

Explanation

In 33250, the heart is exposed through the sternum. A mapping grid of electrodes is placed over the surface of the beating heart. The location of the arrhythmia source is determined. The source is destroyed using electrical current, freezing, or cutting. Any bleeding is controlled with sutures. The chest is closed. In 33251, cardiopulmonary bypass is required. The heart is exposed through the sternum. A mapping grid of electrodes is placed over the surface of the beating heart. The right atrium is opened and a long cut is made around the tricuspid valve until the cut on the outside of the heart is seen. Any other focuses of the arrhythmia are destroyed with electrical current or freezing. The right atrium is closed. Cardiopulmonary bypass is discontinued when heart function returns. Typically this open approach is reserved for patients requiring surgery for additional conditions being replaced by ablation performed via catheter which is threaded through the femoral vein into the area of the heart requiring treatment.

Coding Tips

When this procedure is performed without cardiopulmonary bypass, report 33250; with cardiopulmonary bypass, report 33251. Report 93631 for intraoperative mapping performed by a separate provider. Note diagnosis when reporting ablation procedures. Ablation of supraventricular focus or pathway (Wolff-Parkinson-White syndrome) is reported with 33250–33251, while ablation of ventricular arrhythmogenic focus is reported with 33261. Open operative tissue ablation and reconstruction of atria is reported with 33254–33256. Endoscopic operative tissue ablation and reconstruction of atria is reported with 33265–33266. Ablation procedures are now frequently performed by intracardiac catheter instead of by thoracotomy. For transvenous intracardiac catheter ablation of supraventricular arrhythmogenic focus, see 93653. Insertion of a permanent pacemaker is reported separately, see 33202, 33203, 33207, or 33208.

ICD-10-CM Diagnostic Codes

I45.6	Pre-excitation syndrome
I45.89	Other specified conduction disorders
I47.0	Re-entry ventricular arrhythmia
I47.11	Inappropriate sinus tachycardia, so stated
I47.19	Other supraventricular tachycardia
I47.21	Torsades de pointes
I47.29	Other ventricular tachycardia
I48.0	Paroxysmal atrial fibrillation
I48.11	Longstanding persistent atrial fibrillation
I48.19	Other persistent atrial fibrillation
I48.21	Permanent atrial fibrillation
I48.3	Typical atrial flutter
I48.4	Atypical atrial flutter
I49.01	Ventricular fibrillation
I49.2	Junctional premature depolarization
I49.8	Other specified cardiac arrhythmias

Relative Value Units/Medicare Edits

Non-Facility RVU	Work	PE	MP	Total
33250	25.9	10.88	6.0	42.78
33251	28.92	11.99	7.16	48.07
Facility RVU	**Work**	**PE**	**MP**	**Total**
33250	25.9	10.88	6.0	42.78
33251	28.92	11.99	7.16	48.07

	FUD	Status	MUE	Modifiers				IOM Reference
33250	90	A	1(2)	51	N/A	62*	80	None
33251	90	A	1(2)	51	N/A	62*	80	

* with documentation

Terms To Know

ablation. Removal or destruction of tissue by cutting, electrical energy, chemical substances, or excessive heat application.

arrhythmias. Heart disorder of rhythm or rate, due to an electrical conduction system malfunction.

cardiopulmonary bypass. Venous blood is diverted to a heart-lung machine, which mechanically pumps and oxygenates the blood temporarily so the heart can be bypassed while an open procedure on the heart or coronary arteries is performed. During bypass, the lungs are deflated and immobile.

dysrhythmia. Abnormality or disturbance in rhythm.

paroxysmal supraventricular tachycardia. Rapid heartbeat that starts above the ventricles and occurs sporadically.

Wolff-Parkinson-White syndrome. Pre-excitation associated with paroxysmal tachycardia or atrial fibrillation with a short P-R interval on EKG and an early delta wave. The normal conduction pathway is bypassed.

33254-33256

33254 Operative tissue ablation and reconstruction of atria, limited (eg, modified maze procedure)

33255 Operative tissue ablation and reconstruction of atria, extensive (eg, maze procedure); without cardiopulmonary bypass

33256 with cardiopulmonary bypass

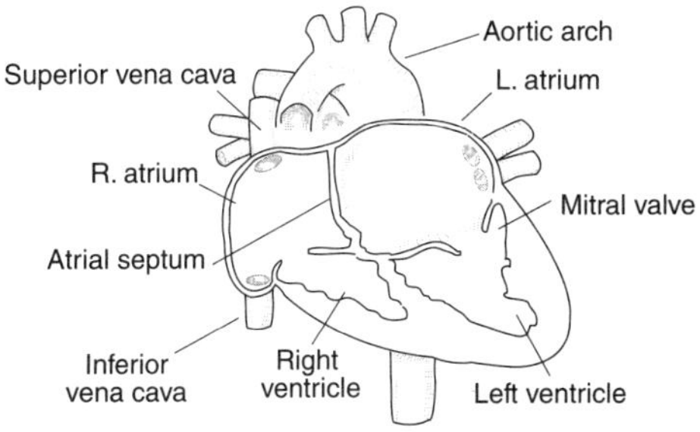

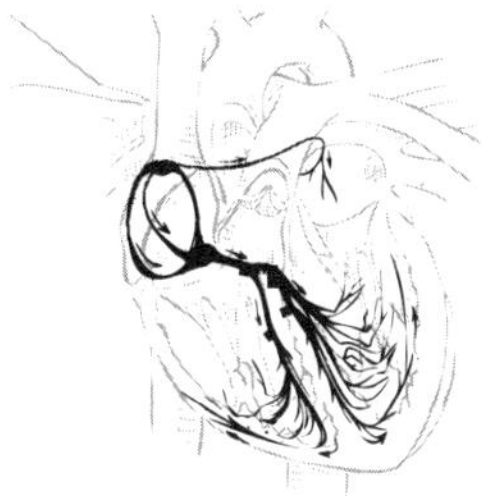

Conduction system of the heart

Explanation

The physician performs operative ablation and reconstruction of the atria to treat atrial fibrillation. Atrial fibrillation is rapid, randomized muscle contraction of the atrial myocardium causing an irregular, rapid heart rate. In a maze procedure, the physician seeks to permanently interrupt aberrant electrical conduction within the atria to restore normal sinus rhythm. The physician performs a midline sternotomy, incising the skin, fascia, muscles, and sternum. The pericardium is incised. For a limited operative ablation and reconstruction (33254), also referred to as a modified maze procedure, an incision is made into the left or right atrium. A combination of surgical incision and/or energy sources such as heat, microwave, laser, ultrasound, or cryoprobe is used to create lesions that will heal into scars that disrupt conduction. In 33255 and 33256, an extensive operative ablation and reconstruction is performed. In an extensive procedure, the right and/or left atrial tissue and/or atrial septum is treated as described in 33254, and additional operative ablation involving the atrioventricular annulus is performed. In any of these procedures, the left atrial appendage may be excised or isolated. In 33256, lines are placed for cardiopulmonary bypass. When cardiopulmonary bypass is achieved, an extensive ablation and reconstruction procedure is performed. The atrial incision lines are reanastomosed. The pericardium is repaired loosely, leaving gaps for blood and fluid to drain into the pleural space. The sternum is reanastomosed with sternal wires and the skin is sutured in layers.

Coding Tips

Excision or isolation of the left atrial appendage by any method, including stapling, oversewing, ligation, or plication, is included in the operative ablation procedure and should not be reported separately. Code 33254–33255 are reported only when there is no concurrently performed procedure requiring median sternotomy or cardiopulmonary bypass. If operative ablation is performed with a concurrent procedure requiring median sternotomy or cardiopulmonary bypass, the operative ablation procedure should be reported with unlisted procedure code 33999. For operative tissue ablation and reconstruction of atria performed endoscopically, see 33265 or 33266. Do not report 33254–33256 with 32100, 32551, 33120, 33130, 33210, 33211, 33390, 33391, 33404–33507, 33510–33523, 33533–33548, 33600–33853, 33858–33864, or 33910–33920.

ICD-10-CM Diagnostic Codes

I47.11	Inappropriate sinus tachycardia, so stated
I47.19	Other supraventricular tachycardia
I48.0	Paroxysmal atrial fibrillation
I48.11	Longstanding persistent atrial fibrillation
I48.19	Other persistent atrial fibrillation
I48.21	Permanent atrial fibrillation
I48.3	Typical atrial flutter
I48.4	Atypical atrial flutter
I49.2	Junctional premature depolarization
I49.8	Other specified cardiac arrhythmias

AMA: 33254 2021,Nov **33255** 2021,Nov **33256** 2021,Nov

Relative Value Units/Medicare Edits

Non-Facility RVU	Work	PE	MP	Total
33254	23.71	10.78	5.72	40.21
33255	29.04	11.98	6.71	47.73
33256	34.9	13.54	8.07	56.51
Facility RVU	**Work**	**PE**	**MP**	**Total**
33254	23.71	10.78	5.72	40.21
33255	29.04	11.98	6.71	47.73
33256	34.9	13.54	8.07	56.51

	FUD	Status	MUE	Modifiers				IOM Reference
33254	90	A	1(2)	51	N/A	62*	80	None
33255	90	A	1(2)	51	N/A	62*	80	
33256	90	A	1(2)	51	N/A	62*	80	

* with documentation

Terms To Know

ablation. Removal or destruction of tissue by cutting, electrical energy, chemical substances, or excessive heat application.

arrhythmias. Heart disorder of rhythm or rate, due to an electrical conduction system malfunction.

cardiopulmonary bypass. Venous blood is diverted to a heart-lung machine, which mechanically pumps and oxygenates the blood temporarily so the heart can be bypassed while an open procedure on the heart or coronary arteries is performed. During bypass, the lungs are deflated and immobile.

33257

\+ **33257** Operative tissue ablation and reconstruction of atria, performed at the time of other cardiac procedure(s), limited (eg, modified maze procedure) (List separately in addition to code for primary procedure)

Explanation

Concurrently with other cardiac procedures, the physician performs operative tissue ablation and reconstruction of the atria to treat atrial fibrillation. Atrial fibrillation is rapid, randomized muscle contraction of the atrial myocardium causing an irregular, rapid heart rate. In this procedure, the physician seeks to permanently interrupt aberrant electrical conduction within the atria to restore normal sinus rhythm. The physician performs a midline sternotomy, incising the skin, fascia, muscles, and sternum. The pericardium is incised. For a limited operative tissue ablation and reconstruction of atria, also referred to as a modified maze procedure, an incision is made into the left or right atrium. A combination of surgical incision and/or energy sources, such as heat, microwave, laser, ultrasound, or cryoprobe, is used to create lesions that will heal into scars that disrupt conduction. The left atrial appendage may be excised or isolated. The atrial incision lines are reanastomosed. The pericardium is repaired loosely, leaving gaps for blood and fluid to drain into the pleural space. The sternum is reanastomosed with sternal wires and the skin is sutured in layers.

Coding Tips

Report 33257 in addition to 33120–33130, 33250–33251, 33261, 33300–33335, 33390–33391, 33404–33496, 33500–33507, 33510–33516, 33533–33548, 33600–33619, 33641–33697, 33702–33732, 33735–33767, 33770, 33877, 33910–33922, 33925–33926, and 33975–33983. Do not report 33257 with 32551, 33210, 33211, 33254–33256, 33265, or 33266. When performed concurrently, 33257 is reported with open cardiac procedures that require sternotomy.

ICD-10-CM Diagnostic Codes

This/these CPT code(s) are add-on code(s). See the primary procedure code that this code is performed with for your ICD-10-CM code selections. Diagnostic code(s) would be the same as the actual procedure performed.

AMA: 33257 2021,Nov

Relative Value Units/Medicare Edits

Non-Facility RVU	Work	PE	MP	Total
33257	9.63	5.32	2.3	17.25
Facility RVU	**Work**	**PE**	**MP**	**Total**
33257	9.63	5.32	2.3	17.25

	FUD	Status	MUE	Modifiers				IOM Reference
33257	N/A	A	1(2)	N/A	N/A	N/A	80	None

* with documentation

Terms To Know

ablation. Removal or destruction of tissue by cutting, electrical energy, chemical substances, or excessive heat application.

reconstruction. Recreating, restoring, or rebuilding a body part or organ.

tissue. Group of similar cells with a similar function that form definite structures and organs. Tissue types include epithelial tissue, muscle tissue, connective tissue, and nervous tissue.

33258

\+ **33258** Operative tissue ablation and reconstruction of atria, performed at the time of other cardiac procedure(s), extensive (eg, maze procedure), without cardiopulmonary bypass (List separately in addition to code for primary procedure)

Explanation

Concurrently with other cardiac procedures, the physician performs operative tissue ablation and reconstruction of the atria to treat atrial fibrillation. Atrial fibrillation is rapid, randomized muscle contraction of the atrial myocardium causing an irregular, rapid heart rate. In this procedure, the physician seeks to permanently interrupt aberrant electrical conduction within the atria to restore normal sinus rhythm. The physician performs a midline sternotomy, incising the skin, fascia, muscles, and sternum. The pericardium is incised. For an extensive operative tissue ablation and reconstruction of the atria, also referred to as a Maze procedure, an incision is made into the left or right atrium. A combination of surgical incision and/or energy sources, such as heat, microwave, laser, ultrasound, or cryoprobe, is used to create lesions that will heal into scars that disrupt conduction. Additional operative ablation involving the atrioventricular annulus is also performed. The left atrial appendage may be excised or isolated. The atrial incision lines are reanastomosed. The pericardium is repaired loosely, leaving gaps for blood and fluid to drain into the pleural space. The sternum is reanastomosed with sternal wires and the skin is sutured in layers.

Coding Tips

Report 33258 with the following codes when cardiopulmonary bypass is not performed: 33130, 33250, 33300, 33310, 33320, 33321, 33330, 33365, 33420, 33501–33503, 33510–33516, 33533–33536, 33690, 33735, 33750, 33755, 33762-33766, 33800–33803, 33820–33824, 33840–33852, 33875, 33877, 33915, 33925, 33981, and 33982. Do not report 33258 with 32551, 33210, 33211, 33254–33256, 33265, or 33266. When performed concurrently, 33258 is reported with open cardiac procedures that require sternotomy.

ICD-10-CM Diagnostic Codes

This/these CPT code(s) are add-on code(s). See the primary procedure code that this code is performed with for your ICD-10-CM code selections. Diagnostic code(s) would be the same as the actual procedure performed.

AMA: 33258 2021,Nov

Relative Value Units/Medicare Edits

Non-Facility RVU	Work	PE	MP	Total
33258	11.0	5.62	2.54	19.16
Facility RVU	**Work**	**PE**	**MP**	**Total**
33258	11.0	5.62	2.54	19.16

	FUD	Status	MUE	Modifiers				IOM Reference
33258	N/A	A	1(2)	N/A	N/A	N/A	80	None

* with documentation

Terms To Know

ablation. Removal or destruction of tissue by cutting, electrical energy, chemical substances, or excessive heat application.

reconstruction. Recreating, restoring, or rebuilding a body part or organ.

Heart and Pericardium

33259

\+ **33259** Operative tissue ablation and reconstruction of atria, performed at the time of other cardiac procedure(s), extensive (eg, maze procedure), with cardiopulmonary bypass (List separately in addition to code for primary procedure)

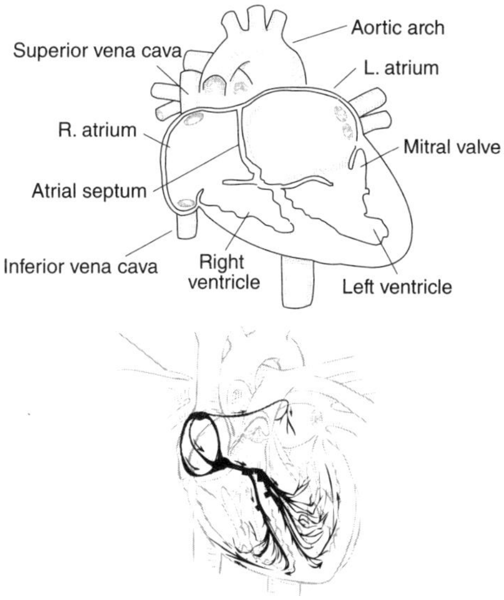

Conduction system of the heart

Aberrant conduction is treated with open heart surgery isolating the pulmonary veins or other anatomically defined triggers in the left or right atrium

Explanation

Concurrently with other cardiac procedures, the physician performs operative tissue ablation and reconstruction of the atria to treat atrial fibrillation. Atrial fibrillation is rapid, randomized muscle contraction of the atrial myocardium causing an irregular, rapid heart rate. In this procedure, the physician seeks to permanently interrupt aberrant electrical conduction within the atria to restore normal sinus rhythm. The physician performs a midline sternotomy, incising the skin, fascia, muscles, and sternum. The pericardium is incised. For an extensive operative tissue ablation and reconstruction of atria with cardiopulmonary bypass, also referred to as a maze procedure, lines are first placed for cardiopulmonary bypass. When cardiopulmonary bypass is achieved, an incision is made into the left or right atrium. A combination of surgical incision and/or energy sources, such as heat, microwave, laser, ultrasound, or cryoprobe, is used to create lesions that will heal into scars that disrupt conduction. Additional operative ablation involving the atrioventricular annulus is also performed. The left atrial appendage may be excised or isolated. The atrial incision lines are reanastomosed. The pericardium is repaired loosely, leaving gaps for blood and fluid to drain into the pleural space. The sternum is reanastomosed with sternal wires and the skin is sutured in layers.

Coding Tips

Report 33259 in addition to the following codes when performed with cardiopulmonary bypass: 33120, 33251, 33261, 33305, 33315, 33322, 33335, 33390–33391, 33404–33417, 33422–33468, 33474–33478, 33496, 33500, 33504–33507, 33510–33516, 33533–33548, 33600–33688, 33692–33726, 33730, 33732, 33736, 33767, 33770, 33783, 33786–33788, 33814, 33853, 33858–33877, 33910, 33916–33922, 33926, 33975–33980, and 33983. Do not report 33259 with 32551, 33210, 33211, 33254–33256, 33265, or 33266. When performed concurrently, 33259 is reported with open cardiac procedures that require sternotomy or cardiopulmonary bypass.

ICD-10-CM Diagnostic Codes

This/these CPT code(s) are add-on code(s). See the primary procedure code that this code is performed with for your ICD-10-CM code selections. Diagnostic code(s) would be the same as the actual procedure performed.

AMA: **33259** 2021,Nov

Relative Value Units/Medicare Edits

Non-Facility RVU	Work	PE	MP	Total
33259	14.14	7.56	3.36	25.06
Facility RVU	**Work**	**PE**	**MP**	**Total**
33259	14.14	7.56	3.36	25.06

	FUD	Status	MUE	Modifiers				IOM Reference
33259	N/A	A	1(2)	N/A	N/A	N/A	80	None

* with documentation

Terms To Know

ablation. Removal or destruction of tissue by cutting, electrical energy, chemical substances, or excessive heat application.

cardiopulmonary bypass. Venous blood is diverted to a heart-lung machine, which mechanically pumps and oxygenates the blood temporarily so the heart can be bypassed while an open procedure on the heart or coronary arteries is performed. During bypass, the lungs are deflated and immobile.

reconstruction. Recreating, restoring, or rebuilding a body part or organ.

tissue. Group of similar cells with a similar function that form definite structures and organs. Tissue types include epithelial tissue, muscle tissue, connective tissue, and nervous tissue.

33261

33261 Operative ablation of ventricular arrhythmogenic focus with cardiopulmonary bypass

Impulse centers that are causing arrhythmia are treated with ablation

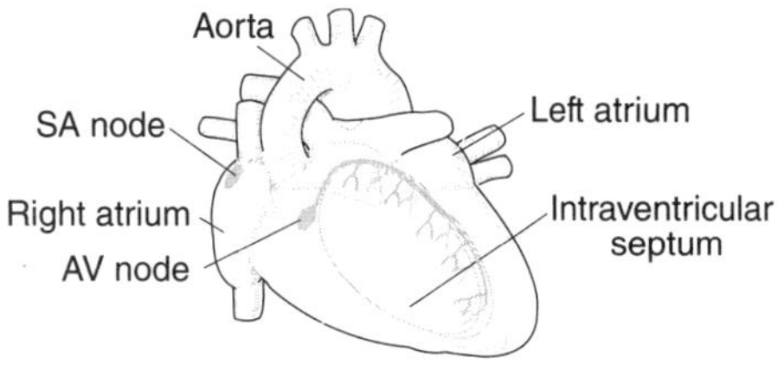

Bypass schematic

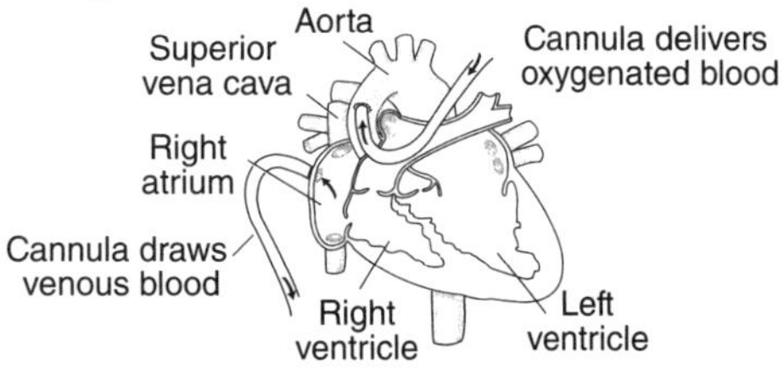

Specialized heart muscle fibers initiate the electrical impulses that contract the atria and the ventricles. The sinoatrial node (SA) is the pacemaker of the heart and initiates the impulse, first contracting the atria. The atrioventricular node (AV) receives the signal from the atria and redistributes it along the intraventricular septum to the muscles that contract the ventricles

Explanation

Following initiation of cardiopulmonary bypass, the physician exposes the heart through the sternum. A mapping grid of electrodes is placed over the surface of the beating heart. The location of the arrhythmia source is determined. The source is destroyed using electrical current, freezing or cutting, though not in the tricuspid valve. Any bleeding is controlled with sutures. The chest is closed.

Coding Tips

To report operative ablation of arrhythmogenic focus by ventricular aneurysmectomy, see 33542. Note diagnosis when reporting ablation procedures. Ablation of ventricular arrhythmogenic focus is reported with 33261, while ablation of supraventricular focus or pathway (Wolff-Parkinson-White syndrome) is reported with 33250–33251. Note also that 33261 involves ventricular ablation below the bundle of His. For open operative tissue ablation and reconstruction of atria, see 33254–33256. For endoscopic operative tissue ablation and reconstruction of atria, see 33265–33266. For transvenous intracardiac catheter ablation of ventricular arrhythmogenic focus, see 93654.

ICD-10-CM Diagnostic Codes

I45.6	Pre-excitation syndrome
I45.89	Other specified conduction disorders
I47.0	Re-entry ventricular arrhythmia
I47.11	Inappropriate sinus tachycardia, so stated
I47.19	Other supraventricular tachycardia
I47.21	Torsades de pointes
I47.29	Other ventricular tachycardia
I48.0	Paroxysmal atrial fibrillation
I48.11	Longstanding persistent atrial fibrillation
I48.19	Other persistent atrial fibrillation
I48.21	Permanent atrial fibrillation
I48.3	Typical atrial flutter
I48.4	Atypical atrial flutter
I49.01	Ventricular fibrillation
I49.02	Ventricular flutter
I49.2	Junctional premature depolarization
I49.8	Other specified cardiac arrhythmias

Relative Value Units/Medicare Edits

Non-Facility RVU	Work	PE	MP	Total
33261	28.92	11.69	6.68	47.29
Facility RVU	**Work**	**PE**	**MP**	**Total**
33261	28.92	11.69	6.68	47.29

	FUD	Status	MUE	Modifiers				IOM Reference
33261	90	A	1(2)	51	N/A	62*	80	None

* with documentation

Terms To Know

ablation. Removal or destruction of tissue by cutting, electrical energy, chemical substances, or excessive heat application.

arrhythmias. Heart disorder of rhythm or rate, due to an electrical conduction system malfunction.

cardiopulmonary bypass. Venous blood is diverted to a heart-lung machine, which mechanically pumps and oxygenates the blood temporarily so the heart can be bypassed while an open procedure on the heart or coronary arteries is performed. During bypass, the lungs are deflated and immobile.

catheter. Flexible tube inserted into an area of the body for introducing or withdrawing fluid.

dysrhythmia. Abnormality or disturbance in rhythm.

lesion. Area of damaged tissue that has lost continuity or function, due to disease or trauma. Lesions may be located on internal structures such as the brain, nerves, or kidneys, or visible on the skin.

Lown (-Ganong)-Levine syndrome. Electrocardiographic disorder indicated by a short P-R interval with normal duration of the QRS complex.

paroxysmal supraventricular tachycardia. Rapid heartbeat that starts above the ventricles and occurs sporadically.

thoracotomy. Surgical procedure for opening the chest wall in order to access the lungs, esophagus, trachea, aorta, heart, and diaphragm.

Wolff-Parkinson-White syndrome. Pre-excitation associated with paroxysmal tachycardia or atrial fibrillation with a short P-R interval on EKG and an early delta wave. The normal conduction pathway is bypassed.

[33267, 33268]

33267 Exclusion of left atrial appendage, open, any method (eg, excision, isolation via stapling, oversewing, ligation, plication, clip)

\+ **33268** Exclusion of left atrial appendage, open, performed at the time of other sternotomy or thoracotomy procedure(s), any method (eg, excision, isolation via stapling, oversewing, ligation, plication, clip) (List separately in addition to code for primary procedure)

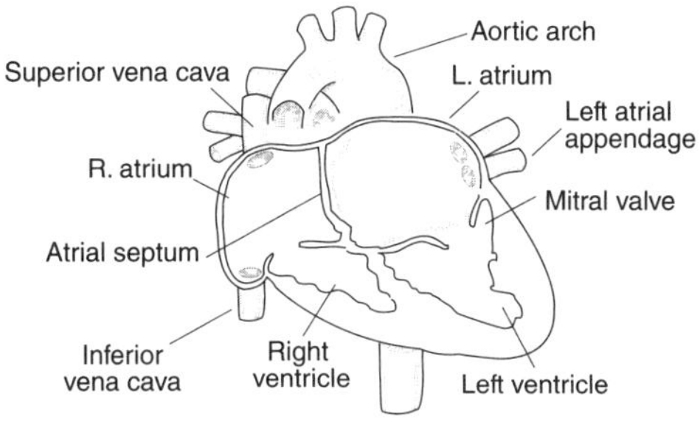

Open exclusion of left atrial appendage

Explanation

The physician excludes the left atrial appendage (LAA) from systemic circulation using an open approach via sternotomy or thoracotomy. Exclusion may be performed by any method (i.e., clip, excision, ligation, oversewing, plication, or stapling). In patients with atrial fibrillation, abnormal electrical impulses prevent the heart from effectively pumping the blood from the atria into the ventricles. Blood collects in the LAA, where clots can form and travel outside the heart to the brain, resulting in stroke. The LAA is the most common site of thrombosis in those with atrial fibrillation. In 33267, the LAA exclusion is the primary procedure. In 33268, the exclusion is performed during the same operative episode as another open cardiac procedure.

Coding Tips

Code 33267 should not be reported with other sternotomy or thoracotomy procedures performed during the same encounter. Code 33268 may be reported with a primary procedure performed via thoracotomy or sternotomy. Surgical LAA exclusion is inherent to 33254-33259, 33265, 33266, 33420, 33422, 33425-33427, and 33430 and should not be reported separately when performed at the same encounter.

ICD-10-CM Diagnostic Codes

I48.0	Paroxysmal atrial fibrillation
I48.11	Longstanding persistent atrial fibrillation
I48.19	Other persistent atrial fibrillation
I48.21	Permanent atrial fibrillation

AMA: 33267 2021,Nov **33268** 2021,Nov

Relative Value Units/Medicare Edits

Non-Facility RVU	Work	PE	MP	Total
33267	18.5	7.94	4.36	30.8
33268	2.5	0.7	0.59	3.79
Facility RVU	**Work**	**PE**	**MP**	**Total**
33267	18.5	7.94	4.36	30.8
33268	2.5	0.7	0.59	3.79

	FUD	Status	MUE	Modifiers				IOM Reference
33267	90	A	1(2)	51	N/A	62*	80	None
33268	N/A	A	1(2)	N/A	N/A	N/A	80	

* with documentation

Terms To Know

LAA. Left atrial appendage.

sternotomy. Incision into the sternum, the bone that forms the front of the chest cavity and connects with the ribs.

thoracotomy. Surgical procedure for opening the chest wall in order to access the lungs, esophagus, trachea, aorta, heart, and diaphragm.

Heart and Pericardium

[33269]

33269 Exclusion of left atrial appendage, thoracoscopic, any method (eg, excision, isolation via stapling, oversewing, ligation, plication, clip)

Explanation

The physician excludes the left atrial appendage (LAA) from systemic circulation using a thoracoscopic approach. Exclusion may be performed by any method (i.e., clip, excision, ligation, oversewing, plication, or stapling). In patients with atrial fibrillation, abnormal electrical impulses prevent the heart from effectively pumping the blood from the atria into the ventricles. Blood collects in the LAA, where clots can form and travel outside the heart to the brain, resulting in stroke. The LAA is the most common site of thrombosis in those with atrial fibrillation. One method utilizes a proprietary clip device. With the patient in a supine position and under appropriate anesthesia, three thoracoscopic ports are placed and access to the left side of the chest is obtained. Pericardial blood vessels are cauterized, and the pericardium is opened to expose the LAA. Using a sizing tool inserted through a lower port, the LAA is measured and the appropriate clip size is selected. The device holding the clip is inserted through the port, manipulated over the LAA, positioned onto the base of the LAA and closed, using echocardiographic guidance to assure complete closure. The clip may be opened and repositioned until adequate closure is obtained. The clip is then released, instruments are removed, and port sites are closed.

Coding Tips

This code may be used to report thoracoscopic LAA exclusion. Codes 33254-33259, 33265, 33266, 33420, 33422, 33425-33427, and 33430 are inherent to surgical LAA exclusion and should not be reported separately when performed at the same encounter.

ICD-10-CM Diagnostic Codes

I48.0	Paroxysmal atrial fibrillation
I48.11	Longstanding persistent atrial fibrillation
I48.19	Other persistent atrial fibrillation
I48.21	Permanent atrial fibrillation

AMA: **33269** 2021,Nov

Relative Value Units/Medicare Edits

Non-Facility RVU	Work	PE	MP	Total
33269	14.31	6.74	3.45	24.5
Facility RVU	**Work**	**PE**	**MP**	**Total**
33269	14.31	6.74	3.45	24.5

	FUD	Status	MUE	Modifiers				IOM Reference
33269	90	A	1(2)	51	N/A	62*	80	None

* with documentation

Terms To Know

cautery. Destruction or burning of tissue by means of a hot instrument, an electric current, or a caustic chemical, such as silver nitrate.

LAA. Left atrial appendage.

plication. Surgical technique involving folding, tucking, or pleating to reduce the size of a hollow structure or organ.

33265-33266

33265 Endoscopy, surgical; operative tissue ablation and reconstruction of atria, limited (eg, modified maze procedure), without cardiopulmonary bypass

33266 operative tissue ablation and reconstruction of atria, extensive (eg, maze procedure), without cardiopulmonary bypass

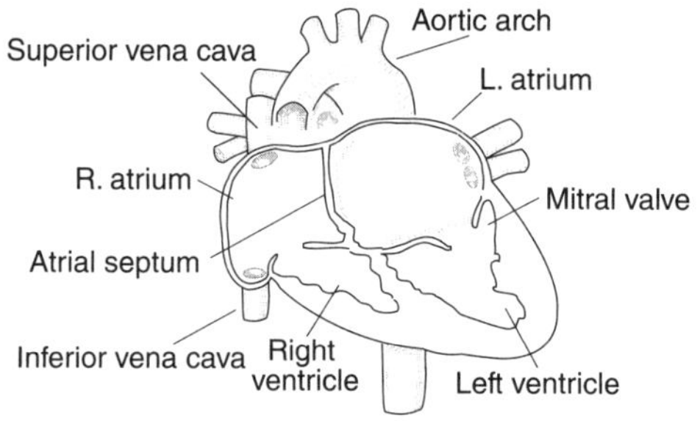

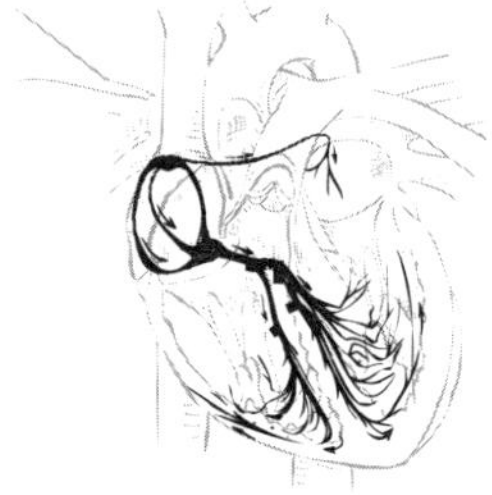

Conduction system of the heart

Aberrant conduction is treated endoscopically through multiple, small chest incisions

Explanation

The physician performs endoscopic operative ablation and reconstruction of the atria to treat atrial fibrillation. Atrial fibrillation is rapid, randomized muscle contraction of the atrial myocardium causing an irregular, rapid heart rate. In a maze procedure, the physician seeks to permanently interrupt aberrant electrical conduction within the atria to restore normal sinus rhythm. Through multiple endoscopic incisions in the chest, the physician accesses and visualizes the outer (epicardial) surface of the heart. For a limited or modified maze procedure performed endoscopically (33265), the pulmonary veins or other anatomically defined triggers are isolated in the left or right atrium and a heat, microwave, laser, ultrasound, or cryoprobe is used to create lesions from the outside of the left atrium that will heal into scars that disrupt conduction. In 33266, the right and/or left atrial tissue and/or atrial septum is treated as described in 33265, and additional operative ablation involving the atrioventricular annulus is performed. In either of these procedures, the left atrial appendage may be excised or isolated. Once sufficient interruption of electrical conduction has been accomplished, the endoscope is removed and access incisions are sutured in layers.

Coding Tips

Excision or isolation of the left atrial appendage by any method, including stapling, oversewing, ligation, or plication, is included in the operative ablation procedure and should not be reported separately. Do not report tube thoracostomy (32551) or temporary pacemaker (33210–33211) separately as these procedures are included in 33265 and 33266. For open operative ablation and reconstruction of atria, see 33254–33256.

ICD-10-CM Diagnostic Codes

I48.0	Paroxysmal atrial fibrillation
I48.11	Longstanding persistent atrial fibrillation

I48.19 Other persistent atrial fibrillation
I48.21 Permanent atrial fibrillation
I48.3 Typical atrial flutter
I48.4 Atypical atrial flutter
I49.2 Junctional premature depolarization
I49.8 Other specified cardiac arrhythmias

AMA: **33265** 2021,Nov **33266** 2021,Nov

Relative Value Units/Medicare Edits

Non-Facility RVU	Work	PE	MP	Total
33265	23.71	10.77	5.7	40.18
33266	33.04	13.2	7.96	54.2
Facility RVU	**Work**	**PE**	**MP**	**Total**
33265	23.71	10.77	5.7	40.18
33266	33.04	13.2	7.96	54.2

	FUD	Status	MUE	Modifiers				IOM Reference
33265	90	A	1(2)	51	N/A	62*	80	None
33266	90	A	1(2)	51	N/A	62*	80	

* with documentation

Terms To Know

ablation. Removal or destruction of tissue by cutting, electrical energy, chemical substances, or excessive heat application.

arrhythmias. Heart disorder of rhythm or rate, due to an electrical conduction system malfunction.

cryosurgery. Application of intense cold, usually produced using liquid nitrogen, to locally freeze diseased or unwanted tissue and induce tissue necrosis without causing harm to adjacent tissue.

endoscopy. Visual inspection of the body using a fiberoptic scope.

laser surgery. Use of concentrated, sharply defined light beams to cut, cauterize, coagulate, seal, or vaporize tissue.

33285-33286

33285 Insertion, subcutaneous cardiac rhythm monitor, including programming
33286 Removal, subcutaneous cardiac rhythm monitor

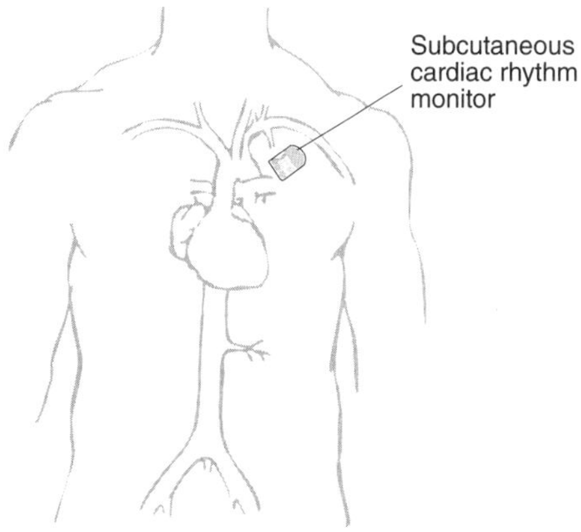

Explanation

The physician implants or removes an electronic device that is capable of recording heartrates and rhythms for over one year (subcutaneous cardiac rhythm monitor, cardiac event recorder, implantable loop recorder or ILR). In 33285, the physician uses a scalpel to make a small parasternal incision and dissects down to the level of subcutaneous tissue located over the left pectoral or mammary area. The monitor is implanted into the subcutaneous tissue. Electrodes that sense heart activity are located on the surface of the monitor, making it unnecessary to place transvenous leads. The device continuously and automatically monitors the heart's electrical activity when sensing the patient's rapid, irregular, or slow heartrate or can also be prompted by the patient in the course of experiencing symptoms. Programming of the device is included in this service. In 33286, the physician removes the monitor when sufficient information regarding the heart's activities has been obtained or when the batteries run out by incising down to the level of the recorder and removing it. In either surgery, the incision is closed with sutures. This type of recorder is capable of storing many separate events. When appropriate, a "programmer" is used by the physician to retrieve the information that can be displayed, stored, or printed.

Coding Tips

Code 33285 includes programming. For subsequent analysis and/or reprogramming, see 93285, 93291, and 93298.

ICD-10-CM Diagnostic Codes

G90.09 Other idiopathic peripheral autonomic neuropathy
I25.2 Old myocardial infarction
I44.0 Atrioventricular block, first degree
I44.1 Atrioventricular block, second degree
I44.2 Atrioventricular block, complete
I45.5 Other specified heart block
I45.6 Pre-excitation syndrome
I47.0 Re-entry ventricular arrhythmia
I47.11 Inappropriate sinus tachycardia, so stated
I47.21 Torsades de pointes

I47.29	Other ventricular tachycardia
I48.0	Paroxysmal atrial fibrillation
I48.11	Longstanding persistent atrial fibrillation
I48.19	Other persistent atrial fibrillation
I48.21	Permanent atrial fibrillation
I48.3	Typical atrial flutter
I48.4	Atypical atrial flutter
I49.01	Ventricular fibrillation
I49.02	Ventricular flutter
I49.1	Atrial premature depolarization
I49.2	Junctional premature depolarization
I49.3	Ventricular premature depolarization
I49.49	Other premature depolarization
I49.5	Sick sinus syndrome
I49.8	Other specified cardiac arrhythmias
I50.1	Left ventricular failure, unspecified
I50.21	Acute systolic (congestive) heart failure
I50.22	Chronic systolic (congestive) heart failure
I50.23	Acute on chronic systolic (congestive) heart failure
I50.31	Acute diastolic (congestive) heart failure
I50.32	Chronic diastolic (congestive) heart failure
I50.33	Acute on chronic diastolic (congestive) heart failure
I50.41	Acute combined systolic (congestive) and diastolic (congestive) heart failure
I50.42	Chronic combined systolic (congestive) and diastolic (congestive) heart failure
I50.43	Acute on chronic combined systolic (congestive) and diastolic (congestive) heart failure
I50.811	Acute right heart failure
I50.812	Chronic right heart failure
I50.813	Acute on chronic right heart failure
I50.814	Right heart failure due to left heart failure
I50.82	Biventricular heart failure
I50.83	High output heart failure
I50.84	End stage heart failure
I50.89	Other heart failure
I97.110	Postprocedural cardiac insufficiency following cardiac surgery
I97.111	Postprocedural cardiac insufficiency following other surgery
I97.130	Postprocedural heart failure following cardiac surgery
I97.131	Postprocedural heart failure following other surgery
I97.190	Other postprocedural cardiac functional disturbances following cardiac surgery
I97.191	Other postprocedural cardiac functional disturbances following other surgery
I97.790	Other intraoperative cardiac functional disturbances during cardiac surgery
I97.791	Other intraoperative cardiac functional disturbances during other surgery
Q24.6	Congenital heart block
R00.2	Palpitations
R42	Dizziness and giddiness
R55	Syncope and collapse
R94.31	Abnormal electrocardiogram [ECG] [EKG]
T82.518A	Breakdown (mechanical) of other cardiac and vascular devices and implants, initial encounter
T82.528A	Displacement of other cardiac and vascular devices and implants, initial encounter
T82.538A	Leakage of other cardiac and vascular devices and implants, initial encounter
T82.598A	Other mechanical complication of other cardiac and vascular devices and implants, initial encounter
T82.7XXA	Infection and inflammatory reaction due to other cardiac and vascular devices, implants and grafts, initial encounter
T82.827A	Fibrosis due to cardiac prosthetic devices, implants and grafts, initial encounter
T82.837A	Hemorrhage due to cardiac prosthetic devices, implants and grafts, initial encounter
T82.847A	Pain due to cardiac prosthetic devices, implants and grafts, initial encounter
T82.867A	Thrombosis due to cardiac prosthetic devices, implants and grafts, initial encounter
T82.897A	Other specified complication of cardiac prosthetic devices, implants and grafts, initial encounter
Z45.09	Encounter for adjustment and management of other cardiac device

Associated HCPCS Codes

C1764	Event recorder, cardiac (implantable)
E0616	Implantable cardiac event recorder with memory, activator, and programmer

AMA: 33285 2019,Oct; 2019,Apr **33286** 2019,Apr

Relative Value Units/Medicare Edits

Non-Facility RVU	Work	PE	MP	Total
33285	1.53	122.46	0.35	124.34
33286	1.5	2.03	0.34	3.87
Facility RVU	**Work**	**PE**	**MP**	**Total**
33285	1.53	0.69	0.35	2.57
33286	1.5	0.68	0.34	2.52

	FUD	Status	MUE	Modifiers				IOM Reference
33285	0	A	1(3)	51	N/A	N/A	N/A	None
33286	0	A	1(3)	51	N/A	N/A	N/A	

* with documentation

Terms To Know

event recorder. Portable, ambulatory heart monitor worn by the patient that makes electrocardiographic recordings of the length and frequency of aberrant cardiac rhythm to help diagnose heart conditions and to assess pacemaker functioning or programming.

implantable cardiovascular monitor. Implantable electronic device that stores cardiovascular physiologic data such as intracardiac pressure waveforms collected from internal sensors or data such as weight and blood pressure collected from external sensors. The information stored in these devices is used as an aid in managing patients with heart failure and other cardiac conditions that are non-rhythm related. The data may be transmitted via local telemetry or remotely to a surveillance technician or an internet-based file server.

33289

33289 Transcatheter implantation of wireless pulmonary artery pressure sensor for long-term hemodynamic monitoring, including deployment and calibration of the sensor, right heart catheterization, selective pulmonary catheterization, radiological supervision and interpretation, and pulmonary artery angiography, when performed

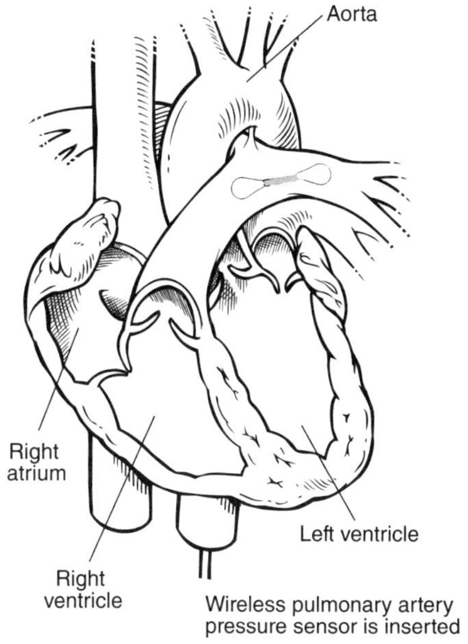

Explanation

The physician places a pulmonary pressure monitoring system. A proprietary device comprised of a battery-free sensor is placed directly in a distal portion of the pulmonary artery of a patient with heart failure to permit ongoing monitoring and measurement of the patient's heartrate, as well as systolic, diastolic, and mean pressures. The system is placed via a corresponding catheter. Pulmonary arterial pressure (PAP) readings transmitted from the sensor to a wireless electronic unit are subsequently transmitted to an online portal that can be accessed by the patient's treating health care provider. Through accurate monitoring of patients diagnosed with heart failure (HF) for exacerbations, it is possible to minimize the need for additional hospitalizations and the associated complications and allow for early pharmacological intervention. Deployment and calibration of the sensor, as well as any associated catheterizations, angiography, and radiological supervision and interpretation, are included in this service, when performed.

Coding Tips

Imaging guidance is included in this procedure and is not reported separately. For remote monitoring of an implantable wireless pulmonary artery pressure sensor, see 93264. Do not report 33289 with 36013-36015, 75741, 75743, 75746, 76000, 93451, 93453, 93456, 93457, 93460, 93461, 93568, 93569, 93573, 93593, 93594, or 93596-93598.

ICD-10-CM Diagnostic Codes

I50.1	Left ventricular failure, unspecified
I50.21	Acute systolic (congestive) heart failure
I50.22	Chronic systolic (congestive) heart failure
I50.23	Acute on chronic systolic (congestive) heart failure
I50.31	Acute diastolic (congestive) heart failure
I50.32	Chronic diastolic (congestive) heart failure
I50.33	Acute on chronic diastolic (congestive) heart failure
I50.41	Acute combined systolic (congestive) and diastolic (congestive) heart failure
I50.42	Chronic combined systolic (congestive) and diastolic (congestive) heart failure
I50.43	Acute on chronic combined systolic (congestive) and diastolic (congestive) heart failure
I50.810	Right heart failure, unspecified
I50.811	Acute right heart failure
I50.812	Chronic right heart failure
I50.813	Acute on chronic right heart failure
I50.814	Right heart failure due to left heart failure
I50.82	Biventricular heart failure
I50.83	High output heart failure
I50.84	End stage heart failure
I50.89	Other heart failure

AMA: 33289 2023,May; 2019,Jun

Relative Value Units/Medicare Edits

Non-Facility RVU	Work	PE	MP	Total
33289	6.0	2.44	1.35	9.79
Facility RVU	**Work**	**PE**	**MP**	**Total**
33289	6.0	2.44	1.35	9.79

	FUD	Status	MUE	Modifiers				IOM Reference
33289	0	A	1(3)	51	N/A	N/A	80*	None

* with documentation

Terms To Know

angiography. Radiographic imaging of the arteries. Imaging may be performed to study the vasculature of any given organ, body system, or area of circulation such as the brain, heart, chest, kidneys, limbs, gastrointestinal tract, aorta, and pulmonary circulation to visualize the formation and the function of the blood vessels to detect problems such as a blockage or stricture. A catheter is inserted through an accessible blood vessel and the artery is injected with a radiopaque contrast material after which x-rays are taken.

calibration. Action or process that involves adjusting, checking, or comparing using a standard of accuracy of an instrument in order to ensure consistent and accurate readings.

distal. ***1)*** Located farther away from a specified reference point or the trunk. ***2)*** Pertaining to the area farthest from the center of the body or the point of origin.

hemodynamic monitoring. Measurement of the blood pressure inside the veins, heart, and arteries as well as blood flow and the amount of oxygen in the blood as a way to see how well the heart is functioning.

transcatheter. Procedure or treatment performed via a catheter.

33300-33305

33300 Repair of cardiac wound; without bypass
33305 with cardiopulmonary bypass

A wound to the heart is repaired

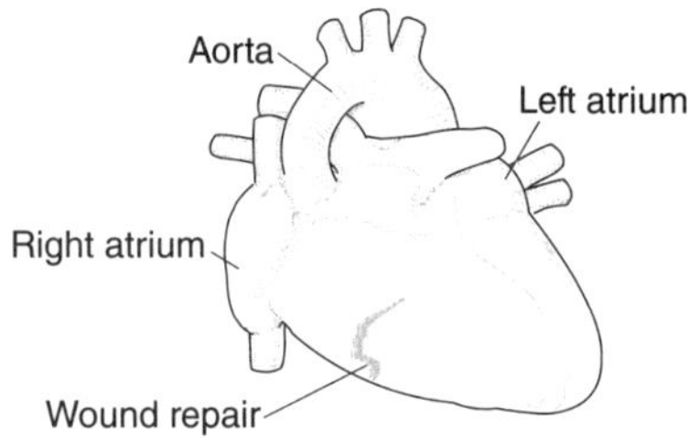

Bypass schematic

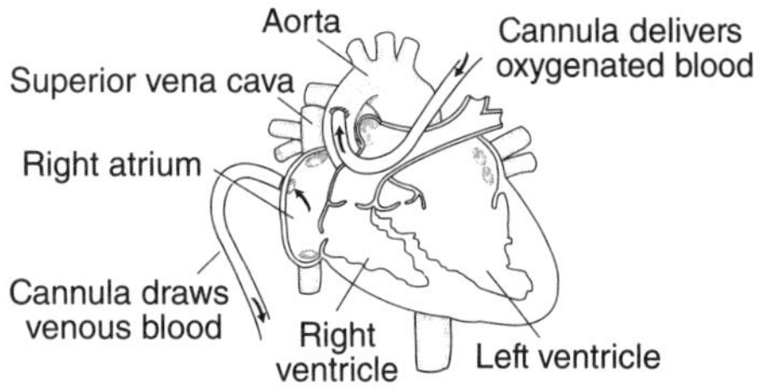

Explanation

The physician gains access to the heart using an incision through the sternum (median sternotomy) or the left anterior chest wall (thoracotomy). A pericardial window may be created if the diagnosis of penetrating cardiac trauma is not confirmed. Once penetrating trauma has been confirmed, the pericardial sac is incised and clotted blood and fluid removed. The entire heart is inspected and wound site(s) identified. Small lacerations are repaired with sutures and reinforced with Teflon felt pledges to anchor the sutures. Lacerations to small coronary vessels are ligated. Lacerations to larger coronary vessels are repaired. Large myocardial wounds may require synthetic grafting to cover the wound. The surgical incision is closed. Chest tubes and/or a mediastinal drainage tube may be left in place following the procedure. Report 33300 when the procedure is performed without cardiopulmonary bypass; report 33305 when cardiopulmonary bypass is required.

Coding Tips

Codes 33300 and 33305 report repair of traumatic wounds, not surgically created wounds. If significant additional time and effort are documented, append modifier 22 and submit a cover letter and operative report. When 33300 or 33305 is performed with another separately identifiable procedure, the highest dollar value code is listed as the primary procedure and subsequent procedures are appended with modifier 51.

ICD-10-CM Diagnostic Codes

I97.51 Accidental puncture and laceration of a circulatory system organ or structure during a circulatory system procedure
I97.52 Accidental puncture and laceration of a circulatory system organ or structure during other procedure
S21.311A Laceration without foreign body of right front wall of thorax with penetration into thoracic cavity, initial encounter
S21.312A Laceration without foreign body of left front wall of thorax with penetration into thoracic cavity, initial encounter
S21.321A Laceration with foreign body of right front wall of thorax with penetration into thoracic cavity, initial encounter
S21.322A Laceration with foreign body of left front wall of thorax with penetration into thoracic cavity, initial encounter
S21.331A Puncture wound without foreign body of right front wall of thorax with penetration into thoracic cavity, initial encounter
S21.332A Puncture wound without foreign body of left front wall of thorax with penetration into thoracic cavity, initial encounter
S21.341A Puncture wound with foreign body of right front wall of thorax with penetration into thoracic cavity, initial encounter
S21.342A Puncture wound with foreign body of left front wall of thorax with penetration into thoracic cavity, initial encounter
S21.351A Open bite of right front wall of thorax with penetration into thoracic cavity, initial encounter
S21.352A Open bite of left front wall of thorax with penetration into thoracic cavity, initial encounter
S21.411A Laceration without foreign body of right back wall of thorax with penetration into thoracic cavity, initial encounter
S21.412A Laceration without foreign body of left back wall of thorax with penetration into thoracic cavity, initial encounter
S21.421A Laceration with foreign body of right back wall of thorax with penetration into thoracic cavity, initial encounter
S21.422A Laceration with foreign body of left back wall of thorax with penetration into thoracic cavity, initial encounter
S21.431A Puncture wound without foreign body of right back wall of thorax with penetration into thoracic cavity, initial encounter
S21.432A Puncture wound without foreign body of left back wall of thorax with penetration into thoracic cavity, initial encounter
S21.441A Puncture wound with foreign body of right back wall of thorax with penetration into thoracic cavity, initial encounter
S21.451A Open bite of right back wall of thorax with penetration into thoracic cavity, initial encounter
S21.452A Open bite of left back wall of thorax with penetration into thoracic cavity, initial encounter
S26.01XA Contusion of heart with hemopericardium, initial encounter
S26.020A Mild laceration of heart with hemopericardium, initial encounter
S26.021A Moderate laceration of heart with hemopericardium, initial encounter
S26.022A Major laceration of heart with hemopericardium, initial encounter
S26.11XA Contusion of heart without hemopericardium, initial encounter
S26.12XA Laceration of heart without hemopericardium, initial encounter

AMA: 33300 2018,Jun

Relative Value Units/Medicare Edits

Non-Facility RVU	Work	PE	MP	Total
33300	44.97	15.96	10.87	71.8
33305	76.93	24.7	18.55	120.18
Facility RVU	**Work**	**PE**	**MP**	**Total**
33300	44.97	15.96	10.87	71.8
33305	76.93	24.7	18.55	120.18

	FUD	Status	MUE	Modifiers				IOM Reference
33300	90	A	1(3)	51	N/A	62*	80	None
33305	90	A	1(3)	51	N/A	62*	80	

* with documentation

 N Newborn: 0 P Pediatric: 0-17 M Maternity: 9-64 A Adult: 15-124 AMA: CPT Assist

33310-33315

33310 Cardiotomy, exploratory (includes removal of foreign body, atrial or ventricular thrombus); without bypass
33315 with cardiopulmonary bypass

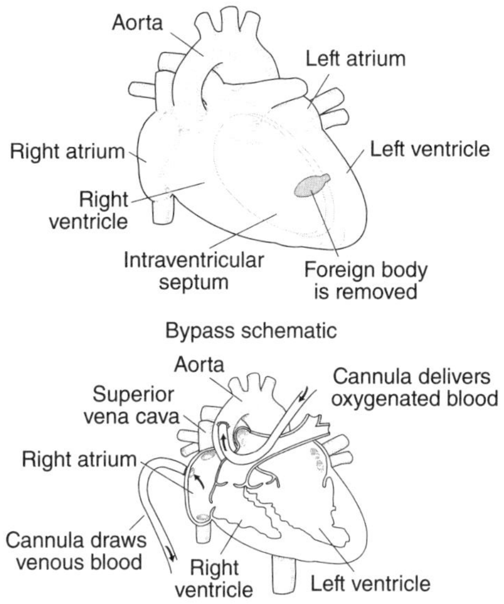

Surgical exploration of the heart is performed, requiring cardiotomy, or incision into heart tissues. A foreign body is removed in the course of the procedure

Explanation

The physician exposes the heart via the sternum. The foreign body is located by feeling the heart. If possible, the object is removed from the surface of the heart. If necessary, a hole is made in one of the ventricles or atria to remove the object or thrombus lodged there. The holes are closed with sutures and small reinforcing patches of Teflon felt. Report 33310 if cardiopulmonary bypass is not initiated; report 33315 if cardiopulmonary bypass is initiated.

Coding Tips

Codes 33310 and 33315 report exploration following trauma to the heart. Removal of foreign body includes objects resulting from penetrating trauma (missiles) or surgical complications (pacing electrodes, catheters, stents). Removal of thrombus includes thrombus due to trauma or complications of surgical procedures. These codes should not be reported for exploration related to congenital anomalies or disease of heart structures. Do not report 33310 or 33315 for removal of thrombus in addition to other cardiac codes unless a separate incision in the heart is required to remove the atrial or ventricular thrombus. When 33515 is performed with other cardiac procedures and requires a separate heart incision, append modifier 59 or an X{EPSU} modifier to 33515. If significant additional time and effort is documented, append modifier 22 and submit a cover letter and operative report. Report any free grafts or flaps separately.

ICD-10-CM Diagnostic Codes

I97.110	Postprocedural cardiac insufficiency following cardiac surgery
I97.111	Postprocedural cardiac insufficiency following other surgery
I97.120	Postprocedural cardiac arrest following cardiac surgery
I97.121	Postprocedural cardiac arrest following other surgery
I97.130	Postprocedural heart failure following cardiac surgery
I97.131	Postprocedural heart failure following other surgery
I97.51	Accidental puncture and laceration of a circulatory system organ or structure during a circulatory system procedure
I97.52	Accidental puncture and laceration of a circulatory system organ or structure during other procedure
I97.710	Intraoperative cardiac arrest during cardiac surgery
I97.711	Intraoperative cardiac arrest during other surgery
I97.89	Other postprocedural complications and disorders of the circulatory system, not elsewhere classified
S26.01XA	Contusion of heart with hemopericardium, initial encounter
S26.020A	Mild laceration of heart with hemopericardium, initial encounter
S26.021A	Moderate laceration of heart with hemopericardium, initial encounter
S26.022A	Major laceration of heart with hemopericardium, initial encounter
S26.09XA	Other injury of heart with hemopericardium, initial encounter
S26.11XA	Contusion of heart without hemopericardium, initial encounter
S26.12XA	Laceration of heart without hemopericardium, initial encounter
S26.19XA	Other injury of heart without hemopericardium, initial encounter
T81.515A	Adhesions due to foreign body accidentally left in body following heart catheterization, initial encounter
T81.525A	Obstruction due to foreign body accidentally left in body following heart catheterization, initial encounter
T81.526A	Obstruction due to foreign body accidentally left in body following aspiration, puncture or other catheterization, initial encounter
T81.535A	Perforation due to foreign body accidentally left in body following heart catheterization, initial encounter
T81.536A	Perforation due to foreign body accidentally left in body following aspiration, puncture or other catheterization, initial encounter
T81.595A	Other complications of foreign body accidentally left in body following heart catheterization, initial encounter
T82.110A	Breakdown (mechanical) of cardiac electrode, initial encounter
T82.120A	Displacement of cardiac electrode, initial encounter
T82.190A	Other mechanical complication of cardiac electrode, initial encounter
T82.513A	Breakdown (mechanical) of balloon (counterpulsation) device, initial encounter
T82.514A	Breakdown (mechanical) of infusion catheter, initial encounter
T82.515A	Breakdown (mechanical) of umbrella device, initial encounter
T82.518A	Breakdown (mechanical) of other cardiac and vascular devices and implants, initial encounter
T82.523A	Displacement of balloon (counterpulsation) device, initial encounter
T82.524A	Displacement of infusion catheter, initial encounter
T82.525A	Displacement of umbrella device, initial encounter
T82.528A	Displacement of other cardiac and vascular devices and implants, initial encounter
T82.533A	Leakage of balloon (counterpulsation) device, initial encounter
T82.534A	Leakage of infusion catheter, initial encounter
T82.535A	Leakage of umbrella device, initial encounter
T82.538A	Leakage of other cardiac and vascular devices and implants, initial encounter
T82.593A	Other mechanical complication of balloon (counterpulsation) device, initial encounter
T82.594A	Other mechanical complication of infusion catheter, initial encounter

T82.595A	Other mechanical complication of umbrella device, initial encounter
T82.598A	Other mechanical complication of other cardiac and vascular devices and implants, initial encounter
T82.898A	Other specified complication of vascular prosthetic devices, implants and grafts, initial encounter

AMA: **33310** 2018,Jun

Relative Value Units/Medicare Edits

Non-Facility RVU	Work	PE	MP	Total
33310	20.34	9.4	4.68	34.42
33315	35.0	12.99	8.41	56.4
Facility RVU	**Work**	**PE**	**MP**	**Total**
33310	20.34	9.4	4.68	34.42
33315	35.0	12.99	8.41	56.4

	FUD	Status	MUE	Modifiers				IOM Reference
33310	90	A	1(2)	51	N/A	62*	80	None
33315	90	A	1(2)	51	N/A	62*	80	

* with documentation

Terms To Know

atria. Two upper chambers of the heart. The left and right atria are divided by the septum, a muscular wall.

cannula. Tube inserted into a blood vessel, duct, or body cavity to facilitate passage.

cardiopulmonary bypass. Venous blood is diverted to a heart-lung machine, which mechanically pumps and oxygenates the blood temporarily so the heart can be bypassed while an open procedure on the heart or coronary arteries is performed. During bypass, the lungs are deflated and immobile.

cardiotomy. Incision of the heart, the cardiac orifice, or the cardiac end of the stomach.

thrombus. Stationary blood clot inside a blood vessel.

33320-33322

33320	Suture repair of aorta or great vessels; without shunt or cardiopulmonary bypass
33321	with shunt bypass
33322	with cardiopulmonary bypass

Schematic of great vessels showing one type of wound repair

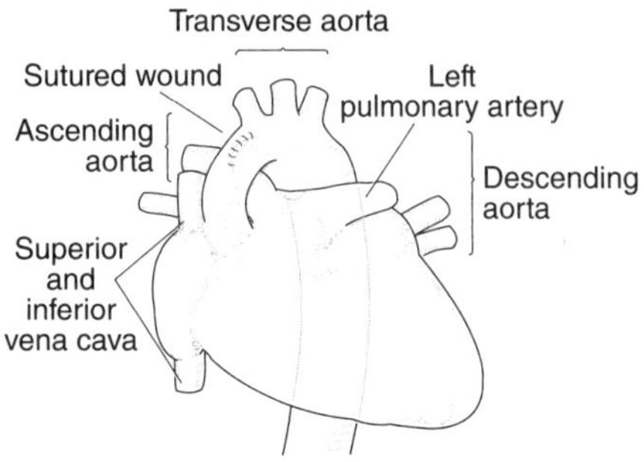

The aorta is typically accessed by a sternotomy incision

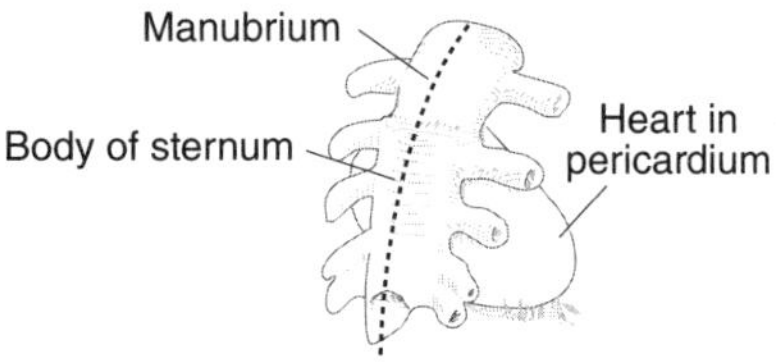

A wound to the aorta or to a great vessel is accessed and repaired using sutures

Explanation

The physician gains access to the mediastinum through an incision through the sternum (median sternotomy) or the chest wall (lateral thoracotomy). The physician repairs the aorta or great vessels while the heart is still beating. The physician closes the surgical incisions and dresses the sternal or chest wall wound. The physician may leave chest tubes and/or a mediastinal drainage tube in place following the procedure. Report 33321 if performed with a shunt bypass; report 33322 if performed with a cardiopulmonary bypass.

Coding Tips

These procedures report repair following trauma to the aorta or great vessels. Repairs related to congenital anomalies or disease should be reported with the appropriate codes for those procedures. If significant additional time and effort are documented, append modifier 22 and submit a cover letter and operative report. When 33320, 33321, or 33322 is performed with another separately identifiable procedure, the highest dollar value code is listed as the primary procedure and subsequent procedures are appended with modifier 51.

ICD-10-CM Diagnostic Codes

I97.51	Accidental puncture and laceration of a circulatory system organ or structure during a circulatory system procedure
I97.52	Accidental puncture and laceration of a circulatory system organ or structure during other procedure
S25.01XA	Minor laceration of thoracic aorta, initial encounter
S25.02XA	Major laceration of thoracic aorta, initial encounter
S25.09XA	Other specified injury of thoracic aorta, initial encounter
S25.21XA	Minor laceration of superior vena cava, initial encounter
S25.22XA	Major laceration of superior vena cava, initial encounter
S25.29XA	Other specified injury of superior vena cava, initial encounter

S25.411A	Minor laceration of right pulmonary blood vessels, initial encounter ☑
S25.412A	Minor laceration of left pulmonary blood vessels, initial encounter ☑
S25.421A	Major laceration of right pulmonary blood vessels, initial encounter ☑
S25.422A	Major laceration of left pulmonary blood vessels, initial encounter ☑
S25.491A	Other specified injury of right pulmonary blood vessels, initial encounter ☑
S25.492A	Other specified injury of left pulmonary blood vessels, initial encounter ☑
S35.01XA	Minor laceration of abdominal aorta, initial encounter
S35.02XA	Major laceration of abdominal aorta, initial encounter
S35.09XA	Other injury of abdominal aorta, initial encounter
S35.11XA	Minor laceration of inferior vena cava, initial encounter
S35.12XA	Major laceration of inferior vena cava, initial encounter
S35.19XA	Other injury of inferior vena cava, initial encounter
T88.8XXA	Other specified complications of surgical and medical care, not elsewhere classified, initial encounter

AMA: **33320** 2018,Jun **33321** 2018,Jun **33322** 2018,Jun

Relative Value Units/Medicare Edits

Non-Facility RVU	Work	PE	MP	Total
33320	18.54	8.52	4.57	31.63
33321	20.81	9.34	4.8	34.95
33322	24.42	10.86	5.98	41.26
Facility RVU	**Work**	**PE**	**MP**	**Total**
33320	18.54	8.52	4.57	31.63
33321	20.81	9.34	4.8	34.95
33322	24.42	10.86	5.98	41.26

	FUD	Status	MUE	Modifiers				IOM Reference
33320	90	A	1(3)	51	N/A	62*	80	None
33321	90	A	1(3)	51	N/A	62*	80	
33322	90	A	1(3)	51	N/A	62*	80	

* with documentation

Terms To Know

anomaly. Irregularity in the structure or position of an organ or tissue.

cardiopulmonary bypass. Venous blood is diverted to a heart-lung machine, which mechanically pumps and oxygenates the blood temporarily so the heart can be bypassed while an open procedure on the heart or coronary arteries is performed. During bypass, the lungs are deflated and immobile.

mediastinum. Collection of organs and tissues that separate the pleural sacs. Located between the sternum and spine above the diaphragm, it contains the heart and great vessels, trachea and bronchi, esophagus, thymus, lymph nodes, and nerves.

33330-33335

33330 Insertion of graft, aorta or great vessels; without shunt, or cardiopulmonary bypass

33335 with cardiopulmonary bypass

A graft is inserted on any of the great vessels

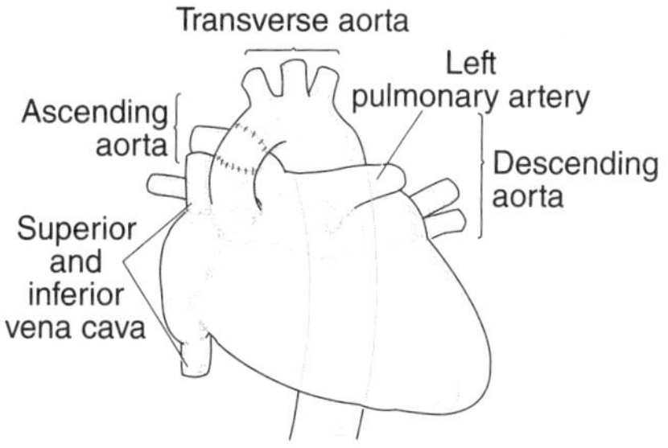

Cardiopulmonary bypass schematic

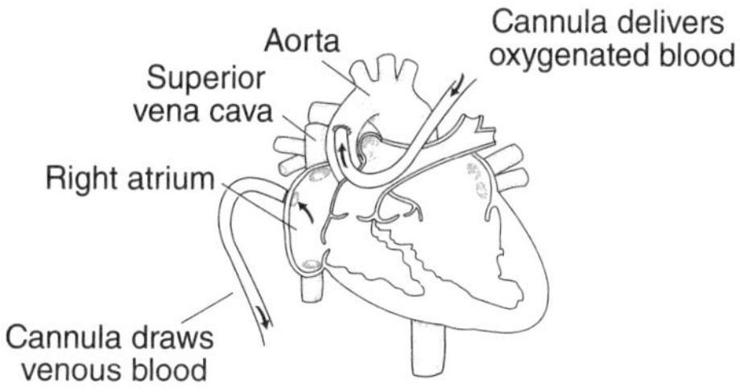

Explanation

In 33330, the physician gains access to the mediastinum through an incision through the sternum (median sternotomy) or the chest wall (lateral thoracotomy). The physician sews in the aortic or great vessel graft while the heart is still beating. In 33335, the physician places cardiopulmonary bypass catheters usually through incisions in the right atrial appendage and aorta or femoral artery. The physician stops the heart by infusing cardioplegia solution into the coronary circulation. The physician sews in the aortic or great vessel graft while the heart is still. The physician takes the patient off cardiopulmonary bypass, closes the surgical incisions and dresses the sternal or chest wall wound. The physician may leave chest tubes and/or a mediastinal drainage tube in place following the procedure.

Coding Tips

These procedures report graft insertion to repair traumatic wounds of the aorta or great vessels. Repairs related to congenital anomalies or disease should be reported with appropriate codes for those procedures. If significant additional time and effort is documented, append modifier 22 and submit a cover letter and operative report. When 33330 or 33335 is performed with another separately identifiable procedure, the highest dollar value code is listed as the primary procedure and subsequent procedures are appended with modifier 51.

ICD-10-CM Diagnostic Codes

I97.51	Accidental puncture and laceration of a circulatory system organ or structure during a circulatory system procedure
I97.52	Accidental puncture and laceration of a circulatory system organ or structure during other procedure
S25.01XA	Minor laceration of thoracic aorta, initial encounter
S25.02XA	Major laceration of thoracic aorta, initial encounter
S25.09XA	Other specified injury of thoracic aorta, initial encounter
S25.21XA	Minor laceration of superior vena cava, initial encounter
S25.22XA	Major laceration of superior vena cava, initial encounter

S25.29XA Other specified injury of superior vena cava, initial encounter

S25.411A Minor laceration of right pulmonary blood vessels, initial encounter ☑

S25.412A Minor laceration of left pulmonary blood vessels, initial encounter ☑

S25.421A Major laceration of right pulmonary blood vessels, initial encounter ☑

S25.422A Major laceration of left pulmonary blood vessels, initial encounter ☑

S25.491A Other specified injury of right pulmonary blood vessels, initial encounter ☑

S25.492A Other specified injury of left pulmonary blood vessels, initial encounter ☑

S35.01XA Minor laceration of abdominal aorta, initial encounter

S35.02XA Major laceration of abdominal aorta, initial encounter

S35.09XA Other injury of abdominal aorta, initial encounter

S35.11XA Minor laceration of inferior vena cava, initial encounter

S35.12XA Major laceration of inferior vena cava, initial encounter

S35.19XA Other injury of inferior vena cava, initial encounter

T88.8XXA Other specified complications of surgical and medical care, not elsewhere classified, initial encounter

AMA: 33330 2018,Jun **33335** 2018,Jun

Relative Value Units/Medicare Edits

Non-Facility RVU	Work	PE	MP	Total
33330	25.29	10.72	5.85	41.86
33335	33.91	13.02	7.84	54.77
Facility RVU	**Work**	**PE**	**MP**	**Total**
33330	25.29	10.72	5.85	41.86
33335	33.91	13.02	7.84	54.77

	FUD	Status	MUE	Modifiers				IOM Reference
33330	90	A	1(3)	51	N/A	62*	80	None
33335	90	A	1(3)	51	N/A	62*	80	

* with documentation

33340

33340 Percutaneous transcatheter closure of the left atrial appendage with endocardial implant, including fluoroscopy, transseptal puncture, catheter placement(s), left atrial angiography, left atrial appendage angiography, when performed, and radiological supervision and interpretation

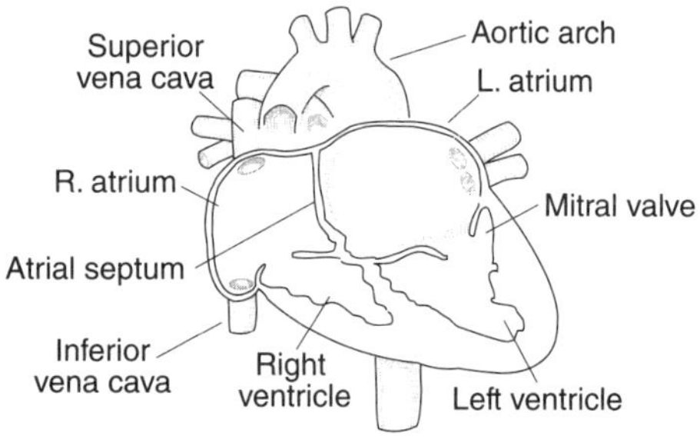

Left atrial appendage is closed with a percutaneously placed endocardial implant

Explanation

A left atrial appendage is closed or occluded using an endocardial implant delivered via catheter. The physician places an introducer sheath in a vein (typically, the femoral vein) using percutaneous puncture. The physician places a lumen catheter through the introducer sheath into the femoral vein and advances it, under fluoroscopic guidance, to the right atrium. The physician exchanges this catheter over a wire for a transseptal puncture needle, dilator, and sheath. The physician advances the transseptal puncture apparatus to the right atrium and punctures the intra-atrial septum (in some cases, the physician may use a patent foramen ovale if present rather than performing a septal puncture). The physician advances the needle, dilator, and transseptal sheath into the left atrium. The occlusive device is positioned over the left atrial appendage and deployed blocking the opening completely. The physician removes the catheters and sheaths from the femoral vessels. Pressure is placed on the wound for 20 to 30 minutes to stem bleeding. This code includes fluoroscopy, transseptal puncture, catheter placement, left atrial and left atrial appendage angiography, and radiological supervision and interpretation.

Coding Tips

Do not report 33340 with 93462. Do not report 33340 with 93452–93453, 93458–93461, or 93595–93598 unless left ventricle catheterization is completed via non-transseptal approach for symptoms separate from left atrial appendage closure procedure. This code should not be reported with 93451, 93453, 93456, 93460–93461, 93593–93594, or 93596–93598 unless right heart catheterization is completed for symptoms separate from left atrial appendage closure procedure.

ICD-10-CM Diagnostic Codes

I48.0 Paroxysmal atrial fibrillation

I48.11 Longstanding persistent atrial fibrillation

I48.19 Other persistent atrial fibrillation

I48.21 Permanent atrial fibrillation

I48.3 Typical atrial flutter

I48.4 Atypical atrial flutter

AMA: 33340 2021,Nov

Relative Value Units/Medicare Edits

Non-Facility RVU	Work	PE	MP	Total
33340	14.0	5.65	3.19	22.84
Facility RVU	**Work**	**PE**	**MP**	**Total**
33340	14.0	5.65	3.19	22.84

	FUD	Status	MUE	Modifiers				IOM Reference
33340	0	A	1(2)	51	N/A	62	80*	None

* with documentation

Terms To Know

angiography. Radiographic imaging of the arteries. Imaging may be performed to study the vasculature of any given organ, body system, or area of circulation such as the brain, heart, chest, kidneys, limbs, gastrointestinal tract, aorta, and pulmonary circulation to visualize the formation and the function of the blood vessels to detect problems such as a blockage or stricture. A catheter is inserted through an accessible blood vessel and the artery is injected with a radiopaque contrast material after which x-rays are taken.

atrial appendage. Also known as an auricular appendage, a pouch connected to the left and right atria of the heart. The left atrial appendage (LAA) is frequently the source of clots causing embolic strokes in patients with atrial fibrillation.

fibrillation. Spontaneous contraction of individual muscle fibers.

implant. Material or device inserted or placed within the body for therapeutic, reconstructive, or diagnostic purposes.

lumen. Space inside an intestine, artery, vein, duct, or tube.

33361-33362

33361 Transcatheter aortic valve replacement (TAVR/TAVI) with prosthetic valve; percutaneous femoral artery approach

33362 open femoral artery approach

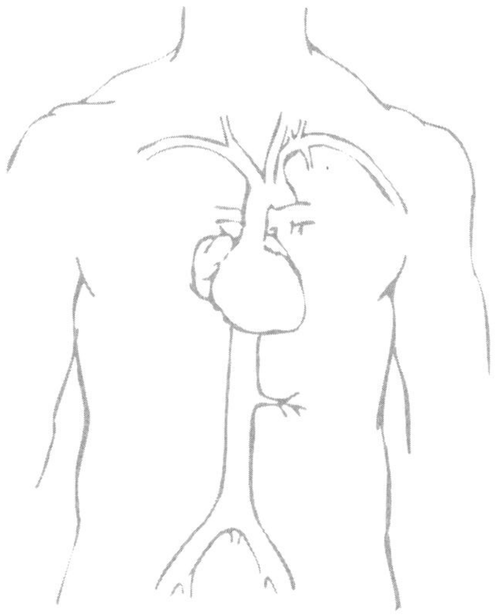

Transcatheter aortic valve is replaced utilizing femoral artery approach

Explanation

Transcatheter aortic valve replacement or implantation (TAVR/TAVI) is performed on patients with symptomatic aortic stenosis that are high risk or not eligible for traditional open chest surgery. A guidewire is placed in the femoral artery in the groin and manipulated into the left ventricle. A catheter is inserted following the guidewire to the aortic valve. A balloon is inflated to compress the native valve. A bioprosthetic valve attached to an expandable stent is deployed over the compressed native valve. The catheter and guidewire are removed. Report 33361 if the catheter access is percutaneous and 33362 when access to the femoral artery is open.

Coding Tips

These procedures are typically performed by two surgeons performing their own components of the procedure. In these instances, append modifier 62. Angiography and radiological supervision to guide the procedure are included in the codes and are not reported separately. Diagnostic coronary angiography performed at the time of the procedure may be reported in certain instances, such as when no prior catheter-based angiography study has been performed or a significant change in the patient's condition has occurred since the time of a prior study. Diagnostic coronary angiography services reported at the same surgical session as TAVR/TAVI services must have modifier 59 appended and must meet specific coverage requirements. Check with local payers for requirements. Percutaneous coronary interventional procedures are reported separately when performed with these codes. For cardiopulmonary bypass with TAVR/TAVI procedures, see 33367–33369. For transcatheter ventricular support with TAVR/TAVI, see the ventricular assist device (VAD) procedure codes (33975–33976, 33990–33993, 33995, 33997) and the balloon pump insertion codes (33967, 33970, 33973). For a transapical approach, see 33366.

ICD-10-CM Diagnostic Codes

I06.0	Rheumatic aortic stenosis
I06.2	Rheumatic aortic stenosis with insufficiency
I08.0	Rheumatic disorders of both mitral and aortic valves
I08.8	Other rheumatic multiple valve diseases

I35.0	Nonrheumatic aortic (valve) stenosis
I35.1	Nonrheumatic aortic (valve) insufficiency
I35.2	Nonrheumatic aortic (valve) stenosis with insufficiency
I35.8	Other nonrheumatic aortic valve disorders
Q23.0	Congenital stenosis of aortic valve

AMA: **33361** 2023,May; 2022,Apr; 2022,Jan **33362** 2023,May; 2022,Apr; 2022,Jan

Relative Value Units/Medicare Edits

Non-Facility RVU	Work	PE	MP	Total
33361	22.47	7.71	5.24	35.42
33362	24.54	8.32	5.74	38.6
Facility RVU	**Work**	**PE**	**MP**	**Total**
33361	22.47	7.71	5.24	35.42
33362	24.54	8.32	5.74	38.6

	FUD	Status	MUE	Modifiers				IOM Reference
33361	0	A	1(2)	51	N/A	62	80*	None
33362	0	A	1(2)	51	N/A	62	80*	

* with documentation

Terms To Know

aortic stenosis. Narrowing of the aortic valve resulting in backflow of blood into the ventricle.

aortic valve. Heart valve, comprising three cusps, that divides the left ventricle and the aorta.

congenital. Present at birth, occurring through heredity or an influence during gestation up to the moment of birth.

percutaneous. Through the skin.

prosthetic. Device that replaces all or part of an internal body organ or body part, or that replaces part of the function of a permanently inoperable or malfunctioning internal body organ or body part.

33363-33364

33363 Transcatheter aortic valve replacement (TAVR/TAVI) with prosthetic valve; open axillary artery approach

33364 open iliac artery approach

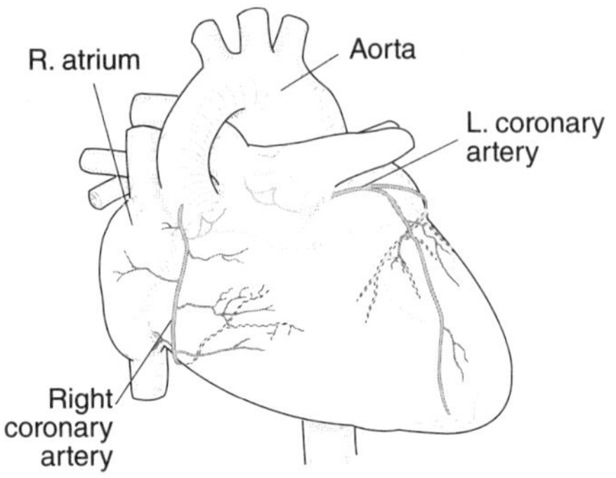

Aortic valves are replaced using a transcatheter approach

Explanation

Transcatheter aortic valve replacement or implantation (TAVR/TAVI) is performed on patients with symptomatic aortic stenosis that are high risk or not eligible for traditional open chest surgery. A guidewire is placed in a peripheral or other artery and manipulated into the left ventricle. A catheter is inserted following the guidewire to the aortic valve. A balloon is inflated to compress the native valve. A porcine valve attached to an expandable stent is deployed over the compressed native valve. The catheter and guidewire are removed. Report 33363 if the catheter access is via an open axillary artery approach and 33364 when access is via an open iliac artery approach.

Coding Tips

These procedures are typically performed by two surgeons performing their own components of the procedure. In these instances, append modifier 62. Angiography and radiological supervision to guide the procedure are included in the codes and are not reported separately. Diagnostic coronary angiography performed at the time of the procedure may be reported in certain instances, such as when no prior catheter-based angiography study has been performed or a significant change in the patient's condition has occurred since the time of a prior study. Diagnostic coronary angiography services reported at the same surgical session as TAVR/TAVI services must have modifier 59 appended and must meet specific coverage requirements. Check with local payers for requirements. Percutaneous coronary interventional procedures are reported separately when performed with these codes. For cardiopulmonary bypass with TAVR/TAVI procedures, see 33367–33369. For transcatheter ventricular support with TAVR/TAVI, see the ventricular assist device (VAD) procedure codes (33975–33976, 33990–33993, 33995, 33997) and the balloon pump insertion codes (33967, 33970, and 33973). For a transapical approach, see 33366.

ICD-10-CM Diagnostic Codes

I06.0	Rheumatic aortic stenosis
I06.2	Rheumatic aortic stenosis with insufficiency
I08.0	Rheumatic disorders of both mitral and aortic valves
I08.8	Other rheumatic multiple valve diseases
I35.0	Nonrheumatic aortic (valve) stenosis
I35.1	Nonrheumatic aortic (valve) insufficiency
I35.2	Nonrheumatic aortic (valve) stenosis with insufficiency
I35.8	Other nonrheumatic aortic valve disorders

Q23.0 Congenital stenosis of aortic valve

AMA: 33363 2023,May; 2022,Apr; 2022,Jan **33364** 2023,May; 2022,Apr; 2022,Jan

Relative Value Units/Medicare Edits

Non-Facility RVU	Work	PE	MP	Total
33363	25.47	8.6	5.99	40.06
33364	25.97	7.9	6.01	39.88
Facility RVU	**Work**	**PE**	**MP**	**Total**
33363	25.47	8.6	5.99	40.06
33364	25.97	7.9	6.01	39.88

	FUD	Status	MUE	Modifiers				IOM Reference
33363	0	A	1(2)	51	N/A	62	80*	None
33364	0	A	1(2)	51	N/A	62	80*	

* with documentation

Terms To Know

angiography. Radiographic imaging of the arteries.

aortic stenosis. Narrowing of the aortic valve resulting in backflow of blood into the ventricle.

aortic valve. Heart valve, comprising three cusps, that divides the left ventricle and the aorta.

prosthetic. Device that replaces all or part of an internal body organ or body part, or that replaces part of the function of a permanently inoperable or malfunctioning internal body organ or body part.

transcatheter. Procedure or treatment performed via a catheter.

33365

33365 Transcatheter aortic valve replacement (TAVR/TAVI) with prosthetic valve; transaortic approach (eg, median sternotomy, mediastinotomy)

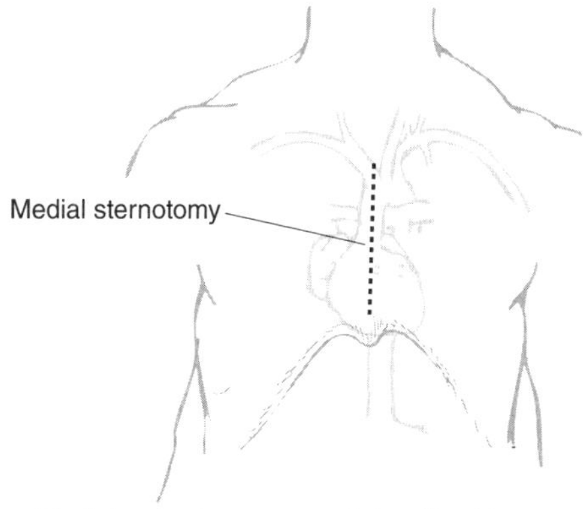

Medial sternotomy approach is utilized for transcatheter aortic value replacement

Explanation

Transcatheter aortic valve replacement or implantation (TAVR/TAVI) is performed on patients with symptomatic aortic stenosis that are high risk or not eligible for traditional open chest surgery. A median sternotomy or mediastinotomy is performed for direct access to the aorta. The aorta is incised and a guidewire is inserted and manipulated into the left ventricle. A catheter is inserted following the guidewire to the aortic valve. A balloon is inflated to compress the native valve. A porcine valve attached to an expandable stent is deployed over the compressed native valve. The catheter and guidewire are removed.

Coding Tips

This procedure is typically performed by two surgeons performing their own components of the procedure. In these instances, append modifier 62. Angiography and radiological supervision to guide the procedure is included in the code and is not reported separately. Diagnostic coronary angiography performed at the time of the procedure may be reported in certain instances, such as when no prior catheter-based angiography study has been performed or a significant change in the patient's condition has occurred since the time of a prior study. Diagnostic coronary angiography services reported at the same surgical session as TAVR/TAVI services must have modifier 59 appended and must meet specific coverage requirements. Check with local payers for requirements. Percutaneous coronary interventional procedures are reported separately when performed with these codes. For cardiopulmonary bypass with TAVR/TAVI procedures, see 33367–33369. For transcatheter ventricular support with TAVR/TAVI, see the ventricular assist device (VAD) procedure codes (33975–33976, 33990–33993, 33995, 33997) and the balloon pump insertion codes (33967, 33970, 33973). For a transapical approach, see 33366.

ICD-10-CM Diagnostic Codes

I06.0	Rheumatic aortic stenosis
I06.2	Rheumatic aortic stenosis with insufficiency
I08.0	Rheumatic disorders of both mitral and aortic valves
I08.8	Other rheumatic multiple valve diseases
I35.0	Nonrheumatic aortic (valve) stenosis
I35.1	Nonrheumatic aortic (valve) insufficiency
I35.2	Nonrheumatic aortic (valve) stenosis with insufficiency
I35.8	Other nonrheumatic aortic valve disorders

Q23.0	Congenital stenosis of aortic valve

AMA: 33365 2023,May; 2022,Apr; 2022,Jan

Relative Value Units/Medicare Edits

Non-Facility RVU	Work	PE	MP	Total
33365	26.59	8.97	6.17	41.73
Facility RVU	**Work**	**PE**	**MP**	**Total**
33365	26.59	8.97	6.17	41.73

	FUD	Status	MUE	Modifiers				IOM Reference
33365	0	A	1(2)	51	N/A	62	80*	None

* with documentation

Terms To Know

aortic valve. Heart valve, comprising three cusps, that divides the left ventricle and the aorta.

median sternotomy. Standard incision for open chest cardiac surgeries, from above the bellybutton to just under the chin, down the center of the chest through the sternum into the thoracic cavity.

mediastinotomy. Incision into the mediastinum for purposes of exploration, foreign body removal, drainage, or biopsy.

prosthetic. Device that replaces all or part of an internal body organ or body part, or that replaces part of the function of a permanently inoperable or malfunctioning internal body organ or body part.

rheumatic heart disease. Manifestation of and sequel to rheumatic fever; any cardiac involvement in rheumatic fever.

33366

33366 Transcatheter aortic valve replacement (TAVR/TAVI) with prosthetic valve; transapical exposure (eg, left thoracotomy)

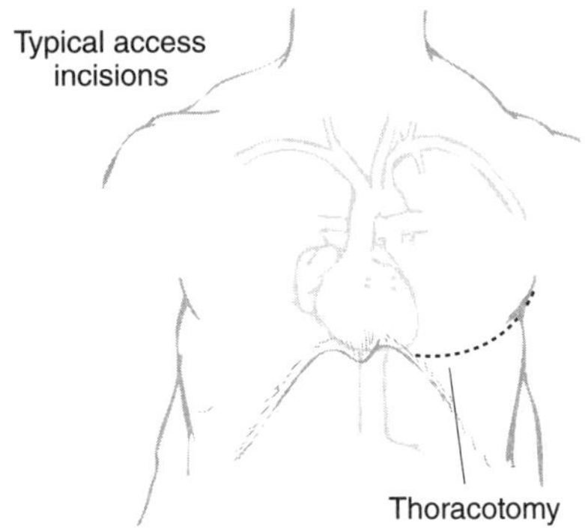

Left thoracotomy approach is used for aortic valve replacement

Explanation

Transcatheter aortic valve replacement or implantation (TAVR/TAVI) is performed on patients with symptomatic aortic stenosis that are high risk or not eligible for traditional open chest surgery. A small incision is made between ribs (usually the fifth or sixth intercostal space) on the lower left side of the patient's chest to achieve direct access to the heart. The pericardium is incised and opened near the left ventricular apex. A guidewire is advanced through the opening into the left ventricle, through the septum, and into the right ventricle. A catheter is inserted following the guidewire to the aortic valve. A balloon is inflated to compress the native valve. A porcine valve attached to an expandable stent is deployed over the compressed native valve. The catheter and guidewire are removed and the pericardium is closed using sutures. A chest tube may be placed. The wound is closed in layers.

Coding Tips

Two surgeons typically perform separate components of this procedure. In this instance, append modifier 62. Angiography and radiological supervision to guide the procedure is included in the procedure and is not reported separately. Diagnostic coronary angiography performed at the time of the procedure may only be reported in certain instances, such as when no prior catheter-based angiography study has been performed or a significant change in the patient's condition has occurred since the time of a prior study. Diagnostic coronary angiography services reported at the same surgical session as TAVR/TAVI services must have modifier 59 appended and must meet specific coverage requirements. Check with local payers for requirements. Percutaneous coronary interventional procedures are reported separately when performed with this procedure. For cardiopulmonary bypass with TAVR/TAVI procedures, see 33367–33369. For transcatheter ventricular support with TAVR/TAVI, see the ventricular assist device (VAD) procedure codes (33975–33976, 33990–33993, 33995, 33997) and the balloon pump insertion codes (33967, 33970, 33973).

ICD-10-CM Diagnostic Codes

I06.0	Rheumatic aortic stenosis
I06.2	Rheumatic aortic stenosis with insufficiency
I08.0	Rheumatic disorders of both mitral and aortic valves
I08.8	Other rheumatic multiple valve diseases
I35.0	Nonrheumatic aortic (valve) stenosis
I35.1	Nonrheumatic aortic (valve) insufficiency
I35.2	Nonrheumatic aortic (valve) stenosis with insufficiency

I35.8 Other nonrheumatic aortic valve disorders
Q23.0 Congenital stenosis of aortic valve

AMA: 33366 2023,May; 2022,Apr; 2022,Jan

Relative Value Units/Medicare Edits

Non-Facility RVU	Work	PE	MP	Total
33366	29.35	9.79	6.78	45.92
Facility RVU	**Work**	**PE**	**MP**	**Total**
33366	29.35	9.79	6.78	45.92

	FUD	Status	MUE	Modifiers				IOM Reference
33366	0	A	1(3)	51	N/A	62	80*	None

* with documentation

Terms To Know

aortic valve. Heart valve, comprising three cusps, that divides the left ventricle and the aorta.

apical. At the top, tip or end of a structure; the opposite of basal.

congenital. Present at birth, occurring through heredity or an influence during gestation up to the moment of birth.

guidewire. Flexible metal instrument designed to lead another instrument in its proper course.

pericardium. Thin and slippery case in which the heart lies that is lined with fluid so that the heart is free to pulse and move as it beats.

stenosis. Narrowing or constriction of a passage.

thoracotomy. Surgical procedure for opening the chest wall in order to access the lungs, esophagus, trachea, aorta, heart, and diaphragm.

33367-33368

+ **33367** Transcatheter aortic valve replacement (TAVR/TAVI) with prosthetic valve; cardiopulmonary bypass support with percutaneous peripheral arterial and venous cannulation (eg, femoral vessels) (List separately in addition to code for primary procedure)
+ **33368** cardiopulmonary bypass support with open peripheral arterial and venous cannulation (eg, femoral, iliac, axillary vessels) (List separately in addition to code for primary procedure)

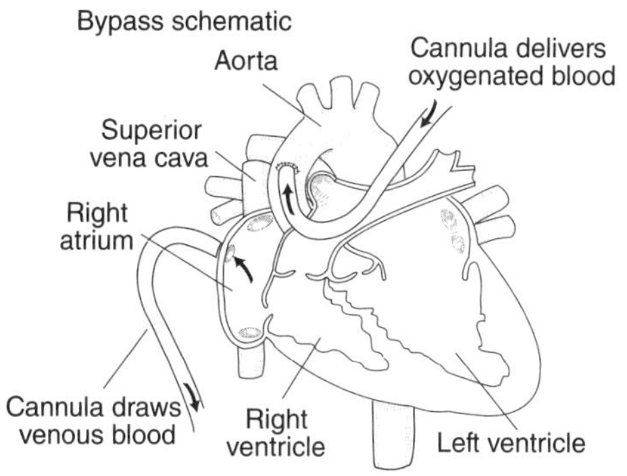

Explanation

The patient's blood is pumped to a bypass machine, oxygenated, and returned to the patient during a transcatheter aortic valve replacement or implantation (TAVR/TAVI). Its purpose is to provide mechanical support for the heart and lungs during the procedure. In 33367, the access for the intake and output of the patient's blood is via percutaneous cannulations of a peripheral artery and vein, typically the femoral vessels. Report 33368 for open peripheral arterial and venous cannulation.

Coding Tips

Report 33367 and 33368 in addition to 33361–33366, 33418, 33477, 0483T-0484T, 0544T-0545T, 0569T-0570T, and 0643T-0644T. Do not report 33367 or 33368 with one another or with 33369. For cerebral embolic protection, see 33370.

ICD-10-CM Diagnostic Codes

This/these CPT code(s) are add-on code(s). See the primary procedure code that this code is performed with for your ICD-10-CM code selections. Diagnostic code(s) would be the same as the actual procedure performed.

Relative Value Units/Medicare Edits

Non-Facility RVU	Work	PE	MP	Total
33367	11.88	3.17	2.74	17.79
33368	14.39	3.84	3.33	21.56
Facility RVU	**Work**	**PE**	**MP**	**Total**
33367	11.88	3.17	2.74	17.79
33368	14.39	3.84	3.33	21.56

	FUD	Status	MUE	Modifiers				IOM Reference
33367	N/A	A	1(2)	N/A	N/A	N/A	80*	None
33368	N/A	A	1(2)	N/A	N/A	N/A	80*	

* with documentation

33369

\+ **33369** Transcatheter aortic valve replacement (TAVR/TAVI) with prosthetic valve; cardiopulmonary bypass support with central arterial and venous cannulation (eg, aorta, right atrium, pulmonary artery) (List separately in addition to code for primary procedure)

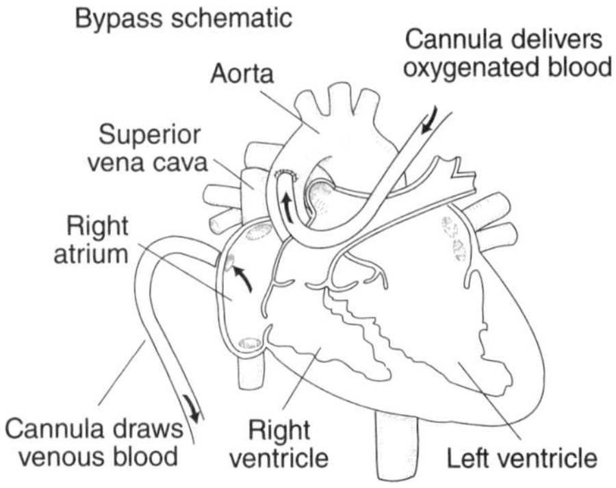

Explanation

The patient's blood is pumped to a bypass machine, oxygenated, and returned to the patient during a transcatheter aortic valve replacement or implantation (TAVR/TAVI). Its purpose is to provide mechanical support for the heart and lungs during the procedure. Access for the intake and output of the patient's blood is via cannulations of a central artery (i.e., aorta, pulmonary artery) and vein.

Coding Tips

Report 33369 in addition to 33361–33366, 33418, 33477, 0483T-0484T, 0544T-0545T, 0569T-0570T, and 0643T-0644T. Do not report 33369 with 33367–33368.

ICD-10-CM Diagnostic Codes

This/these CPT code(s) are add-on code(s). See the primary procedure code that this code is performed with for your ICD-10-CM code selections. Diagnostic code(s) would be the same as the actual procedure performed.

Relative Value Units/Medicare Edits

Non-Facility RVU	Work	PE	MP	Total
33369	19.0	5.07	4.39	28.46
Facility RVU	**Work**	**PE**	**MP**	**Total**
33369	19.0	5.07	4.39	28.46

	FUD	Status	MUE	Modifiers				IOM Reference
33369	N/A	A	1(2)	N/A	N/A	N/A	80*	None

* with documentation

33370

\+ **33370** Transcatheter placement and subsequent removal of cerebral embolic protection device(s), including arterial access, catheterization, imaging, and radiological supervision and interpretation, percutaneous (List separately in addition to code for primary procedure)

Arrows indicate direction of revised blood flow

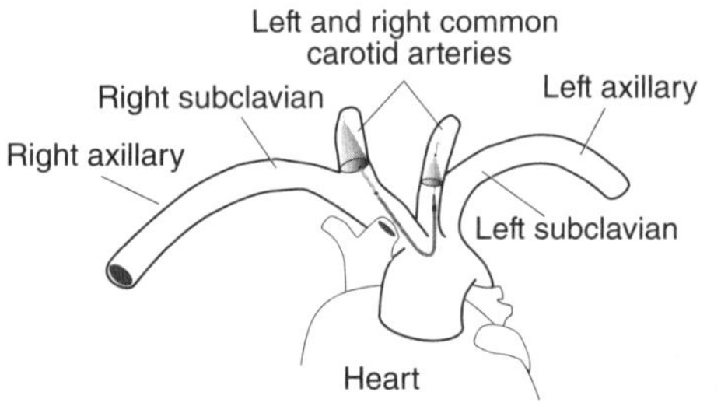

Cerebral embolic protection device is placed in brachiocephalic truck and left common carotid artery

Explanation

A cerebral embolic protection device (CEPD) is a mesh filter designed to collect debris released during transcatheter aortic valve replacement (TAVR) procedures. These devices are intended to reduce the risk of stroke by preventing embolic material from entering the carotid arteries and reaching the cerebral vasculature. A variety of CEPDs exist in various pore sizes, differing in chemical composition and deployment location. They are designed to capture materials such as arterial valve tissue, calcification, foreign matter, and thrombus. This code includes the percutaneous transcatheter placement and subsequent removal, arterial access, catheterization, imaging, and radiological supervision and interpretation.

Coding Tips

Report 33370 in addition to TAVR/TAVI codes 33361-33366. Delivery of embolic protection filters prior to the procedure and placement of additional filters is not reported separately. Replacement or extensive repair of an artery may be reported separately.

ICD-10-CM Diagnostic Codes

This/these CPT code(s) are add-on code(s). See the primary procedure code that this code is performed with for your ICD-10-CM code selections. Diagnostic code(s) would be the same as the actual procedure performed.

AMA: 33370 2022,Apr; 2022,Jan

Relative Value Units/Medicare Edits

Non-Facility RVU	Work	PE	MP	Total
33370	2.5	0.83	0.57	3.9
Facility RVU	**Work**	**PE**	**MP**	**Total**
33370	2.5	0.83	0.57	3.9

	FUD	Status	MUE	Modifiers				IOM Reference
33370	N/A	A	1(2)	N/A	N/A	N/A	80*	None

* with documentation

33390-33391

33390 Valvuloplasty, aortic valve, open, with cardiopulmonary bypass; simple (ie, valvotomy, debridement, debulking, and/or simple commissural resuspension)

33391 complex (eg, leaflet extension, leaflet resection, leaflet reconstruction, or annuloplasty)

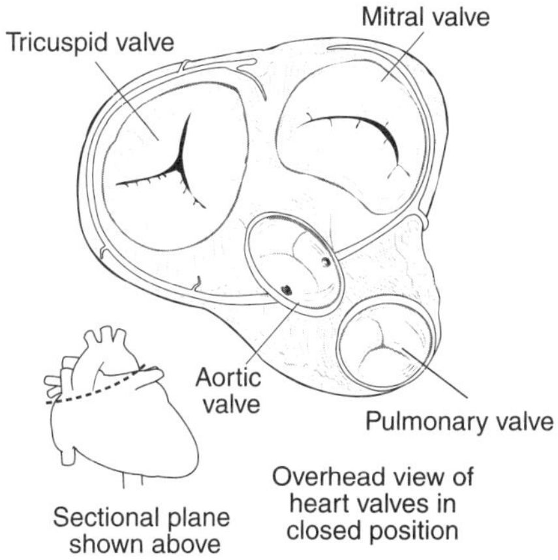

Valvuloplasty of the aortic valve is performed to restore function

Explanation

The physician initiates cardiopulmonary bypass. The aorta is clamped from above the heart and a cold preserving solution is pumped through the heart. The aorta is opened near the valve. The spaces where the heart valve leaflets meet have been fused by inflammation and scarring in diseases requiring this operation. Blunt dilators are passed through the hole and across the aortic valve. Progressively larger dilators are inserted until the valve is wide open. The dilators break the scar tissues that are cut in an open aortic valvoplasty. After the valve is fully dilated, the purse string is tied off. In the simple procedure (33390), cutting into the aortic valve leaflets, debridement utilizing scalpel blades and/or forceps to remove calcium deposits or tumors, and/or simple commissural resuspension may be performed. Commissurotomy requires the physician to stretch or cut the aortic valve due to rigid or fused leaflets. In the complex procedure (33391), extensive repairs to the leaflets may be necessary and/or annuloplasty may also be performed. Annuloplasty requires the physician to attach fibrous tissue to the base of the valve or utilize an implantable ring that prevents blood from accumulating within the left atrium, essentially resizing the valve opening. This procedure assists in maintaining the shape and flexibility of the annulus. The aorta is closed and the clamp is removed. Cardiopulmonary bypass is discontinued when heart function returns.

Coding Tips

These codes should not be reported with each other. Report 33530 in addition to the code for the primary procedure for reoperation on the aortic valve more than one month after the original procedure. For construction of an apical aortic conduit, see 33404. For replacement of an aortic valve, see 33405.

ICD-10-CM Diagnostic Codes

I06.0	Rheumatic aortic stenosis
I06.2	Rheumatic aortic stenosis with insufficiency
I08.0	Rheumatic disorders of both mitral and aortic valves
I08.8	Other rheumatic multiple valve diseases
I35.0	Nonrheumatic aortic (valve) stenosis
I35.1	Nonrheumatic aortic (valve) insufficiency
I35.2	Nonrheumatic aortic (valve) stenosis with insufficiency
I35.8	Other nonrheumatic aortic valve disorders
Q23.0	Congenital stenosis of aortic valve

AMA: **33390** 2018,Jun

Relative Value Units/Medicare Edits

Non-Facility RVU	Work	PE	MP	Total
33390	35.0	13.24	8.24	56.48
33391	41.5	15.6	9.84	66.94
Facility RVU	**Work**	**PE**	**MP**	**Total**
33390	35.0	13.24	8.24	56.48
33391	41.5	15.6	9.84	66.94

	FUD	Status	MUE	Modifiers				IOM Reference
33390	90	A	1(2)	51	N/A	62*	80	None
33391	90	A	1(2)	51	N/A	62*	80	

* with documentation

Terms To Know

annuloplasty. Surgical plication of weakened tissue of the heart, to improve its muscular function. Annuli are thick, fibrous rings and one is found surrounding each of the cardiac chambers. The atrial and ventricular muscle fibers attach to the annuli. In annuloplasty, weakened annuli may be surgically plicated, or tucked, to improve muscular functions.

aortic stenosis. Narrowing of the aortic valve resulting in backflow of blood into the ventricle.

cardiopulmonary bypass. Venous blood is diverted to a heart-lung machine, which mechanically pumps and oxygenates the blood temporarily so the heart can be bypassed while an open procedure on the heart or coronary arteries is performed. During bypass, the lungs are deflated and immobile.

commissurotomy. Surgical division or disruption of any two parts that are joined to form a commissure in order to increase the opening. The procedure most often refers to opening the adherent leaflet bands of fibrous tissue in a stenosed mitral valve.

valvuloplasty. Surgical repair of a valve.

33404

33404 Construction of apical-aortic conduit

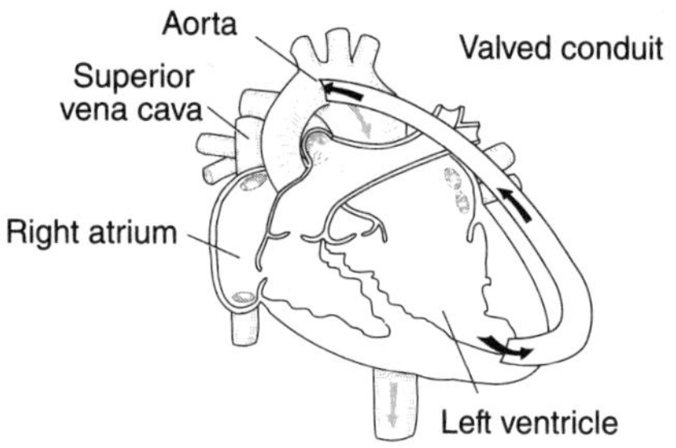

A conduit between the apical tip of the left ventricle and the aorta is established

Explanation

Cardiopulmonary bypass is required. Access to the heart may be achieved by median sternotomy or left thoracotomy. A hole is made in the tip of the left ventricle and another is made in the aorta above the coronary arteries. The conduit is oriented so that the valve in it will only let blood flow out of the heart, but not back in. One end of the conduit is sewn to the hole in the tip of the heart. The other end is sewn to the hole in the aorta. Air is removed from the heart and from the conduit. Cardiopulmonary bypass is discontinued when heart function returns.

Coding Tips

For reoperation on the aortic valve more than one month after the original procedure, report 33530 in addition to the code for the primary procedure. When more than one valve (aortic, mitral, tricuspid, pulmonary) is being repaired or replaced, report each procedure separately and append modifier 51 to the secondary valve procedures. For other valvuloplasty procedures, see 33390–33391. For aortic valve replacement, see 33405–33413. For percutaneous balloon valvuloplasty of the aortic valve, see 92986.

ICD-10-CM Diagnostic Codes

I06.0	Rheumatic aortic stenosis
I06.1	Rheumatic aortic insufficiency
I06.2	Rheumatic aortic stenosis with insufficiency
I06.8	Other rheumatic aortic valve diseases
I35.0	Nonrheumatic aortic (valve) stenosis
I35.1	Nonrheumatic aortic (valve) insufficiency
I35.2	Nonrheumatic aortic (valve) stenosis with insufficiency
I35.8	Other nonrheumatic aortic valve disorders
M31.4	Aortic arch syndrome [Takayasu]
Q23.0	Congenital stenosis of aortic valve
Q25.21	Interruption of aortic arch
Q25.29	Other atresia of aorta
Q25.3	Supravalvular aortic stenosis

Relative Value Units/Medicare Edits

Non-Facility RVU	Work	PE	MP	Total
33404	31.37	12.69	7.27	51.33
Facility RVU	**Work**	**PE**	**MP**	**Total**
33404	31.37	12.69	7.27	51.33

	FUD	Status	MUE	Modifiers				IOM Reference
33404	90	A	1(2)	51	N/A	62*	80	None

* with documentation

Terms To Know

aortic insufficiency. Malfunction of the aortic valve resulting in backflow of blood into the ventricle.

aortic stenosis. Narrowing of the aortic valve resulting in backflow of blood into the ventricle.

aortic valve disorders. Various types of aortic valve dysfunction, two main types being stenosis and insufficiency.

atresia. Congenital closure or absence of a tubular organ or an opening to the body surface.

cardiopulmonary bypass. Venous blood is diverted to a heart-lung machine, which mechanically pumps and oxygenates the blood temporarily so the heart can be bypassed while an open procedure on the heart or coronary arteries is performed. During bypass, the lungs are deflated and immobile.

congenital. Present at birth, occurring through heredity or an influence during gestation up to the moment of birth.

hypothermia with cardiac bypass. Reduction of the body temperature using a bypass system to reduce the oxygen demands of tissue and to protect the myocardium during a procedure.

scar tissue. Fibrous connective tissue that forms around a wounded area or injury, composed mainly of fibroblasts or collagenous fibers.

stenosis. Narrowing or constriction of a passage.

Takayasu's disease. Rare inflammatory disease of the large arteries, especially affecting the aorta, that is usually fatal.

33405-33410

33405 Replacement, aortic valve, open, with cardiopulmonary bypass; with prosthetic valve other than homograft or stentless valve
33406 with allograft valve (freehand)
33410 with stentless tissue valve

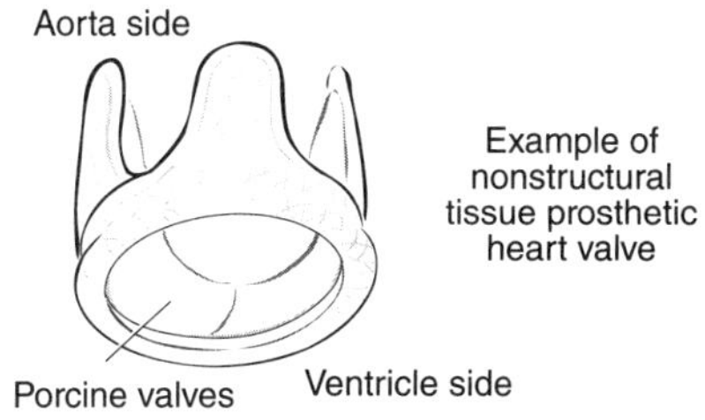

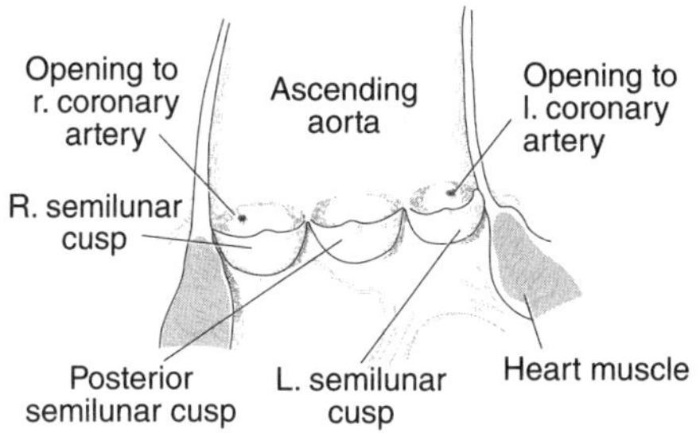

Explanation

Cardiopulmonary bypass is initiated. A clamp is placed on the aorta well above the heart. A cold preserving solution is pumped into the coronary arteries to stop the heart. In 33405, the aorta is opened just above the aortic valve. The valve leaflets are cut out and the annulus of the valve (ring of tissue where the valve leaflets normally attach to the aorta) is cleaned of calcium. The valve annulus size is measured and an appropriate artificial valve is selected. The artificial valve is sewn to the valve annulus. In 33406, an allograft is selected. The tissue valve is trimmed so that it can be sewn to the valve annulus. The aorta above the graft valve is trimmed so that the valve cusps can be suspended when the graft is in place. By doing so, the coronary arteries are not obstructed by the graft. The new valve is sewn in place. The valve annulus size is measured and an appropriate artificial valve is selected. The artificial valve is sewn to the valve annulus. In 33410, the valve annulus size is measured and an appropriate stentless tissue valve is selected, (the stentless valve is unique because unlike other valves it has no rigid external frame or sewing ring) and sutured directly into the aortic wall. The aorta is closed and the clamp is taken off. Cardiopulmonary bypass is discontinued when heart function returns. The wound is closed with layered sutures.

Coding Tips

Report 33530 in addition to the code for the primary procedure for reoperation on the aortic valve more than one month after the original procedure. When more than one valve (aortic, mitral, tricuspid, pulmonary) is being repaired or replaced, report each procedure separately and append modifier 51 to the secondary valve procedures. Do not report these codes with 33440. For valvuloplasty of the aortic valve, see 33390–33391. For construction of an apical aortic conduit, see 33404.

ICD-10-CM Diagnostic Codes

I06.0	Rheumatic aortic stenosis
I06.1	Rheumatic aortic insufficiency
I06.2	Rheumatic aortic stenosis with insufficiency
I06.8	Other rheumatic aortic valve diseases
I08.0	Rheumatic disorders of both mitral and aortic valves
I08.8	Other rheumatic multiple valve diseases
I33.0	Acute and subacute infective endocarditis
I35.0	Nonrheumatic aortic (valve) stenosis
I35.1	Nonrheumatic aortic (valve) insufficiency
I35.2	Nonrheumatic aortic (valve) stenosis with insufficiency
I35.8	Other nonrheumatic aortic valve disorders
Q23.0	Congenital stenosis of aortic valve
Q25.21	Interruption of aortic arch
Q25.29	Other atresia of aorta
Q25.3	Supravalvular aortic stenosis
T82.01XA	Breakdown (mechanical) of heart valve prosthesis, initial encounter
T82.02XA	Displacement of heart valve prosthesis, initial encounter
T82.03XA	Leakage of heart valve prosthesis, initial encounter
T82.09XA	Other mechanical complication of heart valve prosthesis, initial encounter
T82.6XXA	Infection and inflammatory reaction due to cardiac valve prosthesis, initial encounter
T82.817A	Embolism due to cardiac prosthetic devices, implants and grafts, initial encounter
T82.827A	Fibrosis due to cardiac prosthetic devices, implants and grafts, initial encounter
T82.837A	Hemorrhage due to cardiac prosthetic devices, implants and grafts, initial encounter
T82.847A	Pain due to cardiac prosthetic devices, implants and grafts, initial encounter
T82.855A	Stenosis of coronary artery stent, initial encounter
T82.857A	Stenosis of other cardiac prosthetic devices, implants and grafts, initial encounter
T82.867A	Thrombosis due to cardiac prosthetic devices, implants and grafts, initial encounter
T82.897A	Other specified complication of cardiac prosthetic devices, implants and grafts, initial encounter

AMA: **33405** 2019,Nov; 2019,Apr **33406** 2019,Nov; 2019,Apr **33410** 2019,Nov; 2019,Apr

Relative Value Units/Medicare Edits

Non-Facility RVU	Work	PE	MP	Total
33405	41.32	15.52	9.92	66.76
33406	52.68	19.08	13.05	84.81
33410	46.41	17.04	11.23	74.68
Facility RVU	**Work**	**PE**	**MP**	**Total**
33405	41.32	15.52	9.92	66.76
33406	52.68	19.08	13.05	84.81
33410	46.41	17.04	11.23	74.68

	FUD	Status	MUE	Modifiers				IOM Reference
33405	90	A	1(2)	51	N/A	62*	80	None
33406	90	A	1(2)	51	N/A	62*	80	
33410	90	A	1(2)	51	N/A	62*	80	

* with documentation

[33440]

33440 Replacement, aortic valve; by translocation of autologous pulmonary valve and transventricular aortic annulus enlargement of the left ventricular outflow tract with valved conduit replacement of pulmonary valve (Ross-Konno procedure)

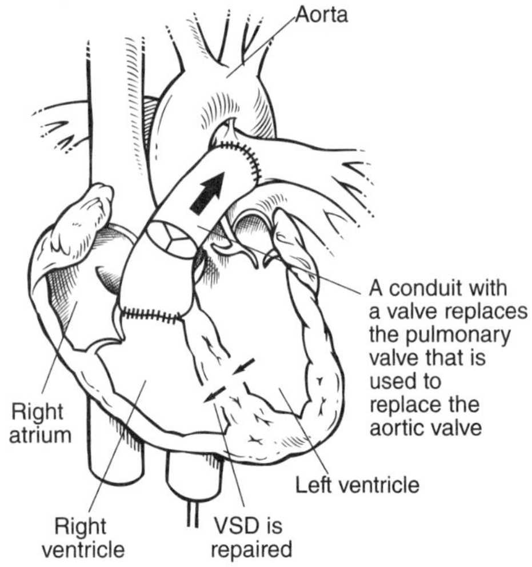

Explanation

Aortoventriculoplasty with pulmonary autograft (Ross-Konno procedure) is a treatment option geared toward younger patients diagnosed with left ventricular outflow tract obstructions who typically require aortic valve replacement reoperation. Cardiopulmonary bypass is initiated. The physician opens the patient using a median sternotomy approach and cold preserving solution is pumped into the coronary arteries to stop the heart. After aortic cross-clamping, the aorta and pulmonary artery are extensively excised and mobilized. Removal of the aortic valve and sinuses of Valsalva are performed. A pulmonary autograft is excised with a muscular tongue of the right ventricular front wall. A Konno technique incision is made in the interventricular septum beginning where the left and right coronary leaflets abut and toward the ventricular septal defect (VSD), if present, resecting the outflow septum. The incision length is based on the morphology of the obstruction and is made as far as needed in order to provide full relief of the left ventricular outflow tract obstruction (LVOTO). The pulmonary autograft is placed into aortic position using great care to precisely position the right ventricular front tongue and avoid injury to the left coronary artery, the pulmonary artery valves, and septal perforator of the left coronary artery. The right and left coronary buttons are implanted back into the autograft avoiding rotation, tension, or kinking. Anastomosis with the ascending aorta is made. Right ventricular (RV) and pulmonary artery (PA) connections are restored via the use of a homograft or bovine jugular vein conduit. Running sutures, including sutures at the base of the root and may include a thin strip of pericardium for reinforcement, are used. An echocardiogram should be performed once the patient has been weaned from bypass.

Coding Tips

For reoperation on the aortic valve more than one month after the original procedure, report 33530 in addition to the code for the primary procedure. Do not report 33440 with 33405-33414, 33416, 33417, 33475, 33608, or 33920. Cardiopulmonary bypass is included in 33440 and should not be reported separately. This code may be reported with codes for mitral valve and atrial septal defect repairs, when performed. For a Ross procedure, see 33413. For a Konno procedure, see 33412.

ICD-10-CM Diagnostic Codes

I06.0	Rheumatic aortic stenosis
I06.1	Rheumatic aortic insufficiency
I06.2	Rheumatic aortic stenosis with insufficiency
I06.8	Other rheumatic aortic valve diseases
I08.0	Rheumatic disorders of both mitral and aortic valves
I08.8	Other rheumatic multiple valve diseases
I35.0	Nonrheumatic aortic (valve) stenosis
I35.1	Nonrheumatic aortic (valve) insufficiency
I35.2	Nonrheumatic aortic (valve) stenosis with insufficiency
I35.8	Other nonrheumatic aortic valve disorders
Q23.0	Congenital stenosis of aortic valve
Q25.21	Interruption of aortic arch
Q25.29	Other atresia of aorta
Q25.3	Supravalvular aortic stenosis
T82.01XA	Breakdown (mechanical) of heart valve prosthesis, initial encounter
T82.02XA	Displacement of heart valve prosthesis, initial encounter
T82.03XA	Leakage of heart valve prosthesis, initial encounter
T82.09XA	Other mechanical complication of heart valve prosthesis, initial encounter
T82.6XXA	Infection and inflammatory reaction due to cardiac valve prosthesis, initial encounter
T82.817A	Embolism due to cardiac prosthetic devices, implants and grafts, initial encounter
T82.827A	Fibrosis due to cardiac prosthetic devices, implants and grafts, initial encounter
T82.837A	Hemorrhage due to cardiac prosthetic devices, implants and grafts, initial encounter
T82.847A	Pain due to cardiac prosthetic devices, implants and grafts, initial encounter
T82.855A	Stenosis of coronary artery stent, initial encounter
T82.857A	Stenosis of other cardiac prosthetic devices, implants and grafts, initial encounter
T82.867A	Thrombosis due to cardiac prosthetic devices, implants and grafts, initial encounter
T82.897A	Other specified complication of cardiac prosthetic devices, implants and grafts, initial encounter

AMA: 33440 2019,Apr

Relative Value Units/Medicare Edits

Non-Facility RVU	Work	PE	MP	Total
33440	64.0	20.6	14.81	99.41
Facility RVU	**Work**	**PE**	**MP**	**Total**
33440	64.0	20.6	14.81	99.41

	FUD	Status	MUE	Modifiers				IOM Reference
33440	90	A	1(2)	51	N/A	62*	80	None

* with documentation

33411-33412

33411 Replacement, aortic valve; with aortic annulus enlargement, noncoronary sinus

33412 with transventricular aortic annulus enlargement (Konno procedure)

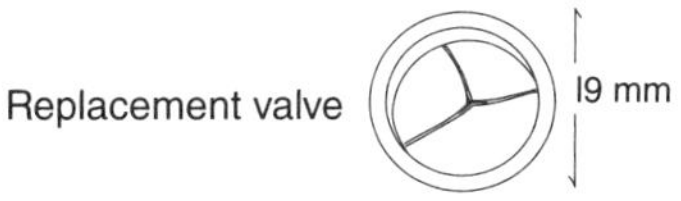

The aortic valve is replaced

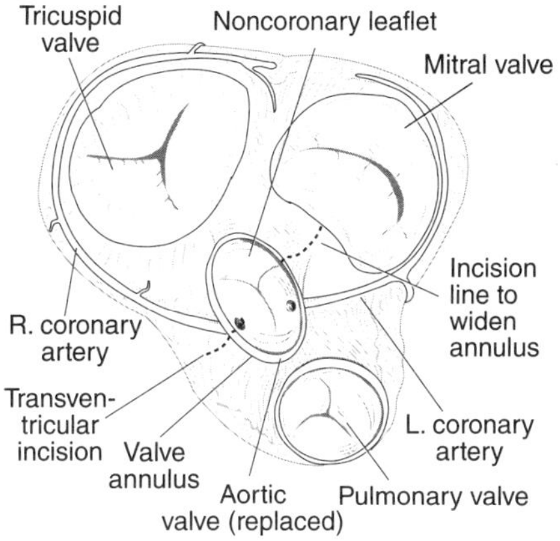

Overhead schematic of major heart valves

Explanation

Cardiopulmonary bypass is initiated. A clamp is placed on the aorta well above the heart. A cold preserving solution is pumped into the coronary arteries to stop the heart. The aorta is opened just above the aortic valve. The valve leaflets (cusps) are cut out and the annulus of the valve (ring of tissue where the valve leaflets normally attach to the aorta) is cleaned of calcium. At this point, a homograft or a xenograft is selected. The tissue valve is trimmed so that it can be sewn to the valve annulus. The aorta above the graft valve is trimmed so that the valve cusps can be suspended when the graft is in place and so the coronary arteries are not obstructed by the graft. When the valve is sized, it must be greater than or equal to 19 mm on a normal sized adult. If a smaller valve is inserted, the heart will slowly fail. Aortic annulus enlargement may be performed utilizing the noncoronary sinus, located just below the aortic valve (Nick's technique). Incision is carried downward posteriorly through the noncoronary aortic sinus across the aortic ring to the origin of the mitral valve. Dacron or other appropriate material is sutured to the fibrous origin of the mitral ring with mattress sutures, which are continued along the anterior and posterior margins of the aortic incision. The valve is sutured to the aortic ring and tied into position. Alternately, the aortic annular enlargement may be performed using the Manougian technique (through the commissure between the left coronary leaflet and the noncoronary leaflet). The aorta is cut longitudinally toward the heart and through the commissure (connecting point where two valve leaflets meet on the aortic wall) between the noncoronary leaflet (no coronary is near this leaflet) and the left coronary leaflet (leaflet near the left coronary artery) and across the valve annulus for a variable distance. The cut may need to extend onto the roof of the left atrium and onto the anterior leaflet of the mitral valve. The end of the cut is determined by the point at which the aortic root accommodates at least a 19 mm valve. The anterior mitral leaflet, left atrial roof, and the aorta are repaired with patches. The new valve is sewn in place. The aorta is closed and the clamp is taken off. Cardiopulmonary bypass is discontinued when heart function returns. In 33412, he physician replaces the aortic valve with transventricular aortic annulus enlargement, also referred to as the Konno procedure. The aorta is incised longitudinally toward a point just to the left of the right coronary artery. The cut is carried across the annulus and for a variable distance onto the right ventricular infundibulum. A triangular patch of pericardium or Dacron (e.g., a gusset) is used to close the incision in the right ventricle and aorta and to enlarge the aortic annulus. The new valve is sewn in place. The aorta is closed and the clamp is taken off. Cardiopulmonary bypass is discontinued when heart function returns.

Coding Tips

For reoperation on the aortic valve more than one month after the original procedure, report 33530 in addition to the code for the primary procedure. When more than one valve (aortic, mitral, tricuspid, pulmonary) is being repaired or replaced, report each procedure separately and append modifier 51 to the secondary valve procedures. Cardiopulmonary bypass is included in these codes and should not be reported separately. Do not report 33412 with 33413. Do not report 33411–33412 with 33440. For valvuloplasty of the aortic valve, see 33390–33391. For construction of the apical aortic conduit, see 33404. For the Ross-Konno procedure, see 33440.

ICD-10-CM Diagnostic Codes

I06.0	Rheumatic aortic stenosis
I06.1	Rheumatic aortic insufficiency
I06.2	Rheumatic aortic stenosis with insufficiency
I06.8	Other rheumatic aortic valve diseases
I08.0	Rheumatic disorders of both mitral and aortic valves
I08.8	Other rheumatic multiple valve diseases
I35.0	Nonrheumatic aortic (valve) stenosis
I35.1	Nonrheumatic aortic (valve) insufficiency
I35.2	Nonrheumatic aortic (valve) stenosis with insufficiency
I35.8	Other nonrheumatic aortic valve disorders
Q23.0	Congenital stenosis of aortic valve
Q25.21	Interruption of aortic arch
Q25.29	Other atresia of aorta
Q25.3	Supravalvular aortic stenosis
T82.01XA	Breakdown (mechanical) of heart valve prosthesis, initial encounter
T82.02XA	Displacement of heart valve prosthesis, initial encounter
T82.03XA	Leakage of heart valve prosthesis, initial encounter
T82.09XA	Other mechanical complication of heart valve prosthesis, initial encounter
T82.6XXA	Infection and inflammatory reaction due to cardiac valve prosthesis, initial encounter
T82.817A	Embolism due to cardiac prosthetic devices, implants and grafts, initial encounter
T82.827A	Fibrosis due to cardiac prosthetic devices, implants and grafts, initial encounter
T82.837A	Hemorrhage due to cardiac prosthetic devices, implants and grafts, initial encounter
T82.847A	Pain due to cardiac prosthetic devices, implants and grafts, initial encounter
T82.855A	Stenosis of coronary artery stent, initial encounter
T82.857A	Stenosis of other cardiac prosthetic devices, implants and grafts, initial encounter
T82.867A	Thrombosis due to cardiac prosthetic devices, implants and grafts, initial encounter
T82.897A	Other specified complication of cardiac prosthetic devices, implants and grafts, initial encounter

AMA: 33411 2023,Mar; 2019,Nov; 2019,Apr **33412** 2019,Nov; 2019,Apr

Relative Value Units/Medicare Edits

Non-Facility RVU	Work	PE	MP	Total
33411	62.07	21.5	14.83	98.4
33412	59.0	19.27	13.67	91.94
Facility RVU	**Work**	**PE**	**MP**	**Total**
33411	62.07	21.5	14.83	98.4
33412	59.0	19.27	13.67	91.94

	FUD	Status	MUE	Modifiers				IOM Reference
33411	90	A	1(2)	51	N/A	N/A	80	None
33412	90	A	1(2)	51	N/A	62*	80	

* with documentation

Terms To Know

aortic insufficiency. Malfunction of the aortic valve resulting in backflow of blood into the ventricle.

aortic stenosis. Narrowing of the aortic valve resulting in backflow of blood into the ventricle.

aortic valve. Heart valve, comprising three cusps, that divides the left ventricle and the aorta.

cardiopulmonary bypass. Venous blood is diverted to a heart-lung machine, which mechanically pumps and oxygenates the blood temporarily so the heart can be bypassed while an open procedure on the heart or coronary arteries is performed. During bypass, the lungs are deflated and immobile.

commissure. Juncture where two corresponding parts come together, especially referring to the union site of adjacent heart valve cusps.

congenital. Present at birth, occurring through heredity or an influence during gestation up to the moment of birth.

33413

33413 Replacement, aortic valve; by translocation of autologous pulmonary valve with allograft replacement of pulmonary valve (Ross procedure)

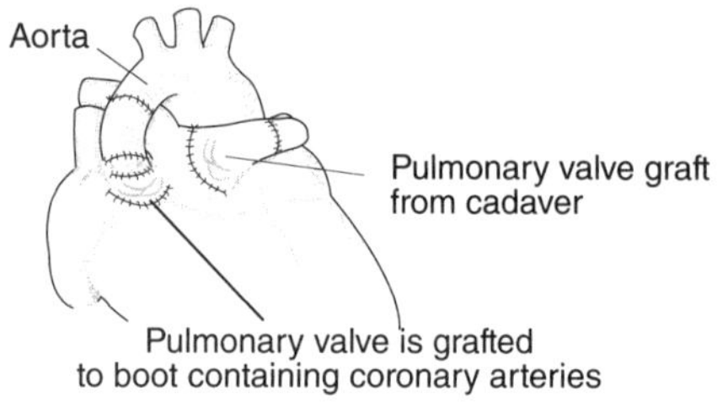

The pulmonary valve is then attached to the aorta and, in effect, becomes the aortic valve. The pulmonary valve is replaced by a graft, usually from a cadaver

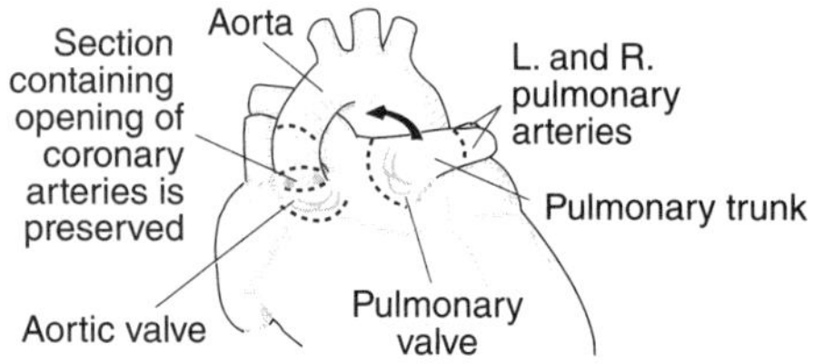

Explanation

Cardiopulmonary bypass is initiated. The aorta and pulmonary artery are separated and the main pulmonary trunk is completely cleaned off. After the heart is stopped, the pulmonary trunk is detached from the branching point of the left and right pulmonary arteries. It is taken off the heart with a small lip of heart muscle. Care is taken when the muscle of interventricular septum is cut. It is possible to damage a large branch of the left anterior descending coronary artery when this muscle is cut. The aorta is opened above the valve. The coronary arteries are detached from the aorta with a surrounding "button" of aortic wall. Next, the aortic valve and its annulus are removed from the heart. A length of the ascending aorta is also removed. The pulmonary artery is sewn to the heart in the aortic position. The commissures and cusps of the pulmonary valve are lined up to be in the same positions as their aortic counterparts were before the aortic valve was removed. The open end of the pulmonary artery is sewn to the ascending aorta. The coronary arteries are re-implanted on the pulmonary artery in positions similar to their positions on the aorta. The pulmonary valve and artery from an organ donor are sewn into the pulmonary position.

Coding Tips

For reoperation on the aortic valve more than one month after the original procedure, report 33530 in addition to the code for the primary procedure. When more than one valve (aortic, mitral, tricuspid, pulmonary) is being repaired or replaced, report each procedure separately and append modifier 51 to the secondary valve procedures. Do not report 33413 with 33412 or 33440. For valvuloplasty of the aortic valve, see 33390–33391. For construction of the apical aortic conduit, see 33404. For the Ross-Konno procedure, see 33440.

ICD-10-CM Diagnostic Codes

I06.0	Rheumatic aortic stenosis
I06.1	Rheumatic aortic insufficiency
I06.2	Rheumatic aortic stenosis with insufficiency
I06.8	Other rheumatic aortic valve diseases
I08.0	Rheumatic disorders of both mitral and aortic valves
I08.8	Other rheumatic multiple valve diseases

I35.0	Nonrheumatic aortic (valve) stenosis
I35.1	Nonrheumatic aortic (valve) insufficiency
I35.2	Nonrheumatic aortic (valve) stenosis with insufficiency
I35.8	Other nonrheumatic aortic valve disorders
Q23.0	Congenital stenosis of aortic valve
Q25.21	Interruption of aortic arch
Q25.29	Other atresia of aorta
Q25.3	Supravalvular aortic stenosis
T82.01XA	Breakdown (mechanical) of heart valve prosthesis, initial encounter
T82.02XA	Displacement of heart valve prosthesis, initial encounter
T82.03XA	Leakage of heart valve prosthesis, initial encounter
T82.09XA	Other mechanical complication of heart valve prosthesis, initial encounter
T82.6XXA	Infection and inflammatory reaction due to cardiac valve prosthesis, initial encounter
T82.817A	Embolism due to cardiac prosthetic devices, implants and grafts, initial encounter
T82.827A	Fibrosis due to cardiac prosthetic devices, implants and grafts, initial encounter
T82.837A	Hemorrhage due to cardiac prosthetic devices, implants and grafts, initial encounter
T82.847A	Pain due to cardiac prosthetic devices, implants and grafts, initial encounter
T82.855A	Stenosis of coronary artery stent, initial encounter
T82.857A	Stenosis of other cardiac prosthetic devices, implants and grafts, initial encounter
T82.867A	Thrombosis due to cardiac prosthetic devices, implants and grafts, initial encounter
T82.897A	Other specified complication of cardiac prosthetic devices, implants and grafts, initial encounter

AMA: 33413 2019,Nov; 2019,Apr

Relative Value Units/Medicare Edits

Non-Facility RVU	Work	PE	MP	Total
33413	59.87	20.49	13.88	94.24
Facility RVU	**Work**	**PE**	**MP**	**Total**
33413	59.87	20.49	13.88	94.24

	FUD	Status	MUE	Modifiers				IOM Reference
33413	90	A	1(2)	51	N/A	62*	80	None

* with documentation

33414

33414 Repair of left ventricular outflow tract obstruction by patch enlargement of the outflow tract

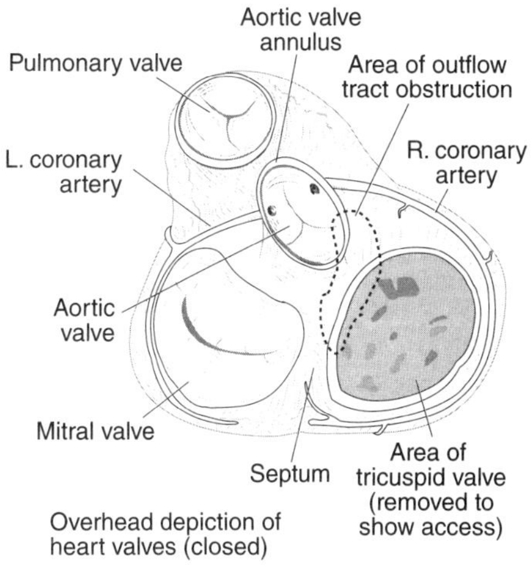

An outflow tract obstruction of the left ventricle is surgically approached

Explanation

The physician enlarges the left ventricular outflow track by patch due to obstruction. The physician performs a midline sternotomy, incising the skin, fascia, muscles, and sternum. The pericardium is incised and lines are placed for cardiopulmonary bypass. Dissection of the aorta is performed within the aorta, right ventricle, and pulmonary artery reaching the aortic annulus. An incision is made in the aorta and the right ventricular outflow tract is opened through the septum. The cusps of the aortic valve are removed. Reconstruction of the left ventricular outflow tract is achieved using a patch of Dacron cut into a diamond shape and the septum is closed to the area of patch placement. The aortic annulus is measured with replacement of aortic valve. An additional patch is attached to broaden the right ventricular outflow tract connecting it to the left ventricular outflow tract patch. The aortic valve prosthesis is connected to the outflow tract patches. The right ventricular outflow tract patch is attached to the right ventriculotomy. The pericardium is repaired loosely, leaving gaps for blood and fluid to drain into the pleural space. The sternum is reanastomosed with sternal wires and the skin is sutured in layers.

Coding Tips

For reoperation on the aortic valve more than one month after the original procedure, report 33530 in addition to the code for the primary procedure. When more than one valve (aortic, mitral, tricuspid, pulmonary) is being repaired or replaced, report each procedure separately and append modifier 51 to the secondary valve procedures. Do not report 33414 with 33440.

ICD-10-CM Diagnostic Codes

I06.0	Rheumatic aortic stenosis
I06.1	Rheumatic aortic insufficiency
I06.2	Rheumatic aortic stenosis with insufficiency
I06.8	Other rheumatic aortic valve diseases
I35.0	Nonrheumatic aortic (valve) stenosis
I35.1	Nonrheumatic aortic (valve) insufficiency
I35.2	Nonrheumatic aortic (valve) stenosis with insufficiency
I35.8	Other nonrheumatic aortic valve disorders
Q23.0	Congenital stenosis of aortic valve
Q25.21	Interruption of aortic arch

Q25.29	Other atresia of aorta
Q25.3	Supravalvular aortic stenosis

AMA: 33414 2023,Mar; 2019,Apr

Relative Value Units/Medicare Edits

Non-Facility RVU	Work	PE	MP	Total
33414	39.37	14.08	9.76	63.21
Facility RVU	**Work**	**PE**	**MP**	**Total**
33414	39.37	14.08	9.76	63.21

	FUD	Status	MUE	Modifiers				IOM Reference
33414	90	A	1(2)	51	N/A	62*	80	None

* with documentation

Terms To Know

anastomosis. Surgically created connection between ducts, blood vessels, or bowel segments to allow flow from one to the other.

aortic insufficiency. Malfunction of the aortic valve resulting in backflow of blood into the ventricle.

aortic stenosis. Narrowing of the aortic valve resulting in backflow of blood into the ventricle.

aortic valve disorders. Various types of aortic valve dysfunction, two main types being stenosis and insufficiency.

atresia. Congenital closure or absence of a tubular organ or an opening to the body surface.

cardiopulmonary bypass. Venous blood is diverted to a heart-lung machine, which mechanically pumps and oxygenates the blood temporarily so the heart can be bypassed while an open procedure on the heart or coronary arteries is performed. During bypass, the lungs are deflated and immobile.

congenital. Present at birth, occurring through heredity or an influence during gestation up to the moment of birth.

pericardium. Thin and slippery case in which the heart lies that is lined with fluid so that the heart is free to pulse and move as it beats.

stenosis. Narrowing or constriction of a passage.

sternotomy. Incision into the sternum, the bone that forms the front of the chest cavity and connects with the ribs.

33415-33416

33415 Resection or incision of subvalvular tissue for discrete subvalvular aortic stenosis

33416 Ventriculomyotomy (-myectomy) for idiopathic hypertrophic subaortic stenosis (eg, asymmetric septal hypertrophy)

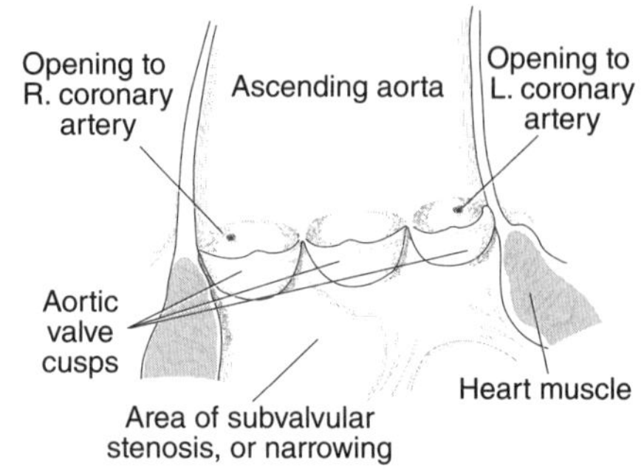

Cutaway schematic of the aortic valve and subvalvular tissues of the septum

Explanation

Cardiopulmonary bypass is initiated. The aorta is opened and the left ventricular outflow tract is assessed below the valve. There is usually a clearly definable ring or shelf below the valve. This is taken off with a tool designed for the purpose. Usually, the left ventricular septal muscle is thickened. A trough of muscle tissue is cut out of the left ventricular septal muscle. The aorta is closed. Cardiopulmonary bypass is discontinued when heart function returns. Report 33416 if there is no ring of subvalvular tissue to remove.

Coding Tips

Note the stenosis site when selecting the code. Subvalvular stenosis, also referred to as subaortic stenosis, is caused by an obstructive lesion in the left ventricle below the aortic valve. Report 33530 in addition to the code for the primary procedure for reoperation on the aortic valve more than one month after the original procedure. For percutaneous transcatheter septal reduction therapy, see 93583. When more than one valve (aortic, mitral, tricuspid, pulmonary) is being repaired or replaced, report each procedure separately and append modifier 51 to the secondary valve procedures. Do not report 33416 with 33440.

ICD-10-CM Diagnostic Codes

I06.0	Rheumatic aortic stenosis
I06.1	Rheumatic aortic insufficiency
I06.2	Rheumatic aortic stenosis with insufficiency
I08.0	Rheumatic disorders of both mitral and aortic valves
I08.2	Rheumatic disorders of both aortic and tricuspid valves
I35.0	Nonrheumatic aortic (valve) stenosis
I35.1	Nonrheumatic aortic (valve) insufficiency
I35.2	Nonrheumatic aortic (valve) stenosis with insufficiency
I35.8	Other nonrheumatic aortic valve disorders
I42.1	Obstructive hypertrophic cardiomyopathy
Q23.0	Congenital stenosis of aortic valve
Q23.1	Congenital insufficiency of aortic valve
Q24.4	Congenital subaortic stenosis
Q25.3	Supravalvular aortic stenosis

AMA: 33416 2019,Apr

Relative Value Units/Medicare Edits

Non-Facility RVU	Work	PE	MP	Total
33415	37.27	13.52	8.83	59.62
33416	36.56	14.24	8.75	59.55
Facility RVU	**Work**	**PE**	**MP**	**Total**
33415	37.27	13.52	8.83	59.62
33416	36.56	14.24	8.75	59.55

	FUD	Status	MUE	Modifiers				IOM Reference
33415	90	A	1(2)	51	N/A	62*	80	None
33416	90	A	1(2)	51	N/A	62*	80	

* with documentation

Terms To Know

aortic insufficiency. Malfunction of the aortic valve resulting in backflow of blood into the ventricle.

aortic stenosis. Narrowing of the aortic valve resulting in backflow of blood into the ventricle.

aortic valve disorders. Various types of aortic valve dysfunction, two main types being stenosis and insufficiency.

atresia. Congenital closure or absence of a tubular organ or an opening to the body surface.

cardiopulmonary bypass. Venous blood is diverted to a heart-lung machine, which mechanically pumps and oxygenates the blood temporarily so the heart can be bypassed while an open procedure on the heart or coronary arteries is performed. During bypass, the lungs are deflated and immobile.

cardiotomy. Incision of the heart, the cardiac orifice, or the cardiac end of the stomach.

congenital. Present at birth, occurring through heredity or an influence during gestation up to the moment of birth.

hypertrophic. Enlarged or overgrown from an increase in cell size of the affected tissue.

incision. Act of cutting into tissue or an organ.

resection. Surgical removal of a part or all of an organ or body part.

stenosis. Narrowing or constriction of a passage.

trabeculae carneae cordis. Bands of muscular tissue that line the walls of the ventricles in the heart.

33417

33417 Aortoplasty (gusset) for supravalvular stenosis

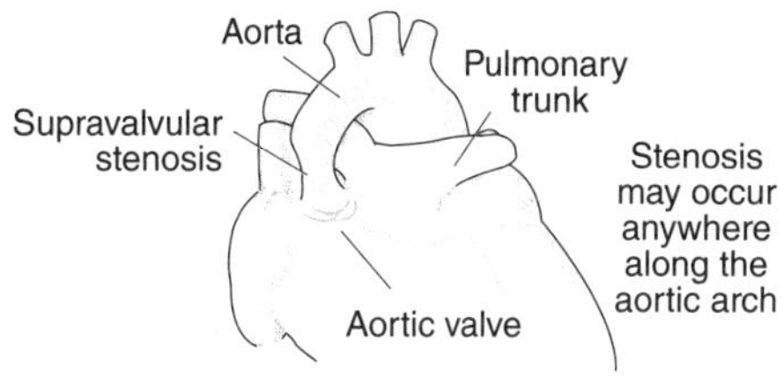

Stenosis, or narrowing, occurs above the aortic valve. Patch graft shown

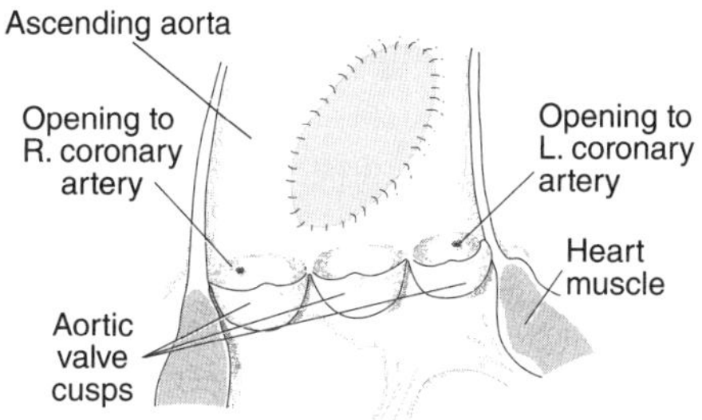

Cutaway schematic of the aortic valve and supravalvular tissues

Explanation

Aortoplasty for supravalvular stenosis is performed with a median sternotomy to gain access. Cardiopulmonary bypass is required. A piece of pericardium or Dacron is prepared. The aorta is clamped beyond the area of narrowing. The heart is stopped with a cold preserving solution. An incision is made into the narrowest point of the ascending aorta and three additional incisions are made that extend into the sinuses of Valsalva. Using patches of pericardium, the sinuses are enlarged. A patch from the noncoronary sinus is extended into the ascending aorta in order to assure symmetrical enlargement. The clamp is released. Cardiopulmonary bypass is discontinued when heart function returns.

Coding Tips

Note the stenosis site when selecting the code. Supravalvular aortic stenosis is a rare condition, occurring above the aortic valve usually caused by a constricting ring of the fibrous tissue at the level of the sinus of Valsalva. Report 33530 in addition to the code for the primary procedure for reoperation on the aortic valve more than one month after the original procedure. When more than one valve (aortic, mitral, tricuspid, pulmonary) is being repaired or replaced, report each procedure separately and append modifier 51 to the secondary valve procedures. Do not report 33417 with 33440.

ICD-10-CM Diagnostic Codes

I06.0	Rheumatic aortic stenosis
I06.1	Rheumatic aortic insufficiency
I06.2	Rheumatic aortic stenosis with insufficiency
I06.8	Other rheumatic aortic valve diseases
I35.0	Nonrheumatic aortic (valve) stenosis
I35.1	Nonrheumatic aortic (valve) insufficiency
I35.2	Nonrheumatic aortic (valve) stenosis with insufficiency
I35.8	Other nonrheumatic aortic valve disorders
Q23.0	Congenital stenosis of aortic valve
Q25.21	Interruption of aortic arch

Q25.29 Other atresia of aorta
Q25.3 Supravalvular aortic stenosis

AMA: **33417** 2019,Apr

Relative Value Units/Medicare Edits

Non-Facility RVU	Work	PE	MP	Total
33417	29.33	12.73	7.27	49.33
Facility RVU	**Work**	**PE**	**MP**	**Total**
33417	29.33	12.73	7.27	49.33

	FUD	Status	MUE	Modifiers				IOM Reference
33417	90	A	1(2)	51	N/A	62*	80	None

* with documentation

Terms To Know

aortic insufficiency. Malfunction of the aortic valve resulting in backflow of blood into the ventricle.

aortic stenosis. Narrowing of the aortic valve resulting in backflow of blood into the ventricle.

aortic valve disorders. Various types of aortic valve dysfunction, two main types being stenosis and insufficiency.

atresia. Congenital closure or absence of a tubular organ or an opening to the body surface.

cardiopulmonary bypass. Venous blood is diverted to a heart-lung machine, which mechanically pumps and oxygenates the blood temporarily so the heart can be bypassed while an open procedure on the heart or coronary arteries is performed. During bypass, the lungs are deflated and immobile.

gusset. Triangular or diamond shaped patch that is placed for reinforcement or expansion.

incision. Act of cutting into tissue or an organ.

pericardium. Thin and slippery case in which the heart lies that is lined with fluid so that the heart is free to pulse and move as it beats.

stenosis. Narrowing or constriction of a passage.

valvuloplasty. Surgical repair of a valve.

33418-33419

33418 Transcatheter mitral valve repair, percutaneous approach, including transseptal puncture when performed; initial prosthesis

\+ **33419** Transcatheter mitral valve repair, percutaneous approach, including transseptal puncture when performed; additional prosthesis(es) during same session (List separately in addition to code for primary procedure)

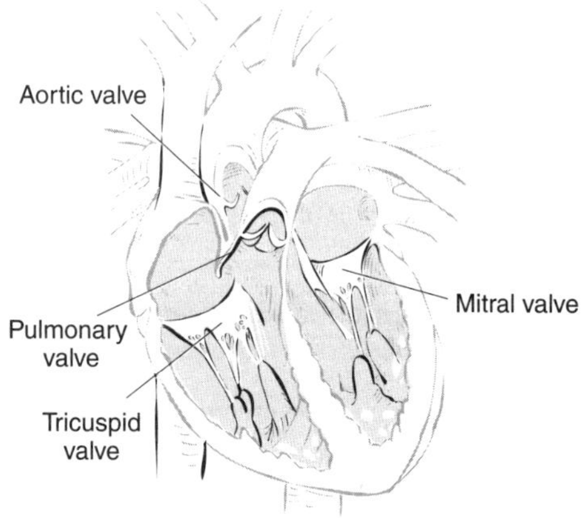

The mitral valve is repaired percutaneously

Explanation

A mitral valve is repaired percutaneously. The procedure is performed under general anesthesia. The physician makes an incision over a lower extremity vessel, usually the femoral vein. A catheter with a specially designed prosthesis or stent is maneuvered through the vessels to the heart under fluoroscopic imaging guidance. Depending on the approach and the device being used, the catheter may be threaded through the inferior vena cava to the right atrium where a septal puncture to access the left atrium and mitral valve is created. Once the device is positioned above the diseased valve, it is secured into place with precautions taken to ensure proper positioning and anchoring. The physician removes the catheter and the surgical wound is closed. Report 33418 for insertion of the initial device and 33419 for any additional devices used during the same operative session.

Coding Tips

Codes 33367 percutaneous bypass, 33368 open peripheral bypass, and 33369 central bypass may be reported in addition to 33418 and 33419 when cardiopulmonary bypass is performed. These codes include percutaneous access, placing sheath, transseptal puncture, advancement of repair device delivery system, repositioning, and deployment of the device, when performed. Report 33419 in addition to 33418 and report only once per encounter. Do not report 33418 with 93462 unless transapical puncture is performed. For transcatheter mitral valve percutaneous approach via coronary sinus, see 0345T. Radiological supervision and interpretation for guidance, including documentation of completion, is included and is not reported separately. Do not report diagnostic heart catheterization with 33418 or 33419 for contrast administration, angiography, road mapping or guidance, to assess regurgitation for guidance, or for hemodynamic measurements occurring before, during, and after the procedure. Other diagnostic cardiac catheterizations may be reported separately when performed for purposes unrelated to TMVR procedures. Diagnostic catheterization and diagnostic coronary angiography codes may be reported separately in cases where a previous examination is not available or the anatomic visualization is poor quality, there has been a clinical change in the patient's condition since the previous examination, or complications arise during the procedure requiring the additional study. Percutaneous coronary procedures may be reported separately, when performed. Codes 33990–33993, 33995, and 33997 for ventricular assist devices and 33967, 33970, and 33973 for balloon pump insertion may be reported separately, when performed.

ICD-10-CM Diagnostic Codes

I05.1	Rheumatic mitral insufficiency
I05.2	Rheumatic mitral stenosis with insufficiency
I05.8	Other rheumatic mitral valve diseases
I08.0	Rheumatic disorders of both mitral and aortic valves
I08.1	Rheumatic disorders of both mitral and tricuspid valves
I08.3	Combined rheumatic disorders of mitral, aortic and tricuspid valves
I08.8	Other rheumatic multiple valve diseases
I34.0	Nonrheumatic mitral (valve) insufficiency
I34.1	Nonrheumatic mitral (valve) prolapse
I34.2	Nonrheumatic mitral (valve) stenosis
I34.81	Nonrheumatic mitral (valve) annulus calcification
I34.89	Other nonrheumatic mitral valve disorders
Q23.2	Congenital mitral stenosis
Q23.3	Congenital mitral insufficiency
Q23.81	Bicuspid aortic valve
Q23.82	Congenital mitral valve cleft leaflet
Q23.88	Other congenital malformations of aortic and mitral valves

AMA: **33418** 2023,May **33419** 2023,May

Relative Value Units/Medicare Edits

Non-Facility RVU	Work	PE	MP	Total
33418	32.25	13.17	7.42	52.84
33419	7.93	2.64	1.81	12.38
Facility RVU	**Work**	**PE**	**MP**	**Total**
33418	32.25	13.17	7.42	52.84
33419	7.93	2.64	1.81	12.38

	FUD	Status	MUE	Modifiers				IOM Reference
33418	90	A	1(3)	51	N/A	62*	80	None
33419	N/A	A	1(2)	N/A	N/A	62*	80	

* with documentation

Terms To Know

angiography. Radiographic imaging of the arteries.

cardiopulmonary bypass. Venous blood is diverted to a heart-lung machine, which mechanically pumps and oxygenates the blood temporarily so the heart can be bypassed while an open procedure on the heart or coronary arteries is performed. During bypass, the lungs are deflated and immobile.

insufficiency. Inadequate closure of the valve that allows abnormal backward blood flow.

mitral valve. Valve with two cusps that is between the left atrium and left ventricle of the heart.

percutaneous. Through the skin.

stenosis. Narrowing or constriction of a passage.

transcatheter. Procedure or treatment performed via a catheter.

33420-33422

33420 Valvotomy, mitral valve; closed heart
33422 open heart, with cardiopulmonary bypass

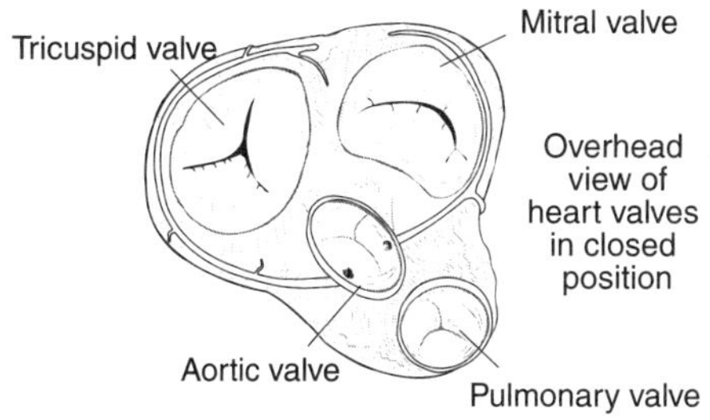

Cutaway view of heart showing left-side valves

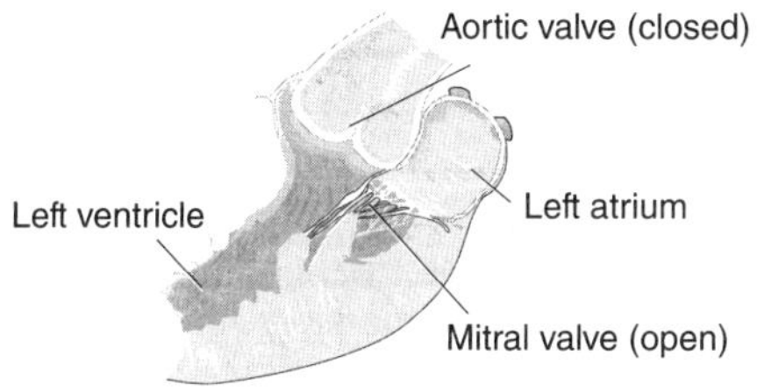

Explanation

In 33420, the chest is opened by median sternotomy or left thoracotomy. The pericardium is opened. An incision is performed within the left atrial appendage where a Tubbs dilator (or gloved physician's finger) is introduced into the left ventricle by way of the apex and opened in the valve. Calcium deposits may be removed from the annulus and leaflets with a bone nibbler. Upon completion of valvotomy, the dilator (or finger) is removed and the incisions are sutured closed. In 33422, the skin and muscle are incised from the sternum to the xiphoid process. The sternum is split and a retractor is utilized to open the chest. An incision is made in the pericardium and cardiopulmonary bypass is initiated. The left atrium is opened from the right side. The mitral valve is exposed. The scar tissue between the lateral ends of the valve leaflets is divided sharply. Cardiopulmonary bypass is discontinued when heart function returns. The pericardium and left atrium are closed. Chest tubes may be inserted to allow drainage.

Coding Tips

For reoperation on the aortic valve more than one month after the original procedure, report 33530 in addition to the code for the primary procedure. When more than one valve (aortic, mitral, tricuspid, pulmonary) is being repaired or replaced, report each procedure separately and append modifier 51 to the secondary valve procedures. For valvuloplasty of the mitral valve with cardiopulmonary bypass, see 33425; with prosthetic ring, see 33426; with radical reconstruction, see 33427. For replacement of the mitral valve with cardiopulmonary bypass, see 33430.

ICD-10-CM Diagnostic Codes

I05.0	Rheumatic mitral stenosis
I05.1	Rheumatic mitral insufficiency
I05.2	Rheumatic mitral stenosis with insufficiency
I05.8	Other rheumatic mitral valve diseases
I08.0	Rheumatic disorders of both mitral and aortic valves
I08.8	Other rheumatic multiple valve diseases
I34.0	Nonrheumatic mitral (valve) insufficiency
I34.1	Nonrheumatic mitral (valve) prolapse

I34.2	Nonrheumatic mitral (valve) stenosis
I34.81	Nonrheumatic mitral (valve) annulus calcification
I34.89	Other nonrheumatic mitral valve disorders
Q23.2	Congenital mitral stenosis
Q23.3	Congenital mitral insufficiency
Q23.82	Congenital mitral valve cleft leaflet
Q23.88	Other congenital malformations of aortic and mitral valves

AMA: **33420** 2021,Nov **33422** 2021,Nov

Relative Value Units/Medicare Edits

Non-Facility RVU	Work	PE	MP	Total
33420	25.79	10.86	5.98	42.63
33422	29.73	12.26	6.86	48.85
Facility RVU	**Work**	**PE**	**MP**	**Total**
33420	25.79	10.86	5.98	42.63
33422	29.73	12.26	6.86	48.85

	FUD	Status	MUE	Modifiers				IOM Reference
33420	90	A	1(2)	51	N/A	62*	N/A	None
33422	90	A	1(2)	51	N/A	62*	80	

* with documentation

Terms To Know

cardiopulmonary bypass. Venous blood is diverted to a heart-lung machine, which mechanically pumps and oxygenates the blood temporarily so the heart can be bypassed while an open procedure on the heart or coronary arteries is performed. During bypass, the lungs are deflated and immobile.

congenital. Present at birth, occurring through heredity or an influence during gestation up to the moment of birth.

mitral valve. Valve with two cusps that is between the left atrium and left ventricle of the heart.

pericardium. Thin and slippery case in which the heart lies that is lined with fluid so that the heart is free to pulse and move as it beats.

prosthesis. Man-made substitute for a missing body part.

scar tissue. Fibrous connective tissue that forms around a wounded area or injury, composed mainly of fibroblasts or collagenous fibers.

stenosis. Narrowing or constriction of a passage.

valvotomy. Cutting through stenosed cardiac valve leaflets or cusp to relieve or repair the obstruction caused by scar tissue and inflammation.

valvuloplasty. Surgical repair of a valve.

33425-33427

33425 Valvuloplasty, mitral valve, with cardiopulmonary bypass;
33426 with prosthetic ring
33427 radical reconstruction, with or without ring

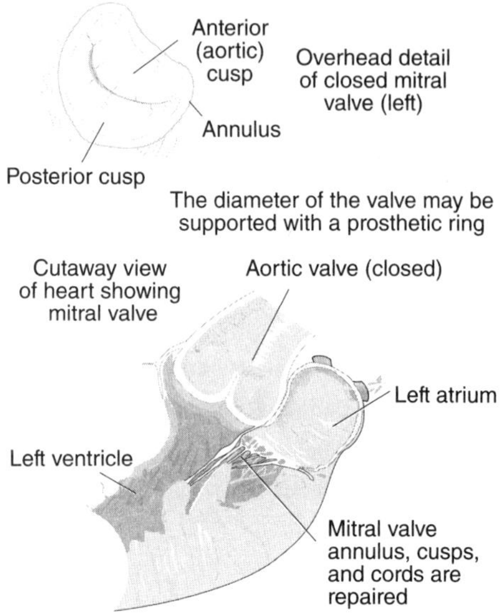

The mitral valve is accessed and surgically repaired

Explanation

This operation is done to improve the ability of the mitral valve to close completely when the ventricle contracts. It is done in patients whose mitral valve has lost the ability to close normally. In almost all cases, this is the result of a mitral valve prolapse in which the mitral leaflets and the cords that tether them on the ventricle have become elongated. Cardiopulmonary bypass is initiated. The left atrium is opened and the mitral valve is exposed. Redundant leaflet tissue is excised and defects in the valve leaflets are closed with sutures. The cords are also shortened with sutures. Valve closure is assessed after the repair. The left atrium is closed and cardiopulmonary bypass is discontinued when heart function returns. Report 33426 if the mitral valve diameter is enlarged requiring placement of a prosthetic ring. Report 33427 if a more extensive repair, including transfer of cords from the posterior leaflet to the anterior leaflet, is performed. A prosthetic ring may be required with extensive reconstruction.

Coding Tips

For reoperation on the mitral valve more than one month after the original procedure, report 33530 in addition to the code for the primary procedure. When more than one valve (aortic, mitral, tricuspid, pulmonary) is being repaired or replaced, report each procedure separately and append modifier 51 to the secondary valve procedures. For valvotomy of the mitral valve, see 33420–33422. For replacement of the mitral valve, see 33430. For percutaneous balloon valvuloplasty of the mitral valve, see 92987.

ICD-10-CM Diagnostic Codes

I05.0	Rheumatic mitral stenosis
I05.1	Rheumatic mitral insufficiency
I05.2	Rheumatic mitral stenosis with insufficiency
I05.8	Other rheumatic mitral valve diseases
I08.0	Rheumatic disorders of both mitral and aortic valves
I08.8	Other rheumatic multiple valve diseases

N Newborn: 0 P Pediatric: 0-17 M Maternity: 9-64 A Adult: 15-124 AMA: CPT Assist

I34.0	Nonrheumatic mitral (valve) insufficiency
I34.1	Nonrheumatic mitral (valve) prolapse
I34.2	Nonrheumatic mitral (valve) stenosis
I34.81	Nonrheumatic mitral (valve) annulus calcification
I34.89	Other nonrheumatic mitral valve disorders
Q23.2	Congenital mitral stenosis
Q23.3	Congenital mitral insufficiency
Q23.82	Congenital mitral valve cleft leaflet
Q23.88	Other congenital malformations of aortic and mitral valves

AMA: 33425 2021,Nov **33426** 2021,Nov; 2021,Apr **33427** 2021,Nov; 2021,Apr

Relative Value Units/Medicare Edits

Non-Facility RVU	Work	PE	MP	Total
33425	49.96	18.28	11.99	80.23
33426	43.28	16.39	10.41	70.08
33427	44.83	16.37	10.46	71.66
Facility RVU	**Work**	**PE**	**MP**	**Total**
33425	49.96	18.28	11.99	80.23
33426	43.28	16.39	10.41	70.08
33427	44.83	16.37	10.46	71.66

	FUD	Status	MUE	Modifiers				IOM Reference
33425	90	A	1(2)	51	N/A	62*	80	None
33426	90	A	1(2)	51	N/A	62*	80	
33427	90	A	1(2)	51	N/A	62*	80	

* with documentation

Terms To Know

cardiopulmonary bypass. Venous blood is diverted to a heart-lung machine, which mechanically pumps and oxygenates the blood temporarily so the heart can be bypassed while an open procedure on the heart or coronary arteries is performed. During bypass, the lungs are deflated and immobile.

congenital. Present at birth, occurring through heredity or an influence during gestation up to the moment of birth.

hypothermia with cardiac bypass. Reduction of the body temperature using a bypass system to reduce the oxygen demands of tissue and to protect the myocardium during a procedure.

mitral valve. Valve with two cusps that is between the left atrium and left ventricle of the heart.

prolapse. Falling, sliding, or sinking of an organ from its normal location in the body.

reconstruction. Recreating, restoring, or rebuilding a body part or organ.

stenosis. Narrowing or constriction of a passage.

33430

33430 Replacement, mitral valve, with cardiopulmonary bypass

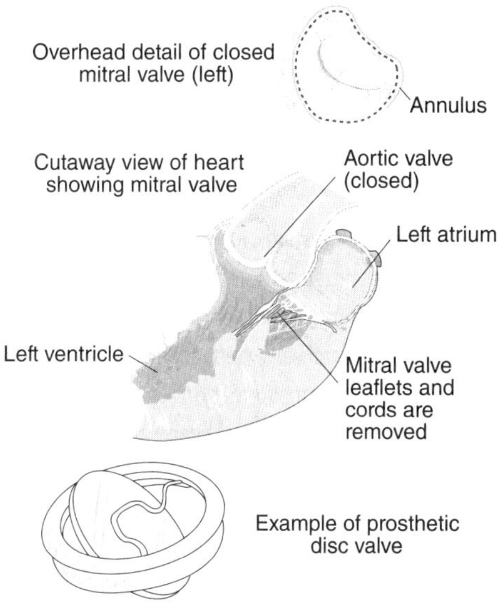

The mitral valve is accessed and surgically removed along with attachment cords. Any of a variety of replacement valves is selected and sutured to the annulus of the former valve

Explanation

The physician performs a sternotomy to gain access to the heart. Cardiopulmonary bypass is initiated. The mitral valve may be accessed by opening the right atrium followed by opening the atrial septum or the left atrium directly, exposing the mitral valve. All leaflet tissue and its attached cords are cut out. Sutures are placed in the mitral annulus. The annulus is sized and an appropriate artificial valve is selected (a totally mechanical valve or a valve with plastic supports and tissue leaflets). The sutures are passed through the sewing ring of the annulus and the sutures are tied down so the sewing ring is adherent to the annulus. The atrial septum (or left atrium) may be sutured closed or left to heal on its own. Cardiopulmonary bypass is discontinued when heart function returns. The sternotomy is closed with wires and the skin is sutured closed.

Coding Tips

For reoperation on the aortic valve more than one month after the original procedure, report 33530 in addition to the code for the primary procedure. When more than one valve (aortic, mitral, tricuspid, pulmonary) is being repaired or replaced, report each procedure separately and append modifier 51 to the secondary valve procedures. For valvuloplasty of the mitral valve, see 33425–33427.

ICD-10-CM Diagnostic Codes

I05.0	Rheumatic mitral stenosis
I05.1	Rheumatic mitral insufficiency
I05.2	Rheumatic mitral stenosis with insufficiency
I05.8	Other rheumatic mitral valve diseases
I08.0	Rheumatic disorders of both mitral and aortic valves
I08.8	Other rheumatic multiple valve diseases
I34.0	Nonrheumatic mitral (valve) insufficiency
I34.1	Nonrheumatic mitral (valve) prolapse
I34.2	Nonrheumatic mitral (valve) stenosis

I34.81	Nonrheumatic mitral (valve) annulus calcification
I34.89	Other nonrheumatic mitral valve disorders
M32.0	Drug-induced systemic lupus erythematosus
M32.11	Endocarditis in systemic lupus erythematosus
M32.12	Pericarditis in systemic lupus erythematosus
M32.13	Lung involvement in systemic lupus erythematosus
M32.14	Glomerular disease in systemic lupus erythematosus
M32.15	Tubulo-interstitial nephropathy in systemic lupus erythematosus
M32.19	Other organ or system involvement in systemic lupus erythematosus
M32.8	Other forms of systemic lupus erythematosus
Q23.2	Congenital mitral stenosis
Q23.3	Congenital mitral insufficiency
Q23.82	Congenital mitral valve cleft leaflet
Q23.88	Other congenital malformations of aortic and mitral valves
T82.01XA	Breakdown (mechanical) of heart valve prosthesis, initial encounter
T82.02XA	Displacement of heart valve prosthesis, initial encounter
T82.03XA	Leakage of heart valve prosthesis, initial encounter
T82.09XA	Other mechanical complication of heart valve prosthesis, initial encounter
T82.6XXA	Infection and inflammatory reaction due to cardiac valve prosthesis, initial encounter
T82.817A	Embolism due to cardiac prosthetic devices, implants and grafts, initial encounter
T82.827A	Fibrosis due to cardiac prosthetic devices, implants and grafts, initial encounter
T82.837A	Hemorrhage due to cardiac prosthetic devices, implants and grafts, initial encounter
T82.847A	Pain due to cardiac prosthetic devices, implants and grafts, initial encounter
T82.855A	Stenosis of coronary artery stent, initial encounter
T82.857A	Stenosis of other cardiac prosthetic devices, implants and grafts, initial encounter
T82.867A	Thrombosis due to cardiac prosthetic devices, implants and grafts, initial encounter
T82.897A	Other specified complication of cardiac prosthetic devices, implants and grafts, initial encounter

AMA: 33430 2024,Oct; 2021,Nov

Relative Value Units/Medicare Edits

Non-Facility RVU	Work	PE	MP	Total
33430	50.93	19.24	12.2	82.37
Facility RVU	**Work**	**PE**	**MP**	**Total**
33430	50.93	19.24	12.2	82.37

	FUD	Status	MUE	Modifiers				IOM Reference
33430	90	A	1(2)	51	N/A	62*	80	None

* with documentation

33460-33464

33460 Valvectomy, tricuspid valve, with cardiopulmonary bypass
33463 Valvuloplasty, tricuspid valve; without ring insertion
33464 with ring insertion

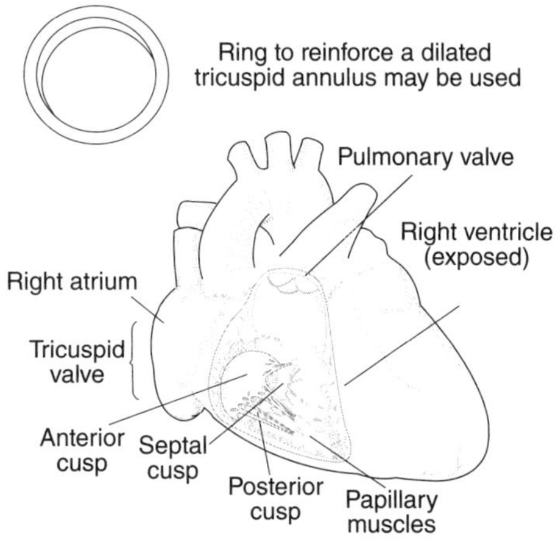

Cutaway view of the heart showing right side valves

Explanation

In 33460, cardiopulmonary bypass is initiated. The right atrium is opened and the tricuspid valve is exposed. The valve tissue and its cords are completely excised. The right atrium is closed. Cardiopulmonary bypass is discontinued when heart function returns. In 33463, cardiopulmonary bypass is initiated with venous uptake tubes in both of the caval veins. The right atrium is opened. Valvuloplasty of the tricuspid valve almost always requires nothing more than reducing the diameter of the tricuspid valve. To accomplish this, a double purse string of sutures is placed around the circumference of the valve and tightened to reduce the valve diameter. The right atrium is closed. Report 33464 if a stiff ring is used to reduce the valve's diameter rather than purse strings.

Coding Tips

For reoperation on the aortic valve more than one month after the original procedure, report 33530 in addition to the code for the primary procedure. When more than one valve (aortic, mitral, tricuspid, pulmonary) is being repaired or replaced, report each procedure separately and append modifier 51 to the secondary valve procedures. For replacement of the tricuspid valve, see 33465. For transcatheter tricuspid valve implantation replacement, see 0646T. For transcatheter tricuspid valve repair, see 0569T-0570T.

ICD-10-CM Diagnostic Codes

I07.0	Rheumatic tricuspid stenosis
I07.1	Rheumatic tricuspid insufficiency
I07.2	Rheumatic tricuspid stenosis and insufficiency
I07.8	Other rheumatic tricuspid valve diseases
I36.0	Nonrheumatic tricuspid (valve) stenosis
I36.1	Nonrheumatic tricuspid (valve) insufficiency
I36.2	Nonrheumatic tricuspid (valve) stenosis with insufficiency
I36.8	Other nonrheumatic tricuspid valve disorders
Q22.4	Congenital tricuspid stenosis
Q22.6	Hypoplastic right heart syndrome
Q22.8	Other congenital malformations of tricuspid valve
T82.01XA	Breakdown (mechanical) of heart valve prosthesis, initial encounter

N Newborn: 0 P Pediatric: 0-17 M Maternity: 9-64 A Adult: 15-124 AMA: CPT Assist

T82.02XA Displacement of heart valve prosthesis, initial encounter

T82.03XA Leakage of heart valve prosthesis, initial encounter

T82.09XA Other mechanical complication of heart valve prosthesis, initial encounter

T82.6XXA Infection and inflammatory reaction due to cardiac valve prosthesis, initial encounter

T82.7XXA Infection and inflammatory reaction due to other cardiac and vascular devices, implants and grafts, initial encounter

T82.817A Embolism due to cardiac prosthetic devices, implants and grafts, initial encounter

T82.827A Fibrosis due to cardiac prosthetic devices, implants and grafts, initial encounter

T82.837A Hemorrhage due to cardiac prosthetic devices, implants and grafts, initial encounter

T82.847A Pain due to cardiac prosthetic devices, implants and grafts, initial encounter

T82.855A Stenosis of coronary artery stent, initial encounter

T82.857A Stenosis of other cardiac prosthetic devices, implants and grafts, initial encounter

T82.867A Thrombosis due to cardiac prosthetic devices, implants and grafts, initial encounter

T82.897A Other specified complication of cardiac prosthetic devices, implants and grafts, initial encounter

AMA: 33463 2018,Jun

Relative Value Units/Medicare Edits

Non-Facility RVU	Work	PE	MP	Total
33460	44.7	15.1	10.37	70.17
33463	57.08	20.06	13.15	90.29
33464	44.62	16.59	10.42	71.63
Facility RVU	**Work**	**PE**	**MP**	**Total**
33460	44.7	15.1	10.37	70.17
33463	57.08	20.06	13.15	90.29
33464	44.62	16.59	10.42	71.63

	FUD	Status	MUE	Modifiers				IOM Reference
33460	90	A	1(2)	51	N/A	62*	80	None
33463	90	A	1(2)	51	N/A	62*	80	
33464	90	A	1(2)	51	N/A	62*	80	

* with documentation

Terms To Know

endocarditis. Inflammatory disease of the interior lining of the heart chamber and heart valves.

tricuspid valve. Valve with three cusps between the right atrium and the right ventricle.

valvectomy. Excision of a valve.

valvuloplasty. Surgical repair of a valve.

33465

33465 Replacement, tricuspid valve, with cardiopulmonary bypass

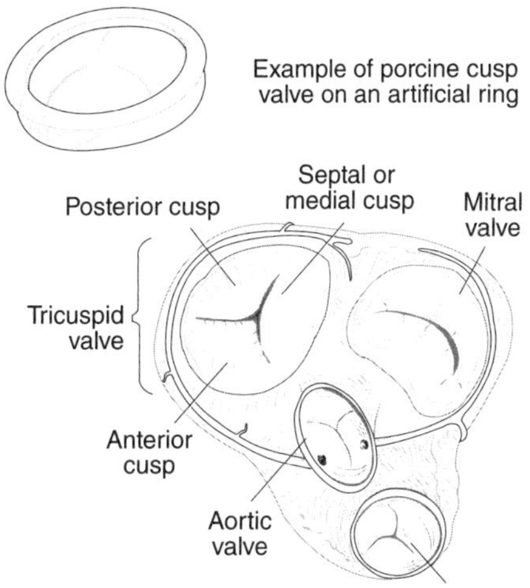

Overhead schematic of heart valves

Explanation

The physician incises the sternum with a cut of about 7 to 9 inches to expose the heart. A minimally invasive procedure could entail a sternal incision of 2 to 4 inches or an incision between the ribs. Cardiopulmonary bypass is initiated with venous uptake tubes in both caval veins. The right atrium is opened and clamps are placed on the aorta. Typically, the tricuspid valve leaflets are left intact; however, when excessive thickening is present, several incisions into the leaflets may be necessary allowing for the best possible fit of the prosthetic. A valve of an appropriate diameter is selected (usually it is a tissue/plastic valve, although a metal valve can also be used). Sutures are placed around the circumference of the tricuspid valve annulus. They are brought through the sewing ring of the valve. The valve is seated so that the sewing ring is resting on the annulus. The sutures are tied tightly. The right atrium is closed. Cardiopulmonary bypass is discontinued when heart function returns.

Coding Tips

For reoperation on the aortic valve more than one month after the original procedure, report 33530 in addition to the code for the primary procedure. When more than one valve (aortic, mitral, tricuspid, pulmonary) is being repaired or replaced, report each procedure separately and append modifier 51 to the secondary valve procedures. For valvectomy of the tricuspid valve, see 33460. For valvuloplasty of the tricuspid valve, see 33463–33464. For transcatheter tricuspid valve implantation replacement, see 0646T. For transcatheter tricuspid valve repair, see 0569T-0570T.

ICD-10-CM Diagnostic Codes

I07.0 Rheumatic tricuspid stenosis

I07.1 Rheumatic tricuspid insufficiency

I07.2 Rheumatic tricuspid stenosis and insufficiency

I07.8 Other rheumatic tricuspid valve diseases

I36.0 Nonrheumatic tricuspid (valve) stenosis

I36.1 Nonrheumatic tricuspid (valve) insufficiency

I36.2 Nonrheumatic tricuspid (valve) stenosis with insufficiency

I36.8 Other nonrheumatic tricuspid valve disorders

Q22.4 Congenital tricuspid stenosis

Q22.6 Hypoplastic right heart syndrome

Q22.8 Other congenital malformations of tricuspid valve
T82.01XA Breakdown (mechanical) of heart valve prosthesis, initial encounter
T82.02XA Displacement of heart valve prosthesis, initial encounter
T82.03XA Leakage of heart valve prosthesis, initial encounter
T82.09XA Other mechanical complication of heart valve prosthesis, initial encounter
T82.6XXA Infection and inflammatory reaction due to cardiac valve prosthesis, initial encounter
T82.817A Embolism due to cardiac prosthetic devices, implants and grafts, initial encounter
T82.827A Fibrosis due to cardiac prosthetic devices, implants and grafts, initial encounter
T82.837A Hemorrhage due to cardiac prosthetic devices, implants and grafts, initial encounter
T82.847A Pain due to cardiac prosthetic devices, implants and grafts, initial encounter
T82.855A Stenosis of coronary artery stent, initial encounter
T82.857A Stenosis of other cardiac prosthetic devices, implants and grafts, initial encounter
T82.867A Thrombosis due to cardiac prosthetic devices, implants and grafts, initial encounter
T82.897A Other specified complication of cardiac prosthetic devices, implants and grafts, initial encounter

Relative Value Units/Medicare Edits

Non-Facility RVU	Work	PE	MP	Total
33465	50.72	18.09	12.08	80.89
Facility RVU	**Work**	**PE**	**MP**	**Total**
33465	50.72	18.09	12.08	80.89

	FUD	Status	MUE	Modifiers				IOM Reference
33465	90	A	1(2)	51	N/A	62*	80	None

* with documentation

Terms To Know

atresia. Congenital closure or absence of a tubular organ or an opening to the body surface.

atria. Two upper chambers of the heart. The left and right atria are divided by the septum, a muscular wall.

cardiopulmonary bypass. Venous blood is diverted to a heart-lung machine, which mechanically pumps and oxygenates the blood temporarily so the heart can be bypassed while an open procedure on the heart or coronary arteries is performed. During bypass, the lungs are deflated and immobile.

tricuspid valve. Valve with three cusps between the right atrium and the right ventricle.

33468

33468 Tricuspid valve repositioning and plication for Ebstein anomaly

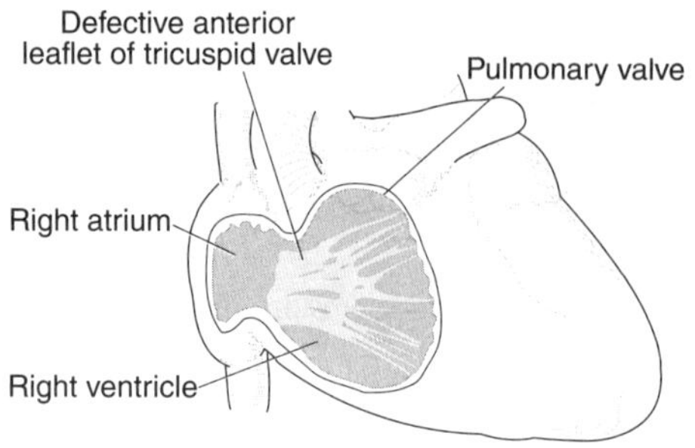

Explanation

In this anomaly, the tricuspid valve annulus is displaced onto the right ventricle, the right ventricle becomes atrophied and the valve leaflets become tethered to the wall of the ventricle. Cardiopulmonary bypass is initiated with venous uptake tubes in both caval veins. The right atrium is opened. The valve is detached from the ventricular wall around its circumference. The edge of the cut valve is sewn circumferentially around the lone port by the true junction of the right atrium and right ventricle. The right atrium is closed. Cardiopulmonary bypass is discontinued when heart function returns.

Coding Tips

For reoperation on the aortic valve more than one month after the original procedure, report 33530 in addition to the code for the primary procedure. When more than one valve (aortic, mitral, tricuspid, pulmonary) is being repaired or replaced, report each procedure separately and append modifier 51 to the secondary valve procedures. For valvuloplasty of the tricuspid valve without ring insertion, see 33463; with ring insertion, see 33464. For replacement of tricuspid valve, see 33465.

ICD-10-CM Diagnostic Codes

Q22.5 Ebstein's anomaly

Relative Value Units/Medicare Edits

Non-Facility RVU	Work	PE	MP	Total
33468	45.13	15.75	11.19	72.07
Facility RVU	**Work**	**PE**	**MP**	**Total**
33468	45.13	15.75	11.19	72.07

	FUD	Status	MUE	Modifiers				IOM Reference
33468	90	A	1(2)	51	N/A	62*	80	None

* with documentation

33474

33474 Valvotomy, pulmonary valve, open heart, with cardiopulmonary bypass

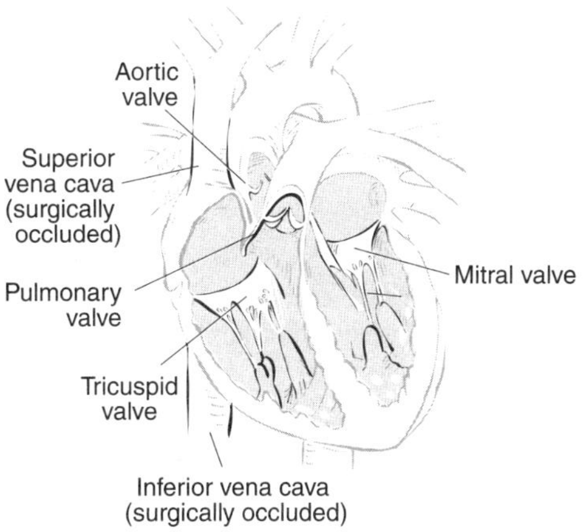

The pulmonary valve is dilated in an open heart surgical session

Explanation

The surgeon creates an incision into the pulmonary valve in order to enlarge the opening to the pulmonary artery, allowing blood to flow more easily into the artery. The heart is exposed through the sternum and the patient is placed on cardiopulmonary bypass. Tourniquets are placed around the superior and inferior caval veins and tightened. An opening is created in the pulmonary artery to allow access to the pulmonary valve. The pulmonary valve in incised. The opening in the pulmonary artery is closed and the tourniquets are released. Cardiopulmonary bypass is discontinued, the sternum is closed with wires or sutures, and the soft tissues are closed with sutures.

Coding Tips

For reoperation on the aortic valve more than one month after the original procedure, report 33530 in addition to the code for the primary procedure. When more than one valve (aortic, mitral, tricuspid, pulmonary) is being repaired or replaced, report each procedure separately and append modifier 51 to the secondary valve procedures. For valvotomy of the pulmonary valve, closed heart, via pulmonary artery, see 33471. For percutaneous balloon valvuloplasty of the pulmonary valve, see 92990.

ICD-10-CM Diagnostic Codes

I37.1	Nonrheumatic pulmonary valve insufficiency
I37.2	Nonrheumatic pulmonary valve stenosis with insufficiency
I37.8	Other nonrheumatic pulmonary valve disorders
Q22.1	Congenital pulmonary valve stenosis
T82.01XA	Breakdown (mechanical) of heart valve prosthesis, initial encounter
T82.02XA	Displacement of heart valve prosthesis, initial encounter
T82.03XA	Leakage of heart valve prosthesis, initial encounter
T82.09XA	Other mechanical complication of heart valve prosthesis, initial encounter
T82.6XXA	Infection and inflammatory reaction due to cardiac valve prosthesis, initial encounter
T82.817A	Embolism due to cardiac prosthetic devices, implants and grafts, initial encounter
T82.827A	Fibrosis due to cardiac prosthetic devices, implants and grafts, initial encounter
T82.837A	Hemorrhage due to cardiac prosthetic devices, implants and grafts, initial encounter
T82.847A	Pain due to cardiac prosthetic devices, implants and grafts, initial encounter
T82.855A	Stenosis of coronary artery stent, initial encounter
T82.857A	Stenosis of other cardiac prosthetic devices, implants and grafts, initial encounter
T82.867A	Thrombosis due to cardiac prosthetic devices, implants and grafts, initial encounter
T82.897A	Other specified complication of cardiac prosthetic devices, implants and grafts, initial encounter

Relative Value Units/Medicare Edits

Non-Facility RVU	Work	PE	MP	Total
33474	39.4	15.06	9.76	64.22
Facility RVU	**Work**	**PE**	**MP**	**Total**
33474	39.4	15.06	9.76	64.22

	FUD	Status	MUE	Modifiers				IOM Reference
33474	90	A	1(2)	51	N/A	62*	80	None

* with documentation

Terms To Know

cardiopulmonary bypass. Venous blood is diverted to a heart-lung machine, which mechanically pumps and oxygenates the blood temporarily so the heart can be bypassed while an open procedure on the heart or coronary arteries is performed. During bypass, the lungs are deflated and immobile.

complication. Condition arising after the beginning of observation and treatment that modifies the course of the patient's illness or the medical care required, or an undesired result or misadventure in medical care.

congenital. Present at birth, occurring through heredity or an influence during gestation up to the moment of birth.

endocarditis. Inflammatory disease of the interior lining of the heart chamber and heart valves.

infection. Presence of microorganisms in body tissues that may result in cellular damage.

occlusion. Constriction, closure, or blockage of a passage.

percutaneous. Through the skin.

stenosis. Narrowing or constriction of a passage.

tourniquet. Device used to apply compressive force to a blood vessel in a limb and slow or prevent blood flow to and from the area.

valvotomy. Cutting through stenosed cardiac valve leaflets or cusp to relieve or repair the obstruction caused by scar tissue and inflammation.

valvuloplasty. Surgical repair of a valve.

33475

33475 Replacement, pulmonary valve

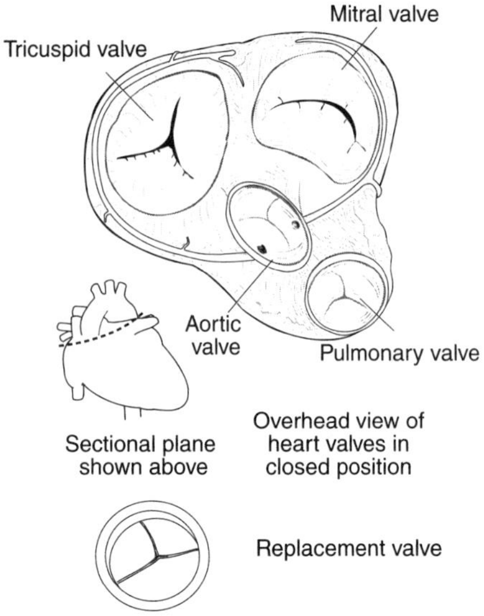

The pulmonary valve is accessed in an open heart surgical session. The valve leaflets are cut out and a replacement valve is secured

Explanation

Cardiopulmonary bypass is initiated with venous uptake tubes in both caval veins. The pulmonary artery is opened and the pulmonary valve leaflets are cut out. Stitches are placed around the circumference of the pulmonary annulus and the valve is sized. An appropriate artificial valve is selected. The stitches are passed through the sewing ring of the valve. The sewing ring is seated against the valve annulus and the stitches are tied. The hole in the pulmonary artery is closed. Cardiopulmonary bypass is discontinued when heart function returns.

Coding Tips

For reoperation on the aortic valve more than one month after the original procedure, report 33530 in addition to the code for the primary procedure. When more than one valve (aortic, mitral, tricuspid, pulmonary) is being repaired or replaced, report each procedure separately and append modifier 51 to the secondary valve procedures. Do not report 33475 with 33440. For valvotomy of the pulmonary valve, closed heart, via the pulmonary artery, see 33471. For valvotomy of the pulmonary valve, open heart, with cardiopulmonary bypass, see 33474. For percutaneous balloon valvuloplasty of the pulmonary valve, see 92990.

ICD-10-CM Diagnostic Codes

I37.0	Nonrheumatic pulmonary valve stenosis
I37.1	Nonrheumatic pulmonary valve insufficiency
I37.2	Nonrheumatic pulmonary valve stenosis with insufficiency
I37.8	Other nonrheumatic pulmonary valve disorders
Q22.1	Congenital pulmonary valve stenosis
T82.01XA	Breakdown (mechanical) of heart valve prosthesis, initial encounter
T82.02XA	Displacement of heart valve prosthesis, initial encounter
T82.03XA	Leakage of heart valve prosthesis, initial encounter
T82.09XA	Other mechanical complication of heart valve prosthesis, initial encounter
T82.6XXA	Infection and inflammatory reaction due to cardiac valve prosthesis, initial encounter
T82.817A	Embolism due to cardiac prosthetic devices, implants and grafts, initial encounter
T82.827A	Fibrosis due to cardiac prosthetic devices, implants and grafts, initial encounter
T82.837A	Hemorrhage due to cardiac prosthetic devices, implants and grafts, initial encounter
T82.847A	Pain due to cardiac prosthetic devices, implants and grafts, initial encounter
T82.855A	Stenosis of coronary artery stent, initial encounter
T82.857A	Stenosis of other cardiac prosthetic devices, implants and grafts, initial encounter
T82.867A	Thrombosis due to cardiac prosthetic devices, implants and grafts, initial encounter
T82.897A	Other specified complication of cardiac prosthetic devices, implants and grafts, initial encounter

AMA: 33475 2019,Apr

Relative Value Units/Medicare Edits

Non-Facility RVU	Work	PE	MP	Total
33475	42.4	15.96	9.85	68.21
Facility RVU	**Work**	**PE**	**MP**	**Total**
33475	42.4	15.96	9.85	68.21

	FUD	Status	MUE	Modifiers				IOM Reference
33475	90	A	1(2)	51	N/A	62*	80	None

* with documentation

Terms To Know

cardiopulmonary bypass. Venous blood is diverted to a heart-lung machine, which mechanically pumps and oxygenates the blood temporarily so the heart can be bypassed while an open procedure on the heart or coronary arteries is performed. During bypass, the lungs are deflated and immobile.

complication. Condition arising after the beginning of observation and treatment that modifies the course of the patient's illness or the medical care required, or an undesired result or misadventure in medical care.

congenital. Present at birth, occurring through heredity or an influence during gestation up to the moment of birth.

endocarditis. Inflammatory disease of the interior lining of the heart chamber and heart valves.

infection. Presence of microorganisms in body tissues that may result in cellular damage.

percutaneous. Through the skin.

stenosis. Narrowing or constriction of a passage.

valvotomy. Cutting through stenosed cardiac valve leaflets or cusp to relieve or repair the obstruction caused by scar tissue and inflammation.

valvuloplasty. Surgical repair of a valve.

33476, 33478

33476 Right ventricular resection for infundibular stenosis, with or without commissurotomy

33478 Outflow tract augmentation (gusset), with or without commissurotomy or infundibular resection

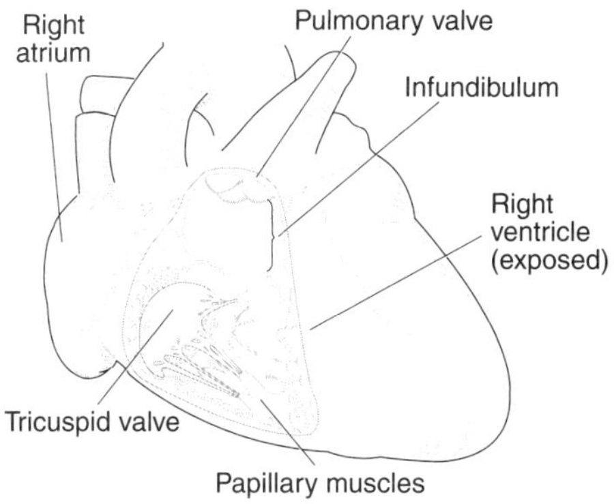

Explanation

Cardiopulmonary bypass is initiated. The right ventricular infundibular muscle is opened and the obstructing muscle bands are cut out. The valve may also need to be opened. If so, the valve is cut open. The hole in the right ventricle is closed with a patch of pericardium. Cardiopulmonary bypass is discontinued when heart function returns. Report 33478 if the operation is performed with a gusset, with or without commissurotomy or infundibular resection.

Coding Tips

For reoperation on the aortic valve more than one month after the original procedure, report 33530 in addition to the code for the primary procedure. When more than one valve (aortic, mitral, tricuspid, pulmonary) is being repaired or replaced, report each procedure separately and append modifier 51 to the secondary valve procedures. For valvotomy of the pulmonary valve, closed heart, via pulmonary artery, see 33471. For valvotomy of the pulmonary valve, open heart, with cardiopulmonary bypass, see 33474. For replacement of the pulmonary valve, see 33475. For percutaneous balloon valvuloplasty of the pulmonary valve, see 92990. Report 33478 with 33768 when a cavopulmonary anastomosis to a second superior vena cava is performed.

ICD-10-CM Diagnostic Codes

Q22.1 Congenital pulmonary valve stenosis

Q24.3 Pulmonary infundibular stenosis

Relative Value Units/Medicare Edits

Non-Facility RVU	Work	PE	MP	Total
33476	26.57	11.95	6.57	45.09
33478	27.54	12.22	6.79	46.55
Facility RVU	Work	PE	MP	Total
33476	26.57	11.95	6.57	45.09
33478	27.54	12.22	6.79	46.55

	FUD	Status	MUE	Modifiers				IOM Reference
33476	90	A	1(2)	51	N/A	62*	80	None
33478	90	A	1(2)	51	N/A	62*	80	

* with documentation

33477

33477 Transcatheter pulmonary valve implantation, percutaneous approach, including pre-stenting of the valve delivery site, when performed

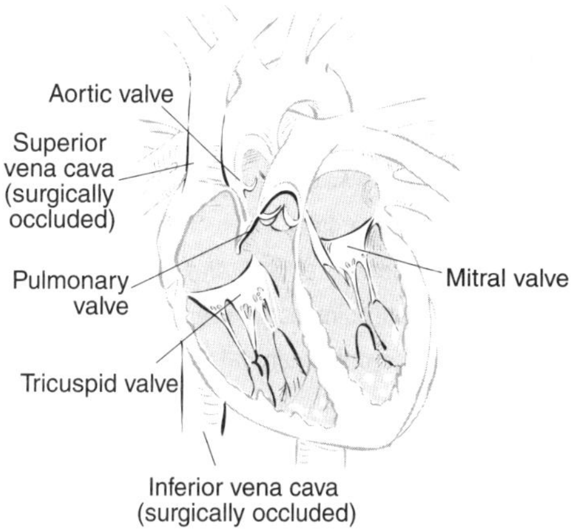

Transcatheter implantation of pulmonary valve

Explanation

Percutaneous placement of a prosthetic pulmonary valve is used primarily to treat patients with stenosis or regurgitation of a previously repaired right ventricular outflow tract (RVOT). The patient is prepped with general anesthesia in addition to endotracheal intubation. The provider inserts a needle through the skin and into an underlying vein, usually a lower extremity vein, although jugular access is also utilized. Angiography and hemodynamic studies are performed and a guidewire is threaded through the needle and advanced into the pulmonary artery. A balloon is inflated in the RVOT conduit to evaluate for coronary compression and an aortogram is performed to visualize the coronary arteries. Pre-stenting is commonly performed with a covered bare metal stent to decrease the risk of fractured stents and more than one stent may be required. The needle is removed and a catheter carrying the prosthetic valve is inserted. The prosthesis is positioned over the diseased pulmonary valve and a balloon is inflated, deploying the prosthetic valve in place. Angiography and hemodynamic evaluations are repeated. The catheter is removed and pressure is applied to stop bleeding at the access site. A single suture may provide hemostasis at the venous access.

Coding Tips

This code should be reported only once per encounter. This procedure includes angiography, cardiac catheterization, contrast injection, imaging guidance, and radiological supervision and interpretation necessary to perform the service. Diagnostic catheterization, diagnostic coronary angiography, and diagnostic pulmonary angiography codes may be reported separately in cases where a previous examination is not available or the anatomic visualization is poor quality, there has been a clinical change in the patient's condition since the previous examination, or complications arise during the procedure requiring the additional study. Cardiopulmonary bypass may be necessary in addition to this procedure. For percutaneous peripheral bypass, see 33367; for open peripheral bypass, see 33368; and for central bypass, see 33369. Do not report 33477 with 76000, 93451, 93453–93461, 93563, 93566–93569, 93573, 93593, 93594, or 93596–93598 for angiography necessary to accomplish the procedure. Do not report 33477 with 37236–37237 or 92997–92998 for angioplasty, valvuloplasty, or stenting within the treatment site. Do not report 93451, 93453, 93454–93461, 93563, 93566–93569, 93573, 93593, 93594, or 93596–93598 with 33477 for angiography, roadmapping, or guidance related to a TPVI procedure. Diagnostic catheterization codes 93451–93453, 93456–93461, and 93593–93598 and diagnostic angiography codes 93454–93461, 93563, 93564, 93568, 93569, and 93573–93575 may be reported

 ● New ▲ Revised + Add On ★ Telemedicine [Resequenced] ☑ Laterality

for services separate from a TPVI if the following is met: 1) No prior study is available and a full diagnostic study is performed; or 2) A prior study is available, but the study has inadequate visualization of anatomy and/or pathology, the patient's condition has changed in respect to the clinical indication since the prior study, or a clinical change occurs during the procedure and requires a more thorough evaluation. For transcatheter ventricular assist during this procedure, see 33990–33993, 33995, or 33997 for VAD; 33946–33989 for ECMO/ECLS; and 33967, 33970, or 33973 for balloon pump insertion.

ICD-10-CM Diagnostic Codes

A52.03	Syphilitic endocarditis
I33.9	Acute and subacute endocarditis, unspecified
I37.0	Nonrheumatic pulmonary valve stenosis
I37.1	Nonrheumatic pulmonary valve insufficiency
I37.2	Nonrheumatic pulmonary valve stenosis with insufficiency
I37.8	Other nonrheumatic pulmonary valve disorders
I97.0	Postcardiotomy syndrome
I97.110	Postprocedural cardiac insufficiency following cardiac surgery
I97.130	Postprocedural heart failure following cardiac surgery
I97.190	Other postprocedural cardiac functional disturbances following cardiac surgery
Q20.0	Common arterial trunk
Q20.1	Double outlet right ventricle
Q20.5	Discordant atrioventricular connection
Q21.3	Tetralogy of Fallot
Q22.0	Pulmonary valve atresia
Q22.1	Congenital pulmonary valve stenosis
Q22.2	Congenital pulmonary valve insufficiency
Q22.3	Other congenital malformations of pulmonary valve
Q24.3	Pulmonary infundibular stenosis

AMA: **33477** 2023,May

Relative Value Units/Medicare Edits

Non-Facility RVU	Work	PE	MP	Total
33477	25.0	9.04	4.33	38.37
Facility RVU	**Work**	**PE**	**MP**	**Total**
33477	25.0	9.04	4.33	38.37

	FUD	Status	MUE	Modifiers				IOM Reference
33477	0	A	1(2)	51	N/A	62*	80*	None

* with documentation

Terms To Know

angiography. Radiographic imaging of the arteries. Imaging may be performed to study the vasculature of any given organ, body system, or area of circulation such as the brain, heart, chest, kidneys, limbs, gastrointestinal tract, aorta, and pulmonary circulation to visualize the formation and the function of the blood vessels to detect problems such as a blockage or stricture. A catheter is inserted through an accessible blood vessel and the artery is injected with a radiopaque contrast material after which x-rays are taken.

catheterization. Use or insertion of a tubular device into a duct, blood vessel, hollow organ, or body cavity for injecting or withdrawing fluids for diagnostic or therapeutic purposes.

33496

33496 Repair of non-structural prosthetic valve dysfunction with cardiopulmonary bypass (separate procedure)

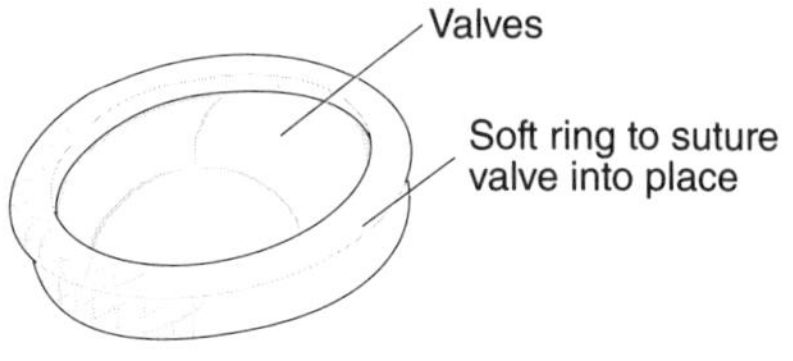

Example of nonstructural prosthetic heart valve

Explanation

This procedure is typically performed to repair an artificial prosthetic valve that is malfunctioning due to leakage around the valve sewing ring or the valve is impeded by blood clot or growth of surrounding tissue (pannus) into the functioning part of the valve. The surgeon exposes the heart through the sternum. Cardiopulmonary bypass is initiated. The prosthetic valve is exposed and the valve is repaired. Cardiopulmonary bypass is discontinued when heart function returns. The sternum is closed with wires or sutures and the soft tissues are closed with sutures.

Coding Tips

This separate procedure by definition is usually a component of a more complex service and is not identified separately. When performed alone or with other unrelated procedures/services, it may be reported. If performed alone, list the code; if performed with other procedures/services, list the code and append modifier 59 or an X{EPSU} modifier. This code is reported for mitral or aortic prosthetic valve repair (e.g., suture of perivalvular prosthetic valve leak, declotting of a prosthetic heart valve). Report 33530 in addition to the code for the primary reoperation procedure on the affected valve more than one month after the original procedure.

ICD-10-CM Diagnostic Codes

T82.01XA	Breakdown (mechanical) of heart valve prosthesis, initial encounter
T82.02XA	Displacement of heart valve prosthesis, initial encounter
T82.03XA	Leakage of heart valve prosthesis, initial encounter
T82.09XA	Other mechanical complication of heart valve prosthesis, initial encounter
T82.221A	Breakdown (mechanical) of biological heart valve graft, initial encounter
T82.222A	Displacement of biological heart valve graft, initial encounter
T82.223A	Leakage of biological heart valve graft, initial encounter
T82.228A	Other mechanical complication of biological heart valve graft, initial encounter
T82.817A	Embolism due to cardiac prosthetic devices, implants and grafts, initial encounter
T82.827A	Fibrosis due to cardiac prosthetic devices, implants and grafts, initial encounter
T82.837A	Hemorrhage due to cardiac prosthetic devices, implants and grafts, initial encounter
T82.847A	Pain due to cardiac prosthetic devices, implants and grafts, initial encounter
T82.857A	Stenosis of other cardiac prosthetic devices, implants and grafts, initial encounter

T82.867A Thrombosis due to cardiac prosthetic devices, implants and grafts, initial encounter

T82.897A Other specified complication of cardiac prosthetic devices, implants and grafts, initial encounter

Z95.2 Presence of prosthetic heart valve

Relative Value Units/Medicare Edits

Non-Facility RVU	Work	PE	MP	Total
33496	29.84	12.14	6.89	48.87
Facility RVU	**Work**	**PE**	**MP**	**Total**
33496	29.84	12.14	6.89	48.87

	FUD	Status	MUE	Modifiers				IOM Reference
33496	90	A	1(3)	51	N/A	62*	80	None

* with documentation

Terms To Know

cardiopulmonary bypass. Venous blood is diverted to a heart-lung machine, which mechanically pumps and oxygenates the blood temporarily so the heart can be bypassed while an open procedure on the heart or coronary arteries is performed. During bypass, the lungs are deflated and immobile.

complication. Condition arising after the beginning of observation and treatment that modifies the course of the patient's illness or the medical care required, or an undesired result or misadventure in medical care.

hypothermia with cardiac bypass. Reduction of the body temperature using a bypass system to reduce the oxygen demands of tissue and to protect the myocardium during a procedure.

prosthesis. Man-made substitute for a missing body part.

suture. Numerous stitching techniques employed in wound closure.

33500-33501

33500 Repair of coronary arteriovenous or arteriocardiac chamber fistula; with cardiopulmonary bypass

33501 without cardiopulmonary bypass

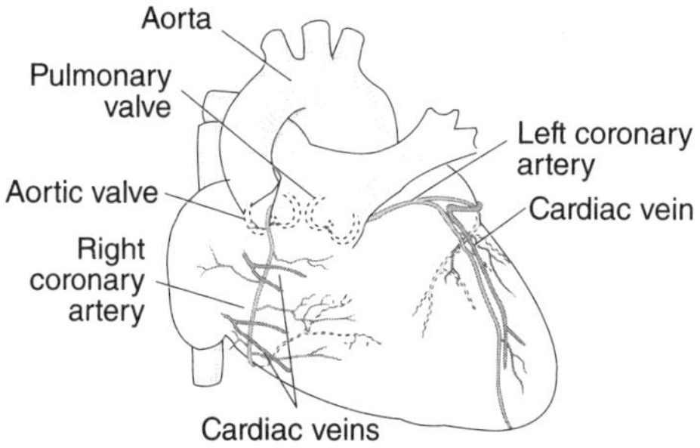

Anatomical variations in coronary vessels are normal; however, a communication between an artery and a vein is a fistula

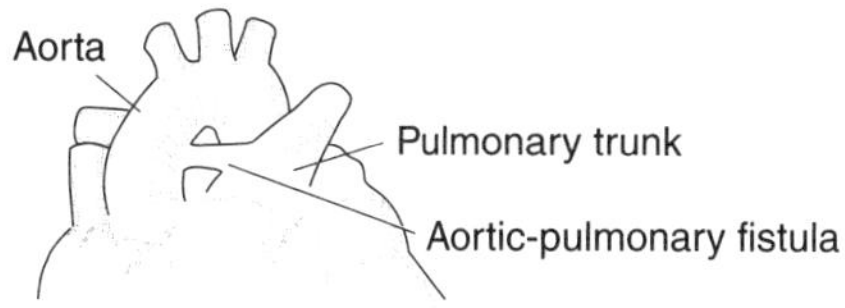

Explanation

The physician repairs a coronary arteriovenous or arteriocardiac chamber fistula. In one technique, a catheter is used to advance a balloon or microcoils for embolization of the artery closest to the site of fistula termination. Open repair may be performed to ligate a complicated fistula or when other cardiac procedures are necessary. Report 33500 when cardiopulmonary bypass is used; 33501 without cardiopulmonary bypass.

Coding Tips

When 33500 or 33501 is performed with another separately identifiable procedure, the highest dollar value code is listed as the primary procedure and subsequent procedures are appended with modifier 51. Do not report endarterectomy or angioplasty separately as they are included in the fistula repair.

ICD-10-CM Diagnostic Codes

I25.41 Coronary artery aneurysm

Q24.5 Malformation of coronary vessels

AMA: **33500** 2021,Dec

Relative Value Units/Medicare Edits

Non-Facility RVU	Work	PE	MP	Total
33500	27.94	11.42	6.47	45.83
33501	19.51	8.83	4.5	32.84
Facility RVU	**Work**	**PE**	**MP**	**Total**
33500	27.94	11.42	6.47	45.83
33501	19.51	8.83	4.5	32.84

	FUD	Status	MUE	Modifiers				IOM Reference
33500	90	A	1(3)	51	N/A	62*	80	None
33501	90	A	1(3)	51	N/A	62	80	

* with documentation

Heart and Pericardium

33502-33504

33502 Repair of anomalous coronary artery from pulmonary artery origin; by ligation
33503 by graft, without cardiopulmonary bypass
33504 by graft, with cardiopulmonary bypass

Schematic showing coronary arteries. Normal configuration is for the left and right branches to originate just above the aortic valve

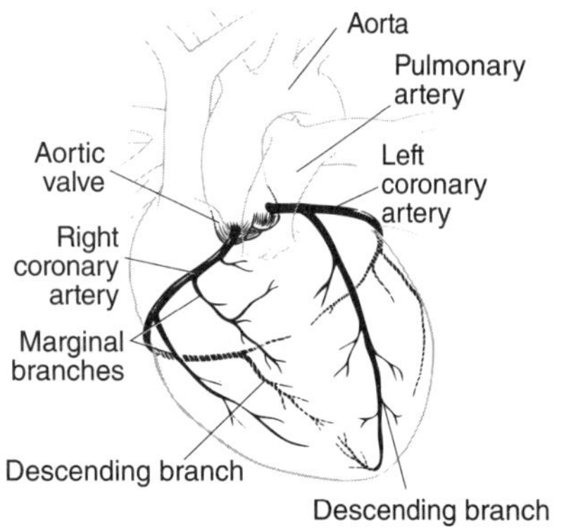

Explanation

In 33502, the physician ligates an anomalous coronary artery arising from the pulmonary artery. Ligation of the anomalous coronary artery has a poor prognosis and may be performed as a temporary measure prior to creation of a double coronary artery system during a subsequent surgical intervention. The anomalous coronary artery is exposed at the site of origin in the pulmonary artery. A suture is placed around the artery and it is ligated. In 33503, the physician repairs an anomalous coronary artery arising from the pulmonary artery using a graft. The anomalous coronary artery is identified and detached. The subsequent hole in the pulmonary artery is sutured closed. An opening is made in the side of the aorta and the free end of the coronary artery is anastomosed to the aorta. Report 33504 if cardiopulmonary bypass is required. This procedure will most always require the cardiopulmonary bypass.

Coding Tips

If significant additional time and effort are documented, append modifier 22 and submit a cover letter and operative report. When 33502, 33503, or 33504 is performed with another separately identifiable procedure, the highest dollar value code is listed as the primary procedure and subsequent procedures are appended with modifier 51. Do not report endarterectomy or angioplasty separately as they are included in the repair of the anomalous artery. Do not append modifier 63 to 33502–33503 as the description of the procedure includes infants up to 4 kg.

ICD-10-CM Diagnostic Codes

Q24.5 Malformation of coronary vessels

Relative Value Units/Medicare Edits

Non-Facility RVU	Work	PE	MP	Total
33502	21.85	10.65	5.4	37.9
33503	22.51	11.33	5.56	39.4
33504	25.46	11.67	6.29	43.42
Facility RVU	**Work**	**PE**	**MP**	**Total**
33502	21.85	10.65	5.4	37.9
33503	22.51	11.33	5.56	39.4
33504	25.46	11.67	6.29	43.42

	FUD	Status	MUE	Modifiers				IOM Reference
33502	90	A	1(3)	51	N/A	62*	80	None
33503	90	A	1(3)	51	N/A	62*	80*	
33504	90	A	1(3)	51	N/A	62*	80	

* with documentation

Terms To Know

angioplasty. Reconstruction or repair of a diseased or damaged blood vessel.

anomaly. Irregularity in the structure or position of an organ or tissue.

cardiopulmonary bypass. Venous blood is diverted to a heart-lung machine, which mechanically pumps and oxygenates the blood temporarily so the heart can be bypassed while an open procedure on the heart or coronary arteries is performed. During bypass, the lungs are deflated and immobile.

congenital. Present at birth, occurring through heredity or an influence during gestation up to the moment of birth.

endarterectomy. Removal of the thickened, endothelial lining of a diseased or damaged artery.

graft. Tissue implant from another part of the body or another person.

33505-33506

33505 Repair of anomalous coronary artery from pulmonary artery origin; with construction of intrapulmonary artery tunnel (Takeuchi procedure)

33506 by translocation from pulmonary artery to aorta

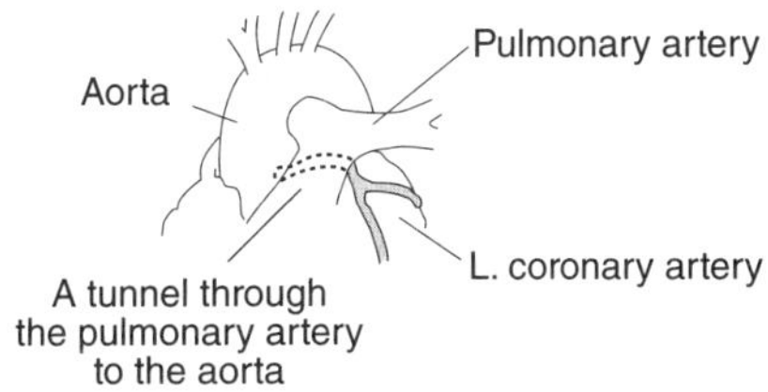

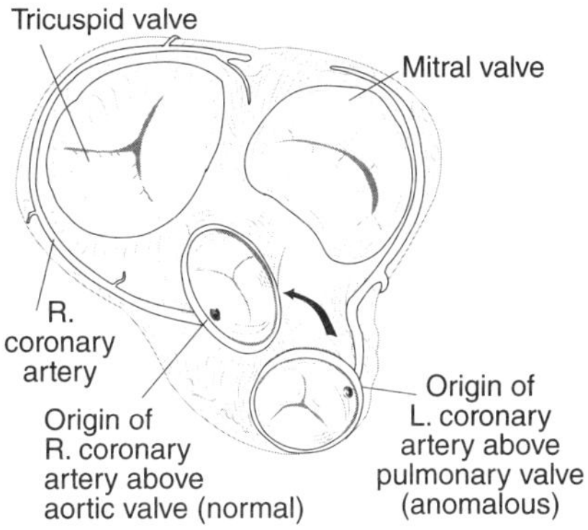

Explanation

In 33505, the physician repairs an anomalous coronary artery arising from the pulmonary artery by construction of an intrapulmonary artery tunnel. Cardiopulmonary bypass is required. This operation is done in cases where the anomalous coronary artery is located far from the aorta on the left lateral side of the pulmonary artery. Openings are made in the aorta and the pulmonary artery at the level of the anomalous coronary artery where the vessels touch each other. The two open areas are sewn together to create a direct aortopulmonary opening. A flap of pulmonary artery wall is created with the anomalous coronary artery at one end. The flap is fashioned into a tunnel with the flap as one side of the tunnel, the back wall of the pulmonary artery as the other side of the tunnel, the hole between the aorta and pulmonary artery as one end, and the anomalous coronary artery as the other end. In this way, blood from the aorta is diverted into the anomalous coronary artery. The hole in the pulmonary artery is closed. Cardiopulmonary bypass is discontinued when heart function returns. This procedure is less common today; surgeons typically repair the defect by direct transfer of the anomalous coronary artery from the pulmonary artery. In 33506, the physician repairs an anomalous coronary artery arising from the pulmonary artery by translocation from the pulmonary artery to the aorta. The anomalous coronary artery arising from the pulmonary artery is detached. The subsequent hole in the pulmonary artery is patched with autologous pericardium. An opening is created in the side of the aorta and the coronary artery is anastomosed into the opening. Cardiopulmonary bypass is almost always required for this operation.

Coding Tips

If significant additional time and effort are documented, append modifier 22 and submit a cover letter and operative report. When 33505 or 33506 is performed with another separately identifiable procedure, the highest dollar value code is listed as the primary procedure and subsequent procedures are appended with modifier 51. Do not report endarterectomy or angioplasty separately as they are included in the repair of the anomalous artery. Do not append modifier 63 to 33505–33506 as the description of the procedure includes infants up to 4 kg.

ICD-10-CM Diagnostic Codes

Q24.5 Malformation of coronary vessels

Relative Value Units/Medicare Edits

Non-Facility RVU	Work	PE	MP	Total
33505	38.4	12.59	9.52	60.51
33506	37.85	13.12	9.38	60.35
Facility RVU	**Work**	**PE**	**MP**	**Total**
33505	38.4	12.59	9.52	60.51
33506	37.85	13.12	9.38	60.35

	FUD	Status	MUE	Modifiers				IOM Reference
33505	90	A	1(3)	51	N/A	62*	80	None
33506	90	A	1(3)	51	N/A	62*	80	

* with documentation

Terms To Know

angioplasty. Reconstruction or repair of a diseased or damaged blood vessel.

anomaly. Irregularity in the structure or position of an organ or tissue.

cardiopulmonary bypass. Venous blood is diverted to a heart-lung machine, which mechanically pumps and oxygenates the blood temporarily so the heart can be bypassed while an open procedure on the heart or coronary arteries is performed. During bypass, the lungs are deflated and immobile.

congenital. Present at birth, occurring through heredity or an influence during gestation up to the moment of birth.

endarterectomy. Removal of the thickened, endothelial lining of a diseased or damaged artery.

33507

33507 Repair of anomalous (eg, intramural) aortic origin of coronary artery by unroofing or translocation

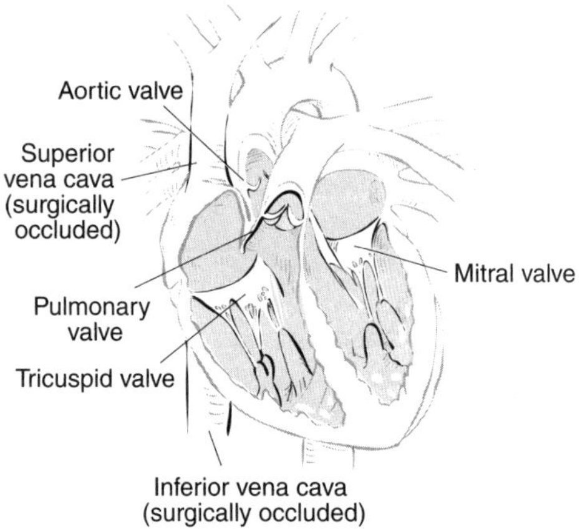

Explanation

The physician repairs an anomalous coronary artery by unroofing or translocation. Common anomalies repaired using this technique include anomalous right coronary artery arising from the left coronary sinus, anomalous left coronary artery arising from the right coronary sinus, and anomalous coronary artery arising from a single ostia. Cardiopulmonary bypass is almost always required. The physician detaches the posterior commissure of the aortic valve. Unroofing of the intramural segment of the coronary artery is accomplished by excision of a triangular portion of the internal aortic wall. The coronary arteries are excised as a single disc and divided into two cuffs. An arterial switch is performed. The posterior commissure of the aortic valve is resuspended to a pericardial patch used to reconstruct the pulmonary artery sinus.

Coding Tips

Endarterectomy and angioplasty are included in the basic procedure and should not be reported separately. For repair of an anomalous coronary artery from pulmonary artery origin, see 33502–33506.

ICD-10-CM Diagnostic Codes

Q24.5 Malformation of coronary vessels

Relative Value Units/Medicare Edits

Non-Facility RVU	Work	PE	MP	Total
33507	31.4	11.5	7.76	50.66
Facility RVU	**Work**	**PE**	**MP**	**Total**
33507	31.4	11.5	7.76	50.66

	FUD	Status	MUE	Modifiers				IOM Reference
33507	90	A	1(3)	51	N/A	62*	80	None

* with documentation

33508

\+ **33508** Endoscopy, surgical, including video-assisted harvest of vein(s) for coronary artery bypass procedure (List separately in addition to code for primary procedure)

Explanation

A surgical vascular endoscopy is done that includes video-assisted harvesting of a vein for a coronary artery bypass. The physician makes a portal incision above the saphenous vein. The endoscope is inserted into the incision and visualization occurs on a video monitor. CO2 gas is insufflated through the endoscope and dissection is made to the vein. A cannula is inserted and a portion of the vein to be removed is released from the surrounding structures. The vein is tied off above and below the portion of the vein to be removed. The vein is removed through the harvesting cannula. The endoscope is removed and the incision is closed with sutures and Steri-strips. The portion of the vein removed is prepared for use in cardiac bypass surgery.

Coding Tips

Report 33508 in addition to 33510–33523. For open harvest of an upper extremity vein, see 35500. For harvest of a femoropopliteal vein not using surgical endoscopy, see 35572.

ICD-10-CM Diagnostic Codes

This/these CPT code(s) are add-on code(s). See the primary procedure code that this code is performed with for your ICD-10-CM code selections. Diagnostic code(s) would be the same as the actual procedure performed.

AMA: 33508 2021,Dec

Relative Value Units/Medicare Edits

Non-Facility RVU	Work	PE	MP	Total
33508	0.31	0.09	0.07	0.47
Facility RVU	**Work**	**PE**	**MP**	**Total**
33508	0.31	0.09	0.07	0.47

	FUD	Status	MUE	Modifiers				IOM Reference
33508	N/A	A	1(2)	N/A	N/A	62*	80	None

* with documentation

Terms To Know

bypass graft. Surgically created alternative blood vessel used to reroute blood flow around an area of obstruction or disease.

cannula. Tube inserted into a blood vessel, duct, or body cavity to facilitate passage.

congestive heart failure. Condition caused by the heart's inability to adequately pump and circulate blood, resulting in fluid accumulation in the lungs and other tissues.

dissection. Separating by cutting tissue or body structures apart.

endoscopy. Visual inspection of the body using a fiberoptic scope.

graft. Tissue implant from another part of the body or another person.

harvest. Removal of cells or tissue from their native site to be used as a graft or transplant to another part of the donor's body or placed into another person.

incision. Act of cutting into tissue or an organ.

33509

33509 Harvest of upper extremity artery, 1 segment, for coronary artery bypass procedure, endoscopic

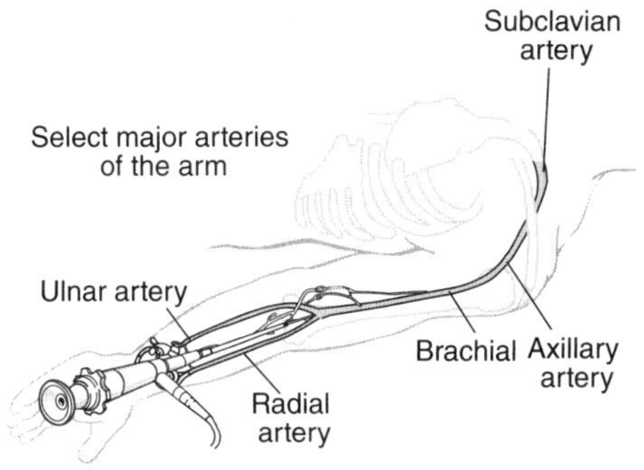

Arthroscopic harvesting of upper extremity artery

Explanation

Using an endoscopic approach, the physician harvests a segment of an artery from an upper extremity (arm) to use for a planned bypass procedure on a coronary artery. A 3 cm longitudinal incision is made just proximal to the wrist crease on the forearm over the radial artery. The physician separates the fascia and identifies the radial artery and its venae comitantes; these are dissected as one pedicle to avoid radial artery trauma. The endoscope is advanced directly over the radial artery, and the port trocar inserted and inflated to form a seal. Following CO_2 insufflation and the establishment of a flow rate to create a tunnel, the physician performs anterior, posterior, and lateral dissection of the artery using the conical dissection tip of the endoscope. The tip is then removed, and the endoscope is placed into a proprietary vessel-harvesting cannula. Using direct energy force, the physician releases the fascia from the distal to the proximal forearm. Radial artery branches are captured between the jaws of the cannula and the artery pedicle divided and ligated. The physician makes a stab incision near the elbow, clamps the radial artery pedicle, and brings it through the stab incision. The radial artery is transected, and the stump ligated. The pedicle is retrieved from the original incision at the wrist. The portion of the radial artery removed is prepared for use in a bypass procedure by flushing with papaverine and clipping the branches.

Coding Tips

This is a unilateral procedure. If performed bilaterally, some payers require that the service be reported twice with modifier 50 appended to the second code while others require identification of the service only once with modifier 50 appended. Check with individual payers. Modifier 50 identifies a procedure performed identically on the opposite side of the body (mirror image). As exempt from modifier 51, 33509 has not been designated in CPT as an add-on service/procedure. However, codes identified as exempt from modifier 51 are not subject to multiple procedure rules. No reimbursement reduction or modifier 51 is applied. To report open harvest of upper extremity artery for coronary artery bypass, see 35600.

ICD-10-CM Diagnostic Codes

I20.0	Unstable angina
I20.1	Angina pectoris with documented spasm
I21.01	ST elevation (STEMI) myocardial infarction involving left main coronary artery
I21.02	ST elevation (STEMI) myocardial infarction involving left anterior descending coronary artery
I21.11	ST elevation (STEMI) myocardial infarction involving right coronary artery
I21.21	ST elevation (STEMI) myocardial infarction involving left circumflex coronary artery
I21.4	Non-ST elevation (NSTEMI) myocardial infarction
I21.A1	Myocardial infarction type 2
I21.B	Myocardial infarction with coronary microvascular dysfunction
I22.0	Subsequent ST elevation (STEMI) myocardial infarction of anterior wall
I22.1	Subsequent ST elevation (STEMI) myocardial infarction of inferior wall
I22.2	Subsequent non-ST elevation (NSTEMI) myocardial infarction
I24.0	Acute coronary thrombosis not resulting in myocardial infarction
I25.110	Atherosclerotic heart disease of native coronary artery with unstable angina pectoris [A]
I25.111	Atherosclerotic heart disease of native coronary artery with angina pectoris with documented spasm [A]
I25.112	Atherosclerotic heart disease of native coronary artery with refractory angina pectoris [A]
I25.3	Aneurysm of heart
I25.41	Coronary artery aneurysm
I25.42	Coronary artery dissection
I25.5	Ischemic cardiomyopathy
I25.6	Silent myocardial ischemia
I25.710	Atherosclerosis of autologous vein coronary artery bypass graft(s) with unstable angina pectoris [A]
I25.711	Atherosclerosis of autologous vein coronary artery bypass graft(s) with angina pectoris with documented spasm [A]
I25.712	Atherosclerosis of autologous vein coronary artery bypass graft(s) with refractory angina pectoris [A]
I25.720	Atherosclerosis of autologous artery coronary artery bypass graft(s) with unstable angina pectoris [A]
I25.721	Atherosclerosis of autologous artery coronary artery bypass graft(s) with angina pectoris with documented spasm [A]
I25.722	Atherosclerosis of autologous artery coronary artery bypass graft(s) with refractory angina pectoris [A]
I25.730	Atherosclerosis of nonautologous biological coronary artery bypass graft(s) with unstable angina pectoris [A]
I25.731	Atherosclerosis of nonautologous biological coronary artery bypass graft(s) with angina pectoris with documented spasm [A]
I25.732	Atherosclerosis of nonautologous biological coronary artery bypass graft(s) with refractory angina pectoris [A]
I25.750	Atherosclerosis of native coronary artery of transplanted heart with unstable angina
I25.751	Atherosclerosis of native coronary artery of transplanted heart with angina pectoris with documented spasm
I25.752	Atherosclerosis of native coronary artery of transplanted heart with refractory angina pectoris [A]
I25.760	Atherosclerosis of bypass graft of coronary artery of transplanted heart with unstable angina [A]
I25.761	Atherosclerosis of bypass graft of coronary artery of transplanted heart with angina pectoris with documented spasm [A]
I25.762	Atherosclerosis of bypass graft of coronary artery of transplanted heart with refractory angina pectoris [A]

I25.790	Atherosclerosis of other coronary artery bypass graft(s) with unstable angina pectoris A
I25.791	Atherosclerosis of other coronary artery bypass graft(s) with angina pectoris with documented spasm A
I25.792	Atherosclerosis of other coronary artery bypass graft(s) with refractory angina pectoris A
I25.810	Atherosclerosis of coronary artery bypass graft(s) without angina pectoris A
I25.811	Atherosclerosis of native coronary artery of transplanted heart without angina pectoris
I25.812	Atherosclerosis of bypass graft of coronary artery of transplanted heart without angina pectoris A
I25.82	Chronic total occlusion of coronary artery
I25.83	Coronary atherosclerosis due to lipid rich plaque A
I25.84	Coronary atherosclerosis due to calcified coronary lesion
I50.21	Acute systolic (congestive) heart failure
I50.22	Chronic systolic (congestive) heart failure
I50.23	Acute on chronic systolic (congestive) heart failure
I50.31	Acute diastolic (congestive) heart failure
I50.32	Chronic diastolic (congestive) heart failure
I50.33	Acute on chronic diastolic (congestive) heart failure
I50.41	Acute combined systolic (congestive) and diastolic (congestive) heart failure
I50.42	Chronic combined systolic (congestive) and diastolic (congestive) heart failure
I50.43	Acute on chronic combined systolic (congestive) and diastolic (congestive) heart failure
I50.811	Acute right heart failure
I50.812	Chronic right heart failure
I50.813	Acute on chronic right heart failure
I50.814	Right heart failure due to left heart failure
I50.82	Biventricular heart failure
I50.83	High output heart failure
I50.84	End stage heart failure
Q24.5	Malformation of coronary vessels
Q26.2	Total anomalous pulmonary venous connection

AMA: 33509 2021,Dec

Relative Value Units/Medicare Edits

Non-Facility RVU	Work	PE	MP	Total
33509	3.34	0.92	0.79	5.05
Facility RVU	**Work**	**PE**	**MP**	**Total**
33509	3.34	0.92	0.79	5.05

	FUD	Status	MUE	Modifiers				IOM Reference
33509	N/A	A	1(3)	N/A	N/A	62*	80	None

* with documentation

33510-33513

33510 Coronary artery bypass, vein only; single coronary venous graft
33511 2 coronary venous grafts
33512 3 coronary venous grafts
33513 4 coronary venous grafts

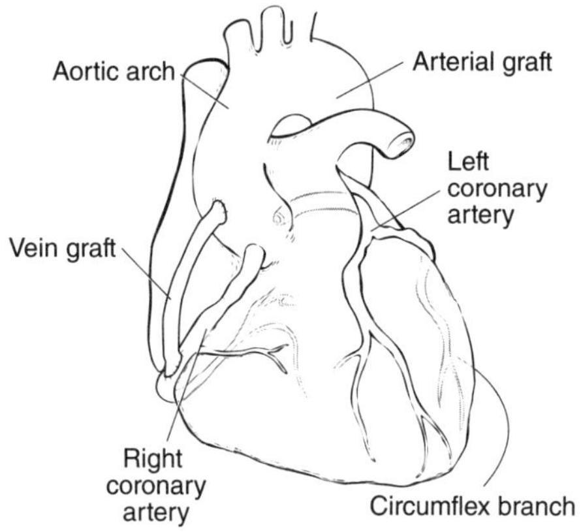

Schematic of a single vein graft bypass

Explanation

Cardiopulmonary bypass is initiated with a single, two-stage venous uptake tube. Saphenous vein is harvested from either leg. Vein may also be taken from the arm, the back of the leg, or from a cadaver. A clamp is placed on the aorta above the heart. Cold preserving solution is pumped through the coronary arteries to stop the heart. A point is chosen on the diseased coronary (arteries) beyond the area of disease and a longitudinal incision is cut in it. The proximal part (the part nearest the thigh) of the vein is trimmed to the same length as the cut in the coronary artery and is cleaned off. The end of the vein is sewn to the side of the coronary artery. A 3 mm to 6 mm hole is punched in the ascending aorta and the other end of the vein graft is sewn to this hole. The clamp on the aorta is released. Cardiopulmonary bypass is discontinued when heart function returns. Report 33511 if two coronary venous grafts are needed; report 33512 if three are needed; report 33513 if four are performed.

Coding Tips

These codes are not to be used to report coronary artery bypass graft (CABG) procedures with arterial grafts and venous grafts during the same procedure. For combined arterial-venous grafts, see 33517–33523 and 33533–33536. Procurement of the saphenous vein graft is included in 33510–33513. When saphenous vein graft procurement is performed by a surgical assistant, append modifier 80 to 33510–33513. Procurement of arm vein is reported separately, see 35500. When coronary endarterectomy of the left anterior descending, circumflex, or right coronary artery is confirmed by the operative report, report 33572 in addition to 33510–33513. For percutaneous ventricular assist device insertion, removal, or repositioning, see 33990-33993, 33995, and 33997. For reoperation more than one month after the original procedure, report 33530 in addition to the code for CABG procedure.

ICD-10-CM Diagnostic Codes

I20.0	Unstable angina
I20.1	Angina pectoris with documented spasm
I20.81	Angina pectoris with coronary microvascular dysfunction
I20.89	Other forms of angina pectoris
I21.01	ST elevation (STEMI) myocardial infarction involving left main coronary artery

I21.02 ST elevation (STEMI) myocardial infarction involving left anterior descending coronary artery

I21.09 ST elevation (STEMI) myocardial infarction involving other coronary artery of anterior wall

I21.11 ST elevation (STEMI) myocardial infarction involving right coronary artery

I21.19 ST elevation (STEMI) myocardial infarction involving other coronary artery of inferior wall

I21.21 ST elevation (STEMI) myocardial infarction involving left circumflex coronary artery

I21.29 ST elevation (STEMI) myocardial infarction involving other sites

I21.4 Non-ST elevation (NSTEMI) myocardial infarction

I21.A1 Myocardial infarction type 2

I21.B Myocardial infarction with coronary microvascular dysfunction

I22.0 Subsequent ST elevation (STEMI) myocardial infarction of anterior wall

I22.1 Subsequent ST elevation (STEMI) myocardial infarction of inferior wall

I22.2 Subsequent non-ST elevation (NSTEMI) myocardial infarction

I22.8 Subsequent ST elevation (STEMI) myocardial infarction of other sites

I24.0 Acute coronary thrombosis not resulting in myocardial infarction

I24.89 Other forms of acute ischemic heart disease

I25.10 Atherosclerotic heart disease of native coronary artery without angina pectoris A

I25.110 Atherosclerotic heart disease of native coronary artery with unstable angina pectoris A

I25.111 Atherosclerotic heart disease of native coronary artery with angina pectoris with documented spasm A

I25.112 Atherosclerotic heart disease of native coronary artery with refractory angina pectoris A

I25.118 Atherosclerotic heart disease of native coronary artery with other forms of angina pectoris A

I25.3 Aneurysm of heart

I25.41 Coronary artery aneurysm

I25.42 Coronary artery dissection

I25.5 Ischemic cardiomyopathy

I25.6 Silent myocardial ischemia

I25.710 Atherosclerosis of autologous vein coronary artery bypass graft(s) with unstable angina pectoris A

I25.711 Atherosclerosis of autologous vein coronary artery bypass graft(s) with angina pectoris with documented spasm A

I25.712 Atherosclerosis of autologous vein coronary artery bypass graft(s) with refractory angina pectoris A

I25.718 Atherosclerosis of autologous vein coronary artery bypass graft(s) with other forms of angina pectoris A

I25.720 Atherosclerosis of autologous artery coronary artery bypass graft(s) with unstable angina pectoris A

I25.721 Atherosclerosis of autologous artery coronary artery bypass graft(s) with angina pectoris with documented spasm A

I25.722 Atherosclerosis of autologous artery coronary artery bypass graft(s) with refractory angina pectoris A

I25.728 Atherosclerosis of autologous artery coronary artery bypass graft(s) with other forms of angina pectoris A

I25.730 Atherosclerosis of nonautologous biological coronary artery bypass graft(s) with unstable angina pectoris A

I25.731 Atherosclerosis of nonautologous biological coronary artery bypass graft(s) with angina pectoris with documented spasm A

I25.732 Atherosclerosis of nonautologous biological coronary artery bypass graft(s) with refractory angina pectoris A

I25.738 Atherosclerosis of nonautologous biological coronary artery bypass graft(s) with other forms of angina pectoris A

I25.750 Atherosclerosis of native coronary artery of transplanted heart with unstable angina

I25.751 Atherosclerosis of native coronary artery of transplanted heart with angina pectoris with documented spasm

I25.752 Atherosclerosis of native coronary artery of transplanted heart with refractory angina pectoris A

I25.758 Atherosclerosis of native coronary artery of transplanted heart with other forms of angina pectoris

I25.760 Atherosclerosis of bypass graft of coronary artery of transplanted heart with unstable angina A

I25.761 Atherosclerosis of bypass graft of coronary artery of transplanted heart with angina pectoris with documented spasm A

I25.762 Atherosclerosis of bypass graft of coronary artery of transplanted heart with refractory angina pectoris A

I25.768 Atherosclerosis of bypass graft of coronary artery of transplanted heart with other forms of angina pectoris A

I25.790 Atherosclerosis of other coronary artery bypass graft(s) with unstable angina pectoris A

I25.791 Atherosclerosis of other coronary artery bypass graft(s) with angina pectoris with documented spasm A

I25.792 Atherosclerosis of other coronary artery bypass graft(s) with refractory angina pectoris A

I25.798 Atherosclerosis of other coronary artery bypass graft(s) with other forms of angina pectoris A

I25.810 Atherosclerosis of coronary artery bypass graft(s) without angina pectoris A

I25.811 Atherosclerosis of native coronary artery of transplanted heart without angina pectoris

I25.812 Atherosclerosis of bypass graft of coronary artery of transplanted heart without angina pectoris A

I25.82 Chronic total occlusion of coronary artery

I25.83 Coronary atherosclerosis due to lipid rich plaque A

I25.84 Coronary atherosclerosis due to calcified coronary lesion

I25.89 Other forms of chronic ischemic heart disease

I45.6 Pre-excitation syndrome

I50.1 Left ventricular failure, unspecified

I50.21 Acute systolic (congestive) heart failure

I50.22 Chronic systolic (congestive) heart failure

I50.23 Acute on chronic systolic (congestive) heart failure

I50.31 Acute diastolic (congestive) heart failure

I50.32 Chronic diastolic (congestive) heart failure

I50.33 Acute on chronic diastolic (congestive) heart failure

I50.41 Acute combined systolic (congestive) and diastolic (congestive) heart failure

I50.42 Chronic combined systolic (congestive) and diastolic (congestive) heart failure

I50.43 Acute on chronic combined systolic (congestive) and diastolic (congestive) heart failure

I50.811 Acute right heart failure

I50.812 Chronic right heart failure

I50.813	Acute on chronic right heart failure
I50.814	Right heart failure due to left heart failure
I50.82	Biventricular heart failure
I50.83	High output heart failure
I50.84	End stage heart failure
Q24.5	Malformation of coronary vessels
Q26.2	Total anomalous pulmonary venous connection

AMA: 33510 2021,Dec; 2018,Jun **33511** 2021,Dec **33512** 2021,Dec **33513** 2021,Dec

Relative Value Units/Medicare Edits

Non-Facility RVU	Work	PE	MP	Total
33510	34.98	13.56	8.34	56.88
33511	38.45	14.82	9.19	62.46
33512	43.98	16.6	10.57	71.15
33513	45.37	16.42	10.86	72.65
Facility RVU	**Work**	**PE**	**MP**	**Total**
33510	34.98	13.56	8.34	56.88
33511	38.45	14.82	9.19	62.46
33512	43.98	16.6	10.57	71.15
33513	45.37	16.42	10.86	72.65

	FUD	Status	MUE	Modifiers				IOM Reference
33510	90	A	1(2)	51	N/A	N/A	80	None
33511	90	A	1(2)	51	N/A	N/A	80	
33512	90	A	1(2)	51	N/A	N/A	80	
33513	90	A	1(2)	51	N/A	N/A	80	

* with documentation

Terms To Know

atherosclerosis. Buildup of yellowish plaques composed of cholesterol and lipoid material within the arteries.

bypass graft. Surgically created alternative blood vessel used to reroute blood flow around an area of obstruction or disease.

cardiopulmonary bypass. Venous blood is diverted to a heart-lung machine, which mechanically pumps and oxygenates the blood temporarily so the heart can be bypassed while an open procedure on the heart or coronary arteries is performed. During bypass, the lungs are deflated and immobile.

harvest. Removal of cells or tissue from their native site to be used as a graft or transplant to another part of the donor's body or placed into another person.

33514-33516

33514 Coronary artery bypass, vein only; 5 coronary venous grafts
33516 6 or more coronary venous grafts

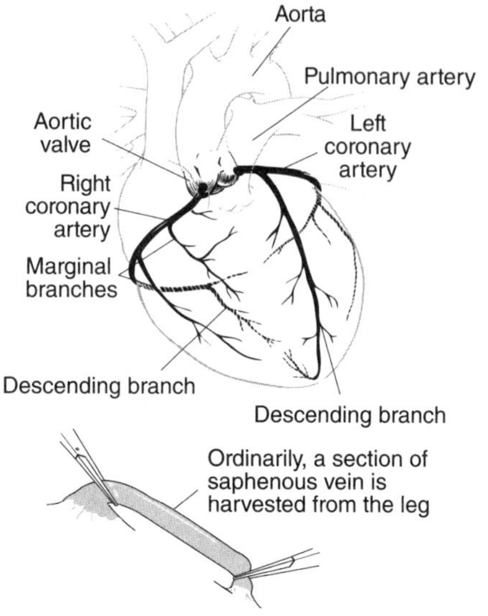

Explanation

Cardiopulmonary bypass is initiated with a single, two-stage venous uptake tube. Saphenous vein is harvested from either leg. Vein may also be taken from the arm, the back of the leg, or from a cadaver. A clamp is placed on the aorta above the heart. Cold preserving solution is pumped through the coronary arteries to stop the heart. A point is chosen on the diseased coronary (arteries) beyond the area of disease and a longitudinal incision is cut in it. The proximal part (the part nearest the thigh) of the vein is trimmed to the same length as the cut in the coronary artery and is cleaned off. The end of the vein is sewn to the side of the coronary artery. A 3 mm to 6 mm hole is punched in the ascending aorta and the other end of the vein graft is sewn to this hole. The clamp on the aorta is released. Cardiopulmonary bypass is discontinued when heart function returns. Report 33514 if five are performed; report 33516 if six or more are performed.

Coding Tips

To report coronary venous grafts, single and up to four, see 33510–33513. These codes are not to be used to report coronary artery bypass graft (CABG) procedures with arterial grafts and venous grafts during the same procedure. For combined arterial-venous grafts, see 33517–33523 and 33533–33536. Procurement of the saphenous vein graft is included in 33514–33516. When saphenous vein graft procurement is performed by a surgical assistant, append modifier 80 to 33514–33516. Procurement of an arm vein is reported separately, see 35500. When coronary endarterectomy of the left anterior descending, circumflex, or right coronary artery is confirmed by the operative report, report 33572 in addition to 33514–33516. For percutaneous ventricular assist device insertion, removal, or repositioning, see 33990-33993, 33995, and 33997. For reoperation more than one month after the original procedure, report 33530 in addition to the code for CABG procedure.

ICD-10-CM Diagnostic Codes

I20.0	Unstable angina
I20.1	Angina pectoris with documented spasm
I20.81	Angina pectoris with coronary microvascular dysfunction
I20.89	Other forms of angina pectoris

I21.01	ST elevation (STEMI) myocardial infarction involving left main coronary artery
I21.02	ST elevation (STEMI) myocardial infarction involving left anterior descending coronary artery
I21.09	ST elevation (STEMI) myocardial infarction involving other coronary artery of anterior wall
I21.11	ST elevation (STEMI) myocardial infarction involving right coronary artery
I21.19	ST elevation (STEMI) myocardial infarction involving other coronary artery of inferior wall
I21.21	ST elevation (STEMI) myocardial infarction involving left circumflex coronary artery
I21.29	ST elevation (STEMI) myocardial infarction involving other sites
I21.4	Non-ST elevation (NSTEMI) myocardial infarction
I21.A1	Myocardial infarction type 2
I21.B	Myocardial infarction with coronary microvascular dysfunction
I22.0	Subsequent ST elevation (STEMI) myocardial infarction of anterior wall
I22.1	Subsequent ST elevation (STEMI) myocardial infarction of inferior wall
I22.2	Subsequent non-ST elevation (NSTEMI) myocardial infarction
I22.8	Subsequent ST elevation (STEMI) myocardial infarction of other sites
I24.0	Acute coronary thrombosis not resulting in myocardial infarction
I24.89	Other forms of acute ischemic heart disease
I25.110	Atherosclerotic heart disease of native coronary artery with unstable angina pectoris [A]
I25.111	Atherosclerotic heart disease of native coronary artery with angina pectoris with documented spasm [A]
I25.112	Atherosclerotic heart disease of native coronary artery with refractory angina pectoris [A]
I25.118	Atherosclerotic heart disease of native coronary artery with other forms of angina pectoris [A]
I25.3	Aneurysm of heart
I25.41	Coronary artery aneurysm
I25.42	Coronary artery dissection
I25.5	Ischemic cardiomyopathy
I25.6	Silent myocardial ischemia
I25.710	Atherosclerosis of autologous vein coronary artery bypass graft(s) with unstable angina pectoris [A]
I25.711	Atherosclerosis of autologous vein coronary artery bypass graft(s) with angina pectoris with documented spasm [A]
I25.712	Atherosclerosis of autologous vein coronary artery bypass graft(s) with refractory angina pectoris [A]
I25.718	Atherosclerosis of autologous vein coronary artery bypass graft(s) with other forms of angina pectoris [A]
I25.720	Atherosclerosis of autologous artery coronary artery bypass graft(s) with unstable angina pectoris [A]
I25.721	Atherosclerosis of autologous artery coronary artery bypass graft(s) with angina pectoris with documented spasm [A]
I25.722	Atherosclerosis of autologous artery coronary artery bypass graft(s) with refractory angina pectoris [A]
I25.728	Atherosclerosis of autologous artery coronary artery bypass graft(s) with other forms of angina pectoris [A]
I25.730	Atherosclerosis of nonautologous biological coronary artery bypass graft(s) with unstable angina pectoris [A]
I25.731	Atherosclerosis of nonautologous biological coronary artery bypass graft(s) with angina pectoris with documented spasm [A]
I25.732	Atherosclerosis of nonautologous biological coronary artery bypass graft(s) with refractory angina pectoris [A]
I25.738	Atherosclerosis of nonautologous biological coronary artery bypass graft(s) with other forms of angina pectoris [A]
I25.750	Atherosclerosis of native coronary artery of transplanted heart with unstable angina
I25.751	Atherosclerosis of native coronary artery of transplanted heart with angina pectoris with documented spasm
I25.752	Atherosclerosis of native coronary artery of transplanted heart with refractory angina pectoris [A]
I25.758	Atherosclerosis of native coronary artery of transplanted heart with other forms of angina pectoris
I25.760	Atherosclerosis of bypass graft of coronary artery of transplanted heart with unstable angina [A]
I25.761	Atherosclerosis of bypass graft of coronary artery of transplanted heart with angina pectoris with documented spasm [A]
I25.762	Atherosclerosis of bypass graft of coronary artery of transplanted heart with refractory angina pectoris [A]
I25.768	Atherosclerosis of bypass graft of coronary artery of transplanted heart with other forms of angina pectoris [A]
I25.790	Atherosclerosis of other coronary artery bypass graft(s) with unstable angina pectoris [A]
I25.791	Atherosclerosis of other coronary artery bypass graft(s) with angina pectoris with documented spasm [A]
I25.792	Atherosclerosis of other coronary artery bypass graft(s) with refractory angina pectoris [A]
I25.798	Atherosclerosis of other coronary artery bypass graft(s) with other forms of angina pectoris [A]
I25.810	Atherosclerosis of coronary artery bypass graft(s) without angina pectoris [A]
I25.811	Atherosclerosis of native coronary artery of transplanted heart without angina pectoris
I25.812	Atherosclerosis of bypass graft of coronary artery of transplanted heart without angina pectoris [A]
I25.82	Chronic total occlusion of coronary artery
I25.83	Coronary atherosclerosis due to lipid rich plaque [A]
I25.84	Coronary atherosclerosis due to calcified coronary lesion
I25.89	Other forms of chronic ischemic heart disease
I45.6	Pre-excitation syndrome
I50.1	Left ventricular failure, unspecified
I50.21	Acute systolic (congestive) heart failure
I50.22	Chronic systolic (congestive) heart failure
I50.23	Acute on chronic systolic (congestive) heart failure
I50.31	Acute diastolic (congestive) heart failure
I50.32	Chronic diastolic (congestive) heart failure
I50.33	Acute on chronic diastolic (congestive) heart failure
I50.41	Acute combined systolic (congestive) and diastolic (congestive) heart failure
I50.42	Chronic combined systolic (congestive) and diastolic (congestive) heart failure
I50.43	Acute on chronic combined systolic (congestive) and diastolic (congestive) heart failure
I50.811	Acute right heart failure
I50.812	Chronic right heart failure

I50.813	Acute on chronic right heart failure
I50.814	Right heart failure due to left heart failure
I50.82	Biventricular heart failure
I50.83	High output heart failure
I50.84	End stage heart failure
Q24.5	Malformation of coronary vessels
Q26.2	Total anomalous pulmonary venous connection

AMA: 33514 2021,Dec **33516** 2021,Dec

Relative Value Units/Medicare Edits

Non-Facility RVU	Work	PE	MP	Total
33514	48.08	17.15	11.15	76.38
33516	49.76	17.75	11.54	79.05
Facility RVU	**Work**	**PE**	**MP**	**Total**
33514	48.08	17.15	11.15	76.38
33516	49.76	17.75	11.54	79.05

	FUD	Status	MUE	Modifiers				IOM Reference
33514	90	A	1(2)	51	N/A	N/A	80	None
33516	90	A	1(2)	51	N/A	N/A	80	

* with documentation

Terms To Know

cadaver. Dead body.

cardiopulmonary bypass. Venous blood is diverted to a heart-lung machine, which mechanically pumps and oxygenates the blood temporarily so the heart can be bypassed while an open procedure on the heart or coronary arteries is performed. During bypass, the lungs are deflated and immobile.

graft. Tissue implant from another part of the body or another person.

harvest. Removal of cells or tissue from their native site to be used as a graft or transplant to another part of the donor's body or placed into another person.

33517-33519

+	**33517**	Coronary artery bypass, using venous graft(s) and arterial graft(s); single vein graft (List separately in addition to code for primary procedure)
+	**33518**	2 venous grafts (List separately in addition to code for primary procedure)
+	**33519**	3 venous grafts (List separately in addition to code for primary procedure)

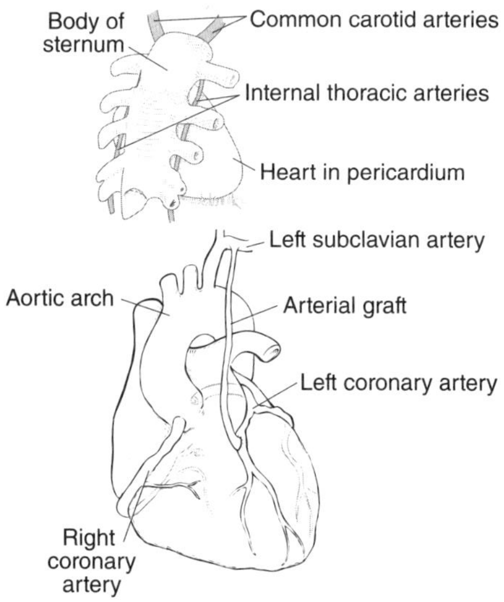

Explanation

The physician initiates cardiopulmonary bypass with a single, two-stage venous uptake tube. The physician harvests saphenous vein from the legs. Other vein grafts may be obtained from the arms, backs of the legs, or cadavers (organ donors). These sources are inferior to the saphenous vein. Arterial grafts may be obtained from the internal mammary artery (along the lateral side of the breastbone), the gastroepiploic artery (from the abdomen), the inferior epigastric artery (from the abdominal wall), or the radial artery (from the nondominant hand). The most commonly used vessel is the internal mammary artery. It is left connected at one end to the subclavian artery from which it arises. Report 33517 for a single vein graft, 33518 if two venous grafts are performed, and 33519 if three venous grafts are performed.

Coding Tips

These codes report combined arterial-venous grafting for coronary bypass and should be reported in addition to the code for the primary procedure. To report combined arterial-venous grafts, it is necessary to report two codes: 1) the appropriate combined arterial-venous graft code (33517–33523); and 2) the appropriate arterial graft code (33533–33536). If venous grafting only is performed, see 33510–33516. If arterial grafting only is performed, see 33533–33536. Procurement of saphenous vein graft is included in 33517–33519. When a surgical assistant performs graft procurement, append modifier 80 to 33517–33519. Report procurement of an upper extremity vein separately, see 35500; for upper extremity artery, see 33509 and 35600. When coronary endarterectomy of the left anterior descending, circumflex, or right coronary artery is confirmed by the operative report, report 33572 in addition to 33513–33516. For percutaneous ventricular assist device insertion, removal, or repositioning, see 33990-33993, 33995, and 33997. For reoperation more than one month after the original procedure, report 33530 in addition to the code for CABG procedure.

ICD-10-CM Diagnostic Codes

This/these CPT code(s) are add-on code(s). See the primary procedure code that this code is performed with for your ICD-10-CM code selections. Diagnostic code(s) would be the same as the actual procedure performed.

AMA: **33517** 2021,Dec **33518** 2021,Dec **33519** 2021,Dec

Relative Value Units/Medicare Edits

Non-Facility RVU	Work	PE	MP	Total
33517	3.61	1.0	0.87	5.48
33518	7.93	2.18	1.89	12.0
33519	10.49	2.88	2.51	15.88
Facility RVU	**Work**	**PE**	**MP**	**Total**
33517	3.61	1.0	0.87	5.48
33518	7.93	2.18	1.89	12.0
33519	10.49	2.88	2.51	15.88

	FUD	Status	MUE	Modifiers				IOM Reference
33517	N/A	A	1(2)	N/A	N/A	N/A	80	None
33518	N/A	A	1(2)	N/A	N/A	N/A	80	
33519	N/A	A	1(2)	N/A	N/A	N/A	80	

* with documentation

Terms To Know

cardiopulmonary bypass. Venous blood is diverted to a heart-lung machine, which mechanically pumps and oxygenates the blood temporarily so the heart can be bypassed while an open procedure on the heart or coronary arteries is performed. During bypass, the lungs are deflated and immobile.

myocardial infarction. Obstruction of circulation to the heart, resulting in necrosis.

occlusion. Constriction, closure, or blockage of a passage.

33521-33523

+ **33521** Coronary artery bypass, using venous graft(s) and arterial graft(s); 4 venous grafts (List separately in addition to code for primary procedure)
+ **33522** 5 venous grafts (List separately in addition to code for primary procedure)
+ **33523** 6 or more venous grafts (List separately in addition to code for primary procedure)

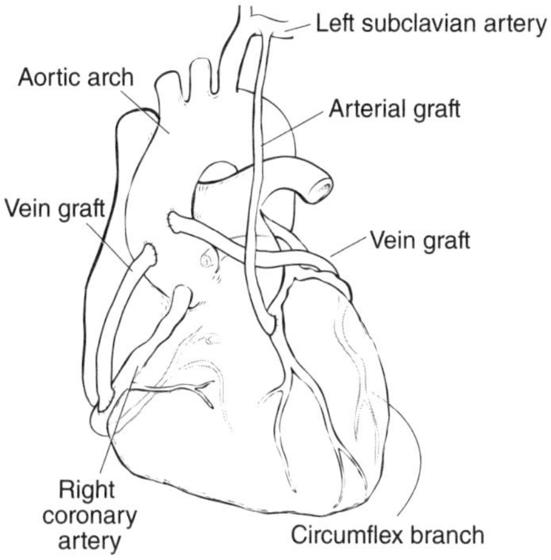

Explanation

The physician initiates cardiopulmonary bypass with a single, two-stage venous uptake tube. The physician harvests saphenous vein from the legs. Other vein grafts may be obtained from the arms, backs of the legs, or cadavers (organ donors). These sources are inferior to the saphenous vein. Arterial grafts may be obtained from the internal mammary artery (along the lateral side of the breastbone), the gastroepiploic artery (from the abdomen), the inferior epigastric artery (from the abdominal wall), or the radial artery (from the nondominant hand). The most commonly used vessel is the internal mammary artery. It is left connected at one end to the subclavian artery from which it arises. Report 33521 if four venous grafts are performed, 33522 if five venous grafts are performed, and 33523 if six or more venous grafts are performed.

Coding Tips

These codes report combined arterial-venous grafting for coronary bypass and should be reported in addition to the code for the primary procedure. To report combined arterial-venous grafts, it is necessary to report two codes: 1) the appropriate combined arterial-venous graft code (33517–33523); and 2) the appropriate arterial graft code (33533–33536). If only venous grafting is performed, see 33510–33516. If only arterial grafting is performed, see 33533–33536. Procurement of saphenous vein graft is included in 33521–33523. When a surgical assistant performs graft procurement, append modifier 80 to 33521–33523. Report procurement of an upper extremity vein separately, see 35500; for upper extremity artery, see 33509 and 35600. When coronary endarterectomy of the left anterior descending, circumflex, or right coronary artery is confirmed by the operative report, report 33572 in addition to 33513–33516. For percutaneous ventricular assist device insertion, removal, or repositioning, see 33990-33993, 33995, and 33997. For reoperation more than one month after the original procedure, report 33530 in addition to the code for CABG procedure.

ICD-10-CM Diagnostic Codes

This/these CPT code(s) are add-on code(s). See the primary procedure code that this code is performed with for your ICD-10-CM code selections. Diagnostic code(s) would be the same as the actual procedure performed.

AMA: **33521** 2021,Dec **33522** 2021,Dec **33523** 2021,Dec

Relative Value Units/Medicare Edits

Non-Facility RVU	Work	PE	MP	Total
33521	12.59	3.44	3.0	19.03
33522	14.14	3.86	3.39	21.39
33523	16.08	4.28	3.71	24.07
Facility RVU	**Work**	**PE**	**MP**	**Total**
33521	12.59	3.44	3.0	19.03
33522	14.14	3.86	3.39	21.39
33523	16.08	4.28	3.71	24.07

	FUD	Status	MUE	Modifiers				IOM Reference
33521	N/A	A	1(2)	N/A	N/A	N/A	80	None
33522	N/A	A	1(2)	N/A	N/A	N/A	80	
33523	N/A	A	1(2)	N/A	N/A	N/A	80	

* with documentation

Terms To Know

cardiopulmonary bypass. Venous blood is diverted to a heart-lung machine, which mechanically pumps and oxygenates the blood temporarily so the heart can be bypassed while an open procedure on the heart or coronary arteries is performed. During bypass, the lungs are deflated and immobile.

graft. Tissue implant from another part of the body or another person.

insufficiency. Inadequate closure of the valve that allows abnormal backward blood flow.

occlusion. Constriction, closure, or blockage of a passage.

venous. Relating to the veins.

33530

\+ **33530** Reoperation, coronary artery bypass procedure or valve procedure, more than 1 month after original operation (List separately in addition to code for primary procedure)

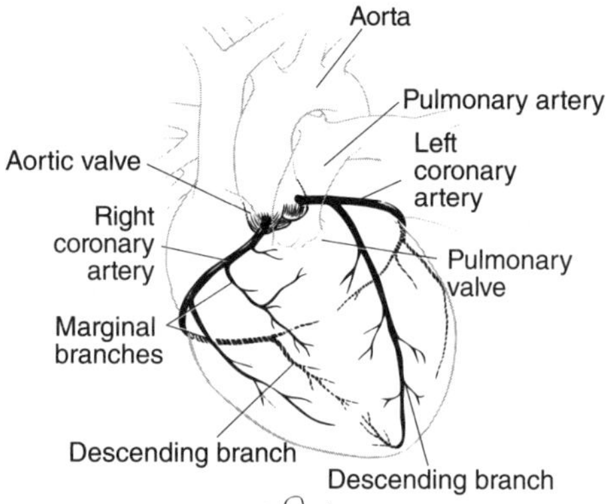

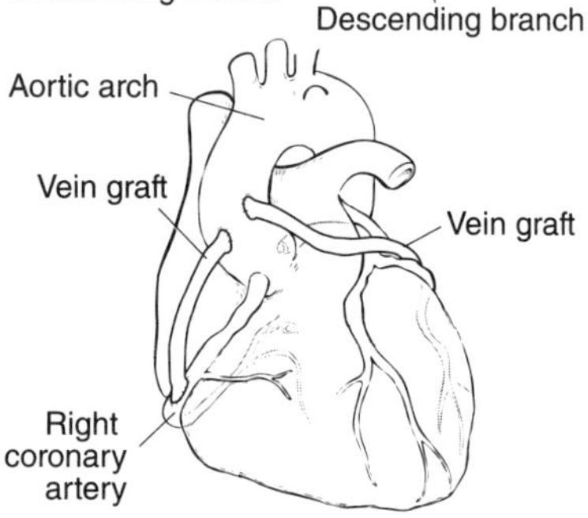

Explanation

For descriptions of the actual therapeutic procedure to be performed, please see the description of that procedure. The breast bone must be split again. Because the heart is invariably tightly adherent to the underside of the sternum in a redo operation, a vibrating saw is used to cut through it. After the sternum is cut, its halves are gently retracted while the tissues that have adhered to its undersurface are carefully cut down. Once the sternum can be opened, the heart is exposed by cutting any chest tissues that have adhered to it since the last operation. It is usually necessary to initiate cardiopulmonary bypass before the heart is completely cleaned off.

Coding Tips

Report 33530 in addition to 33390–33391, 33404–33496, 33510–33536, and 33863.

ICD-10-CM Diagnostic Codes

This/these CPT code(s) are add-on code(s). See the primary procedure code that this code is performed with for your ICD-10-CM code selections. Diagnostic code(s) would be the same as the actual procedure performed.

Relative Value Units/Medicare Edits

Non-Facility RVU	Work	PE	MP	Total
33530	10.13	2.78	2.41	15.32
Facility RVU	**Work**	**PE**	**MP**	**Total**
33530	10.13	2.78	2.41	15.32

	FUD	Status	MUE	Modifiers				IOM Reference
33530	N/A	A	1(2)	N/A	N/A	N/A	80	None

* with documentation

33533-33536

33533 Coronary artery bypass, using arterial graft(s); single arterial graft
33534 2 coronary arterial grafts
33535 3 coronary arterial grafts
33536 4 or more coronary arterial grafts

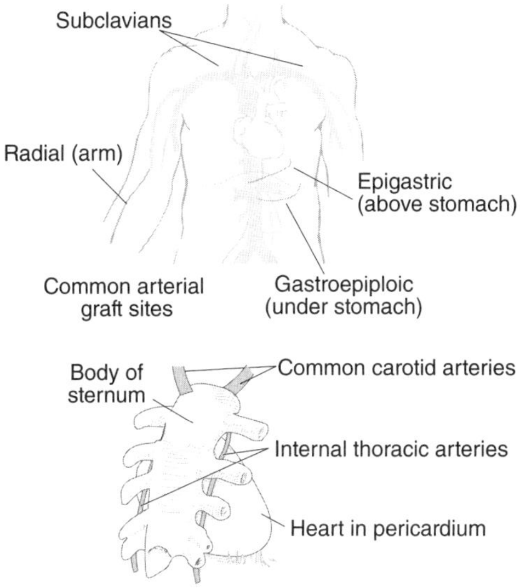

Explanation

Cardiopulmonary bypass is initiated with a single, two-stage venous uptake tube. Arterial grafts may be obtained from the internal mammary artery (along the lateral side of the breast bone), the gastroepiploic artery (from the abdomen), the inferior epigastric artery (from the abdominal wall), or the radial artery (from the non-dominant hand). The most commonly used vessel is the internal mammary artery. It is left connected at one end to the arm artery from which it arises. Report 33534 if two arterial grafts are placed; report 33535 if three are placed; report 33536 if four or more are placed.

Coding Tips

These codes are used to report coronary artery bypass graft (CABG) procedures using either arterial grafts only or combined arterial-venous grafts. To report combined arterial-venous grafts, it is necessary to use two codes: 1) the appropriate arterial graft (33533–33536); and 2) the appropriate combined arterial-venous graft code (33517–33523). Note that 33533–33536 include the use of the internal mammary artery, gastroepiploic artery, epigastric artery, and arterial conduits procured from other sites except the upper extremity. If a surgical assistant performs arterial graft procurement from these sites, report 33533–33536 and append modifier 80 as appropriate. Procurement of an upper extremity artery graft, including the radial artery or other upper extremity artery, is reported separately, see 33509 and 35600. Report 33572 in addition to 33533–33536 when coronary endarterectomy of the left anterior descending, circumflex, or right coronary artery is confirmed by the operative report. For percutaneous ventricular assist device insertion, removal, or repositioning, see 33990-33993, 33995, and 33997. For reoperation more than one month after the original procedure, report 33530 in addition to the code for CABG procedure.

ICD-10-CM Diagnostic Codes

I20.0	Unstable angina
I20.1	Angina pectoris with documented spasm
I20.81	Angina pectoris with coronary microvascular dysfunction
I20.89	Other forms of angina pectoris
I21.01	ST elevation (STEMI) myocardial infarction involving left main coronary artery
I21.02	ST elevation (STEMI) myocardial infarction involving left anterior descending coronary artery
I21.09	ST elevation (STEMI) myocardial infarction involving other coronary artery of anterior wall
I21.11	ST elevation (STEMI) myocardial infarction involving right coronary artery
I21.19	ST elevation (STEMI) myocardial infarction involving other coronary artery of inferior wall
I21.21	ST elevation (STEMI) myocardial infarction involving left circumflex coronary artery
I21.29	ST elevation (STEMI) myocardial infarction involving other sites
I21.4	Non-ST elevation (NSTEMI) myocardial infarction
I21.A1	Myocardial infarction type 2
I21.B	Myocardial infarction with coronary microvascular dysfunction
I22.0	Subsequent ST elevation (STEMI) myocardial infarction of anterior wall
I22.1	Subsequent ST elevation (STEMI) myocardial infarction of inferior wall
I22.2	Subsequent non-ST elevation (NSTEMI) myocardial infarction
I22.8	Subsequent ST elevation (STEMI) myocardial infarction of other sites
I24.0	Acute coronary thrombosis not resulting in myocardial infarction
I24.89	Other forms of acute ischemic heart disease
I25.110	Atherosclerotic heart disease of native coronary artery with unstable angina pectoris A
I25.111	Atherosclerotic heart disease of native coronary artery with angina pectoris with documented spasm A
I25.112	Atherosclerotic heart disease of native coronary artery with refractory angina pectoris A
I25.118	Atherosclerotic heart disease of native coronary artery with other forms of angina pectoris A
I25.3	Aneurysm of heart
I25.41	Coronary artery aneurysm
I25.42	Coronary artery dissection
I25.5	Ischemic cardiomyopathy
I25.6	Silent myocardial ischemia
I25.710	Atherosclerosis of autologous vein coronary artery bypass graft(s) with unstable angina pectoris A
I25.711	Atherosclerosis of autologous vein coronary artery bypass graft(s) with angina pectoris with documented spasm A
I25.712	Atherosclerosis of autologous vein coronary artery bypass graft(s) with refractory angina pectoris A
I25.718	Atherosclerosis of autologous vein coronary artery bypass graft(s) with other forms of angina pectoris A
I25.720	Atherosclerosis of autologous artery coronary artery bypass graft(s) with unstable angina pectoris A
I25.721	Atherosclerosis of autologous artery coronary artery bypass graft(s) with angina pectoris with documented spasm A
I25.722	Atherosclerosis of autologous artery coronary artery bypass graft(s) with refractory angina pectoris A
I25.728	Atherosclerosis of autologous artery coronary artery bypass graft(s) with other forms of angina pectoris A
I25.730	Atherosclerosis of nonautologous biological coronary artery bypass graft(s) with unstable angina pectoris A

 ● New ▲ Revised + Add On ★ Telemedicine [Resequenced] ☑ Laterality

I25.731	Atherosclerosis of nonautologous biological coronary artery bypass graft(s) with angina pectoris with documented spasm [A]
I25.732	Atherosclerosis of nonautologous biological coronary artery bypass graft(s) with refractory angina pectoris [A]
I25.738	Atherosclerosis of nonautologous biological coronary artery bypass graft(s) with other forms of angina pectoris [A]
I25.750	Atherosclerosis of native coronary artery of transplanted heart with unstable angina
I25.751	Atherosclerosis of native coronary artery of transplanted heart with angina pectoris with documented spasm
I25.752	Atherosclerosis of native coronary artery of transplanted heart with refractory angina pectoris [A]
I25.758	Atherosclerosis of native coronary artery of transplanted heart with other forms of angina pectoris
I25.760	Atherosclerosis of bypass graft of coronary artery of transplanted heart with unstable angina [A]
I25.761	Atherosclerosis of bypass graft of coronary artery of transplanted heart with angina pectoris with documented spasm [A]
I25.762	Atherosclerosis of bypass graft of coronary artery of transplanted heart with refractory angina pectoris [A]
I25.768	Atherosclerosis of bypass graft of coronary artery of transplanted heart with other forms of angina pectoris [A]
I25.790	Atherosclerosis of other coronary artery bypass graft(s) with unstable angina pectoris [A]
I25.791	Atherosclerosis of other coronary artery bypass graft(s) with angina pectoris with documented spasm [A]
I25.792	Atherosclerosis of other coronary artery bypass graft(s) with refractory angina pectoris [A]
I25.798	Atherosclerosis of other coronary artery bypass graft(s) with other forms of angina pectoris [A]
I25.810	Atherosclerosis of coronary artery bypass graft(s) without angina pectoris [A]
I25.811	Atherosclerosis of native coronary artery of transplanted heart without angina pectoris
I25.812	Atherosclerosis of bypass graft of coronary artery of transplanted heart without angina pectoris [A]
I25.82	Chronic total occlusion of coronary artery
I25.83	Coronary atherosclerosis due to lipid rich plaque [A]
I25.84	Coronary atherosclerosis due to calcified coronary lesion
I25.89	Other forms of chronic ischemic heart disease
I50.1	Left ventricular failure, unspecified
I50.21	Acute systolic (congestive) heart failure
I50.22	Chronic systolic (congestive) heart failure
I50.23	Acute on chronic systolic (congestive) heart failure
I50.31	Acute diastolic (congestive) heart failure
I50.32	Chronic diastolic (congestive) heart failure
I50.33	Acute on chronic diastolic (congestive) heart failure
I50.41	Acute combined systolic (congestive) and diastolic (congestive) heart failure
I50.42	Chronic combined systolic (congestive) and diastolic (congestive) heart failure
I50.43	Acute on chronic combined systolic (congestive) and diastolic (congestive) heart failure
I50.811	Acute right heart failure
I50.812	Chronic right heart failure
I50.813	Acute on chronic right heart failure
I50.814	Right heart failure due to left heart failure
I50.82	Biventricular heart failure
I50.83	High output heart failure
I50.84	End stage heart failure
Q24.5	Malformation of coronary vessels
Q26.2	Total anomalous pulmonary venous connection

AMA: **33533** 2021,Dec **33534** 2021,Dec **33535** 2021,Dec **33536** 2021,Dec

Relative Value Units/Medicare Edits

Non-Facility RVU	Work	PE	MP	Total
33533	33.75	13.24	8.1	55.09
33534	39.88	15.24	9.57	64.69
33535	44.75	16.48	10.64	71.87
33536	48.43	17.52	11.49	77.44
Facility RVU	**Work**	**PE**	**MP**	**Total**
33533	33.75	13.24	8.1	55.09
33534	39.88	15.24	9.57	64.69
33535	44.75	16.48	10.64	71.87
33536	48.43	17.52	11.49	77.44

	FUD	Status	MUE	Modifiers				IOM Reference
33533	90	A	1(2)	51	N/A	N/A	80	None
33534	90	A	1(2)	51	N/A	N/A	80	
33535	90	A	1(2)	51	N/A	N/A	80	
33536	90	A	1(2)	51	N/A	N/A	80	

* with documentation

Terms To Know

angina. Chest pain that occurs secondary to the inadequate delivery of oxygen to the heart muscle and may be described as a heavy or squeezing pain in the midsternal area of the chest.

bypass. Auxiliary or diverted route to maintain continuous flow.

dissection. (dis. apart; -section, act of cutting) Separating by cutting tissue or body structures apart.

myocardial infarction. Obstruction of circulation to the heart, resulting in necrosis.

33542

33542 Myocardial resection (eg, ventricular aneurysmectomy)

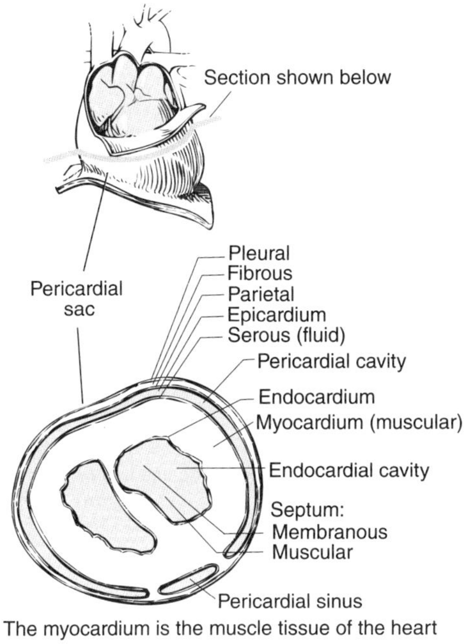

The myocardium is the muscle tissue of the heart

Explanation

This operation is almost always done in conjunction with coronary artery bypass grafting. Prior to placing the bypass grafts, the aneurysm is opened and any clot is removed from the ventricle. The aneurysm is opened widely and damaged tissue is removed from the ventricular wall. The ventricle is repaired by suturing the walls of the ventricle back together directly or with a patch of Gortex, Dacron, or other appropriate material sewn into the defect. All stitches are placed in healthy (not aneurysm) heart tissue and care is taken to avoid the coronary arteries.

Coding Tips

Ventricular aneurysms are usually a complication of myocardial infarction, but may also be caused by bacterial endocarditis or trauma. For ablation of ventricular arrhythmogenic focus to control a ventricular arrhythmia, see 33261. For ventriculomyotomy (-myectomy) for idiopathic hypertrophic subaortic stenosis, see 33416. For excision of an intracardiac tumor without myocardial resection, see 33120. For excision of an external cardiac tumor without myocardial resection, see 33130.

ICD-10-CM Diagnostic Codes

I25.3 Aneurysm of heart

Relative Value Units/Medicare Edits

Non-Facility RVU	Work	PE	MP	Total
33542	48.21	17.26	11.57	77.04
Facility RVU	**Work**	**PE**	**MP**	**Total**
33542	48.21	17.26	11.57	77.04

	FUD	Status	MUE	Modifiers				IOM Reference
33542	90	A	1(2)	51	N/A	62*	80	None

* with documentation

33545

33545 Repair of postinfarction ventricular septal defect, with or without myocardial resection

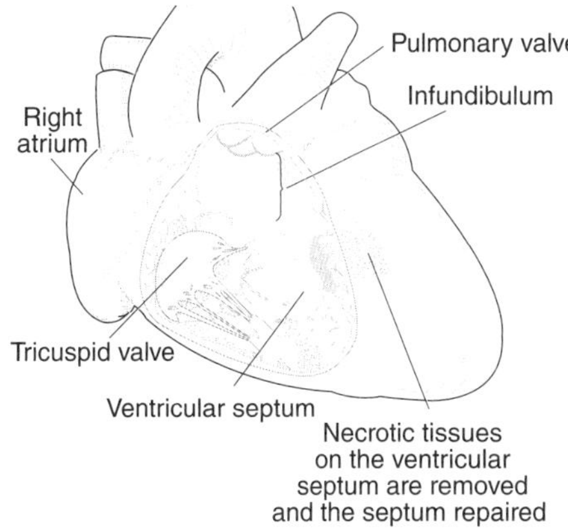

A defect in the ventricular septum caused by myocardial infarction is repaired

Explanation

This operation is always done in conjunction with coronary artery bypass grafting. The heart muscle involved in the infarction extends from the septum onto the surface of the heart. The heart is opened through this dead muscle and all dead muscle on the surface of the heart is cut out as is all the dead muscle in the septum. The septum is reconstructed by sewing in a patch of Gortex, for example, or Dacron. The surface of the heart is closed directly with sutures or with a patch sewn over the hole.

Coding Tips

When 33545 is performed with another separately identifiable procedure, the highest dollar value code is listed as the primary procedure and subsequent procedures are appended with modifier 51. Excision of a ventricular aneurysm is included in 33545. For coronary artery bypass grafting, report 33510–33536 in addition to 33545.

ICD-10-CM Diagnostic Codes

I21.01 ST elevation (STEMI) myocardial infarction involving left main coronary artery

I21.02 ST elevation (STEMI) myocardial infarction involving left anterior descending coronary artery

I21.09 ST elevation (STEMI) myocardial infarction involving other coronary artery of anterior wall

I21.11 ST elevation (STEMI) myocardial infarction involving right coronary artery

I21.19 ST elevation (STEMI) myocardial infarction involving other coronary artery of inferior wall

I21.21 ST elevation (STEMI) myocardial infarction involving left circumflex coronary artery

I21.29 ST elevation (STEMI) myocardial infarction involving other sites

I21.4 Non-ST elevation (NSTEMI) myocardial infarction

I21.A1 Myocardial infarction type 2

I21.B Myocardial infarction with coronary microvascular dysfunction

I22.0 Subsequent ST elevation (STEMI) myocardial infarction of anterior wall

I22.1 Subsequent ST elevation (STEMI) myocardial infarction of inferior wall

Relative Value Units/Medicare Edits

Non-Facility RVU	Work	PE	MP	Total
33545	57.06	19.4	13.22	89.68
Facility RVU	**Work**	**PE**	**MP**	**Total**
33545	57.06	19.4	13.22	89.68

	FUD	Status	MUE	Modifiers				IOM Reference
33545	90	A	1(2)	51	N/A	62*	80	None

* with documentation

Terms To Know

coronary atherosclerosis. Chronic condition marked by thickening and loss of elasticity of the coronary artery, caused by deposits of plaque containing cholesterol, lipoid material, and lipophages.

myocardial infarction. Obstruction of circulation to the heart, resulting in necrosis.

resection. Surgical removal of a part or all of an organ or body part.

tricuspid valve. Valve with three cusps between the right atrium and the right ventricle.

33548

33548 Surgical ventricular restoration procedure, includes prosthetic patch, when performed (eg, ventricular remodeling, SVR, SAVER, Dor procedures)

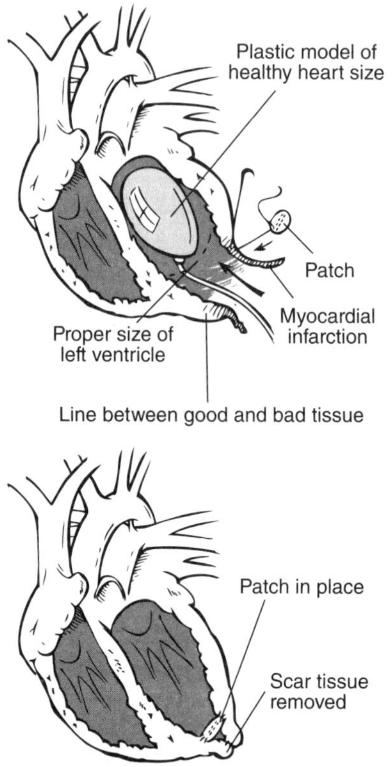

Explanation

The physician performs a surgical ventricular restoration (SVR) procedure to treat congestive heart failure subsequent to a myocardial infarction that has caused scarring or aneurysm of the left ventricle resulting in an enlarged rounded heart. SVR restores the heart to a more normal size and shape thereby improving function. Cardiopulmonary bypass is initiated. The ventricle is collapsed. A small incision is made in the bottom of the left ventricle through the scar tissue. The heart is opened and the area between the scar and the good heart muscle is identified. Using a plastic model of the heart selected based on the body surface area of the patient, the physician reshapes the heart. Rather than closing the defect, the physician sutures a patch over the defect to restore the normal spherical shape of the heart.

Coding Tips

Do not report 33548 with 32551, 33210, 33211, 33310, or 33315. For a Batista procedure or pachopexy, use unlisted code 33999.

ICD-10-CM Diagnostic Codes

I25.3	Aneurysm of heart
I25.41	Coronary artery aneurysm
I25.42	Coronary artery dissection
I25.5	Ischemic cardiomyopathy
I50.1	Left ventricular failure, unspecified
I50.21	Acute systolic (congestive) heart failure
I50.22	Chronic systolic (congestive) heart failure
I50.23	Acute on chronic systolic (congestive) heart failure
I50.31	Acute diastolic (congestive) heart failure

I50.32	Chronic diastolic (congestive) heart failure
I50.33	Acute on chronic diastolic (congestive) heart failure
I50.41	Acute combined systolic (congestive) and diastolic (congestive) heart failure
I50.42	Chronic combined systolic (congestive) and diastolic (congestive) heart failure
I50.43	Acute on chronic combined systolic (congestive) and diastolic (congestive) heart failure
I50.811	Acute right heart failure
I50.812	Chronic right heart failure
I50.813	Acute on chronic right heart failure
I50.814	Right heart failure due to left heart failure
I50.82	Biventricular heart failure
I50.83	High output heart failure
I50.84	End stage heart failure

Relative Value Units/Medicare Edits

Non-Facility RVU	Work	PE	MP	Total
33548	54.14	19.67	12.55	86.36
Facility RVU	**Work**	**PE**	**MP**	**Total**
33548	54.14	19.67	12.55	86.36

	FUD	Status	MUE	Modifiers				IOM Reference
33548	90	A	1(2)	51	N/A	62*	80	None

* with documentation

Terms To Know

aneurysm. Circumscribed dilation or outpouching of an artery wall, often containing blood clots and connecting directly with the lumen of the artery.

atherosclerosis. Buildup of yellowish plaques composed of cholesterol and lipoid material within the arteries.

cardiopulmonary bypass. Venous blood is diverted to a heart-lung machine, which mechanically pumps and oxygenates the blood temporarily so the heart can be bypassed while an open procedure on the heart or coronary arteries is performed. During bypass, the lungs are deflated and immobile.

congestive heart failure. Condition caused by the heart's inability to adequately pump and circulate blood, resulting in fluid accumulation in the lungs and other tissues.

ischemia. Deficiency in blood supply causing tissues to be deprived of oxygen, resulting from trauma, mechanical or functional constriction of blood vessels, or a physical obstruction.

myocardial infarction. Obstruction of circulation to the heart, resulting in necrosis.

occlusion. Constriction, closure, or blockage of a passage.

33572

\+ **33572** Coronary endarterectomy, open, any method, of left anterior descending, circumflex, or right coronary artery performed in conjunction with coronary artery bypass graft procedure, each vessel (List separately in addition to primary procedure)

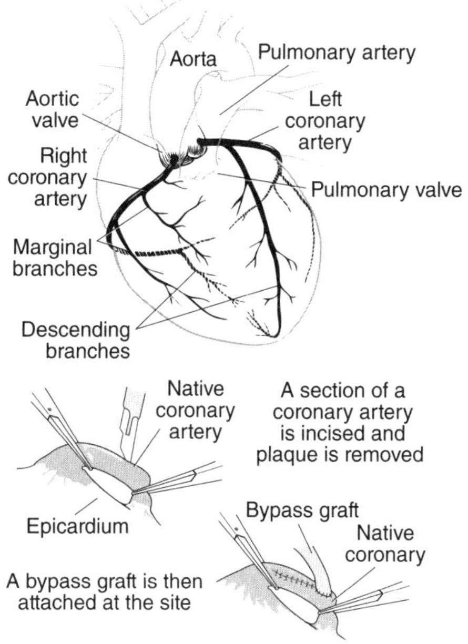

Explanation

This operation is only done when a coronary artery is so full of disease along its length that a good site for sewing on the bypass graft cannot be found. Coronary artery bypass grafts are almost always done along with an endarterectomy. The coronary artery to be cleaned out is opened along its length for a distance greater than that usually opened for a bypass alone, sometimes along its length. The plaque within the artery is separated from the outer layer of the arterial wall with a tool designed for this purpose. The plaque is removed from as much of the artery as is possible. A bypass graft is usually sewn to part of the hole left in the coronary. The rest of the hole is closed directly with suture or a patch of opened vein graft is laid over the open artery and sewn to the coronary artery wall to close the hole.

Coding Tips

Report 33572 in addition to 33510–33516 and 33533–33536. Note that 33572 reports only endarterectomy of the left anterior descending, circumflex, or right coronary artery. Endarterectomy of other coronary arteries is not reported separately. For pulmonary endarterectomy, see 33916. For coronary artery angiography, see 93454–93461.

ICD-10-CM Diagnostic Codes

This/these CPT code(s) are add-on code(s). See the primary procedure code that this code is performed with for your ICD-10-CM code selections. Diagnostic code(s) would be the same as the actual procedure performed.

Relative Value Units/Medicare Edits

Non-Facility RVU	Work	PE	MP	Total
33572	4.44	1.23	1.08	6.75
Facility RVU	**Work**	**PE**	**MP**	**Total**
33572	4.44	1.23	1.08	6.75

	FUD	Status	MUE	Modifiers				IOM Reference
33572	N/A	A	3(2)	N/A	N/A	N/A	80	None

* with documentation

Terms To Know

angioplasty. Reconstruction or repair of a diseased or damaged blood vessel.

bypass graft. Surgically created alternative blood vessel used to reroute blood flow around an area of obstruction or disease.

endarterectomy. Removal of the thickened, endothelial lining of a diseased or damaged artery.

excision. Surgical removal of an organ or tissue.

obstruction. Blockage that prevents normal function of the valve or structure.

plaque. Accumulation of a soft sticky substance on the teeth largely composed of bacteria and its byproducts.

33600-33602

33600 Closure of atrioventricular valve (mitral or tricuspid) by suture or patch

33602 Closure of semilunar valve (aortic or pulmonary) by suture or patch

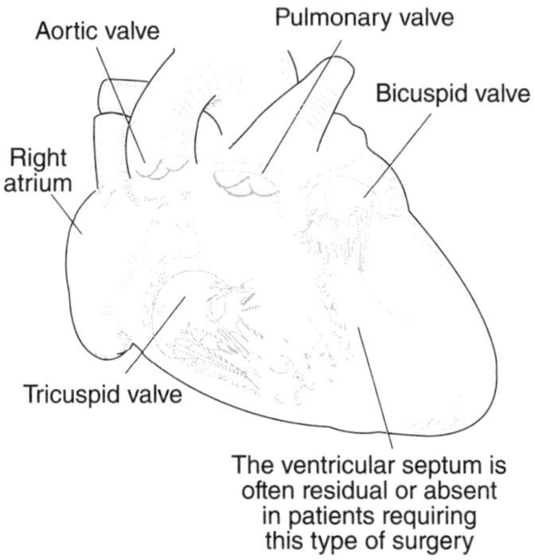

Explanation

Cardiopulmonary bypass is initiated. The appropriate heart chamber (right atrium for the tricuspid valve; left atrium for the mitral valve) is opened and the valve is assessed. The hole in the leaflet is cleaned of any infection. If it can be closed directly without distorting the valve significantly, suture alone is used. If the hole is large, it is closed with a patch made of pericardium. The open heart chamber is closed and cardiopulmonary bypass is discontinued when heart function returns. Report 33602 if the pulmonary artery or aorta are opened to gain access to the valve.

Coding Tips

If significant additional time and effort are documented, append modifier 22 and submit a cover letter and operative report. When 33600 or 33602 is performed with another separately identified procedure, the highest dollar value code is listed as the primary procedure and subsequent procedures are appended with modifier 51. When ligation and takedown of a systemic-to-pulmonary shunt is performed in addition to this procedure, it should be reported separately, see 33924.

ICD-10-CM Diagnostic Codes

I34.0	Nonrheumatic mitral (valve) insufficiency
I34.1	Nonrheumatic mitral (valve) prolapse
I34.2	Nonrheumatic mitral (valve) stenosis
I34.81	Nonrheumatic mitral (valve) annulus calcification
I34.89	Other nonrheumatic mitral valve disorders
I35.0	Nonrheumatic aortic (valve) stenosis
I35.1	Nonrheumatic aortic (valve) insufficiency
I35.2	Nonrheumatic aortic (valve) stenosis with insufficiency
I35.8	Other nonrheumatic aortic valve disorders
I36.0	Nonrheumatic tricuspid (valve) stenosis
I36.1	Nonrheumatic tricuspid (valve) insufficiency
I36.2	Nonrheumatic tricuspid (valve) stenosis with insufficiency
I36.8	Other nonrheumatic tricuspid valve disorders
I37.0	Nonrheumatic pulmonary valve stenosis
I37.1	Nonrheumatic pulmonary valve insufficiency
I37.2	Nonrheumatic pulmonary valve stenosis with insufficiency

I37.8 Other nonrheumatic pulmonary valve disorders
Q20.8 Other congenital malformations of cardiac chambers and connections
Q21.21 Partial atrioventricular septal defect
Q21.22 Transitional atrioventricular septal defect
Q21.23 Complete atrioventricular septal defect
Q21.8 Other congenital malformations of cardiac septa
Q22.0 Pulmonary valve atresia
Q22.2 Congenital pulmonary valve insufficiency
Q22.3 Other congenital malformations of pulmonary valve
Q22.4 Congenital tricuspid stenosis
Q22.5 Ebstein's anomaly
Q22.8 Other congenital malformations of tricuspid valve
Q23.1 Congenital insufficiency of aortic valve

Relative Value Units/Medicare Edits

Non-Facility RVU	Work	PE	MP	Total
33600	30.31	13.0	7.51	50.82
33602	29.34	12.73	7.27	49.34
Facility RVU	**Work**	**PE**	**MP**	**Total**
33600	30.31	13.0	7.51	50.82
33602	29.34	12.73	7.27	49.34

	FUD	Status	MUE	Modifiers				IOM Reference
33600	90	A	1(3)	51	N/A	62*	80	None
33602	90	A	1(3)	51	N/A	62*	80	

* with documentation

Terms To Know

cardiopulmonary bypass. Venous blood is diverted to a heart-lung machine, which mechanically pumps and oxygenates the blood temporarily so the heart can be bypassed while an open procedure on the heart or coronary arteries is performed. During bypass, the lungs are deflated and immobile.

shunt. Surgically created passage between blood vessels or other natural passages, such as an arteriovenous anastomosis, to divert or bypass blood flow from the normal channel.

33606

33606 Anastomosis of pulmonary artery to aorta (Damus-Kaye-Stansel procedure)

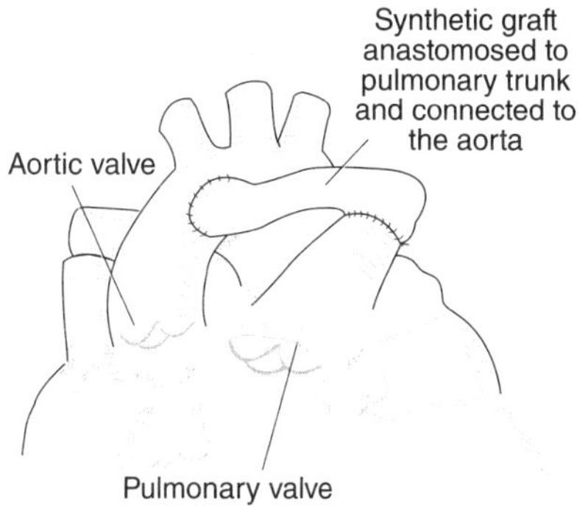

Explanation

The heart is exposed by dividing the breastbone longitudinally. Mechanical, extracorporeal circulation is established and the heart is stopped (cardiopulmonary bypass). The pulmonary artery is cut just before it divides into right and left branches. The pulmonary artery end is connected to the side of the ascending aorta. A piece of Dacron graft is used to construct this connection. This allows the single ventricle to pump blood to the body.

Coding Tips

If significant additional time and effort are documented, append modifier 22 and submit a cover letter and operative report. When 33606 is performed with another separately identifiable procedure, the highest dollar value code is listed as the primary procedure and subsequent procedures are appended with modifier 51. When ligation and takedown of a systemic-to-pulmonary shunt is performed in addition to this procedure, it should be reported separately, see 33924.

ICD-10-CM Diagnostic Codes

Q20.1 Double outlet right ventricle
Q20.3 Discordant ventriculoarterial connection
Q21.3 Tetralogy of Fallot
Q22.0 Pulmonary valve atresia
Q23.4 Hypoplastic left heart syndrome

Relative Value Units/Medicare Edits

Non-Facility RVU	Work	PE	MP	Total
33606	31.53	13.2	7.79	52.52
Facility RVU	**Work**	**PE**	**MP**	**Total**
33606	31.53	13.2	7.79	52.52

	FUD	Status	MUE	Modifiers				IOM Reference
33606	90	A	1(2)	51	N/A	62*	80	None

* with documentation

33608

33608 Repair of complex cardiac anomaly other than pulmonary atresia with ventricular septal defect by construction or replacement of conduit from right or left ventricle to pulmonary artery

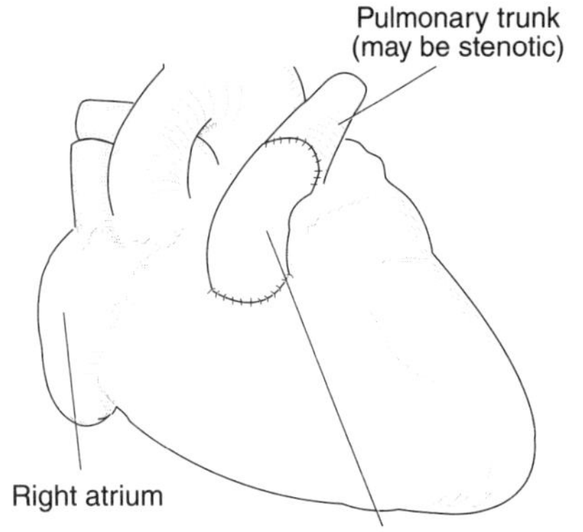

Any of a variety of congenital cardiac malformations may be addressed by creating a shunt from a ventricle to the pulmonary artery

Explanation

Mechanical, extracorporeal circulation is established and the heart is stopped (cardiopulmonary bypass). A hole is made in the pulmonary artery and is enlarged to cross any areas of narrowing. A cadaver ascending aorta is trimmed to the right length. A tube of artery or Dacron is sewn to the valve end of the cadaver aorta. The cadaver artery is connected to the hole in the pulmonary artery. The tube of aorta or Dacron is sewn to the hole in the ventricle to close the hole and allow blood to flow through the new valved tube that now connects the ventricle to the pulmonary artery.

Coding Tips

If significant additional time and effort are documented, append modifier 22 and submit a cover letter and operative report. When 33608 is performed with another separately identifiable procedure, the highest dollar value code is listed as the primary procedure and subsequent procedures are appended with modifier 51. Do not report 33608 with 33440. When ligation and takedown of a systemic-to-pulmonary shunt is performed in addition to this procedure, it should be reported separately, see 33924. For repair of pulmonary atresia with a ventricular septal defect, see 33920. For repair of pulmonary artery arborization anomalies by unifocalization, see 33925–33926.

ICD-10-CM Diagnostic Codes

Q20.1	Double outlet right ventricle
Q20.3	Discordant ventriculoarterial connection
Q21.3	Tetralogy of Fallot

AMA: 33608 2019,Apr

Relative Value Units/Medicare Edits

Non-Facility RVU	Work	PE	MP	Total
33608	31.88	13.43	7.88	53.19
Facility RVU	**Work**	**PE**	**MP**	**Total**
33608	31.88	13.43	7.88	53.19

	FUD	Status	MUE	Modifiers				IOM Reference
33608	90	A	1(2)	51	N/A	62*	80	None

* with documentation

Terms To Know

anomaly. Irregularity in the structure or position of an organ or tissue.

atresia. Congenital closure or absence of a tubular organ or an opening to the body surface.

cadaver. Dead body.

cardiopulmonary bypass. Venous blood is diverted to a heart-lung machine, which mechanically pumps and oxygenates the blood temporarily so the heart can be bypassed while an open procedure on the heart or coronary arteries is performed. During bypass, the lungs are deflated and immobile.

conduit. Surgically created channel for the passage of fluids.

ligation. Tying off a blood vessel or duct with a suture or a soft, thin wire.

tetralogy of Fallot. Specific combination of congenital cardiac defects: obstruction of the right ventricular outflow tract with pulmonary stenosis, interventricular septal defect, malposition of the aorta, overriding the interventricular septum and receiving blood from both the venous and arterial systems, and enlargement of the right ventricle.

ventricular septal defect. Congenital cardiac anomaly resulting in a continual opening in the septum between the ventricles that, in severe cases, causes oxygenated blood to flow back into the lungs, resulting in pulmonary hypertension.

33610

33610 Repair of complex cardiac anomalies (eg, single ventricle with subaortic obstruction) by surgical enlargement of ventricular septal defect

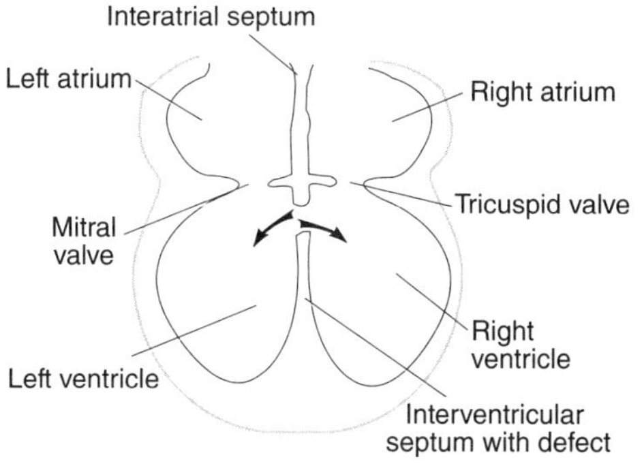

Posterior schematic showing septal defect

In some instances, an interventricular septal defect is desirable, due to anomalies occurring elsewhere in the heart

Explanation

The heart is exposed by dividing the breast bone longitudinally. Mechanical, extra corporeal circulation is established and the heart is stopped (cardiopulmonary bypass). The heart is opened and the hole in the wall between the two ventricles is enlarged so that blood will flow freely across it. A baffle is placed to direct blood that flows across the enlarged ventricular septal defect out the aorta.

Coding Tips

If significant additional time and effort are documented, append modifier 22 and submit a cover letter and operative report. When 33610 is performed with another separately identifiable procedure, the highest dollar value code is listed as the primary procedure and subsequent procedures are appended with modifier 51. Do not append modifier 63 to 33610 as the description or nature of the procedure includes infants up to 4 kg. When ligation and takedown of a systemic-to-pulmonary shunt is performed in addition to this procedure, it should be reported separately, see 33924.

ICD-10-CM Diagnostic Codes

Q20.1 Double outlet right ventricle
Q20.4 Double inlet ventricle

Relative Value Units/Medicare Edits

Non-Facility RVU	Work	PE	MP	Total
33610	31.4	13.3	7.76	52.46
Facility RVU	**Work**	**PE**	**MP**	**Total**
33610	31.4	13.3	7.76	52.46

	FUD	Status	MUE	Modifiers				IOM Reference
33610	90	A	1(2)	51	N/A	62*	80	None

* with documentation

33611-33612

33611 Repair of double outlet right ventricle with intraventricular tunnel repair;
33612 with repair of right ventricular outflow tract obstruction

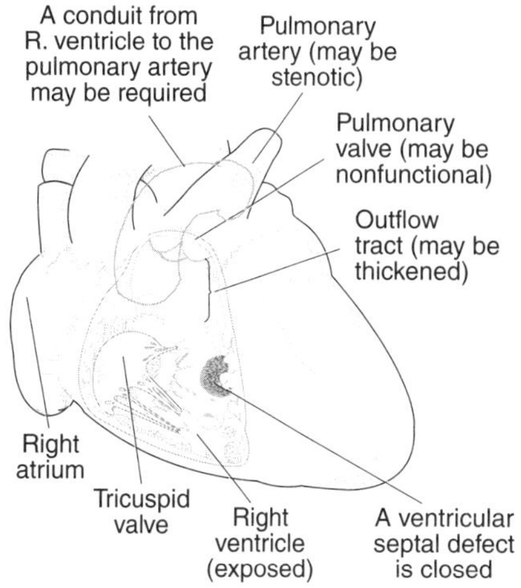

Explanation

Cardiopulmonary bypass is initiated. A hole is made in the right ventricle free wall. This exposes the hole between the right and left ventricles. A patch of pericardium or Dacron is sewn in place to block the hole and directs blood ejected from the left ventricle (i.e., blood coming from the lungs) out the aorta. If the pulmonary artery is of adequate size, blood will flow from the right ventricle to the lungs. If it is inadequate or if the valve does not open, a conduit containing a valve (natural or artificial) is sewn to the hole in the right ventricle free wall. The far end of the conduit is attached to the pulmonary artery. This will allow blood to be pumped from the right ventricle to the lungs. Report 33612 if the obstructing muscles bundles in the outflow part of the right ventricle are excised when the heart is open.

Coding Tips

If significant additional time and effort are documented, append modifier 22 and submit a cover letter and operative report. When 33611 or 33612 is performed with another separately identifiable procedure, the highest dollar value code is listed as the primary procedure and subsequent procedures are appended with modifier 51. Do not append modifier 63 to 33611 as the description or nature of the procedure includes infants up to 4 kg. When ligation and takedown of a systemic-to-pulmonary shunt is performed in addition to this procedure, it should be reported separately, see 33924.

ICD-10-CM Diagnostic Codes

Q20.1 Double outlet right ventricle
Q24.8 Other specified congenital malformations of heart

Relative Value Units/Medicare Edits

Non-Facility RVU	Work	PE	MP	Total
33611	35.57	13.03	8.8	57.4
33612	36.57	13.31	9.06	58.94
Facility RVU	**Work**	**PE**	**MP**	**Total**
33611	35.57	13.03	8.8	57.4
33612	36.57	13.31	9.06	58.94

	FUD	Status	MUE	Modifiers				IOM Reference
33611	90	A	1(2)	51	N/A	62*	80	None
33612	90	A	1(2)	51	N/A	62*	80	

* with documentation

Terms To Know

anomaly. Irregularity in the structure or position of an organ or tissue.

conduit. Surgically created channel for the passage of fluids.

congenital. Present at birth, occurring through heredity or an influence during gestation up to the moment of birth.

ligation. Tying off a blood vessel or duct with a suture or a soft, thin wire.

obstruction. Blockage that prevents normal function of the valve or structure.

pericardium. Thin and slippery case in which the heart lies that is lined with fluid so that the heart is free to pulse and move as it beats.

septum. Anatomical partition or dividing wall.

suture. Numerous stitching techniques employed in wound closure.

ventricular septal defect. Congenital cardiac anomaly resulting in a continual opening in the septum between the ventricles that, in severe cases, causes oxygenated blood to flow back into the lungs, resulting in pulmonary hypertension.

33615

33615 Repair of complex cardiac anomalies (eg, tricuspid atresia) by closure of atrial septal defect and anastomosis of atria or vena cava to pulmonary artery (simple Fontan procedure)

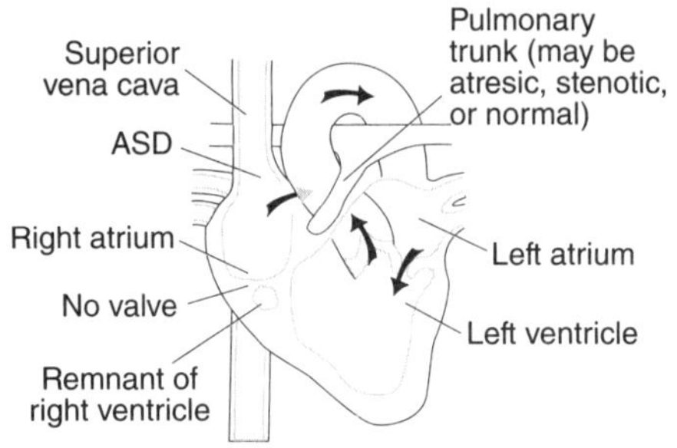

Example of tricuspid atresia with pulmonary atresia (single ventricle)

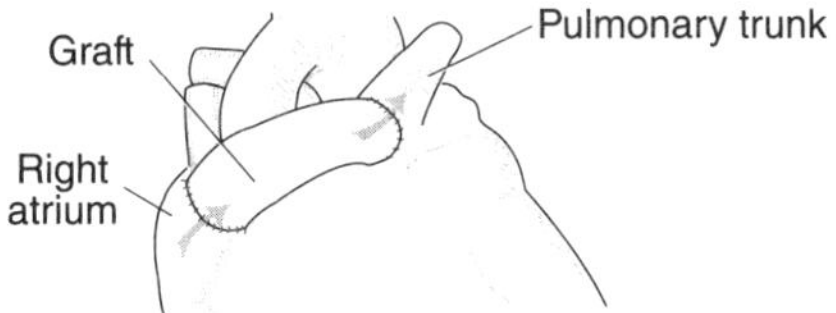

Simple Fontan procedure (no valve placement)

Explanation

The right pulmonary artery (or left in situs inverses) is exposed from the main pulmonary trunk to the hilum of the lung. The superior vena cava is detached from the right atrium. The atrial hole is closed. A hole is made in the top part of the pulmonary artery and the cut end of the superior vena cava is connected to the hole in the pulmonary artery. Pulmonary blood flow comes directly from the venous system and bypasses the heart. Later the process is completed by performing a Fontan operation. This procedure may also be referred to as a simple Fontan or Bidirectional Glenn Shunt (BDG).

Coding Tips

If significant additional time and effort are documented, append modifier 22 and submit a cover letter and operative report. When 33615 is performed with another separately identifiable procedure, the highest dollar value code is listed as the primary procedure and subsequent procedures are appended with modifier 51. For repair of pulmonary atresia with a ventricular septal defect, see 33920. When ligation and takedown of a systemic-to-pulmonary shunt is performed in addition to this procedure, it should be reported separately, see 33924.

ICD-10-CM Diagnostic Codes

Q20.4	Double inlet ventricle
Q21.11	Secundum atrial septal defect
Q21.12	Patent foramen ovale
Q21.13	Coronary sinus atrial septal defect
Q21.14	Superior sinus venosus atrial septal defect
Q21.15	Inferior sinus venosus atrial septal defect
Q21.19	Other specified atrial septal defect
Q21.21	Partial atrioventricular septal defect
Q21.22	Transitional atrioventricular septal defect
Q21.23	Complete atrioventricular septal defect
Q22.0	Pulmonary valve atresia

Q22.4 Congenital tricuspid stenosis
Q22.5 Ebstein's anomaly
Q22.6 Hypoplastic right heart syndrome
Q22.8 Other congenital malformations of tricuspid valve
Q26.2 Total anomalous pulmonary venous connection
Q26.3 Partial anomalous pulmonary venous connection

Relative Value Units/Medicare Edits

Non-Facility RVU	Work	PE	MP	Total
33615	35.89	14.14	8.88	58.91
Facility RVU	**Work**	**PE**	**MP**	**Total**
33615	35.89	14.14	8.88	58.91

	FUD	Status	MUE	Modifiers				IOM Reference
33615	90	A	1(2)	51	N/A	62*	80	None

* with documentation

Terms To Know

anastomosis. Surgically created connection between ducts, blood vessels, or bowel segments to allow flow from one to the other.

anomaly. Irregularity in the structure or position of an organ or tissue.

atrial septal defect. Cardiac anomaly consisting of a patent opening in the atrial septum due to a fusion failure, classified as ostium secundum type, ostium primum defect, or endocardial cushion defect.

congenital. Present at birth, occurring through heredity or an influence during gestation up to the moment of birth.

Fontan procedure. Surgical bypass procedure that corrects tricuspid atresia and other selected congenital conditions by connecting the right atrium directly to the pulmonary artery by anastomosis or by inserting a closed prosthesis between the right atrium and the pulmonary artery and closing the interatrial communication.

ligation. Tying off a blood vessel or duct with a suture or a soft, thin wire.

shunt. Surgically created passage between blood vessels or other natural passages, such as an arteriovenous anastomosis, to divert or bypass blood flow from the normal channel.

stenosis. Narrowing or constriction of a passage.

tricuspid atresia. Congenital absence of the valve that may occur with other defects, such as atrial septal defect, pulmonary atresia, and transposition of great vessels.

33617

33617 Repair of complex cardiac anomalies (eg, single ventricle) by modified Fontan procedure

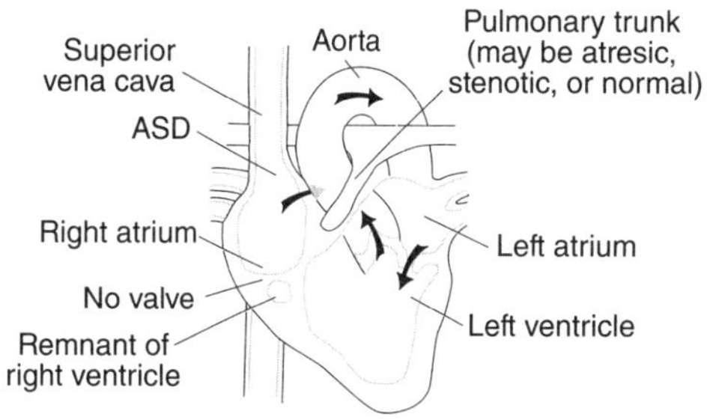

Example of tricuspid atresia with pulmonary atresia (single ventricle)

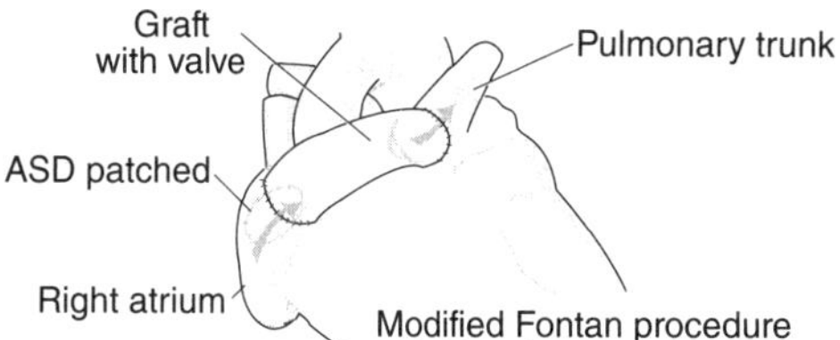

Modified Fontan procedure (with valve placement)

Explanation

This operation is usually considered to be the second stage of a Glen repair. Cardiopulmonary bypass with or without circulatory arrest is required. In this operation, blood flow is directed from the inferior caval vein, through a tunnel created inside the right atrium to the pulmonary artery. All systemic venous return is diverted away from the heart and directly into the pulmonary circulation. The right atrium is widely opened. A large patch of pericardium or Dacron is used for one wall of the tunnel. The lateral wall of the right atrium forms the other half of the tunnel. The tunnel leads from the inferior caval vein, where it joins the right atrium, to the undersurface of the pulmonary artery. The mouth of the tunnel is connected to a hole on the undersurface of the pulmonary artery. Previously, or at the same time, the superior caval vein will already have been directly connected to the upper surface of the pulmonary artery.

Coding Tips

If significant additional time and effort are documented, append modifier 22 and submit a cover letter and operative report. When 33617 is performed with another separately identifiable procedure, the highest dollar value code is listed as the primary procedure and subsequent procedures are appended with modifier 51. When ligation and takedown of a systemic-to-pulmonary shunt is performed with this procedure, it should be reported separately, see 33924. For repair of complex cardiac anomalies (e.g., single ventricle with subaortic obstruction) by surgical enlargement of the interventricular septal defect, see 33610. For repair of a single ventricle with aortic outflow obstruction and aortic arch hypoplasia (hypoplastic left heart syndrome) (e.g., Norwood procedure), see 33619. Report 33617 with 33768 when a cavopulmonary anastomosis to a second superior vena cava is performed.

ICD-10-CM Diagnostic Codes

Q20.4 Double inlet ventricle
Q20.8 Other congenital malformations of cardiac chambers and connections
Q21.4 Aortopulmonary septal defect
Q21.8 Other congenital malformations of cardiac septa

Q21.9	Congenital malformation of cardiac septum, unspecified
Q23.4	Hypoplastic left heart syndrome

Relative Value Units/Medicare Edits

Non-Facility RVU	Work	PE	MP	Total
33617	39.09	15.02	9.68	63.79
Facility RVU	**Work**	**PE**	**MP**	**Total**
33617	39.09	15.02	9.68	63.79

	FUD	Status	MUE	Modifiers				IOM Reference
33617	90	A	1(2)	51	N/A	62*	80	None

* with documentation

Terms To Know

anomaly. Irregularity in the structure or position of an organ or tissue.

atresia. Congenital closure or absence of a tubular organ or an opening to the body surface.

hypoplasia. Condition in which there is underdevelopment of an organ or tissue.

ligation. Tying off a blood vessel or duct with a suture or a soft, thin wire.

obstruction. Blockage that prevents normal function of the valve or structure.

pericardium. Thin and slippery case in which the heart lies that is lined with fluid so that the heart is free to pulse and move as it beats.

suture. Numerous stitching techniques employed in wound closure.

33619

33619 Repair of single ventricle with aortic outflow obstruction and aortic arch hypoplasia (hypoplastic left heart syndrome) (eg, Norwood procedure)

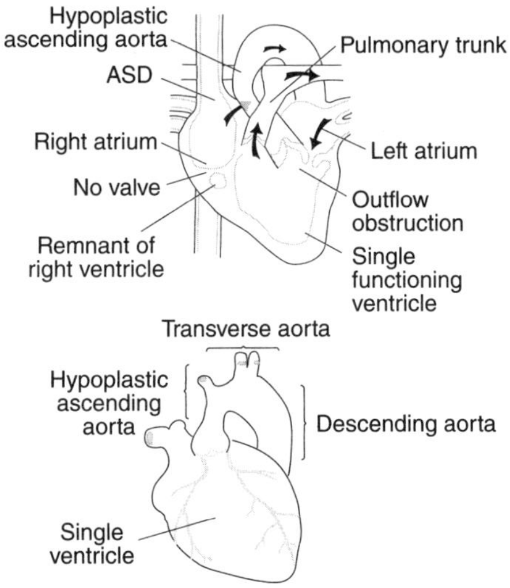

Explanation

Cardiopulmonary bypass and circulatory arrest are required. The small aorta is opened on the inner surface of its arch up to the point where the aortic diameter becomes normal. The pulmonary artery is removed and its connection to the branched pulmonary artery is closed with a patch. A large, rectangular patch of pericardium is used to enlarge the small aorta. The pulmonary valve becomes the systemic arterial valve of the heart and is encircled by the large patch that becomes shaped like a tube as it is sewn along either side of the small ascending aorta and arch that have been opened longitudinally. The coronary arteries are small and still originate in the root of the abnormal aorta.

Coding Tips

If significant additional time and effort are documented, append modifier 22 and submit a cover letter and operative report. When 33619 is performed with another separately identifiable procedure, the highest dollar value code is listed as the primary procedure and subsequent procedures are appended with modifier 51. Do not append modifier 63 to 33619 as the description or nature of the procedure includes infants up to 4 kg. When ligation and takedown of a systemic-to-pulmonary shunt is performed in addition to this procedure, it should be reported separately, see 33924. For repair of complex cardiac anomalies (e.g., single ventricle with subaortic obstruction) by surgical enlargement of the interventricular septal defect, see 33610. For repair of a single ventricle by modified Fontan procedure, see 33617.

ICD-10-CM Diagnostic Codes

Q20.4	Double inlet ventricle
Q20.8	Other congenital malformations of cardiac chambers and connections
Q21.4	Aortopulmonary septal defect
Q21.8	Other congenital malformations of cardiac septa
Q21.9	Congenital malformation of cardiac septum, unspecified
Q23.4	Hypoplastic left heart syndrome

Relative Value Units/Medicare Edits

Non-Facility RVU	Work	PE	MP	Total
33619	48.76	20.18	12.08	81.02
Facility RVU	**Work**	**PE**	**MP**	**Total**
33619	48.76	20.18	12.08	81.02

	FUD	Status	MUE	Modifiers				IOM Reference
33619	90	A	1(2)	51	N/A	62*	80	None

* with documentation

Terms To Know

anomaly. Irregularity in the structure or position of an organ or tissue.

cardiopulmonary bypass. Venous blood is diverted to a heart-lung machine, which mechanically pumps and oxygenates the blood temporarily so the heart can be bypassed while an open procedure on the heart or coronary arteries is performed. During bypass, the lungs are deflated and immobile.

hypoplasia. Condition in which there is underdevelopment of an organ or tissue.

ligation. Tying off a blood vessel or duct with a suture or a soft, thin wire.

obstruction. Blockage that prevents normal function of the valve or structure.

pericardium. Thin and slippery case in which the heart lies that is lined with fluid so that the heart is free to pulse and move as it beats.

33620

33620 Application of right and left pulmonary artery bands (eg, hybrid approach stage 1)

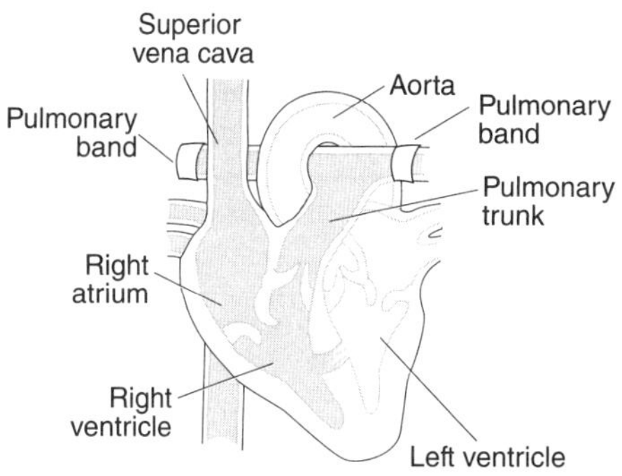

Explanation

The cardiovascular surgeon performs bilateral pulmonary artery banding (bPAB) using a hybrid stage 1 approach, which does not require open heart surgery or circulatory arrest. Hybrid procedures utilize the services of both a cardiovascular surgeon and an interventional cardiologist. This procedure is typically performed on high-risk neonates with hypoplastic left heart syndrome or related congenital anomalies for short-term palliation as part of a staged approach to more definitive surgical repair. Following a median sternotomy, the pulmonary arteries are banded individually in order to restrict some of the pulmonary blood flow. In a separately reportable procedure, the interventional cardiologist may place a stent in the ductus arteriosus under fluoroscopic guidance. Incisions are closed.

Coding Tips

For banding of the main pulmonary artery in connection with a septal defect, see 33690.

ICD-10-CM Diagnostic Codes

Q20.1	Double outlet right ventricle
Q20.2	Double outlet left ventricle
Q20.3	Discordant ventriculoarterial connection
Q20.4	Double inlet ventricle
Q20.5	Discordant atrioventricular connection
Q20.8	Other congenital malformations of cardiac chambers and connections
Q21.0	Ventricular septal defect
Q21.21	Partial atrioventricular septal defect
Q21.22	Transitional atrioventricular septal defect
Q21.23	Complete atrioventricular septal defect
Q21.4	Aortopulmonary septal defect
Q21.8	Other congenital malformations of cardiac septa
Q23.4	Hypoplastic left heart syndrome
Q25.1	Coarctation of aorta
Q25.21	Interruption of aortic arch
Q25.29	Other atresia of aorta

Relative Value Units/Medicare Edits

Non-Facility RVU	Work	PE	MP	Total
33620	30.0	11.11	7.43	48.54
Facility RVU	**Work**	**PE**	**MP**	**Total**
33620	30.0	11.11	7.43	48.54

	FUD	Status	MUE	Modifiers				IOM Reference
33620	90	A	1(2)	51	N/A	62*	80	None

* with documentation

Terms To Know

atresia. Congenital closure or absence of a tubular organ or an opening to the body surface.

conduit. Surgically created channel for the passage of fluids.

congenital anomaly. Abnormality that is present at birth that may be the result of genetic factors, teratogens, or other conditions that affect the fetus in utero. The abnormalities may be readily apparent at birth or may remain undiscovered until some point after birth.

fluoroscopy. Radiology technique that allows visual examination of part of the body or a function of an organ using a device that projects an x-ray image on a fluorescent screen.

hypoplasia. Condition in which there is underdevelopment of an organ or tissue.

hypoplastic left heart syndrome. Hypoplasia or atresia of the left ventricle and aorta or mitral valve with respiratory distress and extreme cyanosis. Cardiac failure and death often result in early infancy.

palliative. Alleviating care or medicine that is intended to provide relief from symptoms, but not cure the disease. Palliative care is employed in cases of terminal illness or severe chronic diseases.

pulmonary artery banding. Surgical constriction of the pulmonary artery to prevent irreversible pulmonary vascular obstructive changes and overflow into the left ventricle.

33621

33621 Transthoracic insertion of catheter for stent placement with catheter removal and closure (eg, hybrid approach stage 1)

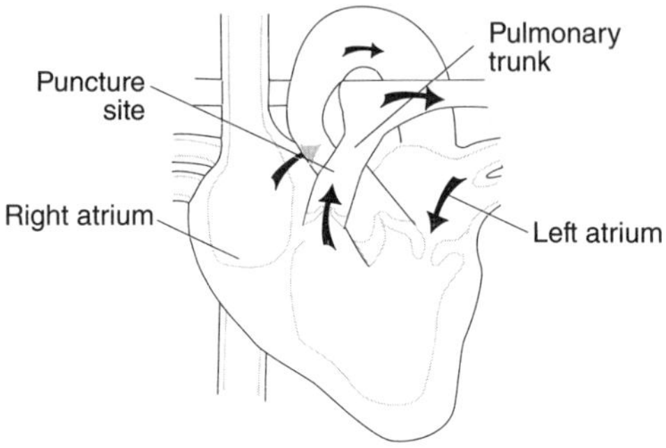

Explanation

The interventional cardiologist performs a transthoracic insertion of a catheter for stent placement using a hybrid stage 1 approach, which does not require open heart surgery or circulatory arrest. Hybrid procedures utilize the services of both an interventional cardiologist and a cardiovascular surgeon. This procedure is typically performed on high-risk neonates with hypoplastic left heart syndrome or related congenital anomalies for short-term palliation as part of a staged approach to more definitive surgical repair. Because pulmonary arteries in a newborn are difficult to access for catheter interventions, access is obtained by direct puncture of the right ventricular outflow tract, typically in the same operative episode as another, separately reportable procedure performed by the cardiovascular surgeon (i.e., pulmonary artery banding, which requires sternotomy). Upon completion of the separately reportable stent placement, the catheter is removed and the incisions are closed.

Coding Tips

Report 33620 in addition to 33621 if both procedures are performed during the same encounter. For stent placement, see 37236.

ICD-10-CM Diagnostic Codes

Q20.1	Double outlet right ventricle
Q20.2	Double outlet left ventricle
Q20.3	Discordant ventriculoarterial connection
Q20.4	Double inlet ventricle
Q20.5	Discordant atrioventricular connection
Q20.8	Other congenital malformations of cardiac chambers and connections
Q21.0	Ventricular septal defect
Q21.21	Partial atrioventricular septal defect
Q21.22	Transitional atrioventricular septal defect
Q21.23	Complete atrioventricular septal defect
Q21.4	Aortopulmonary septal defect
Q21.8	Other congenital malformations of cardiac septa
Q23.4	Hypoplastic left heart syndrome
Q25.1	Coarctation of aorta
Q25.21	Interruption of aortic arch
Q25.29	Other atresia of aorta

Relative Value Units/Medicare Edits

Non-Facility RVU	Work	PE	MP	Total
33621	16.18	7.31	3.99	27.48
Facility RVU	**Work**	**PE**	**MP**	**Total**
33621	16.18	7.31	3.99	27.48

	FUD	Status	MUE	Modifiers				IOM Reference
33621	90	A	1(3)	51	N/A	62*	80	None

* with documentation

Terms To Know

approach. Method or anatomical location used to gain access to a body organ or specific area for procedures. The approach is not coded separately although it may be a specified component of the procedure, such as laparoscopic versus incisional, or spinal procedures in which the amount of dissection required to expose the spine significantly alters with the site of approach.

atresia. Congenital closure or absence of a tubular organ or an opening to the body surface.

catheter. Flexible tube inserted into an area of the body for introducing or withdrawing fluid.

conduit. Surgically created channel for the passage of fluids.

congenital anomaly. Abnormality that is present at birth that may be the result of genetic factors, teratogens, or other conditions that affect the fetus in utero. The abnormalities may be readily apparent at birth or may remain undiscovered until some point after birth.

extracorporeal. Located or taking place outside the body.

hypoplastic left heart syndrome. Hypoplasia or atresia of the left ventricle and aorta or mitral valve with respiratory distress and extreme cyanosis. Cardiac failure and death often result in early infancy.

palliative. Alleviating care or medicine that is intended to provide relief from symptoms, but not cure the disease. Palliative care is employed in cases of terminal illness or severe chronic diseases.

stent. Tube to provide support in a body cavity or lumen.

33622

33622 Reconstruction of complex cardiac anomaly (eg, single ventricle or hypoplastic left heart) with palliation of single ventricle with aortic outflow obstruction and aortic arch hypoplasia, creation of cavopulmonary anastomosis, and removal of right and left pulmonary bands (eg, hybrid approach stage 2, Norwood, bidirectional Glenn, pulmonary artery debanding)

Hypoplastic left heart with single right ventricle

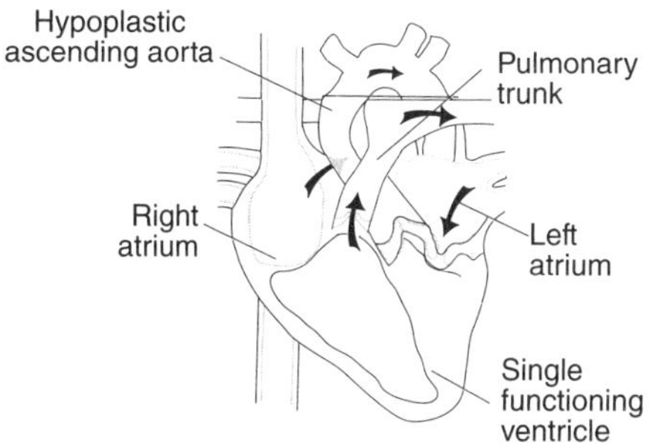

Explanation

While a "hybrid procedure" is one that combines both surgical and transcatheter interventional approaches, a "hybrid approach" may be any of a group of staged procedures that follow (not all procedures classified as hybrid approach are true hybrid procedures). The hybrid approach stage 2 reported by 33622 is part of a planned staged approach that typically follows a hybrid procedure; it is not a hybrid procedure in and of itself. The physician performs a hybrid stage 2 reconstruction of a congenital cardiac abnormality, such as left heart hypoplasia or a single ventricle. The physician gains access to the mediastinum through a sternal incision (median sternotomy). Cardiopulmonary bypass and circulatory arrest are required. For palliation of a single ventricle with aortic outflow obstruction and aortic arch hypoplasia, the physician performs a Norwood procedure. After the bypass pump is turned off, the small aorta is opened on the inner surface of its arch up to the point where the aortic diameter becomes "normal." The physician removes the pulmonary artery bands (placed during a previous surgery). The pulmonary artery is removed and its connection to the branched pulmonary artery is closed with a patch. A large, rectangular patch of pericardium is used to enlarge the small aorta. The pulmonary valve becomes the systemic arterial valve of the heart and is encircled by the large patch that becomes shaped like a tube as it is sewn along either side of the small ascending aorta and arch that have been opened longitudinally. The coronary arteries are small and still originate in the root of the abnormal aorta. The physician creates a cavopulmonary anastomosis. The left superior vena cava is dissected free. The left superior vena cava is divided and anastomosed in end-to-side fashion to the left pulmonary artery. The physician closes the cardiac incisions, takes the patient off cardiopulmonary bypass, closes the remaining surgical incisions, and dresses the sternal or chest wall wound. The physician may leave chest tubes and/or a mediastinal drainage tube in place following the procedure.

Coding Tips

Do not report 33622 with 33619, 33767, 33822, 33840, 33845, 33851, 33853, or 33917. For a bilateral, bidirectional Glenn procedure, report 33768 in addition to 33622.

ICD-10-CM Diagnostic Codes

Q20.1	Double outlet right ventricle
Q20.2	Double outlet left ventricle
Q20.3	Discordant ventriculoarterial connection

Q20.4	Double inlet ventricle
Q20.5	Discordant atrioventricular connection
Q20.6	Isomerism of atrial appendages
Q20.8	Other congenital malformations of cardiac chambers and connections
Q21.0	Ventricular septal defect
Q21.21	Partial atrioventricular septal defect
Q21.22	Transitional atrioventricular septal defect
Q21.23	Complete atrioventricular septal defect
Q21.4	Aortopulmonary septal defect
Q21.8	Other congenital malformations of cardiac septa
Q23.4	Hypoplastic left heart syndrome
Q25.1	Coarctation of aorta

Relative Value Units/Medicare Edits

Non-Facility RVU	Work	PE	MP	Total
33622	64.0	20.85	15.85	100.7
Facility RVU	**Work**	**PE**	**MP**	**Total**
33622	64.0	20.85	15.85	100.7

	FUD	Status	MUE	Modifiers				IOM Reference
33622	90	A	1(2)	51	N/A	62*	80	None

* with documentation

Terms To Know

Glenn procedure. Creation of a shunt by anastomosing the superior vena cava to the pulmonary artery to increase perfusion to both lungs.

hypoplastic left heart syndrome. Hypoplasia or atresia of the left ventricle and aorta or mitral valve with respiratory distress and extreme cyanosis. Cardiac failure and death often result in early infancy.

pericardium. Thin and slippery case in which the heart lies that is lined with fluid so that the heart is free to pulse and move as it beats.

33641

33641 Repair atrial septal defect, secundum, with cardiopulmonary bypass, with or without patch

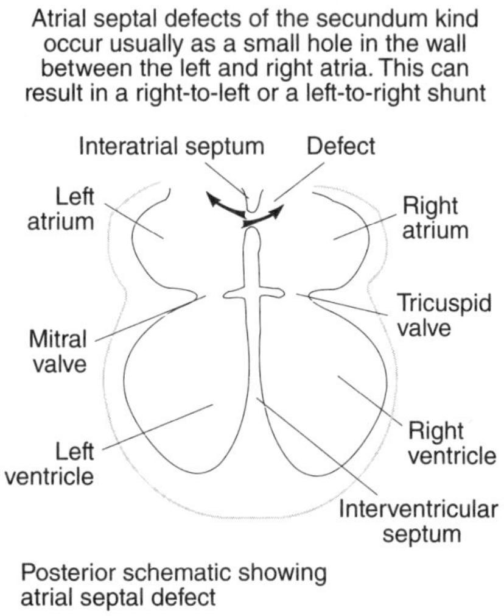

Explanation

Cardiopulmonary bypass is necessary. Two venous tubes are placed for the bypass machine—one draining the superior caval vein and the one draining the inferior caval vein. The right atrium is isolated by the putting tourniquets around the superior vena cava and inferior vena cava and their corresponding tubes. The right atrium is opened and the size and location of the arterial septal defect are assessed. If it is small enough or if the atrial septal tissue is sufficiently redundant, the defect is closed primarily with suture. If not, a patch of pericardium or Dacron is sewn to the edge of the defect to close it.

Coding Tips

Atrial septal defects are normally congenital anomalies; however, they may also be the result of myocardial infarction. Note the diagnosis when selecting codes for repair of atrial septal defects as the code selected is dependent on the exact nature of the defect. For repair of an atrial septal defect with repair of a ventricular septal defect, see 33647. For repair of an ostium primum atrial septal defect, see 33660.

ICD-10-CM Diagnostic Codes

I23.1	Atrial septal defect as current complication following acute myocardial infarction A
I51.0	Cardiac septal defect, acquired A
Q21.11	Secundum atrial septal defect
Q21.12	Patent foramen ovale
Q21.13	Coronary sinus atrial septal defect
Q21.14	Superior sinus venosus atrial septal defect
Q21.15	Inferior sinus venosus atrial septal defect
Q21.19	Other specified atrial septal defect

AMA: 33641 2018,Jun

Heart and Pericardium

Relative Value Units/Medicare Edits

Non-Facility RVU	Work	PE	MP	Total
33641	29.58	11.39	7.33	48.3
Facility RVU	**Work**	**PE**	**MP**	**Total**
33641	29.58	11.39	7.33	48.3

	FUD	Status	MUE	Modifiers				IOM Reference
33641	90	A	1(2)	51	N/A	62*	80	None

* with documentation

Terms To Know

atrial septal defect. Cardiac anomaly consisting of a patent opening in the atrial septum due to a fusion failure, classified as ostium secundum type, ostium primum defect, or endocardial cushion defect.

cardiopulmonary bypass. Venous blood is diverted to a heart-lung machine, which mechanically pumps and oxygenates the blood temporarily so the heart can be bypassed while an open procedure on the heart or coronary arteries is performed. During bypass, the lungs are deflated and immobile.

33645

33645 Direct or patch closure, sinus venosus, with or without anomalous pulmonary venous drainage

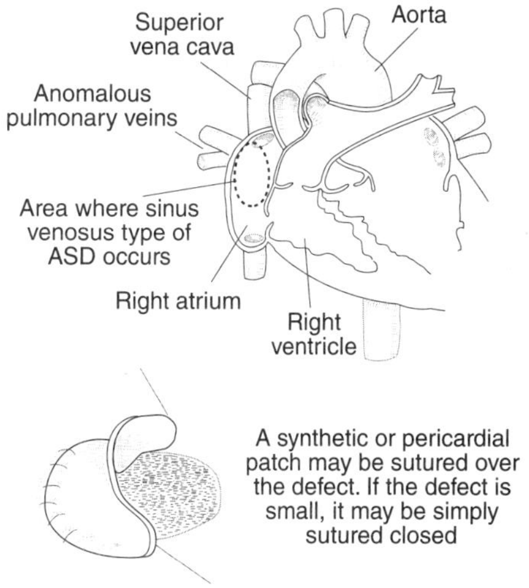

The sinus venosus is the area of the right atrium where the superior vena cava enters the chamber

Explanation

The right atrium is opened and the size and location of the congenital sinus venosus defect is assessed. If it is small enough or if the atrial septal tissue is sufficiently redundant, the defect is closed primarily with suture. If not, a patch of pericardium or Dacron is sewn to the edge of the defect to close it. Care is taken to place the patch so that all pulmonary veins remain patent and there is no obstruction of the superior vena cava, right ventricle, or pulmonary veins by the patch.

Coding Tips

Any repair of pulmonary venous drainage is included in 33645. Do not report 33645 with repair of isolated partial anomalous pulmonary venous return (33724) or repair of pulmonary venous stenosis (33726). Note the diagnosis when selecting codes for repair of septal defects as the code selected is dependent on the exact nature of the defect.

ICD-10-CM Diagnostic Codes

I23.1	Atrial septal defect as current complication following acute myocardial infarction 🅐
I51.0	Cardiac septal defect, acquired 🅐
Q21.11	Secundum atrial septal defect
Q21.12	Patent foramen ovale
Q21.13	Coronary sinus atrial septal defect
Q21.14	Superior sinus venosus atrial septal defect
Q21.15	Inferior sinus venosus atrial septal defect
Q21.19	Other specified atrial septal defect

Relative Value Units/Medicare Edits

Non-Facility RVU	Work	PE	MP	Total
33645	31.3	11.96	7.74	51.0
Facility RVU	**Work**	**PE**	**MP**	**Total**
33645	31.3	11.96	7.74	51.0

	FUD	Status	MUE	Modifiers				IOM Reference
33645	90	A	1(2)	51	N/A	62*	80	None

* with documentation

Terms To Know

atrial septal defect. Cardiac anomaly consisting of a patent opening in the atrial septum due to a fusion failure, classified as ostium secundum type, ostium primum defect, or endocardial cushion defect.

cardiac septal defect, acquired. Abnormal communication between opposite heart chambers due to a defect of the septum. It is not present at birth.

sinus venosus. Atrium, right.

33647

33647 Repair of atrial septal defect and ventricular septal defect, with direct or patch closure

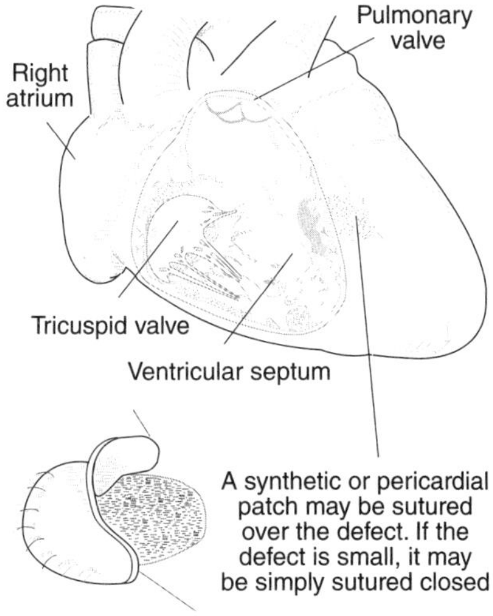

Repair of a ventricular septal defect is accomplished during the same session as a repair of an atrial septal defect

Explanation

Cardiopulmonary bypass is established with the venous uptake tubes in the superior and inferior caval veins. A hole in the right atrium or, if needed, a hole in one of the ventricles is made. The hole in the ventricle is made in the area of scar (if the ventricular septal defect is due to ischemia) or in the anterior part of the right ventricle (if the ventricular septal defect is congenital). All dead heart muscles are cut out (in ischemic ventricular septal defect) and the ventricular septal defect is closed with a patch of Dacron or pericardium. The hole in the atrium or ventricle is closed. Cardiopulmonary bypass is discontinued when heart function is restored.

Coding Tips

Note the diagnosis when selecting codes for repair of septal defects as the code selected is dependent on the exact nature of the defect. Ventricular septal defects are often associated with other cardiac anomalies. Many cardiac procedures include repair of ventricular septal defect in the code description. Code 33647 should not be reported additionally when the procedure specifically includes repair of ventricular septal defect. Do not append modifier 63 to 33647 as the description or nature of the procedure includes infants up to 4 kg. For repair of tricuspid atresia, see 33615. For closure of ventricular septal defect with or without patch, see 33681. For repair of transposition of great arteries, atrial baffle procedure (e.g., Mustard or Senning type) with cardiopulmonary bypass, with closure of ventricular septal defect, see 33776. For repair of transposition of the great arteries, aortic pulmonary artery reconstruction (e.g., Jatene type), with closure of ventricular septal defect, see 33780.

ICD-10-CM Diagnostic Codes

I23.1	Atrial septal defect as current complication following acute myocardial infarction A
I23.2	Ventricular septal defect as current complication following acute myocardial infarction A
I27.89	Other specified pulmonary heart diseases

Heart and Pericardium

I51.0	Cardiac septal defect, acquired [A]
Q21.0	Ventricular septal defect
Q21.11	Secundum atrial septal defect
Q21.12	Patent foramen ovale
Q21.13	Coronary sinus atrial septal defect
Q21.14	Superior sinus venosus atrial septal defect
Q21.15	Inferior sinus venosus atrial septal defect
Q21.19	Other specified atrial septal defect
Q21.21	Partial atrioventricular septal defect
Q21.22	Transitional atrioventricular septal defect
Q21.23	Complete atrioventricular septal defect
Q21.8	Other congenital malformations of cardiac septa
Q21.9	Congenital malformation of cardiac septum, unspecified
Q24.8	Other specified congenital malformations of heart
Q24.9	Congenital malformation of heart, unspecified

Relative Value Units/Medicare Edits

Non-Facility RVU	Work	PE	MP	Total
33647	33.0	12.32	8.16	53.48
Facility RVU	**Work**	**PE**	**MP**	**Total**
33647	33.0	12.32	8.16	53.48

	FUD	Status	MUE	Modifiers				IOM Reference
33647	90	A	1(2)	51	N/A	62*	80	None

* with documentation

Terms To Know

atrial septal defect. Cardiac anomaly consisting of a patent opening in the atrial septum due to a fusion failure, classified as ostium secundum type, ostium primum defect, or endocardial cushion defect.

cardiopulmonary bypass. Venous blood is diverted to a heart-lung machine, which mechanically pumps and oxygenates the blood temporarily so the heart can be bypassed while an open procedure on the heart or coronary arteries is performed. During bypass, the lungs are deflated and immobile.

ostium primum. Temporary opening between the right and left atrium between the lower margin of the septum primum and the atrioventricular canal in a fetal heart. In an adult heart, this condition results in an endocardial cushion defect of a cleft in the basal portion of the atrial septum with abnormal passage of blood through the congenital opening, usually associated with a cleft mitral valve.

ventricular septal defect. Congenital cardiac anomaly resulting in a continual opening in the septum between the ventricles that, in severe cases, causes oxygenated blood to flow back into the lungs, resulting in pulmonary hypertension.

33660-33665

33660 Repair of incomplete or partial atrioventricular canal (ostium primum atrial septal defect), with or without atrioventricular valve repair

33665 Repair of intermediate or transitional atrioventricular canal, with or without atrioventricular valve repair

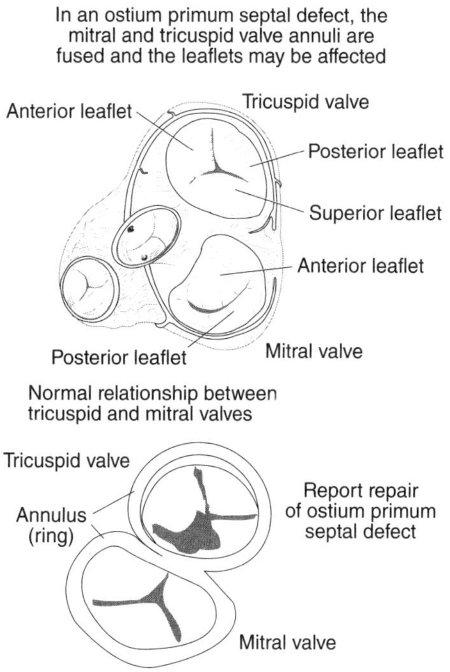

Explanation

Cardiopulmonary bypass is established using venous uptake tubes in both the superior and inferior caval veins. In 33660, the right atrium is opened. A radially oriented cleft or division in the anterior leaflet of the mitral valve is closed with interrupted sutures. Care is taken to assure that the valve closes properly after it is repaired. There is a line of denser valve tissue marking the anatomic line between the two AV valves. The ventricular septal defect is obliterated by sewing this line to the top of the septal muscle. The arterial septal defect is closed with a patch of Dacron or pericardium. The right atrium is closed and cardiopulmonary bypass is discontinued after heart function is restored. In 33665, a hole in the right atrium or, if needed, a hole in one of the ventricles is made. The hole in the ventricle is made in the area of scar tissue (if the ventricular septal defect is due to ischemia) or in the anterior part of the right ventricle (if the ventricular septal defect is congenital). The AV valve anatomy can be highly variable, ranging from normal mitral and tricuspid anatomy with a subvalvular ventricular septal defect to grossly abnormal AV valve leaflet with two separate valves present separated by a line of tissue. The AV valves are repaired. Repair is all that is done if valvular competence can be restored to the left AV valve. If not, the valve is replaced with a mechanical valve on a tissue valve.

Coding Tips

Note the diagnosis when selecting codes for repair of septal defects as the code selected is dependent on the exact nature of the defect. For closure of an atrioventricular valve, see 33600. For repair of an atrial septal defect, secundum, see 33641. For repair of an atrial septal defect and a ventricular septal defect, see 33647. For repair of complete atrioventricular canal, with or without prosthetic valve, see 33670.

Heart and Pericardium

● New ▲ Revised + Add On ★ Telemedicine [Resequenced] ☑ Laterality

ICD-10-CM Diagnostic Codes

Q20.9	Congenital malformation of cardiac chambers and connections, unspecified
Q21.21	Partial atrioventricular septal defect
Q21.22	Transitional atrioventricular septal defect
Q21.23	Complete atrioventricular septal defect
Q21.9	Congenital malformation of cardiac septum, unspecified
Q24.9	Congenital malformation of heart, unspecified

Relative Value Units/Medicare Edits

Non-Facility RVU	Work	PE	MP	Total
33660	31.83	12.01	7.87	51.71
33665	34.85	12.83	8.63	56.31
Facility RVU	**Work**	**PE**	**MP**	**Total**
33660	31.83	12.01	7.87	51.71
33665	34.85	12.83	8.63	56.31

	FUD	Status	MUE	Modifiers				IOM Reference
33660	90	A	1(2)	51	N/A	62*	80	None
33665	90	A	1(2)	51	N/A	62*	80	

* with documentation

Terms To Know

atrial septal defect. Cardiac anomaly consisting of a patent opening in the atrial septum due to a fusion failure, classified as ostium secundum type, ostium primum defect, or endocardial cushion defect.

cardiopulmonary bypass. Venous blood is diverted to a heart-lung machine, which mechanically pumps and oxygenates the blood temporarily so the heart can be bypassed while an open procedure on the heart or coronary arteries is performed. During bypass, the lungs are deflated and immobile.

congenital. Present at birth, occurring through heredity or an influence during gestation up to the moment of birth.

ischemia. Deficiency in blood supply causing tissues to be deprived of oxygen, resulting from trauma, mechanical or functional constriction of blood vessels, or a physical obstruction.

ventricular septal defect. Congenital cardiac anomaly resulting in a continual opening in the septum between the ventricles that, in severe cases, causes oxygenated blood to flow back into the lungs, resulting in pulmonary hypertension.

33670

33670 Repair of complete atrioventricular canal, with or without prosthetic valve

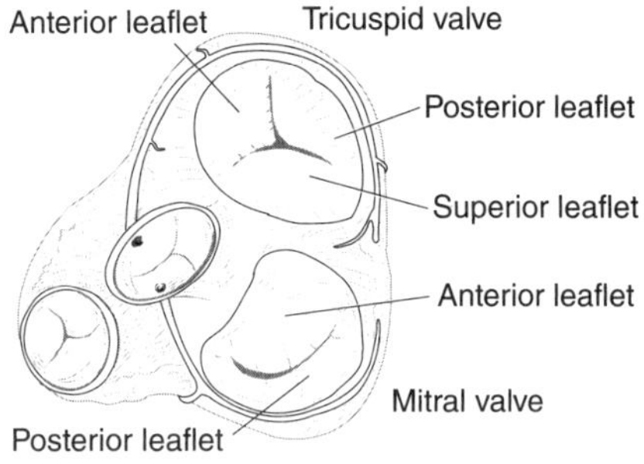

Normal relationship between tricuspid and mitral valves

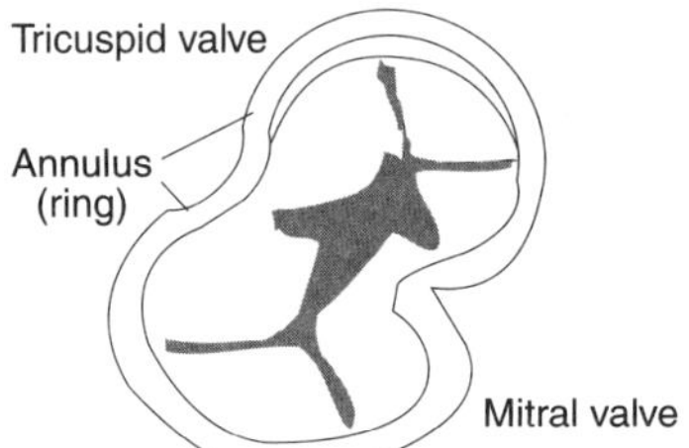

In a complete atrioventricular septal defect, the valves have merged into a single valve. Repair involves closing the VSD and sometimes installing a prosthetic valve

Explanation

Cardiopulmonary bypass is established using venous uptake tubes in the superior and inferior caval veins. The right atrium is opened. A radially oriented cleft or division in the anterior leaflet of the mitral value is closed with the interrupted sutures. Care is taken to assure that the valve closes properly after it is repaired. There is a raphe or line of denser value tissue marking the anatomic line between the two AV valves. The ventricular septal defect is obliterated by sewing this line to the top of the septal muscle. The atrial septal defect is closed with a patch of Dacron or pericardium. The competency of the single AV valve is assessed as is the imaginary line where the plane extending upward from the ventricular septal defect intersects the AV valve. The AV valve leaflets are divided along this line. The ventricular septal defect patch is placed. The valve leaflets are resuspended by sewing them to the ventricular septal defect patch. The competency of the valves is assessed. The atrial septal defect is closed with a patch sewn to the top of the ventricular septal defect patch or an extension of the ventricular septal defect patch is used to close the atrial septal defect (single patch technique). The hole in the right atrium is closed. Cardiopulmonary bypass is discontinued when cardiac function has returned.

Coding Tips

Do not append modifier 63 to 33670 as the description or nature of the procedure includes infants up to 4 kg. For repair of an incomplete or partial atrioventricular canal (ostium primum atrial septal defect), with or without atrial ventricular valve repair, see 33660. For repair of an intermediate or transitional atrioventricular canal, with or without atrioventricular valve repair, see 33665. For repair of an atrial septal defect, secundum, with cardiopulmonary bypass, with or without patch, see 33641. For closure of a ventricular septal defect, with or without patch, see 33681. For repair of transposition of great arteries, atrial baffle procedure (e.g., Mustard or Senning type) with cardiopulmonary bypass, with closure of ventricular septal defect, see 33776. For repair of transposition of the great arteries, aortic pulmonary artery reconstruction (e.g., Jatene type), with closure of ventricular septal defect, see 33780.

ICD-10-CM Diagnostic Codes

Q21.21	Partial atrioventricular septal defect
Q21.22	Transitional atrioventricular septal defect
Q21.23	Complete atrioventricular septal defect

Relative Value Units/Medicare Edits

Non-Facility RVU	Work	PE	MP	Total
33670	36.63	12.21	9.08	57.92
Facility RVU	**Work**	**PE**	**MP**	**Total**
33670	36.63	12.21	9.08	57.92

	FUD	Status	MUE	Modifiers				IOM Reference
33670	90	A	1(2)	51	N/A	62*	80	None

* with documentation

Terms To Know

anomaly. Irregularity in the structure or position of an organ or tissue.

atrial septal defect. Cardiac anomaly consisting of a patent opening in the atrial septum due to a fusion failure, classified as ostium secundum type, ostium primum defect, or endocardial cushion defect.

cardiopulmonary bypass. Venous blood is diverted to a heart-lung machine, which mechanically pumps and oxygenates the blood temporarily so the heart can be bypassed while an open procedure on the heart or coronary arteries is performed. During bypass, the lungs are deflated and immobile.

congenital. Present at birth, occurring through heredity or an influence during gestation up to the moment of birth.

ventricular septal defect. Congenital cardiac anomaly resulting in a continual opening in the septum between the ventricles that, in severe cases, causes oxygenated blood to flow back into the lungs, resulting in pulmonary hypertension.

33675

33675 Closure of multiple ventricular septal defects;

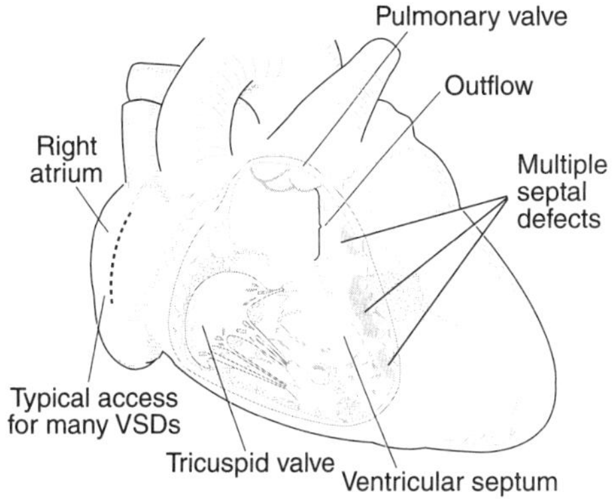

Depiction is of a cutaway view of the right ventricle

Explanation

The physician repairs multiple defects in the tissue separating the right and left ventricles of the heart in an open heart procedure. Cardiopulmonary bypass is established with tubes in both the caval veins. The ventricular septal defects can almost always be accessed and repaired through an incision in the right atrium. Each ventricular septal defect is usually repaired with a patch of Dacron or pericardium, but may be closed using only sutures. The septal defects may be repaired with a pair of patches, one in each ventricle. After the ventricular septal defects are repaired, the access incision in the right atrium is closed with sutures. Cardiopulmonary bypass is discontinued when heart function returns. The chest incision is repaired.

Coding Tips

Aspiration of the pleural space via thoracentesis (32554, 32555), as well as tube thoracostomy (32551), is included and should not be reported separately. Do not report thoracotomy (32100) separately. Temporary transvenous pacemaker placement (33210) is also included and should not be reported separately. Do not report closure of a single ventricular septal defect (33681–33688) separately. For closure of multiple ventricular septal defects with pulmonary valvotomy or infundibular resection, see 33676; with removal of pulmonary artery band, with or without gusset, see 33677. For percutaneous closure, see 93581.

ICD-10-CM Diagnostic Codes

I23.2	Ventricular septal defect as current complication following acute myocardial infarction A
I51.0	Cardiac septal defect, acquired A
Q20.8	Other congenital malformations of cardiac chambers and connections
Q21.0	Ventricular septal defect
Q21.4	Aortopulmonary septal defect
Q21.8	Other congenital malformations of cardiac septa
Q21.9	Congenital malformation of cardiac septum, unspecified
Q24.8	Other specified congenital malformations of heart
Q24.9	Congenital malformation of heart, unspecified

Relative Value Units/Medicare Edits

Non-Facility RVU	Work	PE	MP	Total
33675	35.95	13.15	8.9	58.0
Facility RVU	Work	PE	MP	Total
33675	35.95	13.15	8.9	58.0

	FUD	Status	MUE	Modifiers				IOM Reference
33675	90	A	1(2)	51	N/A	62*	80	None

* with documentation

Terms To Know

atresia. Congenital closure or absence of a tubular organ or an opening to the body surface.

cardiopulmonary bypass. Venous blood is diverted to a heart-lung machine, which mechanically pumps and oxygenates the blood temporarily so the heart can be bypassed while an open procedure on the heart or coronary arteries is performed. During bypass, the lungs are deflated and immobile.

cor biloculare. Congenital anomaly in which the heart is two-chambered, lacking both an atrial and a ventricular septum. Few newborns with this condition live to the first year.

myocardial infarction. Obstruction of circulation to the heart, resulting in necrosis.

ventricular septal defect. Congenital cardiac anomaly resulting in a continual opening in the septum between the ventricles that, in severe cases, causes oxygenated blood to flow back into the lungs, resulting in pulmonary hypertension.

Heart and Pericardium

33676

33676 Closure of multiple ventricular septal defects; with pulmonary valvotomy or infundibular resection (acyanotic)

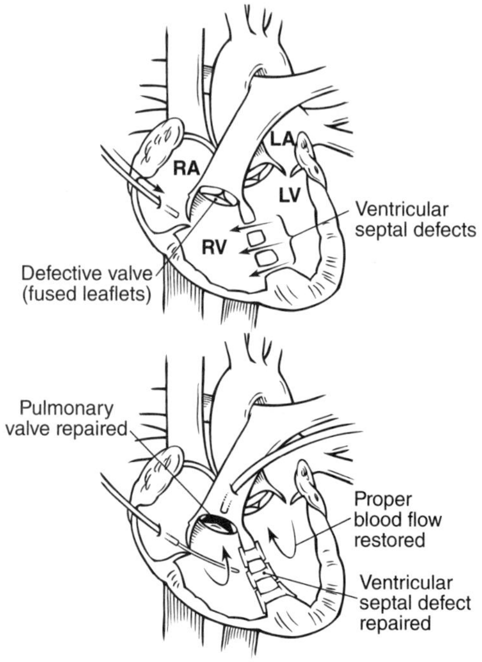

Explanation

The physician repairs multiple defects in the tissue separating the right and left ventricles of the heart, and surgically releases fused leaflets within the pulmonary valve or resects the anterosuperior portion of the right ventricle (infundibulum). The heart is accessed through a midline sternal incision. Cardiopulmonary bypass is established with tubes in both the caval veins. The septal and ventricular defects can almost always be accessed and repaired through an incision in the right atrium, and the pulmonary valve is usually accessed through an incision in the pulmonary artery. Each ventricular septal defect is usually repaired with a patch of Dacron or pericardium, but may be closed using only sutures. The septal defects alternately may be repaired with a pair of patches, applied on each side of the septum. Fused pulmonary valve leaflets are incised and any abnormal tethering of the leaflets to the arterial wall is released. For infundibular resection, obstructions within the right ventricle are excised and the ventricle repaired. After repairs are complete, the access incision in the right atrium is closed with sutures. Cardiopulmonary bypass is discontinued when heart function returns. The chest incision is repaired.

Coding Tips

Aspiration of the pleural space via thoracentesis (32554, 32555), as well as tube thoracostomy (32551), is included and should not be reported separately. Do not report thoracotomy (32100) separately. Temporary transvenous pacemaker placement (33210) is also included and should not be reported separately. Do not report closure of a single ventricular septal defect (33681–33688) separately. For closure of multiple ventricular septal defects only, see 33675; with removal of pulmonary artery band, with or without gusset, see 33677. For percutaneous closure, see 93581.

ICD-10-CM Diagnostic Codes

I23.2 Ventricular septal defect as current complication following acute myocardial infarction A

I51.0	Cardiac septal defect, acquired A
Q20.8	Other congenital malformations of cardiac chambers and connections
Q21.0	Ventricular septal defect
Q21.8	Other congenital malformations of cardiac septa
Q21.9	Congenital malformation of cardiac septum, unspecified
Q22.0	Pulmonary valve atresia
Q22.1	Congenital pulmonary valve stenosis
Q22.2	Congenital pulmonary valve insufficiency
Q22.3	Other congenital malformations of pulmonary valve
Q24.8	Other specified congenital malformations of heart
Q24.9	Congenital malformation of heart, unspecified

Relative Value Units/Medicare Edits

Non-Facility RVU	Work	PE	MP	Total
33676	36.95	13.43	9.16	59.54
Facility RVU	**Work**	**PE**	**MP**	**Total**
33676	36.95	13.43	9.16	59.54

	FUD	Status	MUE	Modifiers				IOM Reference
33676	90	A	1(2)	51	N/A	62*	80	None

* with documentation

Terms To Know

anomaly. Irregularity in the structure or position of an organ or tissue.

congenital. Present at birth, occurring through heredity or an influence during gestation up to the moment of birth.

infundibulectomy. Excision of the anterosuperior portion of the right ventricle of the heart.

valvotomy. Cutting through stenosed cardiac valve leaflets or cusp to relieve or repair the obstruction caused by scar tissue and inflammation.

ventricular septal defect. Congenital cardiac anomaly resulting in a continual opening in the septum between the ventricles that, in severe cases, causes oxygenated blood to flow back into the lungs, resulting in pulmonary hypertension.

33677

33677 Closure of multiple ventricular septal defects; with removal of pulmonary artery band, with or without gusset

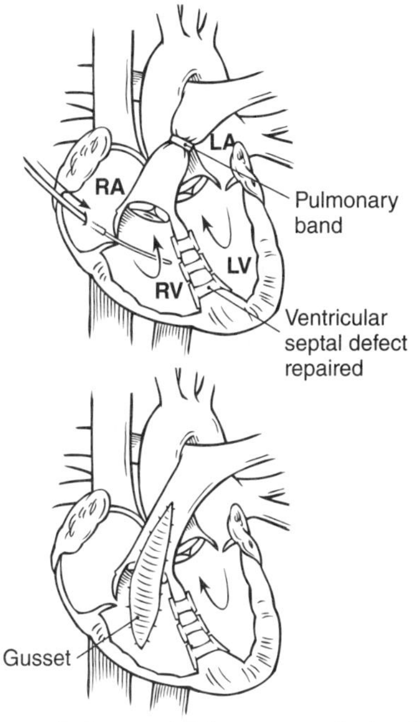

Multiple ventricular septal defects are repaired and a pulmonary artery band is removed, and normal blood flow returns to the heart

Explanation

The physician repairs multiple defects in the tissue separating the right and left ventricles of the heart, removes a previously placed band from the pulmonary artery, and may place a gusset. The heart is accessed through a midline sternal incision. The physician gains access to the mediastinum through an incision through the sternum (median sternotomy). The physician places cardiopulmonary bypass catheters through incisions in the low inferior vena cava, the superior vena cava, and aorta or femoral artery. The physician stops the heart by infusing cardioplegia solution into the coronary circulation. The septal defects can almost always be accessed and repaired through an incision in the right atrium, and the pulmonary valve is usually accessed through an incision in the pulmonary artery. Each ventricular septal defect is usually repaired with a patch of Dacron or pericardium, but may be closed using only sutures. The septal defects alternately may be repaired with a pair of patches applied on each side of the septum. The physician removes the pulmonary artery band (placed during a previous surgery) and dilates the pulmonary artery to normal size. A triangular patch (gusset) may be sutured into the incised pulmonary artery to enlarge its circumference. The physician closes the cardiac incisions, takes the patient off cardiopulmonary bypass, closes the remaining surgical incisions, and dresses the sternal or chest wall wound. The physician may leave chest tubes and/or a mediastinal drainage tube in place following the procedure.

Coding Tips

Aspiration of the pleural space via thoracentesis (32554, 32555), as well as tube thoracostomy (32551), is included and should not be reported separately. Do not report thoracotomy (32100) separately. Temporary transvenous pacemaker placement (33210) is also included and should not be reported separately. Do not report closure of a single ventricular septal defect (33681–33688) separately. For closure of multiple ventricular septal defects only, see 33675; with pulmonary valvotomy or infundibular resection, see 33676. For percutaneous closure, see 93581.

ICD-10-CM Diagnostic Codes

I23.2	Ventricular septal defect as current complication following acute myocardial infarction A
I51.0	Cardiac septal defect, acquired A
Q20.8	Other congenital malformations of cardiac chambers and connections
Q21.0	Ventricular septal defect
Q21.3	Tetralogy of Fallot
Q21.8	Other congenital malformations of cardiac septa
Q21.9	Congenital malformation of cardiac septum, unspecified
Q22.0	Pulmonary valve atresia
Q22.1	Congenital pulmonary valve stenosis
Q22.2	Congenital pulmonary valve insufficiency
Q22.3	Other congenital malformations of pulmonary valve
Q24.8	Other specified congenital malformations of heart
Q24.9	Congenital malformation of heart, unspecified

Relative Value Units/Medicare Edits

Non-Facility RVU	Work	PE	MP	Total
33677	38.45	13.84	9.53	61.82
Facility RVU	**Work**	**PE**	**MP**	**Total**
33677	38.45	13.84	9.53	61.82

	FUD	Status	MUE	Modifiers				IOM Reference
33677	90	A	1(2)	51	N/A	62*	80	None

* with documentation

Terms To Know

anomaly. Irregularity in the structure or position of an organ or tissue.

congenital. Present at birth, occurring through heredity or an influence during gestation up to the moment of birth.

pulmonary artery banding. Surgical constriction of the pulmonary artery to prevent irreversible pulmonary vascular obstructive changes and overflow into the left ventricle.

ventricular septal defect. Congenital cardiac anomaly resulting in a continual opening in the septum between the ventricles that, in severe cases, causes oxygenated blood to flow back into the lungs, resulting in pulmonary hypertension.

33681

33681 Closure of single ventricular septal defect, with or without patch;

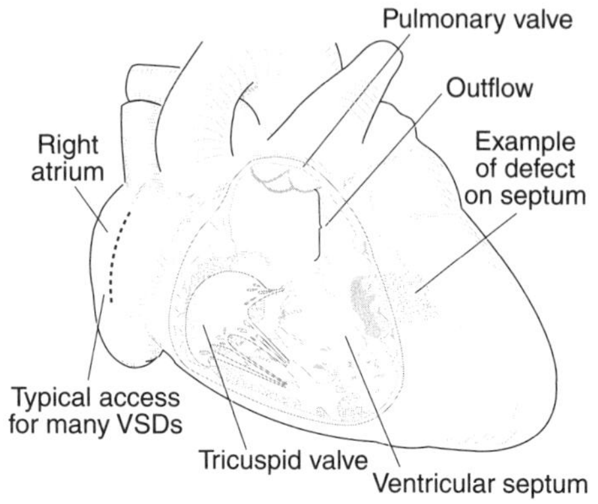

Depiction is of a cutaway view of the right ventricle

A single defect in the ventricular septum is repaired

Explanation

The physician repairs a solitary defect in the tissue separating the right and left ventricles of the heart in an open heart procedure. Cardiopulmonary bypass is established with tubes in both the caval veins. The ventricular septal defect can almost always be accessed and repaired through an incision in the right atrium, except in the case of a supracristal ventricular septal defect, in which the ventricle is higher in the outflow part of the right ventricle. This type of ventricular septal defect is most often accessed and repaired through an incision in the pulmonary artery. All types of ventricular septal defects can be accessed and repaired through an incision in the muscle of the right ventricle, but this causes more damage and is avoided if possible. The ventricular septal defect is usually repaired with a patch of Dacron or pericardium, but may be closed using only sutures. After the ventricular septal defect is closed, the hole that has been created in the right atrium, right ventricle, or pulmonary artery is closed. The chest incision is repaired. Cardiopulmonary bypass is discontinued when heart function returns.

Coding Tips

Ventricular septal defects are often associated with other cardiac anomalies. Many cardiac procedures include repair of a ventricular septal defect in the code description. Code 33681 should not be reported additionally when the procedure description specifically includes repair of ventricular septal defect. For repair of atrial septal defect and ventricular septal defect, with or without direct or patch closure, see 33647.

ICD-10-CM Diagnostic Codes

I23.2	Ventricular septal defect as current complication following acute myocardial infarction A
I51.0	Cardiac septal defect, acquired A
Q20.8	Other congenital malformations of cardiac chambers and connections
Q21.0	Ventricular septal defect
Q21.8	Other congenital malformations of cardiac septa
Q21.9	Congenital malformation of cardiac septum, unspecified
Q22.3	Other congenital malformations of pulmonary valve
Q24.8	Other specified congenital malformations of heart
Q24.9	Congenital malformation of heart, unspecified

Relative Value Units/Medicare Edits

Non-Facility RVU	Work	PE	MP	Total
33681	32.34	14.17	7.99	54.5
Facility RVU	**Work**	**PE**	**MP**	**Total**
33681	32.34	14.17	7.99	54.5

	FUD	Status	MUE	Modifiers				IOM Reference
33681	90	A	1(2)	51	N/A	62*	80	None

* with documentation

Terms To Know

cardiopulmonary bypass. Venous blood is diverted to a heart-lung machine, which mechanically pumps and oxygenates the blood temporarily so the heart can be bypassed while an open procedure on the heart or coronary arteries is performed. During bypass, the lungs are deflated and immobile.

cor biloculare. Congenital anomaly in which the heart is two-chambered, lacking both an atrial and a ventricular septum. Few newborns with this condition live to the first year.

myocardial infarction. Obstruction of circulation to the heart, resulting in necrosis.

ventricular septal defect. Congenital cardiac anomaly resulting in a continual opening in the septum between the ventricles that, in severe cases, causes oxygenated blood to flow back into the lungs, resulting in pulmonary hypertension.

33684

33684 Closure of single ventricular septal defect, with or without patch; with pulmonary valvotomy or infundibular resection (acyanotic)

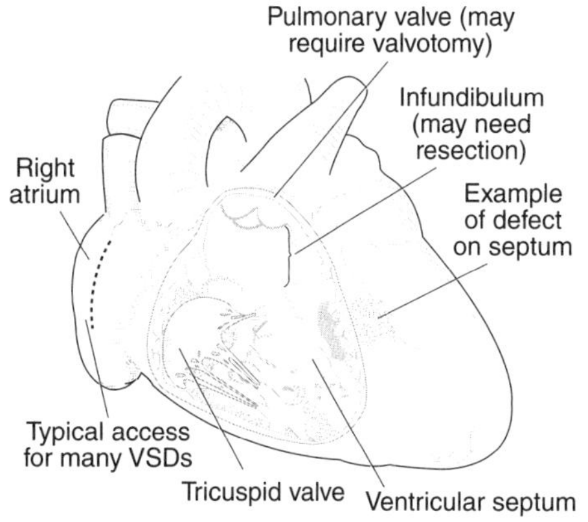

Depiction is of a cutaway view of the right ventricle

Explanation

The physician repairs a solitary defect in the tissue separating the right and left ventricles of the heart in an open heart procedure in conjunction with a pulmonary valvotomy or infundibular resection. Cardiopulmonary bypass is established with venous uptake tubes in both the caval veins. Prior to surgery, it is established by echocardiography, cardiac catheterization, or both that the diameter of the tricuspid valve is large enough to permit a normal cardiac output. If not, the operation is combined with a modified Blalock-Taussig shunt. The right ventricle or pulmonary artery is opened. Through either opening, the infundibular muscle blocking blood flow to the pulmonary artery can be cut out and cuts can be made in the pulmonary valve to reduce the restriction to blood flow that it presents. A singular ventricular septal defect is closed through either of these incisions, if possible. If it is not possible to close the ventricular septal defect with the exposure thus provided, the right atrium is opened and the ventricular septal defect closed. A patch is almost always used. All holes in the heart are closed. Cardiopulmonary bypass is discontinued when heart function is restored.

Coding Tips

When 33684 is performed with another separately identifiable procedure, the highest dollar value code is listed as the primary procedure and subsequent procedures are appended with modifier 51. When ligation and takedown of systemic-to-pulmonary artery shunt is performed in addition to this procedure, it should be reported separately, see 33924. For shunt, subclavian to pulmonary artery (Blalock-Taussig type operation), see 33750. For closure of a ventricular septal defect only, with or without a patch, see 33681.

ICD-10-CM Diagnostic Codes

I23.2	Ventricular septal defect as current complication following acute myocardial infarction A
I51.0	Cardiac septal defect, acquired A
Q20.8	Other congenital malformations of cardiac chambers and connections
Q21.0	Ventricular septal defect
Q21.8	Other congenital malformations of cardiac septa
Q21.9	Congenital malformation of cardiac septum, unspecified
Q22.0	Pulmonary valve atresia

Q22.1	Congenital pulmonary valve stenosis
Q22.2	Congenital pulmonary valve insufficiency
Q22.3	Other congenital malformations of pulmonary valve
Q24.8	Other specified congenital malformations of heart
Q24.9	Congenital malformation of heart, unspecified

Relative Value Units/Medicare Edits

Non-Facility RVU	Work	PE	MP	Total
33684	34.37	12.7	8.5	55.57
Facility RVU	**Work**	**PE**	**MP**	**Total**
33684	34.37	12.7	8.5	55.57

	FUD	Status	MUE	Modifiers				IOM Reference
33684	90	A	1(2)	51	N/A	62*	80	None

* with documentation

Terms To Know

atresia. Congenital closure or absence of a tubular organ or an opening to the body surface.

infundibulectomy. Excision of the anterosuperior portion of the right ventricle of the heart.

myocardial infarction. Obstruction of circulation to the heart, resulting in necrosis.

valvuloplasty. Surgical repair of a valve.

ventricular septal defect. Congenital cardiac anomaly resulting in a continual opening in the septum between the ventricles that, in severe cases, causes oxygenated blood to flow back into the lungs, resulting in pulmonary hypertension.

33688

33688 Closure of single ventricular septal defect, with or without patch; with removal of pulmonary artery band, with or without gusset

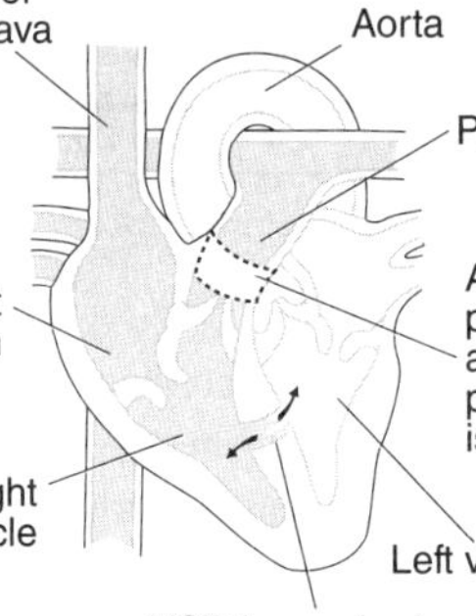

Schematic showing pulmonary band removal and VSD repair

Explanation

The physician repairs a solitary defect in the tissue separating the right and left ventricles of the heart in an open heart procedure in conjunction with removal of a previously placed pulmonary artery (PA) band. The patient is prepared for cardiopulmonary bypass, but it is not established yet. The previously placed pulmonary artery band is dissected out and removed. Stenosis at the site of the pulmonary artery band is assessed before and after band removal with a pressure transducer connected to a needle probe that measures any pressure drop across the area of narrowing. Cardiopulmonary bypass is then established and the ventricular septal defect is repaired. If pulmonary artery pressures proximal to the band site remain high after band removal and ventricular septal defect closure or if the surgeon feels the residual stenosis is too tight, cardiopulmonary bypass is restarted. The surgeon then removes the stenosed segment of pulmonary artery followed by a primary repair or the surgeon makes an incision in the pulmonary artery across the area of narrowing and closes the defect with a patch graft. Heart function is restored and cardiopulmonary bypass is discontinued.

Coding Tips

When ligation and takedown of systemic-to-pulmonary artery shunt is performed in addition to this procedure, it should be reported separately, see 33924. For pulmonary vein repair requiring creation of an atrial septal defect, see 33724. For repair of transposition of great arteries, atrial baffle procedure (e.g., Mustard or Senning type) with cardiopulmonary bypass, with removal of pulmonary band, see 33775. For repair of transposition of the great arteries, aortic pulmonary artery reconstruction (e.g., Jatene type), with removal of pulmonary band, see 33779.

ICD-10-CM Diagnostic Codes

I23.2	Ventricular septal defect as current complication following acute myocardial infarction A
I51.0	Cardiac septal defect, acquired A
Q20.8	Other congenital malformations of cardiac chambers and connections
Q21.0	Ventricular septal defect
Q21.8	Other congenital malformations of cardiac septa
Q21.9	Congenital malformation of cardiac septum, unspecified
Q22.0	Pulmonary valve atresia
Q22.1	Congenital pulmonary valve stenosis

Q22.2	Congenital pulmonary valve insufficiency
Q22.3	Other congenital malformations of pulmonary valve
Q24.8	Other specified congenital malformations of heart
Q24.9	Congenital malformation of heart, unspecified

Relative Value Units/Medicare Edits

Non-Facility RVU	Work	PE	MP	Total
33688	34.75	11.98	8.6	55.33
Facility RVU	**Work**	**PE**	**MP**	**Total**
33688	34.75	11.98	8.6	55.33

	FUD	Status	MUE	Modifiers				IOM Reference
33688	90	A	1(2)	51	N/A	62*	80	None

* with documentation

Terms To Know

cardiopulmonary bypass. Venous blood is diverted to a heart-lung machine, which mechanically pumps and oxygenates the blood temporarily so the heart can be bypassed while an open procedure on the heart or coronary arteries is performed. During bypass, the lungs are deflated and immobile.

stenosis. Narrowing or constriction of a passage.

transposition. Removal or exchange from one side to another; change of position from one place to another.

vena cava. Main venous trunk that empties into the right atrium from both the lower and upper regions, beginning at the junction of the common iliac veins inferiorly and the two brachiocephalic veins superiorly.

ventricular septal defect. Congenital cardiac anomaly resulting in a continual opening in the septum between the ventricles that, in severe cases, causes oxygenated blood to flow back into the lungs, resulting in pulmonary hypertension.

33690

33690 Banding of pulmonary artery

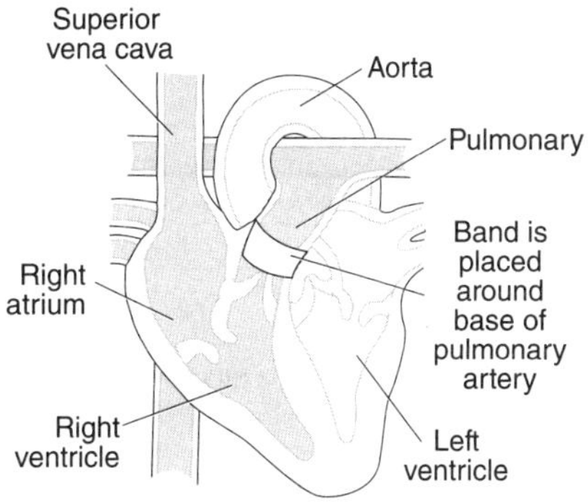

A synthetic band is placed around the base of the pulmonary artery

Explanation

Cardiopulmonary bypass is not required. The pulmonary artery is exposed through a median sternotomy or left thoracotomy. A band of heavy Dacron suture or tape is place around the base of the pulmonary artery. Once the PA pressure distal to the band is less than half of the systemic pressure and the patients arterial saturation is greater than 70 percent, the band is tight enough, but not too tight. The incision is closed.

Coding Tips

Placement of the pulmonary band (banding) is sometimes performed with other procedures on the heart and should be reported separately unless specifically included in the procedure description. When 33690 is performed with another separately identifiable procedure, the highest dollar value code is listed as the primary procedure and subsequent procedures are appended with modifier 51. Do not append modifier 63 to 33690 as the description or nature of the procedure includes infants up to 4 kg. For right and left pulmonary banding within one ventricle, see 33620. For repair of a ventricular septal defect, with or without patch, with removal of pulmonary artery band, with or without gusset, see 33688. For repair of transposition of the great arteries, atrial baffle procedure (e.g., Mustard or Senning type), with cardiopulmonary bypass, with removal of pulmonary band, see 33775. For repair of transposition of the great arteries, aortic pulmonary artery reconstruction (e.g., Jatene type), with removal of pulmonary band, see 33779.

ICD-10-CM Diagnostic Codes

Q20.1	Double outlet right ventricle
Q20.3	Discordant ventriculoarterial connection
Q21.0	Ventricular septal defect
Q21.21	Partial atrioventricular septal defect
Q21.22	Transitional atrioventricular septal defect
Q21.23	Complete atrioventricular septal defect
Q21.9	Congenital malformation of cardiac septum, unspecified
Q22.4	Congenital tricuspid stenosis
Q22.6	Hypoplastic right heart syndrome
Q22.8	Other congenital malformations of tricuspid valve

Relative Value Units/Medicare Edits

Non-Facility RVU	Work	PE	MP	Total
33690	20.36	10.27	5.03	35.66
Facility RVU	**Work**	**PE**	**MP**	**Total**
33690	20.36	10.27	5.03	35.66

	FUD	Status	MUE	Modifiers				IOM Reference
33690	90	A	1(2)	51	N/A	62*	80	None

* with documentation

Terms To Know

atresia. Congenital closure or absence of a tubular organ or an opening to the body surface.

cardiopulmonary bypass. Venous blood is diverted to a heart-lung machine, which mechanically pumps and oxygenates the blood temporarily so the heart can be bypassed while an open procedure on the heart or coronary arteries is performed. During bypass, the lungs are deflated and immobile.

congenital. Present at birth, occurring through heredity or an influence during gestation up to the moment of birth.

gusset. Triangular or diamond shaped patch that is placed for reinforcement or expansion.

incision. Act of cutting into tissue or an organ.

occlusion. Constriction, closure, or blockage of a passage.

stenosis. Narrowing or constriction of a passage.

sternotomy. Incision into the sternum, the bone that forms the front of the chest cavity and connects with the ribs.

thoracotomy. Surgical procedure for opening the chest wall in order to access the lungs, esophagus, trachea, aorta, heart, and diaphragm.

ventricular septal defect. Congenital cardiac anomaly resulting in a continual opening in the septum between the ventricles that, in severe cases, causes oxygenated blood to flow back into the lungs, resulting in pulmonary hypertension.

33692-33694

33692 Complete repair tetralogy of Fallot without pulmonary atresia;
33694 with transannular patch

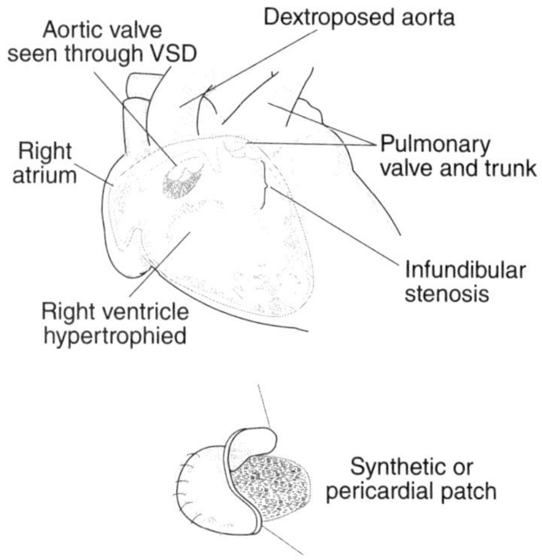

Explanation

In this defect, there are four cardiac anomalies: narrowing of the pulmonary valve annulus and/or the right ventricular infundibulum that restricts normal pulmonary blood flow, a ventricular septal defect, hypertrophy of the right ventricle, and an overriding aorta. In 33692, repair of this defect assumes that the pulmonary valve and right ventricular outflow tract are of adequate size to permit normal pulmonary blood flow. Cardiopulmonary bypass is required. The surgical approach relies on the anatomical location of the VSD, by way of atrial incision or ventriculotomy. The ventricular septal defect is closed with a patch of Dacron allowing normal blood flow from the left ventricle to the aorta. The physician enlarges the pulmonary artery from the right ventricle in order to increase blood flow to the lungs allowing the proper amount of oxygen distribution to the body. Upon completion of the repair, the pericardium is closed and drainage tubes are placed. In 33694, surgical approach may be by right arteriotomy or right ventriculotomy based on the extent of obstruction within the right ventricular outflow tract. Cardiopulmonary bypass is required. Resection of the infundibular muscle is performed first. The ventricular septal defect is sutured closed. A longitudinal incision is made in the pulmonary artery and carried proximally across the pulmonary valve annulus and onto the muscles of the right ventricular outflow tract. The defect is closed with a patch placed across the pulmonary valve annulus. Cardiopulmonary bypass is discontinued when heart function returns.

Coding Tips

When ligation and takedown of systemic-to-pulmonary artery shunt is performed in addition to this procedure, it should be reported separately, see 33924. Do not append modifier 63 to 33694 as the description or nature of the procedure includes infants up to 4 kg. For repair of a complex cardiac anomaly other than pulmonary atresia with ventricular septal defect by construction or replacement of conduit from right to left ventricle to pulmonary artery, see 33608. For complete repair tetralogy of Fallot with pulmonary atresia, including construction of conduit from right ventricle to pulmonary artery and closure of ventricular septal defect, see 33697.

ICD-10-CM Diagnostic Codes

Q21.3 Tetralogy of Fallot

Relative Value Units/Medicare Edits

Non-Facility RVU	Work	PE	MP	Total
33692	36.15	12.36	8.95	57.46
33694	35.57	13.03	8.8	57.4
Facility RVU	**Work**	**PE**	**MP**	**Total**
33692	36.15	12.36	8.95	57.46
33694	35.57	13.03	8.8	57.4

	FUD	Status	MUE	Modifiers				IOM Reference
33692	90	A	1(2)	51	N/A	62*	80	None
33694	90	A	1(2)	51	N/A	62*	80	

* with documentation

Terms To Know

atresia. Congenital closure or absence of a tubular organ or an opening to the body surface.

Blalock-Taussig procedure. Anastomosis of the left subclavian artery to the left pulmonary artery or the right subclavian artery to the right pulmonary artery in order to shunt some of the blood flow from the systemic to the pulmonary circulation.

ligation. Tying off a blood vessel or duct with a suture or a soft, thin wire.

pericardium. Thin and slippery case in which the heart lies that is lined with fluid so that the heart is free to pulse and move as it beats.

Potts-Smith-Gibson procedure. Side-to-side anastomosis of the aorta and left pulmonary artery creating a shunt that enlarges as the child grows.

tetralogy of Fallot. Specific combination of congenital cardiac defects: obstruction of the right ventricular outflow tract with pulmonary stenosis, interventricular septal defect, malposition of the aorta, overriding the interventricular septum and receiving blood from both the venous and arterial systems, and enlargement of the right ventricle.

ventricular septal defect. Congenital cardiac anomaly resulting in a continual opening in the septum between the ventricles that, in severe cases, causes oxygenated blood to flow back into the lungs, resulting in pulmonary hypertension.

Waterston shunt. Surgically created narrow opening to increase pulmonary blood flow in patients with cyanotic heart disease with limited pulmonary circulation. The small opening is created between the ascending aorta and the subjacent right pulmonary artery.

33697

33697 Complete repair tetralogy of Fallot with pulmonary atresia including construction of conduit from right ventricle to pulmonary artery and closure of ventricular septal defect

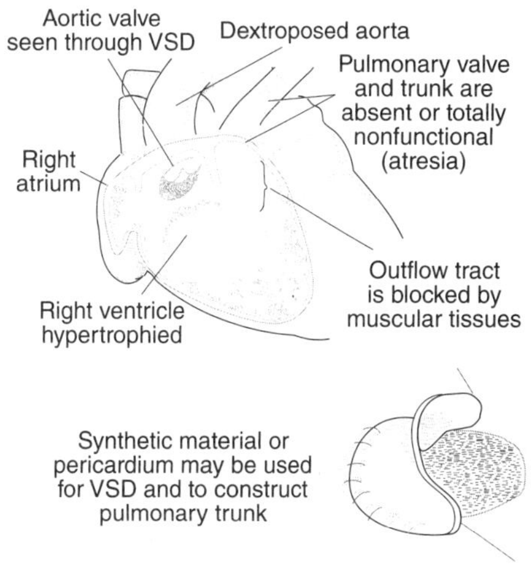

Explanation

The physician completely repairs tetralogy of Fallot with pulmonary atresia, including construction of a conduit from the right ventricle to the pulmonary artery and closure of the ventricular septal defect. Cardiopulmonary bypass is required. A hole is made in the right ventricle and any muscular obstruction in the outflow tract of the right ventricle is removed. The pulmonary artery or its branches are opened longitudinally until normal-sized vessels are encountered. The ventricular septal defect is closed. An aortic graft from a donor is trimmed to form a patch over the opened pulmonary artery. Any excess artery from the donor graft or a patch of pericardium or Dacron is sewn to the graft below the valve to use as a secondary patch for closing the hole in the right ventricle. The graft valve becomes the new pulmonary valve. After the patches and graft are sewn in place and heart function returns, cardiopulmonary bypass is stopped.

Coding Tips

When ligation and takedown of systemic-to-pulmonary artery shunt is performed in addition to this procedure, it should be reported separately, see 33924. For complete repair of tetralogy of Fallot without pulmonary atresia, see 33692; with transannular patch, see 33694. For repair of pulmonary atresia with a ventricular septal defect, see 33920. For closure of a ventricular septal defect, with or without patch, see 33681; with pulmonary valvotomy or infundibular resection (acyanotic), see 33684; with removal of a pulmonary artery band, with or without gusset, see 33688.

ICD-10-CM Diagnostic Codes

Q21.3	Tetralogy of Fallot

Relative Value Units/Medicare Edits

Non-Facility RVU	Work	PE	MP	Total
33697	37.57	13.58	9.31	60.46
Facility RVU	**Work**	**PE**	**MP**	**Total**
33697	37.57	13.58	9.31	60.46

	FUD	Status	MUE	Modifiers				IOM Reference
33697	90	A	1(2)	51	N/A	62*	80	None

* with documentation

Terms To Know

atresia. Congenital closure or absence of a tubular organ or an opening to the body surface.

blue baby. Infant born with bluish discoloration due to cyanosis.

cardiopulmonary bypass. Venous blood is diverted to a heart-lung machine, which mechanically pumps and oxygenates the blood temporarily so the heart can be bypassed while an open procedure on the heart or coronary arteries is performed. During bypass, the lungs are deflated and immobile.

congenital. Present at birth, occurring through heredity or an influence during gestation up to the moment of birth.

graft. Tissue implant from another part of the body or another person.

gusset. Triangular or diamond shaped patch that is placed for reinforcement or expansion.

ligation. Tying off a blood vessel or duct with a suture or a soft, thin wire.

obstruction. Blockage that prevents normal function of the valve or structure.

pericardium. Thin and slippery case in which the heart lies that is lined with fluid so that the heart is free to pulse and move as it beats.

tetralogy of Fallot. Specific combination of congenital cardiac defects: obstruction of the right ventricular outflow tract with pulmonary stenosis, interventricular septal defect, malposition of the aorta, overriding the interventricular septum and receiving blood from both the venous and arterial systems, and enlargement of the right ventricle.

ventricular septal defect. Congenital cardiac anomaly resulting in a continual opening in the septum between the ventricles that, in severe cases, causes oxygenated blood to flow back into the lungs, resulting in pulmonary hypertension.

33702-33710

33702 Repair sinus of Valsalva fistula, with cardiopulmonary bypass;
33710 with repair of ventricular septal defect

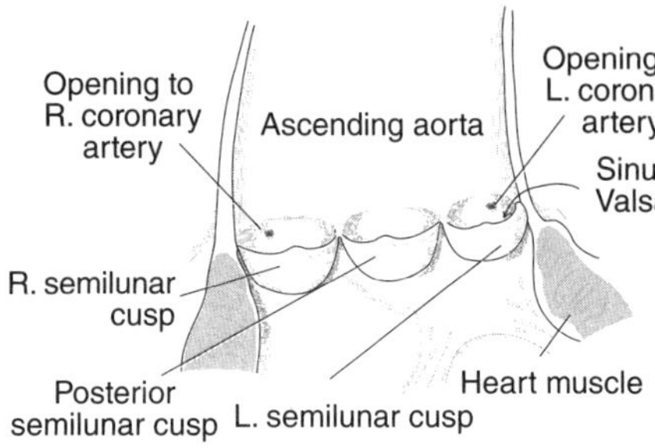

Cutaway depiction of the three cusps of the aortic valve showing location of sinus of Valsalva

Explanation

The physician repairs a sinus of Valsalva fistula. Cardiopulmonary bypass is required. After the heart is stopped, the aorta is opened and the fistula is identified. It is closed with a patch of pericardium. Any aorta valve incompetence is repaired by shortening the redundant valve leaflet diameter with stitches that reef in its free edge. The hole in the aorta is closed. Report 33710 if the sinus of Valsalva fistula is closed through the right atrium or through an incision in the aorta.

Coding Tips

When 33702 or 33710 is performed with another separately identifiable procedure, the highest dollar value code is listed as the primary procedure and subsequent procedures are appended with modifier 51. The patch of the pericardium used for the repair of the fistula is not reported separately. For repair of a sinus of Valsalva aneurysm, see 33720. For aortic valve replacement, see 33405–33413. For repair of a ventricular septal defect alone, see 33681–33688.

ICD-10-CM Diagnostic Codes

Q21.0	Ventricular septal defect
Q25.41	Absence and aplasia of aorta
Q25.42	Hypoplasia of aorta
Q25.44	Congenital dilation of aorta
Q25.45	Double aortic arch
Q25.46	Tortuous aortic arch
Q25.47	Right aortic arch
Q25.48	Anomalous origin of subclavian artery
Q25.49	Other congenital malformations of aorta

Relative Value Units/Medicare Edits

Non-Facility RVU	Work	PE	MP	Total
33702	27.24	11.76	6.73	45.73
33710	37.5	13.56	9.27	60.33
Facility RVU	**Work**	**PE**	**MP**	**Total**
33702	27.24	11.76	6.73	45.73
33710	37.5	13.56	9.27	60.33

	FUD	Status	MUE	Modifiers				IOM Reference
33702	90	A	1(2)	51	N/A	62*	80	None
33710	90	A	1(2)	51	N/A	N/A	80	

* with documentation

Terms To Know

aneurysm. Circumscribed dilation or outpouching of an artery wall, often containing blood clots and connecting directly with the lumen of the artery.

anomaly. Irregularity in the structure or position of an organ or tissue.

cardiopulmonary bypass. Venous blood is diverted to a heart-lung machine, which mechanically pumps and oxygenates the blood temporarily so the heart can be bypassed while an open procedure on the heart or coronary arteries is performed. During bypass, the lungs are deflated and immobile.

congenital. Present at birth, occurring through heredity or an influence during gestation up to the moment of birth.

fistula. Abnormal tube-like passage between two body cavities or organs or from an organ to the outside surface.

graft. Tissue implant from another part of the body or another person.

incision. Act of cutting into tissue or an organ.

pericardium. Thin and slippery case in which the heart lies that is lined with fluid so that the heart is free to pulse and move as it beats.

prosthesis. Man-made substitute for a missing body part.

sinus of Valsalva. Any of three sinuses corresponding to the individual cusps of the aortic valve, located in the most proximal part of the aorta just above the cusps. These structures are contained within the pericardium and appear as distinct but subtle outpouchings or dilations of the aortic wall between each of the semilunar cusps of the valve.

ventricular septal defect. Congenital cardiac anomaly resulting in a continual opening in the septum between the ventricles that, in severe cases, causes oxygenated blood to flow back into the lungs, resulting in pulmonary hypertension.

33720

33720 Repair sinus of Valsalva aneurysm, with cardiopulmonary bypass

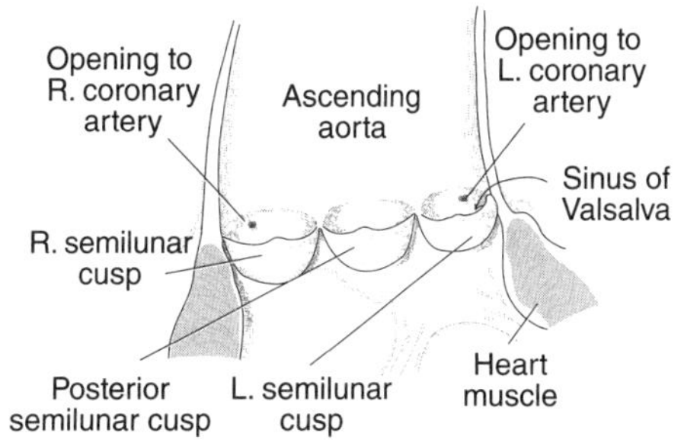

Cutaway depiction of the three cusps of the aortic valve showing location of sinus of Valsalva

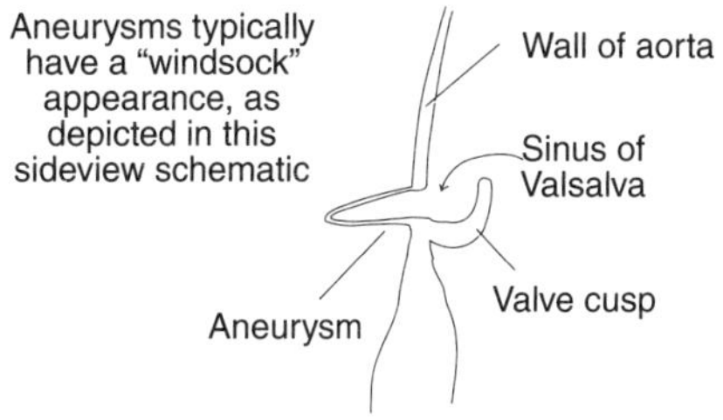

Explanation

Cardiopulmonary bypass is required. The aorta is opened after the heart has stopped. Thrombus (clot) in the aneurysm is removed. The neck of the aneurysm is closed with stitches. The aortic valve is usually incompetent. If the aortic annulus is sufficiently dilated by the aneurysm the aortic valve may need to be replaced with a mechanical aortic valve, a biomechanical valve or a tissue valve from an organ donor. After the valve is repaired or replaced, the aorta is closed. Cardiopulmonary bypass is discontinued after heart function returns.

Coding Tips

When 33720 is performed with another separately identifiable procedure, the highest dollar value code is listed as the primary procedure and subsequent procedures are appended with modifier 51. For aortic valve replacement, see 33405–33413. For repair of ventricular septal defect, see 33681–33688.

ICD-10-CM Diagnostic Codes

Q25.41	Absence and aplasia of aorta
Q25.42	Hypoplasia of aorta
Q25.43	Congenital aneurysm of aorta
Q25.44	Congenital dilation of aorta
Q25.45	Double aortic arch
Q25.46	Tortuous aortic arch
Q25.47	Right aortic arch
Q25.48	Anomalous origin of subclavian artery
Q25.49	Other congenital malformations of aorta

Relative Value Units/Medicare Edits

Non-Facility RVU	Work	PE	MP	Total
33720	27.26	11.77	6.73	45.76
Facility RVU	**Work**	**PE**	**MP**	**Total**
33720	27.26	11.77	6.73	45.76

	FUD	Status	MUE	Modifiers				IOM Reference
33720	90	A	1(2)	51	N/A	62*	80	None

* with documentation

Terms To Know

aneurysm. Circumscribed dilation or outpouching of an artery wall, often containing blood clots and connecting directly with the lumen of the artery.

anomaly. Irregularity in the structure or position of an organ or tissue.

aortic annulus. Aortic valve.

aortic valve. Heart valve, comprising three cusps, that divides the left ventricle and the aorta.

ascending aorta. Thoracic aorta, ascending/arch.

cardiopulmonary bypass. Venous blood is diverted to a heart-lung machine, which mechanically pumps and oxygenates the blood temporarily so the heart can be bypassed while an open procedure on the heart or coronary arteries is performed. During bypass, the lungs are deflated and immobile.

congenital. Present at birth, occurring through heredity or an influence during gestation up to the moment of birth.

dilation. Artificial increase in the diameter of an opening or lumen made by medication or by instrumentation.

extracorporeal. Located or taking place outside the body.

hypothermia with cardiac bypass. Reduction of the body temperature using a bypass system to reduce the oxygen demands of tissue and to protect the myocardium during a procedure.

sinus of Valsalva. Any of three sinuses corresponding to the individual cusps of the aortic valve, located in the most proximal part of the aorta just above the cusps. These structures are contained within the pericardium and appear as distinct but subtle outpouchings or dilations of the aortic wall between each of the semilunar cusps of the valve.

thrombus. Stationary blood clot inside a blood vessel.

ventricular septal defect. Congenital cardiac anomaly resulting in a continual opening in the septum between the ventricles that, in severe cases, causes oxygenated blood to flow back into the lungs, resulting in pulmonary hypertension.

33724

33724 Repair of isolated partial anomalous pulmonary venous return (eg, Scimitar Syndrome)

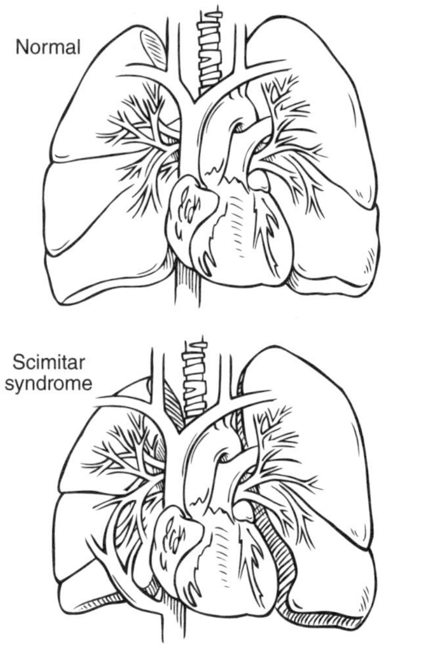

Scimitar syndrome is so named because the aberrant vein casts a shadow shaped like a curved Turkish sword, a scimitar, upon x-ray

Explanation

The physician repairs an isolated partial anomalous venous return (scimitar syndrome) using one of two open techniques. Scimitar syndrome describes a congenital condition in which an aberrant vessel connects the pulmonary vein in the right lung to the inferior vena cava. It can be diagnosed in infancy through adulthood, and symptoms occurring in infancy suggest a more severe form of the disease. Scimitar syndrome is so named because the aberrant vein casts a shadow shaped like a curved Turkish sword, a scimitar, upon x-ray. A midline sternotomy is performed. In one technique, a long pericardial patch graft is used to divert the anomalous pulmonary venous drainage from the inferior vena cava into the left atrium. In the second technique, the anomalous pulmonary vein is divided off the inferior vena cava and reimplanted into the posterior wall of the right atrium. A short pericardial baffle is used to divert flow to the left atrium through an atrial septal defect. Grafts may be required to enlarge remaining vessels. In some cases, a separately reported right pneumonectomy is performed.

Coding Tips

Insertion of a chest tube (32551) is included and should not be reported separately. Temporary transvenous pacemaker placement (33210, 33211) is also included and should not be reported separately. Scimitar syndrome can also be repaired by transcatheter occlusion or embolization. For repair of pulmonary venous stenosis, see 33726. For complete repair of anomalous pulmonary venous return, see 33730.

ICD-10-CM Diagnostic Codes

Q26.3 Partial anomalous pulmonary venous connection

Relative Value Units/Medicare Edits

Non-Facility RVU	Work	PE	MP	Total
33724	27.63	10.87	6.81	45.31
Facility RVU	**Work**	**PE**	**MP**	**Total**
33724	27.63	10.87	6.81	45.31

	FUD	Status	MUE	Modifiers				IOM Reference
33724	90	A	1(2)	51	N/A	62*	80	None

* with documentation

Terms To Know

anomaly. Irregularity in the structure or position of an organ or tissue.

embolization. Placement of a clotting agent, such as a coil, plastic particles, gel, foam, etc., into an area of hemorrhage to stop the bleeding or to block blood flow to a problem area, such as an aneurysm or a tumor.

graft. Tissue implant from another part of the body or another person.

pericardium. Thin and slippery case in which the heart lies that is lined with fluid so that the heart is free to pulse and move as it beats.

sternotomy. Incision into the sternum, the bone that forms the front of the chest cavity and connects with the ribs.

transcatheter. Procedure or treatment performed via a catheter.

33726

33726 Repair of pulmonary venous stenosis

Stenosis is a narrowing or blockage of a passage

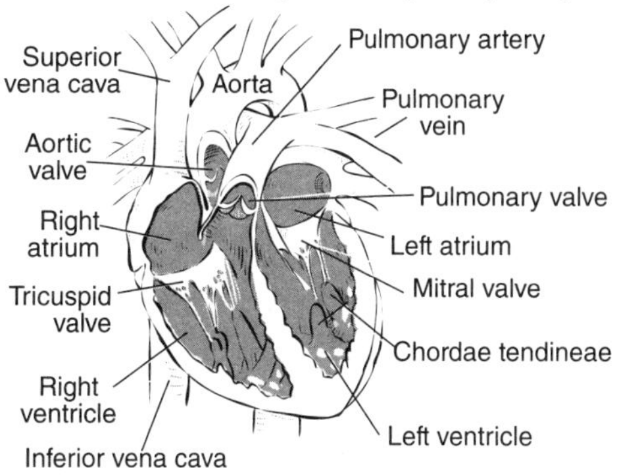

Explanation

The physician gains access to the heart through a midline sternotomy. The physician places cardiopulmonary bypass catheters usually through incisions in the right atrial appendage and aorta or femoral artery. The physician stops the heart by infusing cardioplegia solution into the coronary circulation. Either atria may be incised for exploration to locate and better visualize the defect. The blocked pulmonary vein is opened along its length. The inner layer of the artery is removed. The outer layer of the artery is closed with suture directly or with a patch of pericardium, saphenous vein, or Dacron.

Coding Tips

Insertion of a chest tube (32551) is included and should not be reported separately. Temporary transvenous pacemaker placement (33210, 33211) is also included and should not be reported separately. For partial repair of anomalous pulmonary venous return, see 33724; complete repair, see 33730.

ICD-10-CM Diagnostic Codes

I28.8	Other diseases of pulmonary vessels
Q26.0	Congenital stenosis of vena cava
Q26.1	Persistent left superior vena cava
Q26.2	Total anomalous pulmonary venous connection
Q26.3	Partial anomalous pulmonary venous connection
Q26.4	Anomalous pulmonary venous connection, unspecified
Q26.8	Other congenital malformations of great veins
Q26.9	Congenital malformation of great vein, unspecified

Relative Value Units/Medicare Edits

Non-Facility RVU	Work	PE	MP	Total
33726	37.12	13.47	9.19	59.78
Facility RVU	**Work**	**PE**	**MP**	**Total**
33726	37.12	13.47	9.19	59.78

	FUD	Status	MUE	Modifiers				IOM Reference
33726	90	A	1(2)	51	N/A	62*	80	None

* with documentation

33730

33730 Complete repair of anomalous pulmonary venous return (supracardiac, intracardiac, or infracardiac types)

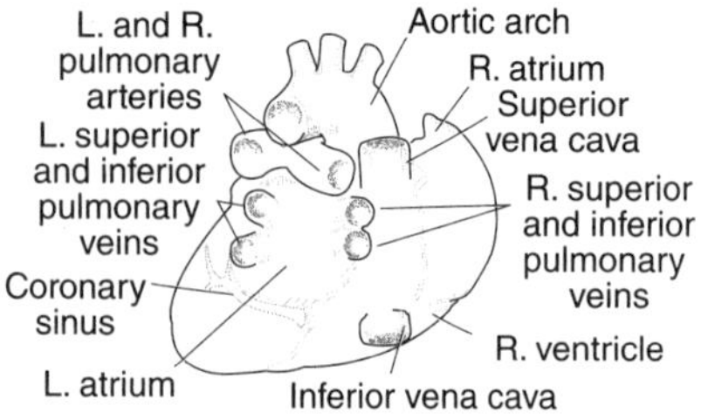

Posterior depiction of normal heart and its major venous returns

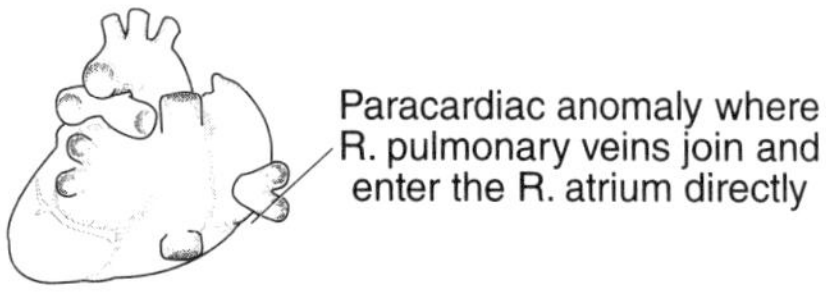

The anomaly typically involves the R. pulmonary veins and a VSD is usually also present

Numerous configurations of anomalous venous drainage occur

Explanation

The physician performs a complete repair of total anomalous pulmonary venous return (TAPVR), a rare congenital defect in which all four pulmonary veins do not connect normally to the left atrium, but rather drain to the right atrium by way of an abnormal connection. Via a midline sternotomy, the physician exposes the heart. Cardiopulmonary bypass is initiated. The abnormal veins are rerouted to the left atrium, most often by connecting them directly to the back wall of the atrium. Any abnormal routes for pulmonary venous drainage are tied off, and any existing atrial septal defect is closed. The heart is restarted, cardiopulmonary bypass is discontinued, and the sternotomy is closed.

Coding Tips

This procedure is performed for total anomalous pulmonary venous return (TAPVR). Do not append modifier 63 to 33730 as the description or nature of the procedure includes infants up to 4 kg. For repair of atrial septal defect, secundum, with cardiopulmonary bypass, with or without patch, see 33641. For direct or patch closure, sinus venosus, with or without anomalous pulmonary venous drainage, see 33645. For repair of an incomplete or partial atrioventricular canal (ostium primum atrial septal defect), with or without atrioventricular valve repair, see 33660. For repair of partial anomalous pulmonary venous return, see 33724. For repair of pulmonary venous stenosis, see 33726.

ICD-10-CM Diagnostic Codes

Q26.2	Total anomalous pulmonary venous connection
Q26.3	Partial anomalous pulmonary venous connection
Q26.4	Anomalous pulmonary venous connection, unspecified
Q26.8	Other congenital malformations of great veins
Q26.9	Congenital malformation of great vein, unspecified

Relative Value Units/Medicare Edits

Non-Facility RVU	Work	PE	MP	Total
33730	36.14	14.06	8.95	59.15
Facility RVU	**Work**	**PE**	**MP**	**Total**
33730	36.14	14.06	8.95	59.15

	FUD	Status	MUE	Modifiers				IOM Reference
33730	90	A	1(2)	51	N/A	62*	80	None

* with documentation

Terms To Know

anomaly. Irregularity in the structure or position of an organ or tissue.

atrial septal defect. Cardiac anomaly consisting of a patent opening in the atrial septum due to a fusion failure, classified as ostium secundum type, ostium primum defect, or endocardial cushion defect.

cardiopulmonary bypass. Venous blood is diverted to a heart-lung machine, which mechanically pumps and oxygenates the blood temporarily so the heart can be bypassed while an open procedure on the heart or coronary arteries is performed. During bypass, the lungs are deflated and immobile.

congenital. Present at birth, occurring through heredity or an influence during gestation up to the moment of birth.

extracorporeal. Located or taking place outside the body.

para-. Indicates near, similar, beside, or past.

sternotomy. Incision into the sternum, the bone that forms the front of the chest cavity and connects with the ribs.

supra. Above.

ventricular septal defect. Congenital cardiac anomaly resulting in a continual opening in the septum between the ventricles that, in severe cases, causes oxygenated blood to flow back into the lungs, resulting in pulmonary hypertension.

33732

33732 Repair of cor triatriatum or supravalvular mitral ring by resection of left atrial membrane

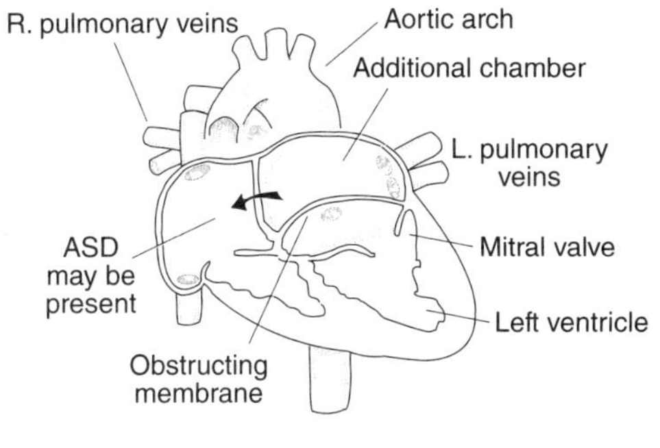

Cardiac anomalies are repaired

Explanation

This lesion is frequently considered to be related to TAPVR, but it is distinctly different. In this anomaly, there is a wall subdividing the left atrium between the pulmonary veins and the mitral valve. This restricts blood flow to the left ventricle and therefore to the rest of the body. Cardiopulmonary bypass is readied. The left atrium is opened and the membrane is cut out. The left atrium is closed. Cardiopulmonary bypass is discontinued when heart function returns.

Coding Tips

When 33732 is performed with another separately identifiable procedure, the highest dollar value code is listed as the primary procedure and subsequent procedures are appended with modifier 51. Do not append modifier 63 to 33732 as the description or nature of the procedure includes infants up to 4 kg. For repair of complex cardiac anomalies (e.g., tricuspid atresia) by closure of atrial septal defect and anastomosis of atria or vena cava (simple Fontan procedures), see 33615. For repair of atrial septal defect, secundum, with cardiopulmonary bypass, with or without patch, see 33641.

ICD-10-CM Diagnostic Codes

Q23.2 Congenital mitral stenosis
Q24.2 Cor triatriatum

Relative Value Units/Medicare Edits

Non-Facility RVU	Work	PE	MP	Total
33732	28.96	12.63	7.17	48.76
Facility RVU	**Work**	**PE**	**MP**	**Total**
33732	28.96	12.63	7.17	48.76

	FUD	Status	MUE	Modifiers				IOM Reference
33732	90	A	1(2)	51	N/A	62*	80	None

* with documentation

Terms To Know

anomaly. Irregularity in the structure or position of an organ or tissue.

congenital. Present at birth, occurring through heredity or an influence during gestation up to the moment of birth.

33735-33736

33735 Atrial septectomy or septostomy; closed heart (Blalock-Hanlon type operation)

33736 open heart with cardiopulmonary bypass

The usual goal of this series of procedures is to surgically create a left-to-right mixing of atrial blood by removal of tissues from the atrial septum (septectomy) or by creation of a hole in the septum

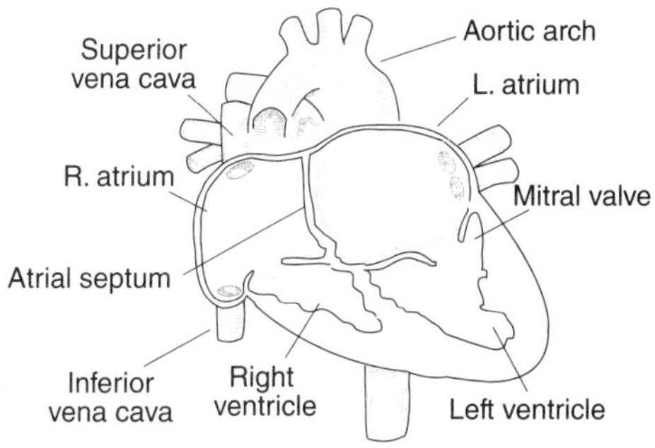

Explanation

These procedures are largely of historical interest only. Code 33735 requires access by lateral thoracotomy. An incision is made in the pericardium with the right pulmonary artery and pulmonary veins tied off. A clamp is utilized at the anterior position of the right atrium and the posterior position of the left atrium. Incisions are made within the right atrium and right pulmonary vein. The atrial septum is removed and incisions are closed. The clamps are removed and ligatures previously placed in the pulmonary veins and right pulmonary artery are released. Alternatively, a purse string may be placed in the right atrial appendage and the appendage is opened in the middle of the purse string. A finger or a dilating tool is passed through the hole in the atrium and the wall between the right and left atria is torn open. The dilating instrument is removed and the purse string is tied to stop the bleeding. The thoracotomy is closed in standard fashion. In 33736, in most pediatric cardiac surgery centers, it has been supplanted by balloon dilation of a naturally occurring hole in the wall between the atrial chambers. No incision is needed for balloon dilation. Operative septostomy/septectomy requires cardiopulmonary bypass with venous uptake tubes in both caval veins. The right atrium is opened and the thin part of the wall between the right and left atria is cut out or opened widely. The goal is to allow free mixing of the blood from the right and left atria. Cardiopulmonary bypass is discontinued when heart function returns.

Coding Tips

Code these procedures with caution as they are used infrequently. Open chest atrial septectomy or septostomy has largely been replaced with balloon dilation of a naturally occurring hole in the wall between the atrial chambers. When ligation and takedown of systemic-to-pulmonary artery shunt is performed in addition to this procedure, it should be reported separately, see 33924. Do not append modifier 63 to 33735–33736 as the description or nature of the procedure includes infants up to 4 kg. For atrial septectomy or septostomy, transvenous method, balloon or blade, see 33741.

ICD-10-CM Diagnostic Codes

Q20.3 Discordant ventriculoarterial connection
Q21.11 Secundum atrial septal defect
Q21.12 Patent foramen ovale
Q21.13 Coronary sinus atrial septal defect
Q21.14 Superior sinus venosus atrial septal defect

Q21.15	Inferior sinus venosus atrial septal defect
Q21.19	Other specified atrial septal defect
Q21.21	Partial atrioventricular septal defect
Q21.22	Transitional atrioventricular septal defect
Q21.23	Complete atrioventricular septal defect
Q22.4	Congenital tricuspid stenosis
Q22.6	Hypoplastic right heart syndrome
Q22.8	Other congenital malformations of tricuspid valve
Q23.81	Bicuspid aortic valve
Q23.82	Congenital mitral valve cleft leaflet
Q23.88	Other congenital malformations of aortic and mitral valves
Q24.8	Other specified congenital malformations of heart
Q26.2	Total anomalous pulmonary venous connection

Relative Value Units/Medicare Edits

Non-Facility RVU	Work	PE	MP	Total
33735	22.2	10.77	5.49	38.46
33736	24.32	11.36	6.01	41.69
Facility RVU	**Work**	**PE**	**MP**	**Total**
33735	22.2	10.77	5.49	38.46
33736	24.32	11.36	6.01	41.69

	FUD	Status	MUE	Modifiers				IOM Reference
33735	90	A	1(2)	51	N/A	N/A	80	None
33736	90	A	1(2)	51	N/A	62*	80	

* with documentation

Terms To Know

Blalock-Hanlon procedure. Atrial septectomy procedure to allow free mixing of the blood from the right and left atria.

occlusion. Constriction, closure, or blockage of a passage.

pulmonary artery banding. Surgical constriction of the pulmonary artery to prevent irreversible pulmonary vascular obstructive changes and overflow into the left ventricle.

Rashkind procedure. Transvenous balloon atrial septectomy or septostomy performed by cardiac catheterization. A balloon catheter is inserted into the heart either to create or enlarge an opening in the interatrial septal wall.

stenosis. Narrowing or constriction of a passage.

tricuspid atresia. Congenital absence of the valve that may occur with other defects, such as atrial septal defect, pulmonary atresia, and transposition of great vessels.

33741

33741 Transcatheter atrial septostomy (TAS) for congenital cardiac anomalies to create effective atrial flow, including all imaging guidance by the proceduralist, when performed, any method (eg, Rashkind, Sang-Park, balloon, cutting balloon, blade)

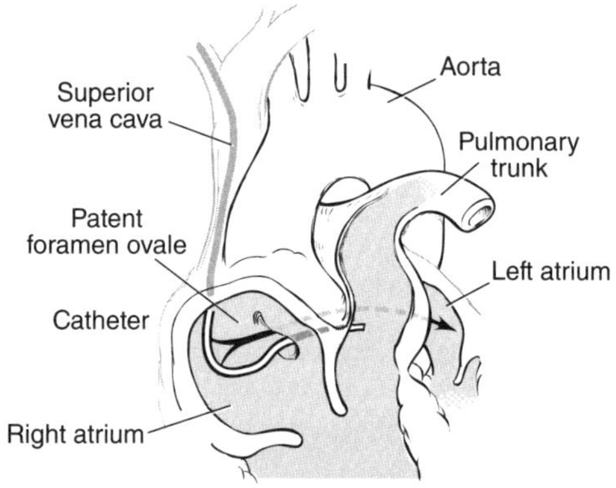

Transcatheter atrial septostomy is performed to create atrial flow

Explanation

The physician performs a transcatheter atrial septostomy (TAS) by various methods to treat specific congenital cardiac anomalies, typically in infants ≤ 4 kg. Various congenital heart defects, particularly those involving transposition of the great vessels, require surgical creation or enlargement of an opening in the interatrial septum (wall) that separates the upper right and left chambers of the heart. In one method, the physician makes a small incision in the arm or leg. Two catheters are placed: a central venous catheter and a second catheter threaded up to the heart. When the foramen ovale has not closed, a deflated balloon (Rashkind-type) is passed through the foramen ovale, inflated, and pulled through the atrial septum, enlarging the opening and improving oxygenation of the blood. When the septum is intact, the deflated balloon is passed from the right atrium through the septum to the left atrium, inflated, and withdrawn, creating an interatrial septal defect and improving oxygenation of the blood. The catheters are removed. Pressure is placed over the incision for 20 to 30 minutes to stem bleeding and the patient is observed for a period afterward. The Park septostomy, or blade method, is an alternative to the Rashkind procedure, and is typically performed on infants older than 1 month of age. The physician makes a small incision in the femoral vein and places a transseptal sheath using standard methods, advancing the sheath to the superior vena cava under fluoroscopic or echocardiographic guidance. Using a transseptal needle to cross the atrial septum, the left atrium is entered. The physician introduces a guidewire into the left atrium and removes the transseptal catheter while leaving the wire in place. A septostomy catheter is advanced over the wire into the left atrium. This catheter has a retracted blade, which the physician extends. The physician pulls the blade slowly across the atrial septum from the left into the right atrium, under fluoroscopic or echocardiographic guidance; several passes with the blade catheter may be made in this fashion. The purpose of this procedure is to increase blood flow across the atrial septum in children with certain forms of cyanotic congenital heart disease. The physician removes the septostomy catheter and venous sheath. Pressure is placed over the incision for 20 to 30 minutes to stem bleeding. The patient is observed for a period afterward. This code includes the percutaneous access, placement of one or more access sheaths, advancement of the transcatheter delivery system, all imaging guidance that is performed, and the creation of effective intracardiac atrial blood flow.

Coding Tips

Code 33741 includes percutaneous access, placing the access sheath(s), advancement of the transcatheter delivery system, and creation of atrial blood flow. Ultrasound guidance for vascular access and fluoroscopic guidance, when performed, is inclusive of this procedure. Diagnostic cardiac catheterization is not usually performed at the same session as 33741 and may be reported when performed. Cardiovascular injection procedures (93563, 93565–93569, 93573–93575) are not usually performed at the same session. Do not report 33741 with 93451–93453, 93456–93461, or 93594–93597 to report fluoroscopic guidance for the intervention or limited hemodynamic and angiographic data used solely to accomplish the intervention. Codes 93451–93453, 93456–93461, and 93593–93597 performed at the same session may be reported separately if: 1) No prior study is available and a full diagnostic study is performed; or 2) A prior study is available, but the study has inadequate visualization of anatomy and/or pathology, the patient's condition has changed in respect to the clinical indication since the prior study, or a clinical change occurs during the procedure and requires a more thorough evaluation. For diagnostic angiography during the same session for separate evaluation from 33741, see 93563, 93565–93569, and 93573–93575. For transseptal puncture, see 93462.

ICD-10-CM Diagnostic Codes

Q20.0	Common arterial trunk
Q20.1	Double outlet right ventricle
Q20.3	Discordant ventriculoarterial connection
Q21.12	Patent foramen ovale
Q21.13	Coronary sinus atrial septal defect
Q21.14	Superior sinus venosus atrial septal defect
Q21.15	Inferior sinus venosus atrial septal defect
Q21.23	Complete atrioventricular septal defect
Q21.3	Tetralogy of Fallot
Q22.0	Pulmonary valve atresia
Q22.4	Congenital tricuspid stenosis
Q22.5	Ebstein's anomaly
Q23.4	Hypoplastic left heart syndrome
Q25.1	Coarctation of aorta
Q25.21	Interruption of aortic arch
Q26.0	Congenital stenosis of vena cava

AMA: 33741 2023,Dec; 2023,May; 2021,Dec; 2020,Nov

Relative Value Units/Medicare Edits

Non-Facility RVU	Work	PE	MP	Total
33741	14.0	4.76	3.23	21.99
Facility RVU	**Work**	**PE**	**MP**	**Total**
33741	14.0	4.76	3.23	21.99

	FUD	Status	MUE	Modifiers				IOM Reference
33741	0	A	1(3)	51	N/A	N/A	80	None

* with documentation

33745-33746

33745 Transcatheter intracardiac shunt (TIS) creation by stent placement for congenital cardiac anomalies to establish effective intracardiac flow, including all imaging guidance by the proceduralist, when performed, left and right heart diagnostic cardiac catheterization for congenital cardiac anomalies, and target zone angioplasty, when performed (eg, atrial septum, Fontan fenestration, right ventricular outflow tract, Mustard/Senning/Warden baffles); initial intracardiac shunt

\+ **33746** each additional intracardiac shunt location (List separately in addition to code for primary procedure)

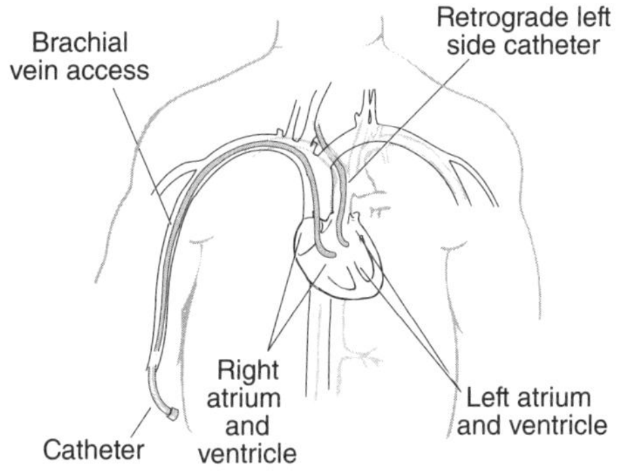

A combined right side catheterization and retrograde left side catheterization is performed to address congenital cardiac anomalies

Transcather intracardia shunt is placed for intracardiac flow

Explanation

The physician treats various congenital cardiac anomalies by placing one or more intracardiac stents to create a shunt that allows for more effective intracardiac blood flow. Under imaging guidance, the physician uses a transcatheter approach to place one or more stents in the same location in 33745. Included in the procedure is intracardiac stent placement, balloon angioplasty of the target zone before or after stent placement, and, when performed, all ultrasound guidance for vascular access, fluoroscopic guidance for the intervention, and complete diagnostic right and left heart catheterization. Report 33746 if additional, different intracardiac locations are treated with stents during the same session.

Coding Tips

Ultrasound guidance for vascular access and fluoroscopic guidance, when performed, is inclusive of this procedure. Diagnostic angiography is usually performed with 33475 but may be reported when performed for an evaluation separate and distinct from the shunt creation. Multiple stents placed in a single location are only reported with a single code. For additional, different intracardiac locations during the same session, see 33746. Do not report 33745 with 93451–93453, 93456–93461, or 93593–93597 to report fluoroscopic guidance for the intervention or limited hemodynamic and angiographic data used solely to accomplish the intervention. For diagnostic cardiac angiography for an evaluation separate from the shunt creation, see 93563, 93565–93569, and 93573–93575.

ICD-10-CM Diagnostic Codes

I42.0	Dilated cardiomyopathy
I42.1	Obstructive hypertrophic cardiomyopathy
I42.2	Other hypertrophic cardiomyopathy
I42.3	Endomyocardial (eosinophilic) disease

Heart and Pericardium

I42.4	Endocardial fibroelastosis
I42.5	Other restrictive cardiomyopathy
I42.6	Alcoholic cardiomyopathy
I42.7	Cardiomyopathy due to drug and external agent
I42.8	Other cardiomyopathies
Q20.0	Common arterial trunk
Q20.1	Double outlet right ventricle
Q20.3	Discordant ventriculoarterial connection
Q21.0	Ventricular septal defect
Q21.11	Secundum atrial septal defect
Q21.12	Patent foramen ovale
Q21.13	Coronary sinus atrial septal defect
Q21.14	Superior sinus venosus atrial septal defect
Q21.15	Inferior sinus venosus atrial septal defect
Q21.19	Other specified atrial septal defect
Q21.21	Partial atrioventricular septal defect
Q21.22	Transitional atrioventricular septal defect
Q21.23	Complete atrioventricular septal defect
Q21.3	Tetralogy of Fallot
Q22.0	Pulmonary valve atresia
Q22.4	Congenital tricuspid stenosis
Q22.5	Ebstein's anomaly
Q23.4	Hypoplastic left heart syndrome
Q25.0	Patent ductus arteriosus
Q25.1	Coarctation of aorta
Q25.21	Interruption of aortic arch
Q25.72	Congenital pulmonary arteriovenous malformation
Q26.0	Congenital stenosis of vena cava

AMA: 33745 2024,Aug; 2023,Dec; 2023,Jun; 2023,May; 2021,Dec; 2020,Nov
33746 2024,Aug; 2023,Dec; 2023,Jun; 2023,May; 2021,Dec; 2020,Nov

Relative Value Units/Medicare Edits

Non-Facility RVU	Work	PE	MP	Total
33745	20.0	6.81	4.61	31.42
33746	8.0	2.72	1.84	12.56
Facility RVU	**Work**	**PE**	**MP**	**Total**
33745	20.0	6.81	4.61	31.42
33746	8.0	2.72	1.84	12.56

	FUD	Status	MUE	Modifiers				IOM Reference
33745	0	A	2(2)	51	N/A	N/A	80	None
33746	N/A	A	1(3)	N/A	N/A	N/A	80	

* with documentation

33750

33750 Shunt; subclavian to pulmonary artery (Blalock-Taussig type operation)

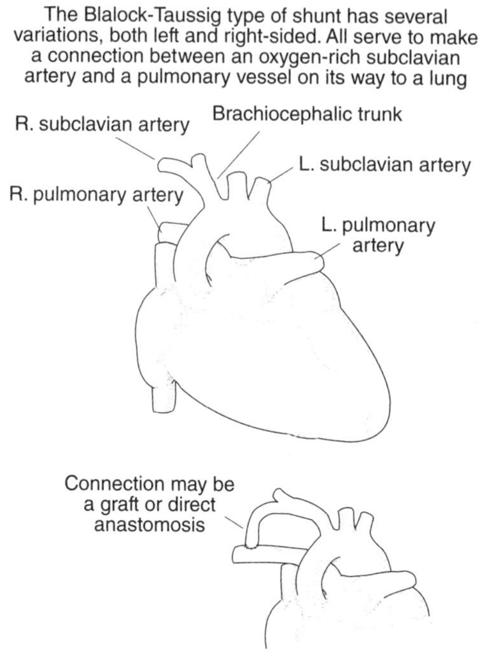

Explanation

In its unmodified form, this operation involves dividing the left subclavian artery, tying off the end of the artery going to the arm, and creating a connection between the end of this artery coming from the heart and the side of the pulmonary artery. The difficulty with this operation is making the connection to the pulmonary artery exactly the right size to supply adequate, but not excessive blood flow to the lungs. Instead, a modified version of the operation is usually performed. The artery to the arm is not divided. Instead, one end of a 3 mm to 5 mm diameter tube of Gortex is sewn to the side of the artery to the arm and the other end is sewn to the side of the pulmonary artery. The size of the tube determines the amount of blood flow to the lungs. Cardiopulmonary bypass is not required. The ductus arteriosus (a connection between the aorta and pulmonary artery that has been supplying blood to the lungs, but usually closes at birth) is tied off.

Coding Tips

This procedure is sometimes performed in addition to 33684. When ligation and takedown of systemic-to-pulmonary artery shunt is performed in addition to this procedure, it should be reported separately, see 33924. Do not append modifier 63 to 33750 as the description or nature of the procedure includes infants up to 4 kg. For shunt, ascending aorta to pulmonary artery (Waterston type operation), see 33755. For descending aorta to pulmonary artery (Potts-Smith type operation), see 33762, and for flow to one lung (classical Glenn procedure), see 33766. For superior vena cava to pulmonary artery for flow to both lungs (bidirectional Glenn procedure), see 33767.

ICD-10-CM Diagnostic Codes

I24.89	Other forms of acute ischemic heart disease
I37.0	Nonrheumatic pulmonary valve stenosis
I37.1	Nonrheumatic pulmonary valve insufficiency
I37.2	Nonrheumatic pulmonary valve stenosis with insufficiency
I37.8	Other nonrheumatic pulmonary valve disorders

Q20.4	Double inlet ventricle
Q20.8	Other congenital malformations of cardiac chambers and connections
Q21.0	Ventricular septal defect
Q21.3	Tetralogy of Fallot
Q21.8	Other congenital malformations of cardiac septa
Q22.0	Pulmonary valve atresia
Q22.1	Congenital pulmonary valve stenosis
Q22.2	Congenital pulmonary valve insufficiency
Q22.3	Other congenital malformations of pulmonary valve
Q22.4	Congenital tricuspid stenosis
Q22.5	Ebstein's anomaly
Q22.6	Hypoplastic right heart syndrome
Q22.8	Other congenital malformations of tricuspid valve
Q24.3	Pulmonary infundibular stenosis
Q24.8	Other specified congenital malformations of heart
Q25.5	Atresia of pulmonary artery
Q25.6	Stenosis of pulmonary artery
Q25.71	Coarctation of pulmonary artery
Q25.72	Congenital pulmonary arteriovenous malformation
Q25.79	Other congenital malformations of pulmonary artery
Q25.8	Other congenital malformations of other great arteries

Relative Value Units/Medicare Edits

Non-Facility RVU	Work	PE	MP	Total
33750	22.22	9.59	5.49	37.3
Facility RVU	**Work**	**PE**	**MP**	**Total**
33750	22.22	9.59	5.49	37.3

	FUD	Status	MUE	Modifiers				IOM Reference
33750	90	A	1(3)	51	N/A	62*	80	None

* with documentation

Terms To Know

atresia. Congenital closure or absence of a tubular organ or an opening to the body surface.

Blalock-Taussig procedure. Anastomosis of the left subclavian artery to the left pulmonary artery or the right subclavian artery to the right pulmonary artery in order to shunt some of the blood flow from the systemic to the pulmonary circulation.

cardiopulmonary bypass. Venous blood is diverted to a heart-lung machine, which mechanically pumps and oxygenates the blood temporarily so the heart can be bypassed while an open procedure on the heart or coronary arteries is performed. During bypass, the lungs are deflated and immobile.

shunt. Surgically created passage between blood vessels or other natural passages, such as an arteriovenous anastomosis, to divert or bypass blood flow from the normal channel.

33755

33755 Shunt; ascending aorta to pulmonary artery (Waterston type operation)

A surgical shunt is created between the ascending aorta and the pulmonary artery

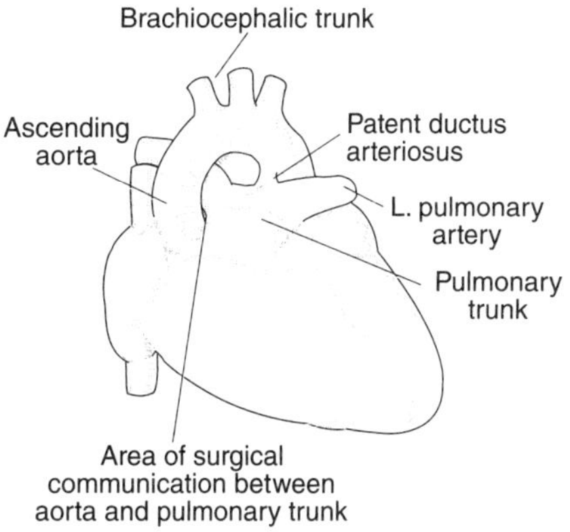

Explanation

This procedure is largely of historic interest. This procedure requires cardiopulmonary bypass. It is designed to allow adequate blood flow to the lungs. After cardiopulmonary bypass is initiated, the aorta is occluded above the heart. A hole may be cut in the aorta with the shunt closed from within by sutures. A more common method utilizes the pulmonary artery detached from the aorta and consequently reattached to the defect of the ascending aorta by sutures. The remaining defect in the pulmonary artery may be closed with sutures, but typically is patched with pericardium or pulmonary homograft. It is difficult to accurately control the diameter of the resulting connection and the resulting flow of blood into the lungs. Cardiopulmonary bypass is discontinued when heart function returns.

Coding Tips

When ligation and takedown of systemic-to-pulmonary artery shunt is performed with this procedure, it should be reported separately, see 33924. Do not append modifier 63 to 33755 as the description or nature of the procedure includes infants up to 4 kg. For shunt, subclavian to pulmonary artery (Blalock-Taussig type operation), see 33750. For descending aorta to pulmonary artery (Potts-Smith type operation), see 33762. For central shunt, with prosthetic graft, see 33764. For superior vena cava to pulmonary artery for flow to one lung (classical Glenn procedure), see 33766. For superior vena cava to pulmonary artery for flow to both lungs (bidirectional Glenn procedure), see 33767.

ICD-10-CM Diagnostic Codes

I24.89	Other forms of acute ischemic heart disease
I37.0	Nonrheumatic pulmonary valve stenosis
I37.1	Nonrheumatic pulmonary valve insufficiency
I37.2	Nonrheumatic pulmonary valve stenosis with insufficiency
I37.8	Other nonrheumatic pulmonary valve disorders
Q20.4	Double inlet ventricle
Q20.8	Other congenital malformations of cardiac chambers and connections
Q21.0	Ventricular septal defect
Q21.3	Tetralogy of Fallot
Q21.8	Other congenital malformations of cardiac septa
Q22.0	Pulmonary valve atresia

Q22.1	Congenital pulmonary valve stenosis
Q22.2	Congenital pulmonary valve insufficiency
Q22.3	Other congenital malformations of pulmonary valve
Q22.4	Congenital tricuspid stenosis
Q22.5	Ebstein's anomaly
Q22.6	Hypoplastic right heart syndrome
Q24.3	Pulmonary infundibular stenosis
Q24.4	Congenital subaortic stenosis
Q24.8	Other specified congenital malformations of heart
Q25.21	Interruption of aortic arch
Q25.3	Supravalvular aortic stenosis
Q25.41	Absence and aplasia of aorta
Q25.42	Hypoplasia of aorta
Q25.43	Congenital aneurysm of aorta
Q25.44	Congenital dilation of aorta
Q25.45	Double aortic arch
Q25.46	Tortuous aortic arch
Q25.47	Right aortic arch
Q25.48	Anomalous origin of subclavian artery
Q25.5	Atresia of pulmonary artery
Q25.6	Stenosis of pulmonary artery
Q25.71	Coarctation of pulmonary artery
Q25.72	Congenital pulmonary arteriovenous malformation
Q25.79	Other congenital malformations of pulmonary artery
Q25.8	Other congenital malformations of other great arteries

Relative Value Units/Medicare Edits

Non-Facility RVU	Work	PE	MP	Total
33755	22.6	10.88	5.59	39.07
Facility RVU	**Work**	**PE**	**MP**	**Total**
33755	22.6	10.88	5.59	39.07

	FUD	Status	MUE	Modifiers				IOM Reference
33755	90	A	1(2)	51	N/A	62*	80	None

* with documentation

Terms To Know

atresia. Congenital closure or absence of a tubular organ or an opening to the body surface.

patent ductus arteriosus. Condition in which the normal channel between the pulmonary artery and the aorta fails to close at birth, causing arterial blood to recirculate in the lungs and inhibiting the blood supply to the aorta.

33762

33762 Shunt; descending aorta to pulmonary artery (Potts-Smith type operation)

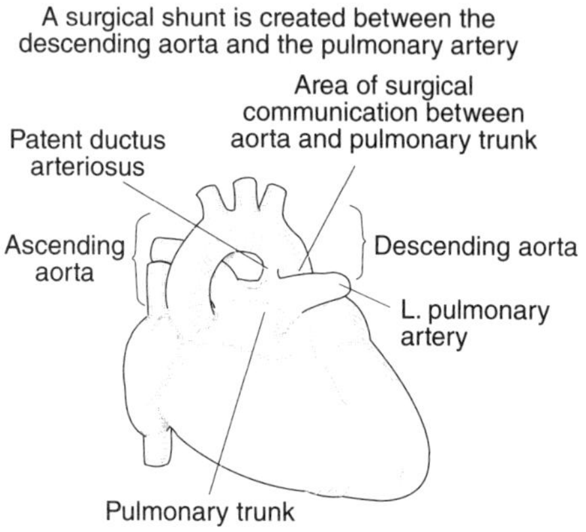

Explanation

This procedure is performed through the left side of the chest. Cardiopulmonary bypass is not required. The pulmonary artery is dissected from its original position to the branches and the aorta is visualized. Occlusion of the pulmonary artery is conducted and incisions are made into both arteries. One end of a 3 mm to 5 mm diameter tube made of polytetrafluoroethylene (PTFE) (e.g., Gortex) is sewn to the side of the descending aorta and the other end is sewn to the pulmonary artery. The ductus arteriosus (a connection between the aorta and pulmonary artery that has been supplying blood to the lungs, but usually closes at birth) is tied off.

Coding Tips

When ligation and takedown of systemic-to-pulmonary artery shunt is performed with this procedure, it should be reported separately, see 33924. Do not append modifier 63 to 33762 as the description or the nature of the procedure includes infants up to 4 kg. For shunt, subclavian to pulmonary artery (Blalock-Taussig type operation), see 33750. For ascending aorta to pulmonary artery (Waterston type operation), see 33755. For central shunt, with prosthetic graft, see 33764. For superior vena cava to pulmonary artery for flow to one lung (classical Glenn procedure), see 33766. For superior vena cava to pulmonary artery for flow to both lungs (bidirectional Glenn procedure), see 33767.

ICD-10-CM Diagnostic Codes

I24.89	Other forms of acute ischemic heart disease
I37.0	Nonrheumatic pulmonary valve stenosis
I37.1	Nonrheumatic pulmonary valve insufficiency
I37.2	Nonrheumatic pulmonary valve stenosis with insufficiency
I37.8	Other nonrheumatic pulmonary valve disorders
Q20.4	Double inlet ventricle
Q20.8	Other congenital malformations of cardiac chambers and connections
Q21.0	Ventricular septal defect
Q21.3	Tetralogy of Fallot
Q21.4	Aortopulmonary septal defect
Q21.8	Other congenital malformations of cardiac septa
Q22.0	Pulmonary valve atresia
Q22.1	Congenital pulmonary valve stenosis
Q22.2	Congenital pulmonary valve insufficiency

Q22.3	Other congenital malformations of pulmonary valve
Q22.4	Congenital tricuspid stenosis
Q22.5	Ebstein's anomaly
Q22.6	Hypoplastic right heart syndrome
Q22.8	Other congenital malformations of tricuspid valve
Q24.3	Pulmonary infundibular stenosis
Q24.4	Congenital subaortic stenosis
Q24.8	Other specified congenital malformations of heart
Q25.3	Supravalvular aortic stenosis
Q25.41	Absence and aplasia of aorta
Q25.42	Hypoplasia of aorta
Q25.43	Congenital aneurysm of aorta
Q25.44	Congenital dilation of aorta
Q25.45	Double aortic arch
Q25.46	Tortuous aortic arch
Q25.47	Right aortic arch
Q25.48	Anomalous origin of subclavian artery
Q25.49	Other congenital malformations of aorta
Q25.5	Atresia of pulmonary artery
Q25.6	Stenosis of pulmonary artery
Q25.71	Coarctation of pulmonary artery
Q25.72	Congenital pulmonary arteriovenous malformation
Q25.79	Other congenital malformations of pulmonary artery
Q25.8	Other congenital malformations of other great arteries

Relative Value Units/Medicare Edits

Non-Facility RVU	Work	PE	MP	Total
33762	22.6	9.7	5.59	37.89
Facility RVU	**Work**	**PE**	**MP**	**Total**
33762	22.6	9.7	5.59	37.89

	FUD	Status	MUE	Modifiers				IOM Reference
33762	90	A	1(2)	51	N/A	62*	80	None

* with documentation

Terms To Know

anastomosis. Surgically created connection between ducts, blood vessels, or bowel segments to allow flow from one to the other.

atresia. Congenital closure or absence of a tubular organ or an opening to the body surface.

patent ductus arteriosus. Condition in which the normal channel between the pulmonary artery and the aorta fails to close at birth, causing arterial blood to recirculate in the lungs and inhibiting the blood supply to the aorta.

33764

33764 Shunt; central, with prosthetic graft

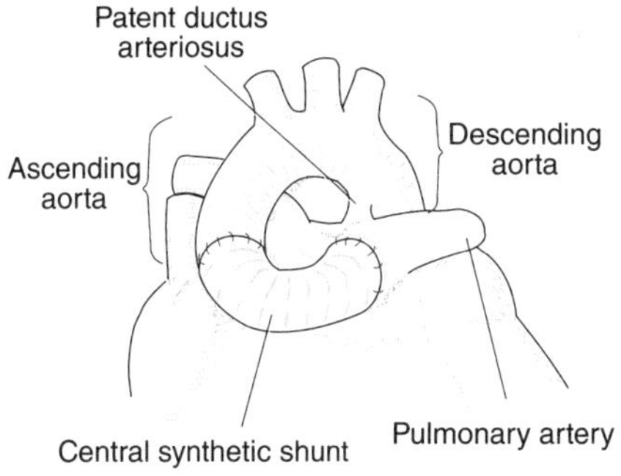

Explanation

The operation is done through an incision in the middle of the breast bone or through an incision in the left chest. Cardiopulmonary bypass is usually not required. One end of a 3 mm to 5 mm diameter tube made of Gortex is sewn to the side of the ascending aorta and the other end is sewn to some part of the pulmonary artery. The ductus arteriosus (a connection between the aorta and pulmonary artery that has been supplying blood to the lungs, but usually closes at birth) is tied off.

Coding Tips

When ligation and takedown of systemic-to-pulmonary artery shunt is performed in addition to this procedure, it should be reported separately, see 33924. For shunt, subclavian to pulmonary artery (Blalock-Taussig type operation), see 33750. For ascending aorta to pulmonary artery (Waterston type operation), see 33755. For descending aorta to pulmonary artery (Potts-Smith type operation), see 33762. For superior vena cava to pulmonary artery for flow to one lung (classical Glenn procedure), see 33766. For superior vena cava to pulmonary artery for flow to both lungs (bidirectional Glenn procedure), see 33767.

ICD-10-CM Diagnostic Codes

I24.89	Other forms of acute ischemic heart disease
I37.0	Nonrheumatic pulmonary valve stenosis
I37.1	Nonrheumatic pulmonary valve insufficiency
I37.2	Nonrheumatic pulmonary valve stenosis with insufficiency
I37.8	Other nonrheumatic pulmonary valve disorders
Q20.4	Double inlet ventricle
Q20.8	Other congenital malformations of cardiac chambers and connections
Q21.0	Ventricular septal defect
Q21.21	Partial atrioventricular septal defect
Q21.22	Transitional atrioventricular septal defect
Q21.23	Complete atrioventricular septal defect
Q21.3	Tetralogy of Fallot
Q21.4	Aortopulmonary septal defect
Q21.8	Other congenital malformations of cardiac septa
Q22.0	Pulmonary valve atresia
Q22.1	Congenital pulmonary valve stenosis
Q22.2	Congenital pulmonary valve insufficiency
Q22.3	Other congenital malformations of pulmonary valve

Q22.4	Congenital tricuspid stenosis
Q22.5	Ebstein's anomaly
Q22.6	Hypoplastic right heart syndrome
Q22.8	Other congenital malformations of tricuspid valve
Q24.3	Pulmonary infundibular stenosis
Q24.8	Other specified congenital malformations of heart
Q25.21	Interruption of aortic arch
Q25.29	Other atresia of aorta
Q25.3	Supravalvular aortic stenosis
Q25.41	Absence and aplasia of aorta
Q25.42	Hypoplasia of aorta
Q25.43	Congenital aneurysm of aorta
Q25.44	Congenital dilation of aorta
Q25.45	Double aortic arch
Q25.46	Tortuous aortic arch
Q25.47	Right aortic arch
Q25.48	Anomalous origin of subclavian artery
Q25.49	Other congenital malformations of aorta
Q25.5	Atresia of pulmonary artery
Q25.6	Stenosis of pulmonary artery
Q25.71	Coarctation of pulmonary artery
Q25.72	Congenital pulmonary arteriovenous malformation
Q25.79	Other congenital malformations of pulmonary artery
Q25.8	Other congenital malformations of other great arteries

Relative Value Units/Medicare Edits

Non-Facility RVU	Work	PE	MP	Total
33764	22.6	10.88	5.59	39.07
Facility RVU	**Work**	**PE**	**MP**	**Total**
33764	22.6	10.88	5.59	39.07

	FUD	Status	MUE	Modifiers				IOM Reference
33764	90	A	1(3)	51	N/A	62*	80	None

* with documentation

Terms To Know

atresia. Congenital closure or absence of a tubular organ or an opening to the body surface.

congenital. Present at birth, occurring through heredity or an influence during gestation up to the moment of birth.

ligation. Tying off a blood vessel or duct with a suture or a soft, thin wire.

patent ductus arteriosus. Condition in which the normal channel between the pulmonary artery and the aorta fails to close at birth, causing arterial blood to recirculate in the lungs and inhibiting the blood supply to the aorta.

33766-33767

33766 Shunt; superior vena cava to pulmonary artery for flow to 1 lung (classical Glenn procedure)

33767 superior vena cava to pulmonary artery for flow to both lungs (bidirectional Glenn procedure)

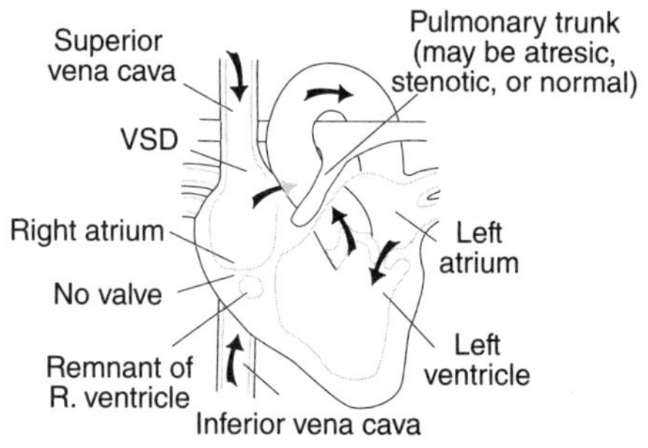

Example of tricuspid atresia with pulmonary atresia (single ventricle)

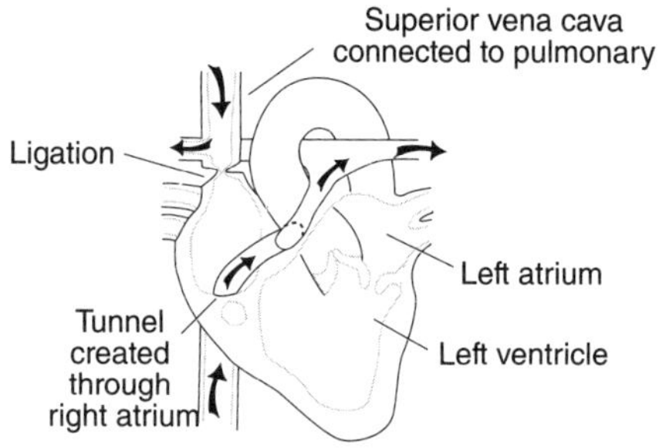

Explanation

In 33766, the operation is performed when there is an irreparable obstruction to blood flow through the right side of the heart. It is usually done as a prelude to a bidirectional or bilateral Glenn procedure, which is usually a prelude to a Fontan procedure. Cardiopulmonary bypass is usually required. The right (or the persistent left) superior caval vein is occluded and its connection with the heart is divided. The heart end of the superior caval vein is closed. The free end of the superior caval vein is sewn to the side of the corresponding pulmonary artery. It is assumed that the corresponding pulmonary artery is isolated from the opposite lung congenitally or surgically. The goal is to permit blood to flow directly from the superior caval vein to the lungs, thereby bypassing the right side of the heart. In 33767, it is assumed that all the pulmonary arteries from both lungs communicate freely. Cardiopulmonary bypass is required. Circulatory arrest and deep cooling of the body are usually employed. The main pulmonary artery is often tied off. The superior caval vein is detached from its connection to the right atrium. The hole left in the right atrium is closed with sutures. The free end of the superior caval vein is sewn to a hole in the side of the pulmonary artery. In this way, blood can flow to the lungs without passing through the right side of the heart. This operation is usually done as a prelude to a Fontan procedure.

Coding Tips

When ligation and takedown of systemic-to-pulmonary artery shunt is performed with this procedure, it should be reported separately, see 33924. For shunt, subclavian to pulmonary artery (Blalock-Taussig type operation), see 33750. For ascending aorta to pulmonary artery (Waterston type operation), see 33755. For descending aorta to pulmonary artery (Potts-Smith type operation), see 33762. For central shunt, with prosthetic graft, see 33764.

ICD-10-CM Diagnostic Codes

I37.0	Nonrheumatic pulmonary valve stenosis
I37.1	Nonrheumatic pulmonary valve insufficiency
I37.2	Nonrheumatic pulmonary valve stenosis with insufficiency
Q20.4	Double inlet ventricle
Q21.0	Ventricular septal defect
Q21.21	Partial atrioventricular septal defect
Q21.22	Transitional atrioventricular septal defect
Q21.23	Complete atrioventricular septal defect
Q21.3	Tetralogy of Fallot
Q21.4	Aortopulmonary septal defect
Q22.0	Pulmonary valve atresia
Q22.1	Congenital pulmonary valve stenosis
Q22.2	Congenital pulmonary valve insufficiency
Q22.4	Congenital tricuspid stenosis
Q22.5	Ebstein's anomaly
Q22.6	Hypoplastic right heart syndrome
Q24.3	Pulmonary infundibular stenosis
Q25.3	Supravalvular aortic stenosis
Q25.41	Absence and aplasia of aorta
Q25.42	Hypoplasia of aorta
Q25.43	Congenital aneurysm of aorta
Q25.44	Congenital dilation of aorta
Q25.45	Double aortic arch
Q25.46	Tortuous aortic arch
Q25.47	Right aortic arch
Q25.48	Anomalous origin of subclavian artery
Q25.5	Atresia of pulmonary artery
Q25.6	Stenosis of pulmonary artery
Q25.71	Coarctation of pulmonary artery
Q25.72	Congenital pulmonary arteriovenous malformation
Q26.0	Congenital stenosis of vena cava
Q26.3	Partial anomalous pulmonary venous connection
R23.0	Cyanosis

Relative Value Units/Medicare Edits

Non-Facility RVU	Work	PE	MP	Total
33766	23.57	9.96	5.82	39.35
33767	25.3	10.44	6.25	41.99
Facility RVU	**Work**	**PE**	**MP**	**Total**
33766	23.57	9.96	5.82	39.35
33767	25.3	10.44	6.25	41.99

	FUD	Status	MUE	Modifiers				IOM Reference
33766	90	A	1(2)	51	N/A	62*	80	None
33767	90	A	1(2)	51	N/A	62*	80	

* with documentation

33768

+ **33768** Anastomosis, cavopulmonary, second superior vena cava (List separately in addition to primary procedure)

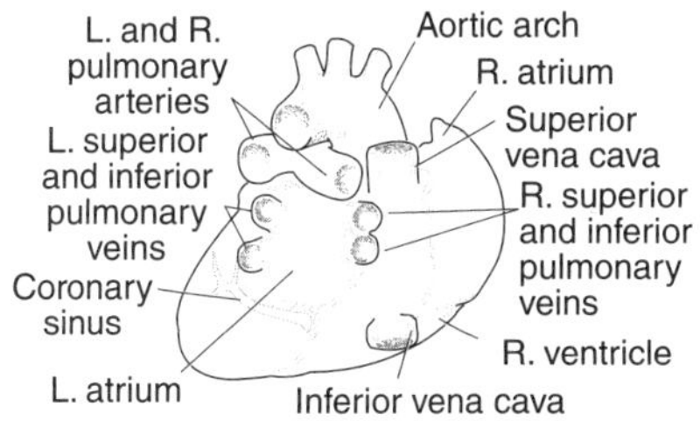

Posterior depiction of normal heart and its major venous returns

An anomalous left superior vena cava is repaired using anastomosis

Explanation

A cavopulmonary anastomosis of an anomalous left superior vena cava is performed in conjunction with separately reportable repair of other cardiac anomalies (e.g., bidirectional Glenn procedure, modified Fontan procedure, outflow tract augmentation). Cavopulmonary anastomosis is required when a left superior vena cava is present. The left superior vena cava is dissected free. The left superior vena cava is divided and anastomosed in end-to-side fashion to the left pulmonary artery.

Coding Tips

Report 33768 in addition to 33478, 33617, 33622, and 33767. Insertion of a chest tube (32551) is included and should not be reported separately. Temporary transvenous pacemaker placement (33210, 33211) is also included and should not be reported separately.

ICD-10-CM Diagnostic Codes

This/these CPT code(s) are add-on code(s). See the primary procedure code that this code is performed with for your ICD-10-CM code selections. Diagnostic code(s) would be the same as the actual procedure performed.

Relative Value Units/Medicare Edits

Non-Facility RVU	Work	PE	MP	Total
33768	8.0	2.2	1.98	12.18
Facility RVU	**Work**	**PE**	**MP**	**Total**
33768	8.0	2.2	1.98	12.18

	FUD	Status	MUE	Modifiers				IOM Reference
33768	N/A	A	1(2)	N/A	N/A	62	80	None

* with documentation

Terms To Know

anastomosis. Surgically created connection between ducts, blood vessels, or bowel segments to allow flow from one to the other.

33770-33771

33770 Repair of transposition of the great arteries with ventricular septal defect and subpulmonary stenosis; without surgical enlargement of ventricular septal defect

33771 with surgical enlargement of ventricular septal defect

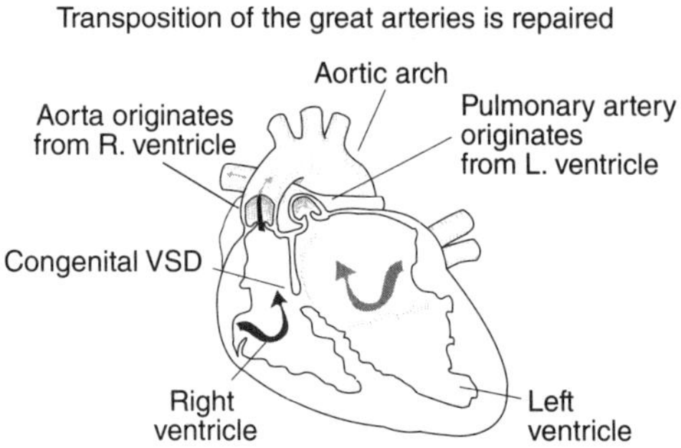

Explanation

The physician gains access to the mediastinum through the sternum (median sternotomy). Cardiopulmonary bypass catheters are usually placed through an incision in the right atrial appendage and aorta or femoral artery and the heart is stopped by infusion of cardioplegia solution into the coronary circulation. A large Dacron patch is applied to direct oxygenated blood from the left ventricle through the large ventricular septal defect into the aortic valve and ascending aorta. The physician ligates the proximal main pulmonary artery or oversews the pulmonic valve. In 33770, a fabric conduit or human cadaveric homograft is placed to direct unoxygenated blood from the right ventricle to the branch pulmonary arteries. The physician may place a bioprosthetic valve in the pulmonary outflow conduit if the pulmonary vascular resistance is elevated. In 33771, a fabric conduit is placed to direct right ventricular flow to the pulmonary artery. The physician may place a bioprosthetic valve in the pulmonary outflow conduit if the pulmonary vascular resistance is elevated. The cardiac incisions are closed, the patient is removed from cardiopulmonary bypass, and the remaining surgical incisions are closed. Chest tubes and/or a mediastinal drainage tube may be inserted for drainage following the procedure.

Coding Tips

Congenital anomalies involving transposition of the great vessels may occur with other anomalies of the heart that also require repair. In addition, repair may be accomplished by a variety of techniques. Review all procedure descriptions in CPT for repair of transposition of the great vessels (33770–33781) prior to selecting a code. When ligation and takedown of systemic-to-pulmonary artery shunt is performed in addition to this procedure, it should be reported separately, see 33924. For repair of transposition of the great arteries, atrial baffle procedure (e.g., Mustard or Senning type), see 33774; with removal of a pulmonary artery band, see 33775; with closure of a ventricular septal defect, see 33776; and with repair of a subpulmonic obstruction, see 33777. For repair of transposition of the great arteries, aortic pulmonary artery reconstruction (e.g., Jatene type), see 33778; with removal of a pulmonary artery band, see 33779; with closure of a ventricular septal defect, see 33780; and with repair of a subpulmonic obstruction, see 33781.

ICD-10-CM Diagnostic Codes

I37.0	Nonrheumatic pulmonary valve stenosis
I37.1	Nonrheumatic pulmonary valve insufficiency
I37.2	Nonrheumatic pulmonary valve stenosis with insufficiency
Q20.1	Double outlet right ventricle
Q20.2	Double outlet left ventricle
Q20.3	Discordant ventriculoarterial connection
Q20.4	Double inlet ventricle
Q20.5	Discordant atrioventricular connection
Q22.0	Pulmonary valve atresia
Q22.1	Congenital pulmonary valve stenosis
Q22.2	Congenital pulmonary valve insufficiency
Q22.4	Congenital tricuspid stenosis
Q22.5	Ebstein's anomaly
Q22.6	Hypoplastic right heart syndrome
Q22.8	Other congenital malformations of tricuspid valve
Q25.41	Absence and aplasia of aorta
Q25.42	Hypoplasia of aorta
Q25.43	Congenital aneurysm of aorta
Q25.44	Congenital dilation of aorta
Q25.45	Double aortic arch
Q25.46	Tortuous aortic arch
Q25.47	Right aortic arch
Q25.48	Anomalous origin of subclavian artery
Q25.72	Congenital pulmonary arteriovenous malformation
Q25.79	Other congenital malformations of pulmonary artery
R23.0	Cyanosis

Relative Value Units/Medicare Edits

Non-Facility RVU	Work	PE	MP	Total
33770	39.07	13.45	9.67	62.19
33771	40.63	13.2	10.08	63.91
Facility RVU	**Work**	**PE**	**MP**	**Total**
33770	39.07	13.45	9.67	62.19
33771	40.63	13.2	10.08	63.91

	FUD	Status	MUE	Modifiers				IOM Reference
33770	90	A	1(2)	51	N/A	62*	80	None
33771	90	A	1(2)	51	N/A	62*	80	

* with documentation

33774-33777

33774 Repair of transposition of the great arteries, atrial baffle procedure (eg, Mustard or Senning type) with cardiopulmonary bypass;
33775 with removal of pulmonary band
33776 with closure of ventricular septal defect
33777 with repair of subpulmonic obstruction

Transposition of the great arteries and other anomalies are repaired

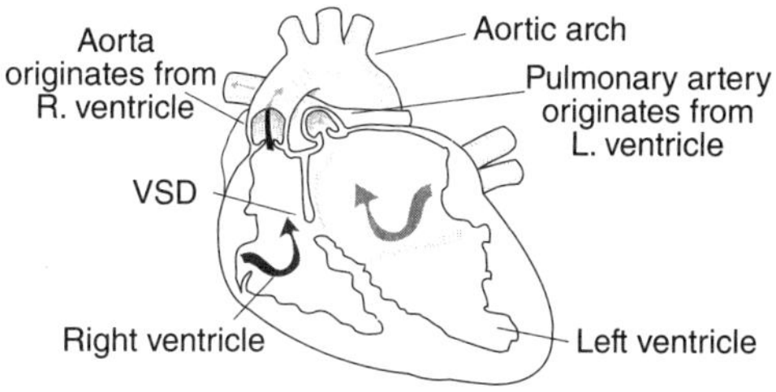

Explanation

The physician gains access to the mediastinum through an incision through the sternum (median sternotomy). Cardiopulmonary bypass catheters are placed through incisions in the low inferior vena cava, the superior vena cava, and aorta or femoral artery and the heart is stopped by infusion of cardioplegia solution into the coronary circulation. In 33774, the physician excises the interatrial septum and sews baffle material (pericardium or Dacron) to direct blood from the pulmonary veins to the right ventricle and the systemic venous drainage to the left ventricle. The pulmonary venous chamber may be enlarged with a woven Dacron or pericardial patch. In 33775, the physician removes the pulmonary artery band (placed during a previous surgery) and dilates the pulmonary artery to normal size. If this is not possible, the pulmonary band and the constricted area of pulmonary artery are removed, and a woven Dacron patch is applied over the hole. The physician excises the interatrial septum and sews baffle material (pericardium or Dacron) to direct blood from the pulmonary veins to the right ventricle and the systemic venous drainage to the left ventricle. The pulmonary venous chamber may be enlarged with a woven Dacron or pericardial patch. In 33776, the ventricular septal defect is closed, usually with a Dacron patch and the interatrial septum is excised. The physician sews baffle material (pericardium or Dacron) to direct blood from the pulmonary veins to the right ventricle and the systemic venous drainage to the left ventricle. The pulmonary venous chamber may be enlarged with a woven Dacron or pericardial patch. In 33777, the physician makes an incision in the right ventricular outflow tract, resects the fibrous muscular tissue causing the subpulmonic obstruction, and sews the ventriculotomy closed. The interatrial septum is excised and baffle material (pericardium or Dacron) is sewn in to direct blood from the pulmonary veins to the right ventricle and the systemic venous drainage to the left ventricle. The pulmonary venous chamber may be enlarged with a woven Dacron or pericardial patch. The cardiac incisions are closed and the patient is taken off cardiopulmonary bypass. The remaining surgical incisions are closed and the sternal or chest wall wounds are dressed. Chest tubes and/or mediastinal drainage tubes may be inserted for drainage following the procedure.

Coding Tips

Congenital anomalies involving transposition of the great vessels may occur with other anomalies of the heart that also require repair. In addition, repair may be accomplished by a variety of techniques. Review all procedure descriptions in CPT for repair of transposition of the great vessels (33770–33781) prior to selecting a code. When ligation and takedown of systemic-to-pulmonary artery shunt is performed in addition to this procedure, it should be reported separately, see 33924. For repair of transposition of the great arteries with ventricular septal defect and subpulmonary stenosis, see 33770–33771.

ICD-10-CM Diagnostic Codes

I37.0	Nonrheumatic pulmonary valve stenosis
I37.1	Nonrheumatic pulmonary valve insufficiency
I37.2	Nonrheumatic pulmonary valve stenosis with insufficiency
Q20.1	Double outlet right ventricle
Q20.2	Double outlet left ventricle
Q20.3	Discordant ventriculoarterial connection
Q20.4	Double inlet ventricle
Q20.5	Discordant atrioventricular connection
Q21.0	Ventricular septal defect
Q21.3	Tetralogy of Fallot
Q21.4	Aortopulmonary septal defect
Q22.0	Pulmonary valve atresia
Q22.1	Congenital pulmonary valve stenosis
Q22.2	Congenital pulmonary valve insufficiency
Q22.4	Congenital tricuspid stenosis
Q22.5	Ebstein's anomaly
Q22.6	Hypoplastic right heart syndrome
Q25.41	Absence and aplasia of aorta
Q25.42	Hypoplasia of aorta
Q25.43	Congenital aneurysm of aorta
Q25.44	Congenital dilation of aorta
Q25.45	Double aortic arch
Q25.46	Tortuous aortic arch
Q25.47	Right aortic arch
Q25.48	Anomalous origin of subclavian artery
Q25.72	Congenital pulmonary arteriovenous malformation
R23.0	Cyanosis

Relative Value Units/Medicare Edits

Non-Facility RVU	Work	PE	MP	Total
33774	31.73	13.63	7.84	53.2
33775	32.99	13.6	8.14	54.73
33776	34.75	14.56	8.6	57.91
33777	34.17	13.12	8.45	55.74
Facility RVU	**Work**	**PE**	**MP**	**Total**
33774	31.73	13.63	7.84	53.2
33775	32.99	13.6	8.14	54.73
33776	34.75	14.56	8.6	57.91
33777	34.17	13.12	8.45	55.74

	FUD	Status	MUE	Modifiers				IOM Reference
33774	90	A	1(2)	51	N/A	62*	80	None
33775	90	A	1(2)	51	N/A	N/A	80	
33776	90	A	1(2)	51	N/A	62*	80	
33777	90	A	1(2)	51	N/A	N/A	80	

* with documentation

33778-33781

33778 Repair of transposition of the great arteries, aortic pulmonary artery reconstruction (eg, Jatene type);
33779 with removal of pulmonary band
33780 with closure of ventricular septal defect
33781 with repair of subpulmonic obstruction

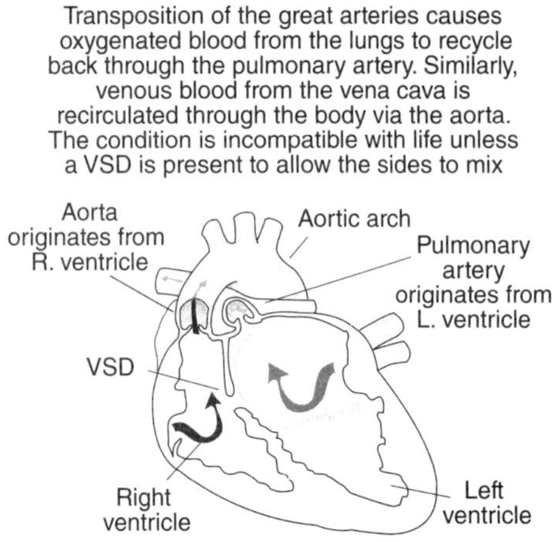

Explanation

The physician gains access to the mediastinum through an incision of the sternum (median sternotomy). Cardiopulmonary bypass catheters are placed through incisions in the low inferior vena cava, the superior vena cava, and aorta or femoral artery and the heart is stopped by infusion of cardioplegia solution into the coronary circulation. In 33778, the physician performs an arterial switch (or Jatene type procedure) for transposition of the great arteries, aortic pulmonary artery reconstruction. The physician removes the coronary ostia from the aortic root and sews them into the root of the pulmonary trunk. The pulmonary trunk and aortic root are each transected and interchanged to direct blood from the pulmonary veins through the left ventricle to the aorta, and the systemic venous drainage to the pulmonary trunk via the right ventricle. In 33779, the physician removes the pulmonary artery band placed during a previous surgery and dilates the pulmonary artery to normal size. If this is not possible, the pulmonary band and constricted area of pulmonary artery are removed and a woven Dacron patch is applied over the hole. The physician removes the coronary ostia from the aortic root and sews into the root of the pulmonary trunk. The pulmonary trunk and aortic root are each transected and interchanged to direct blood from the pulmonary veins through the left ventricle to the aorta, and the systemic venous drainage to the pulmonary trunk via the right ventricle. In 33780, the physician removes the coronary ostia from the aortic root and sews into the root of the pulmonary trunk. The pulmonary trunk and aortic root are each transected and interchanged to direct blood from the pulmonary veins through the left ventricle to the aorta, and the systemic venous drainage to the pulmonary trunk via the right ventricle. The ventricular septal defect is closed, usually with a Dacron patch. In 33781, the physician removes the coronary ostia from the aortic root and sews them into the root of the pulmonary trunk. The pulmonary trunk and aortic root are each transected and interchanged to direct blood from the pulmonary veins through the left ventricle to the aorta, and the systemic venous drainage to the pulmonary trunk via the right ventricle. An incision is made in the right ventricular outflow tract, resection of the fibrous muscular tissue causing the subpulmonic obstruction is performed, and the ventriculotomy is closed. Cardiac incisions are closed and patient is taken off cardiopulmonary bypass. The remaining surgical incisions are closed and the sternal or chest wall wounds are dressed. Chest tubes and/or mediastinal drainage tubes may be inserted following the procedure.

Coding Tips

When ligation and takedown of systemic-to-pulmonary artery shunt is performed in addition to this procedure, it should be reported separately, see 33924. Do not append modifier 63 to 33778 as the description or nature of the procedure includes infants up to 4 kg. For repair of transposition of the great arteries with ventricular septal defect and subpulmonary stenosis, see 33770–33771. For repair of transposition of the great arteries, atrial baffle procedure (e.g., Mustard or Senning type), see 33774; with removal of pulmonary artery band, see 33775; with closure of ventricular septal defect, see 33776; and with repair of subpulmonic obstruction, see 33777.

ICD-10-CM Diagnostic Codes

I37.0	Nonrheumatic pulmonary valve stenosis
I37.1	Nonrheumatic pulmonary valve insufficiency
I37.2	Nonrheumatic pulmonary valve stenosis with insufficiency
I37.8	Other nonrheumatic pulmonary valve disorders
Q20.1	Double outlet right ventricle
Q20.2	Double outlet left ventricle
Q20.3	Discordant ventriculoarterial connection
Q20.4	Double inlet ventricle
Q20.5	Discordant atrioventricular connection
Q20.8	Other congenital malformations of cardiac chambers and connections
Q21.0	Ventricular septal defect
Q21.4	Aortopulmonary septal defect
Q21.8	Other congenital malformations of cardiac septa
Q22.0	Pulmonary valve atresia
Q22.1	Congenital pulmonary valve stenosis
Q22.2	Congenital pulmonary valve insufficiency
Q22.3	Other congenital malformations of pulmonary valve
Q22.4	Congenital tricuspid stenosis
Q22.5	Ebstein's anomaly
Q22.6	Hypoplastic right heart syndrome
Q22.8	Other congenital malformations of tricuspid valve
Q24.8	Other specified congenital malformations of heart
Q25.41	Absence and aplasia of aorta
Q25.42	Hypoplasia of aorta
Q25.43	Congenital aneurysm of aorta
Q25.44	Congenital dilation of aorta
Q25.45	Double aortic arch
Q25.46	Tortuous aortic arch
Q25.47	Right aortic arch
Q25.48	Anomalous origin of subclavian artery
Q25.49	Other congenital malformations of aorta
Q25.72	Congenital pulmonary arteriovenous malformation
Q25.79	Other congenital malformations of pulmonary artery
Q25.8	Other congenital malformations of other great arteries
R23.0	Cyanosis

Relative Value Units/Medicare Edits

Non-Facility RVU	Work	PE	MP	Total
33778	42.75	15.88	10.61	69.24
33779	43.23	14.31	10.7	68.24
33780	43.9	14.79	10.86	69.55
33781	43.21	13.92	10.7	67.83
Facility RVU	**Work**	**PE**	**MP**	**Total**
33778	42.75	15.88	10.61	69.24
33779	43.23	14.31	10.7	68.24
33780	43.9	14.79	10.86	69.55
33781	43.21	13.92	10.7	67.83

	FUD	Status	MUE	Modifiers				IOM Reference
33778	90	A	1(2)	51	N/A	62*	80	None
33779	90	A	1(2)	51	N/A	62*	80	
33780	90	A	1(2)	51	N/A	62*	80	
33781	90	A	1(2)	51	N/A	N/A	80	

* with documentation

Terms To Know

coronary ostia. One or both of the two openings in the aortic sinuses that mark the origins of the left and right coronary arteries.

hypoplastic left heart syndrome. Hypoplasia or atresia of the left ventricle and aorta or mitral valve with respiratory distress and extreme cyanosis. Cardiac failure and death often result in early infancy.

transposition of great vessels. Life-threatening congenital malformation of the two main vessels of the cardiovascular system in which the pulmonary artery branches from the left ventricle and the aorta branches from the right ventricle. This condition causes the blood being returned from the extremities to be shunted back into the systemic circulation without being oxygenated. This condition may appear in differing forms: complete or classical transposition; double outlet right ventricle in which there is incomplete transposition of the vessels or both vessels arise from the right ventricle; and corrected transposition of the great vessels in which a developmental cardiac anomaly inverts the ventricles and valves to compensate for the transposed vessels by producing mirror-image blood flow through the heart.

ventricular septal defect. Congenital cardiac anomaly resulting in a continual opening in the septum between the ventricles that, in severe cases, causes oxygenated blood to flow back into the lungs, resulting in pulmonary hypertension.

33782-33783

33782 Aortic root translocation with ventricular septal defect and pulmonary stenosis repair (ie, Nikaidoh procedure); without coronary ostium reimplantation

33783 with reimplantation of 1 or both coronary ostia

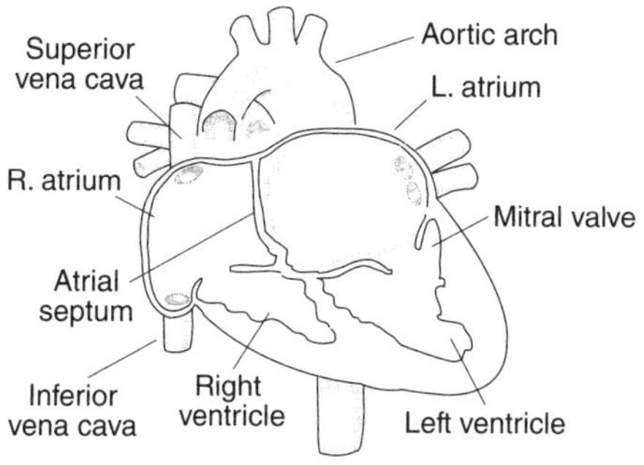

Explanation

The physician repairs anomalies of ventriculoarterial connection, ventricular septal defect (VSD), and pulmonary outflow tract obstruction (stenosis) in the Nikaidoh procedure. A median sternotomy incision is made and cardiopulmonary bypass is initiated. The physician may harvest a piece of pericardium to be used in the reconstruction of the right ventricular outflow tract, and mobilizes the branch pulmonary arteries. The physician harvests the aortic root from the right ventricle, with coronary arteries attached. The outlet septum is divided and the physician excises the pulmonary valve. The left ventricular outflow tract is reconstructed with the posteriorly translocated aortic root and the VSD patch. Using the pericardial patch, the physician reconstructs the right ventricular outflow tract. Report 33782 if no reimplantation of the coronary ostium is performed and 33783 if the physician reimplants one or both coronary ostia.

Coding Tips

For 33782, codes 33412, 33413, 33608, 33681, 33770, 33771, 33778, 33780, and 33920 are not reported separately.

ICD-10-CM Diagnostic Codes

I37.0	Nonrheumatic pulmonary valve stenosis
I37.1	Nonrheumatic pulmonary valve insufficiency
I37.2	Nonrheumatic pulmonary valve stenosis with insufficiency
I37.8	Other nonrheumatic pulmonary valve disorders
Q20.0	Common arterial trunk
Q20.1	Double outlet right ventricle
Q20.2	Double outlet left ventricle
Q20.3	Discordant ventriculoarterial connection
Q20.4	Double inlet ventricle
Q20.5	Discordant atrioventricular connection
Q20.8	Other congenital malformations of cardiac chambers and connections
Q21.0	Ventricular septal defect
Q21.3	Tetralogy of Fallot
Q21.4	Aortopulmonary septal defect
Q22.0	Pulmonary valve atresia
Q22.1	Congenital pulmonary valve stenosis
Q22.2	Congenital pulmonary valve insufficiency
Q22.3	Other congenital malformations of pulmonary valve

Q22.4	Congenital tricuspid stenosis
Q22.5	Ebstein's anomaly
Q22.6	Hypoplastic right heart syndrome
Q24.3	Pulmonary infundibular stenosis
Q24.8	Other specified congenital malformations of heart
Q25.3	Supravalvular aortic stenosis
Q25.41	Absence and aplasia of aorta
Q25.42	Hypoplasia of aorta
Q25.43	Congenital aneurysm of aorta
Q25.44	Congenital dilation of aorta
Q25.45	Double aortic arch
Q25.46	Tortuous aortic arch
Q25.47	Right aortic arch
Q25.48	Anomalous origin of subclavian artery
Q25.5	Atresia of pulmonary artery
Q25.6	Stenosis of pulmonary artery
Q25.71	Coarctation of pulmonary artery
Q25.72	Congenital pulmonary arteriovenous malformation
Q25.79	Other congenital malformations of pulmonary artery

Relative Value Units/Medicare Edits

Non-Facility RVU	Work	PE	MP	Total
33782	60.08	19.78	14.85	94.71
33783	65.08	21.15	16.12	102.35
Facility RVU	**Work**	**PE**	**MP**	**Total**
33782	60.08	19.78	14.85	94.71
33783	65.08	21.15	16.12	102.35

	FUD	Status	MUE	Modifiers				IOM Reference
33782	90	A	1(2)	51	N/A	62*	80	None
33783	90	A	1(2)	51	N/A	62*	80	

* with documentation

Terms To Know

congenital. Present at birth, occurring through heredity or an influence during gestation up to the moment of birth.

coronary ostia. One or both of the two openings in the aortic sinuses that mark the origins of the left and right coronary arteries.

ventricular septal defect. Congenital cardiac anomaly resulting in a continual opening in the septum between the ventricles that, in severe cases, causes oxygenated blood to flow back into the lungs, resulting in pulmonary hypertension.

33786

33786 Total repair, truncus arteriosus (Rastelli type operation)

Two types of truncus arteriosus

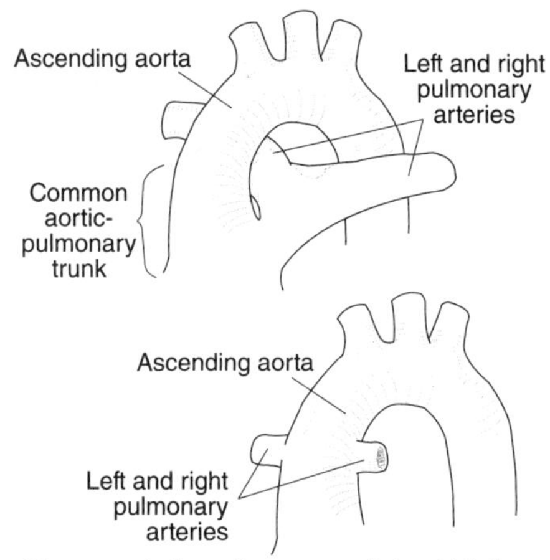

Truncus arteriosus is an anomaly in which the aortic and pulmonary systems are fused into a common trunk. A VSD is always present. Surgical intervention is almost always early in life

Explanation

Total repair, truncus arteriosus (Rastelli type operation) is performed by access to the mediastinum through an incision in the sternum (median sternotomy). Cardiopulmonary bypass catheters are placed usually through incisions in the right atrial appendage and the aorta or femoral artery. The heart is stopped by infusion of cardioplegia solution into the coronary circulation. A large Dacron patch is placed to direct oxygenated blood from the left ventricle through the large ventricular septal defect into the aortic valve and ascending aorta. The proximal main pulmonary artery is ligated or the pulmonic valve is oversewn. A fabric conduit or a human cadaveric homograft is placed to direct unoxygenated blood from the right ventricle to the branch pulmonary arteries after removing them from their origin(s) at the truncal vessel. A pericardial patch is sewn in place to close the defect(s) in the truncal vessel. A bioprosthetic valve may be placed in the pulmonary outflow conduit if the pulmonary vascular resistance is elevated. The cardiac incisions are closed and the patient is taken off cardiopulmonary bypass. The remaining surgical incisions are closed and the sternal or chest wall wounds are dressed. Chest tubes and/or mediastinal drainage tubes may be placed following the procedure.

Coding Tips

When ligation and takedown of systemic-to-pulmonary artery shunt is performed in addition to this procedure, it should be reported separately, see 33924. Do not append modifier 63 to 33786 as the description or nature of the procedure includes infants up to 4 kg. For closure of a ventricular septal defect only, with or without patch, see 33681; with pulmonary valvotomy or infundibular resection (acyanotic), see 33684.

ICD-10-CM Diagnostic Codes

Q20.0	Common arterial trunk
Q20.3	Discordant ventriculoarterial connection
Q20.5	Discordant atrioventricular connection
Q20.8	Other congenital malformations of cardiac chambers and connections
Q22.0	Pulmonary valve atresia
Q22.1	Congenital pulmonary valve stenosis

Q22.2	Congenital pulmonary valve insufficiency
Q22.3	Other congenital malformations of pulmonary valve
Q24.3	Pulmonary infundibular stenosis
Q24.8	Other specified congenital malformations of heart
Q25.21	Interruption of aortic arch
Q25.29	Other atresia of aorta
Q25.41	Absence and aplasia of aorta
Q25.42	Hypoplasia of aorta
Q25.43	Congenital aneurysm of aorta
Q25.44	Congenital dilation of aorta
Q25.45	Double aortic arch
Q25.46	Tortuous aortic arch
Q25.47	Right aortic arch
Q25.48	Anomalous origin of subclavian artery
Q25.49	Other congenital malformations of aorta
Q25.5	Atresia of pulmonary artery
Q25.6	Stenosis of pulmonary artery
Q25.71	Coarctation of pulmonary artery
Q25.72	Congenital pulmonary arteriovenous malformation
Q25.79	Other congenital malformations of pulmonary artery
Q25.8	Other congenital malformations of other great arteries

Relative Value Units/Medicare Edits

Non-Facility RVU	Work	PE	MP	Total
33786	41.87	14.71	10.38	66.96
Facility RVU	**Work**	**PE**	**MP**	**Total**
33786	41.87	14.71	10.38	66.96

	FUD	Status	MUE	Modifiers				IOM Reference
33786	90	A	1(2)	51	N/A	62*	80	None

* with documentation

Terms To Know

anomaly. Irregularity in the structure or position of an organ or tissue.

conduit. Surgically created channel for the passage of fluids.

congenital. Present at birth, occurring through heredity or an influence during gestation up to the moment of birth.

homograft. Graft from one individual to another of the same species.

incision. Act of cutting into tissue or an organ.

suture. Numerous stitching techniques employed in wound closure.

valve. Fold or membrane within a body canal or passageway that prevents backflow of fluids running through it.

33788

33788 Reimplantation of an anomalous pulmonary artery

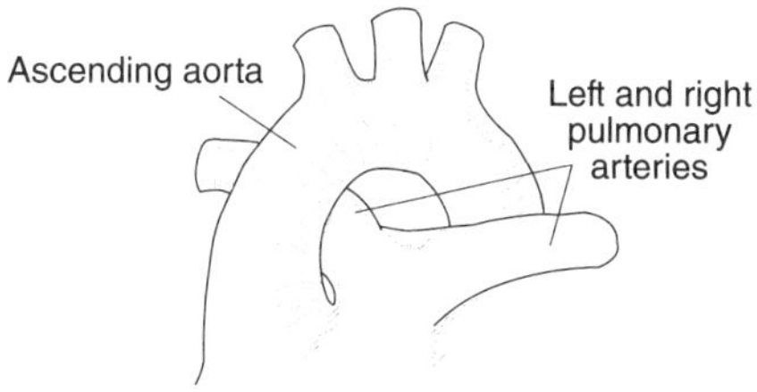

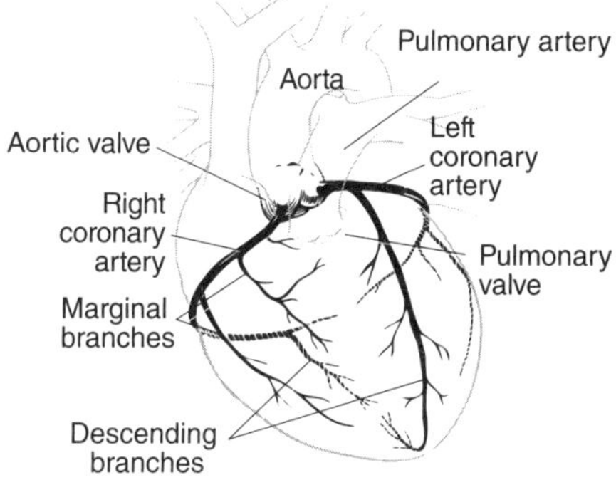

Explanation

Reimplantation of an anomalous pulmonary artery is performed with access to the mediastinum through an incision in the sternum (median sternotomy). Cardiopulmonary bypass catheters are placed usually through incisions in the right atrial appendage and aorta or femoral artery and the heart is stopped by infusion of cardioplegia solution into the coronary circulation. The physician identifies the coronary artery anomaly and reattaches the unperfused pulmonary artery to the pulmonic outflow tract, directly or using a Dacron graft, and ligates the patent ductus arteriosus, if present. The cardiac incisions are closed and the patient is taken off cardiopulmonary bypass. The remaining surgical incisions are closed and the sternal or chest wall wounds are dressed. Chest tubes and/or mediastinal drainage tubes may be inserted following the procedure.

Coding Tips

For pulmonary artery band, see 33690. For complete repair of anomalous venous return (supracardiac, intracardiac, or infracardiac types), see 33730. For partial anomalous returns, see atrial septal defect. For repair of pulmonary artery stenosis by reconstruction with patch or graft, see 33917. For repair of pulmonary atresia with ventricular septal defect, see 33920. For transection of pulmonary artery with cardiopulmonary bypass, see 33922.

ICD-10-CM Diagnostic Codes

Q20.0	Common arterial trunk
Q20.3	Discordant ventriculoarterial connection
Q20.5	Discordant atrioventricular connection
Q20.8	Other congenital malformations of cardiac chambers and connections
Q22.0	Pulmonary valve atresia
Q22.1	Congenital pulmonary valve stenosis
Q22.2	Congenital pulmonary valve insufficiency
Q22.3	Other congenital malformations of pulmonary valve
Q24.3	Pulmonary infundibular stenosis
Q24.8	Other specified congenital malformations of heart
Q25.21	Interruption of aortic arch

Q25.29	Other atresia of aorta
Q25.41	Absence and aplasia of aorta
Q25.42	Hypoplasia of aorta
Q25.43	Congenital aneurysm of aorta
Q25.44	Congenital dilation of aorta
Q25.45	Double aortic arch
Q25.46	Tortuous aortic arch
Q25.47	Right aortic arch
Q25.48	Anomalous origin of subclavian artery
Q25.49	Other congenital malformations of aorta
Q25.5	Atresia of pulmonary artery
Q25.6	Stenosis of pulmonary artery
Q25.71	Coarctation of pulmonary artery
Q25.72	Congenital pulmonary arteriovenous malformation
Q25.79	Other congenital malformations of pulmonary artery
Q25.8	Other congenital malformations of other great arteries

Relative Value Units/Medicare Edits

Non-Facility RVU	Work	PE	MP	Total
33788	27.42	11.03	6.77	45.22
Facility RVU	**Work**	**PE**	**MP**	**Total**
33788	27.42	11.03	6.77	45.22

	FUD	Status	MUE	Modifiers				IOM Reference
33788	90	A	1(2)	51	N/A	62*	80	None

* with documentation

Terms To Know

anomaly. Irregularity in the structure or position of an organ or tissue.

atresia. Congenital closure or absence of a tubular organ or an opening to the body surface.

atrial septal defect. Cardiac anomaly consisting of a patent opening in the atrial septum due to a fusion failure, classified as ostium secundum type, ostium primum defect, or endocardial cushion defect.

ventricular septal defect. Congenital cardiac anomaly resulting in a continual opening in the septum between the ventricles that, in severe cases, causes oxygenated blood to flow back into the lungs, resulting in pulmonary hypertension.

33800

33800 Aortic suspension (aortopexy) for tracheal decompression (eg, for tracheomalacia) (separate procedure)

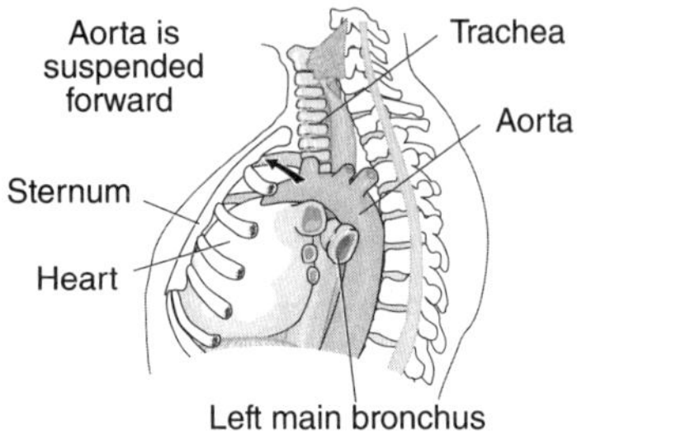

Tissues surrounding an anomalous aortic arch are sutured to those of the sternum to prevent the aorta from pressuring the trachea and causing respiratory compromise. The thymus gland may be removed to allow mobilization of the aorta

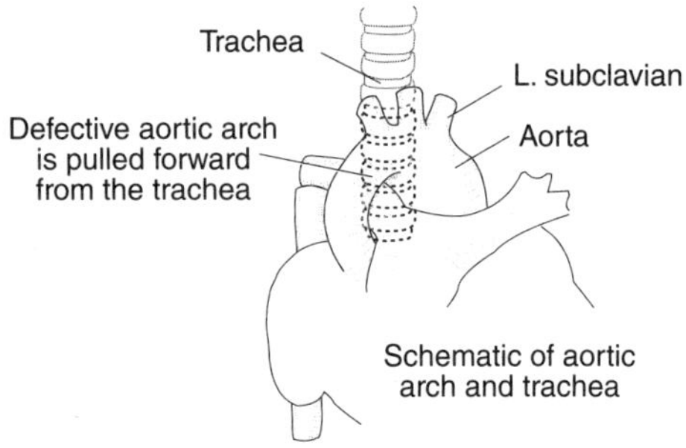

Explanation

Aortopexy for tracheal decompression is performed to open the tracheal lumen thereby preventing collapse. A right lateral thoracotomy or, sometimes, a midline sternotomy is performed to identify the ascending aorta. The thymus is isolated with partial removal performed to allow the ascending aorta to be mobilized and pulled forward. The physician sutures the adventitia of the ascending aorta and base of the innominate artery to the periosteum of the posterior aspect of the sternum or anterior rib. A similar operation may be performed on the descending aorta, depending upon the site of tracheomalacia. The thoracotomy or sternotomy is closed, leaving chest or mediastinal tubes in place.

Coding Tips

Thymectomy is included in this procedure. When 33800 is performed with another separately identifiable procedure, the highest dollar value code is listed as the primary procedure and subsequent procedures are appended with modifier 51. For tracheoplasty, intrathoracic, see 31760.

ICD-10-CM Diagnostic Codes

J39.8	Other specified diseases of upper respiratory tract
Q32.0	Congenital tracheomalacia
Q32.1	Other congenital malformations of trachea
Q34.8	Other specified congenital malformations of respiratory system

Relative Value Units/Medicare Edits

Non-Facility RVU	Work	PE	MP	Total
33800	17.28	7.61	4.27	29.16
Facility RVU	**Work**	**PE**	**MP**	**Total**
33800	17.28	7.61	4.27	29.16

	FUD	Status	MUE	Modifiers				IOM Reference
33800	90	A	1(2)	51	N/A	62	80	None

* with documentation

Terms To Know

anomaly. Irregularity in the structure or position of an organ or tissue.

anterior. Situated in the front area or toward the belly surface of the body; an anatomical reference point used to show the position and relationship of one body structure to another.

congenital. Present at birth, occurring through heredity or an influence during gestation up to the moment of birth.

excision. Surgical removal of an organ or tissue.

incision. Act of cutting into tissue or an organ.

ligate. To tie off a blood vessel or duct with a suture or a soft, thin wire (ligature wire).

mediastinum. Collection of organs and tissues that separate the pleural sacs. Located between the sternum and spine above the diaphragm, it contains the heart and great vessels, trachea and bronchi, esophagus, thymus, lymph nodes, and nerves.

posterior. Located in the back part or caudal end of the body.

sternotomy. Incision into the sternum, the bone that forms the front of the chest cavity and connects with the ribs.

thoracotomy. Surgical procedure for opening the chest wall in order to access the lungs, esophagus, trachea, aorta, heart, and diaphragm.

thymectomy. Excision of the thymus gland, situated in the anterior superior mediastinum.

tracheoplasty. Plastic repair of the trachea, the tube descending from the larynx that branches into the right and left main bronchi.

33802-33803

33802 Division of aberrant vessel (vascular ring);
33803 with reanastomosis

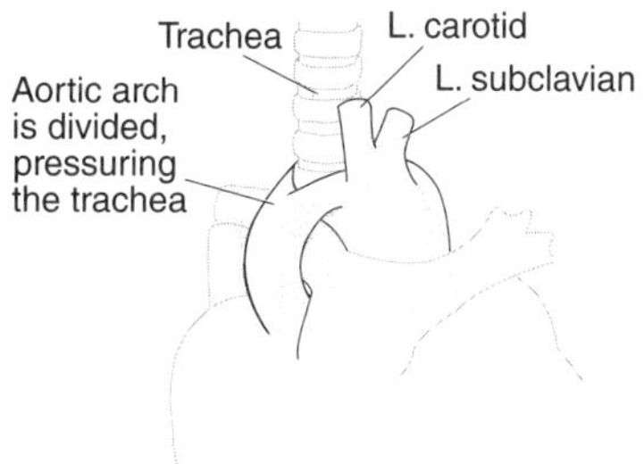

Schematic of aortic arch vascular ring

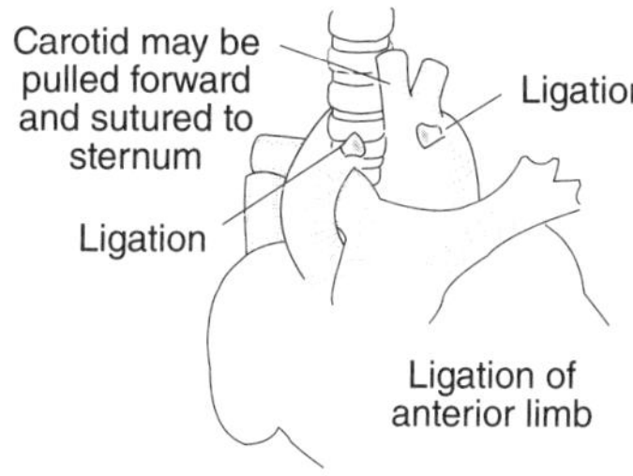

A divided aortic arch is surgically accessed

Explanation

The physician gains access to the mediastinum through an incision through the left chest (posterolateral thoracotomy). The physician identifies the two aortic arches and occludes the smaller left arch with vascular clamps. The physician divides the arch and oversews and possibly ligates the divided ends. The physician dissects away the stumps of the divided left arch and frees them from their mediastinal attachments. The physician attaches traction sutures to the ligated stumps and to the endothoracic fascia anteriorly and posteriorly to minimize obstruction to the esophagus and trachea. The physician closes the remaining surgical incisions and dresses the chest wall wound. The physician may leave a chest tube and/or a mediastinal drainage tube in place following the procedure. Report 33803 if the procedure includes reanastomosis.

Coding Tips

When 33802 or 33803 is performed with another separately identifiable procedure, the highest dollar value code is listed as the primary procedure and subsequent procedures are appended with modifier 51. For repair of transposition of the great arteries, see 33770–33781. For repair of patent ductus arteriosus, see 33820–33824. For excision of coarctation of aorta, see 33840–33851.

ICD-10-CM Diagnostic Codes

I28.8	Other diseases of pulmonary vessels
I77.89	Other specified disorders of arteries and arterioles
Q25.1	Coarctation of aorta
Q25.41	Absence and aplasia of aorta
Q25.42	Hypoplasia of aorta
Q25.43	Congenital aneurysm of aorta
Q25.44	Congenital dilation of aorta
Q25.45	Double aortic arch
Q25.46	Tortuous aortic arch
Q25.47	Right aortic arch
Q25.48	Anomalous origin of subclavian artery

Q25.49	Other congenital malformations of aorta
Q25.6	Stenosis of pulmonary artery
Q25.71	Coarctation of pulmonary artery
Q25.72	Congenital pulmonary arteriovenous malformation
Q25.79	Other congenital malformations of pulmonary artery
Q25.8	Other congenital malformations of other great arteries

Relative Value Units/Medicare Edits

Non-Facility RVU	Work	PE	MP	Total
33802	18.37	9.33	4.54	32.24
33803	20.31	8.69	5.01	34.01
Facility RVU	**Work**	**PE**	**MP**	**Total**
33802	18.37	9.33	4.54	32.24
33803	20.31	8.69	5.01	34.01

	FUD	Status	MUE	Modifiers				IOM Reference
33802	90	A	1(3)	51	N/A	62*	80	None
33803	90	A	1(3)	51	N/A	62*	80	

* with documentation

Terms To Know

anastomosis. Surgically created connection between ducts, blood vessels, or bowel segments to allow flow from one to the other.

anomaly. Irregularity in the structure or position of an organ or tissue.

anterior. Situated in the front area or toward the belly surface of the body; an anatomical reference point used to show the position and relationship of one body structure to another.

congenital. Present at birth, occurring through heredity or an influence during gestation up to the moment of birth.

fascia. Fibrous sheet or band of tissue that envelops organs, muscles, and groupings of muscles.

ligate. To tie off a blood vessel or duct with a suture or a soft, thin wire (ligature wire).

mediastinum. Collection of organs and tissues that separate the pleural sacs. Located between the sternum and spine above the diaphragm, it contains the heart and great vessels, trachea and bronchi, esophagus, thymus, lymph nodes, and nerves.

obstruction. Blockage that prevents normal function of the valve or structure.

occlusion. Constriction, closure, or blockage of a passage.

posterior. Located in the back part or caudal end of the body.

33814

▲ **33814** Obliteration of aortopulmonary septal defect, with cardiopulmonary bypass

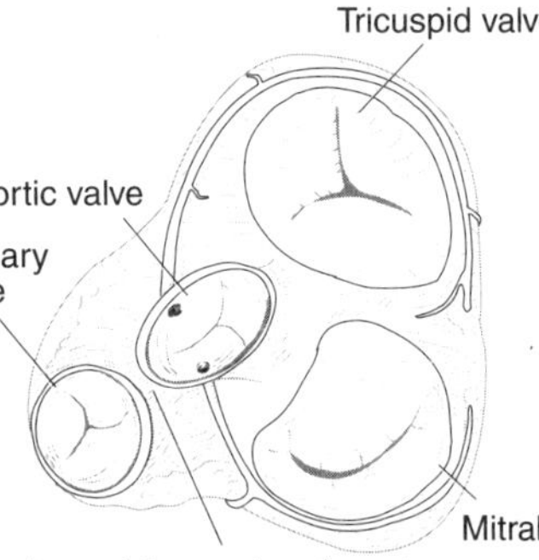

Explanation

The physician performs obliteration of an aortopulmonary septal defect. Access is gained to the mediastinum through an incision through the sternum (median sternotomy). Cardiopulmonary bypass catheters are placed through incisions in the low inferior vena cava, the superior vena cava, and high aorta or femoral artery, and the heart is stopped by infusing cardioplegia solution into the coronary circulation. The physician cross-clamps the aorta and places sump suction in the left atrium to obtain a bloodless surgical field. The aortopulmonary septal defect is exposed by cutting through the ascending aorta or main pulmonary artery. The physician closes the defect with a Dacron fabric patch, closes the aortic or pulmonary arterial incision, closes the remaining surgical incisions, and dresses the sternal wound. The physician may leave chest tubes and/or a mediastinal drainage tube in place following the procedure.

Coding Tips

When 33814 is performed with another separately identifiable procedure, the highest dollar value code is listed as the primary procedure and subsequent procedures are appended with modifier 51. For repair of an atrial septal defect, secundum, with cardiopulmonary bypass, with or without patch, see 33641. For direct or patch closure, sinus venosus, with or without anomalous pulmonary venous drainage, see 33645. For repair of an atrial septal defect and ventricular septal defect, with direct or patch closure, see 33647. For repair of an incomplete or partial atrioventricular canal (ostium primum atrial septal defect), with or without atrioventricular valve repair, see 33660. For closure of a ventricular septal defect, with or without patch graft, see 33681–33688.

ICD-10-CM Diagnostic Codes

Q21.4	Aortopulmonary septal defect
Q21.8	Other congenital malformations of cardiac septa

Relative Value Units/Medicare Edits

Non-Facility RVU	Work	PE	MP	Total
33814	26.57	11.98	6.57	45.12
Facility RVU	**Work**	**PE**	**MP**	**Total**
33814	26.57	11.98	6.57	45.12

	FUD	Status	MUE	Modifiers				IOM Reference
33814	90	A	1(2)	51	N/A	62*	80	None

* with documentation

Terms To Know

atrial septal defect. Cardiac anomaly consisting of a patent opening in the atrial septum due to a fusion failure, classified as ostium secundum type, ostium primum defect, or endocardial cushion defect.

cardiopulmonary bypass. Venous blood is diverted to a heart-lung machine, which mechanically pumps and oxygenates the blood temporarily so the heart can be bypassed while an open procedure on the heart or coronary arteries is performed. During bypass, the lungs are deflated and immobile.

obliterate. Get rid or do away with completely.

ventricular septal defect. Congenital cardiac anomaly resulting in a continual opening in the septum between the ventricles that, in severe cases, causes oxygenated blood to flow back into the lungs, resulting in pulmonary hypertension.

33820-33824

33820 Repair of patent ductus arteriosus; by ligation
33822 by division, younger than 18 years
33824 by division, 18 years and older

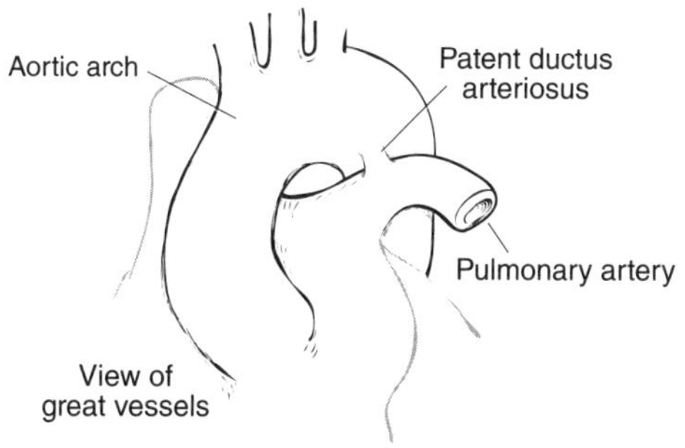

The ductus arteriosus is the natural shunt that bypasses lung circulation in the prenatal phase

Explanation

In 33820, the physician repairs patent ductus arteriosus (PDA) by ligation with access to the mediastinum through an incision of the posterolateral left chest wall (posterolateral thoracotomy). Dissection is performed through the posterior chest wall musculature to expose the superior mediastinum with continued dissection of the tissues surrounding the ductus. Several heavy ligatures are passed around the ductus followed by ligation. The surgical incisions are closed and the chest wall wound is dressed. Chest tubes and/or mediastinal drainage tubes may be inserted following the procedure. In 33822, the repair is performed by division in a patient younger than 18 years of age. The physician dissects away the tissues surrounding the ductus and passes several heavy ligatures around the ductus and ties it off (ligation) at each end. The physician occludes the ductus with vascular clamps and divides the ductus with scissors. The physician closes the aortic end with suture then closes the pulmonary stump. The physician removes the vascular clamps, sutures the pleura closed, closes the remaining surgical incisions, and dresses the chest wall wound. The physician may leave chest tubes and/or a mediastinal drainage tube in place following the procedure. Report 33824 if the patient is 18 years and older.

Coding Tips

When 33820, 33822, or 33824 is performed with another separately identifiable procedure, the highest dollar value code is listed as the primary procedure and subsequent procedures are appended with modifier 51. For excision of coarctation of the aorta, with or without associated patent ductus arteriosus, see 33840–33851. For closure of a ventricular septal defect, see 33681–33688. Use 93582 when closure of patent ductus arteriosus is performed via percutaneous transcatheter.

ICD-10-CM Diagnostic Codes

Q24.8	Other specified congenital malformations of heart
Q25.0	Patent ductus arteriosus
Q25.8	Other congenital malformations of other great arteries
Q28.8	Other specified congenital malformations of circulatory system

Relative Value Units/Medicare Edits

Non-Facility RVU	Work	PE	MP	Total
33820	16.69	7.85	4.12	28.66
33822	17.71	8.13	4.37	30.21
33824	20.23	9.81	4.99	35.03
Facility RVU	**Work**	**PE**	**MP**	**Total**
33820	16.69	7.85	4.12	28.66
33822	17.71	8.13	4.37	30.21
33824	20.23	9.81	4.99	35.03

	FUD	Status	MUE	Modifiers				IOM Reference
33820	90	A	1(2)	51	N/A	N/A	80	None
33822	90	A	1(2)	51	N/A	62*	80	
33824	90	A	1(2)	51	N/A	62*	80	

* with documentation

Terms To Know

ligation. Tying off a blood vessel or duct with a suture or a soft, thin wire.

mediastinum. Collection of organs and tissues that separate the pleural sacs. Located between the sternum and spine above the diaphragm, it contains the heart and great vessels, trachea and bronchi, esophagus, thymus, lymph nodes, and nerves.

musculature. Entire muscle tissue apparatus of the body or a specific part of the body.

occlusion. Constriction, closure, or blockage of a passage.

patent ductus arteriosus. Condition in which the normal channel between the pulmonary artery and the aorta fails to close at birth, causing arterial blood to recirculate in the lungs and inhibiting the blood supply to the aorta.

posterior. Located in the back part or caudal end of the body.

ventricular septal defect. Congenital cardiac anomaly resulting in a continual opening in the septum between the ventricles that, in severe cases, causes oxygenated blood to flow back into the lungs, resulting in pulmonary hypertension.

33840-33851

33840 Excision of coarctation of aorta, with or without associated patent ductus arteriosus; with direct anastomosis

33845 with graft

33851 repair using either left subclavian artery or prosthetic material as gusset for enlargement

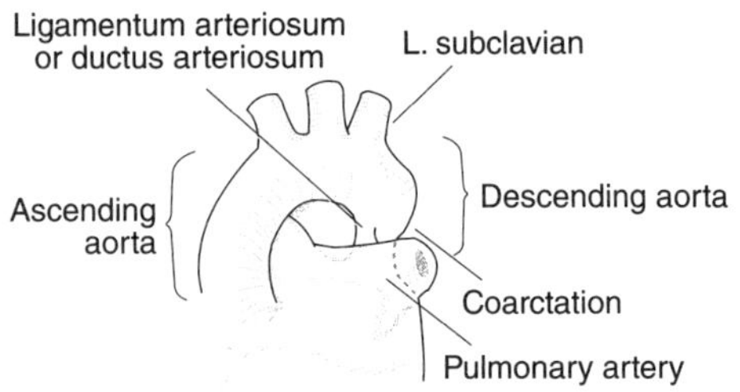

Coarctation is a stenotic narrowing of the descending aorta that is associated with the ductus arteriosum as it turns into the ligamentum arteriosum. This ligament is attached to the heart side of the localized stenosis

Explanation

In 33840–33845, the physician gains access to the mediastinum through an incision through the posterolateral left chest wall (posterolateral thoracotomy). The physician dissects through the posterior chest wall musculature to expose the superior mediastinum, clamping and ligating large collateral vessels as they are encountered. The physician dissects away the tissues surrounding the aorta. The physician clamps the aorta on either side of the coarctation and ties off and divides the ligamentum arteriosum (or patent ductus arteriosus, if present). The physician excises the stricture and sutures the two ends of the aorta to each other. Report 33845 if a graft is placed. In 33851, the physician gains access to the mediastinum through an incision through the posterolateral left chest wall (posterolateral thoracotomy). Dissection through the posterior chest wall musculature to expose the superior mediastinum is performed with clamping and ligating of large collateral vessels as they are encountered. The tissues surrounding the aorta are dissected away and clamps are placed on the aorta at either side of the coarctation and tied off with division of the ligamentum arteriosum (or patent ductus arteriosus, if present). The aorta is opened with a longitudinal incision that extends along the subclavian artery above and for a distance distally. Any extra tissue at the stricture site is excised. The physician sews in the left subclavian artery or a Dacron patch graft to attach and enlarge the aorta at the longitudinal incision. The mediastinal pleura and chest wounds are closed and dressing is applied to the chest wall wound. Chest tubes and/or a mediastinal drainage tube may be placed following the procedure.

Coding Tips

When 33840, 33845, or 33851 is performed with another separately identifiable procedure, the highest dollar value code is listed as the primary procedure and subsequent procedures are appended with modifier 51. For repair of patent ductus arteriosus without excision of coarctation of the aorta, see 33820–33824. For closure of a ventricular septal defect, see 33681–33688.

ICD-10-CM Diagnostic Codes

Q25.0	Patent ductus arteriosus
Q25.1	Coarctation of aorta
Q25.41	Absence and aplasia of aorta
Q25.42	Hypoplasia of aorta
Q25.43	Congenital aneurysm of aorta

Q25.44	Congenital dilation of aorta
Q25.45	Double aortic arch
Q25.46	Tortuous aortic arch
Q25.47	Right aortic arch
Q25.48	Anomalous origin of subclavian artery
Q25.49	Other congenital malformations of aorta

AMA: 33840 2021,Dec **33845** 2021,Dec **33851** 2021,Dec

Relative Value Units/Medicare Edits

Non-Facility RVU	Work	PE	MP	Total
33840	21.34	10.13	5.26	36.73
33845	22.93	10.97	5.67	39.57
33851	21.98	10.31	5.43	37.72
Facility RVU	**Work**	**PE**	**MP**	**Total**
33840	21.34	10.13	5.26	36.73
33845	22.93	10.97	5.67	39.57
33851	21.98	10.31	5.43	37.72

	FUD	Status	MUE	Modifiers				IOM Reference
33840	90	A	1(2)	51	N/A	62*	80	None
33845	90	A	1(2)	51	N/A	62*	80	
33851	90	A	1(2)	51	N/A	62*	80	

* with documentation

Terms To Know

anastomosis. Surgically created connection between ducts, blood vessels, or bowel segments to allow flow from one to the other.

graft. Tissue implant from another part of the body or another person.

posterior. Located in the back part or caudal end of the body.

stenosis. Narrowing or constriction of a passage.

stricture. Narrowing of an anatomical structure.

ventricular septal defect. Congenital cardiac anomaly resulting in a continual opening in the septum between the ventricles that, in severe cases, causes oxygenated blood to flow back into the lungs, resulting in pulmonary hypertension.

33852-33853

33852 Repair of hypoplastic or interrupted aortic arch using autogenous or prosthetic material; without cardiopulmonary bypass

33853 with cardiopulmonary bypass

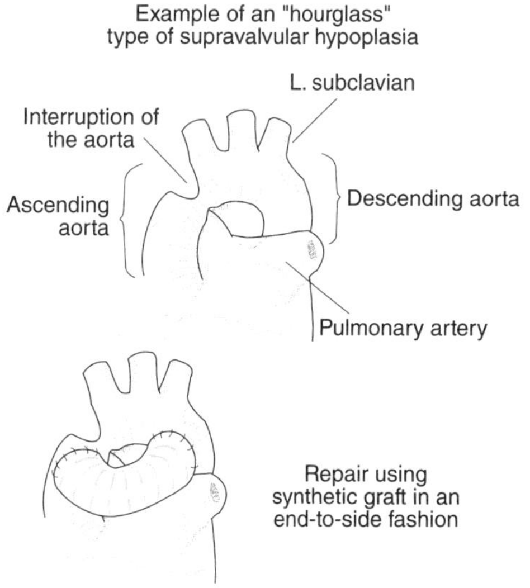

Explanation

The physician surgically attaches the ascending and descending parts of the aorta, where normal connection is too small or interrupted entirely. Access to the mediastinum is achieved through an incision in the sternum (midline sternotomy). The aorta and left carotid artery are clamped to allow completion of the end-to-side attachment of a Dacron mesh graft to the ascending aorta. The physician cross-clamps the graft and releases the proximal clamp and the left carotid artery clamp. End-to-side attachment is performed to secure the distal graft to the descending aorta. The mediastinal pleura and chest are closed with dressing applied to the chest wall wound. Chest tubes and/or a mediastinal drainage tube may be placed following the procedure. Report 33853 when cardiopulmonary bypass is utilized.

Coding Tips

For repair of hypoplastic left heart syndrome (e.g., Norwood type), via excision of coarctation of aorta, see 33619. For excision of coarctation of the aorta with or without associated patent ductus arteriosus, see 33840–33845.

ICD-10-CM Diagnostic Codes

Q25.1	Coarctation of aorta
Q25.21	Interruption of aortic arch
Q25.29	Other atresia of aorta
Q25.3	Supravalvular aortic stenosis
Q25.41	Absence and aplasia of aorta
Q25.42	Hypoplasia of aorta
Q25.43	Congenital aneurysm of aorta
Q25.44	Congenital dilation of aorta
Q25.45	Double aortic arch
Q25.46	Tortuous aortic arch
Q25.47	Right aortic arch
Q25.48	Anomalous origin of subclavian artery
Q25.49	Other congenital malformations of aorta

Relative Value Units/Medicare Edits

Non-Facility RVU	Work	PE	MP	Total
33852	24.41	10.98	6.04	41.43
33853	32.51	13.61	8.04	54.16
Facility RVU	**Work**	**PE**	**MP**	**Total**
33852	24.41	10.98	6.04	41.43
33853	32.51	13.61	8.04	54.16

	FUD	Status	MUE	Modifiers				IOM Reference
33852	90	A	1(2)	51	N/A	N/A	80	None
33853	90	A	1(2)	51	N/A	62*	80	

* with documentation

Terms To Know

atresia. Congenital closure or absence of a tubular organ or an opening to the body surface.

cardiopulmonary bypass. Venous blood is diverted to a heart-lung machine, which mechanically pumps and oxygenates the blood temporarily so the heart can be bypassed while an open procedure on the heart or coronary arteries is performed. During bypass, the lungs are deflated and immobile.

catheter. Flexible tube inserted into an area of the body for introducing or withdrawing fluid.

congenital. Present at birth, occurring through heredity or an influence during gestation up to the moment of birth.

excision. Surgical removal of an organ or tissue.

graft. Tissue implant from another part of the body or another person.

hypoplasia. Condition in which there is underdevelopment of an organ or tissue.

stenosis. Narrowing or constriction of a passage.

33858-33859

33858 Ascending aorta graft, with cardiopulmonary bypass, includes valve suspension, when performed; for aortic dissection

33859 for aortic disease other than dissection (eg, aneurysm)

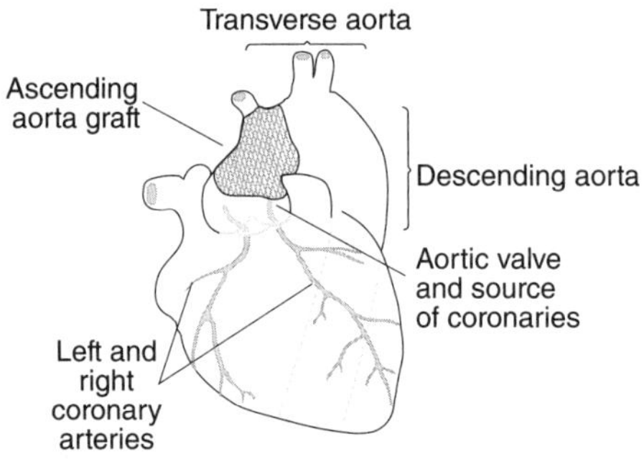

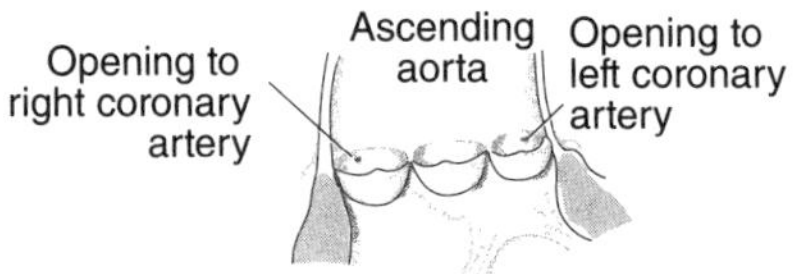

Aortic valve may be suspended with ascending aortic graft

Explanation

In 33858, the surgeon places an ascending aortic graft for aortic dissection and in 33859, for aortic disease other than dissection, such as aneurysm. Following induction of general anesthesia, a median sternotomy is performed. The physician places appropriate arterial and venous cannulation and initiates cardiopulmonary bypass. Following cross-clamp of the distal ascending aorta at the base of the innominate artery, the physician opens the proximal ascending aorta. The affected section of the ascending aorta is removed, the inside and outside of the aortic wall is lined with strips of felt for reinforcement, and a piece of synthetic graft material such as Dacron or PTFE is put in place of the missing piece of the aorta. The patient's aortic valve is preserved, although valve suspension may be performed. The physician closes the sternal incision and dresses the wound. If the patient's ascending aortic disease process includes the aortic arch and requires an aortic hemiarch graft, it is reported separately.

Coding Tips

Thoracic aortic aneurysm repair codes are dependent on aneurysm site: ascending, transverse arch, descending, or thoracoabdominal. Do not report an ascending aortic repair with a beveled anastomosis into the arch with a cross-clamp as a hemiarch graft using 33866. For a transverse arch graft, see 33871. For a descending thoracic aorta graft, see 33875. For repair of a thoracoabdominal aneurysm, see 33877. For direct repair of an aneurysm, a false aneurysm, or excision (partial or total) and graft insertion, with or without patch graft, of the abdominal aorta, see 35081 and 35091; for ruptured aneurysm, abdominal aorta, see 35082.

ICD-10-CM Diagnostic Codes

A52.01	Syphilitic aneurysm of aorta
I71.010	Dissection of ascending aorta
I71.011	Dissection of aortic arch
I71.012	Dissection of descending thoracic aorta
I71.03	Dissection of thoracoabdominal aorta
I71.11	Aneurysm of the ascending aorta, ruptured

N Newborn: 0 P Pediatric: 0-17 M Maternity: 9-64 A Adult: 15-124 AMA: CPT Assist

I71.12 Aneurysm of the aortic arch, ruptured
I71.13 Aneurysm of the descending thoracic aorta, ruptured
I71.21 Aneurysm of the ascending aorta, without rupture
I71.22 Aneurysm of the aortic arch, without rupture
I71.23 Aneurysm of the descending thoracic aorta, without rupture
I79.0 Aneurysm of aorta in diseases classified elsewhere
Q25.43 Congenital aneurysm of aorta

AMA: **33858** 2019,Nov **33859** 2019,Nov

Relative Value Units/Medicare Edits

Non-Facility RVU	Work	PE	MP	Total
33858	63.4	20.84	15.21	99.45
33859	45.13	15.56	10.8	71.49
Facility RVU	**Work**	**PE**	**MP**	**Total**
33858	63.4	20.84	15.21	99.45
33859	45.13	15.56	10.8	71.49

	FUD	Status	MUE	Modifiers				IOM Reference
33858	90	A	1(2)	51	N/A	62*	80	None
33859	90	A	1(2)	51	N/A	62*	80	

* with documentation

Terms To Know

cardiopulmonary bypass. Venous blood is diverted to a heart-lung machine, which mechanically pumps and oxygenates the blood temporarily so the heart can be bypassed while an open procedure on the heart or coronary arteries is performed. During bypass, the lungs are deflated and immobile.

33863-33866

33863 Ascending aorta graft, with cardiopulmonary bypass, with aortic root replacement using valved conduit and coronary reconstruction (eg, Bentall)

33864 Ascending aorta graft, with cardiopulmonary bypass with valve suspension, with coronary reconstruction and valve-sparing aortic root remodeling (eg, David Procedure, Yacoub Procedure)

\+ **33866** Aortic hemiarch graft including isolation and control of the arch vessels, beveled open distal aortic anastomosis extending under one or more of the arch vessels, and total circulatory arrest or isolated cerebral perfusion (List separately in addition to code for primary procedure)

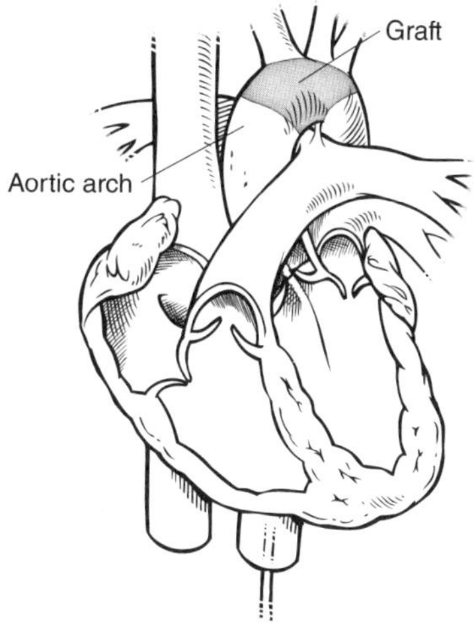

Graft of the aortic hemiarch isolates the arch vessels

Explanation

In 33863, the surgeon places an ascending aortic graft. The aorta is the largest artery in the body, extending from the heart through the chest and down into the abdomen. Cardiopulmonary bypass is required. Deep cooling of the body and circulatory arrest are often required, especially if the transverse arch of the aorta must be replaced. After circulatory arrest or if a cross-clamp can be placed on the aorta before its first branch, the aneurysm (an abnormally widened or weakened section of an artery) is opened. The hole in the aneurysm is lengthened along the aorta until the end of the aneurysm is reached. The aorta is divided at this point. A double layer of felt strips is placed circumferentially around the inner and outer circumference of the normal aorta with the aortic wall sandwiched in between. A Dacron tube graft is sewn to this end of the aorta and its felt layers. The aortic root is also replaced using a valved conduit and coronary reconstruction (e.g., Bentall procedure). In 33864, following induction of general anesthesia, the surgeon accesses the operative field via median sternotomy. Cardiopulmonary bypass is initiated. The coronary ostia are identified, detached from the aorta using dissecting scissors, and mobilized. After exposing the aneurysm site and clamping the artery above and below the aneurysm, the physician makes an incision into the aneurysm and removes any plaque deposits or clotted blood. The arterial section that is affected by the aneurysm is replaced with a synthetic graft. One end of the graft is attached to the arterial wall just above the beginning point of the aneurysm, while the other continues down through the artery to a point below the end of the aneurysm. The proximal coronary arteries are implanted into the aortic vascular graft. The physician performs a valve-sparing aortic root remodeling in which the dilated aortic root is replaced with a Dacron tube (graft) and the native aortic valve is integrated within the graft. The patient is taken off cardiopulmonary bypass and incisions are repaired. This procedure may be referred to as a David or Yacoub procedure in the operative note. When the patient's ascending aortic disease process includes the aortic arch requiring an aortic hemiarch graft, 33866 may be reported in addition to one of the procedures described above. This code describes three distinct elements: complete circulatory arrest or isolated cerebral retro- or antegrade perfusion, transverse arch incision performed under a single or multiple arch vessel(s) such as the left common carotid or innominate, and extending the ascending aortic graft beneath the aortic arch using a slanted or sloped (beveled) anastomosis. All three elements must be performed in order to use this code.

Coding Tips

Thoracic aortic aneurysm repair codes are dependent on aneurysm site: ascending, transverse arch, descending, or thoracoabdominal. Do not report an ascending aortic repair with a beveled anastomosis into the arch with a cross-clamp as a hemiarch graft using 33866. Report 33866 for aortic hemiarch graft when performed with ascending aortic graft codes 33858, 33859, 33863, or 33864. For a transverse arch graft, see 33871. For a descending thoracic aorta graft, see 33875. For repair of a thoracoabdominal aneurysm, see 33877. For direct repair of an aneurysm, a false aneurysm, or excision (partial or total) and graft insertion, with or without patch graft, of the abdominal aorta, see 35081 and 35091; for ruptured aneurysm, abdominal aorta, see 35082. Do not report 33863 with 33405, 33406, 33410–33413, 33858, or 33859. Do not report 33864 with 33858, 33859, or 33863. Do not report 33866 with 33871.

ICD-10-CM Diagnostic Codes

A52.01	Syphilitic aneurysm of aorta
A52.02	Syphilitic aortitis
I06.0	Rheumatic aortic stenosis
I06.1	Rheumatic aortic insufficiency
I06.2	Rheumatic aortic stenosis with insufficiency
I06.8	Other rheumatic aortic valve diseases
I08.0	Rheumatic disorders of both mitral and aortic valves
I08.2	Rheumatic disorders of both aortic and tricuspid valves
I08.3	Combined rheumatic disorders of mitral, aortic and tricuspid valves
I08.8	Other rheumatic multiple valve diseases
I35.0	Nonrheumatic aortic (valve) stenosis
I35.1	Nonrheumatic aortic (valve) insufficiency
I35.2	Nonrheumatic aortic (valve) stenosis with insufficiency
I35.8	Other nonrheumatic aortic valve disorders
I71.010	Dissection of ascending aorta
I71.011	Dissection of aortic arch
I71.012	Dissection of descending thoracic aorta
I71.11	Aneurysm of the ascending aorta, ruptured
I71.12	Aneurysm of the aortic arch, ruptured
I71.13	Aneurysm of the descending thoracic aorta, ruptured
I71.21	Aneurysm of the ascending aorta, without rupture
I71.22	Aneurysm of the aortic arch, without rupture
I71.23	Aneurysm of the descending thoracic aorta, without rupture
I79.0	Aneurysm of aorta in diseases classified elsewhere
Q23.0	Congenital stenosis of aortic valve
Q23.1	Congenital insufficiency of aortic valve
Q23.81	Bicuspid aortic valve
Q23.88	Other congenital malformations of aortic and mitral valves
Q25.1	Coarctation of aorta
Q25.3	Supravalvular aortic stenosis
Q25.41	Absence and aplasia of aorta
Q25.42	Hypoplasia of aorta
Q25.43	Congenital aneurysm of aorta
Q25.44	Congenital dilation of aorta
Q25.45	Double aortic arch
Q25.46	Tortuous aortic arch
Q25.47	Right aortic arch
Q25.48	Anomalous origin of subclavian artery
Q25.49	Other congenital malformations of aorta
Q25.8	Other congenital malformations of other great arteries
Q87.410	Marfan syndrome with aortic dilation

AMA: **33863** 2019,Nov **33864** 2019,Nov **33866** 2019,Nov

Relative Value Units/Medicare Edits

Non-Facility RVU	Work	PE	MP	Total
33863	58.79	19.32	14.07	92.18
33864	60.08	19.58	14.48	94.14
33866	17.75	4.88	4.25	26.88
Facility RVU	**Work**	**PE**	**MP**	**Total**
33863	58.79	19.32	14.07	92.18
33864	60.08	19.58	14.48	94.14
33866	17.75	4.88	4.25	26.88

	FUD	Status	MUE	Modifiers				IOM Reference
33863	90	A	1(2)	51	N/A	62*	80	None
33864	90	A	1(2)	51	N/A	62*	80	
33866	N/A	A	1(2)	N/A	N/A	N/A	80*	

* with documentation

33871

33871 Transverse aortic arch graft, with cardiopulmonary bypass, with profound hypothermia, total circulatory arrest and isolated cerebral perfusion with reimplantation of arch vessel(s) (eg, island pedicle or individual arch vessel reimplantation)

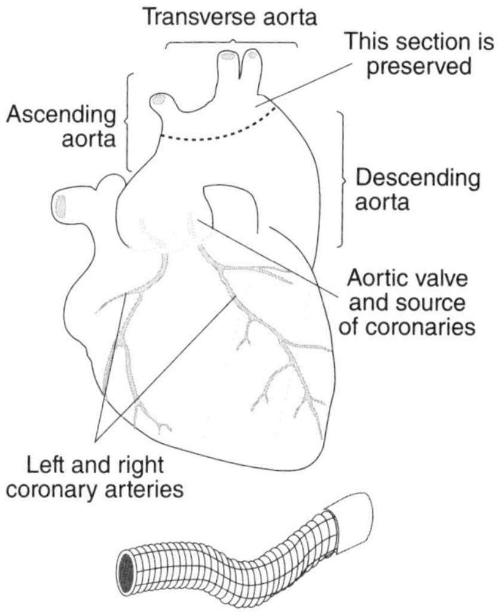

An aortic graft is placed and the transverse section containing the great arteries is sutured to it

Explanation

The physician performs a transverse aortic arch graft in which the entire aortic arch is replaced. This operation requires cardiopulmonary bypass, profound hypothermia, total circulatory arrest, and isolated cerebral perfusion. The patient's body temperature is lowered to 18 to 21 degrees centigrade and the bypass pump is stopped. The aneurysm is opened along its length and a patch of aortic wall containing the openings of the arteries to the head and arms is cut out. Each of these vessels will have been surrounded by tourniquets that were tightened before the bypass pump was stopped. The hole in the aneurysm is lengthened along the aorta until the end of the aneurysm is reached. The aorta is divided at this point. A double layer of felt strips is placed circumferentially around the inner and outer circumference of the normal aorta with the aortic wall sandwiched between. A Dacron tube graft is sewn to this end of the aorta and its felt layers. The aortic root where the aorta emerges from the heart is assessed. This area is where the aortic valve is located. If the valve closes normally, the aortic root size is reduced using stitches that also sew a double layer of felt to the aorta as previously described. Arch vessels are reimplanted individually or using an island pedicle. The physician closes the sternal incision and dresses the wound.

Coding Tips

Thoracic aortic aneurysm repair codes are dependent on aneurysm site: ascending, transverse arch, descending, or thoracoabdominal. For ascending aorta graft, see 33858, 33859, 33863, or 33864. For aortic hemiarch graft performed with ascending aortic graft, see 33866. For descending thoracic aorta graft, see 33875. For repair of a thoracoabdominal aneurysm, see 33877. For direct repair of an aneurysm, false aneurysm, or excision (partial or total) and graft insertion, with or without patch graft, of the abdominal aorta, see 35081–35103. Do not report 33871 with 33866.

ICD-10-CM Diagnostic Codes

A52.01	Syphilitic aneurysm of aorta
I71.010	Dissection of ascending aorta
I71.011	Dissection of aortic arch
I71.012	Dissection of descending thoracic aorta
I71.03	Dissection of thoracoabdominal aorta
I71.11	Aneurysm of the ascending aorta, ruptured
I71.12	Aneurysm of the aortic arch, ruptured
I71.13	Aneurysm of the descending thoracic aorta, ruptured
I71.21	Aneurysm of the ascending aorta, without rupture
I71.22	Aneurysm of the aortic arch, without rupture
I71.23	Aneurysm of the descending thoracic aorta, without rupture
I71.51	Supraceliac aneurysm of the thoracoabdominal aorta, ruptured
I71.52	Paravisceral aneurysm of the thoracoabdominal aorta, ruptured
I71.61	Supraceliac aneurysm of the thoracoabdominal aorta, without rupture
I71.62	Paravisceral aneurysm of the thoracoabdominal aorta, without rupture
I79.0	Aneurysm of aorta in diseases classified elsewhere
Q25.43	Congenital aneurysm of aorta

AMA: **33871** 2019,Nov

Relative Value Units/Medicare Edits

Non-Facility RVU	Work	PE	MP	Total
33871	60.88	19.92	14.62	95.42
Facility RVU	**Work**	**PE**	**MP**	**Total**
33871	60.88	19.92	14.62	95.42

	FUD	Status	MUE	Modifiers				IOM Reference
33871	90	A	1(2)	51	N/A	62*	80	None

* with documentation

Terms To Know

cardiopulmonary bypass. Venous blood is diverted to a heart-lung machine, which mechanically pumps and oxygenates the blood temporarily so the heart can be bypassed while an open procedure on the heart or coronary arteries is performed. During bypass, the lungs are deflated and immobile.

transverse. Crosswise at right angles to the long axis of a structure or part.

33875-33877

33875 Descending thoracic aorta graft, with or without bypass
33877 Repair of thoracoabdominal aortic aneurysm with graft, with or without cardiopulmonary bypass

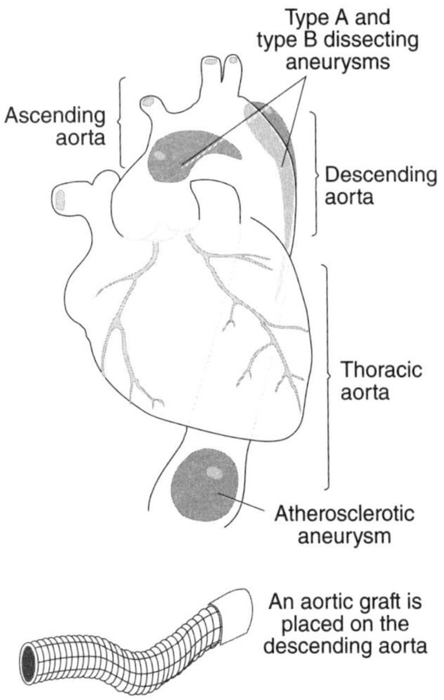

Explanation

A segment of the intrathoracic descending aorta is replaced with a tube of Dacron. This is done through an incision in the left chest cavity. The great concern in performing this operation is possible damage to the spinal cord. Preserving the spinal cord can be accomplished using a cardiopulmonary bypass circuit from above the aneurysm to below it, using deep cooling of the body and stopping the bypass machine, using perfusion of one or more spinal artery branches with blood pumped through it or using the "clamp and go" method in which no effort, except a speedy operation, is used to preserve the spinal cord. No matter what spinal cord preservation method is chosen, clamps are placed across the aorta above and below the aneurysm. The aneurysm is cut out and the ends of any small branches are closed with sutures. One end of a Dacron tube graft is sewn to the end of the aorta above the aneurysm and the other end of the graft is sewn to the aorta below the aneurysm. The clamps on the aorta are released. Report 33877 if aorta is exposed through the left chest.

Coding Tips

Thoracic aortic aneurysm repair codes are dependent on aneurysm site: ascending, transverse arch, descending, or thoracoabdominal. For ascending aorta graft, see 33858–33864. For transverse arch graft, see 33871. For direct repair of aneurysm, false aneurysm, or excision (partial or total) and graft insertion, with or without patch graft, of the abdominal aorta, see 35081–35103. Aneurysms of the thoracic aorta can also be performed endoscopically. For endoscopic repair of the descending thoracic aorta, see 33880–33891. For endoscopic repair of abdominal aortic aneurysm, see 34701–34848.

ICD-10-CM Diagnostic Codes

A52.01	Syphilitic aneurysm of aorta
A52.02	Syphilitic aortitis
I06.0	Rheumatic aortic stenosis
I06.1	Rheumatic aortic insufficiency
I06.2	Rheumatic aortic stenosis with insufficiency
I08.0	Rheumatic disorders of both mitral and aortic valves
I08.2	Rheumatic disorders of both aortic and tricuspid valves
I08.3	Combined rheumatic disorders of mitral, aortic and tricuspid valves
I08.8	Other rheumatic multiple valve diseases
I35.0	Nonrheumatic aortic (valve) stenosis
I35.1	Nonrheumatic aortic (valve) insufficiency
I35.2	Nonrheumatic aortic (valve) stenosis with insufficiency
I35.8	Other nonrheumatic aortic valve disorders
I71.010	Dissection of ascending aorta
I71.011	Dissection of aortic arch
I71.012	Dissection of descending thoracic aorta
I71.03	Dissection of thoracoabdominal aorta
I71.11	Aneurysm of the ascending aorta, ruptured
I71.12	Aneurysm of the aortic arch, ruptured
I71.13	Aneurysm of the descending thoracic aorta, ruptured
I71.21	Aneurysm of the ascending aorta, without rupture
I71.22	Aneurysm of the aortic arch, without rupture
I71.23	Aneurysm of the descending thoracic aorta, without rupture
I71.51	Supraceliac aneurysm of the thoracoabdominal aorta, ruptured
I71.52	Paravisceral aneurysm of the thoracoabdominal aorta, ruptured
I71.61	Supraceliac aneurysm of the thoracoabdominal aorta, without rupture
I71.62	Paravisceral aneurysm of the thoracoabdominal aorta, without rupture
I74.11	Embolism and thrombosis of thoracic aorta
I74.19	Embolism and thrombosis of other parts of aorta
I77.810	Thoracic aortic ectasia
I77.812	Thoracoabdominal aortic ectasia
I77.89	Other specified disorders of arteries and arterioles
I79.0	Aneurysm of aorta in diseases classified elsewhere
Q23.0	Congenital stenosis of aortic valve
Q23.1	Congenital insufficiency of aortic valve
Q23.81	Bicuspid aortic valve
Q23.88	Other congenital malformations of aortic and mitral valves
Q25.1	Coarctation of aorta
Q25.3	Supravalvular aortic stenosis
Q25.41	Absence and aplasia of aorta
Q25.42	Hypoplasia of aorta
Q25.43	Congenital aneurysm of aorta
Q25.44	Congenital dilation of aorta
Q25.45	Double aortic arch
Q25.46	Tortuous aortic arch
Q25.47	Right aortic arch
Q25.48	Anomalous origin of subclavian artery
Q25.49	Other congenital malformations of aorta
Q25.8	Other congenital malformations of other great arteries
Q87.410	Marfan syndrome with aortic dilation
Q87.418	Marfan syndrome with other cardiovascular manifestations
S25.01XA	Minor laceration of thoracic aorta, initial encounter
S25.02XA	Major laceration of thoracic aorta, initial encounter

S25.09XA Other specified injury of thoracic aorta, initial encounter
S26.01XA Contusion of heart with hemopericardium, initial encounter
S26.020A Mild laceration of heart with hemopericardium, initial encounter
S26.021A Moderate laceration of heart with hemopericardium, initial encounter
S26.022A Major laceration of heart with hemopericardium, initial encounter
S26.09XA Other injury of heart with hemopericardium, initial encounter
S26.11XA Contusion of heart without hemopericardium, initial encounter
S26.12XA Laceration of heart without hemopericardium, initial encounter
S26.19XA Other injury of heart without hemopericardium, initial encounter

AMA: **33875** 2019,Nov **33877** 2019,Nov

Relative Value Units/Medicare Edits

Non-Facility RVU	Work	PE	MP	Total
33875	50.72	17.57	12.25	80.54
33877	69.03	19.79	16.81	105.63
Facility RVU	**Work**	**PE**	**MP**	**Total**
33875	50.72	17.57	12.25	80.54
33877	69.03	19.79	16.81	105.63

	FUD	Status	MUE	Modifiers				IOM Reference
33875	90	A	1(2)	51	N/A	62	80	None
33877	90	A	1(2)	51	N/A	62	80	

* with documentation

Terms To Know

aneurysm. Circumscribed dilation or outpouching of an artery wall, often containing blood clots and connecting directly with the lumen of the artery.

cardiopulmonary bypass. Venous blood is diverted to a heart-lung machine, which mechanically pumps and oxygenates the blood temporarily so the heart can be bypassed while an open procedure on the heart or coronary arteries is performed. During bypass, the lungs are deflated and immobile.

33880-33881

33880 Endovascular repair of descending thoracic aorta (eg, aneurysm, pseudoaneurysm, dissection, penetrating ulcer, intramural hematoma, or traumatic disruption); involving coverage of left subclavian artery origin, initial endoprosthesis plus descending thoracic aortic extension(s), if required, to level of celiac artery origin

33881 not involving coverage of left subclavian artery origin, initial endoprosthesis plus descending thoracic aortic extension(s), if required, to level of celiac artery origin

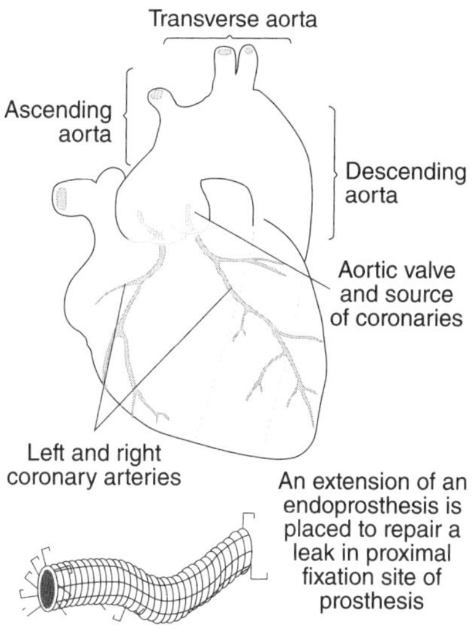

This procedure is performed by threading the prosthesis through the patient's vessels rather than through an open approach

Explanation

The physician repairs the descending thoracic aorta by placing an endoprosthesis from within the artery. Endovascular repair may be performed for an aneurysm, pseudoaneurysm, dissection, penetrating ulcer, intramural hematoma, or traumatic disruption. The defect in the descending thoracic aorta is identified using aortography. The endoprosthesis, contained inside a holding device, is introduced into the artery under fluoroscopy and positioned at the target zone area of repair. Extension prostheses may be required to the level of the celiac artery origin. When the endoprosthesis is in position, it is deployed within the artery at the target site in the descending thoracic aorta, covering the origin of the left subclavian artery in 33880. A balloon angioplasty may be necessary to achieve proper positioning and functioning of the endoprosthesis. The placement position is confirmed, the catheter is removed, and the arteriotomy site is closed. Report 33880 when the repair covers the left subclavian artery origin and 33881 when the repair does not cover the left subclavian artery origin.

Coding Tips

These codes include all device introduction, manipulation, positioning, and deployment. Balloon angioplasty and/or stent deployment is not reported separately. Open arterial exposure, introduction of guidewires and catheters, and extensive repair or replacement of an artery should be reported separately. Report transposition of subclavian to carotid (33889) and carotid-carotid bypass (33891) separately. These codes include distal extensions in the distal thoracic aorta, but proximal extensions (33883–33884) are reported separately. For radiological supervision and interpretation, see 75956–75957.

ICD-10-CM Diagnostic Codes

A52.01 Syphilitic aneurysm of aorta
A52.02 Syphilitic aortitis
I71.010 Dissection of ascending aorta
I71.011 Dissection of aortic arch
I71.012 Dissection of descending thoracic aorta
I71.03 Dissection of thoracoabdominal aorta
I71.11 Aneurysm of the ascending aorta, ruptured
I71.12 Aneurysm of the aortic arch, ruptured
I71.13 Aneurysm of the descending thoracic aorta, ruptured
I71.21 Aneurysm of the ascending aorta, without rupture
I71.22 Aneurysm of the aortic arch, without rupture
I71.23 Aneurysm of the descending thoracic aorta, without rupture
I71.51 Supraceliac aneurysm of the thoracoabdominal aorta, ruptured
I71.52 Paravisceral aneurysm of the thoracoabdominal aorta, ruptured
I71.61 Supraceliac aneurysm of the thoracoabdominal aorta, without rupture
I71.62 Paravisceral aneurysm of the thoracoabdominal aorta, without rupture
I74.11 Embolism and thrombosis of thoracic aorta
I74.19 Embolism and thrombosis of other parts of aorta
I77.810 Thoracic aortic ectasia
I77.812 Thoracoabdominal aortic ectasia
I77.89 Other specified disorders of arteries and arterioles
I79.0 Aneurysm of aorta in diseases classified elsewhere
Q25.41 Absence and aplasia of aorta
Q25.42 Hypoplasia of aorta
Q25.43 Congenital aneurysm of aorta
Q25.44 Congenital dilation of aorta
Q25.45 Double aortic arch
Q25.46 Tortuous aortic arch
Q25.47 Right aortic arch
Q25.48 Anomalous origin of subclavian artery
Q25.49 Other congenital malformations of aorta
Q25.8 Other congenital malformations of other great arteries
S25.01XA Minor laceration of thoracic aorta, initial encounter
S25.02XA Major laceration of thoracic aorta, initial encounter
S25.09XA Other specified injury of thoracic aorta, initial encounter
S25.112A Minor laceration of left innominate or subclavian artery, initial encounter ☑
S25.122A Major laceration of left innominate or subclavian artery, initial encounter ☑
S25.192A Other specified injury of left innominate or subclavian artery, initial encounter ☑
S26.01XA Contusion of heart with hemopericardium, initial encounter
S26.020A Mild laceration of heart with hemopericardium, initial encounter
S26.021A Moderate laceration of heart with hemopericardium, initial encounter
S26.022A Major laceration of heart with hemopericardium, initial encounter
S26.09XA Other injury of heart with hemopericardium, initial encounter
S26.11XA Contusion of heart without hemopericardium, initial encounter
S26.12XA Laceration of heart without hemopericardium, initial encounter
S26.19XA Other injury of heart without hemopericardium, initial encounter
S35.211A Minor laceration of celiac artery, initial encounter
S35.212A Major laceration of celiac artery, initial encounter
S35.218A Other injury of celiac artery, initial encounter

Relative Value Units/Medicare Edits

Non-Facility RVU	Work	PE	MP	Total
33880	34.58	9.34	8.34	52.26
33881	29.58	8.16	7.15	44.89
Facility RVU	**Work**	**PE**	**MP**	**Total**
33880	34.58	9.34	8.34	52.26
33881	29.58	8.16	7.15	44.89

	FUD	Status	MUE	Modifiers				IOM Reference
33880	90	A	1(2)	51	N/A	62	80	None
33881	90	A	1(2)	51	N/A	62	80	

* with documentation

Terms To Know

aneurysm. Circumscribed dilation or outpouching of an artery wall, often containing blood clots and connecting directly with the lumen of the artery.

angioplasty. Reconstruction or repair of a diseased or damaged blood vessel.

angioplasty balloon. Balloon-tipped medical device used to clear the blockage of an artery. After insertion into the clogged artery, the balloon is inflated to expand a narrowing arterial section.

balloon catheter. Any catheter equipped with an inflatable balloon at the end to hold it in place in a body cavity or to be used for dilation of a vessel lumen.

embolism. Obstruction of a blood vessel resulting from a clot or foreign substance.

thrombosis. Condition arising from the presence or formation of blood clots within a blood vessel that may cause vascular obstruction and insufficient oxygenation.

33883-33884

33883 Placement of proximal extension prosthesis for endovascular repair of descending thoracic aorta (eg, aneurysm, pseudoaneurysm, dissection, penetrating ulcer, intramural hematoma, or traumatic disruption); initial extension

\+ **33884** each additional proximal extension (List separately in addition to code for primary procedure)

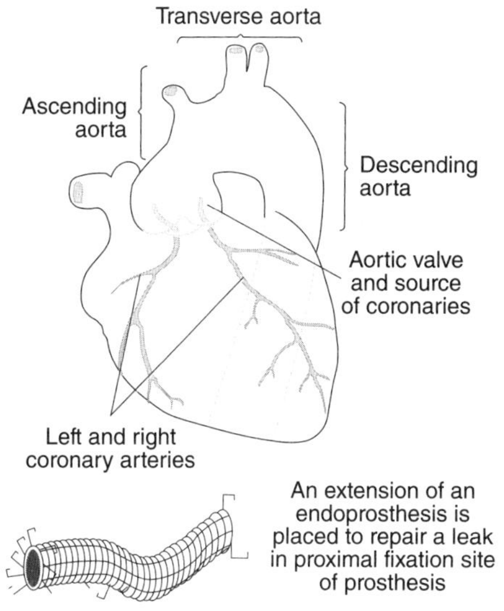

This procedure is performed by threading the prosthesis through the patient's vessels rather than through an open approach

Explanation

A leak, called an endoleak, may occur at the proximal fixation sites of a grafted descending thoracic aorta defect through the body of the graft or from patent arteries within the defect and may require endovascular repair. A proximal extension prosthesis is placed endovascularly to repair an endoleak in a grafted descending thoracic aortic aneurysm, pseudoaneurysm, dissection, penetrating ulcer, intramural hematoma, or traumatic disruption. The target site is identified by aortography and the proper extension prosthesis is selected. Under fluoroscopy, the extension prosthesis, contained inside a long plastic holding capsule, is threaded through the arteries to the site of the leak. Once the extension prosthesis is in place, the holding capsule is removed. The extension prosthesis, activated by heat, expands like a spring and becomes anchored to the artery wall at the site of the endoleak. If full expansion of the prosthesis does not occur automatically, a balloon catheter is threaded to the graft site and inflated within the endovascular prosthesis until full expansion is achieved. The placement position is confirmed, the catheter is removed, and the arteriotomy site is closed. Report 33883 for an initial proximal extension and 33884 for each additional proximal extension.

Coding Tips

Report 33884 in addition to 33883. These codes include all device introduction, manipulation, positioning, and deployment. Balloon angioplasty and/or stent deployment is not reported separately. Open arterial exposure, introduction of guidewires and catheters, and extensive repair or replacement of an artery should be reported separately. For radiological supervision and interpretation, see 75958.

ICD-10-CM Diagnostic Codes

A52.01	Syphilitic aneurysm of aorta
A52.02	Syphilitic aortitis
I71.010	Dissection of ascending aorta
I71.011	Dissection of aortic arch
I71.012	Dissection of descending thoracic aorta
I71.03	Dissection of thoracoabdominal aorta
I71.13	Aneurysm of the descending thoracic aorta, ruptured
I71.21	Aneurysm of the ascending aorta, without rupture
I71.22	Aneurysm of the aortic arch, without rupture
I71.23	Aneurysm of the descending thoracic aorta, without rupture
I74.11	Embolism and thrombosis of thoracic aorta
I74.19	Embolism and thrombosis of other parts of aorta
I77.810	Thoracic aortic ectasia
I77.812	Thoracoabdominal aortic ectasia
I77.89	Other specified disorders of arteries and arterioles
I79.0	Aneurysm of aorta in diseases classified elsewhere
Q25.41	Absence and aplasia of aorta
Q25.42	Hypoplasia of aorta
Q25.43	Congenital aneurysm of aorta
Q25.44	Congenital dilation of aorta
Q25.45	Double aortic arch
Q25.46	Tortuous aortic arch
Q25.47	Right aortic arch
Q25.48	Anomalous origin of subclavian artery
Q25.49	Other congenital malformations of aorta
Q25.8	Other congenital malformations of other great arteries
S25.01XA	Minor laceration of thoracic aorta, initial encounter
S25.02XA	Major laceration of thoracic aorta, initial encounter
S25.09XA	Other specified injury of thoracic aorta, initial encounter
S26.01XA	Contusion of heart with hemopericardium, initial encounter
S26.020A	Mild laceration of heart with hemopericardium, initial encounter
S26.021A	Moderate laceration of heart with hemopericardium, initial encounter
S26.022A	Major laceration of heart with hemopericardium, initial encounter
S26.09XA	Other injury of heart with hemopericardium, initial encounter
S26.11XA	Contusion of heart without hemopericardium, initial encounter
S26.12XA	Laceration of heart without hemopericardium, initial encounter
S26.19XA	Other injury of heart without hemopericardium, initial encounter

Relative Value Units/Medicare Edits

Non-Facility RVU	Work	PE	MP	Total
33883	21.09	6.44	5.05	32.58
33884	8.2	1.28	2.04	11.52
Facility RVU	**Work**	**PE**	**MP**	**Total**
33883	21.09	6.44	5.05	32.58
33884	8.2	1.28	2.04	11.52

	FUD	Status	MUE	Modifiers				IOM Reference
33883	90	A	1(2)	51	N/A	62	80	None
33884	N/A	A	2(3)	N/A	N/A	62	80	

* with documentation

33886

33886 Placement of distal extension prosthesis(s) delayed after endovascular repair of descending thoracic aorta

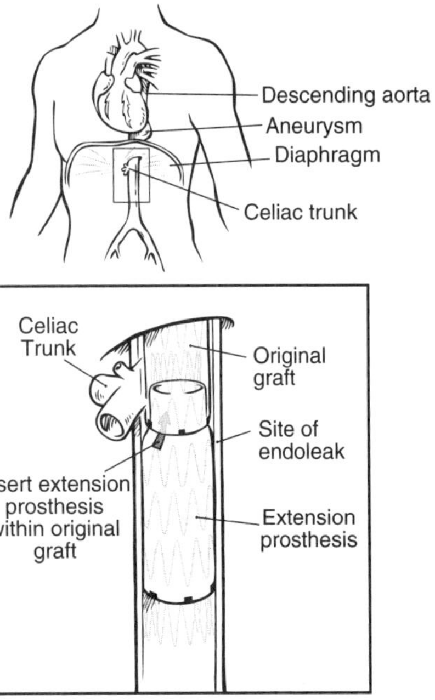

Repair of endoleak in descending thoracic aorta

Explanation

A leak, called an endoleak, may occur at the distal fixation sites of a previously grafted descending thoracic aorta defect through the body of the graft or from patent arteries within the defect and may require endovascular repair. One or more distal extension prosthesis modules are placed endovascularly to the level of the celiac artery to repair an endoleak in a previously grafted descending thoracic aortic aneurysm, pseudoaneurysm, dissection, penetrating ulcer, intramural hematoma, or traumatic disruption. The target site is identified by aortography and the proper extension prosthesis is selected. Under fluoroscopy, the extension prosthesis, contained inside a long plastic holding capsule, is threaded through the arteries to the site of the leak. Once the extension prosthesis is in place, the holding capsule is removed. The extension prosthesis, activated by heat, expands like a spring and becomes anchored to the artery wall at the site of the endoleak. If full expansion of the prosthesis does not occur automatically, a balloon catheter is threaded to the graft site and inflated within the endovascular prosthesis until full expansion is achieved. The placement position is confirmed, the catheter is removed, and the arteriotomy site is closed. This code is reported only once regardless of the number of extension modules deployed.

Coding Tips

This code includes all device introduction, manipulation, positioning, and deployment. Balloon angioplasty and/or stent deployment is not reported separately. Do not report 33886 with 33880 or 33881. Report 33886 once, regardless of the number of modules deployed. Open arterial exposure, introduction of guidewires and catheters, and extensive repair or replacement of an artery should be reported separately. For radiological supervision and interpretation, see 75959.

ICD-10-CM Diagnostic Codes

A52.01 Syphilitic aneurysm of aorta
A52.02 Syphilitic aortitis
I71.012 Dissection of descending thoracic aorta
I71.03 Dissection of thoracoabdominal aorta
I71.13 Aneurysm of the descending thoracic aorta, ruptured
I71.23 Aneurysm of the descending thoracic aorta, without rupture
I71.51 Supraceliac aneurysm of the thoracoabdominal aorta, ruptured
I71.52 Paravisceral aneurysm of the thoracoabdominal aorta, ruptured
I71.61 Supraceliac aneurysm of the thoracoabdominal aorta, without rupture
I71.62 Paravisceral aneurysm of the thoracoabdominal aorta, without rupture
I74.11 Embolism and thrombosis of thoracic aorta
I74.19 Embolism and thrombosis of other parts of aorta
I77.810 Thoracic aortic ectasia
I77.812 Thoracoabdominal aortic ectasia
I77.89 Other specified disorders of arteries and arterioles
I79.0 Aneurysm of aorta in diseases classified elsewhere
Q25.41 Absence and aplasia of aorta
Q25.42 Hypoplasia of aorta
Q25.43 Congenital aneurysm of aorta
Q25.44 Congenital dilation of aorta
Q25.45 Double aortic arch
Q25.46 Tortuous aortic arch
Q25.47 Right aortic arch
Q25.48 Anomalous origin of subclavian artery
Q25.49 Other congenital malformations of aorta
S25.01XA Minor laceration of thoracic aorta, initial encounter
S25.02XA Major laceration of thoracic aorta, initial encounter
S25.09XA Other specified injury of thoracic aorta, initial encounter
S26.01XA Contusion of heart with hemopericardium, initial encounter
S26.020A Mild laceration of heart with hemopericardium, initial encounter
S26.021A Moderate laceration of heart with hemopericardium, initial encounter
S26.022A Major laceration of heart with hemopericardium, initial encounter
S26.09XA Other injury of heart with hemopericardium, initial encounter
S26.11XA Contusion of heart without hemopericardium, initial encounter
S26.12XA Laceration of heart without hemopericardium, initial encounter
S26.19XA Other injury of heart without hemopericardium, initial encounter

Relative Value Units/Medicare Edits

Non-Facility RVU	Work	PE	MP	Total
33886	18.09	5.65	4.39	28.13
Facility RVU	**Work**	**PE**	**MP**	**Total**
33886	18.09	5.65	4.39	28.13

	FUD	Status	MUE	Modifiers				IOM Reference
33886	90	A	1(2)	51	N/A	62	80	None

* with documentation

33889

33889 Open subclavian to carotid artery transposition performed in conjunction with endovascular repair of descending thoracic aorta, by neck incision, unilateral

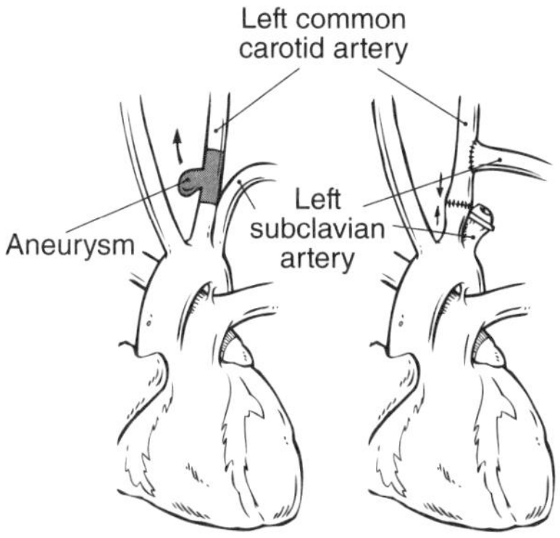

The left subclavian artery is anastomosed to the side of the left common carotid artery

Explanation

The physician performs a unilateral open subclavian to carotid artery transposition in conjunction with endovascular repair of the descending aorta. The physician performs a 2 to 3 cm supraclavicular incision to gain access to the carotid and subclavian arteries. The clavicular section of the sternocleidomastoid muscle is partially divided exposing the phrenic nerve, which is identified and avoided. The physician clears the adventitia of the chosen translocation site in the wall of the common carotid artery. The section of artery where the aneurysm occurs is isolated and dissected from adjacent structures. Vessel clamps are affixed above and below the defect. The repair is accomplished by excising the segment containing the aneurysm. The vessel ends are sutured in an end-to-end fashion. Next, the subclavian artery is transposed and anastomosed to the common carotid artery in an end-to-side fashion. Vessel clamps are removed and the incision is closed with layered sutures.

Coding Tips

Report 33889 in addition to 33880 or 33881 when an open subclavian-to-carotid artery transposition is performed during the same surgical session as the endovascular repair of the descending thoracic aorta. Do not report 33889 with 35694.

ICD-10-CM Diagnostic Codes

G45.1	Carotid artery syndrome (hemispheric)
I63.031	Cerebral infarction due to thrombosis of right carotid artery ☑
I63.131	Cerebral infarction due to embolism of right carotid artery ☑
I63.81	Other cerebral infarction due to occlusion or stenosis of small artery
I63.89	Other cerebral infarction
I65.21	Occlusion and stenosis of right carotid artery ☑
I70.0	Atherosclerosis of aorta [A]
I70.8	Atherosclerosis of other arteries [A]
I71.012	Dissection of descending thoracic aorta
I71.13	Aneurysm of the descending thoracic aorta, ruptured
I71.23	Aneurysm of the descending thoracic aorta, without rupture
I72.0	Aneurysm of carotid artery
I72.6	Aneurysm of vertebral artery
I77.1	Stricture of artery
I77.71	Dissection of carotid artery
I77.76	Dissection of artery of upper extremity
Q25.21	Interruption of aortic arch
Q25.3	Supravalvular aortic stenosis
Q25.41	Absence and aplasia of aorta
Q25.42	Hypoplasia of aorta
Q25.43	Congenital aneurysm of aorta
Q25.44	Congenital dilation of aorta
Q25.45	Double aortic arch
Q25.46	Tortuous aortic arch
Q25.47	Right aortic arch
Q25.48	Anomalous origin of subclavian artery
Q25.49	Other congenital malformations of aorta
Q25.8	Other congenital malformations of other great arteries
S15.011A	Minor laceration of right carotid artery, initial encounter ☑
S15.012A	Minor laceration of left carotid artery, initial encounter ☑
S15.021A	Major laceration of right carotid artery, initial encounter ☑
S15.022A	Major laceration of left carotid artery, initial encounter ☑
S15.091A	Other specified injury of right carotid artery, initial encounter ☑
S15.092A	Other specified injury of left carotid artery, initial encounter ☑

Relative Value Units/Medicare Edits

Non-Facility RVU	Work	PE	MP	Total
33889	15.92	3.37	3.93	23.22
Facility RVU	**Work**	**PE**	**MP**	**Total**
33889	15.92	3.37	3.93	23.22

	FUD	Status	MUE	Modifiers				IOM Reference
33889	0	A	1(2)	51	50	62	80	None

* with documentation

Terms To Know

aneurysm. Circumscribed dilation or outpouching of an artery wall, often containing blood clots and connecting directly with the lumen of the artery.

stenosis. Narrowing or constriction of a passage.

stricture. Narrowing of an anatomical structure.

33891

33891 Bypass graft, with other than vein, transcervical retropharyngeal carotid-carotid, performed in conjunction with endovascular repair of descending thoracic aorta, by neck incision

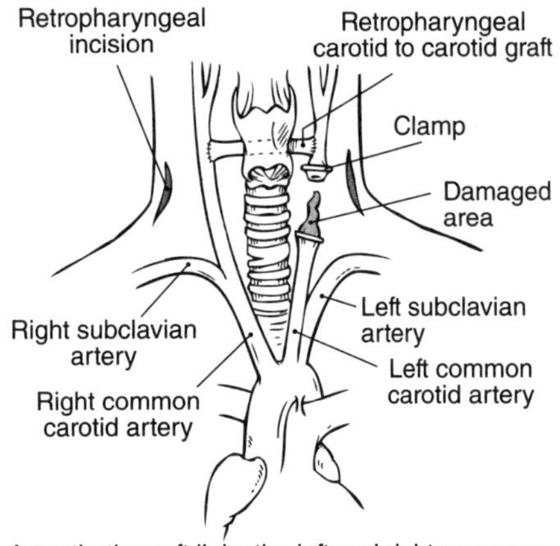

A synthetic graft links the left and right common carotid arteries as an adjunct to an endovascular repair of the descending thoracic aorta

Explanation

The physician performs a transcervical retropharyngeal carotid-to-carotid bypass graft with other than vein in conjunction with endovascular repair of the descending thoracic aorta. Through incisions in the neck, the physician isolates and dissects the common carotid arteries, separating them from adjacent critical structures. The physician creates a bypass around a section of carotid artery that is damaged or blocked using a synthetic vein graft and one of two methods of repair. After vessel clamps have been affixed above and below the damaged area, the ends of the synthetic vein graft are sutured into the side of the carotid arterial wall (end-to-side). In the second method, the carotid artery may be cut above the damaged area and sutured to one end of a synthetic vein graft, which is sutured to the side of the carotid artery on the opposite side of the neck (end-to-end). In either case, the blocked or damaged section of artery is not removed. When the clamps are removed, the synthetic vein graft forms a new path through which blood can easily bypass the blocked or damaged area. After the graft procedure is completed, the skin incisions are repaired with layered sutures.

Coding Tips

Report 33891 in addition to 33880 and 33881 when an open carotid-to-carotid artery bypass graft with other than vein is performed during the same surgical session as the endovascular repair of the descending thoracic aorta. Do not report 33891 with 35509 or 35601.

ICD-10-CM Diagnostic Codes

G45.1	Carotid artery syndrome (hemispheric)
G45.8	Other transient cerebral ischemic attacks and related syndromes
I63.031	Cerebral infarction due to thrombosis of right carotid artery ☑
I63.032	Cerebral infarction due to thrombosis of left carotid artery ☑
I63.131	Cerebral infarction due to embolism of right carotid artery ☑
I63.132	Cerebral infarction due to embolism of left carotid artery ☑
I63.19	Cerebral infarction due to embolism of other precerebral artery
I63.81	Other cerebral infarction due to occlusion or stenosis of small artery
I63.89	Other cerebral infarction
I65.21	Occlusion and stenosis of right carotid artery ☑
I65.22	Occlusion and stenosis of left carotid artery ☑
I65.23	Occlusion and stenosis of bilateral carotid arteries ☑
I70.0	Atherosclerosis of aorta [A]
I70.8	Atherosclerosis of other arteries [A]
I71.010	Dissection of ascending aorta
I71.012	Dissection of descending thoracic aorta
I71.13	Aneurysm of the descending thoracic aorta, ruptured
I71.23	Aneurysm of the descending thoracic aorta, without rupture
I72.0	Aneurysm of carotid artery
I72.5	Aneurysm of other precerebral arteries
I72.6	Aneurysm of vertebral artery
I72.8	Aneurysm of other specified arteries
I77.1	Stricture of artery
I77.71	Dissection of carotid artery
I77.75	Dissection of other precerebral arteries
I77.76	Dissection of artery of upper extremity
I77.77	Dissection of artery of lower extremity
Q25.21	Interruption of aortic arch
Q25.41	Absence and aplasia of aorta
Q25.42	Hypoplasia of aorta
Q25.43	Congenital aneurysm of aorta
Q25.44	Congenital dilation of aorta
Q25.45	Double aortic arch
Q25.46	Tortuous aortic arch
Q25.47	Right aortic arch
S15.011A	Minor laceration of right carotid artery, initial encounter ☑
S15.012A	Minor laceration of left carotid artery, initial encounter ☑
S15.021A	Major laceration of right carotid artery, initial encounter ☑
S15.022A	Major laceration of left carotid artery, initial encounter ☑
S15.091A	Other specified injury of right carotid artery, initial encounter ☑
S15.092A	Other specified injury of left carotid artery, initial encounter ☑

Relative Value Units/Medicare Edits

Non-Facility RVU	Work	PE	MP	Total
33891	20.0	3.11	4.97	28.08
Facility RVU	**Work**	**PE**	**MP**	**Total**
33891	20.0	3.11	4.97	28.08

	FUD	Status	MUE	Modifiers				IOM Reference
33891	0	A	1(2)	51	50	62	80	None

* with documentation

33894-33895

33894 Endovascular stent repair of coarctation of the ascending, transverse, or descending thoracic or abdominal aorta, involving stent placement; across major side branches

33895 Endovascular stent repair of coarctation of the ascending, transverse, or descending thoracic or abdominal aorta, involving stent placement; not crossing major side branches

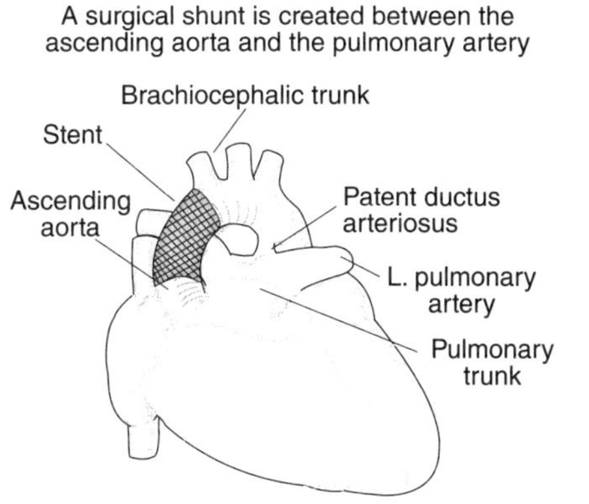

Stent placement for coarctation of ascending aorta

Explanation

The physician places an endovascular stent to repair a narrowing (coarctation) of the ascending, descending, or transverse thoracic or abdominal aorta. The aorta, the largest artery in the body, moves oxygen enriched blood from the heart to the rest of the body. Coarctation of the aorta (CoA), which is usually present at birth, forces the heart to work harder to pump blood through the aorta. Following anesthesia, the physician gains arterial access, typically via the femoral artery. A second arterial access via the brachial or radial artery may also be required for antegrade catheterization of the aortic coarctation. IV heparin is administered, and a multipurpose catheter is advanced into the descending aorta, followed by a soft-tipped glide wire through the CoA site. The catheter is replaced over the wire by a pigtail or multitrack catheter and peak pressure gradient (PPG) is obtained. Angiography is obtained and measurements are made at various points of the aorta to determine the most appropriate stent and balloon size. The soft-tipped wire is exchanged for a stiffer exchange wire, which is secured in the ascending aorta or right subclavian artery. The physician advances a long sheath from the femoral artery site and places it across the CoA segment for stent deployment. The stent is hand-crimped on the balloon catheter and the stent/balloon assembly is advanced through the sheath over the stiff wire and positioned across the CoA site. The physician withdraws the sheath enough to uncover the stent/balloon and confirms the correct position, repositioning the stent, if necessary, prior to inflation. Balloons are deflated and the balloon catheter removed over the wire while the sheath is maintained in position. Following stent deployment, another PPG across the CoA is obtained, and a final angiogram is performed to evaluate the final result and to assure there are no complications such as aortic wall injury. Report 33894 if the procedure is performed across major aortic side branches; report 33895 if no major side branches are crossed.

Coding Tips

These codes include fluoroscopic guidance for the intervention, catheter/wire introduction and manipulation, diagnostic congenital left heart catheterization, and angiography of the target lesion. Temporary pacemaker insertion for rapid pacing to facilitate stent positioning or balloon angioplasty within the treatment area before or after the stent deployment is not reported separately. For balloon angioplasty of an additional coarctation of the aorta outside of the treatment area for the coarctation stent, see 33897. Report 37236 or 37246 for balloon angioplasty or stenting of the aorta for lesions other than coarctation of the aorta in a segment separate from the coarctation treatment zone. Carotid, iliac, innominate, subclavian, visceral, or pulmonary artery balloon angioplasty or stenting, or arterial or venous embolization, may be reported separately when performed before or after the coarctation stent placement. Do not report these codes with 33210, 34701-34706, 36200, 75600, 75605, 75625, 93567, or 93595-93597. Do not report these codes with 33897, 37236, or 37246 for aortic balloon angioplasty or stenting within the coarctation stent treatment area. For additional diagnostic right heart catheterization at the same setting, see 93593 and 93594.

ICD-10-CM Diagnostic Codes

Q25.1 Coarctation of aorta

AMA: **33894** 2023,Jun; 2023,May; 2021,Dec **33895** 2023,Jun; 2023,May; 2021,Dec

Relative Value Units/Medicare Edits

Non-Facility RVU	Work	PE	MP	Total
33894	18.27	6.22	4.22	28.71
33895	14.54	4.95	3.36	22.85
Facility RVU	**Work**	**PE**	**MP**	**Total**
33894	18.27	6.22	4.22	28.71
33895	14.54	4.95	3.36	22.85

	FUD	Status	MUE	Modifiers				IOM Reference
33894	0	A	1(3)	51	N/A	N/A	80*	None
33895	0	A	1(3)	51	N/A	N/A	80*	

* with documentation

Terms To Know

angiography. Radiographic imaging of the arteries. Imaging may be performed to study the vasculature of any given organ, body system, or area of circulation such as the brain, heart, chest, kidneys, limbs, gastrointestinal tract, aorta, and pulmonary circulation to visualize the formation and the function of the blood vessels to detect problems such as a blockage or stricture. A catheter is inserted through an accessible blood vessel and the artery is injected with a radiopaque contrast material after which x-rays are taken.

coarctation of aorta. Localized deformation of the aortic media that causes a severe constriction of the vessel, resulting in high blood pressure in the arms and low pressure in the legs. This condition must be treated to prevent a cerebrovascular accident, endocarditis, congestive heart failure, or rupture of the aorta.

stent. Tube to provide support in a body cavity or lumen.

33897

33897 Percutaneous transluminal angioplasty of native or recurrent coarctation of the aorta

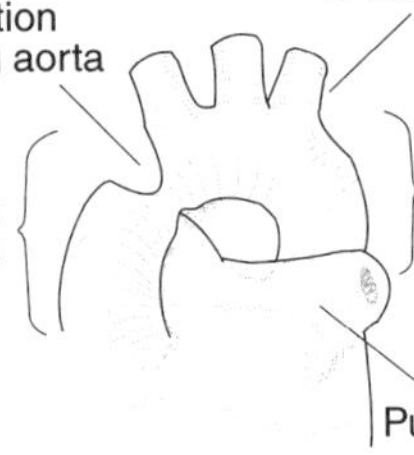

Angioplasty of coarctation of aorta

Explanation

The physician performs percutaneous transluminal angioplasty (PTA) of a native or recurrent coarctation of the aorta (CoA). Cardiac catheterization and selective angiography are first performed to confirm the clinical diagnosis, exclude other defects, and evaluate the suitability for balloon angioplasty. The aorta, the largest artery in the body, moves oxygen-enriched blood from the heart to the rest of the body. Coarctation, which is usually present at birth, forces the heart to work harder to pump blood through the aorta. Following appropriate sedation, the physician gains access percutaneously via the femoral artery, introduces the catheter, and positions it across the aortic coarctation. A guidewire is passed through the catheter into the ascending aorta, where the tip is positioned. The physician then positions a balloon angioplasty catheter across the coarctation and inflates it with diluted contrast material while monitoring the pressure of inflation. The balloon is inflated for five second intervals; typically, a total of two to four inflations are performed approximately five minutes apart. Aortography is performed, as well as pressure gradient measurements across the CoA. Heartrate, systemic pressure, and cardiac index are recorded before and approximately 15 minutes following balloon dilation to confirm that the change in pressure gradient is dilation-related and not merely a change in patient status.

Coding Tips

Report 37236 or 37246 for balloon angioplasty or stenting of the aorta for lesions other than coarctation of the aorta in a segment separate from the coarctation treatment zone. Do not report 33897 with 33210, 34701-34706, 36200, 75600, 75605, 75625, 93567, or 93595-93597. Do not report 33897 with 37236 or 37246 for aortic balloon angioplasty or stenting within the coarctation stent treatment area. Do not report 33897 with 33894 or 33895 for aortic balloon angioplasty within the coarctation stent treatment area. For additional diagnostic right heart catheterization at the same setting, see 93593 and 93594.

ICD-10-CM Diagnostic Codes

Q25.1 Coarctation of aorta

AMA: 33897 2023,Jun; 2021,Dec

Relative Value Units/Medicare Edits

Non-Facility RVU	Work	PE	MP	Total
33897	10.81	3.68	2.49	16.98
Facility RVU	**Work**	**PE**	**MP**	**Total**
33897	10.81	3.68	2.49	16.98

	FUD	Status	MUE	Modifiers				IOM Reference
33897	0	A	1(3)	51	N/A	N/A	80*	None

* with documentation

Terms To Know

coarctation of aorta. Localized deformation of the aortic media that causes a severe constriction of the vessel, resulting in high blood pressure in the arms and low pressure in the legs. This condition must be treated to prevent a cerebrovascular accident, endocarditis, congestive heart failure, or rupture of the aorta.

transluminal balloon angioplasty. Balloon-tipped catheter is placed within a narrowed artery or vein and the balloon is inflated to stretch the vessel to a larger diameter for increased blood flow.

33900-33904

33900 Percutaneous pulmonary artery revascularization by stent placement, initial; normal native connections, unilateral

33901 Percutaneous pulmonary artery revascularization by stent placement, initial; normal native connections, bilateral

33902 Percutaneous pulmonary artery revascularization by stent placement, initial; abnormal connections, unilateral

33903 Percutaneous pulmonary artery revascularization by stent placement, initial; abnormal connections, bilateral

\+ **33904** Percutaneous pulmonary artery revascularization by stent placement, each additional vessel or separate lesion, normal or abnormal connections (List separately in addition to code for primary procedure)

Additional stent is deployed percutaneously into the pulmonary artery

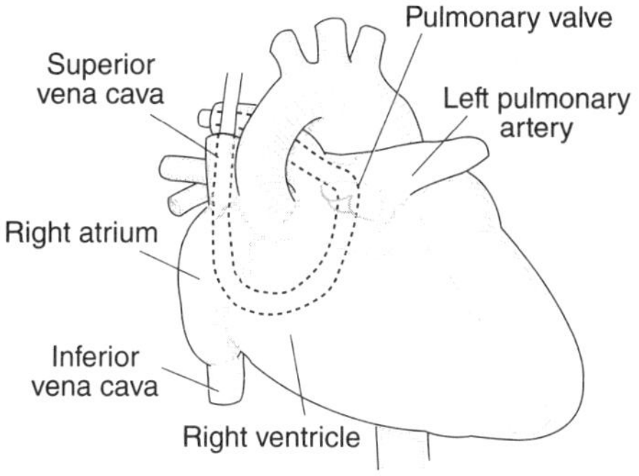

Explanation

The physician performs revascularization of the pulmonary artery by percutaneous stent placement. This procedure may be used for patients with pulmonary artery stenosis, which is a narrowing of the pulmonary artery, the large blood vessel that connects the heart's right ventricle to the lungs. With the patient under appropriate anesthesia, an introducer sheath is placed into a vein (typically the femoral vein) using a percutaneous puncture and advanced to the target location. A catheter with a balloon and stent attached is inserted and threaded with a guidewire into the vessel. The wire is removed. The catheter is fed through the vascular system to the stenotic segment of the pulmonary artery. Position of the balloon and stent is confirmed angiographically. The provider employs balloon dilation as necessary to reach optimal stent diameter within the region of stenosis. Several inflations may be performed along the narrowed area. The catheter is slowly withdrawn after deflation. Pressure is applied to the puncture site to stop the bleeding after the catheter is removed. Report 33900 for an initial unilateral stent placement on a patient with normal native connections (those in which the blood flow follows the expected course through the great vessels and heart chambers); report 33901 for bilateral placement. Report 33902 for unilateral stent placement on a patient with abnormal connections (those in which alternative blood flow connections exist, as in patients with aberrant cardiac anatomy); report 33903 for bilateral placement. Report 33904 for stent placement in each additional vessel or separate lesion, whether the connections are normal or abnormal.

Coding Tips

These procedures include vascular access, catheter and guidewire manipulation, fluoroscopic guidance, post-diagnostic angiography for roadmapping, post-implant evaluation, stent positioning and balloon inflation for stent delivery, and radiologic supervision and interpretation necessary to perform the procedure. Do not report 33900–33904 with 93451–93461, 93563, 93566–93568, 93593, 93594, or 93596–93598 for contrast injections, angiography, roadmapping and/or fluoroscopic guidance, or catheterization for hemodynamic measurements related to a TPVI procedure. Cardiopulmonary bypass may be necessary in addition to this procedure. For percutaneous peripheral bypass, see 33367; for open peripheral bypass, see 33368; and for central bypass, see 33369. Diagnostic catheterization codes (93451–93453, 93456–93461, 93593–93598) and diagnostic coronary and pulmonary angiography codes (93454–93461, 93563–93568) may be reported separately with 33900–33904 in cases where a previous examination is not available or the anatomic visualization is poor quality, there has been a clinical change in the patient's condition since the previous examination, or complications arise during the procedure requiring the additional study. Do not report 33900–33904 with 76000, 93451–93461, 93563–93568, 93593, 93594, or 93596–93598 for catheterization and angiography intrinsic to the procedure. Do not report 92997 or 92998 before or after stent deployment, for same target lesion as stent implant. Report 33900–33904 in addition to 92997 or 92998 for a separate lesion in a different artery.

ICD-10-CM Diagnostic Codes

I28.8	Other diseases of pulmonary vessels
Q21.3	Tetralogy of Fallot
Q24.3	Pulmonary infundibular stenosis
Q25.5	Atresia of pulmonary artery
Q25.6	Stenosis of pulmonary artery
Q25.71	Coarctation of pulmonary artery
Q25.72	Congenital pulmonary arteriovenous malformation

AMA: 33900 2023,Jun; 2023,May **33901** 2023,Jun; 2023,May **33902** 2023,Jun; 2023,May **33903** 2023,Jun; 2023,May **33904** 2023,Jun; 2023,May

Relative Value Units/Medicare Edits

Non-Facility RVU	Work	PE	MP	Total
33900	11.03	3.87	2.06	16.96
33901	14.5	5.08	2.71	22.29
33902	14.0	4.91	2.61	21.52
33903	16.5	5.79	3.07	25.36
33904	5.53	1.94	1.05	8.52
Facility RVU	**Work**	**PE**	**MP**	**Total**
33900	11.03	3.87	2.06	16.96
33901	14.5	5.08	2.71	22.29
33902	14.0	4.91	2.61	21.52
33903	16.5	5.79	3.07	25.36
33904	5.53	1.94	1.05	8.52

	FUD	Status	MUE	Modifiers				IOM Reference
33900	0	A	1(2)	51	N/A	N/A	80*	None
33901	0	A	1(2)	51	N/A	N/A	80*	
33902	0	A	1(2)	51	N/A	N/A	80*	
33903	0	A	1(2)	51	N/A	N/A	80*	
33904	N/A	A	1(3)	N/A	N/A	N/A	80*	

* with documentation

33910-33915

33910 Pulmonary artery embolectomy; with cardiopulmonary bypass
33915 without cardiopulmonary bypass

Bypass schematic

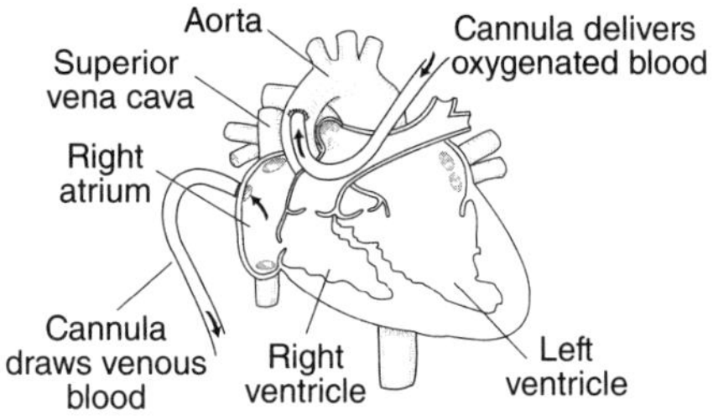

Cutaway depiction of right side of heart

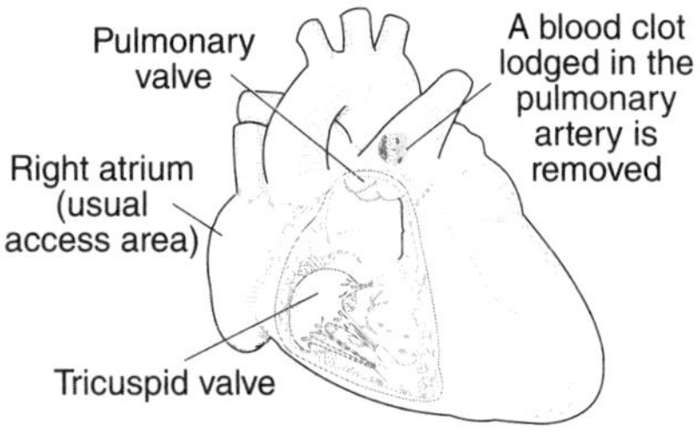

A blood clot (embolism) has broken free and traveled the venous route to the right side of the heart where it has lodged in the pulmonary artery

Explanation

This operation is only done for patients who are in extremis following a pulmonary artery embolism (i.e., a blood clot originating in one of the large veins in the leg breaks loose and travels into the heart via the caval vein where it obstructs blood flow to the lungs). Survival is low. If cardiopulmonary bypass is used, the physician opens the right atrium widely. If cardiopulmonary bypass is not used, the right atrium is opened through a hole in the middle of a purse string. The clot is "milked" out of the pulmonary artery into the right atrium and out the hole. Report 33910 if cardiopulmonary bypass is required and the right atrium is opened widely. Report 33910 if cardiopulmonary bypass is initiated. Report 33915 if cardiopulmonary bypass is not initiated.

Coding Tips

If significant additional time and effort are documented, append modifier 22 and submit a cover letter and operative report. When 33910 or 33915 is performed with another separately identifiable procedure, the highest dollar value code is listed as the primary procedure and subsequent procedures are appended with modifier 51. For embolectomy of other arteries, see 34001–34203.

ICD-10-CM Diagnostic Codes

I26.01	Septic pulmonary embolism with acute cor pulmonale
I26.02	Saddle embolus of pulmonary artery with acute cor pulmonale
I26.09	Other pulmonary embolism with acute cor pulmonale
I26.90	Septic pulmonary embolism without acute cor pulmonale
I26.92	Saddle embolus of pulmonary artery without acute cor pulmonale
I26.93	Single subsegmental thrombotic pulmonary embolism without acute cor pulmonale
I26.94	Multiple subsegmental thrombotic pulmonary emboli without acute cor pulmonale
I26.99	Other pulmonary embolism without acute cor pulmonale
I27.82	Chronic pulmonary embolism
I27.89	Other specified pulmonary heart diseases
T81.718A	Complication of other artery following a procedure, not elsewhere classified, initial encounter
T82.817A	Embolism due to cardiac prosthetic devices, implants and grafts, initial encounter
T82.818A	Embolism due to vascular prosthetic devices, implants and grafts, initial encounter

AMA: 33910 2023,Jan **33915** 2023,Jan

Relative Value Units/Medicare Edits

Non-Facility RVU	Work	PE	MP	Total
33910	48.21	17.14	11.18	76.53
33915	24.95	9.63	5.76	40.34
Facility RVU	**Work**	**PE**	**MP**	**Total**
33910	48.21	17.14	11.18	76.53
33915	24.95	9.63	5.76	40.34

	FUD	Status	MUE	Modifiers				IOM Reference
33910	90	A	1(3)	51	N/A	62*	80	None
33915	90	A	1(3)	51	N/A	62*	80	

* with documentation

Terms To Know

cardiopulmonary bypass. Venous blood is diverted to a heart-lung machine, which mechanically pumps and oxygenates the blood temporarily so the heart can be bypassed while an open procedure on the heart or coronary arteries is performed. During bypass, the lungs are deflated and immobile.

embolectomy. Surgical excision of a blood clot or other foreign material that broke away from its original source and traveled in the blood stream, becoming lodged in a blood vessel and blocking circulation.

embolism. Obstruction of a blood vessel resulting from a clot or foreign substance.

iatrogenic. Adversely induced in the patient; caused by medical treatment.

incision. Act of cutting into tissue or an organ.

infarction. Area of necrosis in tissue, due to ischemia from lack of circulation, usually from a thrombus or an embolus.

33916-33917

33916 Pulmonary endarterectomy, with or without embolectomy, with cardiopulmonary bypass

33917 Repair of pulmonary artery stenosis by reconstruction with patch or graft

The inner tissues of the lumen are removed and the artery is repaired directly or with a patch

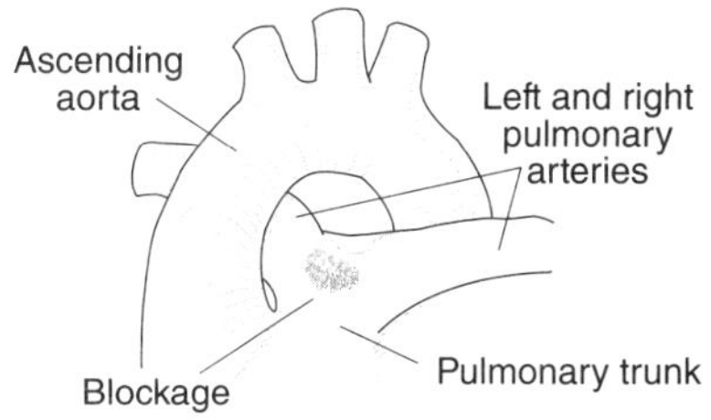

A stenotic (narrowed) pulmonary artery is repaired using a patch or graft

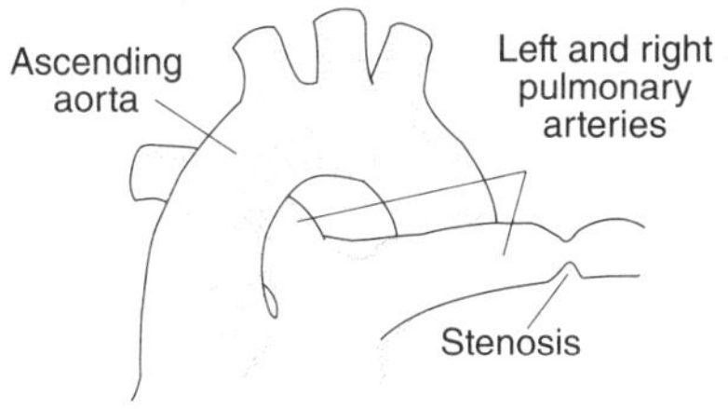

Repair of a blockage in the greater pulmonary arteries is accomplished by opening the artery along its length overlying the blockage. If an embolism is present it is removed

Explanation

In 33916, a pulmonary endarterectomy is performed to treat patients diagnosed with chronic thromboembolic pulmonary hypertension. Cardiopulmonary bypass and hypothermia is required in order to perform this procedure. Only the main and branch pulmonary arteries can be treated. Via a median sternotomy, the pulmonary arteries are opened along their lengths. If present, any thrombotic or embolic material is extracted. The inner layer of each artery is removed. Once the endarterectomies are complete, the arteries are closed with suture directly or with a patch of pericardium, saphenous vein or Dacron. Homeostasis is achieved and the chest is closed in layers using standard techniques. In 33917, the physician reconstructs the pulmonary artery to correct any outflow tract obstruction caused by stenosis. Cardiopulmonary bypass is required. Via a median sternotomy, the stenotic pulmonary artery is opened longitudinally until healthy artery is encountered. The diseased vessel is removed. A patch is trimmed to reconstruct the defect in the artery or grafting may be performed if the defect is too complex or large for a patch. After the patch or graft is placed, homeostasis is achieved and the chest is closed in layers using standard techniques.

Coding Tips

The insertion of grafts or implanted materials is considered part of this procedure and is not reported separately. If significant additional time and effort are documented, append modifier 22 and submit a cover letter and operative report. When 33916 or 33917 is performed with another separately identifiable procedure, the highest dollar value code is listed as the primary procedure and subsequent procedures are appended with modifier 51. For coronary endarterectomy, see 33572.

ICD-10-CM Diagnostic Codes

I26.01	Septic pulmonary embolism with acute cor pulmonale
I26.02	Saddle embolus of pulmonary artery with acute cor pulmonale
I26.90	Septic pulmonary embolism without acute cor pulmonale
I26.92	Saddle embolus of pulmonary artery without acute cor pulmonale
I26.93	Single subsegmental thrombotic pulmonary embolism without acute cor pulmonale
I26.94	Multiple subsegmental thrombotic pulmonary emboli without acute cor pulmonale
I27.0	Primary pulmonary hypertension
I27.21	Secondary pulmonary arterial hypertension
I27.22	Pulmonary hypertension due to left heart disease
I27.23	Pulmonary hypertension due to lung diseases and hypoxia
I27.24	Chronic thromboembolic pulmonary hypertension
I27.82	Chronic pulmonary embolism
I27.83	Eisenmenger's syndrome
I37.0	Nonrheumatic pulmonary valve stenosis
I37.2	Nonrheumatic pulmonary valve stenosis with insufficiency
Q22.1	Congenital pulmonary valve stenosis
Q22.2	Congenital pulmonary valve insufficiency
Q24.3	Pulmonary infundibular stenosis
Q25.6	Stenosis of pulmonary artery
Q25.72	Congenital pulmonary arteriovenous malformation
S25.411A	Minor laceration of right pulmonary blood vessels, initial encounter ☑
S25.412A	Minor laceration of left pulmonary blood vessels, initial encounter ☑
S25.421A	Major laceration of right pulmonary blood vessels, initial encounter ☑
S25.422A	Major laceration of left pulmonary blood vessels, initial encounter ☑
T81.718A	Complication of other artery following a procedure, not elsewhere classified, initial encounter
T82.817A	Embolism due to cardiac prosthetic devices, implants and grafts, initial encounter
T82.818A	Embolism due to vascular prosthetic devices, implants and grafts, initial encounter

AMA: **33916** 2023,Jan

Relative Value Units/Medicare Edits

Non-Facility RVU	Work	PE	MP	Total
33916	78.0	25.69	18.45	122.14
33917	25.3	11.63	6.25	43.18
Facility RVU	**Work**	**PE**	**MP**	**Total**
33916	78.0	25.69	18.45	122.14
33917	25.3	11.63	6.25	43.18

	FUD	Status	MUE	Modifiers				IOM Reference
33916	90	A	1(3)	51	N/A	62*	80	None
33917	90	A	1(2)	51	N/A	62*	80	

* with documentation

33920

33920 Repair of pulmonary atresia with ventricular septal defect, by construction or replacement of conduit from right or left ventricle to pulmonary artery

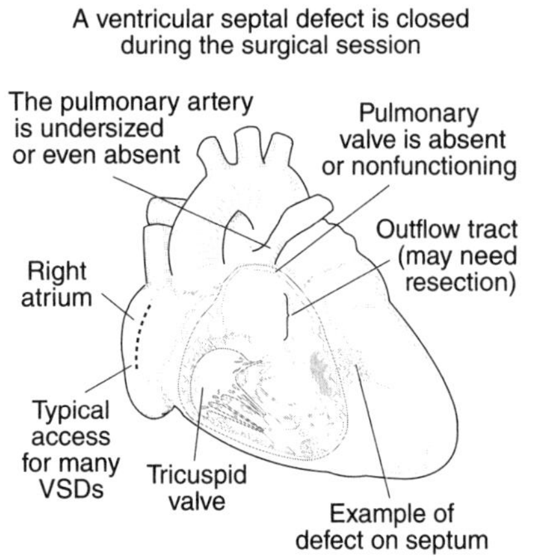

Pulmonary atresia (the absence of an outlet) is surgically treated by constructing a connection from a ventricle (usually the right) to a point on the pulmonary artery that is of normal diameter

Explanation

Cardiopulmonary bypass is required. A hole is made in the right ventricle and any muscular obstruction in the outflow tract of the right ventricle is removed. The pulmonary artery or its branches are opened longitudinally until normal-sized vessels are encountered. The ventricular septal defect is closed. An aortic graft from an organ donor is trimmed to form a patch over the opened pulmonary artery. Any excess artery from the donor graft or a patch of pericardium or Dacron is sewn to the graft below the valve to use as a secondary patch for closing the hole in the right ventricle. The graft valve becomes the new pulmonary valve. After the patches and graft are sewn in place, cardiopulmonary bypass is stopped when heart function returns.

Coding Tips

The insertion of grafts or implanted materials is considered part of this procedure and is not reported separately. If significant additional time and effort are documented, append modifier 22 and submit a cover letter and operative report. When 33920 is performed with another separately identifiable procedure, the highest dollar value code is listed as the primary procedure and subsequent procedures are appended with modifier 51. When ligation and takedown of systemic-to-pulmonary artery shunt is performed in addition to this procedure, it should be reported separately, see 33924. Do not report 33920 with 33440. For repair of other complex cardiac anomalies by construction or replacement of right or left ventricle to pulmonary artery conduit, see 33608. For closure of a ventricular septal defect only, with or without patch, see 33681–33688.

ICD-10-CM Diagnostic Codes

Q21.0	Ventricular septal defect
Q21.8	Other congenital malformations of cardiac septa
Q22.0	Pulmonary valve atresia
Q22.3	Other congenital malformations of pulmonary valve
Q25.5	Atresia of pulmonary artery
Q25.79	Other congenital malformations of pulmonary artery

AMA: 33920 2019,Apr

Relative Value Units/Medicare Edits

Non-Facility RVU	Work	PE	MP	Total
33920	32.74	12.48	8.09	53.31
Facility RVU	**Work**	**PE**	**MP**	**Total**
33920	32.74	12.48	8.09	53.31

	FUD	Status	MUE	Modifiers				IOM Reference
33920	90	A	1(2)	51	N/A	62*	80	None

* with documentation

Terms To Know

anomaly. Irregularity in the structure or position of an organ or tissue.

atresia. Congenital closure or absence of a tubular organ or an opening to the body surface.

cardiopulmonary bypass. Venous blood is diverted to a heart-lung machine, which mechanically pumps and oxygenates the blood temporarily so the heart can be bypassed while an open procedure on the heart or coronary arteries is performed. During bypass, the lungs are deflated and immobile.

conduit. Surgically created channel for the passage of fluids.

congenital. Present at birth, occurring through heredity or an influence during gestation up to the moment of birth.

graft. Tissue implant from another part of the body or another person.

ligation. Tying off a blood vessel or duct with a suture or a soft, thin wire.

obstruction. Blockage that prevents normal function of the valve or structure.

shunt. Surgically created passage between blood vessels or other natural passages, such as an arteriovenous anastomosis, to divert or bypass blood flow from the normal channel.

stenosis. Narrowing or constriction of a passage.

ventricular septal defect. Congenital cardiac anomaly resulting in a continual opening in the septum between the ventricles that, in severe cases, causes oxygenated blood to flow back into the lungs, resulting in pulmonary hypertension.

33922

33922 Transection of pulmonary artery with cardiopulmonary bypass

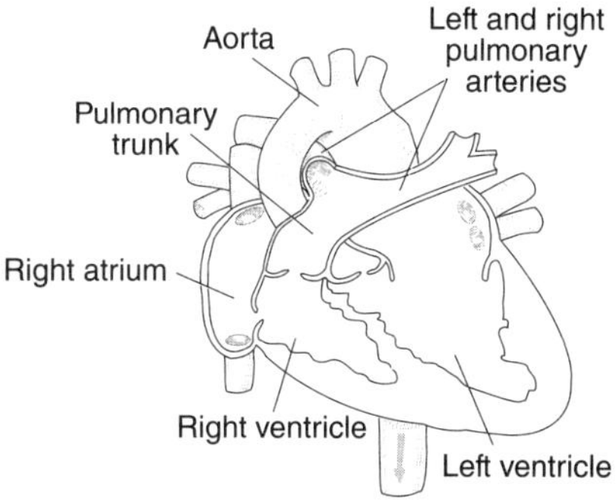

A pulmonary artery is transected and a diseased portion removed. The ends are then anastomosed together. Cardiopulmonary bypass is employed

Explanation

Cardiopulmonary bypass is required. After it is started, cuts are made all the way across the pulmonary artery just above and just below the part of the artery containing the disease. The pulmonary artery is closed directly or is closed using a piece of the pulmonary artery or a piece of the aorta from an organ donor that is placed as an interposition graft.

Coding Tips

The insertion of grafts or implanted materials is considered part of this procedure and is not reported separately. If significant additional time and effort are documented, append modifier 22 and submit a cover letter and operative report. When 33922 is performed with another separately identifiable procedure, the highest dollar value code is listed as the primary procedure and subsequent procedures are appended with modifier 51. Do not append modifier 63 to 33922 as the description or nature of the procedure includes infants up to 4 kg. When ligation and takedown of systemic-to-pulmonary artery shunt is performed in addition to this procedure, it should be reported separately, see 33924.

ICD-10-CM Diagnostic Codes

I28.1	Aneurysm of pulmonary artery
I28.8	Other diseases of pulmonary vessels
Q22.0	Pulmonary valve atresia
Q22.3	Other congenital malformations of pulmonary valve
Q25.5	Atresia of pulmonary artery
Q25.6	Stenosis of pulmonary artery
Q25.71	Coarctation of pulmonary artery
Q25.72	Congenital pulmonary arteriovenous malformation
Q25.79	Other congenital malformations of pulmonary artery
Q25.8	Other congenital malformations of other great arteries
S25.411A	Minor laceration of right pulmonary blood vessels, initial encounter ☑
S25.412A	Minor laceration of left pulmonary blood vessels, initial encounter ☑
S25.421A	Major laceration of right pulmonary blood vessels, initial encounter ☑
S25.422A	Major laceration of left pulmonary blood vessels, initial encounter ☑
S25.491A	Other specified injury of right pulmonary blood vessels, initial encounter ☑
S25.492A	Other specified injury of left pulmonary blood vessels, initial encounter ☑

Relative Value Units/Medicare Edits

Non-Facility RVU	Work	PE	MP	Total
33922	24.22	10.93	6.0	41.15
Facility RVU	**Work**	**PE**	**MP**	**Total**
33922	24.22	10.93	6.0	41.15

	FUD	Status	MUE	Modifiers				IOM Reference
33922	90	A	1(2)	51	N/A	62*	80	None

* with documentation

Terms To Know

anastomosis. Surgically created connection between ducts, blood vessels, or bowel segments to allow flow from one to the other.

anomaly. Irregularity in the structure or position of an organ or tissue.

cardiopulmonary bypass. Venous blood is diverted to a heart-lung machine, which mechanically pumps and oxygenates the blood temporarily so the heart can be bypassed while an open procedure on the heart or coronary arteries is performed. During bypass, the lungs are deflated and immobile.

congenital. Present at birth, occurring through heredity or an influence during gestation up to the moment of birth.

graft. Tissue implant from another part of the body or another person.

hypothermia with cardiac bypass. Reduction of the body temperature using a bypass system to reduce the oxygen demands of tissue and to protect the myocardium during a procedure.

ligation. Tying off a blood vessel or duct with a suture or a soft, thin wire.

transection. Transverse dissection; to cut across a long axis; cross section.

33924

\+ **33924** Ligation and takedown of a systemic-to-pulmonary artery shunt, performed in conjunction with a congenital heart procedure (List separately in addition to code for primary procedure)

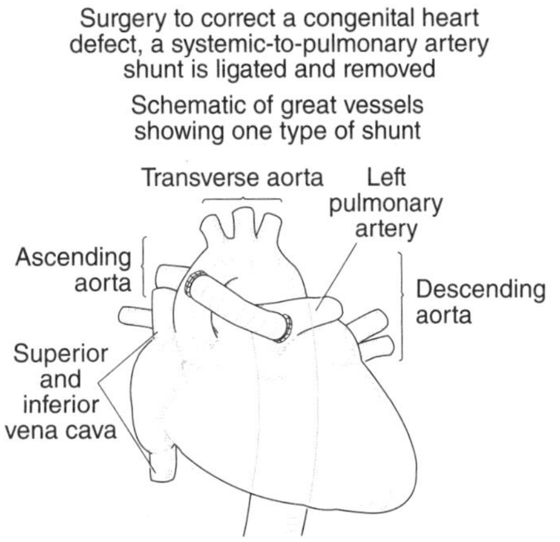

Explanation

During a separately reportable congenital heart procedure, the physician ligates and takes down a previously formed systemic-to-pulmonary artery shunt. The shunt is ligated and the systemic arteries are returned to their correct anatomic position.

Coding Tips

Report 33924 in addition to 33474–33478, 33600–33617, 33622, 33684–33688, 33692–33697, 33735–33767, 33770–33783, 33786, 33917, 33920, 33922, 33925, 33926, 33935, and 33945.

ICD-10-CM Diagnostic Codes

This/these CPT code(s) are add-on code(s). See the primary procedure code that this code is performed with for your ICD-10-CM code selections. Diagnostic code(s) would be the same as the actual procedure performed.

Relative Value Units/Medicare Edits

Non-Facility RVU	Work	PE	MP	Total
33924	5.49	1.5	1.35	8.34
Facility RVU	**Work**	**PE**	**MP**	**Total**
33924	5.49	1.5	1.35	8.34

	FUD	Status	MUE	Modifiers				IOM Reference
33924	N/A	A	1(2)	N/A	N/A	62*	80	None

* with documentation

Terms To Know

congenital. Present at birth, occurring through heredity or an influence during gestation up to the moment of birth.

ligation. Tying off a blood vessel or duct with a suture or a soft, thin wire.

33925-33926

33925 Repair of pulmonary artery arborization anomalies by unifocalization; without cardiopulmonary bypass

33926 with cardiopulmonary bypass

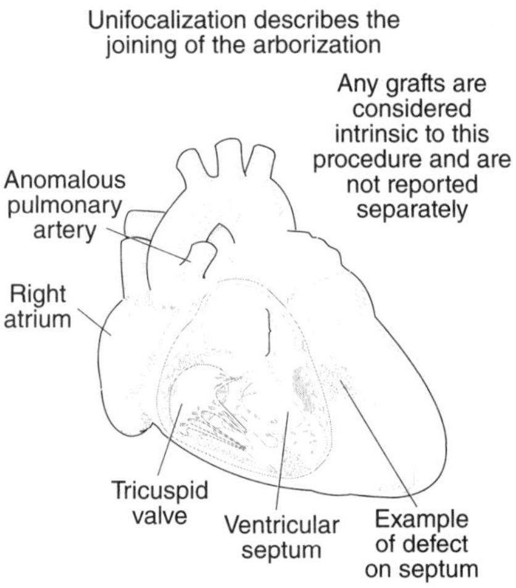

Explanation

The physician repairs pulmonary artery arborization anomalies (i.e., stenosis of unbranched and intrapulmonary arteries) by unifocalization, a surgical technique in which the various sources of pulmonary blood supply can be perfused from a single source. In patients with pulmonary atresia or with a ventricular septal defect (VSD), the pulmonary blood supply often comes from multiple sources, particularly major aortopulmonary collateral arteries (MAPCA), which often arise from the aorta and its direct branches. Unifocalization, which may be performed as a single operation or as a staged procedure, interrupts the extracardiac sources of pulmonary arterial blood flow; restores segmental, lobar, and pulmonary arterial confluence; replaces missing central pulmonary arterial branches; and creates a central, accessible source of pulmonary arterial blood flow. The physician accesses the mediastinum through an extended median sternotomy or a bilateral transsternal thoracotomy. The major aortopulmonary collateral arteries are identified, mobilized, and dissected, using a variety of techniques, from the upper descending aorta, the aortic arch, brachiocephalic vessels, or coronary arteries, and anastomosed to the native pulmonary artery. Ligation of the collateral arteries at their origin is performed to achieve controlled perfusion. As each artery is ligated, desaturation is assessed by pulse oximetry. If desaturation approaches a compromising level, the surgeon may proceed with cardiopulmonary bypass at this point. Report 33925 when the procedure is performed without cardiopulmonary bypass and 33926 when it is performed with cardiopulmonary bypass.

Coding Tips

If significant additional time and effort is documented, append modifier 22 and submit a cover letter and operative report. For repair of other complex cardiac anomalies by construction or replacement of right or left ventricle to pulmonary artery conduit, see 33608.

ICD-10-CM Diagnostic Codes

I28.8	Other diseases of pulmonary vessels
I77.1	Stricture of artery
Q21.0	Ventricular septal defect
Q21.21	Partial atrioventricular septal defect
Q21.22	Transitional atrioventricular septal defect

Q21.23	Complete atrioventricular septal defect
Q21.3	Tetralogy of Fallot
Q21.4	Aortopulmonary septal defect
Q21.8	Other congenital malformations of cardiac septa
Q25.5	Atresia of pulmonary artery
Q25.6	Stenosis of pulmonary artery
Q25.71	Coarctation of pulmonary artery
Q25.72	Congenital pulmonary arteriovenous malformation
Q25.79	Other congenital malformations of pulmonary artery

Relative Value Units/Medicare Edits

Non-Facility RVU	Work	PE	MP	Total
33925	31.3	11.47	7.74	50.51
33926	44.73	15.15	11.1	70.98
Facility RVU	**Work**	**PE**	**MP**	**Total**
33925	31.3	11.47	7.74	50.51
33926	44.73	15.15	11.1	70.98

	FUD	Status	MUE	Modifiers				IOM Reference
33925	90	A	1(2)	51	N/A	62*	80	None
33926	90	A	1(2)	51	N/A	62*	80	

* with documentation

Terms To Know

anomaly. Irregularity in the structure or position of an organ or tissue.

cardiopulmonary bypass. Venous blood is diverted to a heart-lung machine, which mechanically pumps and oxygenates the blood temporarily so the heart can be bypassed while an open procedure on the heart or coronary arteries is performed. During bypass, the lungs are deflated and immobile.

tetralogy of Fallot. Specific combination of congenital cardiac defects: obstruction of the right ventricular outflow tract with pulmonary stenosis, interventricular septal defect, malposition of the aorta, overriding the interventricular septum and receiving blood from both the venous and arterial systems, and enlargement of the right ventricle.

ventricular septal defect. Congenital cardiac anomaly resulting in a continual opening in the septum between the ventricles that, in severe cases, causes oxygenated blood to flow back into the lungs, resulting in pulmonary hypertension.

33927-33929

33927 Implantation of a total replacement heart system (artificial heart) with recipient cardiectomy

33928 Removal and replacement of total replacement heart system (artificial heart)

\+ **33929** Removal of a total replacement heart system (artificial heart) for heart transplantation (List separately in addition to code for primary procedure)

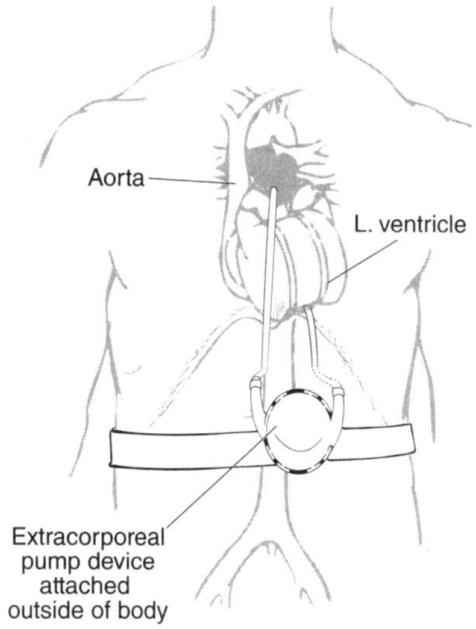

Implantable replacement heart system with removal of native heart

Explanation

In 33927, the physician implants a total replacement heart system, or artificial heart, as a temporary measure until transplantation or to prolong life for patients not eligible for transplant. One artificial heart system, described here, is a self-contained, electrohydraulic action heart, charged from a battery source through the skin. Once attached, the natural atria pump blood into the artificial ventricles of the replacement heart and the hydraulic pump moves the blood into circulation. The patient is prepared for open heart surgery, and an extended median sternotomy is made. A subcutaneous/submuscular pocket is created in the patient's abdominal area for the internal battery and the heart's pumping controller unit, and these internal components are placed between muscle layers. A separate incision is made over the chest wall for placement of the internal transcutaneous energy transmission coil, which is sutured into an appropriate position where the external coil may lie flat over it without much interposing tissue. Cardiopulmonary bypass is initiated, the aorta is cross-clamped, and cardiectomy is undertaken to remove the native ventricles and transect the great vessels. Outflow grafts are anastomosed to the pulmonary artery and the aorta. The artificial ventricles are anastomosed to the native atrial cuffs and all air is removed from the system. The aortic cross-clamp is released and cardiopulmonary bypass weaned onto the artificial heart support. The internal components are connected to the artificial heart and energy is transferred through the transcutaneous coils, where external battery packs transmit power across the skin to keep the internal battery charged. In 33928, the physician removes and replaces a total replacement heart system or artificial heart. The thoracic unit is the pump that consists of the artificial ventricles, which are attached to the natural atria, containing their corresponding valves, and the motor-driven hydraulic pumping system, or the pneumatic air pressure valves, depending on the system. Removal and replacement of this component requires open chest access in a procedure following the same kind of steps for implantation (see 33927). Internal components include the implanted rechargeable battery, which is continually charged by external battery packs, the internal transcutaneous coil for receiving the battery charge across the skin, or the control unit, which monitors and controls the pumping speed of the artificial heart. These components are removed and replaced back in their prepared subcutaneous/submuscular pockets and tunneled back to their connection with the thoracic unit. Report 33929 for removal of a total replacement heart system or artificial heart for heart transplantation.

Coding Tips

Report 33929 in addition to 33945. For implantation with replacement of a total heart system with recipient cardiectomy, see 33927. For implant of a ventricular assist device, see 33975, 33976, 33979, 33990, 33991, and 33995. For revision or replacement of components only, see 33999.

ICD-10-CM Diagnostic Codes

I50.1	Left ventricular failure, unspecified
I50.21	Acute systolic (congestive) heart failure
I50.22	Chronic systolic (congestive) heart failure
I50.23	Acute on chronic systolic (congestive) heart failure
I50.31	Acute diastolic (congestive) heart failure
I50.32	Chronic diastolic (congestive) heart failure
I50.33	Acute on chronic diastolic (congestive) heart failure
I50.41	Acute combined systolic (congestive) and diastolic (congestive) heart failure
I50.42	Chronic combined systolic (congestive) and diastolic (congestive) heart failure
I50.43	Acute on chronic combined systolic (congestive) and diastolic (congestive) heart failure
I50.810	Right heart failure, unspecified
I50.811	Acute right heart failure
I50.812	Chronic right heart failure
I50.813	Acute on chronic right heart failure
I50.814	Right heart failure due to left heart failure
I50.82	Biventricular heart failure
I50.83	High output heart failure
I50.84	End stage heart failure
I50.89	Other heart failure
T82.512A	Breakdown (mechanical) of artificial heart, initial encounter
T82.522A	Displacement of artificial heart, initial encounter
T82.532A	Leakage of artificial heart, initial encounter
T82.592A	Other mechanical complication of artificial heart, initial encounter
T86.21	Heart transplant rejection
T86.22	Heart transplant failure
T86.23	Heart transplant infection
Z76.82	Awaiting organ transplant status
Z95.812	Presence of fully implantable artificial heart

AMA: 33927 2018,Jun **33928** 2018,Jun **33929** 2018,Jun

Relative Value Units/Medicare Edits

Non-Facility RVU	Work	PE	MP	Total
33927	49.0	13.46	12.14	74.6
33928	0.0	0.0	0.0	0.0
33929	0.0	0.0	0.0	0.0
Facility RVU	**Work**	**PE**	**MP**	**Total**
33927	49.0	13.46	12.14	74.6
33928	0.0	0.0	0.0	0.0
33929	0.0	0.0	0.0	0.0

	FUD	Status	MUE	Modifiers				IOM Reference
33927	N/A	A	1(3)	51	N/A	N/A	80	None
33928	N/A	C	1(3)	51	N/A	N/A	80	
33929	N/A	C	1(3)	N/A	N/A	N/A	80	

* with documentation

Terms To Know

cardiectomy. Surgical removal of the heart, may be for transplant or replacement with mechanical heart.

ventricular assist device. Temporary measure used to support the heart by substituting for left and/or right heart function. The device replaces the work of the left and/or right ventricle when a patient has a damaged or weakened heart. A left ventricular assist device (VAD) helps the heart pump blood through the rest of the body. A right VAD helps the heart pump blood to the lungs to become oxygenated again. Catheters are inserted to circulate the blood through external tubing to a pump machine located outside of the body and back to the correct artery.

33930

33930 Donor cardiectomy-pneumonectomy (including cold preservation)

Explanation

The physician performs a donor cardiectomy-pneumonectomy by removing the heart and lung from a donor cadaver for transplantation. This is usually performed when other organs such as the liver, kidneys, intestines, or pancreas are also acquired from the organ donor. The chest cavity is accessed and cold preserving solutions are infused into the aorta and pulmonary arteries. After enough solution has been given, the heart and lungs are removed by transection, en bloc. This includes the aorta well above the heart, the right atrium, the atrial septum, and the left atrium, completely and as close to the patient's spine (or as posteriorly) as possible. The heart/lung block is preserved for transplantation into the recipient. The organ remains under refrigeration, specially packed in a sealable container with some preserving solution and kept on ice in a suitable carrier.

Coding Tips

Combined heart and lung transplantation involves three distinct components. Code 33930 reports only the cadaver cardiectomy-pneumonectomy. Backbench work (33933), which involves preparation of the cadaver donor heart and lung allograft prior to transplant, is reported separately. Transplant of the cadaver donor heart and lung including recipient cardiectomy-pneumonectomy and care of the recipient (33935) is also reported separately. Any additional repair or resection procedures on the donor heart or lung are also reported separately, see 33300, 33310, 33320, 33390, 33463, 33464, 33510, 33641, 35216, 35276, or 35685. Donor cardiectomy-pneumonectomy and any backbench work, repair, or resection procedures on the donor heart are usually the financial responsibility of the recipient.

ICD-10-CM Diagnostic Codes

Z52.89 Donor of other specified organs or tissues

AMA: 33930 2018,Jun

Relative Value Units/Medicare Edits

Non-Facility RVU	Work	PE	MP	Total
33930	0.0	0.0	0.0	0.0
Facility RVU	**Work**	**PE**	**MP**	**Total**
33930	0.0	0.0	0.0	0.0

	FUD	Status	MUE	Modifiers				IOM Reference
33930	N/A	X	1(2)	N/A	N/A	N/A	N/A	None

* with documentation

Terms To Know

allograft. Graft from one individual to another of the same species.

cardiectomy. Surgical removal of the heart, may be for transplant or replacement with mechanical heart.

donor. Person from whom tissues or organs are removed for transplantation.

pneumonectomy. Surgical removal of a lung or lung tissue.

transplant. Insertion of an organ or tissue from one person or site into another.

33933

33933 Backbench standard preparation of cadaver donor heart/lung allograft prior to transplantation, including dissection of allograft from surrounding soft tissues to prepare aorta, superior vena cava, inferior vena cava, and trachea for implantation

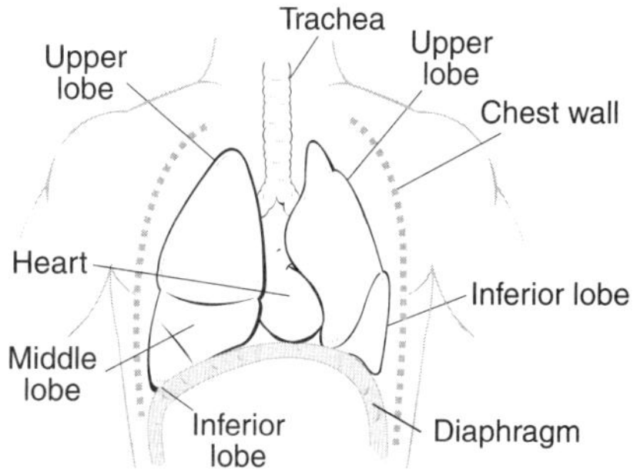

Backbench preparation is performed on the heart and lungs from a cadaver in preparation for transplantation

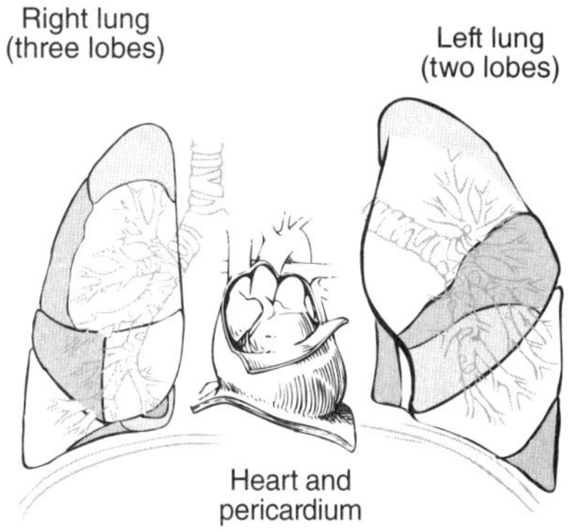

Explanation

The physician performs a standard backbench preparation of the heart and lungs following procurement from a cadaver donor. Backbench or back table preparation refers to procedures performed on the donor organs following procurement to prepare the donor organs for transplant. The heart and lungs are removed en bloc. The heart and lungs are inspected following procurement to identify any injury or abnormality not noted prior to procurement. The physician prepares the heart and lungs by dissecting free any residual soft tissue. Attention is focused on the aorta, superior vena cava, inferior vena cava, and the trachea. The aorta, which was divided at the aortic arch, is inspected and residual tissue removed. The superior vena cava is inspected and residual tissue removed. The inferior vena cava is inspected to assure adequate length has been preserved. Any residual tissue is removed from the inferior vena cava. The trachea, which was divided as far above the carina as possible, is inspected and residual tissue removed. When all residual soft tissue has been removed and the vessels prepared, the heart and lungs are ready for transplant.

Coding Tips

Combined heart and lung transplantation involves three distinct components. Code 33933 includes only backbench work to prepare the cadaver donor heart and lung allograft prior to transplant. Cadaver cardiectomy-pneumonectomy (33930) is reported separately. Transplant of the cadaver donor heart and lung including recipient cardiectomy-pneumonectomy and care of the recipient (33935) is also reported separately. Any additional repair or resection procedures on the donor heart are also reported separately, see 33300, 33310, 33320, 33390, 33463, 33464, 33510, 33641, 35216, 35276, or 35685. Donor cardiectomy-pneumonectomy and any backbench work, repair, or resection procedures on the donor heart are usually the financial responsibility of the recipient.

ICD-10-CM Diagnostic Codes

This code is not identified as an add-on code by CPT® but is performed at the same time as another primary procedure. Refer to the corresponding primary procedure code for ICD-10-CM diagnosis code links.

AMA: **33933** 2018,Jun

Relative Value Units/Medicare Edits

Non-Facility RVU	Work	PE	MP	Total
33933	0.0	0.0	0.0	0.0
Facility RVU	**Work**	**PE**	**MP**	**Total**
33933	0.0	0.0	0.0	0.0

	FUD	Status	MUE	Modifiers				IOM Reference
33933	N/A	C	1(2)	51	N/A	62*	80	None

* with documentation

Terms To Know

allograft. Graft from one individual to another of the same species.

backbench preparation. Procedures performed on a donor organ following procurement to prepare the organ for transplant into the recipient. Excess fat and other tissue may be removed, the organ may be perfused, and vital arteries may be sized, repaired, or modified to fit the patient. These procedures are done on a back table in the operating room before transplantation can begin.

cadaver. Dead body.

carina. Ridge at the junction of the trachea and the bronchi formed by a projection of the lowest tracheal cartilage separating the openings of the two bronchi.

en bloc. In total.

resection. Surgical removal of a part or all of an organ or body part.

vena cava. Main venous trunk that empties into the right atrium from both the lower and upper regions, beginning at the junction of the common iliac veins inferiorly and the two brachiocephalic veins superiorly.

33935

33935 Heart-lung transplant with recipient cardiectomy-pneumonectomy

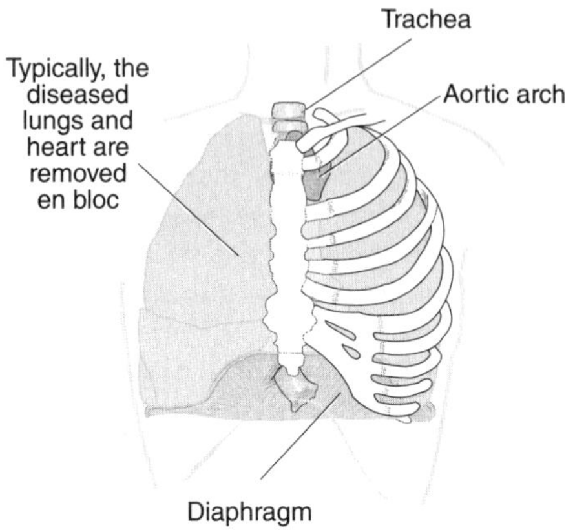

The diseased heart and lung are removed from the patient and the donor organs are placed and surgically connected

Explanation

The patient is placed on cardiopulmonary bypass and the heart and lungs are removed. The donor's organs are placed by sewing the left atrium of the donor to the left atrium of the recipient's first, and then sewing together the atrial septums and the right atrium. The donor aorta is trimmed to an appropriate length and sewn to the ascending aorta of the recipient. Immunosuppressive drugs may be given to the patient before, during, and after surgery. Cardiopulmonary bypass is discontinued when function returns to the donor heart.

Coding Tips

Combined heart and lung transplantation involves three distinct components. Code 33935 includes only transplant of the cadaver donor heart and lung including recipient cardiectomy-pneumonectomy and care of the recipient. Cadaver cardiectomy-pneumonectomy (33930) is reported separately. Backbench work (33933), which involves preparation of the cadaver donor heart and lung allograft prior to transplant, is also reported separately. Any additional repair or resection procedures on the donor heart are also reported separately, see 33300, 33310, 33320, 33390, 33463, 33464, 33510, 33641, 35216, 35276, or 35685. Donor cardiectomy-pneumonectomy and any backbench work, repair, or resection procedures on the donor heart are usually the financial responsibility of the recipient.

ICD-10-CM Diagnostic Codes

C34.11	Malignant neoplasm of upper lobe, right bronchus or lung ☑
C34.12	Malignant neoplasm of upper lobe, left bronchus or lung ☑
C34.2	Malignant neoplasm of middle lobe, bronchus or lung
C34.31	Malignant neoplasm of lower lobe, right bronchus or lung ☑
C34.32	Malignant neoplasm of lower lobe, left bronchus or lung ☑
C38.0	Malignant neoplasm of heart
C38.8	Malignant neoplasm of overlapping sites of heart, mediastinum and pleura
C78.01	Secondary malignant neoplasm of right lung ☑
C78.02	Secondary malignant neoplasm of left lung ☑
E84.0	Cystic fibrosis with pulmonary manifestations
I11.0	Hypertensive heart disease with heart failure
I25.3	Aneurysm of heart

Heart and Pericardium

I25.82	Chronic total occlusion of coronary artery
I27.0	Primary pulmonary hypertension
I27.21	Secondary pulmonary arterial hypertension
I27.22	Pulmonary hypertension due to left heart disease
I27.23	Pulmonary hypertension due to lung diseases and hypoxia
I27.24	Chronic thromboembolic pulmonary hypertension
I27.83	Eisenmenger's syndrome
I40.0	Infective myocarditis
I40.1	Isolated myocarditis
I42.0	Dilated cardiomyopathy
I42.1	Obstructive hypertrophic cardiomyopathy
I42.3	Endomyocardial (eosinophilic) disease
I42.4	Endocardial fibroelastosis
I50.1	Left ventricular failure, unspecified
I50.21	Acute systolic (congestive) heart failure
I50.22	Chronic systolic (congestive) heart failure
I50.23	Acute on chronic systolic (congestive) heart failure
I50.31	Acute diastolic (congestive) heart failure
I50.32	Chronic diastolic (congestive) heart failure
I50.33	Acute on chronic diastolic (congestive) heart failure
I50.41	Acute combined systolic (congestive) and diastolic (congestive) heart failure
I50.42	Chronic combined systolic (congestive) and diastolic (congestive) heart failure
I50.43	Acute on chronic combined systolic (congestive) and diastolic (congestive) heart failure
I50.811	Acute right heart failure
I50.812	Chronic right heart failure
I50.813	Acute on chronic right heart failure
I50.814	Right heart failure due to left heart failure
I50.82	Biventricular heart failure
I50.83	High output heart failure
I50.84	End stage heart failure
I51.5	Myocardial degeneration
I51.7	Cardiomegaly
J43.0	Unilateral pulmonary emphysema [MacLeod's syndrome]
J44.0	Chronic obstructive pulmonary disease with (acute) lower respiratory infection
J44.1	Chronic obstructive pulmonary disease with (acute) exacerbation
J47.0	Bronchiectasis with acute lower respiratory infection
J47.1	Bronchiectasis with (acute) exacerbation
J70.1	Chronic and other pulmonary manifestations due to radiation
J70.3	Chronic drug-induced interstitial lung disorders
J81.1	Chronic pulmonary edema
J84.112	Idiopathic pulmonary fibrosis
J84.113	Idiopathic non-specific interstitial pneumonitis
J84.114	Acute interstitial pneumonitis
J84.115	Respiratory bronchiolitis interstitial lung disease
J84.116	Cryptogenic organizing pneumonia
J84.117	Desquamative interstitial pneumonia
J84.170	Interstitial lung disease with progressive fibrotic phenotype in diseases classified elsewhere
J84.178	Other interstitial pulmonary diseases with fibrosis in diseases classified elsewhere
J84.2	Lymphoid interstitial pneumonia
J96.11	Chronic respiratory failure with hypoxia
J96.12	Chronic respiratory failure with hypercapnia
J96.21	Acute and chronic respiratory failure with hypoxia
J96.22	Acute and chronic respiratory failure with hypercapnia
J98.11	Atelectasis
J98.2	Interstitial emphysema
Q20.6	Isomerism of atrial appendages
Q24.4	Congenital subaortic stenosis
Q24.5	Malformation of coronary vessels
Q24.6	Congenital heart block
Q33.0	Congenital cystic lung
Q33.3	Agenesis of lung
Q33.4	Congenital bronchiectasis
Q33.6	Congenital hypoplasia and dysplasia of lung

AMA: 33935 2018,Jun

Relative Value Units/Medicare Edits

Non-Facility RVU	Work	PE	MP	Total
33935	91.78	31.07	21.24	144.09
Facility RVU	**Work**	**PE**	**MP**	**Total**
33935	91.78	31.07	21.24	144.09

	FUD	Status	MUE	Modifiers				IOM Reference
33935	90	R	1(2)	51	N/A	62*	80	None

* with documentation

Terms To Know

cardiectomy. Surgical removal of the heart, may be for transplant or replacement with mechanical heart.

pneumonectomy. Surgical removal of a lung or lung tissue.

33940

33940 Donor cardiectomy (including cold preservation)

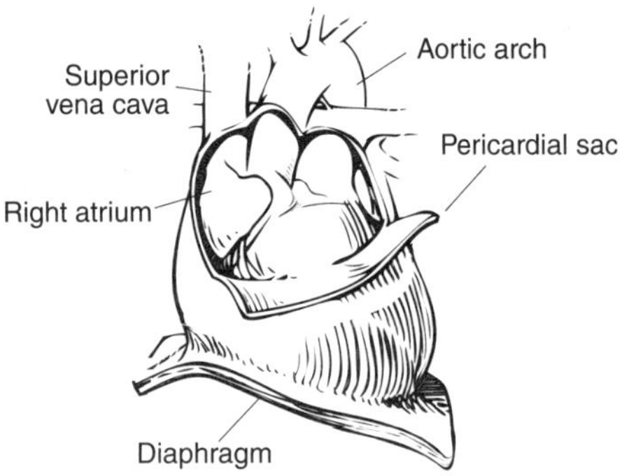

A cadaver donor heart is removed and additional work is performed to prepare and maintain the harvested heart in anticipation of a transplant

Explanation

The physician performs a donor cardiectomy by removing the heart from a donor cadaver for transplantation. This is usually performed when other organs such as the liver, kidneys, intestines, or pancreas are also acquired from the organ donor. The chest cavity is accessed and cold preserving solutions are infused into the aorta. After enough solution has been given, the heart is removed by transection, en bloc. This includes the aorta well above the heart, the right atrium, the atrial septum, and the left atrium, completely and as close to the patient's spine (or as posteriorly) as possible. The heart is preserved for transplantation into the recipient. The organ remains under refrigeration, specially packed in a sealable container with some preserving solution and kept on ice in a suitable carrier to maintain hypothermia.

Coding Tips

Heart transplantation involves three distinct components. Code 33940 reports only the cadaver cardiectomy. Backbench work (33944), which involves preparation of the cadaver donor heart allograft prior to transplant, is reported separately. Transplant of the cadaver donor heart with or without recipient cardiectomy and care of the recipient (33945) is also reported separately. Any additional repair or resection procedures on the donor heart are also reported separately, see 33300, 33310, 33320, 33390, 33463, 33464, 33510, 33641, 35216, 35276, or 35685. Donor cardiectomy and any backbench work, repair, or resection procedures on the donor heart are usually the financial responsibility of the recipient.

ICD-10-CM Diagnostic Codes

Z52.89 Donor of other specified organs or tissues

AMA: **33940** 2018,Jun

Relative Value Units/Medicare Edits

Non-Facility RVU	Work	PE	MP	Total
33940	0.0	0.0	0.0	0.0
Facility RVU	**Work**	**PE**	**MP**	**Total**
33940	0.0	0.0	0.0	0.0

	FUD	Status	MUE	Modifiers				IOM Reference
33940	N/A	X	1(2)	N/A	N/A	N/A	N/A	None

* with documentation

33944

33944 Backbench standard preparation of cadaver donor heart allograft prior to transplantation, including dissection of allograft from surrounding soft tissues to prepare aorta, superior vena cava, inferior vena cava, pulmonary artery, and left atrium for implantation

Explanation

The physician performs a standard backbench preparation of the heart following procurement from a cadaver donor. Backbench or back table preparation refers to procedures performed on the donor organs following procurement to prepare the donor organs for transplant. The heart is removed or the heart and lungs are removed en bloc. If the heart and lungs are removed en bloc, back table separation of the heart and lungs is performed. The heart is inspected following procurement to identify any injury or abnormality not noted prior to procurement. The physician prepares the heart by dissecting free any residual soft tissue. Attention is focused on the aorta, superior vena cava, inferior vena cava, and the left atrium. The aorta, which was divided at the aortic arch, is inspected and residual tissue removed. The superior vena cava is inspected and residual tissue removed. The inferior vena cava is inspected to assure adequate length has been preserved. Any residual tissue is removed. The left atrium is inspected and residual tissue removed. When all residual soft tissue has been removed and the vessels prepared, the heart is ready for transplant.

Coding Tips

Heart transplantation involves three distinct components. Code 33944 includes only backbench work to prepare the cadaver donor heart allograft prior to transplant. Cadaver cardiectomy (33940) is reported separately. Transplant of the cadaver donor heart with or without recipient cardiectomy and care of the recipient (33945) is also reported separately. Any additional repair or resection procedures on the donor heart are also reported separately, see 33300, 33310, 33320, 33390, 33463, 33464, 33510, 33641, 35216, 35276, or 35685. Donor cardiectomy and any backbench work, repair, or resection procedures on the donor heart are usually the financial responsibility of the recipient.

ICD-10-CM Diagnostic Codes

This code is not identified as an add-on code by CPT® but is performed at the same time as another primary procedure. Refer to the corresponding primary procedure code for ICD-10-CM diagnosis code links.

AMA: **33944** 2018,Jun

Relative Value Units/Medicare Edits

Non-Facility RVU	Work	PE	MP	Total
33944	0.0	0.0	0.0	0.0
Facility RVU	**Work**	**PE**	**MP**	**Total**
33944	0.0	0.0	0.0	0.0

	FUD	Status	MUE	Modifiers				IOM Reference
33944	N/A	C	1(2)	51	N/A	62*	80	None

* with documentation

Terms To Know

allograft. Graft from one individual to another of the same species.

cadaver. Dead body.

33945

33945 Heart transplant, with or without recipient cardiectomy

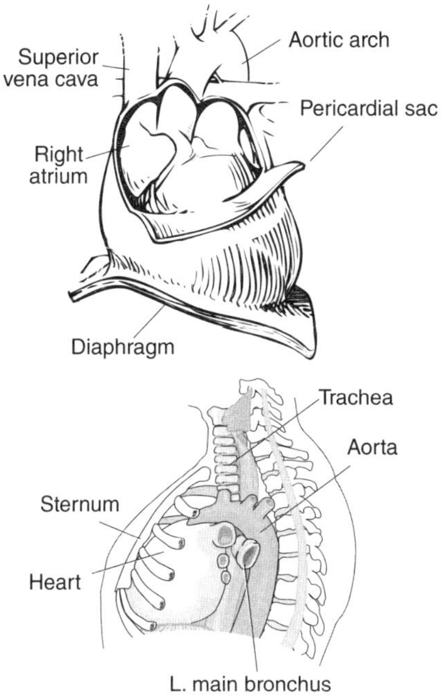

A cadaver donor heart has been prepared and maintained. The recipient's diseased heart may or may not be removed as part of the transplant procedure

Explanation

The patient is placed on cardiopulmonary bypass. Cardiac transplantation may be performed by one of two techniques: total orthotopic heart replacement or heterotopic implantation. A total orthotopic heart replacement involves excising the ventricles, atrial appendages, and most of the coronary sinus from the donor heart. The recipient heart is then opened. The atria, aorta, and pulmonary artery of the recipient heart are anastomosed to the donor heart. The sinoatrial nodes of both the donor and recipient heart are left intact. In a heterotopic implantation, the donor's organs are placed by sewing the left atrium of the donor heart to the left atrium of the recipient, and then sewing together the atrial septum and the right atrium. The donor aorta is trimmed to an appropriate length and sewn to the ascending aorta of the recipient. Immunosuppressive drugs may be given to the patient before, during, and after the operation. Cardiopulmonary bypass is discontinued when the donor heart begins functioning in the recipient.

Coding Tips

Heart transplantation involves three distinct components. Code 33945 includes only transplant of the cadaver donor heart with or without recipient cardiectomy and care of the recipient. Cadaver cardiectomy (33940) is reported separately. Backbench work (33944), which involves preparation of the cadaver donor heart allograft prior to transplant, is also reported separately. Any additional repair or resection procedures on the donor heart are also reported separately, see 33300, 33310, 33320, 33390, 33463, 33464, 33510, 33641, 35216, 35276, or 35685. Donor cardiectomy and any backbench work, repair, or resection procedures on the donor heart are usually the financial responsibility of the recipient.

ICD-10-CM Diagnostic Codes

C38.0	Malignant neoplasm of heart
C38.8	Malignant neoplasm of overlapping sites of heart, mediastinum and pleura
I09.81	Rheumatic heart failure
I11.0	Hypertensive heart disease with heart failure
I27.0	Primary pulmonary hypertension
I27.21	Secondary pulmonary arterial hypertension
I27.22	Pulmonary hypertension due to left heart disease
I27.23	Pulmonary hypertension due to lung diseases and hypoxia
I27.24	Chronic thromboembolic pulmonary hypertension
I27.29	Other secondary pulmonary hypertension
I27.83	Eisenmenger's syndrome
I27.89	Other specified pulmonary heart diseases
I27.9	Pulmonary heart disease, unspecified
I40.0	Infective myocarditis
I40.1	Isolated myocarditis
I40.8	Other acute myocarditis
I42.0	Dilated cardiomyopathy
I42.1	Obstructive hypertrophic cardiomyopathy
I42.3	Endomyocardial (eosinophilic) disease
I42.4	Endocardial fibroelastosis
I42.5	Other restrictive cardiomyopathy
I42.8	Other cardiomyopathies
I43	Cardiomyopathy in diseases classified elsewhere
I50.1	Left ventricular failure, unspecified
I50.21	Acute systolic (congestive) heart failure
I50.22	Chronic systolic (congestive) heart failure
I50.23	Acute on chronic systolic (congestive) heart failure
I50.31	Acute diastolic (congestive) heart failure
I50.32	Chronic diastolic (congestive) heart failure
I50.33	Acute on chronic diastolic (congestive) heart failure
I50.41	Acute combined systolic (congestive) and diastolic (congestive) heart failure
I50.42	Chronic combined systolic (congestive) and diastolic (congestive) heart failure
I50.43	Acute on chronic combined systolic (congestive) and diastolic (congestive) heart failure
I50.811	Acute right heart failure
I50.812	Chronic right heart failure
I50.813	Acute on chronic right heart failure
I50.814	Right heart failure due to left heart failure
I50.82	Biventricular heart failure
I50.83	High output heart failure
I50.84	End stage heart failure
I50.9	Heart failure, unspecified
I51.5	Myocardial degeneration
I51.7	Cardiomegaly
I51.89	Other ill-defined heart diseases
Q20.6	Isomerism of atrial appendages
Q20.8	Other congenital malformations of cardiac chambers and connections
Q21.8	Other congenital malformations of cardiac septa
Q24.4	Congenital subaortic stenosis
Q24.5	Malformation of coronary vessels

Q24.6	Congenital heart block
Q24.8	Other specified congenital malformations of heart
Q24.9	Congenital malformation of heart, unspecified
T86.21	Heart transplant rejection
T86.22	Heart transplant failure

AMA: 33945 2018,Jun

Relative Value Units/Medicare Edits

Non-Facility RVU	Work	PE	MP	Total
33945	89.5	31.71	21.52	142.73
Facility RVU	**Work**	**PE**	**MP**	**Total**
33945	89.5	31.71	21.52	142.73

	FUD	Status	MUE	Modifiers				IOM Reference
33945	90	R	1(2)	51	N/A	62*	80	None

* with documentation

Terms To Know

atherosclerosis. Buildup of yellowish plaques composed of cholesterol and lipoid material within the arteries.

cadaver. Dead body.

cardiectomy. Surgical removal of the heart, may be for transplant or replacement with mechanical heart.

cardiomyopathy. General term used to describe a number of conditions of the heart muscle.

cardiopulmonary bypass. Venous blood is diverted to a heart-lung machine, which mechanically pumps and oxygenates the blood temporarily so the heart can be bypassed while an open procedure on the heart or coronary arteries is performed. During bypass, the lungs are deflated and immobile.

congestive heart failure. Condition caused by the heart's inability to adequately pump and circulate blood, resulting in fluid accumulation in the lungs and other tissues.

rheumatic heart disease. Manifestation of and sequel to rheumatic fever; any cardiac involvement in rheumatic fever.

transplant. Insertion of an organ or tissue from one person or site into another.

33946-33947

33946 Extracorporeal membrane oxygenation (ECMO)/extracorporeal life support (ECLS) provided by physician; initiation, veno-venous

33947 initiation, veno-arterial

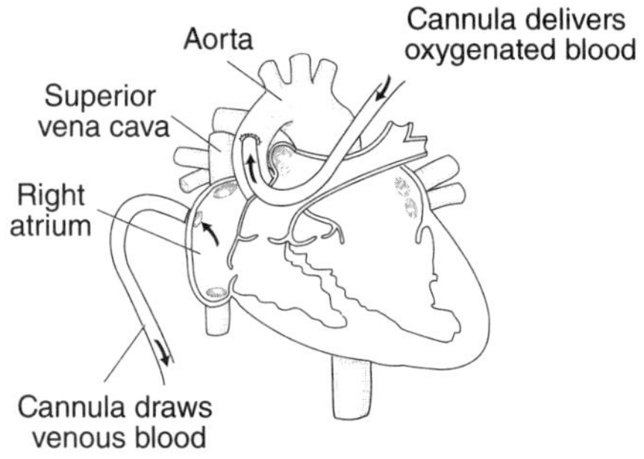

Explanation

The physician initiates veno-venous or veno-arterial extracorporeal membrane oxygenation (ECMO)/extracorporeal life support (ECLS). In ECMO/ECLS, the patient's blood is pumped to a machine, oxygenated, and returned to the patient, similar to a cardiopulmonary bypass but modified for prolonged use (days to weeks) at the bedside. Its purpose is to provide mechanical support for the heart and lungs in order to allow time for recovery. Report 33946 for initiation of veno-venous ECMO/ECLS, which exchanges blood between large veins through a single double-lumen cannula. Report 33947 for initiation of veno-arterial ECMO/ECLS, which exchanges oxygen poor blood from a central vein or right atrium with oxygen rich blood pumped back into the patient within the arterial circulation through two cannulae: one into a vein and the other into an artery.

Coding Tips

These services are reported separately in addition to daily management, hospital observation, inpatient, or critical care codes. The physician providing all components of ECMO/ECLS should report all codes for services provided. When performed by different providers, each should bill for the service performed. If extensive repair or replacement of an artery is required and performed, report 35266, 35286, 35371, or 35665 in addition to 33946 and 33947. Do not report 33946 or 33947 with daily management codes 33948 and 33949 or repositioning codes 33957–33959 and 33962–33964. Codes 33946 and 33947 are separate services from daily overall management of a patient. The daily overall management may be reported with relevant inpatient or observation codes (99221–99223, 99231–99236, critical care or intensive care codes (99291, 99292, 99468, 99469, 99471, 99472, 99475–99480), or evaluation and management codes. Do not append modifier 63 to 33946 and 33947 as the description or nature of the procedure includes infants up to 4 kg. For cannula insertion, see 33951–33956.

ICD-10-CM Diagnostic Codes

I40.0	Infective myocarditis
I40.1	Isolated myocarditis
I50.21	Acute systolic (congestive) heart failure
I50.22	Chronic systolic (congestive) heart failure
I50.23	Acute on chronic systolic (congestive) heart failure
I50.31	Acute diastolic (congestive) heart failure

I50.32	Chronic diastolic (congestive) heart failure
I50.33	Acute on chronic diastolic (congestive) heart failure
I50.41	Acute combined systolic (congestive) and diastolic (congestive) heart failure
I50.42	Chronic combined systolic (congestive) and diastolic (congestive) heart failure
I50.43	Acute on chronic combined systolic (congestive) and diastolic (congestive) heart failure
I50.811	Acute right heart failure
I50.812	Chronic right heart failure
I50.813	Acute on chronic right heart failure
I50.814	Right heart failure due to left heart failure
I50.82	Biventricular heart failure
I50.83	High output heart failure
I50.84	End stage heart failure
I97.0	Postcardiotomy syndrome
I97.110	Postprocedural cardiac insufficiency following cardiac surgery
I97.120	Postprocedural cardiac arrest following cardiac surgery
I97.130	Postprocedural heart failure following cardiac surgery
J80	Acute respiratory distress syndrome
J84.170	Interstitial lung disease with progressive fibrotic phenotype in diseases classified elsewhere
J84.178	Other interstitial pulmonary diseases with fibrosis in diseases classified elsewhere
J93.0	Spontaneous tension pneumothorax
J93.11	Primary spontaneous pneumothorax
J93.12	Secondary spontaneous pneumothorax
J93.81	Chronic pneumothorax
J95.1	Acute pulmonary insufficiency following thoracic surgery
J95.3	Chronic pulmonary insufficiency following surgery
J95.822	Acute and chronic postprocedural respiratory failure
J95.851	Ventilator associated pneumonia
J95.87	Transfusion-associated dyspnea (TAD)
J96.01	Acute respiratory failure with hypoxia
J96.02	Acute respiratory failure with hypercapnia
J96.11	Chronic respiratory failure with hypoxia
J96.12	Chronic respiratory failure with hypercapnia
J96.21	Acute and chronic respiratory failure with hypoxia
J96.22	Acute and chronic respiratory failure with hypercapnia
P22.0	Respiratory distress syndrome of newborn N
P25.0	Interstitial emphysema originating in the perinatal period N
P25.1	Pneumothorax originating in the perinatal period N
P28.5	Respiratory failure of newborn N
P28.81	Respiratory arrest of newborn N
P29.0	Neonatal cardiac failure N
P29.2	Neonatal hypertension N
P29.30	Pulmonary hypertension of newborn
P29.4	Transient myocardial ischemia in newborn N
P29.81	Cardiac arrest of newborn N
Q22.2	Congenital pulmonary valve insufficiency
R06.03	Acute respiratory distress
R09.2	Respiratory arrest
R57.0	Cardiogenic shock
S27.0XXA	Traumatic pneumothorax, initial encounter
S27.1XXA	Traumatic hemothorax, initial encounter
S27.2XXA	Traumatic hemopneumothorax, initial encounter
T81.11XA	Postprocedural cardiogenic shock, initial encounter

Relative Value Units/Medicare Edits

Non-Facility RVU	Work	PE	MP	Total
33946	6.0	1.78	1.29	9.07
33947	6.63	1.97	1.44	10.04
Facility RVU	**Work**	**PE**	**MP**	**Total**
33946	6.0	1.78	1.29	9.07
33947	6.63	1.97	1.44	10.04

	FUD	Status	MUE	Modifiers				IOM Reference
33946	N/A	A	1(2)	N/A	N/A	N/A	N/A	None
33947	N/A	A	1(2)	N/A	N/A	N/A	N/A	

* with documentation

Terms To Know

anomaly. Irregularity in the structure or position of an organ or tissue.

cardiogenic shock. Shock caused by an inadequate supply of oxygen to the body's tissues due to a malfunction of the pumping action of the heart.

congenital anomaly. Abnormality that is present at birth that may be the result of genetic factors, teratogens, or other conditions that affect the fetus in utero. The abnormalities may be readily apparent at birth or may remain undiscovered until some point after birth.

extracorporeal. Located or taking place outside the body.

meconium aspiration syndrome. Newborn respiratory complications resulting from the passage and subsequent aspiration of meconium (fetal intestinal waste material) prior to or during delivery.

respiratory distress syndrome. Premature neonates with respiratory distress and associated with reduced amounts of lung surfactant. Frequently fatal.

33948-33949

33948 Extracorporeal membrane oxygenation (ECMO)/extracorporeal life support (ECLS) provided by physician; daily management, each day, veno-venous

33949 daily management, each day, veno-arterial

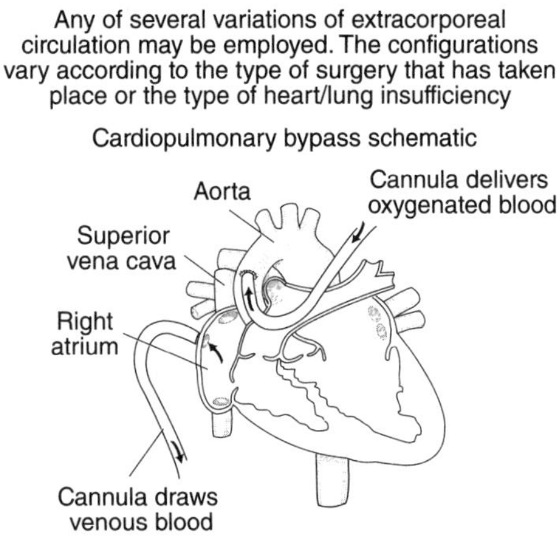

Explanation

The physician performs daily management of extracorporeal membrane oxygenation (ECMO)/extracorporeal life support (ECLS). In ECMO/ECLS, the patient's blood is pumped to a machine, oxygenated, and returned to the patient, similar to a cardiopulmonary bypass but modified for prolonged use (days to weeks) at the bedside. Its purpose is to provide mechanical support for the heart and lungs in order to allow time for recovery. Patients receiving ECMO/ECLS require daily management to monitor for infections of the skin along cannulas and to identify any evidence of clotting in the legs or any deposits visualized within the pump. Report 33948 for daily management of veno-venous ECMO/ECLS, which exchanges blood between large veins through a single double-lumen cannula. Report 33949 for daily management of veno-arterial ECMO/ECLS, which exchanges oxygen poor blood from a central vein or right atrium with oxygen rich blood pumped back into the patient within the arterial circulation through two cannulae: one into a vein and the other into an artery.

Coding Tips

These services are separately reported in addition to daily overall management reported with hospital observation, inpatient, or critical care codes. Codes 33946 and 33947 are separate services from daily overall management of a patient. The daily overall management may be reported with relevant inpatient or observation codes (99221–99223, 99231–99236), critical care or intensive care codes (99291, 99292, 99468, 99469, 99471, 99472, 99475–99480), and evaluation and management codes. Do not append modifier 63 to 33948 and 33949 as the description or nature of the procedure includes infants up to 4 kg. Do not report 33948 and 33949 with 33946 or 33947.

ICD-10-CM Diagnostic Codes

I40.0	Infective myocarditis
I40.1	Isolated myocarditis
I50.21	Acute systolic (congestive) heart failure
I50.22	Chronic systolic (congestive) heart failure
I50.23	Acute on chronic systolic (congestive) heart failure
I50.31	Acute diastolic (congestive) heart failure
I50.32	Chronic diastolic (congestive) heart failure
I50.33	Acute on chronic diastolic (congestive) heart failure
I50.41	Acute combined systolic (congestive) and diastolic (congestive) heart failure
I50.42	Chronic combined systolic (congestive) and diastolic (congestive) heart failure
I50.43	Acute on chronic combined systolic (congestive) and diastolic (congestive) heart failure
I50.811	Acute right heart failure
I50.812	Chronic right heart failure
I50.813	Acute on chronic right heart failure
I50.814	Right heart failure due to left heart failure
I50.82	Biventricular heart failure
I50.83	High output heart failure
I50.84	End stage heart failure
I97.0	Postcardiotomy syndrome
I97.110	Postprocedural cardiac insufficiency following cardiac surgery
I97.120	Postprocedural cardiac arrest following cardiac surgery
I97.130	Postprocedural heart failure following cardiac surgery
J80	Acute respiratory distress syndrome
J84.170	Interstitial lung disease with progressive fibrotic phenotype in diseases classified elsewhere
J84.178	Other interstitial pulmonary diseases with fibrosis in diseases classified elsewhere
J93.0	Spontaneous tension pneumothorax
J93.11	Primary spontaneous pneumothorax
J93.12	Secondary spontaneous pneumothorax
J93.81	Chronic pneumothorax
J95.1	Acute pulmonary insufficiency following thoracic surgery
J95.3	Chronic pulmonary insufficiency following surgery
J95.822	Acute and chronic postprocedural respiratory failure
J95.851	Ventilator associated pneumonia
J95.87	Transfusion-associated dyspnea (TAD)
J96.01	Acute respiratory failure with hypoxia
J96.02	Acute respiratory failure with hypercapnia
J96.11	Chronic respiratory failure with hypoxia
J96.12	Chronic respiratory failure with hypercapnia
J96.21	Acute and chronic respiratory failure with hypoxia
J96.22	Acute and chronic respiratory failure with hypercapnia
P22.0	Respiratory distress syndrome of newborn N
P25.0	Interstitial emphysema originating in the perinatal period N
P25.1	Pneumothorax originating in the perinatal period N
P28.5	Respiratory failure of newborn N
P28.81	Respiratory arrest of newborn N
P29.0	Neonatal cardiac failure N
P29.2	Neonatal hypertension N
P29.30	Pulmonary hypertension of newborn
P29.4	Transient myocardial ischemia in newborn N
P29.81	Cardiac arrest of newborn N
Q22.2	Congenital pulmonary valve insufficiency
R06.03	Acute respiratory distress
R09.2	Respiratory arrest
R57.0	Cardiogenic shock
S27.0XXA	Traumatic pneumothorax, initial encounter
S27.1XXA	Traumatic hemothorax, initial encounter

S27.2XXA Traumatic hemopneumothorax, initial encounter
T81.11XA Postprocedural cardiogenic shock, initial encounter

Relative Value Units/Medicare Edits

Non-Facility RVU	Work	PE	MP	Total
33948	4.73	1.44	0.8	6.97
33949	4.6	1.4	0.81	6.81
Facility RVU	**Work**	**PE**	**MP**	**Total**
33948	4.73	1.44	0.8	6.97
33949	4.6	1.4	0.81	6.81

	FUD	Status	MUE	Modifiers				IOM Reference
33948	N/A	A	1(2)	N/A	N/A	N/A	N/A	None
33949	N/A	A	1(2)	N/A	N/A	N/A	N/A	

* with documentation

Terms To Know

hypercapnia. Excess carbon dioxide in the blood.

hypoxia. Organ or tissue receiving an oxygen supply that is below the necessary oxygen levels, even when there is adequate blood perfusion.

myocarditis. Inflammation of the middle layer of the heart, which is composed of muscle tissue.

pneumothorax. Collapsed lung due to air or gas trapped in the pleural space formed by the membrane that encloses the lungs and lines the thoracic cavity.

33951-33952

33951 Extracorporeal membrane oxygenation (ECMO)/extracorporeal life support (ECLS) provided by physician; insertion of peripheral (arterial and/or venous) cannula(e), percutaneous, birth through 5 years of age (includes fluoroscopic guidance, when performed)

33952 insertion of peripheral (arterial and/or venous) cannula(e), percutaneous, 6 years and older (includes fluoroscopic guidance, when performed)

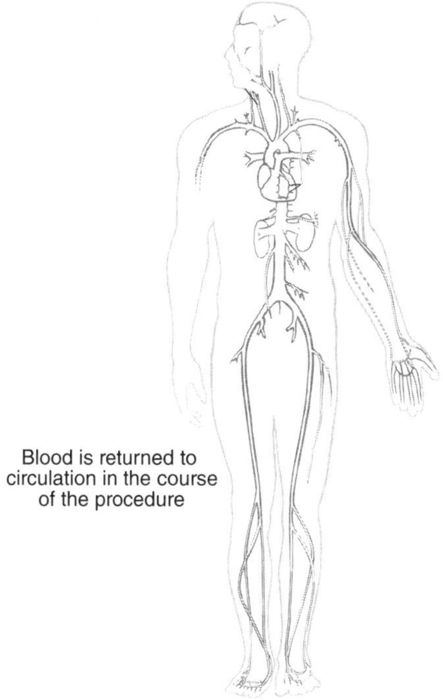

Explanation

The physician inserts a peripheral cannula for extracorporeal membrane oxygenation (ECMO)/extracorporeal life support (ECLS) percutaneously. When veno-arterial ECMO/ECLS is performed, a cannula is typically placed in the inferior vena cava or right atrium allowing for drainage. This cannula is introduced at the internal jugular or femoral vein. The blood is pumped back into the patient through a cannula placed within the femoral artery. When veno-venous ECMO/ECLS is performed, two or more cannulae are used within the large veins (jugular, femoral, or both) to assist with draining and oxygenated blood flow. A relatively new dual-chamber cannula is being utilized in some facilities for improved drainage, to reduce the risk of complications, and to improve the ability to move the patient. Report 33951 for peripheral insertion of a cannula performed percutaneously on patients from birth through age 5 and 33952 for patients age 6 years and older. Fluoroscopic guidance is included in these procedures when performed.

Coding Tips

For initiation and daily management/maintenance of extracorporeal circulation, see 33946, 33947, 33948, and 33949. The physician providing all components of ECMO/ECLS should report all codes for services provided. When performed by different providers, each should bill for the service performed. If cannula is taken from one vessel and inserted into another, report the removal (33965–33969, 33984–33986, and 33955–33956) and insertion (33951–33955) codes. However, if cannula(e) is removed and reinserted into the same vessel, report only the insertion codes. If extensive repair or replacement of an artery is required and performed, report 35266, 35286, 35371, or 35665 in addition to 33951 and 33952. Do not report repositioning of cannula (33957–33959 and 33962–33964) with 33951 and 33952.

ICD-10-CM Diagnostic Codes

I40.0	Infective myocarditis
I40.1	Isolated myocarditis
I50.21	Acute systolic (congestive) heart failure
I50.22	Chronic systolic (congestive) heart failure
I50.23	Acute on chronic systolic (congestive) heart failure
I50.31	Acute diastolic (congestive) heart failure
I50.32	Chronic diastolic (congestive) heart failure
I50.33	Acute on chronic diastolic (congestive) heart failure
I50.41	Acute combined systolic (congestive) and diastolic (congestive) heart failure
I50.42	Chronic combined systolic (congestive) and diastolic (congestive) heart failure
I50.43	Acute on chronic combined systolic (congestive) and diastolic (congestive) heart failure
I50.811	Acute right heart failure
I50.812	Chronic right heart failure
I50.813	Acute on chronic right heart failure
I50.814	Right heart failure due to left heart failure
I50.82	Biventricular heart failure
I50.83	High output heart failure
I50.84	End stage heart failure
I97.0	Postcardiotomy syndrome
I97.110	Postprocedural cardiac insufficiency following cardiac surgery
I97.120	Postprocedural cardiac arrest following cardiac surgery
I97.130	Postprocedural heart failure following cardiac surgery
J80	Acute respiratory distress syndrome
J84.170	Interstitial lung disease with progressive fibrotic phenotype in diseases classified elsewhere
J84.178	Other interstitial pulmonary diseases with fibrosis in diseases classified elsewhere
J93.0	Spontaneous tension pneumothorax
J93.11	Primary spontaneous pneumothorax
J93.12	Secondary spontaneous pneumothorax
J93.81	Chronic pneumothorax
J95.1	Acute pulmonary insufficiency following thoracic surgery
J95.3	Chronic pulmonary insufficiency following surgery
J95.822	Acute and chronic postprocedural respiratory failure
J95.851	Ventilator associated pneumonia
J95.87	Transfusion-associated dyspnea (TAD)
J96.01	Acute respiratory failure with hypoxia
J96.02	Acute respiratory failure with hypercapnia
J96.11	Chronic respiratory failure with hypoxia
J96.12	Chronic respiratory failure with hypercapnia
J96.21	Acute and chronic respiratory failure with hypoxia
J96.22	Acute and chronic respiratory failure with hypercapnia
P22.0	Respiratory distress syndrome of newborn N
P25.0	Interstitial emphysema originating in the perinatal period N
P25.1	Pneumothorax originating in the perinatal period N
P28.5	Respiratory failure of newborn N
P28.81	Respiratory arrest of newborn N
P29.0	Neonatal cardiac failure N
P29.2	Neonatal hypertension N
P29.30	Pulmonary hypertension of newborn
P29.4	Transient myocardial ischemia in newborn N
P29.81	Cardiac arrest of newborn N
Q22.2	Congenital pulmonary valve insufficiency
R06.03	Acute respiratory distress
R09.2	Respiratory arrest
R57.0	Cardiogenic shock
S27.0XXA	Traumatic pneumothorax, initial encounter
S27.1XXA	Traumatic hemothorax, initial encounter
S27.2XXA	Traumatic hemopneumothorax, initial encounter
T81.11XA	Postprocedural cardiogenic shock, initial encounter

Relative Value Units/Medicare Edits

Non-Facility RVU	Work	PE	MP	Total
33951	8.15	2.29	1.87	12.31
33952	8.15	2.51	1.84	12.5
Facility RVU	**Work**	**PE**	**MP**	**Total**
33951	8.15	2.29	1.87	12.31
33952	8.15	2.51	1.84	12.5

	FUD	Status	MUE	Modifiers				IOM Reference
33951	0	A	1(3)	51	N/A	N/A	80*	None
33952	0	A	1(3)	51	N/A	N/A	80*	

* with documentation

Terms To Know

asphyxia. Insufficient intake of oxygen, resulting in pathological changes brought on by a lack of oxygen perfusion to the tissues or excessive carbon dioxide in the blood.

cannula. Tube inserted into a blood vessel, duct, or body cavity to facilitate passage.

extracorporeal. Located or taking place outside the body.

fluoroscopy. Radiology technique that allows visual examination of part of the body or a function of an organ using a device that projects an x-ray image on a fluorescent screen.

meconium aspiration syndrome. Newborn respiratory complications resulting from the passage and subsequent aspiration of meconium (fetal intestinal waste material) prior to or during delivery.

33953-33954

33953 Extracorporeal membrane oxygenation (ECMO)/extracorporeal life support (ECLS) provided by physician; insertion of peripheral (arterial and/or venous) cannula(e), open, birth through 5 years of age

33954 insertion of peripheral (arterial and/or venous) cannula(e), open, 6 years and older

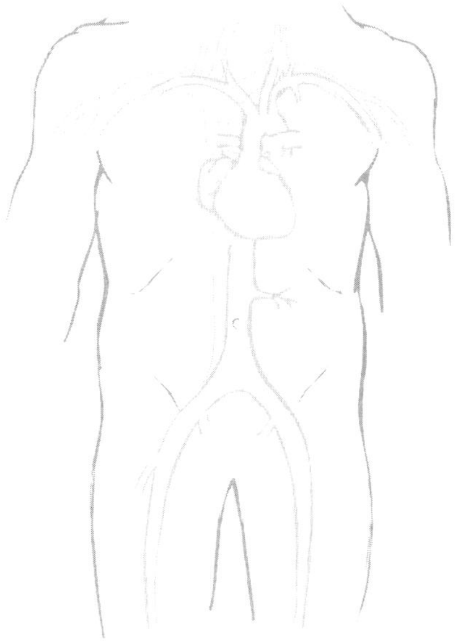

Open insertion of a cannula into a peripheral artery or vein, such as the femoral artery

Explanation

The physician inserts a peripheral cannula for extracorporeal membrane oxygenation (ECMO)/extracorporeal life support (ECLS) using an open approach. When veno-arterial ECMO/ECLS is performed, a cannula is typically placed in the inferior vena cava or right atrium allowing for drainage. This cannula is introduced at the internal jugular or femoral vein. The blood is pumped back into the patient through a cannula placed within the femoral artery. When veno-venous ECMO/ECLS is performed, two or more cannulae are used within the large veins (jugular, femoral, or both) to assist with draining and oxygenated blood flow. A relatively new dual-chamber cannula is being utilized in some facilities for improved drainage, to reduce the risk of complications, and to improve the ability to move the patient. Report 33953 for peripheral insertion of a cannula using an open approach on patients from birth through age 5 and 33954 for patients age 6 years and older.

Coding Tips

For initiation and daily management/maintenance of extracorporeal circulation, see 33946, 33947, 33948, and 33949. The physician providing all components of ECMO/ECLS should report all codes for services provided. When performed by different providers, each should bill for the service performed. If cannula is taken from one vessel and inserted into another, report the removal (33965–33969, 33984–33986, and 33955–33956) and insertion (33951–33955) codes. However, if cannula(e) is removed and reinserted into the same vessel, report only the insertion codes. If extensive repair or replacement of an artery is required and performed, report 35266, 35286, 35371, or 35665 in addition to 33953 and 33954. Do not report 33953 or 33954 with 34714-34716, 34812, 34820, 34833, and 34834.

ICD-10-CM Diagnostic Codes

I40.0	Infective myocarditis
I40.1	Isolated myocarditis
I50.21	Acute systolic (congestive) heart failure
I50.22	Chronic systolic (congestive) heart failure
I50.23	Acute on chronic systolic (congestive) heart failure
I50.31	Acute diastolic (congestive) heart failure
I50.32	Chronic diastolic (congestive) heart failure
I50.33	Acute on chronic diastolic (congestive) heart failure
I50.41	Acute combined systolic (congestive) and diastolic (congestive) heart failure
I50.42	Chronic combined systolic (congestive) and diastolic (congestive) heart failure
I50.43	Acute on chronic combined systolic (congestive) and diastolic (congestive) heart failure
I50.811	Acute right heart failure
I50.812	Chronic right heart failure
I50.813	Acute on chronic right heart failure
I50.814	Right heart failure due to left heart failure
I50.82	Biventricular heart failure
I50.83	High output heart failure
I50.84	End stage heart failure
I97.0	Postcardiotomy syndrome
I97.110	Postprocedural cardiac insufficiency following cardiac surgery
I97.120	Postprocedural cardiac arrest following cardiac surgery
I97.130	Postprocedural heart failure following cardiac surgery
J80	Acute respiratory distress syndrome
J84.170	Interstitial lung disease with progressive fibrotic phenotype in diseases classified elsewhere
J84.178	Other interstitial pulmonary diseases with fibrosis in diseases classified elsewhere
J93.0	Spontaneous tension pneumothorax
J93.11	Primary spontaneous pneumothorax
J93.12	Secondary spontaneous pneumothorax
J93.81	Chronic pneumothorax
J95.1	Acute pulmonary insufficiency following thoracic surgery
J95.3	Chronic pulmonary insufficiency following surgery
J95.822	Acute and chronic postprocedural respiratory failure
J95.851	Ventilator associated pneumonia
J95.87	Transfusion-associated dyspnea (TAD)
J96.01	Acute respiratory failure with hypoxia
J96.02	Acute respiratory failure with hypercapnia
J96.11	Chronic respiratory failure with hypoxia
J96.12	Chronic respiratory failure with hypercapnia
J96.21	Acute and chronic respiratory failure with hypoxia
J96.22	Acute and chronic respiratory failure with hypercapnia
P22.0	Respiratory distress syndrome of newborn N
P25.0	Interstitial emphysema originating in the perinatal period N
P25.1	Pneumothorax originating in the perinatal period N
P28.5	Respiratory failure of newborn N
P28.81	Respiratory arrest of newborn N
P29.0	Neonatal cardiac failure N
P29.2	Neonatal hypertension N
P29.30	Pulmonary hypertension of newborn
P29.4	Transient myocardial ischemia in newborn N
P29.81	Cardiac arrest of newborn N

Q22.2	Congenital pulmonary valve insufficiency
R06.03	Acute respiratory distress
R09.2	Respiratory arrest
R57.0	Cardiogenic shock
S27.0XXA	Traumatic pneumothorax, initial encounter
S27.1XXA	Traumatic hemothorax, initial encounter
S27.2XXA	Traumatic hemopneumothorax, initial encounter
T81.11XA	Postprocedural cardiogenic shock, initial encounter

Relative Value Units/Medicare Edits

Non-Facility RVU	Work	PE	MP	Total
33953	9.11	2.54	2.1	13.75
33954	9.11	2.64	2.17	13.92
Facility RVU	**Work**	**PE**	**MP**	**Total**
33953	9.11	2.54	2.1	13.75
33954	9.11	2.64	2.17	13.92

	FUD	Status	MUE	Modifiers				IOM Reference
33953	0	A	1(3)	51	N/A	N/A	80*	None
33954	0	A	1(3)	51	N/A	N/A	80*	

* with documentation

Terms To Know

asphyxia. Insufficient intake of oxygen, resulting in pathological changes brought on by a lack of oxygen perfusion to the tissues or excessive carbon dioxide in the blood.

cannula. Tube inserted into a blood vessel, duct, or body cavity to facilitate passage.

cardiogenic shock. Shock caused by an inadequate supply of oxygen to the body's tissues due to a malfunction of the pumping action of the heart.

congenital. Present at birth, occurring through heredity or an influence during gestation up to the moment of birth.

extracorporeal. Located or taking place outside the body.

meconium aspiration syndrome. Newborn respiratory complications resulting from the passage and subsequent aspiration of meconium (fetal intestinal waste material) prior to or during delivery.

vena cava. Main venous trunk that empties into the right atrium from both the lower and upper regions, beginning at the junction of the common iliac veins inferiorly and the two brachiocephalic veins superiorly.

33955-33956

33955 Extracorporeal membrane oxygenation (ECMO)/extracorporeal life support (ECLS) provided by physician; insertion of central cannula(e) by sternotomy or thoracotomy, birth through 5 years of age

33956 insertion of central cannula(e) by sternotomy or thoracotomy, 6 years and older

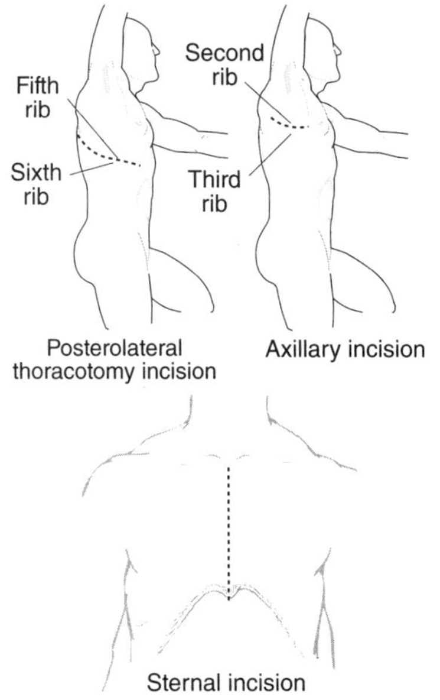

Any of a number of access incisions may be used

Explanation

The physician inserts central cannulae for extracorporeal membrane oxygenation (ECMO)/extracorporeal life support (ECLS) via sternotomy or thoracotomy. A cannula is placed in the inferior vena cava or right atrium allowing for drainage. This cannula is introduced at the internal jugular or femoral vein accomplished by sternotomy or thoracotomy. The blood is pumped back into the patient through a cannula surgically placed within the ascending aorta, referred to as central ECMO/ECLS. This form of introduction is typically utilized following cardiopulmonary bypass since the location of cannulae placement would be the same as location during surgery. When veno-venous ECMO/ECLS is performed, two or more cannulae are used within the large veins (jugular, femoral, or both) to assist with draining and oxygenated blood flow. A relatively new dual-chamber cannula is being utilized in some facilities for improved drainage, to reduce the risk of complications, and to improve the ability to move the patient. Report 33955 for centrally inserted cannulae by sternotomy or thoracotomy performed on patients from birth through age 5 and 33956 for patients age 6 years and older.

Coding Tips

For initiation and daily management/maintenance of extracorporeal circulation, see 33946, 33947, 33948, and 33949. The physician providing all components of ECMO/ECLS should report all codes for services provided. When performed by different providers, each should bill for the service performed. If cannula is taken from one vessel and inserted into another, report the removal (33965–33969, 33984–33986), and insertion (33951–33955) codes. However, if cannula(e) is removed and reinserted into the same vessel, report only the insertion codes. If extensive repair or replacement of an artery is required and performed, report 35266, 35286, 35371, or 35665 in addition to 33955 and 33956. Do not report 33955 or 33956 with 32100 or 39010.

ICD-10-CM Diagnostic Codes

I40.0	Infective myocarditis
I40.1	Isolated myocarditis
I50.21	Acute systolic (congestive) heart failure
I50.22	Chronic systolic (congestive) heart failure
I50.23	Acute on chronic systolic (congestive) heart failure
I50.31	Acute diastolic (congestive) heart failure
I50.32	Chronic diastolic (congestive) heart failure
I50.33	Acute on chronic diastolic (congestive) heart failure
I50.41	Acute combined systolic (congestive) and diastolic (congestive) heart failure
I50.42	Chronic combined systolic (congestive) and diastolic (congestive) heart failure
I50.43	Acute on chronic combined systolic (congestive) and diastolic (congestive) heart failure
I50.811	Acute right heart failure
I50.812	Chronic right heart failure
I50.813	Acute on chronic right heart failure
I50.814	Right heart failure due to left heart failure
I50.82	Biventricular heart failure
I50.83	High output heart failure
I50.84	End stage heart failure
I97.0	Postcardiotomy syndrome
I97.110	Postprocedural cardiac insufficiency following cardiac surgery
I97.120	Postprocedural cardiac arrest following cardiac surgery
I97.130	Postprocedural heart failure following cardiac surgery
J80	Acute respiratory distress syndrome
J84.170	Interstitial lung disease with progressive fibrotic phenotype in diseases classified elsewhere
J84.178	Other interstitial pulmonary diseases with fibrosis in diseases classified elsewhere
J93.0	Spontaneous tension pneumothorax
J93.11	Primary spontaneous pneumothorax
J93.12	Secondary spontaneous pneumothorax
J93.81	Chronic pneumothorax
J95.1	Acute pulmonary insufficiency following thoracic surgery
J95.3	Chronic pulmonary insufficiency following surgery
J95.822	Acute and chronic postprocedural respiratory failure
J95.851	Ventilator associated pneumonia
J95.87	Transfusion-associated dyspnea (TAD)
J96.01	Acute respiratory failure with hypoxia
J96.02	Acute respiratory failure with hypercapnia
J96.11	Chronic respiratory failure with hypoxia
J96.12	Chronic respiratory failure with hypercapnia
J96.21	Acute and chronic respiratory failure with hypoxia
J96.22	Acute and chronic respiratory failure with hypercapnia
P22.0	Respiratory distress syndrome of newborn N
P25.0	Interstitial emphysema originating in the perinatal period N
P25.1	Pneumothorax originating in the perinatal period N
P28.5	Respiratory failure of newborn N
P28.81	Respiratory arrest of newborn N
P29.0	Neonatal cardiac failure N
P29.2	Neonatal hypertension N
P29.30	Pulmonary hypertension of newborn
P29.4	Transient myocardial ischemia in newborn N
P29.81	Cardiac arrest of newborn N
Q22.2	Congenital pulmonary valve insufficiency
R06.03	Acute respiratory distress
R09.2	Respiratory arrest
R57.0	Cardiogenic shock
S27.0XXA	Traumatic pneumothorax, initial encounter
S27.1XXA	Traumatic hemothorax, initial encounter
S27.2XXA	Traumatic hemopneumothorax, initial encounter
T81.11XA	Postprocedural cardiogenic shock, initial encounter

Relative Value Units/Medicare Edits

Non-Facility RVU	Work	PE	MP	Total
33955	16.0	4.38	3.7	24.08
33956	16.0	4.59	3.87	24.46
Facility RVU	**Work**	**PE**	**MP**	**Total**
33955	16.0	4.38	3.7	24.08
33956	16.0	4.59	3.87	24.46

	FUD	Status	MUE	Modifiers				IOM Reference
33955	0	A	1(3)	51	N/A	62*	80*	None
33956	0	A	1(3)	51	N/A	62*	80*	

* with documentation

Terms To Know

asphyxia. Insufficient intake of oxygen, resulting in pathological changes brought on by a lack of oxygen perfusion to the tissues or excessive carbon dioxide in the blood.

cannula. Tube inserted into a blood vessel, duct, or body cavity to facilitate passage.

cardiogenic shock. Shock caused by an inadequate supply of oxygen to the body's tissues due to a malfunction of the pumping action of the heart.

congenital. Present at birth, occurring through heredity or an influence during gestation up to the moment of birth.

extracorporeal. Located or taking place outside the body.

meconium aspiration syndrome. Newborn respiratory complications resulting from the passage and subsequent aspiration of meconium (fetal intestinal waste material) prior to or during delivery.

vena cava. Main venous trunk that empties into the right atrium from both the lower and upper regions, beginning at the junction of the common iliac veins inferiorly and the two brachiocephalic veins superiorly.

 ● New ▲ Revised + Add On ★ Telemedicine [Resequenced] ☑ Laterality

33957-33958

33957 Extracorporeal membrane oxygenation (ECMO)/extracorporeal life support (ECLS) provided by physician; reposition peripheral (arterial and/or venous) cannula(e), percutaneous, birth through 5 years of age (includes fluoroscopic guidance, when performed)

33958 reposition peripheral (arterial and/or venous) cannula(e), percutaneous, 6 years and older (includes fluoroscopic guidance, when performed)

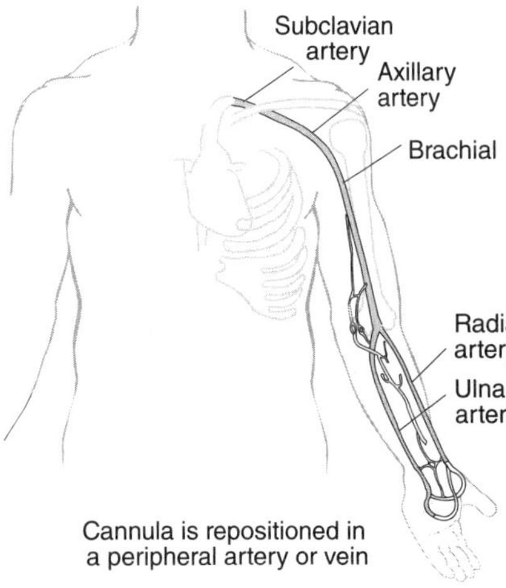

Cannula is repositioned in a peripheral artery or vein

Explanation

The physician repositions a peripheral cannula used for extracorporeal membrane oxygenation (ECMO)/extracorporeal life support (ECLS) percutaneously. Repositioning of the cannula may be necessary in the event of technical and/or vascular complications, such as blood flow obstruction, movement of the cannula from the original position, and/or bleeding issues resulting from the use of heparin during ECMO/ECLS. Oftentimes this requires a pull back of the cannula until it is back in an optimal position; however, in some cases, repositioning may require another procedure to achieve an appropriate position based on the specific location of the cannula and the complication. Report 33957 for percutaneous repositioning performed on a peripheral vessel for patients from birth through age 5 and 33958 for patients age 6 years and older. These codes include fluoroscopic guidance when performed.

Coding Tips

Do not report daily management codes 33948 and 33949 or repositioning codes 33957–33959 and 33962–33964 with 33946 or 33947. Repositioning of the cannula is not reported separately during the same encounter as insertion (33951–33955). Fluoroscopic guidance is included and is not reported separately. Do not report 33957 or 33958 with 34713, 34812, 34820, or 34834.

ICD-10-CM Diagnostic Codes

T82.310A Breakdown (mechanical) of aortic (bifurcation) graft (replacement), initial encounter
T82.311A Breakdown (mechanical) of carotid arterial graft (bypass), initial encounter
T82.312A Breakdown (mechanical) of femoral arterial graft (bypass), initial encounter
T82.318A Breakdown (mechanical) of other vascular grafts, initial encounter
T82.320A Displacement of aortic (bifurcation) graft (replacement), initial encounter
T82.321A Displacement of carotid arterial graft (bypass), initial encounter
T82.322A Displacement of femoral arterial graft (bypass), initial encounter
T82.328A Displacement of other vascular grafts, initial encounter
T82.330A Leakage of aortic (bifurcation) graft (replacement), initial encounter
T82.331A Leakage of carotid arterial graft (bypass), initial encounter
T82.332A Leakage of femoral arterial graft (bypass), initial encounter
T82.338A Leakage of other vascular grafts, initial encounter
T82.390A Other mechanical complication of aortic (bifurcation) graft (replacement), initial encounter
T82.391A Other mechanical complication of carotid arterial graft (bypass), initial encounter
T82.392A Other mechanical complication of femoral arterial graft (bypass), initial encounter
T82.398A Other mechanical complication of other vascular grafts, initial encounter
T82.528A Displacement of other cardiac and vascular devices and implants, initial encounter
T82.538A Leakage of other cardiac and vascular devices and implants, initial encounter
T82.598A Other mechanical complication of other cardiac and vascular devices and implants, initial encounter
T82.818A Embolism due to vascular prosthetic devices, implants and grafts, initial encounter
T82.828A Fibrosis due to vascular prosthetic devices, implants and grafts, initial encounter
T82.838A Hemorrhage due to vascular prosthetic devices, implants and grafts, initial encounter
T82.848A Pain due to vascular prosthetic devices, implants and grafts, initial encounter
T82.856A Stenosis of peripheral vascular stent, initial encounter
T82.858A Stenosis of other vascular prosthetic devices, implants and grafts, initial encounter
T82.868A Thrombosis due to vascular prosthetic devices, implants and grafts, initial encounter
T82.898A Other specified complication of vascular prosthetic devices, implants and grafts, initial encounter
T88.8XXA Other specified complications of surgical and medical care, not elsewhere classified, initial encounter

Relative Value Units/Medicare Edits

Non-Facility RVU	Work	PE	MP	Total
33957	3.51	1.05	0.8	5.36
33958	3.51	1.05	0.8	5.36
Facility RVU	**Work**	**PE**	**MP**	**Total**
33957	3.51	1.05	0.8	5.36
33958	3.51	1.05	0.8	5.36

	FUD	Status	MUE	Modifiers				IOM Reference
33957	0	A	1(3)	51	N/A	N/A	80*	None
33958	0	A	1(3)	51	N/A	N/A	80*	

* with documentation

N Newborn: 0 P Pediatric: 0-17 M Maternity: 9-64 A Adult: 15-124 AMA: CPT Assist

33959 [33962]

33959 Extracorporeal membrane oxygenation (ECMO)/extracorporeal life support (ECLS) provided by physician; reposition peripheral (arterial and/or venous) cannula(e), open, birth through 5 years of age (includes fluoroscopic guidance, when performed)

33962 Extracorporeal membrane oxygenation (ECMO)/extracorporeal life support (ECLS) provided by physician; reposition peripheral (arterial and/or venous) cannula(e), open, 6 years and older (includes fluoroscopic guidance, when performed)

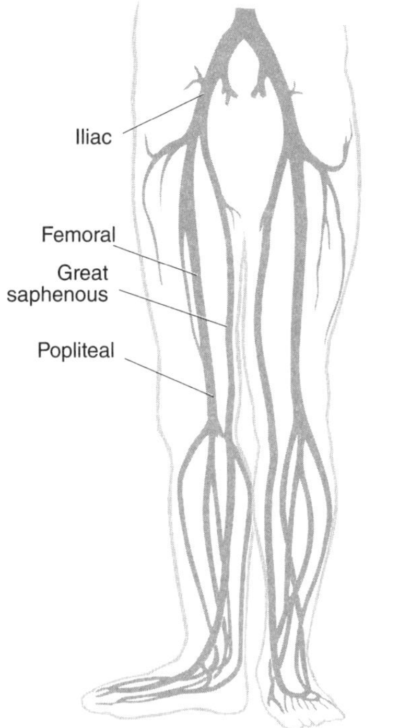

A single segment of femoropopliteal vein is harvested for a vascular reconstruction

Explanation

The physician repositions a peripheral cannula used for extracorporeal membrane oxygenation (ECMO)/extracorporeal life support (ECLS) via an open approach. Repositioning of the cannula may be necessary in the event of technical and/or vascular complications, such as blood flow obstruction, movement of the cannula from the original position, and/or bleeding issues resulting from the use of heparin during ECMO/ECLS. Oftentimes this requires a pull back of the cannula until it is back in an optimal position; however, in some cases, repositioning may require another procedure to achieve an appropriate position based on the specific location of the cannula and the complication. Report 33959 if the reposition is performed by open approach on a peripheral vessel for patients from birth through age 5 and 33962 for patients age 6 years and older. These codes include fluoroscopic guidance when performed.

Coding Tips

Do not report daily management codes 33948 and 33949 or repositioning codes 33957–33959 and 33962–33964 with 33946 and 33947. Repositioning of cannula is not reported separately during the same encounter as insertion (33951–33955). Fluoroscopic guidance is included and is not reported separately. Do not report 33959 or 33962 with 34714-34716, 34812, 34820, or 34834.

ICD-10-CM Diagnostic Codes

T82.310A Breakdown (mechanical) of aortic (bifurcation) graft (replacement), initial encounter

T82.311A Breakdown (mechanical) of carotid arterial graft (bypass), initial encounter

T82.312A Breakdown (mechanical) of femoral arterial graft (bypass), initial encounter

T82.318A Breakdown (mechanical) of other vascular grafts, initial encounter

T82.320A Displacement of aortic (bifurcation) graft (replacement), initial encounter

T82.321A Displacement of carotid arterial graft (bypass), initial encounter

T82.322A Displacement of femoral arterial graft (bypass), initial encounter

T82.330A Leakage of aortic (bifurcation) graft (replacement), initial encounter

T82.331A Leakage of carotid arterial graft (bypass), initial encounter

T82.332A Leakage of femoral arterial graft (bypass), initial encounter

T82.338A Leakage of other vascular grafts, initial encounter

T82.518A Breakdown (mechanical) of other cardiac and vascular devices and implants, initial encounter

T82.528A Displacement of other cardiac and vascular devices and implants, initial encounter

T82.538A Leakage of other cardiac and vascular devices and implants, initial encounter

T82.818A Embolism due to vascular prosthetic devices, implants and grafts, initial encounter

T82.828A Fibrosis due to vascular prosthetic devices, implants and grafts, initial encounter

T82.838A Hemorrhage due to vascular prosthetic devices, implants and grafts, initial encounter

T82.848A Pain due to vascular prosthetic devices, implants and grafts, initial encounter

T82.858A Stenosis of other vascular prosthetic devices, implants and grafts, initial encounter

T82.868A Thrombosis due to vascular prosthetic devices, implants and grafts, initial encounter

Relative Value Units/Medicare Edits

Non-Facility RVU	Work	PE	MP	Total
33959	4.47	1.31	1.05	6.83
33962	4.47	1.31	1.05	6.83
Facility RVU	**Work**	**PE**	**MP**	**Total**
33959	4.47	1.31	1.05	6.83
33962	4.47	1.31	1.05	6.83

	FUD	Status	MUE	Modifiers				IOM Reference
33959	0	A	1(3)	51	N/A	N/A	80*	None
33962	0	A	1(3)	51	N/A	N/A	80*	

* with documentation

Heart and Pericardium

 ● New ▲ Revised + Add On ★ Telemedicine [Resequenced] ☑ Laterality

[33963, 33964]

33963 Extracorporeal membrane oxygenation (ECMO)/extracorporeal life support (ECLS) provided by physician; reposition of central cannula(e) by sternotomy or thoracotomy, birth through 5 years of age (includes fluoroscopic guidance, when performed)

33964 Extracorporeal membrane oxygenation (ECMO)/extracorporeal life support (ECLS) provided by physician; reposition central cannula(e) by sternotomy or thoracotomy, 6 years and older (includes fluoroscopic guidance, when performed)

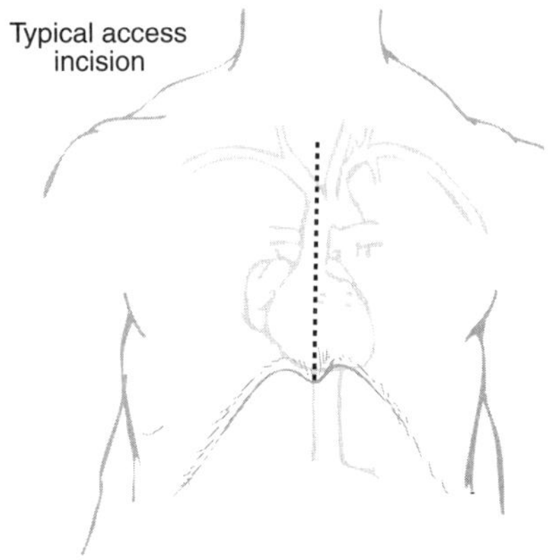

Central cannula is repositioned by sternotomy or thoracotomy

Explanation

The physician repositions a central cannula used for extracorporeal membrane oxygenation (ECMO)/extracorporeal life support (ECLS) via a sternotomy or thoracotomy. Repositioning of the cannula may be necessary in the event of technical and/or vascular complications, such as blood flow obstruction, movement of the cannula from the original position, and/or bleeding issues resulting from the use of heparin during ECMO/ECLS. Oftentimes this requires a pull back of the cannula until it is back in an optimal position; however, in some cases, repositioning may require another procedure to achieve an appropriate position based on the specific location of the cannula and the complication. Report 33963 for repositioning of a central cannula by sternotomy or thoracotomy performed on patients from birth through age 5 and 33964 for patients age 6 years and older. These codes include fluoroscopic guidance when performed.

Coding Tips

Do not report daily management codes 33948 and 33949 or repositioning codes 33957–33959 and 33962–33964 with 33946 and 33947. Repositioning of cannula in not reported separately during the same encounter as insertion (33951–33955). Fluoroscopic guidance is included and is not reported separately. Do not report 33963 or 33964 with 32100 or 39010.

ICD-10-CM Diagnostic Codes

T82.310A Breakdown (mechanical) of aortic (bifurcation) graft (replacement), initial encounter
T82.311A Breakdown (mechanical) of carotid arterial graft (bypass), initial encounter
T82.312A Breakdown (mechanical) of femoral arterial graft (bypass), initial encounter
T82.318A Breakdown (mechanical) of other vascular grafts, initial encounter
T82.320A Displacement of aortic (bifurcation) graft (replacement), initial encounter
T82.321A Displacement of carotid arterial graft (bypass), initial encounter
T82.322A Displacement of femoral arterial graft (bypass), initial encounter
T82.328A Displacement of other vascular grafts, initial encounter
T82.330A Leakage of aortic (bifurcation) graft (replacement), initial encounter
T82.331A Leakage of carotid arterial graft (bypass), initial encounter
T82.332A Leakage of femoral arterial graft (bypass), initial encounter
T82.338A Leakage of other vascular grafts, initial encounter
T82.390A Other mechanical complication of aortic (bifurcation) graft (replacement), initial encounter
T82.391A Other mechanical complication of carotid arterial graft (bypass), initial encounter
T82.392A Other mechanical complication of femoral arterial graft (bypass), initial encounter
T82.398A Other mechanical complication of other vascular grafts, initial encounter
T82.518A Breakdown (mechanical) of other cardiac and vascular devices and implants, initial encounter
T82.528A Displacement of other cardiac and vascular devices and implants, initial encounter
T82.538A Leakage of other cardiac and vascular devices and implants, initial encounter
T82.598A Other mechanical complication of other cardiac and vascular devices and implants, initial encounter
T82.818A Embolism due to vascular prosthetic devices, implants and grafts, initial encounter
T82.828A Fibrosis due to vascular prosthetic devices, implants and grafts, initial encounter
T82.838A Hemorrhage due to vascular prosthetic devices, implants and grafts, initial encounter
T82.848A Pain due to vascular prosthetic devices, implants and grafts, initial encounter
T82.856A Stenosis of peripheral vascular stent, initial encounter
T82.858A Stenosis of other vascular prosthetic devices, implants and grafts, initial encounter
T82.868A Thrombosis due to vascular prosthetic devices, implants and grafts, initial encounter
T82.898A Other specified complication of vascular prosthetic devices, implants and grafts, initial encounter
T88.8XXA Other specified complications of surgical and medical care, not elsewhere classified, initial encounter

Relative Value Units/Medicare Edits

Non-Facility RVU	Work	PE	MP	Total
33963	9.0	2.51	2.08	13.59
33964	9.5	2.65	2.2	14.35
Facility RVU	**Work**	**PE**	**MP**	**Total**
33963	9.0	2.51	2.08	13.59
33964	9.5	2.65	2.2	14.35

	FUD	Status	MUE	Modifiers				IOM Reference
33963	0	A	1(3)	51	N/A	62*	80*	None
33964	0	A	1(3)	51	N/A	62*	80*	

* with documentation

[33965, 33966]

33965 Extracorporeal membrane oxygenation (ECMO)/extracorporeal life support (ECLS) provided by physician; removal of peripheral (arterial and/or venous) cannula(e), percutaneous, birth through 5 years of age

33966 Extracorporeal membrane oxygenation (ECMO)/extracorporeal life support (ECLS) provided by physician; removal of peripheral (arterial and/or venous) cannula(e), percutaneous, 6 years and older

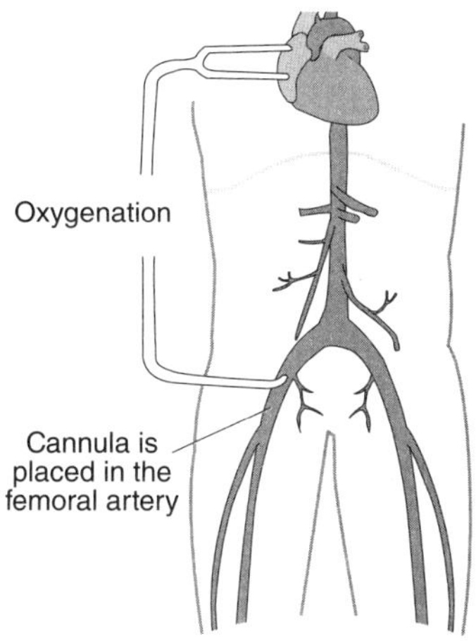

Percutaneous removal of a cannula from a peripheral artery or vein

Explanation

When extracorporeal membrane oxygenation (ECMO)/extracorporeal life support (ECLS) therapy is complete, the physician removes the cannula. Cannulae introduced percutaneously are simply pulled out like any other percutaneous placed catheter. Pressure is applied to the site for a limited time to stop bleeding. Report 33965 for removal of a peripheral percutaneous cannula for patients from birth through age 5 and 33966 for patients age 6 and older.

Coding Tips

If cannula is taken from one vessel and inserted into another, report the removal (33965–33969, 33984–33986, and 33955–33956) and insertion (33951–33955) codes. However, if cannula(e) is removed and reinserted into the same vessel, report only the insertion codes. If extensive repair or replacement of an artery is required and performed, report 35266, 35286, 35371, or 35665 in addition to 33965 and 33966.

ICD-10-CM Diagnostic Codes

T80.1XXA Vascular complications following infusion, transfusion and therapeutic injection, initial encounter

T80.211A Bloodstream infection due to central venous catheter, initial encounter

T80.212A Local infection due to central venous catheter, initial encounter

T80.29XA Infection following other infusion, transfusion and therapeutic injection, initial encounter

T82.310A Breakdown (mechanical) of aortic (bifurcation) graft (replacement), initial encounter

T82.311A Breakdown (mechanical) of carotid arterial graft (bypass), initial encounter

T82.312A Breakdown (mechanical) of femoral arterial graft (bypass), initial encounter

T82.320A Displacement of aortic (bifurcation) graft (replacement), initial encounter

T82.321A Displacement of carotid arterial graft (bypass), initial encounter

T82.322A Displacement of femoral arterial graft (bypass), initial encounter

T82.330A Leakage of aortic (bifurcation) graft (replacement), initial encounter

T82.331A Leakage of carotid arterial graft (bypass), initial encounter

T82.332A Leakage of femoral arterial graft (bypass), initial encounter

T82.338A Leakage of other vascular grafts, initial encounter

T82.518A Breakdown (mechanical) of other cardiac and vascular devices and implants, initial encounter

T82.528A Displacement of other cardiac and vascular devices and implants, initial encounter

T82.538A Leakage of other cardiac and vascular devices and implants, initial encounter

T82.818A Embolism due to vascular prosthetic devices, implants and grafts, initial encounter

T82.828A Fibrosis due to vascular prosthetic devices, implants and grafts, initial encounter

T82.838A Hemorrhage due to vascular prosthetic devices, implants and grafts, initial encounter

T82.848A Pain due to vascular prosthetic devices, implants and grafts, initial encounter

T82.856A Stenosis of peripheral vascular stent, initial encounter

T82.858A Stenosis of other vascular prosthetic devices, implants and grafts, initial encounter

T82.868A Thrombosis due to vascular prosthetic devices, implants and grafts, initial encounter

Relative Value Units/Medicare Edits

Non-Facility RVU	Work	PE	MP	Total
33965	3.51	1.05	0.8	5.36
33966	4.5	1.4	1.04	6.94
Facility RVU	**Work**	**PE**	**MP**	**Total**
33965	3.51	1.05	0.8	5.36
33966	4.5	1.4	1.04	6.94

	FUD	Status	MUE	Modifiers				IOM Reference
33965	0	A	1(3)	51	N/A	N/A	80*	None
33966	0	A	1(3)	51	N/A	N/A	80*	

* with documentation

[33969, 33984]

33969 Extracorporeal membrane oxygenation (ECMO)/extracorporeal life support (ECLS) provided by physician; removal of peripheral (arterial and/or venous) cannula(e), open, birth through 5 years of age

33984 Extracorporeal membrane oxygenation (ECMO)/extracorporeal life support (ECLS) provided by physician; removal of peripheral (arterial and/or venous) cannula(e), open, 6 years and older

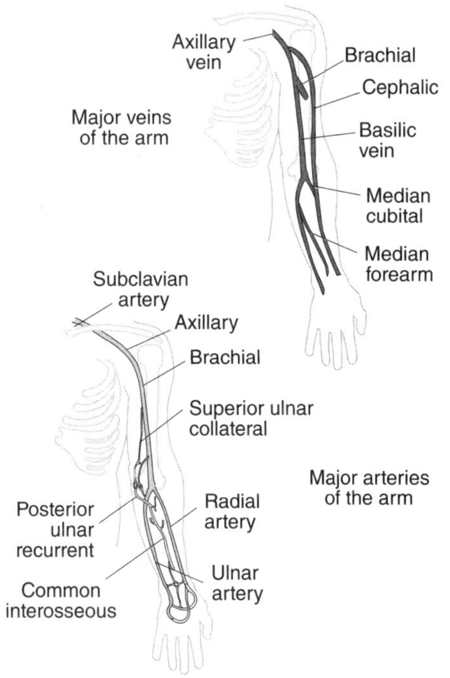

Explanation

When extracorporeal membrane oxygenation (ECMO)/extracorporeal life support (ECLS) therapy is complete, the physician removes the cannula. Cannulae placed via an open procedure require surgical intervention, sometimes performed bedside. The vessels cannulated are repaired and the skin is closed with stitches. Some patients require continued ventilation upon discontinuation of ECMO/ECLS therapy. Report 33969 for removal of a peripheral cannula performed by open approach for patients from birth through age 5 and 33984 for patients age 6 and older.

Coding Tips

If cannula is taken from one vessel and inserted into another, report the removal (33965–33969, 33984–33986, and 33955–33956) and insertion (33951–33955) codes. However, if cannula(e) is removed and reinserted into the same vessel, report only the insertion codes. If extensive repair or replacement of an artery is required and performed, report 35266, 35286, 35371, or 35665 in addition to 33965 and 33966. Do not report 33969 or 33984 with 34714-34716, 34812, 34820, 34834, 35201, 35206, 35211, or 35226.

ICD-10-CM Diagnostic Codes

T80.1XXA Vascular complications following infusion, transfusion and therapeutic injection, initial encounter

T80.211A Bloodstream infection due to central venous catheter, initial encounter

T80.212A Local infection due to central venous catheter, initial encounter

T80.29XA Infection following other infusion, transfusion and therapeutic injection, initial encounter

T82.310A Breakdown (mechanical) of aortic (bifurcation) graft (replacement), initial encounter

T82.311A Breakdown (mechanical) of carotid arterial graft (bypass), initial encounter

T82.312A Breakdown (mechanical) of femoral arterial graft (bypass), initial encounter

T82.318A Breakdown (mechanical) of other vascular grafts, initial encounter

T82.320A Displacement of aortic (bifurcation) graft (replacement), initial encounter

T82.321A Displacement of carotid arterial graft (bypass), initial encounter

T82.322A Displacement of femoral arterial graft (bypass), initial encounter

T82.328A Displacement of other vascular grafts, initial encounter

T82.330A Leakage of aortic (bifurcation) graft (replacement), initial encounter

T82.331A Leakage of carotid arterial graft (bypass), initial encounter

T82.332A Leakage of femoral arterial graft (bypass), initial encounter

T82.518A Breakdown (mechanical) of other cardiac and vascular devices and implants, initial encounter

T82.528A Displacement of other cardiac and vascular devices and implants, initial encounter

T82.538A Leakage of other cardiac and vascular devices and implants, initial encounter

T82.818A Embolism due to vascular prosthetic devices, implants and grafts, initial encounter

T82.828A Fibrosis due to vascular prosthetic devices, implants and grafts, initial encounter

T82.838A Hemorrhage due to vascular prosthetic devices, implants and grafts, initial encounter

T82.848A Pain due to vascular prosthetic devices, implants and grafts, initial encounter

T82.856A Stenosis of peripheral vascular stent, initial encounter

T82.858A Stenosis of other vascular prosthetic devices, implants and grafts, initial encounter

T82.868A Thrombosis due to vascular prosthetic devices, implants and grafts, initial encounter

Relative Value Units/Medicare Edits

Non-Facility RVU	Work	PE	MP	Total
33969	5.22	1.5	1.21	7.93
33984	5.46	1.53	1.31	8.3
Facility RVU	**Work**	**PE**	**MP**	**Total**
33969	5.22	1.5	1.21	7.93
33984	5.46	1.53	1.31	8.3

	FUD	Status	MUE	Modifiers				IOM Reference
33969	0	A	1(3)	51	N/A	N/A	80*	None
33984	0	A	1(3)	51	N/A	N/A	80*	

* with documentation

[33985, 33986]

33985 Extracorporeal membrane oxygenation (ECMO)/extracorporeal life support (ECLS) provided by physician; removal of central cannula(e) by sternotomy or thoracotomy, birth through 5 years of age

33986 Extracorporeal membrane oxygenation (ECMO)/extracorporeal life support (ECLS) provided by physician; removal of central cannula(e) by sternotomy or thoracotomy, 6 years and older

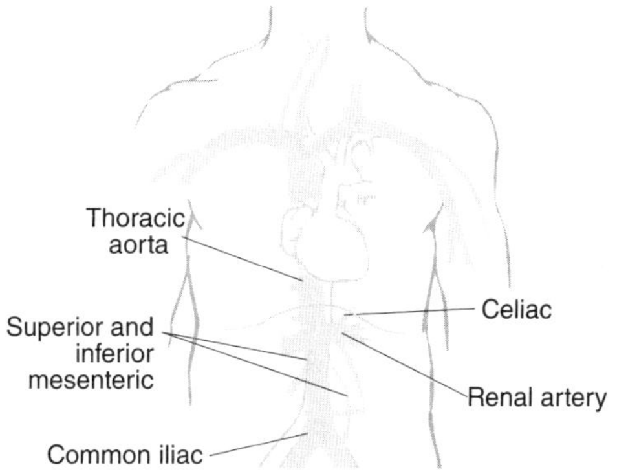

Removal of central cannula through sternotomy or thoracotomy

Explanation

When extracorporeal membrane oxygenation (ECMO)/extracorporeal life support (ECLS) therapy is complete, the physician removes the cannula. Cannulae placed via sternotomy or thoracotomy requires surgical intervention. The vessels cannulated are repaired and the skin is closed with stitches. Some patients require continued ventilation upon discontinuation of ECMO therapy. Report 33985 for removal of a central cannula performed by sternotomy or thoracotomy for patients from birth through age 5 and 33986 for patients age 6 and older.

Coding Tips

If cannula is taken from one vessel and inserted into another, report the removal (33965–33969, 33984–33986, and 33955–33956) and insertion (33951–33955) codes. However, if cannula(e) is removed and reinserted into the same vessel, report only the insertion codes. If extensive repair or replacement of an artery is required and performed, report 35266, 35286, 35371, or 35665 in addition to 33965 and 33966. Do not report 33985 or 33986 with 35211.

ICD-10-CM Diagnostic Codes

T80.1XXA Vascular complications following infusion, transfusion and therapeutic injection, initial encounter
T80.211A Bloodstream infection due to central venous catheter, initial encounter
T80.212A Local infection due to central venous catheter, initial encounter
T80.29XA Infection following other infusion, transfusion and therapeutic injection, initial encounter
T82.310A Breakdown (mechanical) of aortic (bifurcation) graft (replacement), initial encounter
T82.311A Breakdown (mechanical) of carotid arterial graft (bypass), initial encounter
T82.312A Breakdown (mechanical) of femoral arterial graft (bypass), initial encounter
T82.321A Displacement of carotid arterial graft (bypass), initial encounter
T82.322A Displacement of femoral arterial graft (bypass), initial encounter
T82.330A Leakage of aortic (bifurcation) graft (replacement), initial encounter
T82.331A Leakage of carotid arterial graft (bypass), initial encounter
T82.332A Leakage of femoral arterial graft (bypass), initial encounter
T82.510A Breakdown (mechanical) of surgically created arteriovenous fistula, initial encounter
T82.511A Breakdown (mechanical) of surgically created arteriovenous shunt, initial encounter
T82.513A Breakdown (mechanical) of balloon (counterpulsation) device, initial encounter
T82.518A Breakdown (mechanical) of other cardiac and vascular devices and implants, initial encounter
T82.528A Displacement of other cardiac and vascular devices and implants, initial encounter
T82.538A Leakage of other cardiac and vascular devices and implants, initial encounter
T82.818A Embolism due to vascular prosthetic devices, implants and grafts, initial encounter
T82.828A Fibrosis due to vascular prosthetic devices, implants and grafts, initial encounter
T82.838A Hemorrhage due to vascular prosthetic devices, implants and grafts, initial encounter
T82.848A Pain due to vascular prosthetic devices, implants and grafts, initial encounter
T82.856A Stenosis of peripheral vascular stent, initial encounter
T82.868A Thrombosis due to vascular prosthetic devices, implants and grafts, initial encounter

Relative Value Units/Medicare Edits

Non-Facility RVU	Work	PE	MP	Total
33985	9.89	2.75	2.28	14.92
33986	10.0	2.92	2.4	15.32
Facility RVU	**Work**	**PE**	**MP**	**Total**
33985	9.89	2.75	2.28	14.92
33986	10.0	2.92	2.4	15.32

	FUD	Status	MUE	Modifiers				IOM Reference
33985	0	A	1(3)	51	N/A	62*	80*	None
33986	0	A	1(3)	51	N/A	62*	80*	

* with documentation

Heart and Pericardium

[33987]

\+ **33987** Arterial exposure with creation of graft conduit (eg, chimney graft) to facilitate arterial perfusion for ECMO/ECLS (List separately in addition to code for primary procedure)

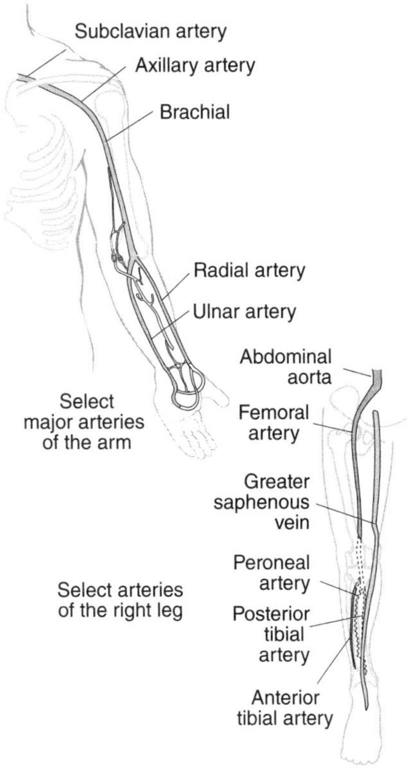

Explanation

The physician inserts a cannula(e) to provide prolonged extracorporeal circulation for cardiopulmonary insufficiency. The artery is exposed to create a graft that will broaden the vessel upwards (similar to a chimney) from the main artery being utilized. The graft is placed next to the artery often allowing for improved blood flow to smaller branches. Creating this type of graft requires special attention to the length needed to effectively use this technique. This cannula carries blood that is low in oxygen and high in carbon dioxide into the extracorporeal membrane oxygenation (ECMO) circuit. In veno-venous ECMO, if a double lumen cannula was inserted, blood that has passed through the membrane oxygenator that is now high in oxygen and low in carbon dioxide (oxygenated blood) is rewarmed to body temperature and returned via the same cannula. If a single lumen cannula is used, a second cannula is inserted into a second vein (venovenous ECMO) or a main artery (venoarterial ECMO), usually the femoral but in children the carotid may be used. This second cannula passes from the ECMO circuit carrying oxygenated, rewarmed blood back to the vein or artery.

Coding Tips

Report 33987 in addition to 33953–33956. Do not report 33987 with 34714, 34716, or 34833.

ICD-10-CM Diagnostic Codes

This/these CPT code(s) are add-on code(s). See the primary procedure code that this code is performed with for your ICD-10-CM code selections. Diagnostic code(s) would be the same as the actual procedure performed.

Relative Value Units/Medicare Edits

Non-Facility RVU	Work	PE	MP	Total
33987	4.04	1.08	0.94	6.06
Facility RVU	**Work**	**PE**	**MP**	**Total**
33987	4.04	1.08	0.94	6.06

	FUD	Status	MUE	Modifiers				IOM Reference
33987	N/A	A	1(3)	N/A	N/A	62*	80*	None

* with documentation

Terms To Know

conduit. Surgically created channel for the passage of fluids.

extracorporeal membrane oxygenation. Procedure done for cardiopulmonary insufficiency that shunts the circulating venous blood through catheters inserted into the right atrium to the outside of the body where it is oxygenated, bypassing the lungs, then returned to the body through another cannula inserted in the femoral artery.

graft. Tissue implant from another part of the body or another person.

perfusion. Act of pouring over or through, especially the passage of a fluid through the vessels of a specific organ.

[33988, 33989]

33988 Insertion of left heart vent by thoracic incision (eg, sternotomy, thoracotomy) for ECMO/ECLS

33989 Removal of left heart vent by thoracic incision (eg, sternotomy, thoracotomy) for ECMO/ECLS

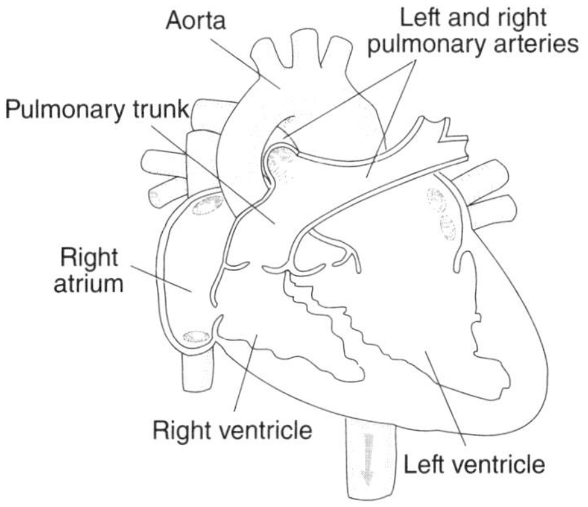

A vent cannula is inserted into the left ventricle of the heart

Explanation

The physician inserts a cannula(e) to provide extracorporeal membrane oxygenation (ECMO) or extracorporeal life support services (ECLS). A small incision is made to access the vessel. A single or double lumen cannula is inserted and passed into the inferior vena cava or right atrium. This cannula carries blood that is low in oxygen and high in carbon dioxide into the ECMO circuit. If a single lumen cannula is used, a second cannula is inserted into a main artery (venoarterial ECMO), usually the femoral but in children the carotid may be used. This second cannula passes from the ECMO circuit carrying oxygenated, rewarmed blood back to the vein or artery. This process reduces the amount of work the cardiac muscle must provide and if recovery is anticipated, ventricle expansion should be minimal and is often achieved by placing a catheter (to vent) in the left ventricle for draining. ECMO with ventricular decompression can be attained by insertion of a vent catheter directly into the left ventricle. Through an open incision into the thorax, the vent cannula is most commonly inserted into the pulmonary artery and positioned in the left ventricle. Report 33988 for insertion of the left heart vent and 33989 for removal of the left heart vent.

Coding Tips

The physician providing all components of ECMO/ECLS should report all codes for services provided. When performed by different providers, each should bill for the service performed. All services pertaining to cannulation, initiation, management, and discontinuation of the ECMO/ECLS circuit and parameters are separate from the daily overall management of the patient. Daily overall management is reported with hospital observation, inpatient, or critical care codes.

ICD-10-CM Diagnostic Codes

I40.0	Infective myocarditis
I40.1	Isolated myocarditis
I50.21	Acute systolic (congestive) heart failure
I50.22	Chronic systolic (congestive) heart failure
I50.23	Acute on chronic systolic (congestive) heart failure
I50.31	Acute diastolic (congestive) heart failure
I50.32	Chronic diastolic (congestive) heart failure
I50.33	Acute on chronic diastolic (congestive) heart failure
I50.41	Acute combined systolic (congestive) and diastolic (congestive) heart failure
I50.42	Chronic combined systolic (congestive) and diastolic (congestive) heart failure
I50.43	Acute on chronic combined systolic (congestive) and diastolic (congestive) heart failure
I50.811	Acute right heart failure
I50.812	Chronic right heart failure
I50.813	Acute on chronic right heart failure
I50.814	Right heart failure due to left heart failure
I50.82	Biventricular heart failure
I50.83	High output heart failure
I50.84	End stage heart failure
I97.0	Postcardiotomy syndrome
I97.110	Postprocedural cardiac insufficiency following cardiac surgery
I97.120	Postprocedural cardiac arrest following cardiac surgery
I97.130	Postprocedural heart failure following cardiac surgery
I97.710	Intraoperative cardiac arrest during cardiac surgery
J80	Acute respiratory distress syndrome
J85.1	Abscess of lung with pneumonia
J93.0	Spontaneous tension pneumothorax
J93.11	Primary spontaneous pneumothorax
J93.12	Secondary spontaneous pneumothorax
J93.81	Chronic pneumothorax
J95.821	Acute postprocedural respiratory failure
J95.822	Acute and chronic postprocedural respiratory failure
J96.01	Acute respiratory failure with hypoxia
J96.02	Acute respiratory failure with hypercapnia
J96.11	Chronic respiratory failure with hypoxia
J96.12	Chronic respiratory failure with hypercapnia
J96.21	Acute and chronic respiratory failure with hypoxia
J96.22	Acute and chronic respiratory failure with hypercapnia
P22.0	Respiratory distress syndrome of newborn N
P24.01	Meconium aspiration with respiratory symptoms N
P24.11	Neonatal aspiration of (clear) amniotic fluid and mucus with respiratory symptoms N
P24.21	Neonatal aspiration of blood with respiratory symptoms N
P25.1	Pneumothorax originating in the perinatal period N
P25.2	Pneumomediastinum originating in the perinatal period N
P25.3	Pneumopericardium originating in the perinatal period N
P28.5	Respiratory failure of newborn N
P28.81	Respiratory arrest of newborn N
P29.0	Neonatal cardiac failure N
P29.30	Pulmonary hypertension of newborn
P29.4	Transient myocardial ischemia in newborn N
P29.81	Cardiac arrest of newborn N
R06.03	Acute respiratory distress
R09.2	Respiratory arrest
R57.0	Cardiogenic shock
S27.0XXA	Traumatic pneumothorax, initial encounter
S27.1XXA	Traumatic hemothorax, initial encounter
S27.2XXA	Traumatic hemopneumothorax, initial encounter

T79.4XXA Traumatic shock, initial encounter
T81.11XA Postprocedural cardiogenic shock, initial encounter

Relative Value Units/Medicare Edits

Non-Facility RVU	Work	PE	MP	Total
33988	15.0	4.11	3.47	22.58
33989	9.5	2.65	2.2	14.35
Facility RVU	**Work**	**PE**	**MP**	**Total**
33988	15.0	4.11	3.47	22.58
33989	9.5	2.65	2.2	14.35

	FUD	Status	MUE	Modifiers				IOM Reference
33988	0	A	1(3)	51	N/A	62*	80*	None
33989	0	A	1(3)	51	N/A	62*	80*	

* with documentation

Terms To Know

cannula. Tube inserted into a blood vessel, duct, or body cavity to facilitate passage.

catheter. Flexible tube inserted into an area of the body for introducing or withdrawing fluid.

critical care. Treatment of critically ill patients in a variety of medical emergencies that requires the constant attendance of the physician (e.g., cardiac arrest, shock, bleeding, respiratory failure, postoperative complications, critically ill neonate).

lumen. Space inside an intestine, artery, vein, duct, or tube.

thoracentesis. Surgical puncture of the chest cavity with a specialized needle or hollow tubing to aspirate fluid from within the pleural space for diagnostic or therapeutic reasons.

vena cava. Main venous trunk that empties into the right atrium from both the lower and upper regions, beginning at the junction of the common iliac veins inferiorly and the two brachiocephalic veins superiorly.

33967

33967 Insertion of intra-aortic balloon assist device, percutaneous

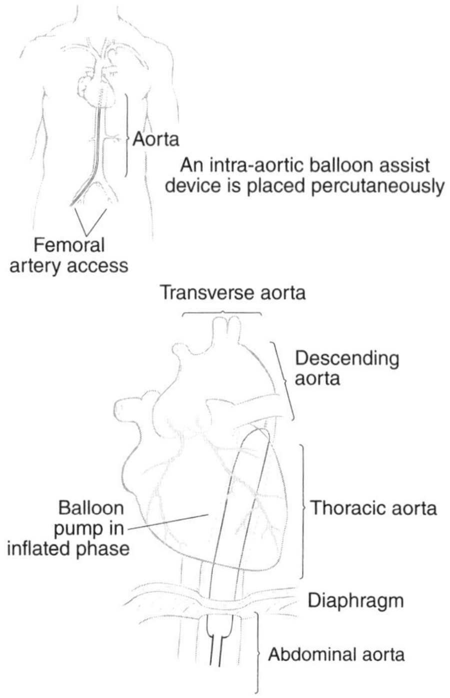

Explanation

An intra-aortic balloon catheter, usually with a 40 cc volume capacity, is inserted into the femoral artery and advanced under fluoroscopy to the distal portion of the aortic arch. After correct placement of the intra-aortic balloon assist device (IAB) in the descending aorta with its tip at the distal aortic arch, the balloon is connected to a drive console. The console consists of a pressurized gas reservoir, a monitor for ECG and pressure wave recording, adjustments for inflation/deflation timing, triggering selection switches, and battery back-up power sources. Helium or carbon dioxide is used for inflation. Inflation and deflation are synchronized to the patient's cardiac cycle. Inflation at the onset of diastole results in proximal and distal displacement of blood volume in the aorta. Deflation occurs just prior to the onset of systole. Once the patient's cardiac performance improves, weaning from the intra-aortic balloon catheter pump (IABP) begins by gradually decreasing the balloon augmentation ratio under control of hemodynamic stability.

Coding Tips

When 33967 is performed with another separately identifiable procedure, the highest dollar value code is listed as the primary procedure and subsequent procedures are appended with modifier 51. If the approach is open through the femoral artery, see 33970. For insertion through the ascending aorta, see 33973. For removal of an intra-aortic balloon assist device, percutaneous, see 33968.

ICD-10-CM Diagnostic Codes

I11.0 Hypertensive heart disease with heart failure
I16.0 Hypertensive urgency
I16.1 Hypertensive emergency
I20.0 Unstable angina
I20.1 Angina pectoris with documented spasm
I20.81 Angina pectoris with coronary microvascular dysfunction

I20.89	Other forms of angina pectoris
I21.01	ST elevation (STEMI) myocardial infarction involving left main coronary artery
I21.02	ST elevation (STEMI) myocardial infarction involving left anterior descending coronary artery
I21.09	ST elevation (STEMI) myocardial infarction involving other coronary artery of anterior wall
I21.11	ST elevation (STEMI) myocardial infarction involving right coronary artery
I21.19	ST elevation (STEMI) myocardial infarction involving other coronary artery of inferior wall
I21.21	ST elevation (STEMI) myocardial infarction involving left circumflex coronary artery
I21.29	ST elevation (STEMI) myocardial infarction involving other sites
I21.4	Non-ST elevation (NSTEMI) myocardial infarction
I21.A1	Myocardial infarction type 2
I22.0	Subsequent ST elevation (STEMI) myocardial infarction of anterior wall
I22.1	Subsequent ST elevation (STEMI) myocardial infarction of inferior wall
I22.2	Subsequent non-ST elevation (NSTEMI) myocardial infarction
I22.8	Subsequent ST elevation (STEMI) myocardial infarction of other sites
I24.81	Acute coronary microvascular dysfunction
I24.89	Other forms of acute ischemic heart disease
I25.10	Atherosclerotic heart disease of native coronary artery without angina pectoris [A]
I25.112	Atherosclerotic heart disease of native coronary artery with refractory angina pectoris [A]
I25.2	Old myocardial infarction
I25.3	Aneurysm of heart
I25.41	Coronary artery aneurysm
I25.42	Coronary artery dissection
I25.5	Ischemic cardiomyopathy
I25.6	Silent myocardial ischemia
I25.712	Atherosclerosis of autologous vein coronary artery bypass graft(s) with refractory angina pectoris [A]
I25.722	Atherosclerosis of autologous artery coronary artery bypass graft(s) with refractory angina pectoris [A]
I25.732	Atherosclerosis of nonautologous biological coronary artery bypass graft(s) with refractory angina pectoris [A]
I25.762	Atherosclerosis of bypass graft of coronary artery of transplanted heart with refractory angina pectoris [A]
I25.792	Atherosclerosis of other coronary artery bypass graft(s) with refractory angina pectoris [A]
I34.0	Nonrheumatic mitral (valve) insufficiency
I34.1	Nonrheumatic mitral (valve) prolapse
I34.2	Nonrheumatic mitral (valve) stenosis
I34.81	Nonrheumatic mitral (valve) annulus calcification
I35.0	Nonrheumatic aortic (valve) stenosis
I35.1	Nonrheumatic aortic (valve) insufficiency
I35.2	Nonrheumatic aortic (valve) stenosis with insufficiency
I35.8	Other nonrheumatic aortic valve disorders
I42.0	Dilated cardiomyopathy
I42.5	Other restrictive cardiomyopathy
I42.8	Other cardiomyopathies
I46.2	Cardiac arrest due to underlying cardiac condition
I46.8	Cardiac arrest due to other underlying condition
I47.0	Re-entry ventricular arrhythmia
I47.11	Inappropriate sinus tachycardia, so stated
I47.21	Torsades de pointes
I47.29	Other ventricular tachycardia
I50.1	Left ventricular failure, unspecified
I50.21	Acute systolic (congestive) heart failure
I50.22	Chronic systolic (congestive) heart failure
I50.23	Acute on chronic systolic (congestive) heart failure
I50.31	Acute diastolic (congestive) heart failure
I50.32	Chronic diastolic (congestive) heart failure
I50.33	Acute on chronic diastolic (congestive) heart failure
I50.41	Acute combined systolic (congestive) and diastolic (congestive) heart failure
I50.42	Chronic combined systolic (congestive) and diastolic (congestive) heart failure
I50.43	Acute on chronic combined systolic (congestive) and diastolic (congestive) heart failure
I50.811	Acute right heart failure
I50.812	Chronic right heart failure
I50.813	Acute on chronic right heart failure
I50.814	Right heart failure due to left heart failure
I50.82	Biventricular heart failure
I50.83	High output heart failure
I50.84	End stage heart failure
I51.5	Myocardial degeneration
I97.0	Postcardiotomy syndrome
I97.110	Postprocedural cardiac insufficiency following cardiac surgery
I97.111	Postprocedural cardiac insufficiency following other surgery
I97.120	Postprocedural cardiac arrest following cardiac surgery
I97.121	Postprocedural cardiac arrest following other surgery
I97.130	Postprocedural heart failure following cardiac surgery
I97.131	Postprocedural heart failure following other surgery
I97.190	Other postprocedural cardiac functional disturbances following cardiac surgery
I97.191	Other postprocedural cardiac functional disturbances following other surgery
I97.710	Intraoperative cardiac arrest during cardiac surgery
I97.711	Intraoperative cardiac arrest during other surgery
I97.790	Other intraoperative cardiac functional disturbances during cardiac surgery
I97.791	Other intraoperative cardiac functional disturbances during other surgery
I97.88	Other intraoperative complications of the circulatory system, not elsewhere classified
I97.89	Other postprocedural complications and disorders of the circulatory system, not elsewhere classified
Q21.0	Ventricular septal defect
Q21.11	Secundum atrial septal defect
Q21.12	Patent foramen ovale
Q21.13	Coronary sinus atrial septal defect
Q21.14	Superior sinus venosus atrial septal defect

Q21.15	Inferior sinus venosus atrial septal defect
Q21.21	Partial atrioventricular septal defect
Q21.22	Transitional atrioventricular septal defect
Q21.23	Complete atrioventricular septal defect
Q21.3	Tetralogy of Fallot
Q21.4	Aortopulmonary septal defect
Q21.8	Other congenital malformations of cardiac septa
Q23.0	Congenital stenosis of aortic valve
Q23.1	Congenital insufficiency of aortic valve
Q23.2	Congenital mitral stenosis
Q23.3	Congenital mitral insufficiency
Q23.81	Bicuspid aortic valve
Q23.88	Other congenital malformations of aortic and mitral valves
Q24.4	Congenital subaortic stenosis
Q24.5	Malformation of coronary vessels
Q24.6	Congenital heart block
Q24.8	Other specified congenital malformations of heart
R09.2	Respiratory arrest
R09.89	Other specified symptoms and signs involving the circulatory and respiratory systems
R57.0	Cardiogenic shock

AMA: 33967 2022,Jul

Relative Value Units/Medicare Edits

Non-Facility RVU	Work	PE	MP	Total
33967	4.84	1.62	1.11	7.57
Facility RVU	**Work**	**PE**	**MP**	**Total**
33967	4.84	1.62	1.11	7.57

	FUD	Status	MUE	Modifiers				IOM Reference
33967	0	A	1(3)	51	N/A	N/A	80*	None

* with documentation

Terms To Know

augmentation. Add to or increase the substance of a body site, usually performed as plastic reconstructive measures. Augmentation may involve the use of an implant or prosthesis, especially within soft tissue or grafting procedures, such as bone tissue.

balloon assist device. Circulation assist device consisting of a balloon placed in the thoracic aorta that inflates and deflates in coordination with the beating of the heart.

distal. *1)* Located farther away from a specified reference point or the trunk. *2)* Pertaining to the area farthest from the center of the body or the point of origin.

percutaneous. Through the skin.

reservoir. Space or body cavity for storage of liquid.

transverse. Crosswise at right angles to the long axis of a structure or part.

33968

33968 Removal of intra-aortic balloon assist device, percutaneous

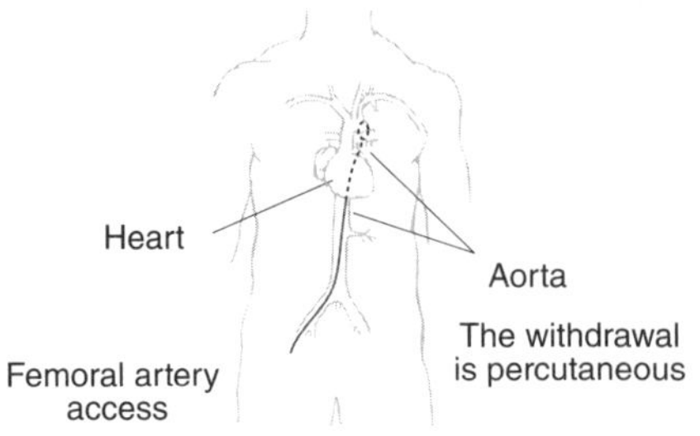

A balloon assist device in the aortic region is removed percutaneously

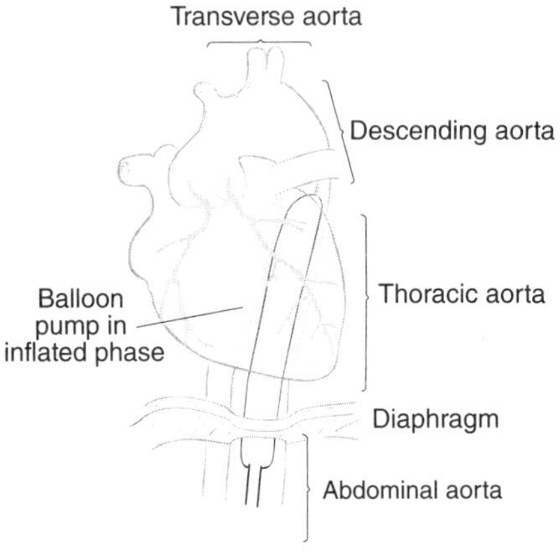

Explanation

The physician removes an intra-aortic balloon assist device (IABP). In a previous separately reportable procedure an IABP was inserted. When the patient is stabilized they are weaned off of the IAPB. The pump is turned off and the IABP catheter with the attached balloon is withdrawn from the femoral artery. Pressure is placed over the wound in the groin for a specified period of time. A light dressing is applied. The patient may be placed at bed rest and observed for several hours to avoid problems that could arise from bleeding or a hematoma at the puncture site.

Coding Tips

The approach may be percutaneous, open through the femoral artery, or open through the ascending aorta; the approach is key to correct coding of insertion and removal of intra-aortic balloon assist device. For insertion and removal through the femoral artery, open approach, see 33970–33971. For insertion and removal through the ascending aorta, see 33973–33974. For percutaneous insertion, see 33967.

ICD-10-CM Diagnostic Codes

T82.513A	Breakdown (mechanical) of balloon (counterpulsation) device, initial encounter
T82.518A	Breakdown (mechanical) of other cardiac and vascular devices and implants, initial encounter
T82.523A	Displacement of balloon (counterpulsation) device, initial encounter
T82.528A	Displacement of other cardiac and vascular devices and implants, initial encounter
T82.533A	Leakage of balloon (counterpulsation) device, initial encounter
T82.538A	Leakage of other cardiac and vascular devices and implants, initial encounter

T82.593A	Other mechanical complication of balloon (counterpulsation) device, initial encounter
T82.598A	Other mechanical complication of other cardiac and vascular devices and implants, initial encounter
T82.7XXA	Infection and inflammatory reaction due to other cardiac and vascular devices, implants and grafts, initial encounter
T82.817A	Embolism due to cardiac prosthetic devices, implants and grafts, initial encounter
T82.827A	Fibrosis due to cardiac prosthetic devices, implants and grafts, initial encounter
T82.837A	Hemorrhage due to cardiac prosthetic devices, implants and grafts, initial encounter
T82.847A	Pain due to cardiac prosthetic devices, implants and grafts, initial encounter
T82.855A	Stenosis of coronary artery stent, initial encounter
T82.857A	Stenosis of other cardiac prosthetic devices, implants and grafts, initial encounter
T82.867A	Thrombosis due to cardiac prosthetic devices, implants and grafts, initial encounter
T82.897A	Other specified complication of cardiac prosthetic devices, implants and grafts, initial encounter
T82.898A	Other specified complication of vascular prosthetic devices, implants and grafts, initial encounter
Z45.09	Encounter for adjustment and management of other cardiac device

Relative Value Units/Medicare Edits

Non-Facility RVU	Work	PE	MP	Total
33968	0.64	0.21	0.14	0.99
Facility RVU	**Work**	**PE**	**MP**	**Total**
33968	0.64	0.21	0.14	0.99

	FUD	Status	MUE	Modifiers				IOM Reference
33968	0	A	1(3)	N/A	N/A	N/A	N/A	None

* with documentation

Terms To Know

ascending aorta. Thoracic aorta, ascending/arch.

graft. Tissue implant from another part of the body or another person.

hematoma. Tumor-like collection of blood in some part of the body caused by a break in a blood vessel wall, usually as a result of trauma.

intra-aortic balloon pump. Internal cardiac assist device usually inserted through the femoral artery into the descending aorta, either percutaneously or by open approach, and connected to a drive console that monitors the patient's condition as the balloon is synchronously inflated and deflated to improve cardiac performance.

33970-33971

33970 Insertion of intra-aortic balloon assist device through the femoral artery, open approach

33971 Removal of intra-aortic balloon assist device including repair of femoral artery, with or without graft

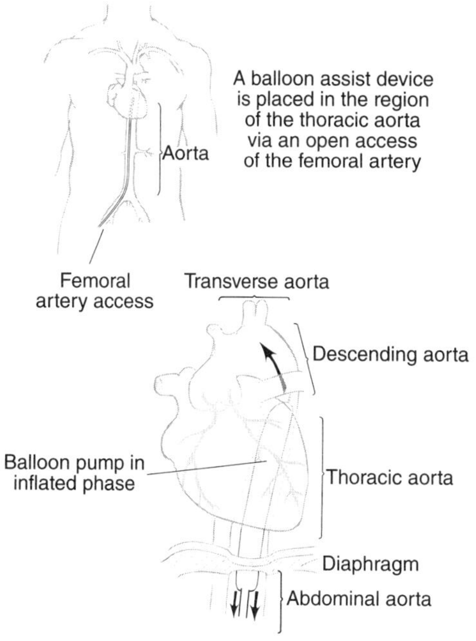

Removal of the device with repair to the artery

Explanation

This operation is done to help support the function of the left ventricle of the heart. In 33970, the left or right femoral artery is exposed in the groin. After the vessel is occluded above and below the proposed insertion site, the artery is opened transversely. In some cases, the end of a small tube of Gortex may be sewn to the side of the artery. The tip of the balloon catheter is inserted into the artery (or Gortex tube). The clamp occluding the artery upstream is released and the balloon catheter is advanced through the femoral artery and into the aorta above the level of the kidney arteries, but not beyond the left arm artery. It is connected to a pump and the pump is turned on. The pump inflates and deflates the balloon during each heartbeat cycle. In 33971, the previously placed balloon pump is withdrawn and the artery is occluded above and below the hole. If a Gortex sleeve has been used, it is simply tied off and no other repair is needed. If the balloon was directly introduced into the artery, the hole is sewn shut. If sewing the hole shut narrows the artery significantly, the hole can be patched with a piece of saphenous vein or Dacron. If the arterial diameter has been damaged, the segment of artery containing the hole can be removed and the artery replaced with an interposition graft of saphenous vein or Dacron tube.

Coding Tips

The approach may be percutaneous, open through the femoral artery, or open through the ascending aorta; the approach is key to correct coding of insertion and removal of the intra-aortic balloon assist device. For insertion and removal through the ascending aorta, see 33973–33974. For percutaneous insertion, see 33967. For removal of an intra-aortic balloon assist device, percutaneous, see 33968.

ICD-10-CM Diagnostic Codes

I11.0	Hypertensive heart disease with heart failure

I16.0	Hypertensive urgency
I16.1	Hypertensive emergency
I20.0	Unstable angina
I20.1	Angina pectoris with documented spasm
I20.81	Angina pectoris with coronary microvascular dysfunction
I20.89	Other forms of angina pectoris
I21.01	ST elevation (STEMI) myocardial infarction involving left main coronary artery
I21.02	ST elevation (STEMI) myocardial infarction involving left anterior descending coronary artery
I21.09	ST elevation (STEMI) myocardial infarction involving other coronary artery of anterior wall
I21.11	ST elevation (STEMI) myocardial infarction involving right coronary artery
I21.19	ST elevation (STEMI) myocardial infarction involving other coronary artery of inferior wall
I21.21	ST elevation (STEMI) myocardial infarction involving left circumflex coronary artery
I21.29	ST elevation (STEMI) myocardial infarction involving other sites
I21.4	Non-ST elevation (NSTEMI) myocardial infarction
I21.A1	Myocardial infarction type 2
I22.0	Subsequent ST elevation (STEMI) myocardial infarction of anterior wall
I22.1	Subsequent ST elevation (STEMI) myocardial infarction of inferior wall
I22.2	Subsequent non-ST elevation (NSTEMI) myocardial infarction
I22.8	Subsequent ST elevation (STEMI) myocardial infarction of other sites
I24.81	Acute coronary microvascular dysfunction
I24.89	Other forms of acute ischemic heart disease
I25.10	Atherosclerotic heart disease of native coronary artery without angina pectoris A
I25.2	Old myocardial infarction
I25.3	Aneurysm of heart
I25.41	Coronary artery aneurysm
I25.42	Coronary artery dissection
I25.5	Ischemic cardiomyopathy
I25.6	Silent myocardial ischemia
I34.0	Nonrheumatic mitral (valve) insufficiency
I34.1	Nonrheumatic mitral (valve) prolapse
I34.2	Nonrheumatic mitral (valve) stenosis
I34.81	Nonrheumatic mitral (valve) annulus calcification
I35.0	Nonrheumatic aortic (valve) stenosis
I35.1	Nonrheumatic aortic (valve) insufficiency
I35.2	Nonrheumatic aortic (valve) stenosis with insufficiency
I35.8	Other nonrheumatic aortic valve disorders
I42.0	Dilated cardiomyopathy
I42.5	Other restrictive cardiomyopathy
I42.8	Other cardiomyopathies
I46.2	Cardiac arrest due to underlying cardiac condition
I46.8	Cardiac arrest due to other underlying condition
I47.0	Re-entry ventricular arrhythmia
I47.11	Inappropriate sinus tachycardia, so stated
I47.21	Torsades de pointes
I47.29	Other ventricular tachycardia
I50.1	Left ventricular failure, unspecified
I50.21	Acute systolic (congestive) heart failure
I50.22	Chronic systolic (congestive) heart failure
I50.23	Acute on chronic systolic (congestive) heart failure
I50.31	Acute diastolic (congestive) heart failure
I50.32	Chronic diastolic (congestive) heart failure
I50.33	Acute on chronic diastolic (congestive) heart failure
I50.41	Acute combined systolic (congestive) and diastolic (congestive) heart failure
I50.42	Chronic combined systolic (congestive) and diastolic (congestive) heart failure
I50.43	Acute on chronic combined systolic (congestive) and diastolic (congestive) heart failure
I50.811	Acute right heart failure
I50.812	Chronic right heart failure
I50.813	Acute on chronic right heart failure
I50.814	Right heart failure due to left heart failure
I50.82	Biventricular heart failure
I50.83	High output heart failure
I50.84	End stage heart failure
I51.5	Myocardial degeneration
I97.0	Postcardiotomy syndrome
I97.110	Postprocedural cardiac insufficiency following cardiac surgery
I97.111	Postprocedural cardiac insufficiency following other surgery
I97.120	Postprocedural cardiac arrest following cardiac surgery
I97.121	Postprocedural cardiac arrest following other surgery
I97.130	Postprocedural heart failure following cardiac surgery
I97.131	Postprocedural heart failure following other surgery
I97.190	Other postprocedural cardiac functional disturbances following cardiac surgery
I97.191	Other postprocedural cardiac functional disturbances following other surgery
I97.710	Intraoperative cardiac arrest during cardiac surgery
I97.711	Intraoperative cardiac arrest during other surgery
I97.790	Other intraoperative cardiac functional disturbances during cardiac surgery
I97.791	Other intraoperative cardiac functional disturbances during other surgery
I97.88	Other intraoperative complications of the circulatory system, not elsewhere classified
I97.89	Other postprocedural complications and disorders of the circulatory system, not elsewhere classified
Q21.0	Ventricular septal defect
Q21.11	Secundum atrial septal defect
Q21.13	Coronary sinus atrial septal defect
Q21.21	Partial atrioventricular septal defect
Q21.22	Transitional atrioventricular septal defect
Q21.23	Complete atrioventricular septal defect
Q21.3	Tetralogy of Fallot
Q21.4	Aortopulmonary septal defect
Q21.8	Other congenital malformations of cardiac septa
Q23.0	Congenital stenosis of aortic valve
Q23.1	Congenital insufficiency of aortic valve

Q23.2	Congenital mitral stenosis
Q23.3	Congenital mitral insufficiency
Q23.81	Bicuspid aortic valve
Q23.82	Congenital mitral valve cleft leaflet
Q23.88	Other congenital malformations of aortic and mitral valves
Q24.4	Congenital subaortic stenosis
Q24.5	Malformation of coronary vessels
Q24.6	Congenital heart block
Q24.8	Other specified congenital malformations of heart
R09.2	Respiratory arrest
R57.0	Cardiogenic shock
T82.513A	Breakdown (mechanical) of balloon (counterpulsation) device, initial encounter
T82.523A	Displacement of balloon (counterpulsation) device, initial encounter
T82.533A	Leakage of balloon (counterpulsation) device, initial encounter
T82.593A	Other mechanical complication of balloon (counterpulsation) device, initial encounter
T82.7XXA	Infection and inflammatory reaction due to other cardiac and vascular devices, implants and grafts, initial encounter
T82.818A	Embolism due to vascular prosthetic devices, implants and grafts, initial encounter
T82.828A	Fibrosis due to vascular prosthetic devices, implants and grafts, initial encounter
T82.838A	Hemorrhage due to vascular prosthetic devices, implants and grafts, initial encounter
T82.848A	Pain due to vascular prosthetic devices, implants and grafts, initial encounter
T82.858A	Stenosis of other vascular prosthetic devices, implants and grafts, initial encounter
T82.868A	Thrombosis due to vascular prosthetic devices, implants and grafts, initial encounter

AMA: 33970 2022,Jul

Relative Value Units/Medicare Edits

Non-Facility RVU	Work	PE	MP	Total
33970	6.74	2.05	1.53	10.32
33971	11.99	6.16	2.79	20.94
Facility RVU	**Work**	**PE**	**MP**	**Total**
33970	6.74	2.05	1.53	10.32
33971	11.99	6.16	2.79	20.94

	FUD	Status	MUE	Modifiers				IOM Reference
33970	0	A	1(3)	51	N/A	62*	80	None
33971	90	A	1(3)	51	N/A	N/A	N/A	

* with documentation

33973-33974

33973 Insertion of intra-aortic balloon assist device through the ascending aorta

33974 Removal of intra-aortic balloon assist device from the ascending aorta, including repair of the ascending aorta, with or without graft

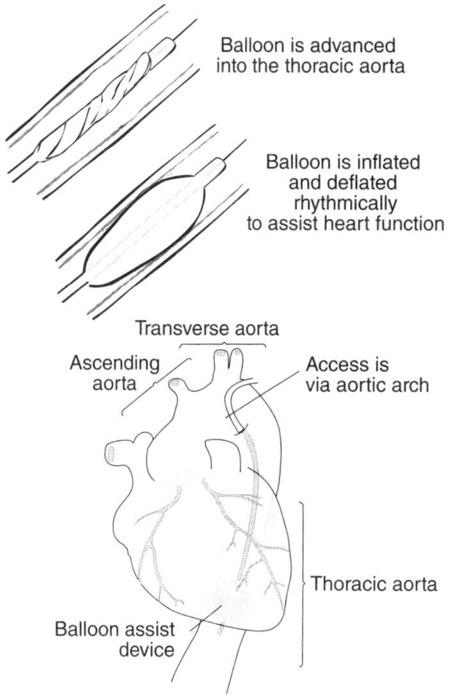

Explanation

The procedure is done when 1) the femoral arteries cannot be readily exposed in the operating room because of patient positioning; 2) the arteries are occluded by atherosclerosis or trauma; 3) there will be a need to reopen the patient's chest soon. In 33973, a balloon placed in this fashion must be removed in the operating room and the chest must be reopened. A purse string is placed in the aorta. A hole is made in the aorta in the middle of the purse string. The balloon is inserted through this hole until it lies beyond the left arm artery but above the kidney arteries. The purse string is tightened with a tourniquet. The chest incision is not closed. The balloon is driven by a pump outside the patient. In 33974, the physician removes an ascending aortic intra-aortic balloon assist device during performance of a primary procedure. If the sternum is open, the physician removes the aortic balloon while tightening purse-string sutures around the hole. When hemostasis is assured, the pericardium is repaired loosely with or without graft, leaving gaps for blood and fluid to drain into the pleural space. The sternum is reanastomosed with sternal wires and the skin is sutured in layers. If the sternum is closed, a Dacron-tube graft (reported separately) is used as a vehicle for balloon removal. As the balloon is removed, the Dacron-tube graft tightens around the aortic incision to create aortic hemostasis.

Coding Tips

The approach may be percutaneous, open through the femoral artery, or open through the ascending aorta; the approach is key to correct coding of insertion and removal of the intra-aortic balloon assist device. For open approach through the femoral artery, see 33970–33971. For percutaneous insertion, see 33967. For percutaneous removal, see 33968.

ICD-10-CM Diagnostic Codes

I11.0	Hypertensive heart disease with heart failure
I20.0	Unstable angina
I20.1	Angina pectoris with documented spasm
I20.81	Angina pectoris with coronary microvascular dysfunction
I20.89	Other forms of angina pectoris
I21.01	ST elevation (STEMI) myocardial infarction involving left main coronary artery
I21.02	ST elevation (STEMI) myocardial infarction involving left anterior descending coronary artery
I21.09	ST elevation (STEMI) myocardial infarction involving other coronary artery of anterior wall
I21.11	ST elevation (STEMI) myocardial infarction involving right coronary artery
I21.19	ST elevation (STEMI) myocardial infarction involving other coronary artery of inferior wall
I21.21	ST elevation (STEMI) myocardial infarction involving left circumflex coronary artery
I21.29	ST elevation (STEMI) myocardial infarction involving other sites
I21.4	Non-ST elevation (NSTEMI) myocardial infarction
I22.0	Subsequent ST elevation (STEMI) myocardial infarction of anterior wall
I22.1	Subsequent ST elevation (STEMI) myocardial infarction of inferior wall
I22.2	Subsequent non-ST elevation (NSTEMI) myocardial infarction
I22.8	Subsequent ST elevation (STEMI) myocardial infarction of other sites
I24.81	Acute coronary microvascular dysfunction
I24.89	Other forms of acute ischemic heart disease
I25.2	Old myocardial infarction
I25.3	Aneurysm of heart
I25.41	Coronary artery aneurysm
I25.42	Coronary artery dissection
I25.5	Ischemic cardiomyopathy
I25.6	Silent myocardial ischemia
I34.0	Nonrheumatic mitral (valve) insufficiency
I34.1	Nonrheumatic mitral (valve) prolapse
I34.2	Nonrheumatic mitral (valve) stenosis
I34.81	Nonrheumatic mitral (valve) annulus calcification
I34.89	Other nonrheumatic mitral valve disorders
I35.0	Nonrheumatic aortic (valve) stenosis
I35.1	Nonrheumatic aortic (valve) insufficiency
I35.2	Nonrheumatic aortic (valve) stenosis with insufficiency
I35.8	Other nonrheumatic aortic valve disorders
I42.0	Dilated cardiomyopathy
I42.5	Other restrictive cardiomyopathy
I42.8	Other cardiomyopathies
I46.2	Cardiac arrest due to underlying cardiac condition
I46.8	Cardiac arrest due to other underlying condition
I47.0	Re-entry ventricular arrhythmia
I47.11	Inappropriate sinus tachycardia, so stated
I47.21	Torsades de pointes
I47.29	Other ventricular tachycardia
I50.1	Left ventricular failure, unspecified
I50.21	Acute systolic (congestive) heart failure
I50.22	Chronic systolic (congestive) heart failure
I50.23	Acute on chronic systolic (congestive) heart failure
I50.31	Acute diastolic (congestive) heart failure
I50.32	Chronic diastolic (congestive) heart failure
I50.33	Acute on chronic diastolic (congestive) heart failure
I50.41	Acute combined systolic (congestive) and diastolic (congestive) heart failure
I50.42	Chronic combined systolic (congestive) and diastolic (congestive) heart failure
I50.43	Acute on chronic combined systolic (congestive) and diastolic (congestive) heart failure
I51.5	Myocardial degeneration
I97.0	Postcardiotomy syndrome
I97.110	Postprocedural cardiac insufficiency following cardiac surgery
I97.111	Postprocedural cardiac insufficiency following other surgery
I97.120	Postprocedural cardiac arrest following cardiac surgery
I97.121	Postprocedural cardiac arrest following other surgery
I97.130	Postprocedural heart failure following cardiac surgery
I97.131	Postprocedural heart failure following other surgery
I97.190	Other postprocedural cardiac functional disturbances following cardiac surgery
I97.191	Other postprocedural cardiac functional disturbances following other surgery
I97.710	Intraoperative cardiac arrest during cardiac surgery
I97.711	Intraoperative cardiac arrest during other surgery
I97.790	Other intraoperative cardiac functional disturbances during cardiac surgery
I97.791	Other intraoperative cardiac functional disturbances during other surgery
I97.88	Other intraoperative complications of the circulatory system, not elsewhere classified
I97.89	Other postprocedural complications and disorders of the circulatory system, not elsewhere classified
Q21.0	Ventricular septal defect
Q21.11	Secundum atrial septal defect
Q21.12	Patent foramen ovale
Q21.13	Coronary sinus atrial septal defect
Q21.14	Superior sinus venosus atrial septal defect
Q21.15	Inferior sinus venosus atrial septal defect
Q21.21	Partial atrioventricular septal defect
Q21.22	Transitional atrioventricular septal defect
Q21.23	Complete atrioventricular septal defect
Q21.3	Tetralogy of Fallot
Q21.4	Aortopulmonary septal defect
Q21.8	Other congenital malformations of cardiac septa
Q23.0	Congenital stenosis of aortic valve
Q23.1	Congenital insufficiency of aortic valve
Q23.2	Congenital mitral stenosis
Q23.3	Congenital mitral insufficiency
Q23.81	Bicuspid aortic valve
Q23.82	Congenital mitral valve cleft leaflet
Q23.88	Other congenital malformations of aortic and mitral valves
Q24.4	Congenital subaortic stenosis

Q24.5	Malformation of coronary vessels
Q24.6	Congenital heart block
Q24.8	Other specified congenital malformations of heart
R09.2	Respiratory arrest
R57.0	Cardiogenic shock
T82.513A	Breakdown (mechanical) of balloon (counterpulsation) device, initial encounter
T82.523A	Displacement of balloon (counterpulsation) device, initial encounter
T82.533A	Leakage of balloon (counterpulsation) device, initial encounter
T82.593A	Other mechanical complication of balloon (counterpulsation) device, initial encounter
T82.7XXA	Infection and inflammatory reaction due to other cardiac and vascular devices, implants and grafts, initial encounter
T82.818A	Embolism due to vascular prosthetic devices, implants and grafts, initial encounter
T82.828A	Fibrosis due to vascular prosthetic devices, implants and grafts, initial encounter
T82.838A	Hemorrhage due to vascular prosthetic devices, implants and grafts, initial encounter
T82.848A	Pain due to vascular prosthetic devices, implants and grafts, initial encounter
T82.858A	Stenosis of other vascular prosthetic devices, implants and grafts, initial encounter
T82.868A	Thrombosis due to vascular prosthetic devices, implants and grafts, initial encounter
T82.898A	Other specified complication of vascular prosthetic devices, implants and grafts, initial encounter

AMA: 33973 2022,Jul

Relative Value Units/Medicare Edits

Non-Facility RVU	Work	PE	MP	Total
33973	9.75	2.6	2.24	14.59
33974	15.03	7.8	3.48	26.31
Facility RVU	**Work**	**PE**	**MP**	**Total**
33973	9.75	2.6	2.24	14.59
33974	15.03	7.8	3.48	26.31

	FUD	Status	MUE	Modifiers				IOM Reference
33973	0	A	1(3)	51	N/A	62*	80	None
33974	90	A	1(3)	51	N/A	N/A	N/A	

* with documentation

33975-33976

33975 Insertion of ventricular assist device; extracorporeal, single ventricle
33976 extracorporeal, biventricular

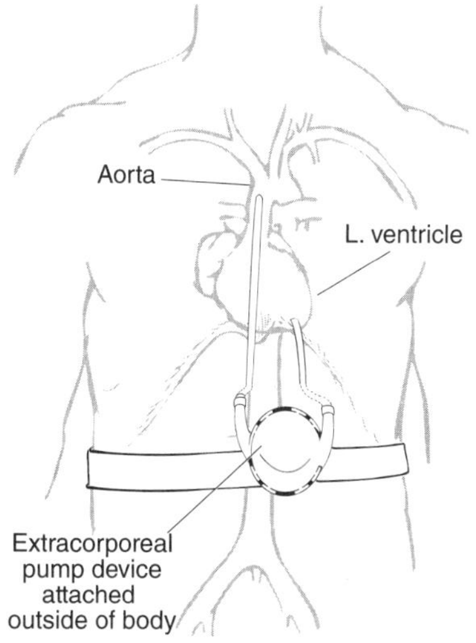

A single ventricle assist device is located outside of the body and its lines attached to the heart and aorta

The configurations vary according to which side of the heart is failing

Explanation

Cardiopulmonary bypass is required. For right ventricular failure, a pump uptake tube is placed in the right ventricular apex. A pump delivery tube is placed in the pulmonary artery. The pump is turned on and the patient is weaned off cardiopulmonary bypass. For left ventricular failure, the pump uptake tube is placed in one of the pulmonary veins or in the left ventricle apex. The arterial delivery tube is placed in the aorta. The pump is turned on and the patient is removed from cardiopulmonary bypass. The implanted pump is placed in a pocket formed in the upper abdominal wall, but outside the abdominal cavity. Tubes for the pump drive are brought out through separate incisions in the skin. The pump is started and the patient is weaned off cardiopulmonary bypass. The device is removed when the patient's ventricle recovers, a total artificial heart is placed or the patient undergoes heart transplantation. Report 33976 if biventricular support is needed.

Coding Tips

These codes are used to report initial insertion or replacement of the entire ventricular assist device. Removal of the device being replaced is included and should not be reported separately. For percutaneous implantation of a ventricular assist device, see 33990–33991; for the removal of the device, see 33992. For heart transplant, with or without recipient cardiectomy, see 33945.

ICD-10-CM Diagnostic Codes

I09.81	Rheumatic heart failure
I11.0	Hypertensive heart disease with heart failure
I16.0	Hypertensive urgency
I16.1	Hypertensive emergency
I20.0	Unstable angina
I20.1	Angina pectoris with documented spasm
I21.01	ST elevation (STEMI) myocardial infarction involving left main coronary artery

Heart and Pericardium

I21.02 ST elevation (STEMI) myocardial infarction involving left anterior descending coronary artery
I21.11 ST elevation (STEMI) myocardial infarction involving right coronary artery
I21.21 ST elevation (STEMI) myocardial infarction involving left circumflex coronary artery
I21.4 Non-ST elevation (NSTEMI) myocardial infarction
I21.A1 Myocardial infarction type 2
I21.B Myocardial infarction with coronary microvascular dysfunction
I22.0 Subsequent ST elevation (STEMI) myocardial infarction of anterior wall
I22.1 Subsequent ST elevation (STEMI) myocardial infarction of inferior wall
I22.2 Subsequent non-ST elevation (NSTEMI) myocardial infarction
I25.2 Old myocardial infarction
I25.3 Aneurysm of heart
I25.41 Coronary artery aneurysm
I25.42 Coronary artery dissection
I25.5 Ischemic cardiomyopathy
I25.6 Silent myocardial ischemia
I34.0 Nonrheumatic mitral (valve) insufficiency
I34.1 Nonrheumatic mitral (valve) prolapse
I34.2 Nonrheumatic mitral (valve) stenosis
I34.81 Nonrheumatic mitral (valve) annulus calcification
I35.0 Nonrheumatic aortic (valve) stenosis
I35.1 Nonrheumatic aortic (valve) insufficiency
I35.2 Nonrheumatic aortic (valve) stenosis with insufficiency
I40.0 Infective myocarditis
I40.1 Isolated myocarditis
I41 Myocarditis in diseases classified elsewhere
I42.0 Dilated cardiomyopathy
I42.1 Obstructive hypertrophic cardiomyopathy
I42.7 Cardiomyopathy due to drug and external agent
I43 Cardiomyopathy in diseases classified elsewhere
I46.2 Cardiac arrest due to underlying cardiac condition
I46.8 Cardiac arrest due to other underlying condition
I47.0 Re-entry ventricular arrhythmia
I47.11 Inappropriate sinus tachycardia, so stated
I47.19 Other supraventricular tachycardia
I47.21 Torsades de pointes
I50.21 Acute systolic (congestive) heart failure
I50.22 Chronic systolic (congestive) heart failure
I50.23 Acute on chronic systolic (congestive) heart failure
I50.31 Acute diastolic (congestive) heart failure
I50.32 Chronic diastolic (congestive) heart failure
I50.33 Acute on chronic diastolic (congestive) heart failure
I50.41 Acute combined systolic (congestive) and diastolic (congestive) heart failure
I50.42 Chronic combined systolic (congestive) and diastolic (congestive) heart failure
I50.43 Acute on chronic combined systolic (congestive) and diastolic (congestive) heart failure
I50.811 Acute right heart failure
I50.812 Chronic right heart failure
I50.813 Acute on chronic right heart failure
I50.814 Right heart failure due to left heart failure
I50.82 Biventricular heart failure
I50.83 High output heart failure
I50.84 End stage heart failure
I51.5 Myocardial degeneration
I97.110 Postprocedural cardiac insufficiency following cardiac surgery
I97.111 Postprocedural cardiac insufficiency following other surgery
I97.120 Postprocedural cardiac arrest following cardiac surgery
I97.121 Postprocedural cardiac arrest following other surgery
I97.130 Postprocedural heart failure following cardiac surgery
I97.131 Postprocedural heart failure following other surgery
I97.710 Intraoperative cardiac arrest during cardiac surgery
I97.711 Intraoperative cardiac arrest during other surgery
Q21.0 Ventricular septal defect
Q21.11 Secundum atrial septal defect
Q21.13 Coronary sinus atrial septal defect
Q21.14 Superior sinus venosus atrial septal defect
Q21.15 Inferior sinus venosus atrial septal defect
Q21.21 Partial atrioventricular septal defect
Q21.22 Transitional atrioventricular septal defect
Q21.23 Complete atrioventricular septal defect
Q21.3 Tetralogy of Fallot
Q21.4 Aortopulmonary septal defect
Q23.0 Congenital stenosis of aortic valve
Q23.1 Congenital insufficiency of aortic valve
Q23.2 Congenital mitral stenosis
Q23.3 Congenital mitral insufficiency
Q23.81 Bicuspid aortic valve
Q23.82 Congenital mitral valve cleft leaflet
Q23.88 Other congenital malformations of aortic and mitral valves
Q24.4 Congenital subaortic stenosis
Q24.5 Malformation of coronary vessels
Q24.6 Congenital heart block
R09.2 Respiratory arrest

AMA: 33975 2018,Jun **33976** 2018,Jun

Relative Value Units/Medicare Edits

Non-Facility RVU	Work	PE	MP	Total
33975	25.0	7.14	6.02	38.16
33976	30.75	8.2	7.12	46.07
Facility RVU	**Work**	**PE**	**MP**	**Total**
33975	25.0	7.14	6.02	38.16
33976	30.75	8.2	7.12	46.07

	FUD	Status	MUE	Modifiers				IOM Reference
33975	N/A	A	1(3)	51	N/A	N/A	80	None
33976	N/A	A	1(3)	51	N/A	N/A	80	

* with documentation

33977-33978

33977 Removal of ventricular assist device; extracorporeal, single ventricle
33978 extracorporeal, biventricular

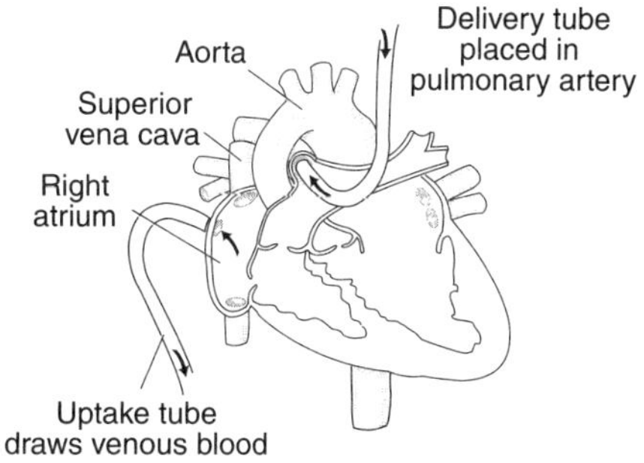

Depiction of right ventricular circulation support

Explanation

Cardiopulmonary bypass is required. The pump is stopped. All the tubes are removed and any holes in the heart or vessels are closed. The device is removed from the patient's body. Cardiopulmonary bypass is discontinued when the patient's heart function returns. An intra-aortic balloon pump is often required to allow discontinuation of bypass. All wounds are closed. Report 33978 if biventricular support is needed.

Coding Tips

These codes are used to report removal of the entire ventricular assist device. Removal of the device is included when the entire ventricular assist device is replaced and should not be reported separately. For percutaneous implantation of a ventricular assist device, see 33990–33991; for removal of the device, see 33992. For heart transplant, with or without recipient cardiectomy, see 33945.

ICD-10-CM Diagnostic Codes

T82.518A Breakdown (mechanical) of other cardiac and vascular devices and implants, initial encounter
T82.528A Displacement of other cardiac and vascular devices and implants, initial encounter
T82.538A Leakage of other cardiac and vascular devices and implants, initial encounter
T82.598A Other mechanical complication of other cardiac and vascular devices and implants, initial encounter
T82.7XXA Infection and inflammatory reaction due to other cardiac and vascular devices, implants and grafts, initial encounter
T82.817A Embolism due to cardiac prosthetic devices, implants and grafts, initial encounter
T82.827A Fibrosis due to cardiac prosthetic devices, implants and grafts, initial encounter
T82.837A Hemorrhage due to cardiac prosthetic devices, implants and grafts, initial encounter
T82.847A Pain due to cardiac prosthetic devices, implants and grafts, initial encounter
T82.855A Stenosis of coronary artery stent, initial encounter
T82.857A Stenosis of other cardiac prosthetic devices, implants and grafts, initial encounter
T82.867A Thrombosis due to cardiac prosthetic devices, implants and grafts, initial encounter
T82.897A Other specified complication of cardiac prosthetic devices, implants and grafts, initial encounter
T82.898A Other specified complication of vascular prosthetic devices, implants and grafts, initial encounter
Z45.09 Encounter for adjustment and management of other cardiac device
Z95.811 Presence of heart assist device

Relative Value Units/Medicare Edits

Non-Facility RVU	Work	PE	MP	Total
33977	20.86	7.18	4.88	32.92
33978	25.0	8.03	5.77	38.8
Facility RVU	**Work**	**PE**	**MP**	**Total**
33977	20.86	7.18	4.88	32.92
33978	25.0	8.03	5.77	38.8

	FUD	Status	MUE	Modifiers				IOM Reference
33977	N/A	A	1(3)	51	N/A	N/A	80	None
33978	N/A	A	1(3)	51	N/A	N/A	80	

* with documentation

Terms To Know

cardiopulmonary bypass. Venous blood is diverted to a heart-lung machine, which mechanically pumps and oxygenates the blood temporarily so the heart can be bypassed while an open procedure on the heart or coronary arteries is performed. During bypass, the lungs are deflated and immobile.

complication. Condition arising after the beginning of observation and treatment that modifies the course of the patient's illness or the medical care required, or an undesired result or misadventure in medical care.

extracorporeal. Located or taking place outside the body.

graft. Tissue implant from another part of the body or another person.

implant. Material or device inserted or placed within the body for therapeutic, reconstructive, or diagnostic purposes.

infection. Presence of microorganisms in body tissues that may result in cellular damage.

intra-aortic balloon pump. Internal cardiac assist device usually inserted through the femoral artery into the descending aorta, either percutaneously or by open approach, and connected to a drive console that monitors the patient's condition as the balloon is synchronously inflated and deflated to improve cardiac performance.

percutaneous. Through the skin.

33979-33980

33979 Insertion of ventricular assist device, implantable intracorporeal, single ventricle

33980 Removal of ventricular assist device, implantable intracorporeal, single ventricle

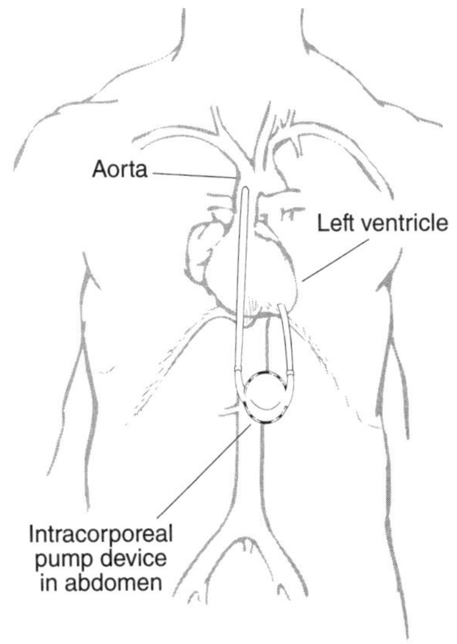

A single ventricular assist device

Explanation

The physician makes a midline incision extending from the sternal notch to the umbilicus. Sternotomy is performed prior to creation of the pocket. The preperitoneal fat is dissected from the undersurface of the rectus sheath using low-power cautery. Superiorly the dissection is carried to the undersurface of the diaphragm until the apex of the heart can be palpated just lateral to the inferior phrenic artery and vein and carried well back into the retroperitoneum. The preperitoneal space is opened to allow room for the device outflow valve and graft conduit. The muscular attachment of the right hemidiaphragm to the medial edge of the sternum is divided to allow room for the graft. A small incision is made and a tunneling device is passed subcutaneously inferiorly around the umbilicus, and into the pocket through the rectus sheath at its most inferior aspect. The tunneler is screwed onto the end of the drive line, which is pulled back through the tunnel to the skin. The drive line is not attached to the skin. Cardiopulmonary bypass is instituted using standard aortic and dual stage venous cannulae. The apex of the left ventricle is elevated. The physician cores out a piece of ventricle and places the apical cuff sutures. An apical vent is passed into the left ventricle. Pledgeted 2-0 Ethibond sutures are placed circumferentially partial thickness into the myocardium and passed through the sewing ring of the apical cuff. Once the apical cuff is secure, a cruciate incision in the diaphragm opposite the ventricular apex is made just lateral to the inferior phrenic vessels, and the inflow cannula is brought into the chest. The inflow cannula is inserted through the apical cuff until the sintered titanium surface is within the cuff. The Dacron tie of the inflow cuff is secured and an additional plastic band and Dacron tie are used to reinforce the connection and flatten out the silicone cuff. Blood is allowed to passively fill the device and exit via the outflow valve. A partial occluding clamp is placed on the right lateral aspect of the ascending aorta and a longitudinal aortotomy is performed. The periaortic adventitia is left in place and a strip of pericardium is incorporated into the anastomosis. The apex and heel of the anastomosis are reinforced with interrupted 4-0 Prolene pledgeted horizontal mattress stitches. Inotropic support is started before separating from bypass and activating the LVAD. The device is switched to automatic mode after the cessation of cardiopulmonary bypass. Transesophageal echocardiography is used to ensure adequate ventricular decompression and a bubble study is performed to rule out a patent foramen ovale. A thermodilution cardiac output is performed and compared to the output from the LVAD. In the presence of severe coagulopathy, the chest may need to be packed open. The device is removed (33980) when the patient's ventricle recovers, an artificial heart is placed, or the patient undergoes heart transplantation.

Coding Tips

Code 33979 includes replacement of the pump and cannulas. Removal of the device being replaced is included and should not be reported separately. For percutaneous implantation of a ventricular assist device, see 33990–33991; for removal of the device, see 33992.

ICD-10-CM Diagnostic Codes

I09.81	Rheumatic heart failure
I11.0	Hypertensive heart disease with heart failure
I16.0	Hypertensive urgency
I16.1	Hypertensive emergency
I20.0	Unstable angina
I20.1	Angina pectoris with documented spasm
I20.81	Angina pectoris with coronary microvascular dysfunction
I20.89	Other forms of angina pectoris
I21.01	ST elevation (STEMI) myocardial infarction involving left main coronary artery
I21.02	ST elevation (STEMI) myocardial infarction involving left anterior descending coronary artery
I21.09	ST elevation (STEMI) myocardial infarction involving other coronary artery of anterior wall
I21.11	ST elevation (STEMI) myocardial infarction involving right coronary artery
I21.19	ST elevation (STEMI) myocardial infarction involving other coronary artery of inferior wall
I21.21	ST elevation (STEMI) myocardial infarction involving left circumflex coronary artery
I21.29	ST elevation (STEMI) myocardial infarction involving other sites
I21.4	Non-ST elevation (NSTEMI) myocardial infarction
I21.A1	Myocardial infarction type 2
I21.B	Myocardial infarction with coronary microvascular dysfunction
I22.0	Subsequent ST elevation (STEMI) myocardial infarction of anterior wall
I22.1	Subsequent ST elevation (STEMI) myocardial infarction of inferior wall
I22.2	Subsequent non-ST elevation (NSTEMI) myocardial infarction
I22.8	Subsequent ST elevation (STEMI) myocardial infarction of other sites
I24.89	Other forms of acute ischemic heart disease
I25.2	Old myocardial infarction
I25.3	Aneurysm of heart
I25.41	Coronary artery aneurysm
I25.42	Coronary artery dissection
I25.5	Ischemic cardiomyopathy
I25.6	Silent myocardial ischemia
I25.89	Other forms of chronic ischemic heart disease
I34.0	Nonrheumatic mitral (valve) insufficiency
I34.1	Nonrheumatic mitral (valve) prolapse
I34.2	Nonrheumatic mitral (valve) stenosis

I34.81 Nonrheumatic mitral (valve) annulus calcification
I35.0 Nonrheumatic aortic (valve) stenosis
I35.1 Nonrheumatic aortic (valve) insufficiency
I35.2 Nonrheumatic aortic (valve) stenosis with insufficiency
I35.8 Other nonrheumatic aortic valve disorders
I40.0 Infective myocarditis
I40.1 Isolated myocarditis
I41 Myocarditis in diseases classified elsewhere
I42.0 Dilated cardiomyopathy
I42.1 Obstructive hypertrophic cardiomyopathy
I42.2 Other hypertrophic cardiomyopathy
I42.5 Other restrictive cardiomyopathy
I42.7 Cardiomyopathy due to drug and external agent
I42.8 Other cardiomyopathies
I43 Cardiomyopathy in diseases classified elsewhere
I46.2 Cardiac arrest due to underlying cardiac condition
I46.8 Cardiac arrest due to other underlying condition
I47.0 Re-entry ventricular arrhythmia
I47.11 Inappropriate sinus tachycardia, so stated
I47.21 Torsades de pointes
I50.1 Left ventricular failure, unspecified
I50.21 Acute systolic (congestive) heart failure
I50.22 Chronic systolic (congestive) heart failure
I50.23 Acute on chronic systolic (congestive) heart failure
I50.31 Acute diastolic (congestive) heart failure
I50.32 Chronic diastolic (congestive) heart failure
I50.33 Acute on chronic diastolic (congestive) heart failure
I50.41 Acute combined systolic (congestive) and diastolic (congestive) heart failure
I50.42 Chronic combined systolic (congestive) and diastolic (congestive) heart failure
I50.43 Acute on chronic combined systolic (congestive) and diastolic (congestive) heart failure
I50.811 Acute right heart failure
I50.812 Chronic right heart failure
I50.813 Acute on chronic right heart failure
I50.814 Right heart failure due to left heart failure
I50.82 Biventricular heart failure
I50.83 High output heart failure
I50.84 End stage heart failure
I51.5 Myocardial degeneration
I97.110 Postprocedural cardiac insufficiency following cardiac surgery
I97.111 Postprocedural cardiac insufficiency following other surgery
I97.120 Postprocedural cardiac arrest following cardiac surgery
I97.121 Postprocedural cardiac arrest following other surgery
I97.130 Postprocedural heart failure following cardiac surgery
I97.131 Postprocedural heart failure following other surgery
I97.710 Intraoperative cardiac arrest during cardiac surgery
I97.711 Intraoperative cardiac arrest during other surgery
I97.790 Other intraoperative cardiac functional disturbances during cardiac surgery
I97.791 Other intraoperative cardiac functional disturbances during other surgery
Q21.0 Ventricular septal defect
Q21.11 Secundum atrial septal defect
Q21.12 Patent foramen ovale
Q21.13 Coronary sinus atrial septal defect
Q21.21 Partial atrioventricular septal defect
Q21.22 Transitional atrioventricular septal defect
Q21.23 Complete atrioventricular septal defect
Q21.3 Tetralogy of Fallot
Q21.4 Aortopulmonary septal defect
Q23.0 Congenital stenosis of aortic valve
Q23.1 Congenital insufficiency of aortic valve
Q23.2 Congenital mitral stenosis
Q23.3 Congenital mitral insufficiency
Q23.88 Other congenital malformations of aortic and mitral valves
Q24.4 Congenital subaortic stenosis
Q24.5 Malformation of coronary vessels
Q24.6 Congenital heart block
R57.0 Cardiogenic shock
T82.518A Breakdown (mechanical) of other cardiac and vascular devices and implants, initial encounter
T82.528A Displacement of other cardiac and vascular devices and implants, initial encounter
T82.538A Leakage of other cardiac and vascular devices and implants, initial encounter
T82.7XXA Infection and inflammatory reaction due to other cardiac and vascular devices, implants and grafts, initial encounter
T82.817A Embolism due to cardiac prosthetic devices, implants and grafts, initial encounter
T82.827A Fibrosis due to cardiac prosthetic devices, implants and grafts, initial encounter
T82.837A Hemorrhage due to cardiac prosthetic devices, implants and grafts, initial encounter
T82.847A Pain due to cardiac prosthetic devices, implants and grafts, initial encounter

AMA: **33979** 2018,Jun

Relative Value Units/Medicare Edits

Non-Facility RVU	Work	PE	MP	Total
33979	37.5	10.36	9.0	56.86
33980	33.5	10.66	8.08	52.24
Facility RVU	**Work**	**PE**	**MP**	**Total**
33979	37.5	10.36	9.0	56.86
33980	33.5	10.66	8.08	52.24

	FUD	Status	MUE	Modifiers				IOM Reference
33979	N/A	A	1(3)	51	N/A	N/A	80	None
33980	N/A	A	1(3)	51	N/A	N/A	80	

* with documentation

Heart and Pericardium

33981

33981 Replacement of extracorporeal ventricular assist device, single or biventricular, pump(s), single or each pump

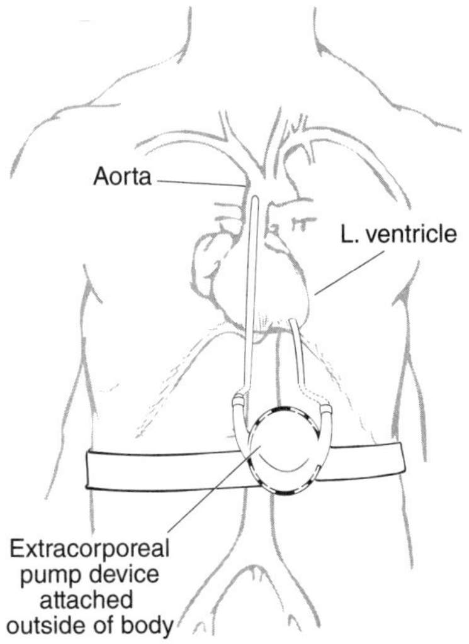

A single ventricle assist device is located outside of the body and its lines attached to the heart and aorta

Explanation

The physician replaces the blood pump component of an extracorporeal ventricular assist device (VAD). The previously implanted pump, which was placed in a pocket formed in the upper abdominal wall (but outside the abdominal cavity), is removed. Pump replacement includes removal of the existing pump, insertion of a new pump, connection, de-airing, and new pump initiation. Report 33981 for one or more pumps; this code reports pump replacement of single or biventricular VAD systems.

Coding Tips

Replacement of the pump includes removal of the previous pump, insertion of a new pump, and connection, de-airing, and initiation of the pump. For replacement of a ventricular assist device, extracorporeal, using percutaneous transseptal access, see 33999.

ICD-10-CM Diagnostic Codes

I09.81	Rheumatic heart failure
I11.0	Hypertensive heart disease with heart failure
I16.0	Hypertensive urgency
I16.1	Hypertensive emergency
I20.0	Unstable angina
I20.1	Angina pectoris with documented spasm
I20.81	Angina pectoris with coronary microvascular dysfunction
I20.89	Other forms of angina pectoris
I21.01	ST elevation (STEMI) myocardial infarction involving left main coronary artery
I21.02	ST elevation (STEMI) myocardial infarction involving left anterior descending coronary artery
I21.09	ST elevation (STEMI) myocardial infarction involving other coronary artery of anterior wall
I21.11	ST elevation (STEMI) myocardial infarction involving right coronary artery
I21.19	ST elevation (STEMI) myocardial infarction involving other coronary artery of inferior wall
I21.21	ST elevation (STEMI) myocardial infarction involving left circumflex coronary artery
I21.29	ST elevation (STEMI) myocardial infarction involving other sites
I21.4	Non-ST elevation (NSTEMI) myocardial infarction
I21.A1	Myocardial infarction type 2
I21.B	Myocardial infarction with coronary microvascular dysfunction
I22.0	Subsequent ST elevation (STEMI) myocardial infarction of anterior wall
I22.1	Subsequent ST elevation (STEMI) myocardial infarction of inferior wall
I22.2	Subsequent non-ST elevation (NSTEMI) myocardial infarction
I22.8	Subsequent ST elevation (STEMI) myocardial infarction of other sites
I24.89	Other forms of acute ischemic heart disease
I25.2	Old myocardial infarction
I25.3	Aneurysm of heart
I25.41	Coronary artery aneurysm
I25.42	Coronary artery dissection
I25.5	Ischemic cardiomyopathy
I25.6	Silent myocardial ischemia
I34.0	Nonrheumatic mitral (valve) insufficiency
I34.1	Nonrheumatic mitral (valve) prolapse
I34.2	Nonrheumatic mitral (valve) stenosis
I34.81	Nonrheumatic mitral (valve) annulus calcification
I35.0	Nonrheumatic aortic (valve) stenosis
I35.1	Nonrheumatic aortic (valve) insufficiency
I35.2	Nonrheumatic aortic (valve) stenosis with insufficiency
I35.8	Other nonrheumatic aortic valve disorders
I42.0	Dilated cardiomyopathy
I42.5	Other restrictive cardiomyopathy
I42.8	Other cardiomyopathies
I46.2	Cardiac arrest due to underlying cardiac condition
I46.8	Cardiac arrest due to other underlying condition
I47.0	Re-entry ventricular arrhythmia
I47.11	Inappropriate sinus tachycardia, so stated
I47.21	Torsades de pointes
I47.29	Other ventricular tachycardia
I50.1	Left ventricular failure, unspecified
I50.21	Acute systolic (congestive) heart failure
I50.22	Chronic systolic (congestive) heart failure
I50.23	Acute on chronic systolic (congestive) heart failure
I50.31	Acute diastolic (congestive) heart failure
I50.32	Chronic diastolic (congestive) heart failure
I50.33	Acute on chronic diastolic (congestive) heart failure
I50.41	Acute combined systolic (congestive) and diastolic (congestive) heart failure
I50.42	Chronic combined systolic (congestive) and diastolic (congestive) heart failure
I50.43	Acute on chronic combined systolic (congestive) and diastolic (congestive) heart failure
I50.811	Acute right heart failure
I50.812	Chronic right heart failure

I50.813 Acute on chronic right heart failure
I50.814 Right heart failure due to left heart failure
I50.82 Biventricular heart failure
I50.83 High output heart failure
I50.84 End stage heart failure
I51.5 Myocardial degeneration
I97.110 Postprocedural cardiac insufficiency following cardiac surgery
I97.111 Postprocedural cardiac insufficiency following other surgery
I97.120 Postprocedural cardiac arrest following cardiac surgery
I97.121 Postprocedural cardiac arrest following other surgery
I97.130 Postprocedural heart failure following cardiac surgery
I97.131 Postprocedural heart failure following other surgery
I97.190 Other postprocedural cardiac functional disturbances following cardiac surgery
I97.191 Other postprocedural cardiac functional disturbances following other surgery
I97.710 Intraoperative cardiac arrest during cardiac surgery
I97.711 Intraoperative cardiac arrest during other surgery
I97.790 Other intraoperative cardiac functional disturbances during cardiac surgery
I97.791 Other intraoperative cardiac functional disturbances during other surgery
I97.88 Other intraoperative complications of the circulatory system, not elsewhere classified
I97.89 Other postprocedural complications and disorders of the circulatory system, not elsewhere classified
Q21.0 Ventricular septal defect
Q21.11 Secundum atrial septal defect
Q21.12 Patent foramen ovale
Q21.13 Coronary sinus atrial septal defect
Q21.14 Superior sinus venosus atrial septal defect
Q21.15 Inferior sinus venosus atrial septal defect
Q21.21 Partial atrioventricular septal defect
Q21.22 Transitional atrioventricular septal defect
Q21.23 Complete atrioventricular septal defect
Q21.3 Tetralogy of Fallot
Q21.4 Aortopulmonary septal defect
Q21.8 Other congenital malformations of cardiac septa
Q23.0 Congenital stenosis of aortic valve
Q23.1 Congenital insufficiency of aortic valve
Q23.2 Congenital mitral stenosis
Q23.3 Congenital mitral insufficiency
Q23.81 Bicuspid aortic valve
Q23.82 Congenital mitral valve cleft leaflet
Q23.88 Other congenital malformations of aortic and mitral valves
Q24.4 Congenital subaortic stenosis
Q24.5 Malformation of coronary vessels
Q24.6 Congenital heart block
Q24.8 Other specified congenital malformations of heart
R09.2 Respiratory arrest
R09.89 Other specified symptoms and signs involving the circulatory and respiratory systems
R57.0 Cardiogenic shock
T82.518A Breakdown (mechanical) of other cardiac and vascular devices and implants, initial encounter
T82.528A Displacement of other cardiac and vascular devices and implants, initial encounter
T82.538A Leakage of other cardiac and vascular devices and implants, initial encounter
T82.598A Other mechanical complication of other cardiac and vascular devices and implants, initial encounter
T82.7XXA Infection and inflammatory reaction due to other cardiac and vascular devices, implants and grafts, initial encounter
T82.817A Embolism due to cardiac prosthetic devices, implants and grafts, initial encounter
T82.827A Fibrosis due to cardiac prosthetic devices, implants and grafts, initial encounter
T82.837A Hemorrhage due to cardiac prosthetic devices, implants and grafts, initial encounter
T82.847A Pain due to cardiac prosthetic devices, implants and grafts, initial encounter
T82.857A Stenosis of other cardiac prosthetic devices, implants and grafts, initial encounter
T82.867A Thrombosis due to cardiac prosthetic devices, implants and grafts, initial encounter
T82.897A Other specified complication of cardiac prosthetic devices, implants and grafts, initial encounter
Z45.09 Encounter for adjustment and management of other cardiac device
Z95.811 Presence of heart assist device

Relative Value Units/Medicare Edits

Non-Facility RVU	Work	PE	MP	Total
33981	16.11	4.29	3.72	24.12
Facility RVU	**Work**	**PE**	**MP**	**Total**
33981	16.11	4.29	3.72	24.12

	FUD	Status	MUE	Modifiers				IOM Reference
33981	N/A	A	1(3)	51	N/A	N/A	80	None

* with documentation

33982-33983

33982 Replacement of ventricular assist device pump(s); implantable intracorporeal, single ventricle, without cardiopulmonary bypass

33983 implantable intracorporeal, single ventricle, with cardiopulmonary bypass

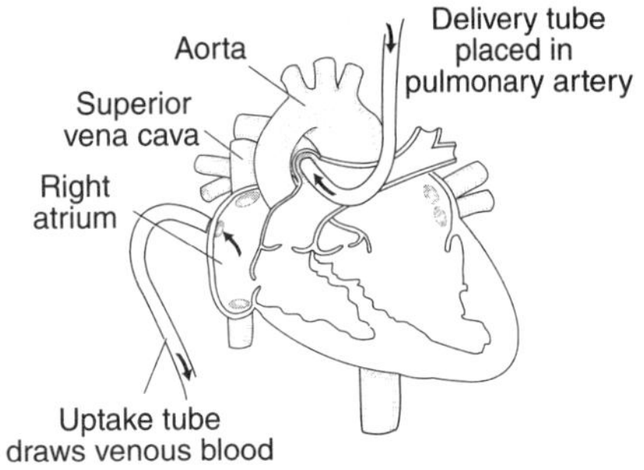

Depiction of right ventricular circulation support

Explanation

The physician replaces the blood pump component of an implantable, intracorporeal, single ventricle VAD (ventricular assist device). This may be accomplished without cardiopulmonary bypass (33982) or with cardiopulmonary bypass (33983). Pump replacement includes removal of the existing pump, insertion of a new pump, connection, de-airing, and new pump initiation.

Coding Tips

Replacement of the new pump includes removal of the previous pump, insertion of the new pump, and connection, de-airing, and initiation of the pump. For replacement of a ventricular assist device, extracorporeal, using percutaneous transseptal access, see 33999.

ICD-10-CM Diagnostic Codes

I11.0	Hypertensive heart disease with heart failure
I16.0	Hypertensive urgency
I16.1	Hypertensive emergency
I20.0	Unstable angina
I20.1	Angina pectoris with documented spasm
I20.81	Angina pectoris with coronary microvascular dysfunction
I21.01	ST elevation (STEMI) myocardial infarction involving left main coronary artery
I21.02	ST elevation (STEMI) myocardial infarction involving left anterior descending coronary artery
I21.11	ST elevation (STEMI) myocardial infarction involving right coronary artery
I21.21	ST elevation (STEMI) myocardial infarction involving left circumflex coronary artery
I21.4	Non-ST elevation (NSTEMI) myocardial infarction
I21.A1	Myocardial infarction type 2
I22.0	Subsequent ST elevation (STEMI) myocardial infarction of anterior wall
I22.1	Subsequent ST elevation (STEMI) myocardial infarction of inferior wall
I22.2	Subsequent non-ST elevation (NSTEMI) myocardial infarction
I25.2	Old myocardial infarction
I25.3	Aneurysm of heart
I25.41	Coronary artery aneurysm
I25.42	Coronary artery dissection
I25.5	Ischemic cardiomyopathy
I25.6	Silent myocardial ischemia
I34.0	Nonrheumatic mitral (valve) insufficiency
I34.1	Nonrheumatic mitral (valve) prolapse
I34.2	Nonrheumatic mitral (valve) stenosis
I34.81	Nonrheumatic mitral (valve) annulus calcification
I35.0	Nonrheumatic aortic (valve) stenosis
I35.1	Nonrheumatic aortic (valve) insufficiency
I35.2	Nonrheumatic aortic (valve) stenosis with insufficiency
I42.0	Dilated cardiomyopathy
I46.2	Cardiac arrest due to underlying cardiac condition
I46.8	Cardiac arrest due to other underlying condition
I47.0	Re-entry ventricular arrhythmia
I47.21	Torsades de pointes
I50.21	Acute systolic (congestive) heart failure
I50.22	Chronic systolic (congestive) heart failure
I50.23	Acute on chronic systolic (congestive) heart failure
I50.31	Acute diastolic (congestive) heart failure
I50.32	Chronic diastolic (congestive) heart failure
I50.33	Acute on chronic diastolic (congestive) heart failure
I50.41	Acute combined systolic (congestive) and diastolic (congestive) heart failure
I50.42	Chronic combined systolic (congestive) and diastolic (congestive) heart failure
I50.43	Acute on chronic combined systolic (congestive) and diastolic (congestive) heart failure
I50.811	Acute right heart failure
I50.812	Chronic right heart failure
I50.813	Acute on chronic right heart failure
I50.814	Right heart failure due to left heart failure
I50.82	Biventricular heart failure
I50.83	High output heart failure
I50.84	End stage heart failure
I51.5	Myocardial degeneration
I97.110	Postprocedural cardiac insufficiency following cardiac surgery
I97.111	Postprocedural cardiac insufficiency following other surgery
I97.120	Postprocedural cardiac arrest following cardiac surgery
I97.121	Postprocedural cardiac arrest following other surgery
I97.130	Postprocedural heart failure following cardiac surgery
I97.131	Postprocedural heart failure following other surgery
I97.710	Intraoperative cardiac arrest during cardiac surgery
I97.711	Intraoperative cardiac arrest during other surgery
Q21.0	Ventricular septal defect
Q21.21	Partial atrioventricular septal defect
Q21.22	Transitional atrioventricular septal defect
Q21.23	Complete atrioventricular septal defect
Q21.3	Tetralogy of Fallot
Q21.4	Aortopulmonary septal defect
Q23.0	Congenital stenosis of aortic valve
Q23.1	Congenital insufficiency of aortic valve
Q23.2	Congenital mitral stenosis

Q23.3	Congenital mitral insufficiency
Q23.81	Bicuspid aortic valve
Q23.82	Congenital mitral valve cleft leaflet
Q23.88	Other congenital malformations of aortic and mitral valves
Q24.4	Congenital subaortic stenosis
Q24.5	Malformation of coronary vessels
Q24.6	Congenital heart block
R09.2	Respiratory arrest
T82.518A	Breakdown (mechanical) of other cardiac and vascular devices and implants, initial encounter
T82.528A	Displacement of other cardiac and vascular devices and implants, initial encounter
T82.538A	Leakage of other cardiac and vascular devices and implants, initial encounter
T82.7XXA	Infection and inflammatory reaction due to other cardiac and vascular devices, implants and grafts, initial encounter
T82.817A	Embolism due to cardiac prosthetic devices, implants and grafts, initial encounter
T82.827A	Fibrosis due to cardiac prosthetic devices, implants and grafts, initial encounter
T82.837A	Hemorrhage due to cardiac prosthetic devices, implants and grafts, initial encounter
T82.847A	Pain due to cardiac prosthetic devices, implants and grafts, initial encounter
T82.857A	Stenosis of other cardiac prosthetic devices, implants and grafts, initial encounter
T82.867A	Thrombosis due to cardiac prosthetic devices, implants and grafts, initial encounter
Z45.09	Encounter for adjustment and management of other cardiac device
Z95.811	Presence of heart assist device

Relative Value Units/Medicare Edits

Non-Facility RVU	Work	PE	MP	Total
33982	37.86	10.09	8.77	56.72
33983	44.54	11.88	10.33	66.75
Facility RVU	**Work**	**PE**	**MP**	**Total**
33982	37.86	10.09	8.77	56.72
33983	44.54	11.88	10.33	66.75

	FUD	Status	MUE	Modifiers				IOM Reference
33982	N/A	A	1(3)	51	N/A	N/A	80	None
33983	N/A	A	1(3)	51	N/A	N/A	80	

* with documentation

33990-33991 [33995]

33995 Insertion of ventricular assist device, percutaneous, including radiological supervision and interpretation; right heart, venous access only

33990 left heart, arterial access only

33991 left heart, both arterial and venous access, with transseptal puncture

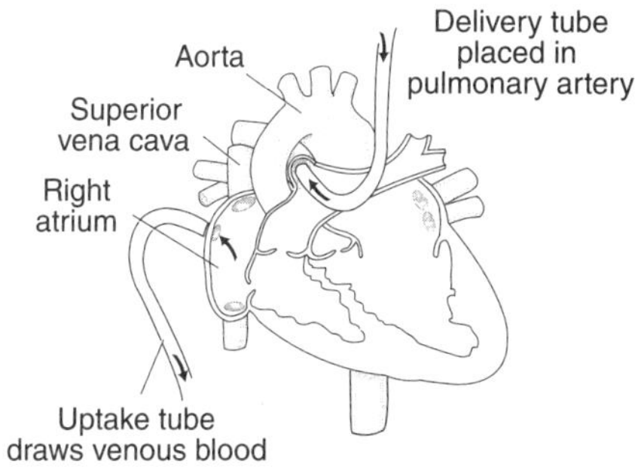

Depiction of right ventricular circulation support

Explanation

The physician performs a percutaneous insertion of a ventricular assist device (VAD) into the left, right, or both ventricles (lower chambers) of the heart. This mechanical pump assists in pushing blood from the ventricles. The procedure may be temporary for some until the heart regains the ability to pump blood on its own again (bridge to recovery), for patients awaiting heart transplant (bridge to transplant), or permanent in those who are ineligible for heart transplantation due to age or medical conditions (destination therapy). A percutaneous right ventricular assist device (RVAD) is reported with 33995. One approach described by this code involves placing two venous cannulas (typically two femoral venous cannulas or one femoral and one internal jugular venous cannula). One is positioned in the right atrium and another in the pulmonary artery. An extracorporeal centrifugal pump is used, with the inflow from the right atrial cannula and the outflow to the pulmonary artery. A left ventricular assist device (LVAD) bypasses the left ventricle during the blood oxygenation cycle, making the ventricle work less during the systolic phase. In percutaneous placement of an LVAD, a catheter is inserted in the patient's femoral vein and maneuvered to the left atrium. A centrifugal assist device is placed outside the body, usually on the patient's thigh. The catheter is attached to the device. Oxygenated blood is pumped from the left atrium to the device and distributed to one or both femoral arteries via catheter. Report 33990 when the LVAD is inserted with a single arterial access. Report 33991 if the septum is punctured for left atrial access and the procedure includes both arterial and venous access. These codes include radiological supervision and interpretation.

Coding Tips

When medically necessary, report moderate (conscious) sedation provided by the performing physician with 99151-99153. When provided by another physician, report 99155-99157. For repositioning of the percutaneous ventricular assist device, see 33993. For removal of the percutaneous ventricular assist device, see 33992. For insertion of implantable intracorporeal ventricular assist devices, see 33979.

ICD-10-CM Diagnostic Codes

I09.81	Rheumatic heart failure
I11.0	Hypertensive heart disease with heart failure

I16.0	Hypertensive urgency
I16.1	Hypertensive emergency
I20.0	Unstable angina
I20.1	Angina pectoris with documented spasm
I20.81	Angina pectoris with coronary microvascular dysfunction
I21.01	ST elevation (STEMI) myocardial infarction involving left main coronary artery
I21.02	ST elevation (STEMI) myocardial infarction involving left anterior descending coronary artery
I21.09	ST elevation (STEMI) myocardial infarction involving other coronary artery of anterior wall
I21.11	ST elevation (STEMI) myocardial infarction involving right coronary artery
I21.19	ST elevation (STEMI) myocardial infarction involving other coronary artery of inferior wall
I21.21	ST elevation (STEMI) myocardial infarction involving left circumflex coronary artery
I21.29	ST elevation (STEMI) myocardial infarction involving other sites
I21.4	Non-ST elevation (NSTEMI) myocardial infarction
I21.A1	Myocardial infarction type 2
I21.B	Myocardial infarction with coronary microvascular dysfunction
I22.0	Subsequent ST elevation (STEMI) myocardial infarction of anterior wall
I22.1	Subsequent ST elevation (STEMI) myocardial infarction of inferior wall
I22.2	Subsequent non-ST elevation (NSTEMI) myocardial infarction
I22.8	Subsequent ST elevation (STEMI) myocardial infarction of other sites
I24.89	Other forms of acute ischemic heart disease
I25.2	Old myocardial infarction
I25.3	Aneurysm of heart
I25.41	Coronary artery aneurysm
I25.42	Coronary artery dissection
I25.5	Ischemic cardiomyopathy
I25.6	Silent myocardial ischemia
I25.89	Other forms of chronic ischemic heart disease
I34.0	Nonrheumatic mitral (valve) insufficiency
I34.1	Nonrheumatic mitral (valve) prolapse
I34.2	Nonrheumatic mitral (valve) stenosis
I34.81	Nonrheumatic mitral (valve) annulus calcification
I35.0	Nonrheumatic aortic (valve) stenosis
I35.1	Nonrheumatic aortic (valve) insufficiency
I35.2	Nonrheumatic aortic (valve) stenosis with insufficiency
I35.8	Other nonrheumatic aortic valve disorders
I40.0	Infective myocarditis
I40.1	Isolated myocarditis
I41	Myocarditis in diseases classified elsewhere
I42.0	Dilated cardiomyopathy
I42.1	Obstructive hypertrophic cardiomyopathy
I42.2	Other hypertrophic cardiomyopathy
I42.5	Other restrictive cardiomyopathy
I42.7	Cardiomyopathy due to drug and external agent
I42.8	Other cardiomyopathies
I43	Cardiomyopathy in diseases classified elsewhere
I46.2	Cardiac arrest due to underlying cardiac condition
I46.8	Cardiac arrest due to other underlying condition
I47.0	Re-entry ventricular arrhythmia
I47.11	Inappropriate sinus tachycardia, so stated
I47.21	Torsades de pointes
I47.29	Other ventricular tachycardia
I50.1	Left ventricular failure, unspecified
I50.21	Acute systolic (congestive) heart failure
I50.22	Chronic systolic (congestive) heart failure
I50.23	Acute on chronic systolic (congestive) heart failure
I50.31	Acute diastolic (congestive) heart failure
I50.32	Chronic diastolic (congestive) heart failure
I50.33	Acute on chronic diastolic (congestive) heart failure
I50.41	Acute combined systolic (congestive) and diastolic (congestive) heart failure
I50.42	Chronic combined systolic (congestive) and diastolic (congestive) heart failure
I50.43	Acute on chronic combined systolic (congestive) and diastolic (congestive) heart failure
I50.811	Acute right heart failure
I50.812	Chronic right heart failure
I50.813	Acute on chronic right heart failure
I50.814	Right heart failure due to left heart failure
I50.82	Biventricular heart failure
I50.83	High output heart failure
I50.84	End stage heart failure
I51.5	Myocardial degeneration
I97.110	Postprocedural cardiac insufficiency following cardiac surgery
I97.111	Postprocedural cardiac insufficiency following other surgery
I97.120	Postprocedural cardiac arrest following cardiac surgery
I97.121	Postprocedural cardiac arrest following other surgery
I97.130	Postprocedural heart failure following cardiac surgery
I97.131	Postprocedural heart failure following other surgery
I97.190	Other postprocedural cardiac functional disturbances following cardiac surgery
I97.191	Other postprocedural cardiac functional disturbances following other surgery
I97.710	Intraoperative cardiac arrest during cardiac surgery
I97.711	Intraoperative cardiac arrest during other surgery
I97.790	Other intraoperative cardiac functional disturbances during cardiac surgery
I97.791	Other intraoperative cardiac functional disturbances during other surgery
I97.88	Other intraoperative complications of the circulatory system, not elsewhere classified
I97.89	Other postprocedural complications and disorders of the circulatory system, not elsewhere classified
Q21.0	Ventricular septal defect
Q21.21	Partial atrioventricular septal defect
Q21.22	Transitional atrioventricular septal defect
Q21.23	Complete atrioventricular septal defect
Q21.3	Tetralogy of Fallot
Q21.4	Aortopulmonary septal defect
Q21.8	Other congenital malformations of cardiac septa

Q23.0	Congenital stenosis of aortic valve
Q23.1	Congenital insufficiency of aortic valve
Q23.2	Congenital mitral stenosis
Q23.3	Congenital mitral insufficiency
Q23.81	Bicuspid aortic valve
Q23.82	Congenital mitral valve cleft leaflet
Q23.88	Other congenital malformations of aortic and mitral valves
Q24.4	Congenital subaortic stenosis
Q24.5	Malformation of coronary vessels
Q24.6	Congenital heart block
Q24.8	Other specified congenital malformations of heart
R57.0	Cardiogenic shock

AMA: **33990** 2022,Jul; 2021,Dec; 2020,Dec; 2018,Jun **33991** 2022,Jul; 2021,Dec; 2020,Dec; 2018,Jun **33995** 2021,Dec; 2020,Dec

Relative Value Units/Medicare Edits

Non-Facility RVU	Work	PE	MP	Total
33995	6.75	2.16	1.47	10.38
33990	6.75	2.26	1.54	10.55
33991	8.84	2.36	2.04	13.24
Facility RVU	**Work**	**PE**	**MP**	**Total**
33995	6.75	2.16	1.47	10.38
33990	6.75	2.26	1.54	10.55
33991	8.84	2.36	2.04	13.24

	FUD	Status	MUE	Modifiers				IOM Reference
33995	0	A	1(3)	51	N/A	N/A	80	None
33990	0	A	1(3)	51	N/A	N/A	80	
33991	0	A	1(3)	51	N/A	N/A	80	

* with documentation

Terms To Know

cardiogenic shock. Shock caused by an inadequate supply of oxygen to the body's tissues due to a malfunction of the pumping action of the heart.

hypertrophic. Enlarged or overgrown from an increase in cell size of the affected tissue.

idiopathic. Having no known cause.

percutaneous. Through the skin.

rheumatic heart disease. Manifestation of and sequel to rheumatic fever; any cardiac involvement in rheumatic fever.

ventricular assist device. Temporary measure used to support the heart by substituting for left and/or right heart function. The device replaces the work of the left and/or right ventricle when a patient has a damaged or weakened heart. A left ventricular assist device (VAD) helps the heart pump blood through the rest of the body. A right VAD helps the heart pump blood to the lungs to become oxygenated again. Catheters are inserted to circulate the blood through external tubing to a pump machine located outside of the body and back to the correct artery.

33992

33992 Removal of percutaneous left heart ventricular assist device, arterial or arterial and venous cannula(s), at separate and distinct session from insertion

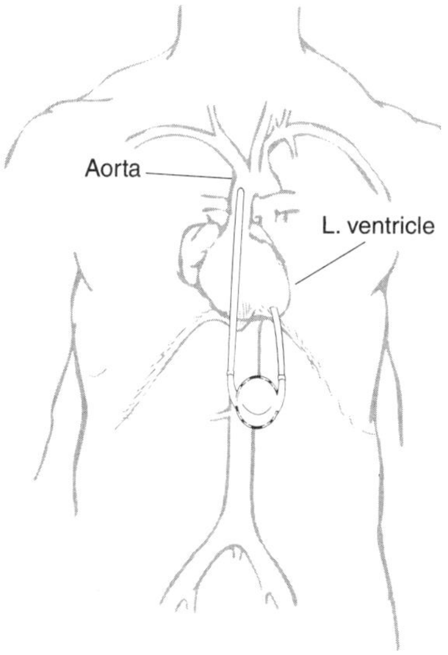

Ventricular assist device is removed percutaneously

Explanation

A left ventricular assist device (LVAD) bypasses the left ventricle during the blood oxygenation cycle making the ventricle work less during the systolic phase. The device is removed when the patient's ventricle recovers, an artificial heart is placed, or the patient undergoes heart transplantation. The arterial or arterial and venous cannulas are removed, and the external centrifugal assist device is discontinued and removed. This code can only be reported for the removal of an LVAD during a different operative encounter than the insertion, and is only used for a percutaneous LVAD, not an implantable LVAD.

Coding Tips

When medically necessary, report moderate (conscious) sedation provided by the performing physician with 99151-99153. When provided by another physician, report 99155-99157. For insertion of a percutaneous ventricular assist device, see 33990–33991. For repositioning of a percutaneous ventricular assist device, see 33993. For removal of implantable intracorporeal ventricular assist devices, see 33980. For removal of extracorporeal ventricular assist devices, see 33977–33978.

ICD-10-CM Diagnostic Codes

T82.518A	Breakdown (mechanical) of other cardiac and vascular devices and implants, initial encounter
T82.528A	Displacement of other cardiac and vascular devices and implants, initial encounter
T82.538A	Leakage of other cardiac and vascular devices and implants, initial encounter
T82.598A	Other mechanical complication of other cardiac and vascular devices and implants, initial encounter
T82.7XXA	Infection and inflammatory reaction due to other cardiac and vascular devices, implants and grafts, initial encounter
T82.817A	Embolism due to cardiac prosthetic devices, implants and grafts, initial encounter
T82.827A	Fibrosis due to cardiac prosthetic devices, implants and grafts, initial encounter

T82.837A	Hemorrhage due to cardiac prosthetic devices, implants and grafts, initial encounter
T82.847A	Pain due to cardiac prosthetic devices, implants and grafts, initial encounter
T82.857A	Stenosis of other cardiac prosthetic devices, implants and grafts, initial encounter
T82.867A	Thrombosis due to cardiac prosthetic devices, implants and grafts, initial encounter
T82.897A	Other specified complication of cardiac prosthetic devices, implants and grafts, initial encounter
Z45.09	Encounter for adjustment and management of other cardiac device
Z95.811	Presence of heart assist device

AMA: 33992 2022,Jul; 2021,Dec; 2020,Dec

Relative Value Units/Medicare Edits

Non-Facility RVU	Work	PE	MP	Total
33992	3.55	1.14	0.81	5.5
Facility RVU	**Work**	**PE**	**MP**	**Total**
33992	3.55	1.14	0.81	5.5

	FUD	Status	MUE	Modifiers				IOM Reference
33992	0	A	1(2)	51	N/A	N/A	80	None

* with documentation

Terms To Know

extracorporeal. Located or taking place outside the body.

moderate sedation. Medically controlled state of depressed consciousness, with or without analgesia, while maintaining the patient's airway, protective reflexes, and ability to respond to stimulation or verbal commands.

percutaneous. Through the skin.

ventricular assist device. Temporary measure used to support the heart by substituting for left and/or right heart function. The device replaces the work of the left and/or right ventricle when a patient has a damaged or weakened heart. A left ventricular assist device (VAD) helps the heart pump blood through the rest of the body. A right VAD helps the heart pump blood to the lungs to become oxygenated again. Catheters are inserted to circulate the blood through external tubing to a pump machine located outside of the body and back to the correct artery.

[33997]

33997 Removal of percutaneous right heart ventricular assist device, venous cannula, at separate and distinct session from insertion

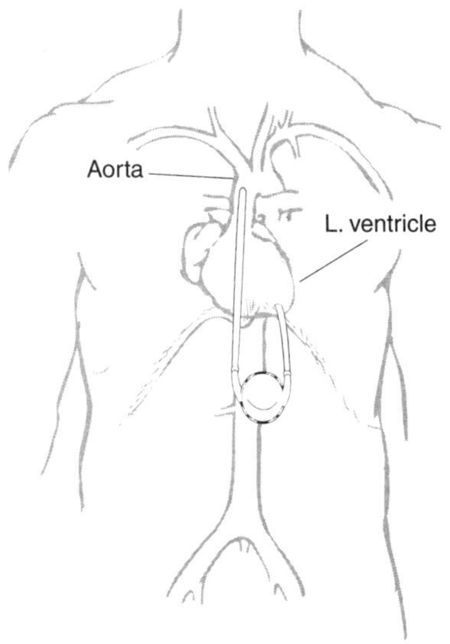

Ventricular assist device is removed percutaneously

Explanation

A right ventricular assist device (RVAD) assists the right ventricle in pumping blood to the pulmonary artery and is typically only used for short-term, right ventricular support following left ventricular assist device (LVAD) surgery or other heart surgery. The device is removed when the patient's right ventricle recovers sufficiently. The venous cannula is removed, and the external centrifugal assist device is discontinued and removed. This code can only be reported for the removal of an RVAD during a different operative encounter than the insertion, and is only used for a percutaneous RVAD, not an implantable RVAD.

Coding Tips

When medically necessary, report moderate (conscious) sedation provided by the performing physician with 99151-99153. When provided by another physician, report 99155-99157. For removal of a left or right heart ventricular assist device, open approach, see 35206, 35226, 35286, and 35371.

ICD-10-CM Diagnostic Codes

T82.518A	Breakdown (mechanical) of other cardiac and vascular devices and implants, initial encounter
T82.528A	Displacement of other cardiac and vascular devices and implants, initial encounter
T82.538A	Leakage of other cardiac and vascular devices and implants, initial encounter
T82.598A	Other mechanical complication of other cardiac and vascular devices and implants, initial encounter
T82.7XXA	Infection and inflammatory reaction due to other cardiac and vascular devices, implants and grafts, initial encounter
T82.817A	Embolism due to cardiac prosthetic devices, implants and grafts, initial encounter
T82.827A	Fibrosis due to cardiac prosthetic devices, implants and grafts, initial encounter
T82.837A	Hemorrhage due to cardiac prosthetic devices, implants and grafts, initial encounter

T82.847A	Pain due to cardiac prosthetic devices, implants and grafts, initial encounter
T82.857A	Stenosis of other cardiac prosthetic devices, implants and grafts, initial encounter
T82.867A	Thrombosis due to cardiac prosthetic devices, implants and grafts, initial encounter
T82.897A	Other specified complication of cardiac prosthetic devices, implants and grafts, initial encounter
T88.8XXA	Other specified complications of surgical and medical care, not elsewhere classified, initial encounter
Z45.09	Encounter for adjustment and management of other cardiac device
Z95.811	Presence of heart assist device

AMA: **33997** 2021,Dec; 2020,Dec

Relative Value Units/Medicare Edits

Non-Facility RVU	Work	PE	MP	Total
33997	3.0	1.02	0.7	4.72
Facility RVU	**Work**	**PE**	**MP**	**Total**
33997	3.0	1.02	0.7	4.72

	FUD	Status	MUE	Modifiers				IOM Reference
33997	0	A	1(3)	51	N/A	N/A	80	None

* with documentation

Terms To Know

cannula. Tube inserted into a blood vessel, duct, or body cavity to facilitate passage.

ventricular assist device. Temporary measure used to support the heart by substituting for left and/or right heart function. The device replaces the work of the left and/or right ventricle when a patient has a damaged or weakened heart. A left ventricular assist device (VAD) helps the heart pump blood through the rest of the body. A right VAD helps the heart pump blood to the lungs to become oxygenated again. Catheters are inserted to circulate the blood through external tubing to a pump machine located outside of the body and back to the correct artery.

33993

33993 Repositioning of percutaneous right or left heart ventricular assist device with imaging guidance at separate and distinct session from insertion

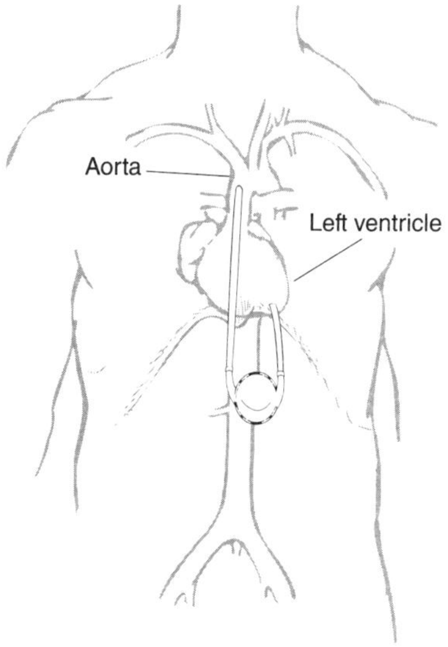

Ventricular assist device is repositioned percutaneously

Explanation

A left ventricular assist device (LVAD) is the most common type of VAD, helping the left ventricle pump blood to the aorta. A right ventricular assist device (RVAD) assists the right ventricle in pumping blood to the pulmonary artery and is typically used only for short-term, right ventricular support following LVAD surgery or other cardiac surgery. Report 33993 when the components of a percutaneously placed LVAD or RVAD need to be repositioned at any time other than during the surgical encounter for insertion. This code includes imaging guidance.

Coding Tips

When medically necessary, report moderate (conscious) sedation provided by the performing physician with 99151-99153. When provided by another physician, report 99155-99157. Imaging guidance is considered part of this procedure and is not reported separately. For insertion of the percutaneous ventricular assist device, see 33990–33991. For removal of the percutaneous ventricular assist device, see 33992.

ICD-10-CM Diagnostic Codes

T82.528A	Displacement of other cardiac and vascular devices and implants, initial encounter
T82.897A	Other specified complication of cardiac prosthetic devices, implants and grafts, initial encounter
Z45.09	Encounter for adjustment and management of other cardiac device
Z95.811	Presence of heart assist device

AMA: **33993** 2022,Jul; 2021,Dec; 2020,Dec

Relative Value Units/Medicare Edits

Non-Facility RVU	Work	PE	MP	Total
33993	3.1	1.1	0.66	4.86
Facility RVU	**Work**	**PE**	**MP**	**Total**
33993	3.1	1.1	0.66	4.86

	FUD	Status	MUE	Modifiers				IOM Reference
33993	0	A	1(3)	51	N/A	N/A	80	None

* with documentation

Terms To Know

conscious sedation. Medically controlled state of depressed consciousness, with or without analgesia, while maintaining the patient's airway, protective reflexes, and ability to respond to stimulation or verbal commands.

LVAD. Left ventricular assist device. Temporarily implanted device that helps the left ventricle of a damaged heart continue to pump an adequate supply of blood to meet the body's needs, generally used as a temporary measure while awaiting transplantation.

34001

34001 Embolectomy or thrombectomy, with or without catheter; carotid, subclavian or innominate artery, by neck incision

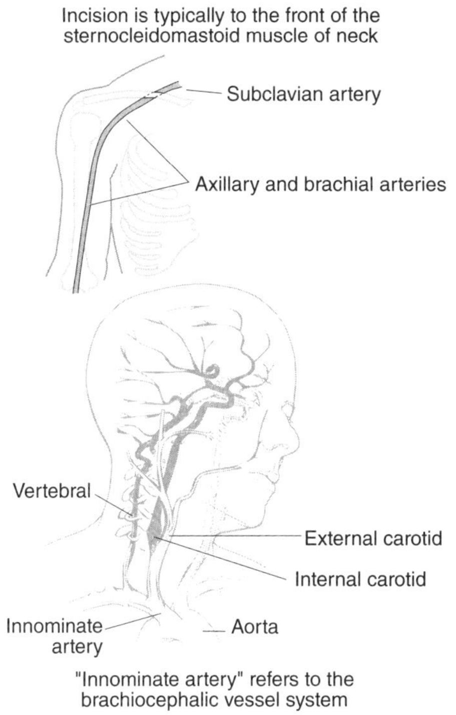

Explanation

To remove a blood clot in the carotid, subclavian, or innominate artery, the physician makes an incision in the skin of the neck usually in front of the sternocleidomastoid muscle over the site of the clot or immediately above it. The artery is isolated and dissected from critical structures. The artery may be clamped above and below the clot and incised. The physician removes the blood clot and sutures the artery. The clamps are removed. If a catheter is required, it is threaded past the clot and a small balloon at its tip is inflated. The catheter is withdrawn, capturing and retrieving the clot. The physician may make several passes to remove the entire clot. The blood vessel is repaired with sutures and the skin incision is repaired with layered closure.

Coding Tips

Establishing both inflow and outflow by any method is included. That portion of the operative arteriogram performed by the surgeon is also included. Angioscopy performed during therapeutic intervention should be reported in addition to the code for the primary procedure; see 35400. For arterial embolectomy or thrombectomy, innominate, subclavian, by thoracic incision, see 34051; by arm incision, see 34101. For venous thrombectomy subclavian by neck incision, see 34471; by arm incision, see 34490. For thrombectomy of an arterial graft, see 35875–35876.

ICD-10-CM Diagnostic Codes

G45.0	Vertebro-basilar artery syndrome
G45.1	Carotid artery syndrome (hemispheric)
G45.2	Multiple and bilateral precerebral artery syndromes
G45.3	Amaurosis fugax
G45.8	Other transient cerebral ischemic attacks and related syndromes
G45.9	Transient cerebral ischemic attack, unspecified
I63.031	Cerebral infarction due to thrombosis of right carotid artery ☑
I63.032	Cerebral infarction due to thrombosis of left carotid artery ☑
I63.033	Cerebral infarction due to thrombosis of bilateral carotid arteries ☑
I63.09	Cerebral infarction due to thrombosis of other precerebral artery
I63.131	Cerebral infarction due to embolism of right carotid artery ☑
I63.132	Cerebral infarction due to embolism of left carotid artery ☑
I63.133	Cerebral infarction due to embolism of bilateral carotid arteries ☑
I65.21	Occlusion and stenosis of right carotid artery ☑
I65.22	Occlusion and stenosis of left carotid artery ☑
I65.23	Occlusion and stenosis of bilateral carotid arteries ☑
I65.8	Occlusion and stenosis of other precerebral arteries
I67.2	Cerebral atherosclerosis [A]
I67.81	Acute cerebrovascular insufficiency
I67.841	Reversible cerebrovascular vasoconstriction syndrome
I67.848	Other cerebrovascular vasospasm and vasoconstriction
I67.89	Other cerebrovascular disease
I76	Septic arterial embolism

AMA: 34001 2022,Jun

Relative Value Units/Medicare Edits

Non-Facility RVU	Work	PE	MP	Total
34001	17.88	4.51	4.44	26.83
Facility RVU	**Work**	**PE**	**MP**	**Total**
34001	17.88	4.51	4.44	26.83

	FUD	Status	MUE	Modifiers				IOM Reference
34001	90	A	1(3)	51	50	62*	80	None

* with documentation

Terms To Know

embolism. Obstruction of a blood vessel resulting from a clot or foreign substance.

thrombosis. Condition arising from the presence or formation of blood clots within a blood vessel that may cause vascular obstruction and insufficient oxygenation.

34051

34051 Embolectomy or thrombectomy, with or without catheter; innominate, subclavian artery, by thoracic incision

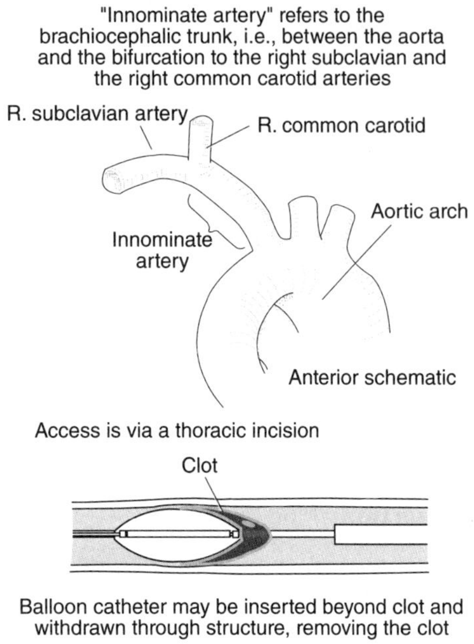

Explanation

The physician exposes the innominate or subclavian artery by making an incision in the anterior chest (midline sternotomy or lateral thoracotomy). The physician identifies the embolus or thrombus and occludes the artery proximal to the clot. The physician makes a small incision in the artery proximal to the clot and withdraws it using ring forceps, or by passing a Fogarty balloon catheter beyond the clot, inflating and withdrawing the balloon. The physician establishes proof of patency by injecting contrast in the artery under fluoroscope. The physician sutures the arteriotomy closed, removes the vascular clamp or tie, and closes the chest wall. The physician may leave chest tubes and/or a mediastinal drainage tube in place following the procedure.

Coding Tips

Establishing both inflow and outflow by any method is included. That portion of the operative arteriogram performed by the surgeon is also included. Angioscopy performed during therapeutic intervention should be reported in addition to the code for the primary procedure; see 35400.

ICD-10-CM Diagnostic Codes

G45.0	Vertebro-basilar artery syndrome
G45.2	Multiple and bilateral precerebral artery syndromes
G45.8	Other transient cerebral ischemic attacks and related syndromes
G45.9	Transient cerebral ischemic attack, unspecified
I63.09	Cerebral infarction due to thrombosis of other precerebral artery
I63.19	Cerebral infarction due to embolism of other precerebral artery
I63.29	Cerebral infarction due to unspecified occlusion or stenosis of other precerebral arteries
I63.9	Cerebral infarction, unspecified
I76	Septic arterial embolism

AMA: 34051 2022,Jun

Relative Value Units/Medicare Edits

Non-Facility RVU	Work	PE	MP	Total
34051	16.99	8.39	3.92	29.3
Facility RVU	**Work**	**PE**	**MP**	**Total**
34051	16.99	8.39	3.92	29.3

	FUD	Status	MUE	Modifiers				IOM Reference
34051	90	A	1(3)	51	50	62*	80	None

* with documentation

Terms To Know

angioscopy. Visualization of capillary blood vessels with a microscope, or the inside of a blood vessel with a fiberoptic-equipped catheter.

embolism. Obstruction of a blood vessel resulting from a clot or foreign substance.

hemiplegia. Paralysis of one side of the body.

occlusion. Constriction, closure, or blockage of a passage.

thrombosis. Condition arising from the presence or formation of blood clots within a blood vessel that may cause vascular obstruction and insufficient oxygenation.

34101-34111

34101 Embolectomy or thrombectomy, with or without catheter; axillary, brachial, innominate, subclavian artery, by arm incision
34111 radial or ulnar artery, by arm incision

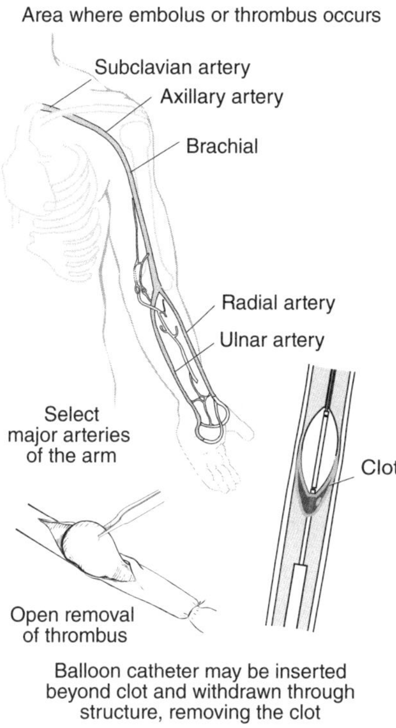

Explanation

In 34101, to remove a blood clot in the axillary, brachial, innominate, or subclavian artery, the physician makes an incision in the skin of the arm at the site of the blood clot or above it. In 34111, to remove a blood clot in the radial or ulnar artery, the physician makes an incision in the skin of the arm, over the site of the clot or immediately above it. The artery is isolated and dissected from adjacent critical structures. The artery may be clamped above and below the clot, and incised. The physician removes the blood clot and repairs the artery. The clamps are removed. If a catheter is required, it is threaded past the clot and a small balloon at its tip is inflated. The catheter is withdrawn, capturing and retrieving the clot. The physician may make several passes to remove all of the clot. The blood vessel is repaired with sutures and the skin incision is repaired with a layered closure.

Coding Tips

Establishing both inflow and outflow by any method is included. The portion of the operative arteriogram performed by the surgeon is also included. Angioscopy performed during therapeutic intervention should be reported in addition to the code for the primary procedure; see 35400. For arterial embolectomy or thrombectomy, carotid, innominate, subclavian, by thoracic incision, see 34001; innominate, subclavian, by thoracic incision, see 34051. For venous thrombectomy, subclavian, by neck incision, see 34471; axillary and subclavian by arm incision, see 34490. For thrombectomy of an arterial graft, see 35875–35876.

ICD-10-CM Diagnostic Codes

G45.2	Multiple and bilateral precerebral artery syndromes
I63.09	Cerebral infarction due to thrombosis of other precerebral artery
I63.19	Cerebral infarction due to embolism of other precerebral artery
I65.8	Occlusion and stenosis of other precerebral arteries
I73.89	Other specified peripheral vascular diseases
I73.9	Peripheral vascular disease, unspecified
I74.2	Embolism and thrombosis of arteries of the upper extremities
I75.011	Atheroembolism of right upper extremity ☑
I75.012	Atheroembolism of left upper extremity ☑
I75.013	Atheroembolism of bilateral upper extremities ☑
I76	Septic arterial embolism

AMA: 34101 2022,Jun **34111** 2022,Jun

Relative Value Units/Medicare Edits

Non-Facility RVU	Work	PE	MP	Total
34101	10.93	3.86	2.71	17.5
34111	10.93	3.84	2.71	17.48
Facility RVU	**Work**	**PE**	**MP**	**Total**
34101	10.93	3.86	2.71	17.5
34111	10.93	3.84	2.71	17.48

	FUD	Status	MUE	Modifiers				IOM Reference
34101	90	A	1(3)	51	50	62*	80	None
34111	90	A	2(3)	51	50	62*	80	

* with documentation

Terms To Know

angioscopy. Visualization of capillary blood vessels with a microscope, or the inside of a blood vessel with a fiberoptic-equipped catheter.

catheter. Flexible tube inserted into an area of the body for introducing or withdrawing fluid.

dissect. Cut apart or separate tissue for surgical purposes or for visual or microscopic study.

embolism. Obstruction of a blood vessel resulting from a clot or foreign substance.

thrombosis. Condition arising from the presence or formation of blood clots within a blood vessel that may cause vascular obstruction and insufficient oxygenation.

34151

34151 Embolectomy or thrombectomy, with or without catheter; renal, celiac, mesentery, aortoiliac artery, by abdominal incision

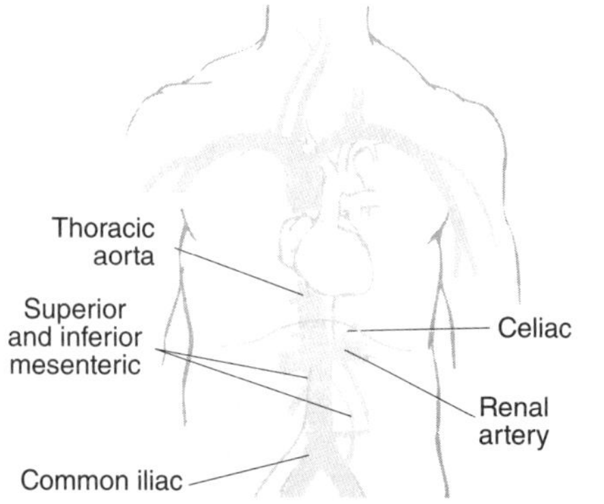

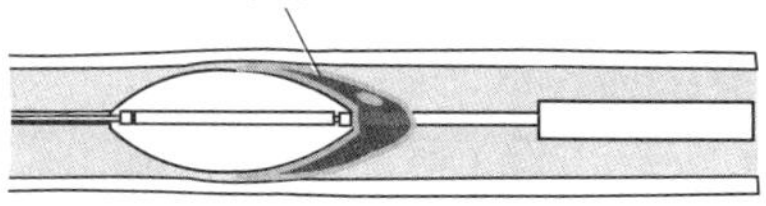

Balloon catheter may be inserted beyond clot and withdrawn through structure, removing the clot

Explanation

To remove a blood clot in the renal, celiac, mesentery, aortoiliac artery, the physician makes an incision in the skin of the abdomen over the site of the clot or immediately above or below it. The vein is isolated and dissected from adjacent critical structures. The artery may be clamped above and below the clot and incised. The physician removes the blood clot. The clamps are removed. If a catheter is required, it is threaded past the clot and a small balloon at its tip is inflated. The catheter is withdrawn, capturing and retrieving the clot. The physician may make several passes to remove all of the clot. The blood vessel is repaired with sutures and the skin incision is repaired with a layered closure.

Coding Tips

Establishing both inflow and outflow by any method is included. The portion of the operative arteriogram performed by the surgeon is also included. Angioscopy performed during therapeutic intervention should be reported in addition to the code for the primary procedure; see 35400. For thrombectomy of an arterial or venous graft, see 35875–35876.

ICD-10-CM Diagnostic Codes

I70.1	Atherosclerosis of renal artery A
I74.01	Saddle embolus of abdominal aorta
I74.09	Other arterial embolism and thrombosis of abdominal aorta
I74.19	Embolism and thrombosis of other parts of aorta
I74.5	Embolism and thrombosis of iliac artery
I75.81	Atheroembolism of kidney
I76	Septic arterial embolism
K55.011	Focal (segmental) acute (reversible) ischemia of small intestine
K55.012	Diffuse acute (reversible) ischemia of small intestine
K55.021	Focal (segmental) acute infarction of small intestine
K55.022	Diffuse acute infarction of small intestine
K55.031	Focal (segmental) acute (reversible) ischemia of large intestine
K55.032	Diffuse acute (reversible) ischemia of large intestine
K55.041	Focal (segmental) acute infarction of large intestine
K55.042	Diffuse acute infarction of large intestine
K55.1	Chronic vascular disorders of intestine
K55.8	Other vascular disorders of intestine
N28.0	Ischemia and infarction of kidney

AMA: **34151** 2022,Jun

Relative Value Units/Medicare Edits

Non-Facility RVU	Work	PE	MP	Total
34151	26.52	7.71	6.54	40.77
Facility RVU	**Work**	**PE**	**MP**	**Total**
34151	26.52	7.71	6.54	40.77

	FUD	Status	MUE	Modifiers				IOM Reference
34151	90	A	1(3)	51	50	62*	80	None

* with documentation

Terms To Know

angioscopy. Visualization of capillary blood vessels with a microscope, or the inside of a blood vessel with a fiberoptic-equipped catheter.

atherosclerosis. Buildup of yellowish plaques composed of cholesterol and lipoid material within the arteries.

catheter. Flexible tube inserted into an area of the body for introducing or withdrawing fluid.

complication. Condition arising after the beginning of observation and treatment that modifies the course of the patient's illness or the medical care required, or an undesired result or misadventure in medical care.

embolism. Obstruction of a blood vessel resulting from a clot or foreign substance.

34201

34201 Embolectomy or thrombectomy, with or without catheter; femoropopliteal, aortoiliac artery, by leg incision

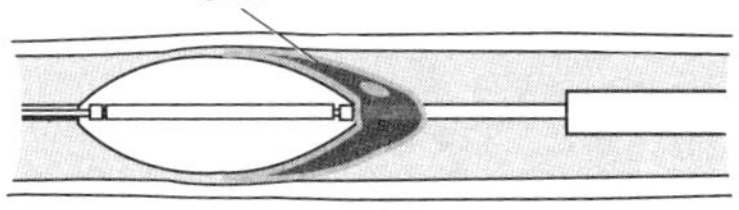

Balloon catheter may be inserted beyond clot and withdrawn through structure, removing the clot

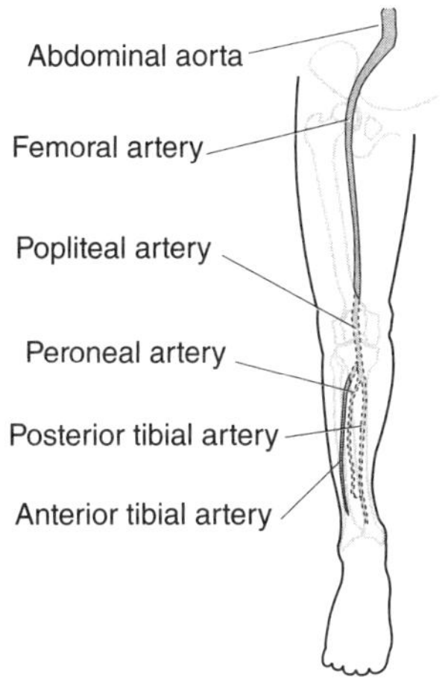

Explanation

To remove a blood clot in the femoropopliteal or aortoiliac artery, the physician makes an incision in the skin of the leg over the femoral artery. The artery is isolated and dissected from adjacent critical structures. The artery may be clamped above and below the clot and incised. The physician removes the blood clot and repairs the vessel. The clamps are removed. If a catheter is required, it is threaded past the clot and a small balloon at its tip is inflated. The catheter is withdrawn, capturing and retrieving the clot. The physician may make several passes to remove all of the clot. The blood vessel is repaired with sutures and the skin incision is repaired with a layered closure.

Coding Tips

Establishing both inflow and outflow by any method is included. The portion of the operative arteriogram performed by the surgeon is also included. Angioscopy performed during therapeutic intervention should be reported in addition to the code for the primary procedure; see 35400. For venous thrombectomy of the vena cava, iliac, or femoropopliteal vein by leg incision, see 34421. For thrombectomy of an arterial or venous graft, see 35875–35876.

ICD-10-CM Diagnostic Codes

I74.01	Saddle embolus of abdominal aorta
I74.09	Other arterial embolism and thrombosis of abdominal aorta
I74.19	Embolism and thrombosis of other parts of aorta
I74.3	Embolism and thrombosis of arteries of the lower extremities
I74.5	Embolism and thrombosis of iliac artery
I75.021	Atheroembolism of right lower extremity ☑
I75.022	Atheroembolism of left lower extremity ☑
I75.023	Atheroembolism of bilateral lower extremities ☑

AMA: 34201 2022,Jun

Relative Value Units/Medicare Edits

Non-Facility RVU	Work	PE	MP	Total
34201	19.48	5.62	4.83	29.93
Facility RVU	**Work**	**PE**	**MP**	**Total**
34201	19.48	5.62	4.83	29.93

	FUD	Status	MUE	Modifiers				IOM Reference
34201	90	A	1(3)	51	50	62*	80	None

* with documentation

Terms To Know

angioscopy. Visualization of capillary blood vessels with a microscope, or the inside of a blood vessel with a fiberoptic-equipped catheter.

catheter. Flexible tube inserted into an area of the body for introducing or withdrawing fluid.

embolism. Obstruction of a blood vessel resulting from a clot or foreign substance.

graft. Tissue implant from another part of the body or another person.

incision. Act of cutting into tissue or an organ.

thrombectomy. Removal of a clot (thrombus) from a blood vessel utilizing various methods.

34203

34203 Embolectomy or thrombectomy, with or without catheter; popliteal-tibio-peroneal artery, by leg incision

Explanation

To remove a blood clot in the popliteal-tibio-peroneal artery, the physician makes an incision in the skin of the leg over the femoral or popliteal artery. The artery is isolated and dissected from adjacent critical structures. The artery may be clamped above and below the clot and incised. The physician removes the blood clot. The clamps are removed. If a catheter is required, it is threaded past the clot and a small balloon at its tip is inflated. The catheter is withdrawn, capturing and retrieving the clot. The physician may make several passes to remove all of the clot. The blood vessel is repaired with sutures and the skin incision is repaired with a layered closure.

Coding Tips

Establishing both inflow and outflow by any method is included. The portion of the operative arteriogram performed by the surgeon is also included. Angioscopy performed during therapeutic intervention should be reported in addition to the code for the primary procedure; see 35400. For thrombectomy of an arterial or venous graft, see 35875–35876.

ICD-10-CM Diagnostic Codes

I74.3	Embolism and thrombosis of arteries of the lower extremities
I75.021	Atheroembolism of right lower extremity ☑
I75.022	Atheroembolism of left lower extremity ☑
I75.023	Atheroembolism of bilateral lower extremities ☑

AMA: 34203 2022,Jun

Relative Value Units/Medicare Edits

Non-Facility RVU	Work	PE	MP	Total
34203	17.86	5.53	4.42	27.81
Facility RVU	**Work**	**PE**	**MP**	**Total**
34203	17.86	5.53	4.42	27.81

	FUD	Status	MUE	Modifiers				IOM Reference
34203	90	A	1(2)	51	50	62*	80	None

* with documentation

Terms To Know

angioscopy. Visualization of capillary blood vessels with a microscope, or the inside of a blood vessel with a fiberoptic-equipped catheter.

arteriogram. Radiograph of arteries.

embolism. Obstruction of a blood vessel resulting from a clot or foreign substance.

thrombectomy. Removal of a clot (thrombus) from a blood vessel utilizing various methods.

thrombosis. Condition arising from the presence or formation of blood clots within a blood vessel that may cause vascular obstruction and insufficient oxygenation.

34401

34401 Thrombectomy, direct or with catheter; vena cava, iliac vein, by abdominal incision

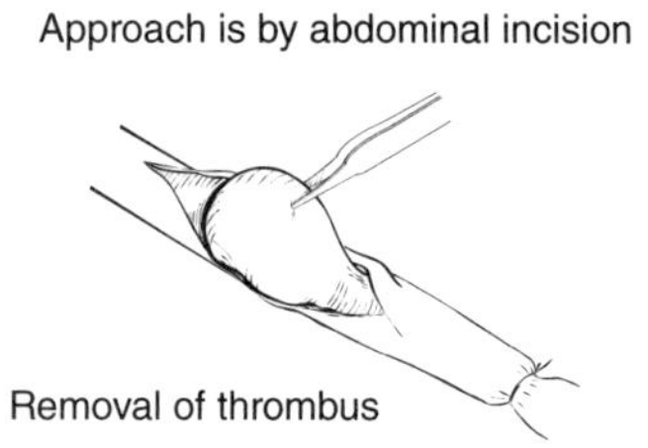

A thrombus in the vena cava and/or iliac vein is removed by an abdominal incision

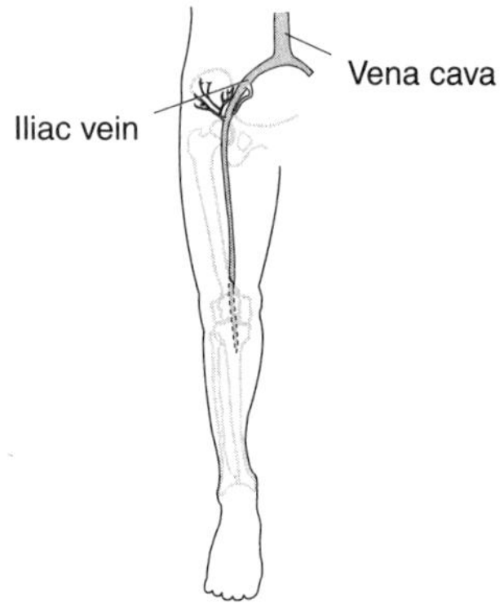

Explanation

The physician exposes the vena cava or iliac vein by making an abdominal incision. The physician identifies the thrombus by venogram and may perform a contralateral femoral venogram to rule out inferior vena caval involvement. The physician makes an incision in the vena cava or iliac vein. The physician withdraws the clot by passing a Fogarty balloon catheter beyond the clot, inflating and withdrawing the balloon. The physician may attempt to reduce the risk of pulmonary embolism by increasing intrathoracic pressure in a ventilated patient. The physician may establish proof of patency by repeat venography. The physician sutures the venotomy closed and closes the wound.

Coding Tips

Establishing both inflow and outflow by any method is included. The portion of the operative arteriogram performed by the surgeon is also included. Angioscopy performed during therapeutic intervention should be reported in addition to the code for the primary procedure; see 35400. For arterial thrombectomy aortoiliac by abdominal incision, see 34151; by leg incision, see 34201. For venous thrombectomy of the vena cava or the iliac or femoropopliteal vein by leg incision, see 34421; by abdominal and leg incision, see 34451. For thrombectomy of an arterial or venous graft, see 35875–35876.

ICD-10-CM Diagnostic Codes

I80.211	Phlebitis and thrombophlebitis of right iliac vein ☑
I80.212	Phlebitis and thrombophlebitis of left iliac vein ☑
I80.213	Phlebitis and thrombophlebitis of iliac vein, bilateral ☑
I82.220	Acute embolism and thrombosis of inferior vena cava
I82.221	Chronic embolism and thrombosis of inferior vena cava
I82.421	Acute embolism and thrombosis of right iliac vein ☑
I82.422	Acute embolism and thrombosis of left iliac vein ☑
I82.423	Acute embolism and thrombosis of iliac vein, bilateral ☑
I82.521	Chronic embolism and thrombosis of right iliac vein ☑

N Newborn: 0 P Pediatric: 0-17 M Maternity: 9-64 A Adult: 15-124 AMA: CPT Assist

I82.522 Chronic embolism and thrombosis of left iliac vein ☑
I82.523 Chronic embolism and thrombosis of iliac vein, bilateral ☑
T81.72XA Complication of vein following a procedure, not elsewhere classified, initial encounter

AMA: **34401** 2022,Jun

Relative Value Units/Medicare Edits

Non-Facility RVU	Work	PE	MP	Total
34401	26.52	11.65	5.87	44.04
Facility RVU	**Work**	**PE**	**MP**	**Total**
34401	26.52	11.65	5.87	44.04

	FUD	Status	MUE	Modifiers				IOM Reference
34401	90	A	1(3)	51	50	62*	80	None

* with documentation

Terms To Know

embolism. Obstruction of a blood vessel resulting from a clot or foreign substance.

thrombectomy. Removal of a clot (thrombus) from a blood vessel utilizing various methods.

thrombosis. Condition arising from the presence or formation of blood clots within a blood vessel that may cause vascular obstruction and insufficient oxygenation.

vena cava. Main venous trunk that empties into the right atrium from both the lower and upper regions, beginning at the junction of the common iliac veins inferiorly and the two brachiocephalic veins superiorly.

34421-34451

34421 Thrombectomy, direct or with catheter; vena cava, iliac, femoropopliteal vein, by leg incision
34451 vena cava, iliac, femoropopliteal vein, by abdominal and leg incision

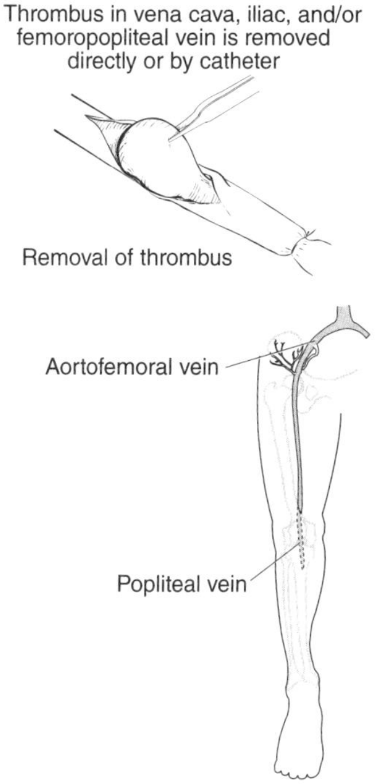

Explanation

In 34421, to remove a blood clot in the vena cava, iliac, or femoropopliteal vein, the physician makes an incision in the skin of the upper leg over the site of the clot or immediately above or below it. The vein is isolated and dissected from adjacent critical structures. The vein may be clamped above and below the clot and incised. The physician removes the blood clot. The clamps are removed. If a catheter is required, it is threaded past the clot and a small balloon at its tip is inflated. The catheter is withdrawn, capturing and retrieving the clot. The physician may make several passes to remove all of the clot. The blood vessel is repaired with sutures and the skin incision is repaired with a layered closure. In 34451, the physician exposes the vena cava, iliac, or femoropopliteal veins by making abdominal and leg incisions. The physician identifies the thrombus by venogram and may perform a contralateral femoral venogram to rule out inferior vena caval involvement. An incision is made over the site of the clot or immediately above or below it. The vein is isolated and dissected from adjacent critical structures. The vein may be clamped above and below the clot and incised. The physician removes the blood clot. The clamps are removed. The physician may cut down and introduce a Fogarty catheter via the popliteal vein, advancing the catheter toward the femoral vein while extruding thrombus through the femoral venotomy. The physician withdraws the clot by passing a Fogarty balloon catheter beyond the clot, inflating, and withdrawing the balloon. The physician may establish proof of patency by repeat venography. The physician sutures the venotomy closed and closes the wound.

Coding Tips

Establishing both inflow and outflow by any method is included. The portion of the operative arteriogram performed by the surgeon is also included. Angioscopy performed during therapeutic intervention should be reported in addition to the code for the primary procedure; see 35400. For arterial

● New ▲ Revised + Add On ★ Telemedicine [Resequenced] ☑ Laterality

thrombectomy of the aortoiliac artery by abdominal incision, see 34151; aortoiliac, femoropopliteal by leg incision, see 34201.

ICD-10-CM Diagnostic Codes

I80.11	Phlebitis and thrombophlebitis of right femoral vein ☑
I80.211	Phlebitis and thrombophlebitis of right iliac vein ☑
I80.221	Phlebitis and thrombophlebitis of right popliteal vein ☑
I82.220	Acute embolism and thrombosis of inferior vena cava
I82.221	Chronic embolism and thrombosis of inferior vena cava
I82.411	Acute embolism and thrombosis of right femoral vein ☑
I82.421	Acute embolism and thrombosis of right iliac vein ☑
I82.431	Acute embolism and thrombosis of right popliteal vein ☑
I82.491	Acute embolism and thrombosis of other specified deep vein of right lower extremity ☑
I82.511	Chronic embolism and thrombosis of right femoral vein ☑
I82.521	Chronic embolism and thrombosis of right iliac vein ☑
I82.531	Chronic embolism and thrombosis of right popliteal vein ☑
I82.591	Chronic embolism and thrombosis of other specified deep vein of right lower extremity ☑
T81.72XA	Complication of vein following a procedure, not elsewhere classified, initial encounter

AMA: 34421 2022,Jun **34451** 2022,Jun

Relative Value Units/Medicare Edits

Non-Facility RVU	Work	PE	MP	Total
34421	13.37	3.72	3.33	20.42
34451	28.52	6.45	7.11	42.08
Facility RVU	**Work**	**PE**	**MP**	**Total**
34421	13.37	3.72	3.33	20.42
34451	28.52	6.45	7.11	42.08

	FUD	Status	MUE	Modifiers				IOM Reference
34421	90	A	1(3)	51	50	62*	80	None
34451	90	A	1(3)	51	50	62*	80	

* with documentation

Terms To Know

angioscopy. Visualization of capillary blood vessels with a microscope, or the inside of a blood vessel with a fiberoptic-equipped catheter.

contralateral. Located on, or affecting, the opposite side of the body, usually as it relates to a bilateral body part.

embolism. Obstruction of a blood vessel resulting from a clot or foreign substance.

thrombosis. Condition arising from the presence or formation of blood clots within a blood vessel that may cause vascular obstruction and insufficient oxygenation.

vena cava. Main venous trunk that empties into the right atrium from both the lower and upper regions, beginning at the junction of the common iliac veins inferiorly and the two brachiocephalic veins superiorly.

34471-34490

34471 Thrombectomy, direct or with catheter; subclavian vein, by neck incision

34490 axillary and subclavian vein, by arm incision

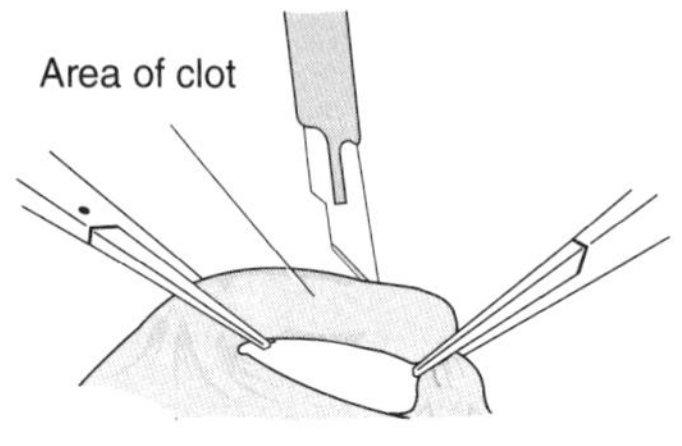

A thrombus may be approached directly by incision

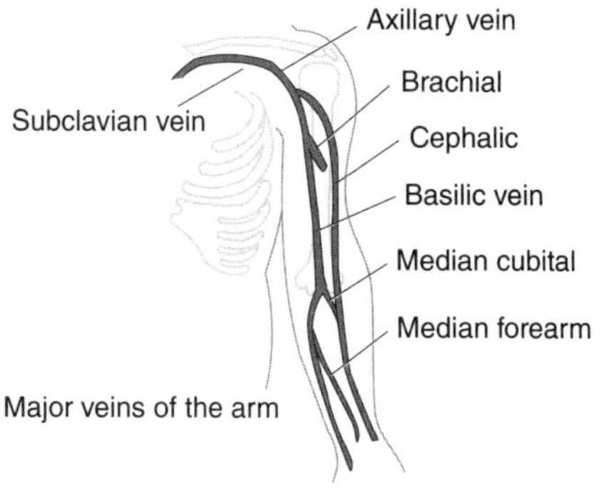

Major veins of the arm

Explanation

In 34471, to remove a blood clot in the subclavian vein, the physician makes an incision in the skin of the neck over the site of the clot or immediately above or below it. In 34490, to remove a blood clot in the axillary and subclavian vein, the physician makes an incision in the skin of the arm over the site of the clot or immediately above or below it. The vein is isolated and dissected from adjacent critical structures. The vein may be clamped above and below the clot and incised. The physician removes the blood clot. The clamps are removed. If a catheter is required, it is threaded past the clot and a small balloon at its tip is inflated. The catheter is withdrawn, capturing and retrieving the clot. The physician may make several passes to remove the entire clot. The blood vessel is repaired with sutures and the skin incision is repaired with a layered closure.

Coding Tips

Establishing both inflow and outflow by any method is included. The portion of the operative arteriogram performed by the surgeon is also included. Angioscopy performed during therapeutic intervention should be reported in addition to the code for the primary procedure; see 35400. For arterial embolectomy/thrombectomy of the subclavian vein, by neck incision, see 34001; by thoracic incision, see 34051. For arterial embolectomy/thrombectomy of the axillary or subclavian artery by arm incision, see 34101. For thrombectomy of an arterial or venous graft, see 35875–35876.

ICD-10-CM Diagnostic Codes

I82.A11	Acute embolism and thrombosis of right axillary vein ☑
I82.A12	Acute embolism and thrombosis of left axillary vein ☑
I82.A13	Acute embolism and thrombosis of axillary vein, bilateral ☑
I82.A21	Chronic embolism and thrombosis of right axillary vein ☑
I82.A22	Chronic embolism and thrombosis of left axillary vein ☑
I82.A23	Chronic embolism and thrombosis of axillary vein, bilateral ☑

I82.B11 Acute embolism and thrombosis of right subclavian vein ☑
I82.B12 Acute embolism and thrombosis of left subclavian vein ☑
I82.B13 Acute embolism and thrombosis of subclavian vein, bilateral ☑
I82.B21 Chronic embolism and thrombosis of right subclavian vein ☑
I82.B22 Chronic embolism and thrombosis of left subclavian vein ☑
I82.B23 Chronic embolism and thrombosis of subclavian vein, bilateral ☑
T81.72XA Complication of vein following a procedure, not elsewhere classified, initial encounter

AMA: **34471** 2022,Jun **34490** 2022,Jun

Relative Value Units/Medicare Edits

Non-Facility RVU	Work	PE	MP	Total
34471	21.11	5.3	5.25	31.66
34490	10.91	3.3	2.71	16.92
Facility RVU	**Work**	**PE**	**MP**	**Total**
34471	21.11	5.3	5.25	31.66
34490	10.91	3.3	2.71	16.92

	FUD	Status	MUE	Modifiers				IOM Reference
34471	90	A	1(2)	51	50	62*	N/A	None
34490	90	A	1(2)	51	50	N/A	N/A	

* with documentation

Terms To Know

angioscopy. Visualization of capillary blood vessels with a microscope, or the inside of a blood vessel with a fiberoptic-equipped catheter.

arteriogram. Radiograph of arteries.

embolism. Obstruction of a blood vessel resulting from a clot or foreign substance.

thrombosis. Condition arising from the presence or formation of blood clots within a blood vessel that may cause vascular obstruction and insufficient oxygenation.

34501

34501 Valvuloplasty, femoral vein

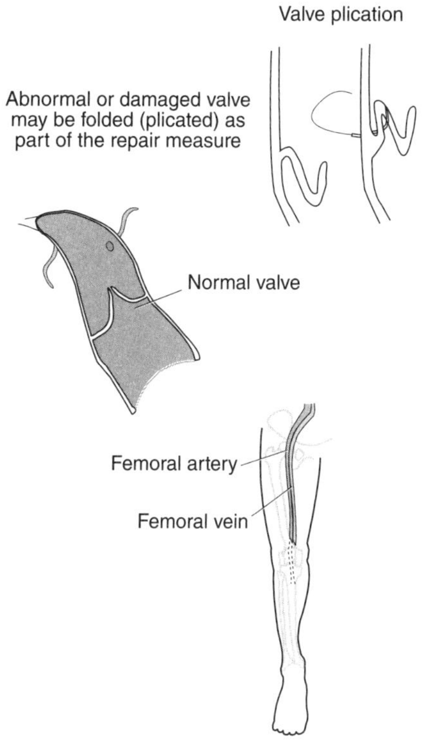

Explanation

The physician makes an incision in the skin overlying the site of the incompetent valve. The femoral vein is isolated and dissected from adjacent critical structures. The physician affixes vessel clamps above and below the malfunctioning valve. The physician opens the vein and repairs the valve leaflets by suture plication (tacking the excess valve material). The vein is repaired with sutures. The clamps are removed and the skin incision is repaired with a layered closure.

Coding Tips

Establishing both inflow and outflow by any method is included. The portion of the operative arteriogram performed by the surgeon is also included. Angioscopy performed during therapeutic intervention should be reported in addition to the code for the primary procedure, see 35400. For venous valve transposition, any vein donor, see 34510. For insertion of a bioprosthetic valve of the femoral vein, see 0744T.

ICD-10-CM Diagnostic Codes

I80.11 Phlebitis and thrombophlebitis of right femoral vein ☑
I82.411 Acute embolism and thrombosis of right femoral vein ☑
I82.511 Chronic embolism and thrombosis of right femoral vein ☑
I83.011 Varicose veins of right lower extremity with ulcer of thigh Ⓐ ☑
I83.012 Varicose veins of right lower extremity with ulcer of calf Ⓐ ☑
I83.013 Varicose veins of right lower extremity with ulcer of ankle Ⓐ ☑
I83.014 Varicose veins of right lower extremity with ulcer of heel and midfoot Ⓐ ☑
I83.015 Varicose veins of right lower extremity with ulcer other part of foot Ⓐ ☑

I83.018	Varicose veins of right lower extremity with ulcer other part of lower leg [A] ☑
I83.11	Varicose veins of right lower extremity with inflammation [A] ☑
I83.211	Varicose veins of right lower extremity with both ulcer of thigh and inflammation [A] ☑
I83.212	Varicose veins of right lower extremity with both ulcer of calf and inflammation [A] ☑
I83.213	Varicose veins of right lower extremity with both ulcer of ankle and inflammation [A] ☑
I83.214	Varicose veins of right lower extremity with both ulcer of heel and midfoot and inflammation [A] ☑
I83.215	Varicose veins of right lower extremity with both ulcer other part of foot and inflammation [A] ☑
I83.218	Varicose veins of right lower extremity with both ulcer of other part of lower extremity and inflammation [A] ☑
I83.811	Varicose veins of right lower extremity with pain [A] ☑
I83.891	Varicose veins of right lower extremity with other complications [A] ☑
I83.91	Asymptomatic varicose veins of right lower extremity [A] ☑
I87.001	Postthrombotic syndrome without complications of right lower extremity ☑
I87.011	Postthrombotic syndrome with ulcer of right lower extremity ☑
I87.021	Postthrombotic syndrome with inflammation of right lower extremity ☑
I87.031	Postthrombotic syndrome with ulcer and inflammation of right lower extremity ☑
I87.091	Postthrombotic syndrome with other complications of right lower extremity ☑
I87.2	Venous insufficiency (chronic) (peripheral)
Q27.32	Arteriovenous malformation of vessel of lower limb
S75.111A	Minor laceration of femoral vein at hip and thigh level, right leg, initial encounter ☑
S75.121A	Major laceration of femoral vein at hip and thigh level, right leg, initial encounter ☑
S75.191A	Other specified injury of femoral vein at hip and thigh level, right leg, initial encounter ☑

Relative Value Units/Medicare Edits

Non-Facility RVU	Work	PE	MP	Total
34501	16.85	5.29	4.19	26.33
Facility RVU	**Work**	**PE**	**MP**	**Total**
34501	16.85	5.29	4.19	26.33

	FUD	Status	MUE	Modifiers				IOM Reference
34501	90	A	1(2)	51	50	62*	80	None

* with documentation

34502

34502 Reconstruction of vena cava, any method

Explanation

The physician exposes the inferior vena cava by making an incision in the anterior abdomen. Clamps are placed on the vena cava proximally and any defects are sutured closed. Abnormal vena caval tissue may be replaced or bypassed with synthetic graft material. An injection of intravenous contrast may be administered under fluoroscopy to demonstrate appropriate flow. The clamps are removed and the abdominal wall incision is closed. A surgical drain may be left in place at the conclusion of the procedure.

Coding Tips

Establishing both inflow and outflow by any method is included. The portion of the operative arteriogram performed by the surgeon is also included. Angioscopy performed during therapeutic intervention should be reported in addition to the code for the primary procedure; see 35400. For resection with reconstruction of the vena cava, see 37799.

ICD-10-CM Diagnostic Codes

I82.210	Acute embolism and thrombosis of superior vena cava
I82.211	Chronic embolism and thrombosis of superior vena cava
I82.220	Acute embolism and thrombosis of inferior vena cava
I82.221	Chronic embolism and thrombosis of inferior vena cava
I87.1	Compression of vein
I87.2	Venous insufficiency (chronic) (peripheral)
Q26.0	Congenital stenosis of vena cava
Q26.1	Persistent left superior vena cava
Q26.8	Other congenital malformations of great veins
S25.21XA	Minor laceration of superior vena cava, initial encounter
S25.22XA	Major laceration of superior vena cava, initial encounter
S25.29XA	Other specified injury of superior vena cava, initial encounter
S35.11XA	Minor laceration of inferior vena cava, initial encounter
S35.12XA	Major laceration of inferior vena cava, initial encounter
S35.19XA	Other injury of inferior vena cava, initial encounter
T81.72XA	Complication of vein following a procedure, not elsewhere classified, initial encounter

Relative Value Units/Medicare Edits

Non-Facility RVU	Work	PE	MP	Total
34502	28.07	11.0	6.51	45.58
Facility RVU	**Work**	**PE**	**MP**	**Total**
34502	28.07	11.0	6.51	45.58

	FUD	Status	MUE	Modifiers				IOM Reference
34502	90	A	1(2)	51	N/A	N/A	80	None

* with documentation

Terms To Know

reconstruction. Recreating, restoring, or rebuilding a body part or organ.

vena cava. Main venous trunk that empties into the right atrium from both the lower and upper regions, beginning at the junction of the common iliac veins inferiorly and the two brachiocephalic veins superiorly.

34510

34510 Venous valve transposition, any vein donor

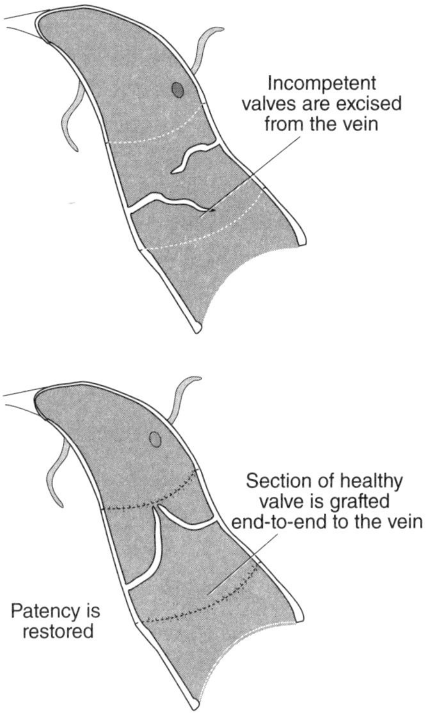

Explanation

The physician makes an incision in the skin overlying the site of the malfunctioning valve. The vein is isolated and dissected from adjacent critical structures. The physician affixes vessel clamps above and below the vein and excises the section of vein containing the malfunctioning valve. A section of harvested vein containing functional valves is sutured end-to-end to the vein. The clamps are removed and the skin incision is repaired with a layered closure.

Coding Tips

Establishing both inflow and outflow by any method is included. The portion of the operative arteriogram performed by the surgeon is also included. Angioscopy performed during therapeutic intervention should be reported in addition to the code for the primary procedure, see 35400. For crossover vein graft to venous system, see 34520. For insertion of a bioprosthetic valve of the femoral vein, see 0744T.

ICD-10-CM Diagnostic Codes

I80.291 Phlebitis and thrombophlebitis of other deep vessels of right lower extremity ☑
I82.491 Acute embolism and thrombosis of other specified deep vein of right lower extremity ☑
I82.591 Chronic embolism and thrombosis of other specified deep vein of right lower extremity ☑
I83.011 Varicose veins of right lower extremity with ulcer of thigh A ☑
I83.012 Varicose veins of right lower extremity with ulcer of calf A ☑
I83.013 Varicose veins of right lower extremity with ulcer of ankle A ☑
I83.014 Varicose veins of right lower extremity with ulcer of heel and midfoot A ☑
I83.015 Varicose veins of right lower extremity with ulcer other part of foot A ☑
I83.018 Varicose veins of right lower extremity with ulcer other part of lower leg A ☑
I83.11 Varicose veins of right lower extremity with inflammation A ☑
I83.211 Varicose veins of right lower extremity with both ulcer of thigh and inflammation A ☑
I83.212 Varicose veins of right lower extremity with both ulcer of calf and inflammation A ☑
I83.213 Varicose veins of right lower extremity with both ulcer of ankle and inflammation A ☑
I83.214 Varicose veins of right lower extremity with both ulcer of heel and midfoot and inflammation A ☑
I83.215 Varicose veins of right lower extremity with both ulcer other part of foot and inflammation A ☑
I83.218 Varicose veins of right lower extremity with both ulcer of other part of lower extremity and inflammation A ☑
I83.811 Varicose veins of right lower extremity with pain A ☑
I83.891 Varicose veins of right lower extremity with other complications A ☑
I83.91 Asymptomatic varicose veins of right lower extremity A ☑
I87.001 Postthrombotic syndrome without complications of right lower extremity ☑
I87.011 Postthrombotic syndrome with ulcer of right lower extremity ☑
I87.021 Postthrombotic syndrome with inflammation of right lower extremity ☑
I87.031 Postthrombotic syndrome with ulcer and inflammation of right lower extremity ☑
I87.091 Postthrombotic syndrome with other complications of right lower extremity ☑
I87.1 Compression of vein
I87.2 Venous insufficiency (chronic) (peripheral)
I87.301 Chronic venous hypertension (idiopathic) without complications of right lower extremity ☑
I87.311 Chronic venous hypertension (idiopathic) with ulcer of right lower extremity ☑
I87.321 Chronic venous hypertension (idiopathic) with inflammation of right lower extremity ☑
I87.331 Chronic venous hypertension (idiopathic) with ulcer and inflammation of right lower extremity ☑
I87.391 Chronic venous hypertension (idiopathic) with other complications of right lower extremity ☑
Q27.32 Arteriovenous malformation of vessel of lower limb

Relative Value Units/Medicare Edits

Non-Facility RVU	Work	PE	MP	Total
34510	19.91	5.11	4.95	29.97
Facility RVU	**Work**	**PE**	**MP**	**Total**
34510	19.91	5.11	4.95	29.97

	FUD	Status	MUE	Modifiers				IOM Reference
34510	90	A	2(3)	51	50	62*	80	None

* with documentation

34520

34520 Cross-over vein graft to venous system

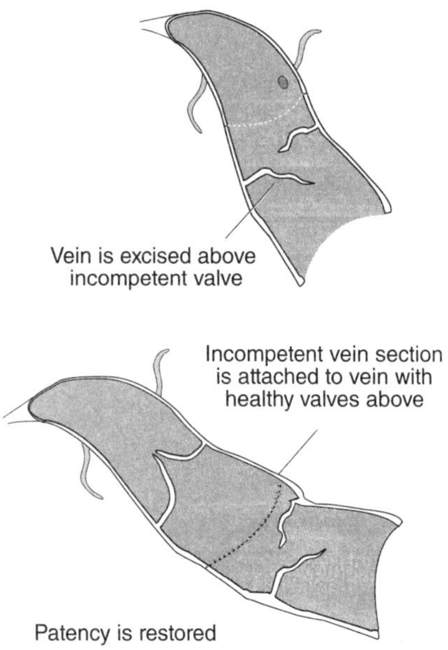

Explanation

The physician makes an incision in the skin overlying the site of the incompetent valve. The incompetent vein is isolated and dissected from adjacent critical structures. The physician affixes vessel clamps above and below the vein. The divided section of incompetent vein is connected to a nearby vein with functioning valves, placing competent values above the incompetent vein. Both the vein and the skin incision are closed with sutures.

Coding Tips

Establishing both inflow and outflow by any method is included. The portion of the operative arteriogram performed by the surgeon is also included. Angioscopy performed during therapeutic intervention should be reported in addition to the code for the primary procedure; see 35400. For venous valve transposition, any vein donor, see 34510.

ICD-10-CM Diagnostic Codes

I80.11	Phlebitis and thrombophlebitis of right femoral vein ☑
I80.211	Phlebitis and thrombophlebitis of right iliac vein ☑
I80.291	Phlebitis and thrombophlebitis of other deep vessels of right lower extremity ☑
I82.411	Acute embolism and thrombosis of right femoral vein ☑
I82.421	Acute embolism and thrombosis of right iliac vein ☑
I82.511	Chronic embolism and thrombosis of right femoral vein ☑
I82.521	Chronic embolism and thrombosis of right iliac vein ☑
I82.591	Chronic embolism and thrombosis of other specified deep vein of right lower extremity ☑
I83.011	Varicose veins of right lower extremity with ulcer of thigh [A] ☑
I83.012	Varicose veins of right lower extremity with ulcer of calf [A] ☑
I83.013	Varicose veins of right lower extremity with ulcer of ankle [A] ☑
I83.014	Varicose veins of right lower extremity with ulcer of heel and midfoot [A] ☑
I83.015	Varicose veins of right lower extremity with ulcer other part of foot [A] ☑
I83.11	Varicose veins of right lower extremity with inflammation [A] ☑
I83.211	Varicose veins of right lower extremity with both ulcer of thigh and inflammation [A] ☑
I83.212	Varicose veins of right lower extremity with both ulcer of calf and inflammation [A] ☑
I83.213	Varicose veins of right lower extremity with both ulcer of ankle and inflammation [A] ☑
I83.214	Varicose veins of right lower extremity with both ulcer of heel and midfoot and inflammation [A] ☑
I83.218	Varicose veins of right lower extremity with both ulcer of other part of lower extremity and inflammation [A] ☑
I83.811	Varicose veins of right lower extremity with pain [A] ☑
I83.91	Asymptomatic varicose veins of right lower extremity [A] ☑
I87.001	Postthrombotic syndrome without complications of right lower extremity ☑
I87.011	Postthrombotic syndrome with ulcer of right lower extremity ☑
I87.021	Postthrombotic syndrome with inflammation of right lower extremity ☑
I87.031	Postthrombotic syndrome with ulcer and inflammation of right lower extremity ☑
I87.091	Postthrombotic syndrome with other complications of right lower extremity ☑
I87.1	Compression of vein
I87.2	Venous insufficiency (chronic) (peripheral)
I87.301	Chronic venous hypertension (idiopathic) without complications of right lower extremity ☑
I87.311	Chronic venous hypertension (idiopathic) with ulcer of right lower extremity ☑
I87.321	Chronic venous hypertension (idiopathic) with inflammation of right lower extremity ☑
I87.331	Chronic venous hypertension (idiopathic) with ulcer and inflammation of right lower extremity ☑
Q26.0	Congenital stenosis of vena cava
Q26.1	Persistent left superior vena cava
Q27.32	Arteriovenous malformation of vessel of lower limb
S35.514A	Injury of right iliac vein, initial encounter ☑
S75.121A	Major laceration of femoral vein at hip and thigh level, right leg, initial encounter ☑

AMA: 34520 2023,Mar

Relative Value Units/Medicare Edits

Non-Facility RVU	Work	PE	MP	Total
34520	19.18	5.1	4.75	29.03
Facility RVU	**Work**	**PE**	**MP**	**Total**
34520	19.18	5.1	4.75	29.03

	FUD	Status	MUE	Modifiers				IOM Reference
34520	90	A	1(3)	51	50	62*	80	None

* with documentation

34530

34530 Saphenopopliteal vein anastomosis

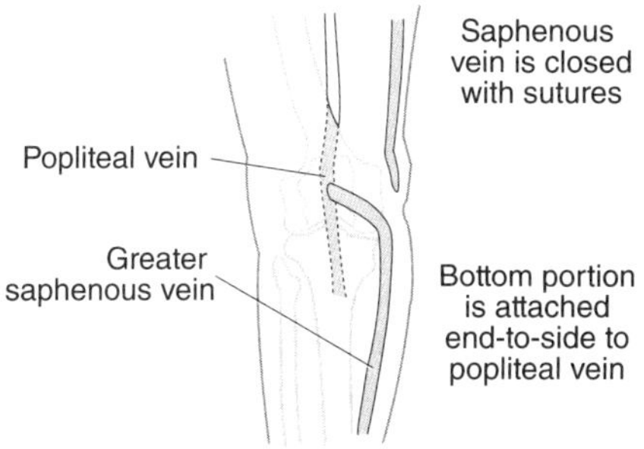

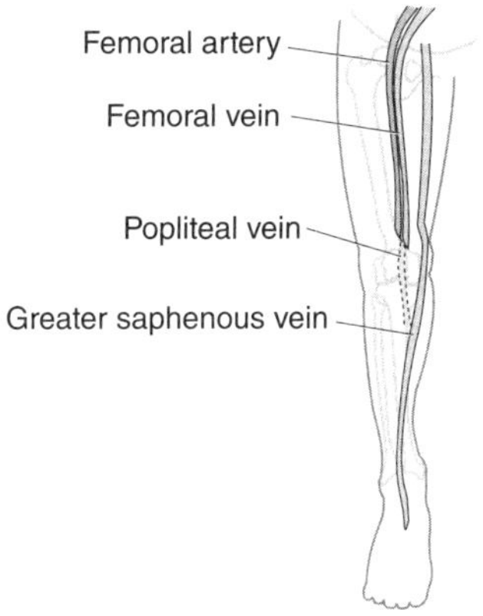

Explanation

The physician makes an incision in the skin overlying the site of the greater saphenous vein just below the knee. The vein is isolated and dissected from adjacent critical structures. The physician affixes vessel clamps above and below the incision site. The dissected section of saphenous vein is connected to the popliteal vein in an end-to-side anastomosis. The other end of the saphenous vein is closed with sutures. Once the saphenous vein and the popliteal vein are connected, the clamps are removed and the skin incision is repaired with layered closure.

Coding Tips

Establishing both inflow and outflow by any method is included. The portion of the operative arteriogram performed by the surgeon is also included. Angioscopy performed during therapeutic intervention should be reported in addition to the code for the primary procedure; see 35400. For venous valve transposition, any vein donor, see 34510. For crossover vein graft, see 34520. For direct repair of a blood vessel other than for fistula, see 35226, 35256, and 35286.

ICD-10-CM Diagnostic Codes

I80.221	Phlebitis and thrombophlebitis of right popliteal vein ☑
I82.431	Acute embolism and thrombosis of right popliteal vein ☑
I83.011	Varicose veins of right lower extremity with ulcer of thigh A ☑
I83.012	Varicose veins of right lower extremity with ulcer of calf A ☑
I83.013	Varicose veins of right lower extremity with ulcer of ankle A ☑
I83.014	Varicose veins of right lower extremity with ulcer of heel and midfoot A ☑
I83.015	Varicose veins of right lower extremity with ulcer other part of foot A ☑
I83.11	Varicose veins of right lower extremity with inflammation A ☑
I83.211	Varicose veins of right lower extremity with both ulcer of thigh and inflammation A ☑
I83.212	Varicose veins of right lower extremity with both ulcer of calf and inflammation A ☑
I83.213	Varicose veins of right lower extremity with both ulcer of ankle and inflammation A ☑
I83.214	Varicose veins of right lower extremity with both ulcer of heel and midfoot and inflammation A ☑
I83.215	Varicose veins of right lower extremity with both ulcer other part of foot and inflammation A ☑
I83.811	Varicose veins of right lower extremity with pain A ☑
I83.891	Varicose veins of right lower extremity with other complications A ☑
I87.011	Postthrombotic syndrome with ulcer of right lower extremity ☑
I87.021	Postthrombotic syndrome with inflammation of right lower extremity ☑
I87.031	Postthrombotic syndrome with ulcer and inflammation of right lower extremity ☑
I87.091	Postthrombotic syndrome with other complications of right lower extremity ☑
I87.1	Compression of vein
I87.2	Venous insufficiency (chronic) (peripheral)
I87.311	Chronic venous hypertension (idiopathic) with ulcer of right lower extremity ☑
I87.321	Chronic venous hypertension (idiopathic) with inflammation of right lower extremity ☑
I87.331	Chronic venous hypertension (idiopathic) with ulcer and inflammation of right lower extremity ☑
I87.391	Chronic venous hypertension (idiopathic) with other complications of right lower extremity ☑
Q27.32	Arteriovenous malformation of vessel of lower limb
S75.221A	Major laceration of greater saphenous vein at hip and thigh level, right leg, initial encounter ☑
S85.311A	Laceration of greater saphenous vein at lower leg level, right leg, initial encounter ☑
S85.411A	Laceration of lesser saphenous vein at lower leg level, right leg, initial encounter ☑
S85.511A	Laceration of popliteal vein, right leg, initial encounter ☑

Relative Value Units/Medicare Edits

Non-Facility RVU	Work	PE	MP	Total
34530	17.93	5.28	4.45	27.66
Facility RVU	**Work**	**PE**	**MP**	**Total**
34530	17.93	5.28	4.45	27.66

	FUD	Status	MUE	Modifiers				IOM Reference
34530	90	A	1(2)	51	50	62*	80	None

* with documentation

34701-34702

34701 Endovascular repair of infrarenal aorta by deployment of an aorto-aortic tube endograft including pre-procedure sizing and device selection, all nonselective catheterization(s), all associated radiological supervision and interpretation, all endograft extension(s) placed in the aorta from the level of the renal arteries to the aortic bifurcation, and all angioplasty/stenting performed from the level of the renal arteries to the aortic bifurcation; for other than rupture (eg, for aneurysm, pseudoaneurysm, dissection, penetrating ulcer)

34702 for rupture including temporary aortic and/or iliac balloon occlusion, when performed (eg, for aneurysm, pseudoaneurysm, dissection, penetrating ulcer, traumatic disruption)

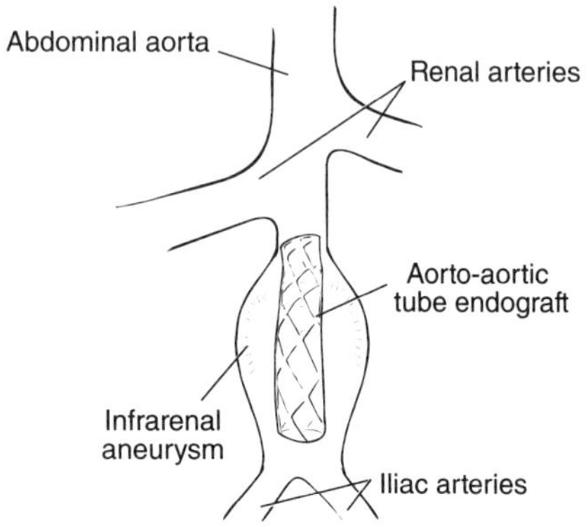

Explanation

The physician introduces, positions, and deploys an endograft to treat abdominal aortic conditions, with or without rupture, such as an aneurysm, pseudoaneurysm, dissection, penetrating ulcer, or traumatic disruption located in the infrarenal abdominal aorta that may or may not extend into the iliac arteries. A covered stent may be referred to using terms such as endovascular graft, endoprosthesis, endograft, or stent graft. The infrarenal aortic endograft may be an aortic tube device, a bifurcated unibody device, a modular bifurcated docking system with docking limbs, or an aorto-uni-iliac device. The abdominal aortic treatment zone is defined as the infrarenal aorta. This procedure requires a vascular surgeon and a radiologist. In 34701, an incision is made over the femoral artery, which is normally used for access, and a guidewire is threaded into the blood vessel. A catheter with a stent-transporting tip is advanced over the guidewire into the vessel. The catheter carries the aortic tube prosthesis, approximately 6 inches long and contained inside a holding capsule, through the arterial tree to the site of the aortic infrarenal aneurysm. Once the stent is in proper position, the holding capsule is removed and the stent is deployed, expanding like a spring to anchor itself to normal walls of the aorta above and below the aneurysm. The device serves as a substitute channel for blood flow. If full expansion of the prosthesis does not occur, or leaks are present, a balloon catheter is threaded to the graft site and inflated within the prosthesis until full expansion is achieved and leaking is stopped. The catheter/guidewire is removed and the arteriotomy site is closed. The aneurysm, excluded from the blood flow, typically shrinks over time. The treatment zone for endograft procedures is defined by those vessels that contain an endograft (main body, docking limbs, and/or extensions) deployed during that operative session. Report 34702 when endovascular repair is performed on a ruptured aneurysm in the aorta. Rupture is defined as clinical and/or radiographic evidence of acute hemorrhage. A chronic, contained rupture is considered a pseudoaneurysm and its endovascular treatment is reported with 34701. Nonselective catheterization is included in these codes. Balloon angioplasty and/or stenting at the sealing zone of an endograft is an integral part of the procedure. Fluoroscopic guidance and radiological supervision and interpretation in conjunction with endograft repair is not reported separately, and includes all intraprocedural imaging (e.g., angiography, rotational CT) of the aorta and its branches prior to deployment of the endovascular device, fluoroscopic guidance, and roadmapping used in the delivery of the endovascular components, and intraprocedural and completion angiography (e.g., confirm position, detect endoleak, evaluate runoff) performed at the time of the endovascular infrarenal aorta repair.

Coding Tips

Preprocedure sizing and device selection, all nonselective catheterizations, radiological supervision and interpretation, endograft extensions, and angioplasty stenting are included in these procedures and should not be reported separately. For repair requiring a decompressive laparotomy for abdominal compartment syndrome, report 49000 in addition to 34702. Report 34709 in addition to 34701 or 34702 for placement of an extension prosthesis that terminates in the abdominal aorta proximal to the renal arteries. For covered stent placements for atherosclerotic occlusive disease of the abdominal aorta, see 37236 and 37237. For repair of infrarenal aorta and/or iliac arteries by deployment of an aorto-uni-iliac endograft, see 34703 and 34704. For repair of infrarenal aorta and/or iliac arteries by deployment of an aorto-bi-iliac endograft, see 34705 and 34706.

ICD-10-CM Diagnostic Codes

A52.01	Syphilitic aneurysm of aorta
I71.02	Dissection of abdominal aorta
I71.33	Infrarenal abdominal aortic aneurysm, ruptured
I71.43	Infrarenal abdominal aortic aneurysm, without rupture
I77.811	Abdominal aortic ectasia
I77.89	Other specified disorders of arteries and arterioles
Q25.43	Congenital aneurysm of aorta
Q25.44	Congenital dilation of aorta
Q25.49	Other congenital malformations of aorta
Q79.61	Classical Ehlers-Danlos syndrome
Q79.62	Hypermobile Ehlers-Danlos syndrome
Q79.63	Vascular Ehlers-Danlos syndrome
Q79.69	Other Ehlers-Danlos syndromes
Q87.410	Marfan syndrome with aortic dilation
S35.02XA	Major laceration of abdominal aorta, initial encounter
S35.09XA	Other injury of abdominal aorta, initial encounter

AMA: 34701 2023,Jun; 2021,Dec; 2019,Nov **34702** 2023,Jun; 2021,Dec; 2019,Nov

Relative Value Units/Medicare Edits

Non-Facility RVU	Work	PE	MP	Total
34701	23.71	6.68	5.72	36.11
34702	36.0	9.08	8.85	53.93
Facility RVU	**Work**	**PE**	**MP**	**Total**
34701	23.71	6.68	5.72	36.11
34702	36.0	9.08	8.85	53.93

	FUD	Status	MUE	Modifiers				IOM Reference
34701	90	A	1(2)	51	N/A	62	80	None
34702	90	A	1(2)	51	N/A	62	80	

* with documentation

34703-34706

34703 Endovascular repair of infrarenal aorta and/or iliac artery(ies) by deployment of an aorto-uni-iliac endograft including pre-procedure sizing and device selection, all nonselective catheterization(s), all associated radiological supervision and interpretation, all endograft extension(s) placed in the aorta from the level of the renal arteries to the iliac bifurcation, and all angioplasty/stenting performed from the level of the renal arteries to the iliac bifurcation; for other than rupture (eg, for aneurysm, pseudoaneurysm, dissection, penetrating ulcer)

34704 for rupture including temporary aortic and/or iliac balloon occlusion, when performed (eg, for aneurysm, pseudoaneurysm, dissection, penetrating ulcer, traumatic disruption)

34705 Endovascular repair of infrarenal aorta and/or iliac artery(ies) by deployment of an aorto-bi-iliac endograft including pre-procedure sizing and device selection, all nonselective catheterization(s), all associated radiological supervision and interpretation, all endograft extension(s) placed in the aorta from the level of the renal arteries to the iliac bifurcation, and all angioplasty/stenting performed from the level of the renal arteries to the iliac bifurcation; for other than rupture (eg, for aneurysm, pseudoaneurysm, dissection, penetrating ulcer)

34706 for rupture including temporary aortic and/or iliac balloon occlusion, when performed (eg, for aneurysm, pseudoaneurysm, dissection, penetrating ulcer, traumatic disruption)

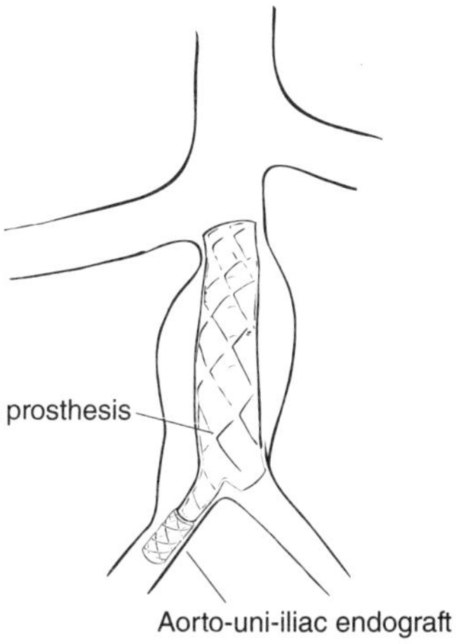

Explanation

The physician introduces, positions, and deploys an endograft to treat abdominal aortic conditions, with or without rupture, such as an aneurysm, pseudoaneurysm, dissection, penetrating ulcer, or traumatic disruption located in the infrarenal abdominal aorta that may or may not extend into the iliac arteries. A covered stent may be referred to as an endovascular graft, endoprosthesis, endograft, or stent graft. The infrarenal aortic endograft may be an aortic tube device, a bifurcated unibody device, a modular bifurcated docking system with docking limbs, or an aorto-uni-iliac device. In 34703 and 34704, the abdominal aortic treatment zone is typically defined as the infrarenal aorta and ipsilateral common iliac artery. In 34705 and 34706, the abdominal aortic treatment zone is typically defined as the infrarenal aorta and both common iliac arteries. These procedures require a vascular surgeon and a radiologist. In 34703, under general anesthesia, a small incision is made in the groin over one femoral artery or both femoral arteries through which the endovascular devices are inserted. If contralateral femoral access is necessary, a percutaneous sheath may be placed. An aorta-uni-iliac prosthetic graft device contained inside a plastic holding capsule is threaded through the arteries to the site of the infrarenal aneurysm. The endograft is deployed by slowly removing the holding capsule away from the endograft, with continual monitoring of exact positioning. Once the prosthesis is in place, the holding capsule is removed. Balloon angioplasty is performed at the ends of the prosthesis to expand and seat the graft. Stents are deployed within the body of the endograft to maintain expansion forces. The aorta-uni-iliac prosthetic endograft is supported along its length by a series of metal rings sutured to the graft and is held in place by the radial force applied by the rings to the patient's aorta. Once in place, the arteriotomy site is closed. Report 34705 for simultaneous bilateral iliac artery aneurysm repairs with aorto-bi-iliac endograft. Report 34704 and 34706 when endovascular repair is performed on a ruptured aneurysm in the aorta or iliac arteries. Rupture is defined as clinical and/or radiographic evidence of acute hemorrhage. A chronic, contained rupture is considered a pseudoaneurysm and its endovascular treatment is reported with 34703 and 34705. Nonselective catheterization is included in 34703, 34704, 34705, and 34706. Balloon angioplasty and/or stenting at the sealing zone of an endograft is an integral part of the procedure. Fluoroscopic guidance and radiological supervision and interpretation in conjunction with endograft repair is not separately reported, and includes all intraprocedural imaging (e.g., angiography, rotational CT) of the aorta and its branches prior to deployment of the endovascular device, fluoroscopic guidance and roadmapping used in the delivery of the endovascular components, and intraprocedural and completion angiography (e.g., confirm position, detect endoleak, evaluate runoff) performed at the time of the endovascular infrarenal aorta and/or iliac repair.

Coding Tips

Preprocedure sizing and device selection, all nonselective catheterizations, radiological supervision and interpretation, endograft extensions, and angioplasty stenting are included in these procedures and should not be reported separately. For decompressive laparotomy, report 49000 in addition to 34704 or 34706, as appropriate. Report 34709 in addition to 34703, 34704, 34705, or 34706 for placement of an extension prosthesis that terminates in the internal iliac, external iliac, or common femoral arteries. For treatment of atherosclerotic occlusive disease in the iliac arteries with covered stents, see 37221 and 37223. For covered stent placement for atherosclerotic occlusive disease in the aorta, see 37236 and 37237. For simultaneous bilateral iliac artery aneurysm repairs with aorto-bi-iliac endograft, see 34705 and 34706. For repair of an infrarenal aorta by deployment of an aorto-aortic tube endograft, see 34701 and 34702. For isolated bilateral iliac artery repair, see 34707 or 34708 and append modifier 50.

ICD-10-CM Diagnostic Codes

A52.01	Syphilitic aneurysm of aorta
I71.02	Dissection of abdominal aorta
I71.33	Infrarenal abdominal aortic aneurysm, ruptured
I71.43	Infrarenal abdominal aortic aneurysm, without rupture
I72.3	Aneurysm of iliac artery
I77.72	Dissection of iliac artery
I77.811	Abdominal aortic ectasia
I77.89	Other specified disorders of arteries and arterioles
Q25.43	Congenital aneurysm of aorta
Q25.44	Congenital dilation of aorta
Q25.49	Other congenital malformations of aorta
Q25.8	Other congenital malformations of other great arteries
Q79.61	Classical Ehlers-Danlos syndrome
Q79.63	Vascular Ehlers-Danlos syndrome
Q87.410	Marfan syndrome with aortic dilation
Q87.418	Marfan syndrome with other cardiovascular manifestations

S35.02XA Major laceration of abdominal aorta, initial encounter
S35.09XA Other injury of abdominal aorta, initial encounter
S35.511A Injury of right iliac artery, initial encounter ☑
S35.512A Injury of left iliac artery, initial encounter ☑
S35.59XA Injury of other iliac blood vessels, initial encounter

AMA: 34703 2023,Jun; 2021,Dec; 2019,Nov **34704** 2023,Jun; 2021,Dec; 2019,Nov **34705** 2023,Jun; 2021,Dec; 2019,Nov **34706** 2023,Jun; 2021,Dec; 2019,Nov

Relative Value Units/Medicare Edits

Non-Facility RVU	Work	PE	MP	Total
34703	26.52	7.16	6.43	40.11
34704	45.0	10.97	10.89	66.86
34705	29.58	7.85	7.17	44.6
34706	45.0	10.51	10.96	66.47
Facility RVU	**Work**	**PE**	**MP**	**Total**
34703	26.52	7.16	6.43	40.11
34704	45.0	10.97	10.89	66.86
34705	29.58	7.85	7.17	44.6
34706	45.0	10.51	10.96	66.47

	FUD	Status	MUE	Modifiers				IOM Reference
34703	90	A	1(2)	51	N/A	62	80	None
34704	90	A	1(2)	51	N/A	62	80	
34705	90	A	1(2)	51	N/A	62	80	
34706	90	A	1(2)	51	N/A	62	80	

* with documentation

Terms To Know

aneurysm. Circumscribed dilation or outpouching of an artery wall, often containing blood clots and connecting directly with the lumen of the artery.

dissection. (dis. apart; -section, act of cutting) Separating by cutting tissue or body structures apart.

endometriosis interna. Abnormal presence of endometrial glands and tissue within the myometrium, the smooth muscle walls of the uterus, causing hypertrophy of the myometrium. At menses, blood is trapped within the muscle of the uterus, causing pain and cramping.

endoprosthesis. Intravascular device in the form of a hollow stent placed within a duct or artery to provide passage through an obstructed area, such as in a bile duct, or to act as a replacement for damaged arterial walls, as in treating an aneurysm.

fluoroscopy. Radiology technique that allows visual examination of part of the body or a function of an organ using a device that projects an x-ray image on a fluorescent screen.

34707-34708

34707 Endovascular repair of iliac artery by deployment of an ilio-iliac tube endograft including pre-procedure sizing and device selection, all nonselective catheterization(s), all associated radiological supervision and interpretation, and all endograft extension(s) proximally to the aortic bifurcation and distally to the iliac bifurcation, and treatment zone angioplasty/stenting, when performed, unilateral; for other than rupture (eg, for aneurysm, pseudoaneurysm, dissection, arteriovenous malformation)

34708 for rupture including temporary aortic and/or iliac balloon occlusion, when performed (eg, for aneurysm, pseudoaneurysm, dissection, arteriovenous malformation, traumatic disruption)

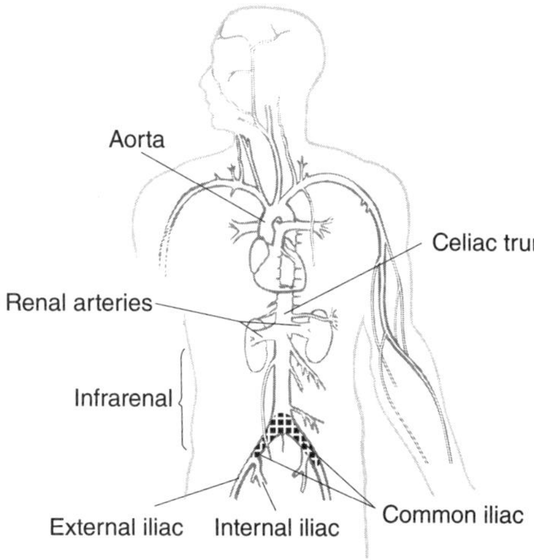

Ilio-iliac tube endograft

Explanation

The physician introduces, positions, and deploys an ilio-iliac endograft for treatment of isolated arterial pathology (with or without rupture), such as an aneurysm, pseudoaneurysm, dissection, arteriovenous malformation, or trauma involving the iliac artery. The treatment zone is defined as the portion of the iliac artery (e.g., common, internal, external iliac arteries) involved. The procedure requires a vascular surgeon and a radiologist. The patient receives medication (Heparin) to help prevent blood clots prior to the procedure. In 34707, under general anesthesia, the physician makes a small incision near the patient's hip bone area to enter the iliac artery. A proprietary device is used, which is comprised of two main components: a trunk component and a contralateral leg component. The endoprosthesis, contained inside a holding device, is introduced into the artery under fluoroscopy and positioned at the target zone area of repair by threading guidewires and catheters. Nonselective catheterization is included. Report 34708 when endovascular repair is performed on a ruptured aneurysm in the iliac artery. Rupture is defined as clinical and/or radiographic evidence of acute hemorrhage. A chronic, contained rupture is considered a pseudoaneurysm, and its endovascular treatment is reported with 34707. Balloon angioplasty and/or stenting at the treatment zone of an endograft is an integral part of the procedure. Fluoroscopic guidance and radiological supervision and interpretation, in conjunction with endograft repair, are not reported separately. Included are all intraprocedural imaging (e.g., angiography, rotational CT) of the iliac artery prior to deployment of the endovascular device, fluoroscopic guidance and roadmapping used in the delivery of the endovascular components, and intraprocedural and completion angiography (e.g., confirm position, detect endoleak, evaluate runoff) performed at the time of the endovascular iliac repair.

Coding Tips

Preprocedure sizing and device selection, all nonselective catheterizations, radiological supervision and interpretation, endograft extensions, and angioplasty stenting are included in the procedure and should not be reported separately. Report 34709 in addition to 34707 or 34708 for placement of an extension prosthesis that terminates in the internal iliac, external iliac, or common femoral arteries. For isolated bilateral iliac artery repair, append modifier 50. For decompressive laparotomy, report 49000 in addition to 34708. For covered stent placements for atherosclerotic occlusive disease of the abdominal aorta, see 37236 and 37237; iliac artery, see 37221 and 37223. For simultaneous bilateral iliac artery aneurysm repairs with aorto-bi-iliac endograft, see 34705 and 34706. For repair of an infrarenal aorta by deployment of an aorto-aortic tube endograft, see 34701 and 34702.

ICD-10-CM Diagnostic Codes

I72.3	Aneurysm of iliac artery
I77.72	Dissection of iliac artery
I77.89	Other specified disorders of arteries and arterioles
Q25.8	Other congenital malformations of other great arteries
S35.511A	Injury of right iliac artery, initial encounter ☑
S35.512A	Injury of left iliac artery, initial encounter ☑
S35.59XA	Injury of other iliac blood vessels, initial encounter

AMA: 34707 2019,Nov **34708** 2019,Nov

Relative Value Units/Medicare Edits

Non-Facility RVU	Work	PE	MP	Total
34707	22.28	6.23	5.41	33.92
34708	36.5	7.56	9.11	53.17
Facility RVU	**Work**	**PE**	**MP**	**Total**
34707	22.28	6.23	5.41	33.92
34708	36.5	7.56	9.11	53.17

	FUD	Status	MUE	Modifiers				IOM Reference
34707	90	A	1(2)	51	50	62	80	None
34708	90	A	1(2)	51	50	62	80	

* with documentation

Terms To Know

aneurysm. Circumscribed dilation or outpouching of an artery wall, often containing blood clots and connecting directly with the lumen of the artery.

arteriovenous malformation. Connecting passage between an artery and a vein.

endoprosthesis. Intravascular device in the form of a hollow stent placed within a duct or artery to provide passage through an obstructed area, such as in a bile duct, or to act as a replacement for damaged arterial walls, as in treating an aneurysm.

[34717]

\+ **34717** Endovascular repair of iliac artery at the time of aorto-iliac artery endograft placement by deployment of an iliac branched endograft including pre-procedure sizing and device selection, all ipsilateral selective iliac artery catheterization(s), all associated radiological supervision and interpretation, and all endograft extension(s) proximally to the aortic bifurcation and distally in the internal iliac, external iliac, and common femoral artery(ies), and treatment zone angioplasty/stenting, when performed, for rupture or other than rupture (eg, for aneurysm, pseudoaneurysm, dissection, arteriovenous malformation, penetrating ulcer, traumatic disruption), unilateral (List separately in addition to code for primary procedure)

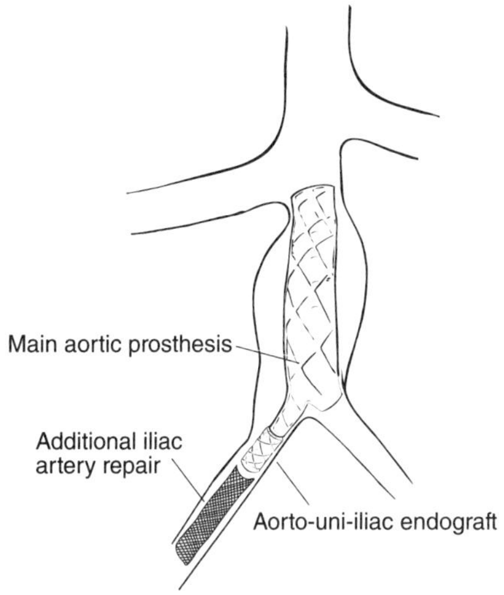

Explanation

At the time of aorto-iliac artery endograft placement, the physician repairs a unilateral iliac artery rupture, aneurysm, pseudoaneurysm, arteriovenous (AV) malformation, dissection, penetrating ulcer, or traumatic disruption by placing an iliac branched endograft. The endograft, contained inside a holding device, is introduced into the artery under fluoroscopy and positioned at the target zone area of repair. This may require open access exposure of the artery or may be accomplished by threading guidewires and catheters through to the site. Once the endoprosthesis is in place, it is deployed within the artery at the targeted site. The position of the endoprosthesis is confirmed, any endoleaks are identified, and the status of runoff vessels is evaluated for any related stenosis, dissection, thrombosis, or embolism. All selective ipsilateral catheterization(s) necessary for device placement, device selection and preprocedural sizing, endograft extension(s), angioplasty or stenting within the treatment zone, as well as radiological supervision and interpretation are included in this procedure. Report 34717, once per side, in addition to the code for the primary procedure.

Coding Tips

Report 34717 in addition to 34703–34706. Code 34717 should be reported twice when performed bilaterally. Do not report with modifier 50 per CPT guidelines. Medicare may still require the use of modifier 50. Do not report 34717 with 34709 on the same side. Do not report 34717 with 34710 or 34711. Selective arterial catheterization of the internal and external iliac arteries on the same side as the iliac branched endograft should not be reported separately. Selective catheterization of the renal artery, opposite hypogastric artery, and other artery families outside of the treatment area of the graft may be reported separately. For placement of an iliac branched endograft at a setting separate from the aorto-iliac endograft placement, see 34718.

ICD-10-CM Diagnostic Codes

This/these CPT code(s) are add-on code(s). See the primary procedure code that this code is performed with for your ICD-10-CM code selections.

AMA: 34717 2019,Nov

Relative Value Units/Medicare Edits

Non-Facility RVU	Work	PE	MP	Total
34717	9.0	1.71	2.2	12.91
Facility RVU	Work	PE	MP	Total
34717	9.0	1.71	2.2	12.91

	FUD	Status	MUE	Modifiers				IOM Reference
34717	N/A	A	2(2)	N/A	N/A	62	80	None

* with documentation

Terms To Know

angioplasty. Reconstruction or repair of a diseased or damaged blood vessel.

distal. *1)* Located farther away from a specified reference point or the trunk. *2)* Pertaining to the area farthest from the center of the body or the point of origin.

ipsilateral. Located on, or affecting, the same side of the body, usually as it relates to a bilateral body part.

proximal. Located closest to a specified reference point, usually the midline or trunk.

34709

\+ **34709** Placement of extension prosthesis(es) distal to the common iliac artery(ies) or proximal to the renal artery(ies) for endovascular repair of infrarenal abdominal aortic or iliac aneurysm, false aneurysm, dissection, penetrating ulcer, including pre-procedure sizing and device selection, all nonselective catheterization(s), all associated radiological supervision and interpretation, and treatment zone angioplasty/stenting, when performed, per vessel treated (List separately in addition to code for primary procedure)

Explanation

The physician places an extension prosthesis distal to the common iliac artery or proximal to the renal artery for endovascular repair of an infrarenal abdominal aortic or iliac aneurysm, pseudoaneurysm, dissection or penetrating ulcer that terminates in the internal iliac, external iliac, or common femoral arteries or in the abdominal aorta proximal to the renal arteries. Using separately reportable aortography, the target site is identified. The proper extension prosthesis is selected. Under separately reportable fluoroscopy, the extension prosthesis, contained inside a long plastic holding capsule, is threaded through the arteries to the leak site. Once the extension prosthesis is in place, the holding capsule is removed. The extension prosthesis, activated by heat, expands like a spring and becomes anchored to the artery wall at the site of the endoleak. If full expansion of the prosthesis does not occur automatically, a balloon catheter is threaded to the graft site and inflated within the endovascular prosthesis until full expansion is achieved. The catheter is removed and the arteriotomy site is closed.

Coding Tips

Report 34709 in addition to 34701-34708. Report 34709 only once per vessel treated. Do not report 34709 for placement of a docking limb extending into the external iliac artery. Selective catheterization of the renal arteries, hypogastric arteries, and/or arterial families outside of the treatment area may be reported separately. For endograft placement into a renal artery covered by a proximal extension, see 37236 and 37237.

ICD-10-CM Diagnostic Codes

This/these CPT code(s) are add-on code(s). See the primary procedure code that this code is performed with for your ICD-10-CM code selections. Diagnostic code(s) would be the same as the actual procedure performed.

AMA: 34709 2019,Nov

Relative Value Units/Medicare Edits

Non-Facility RVU	Work	PE	MP	Total
34709	6.5	1.32	1.57	9.39
Facility RVU	Work	PE	MP	Total
34709	6.5	1.32	1.57	9.39

	FUD	Status	MUE	Modifiers				IOM Reference
34709	N/A	A	3(3)	N/A	N/A	62	80	None

* with documentation

Terms To Know

aneurysm. Circumscribed dilation or outpouching of an artery wall, often containing blood clots and connecting directly with the lumen of the artery.

[34718]

34718 Endovascular repair of iliac artery, not associated with placement of an aorto-iliac artery endograft at the same session, by deployment of an iliac branched endograft, including pre-procedure sizing and device selection, all ipsilateral selective iliac artery catheterization(s), all associated radiological supervision and interpretation, and all endograft extension(s) proximally to the aortic bifurcation and distally in the internal iliac, external iliac, and common femoral artery(ies), and treatment zone angioplasty/stenting, when performed, for other than rupture (eg, for aneurysm, pseudoaneurysm, dissection, arteriovenous malformation, penetrating ulcer), unilateral

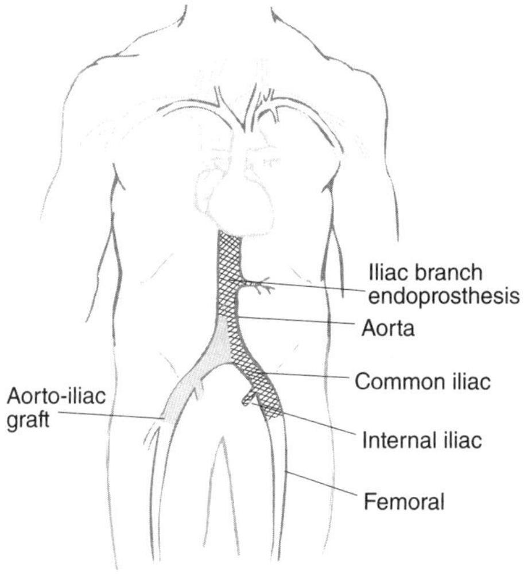

Iliac vessels

Explanation

The physician repairs a unilateral iliac artery aneurysm, pseudoaneurysm, arteriovenous (AV) malformation, dissection, or penetrating ulcer by placing an iliac branched endograft. The endograft, contained inside a holding device, is introduced into the artery under fluoroscopy and positioned at the target zone area of repair. This may require open access exposure of the artery or may be accomplished by threading guidewires and catheters through to the site. Once the endoprosthesis is in place, it is deployed within the artery at the targeted site. The position of the endoprosthesis is confirmed, any endoleaks are identified, and the status of runoff vessels is evaluated for any related stenosis, dissection, thrombosis, or embolism. All selective ipsilateral catheterization(s) necessary for device placement, device selection and preprocedural sizing, endograft extension(s), angioplasty or stenting within the treatment zone, as well as radiological supervision and interpretation is included in this procedure. Placement of an aorto-iliac artery endograft is not performed during this session.

Coding Tips

These are unilateral procedures. If performed bilaterally, some payers require that the service be reported twice with modifier 50 appended to the second code while others require identification of the service only once with modifier 50 appended. Check with individual payers. Modifier 50 identifies a procedure performed identically on the opposite side of the body (mirror image). Do not report 34718 with 34701–34709 or 34717. Do not report 34718 with 34710 or 34711 on the same side. Selective arterial catheterization of the internal and external iliac arteries on the same side as the iliac branched endograft should not be reported separately. Selective catheterization of the renal artery, opposite hypogastric artery, and other artery families outside of the treatment area of the graft may be reported separately. For placement of an iliac branched endograft in the same setting as an aorto-iliac endograft placement, see 34717. For placement of an isolated iliac branched endograft for rupture, see 37799.

ICD-10-CM Diagnostic Codes

I72.3	Aneurysm of iliac artery
I77.2	Rupture of artery
I77.72	Dissection of iliac artery
Q27.32	Arteriovenous malformation of vessel of lower limb
S35.511A	Injury of right iliac artery, initial encounter ☑
S35.512A	Injury of left iliac artery, initial encounter ☑
S35.513A	Injury of unspecified iliac artery, initial encounter

AMA: 34718 2019,Nov

Relative Value Units/Medicare Edits

Non-Facility RVU	Work	PE	MP	Total
34718	24.0	6.31	5.87	36.18
Facility RVU	**Work**	**PE**	**MP**	**Total**
34718	24.0	6.31	5.87	36.18

	FUD	Status	MUE	Modifiers				IOM Reference
34718	90	A	2(2)	51	N/A	62	80	None

* with documentation

Terms To Know

angioplasty. Reconstruction or repair of a diseased or damaged blood vessel.

bifurcated. Having two branches or divisions, such as the left pulmonary veins that split off from the left atrium to carry oxygenated blood away from the heart.

distal. *1)* Located farther away from a specified reference point or the trunk. *2)* Pertaining to the area farthest from the center of the body or the point of origin.

ipsilateral. Located on, or affecting, the same side of the body, usually as it relates to a bilateral body part.

selective placement. Introduction and manipulation of a catheter or guidewire within a vascular tree or family into a specified target area that is identified and monitored by radiographic imaging in order to carry out a diagnostic or therapeutic procedure.

34710-34711

34710 Delayed placement of distal or proximal extension prosthesis for endovascular repair of infrarenal abdominal aortic or iliac aneurysm, false aneurysm, dissection, endoleak, or endograft migration, including pre-procedure sizing and device selection, all nonselective catheterization(s), all associated radiological supervision and interpretation, and treatment zone angioplasty/stenting, when performed; initial vessel treated

\+ **34711** each additional vessel treated (List separately in addition to code for primary procedure)

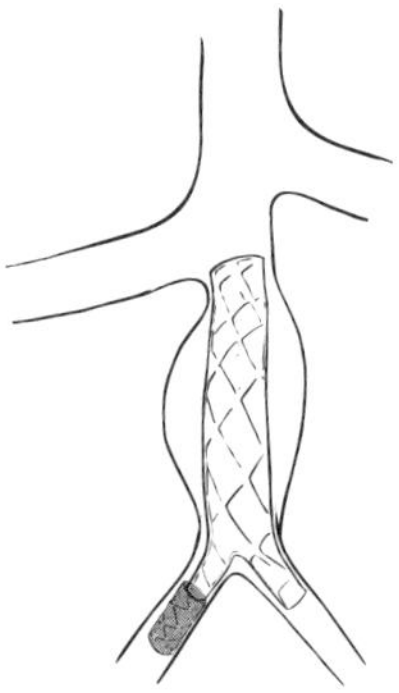

Extension prosthesis

Explanation

The physician performs delayed endovascular placement of a distal or proximal extension prosthesis to repair an infrarenal abdominal aortic or iliac aneurysm, pseudoaneurysm, dissection, endoleak, or endograft migration. A leak may occur at fixation sites of a grafted aneurysm through the body of the graft or from patent arteries within the aneurysm sac and may require endovascular reparation. Using separately reportable aortography, the target site is identified. The proper extension prosthesis is selected. Under separately reportable fluoroscopy, the extension prosthesis, contained inside a long plastic holding capsule, is threaded through the arteries to the leak site. Once the extension prosthesis is in place, the holding capsule is removed. The extension prosthesis, activated by heat, expands like a spring and becomes anchored to the artery wall at the site of the endoleak. If full expansion of the prosthesis does not occur automatically, a balloon catheter is threaded to the graft site and inflated within the endovascular prosthesis until full expansion is achieved. The catheter is removed and the arteriotomy site is closed. These procedures include all nonselective catheterizations, sizing, and device selection prior to the procedure; radiological supervision and interpretation; and treatment zone angioplasty or stenting, when performed. These codes may only be reported once per vessel treated (e.g., multiple endograft extensions placed in a single vessel may only be reported once). Report 34710 for placement of an extension prosthesis in the initial vessel and 34711 for placement of an extension prosthesis in each additional vessel.

Coding Tips

These are unilateral procedures. If performed bilaterally, some payers require that the service be reported twice with modifier 50 appended to the second code while others require identification of the service only once with modifier 50 appended. Check with individual payers. Modifier 50 identifies a procedure performed identically on the opposite side of the body (mirror image). Report 34711 in addition to 34710. These codes may only be reported once per operative session. For decompressive laparotomy, report 49000 in addition to 34710. For delayed revision using a transcatheter enhanced fixation device, see 34712. Do not report 34710 or 34711 with 34701-34709 or 34841-34848. Do not report these codes in addition to 34718 for the same side. For endovascular repair of an iliac artery bifurcation, see 34717-34718. For intravascular ultrasound performed during an endovascular aneurysm repair, see 37252 and 37253. For isolated bilateral iliac artery repair, see 34707 and 34708 and append modifier 50. For open artery exposure, use 34714-34716, 34812, 34820, 34833, or 34834 in addition to 34701-34708, 34710, 34712, or 34718, when applicable. For percutaneous arterial closure, use 34713 in addition to 34701-34708, 34710, 34712, or 34718, when applicable. For simultaneous bilateral iliac artery aneurysm repairs with an aorto-bi-iliac endograft, report 34705 or 34706, when applicable.

ICD-10-CM Diagnostic Codes

A52.01	Syphilitic aneurysm of aorta
I71.02	Dissection of abdominal aorta
I71.33	Infrarenal abdominal aortic aneurysm, ruptured
I71.43	Infrarenal abdominal aortic aneurysm, without rupture
I72.3	Aneurysm of iliac artery
I77.72	Dissection of iliac artery
I77.811	Abdominal aortic ectasia
I77.89	Other specified disorders of arteries and arterioles
Q25.43	Congenital aneurysm of aorta
Q25.44	Congenital dilation of aorta
Q25.49	Other congenital malformations of aorta
Q25.8	Other congenital malformations of other great arteries
Q25.9	Congenital malformation of great arteries, unspecified
Q79.61	Classical Ehlers-Danlos syndrome
Q79.62	Hypermobile Ehlers-Danlos syndrome
Q79.63	Vascular Ehlers-Danlos syndrome
Q79.69	Other Ehlers-Danlos syndromes
Q87.410	Marfan syndrome with aortic dilation
Q87.418	Marfan syndrome with other cardiovascular manifestations
S35.01XA	Minor laceration of abdominal aorta, initial encounter
S35.02XA	Major laceration of abdominal aorta, initial encounter
S35.09XA	Other injury of abdominal aorta, initial encounter
S35.511A	Injury of right iliac artery, initial encounter ☑
S35.59XA	Injury of other iliac blood vessels, initial encounter

AMA: **34710** 2019,Nov **34711** 2019,Nov

Relative Value Units/Medicare Edits

Non-Facility RVU	Work	PE	MP	Total
34710	15.0	4.67	3.63	23.3
34711	6.0	1.11	1.47	8.58
Facility RVU	**Work**	**PE**	**MP**	**Total**
34710	15.0	4.67	3.63	23.3
34711	6.0	1.11	1.47	8.58

	FUD	Status	MUE	Modifiers				IOM Reference
34710	90	A	1(2)	51	N/A	62	80	None
34711	N/A	A	2(3)	N/A	N/A	62	80	

* with documentation

34712

34712 Transcatheter delivery of enhanced fixation device(s) to the endograft (eg, anchor, screw, tack) and all associated radiological supervision and interpretation

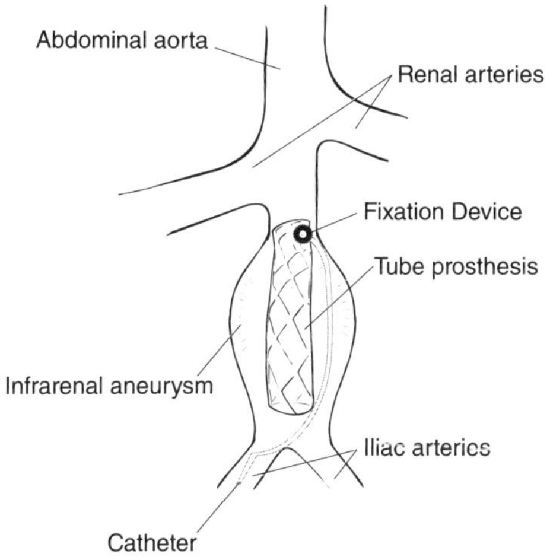

Explanation

The physician performs transcatheter delivery of accessory-enhanced fixation devices, such as an anchor, screw, or tack, to the endograft. Commonly referred to as a bioprosthesis, this procedure is used for patients with abdominal aortic and/or iliac artery conditions, such as an aneurysm with complex anatomies, or for patients who are experiencing an endoleak. Proprietary devices ensure a safe and effective treatment solution for these types of repairs. They enhance durability to the level of a surgical anastomosis and address concerns for future complications. They are used to improve fixation and sealing of an endovascular graft, either in primary cases or to fix endoleaks and stent migration. The devices lock the endograft to the abdominal aorta and/or iliac artery to secure the patient's future and maximize outcomes in challenging patients. The fixation devices quickly identify, aim, and activate a sealing mechanism to close up endoleaks. Endoanchors are used to repair an endovascular graft in cases where the original graft has moved away from the implant site and developed endoleaks. In such cases, augmented fixation and/or sealing is required to regain or maintain effective aneurysm exclusion. These devices can be placed during the initial endoprosthesis placement procedure or for a subsequent repair procedure. Percutaneous access using a sheath smaller than 12 French is included in 34712 and is not reported separately. Radiologic supervision and interpretation are included in this procedure.

Coding Tips

Report this code only once per operative session. Radiological supervision and interpretation is included and should not be reported separately. For vascular access requiring the use of closure devices for sheaths of 12 French or larger, or access requiring open surgical arterial exposure, see 34713-34716, 34812, 34820, 34833, and 34834. Percutaneous access using a sheath smaller than 12 French is included in 34712 and should not be reported separately.

ICD-10-CM Diagnostic Codes

A52.01 Syphilitic aneurysm of aorta
I71.02 Dissection of abdominal aorta
I71.31 Pararenal abdominal aortic aneurysm, ruptured
I71.32 Juxtarenal abdominal aortic aneurysm, ruptured
I71.33 Infrarenal abdominal aortic aneurysm, ruptured
I71.41 Pararenal abdominal aortic aneurysm, without rupture
I71.42 Juxtarenal abdominal aortic aneurysm, without rupture
I71.43 Infrarenal abdominal aortic aneurysm, without rupture
I72.3 Aneurysm of iliac artery
I77.72 Dissection of iliac artery
I77.811 Abdominal aortic ectasia
I77.89 Other specified disorders of arteries and arterioles
Q25.43 Congenital aneurysm of aorta
Q25.44 Congenital dilation of aorta
Q25.49 Other congenital malformations of aorta
Q25.8 Other congenital malformations of other great arteries
Q25.9 Congenital malformation of great arteries, unspecified
Q79.61 Classical Ehlers-Danlos syndrome
Q79.62 Hypermobile Ehlers-Danlos syndrome
Q79.63 Vascular Ehlers-Danlos syndrome
Q87.410 Marfan syndrome with aortic dilation
Q87.418 Marfan syndrome with other cardiovascular manifestations
S35.01XA Minor laceration of abdominal aorta, initial encounter
S35.02XA Major laceration of abdominal aorta, initial encounter
S35.09XA Other injury of abdominal aorta, initial encounter
S35.511A Injury of right iliac artery, initial encounter ☑
S35.512A Injury of left iliac artery, initial encounter ☑
S35.59XA Injury of other iliac blood vessels, initial encounter

Relative Value Units/Medicare Edits

Non-Facility RVU	Work	PE	MP	Total
34712	12.0	4.34	2.86	19.2
Facility RVU	**Work**	**PE**	**MP**	**Total**
34712	12.0	4.34	2.86	19.2

	FUD	Status	MUE	Modifiers				IOM Reference
34712	90	A	1(2)	51	N/A	62	80	None

* with documentation

Terms To Know

fixation. Act or condition of being attached, secured, fastened, or held in position.

transcatheter. Procedure or treatment performed via a catheter.

 ● New ▲ Revised + Add On ★ Telemedicine [Resequenced] ☑ Laterality

34713-34714 [34812]

+ **34713** Percutaneous access and closure of femoral artery for delivery of endograft through a large sheath (12 French or larger), including ultrasound guidance, when performed, unilateral (List separately in addition to code for primary procedure)
+ **34812** Open femoral artery exposure for delivery of endovascular prosthesis, by groin incision, unilateral (List separately in addition to code for primary procedure)
+ **34714** Open femoral artery exposure with creation of conduit for delivery of endovascular prosthesis or for establishment of cardiopulmonary bypass, by groin incision, unilateral (List separately in addition to code for primary procedure)

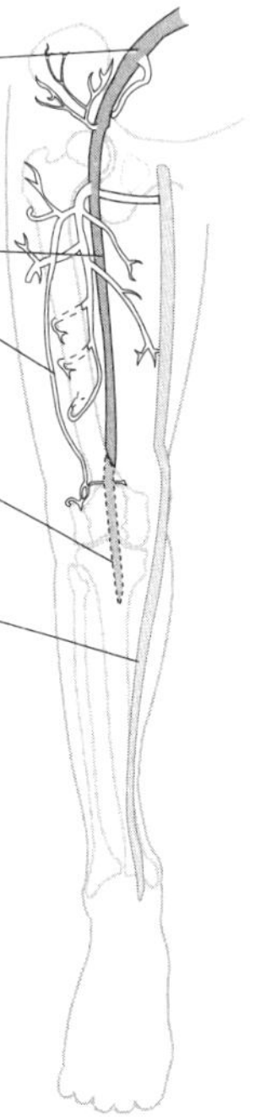

Explanation

The femoral artery may be accessed percutaneously or by open incision. For percutaneous access the femoral artery is identified using ultrasound guidance and the guide catheter is percutaneously inserted with subsequent insertion of a large arterial sheath (i.e., 12 French or larger). Closure may involve the use of an arterial closure device (ACD). Several types of ACDs may be used for closure including a small balloon that ensures sealant coverage of the arteriotomy, four needles that anchor and close suture material upon removal, or a collagen sponge with polymer that forms a self-tightening suture seal. Alternately, the femoral artery may be examined via an open technique. With the patient in the supine position, the physician exposes the femoral artery through an incision in the groin area revealing the femoral artery on one side while underlying subcutaneous layers and muscles incised to reach the artery are placed out of the way as hemostasis is achieved in preparation for delivery of the endograft, endovascular prosthesis, or creation of a conduit. Closure may be by direct suture. Report 34713 for percutaneous access and closure of a femoral arteriotomy for delivery of an endovascular prosthesis. Ultrasound guidance is included. Report 34812 for open femoral artery exposure with delivery of an endovascular prosthesis and repair and closure of the femoral artery. Report 34714 for open femoral artery exposure with endovascular device delivery or establishment of cardiopulmonary bypass that requires creation of a prosthetic conduit utilizing a femoral artery.

Coding Tips

These codes should only be reported once per side and should be reported twice when performed bilaterally. Do not report with modifier 50 per CPT guidelines. Medicare may still require the use of modifier 50. Report 34713 and 34812 in addition to 33880, 33881, 33883, 33884, 33886, 34701-34708, 34710, 34712, 34718, and 34841-34848. Code 34812 may be reported with 33990 or 33991. Do not report 34713 with the prior list of codes if a sheath smaller than 12 French was used or for percutaneous access and closure of the femoral artery in addition to 37221, 37223, 37236, or 37237. Do not report 34812 with 33953, 33954, 33959, 33962, 33969, 33984, or 33987. Code 34714 may be reported with an extensive number of primary procedures ranging from 32852-34848. Refer to the CPT manual for details. Do not report 34714 with 33362, 33953, 33954, 33959, 33962, 33969, 33984, or 34812 when performed on the same side.

ICD-10-CM Diagnostic Codes

This/these CPT code(s) are add-on code(s). See the primary procedure code that this code is performed with for your ICD-10-CM code selections. Diagnostic code(s) would be the same as the actual procedure performed.

AMA: **34713** 2022,Oct

Relative Value Units/Medicare Edits

Non-Facility RVU	Work	PE	MP	Total
34713	2.5	0.49	0.6	3.59
34812	4.13	0.85	1.03	6.01
34714	5.25	1.35	1.27	7.87
Facility RVU	**Work**	**PE**	**MP**	**Total**
34713	2.5	0.49	0.6	3.59
34812	4.13	0.85	1.03	6.01
34714	5.25	1.35	1.27	7.87

	FUD	Status	MUE	Modifiers				IOM Reference
34713	N/A	A	1(3)	N/A	50	62	80	None
34812	N/A	A	1(3)	N/A	50	62	80	
34714	N/A	A	1(3)	N/A	50	62	80	

* with documentation

[34820]

\+ **34820** Open iliac artery exposure for delivery of endovascular prosthesis or iliac occlusion during endovascular therapy, by abdominal or retroperitoneal incision, unilateral (List separately in addition to code for primary procedure)

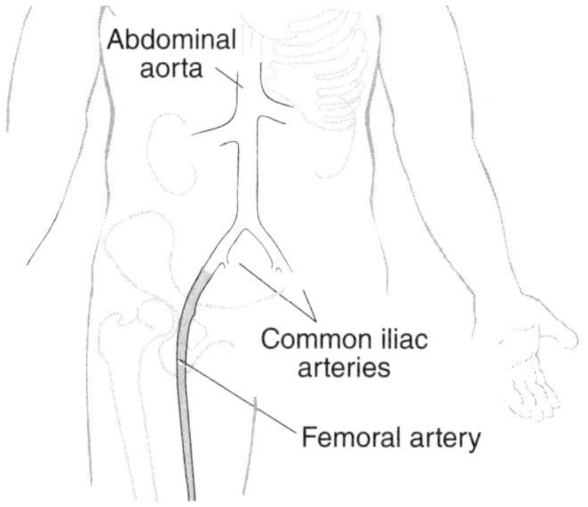

An iliac artery is surgically exposed to deliver an endovascular prosthesis or to occlude an iliac artery. The procedure occurs during endovascular therapy and access is abdominal or retroperitoneal

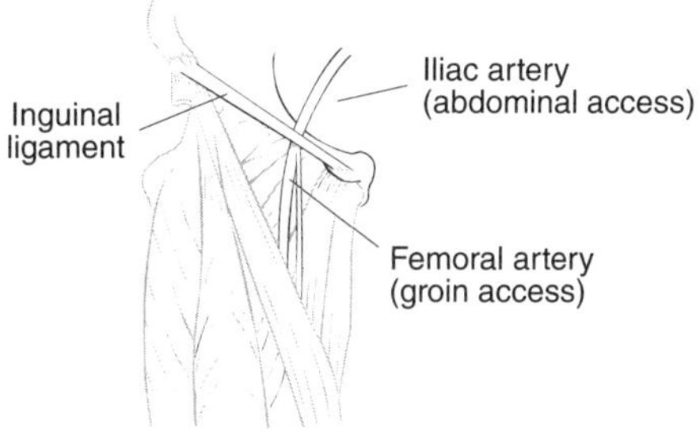

Explanation

The physician makes an abdominal or retroperitoneal incision to expose the iliac artery on one side to facilitate the delivery of an endovascular prosthesis or to perform temporary iliac artery occlusion during a procedure for endovascular therapy. The patient is placed supine and the buttocks are elevated. An incision is made parallel with and just above the inguinal ligament. The incision is in the middle third of a proximally curved line extending from the anterior superior iliac spine to the pubic symphysis. Hemostasis of vessels is achieved and the aponeuroses of the external and internal oblique and the transversus muscles are incised parallel to the inguinal ligament. The structures are reflected upward and medially, the transversalis fascia is opened, and the retroperitoneal space is entered. The iliac artery is exposed in preparation for delivering an endovascular prosthesis and its sheath is opened with tape placed about it. If the artery has been exposed for the purpose of placing a temporary occlusion device, the clamp is placed.

Coding Tips

Depending on the type of exposure required, this service may be performed by a surgeon other than the one performing the endovascular repair. Code 34820 should only be reported once per side and should be reported twice when performed bilaterally. Do not report with modifier 50 per CPT guidelines. Medicare may still require the use of modifier 50. Report 34820 in addition to 33880, 33881, 33883, 33884, 33886, 33990, 33991, 34701-34708, 34710, 34712, 34718, or 34841-34848. Do not report 34820 with 33953, 33954, 33959, 33962, 33969, or 33984.

ICD-10-CM Diagnostic Codes

This/these CPT code(s) are add-on code(s). See the primary procedure code that this code is performed with for your ICD-10-CM code selections. Diagnostic code(s) would be the same as the actual procedure performed.

Relative Value Units/Medicare Edits

Non-Facility RVU	Work	PE	MP	Total
34820	7.0	1.09	1.73	9.82
Facility RVU	**Work**	**PE**	**MP**	**Total**
34820	7.0	1.09	1.73	9.82

	FUD	Status	MUE	Modifiers				IOM Reference
34820	N/A	A	1(3)	N/A	50	62	80	None

* with documentation

Terms To Know

aneurysm. Circumscribed dilation or outpouching of an artery wall, often containing blood clots and connecting directly with the lumen of the artery.

atherosclerosis. Buildup of yellowish plaques composed of cholesterol and lipoid material within the arteries.

catheter. Flexible tube inserted into an area of the body for introducing or withdrawing fluid.

fluoroscopy. Radiology technique that allows visual examination of part of the body or a function of an organ using a device that projects an x-ray image on a fluorescent screen.

occlusion. Constriction, closure, or blockage of a passage.

sheath. Covering enclosing an organ or part.

stent. Tube to provide support in a body cavity or lumen.

[34833, 34834]

+ **34833** Open iliac artery exposure with creation of conduit for delivery of endovascular prosthesis or for establishment of cardiopulmonary bypass, by abdominal or retroperitoneal incision, unilateral (List separately in addition to code for primary procedure)
+ **34834** Open brachial artery exposure for delivery of endovascular prosthesis, unilateral (List separately in addition to code for primary procedure)

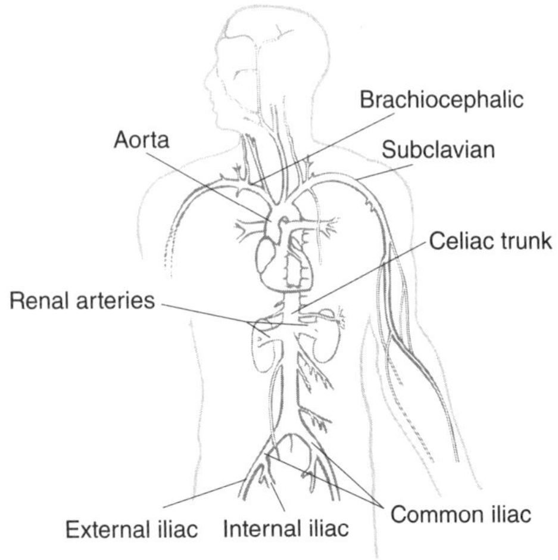

Explanation

In 34833, a conduit is created for the delivery of an endovascular prosthesis or for the establishment of cardiopulmonary bypass via transabdominal or retroperitoneal incision. A skin incision is made parallel with and just above the inguinal ligament. The skin is incised and the retroperitoneal space is entered to access the iliac artery. Bowels, blood vessels, and other soft tissue are mobilized from the area to give clear access to the iliac artery. With adequate exposure, loops are passed around the vessel proximally and distally. Anticoagulation is achieved and vascular clamps are applied. An arteriotomy is made for creation of the conduit, which is formed by placing a tubular piece of bypass graft material that has been fashioned into the right size onto the iliac artery and suturing it together. The conduit is clamped and the vascular clamps are removed from the iliac artery. Additional sutures are placed as needed. Through the newly created conduit, endovascular repair by deployment of a prosthesis may be undertaken. After the repair is complete, the conduit may be closed in one of two ways. The open end of the conduit may be sewn to the distal external iliac artery, and thereby left in place as a channel for external iliac bypass graft, or it may be cut close to the iliac artery and simply oversewn with sutures. This code reports the creation of the conduit, not the endovascular repair. In 34834, open brachial artery exposure is done for delivery of an endovascular prosthesis. An incision is made in the skin of the upper arm and nerves, blood vessels, and other soft tissues are mobilized from the area to give clear access to the brachial artery. With adequate exposure, loops are passed around the vessel proximally and distally. Anticoagulation is achieved and vascular clamps are alternately applied and removed as needed for introduction of guidewires, sheaths, and catheters through the brachial artery for accomplishing deployment of an aortic or iliac endovascular prosthesis. After the endovascular repair is complete, the opening remaining in the brachial artery is closed with fine sutures after irrigation and trimming of the edges has been done. Hemostasis is achieved and the wound is irrigated and closed. This code reports the open brachial artery exposure, not the endovascular repair.

Coding Tips

Depending on the type of exposure required, this service may be performed by a surgeon other than the one performing the endovascular repair. These codes should only be reported once per side and should be reported twice when performed bilaterally. Do not report with modifier 50 per CPT guidelines. Medicare may still require the use of modifier 50. Code 34833 may be reported with an extensive number of primary procedures ranging from 32852-34848. Refer to the CPT manual for details. Do not report 34833 with 33364, 33953, 33954, 33959, 33962, 33969, 33984, or 34820 when performed on the same side. Report 34834 in addition to 33880-33884, 33886, 33990, 33991, 34701-34708, 34710, 34712, 34718, or 34841-34848. Do not report 34834 with 33953, 33954, 33959, 33962, 33969, or 33984.

ICD-10-CM Diagnostic Codes

This/these CPT code(s) are add-on code(s). See the primary procedure code that this code is performed with for your ICD-10-CM code selections. Diagnostic code(s) would be the same as the actual procedure performed.

Relative Value Units/Medicare Edits

Non-Facility RVU	Work	PE	MP	Total
34833	8.16	1.27	2.03	11.46
34834	2.65	0.46	0.66	3.77
Facility RVU	**Work**	**PE**	**MP**	**Total**
34833	8.16	1.27	2.03	11.46
34834	2.65	0.46	0.66	3.77

	FUD	Status	MUE	Modifiers				IOM Reference
34833	N/A	A	1(2)	N/A	50	62	80	None
34834	N/A	A	1(2)	N/A	50	62	80	

* with documentation

Terms To Know

cardiopulmonary bypass. Venous blood is diverted to a heart-lung machine, which mechanically pumps and oxygenates the blood temporarily so the heart can be bypassed while an open procedure on the heart or coronary arteries is performed. During bypass, the lungs are deflated and immobile.

catheter. Flexible tube inserted into an area of the body for introducing or withdrawing fluid.

conduit. Surgically created channel for the passage of fluids.

guidewire. Flexible metal instrument designed to lead another instrument in its proper course.

retroperitoneal. Located behind the peritoneum, the membrane that lines the abdominopelvic walls and forms a covering for the internal organs.

sheath. Covering enclosing an organ or part.

transabdominal. Across or through the belly or abdomen.

34715-34716

+ 34715 Open axillary/subclavian artery exposure for delivery of endovascular prosthesis by infraclavicular or supraclavicular incision, unilateral (List separately in addition to code for primary procedure)

+ 34716 Open axillary/subclavian artery exposure with creation of conduit for delivery of endovascular prosthesis or for establishment of cardiopulmonary bypass, by infraclavicular or supraclavicular incision, unilateral (List separately in addition to code for primary procedure)

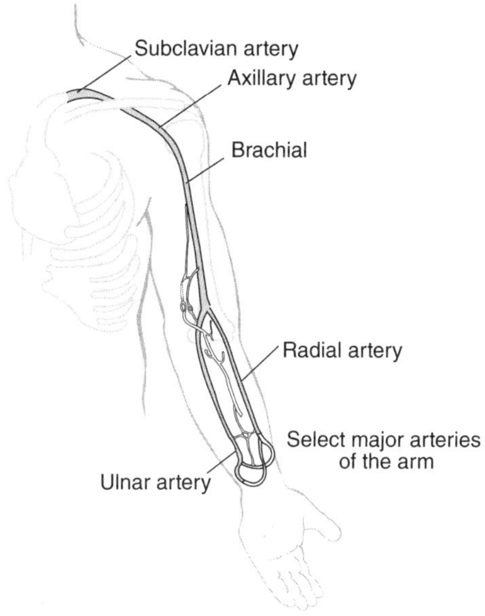

Explanation

The physician exposes the axillary or subclavian artery for delivery of an endovascular prosthesis and performs closure of the artery with an arterial closure device (ACD). In one method, an ACD is inserted through the existing procedural sheath. A small balloon is inflated within the artery and pulled back to the arterial wall, serving as an anchor to ensure proper placement, and is inflated. The balloon is deflated and removed through the tract, leaving behind only the expanded sealant, which seals the arteriotomy. In an alternate method, an ACD utilizes four needles (two sutures) directed outward from within the arterial lumen. It is advanced over a guidewire until blood return indicates proper placement. When the physician pulls the device handle, the needles are deployed and pulled through the arterial wall. The needles remain contained within the device shaft and are removed by pulling them up through the device shaft, leaving behind the suture ends, which are then tied and the device is removed. Yet another method uses an ACD composed of collagen sponge and polymer anchor joined together with a self-tightening suture that seals and sandwiches the arteriotomy for a more complete closure. The device stops the flow of blood mechanically, which is supported by the platelet-inducing properties of the collagen. Report 34715 for delivery of an endovascular prosthesis by axillary or subclavian exposure through an infraclavicular or supraclavicular or sternotomy incision during endovascular aneurysm repair. The patient is placed in supine position and open incision is made. Hemostasis of vessels is achieved. The underlying subcutaneous layers and muscles are incised to reach the artery and reflected out of the way. The axillary or subclavian artery is exposed in preparation for delivery of the endovascular prosthesis and its sheath is opened with tape placed about it. Report 34716 for endovascular device delivery or establishment of cardiopulmonary bypass that requires creation of a prosthetic conduit utilizing axillary or subclavian artery exposure through an infraclavicular or supraclavicular or sternotomy incision during endovascular aneurysm repair or cardiac procedures requiring cardiopulmonary bypass.

Coding Tips

These codes should only be reported once per side and should be reported twice when performed bilaterally. Do not report with modifier 50 per CPT guidelines. Medicare may still require the use of modifier 50. Report 34715 in addition to 33880-33884, 33886, 33990, 33991, 34701-34708, 34710, 34712, 34718, or 34841-34848. Do not report 34715 with 33363, 33953, 33954, 33959, 33962, 33969, or 33984. Code 34716 may be reported with an extensive number of primary procedures ranging from 32852-34848. Refer to the CPT manual for details.

ICD-10-CM Diagnostic Codes

This/these CPT code(s) are add-on code(s). See the primary procedure code that this code is performed with for your ICD-10-CM code selections. Diagnostic code(s) would be the same as the actual procedure performed.

Relative Value Units/Medicare Edits

Non-Facility RVU	Work	PE	MP	Total
34715	6.0	1.22	1.49	8.71
34716	7.19	1.96	1.72	10.87
Facility RVU	**Work**	**PE**	**MP**	**Total**
34715	6.0	1.22	1.49	8.71
34716	7.19	1.96	1.72	10.87

	FUD	Status	MUE	Modifiers				IOM Reference
34715	N/A	A	1(3)	N/A	50	62	80	None
34716	N/A	A	1(3)	N/A	50	62	80	

* with documentation

Terms To Know

arteriotomy. Incision into an artery.

endovascular therapy. Intravascular catheters, scopes, stents, balloons, and other devices or methods used to treat vascular disease.

34808

+ **34808** Endovascular placement of iliac artery occlusion device (List separately in addition to code for primary procedure)

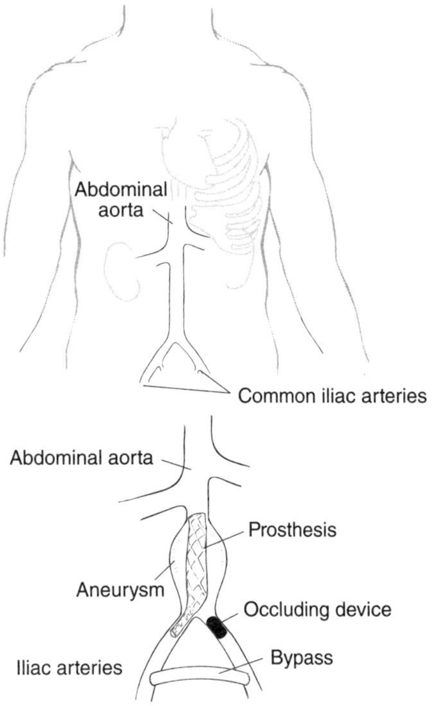

A device is placed endovascularly into an iliac artery in order to occlude blood flow

Explanation

Endovascular placement of an iliac artery occlusion device is performed during separately reportable repair of an abdominal aortic aneurysm and/or endovascular graft procedure. As part of the repair, the iliac artery is occluded. Under separately reportable fluoroscopy, an iliac artery occlusion device is threaded through the arteries and placed distal to the aneurysm. When the aneurysmal repair is complete, the endovascular occlusion device may be left in the artery. Catheters and devices used for access and to deploy the occlusion device are removed and any bleeding controlled.

Coding Tips

Report 34808 in addition to 34701-34704, 34707-34710, 34813, or 34841-34844. When an open approach is required, report the appropriate arterial exposure code (34714, 34812, 34820, 34833) in addition to the endovascular placement of the occlusion device.

ICD-10-CM Diagnostic Codes

This/these CPT code(s) are add-on code(s). See the primary procedure code that this code is performed with for your ICD-10-CM code selections. Diagnostic code(s) would be the same as the actual procedure performed.

Relative Value Units/Medicare Edits

Non-Facility RVU	Work	PE	MP	Total
34808	4.12	0.76	1.03	5.91
Facility RVU	**Work**	**PE**	**MP**	**Total**
34808	4.12	0.76	1.03	5.91

	FUD	Status	MUE	Modifiers				IOM Reference
34808	N/A	A	1(3)	N/A	N/A	62	80	None

* with documentation

Terms To Know

aneurysm. Circumscribed dilation or outpouching of an artery wall, often containing blood clots and connecting directly with the lumen of the artery.

fluoroscopy. Radiology technique that allows visual examination of part of the body or a function of an organ using a device that projects an x-ray image on a fluorescent screen.

graft. Tissue implant from another part of the body or another person.

occlusion. Constriction, closure, or blockage of a passage.

suture. Numerous stitching techniques employed in wound closure.

buried suture. Continuous or interrupted suture placed under the skin for a layered closure.

continuous suture. Running stitch with tension evenly distributed across a single strand to provide a leakproof closure line.

interrupted suture. Series of single stitches with tension isolated at each stitch, in which all stitches are not affected if one becomes loose, and the isolated sutures cannot act as a wick to transport an infection.

purse-string suture. Continuous suture placed around a tubular structure and tightened, to reduce or close the lumen.

retention suture. Secondary stitching that bridges the primary suture, providing support for the primary repair; a plastic or rubber bolster may be placed over the primary repair and under the retention sutures.

34813

+ **34813** Placement of femoral-femoral prosthetic graft during endovascular aortic aneurysm repair (List separately in addition to code for primary procedure)

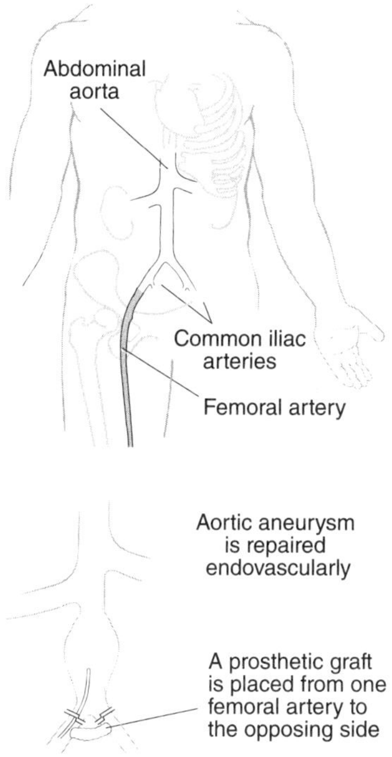

Explanation

During separately reportable endovascular repair of an aortic aneurysm, a diseased or damaged femoral artery is repaired by placing a prosthetic femoral-femoral graft. Through incisions in the skin of the upper thighs, the physician isolates and dissects a section of the affected femoral artery. Once vessel clamps have been affixed above and below the area of damaged vessel to be anastomosed, the femoral artery is cut above and below the diseased or damaged area and the new distal and proximal ends are sutured to the ends of the prosthetic graft, which now replaces the section of diseased or damaged artery. When the clamps are removed, the blood flows unobstructed through the femoral artery. After the graft is complete, the skin incisions are repaired with layered closures.

Coding Tips

Report 34813 in addition to 34812 as appropriate. For femoral artery grafting, see 35521, 35533, 35539, 35540, 35556, 35558, 35566, 35621, 35646, 35654–35661, 35666, and 35700.

ICD-10-CM Diagnostic Codes

This/these CPT code(s) are add-on code(s). See the primary procedure code that this code is performed with for your ICD-10-CM code selections. Diagnostic code(s) would be the same as the actual procedure performed.

Relative Value Units/Medicare Edits

Non-Facility RVU	Work	PE	MP	Total
34813	4.79	0.87	1.19	6.85
Facility RVU	**Work**	**PE**	**MP**	**Total**
34813	4.79	0.87	1.19	6.85

	FUD	Status	MUE	Modifiers				IOM Reference
34813	N/A	A	1(2)	N/A	N/A	62	80	None

* with documentation

Terms To Know

anastomosis. Surgically created connection between ducts, blood vessels, or bowel segments to allow flow from one to the other.

aneurysm. Circumscribed dilation or outpouching of an artery wall, often containing blood clots and connecting directly with the lumen of the artery.

atherosclerosis. Buildup of yellowish plaques composed of cholesterol and lipoid material within the arteries.

bypass. Auxiliary or diverted route to maintain continuous flow.

distal. *1)* Located farther away from a specified reference point or the trunk. *2)* Pertaining to the area farthest from the center of the body or the point of origin.

graft. Tissue implant from another part of the body or another person.

incision. Act of cutting into tissue or an organ.

proximal. Located closest to a specified reference point, usually the midline or trunk.

stricture. Narrowing of an anatomical structure.

34830-34832

34830 Open repair of infrarenal aortic aneurysm or dissection, plus repair of associated arterial trauma, following unsuccessful endovascular repair; tube prosthesis

34831 aorto-bi-iliac prosthesis

34832 aorto-bifemoral prosthesis

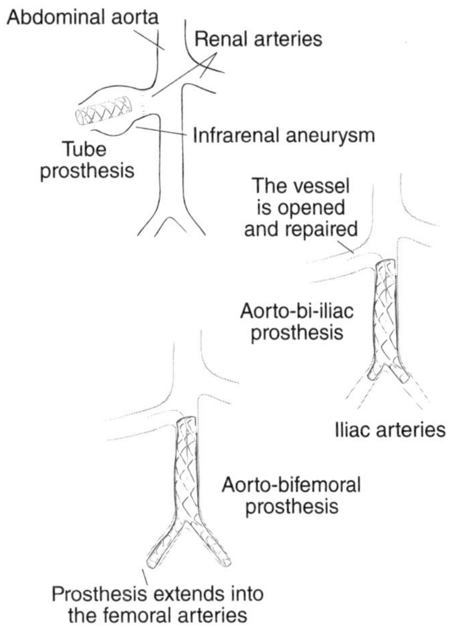

An infrarenal aortic aneurysm or dissection is treated in an open surgical session following an unsuccessful endovascular treatment attempt. A tube prosthesis is placed and any associated arterial trauma is repaired

Explanation

An attempted endovascular repair of an aortic aneurysm originating below the renal arteries (infrarenal) fails, necessitating open repair of the aneurysm as well as repair of any trauma associated with the endovascular attempt. An incision is made in the abdomen from just below the diaphragm to the umbilicus. The aorta is exposed, the aneurysm identified, and the aorta and other arteries inspected for injury resulting from the failed endovascular procedure. Repair of the aneurysm is accomplished by temporarily clamping the aorta both above and below the aneurysm. It is usually possible to place the upper clamp just below the origins of the renal arteries so that the kidneys continue to receive blood flow throughout the operation. Blood flow to the legs is interrupted while the aorta is clamped. The aneurysm is opened lengthwise and any thrombi (blood clots) removed. The aneurysm wall is not removed. The aorta is cut above and below the aneurysm and a prosthetic graft made of synthetic material is sutured in place between the two ends. The aneurysm wall is wrapped around the synthetic graft. The clamps are removed allowing blood to flow through the graft and into the vessels of the lower extremities. The surgical wound is closed. Repair using a tube prosthesis is reported with 34830; repair with an aorto-bi-iliac prosthesis is reported with 34831; and repair with an aorto-bifemoral prosthesis is reported with 34832.

Coding Tips

These codes should be used only when an endovascular repair has been attempted but has been unsuccessful. To report direct repair of an abdominal aortic aneurysm not preceded by attempted endovascular repair, see 35081–35103.

ICD-10-CM Diagnostic Codes

A52.01	Syphilitic aneurysm of aorta
I71.02	Dissection of abdominal aorta
I71.33	Infrarenal abdominal aortic aneurysm, ruptured
I71.43	Infrarenal abdominal aortic aneurysm, without rupture
Q25.43	Congenital aneurysm of aorta
Q25.44	Congenital dilation of aorta
Q25.47	Right aortic arch
Q25.48	Anomalous origin of subclavian artery
Q25.49	Other congenital malformations of aorta
Q25.8	Other congenital malformations of other great arteries
Q79.61	Classical Ehlers-Danlos syndrome
Q79.62	Hypermobile Ehlers-Danlos syndrome
Q79.63	Vascular Ehlers-Danlos syndrome
Q87.410	Marfan syndrome with aortic dilation
Q87.418	Marfan syndrome with other cardiovascular manifestations
S35.01XA	Minor laceration of abdominal aorta, initial encounter
S35.02XA	Major laceration of abdominal aorta, initial encounter
S35.09XA	Other injury of abdominal aorta, initial encounter

Relative Value Units/Medicare Edits

Non-Facility RVU	Work	PE	MP	Total
34830	35.23	7.58	8.79	51.6
34831	37.98	8.97	9.48	56.43
34832	37.98	8.01	9.48	55.47
Facility RVU	**Work**	**PE**	**MP**	**Total**
34830	35.23	7.58	8.79	51.6
34831	37.98	8.97	9.48	56.43
34832	37.98	8.01	9.48	55.47

	FUD	Status	MUE	Modifiers				IOM Reference
34830	90	A	1(2)	51	N/A	62	80	None
34831	90	A	1(2)	51	N/A	62	80	
34832	90	A	1(2)	51	N/A	62	80	

* with documentation

Terms To Know

aneurysm. Circumscribed dilation or outpouching of an artery wall, often containing blood clots and connecting directly with the lumen of the artery.

34839

34839 Physician planning of a patient-specific fenestrated visceral aortic endograft requiring a minimum of 90 minutes of physician time

Explanation

The physician spends at least 90 minutes planning for the placement of a fenestrated visceral aortic endograft, which requires detailed preparation prior to implantation. The planning includes review of radiological imaging enhanced by computer software to assist in the production of the device. Before placement, the physician needs to determine the size parameters of the graft that will conform to the branches of the aorta. These dimensions allow the physician to cut holes (fenestrations) in the device at each visceral artery orifice to allow side branch perfusion of these vessels. Precise planning must allow for adequate blood flow upon completion of placement. The physician must document at least 90 minutes of planning in the medical record.

Coding Tips

This code is reported the date the planning is completed. Do not report 34839 with 76376 or 76377. Do not report 34839 with 34841–34848 when performed the day before or the day of the fenestrated endovascular repair.

ICD-10-CM Diagnostic Codes

A52.01	Syphilitic aneurysm of aorta
I71.02	Dissection of abdominal aorta
I71.03	Dissection of thoracoabdominal aorta
I71.11	Aneurysm of the ascending aorta, ruptured
I71.12	Aneurysm of the aortic arch, ruptured
I71.13	Aneurysm of the descending thoracic aorta, ruptured
I71.21	Aneurysm of the ascending aorta, without rupture
I71.22	Aneurysm of the aortic arch, without rupture
I71.23	Aneurysm of the descending thoracic aorta, without rupture
I71.31	Pararenal abdominal aortic aneurysm, ruptured
I71.32	Juxtarenal abdominal aortic aneurysm, ruptured
I71.33	Infrarenal abdominal aortic aneurysm, ruptured
I71.51	Supraceliac aneurysm of the thoracoabdominal aorta, ruptured
I71.52	Paravisceral aneurysm of the thoracoabdominal aorta, ruptured
I71.61	Supraceliac aneurysm of the thoracoabdominal aorta, without rupture
I71.62	Paravisceral aneurysm of the thoracoabdominal aorta, without rupture
I72.2	Aneurysm of renal artery
I72.8	Aneurysm of other specified arteries
I77.73	Dissection of renal artery
I77.79	Dissection of other specified artery
I79.0	Aneurysm of aorta in diseases classified elsewhere
Q25.41	Absence and aplasia of aorta
Q25.42	Hypoplasia of aorta
Q25.43	Congenital aneurysm of aorta
Q25.44	Congenital dilation of aorta
Q25.45	Double aortic arch
Q25.46	Tortuous aortic arch
Q25.47	Right aortic arch
Q25.48	Anomalous origin of subclavian artery
Q25.49	Other congenital malformations of aorta
Q25.8	Other congenital malformations of other great arteries
S35.01XA	Minor laceration of abdominal aorta, initial encounter
S35.02XA	Major laceration of abdominal aorta, initial encounter
S35.09XA	Other injury of abdominal aorta, initial encounter
S35.211A	Minor laceration of celiac artery, initial encounter
S35.212A	Major laceration of celiac artery, initial encounter
S35.218A	Other injury of celiac artery, initial encounter
S35.221A	Minor laceration of superior mesenteric artery, initial encounter
S35.222A	Major laceration of superior mesenteric artery, initial encounter
S35.228A	Other injury of superior mesenteric artery, initial encounter
S35.291A	Minor laceration of branches of celiac and mesenteric artery, initial encounter
S35.292A	Major laceration of branches of celiac and mesenteric artery, initial encounter
S35.298A	Other injury of branches of celiac and mesenteric artery, initial encounter
S35.411A	Laceration of right renal artery, initial encounter ☑
S35.412A	Laceration of left renal artery, initial encounter ☑
S35.491A	Other specified injury of right renal artery, initial encounter ☑
S35.492A	Other specified injury of left renal artery, initial encounter ☑
S35.8X1A	Laceration of other blood vessels at abdomen, lower back and pelvis level, initial encounter
S35.8X8A	Other specified injury of other blood vessels at abdomen, lower back and pelvis level, initial encounter

Relative Value Units/Medicare Edits

Non-Facility RVU	Work	PE	MP	Total
34839	0.0	0.0	0.0	0.0
Facility RVU	**Work**	**PE**	**MP**	**Total**
34839	0.0	0.0	0.0	0.0

	FUD	Status	MUE	Modifiers				IOM Reference
34839	N/A	B	1(2)	N/A	N/A	N/A	80*	None

* with documentation

Terms To Know

aneurysm. Circumscribed dilation or outpouching of an artery wall, often containing blood clots and connecting directly with the lumen of the artery.

dissection. (dis. apart; -section, act of cutting) Separating by cutting tissue or body structures apart.

fenestration. Presence of small openings from piercing or perforations.

graft. Tissue implant from another part of the body or another person.

vascular. Pertaining to blood vessels.

34841-34844

34841 Endovascular repair of visceral aorta (eg, aneurysm, pseudoaneurysm, dissection, penetrating ulcer, intramural hematoma, or traumatic disruption) by deployment of a fenestrated visceral aortic endograft and all associated radiological supervision and interpretation, including target zone angioplasty, when performed; including one visceral artery endoprosthesis (superior mesenteric, celiac or renal artery)

34842 including two visceral artery endoprostheses (superior mesenteric, celiac and/or renal artery[s])

34843 including three visceral artery endoprostheses (superior mesenteric, celiac and/or renal artery[s])

34844 including four or more visceral artery endoprostheses (superior mesenteric, celiac and/or renal artery[s])

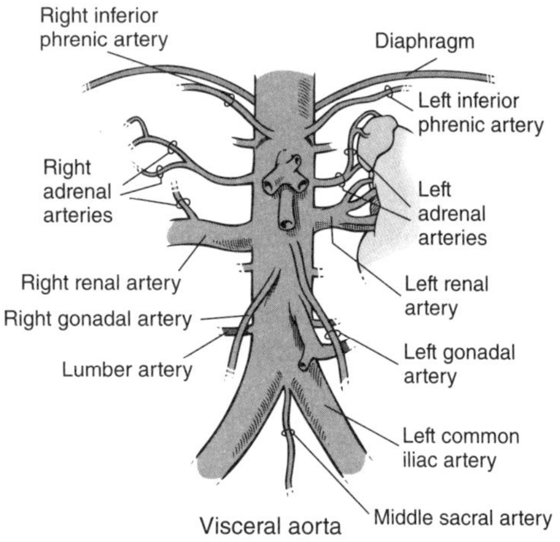

Explanation

Endovascular repair of an abdominal aortic aneurysm, pseudoaneurysm, or dissection, using a prosthesis, and involving visceral branches (superior mesenteric, celiac, and/or renal artery) requires the skills of a vascular surgeon and a radiologist. A small incision is made in the groin over both femoral arteries. Under fluoroscopic guidance, the physician inserts an aortic component through one femoral artery. These are contained inside a plastic holding capsule that is threaded through the arteries to the site of the aneurysm. The physician places the necessary extension prostheses and cuts fenestrations (holes) at each visceral artery orifice to allow side branch perfusion of these vessels. Next, catheters are used to place overlapping stents at each fenestration and vessel orifice to secure the junction. Once the graft components and stents are in place, the holding capsule and catheters are removed and the arteriotomy site is closed. Report 34841 when one visceral artery is included, 34842 for two, 34843 for three, and 34844 for four or more arteries.

Coding Tips

Do not report introduction of catheters and guidewires into the aorta and visceral and/or renal arteries separately in addition to these procedures. Balloon angioplasty within the target zone of the endograft is also not reported separately, whether prior to or after graft deployment. Fluoroscopic guidance is included in these procedures and not reported separately. Catheterization of the hypogastric arteries, arterial families outside of the treatment zone of the graft, exposure of the access vessels, extensive repair of the access vessels, and other separate interventional procedures outside of the target treatment zone performed at the time of this service may be reported separately. For endovascular treatment of the descending thoracic aorta, see 33880–33886 and 75956–75959. For endovascular infrarenal abdominal aortic aneurysm repair without the use of a graft, see 34701–34706. Do not report these codes with 34701–34706 or 34845–34848. Do not report these codes in addition to 34839 when planning is performed the day before or the day of the fenestrated repair. These codes should not be reported with 37236 or 37237 when covered or bare metal stents are placed into the visceral branches of the endoprosthesis target zone.

ICD-10-CM Diagnostic Codes

A52.01	Syphilitic aneurysm of aorta
I71.02	Dissection of abdominal aorta
I71.03	Dissection of thoracoabdominal aorta
I71.31	Pararenal abdominal aortic aneurysm, ruptured
I71.32	Juxtarenal abdominal aortic aneurysm, ruptured
I71.51	Supraceliac aneurysm of the thoracoabdominal aorta, ruptured
I71.52	Paravisceral aneurysm of the thoracoabdominal aorta, ruptured
I71.61	Supraceliac aneurysm of the thoracoabdominal aorta, without rupture
I71.62	Paravisceral aneurysm of the thoracoabdominal aorta, without rupture
Q25.43	Congenital aneurysm of aorta
Q25.44	Congenital dilation of aorta
Q25.49	Other congenital malformations of aorta
S35.01XA	Minor laceration of abdominal aorta, initial encounter
S35.02XA	Major laceration of abdominal aorta, initial encounter
S35.09XA	Other injury of abdominal aorta, initial encounter
T82.818A	Embolism due to vascular prosthetic devices, implants and grafts, initial encounter
T82.858A	Stenosis of other vascular prosthetic devices, implants and grafts, initial encounter
T82.868A	Thrombosis due to vascular prosthetic devices, implants and grafts, initial encounter

Relative Value Units/Medicare Edits

Non-Facility RVU	Work	PE	MP	Total
34841	0.0	0.0	0.0	0.0
34842	0.0	0.0	0.0	0.0
34843	0.0	0.0	0.0	0.0
34844	0.0	0.0	0.0	0.0
Facility RVU	**Work**	**PE**	**MP**	**Total**
34841	0.0	0.0	0.0	0.0
34842	0.0	0.0	0.0	0.0
34843	0.0	0.0	0.0	0.0
34844	0.0	0.0	0.0	0.0

	FUD	Status	MUE	Modifiers				IOM Reference
34841	N/A	C	1(2)	51	N/A	62	80	None
34842	N/A	C	1(2)	51	N/A	62	80	
34843	N/A	C	1(2)	51	N/A	62	80	
34844	N/A	C	1(2)	51	N/A	62	80	

* with documentation

34845-34848

34845 Endovascular repair of visceral aorta and infrarenal abdominal aorta (eg, aneurysm, pseudoaneurysm, dissection, penetrating ulcer, intramural hematoma, or traumatic disruption) with a fenestrated visceral aortic endograft and concomitant unibody or modular infrarenal aortic endograft and all associated radiological supervision and interpretation, including target zone angioplasty, when performed; including one visceral artery endoprosthesis (superior mesenteric, celiac or renal artery)

34846 including two visceral artery endoprostheses (superior mesenteric, celiac and/or renal artery[s])

34847 including three visceral artery endoprostheses (superior mesenteric, celiac and/or renal artery[s])

34848 including four or more visceral artery endoprostheses (superior mesenteric, celiac and/or renal artery[s])

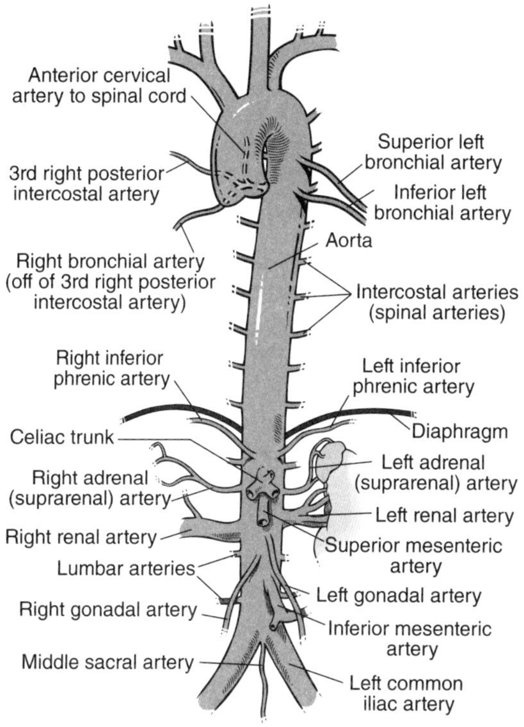

Explanation

Endovascular repair of an abdominal aortic aneurysm, pseudoaneurysm, or dissection, using a prosthesis, and involving visceral branches (superior mesenteric, celiac, and/or renal artery) requires the skills of a vascular surgeon and a radiologist. A small incision is made in the groin over both femoral arteries through which the endovascular devices are inserted. Under fluoroscopic guidance, the physician inserts the aortic component and one iliac limb through one femoral artery. These are contained inside a plastic holding capsule that is threaded through the arteries to the site of the aneurysm. Next, the physician inserts the opposite iliac limb by contralateral femoral artery access. The physician mates the aortic and iliac limb inserted into the first femoral artery to the opposite iliac limb inserted by contralateral femoral artery access. Since this repair extends above the visceral vessels, a visceral extension prosthesis is required. The physician places the extension prosthesis and cuts fenestrations (holes) at each visceral artery orifice to allow side branch perfusion of these vessels. Catheters are used to place overlapping stents at each fenestration and vessel orifice to secure the junction. Once the graft components and stents are in place, the holding capsule and catheters are removed and the arteriotomy site is closed. Report 34845 when one visceral artery is included, 34846 for two, 34847 for three, and 34848 for four or more arteries.

Coding Tips

Do not report introduction of catheters and guidewires into the aorta and visceral and/or renal arteries separately with these procedures. Balloon angioplasty within the target zone of the endograft is also not reported separately, whether prior to or after graft deployment. Fluoroscopic guidance with these procedures is included and is not reported separately. Catheterization of the hypogastric arteries, arterial families outside of the treatment zone of the graft, exposure of the access vessels, extensive repair of the access vessels, and other separate interventional procedures outside of the target treatment zone performed at the time of this service may be reported separately. For endovascular treatment of the descending thoracic aorta, see 33880–33886 and 75956–75959. For endovascular infrarenal abdominal aortic aneurysm repair without the use of a graft, see 34701–34706. Do not report these codes with 34701–34706, 34841–34844, 35081, or 35102. Do not report these codes with 37220–37223 for endovascular revascularization except when performed outside of the area treated with the endoprosthesis. Do not report these codes with 34839 when planning occurs the day before or the day of repair. For placement of distal extension prosthesis terminating in the internal or external iliac or common femoral artery, see 34709-34711 or 34718. These codes should not be reported with 37236 or 37237 when covered or bare metal stents are placed into the visceral branches of the endoprosthesis target zone.

ICD-10-CM Diagnostic Codes

A52.01	Syphilitic aneurysm of aorta
I71.02	Dissection of abdominal aorta
I71.03	Dissection of thoracoabdominal aorta
I71.31	Pararenal abdominal aortic aneurysm, ruptured
I71.32	Juxtarenal abdominal aortic aneurysm, ruptured
I71.33	Infrarenal abdominal aortic aneurysm, ruptured
I71.51	Supraceliac aneurysm of the thoracoabdominal aorta, ruptured
I71.52	Paravisceral aneurysm of the thoracoabdominal aorta, ruptured
I71.61	Supraceliac aneurysm of the thoracoabdominal aorta, without rupture
I71.62	Paravisceral aneurysm of the thoracoabdominal aorta, without rupture
I79.0	Aneurysm of aorta in diseases classified elsewhere
Q25.41	Absence and aplasia of aorta
Q25.42	Hypoplasia of aorta
Q25.43	Congenital aneurysm of aorta
Q25.44	Congenital dilation of aorta
Q25.48	Anomalous origin of subclavian artery
Q25.49	Other congenital malformations of aorta
S35.01XA	Minor laceration of abdominal aorta, initial encounter
S35.02XA	Major laceration of abdominal aorta, initial encounter
S35.09XA	Other injury of abdominal aorta, initial encounter

AMA: **34845** 2022,Oct **34846** 2022,Oct **34847** 2022,Oct **34848** 2022,Oct

Relative Value Units/Medicare Edits

Non-Facility RVU	Work	PE	MP	Total
34845	0.0	0.0	0.0	0.0
34846	0.0	0.0	0.0	0.0
34847	0.0	0.0	0.0	0.0
34848	0.0	0.0	0.0	0.0
Facility RVU	**Work**	**PE**	**MP**	**Total**
34845	0.0	0.0	0.0	0.0
34846	0.0	0.0	0.0	0.0
34847	0.0	0.0	0.0	0.0
34848	0.0	0.0	0.0	0.0

	FUD	Status	MUE	Modifiers				IOM Reference
34845	N/A	C	1(2)	51	N/A	62	80	None
34846	N/A	C	1(2)	51	N/A	62	80	
34847	N/A	C	1(2)	51	N/A	62	80	
34848	N/A	C	1(2)	51	N/A	62	80	

* with documentation

Terms To Know

aneurysm. Circumscribed dilation or outpouching of an artery wall, often containing blood clots and connecting directly with the lumen of the artery.

angioplasty. Reconstruction or repair of a diseased or damaged blood vessel.

dissection. (dis. apart; -section, act of cutting) Separating by cutting tissue or body structures apart.

endoprosthesis. Intravascular device in the form of a hollow stent placed within a duct or artery to provide passage through an obstructed area, such as in a bile duct, or to act as a replacement for damaged arterial walls, as in treating an aneurysm.

pseudoaneurysm. False aneurysm produced by a dilated vessel wall, or a ruptured blood vessel that has formed a clot that pulsates, mimicking a true aneurysm.

vascular. Pertaining to blood vessels.

35001-35002

35001 Direct repair of aneurysm, pseudoaneurysm, or excision (partial or total) and graft insertion, with or without patch graft; for aneurysm and associated occlusive disease, carotid, subclavian artery, by neck incision

35002 for ruptured aneurysm, carotid, subclavian artery, by neck incision

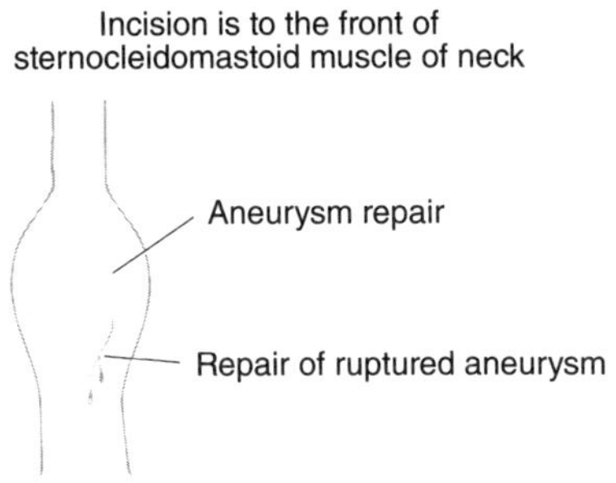

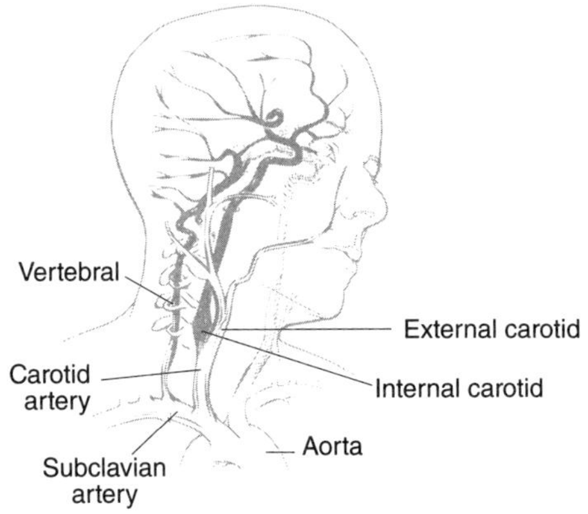

Explanation

The physician makes an incision in the neck in front of the sternocleidomastoid muscle. The section of the carotid or subclavian artery (35001) or the ruptured section (35002) is isolated and dissected from adjacent critical structures. Vessel clamps are affixed above and below the defect. The repair may be accomplished by removing the segment of artery containing the aneurysm and suturing the exposed ends of the vessel in an end-to-end fashion or the aneurysm may be bypassed with a venous or synthetic graft. If a large section is removed, a harvested or synthetic graft is inserted into the defect, or a patch may be sutured into place to open up the diameter of the vessel. The skin incision is repaired with a layered closure.

Coding Tips

Preparation of the artery for anastomosis, including endarterectomy, is integral to the procedure and should not be reported separately. Establishing inflow and outflow by any method is included. The portion of the operative arteriogram performed by the surgeon is also included. Angioscopy performed during therapeutic intervention should be reported in addition to the code for the primary procedure; see 35400. Harvested vein or synthetic material may be used for the graft. Any graft harvest is not reported separately. For direct repairs associated with occlusive disease only, see 35201, 35231, and 35261.

ICD-10-CM Diagnostic Codes

G45.1	Carotid artery syndrome (hemispheric)
G45.2	Multiple and bilateral precerebral artery syndromes
G45.3	Amaurosis fugax

G45.8	Other transient cerebral ischemic attacks and related syndromes
G45.9	Transient cerebral ischemic attack, unspecified
I63.031	Cerebral infarction due to thrombosis of right carotid artery ☑
I63.032	Cerebral infarction due to thrombosis of left carotid artery ☑
I63.09	Cerebral infarction due to thrombosis of other precerebral artery
I63.131	Cerebral infarction due to embolism of right carotid artery ☑
I63.132	Cerebral infarction due to embolism of left carotid artery ☑
I63.19	Cerebral infarction due to embolism of other precerebral artery
I65.21	Occlusion and stenosis of right carotid artery ☑
I65.22	Occlusion and stenosis of left carotid artery ☑
I65.23	Occlusion and stenosis of bilateral carotid arteries ☑
I65.8	Occlusion and stenosis of other precerebral arteries
I72.0	Aneurysm of carotid artery
I72.6	Aneurysm of vertebral artery
I77.1	Stricture of artery
I77.2	Rupture of artery
I77.71	Dissection of carotid artery
I77.76	Dissection of artery of upper extremity
I77.77	Dissection of artery of lower extremity
I77.79	Dissection of other specified artery
I77.89	Other specified disorders of arteries and arterioles

Relative Value Units/Medicare Edits

Non-Facility RVU	Work	PE	MP	Total
35001	20.81	6.88	5.24	32.93
35002	22.23	5.62	5.54	33.39
Facility RVU	**Work**	**PE**	**MP**	**Total**
35001	20.81	6.88	5.24	32.93
35002	22.23	5.62	5.54	33.39

	FUD	Status	MUE	Modifiers				IOM Reference
35001	90	A	1(2)	51	50	62*	80	None
35002	90	A	1(2)	51	50	62*	80	

* with documentation

Terms To Know

anastomosis. Surgically created connection between ducts, blood vessels, or bowel segments to allow flow from one to the other.

35005

35005 Direct repair of aneurysm, pseudoaneurysm, or excision (partial or total) and graft insertion, with or without patch graft; for aneurysm, pseudoaneurysm, and associated occlusive disease, vertebral artery

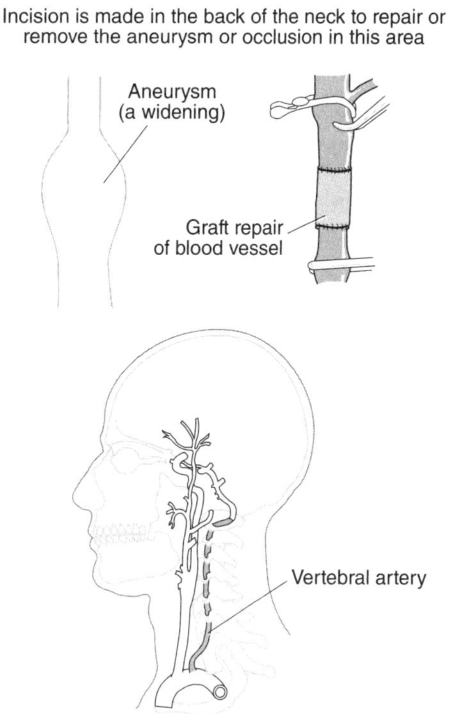

Explanation

The physician makes an incision in the skin overlying the neck. The enlarged or blocked section of the vertebral artery is isolated and dissected from muscles and adjacent critical structures. A portion of a cervical vertebra may be removed to access the defect. Vessel clamps are affixed above and below the defect, which may be repaired or removed. The repair may be accomplished by removing the segment of artery containing the aneurysm and suturing the exposed ends of the vessel in an end-to-end fashion or the aneurysm may be bypassed with a venous or synthetic graft. If a large section is removed, a harvested or synthetic graft is inserted into the defect. Instead of a complete graft, a patch may be sutured into place to open up the diameter of the vessel. Once the vessel is repaired, the clamps are removed. The skin incision is repaired with a layered closure.

Coding Tips

Preparation of the artery for anastomosis, including endarterectomy, is integral to the procedure and should not be reported separately. Establishing both inflow and outflow by any method is included. The portion of the operative arteriogram performed by the surgeon is also included. Angioscopy performed during therapeutic intervention should be reported in addition to the code for the primary procedure, see 35400. Harvested vein or synthetic material may be used for the graft. Any graft harvest is not reported separately. For direct repairs associated with occlusive disease only, see 35201, 35231, and 35261.

ICD-10-CM Diagnostic Codes

G45.8	Other transient cerebral ischemic attacks and related syndromes
I63.011	Cerebral infarction due to thrombosis of right vertebral artery ☑
I63.012	Cerebral infarction due to thrombosis of left vertebral artery ☑

I63.013 Cerebral infarction due to thrombosis of bilateral vertebral arteries ☑
I63.111 Cerebral infarction due to embolism of right vertebral artery ☑
I63.112 Cerebral infarction due to embolism of left vertebral artery ☑
I63.113 Cerebral infarction due to embolism of bilateral vertebral arteries ☑
I65.01 Occlusion and stenosis of right vertebral artery ☑
I65.02 Occlusion and stenosis of left vertebral artery ☑
I65.03 Occlusion and stenosis of bilateral vertebral arteries ☑
I77.74 Dissection of vertebral artery
I77.89 Other specified disorders of arteries and arterioles

Relative Value Units/Medicare Edits

Non-Facility RVU	Work	PE	MP	Total
35005	19.29	5.16	4.79	29.24
Facility RVU	**Work**	**PE**	**MP**	**Total**
35005	19.29	5.16	4.79	29.24

	FUD	Status	MUE	Modifiers				IOM Reference
35005	90	A	1(2)	51	50	62*	80	None

* with documentation

Terms To Know

aneurysm. Circumscribed dilation or outpouching of an artery wall, often containing blood clots and connecting directly with the lumen of the artery.

dissection. Separating by cutting tissue or body structures apart.

embolism. Obstruction of a blood vessel resulting from a clot or foreign substance.

pseudoaneurysm. False aneurysm produced by a dilated vessel wall, or a ruptured blood vessel that has formed a clot that pulsates, mimicking a true aneurysm.

stenosis. Narrowing or constriction of a passage.

35011-35013

35011 Direct repair of aneurysm, pseudoaneurysm, or excision (partial or total) and graft insertion, with or without patch graft; for aneurysm and associated occlusive disease, axillary-brachial artery, by arm incision

35013 for ruptured aneurysm, axillary-brachial artery, by arm incision

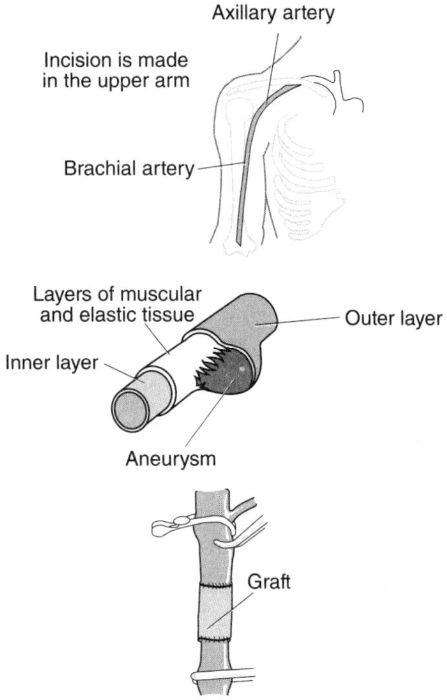

Explanation

The physician makes an incision in the skin of the arm or axilla. The enlarged or blocked section of the axillary or brachial artery (35011) or the ruptured section (35013) is isolated and dissected from adjacent critical structures. Vessel clamps are affixed above and below the defect, which may be repaired or removed. The repair may be accomplished by removing the segment of artery containing the aneurysm and suturing the exposed ends of the vessel in an end-to-end fashion or the aneurysm may be bypassed with a venous or synthetic graft. If a large section is removed, a harvested or synthetic graft is inserted into the defect. Instead of a complete graft, a patch may be sutured into place to open up the diameter of the vessel. Once the vessel is repaired, the clamps are removed. The skin incision is repaired with a layered closure.

Coding Tips

Preparation of the artery for anastomosis, including endarterectomy, is integral to the procedure and should not be reported separately. Establishing both inflow and outflow by any method is included. The portion of the operative arteriogram performed by the surgeon is also included. Angioscopy performed during therapeutic intervention should be reported in addition to the code for the primary procedure; see 35400. Harvested vein or synthetic material may be used for the graft. Any graft harvest is not reported separately. For direct repairs associated with occlusive disease only, see 35206, 35236, and 35266.

ICD-10-CM Diagnostic Codes

I70.8 Atherosclerosis of other arteries [A]
I70.92 Chronic total occlusion of artery of the extremities [A]
I72.1 Aneurysm of artery of upper extremity

I72.8	Aneurysm of other specified arteries
I74.2	Embolism and thrombosis of arteries of the upper extremities
I75.011	Atheroembolism of right upper extremity ☑
I75.012	Atheroembolism of left upper extremity ☑
I75.013	Atheroembolism of bilateral upper extremities ☑
I77.1	Stricture of artery
I77.2	Rupture of artery
I77.79	Dissection of other specified artery

Relative Value Units/Medicare Edits

Non-Facility RVU	Work	PE	MP	Total
35011	18.58	6.45	4.65	29.68
35013	23.23	8.2	5.82	37.25
Facility RVU	**Work**	**PE**	**MP**	**Total**
35011	18.58	6.45	4.65	29.68
35013	23.23	8.2	5.82	37.25

	FUD	Status	MUE	Modifiers				IOM Reference
35011	90	A	1(2)	51	50	62*	80	None
35013	90	A	1(2)	51	50	62*	80	

* with documentation

Terms To Know

anastomosis. Surgically created connection between ducts, blood vessels, or bowel segments to allow flow from one to the other.

aneurysm. Circumscribed dilation or outpouching of an artery wall, often containing blood clots and connecting directly with the lumen of the artery.

angioscopy. Visualization of capillary blood vessels with a microscope, or the inside of a blood vessel with a fiberoptic-equipped catheter.

atherosclerosis. Buildup of yellowish plaques composed of cholesterol and lipoid material within the arteries.

claudication. Lameness, pain, and weakness occurring in the arms or legs during exercise due to muscles not receiving the needed oxygen and nutrients.

embolism. Obstruction of a blood vessel resulting from a clot or foreign substance.

pseudoaneurysm. False aneurysm produced by a dilated vessel wall, or a ruptured blood vessel that has formed a clot that pulsates, mimicking a true aneurysm.

stricture. Narrowing of an anatomical structure.

35021-35022

35021 Direct repair of aneurysm, pseudoaneurysm, or excision (partial or total) and graft insertion, with or without patch graft; for aneurysm, pseudoaneurysm, and associated occlusive disease, innominate, subclavian artery, by thoracic incision

35022 for ruptured aneurysm, innominate, subclavian artery, by thoracic incision

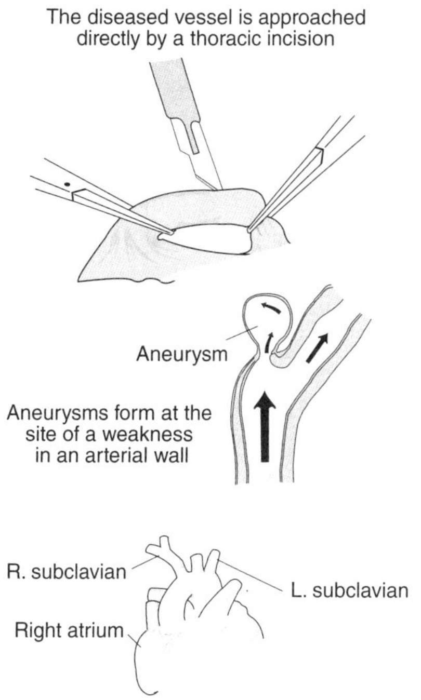

Explanation

The physician exposes the innominate or subclavian artery by median sternotomy or lateral thoracotomy. In 35021, the physician anticoagulates the patient with heparin, clamps the aortic arch widely around the origin of the innominate artery, and clamps the right common carotid and right subclavian arteries. The physician excises the aneurysmal tissue. In 35022, the physician clamps the aortic arch widely around the origin of the innominate artery, and clamps the right common carotid and right subclavian arteries. The physician excises the ruptured aneurysmal tissue. In both procedures, the physician may use a woven Dacron patch graft or harvested vein to repair the aneurysmal artery. The physician unclamps the aorta, as well as the right common carotid and right subclavian arteries. The physician closes the sternotomy or thoracotomy, leaving a chest tube in place.

Coding Tips

Preparation of the artery for anastomosis, including endarterectomy, is integral to the procedure and should not be reported separately. Establishing both inflow and outflow by any method is included. The portion of the operative arteriogram performed by the surgeon is also included. Angioscopy performed during therapeutic intervention should be reported in addition to the code for the primary procedure; see 35400. Harvested vein or synthetic material may be used for the graft. Any graft harvest is not reported separately. For direct repairs associated with occlusive disease only, see 35211, 35216, 35241, 35246, 35271, and 35276.

ICD-10-CM Diagnostic Codes

G45.2	Multiple and bilateral precerebral artery syndromes
G45.3	Amaurosis fugax

G45.8	Other transient cerebral ischemic attacks and related syndromes
I63.09	Cerebral infarction due to thrombosis of other precerebral artery
I63.19	Cerebral infarction due to embolism of other precerebral artery
I63.29	Cerebral infarction due to unspecified occlusion or stenosis of other precerebral arteries
I63.81	Other cerebral infarction due to occlusion or stenosis of small artery
I63.89	Other cerebral infarction
I67.850	Cerebral autosomal dominant arteriopathy with subcortical infarcts and leukoencephalopathy
I67.858	Other hereditary cerebrovascular disease
I70.8	Atherosclerosis of other arteries [A]
I72.8	Aneurysm of other specified arteries
I77.1	Stricture of artery
I77.2	Rupture of artery
I77.79	Dissection of other specified artery
I77.89	Other specified disorders of arteries and arterioles
Q28.1	Other malformations of precerebral vessels
Q28.8	Other specified congenital malformations of circulatory system

Relative Value Units/Medicare Edits

Non-Facility RVU	Work	PE	MP	Total
35021	22.17	9.76	5.13	37.06
35022	25.7	10.71	5.96	42.37
Facility RVU	**Work**	**PE**	**MP**	**Total**
35021	22.17	9.76	5.13	37.06
35022	25.7	10.71	5.96	42.37

	FUD	Status	MUE	Modifiers				IOM Reference
35021	90	A	1(2)	51	50	62*	80	None
35022	90	A	1(2)	51	50	62*	80	

* with documentation

Terms To Know

anastomosis. Surgically created connection between ducts, blood vessels, or bowel segments to allow flow from one to the other.

aneurysm. Circumscribed dilation or outpouching of an artery wall, often containing blood clots and connecting directly with the lumen of the artery.

atherosclerosis. Buildup of yellowish plaques composed of cholesterol and lipoid material within the arteries.

median sternotomy. Standard incision for open chest cardiac surgeries, from above the bellybutton to just under the chin, down the center of the chest through the sternum into the thoracic cavity.

pseudoaneurysm. False aneurysm produced by a dilated vessel wall, or a ruptured blood vessel that has formed a clot that pulsates, mimicking a true aneurysm.

rupture. Tearing or breaking open of tissue.

thoracotomy. Surgical procedure for opening the chest wall in order to access the lungs, esophagus, trachea, aorta, heart, and diaphragm.

35045

35045 Direct repair of aneurysm, pseudoaneurysm, or excision (partial or total) and graft insertion, with or without patch graft; for aneurysm, pseudoaneurysm, and associated occlusive disease, radial or ulnar artery

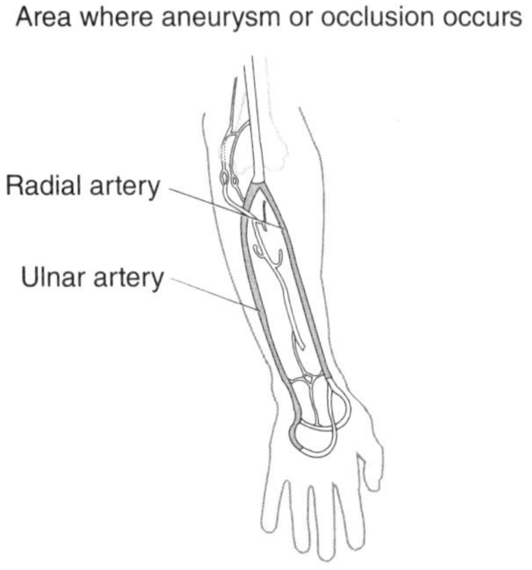

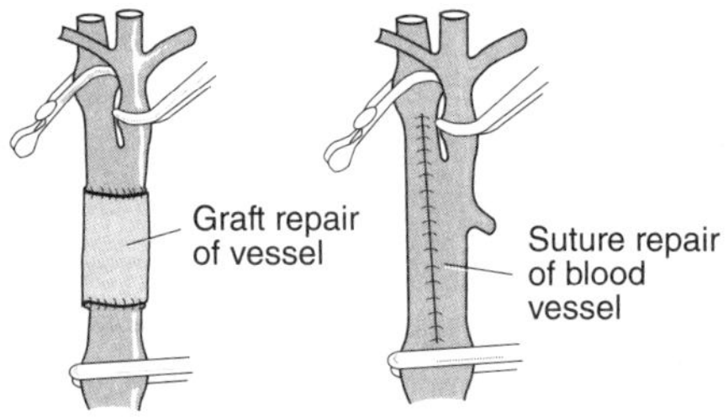

Explanation

The physician makes an incision in the skin overlying the arm. The enlarged or blocked section of the radial or ulnar artery is isolated and dissected from adjacent critical structures. Vessel clamps are affixed above and below the defect, which may be repaired or removed. The repair may be accomplished by removing the segment of artery containing the aneurysm and suturing the exposed ends of the vessel in an end-to-end fashion or the aneurysm may be bypassed with a venous or synthetic graft. If a large section is removed, a harvested or synthetic graft is inserted into the defect. Instead of a complete graft, a patch may be sutured into place to open up the diameter of the vessel. Once the vessel is repaired, the clamps are removed. The skin incision is repaired with a layered closure.

Coding Tips

Preparation of the artery for anastomosis, including endarterectomy, is integral to the procedure and should not be reported separately. Establishing both inflow and outflow by any method is included. The portion of the operative arteriogram performed by the surgeon is also included. Angioscopy performed during therapeutic intervention should be reported in addition to the code for the primary procedure; see 35400. Harvested vein or synthetic material may be used for the graft. Any graft harvest is not reported separately. For direct repairs associated with occlusive disease only, see 35206, 35236, and 35266.

ICD-10-CM Diagnostic Codes

I70.8	Atherosclerosis of other arteries [A]
I70.92	Chronic total occlusion of artery of the extremities [A]
I72.1	Aneurysm of artery of upper extremity

I72.8	Aneurysm of other specified arteries	
I74.2	Embolism and thrombosis of arteries of the upper extremities	
I75.011	Atheroembolism of right upper extremity ☑	
I75.012	Atheroembolism of left upper extremity ☑	
I75.013	Atheroembolism of bilateral upper extremities ☑	
I77.1	Stricture of artery	
I77.2	Rupture of artery	
I77.79	Dissection of other specified artery	
I77.89	Other specified disorders of arteries and arterioles	

Relative Value Units/Medicare Edits

Non-Facility RVU	Work	PE	MP	Total
35045	18.01	6.11	4.37	28.49
Facility RVU	**Work**	**PE**	**MP**	**Total**
35045	18.01	6.11	4.37	28.49

	FUD	Status	MUE	Modifiers				IOM Reference
35045	90	A	1(3)	51	50	62*	80	None

* with documentation

Terms To Know

anastomosis. Surgically created connection between ducts, blood vessels, or bowel segments to allow flow from one to the other.

aneurysm. Circumscribed dilation or outpouching of an artery wall, often containing blood clots and connecting directly with the lumen of the artery.

atherosclerosis. Buildup of yellowish plaques composed of cholesterol and lipoid material within the arteries.

suture. Numerous stitching techniques employed in wound closure.

buried suture. Continuous or interrupted suture placed under the skin for a layered closure.

continuous suture. Running stitch with tension evenly distributed across a single strand to provide a leakproof closure line.

interrupted suture. Series of single stitches with tension isolated at each stitch, in which all stitches are not affected if one becomes loose, and the isolated sutures cannot act as a wick to transport an infection.

purse-string suture. Continuous suture placed around a tubular structure and tightened, to reduce or close the lumen.

retention suture. Secondary stitching that bridges the primary suture, providing support for the primary repair; a plastic or rubber bolster may be placed over the primary repair and under the retention sutures.

35081

35081 Direct repair of aneurysm, pseudoaneurysm, or excision (partial or total) and graft insertion, with or without patch graft; for aneurysm, pseudoaneurysm, and associated occlusive disease, abdominal aorta

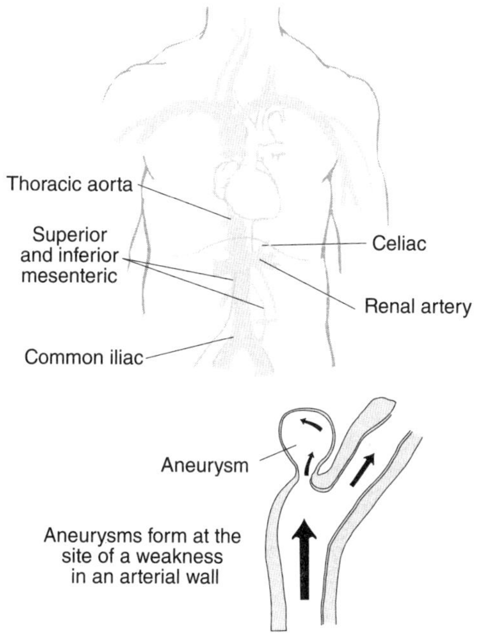

The aneurysm or occlusion of the abdominal aorta is repaired with a graft insertion. A patch graft may be required

Explanation

The physician exposes the abdominal aorta using a transperitoneal approach, placing a long incision in the mid abdomen. The physician retracts the transverse colon and small bowel to allow dissection and exposure of the aorta. The physician places an umbilical tape or rubber catheter around the aorta proximal to the aneurysm. The physician exposes the iliac arteries and achieves control of blood flow with umbilical tape or rubber catheters. The physician anticoagulates the patient and cross-clamps the iliac arteries and proximal aorta. The physician opens and clears the aneurysm, controls collateral bleeding from the lumbar arteries with suture, and sutures a Y-shaped knitted Dacron graft to the proximal aorta. The physician sutures the distal ends of the graft to the iliac arteries. The physician may anastomose the inferior mesenteric arteries and any aberrant or accessory renal arteries to the Dacron graft. The physician sutures the remaining aneurysmal shell around the graft and closes the retroperitoneum. The physician closes the abdominal wound, leaving drains in place.

Coding Tips

Preparation of the artery for anastomosis, including endarterectomy, is integral to the procedure and should not be reported separately. Establishing both inflow and outflow by any method is included. The portion of the operative arteriogram performed by the surgeon is also included. Angioscopy performed during therapeutic intervention should be reported in addition to the code for the primary procedure; see 35400. Harvested vein or synthetic material may be used for the graft. Any graft harvest is not reported separately. For thoracic aortic aneurysm, see 33858–33875. For direct repairs associated with occlusive disease only, see 35221, 35251, and 35281.

ICD-10-CM Diagnostic Codes

I70.0	Atherosclerosis of aorta [A]

I71.02	Dissection of abdominal aorta
I71.61	Supraceliac aneurysm of the thoracoabdominal aorta, without rupture
I71.62	Paravisceral aneurysm of the thoracoabdominal aorta, without rupture
I74.01	Saddle embolus of abdominal aorta
I74.09	Other arterial embolism and thrombosis of abdominal aorta
I76	Septic arterial embolism
I77.1	Stricture of artery
I77.89	Other specified disorders of arteries and arterioles
Q25.43	Congenital aneurysm of aorta
Q25.44	Congenital dilation of aorta
Q79.61	Classical Ehlers-Danlos syndrome
Q79.62	Hypermobile Ehlers-Danlos syndrome
Q79.63	Vascular Ehlers-Danlos syndrome
Q87.410	Marfan syndrome with aortic dilation

Relative Value Units/Medicare Edits

Non-Facility RVU	Work	PE	MP	Total
35081	33.53	8.81	8.33	50.67
Facility RVU	**Work**	**PE**	**MP**	**Total**
35081	33.53	8.81	8.33	50.67

	FUD	Status	MUE	Modifiers				IOM Reference
35081	90	A	1(2)	51	N/A	62*	80	None

* with documentation

Terms To Know

aneurysm. Circumscribed dilation or outpouching of an artery wall, often containing blood clots and connecting directly with the lumen of the artery.

atherosclerosis. Buildup of yellowish plaques composed of cholesterol and lipoid material within the arteries.

embolism. Obstruction of a blood vessel resulting from a clot or foreign substance.

pseudoaneurysm. False aneurysm produced by a dilated vessel wall, or a ruptured blood vessel that has formed a clot that pulsates, mimicking a true aneurysm.

35082

35082 Direct repair of aneurysm, pseudoaneurysm, or excision (partial or total) and graft insertion, with or without patch graft; for ruptured aneurysm, abdominal aorta

Access is via an abdominal incision

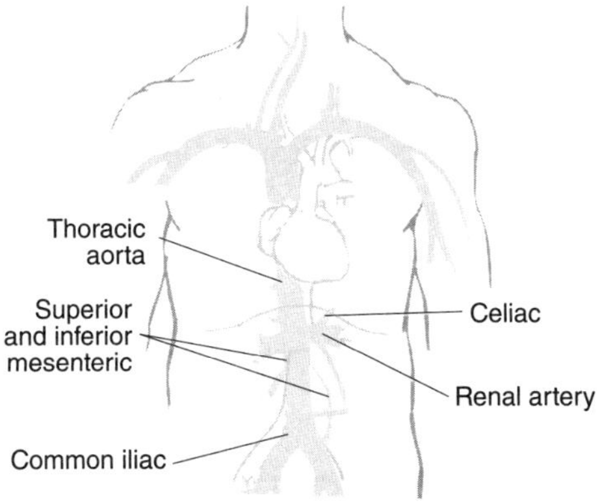

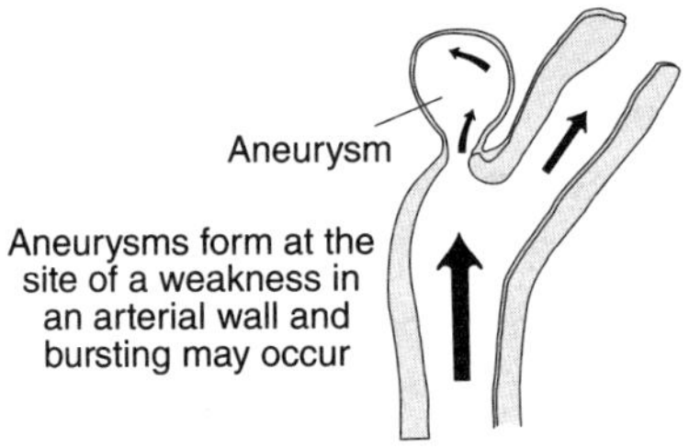

A burst aneurysm or occlusion of the abdominal aorta is repaired with a graft insertion. A patch graft may be required

Explanation

The physician quickly exposes the abdominal aorta using a transperitoneal approach, placing a long incision in the midabdomen, and retracts the transverse colon and small bowel to allow dissection and exposure of the aorta. Bleeding control is achieved by pushing the liver aside and compressing the aorta manually against the spine. The aorta is cross-clamped proximal to the dissection. The physician exposes the iliac arteries and achieves control of blood flow with umbilical tape or rubber catheters. If bleeding is controlled, the patient receives anticoagulation while the iliac arteries and proximal aorta are cross-clamped. The physician opens and clears the aneurysm, controls collateral bleeding from the lumbar arteries with suture, and sutures a Y-shaped knitted Dacron graft to the proximal aorta. The distal ends of the graft are sutured to the iliac arteries with the remaining aneurysmal shell around the graft. The retroperitoneum and abdominal wounds are closed, leaving drains in place.

Coding Tips

Preparation of the artery for anastomosis, including endarterectomy, is integral to the procedure and should not be reported separately. Establishing both inflow and outflow by any method is included. The portion of the operative arteriogram performed by the surgeon is also included. Angioscopy performed during therapeutic intervention should be reported in addition to the code for the primary procedure; see 35400. Harvested vein or synthetic material may be used for the graft. Any graft harvest is not reported separately. For thoracic aortic aneurysm, see 33858–33875. For direct repairs associated with occlusive disease only, see 35221, 35251, and 35281.

ICD-10-CM Diagnostic Codes

I71.31	Pararenal abdominal aortic aneurysm, ruptured
I71.32	Juxtarenal abdominal aortic aneurysm, ruptured
I71.33	Infrarenal abdominal aortic aneurysm, ruptured
I71.51	Supraceliac aneurysm of the thoracoabdominal aorta, ruptured
I71.52	Paravisceral aneurysm of the thoracoabdominal aorta, ruptured
I74.01	Saddle embolus of abdominal aorta
S35.02XA	Major laceration of abdominal aorta, initial encounter

Relative Value Units/Medicare Edits

Non-Facility RVU	Work	PE	MP	Total
35082	42.09	10.72	10.44	63.25
Facility RVU	**Work**	**PE**	**MP**	**Total**
35082	42.09	10.72	10.44	63.25

	FUD	Status	MUE	Modifiers				IOM Reference
35082	90	A	1(2)	51	N/A	62*	80	None

* with documentation

Terms To Know

anastomosis. Surgically created connection between ducts, blood vessels, or bowel segments to allow flow from one to the other.

aneurysm. Circumscribed dilation or outpouching of an artery wall, often containing blood clots and connecting directly with the lumen of the artery.

angioscopy. Visualization of capillary blood vessels with a microscope, or the inside of a blood vessel with a fiberoptic-equipped catheter.

arteriogram. Radiograph of arteries.

atherosclerosis. Buildup of yellowish plaques composed of cholesterol and lipoid material within the arteries.

35091

35091 Direct repair of aneurysm, pseudoaneurysm, or excision (partial or total) and graft insertion, with or without patch graft; for aneurysm, pseudoaneurysm, and associated occlusive disease, abdominal aorta involving visceral vessels (mesenteric, celiac, renal)

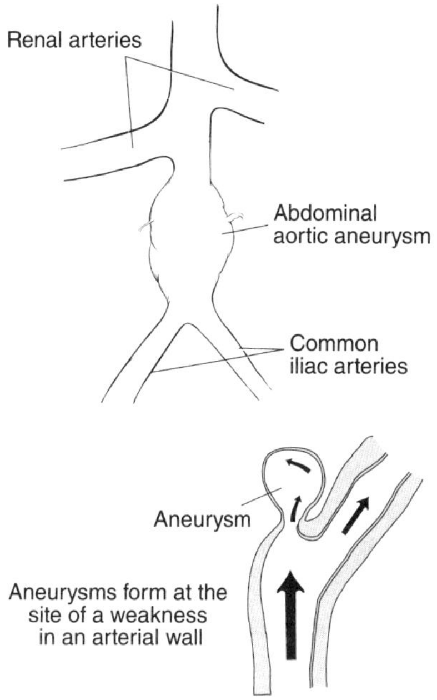

An aneurysm or occlusion of the abdominal aorta is repaired with a graft insertion. Mesenteric, celiac, or renal vessels may be involved and a patch graft may be required

Explanation

The physician exposes the abdominal aorta using a transperitoneal approach, placing a long incision in the midabdomen. The physician retracts the transverse colon and small bowel to allow dissection and exposure of the aorta. The physician places an umbilical tape or rubber catheter around the aorta proximal to the aneurysm. The physician exposes the iliac arteries and achieves control of blood flow with umbilical tape or rubber catheters. The physician anticoagulates the patient and cross-clamps the iliac arteries and proximal aorta. The physician opens and clears the aneurysm, controls collateral bleeding from the lumbar arteries with suture, and sutures a Y-shaped knitted Dacron graft to the proximal aorta. The physician sutures the distal ends of the graft to the iliac arteries. The physician will anastomose the inferior mesenteric arteries and any aberrant or accessory renal arteries to the Dacron graft, when applicable. The physician sutures the remaining aneurysmal shell around the graft and closes the retroperitoneum. The physician closes the abdominal wound, leaving drains in place.

Coding Tips

Preparation of the artery for anastomosis, including endarterectomy, is integral to the procedure and should not be reported separately. Establishing both inflow and outflow by any method is included. The portion of the operative arteriogram performed by the surgeon is also included. Angioscopy performed during therapeutic intervention should be reported in addition to the code for the primary procedure; see 35400. Harvested vein or synthetic material may be used for the graft. Any graft harvest is not reported separately. For thoracic aortic aneurysm, see 33858–33875. For direct repairs associated with occlusive disease only, see 35221, 35251, and 35281.

ICD-10-CM Diagnostic Codes

I70.0	Atherosclerosis of aorta A
I70.1	Atherosclerosis of renal artery A
I71.02	Dissection of abdominal aorta
I72.2	Aneurysm of renal artery
I77.1	Stricture of artery
I77.73	Dissection of renal artery
K55.011	Focal (segmental) acute (reversible) ischemia of small intestine
K55.012	Diffuse acute (reversible) ischemia of small intestine
K55.021	Focal (segmental) acute infarction of small intestine
K55.022	Diffuse acute infarction of small intestine
K55.031	Focal (segmental) acute (reversible) ischemia of large intestine
K55.032	Diffuse acute (reversible) ischemia of large intestine
K55.041	Focal (segmental) acute infarction of large intestine
K55.042	Diffuse acute infarction of large intestine
K55.1	Chronic vascular disorders of intestine
K55.8	Other vascular disorders of intestine
N28.0	Ischemia and infarction of kidney
Q25.43	Congenital aneurysm of aorta
Q25.44	Congenital dilation of aorta
Q79.61	Classical Ehlers-Danlos syndrome
Q79.62	Hypermobile Ehlers-Danlos syndrome
Q79.63	Vascular Ehlers-Danlos syndrome
Q87.410	Marfan syndrome with aortic dilation

Relative Value Units/Medicare Edits

Non-Facility RVU	Work	PE	MP	Total
35091	35.35	7.92	8.77	52.04
Facility RVU	**Work**	**PE**	**MP**	**Total**
35091	35.35	7.92	8.77	52.04

	FUD	Status	MUE	Modifiers				IOM Reference
35091	90	A	1(2)	51	50	62*	80	None

* with documentation

Terms To Know

anastomosis. Surgically created connection between ducts, blood vessels, or bowel segments to allow flow from one to the other.

aneurysm. Circumscribed dilation or outpouching of an artery wall, often containing blood clots and connecting directly with the lumen of the artery.

atherosclerosis. Buildup of yellowish plaques composed of cholesterol and lipoid material within the arteries.

pseudoaneurysm. False aneurysm produced by a dilated vessel wall, or a ruptured blood vessel that has formed a clot that pulsates, mimicking a true aneurysm.

35092

35092 Direct repair of aneurysm, pseudoaneurysm, or excision (partial or total) and graft insertion, with or without patch graft; for ruptured aneurysm, abdominal aorta involving visceral vessels (mesenteric, celiac, renal)

Report direct repair of a ruptured aneurysm of the abdominal aorta involving visceral vessels, such as celiac, renal, and/or mesenteric

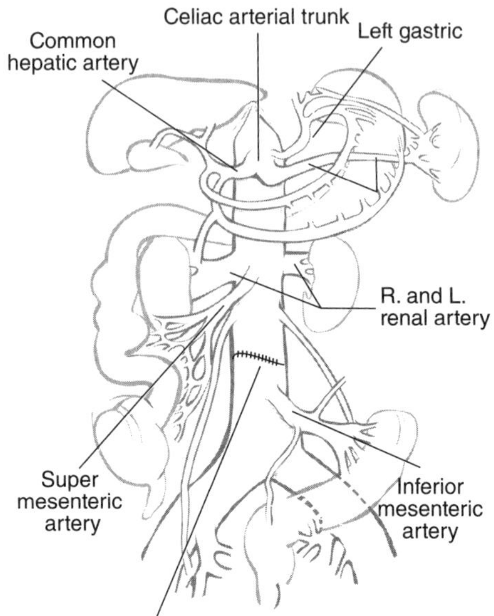

Explanation

The physician quickly exposes the abdominal aorta using a transperitoneal approach, placing a long incision in the midabdomen and retracting the transverse colon and small bowel to allow dissection and exposure of the aorta. Control of bleeding is achieved by pushing the liver aside and compressing the aorta manually against the spine. The aorta is cross-clamped proximal to the dissection and the iliac arteries are exposed. Control of blood flow is done with umbilical tape or rubber catheters. If bleeding is controlled, the iliac arteries and proximal aorta are cross-clamped. The physician opens and clears the aneurysm, controls collateral bleeding from the lumbar arteries with suture, then sutures a Y-shaped knitted Dacron graft to the proximal aorta. The distal ends of the graft are sutured to the iliac arteries. The physician may anastomose the celiac, inferior mesenteric, and/or renal arteries to the Dacron graft. The remaining aneurysmal shell is sutured around the graft. The retroperitoneum and abdominal wounds are closed, leaving drains in place.

Coding Tips

Preparation of the artery for anastomosis, including endarterectomy, is integral to the procedure and should not be reported separately. Establishing both inflow and outflow by any method is included. The portion of the operative arteriogram performed by the surgeon is also included. Angioscopy performed during therapeutic intervention should be reported in addition to the code for the primary procedure; see 35400. Harvested vein or synthetic material may be used for the graft. Any graft harvest is not reported separately. For thoracic aortic aneurysm, see 33858–33875. For direct repairs associated with occlusive disease only, see 35221, 35251, and 35281.

ICD-10-CM Diagnostic Codes

I71.31	Pararenal abdominal aortic aneurysm, ruptured

I71.32	Juxtarenal abdominal aortic aneurysm, ruptured
I71.33	Infrarenal abdominal aortic aneurysm, ruptured
I71.51	Supraceliac aneurysm of the thoracoabdominal aorta, ruptured
I71.52	Paravisceral aneurysm of the thoracoabdominal aorta, ruptured
I72.2	Aneurysm of renal artery
I72.8	Aneurysm of other specified arteries

Relative Value Units/Medicare Edits

Non-Facility RVU	Work	PE	MP	Total
35092	50.97	12.28	12.68	75.93
Facility RVU	**Work**	**PE**	**MP**	**Total**
35092	50.97	12.28	12.68	75.93

	FUD	Status	MUE	Modifiers				IOM Reference
35092	90	A	1(2)	51	50	62*	80	None

* with documentation

Terms To Know

aneurysm. Circumscribed dilation or outpouching of an artery wall, often containing blood clots and connecting directly with the lumen of the artery.

endarterectomy. Removal of the thickened, endothelial lining of a diseased or damaged artery.

pseudoaneurysm. False aneurysm produced by a dilated vessel wall, or a ruptured blood vessel that has formed a clot that pulsates, mimicking a true aneurysm.

35102

35102 Direct repair of aneurysm, pseudoaneurysm, or excision (partial or total) and graft insertion, with or without patch graft; for aneurysm, pseudoaneurysm, and associated occlusive disease, abdominal aorta involving iliac vessels (common, hypogastric, external)

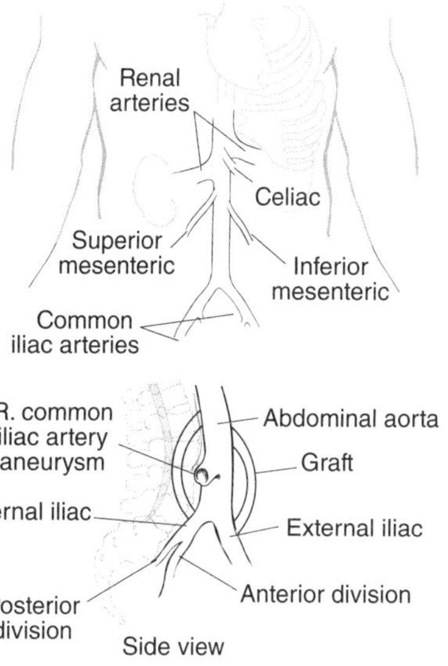

Explanation

The physician exposes the abdominal aorta using a transperitoneal approach, placing a long incision in the midabdomen, and retracting the transverse colon and small bowel to allow dissection and exposure of the aorta. Umbilical tape or a rubber catheter is placed around the aorta proximal to the aneurysm. The iliac arteries are exposed and control of blood flow is achieved with umbilical tape or rubber catheters. The physician anticoagulates the patient and cross-clamps the iliac arteries and proximal aorta. The physician opens and clears the aneurysm, controls collateral bleeding from the lumbar arteries with suture, then sutures a Y-shaped knitted Dacron graft to the proximal aorta. The distal ends of the graft are sutured to the iliac arteries. The physician may anastomose grafts from other involved iliac vessels (common, hypogastric, external) to the Dacron graft. The remaining aneurysmal shell is sutured around the graft. The retroperitoneal and abdominal wounds are closed, leaving drains in place.

Coding Tips

Preparation of the artery for anastomosis, including endarterectomy, is integral to the procedure and should not be reported separately. Establishing both inflow and outflow by any method is included. The portion of the operative arteriogram performed by the surgeon is also included. Angioscopy performed during therapeutic intervention should be reported in addition to the code for the primary procedure; see 35400. Harvested vein or synthetic material may be used for the graft. Any graft harvest is not reported separately. For thoracic aortic aneurysm, see 33858–33875. For direct repairs associated with occlusive disease only, see 35221, 35251, and 35281.

ICD-10-CM Diagnostic Codes

I70.0	Atherosclerosis of aorta A
I71.41	Pararenal abdominal aortic aneurysm, without rupture
I71.42	Juxtarenal abdominal aortic aneurysm, without rupture
I71.43	Infrarenal abdominal aortic aneurysm, without rupture
I71.61	Supraceliac aneurysm of the thoracoabdominal aorta, without rupture

I71.62	Paravisceral aneurysm of the thoracoabdominal aorta, without rupture
I72.3	Aneurysm of iliac artery
I73.89	Other specified peripheral vascular diseases
I74.01	Saddle embolus of abdominal aorta
I74.09	Other arterial embolism and thrombosis of abdominal aorta
I74.19	Embolism and thrombosis of other parts of aorta
I74.5	Embolism and thrombosis of iliac artery
I76	Septic arterial embolism
I77.1	Stricture of artery
I77.72	Dissection of iliac artery
I77.89	Other specified disorders of arteries and arterioles

Relative Value Units/Medicare Edits

Non-Facility RVU	Work	PE	MP	Total
35102	36.53	9.48	9.08	55.09
Facility RVU	**Work**	**PE**	**MP**	**Total**
35102	36.53	9.48	9.08	55.09

	FUD	Status	MUE	Modifiers				IOM Reference
35102	90	A	1(2)	51	50	62*	80	None

* with documentation

Terms To Know

anastomosis. Surgically created connection between ducts, blood vessels, or bowel segments to allow flow from one to the other.

atherosclerosis. Buildup of yellowish plaques composed of cholesterol and lipoid material within the arteries.

35103

35103 Direct repair of aneurysm, pseudoaneurysm, or excision (partial or total) and graft insertion, with or without patch graft; for ruptured aneurysm, abdominal aorta involving iliac vessels (common, hypogastric, external)

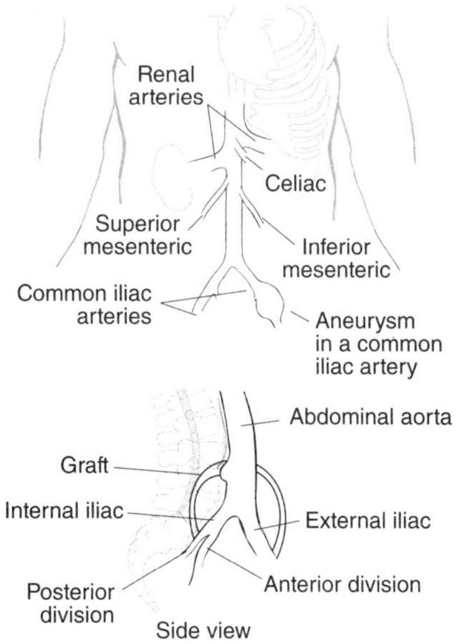

Explanation

The physician quickly exposes the abdominal aorta using a transperitoneal approach, placing a long incision in the midabdomen. The transverse colon and small bowel are retracted to allow dissection and exposure of the aorta. The physician quickly achieves control of bleeding by pushing the liver aside and compressing the aorta manually against the spine. The aorta is cross-clamped proximal to the dissection and the iliac arteries are exposed. Control of blood flow is achieved with umbilical tape or rubber catheters. Anticoagulation is provided (if bleeding is controlled) and the iliac arteries and proximal aorta are cross-clamped. The physician opens and clears the aneurysm, controls collateral bleeding from the lumbar arteries with suture, and sutures a Y-shaped knitted Dacron graft to the proximal aorta. The distal ends of the graft are sutured to the iliac arteries. The physician may anastomose grafts from other involved iliac vessels (common, hypogastric, external) to the Dacron graft. The remaining aneurysmal shell is sutured around the graft. The retroperitoneal and abdominal wounds are closed, leaving drains in place.

Coding Tips

Preparation of the artery for anastomosis, including endarterectomy, is integral to the procedure and should not be reported separately. Establishing both inflow and outflow by any method is included. The portion of the operative arteriogram performed by the surgeon is also included. Angioscopy performed during therapeutic intervention should be reported in addition to the code for the primary procedure; see 35400. Harvested vein or synthetic material may be used for the graft. Any graft harvest is not reported separately. For thoracic aortic aneurysm, see 33858–33875. For direct repairs associated with occlusive disease only, see 35221, 35251, and 35281.

ICD-10-CM Diagnostic Codes

I70.0	Atherosclerosis of aorta A
I71.02	Dissection of abdominal aorta
I71.31	Pararenal abdominal aortic aneurysm, ruptured
I71.32	Juxtarenal abdominal aortic aneurysm, ruptured

I71.33	Infrarenal abdominal aortic aneurysm, ruptured
I71.51	Supraceliac aneurysm of the thoracoabdominal aorta, ruptured
I71.52	Paravisceral aneurysm of the thoracoabdominal aorta, ruptured
I72.3	Aneurysm of iliac artery
I73.89	Other specified peripheral vascular diseases
I74.01	Saddle embolus of abdominal aorta
I74.09	Other arterial embolism and thrombosis of abdominal aorta
I74.19	Embolism and thrombosis of other parts of aorta
I74.5	Embolism and thrombosis of iliac artery
I76	Septic arterial embolism
I77.1	Stricture of artery
I77.72	Dissection of iliac artery

Relative Value Units/Medicare Edits

Non-Facility RVU	Work	PE	MP	Total
35103	43.62	10.33	10.9	64.85
Facility RVU	**Work**	**PE**	**MP**	**Total**
35103	43.62	10.33	10.9	64.85

	FUD	Status	MUE	Modifiers				IOM Reference
35103	90	A	1(2)	51	50	62*	80	None

* with documentation

Terms To Know

anastomosis. Surgically created connection between ducts, blood vessels, or bowel segments to allow flow from one to the other.

arteriogram. Radiograph of arteries.

atherosclerosis. Buildup of yellowish plaques composed of cholesterol and lipoid material within the arteries.

complication. Condition arising after the beginning of observation and treatment that modifies the course of the patient's illness or the medical care required, or an undesired result or misadventure in medical care.

pseudoaneurysm. False aneurysm produced by a dilated vessel wall, or a ruptured blood vessel that has formed a clot that pulsates, mimicking a true aneurysm.

35111-35112

35111 Direct repair of aneurysm, pseudoaneurysm, or excision (partial or total) and graft insertion, with or without patch graft; for aneurysm, pseudoaneurysm, and associated occlusive disease, splenic artery

35112 for ruptured aneurysm, splenic artery

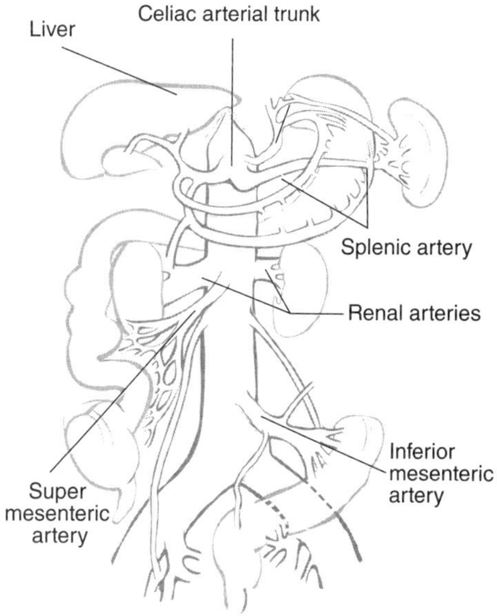

Explanation

The physician exposes the splenic artery using an abdominal incision. If the aneurysm involves the proximal or distal (hilar) splenic artery, in 35111, the physician may repair the aneurysm using harvested venous material or synthetic graft material or simply tie off the diseased artery and vein. In 35112, the physician may repair the aneurysm using harvested venous material or synthetic graft material or simply tie off the diseased artery and vein. If the aneurysm involves the middle splenic artery, which is surrounded by pancreatic tissue, the artery may be tied off to avoid dissection of the pancreas. The abdominal wound is closed, leaving drains in place.

Coding Tips

Preparation of the artery for anastomosis, including endarterectomy, is integral to the procedure and should not be reported separately. Establishing both inflow and outflow by any method is included. That portion of the operative arteriogram performed by the surgeon is also included. Angioscopy performed during therapeutic intervention should be reported in addition to the code for the primary procedure; see 35400. Harvested vein or synthetic material may be used for the graft. Any graft harvest is not reported separately. For direct repairs associated with occlusive disease only, see 35221, 35251, and 35281.

ICD-10-CM Diagnostic Codes

D73.5	Infarction of spleen
I72.8	Aneurysm of other specified arteries
I73.89	Other specified peripheral vascular diseases
I74.19	Embolism and thrombosis of other parts of aorta
I74.8	Embolism and thrombosis of other arteries
I76	Septic arterial embolism
I77.1	Stricture of artery
I77.79	Dissection of other specified artery
I77.89	Other specified disorders of arteries and arterioles

S35.291A	Minor laceration of branches of celiac and mesenteric artery, initial encounter
S35.292A	Major laceration of branches of celiac and mesenteric artery, initial encounter
S35.298A	Other injury of branches of celiac and mesenteric artery, initial encounter
S36.020A	Minor contusion of spleen, initial encounter
S36.021A	Major contusion of spleen, initial encounter
S36.030A	Superficial (capsular) laceration of spleen, initial encounter
S36.031A	Moderate laceration of spleen, initial encounter
S36.032A	Major laceration of spleen, initial encounter

Relative Value Units/Medicare Edits

Non-Facility RVU	Work	PE	MP	Total
35111	26.28	6.11	6.55	38.94
35112	32.57	7.17	8.11	47.85
Facility RVU	Work	PE	MP	Total
35111	26.28	6.11	6.55	38.94
35112	32.57	7.17	8.11	47.85

	FUD	Status	MUE	Modifiers				IOM Reference
35111	90	A	1(2)	51	N/A	62*	80	None
35112	90	A	1(2)	51	50	62*	80	

* with documentation

Terms To Know

aneurysm. Circumscribed dilation or outpouching of an artery wall, often containing blood clots and connecting directly with the lumen of the artery.

late effect. Abnormality, dysfunction, or other residual condition produced after the acute phase of an illness, injury, or disease is over. There is no time limit on when late effects can appear.

pseudoaneurysm. False aneurysm produced by a dilated vessel wall, or a ruptured blood vessel that has formed a clot that pulsates, mimicking a true aneurysm.

35121-35122

35121 Direct repair of aneurysm, pseudoaneurysm, or excision (partial or total) and graft insertion, with or without patch graft; for aneurysm, pseudoaneurysm, and associated occlusive disease, hepatic, celiac, renal, or mesenteric artery

35122 for ruptured aneurysm, hepatic, celiac, renal, or mesenteric artery

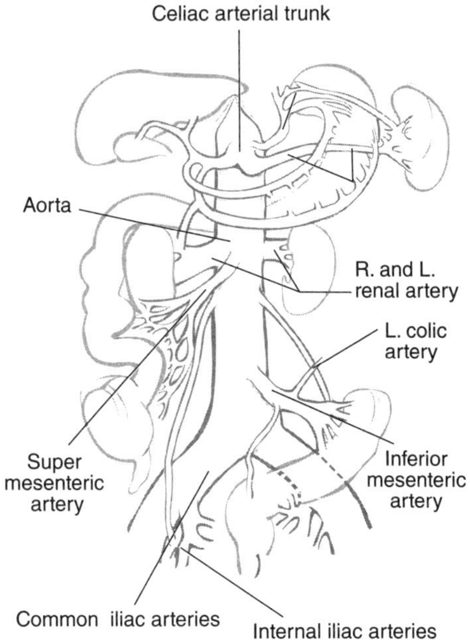

Explanation

In 35121, the physician exposes the involved hepatic, celiac, renal, or mesenteric artery using an abdominal incision, retracting and dissecting past large and small bowel. If the aneurysm involves an artery whose vascular distribution has adequate collaterals (the common hepatic artery, for example), the physician may simply tie off the diseased artery. Otherwise, the physician repairs the aneurysm, often using harvested vein graft, harvested internal iliac artery graft, or synthetic graft material. The physician closes the abdominal wound, leaving drains in place. In 35122, the physician quickly exposes the involved hepatic, celiac, renal, or mesenteric artery using an abdominal incision, retracting and dissecting past large and small bowel. Bleeding is controlled by clamping or compressing the involved artery proximal to the rupture. If the aneurysm involves an artery whose vascular distribution has adequate collaterals (e.g., the common hepatic artery), the physician may simply tie off the diseased artery. Otherwise, the aneurysm is repaired, often using harvested vein graft, harvested internal iliac artery graft, or synthetic graft material. The abdominal wound is closed, leaving drains in place.

Coding Tips

Preparation of the artery for anastomosis, including endarterectomy, is integral to the procedure and should not be reported separately. Establishing both inflow and outflow by any method is included. That portion of the operative arteriogram performed by the surgeon is also included. Angioscopy performed during therapeutic intervention should be reported in addition to the code for the primary procedure; see 35400. Harvested vein or synthetic material may be used for the graft. Any graft harvest is not reported separately. For direct repairs associated with occlusive disease only, see 35221, 35251, and 35281.

ICD-10-CM Diagnostic Codes

I70.1	Atherosclerosis of renal artery A

 N Newborn: 0 P Pediatric: 0-17 M Maternity: 9-64 A Adult: 15-124 AMA: CPT Assist

I70.8 Atherosclerosis of other arteries A
I72.2 Aneurysm of renal artery
I72.8 Aneurysm of other specified arteries
I77.1 Stricture of artery
I77.73 Dissection of renal artery
I77.79 Dissection of other specified artery
K55.011 Focal (segmental) acute (reversible) ischemia of small intestine
K55.012 Diffuse acute (reversible) ischemia of small intestine
K55.021 Focal (segmental) acute infarction of small intestine
K55.022 Diffuse acute infarction of small intestine
K55.031 Focal (segmental) acute (reversible) ischemia of large intestine
K55.032 Diffuse acute (reversible) ischemia of large intestine
K55.041 Focal (segmental) acute infarction of large intestine
K55.042 Diffuse acute infarction of large intestine
K55.1 Chronic vascular disorders of intestine
K55.8 Other vascular disorders of intestine
N28.0 Ischemia and infarction of kidney

Relative Value Units/Medicare Edits

Non-Facility RVU	Work	PE	MP	Total
35121	31.52	6.91	7.85	46.28
35122	37.89	8.0	9.46	55.35
Facility RVU	**Work**	**PE**	**MP**	**Total**
35121	31.52	6.91	7.85	46.28
35122	37.89	8.0	9.46	55.35

	FUD	Status	MUE	Modifiers				IOM Reference
35121	90	A	1(3)	51	50	N/A	80	None
35122	90	A	1(3)	51	50	62*	80	

* with documentation

Terms To Know

anastomosis. Surgically created connection between ducts, blood vessels, or bowel segments to allow flow from one to the other.

aneurysm. Circumscribed dilation or outpouching of an artery wall, often containing blood clots and connecting directly with the lumen of the artery.

pseudoaneurysm. False aneurysm produced by a dilated vessel wall, or a ruptured blood vessel that has formed a clot that pulsates, mimicking a true aneurysm.

35131-35132

35131 Direct repair of aneurysm, pseudoaneurysm, or excision (partial or total) and graft insertion, with or without patch graft; for aneurysm, pseudoaneurysm, and associated occlusive disease, iliac artery (common, hypogastric, external)

35132 for ruptured aneurysm, iliac artery (common, hypogastric, external)

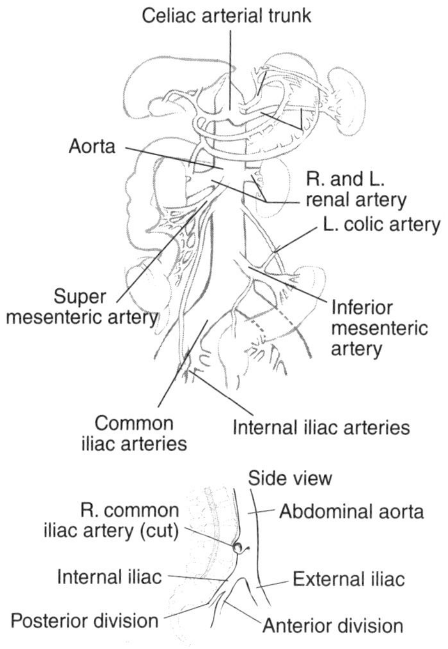

Explanation

The physician exposes the involved iliac arterial branch(es) (common, hypogastric, external) using a low abdominal incision. In 35131, the aneurysm is repaired by clamping off the affected artery proximally and distally and replacing the affected arterial segment with harvested venous material or synthetic graft material such as Dacron mesh. In 35132, bleeding is controlled by clamping or compressing the proximal segment of the affected artery. The ruptured aneurysm is repaired by clamping off the affected artery proximally and distally and replacing the affected arterial segment with harvested venous material or synthetic graft material such as Dacron mesh. The arterial patency is confirmed with a Doppler probe or by angiography. The abdominal wound is closed, leaving drains in place.

Coding Tips

Preparation of the artery for anastomosis, including endarterectomy, is integral to the procedure and should not be reported separately. Establishing both inflow and outflow by any method is included. That portion of the operative arteriogram performed by the surgeon is also included. Angioscopy performed during therapeutic intervention should be reported in addition to the code for the primary procedure; see 35400. Harvested vein or synthetic material may be used for the graft. Any graft harvest is not reported separately. For direct repairs associated with occlusive disease only, see 35221, 35251, and 35281.

ICD-10-CM Diagnostic Codes

I72.3 Aneurysm of iliac artery
I74.5 Embolism and thrombosis of iliac artery
I77.1 Stricture of artery
I77.72 Dissection of iliac artery

Relative Value Units/Medicare Edits

Non-Facility RVU	Work	PE	MP	Total
35131	26.4	7.52	6.56	40.48
35132	32.57	7.17	8.11	47.85
Facility RVU	**Work**	**PE**	**MP**	**Total**
35131	26.4	7.52	6.56	40.48
35132	32.57	7.17	8.11	47.85

	FUD	Status	MUE	Modifiers				IOM Reference
35131	90	A	1(2)	51	50	62*	80	None
35132	90	A	1(2)	51	50	62*	80	

* with documentation

Terms To Know

anastomosis. Surgically created connection between ducts, blood vessels, or bowel segments to allow flow from one to the other.

aneurysm. Circumscribed dilation or outpouching of an artery wall, often containing blood clots and connecting directly with the lumen of the artery.

anomaly. Irregularity in the structure or position of an organ or tissue.

atherosclerosis. Buildup of yellowish plaques composed of cholesterol and lipoid material within the arteries.

congenital. Present at birth, occurring through heredity or an influence during gestation up to the moment of birth.

digital subtraction angiography. Diagnostic imaging technique that applies computer technology to fluoroscopy for the purpose of visualizing the same vascular structures observable with conventional angiography.

excision. Surgical removal of an organ or tissue.

graft. Tissue implant from another part of the body or another person.

late effect. Abnormality, dysfunction, or other residual condition produced after the acute phase of an illness, injury, or disease is over. There is no time limit on when late effects can appear.

pseudoaneurysm. False aneurysm produced by a dilated vessel wall, or a ruptured blood vessel that has formed a clot that pulsates, mimicking a true aneurysm.

35141-35142

35141 Direct repair of aneurysm, pseudoaneurysm, or excision (partial or total) and graft insertion, with or without patch graft; for aneurysm, pseudoaneurysm, and associated occlusive disease, common femoral artery (profunda femoris, superficial femoral)

35142 for ruptured aneurysm, common femoral artery (profunda femoris, superficial femoral)

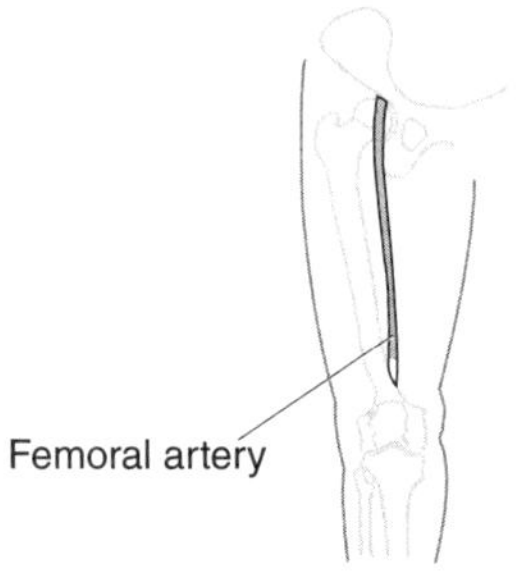

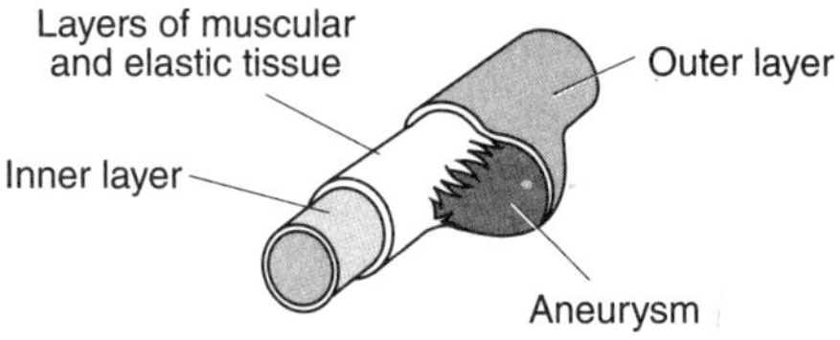

Area of aneurysm or occlusion

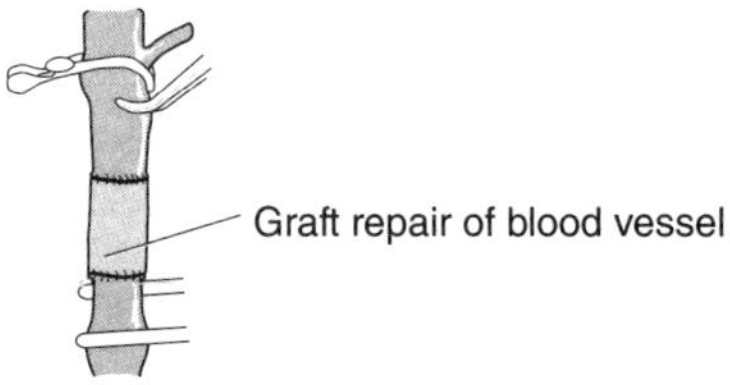

Explanation

The physician makes an incision in the skin of the leg. The enlarged or blocked section of the femoral artery (35141) or ruptured section (35142) is isolated and dissected from adjacent critical structures. Vessel clamps are affixed above and below the defect, which may be repaired or removed. The repair may be accomplished by removing the segment of artery containing the aneurysm and suturing the exposed ends of the vessel in an end-to-end fashion or the aneurysm may be bypassed with a venous or synthetic graft. If a large section is removed, a harvested or synthetic graft is inserted into the defect. Instead of a complete graft, a patch may be sutured into place to open up the diameter of the vessel. Once the vessel is repaired, the clamps are removed. The skin incision is repaired with a layered closure.

Coding Tips

Preparation of the artery for anastomosis, including endarterectomy, is integral to the procedure and should not be reported separately. Establishing both inflow and outflow by any method is included. That portion of the operative arteriogram performed by the surgeon is also included. Angioscopy performed during therapeutic intervention should be reported in addition to the code for the primary procedure; see 35400. Harvested vein or synthetic material may be used for the graft. Any graft harvest is not reported separately. For direct repairs associated with occlusive disease only, see 35226, 35256, and 35286.

ICD-10-CM Diagnostic Codes

I70.211 Atherosclerosis of native arteries of extremities with intermittent claudication, right leg A ☑
I70.212 Atherosclerosis of native arteries of extremities with intermittent claudication, left leg A ☑
I70.213 Atherosclerosis of native arteries of extremities with intermittent claudication, bilateral legs A ☑
I70.221 Atherosclerosis of native arteries of extremities with rest pain, right leg A ☑
I70.222 Atherosclerosis of native arteries of extremities with rest pain, left leg A ☑
I70.223 Atherosclerosis of native arteries of extremities with rest pain, bilateral legs A ☑
I72.4 Aneurysm of artery of lower extremity
I74.3 Embolism and thrombosis of arteries of the lower extremities
I75.021 Atheroembolism of right lower extremity ☑
I75.022 Atheroembolism of left lower extremity ☑
I75.023 Atheroembolism of bilateral lower extremities ☑
I76 Septic arterial embolism

Relative Value Units/Medicare Edits

Non-Facility RVU	Work	PE	MP	Total
35141	20.91	5.9	5.19	32.0
35142	25.16	7.23	6.26	38.65
Facility RVU	**Work**	**PE**	**MP**	**Total**
35141	20.91	5.9	5.19	32.0
35142	25.16	7.23	6.26	38.65

	FUD	Status	MUE	Modifiers				IOM Reference
35141	90	A	1(2)	51	50	62*	80	None
35142	90	A	1(2)	51	50	62*	80	

* with documentation

Terms To Know

anastomosis. Surgically created connection between ducts, blood vessels, or bowel segments to allow flow from one to the other.

aneurysm. Circumscribed dilation or outpouching of an artery wall, often containing blood clots and connecting directly with the lumen of the artery.

pseudoaneurysm. False aneurysm produced by a dilated vessel wall, or a ruptured blood vessel that has formed a clot that pulsates, mimicking a true aneurysm.

35151-35152

35151 Direct repair of aneurysm, pseudoaneurysm, or excision (partial or total) and graft insertion, with or without patch graft; for aneurysm, pseudoaneurysm, and associated occlusive disease, popliteal artery
35152 for ruptured aneurysm, popliteal artery

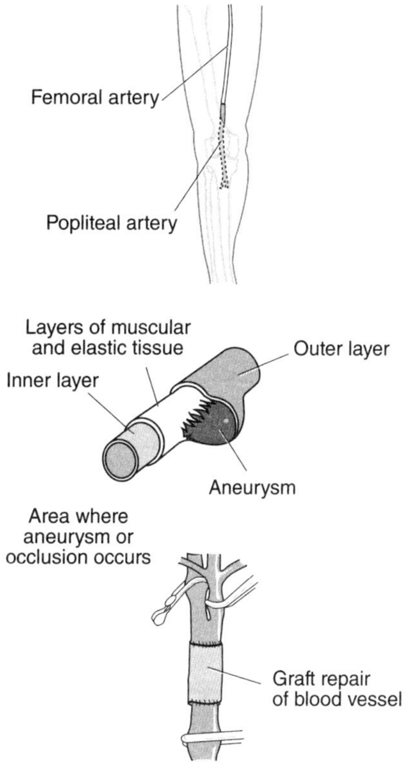

Explanation

The physician makes an incision in the skin over the leg. The enlarged or blocked section of the popliteal artery (35151) or the ruptured section (35152) is isolated and dissected from adjacent critical structures. Vessel clamps are affixed above and below the defect, which may be repaired or removed. The repair may be accomplished by removing the segment of artery containing the aneurysm and suturing the exposed ends of the vessel in an end-to-end fashion or the aneurysm may be bypassed with a venous or synthetic graft. If a large section is removed, a harvested or synthetic graft is inserted into the defect. Instead of a complete graft, a patch may be sutured into place to open up the diameter of the vessel. Once the vessel is repaired, the clamps are removed. The skin incision is repaired with a layered closure.

Coding Tips

Preparation of the artery for anastomosis, including endarterectomy, is integral to the procedure and should not be reported separately. Establishing both inflow and outflow by any method is included. That portion of the operative arteriogram performed by the surgeon is also included. Angioscopy performed during therapeutic intervention should be reported in addition to the code for the primary procedure; see 35400. Harvested vein or synthetic material may be used for the graft. Any graft harvest is not reported separately. For direct repairs associated with occlusive disease only, see 35226, 35256, and 35286.

ICD-10-CM Diagnostic Codes

I70.211 Atherosclerosis of native arteries of extremities with intermittent claudication, right leg A ☑

I70.212	Atherosclerosis of native arteries of extremities with intermittent claudication, left leg A ☑
I70.213	Atherosclerosis of native arteries of extremities with intermittent claudication, bilateral legs A ☑
I70.221	Atherosclerosis of native arteries of extremities with rest pain, right leg A ☑
I70.222	Atherosclerosis of native arteries of extremities with rest pain, left leg A ☑
I70.223	Atherosclerosis of native arteries of extremities with rest pain, bilateral legs A ☑
I72.4	Aneurysm of artery of lower extremity
I74.3	Embolism and thrombosis of arteries of the lower extremities
I75.021	Atheroembolism of right lower extremity ☑
I75.022	Atheroembolism of left lower extremity ☑
I75.023	Atheroembolism of bilateral lower extremities ☑
I77.1	Stricture of artery
I77.79	Dissection of other specified artery

Relative Value Units/Medicare Edits

Non-Facility RVU	Work	PE	MP	Total
35151	23.72	6.74	5.92	36.38
35152	27.66	6.41	6.87	40.94
Facility RVU	**Work**	**PE**	**MP**	**Total**
35151	23.72	6.74	5.92	36.38
35152	27.66	6.41	6.87	40.94

	FUD	Status	MUE	Modifiers				IOM Reference
35151	90	A	1(2)	51	50	62*	80	None
35152	90	A	1(2)	51	50	62*	80	

* with documentation

Terms To Know

aneurysm. Circumscribed dilation or outpouching of an artery wall, often containing blood clots and connecting directly with the lumen of the artery.

pseudoaneurysm. False aneurysm produced by a dilated vessel wall, or a ruptured blood vessel that has formed a clot that pulsates, mimicking a true aneurysm.

35180

35180 Repair, congenital arteriovenous fistula; head and neck

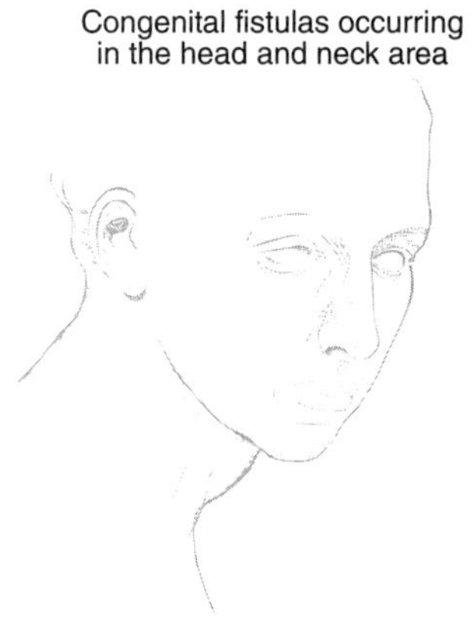

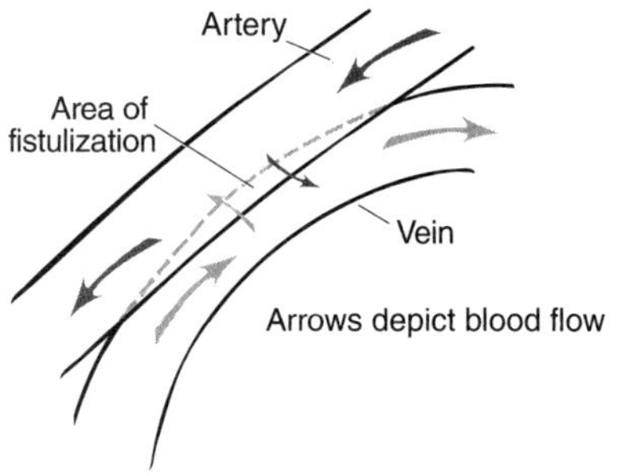

Explanation

The physician makes an incision in the skin of the head or neck over the site of the unnatural opening, a congenital fistula, that exists between an artery and vein. The fistula is isolated and dissected from adjacent critical structures, and vessel clamps are applied to the vein and the artery. The walls of the artery and vein creating the fistula are each sutured closed. A graft or patch graft may be required to complete the repair. The fistula is tied off, or it may be excised. Once the fistula has been eliminated, the clamps are removed and the skin incision is repaired with a layered closure.

Coding Tips

Fistula repair may be performed in stages during multiple operative or invasive radiology sessions. Report each separate session according to the procedure performed. Establishing both inflow and outflow by any method is included. That portion of the operative arteriogram performed by the surgeon is also included. Angioscopy performed during therapeutic intervention should be reported in addition to the code for the primary procedure; see 35400. For repair of an acquired or traumatic arteriovenous fistula, head and neck, see 35188. For repair of blood vessel other than for fistula, neck, see 35201, 35231, and 35261.

ICD-10-CM Diagnostic Codes

I60.01	Nontraumatic subarachnoid hemorrhage from right carotid siphon and bifurcation ☑
I60.02	Nontraumatic subarachnoid hemorrhage from left carotid siphon and bifurcation ☑
I60.11	Nontraumatic subarachnoid hemorrhage from right middle cerebral artery ☑
I60.12	Nontraumatic subarachnoid hemorrhage from left middle cerebral artery ☑

I60.31	Nontraumatic subarachnoid hemorrhage from right posterior communicating artery ☑
I60.32	Nontraumatic subarachnoid hemorrhage from left posterior communicating artery ☑
I60.4	Nontraumatic subarachnoid hemorrhage from basilar artery
I60.51	Nontraumatic subarachnoid hemorrhage from right vertebral artery ☑
I60.52	Nontraumatic subarachnoid hemorrhage from left vertebral artery ☑
I60.6	Nontraumatic subarachnoid hemorrhage from other intracranial arteries
I60.8	Other nontraumatic subarachnoid hemorrhage
I61.0	Nontraumatic intracerebral hemorrhage in hemisphere, subcortical
I61.1	Nontraumatic intracerebral hemorrhage in hemisphere, cortical
I61.3	Nontraumatic intracerebral hemorrhage in brain stem
I61.4	Nontraumatic intracerebral hemorrhage in cerebellum
I61.5	Nontraumatic intracerebral hemorrhage, intraventricular
I61.6	Nontraumatic intracerebral hemorrhage, multiple localized
I61.8	Other nontraumatic intracerebral hemorrhage
I62.01	Nontraumatic acute subdural hemorrhage
I62.02	Nontraumatic subacute subdural hemorrhage
I62.03	Nontraumatic chronic subdural hemorrhage
I62.1	Nontraumatic extradural hemorrhage
I67.0	Dissection of cerebral arteries, nonruptured
I67.1	Cerebral aneurysm, nonruptured
I67.89	Other cerebrovascular disease
Q25.8	Other congenital malformations of other great arteries
Q26.8	Other congenital malformations of great veins
Q27.8	Other specified congenital malformations of peripheral vascular system
Q28.0	Arteriovenous malformation of precerebral vessels
Q28.1	Other malformations of precerebral vessels
Q28.2	Arteriovenous malformation of cerebral vessels
Q28.3	Other malformations of cerebral vessels
Q28.8	Other specified congenital malformations of circulatory system

Relative Value Units/Medicare Edits

Non-Facility RVU	Work	PE	MP	Total
35180	15.1	4.21	3.75	23.06
Facility RVU	**Work**	**PE**	**MP**	**Total**
35180	15.1	4.21	3.75	23.06

	FUD	Status	MUE	Modifiers				IOM Reference
35180	90	A	2(3)	51	N/A	62*	80	None

* with documentation

35182

35182 Repair, congenital arteriovenous fistula; thorax and abdomen

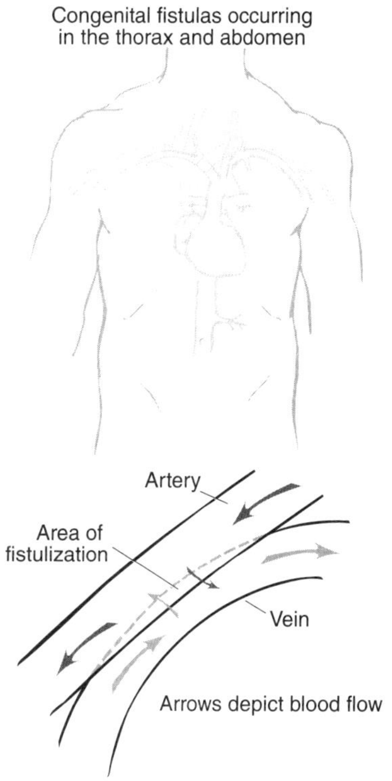

Explanation

The congenital arteriovenous fistula is exposed by choosing an incision appropriate to the fistula site. The physician examines the fistulous connection and repairs it by ligation (tying it off) or may repair the fistula by clamping the connection from both sides, dividing the connection with scissors, and closing each side with suture. A synthetic graft material or vein material harvested from the patient may be sewn in to enlarge the arterial or venous lumen. The vessel patency is confirmed with a Doppler probe or angiography prior to closing the wound. The physician may leave surgical drains in place.

Coding Tips

Fistula repair may be performed in stages during multiple operative or invasive radiology sessions. Report each separate session according to the procedure performed. Establishing both inflow and outflow by any method is included. That portion of the operative arteriogram performed by the surgeon is also included. Angioscopy performed during therapeutic intervention should be reported in addition to the code for the primary procedure; see 35400. For repair of an acquired or traumatic arteriovenous fistula, thorax and abdomen, see 35189. For repair of blood vessel other than for fistula, see 35211–35221, 35241–35251, and 35271–35281.

ICD-10-CM Diagnostic Codes

Q24.5	Malformation of coronary vessels
Q25.41	Absence and aplasia of aorta
Q25.42	Hypoplasia of aorta
Q25.43	Congenital aneurysm of aorta
Q25.44	Congenital dilation of aorta
Q25.45	Double aortic arch
Q25.46	Tortuous aortic arch
Q25.47	Right aortic arch

Q25.48	Anomalous origin of subclavian artery
Q25.49	Other congenital malformations of aorta
Q25.72	Congenital pulmonary arteriovenous malformation
Q25.79	Other congenital malformations of pulmonary artery
Q25.8	Other congenital malformations of other great arteries
Q26.6	Portal vein-hepatic artery fistula
Q26.8	Other congenital malformations of great veins
Q27.2	Other congenital malformations of renal artery
Q27.33	Arteriovenous malformation of digestive system vessel
Q27.34	Arteriovenous malformation of renal vessel
Q27.8	Other specified congenital malformations of peripheral vascular system

Relative Value Units/Medicare Edits

Non-Facility RVU	Work	PE	MP	Total
35182	31.71	13.36	7.84	52.91
Facility RVU	**Work**	**PE**	**MP**	**Total**
35182	31.71	13.36	7.84	52.91

	FUD	Status	MUE	Modifiers				IOM Reference
35182	90	A	2(3)	51	N/A	62*	80	None

* with documentation

Terms To Know

acquired. Produced by outside influences and not by genetics or birth defect.

angioscopy. Visualization of capillary blood vessels with a microscope, or the inside of a blood vessel with a fiberoptic-equipped catheter.

anomaly. Irregularity in the structure or position of an organ or tissue.

arteriogram. Radiograph of arteries.

congenital. Present at birth, occurring through heredity or an influence during gestation up to the moment of birth.

digital subtraction angiography. Diagnostic imaging technique that applies computer technology to fluoroscopy for the purpose of visualizing the same vascular structures observable with conventional angiography.

excision. Surgical removal of an organ or tissue.

fistula. Abnormal tube-like passage between two body cavities or organs or from an organ to the outside surface.

graft. Tissue implant from another part of the body or another person.

incision. Act of cutting into tissue or an organ.

ligation. Tying off a blood vessel or duct with a suture or a soft, thin wire.

35184

35184 Repair, congenital arteriovenous fistula; extremities

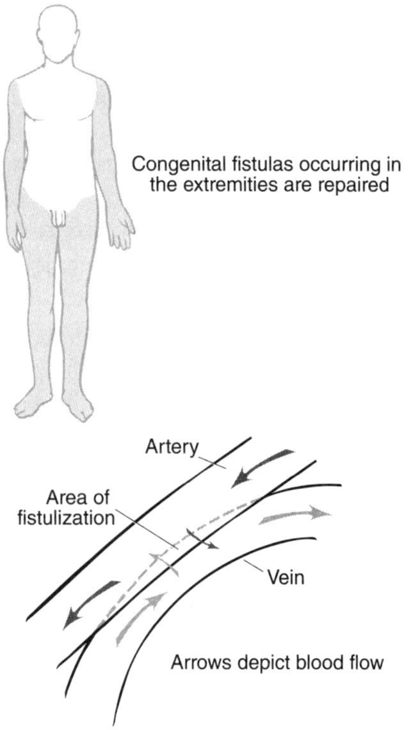

Explanation

The physician makes an incision in the skin of an extremity over the site of the unnatural opening, a congenital fistula, that exists between an artery and vein. The fistula is isolated and dissected from adjacent critical structures, and vessel clamps are applied to the vein and the artery. The walls of the artery and vein creating the fistula are each sutured closed. A graft or patch graft may be required to complete the repair. The fistula is tied off, or it may be excised. Once the fistula has been eliminated, the clamps are removed and the skin incision is repaired with a layered closure.

Coding Tips

Fistula repair may be performed in stages during multiple operative or invasive radiology sessions. Report each separate session according to the procedure performed. Establishing both inflow and outflow by any method is included. That portion of the operative arteriogram performed by the surgeon is also included. Angioscopy performed during therapeutic intervention should be reported in addition to the code for the primary procedure; see 35400. For repair of an acquired or traumatic arteriovenous fistula, extremities, see 35190. For repair of blood vessel other than for fistula, see 35206, 35226, 35236, 35256, 35266, and 35286. For revision of an arteriovenous fistula, with or without thrombectomy, autogenous or nonautogenous graft (separate procedure), see 36832.

ICD-10-CM Diagnostic Codes

Q27.31	Arteriovenous malformation of vessel of upper limb
Q27.32	Arteriovenous malformation of vessel of lower limb

Relative Value Units/Medicare Edits

Non-Facility RVU	Work	PE	MP	Total
35184	18.82	4.81	4.67	28.3
Facility RVU	**Work**	**PE**	**MP**	**Total**
35184	18.82	4.81	4.67	28.3

	FUD	Status	MUE	Modifiers				IOM Reference
35184	90	A	2(3)	51	N/A	62*	80	None

* with documentation

Terms To Know

acquired. Produced by outside influences and not by genetics or birth defect.

angioscopy. Visualization of capillary blood vessels with a microscope, or the inside of a blood vessel with a fiberoptic-equipped catheter.

anomaly. Irregularity in the structure or position of an organ or tissue.

arteriogram. Radiograph of arteries.

arteriovenous fistula. Connecting passage between an artery and a vein.

autogenous transplant. Tissue, such as bone, that is harvested from the patient and used for transplantation back into the same patient.

congenital. Present at birth, occurring through heredity or an influence during gestation up to the moment of birth.

graft. Tissue implant from another part of the body or another person.

suture. Numerous stitching techniques employed in wound closure.

thrombectomy. Removal of a clot (thrombus) from a blood vessel utilizing various methods.

35188-35189

35188 Repair, acquired or traumatic arteriovenous fistula; head and neck
35189 thorax and abdomen

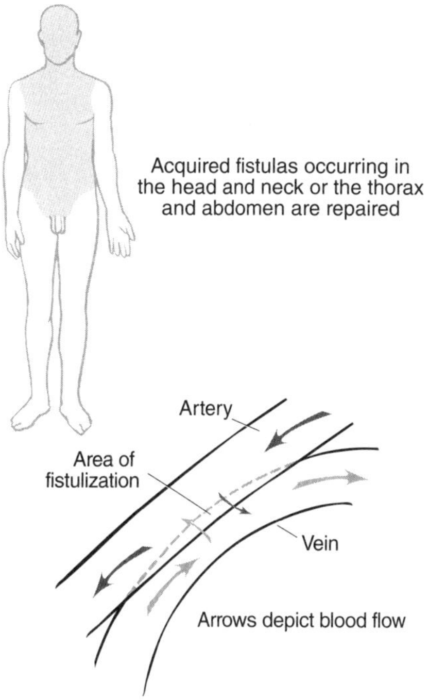

Explanation

The physician makes an incision in the skin of the head or neck over the site of the unnatural opening, a fistula, created through trauma. The fistula connects an artery to a vein. The fistula is isolated and dissected from adjacent critical structures, and vessel clamps are applied to the vein and the artery. The walls of the artery and vein creating the fistula are each repaired and closed. A graft or patch graft may be required to complete the repair. The fistula is tied off or excised. Once the fistula has been eliminated, the clamps are removed and the skin incision is repaired with a layered closure. Report 35189 if either fistula is in the thorax or abdomen.

Coding Tips

Fistula repair may be performed in stages during multiple operative or invasive radiology sessions. Report each separate session according to the procedure performed. Establishing inflow and outflow by any method is included. That portion of the operative arteriogram performed by the surgeon is also included. Angioscopy performed during therapeutic intervention should be reported in addition to the code for the primary procedure, see 35400. For repair of a congenital arteriovenous fistula, head and neck, see 35180; thorax and abdomen, see 35182. For repair of a blood vessel other than for fistula, see 35201, 35211–35221, 35231, 35241–35251, 35261, and 35271–35281.

ICD-10-CM Diagnostic Codes

I77.0	Arteriovenous fistula, acquired
S15.021A	Major laceration of right carotid artery, initial encounter ☑
S15.121A	Major laceration of right vertebral artery, initial encounter ☑
S15.221A	Major laceration of right external jugular vein, initial encounter ☑
S15.321A	Major laceration of right internal jugular vein, initial encounter ☑
S25.121A	Major laceration of right innominate or subclavian artery, initial encounter ☑
S25.22XA	Major laceration of superior vena cava, initial encounter

S25.321A Major laceration of right innominate or subclavian vein, initial encounter ☑
S25.322A Major laceration of left innominate or subclavian vein, initial encounter ☑
S25.421A Major laceration of right pulmonary blood vessels, initial encounter ☑
S25.422A Major laceration of left pulmonary blood vessels, initial encounter ☑
S25.511A Laceration of intercostal blood vessels, right side, initial encounter ☑
S25.512A Laceration of intercostal blood vessels, left side, initial encounter ☑
S25.811A Laceration of other blood vessels of thorax, right side, initial encounter ☑
S25.812A Laceration of other blood vessels of thorax, left side, initial encounter ☑
S35.02XA Major laceration of abdominal aorta, initial encounter
S35.12XA Major laceration of inferior vena cava, initial encounter
S35.212A Major laceration of celiac artery, initial encounter
S35.222A Major laceration of superior mesenteric artery, initial encounter
S35.232A Major laceration of inferior mesenteric artery, initial encounter
S35.292A Major laceration of branches of celiac and mesenteric artery, initial encounter
S35.311A Laceration of portal vein, initial encounter
S35.321A Laceration of splenic vein, initial encounter
S35.331A Laceration of superior mesenteric vein, initial encounter
S35.341A Laceration of inferior mesenteric vein, initial encounter
S35.411A Laceration of right renal artery, initial encounter ☑
S35.414A Laceration of right renal vein, initial encounter ☑
S35.511A Injury of right iliac artery, initial encounter ☑
S35.514A Injury of right iliac vein, initial encounter ☑

Relative Value Units/Medicare Edits

Non-Facility RVU	Work	PE	MP	Total
35188	18.0	13.62	7.5	39.12
35189	29.98	6.77	7.48	44.23
Facility RVU	**Work**	**PE**	**MP**	**Total**
35188	18.0	13.62	7.5	39.12
35189	29.98	6.77	7.48	44.23

	FUD	Status	MUE	Modifiers				IOM Reference
35188	90	A	2(3)	51	N/A	62*	80	None
35189	90	A	1(3)	51	N/A	62*	80	

* with documentation

Terms To Know

aneurysm. Circumscribed dilation or outpouching of an artery wall, often containing blood clots and connecting directly with the lumen of the artery.

angioscopy. Visualization of capillary blood vessels with a microscope, or the inside of a blood vessel with a fiberoptic-equipped catheter.

arteriogram. Radiograph of arteries.

graft. Tissue implant from another part of the body or another person.

35190

35190 Repair, acquired or traumatic arteriovenous fistula; extremities

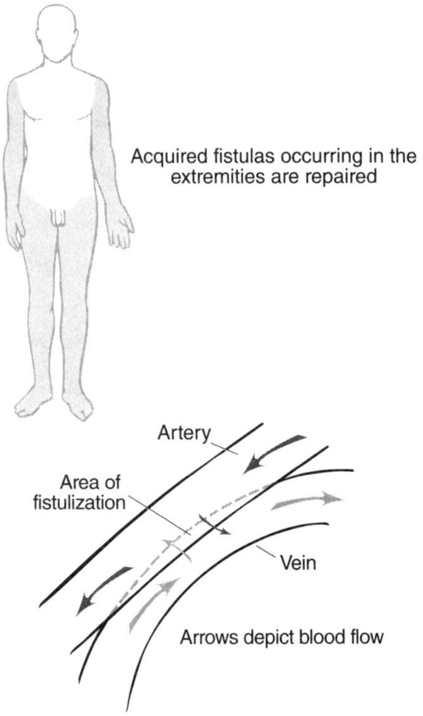

Explanation

The physician makes an incision in the skin of an extremity at the site of the unnatural opening, a fistula, created through trauma. It connects an artery to a vein. The fistula is isolated and dissected from adjacent critical structures, and vessel clamps are applied to the vein and the artery. The walls of the artery and vein creating the fistula are each repaired and closed. A graft or patch graft may be required to complete the repair. The fistula is tied off or excised. Once the fistula has been eliminated, the clamps are removed and the skin incision is repaired with a layered closure.

Coding Tips

Fistula repair may be performed in stages during multiple operative or invasive radiology sessions. Report each separate session according to the procedure performed. Establishing both inflow and outflow by any method is included. That portion of the operative arteriogram performed by the surgeon is also included. Angioscopy performed during therapeutic intervention should be reported in addition to the code for the primary procedure; see 35400. For repair of a congenital arteriovenous fistula, extremities, see 35184. For repair of blood vessel other than for fistula, see 35206, 35236, and 35286. For revision of a surgically created arteriovenous fistula, with or without thrombectomy, autogenous or non-autogenous graft (separate procedure), see 36832.

ICD-10-CM Diagnostic Codes

I77.0 Arteriovenous fistula, acquired
I77.2 Rupture of artery
S45.011A Laceration of axillary artery, right side, initial encounter ☑
S45.111A Laceration of brachial artery, right side, initial encounter ☑
S45.211A Laceration of axillary or brachial vein, right side, initial encounter ☑
S45.311A Laceration of superficial vein at shoulder and upper arm level, right arm, initial encounter ☑

S55.011A Laceration of ulnar artery at forearm level, right arm, initial encounter ☑
S55.111A Laceration of radial artery at forearm level, right arm, initial encounter ☑
S55.211A Laceration of vein at forearm level, right arm, initial encounter ☑
S65.011A Laceration of ulnar artery at wrist and hand level of right arm, initial encounter ☑
S65.111A Laceration of radial artery at wrist and hand level of right arm, initial encounter ☑
S75.021A Major laceration of femoral artery, right leg, initial encounter ☑
S75.121A Major laceration of femoral vein at hip and thigh level, right leg, initial encounter ☑
S75.221A Major laceration of greater saphenous vein at hip and thigh level, right leg, initial encounter ☑
S85.011A Laceration of popliteal artery, right leg, initial encounter ☑
S85.141A Laceration of anterior tibial artery, right leg, initial encounter ☑
S85.171A Laceration of posterior tibial artery, right leg, initial encounter ☑
S85.211A Laceration of peroneal artery, right leg, initial encounter ☑
S85.311A Laceration of greater saphenous vein at lower leg level, right leg, initial encounter ☑
S85.511A Laceration of popliteal vein, right leg, initial encounter ☑

Relative Value Units/Medicare Edits

Non-Facility RVU	Work	PE	MP	Total
35190	13.42	5.54	3.33	22.29
Facility RVU	**Work**	**PE**	**MP**	**Total**
35190	13.42	5.54	3.33	22.29

	FUD	Status	MUE	Modifiers				IOM Reference
35190	90	A	2(3)	51	N/A	62*	80	None

* with documentation

Terms To Know

arteriogram. Radiograph of arteries.

embolism. Obstruction of a blood vessel resulting from a clot or foreign substance.

fistula. Abnormal tube-like passage between two body cavities or organs or from an organ to the outside surface.

graft. Tissue implant from another part of the body or another person.

thrombectomy. Removal of a clot (thrombus) from a blood vessel utilizing various methods.

thrombosis. Condition arising from the presence or formation of blood clots within a blood vessel that may cause vascular obstruction and insufficient oxygenation.

35201

35201 Repair blood vessel, direct; neck

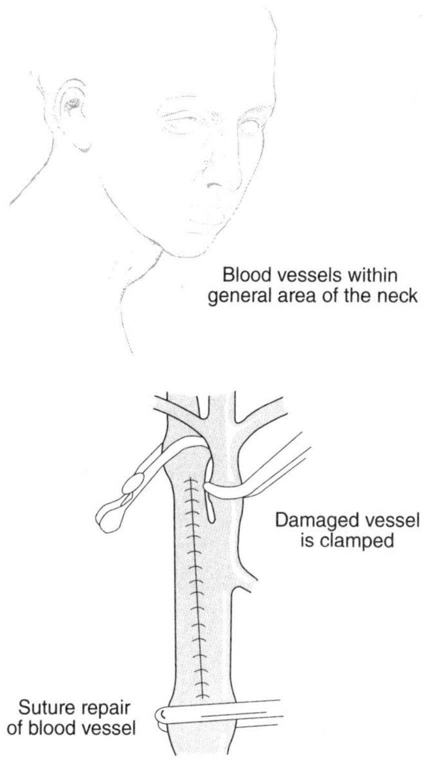

Explanation

The physician makes an incision in the skin of the neck over the site of an injured blood vessel. The vessel is isolated and dissected from adjacent critical structures, and vessel clamps are applied. The edges of the injured vessel may be trimmed to ease repair. A patch graft may be sutured over the defect or the hole in the vessel may be repaired with sutures. The clamps are removed and the skin incision is repaired with a layered closure.

Coding Tips

Establishing both inflow and outflow by any method is included. That portion of the operative arteriogram performed by the surgeon is also included. Angioscopy performed during therapeutic intervention should be reported in addition to the code for the primary procedure, see 35400. Any graft harvest is not reported separately. For repair of aneurysm carotid, subclavian, see 35001–35002. For repair of a blood vessel of the neck with vein graft, see 35231; with synthetic graft, see 35261. For repair of a congenital arteriovenous fistula, see 35180. For repair of an acquired or traumatic arteriovenous fistula, see 35188. Do not report 35201 with 33969, 33984, 33985, or 33986.

ICD-10-CM Diagnostic Codes

G45.0 Vertebro-basilar artery syndrome
G45.1 Carotid artery syndrome (hemispheric)
G45.2 Multiple and bilateral precerebral artery syndromes
I65.01 Occlusion and stenosis of right vertebral artery ☑
I65.02 Occlusion and stenosis of left vertebral artery ☑
I65.03 Occlusion and stenosis of bilateral vertebral arteries ☑
I65.21 Occlusion and stenosis of right carotid artery ☑
I65.22 Occlusion and stenosis of left carotid artery ☑
I65.23 Occlusion and stenosis of bilateral carotid arteries ☑

I77.71	Dissection of carotid artery
S15.011A	Minor laceration of right carotid artery, initial encounter ☑
S15.012A	Minor laceration of left carotid artery, initial encounter ☑
S15.021A	Major laceration of right carotid artery, initial encounter ☑
S15.022A	Major laceration of left carotid artery, initial encounter ☑
S15.091A	Other specified injury of right carotid artery, initial encounter ☑
S15.111A	Minor laceration of right vertebral artery, initial encounter ☑
S15.112A	Minor laceration of left vertebral artery, initial encounter ☑
S15.121A	Major laceration of right vertebral artery, initial encounter ☑
S15.122A	Major laceration of left vertebral artery, initial encounter ☑
S15.191A	Other specified injury of right vertebral artery, initial encounter ☑
S15.211A	Minor laceration of right external jugular vein, initial encounter ☑
S15.212A	Minor laceration of left external jugular vein, initial encounter ☑
S15.221A	Major laceration of right external jugular vein, initial encounter ☑
S15.222A	Major laceration of left external jugular vein, initial encounter ☑
S15.291A	Other specified injury of right external jugular vein, initial encounter ☑
S15.311A	Minor laceration of right internal jugular vein, initial encounter ☑
S15.312A	Minor laceration of left internal jugular vein, initial encounter ☑
S15.321A	Major laceration of right internal jugular vein, initial encounter ☑
S15.322A	Major laceration of left internal jugular vein, initial encounter ☑
S15.391A	Other specified injury of right internal jugular vein, initial encounter ☑
S15.8XXA	Injury of other specified blood vessels at neck level, initial encounter
S25.311A	Minor laceration of right innominate or subclavian vein, initial encounter ☑
S25.312A	Minor laceration of left innominate or subclavian vein, initial encounter ☑
S25.321A	Major laceration of right innominate or subclavian vein, initial encounter ☑
S25.322A	Major laceration of left innominate or subclavian vein, initial encounter ☑
S25.391A	Other specified injury of right innominate or subclavian vein, initial encounter ☑

AMA: 35201 2019,Dec

Relative Value Units/Medicare Edits

Non-Facility RVU	Work	PE	MP	Total
35201	16.93	6.59	4.0	27.52
Facility RVU	**Work**	**PE**	**MP**	**Total**
35201	16.93	6.59	4.0	27.52

	FUD	Status	MUE	Modifiers				IOM Reference
35201	90	A	2(3)	51	50	62*	80	None

* with documentation

35206

35206 Repair blood vessel, direct; upper extremity

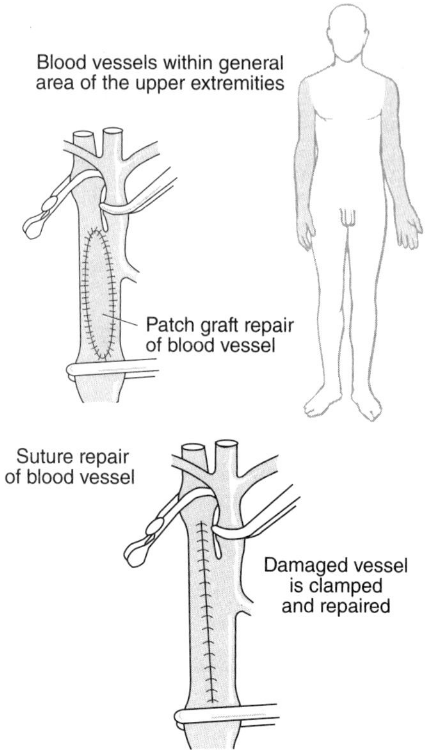

Explanation

The physician makes an incision in the skin of an upper extremity over the site of an injured blood vessel. The vessel is isolated and dissected from adjacent critical structures, and vessel clamps are applied. The edges of the injured vessel may be trimmed to ease repair. A patch graft may be sutured over the defect or the hole in the vessel may be repaired with sutures. The clamps are removed and the skin incision is repaired with a layered closure.

Coding Tips

Establishing both inflow and outflow by any method is included. That portion of the operative arteriogram performed by the surgeon is also included. Angioscopy performed during therapeutic intervention should be reported in addition to the code for the primary procedure; see 35400. Any graft harvest is not reported separately. For repair of an axillary-brachial aneurysm, see 35011–35013; ulnar, radial aneurysm, see 35045. For repair of a blood vessel of an upper extremity with vein graft, see 35236; with synthetic graft, see 35266. For repair of a congenital arteriovenous fistula, see 35184. For repair of an acquired or traumatic arteriovenous fistula, see 35190. Do not report 35206 with 33969, 33984, 33985, 33986.

ICD-10-CM Diagnostic Codes

I77.1	Stricture of artery
I77.2	Rupture of artery
S45.011A	Laceration of axillary artery, right side, initial encounter ☑
S45.091A	Other specified injury of axillary artery, right side, initial encounter ☑
S45.111A	Laceration of brachial artery, right side, initial encounter ☑
S45.191A	Other specified injury of brachial artery, right side, initial encounter ☑

S45.211A Laceration of axillary or brachial vein, right side, initial encounter ☑

S45.291A Other specified injury of axillary or brachial vein, right side, initial encounter ☑

S45.311A Laceration of superficial vein at shoulder and upper arm level, right arm, initial encounter ☑

S45.391A Other specified injury of superficial vein at shoulder and upper arm level, right arm, initial encounter ☑

S45.811A Laceration of other specified blood vessels at shoulder and upper arm level, right arm, initial encounter ☑

S55.011A Laceration of ulnar artery at forearm level, right arm, initial encounter ☑

S55.091A Other specified injury of ulnar artery at forearm level, right arm, initial encounter ☑

S55.111A Laceration of radial artery at forearm level, right arm, initial encounter ☑

S55.191A Other specified injury of radial artery at forearm level, right arm, initial encounter ☑

S55.211A Laceration of vein at forearm level, right arm, initial encounter ☑

S55.291A Other specified injury of vein at forearm level, right arm, initial encounter ☑

S55.811A Laceration of other blood vessels at forearm level, right arm, initial encounter ☑

S55.891A Other specified injury of other blood vessels at forearm level, right arm, initial encounter ☑

S65.011A Laceration of ulnar artery at wrist and hand level of right arm, initial encounter ☑

S65.091A Other specified injury of ulnar artery at wrist and hand level of right arm, initial encounter ☑

S65.111A Laceration of radial artery at wrist and hand level of right arm, initial encounter ☑

S65.191A Other specified injury of radial artery at wrist and hand level of right arm, initial encounter ☑

S65.811A Laceration of other blood vessels at wrist and hand level of right arm, initial encounter ☑

AMA: 35206 2020,Dec; 2019,Dec

Relative Value Units/Medicare Edits

Non-Facility RVU	Work	PE	MP	Total
35206	13.84	6.32	3.22	23.38
Facility RVU	**Work**	**PE**	**MP**	**Total**
35206	13.84	6.32	3.22	23.38

	FUD	Status	MUE	Modifiers				IOM Reference
35206	90	A	2(3)	51	50	62*	80	None

* with documentation

35207

35207 Repair blood vessel, direct; hand, finger

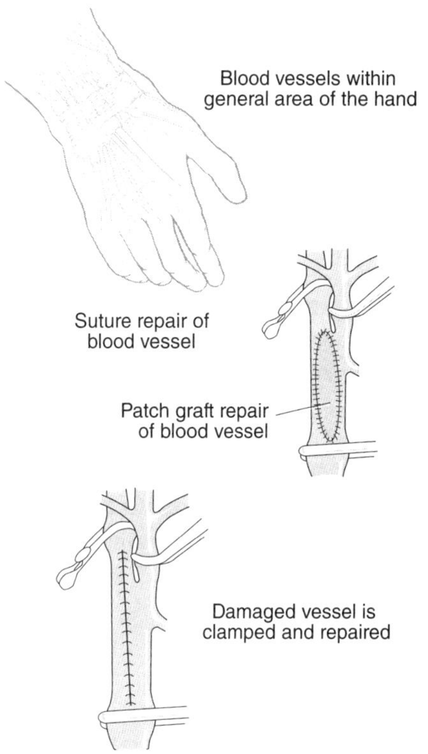

Explanation

The physician makes an incision in the skin of the hand or finger over the site of an injured blood vessel. The vessel is isolated and dissected from adjacent critical structures, and vessel clamps are applied. The edges of the injured vessel may be trimmed to ease repair. A patch graft may be sutured over the defect or the hole in the vessel may be repaired with sutures. The clamps are removed and the skin incision is repaired with a layered closure.

Coding Tips

Establishing both inflow and outflow by any method is included. That portion of the operative arteriogram performed by the surgeon is also included. Angioscopy performed during therapeutic intervention should be reported in addition to the code for the primary procedure; see 35400. Any graft harvest is not reported separately. For repair of a congenital arteriovenous fistula, see 35184. For repair of an acquired or traumatic arteriovenous fistula, see 35190.

ICD-10-CM Diagnostic Codes

I77.1 Stricture of artery

I77.2 Rupture of artery

S65.011A Laceration of ulnar artery at wrist and hand level of right arm, initial encounter ☑

S65.091A Other specified injury of ulnar artery at wrist and hand level of right arm, initial encounter ☑

S65.111A Laceration of radial artery at wrist and hand level of right arm, initial encounter ☑

S65.191A Other specified injury of radial artery at wrist and hand level of right arm, initial encounter ☑

S65.411A Laceration of blood vessel of right thumb, initial encounter ☑

 ● New ▲ Revised + Add On ★ Telemedicine [Resequenced] ☑ Laterality

S65.491A Other specified injury of blood vessel of right thumb, initial encounter A

S65.510A Laceration of blood vessel of right index finger, initial encounter A

S65.512A Laceration of blood vessel of right middle finger, initial encounter A

S65.514A Laceration of blood vessel of right ring finger, initial encounter A

S65.516A Laceration of blood vessel of right little finger, initial encounter A

S65.590A Other specified injury of blood vessel of right index finger, initial encounter A

S65.592A Other specified injury of blood vessel of right middle finger, initial encounter A

S65.594A Other specified injury of blood vessel of right ring finger, initial encounter A

S65.596A Other specified injury of blood vessel of right little finger, initial encounter A

S65.811A Laceration of other blood vessels at wrist and hand level of right arm, initial encounter A

S65.891A Other specified injury of other blood vessels at wrist and hand level of right arm, initial encounter A

S69.81XA Other specified injuries of right wrist, hand and finger(s), initial encounter A

AMA: 35207 2019,Dec

Relative Value Units/Medicare Edits

Non-Facility RVU	Work	PE	MP	Total
35207	10.94	9.73	2.08	22.75
Facility RVU	**Work**	**PE**	**MP**	**Total**
35207	10.94	9.73	2.08	22.75

	FUD	Status	MUE	Modifiers				IOM Reference
35207	90	A	3(3)	51	50	62*	N/A	None

* with documentation

35211-35216

35211 Repair blood vessel, direct; intrathoracic, with bypass
35216 intrathoracic, without bypass

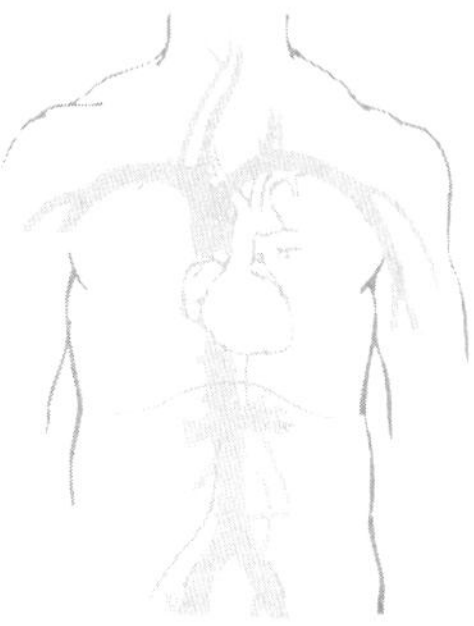

Procedures are within the thorax

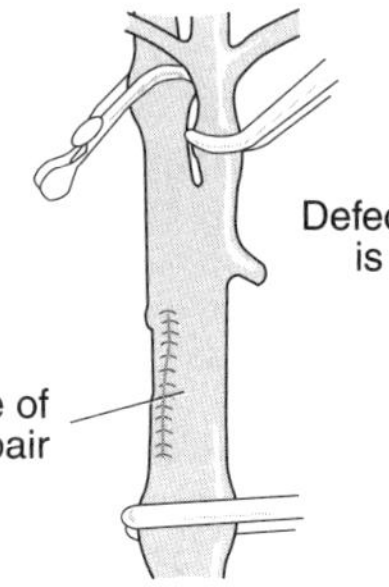

Explanation

The abnormal blood vessel (arterial or venous) is exposed by choosing a thoracic incision appropriate to the involved vessel. In 35211, the physician places cardiopulmonary bypass catheters (through incisions in the low inferior vena cava, the superior vena cava, and high aorta or femoral artery). The heart is stopped by infusing cardioplegia solution into the coronary circulation. The abnormal vessel is examined and repaired by ligation (tying it off) or may be repaired by clamping it proximally and distally to the defect, and suturing the defect closed. The physician may repair the vessel by sewing in synthetic graft material or vein material harvested from the patient in order to enlarge the lumen of the repaired vessel (patch graft). Vessel patency is confirmed with a Doppler probe or angiography prior to taking the patient off cardiopulmonary bypass and closing the wound. The physician leaves chest and, possibly, mediastinal drains in place. Report 35216 when the procedure is performed without the use of cardiopulmonary bypass.

Coding Tips

Establishing both inflow and outflow by any method is included. That portion of the operative arteriogram performed by the surgeon is also included. Angioscopy performed during therapeutic intervention should be reported in addition to the code for the primary procedure; see 35400. Any graft harvest is not reported separately. For repair of a thoracic aortic aneurysm, see 33858–33875. For repair of an innominate, subclavian aneurysm by thoracic incision, see 35021–35022. For vein graft repair of an intrathoracic blood vessel, see 35241–35246; with graft other than vein, see 35271–35276. Do not report these codes with 33969, 33984, 33985, or 33986.

ICD-10-CM Diagnostic Codes

I77.1 Stricture of artery

I77.2 Rupture of artery

I80.8 Phlebitis and thrombophlebitis of other sites

I87.1 Compression of vein

S21.121A	Laceration with foreign body of right front wall of thorax without penetration into thoracic cavity, initial encounter
S21.141A	Puncture wound with foreign body of right front wall of thorax without penetration into thoracic cavity, initial encounter
S25.01XA	Minor laceration of thoracic aorta, initial encounter
S25.02XA	Major laceration of thoracic aorta, initial encounter
S25.111A	Minor laceration of right innominate or subclavian artery, initial encounter ☑
S25.121A	Major laceration of right innominate or subclavian artery, initial encounter ☑
S25.191A	Other specified injury of right innominate or subclavian artery, initial encounter ☑
S25.21XA	Minor laceration of superior vena cava, initial encounter
S25.22XA	Major laceration of superior vena cava, initial encounter
S25.311A	Minor laceration of right innominate or subclavian vein, initial encounter ☑
S25.321A	Major laceration of right innominate or subclavian vein, initial encounter ☑
S25.391A	Other specified injury of right innominate or subclavian vein, initial encounter ☑
S25.411A	Minor laceration of right pulmonary blood vessels, initial encounter ☑
S25.421A	Major laceration of right pulmonary blood vessels, initial encounter ☑
S25.491A	Other specified injury of right pulmonary blood vessels, initial encounter ☑
S25.511A	Laceration of intercostal blood vessels, right side, initial encounter ☑
S25.591A	Other specified injury of intercostal blood vessels, right side, initial encounter ☑
S35.11XA	Minor laceration of inferior vena cava, initial encounter
S35.12XA	Major laceration of inferior vena cava, initial encounter

AMA: 35216 2018,Jun

Relative Value Units/Medicare Edits

Non-Facility RVU	Work	PE	MP	Total
35211	24.58	10.59	5.92	41.09
35216	36.61	16.89	8.65	62.15
Facility RVU	**Work**	**PE**	**MP**	**Total**
35211	24.58	10.59	5.92	41.09
35216	36.61	16.89	8.65	62.15

	FUD	Status	MUE	Modifiers				IOM Reference
35211	90	A	3(3)	51	50	62*	80	None
35216	90	A	2(3)	51	50	62*	80	

* with documentation

35221

35221 Repair blood vessel, direct; intra-abdominal

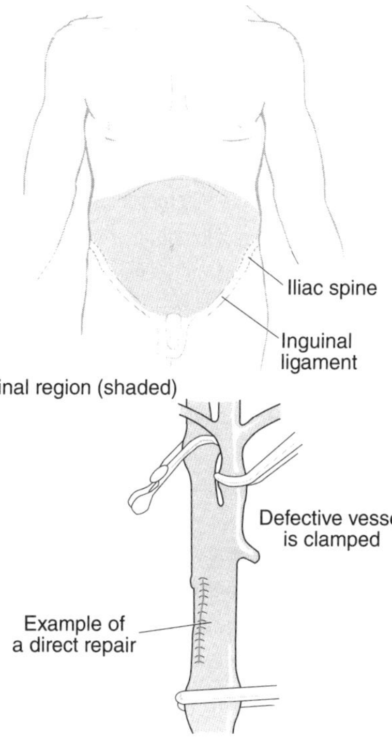

Explanation

The physician exposes the abnormal blood vessel (arterial or venous) by choosing an abdominal incision appropriate to the involved vessel. The abnormal vessel is examined and repaired by ligation (tying it off) or may be repaired by clamping it proximally and distally to the defect. The defect is sutured closed. A patch graft may be sutured over any remaining defect. Vessel patency is confirmed with a Doppler probe or angiography prior to closing the wound, leaving surgical drains in place.

Coding Tips

Establishing both inflow and outflow by any method is included. That portion of the operative arteriogram performed by the surgeon is also included. Angioscopy performed during therapeutic intervention should be reported in addition to the code for the primary procedure; see 35400. Any graft harvest is not reported separately. For repair of an intra-abdominal aneurysm, see 35081–35132. For repair of an intra-abdominal blood vessel with vein graft, see 35251; with graft other than vein, see 35281.

ICD-10-CM Diagnostic Codes

I70.1	Atherosclerosis of renal artery 🅰
I77.1	Stricture of artery
I77.811	Abdominal aortic ectasia
I77.812	Thoracoabdominal aortic ectasia
I82.0	Budd-Chiari syndrome
K55.011	Focal (segmental) acute (reversible) ischemia of small intestine
K55.012	Diffuse acute (reversible) ischemia of small intestine
K55.021	Focal (segmental) acute infarction of small intestine
K55.022	Diffuse acute infarction of small intestine
K55.031	Focal (segmental) acute (reversible) ischemia of large intestine
K55.032	Diffuse acute (reversible) ischemia of large intestine

K55.041 Focal (segmental) acute infarction of large intestine
K55.042 Diffuse acute infarction of large intestine
S35.01XA Minor laceration of abdominal aorta, initial encounter
S35.02XA Major laceration of abdominal aorta, initial encounter
S35.211A Minor laceration of celiac artery, initial encounter
S35.212A Major laceration of celiac artery, initial encounter
S35.218A Other injury of celiac artery, initial encounter
S35.221A Minor laceration of superior mesenteric artery, initial encounter
S35.222A Major laceration of superior mesenteric artery, initial encounter
S35.228A Other injury of superior mesenteric artery, initial encounter
S35.231A Minor laceration of inferior mesenteric artery, initial encounter
S35.232A Major laceration of inferior mesenteric artery, initial encounter
S35.238A Other injury of inferior mesenteric artery, initial encounter
S35.291A Minor laceration of branches of celiac and mesenteric artery, initial encounter
S35.292A Major laceration of branches of celiac and mesenteric artery, initial encounter
S35.298A Other injury of branches of celiac and mesenteric artery, initial encounter
S35.311A Laceration of portal vein, initial encounter
S35.318A Other specified injury of portal vein, initial encounter
S35.321A Laceration of splenic vein, initial encounter
S35.328A Other specified injury of splenic vein, initial encounter
S35.331A Laceration of superior mesenteric vein, initial encounter
S35.338A Other specified injury of superior mesenteric vein, initial encounter
S35.341A Laceration of inferior mesenteric vein, initial encounter
S35.348A Other specified injury of inferior mesenteric vein, initial encounter
S35.411A Laceration of right renal artery, initial encounter ☑
S35.414A Laceration of right renal vein, initial encounter ☑
S35.491A Other specified injury of right renal artery, initial encounter ☑
S35.494A Other specified injury of right renal vein, initial encounter ☑
S35.511A Injury of right iliac artery, initial encounter ☑
S35.514A Injury of right iliac vein, initial encounter ☑
S35.531A Injury of right uterine artery, initial encounter ☑
S35.534A Injury of right uterine vein, initial encounter ☑

AMA: **35221** 2024,Oct

Relative Value Units/Medicare Edits

Non-Facility RVU	Work	PE	MP	Total
35221	26.62	10.37	6.52	43.51
Facility RVU	**Work**	**PE**	**MP**	**Total**
35221	26.62	10.37	6.52	43.51

	FUD	Status	MUE	Modifiers				IOM Reference
35221	90	A	3(3)	51	50	62*	80	None

* with documentation

35226

35226 Repair blood vessel, direct; lower extremity

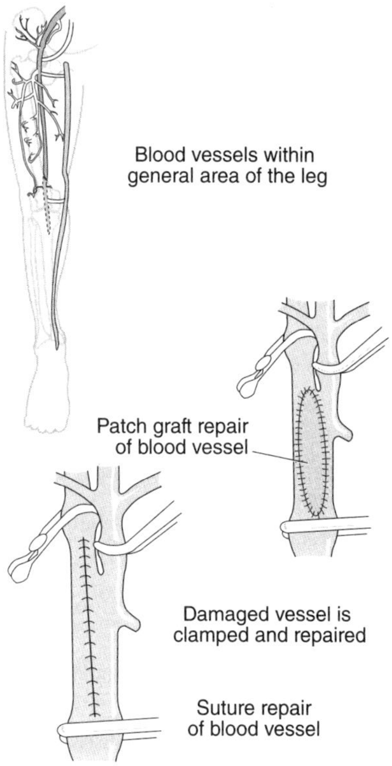

Explanation

The physician makes an incision in the skin of a lower extremity over the site of an injured blood vessel. The vessel is isolated and dissected from adjacent critical structures, and vessel clamps are applied. The edges of the injured vessel may be trimmed to ease repair. A patch graft may be sutured over the defect or the hole in the vessel may be repaired with sutures. The clamps are removed and the skin incision is repaired with a layered closure.

Coding Tips

Establishing both inflow and outflow by any method is included. That portion of the operative arteriogram performed by the surgeon is also included. Simple direct repair of a vessel is included in most primary cardiac procedures. Do not report 35226 separately for direct vessel repair following removal of the cannula during a cardiac procedure. Angioscopy performed during therapeutic intervention should be reported in addition to the code for the primary procedure, see 35400. Any graft harvest is not reported separately. For repair of an aneurysm, lower extremity, see 35141–35152. For repair of a blood vessel of a lower extremity with vein graft, see 35256; with synthetic graft, see 35286. For repair of a congenital arteriovenous fistula, see 35184. For repair of an acquired or traumatic arteriovenous fistula, see 35190. Do not report 35226 with 33969, 33984, 33985, or 33986.

ICD-10-CM Diagnostic Codes

I70.92 Chronic total occlusion of artery of the extremities [A]
I77.2 Rupture of artery
I80.01 Phlebitis and thrombophlebitis of superficial vessels of right lower extremity ☑
I80.02 Phlebitis and thrombophlebitis of superficial vessels of left lower extremity ☑

I80.03 Phlebitis and thrombophlebitis of superficial vessels of lower extremities, bilateral ☑
I80.11 Phlebitis and thrombophlebitis of right femoral vein ☑
I80.12 Phlebitis and thrombophlebitis of left femoral vein ☑
I80.13 Phlebitis and thrombophlebitis of femoral vein, bilateral ☑
I80.221 Phlebitis and thrombophlebitis of right popliteal vein ☑
I80.222 Phlebitis and thrombophlebitis of left popliteal vein ☑
I80.223 Phlebitis and thrombophlebitis of popliteal vein, bilateral ☑
I80.231 Phlebitis and thrombophlebitis of right tibial vein ☑
I80.232 Phlebitis and thrombophlebitis of left tibial vein ☑
I80.233 Phlebitis and thrombophlebitis of tibial vein, bilateral ☑
S75.021A Major laceration of femoral artery, right leg, initial encounter ☑
S75.022A Major laceration of femoral artery, left leg, initial encounter ☑
S75.221A Major laceration of greater saphenous vein at hip and thigh level, right leg, initial encounter ☑
S75.222A Major laceration of greater saphenous vein at hip and thigh level, left leg, initial encounter ☑
S85.011A Laceration of popliteal artery, right leg, initial encounter ☑
S85.012A Laceration of popliteal artery, left leg, initial encounter ☑
S85.141A Laceration of anterior tibial artery, right leg, initial encounter ☑
S85.142A Laceration of anterior tibial artery, left leg, initial encounter ☑
S85.171A Laceration of posterior tibial artery, right leg, initial encounter ☑
S85.172A Laceration of posterior tibial artery, left leg, initial encounter ☑
S85.211A Laceration of peroneal artery, right leg, initial encounter ☑
S85.212A Laceration of peroneal artery, left leg, initial encounter ☑
S85.311A Laceration of greater saphenous vein at lower leg level, right leg, initial encounter ☑
S85.312A Laceration of greater saphenous vein at lower leg level, left leg, initial encounter ☑
S85.411A Laceration of lesser saphenous vein at lower leg level, right leg, initial encounter ☑
S85.412A Laceration of lesser saphenous vein at lower leg level, left leg, initial encounter ☑
S85.511A Laceration of popliteal vein, right leg, initial encounter ☑
S85.512A Laceration of popliteal vein, left leg, initial encounter ☑
S95.011A Laceration of dorsal artery of right foot, initial encounter ☑
S95.012A Laceration of dorsal artery of left foot, initial encounter ☑
S95.211A Laceration of dorsal vein of right foot, initial encounter ☑
S95.212A Laceration of dorsal vein of left foot, initial encounter ☑

AMA: 35226 2020,Dec; 2019,Jul

Relative Value Units/Medicare Edits

Non-Facility RVU	Work	PE	MP	Total
35226	15.3	5.33	3.72	24.35
Facility RVU	**Work**	**PE**	**MP**	**Total**
35226	15.3	5.33	3.72	24.35

	FUD	Status	MUE	Modifiers				IOM Reference
35226	90	A	3(3)	51	50	62*	80	None

* with documentation

35231

35231 Repair blood vessel with vein graft; neck

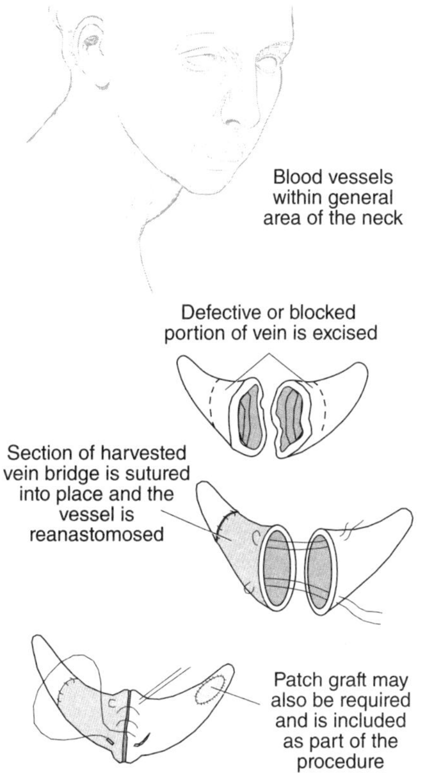

Explanation

The physician makes an incision in the skin in the neck over the site of an injured blood vessel. The vessel is isolated and dissected from adjacent critical structures, and vessel clamps are applied. The defect is too extensive to repair directly, so the physician removes a short length of vein. The physician repairs the injured vessel with a length of vein harvested from another site in the body or with cadaver vein. The vein is sutured end-to-end to the vessel, replacing the excised portion, or is used as a patch to repair a large hole in the side of the vessel. A patch graft may be sutured over any remaining defect. The clamps are removed and the skin incision is repaired with a layered closure.

Coding Tips

Establishing both inflow and outflow by any method is included. That portion of the operative arteriogram performed by the surgeon is also included. Angioscopy performed during therapeutic intervention should be reported in addition to the code for the primary procedure; see 35400. Any graft harvest is not reported separately. For repair of aneurysm carotid, subclavian, see 35001–35002. For direct repair of a blood vessel, neck, see 35201. For repair of a blood vessel of neck with synthetic graft, see 35261. For repair of a congenital arteriovenous fistula, see 35180. For repair of an acquired or traumatic arteriovenous fistula, see 35188.

ICD-10-CM Diagnostic Codes

G45.0 Vertebro-basilar artery syndrome
G45.1 Carotid artery syndrome (hemispheric)
G45.2 Multiple and bilateral precerebral artery syndromes
G45.8 Other transient cerebral ischemic attacks and related syndromes
I65.01 Occlusion and stenosis of right vertebral artery ☑
I65.1 Occlusion and stenosis of basilar artery

I65.21 Occlusion and stenosis of right carotid artery ☑
I65.8 Occlusion and stenosis of other precerebral arteries
I67.0 Dissection of cerebral arteries, nonruptured
I77.1 Stricture of artery
I77.2 Rupture of artery
I77.71 Dissection of carotid artery
I77.79 Dissection of other specified artery
I77.89 Other specified disorders of arteries and arterioles
S15.011A Minor laceration of right carotid artery, initial encounter ☑
S15.021A Major laceration of right carotid artery, initial encounter ☑
S15.091A Other specified injury of right carotid artery, initial encounter ☑
S15.111A Minor laceration of right vertebral artery, initial encounter ☑
S15.121A Major laceration of right vertebral artery, initial encounter ☑
S15.191A Other specified injury of right vertebral artery, initial encounter ☑
S15.211A Minor laceration of right external jugular vein, initial encounter ☑
S15.221A Major laceration of right external jugular vein, initial encounter ☑
S15.291A Other specified injury of right external jugular vein, initial encounter ☑
S15.311A Minor laceration of right internal jugular vein, initial encounter ☑
S15.321A Major laceration of right internal jugular vein, initial encounter ☑
S15.391A Other specified injury of right internal jugular vein, initial encounter ☑
S25.111A Minor laceration of right innominate or subclavian artery, initial encounter ☑
S25.121A Major laceration of right innominate or subclavian artery, initial encounter ☑
S25.191A Other specified injury of right innominate or subclavian artery, initial encounter ☑
S25.311A Minor laceration of right innominate or subclavian vein, initial encounter ☑
S25.321A Major laceration of right innominate or subclavian vein, initial encounter ☑
S25.391A Other specified injury of right innominate or subclavian vein, initial encounter ☑

AMA: **35231** 2019,Dec; 2019,Jul

Relative Value Units/Medicare Edits

Non-Facility RVU	Work	PE	MP	Total
35231	21.16	12.0	3.88	37.04
Facility RVU	**Work**	**PE**	**MP**	**Total**
35231	21.16	12.0	3.88	37.04

	FUD	Status	MUE	Modifiers				IOM Reference
35231	90	A	2(3)	51	50	62*	80	None

* with documentation

35236

35236 Repair blood vessel with vein graft; upper extremity

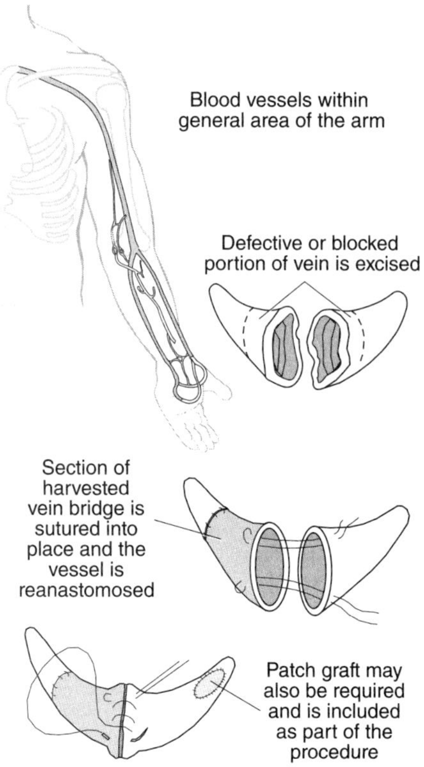

Explanation

The physician makes an incision in the skin of an upper extremity over the site of an injured blood vessel. The vessel is isolated and dissected from adjacent critical structures, and vessel clamps are applied. The defect is too extensive to repair directly, so the physician removes a short length of vein. The physician repairs the injured vessel with a length of vein harvested from another site in the body or with cadaver vein. The vein is sutured end-to-end to the vessel, replacing the excised portion, or is used as a patch to repair a large hole in the side of the vessel. A patch graft may be sutured over any remaining defect. The clamps are removed and the skin incision is repaired with a layered closure.

Coding Tips

Establishing both inflow and outflow by any method is included. That portion of the operative arteriogram performed by the surgeon is also included. Angioscopy performed during therapeutic intervention should be reported in addition to the code for the primary procedure; see 35400. Any graft harvest is not reported separately. For repair of an axillary-brachial aneurysm, see 35011–35013; for repair ulnar, radial aneurysm, see 35045. For direct repair of a blood vessel, upper extremity, see 35206. For repair of a blood vessel of the upper extremity with a synthetic graft, see 35266. For repair of a congenital arteriovenous fistula, see 35184. For repair of an acquired or traumatic arteriovenous fistula, see 35190.

ICD-10-CM Diagnostic Codes

I77.2 Rupture of artery
S45.011A Laceration of axillary artery, right side, initial encounter ☑
S45.091A Other specified injury of axillary artery, right side, initial encounter ☑
S45.111A Laceration of brachial artery, right side, initial encounter ☑

S45.191A Other specified injury of brachial artery, right side, initial encounter ☑
S45.211A Laceration of axillary or brachial vein, right side, initial encounter ☑
S45.291A Other specified injury of axillary or brachial vein, right side, initial encounter ☑
S45.311A Laceration of superficial vein at shoulder and upper arm level, right arm, initial encounter ☑
S45.391A Other specified injury of superficial vein at shoulder and upper arm level, right arm, initial encounter ☑
S45.811A Laceration of other specified blood vessels at shoulder and upper arm level, right arm, initial encounter ☑
S55.011A Laceration of ulnar artery at forearm level, right arm, initial encounter ☑
S55.091A Other specified injury of ulnar artery at forearm level, right arm, initial encounter ☑
S55.111A Laceration of radial artery at forearm level, right arm, initial encounter ☑
S55.191A Other specified injury of radial artery at forearm level, right arm, initial encounter ☑
S55.211A Laceration of vein at forearm level, right arm, initial encounter ☑
S55.291A Other specified injury of vein at forearm level, right arm, initial encounter ☑
S55.811A Laceration of other blood vessels at forearm level, right arm, initial encounter ☑
S65.011A Laceration of ulnar artery at wrist and hand level of right arm, initial encounter ☑
S65.091A Other specified injury of ulnar artery at wrist and hand level of right arm, initial encounter ☑
S65.111A Laceration of radial artery at wrist and hand level of right arm, initial encounter ☑
S65.191A Other specified injury of radial artery at wrist and hand level of right arm, initial encounter ☑
S65.411A Laceration of blood vessel of right thumb, initial encounter ☑
S65.510A Laceration of blood vessel of right index finger, initial encounter ☑
S65.512A Laceration of blood vessel of right middle finger, initial encounter ☑
S65.514A Laceration of blood vessel of right ring finger, initial encounter ☑
S65.516A Laceration of blood vessel of right little finger, initial encounter ☑
S65.811A Laceration of other blood vessels at wrist and hand level of right arm, initial encounter ☑

AMA: 35236 2019,Dec; 2019,Jul

Relative Value Units/Medicare Edits

Non-Facility RVU	Work	PE	MP	Total
35236	18.02	7.17	4.25	29.44
Facility RVU	**Work**	**PE**	**MP**	**Total**
35236	18.02	7.17	4.25	29.44

	FUD	Status	MUE	Modifiers				IOM Reference
35236	90	A	2(3)	51	50	62*	80	None

* with documentation

35241-35246

35241 Repair blood vessel with vein graft; intrathoracic, with bypass
35246 intrathoracic, without bypass

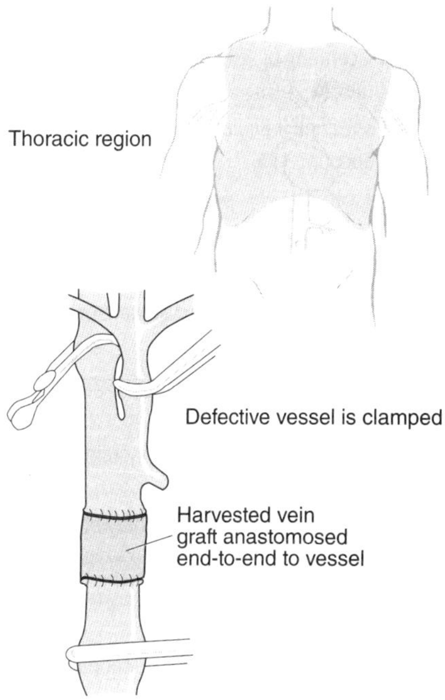

Explanation

The physician exposes the abnormal blood vessel (arterial or venous) by choosing a thoracic incision appropriate to the involved vessel. The physician places cardiopulmonary bypass catheters (in 35241) through incisions in the low inferior vena cava, the superior vena cava, and high aorta or femoral artery. The physician stops the heart by infusing cardioplegia solution into the coronary circulation. For both procedures, the physician examines the abnormal vessel and repairs it by clamping proximally and distally to the defect, and sewing in venous graft material harvested from the patient in order to bypass the abnormal area of the vessel (bypass graft). The physician confirms vessel patency with Doppler probe or angiography prior to taking the patient off cardiopulmonary bypass (in 35241) and closing the wound. The physician leaves chest and, possibly, mediastinal drains in place. Report 35246 when the procedure is performed without cardiopulmonary bypass.

Coding Tips

Establishing both inflow and outflow by any method is included. That portion of the operative arteriogram performed by the surgeon is also included. Angioscopy performed during therapeutic intervention should be reported in addition to the code for the primary procedure; see 35400. Any graft harvest is not reported separately. For repair of a thoracic aortic aneurysm, see 33858–33875. For repair of an innominate, subclavian aneurysm by thoracic incision, see 35021–35022. For a direct repair of an intrathoracic blood vessel, see 35211–35216; with graft other than vein, see 35271–35276.

ICD-10-CM Diagnostic Codes

I77.2 Rupture of artery
I77.5 Necrosis of artery
I77.810 Thoracic aortic ectasia
I77.812 Thoracoabdominal aortic ectasia
I77.89 Other specified disorders of arteries and arterioles
I80.8 Phlebitis and thrombophlebitis of other sites

I87.1	Compression of vein
S25.01XA	Minor laceration of thoracic aorta, initial encounter
S25.02XA	Major laceration of thoracic aorta, initial encounter
S25.09XA	Other specified injury of thoracic aorta, initial encounter
S25.111A	Minor laceration of right innominate or subclavian artery, initial encounter ☑
S25.121A	Major laceration of right innominate or subclavian artery, initial encounter ☑
S25.191A	Other specified injury of right innominate or subclavian artery, initial encounter ☑
S25.21XA	Minor laceration of superior vena cava, initial encounter
S25.22XA	Major laceration of superior vena cava, initial encounter
S25.29XA	Other specified injury of superior vena cava, initial encounter
S25.311A	Minor laceration of right innominate or subclavian vein, initial encounter ☑
S25.321A	Major laceration of right innominate or subclavian vein, initial encounter ☑
S25.391A	Other specified injury of right innominate or subclavian vein, initial encounter ☑
S25.411A	Minor laceration of right pulmonary blood vessels, initial encounter ☑
S25.421A	Major laceration of right pulmonary blood vessels, initial encounter ☑
S25.491A	Other specified injury of right pulmonary blood vessels, initial encounter ☑
S25.511A	Laceration of intercostal blood vessels, right side, initial encounter ☑
S25.591A	Other specified injury of intercostal blood vessels, right side, initial encounter ☑
S25.811A	Laceration of other blood vessels of thorax, right side, initial encounter ☑
S35.11XA	Minor laceration of inferior vena cava, initial encounter
S35.12XA	Major laceration of inferior vena cava, initial encounter
S35.19XA	Other injury of inferior vena cava, initial encounter

AMA: 35241 2019,Jul **35246** 2019,Jul

Relative Value Units/Medicare Edits

Non-Facility RVU	Work	PE	MP	Total
35241	25.58	10.68	5.93	42.19
35246	28.23	11.11	6.53	45.87
Facility RVU	**Work**	**PE**	**MP**	**Total**
35241	25.58	10.68	5.93	42.19
35246	28.23	11.11	6.53	45.87

	FUD	Status	MUE	Modifiers				IOM Reference
35241	90	A	2(3)	51	50	62*	80	None
35246	90	A	2(3)	51	50	62*	80	

* with documentation

35251

35251 Repair blood vessel with vein graft; intra-abdominal

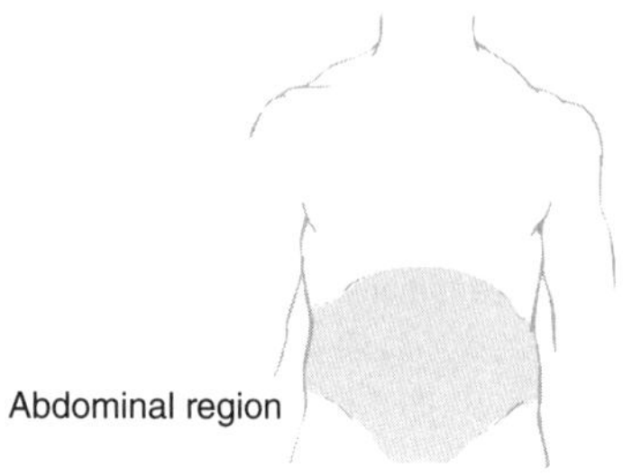

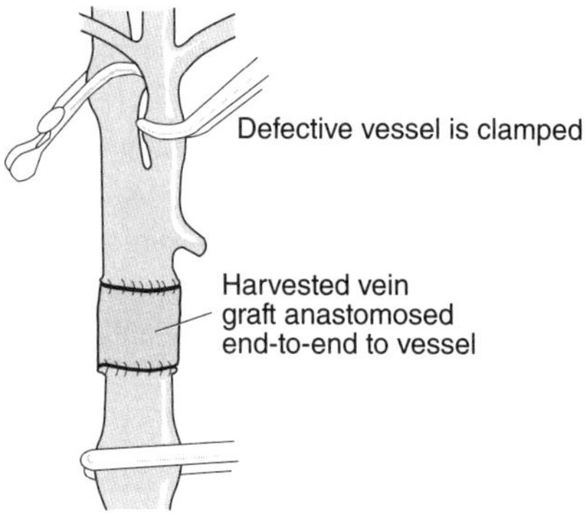

Explanation

The physician exposes the abnormal blood vessel (arterial or venous) by choosing an abdominal incision appropriate to the involved vessel. The physician examines the abnormal vessel and repairs it by clamping proximally and distally to the defect, and sewing in vein material harvested from the patient (patch graft). The physician confirms vessel patency with Doppler probe or angiography prior to closing the wound. The physician leaves surgical drains in place.

Coding Tips

Establishing both inflow and outflow by any method is included. That portion of the operative arteriogram performed by the surgeon is also included. Angioscopy performed during therapeutic intervention should be reported in addition to the code for the primary procedure; see 35400. Any graft harvest is not reported separately. For repair of an intra-abdominal aneurysm, see 35081–35132. For direct repair of an intra-abdominal blood vessel, see 35221. For repair of an intra-abdominal blood vessel with graft other than vein, see 35281.

ICD-10-CM Diagnostic Codes

I77.811	Abdominal aortic ectasia
I77.812	Thoracoabdominal aortic ectasia
I82.0	Budd-Chiari syndrome
K55.011	Focal (segmental) acute (reversible) ischemia of small intestine
K55.012	Diffuse acute (reversible) ischemia of small intestine
K55.021	Focal (segmental) acute infarction of small intestine
K55.022	Diffuse acute infarction of small intestine
K55.031	Focal (segmental) acute (reversible) ischemia of large intestine
K55.032	Diffuse acute (reversible) ischemia of large intestine
K55.041	Focal (segmental) acute infarction of large intestine
K55.042	Diffuse acute infarction of large intestine
S35.01XA	Minor laceration of abdominal aortic, initial encounter

S35.02XA Major laceration of abdominal aorta, initial encounter
S35.211A Minor laceration of celiac artery, initial encounter
S35.212A Major laceration of celiac artery, initial encounter
S35.218A Other injury of celiac artery, initial encounter
S35.221A Minor laceration of superior mesenteric artery, initial encounter
S35.222A Major laceration of superior mesenteric artery, initial encounter
S35.228A Other injury of superior mesenteric artery, initial encounter
S35.231A Minor laceration of inferior mesenteric artery, initial encounter
S35.232A Major laceration of inferior mesenteric artery, initial encounter
S35.238A Other injury of inferior mesenteric artery, initial encounter
S35.291A Minor laceration of branches of celiac and mesenteric artery, initial encounter
S35.292A Major laceration of branches of celiac and mesenteric artery, initial encounter
S35.298A Other injury of branches of celiac and mesenteric artery, initial encounter
S35.311A Laceration of portal vein, initial encounter
S35.318A Other specified injury of portal vein, initial encounter
S35.321A Laceration of splenic vein, initial encounter
S35.328A Other specified injury of splenic vein, initial encounter
S35.331A Laceration of superior mesenteric vein, initial encounter
S35.338A Other specified injury of superior mesenteric vein, initial encounter
S35.341A Laceration of inferior mesenteric vein, initial encounter
S35.348A Other specified injury of inferior mesenteric vein, initial encounter
S35.411A Laceration of right renal artery, initial encounter ☑
S35.414A Laceration of right renal vein, initial encounter ☑
S35.491A Other specified injury of right renal artery, initial encounter ☑
S35.494A Other specified injury of right renal vein, initial encounter ☑
S35.511A Injury of right iliac artery, initial encounter ☑
S35.514A Injury of right iliac vein, initial encounter ☑
S35.531A Injury of right uterine artery, initial encounter ☑
S35.534A Injury of right uterine vein, initial encounter ☑
S35.59XA Injury of other iliac blood vessels, initial encounter
S35.8X1A Laceration of other blood vessels at abdomen, lower back and pelvis level, initial encounter

AMA: **35251** 2019,Jul

Relative Value Units/Medicare Edits

Non-Facility RVU	Work	PE	MP	Total
35251	31.91	11.49	7.85	51.25
Facility RVU	**Work**	**PE**	**MP**	**Total**
35251	31.91	11.49	7.85	51.25

	FUD	Status	MUE	Modifiers				IOM Reference
35251	90	A	2(3)	51	50	62*	80	None

* with documentation

35256

35256 Repair blood vessel with vein graft; lower extremity

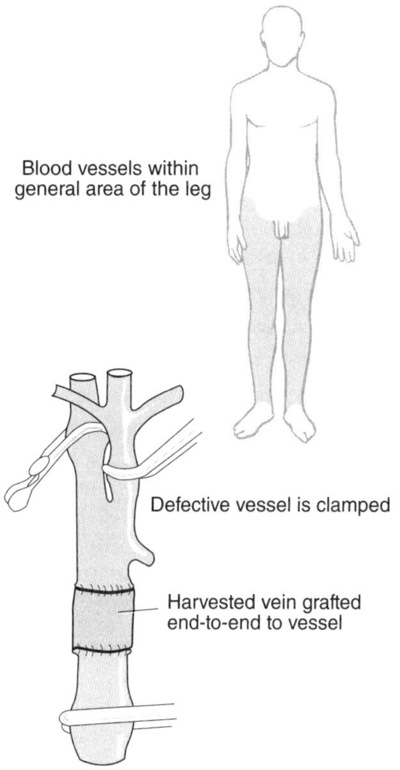

Explanation

The physician makes an incision in the skin of a lower extremity over the site of an injured blood vessel. The vessel is isolated and dissected from adjacent critical structures, and vessel clamps are applied. The physician repairs the injured vessel by sewing in vein material harvested from the patient (patch graft). The clamps are removed and the skin incision is repaired with a layered closure.

Coding Tips

Establishing both inflow and outflow by any method is included. That portion of the operative arteriogram performed by the surgeon is also included. Angioscopy performed during therapeutic intervention should be reported in addition to the code for the primary procedure; see 35400. Any graft harvest is not reported separately. For repair of an aneurysm, lower extremity, see 35141–35152. For direct repair of a blood vessel, lower extremity, see 35226. For repair of a lower extremity blood vessel with graft other than vein, see 35286. For repair of a congenital arteriovenous fistula, see 35184. For repair of an acquired or traumatic arteriovenous fistula, see 35190.

ICD-10-CM Diagnostic Codes

I70.92 Chronic total occlusion of artery of the extremities A
I77.2 Rupture of artery
I80.01 Phlebitis and thrombophlebitis of superficial vessels of right lower extremity ☑
I80.02 Phlebitis and thrombophlebitis of superficial vessels of left lower extremity ☑
I80.03 Phlebitis and thrombophlebitis of superficial vessels of lower extremities, bilateral ☑
I80.11 Phlebitis and thrombophlebitis of right femoral vein ☑

I80.12 Phlebitis and thrombophlebitis of left femoral vein ☑
I80.13 Phlebitis and thrombophlebitis of femoral vein, bilateral ☑
I80.221 Phlebitis and thrombophlebitis of right popliteal vein ☑
I80.222 Phlebitis and thrombophlebitis of left popliteal vein ☑
I80.223 Phlebitis and thrombophlebitis of popliteal vein, bilateral ☑
I80.231 Phlebitis and thrombophlebitis of right tibial vein ☑
I80.232 Phlebitis and thrombophlebitis of left tibial vein ☑
I80.233 Phlebitis and thrombophlebitis of tibial vein, bilateral ☑
S75.021A Major laceration of femoral artery, right leg, initial encounter ☑
S75.022A Major laceration of femoral artery, left leg, initial encounter ☑
S75.221A Major laceration of greater saphenous vein at hip and thigh level, right leg, initial encounter ☑
S75.222A Major laceration of greater saphenous vein at hip and thigh level, left leg, initial encounter ☑
S85.011A Laceration of popliteal artery, right leg, initial encounter ☑
S85.012A Laceration of popliteal artery, left leg, initial encounter ☑
S85.141A Laceration of anterior tibial artery, right leg, initial encounter ☑
S85.142A Laceration of anterior tibial artery, left leg, initial encounter ☑
S85.171A Laceration of posterior tibial artery, right leg, initial encounter ☑
S85.172A Laceration of posterior tibial artery, left leg, initial encounter ☑
S85.211A Laceration of peroneal artery, right leg, initial encounter ☑
S85.212A Laceration of peroneal artery, left leg, initial encounter ☑
S85.311A Laceration of greater saphenous vein at lower leg level, right leg, initial encounter ☑
S85.312A Laceration of greater saphenous vein at lower leg level, left leg, initial encounter ☑
S85.411A Laceration of lesser saphenous vein at lower leg level, right leg, initial encounter ☑
S85.412A Laceration of lesser saphenous vein at lower leg level, left leg, initial encounter ☑
S85.511A Laceration of popliteal vein, right leg, initial encounter ☑
S85.512A Laceration of popliteal vein, left leg, initial encounter ☑
S95.011A Laceration of dorsal artery of right foot, initial encounter ☑
S95.012A Laceration of dorsal artery of left foot, initial encounter ☑
S95.211A Laceration of dorsal vein of right foot, initial encounter ☑
S95.212A Laceration of dorsal vein of left foot, initial encounter ☑

AMA: **35256** 2019,Dec; 2019,Jul

Relative Value Units/Medicare Edits

Non-Facility RVU	Work	PE	MP	Total
35256	19.06	6.02	4.61	29.69
Facility RVU	**Work**	**PE**	**MP**	**Total**
35256	19.06	6.02	4.61	29.69

	FUD	Status	MUE	Modifiers				IOM Reference
35256	90	A	2(3)	51	50	62*	80	None

* with documentation

35261

35261 Repair blood vessel with graft other than vein; neck

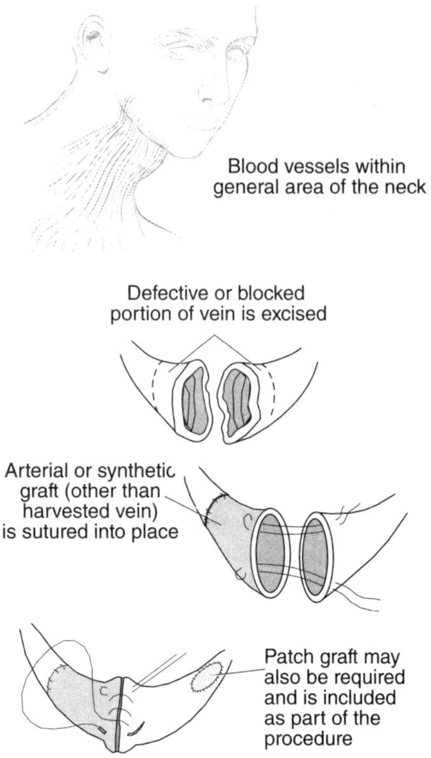

Explanation

The physician makes an incision in the skin of the neck over the site of an injured blood vessel. The vessel is isolated and dissected from adjacent critical structures and vessel clamps are applied. If the defect is too extensive to repair directly, the physician repairs the injured vessel with a length of synthetic graft material (patch graft). The clamps are removed and the skin incision is repaired with layered closure.

Coding Tips

Establishing both inflow and outflow by any method is included. That portion of the operative arteriogram performed by the surgeon is also included. Angioscopy performed during therapeutic intervention should be reported in addition to the code for the primary procedure; see 35400. Any graft harvest is not reported separately. For repair of an aneurysm, carotid, subclavian, see 35001–35002. For direct repair of a blood vessel, neck, see 35201. For repair of a blood vessel of neck with vein graft, see 35231. For repair of a congenital arteriovenous fistula, see 35180. For repair of an acquired or traumatic arteriovenous fistula, see 35188.

ICD-10-CM Diagnostic Codes

G45.0 Vertebro-basilar artery syndrome
G45.1 Carotid artery syndrome (hemispheric)
G45.2 Multiple and bilateral precerebral artery syndromes
G45.3 Amaurosis fugax
G45.8 Other transient cerebral ischemic attacks and related syndromes
G45.9 Transient cerebral ischemic attack, unspecified
I63.011 Cerebral infarction due to thrombosis of right vertebral artery ☑
I63.02 Cerebral infarction due to thrombosis of basilar artery
I63.031 Cerebral infarction due to thrombosis of right carotid artery ☑

I63.111 Cerebral infarction due to embolism of right vertebral artery ☑
I63.12 Cerebral infarction due to embolism of basilar artery
I63.131 Cerebral infarction due to embolism of right carotid artery ☑
I65.01 Occlusion and stenosis of right vertebral artery ☑
I65.1 Occlusion and stenosis of basilar artery
I65.21 Occlusion and stenosis of right carotid artery ☑
I65.8 Occlusion and stenosis of other precerebral arteries
I67.81 Acute cerebrovascular insufficiency
I67.841 Reversible cerebrovascular vasoconstriction syndrome
I67.848 Other cerebrovascular vasospasm and vasoconstriction
I67.89 Other cerebrovascular disease
I72.0 Aneurysm of carotid artery
I77.1 Stricture of artery
I77.2 Rupture of artery
I77.71 Dissection of carotid artery
I77.79 Dissection of other specified artery
S15.011A Minor laceration of right carotid artery, initial encounter ☑
S15.021A Major laceration of right carotid artery, initial encounter ☑
S15.091A Other specified injury of right carotid artery, initial encounter ☑
S15.111A Minor laceration of right vertebral artery, initial encounter ☑
S15.121A Major laceration of right vertebral artery, initial encounter ☑
S15.191A Other specified injury of right vertebral artery, initial encounter ☑
S15.211A Minor laceration of right external jugular vein, initial encounter ☑
S15.221A Major laceration of right external jugular vein, initial encounter ☑
S15.291A Other specified injury of right external jugular vein, initial encounter ☑
S15.311A Minor laceration of right internal jugular vein, initial encounter ☑
S15.321A Major laceration of right internal jugular vein, initial encounter ☑
S15.391A Other specified injury of right internal jugular vein, initial encounter ☑
S15.8XXA Injury of other specified blood vessels at neck level, initial encounter

AMA: 35261 2019,Dec; 2019,Jul

Relative Value Units/Medicare Edits

Non-Facility RVU	Work	PE	MP	Total
35261	18.96	5.13	4.7	28.79
Facility RVU	**Work**	**PE**	**MP**	**Total**
35261	18.96	5.13	4.7	28.79

	FUD	Status	MUE	Modifiers				IOM Reference
35261	90	A	1(3)	51	50	62*	80	None

* with documentation

35266

35266 Repair blood vessel with graft other than vein; upper extremity

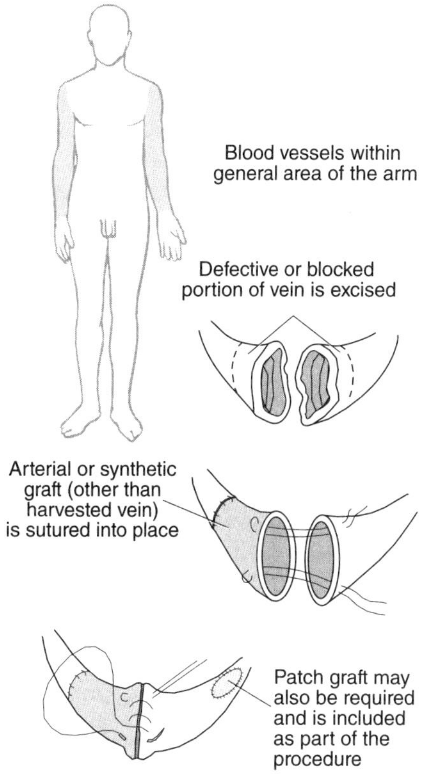

Explanation

The physician makes an incision in the skin of an upper extremity over the site of an injured blood vessel. The vessel is isolated and dissected from adjacent critical structures and vessel clamps are applied. If the defect is too extensive to repair directly, the physician repairs the injured vessel with a length of synthetic graft material (patch graft). The clamps are removed and the skin incision is repaired with layered closure.

Coding Tips

Establishing both inflow and outflow by any method is included. That portion of the operative arteriogram performed by the surgeon is also included. Angioscopy performed during therapeutic intervention should be reported in addition to the code for the primary procedure; see 35400. Any graft harvest is not reported separately. For repair of an axillary-brachial aneurysm, see 35011–35013; for repair ulnar, radial aneurysm, see 35045. For direct repair of a blood vessel, upper extremity, see 35206. For repair of a blood vessel, upper extremity, with vein graft, see 35236. For repair of a congenital arteriovenous fistula, see 35184. For repair of an acquired or traumatic arteriovenous fistula, see 35190.

ICD-10-CM Diagnostic Codes

I70.92 Chronic total occlusion of artery of the extremities A
I77.2 Rupture of artery
S45.011A Laceration of axillary artery, right side, initial encounter ☑
S45.091A Other specified injury of axillary artery, right side, initial encounter ☑
S45.111A Laceration of brachial artery, right side, initial encounter ☑
S45.191A Other specified injury of brachial artery, right side, initial encounter ☑

 ● New ▲ Revised + Add On ★ Telemedicine [Resequenced] ☑ Laterality

S45.211A Laceration of axillary or brachial vein, right side, initial encounter ☑
S45.291A Other specified injury of axillary or brachial vein, right side, initial encounter ☑
S45.311A Laceration of superficial vein at shoulder and upper arm level, right arm, initial encounter ☑
S45.391A Other specified injury of superficial vein at shoulder and upper arm level, right arm, initial encounter ☑
S45.811A Laceration of other specified blood vessels at shoulder and upper arm level, right arm, initial encounter ☑
S55.011A Laceration of ulnar artery at forearm level, right arm, initial encounter ☑
S55.091A Other specified injury of ulnar artery at forearm level, right arm, initial encounter ☑
S55.111A Laceration of radial artery at forearm level, right arm, initial encounter ☑
S55.191A Other specified injury of radial artery at forearm level, right arm, initial encounter ☑
S55.211A Laceration of vein at forearm level, right arm, initial encounter ☑
S55.291A Other specified injury of vein at forearm level, right arm, initial encounter ☑
S55.811A Laceration of other blood vessels at forearm level, right arm, initial encounter ☑
S65.011A Laceration of ulnar artery at wrist and hand level of right arm, initial encounter ☑
S65.091A Other specified injury of ulnar artery at wrist and hand level of right arm, initial encounter ☑
S65.111A Laceration of radial artery at wrist and hand level of right arm, initial encounter ☑
S65.191A Other specified injury of radial artery at wrist and hand level of right arm, initial encounter ☑
S65.411A Laceration of blood vessel of right thumb, initial encounter ☑
S65.510A Laceration of blood vessel of right index finger, initial encounter ☑
S65.512A Laceration of blood vessel of right middle finger, initial encounter ☑
S65.514A Laceration of blood vessel of right ring finger, initial encounter ☑
S65.516A Laceration of blood vessel of right little finger, initial encounter ☑
S65.811A Laceration of other blood vessels at wrist and hand level of right arm, initial encounter ☑

AMA: 35266 2019,Dec; 2019,Jul

Relative Value Units/Medicare Edits

Non-Facility RVU	Work	PE	MP	Total
35266	15.83	5.79	3.84	25.46
Facility RVU	**Work**	**PE**	**MP**	**Total**
35266	15.83	5.79	3.84	25.46

	FUD	Status	MUE	Modifiers				IOM Reference
35266	90	A	2(3)	51	50	62*	80	None

* with documentation

35271-35276

35271 Repair blood vessel with graft other than vein; intrathoracic, with bypass
35276 intrathoracic, without bypass

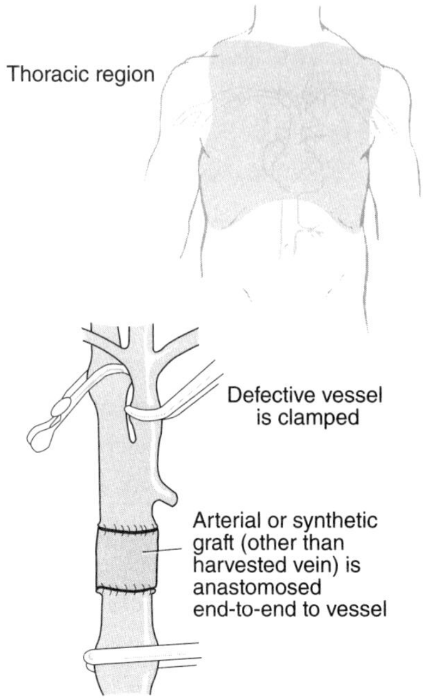

Explanation

In 35271, the physician exposes the abnormal blood vessel (arterial or venous) by choosing a thoracic incision appropriate to the involved vessel. The physician places cardiopulmonary bypass catheters (through incisions in the low inferior vena cava, the superior vena cava, and high aorta or femoral artery). The physician stops the heart by infusing cardioplegia solution into the coronary circulation. The physician examines the abnormal vessel and repairs it by clamping proximally and distally to the defect and sewing in synthetic graft material in order to cover the defect. The physician confirms vessel patency with Doppler probe or angiography prior to taking the patient off cardiopulmonary bypass and closing the wound. The physician leaves chest and, possibly, mediastinal drains in place. In 35276, the physician exposes the abnormal blood vessel (arterial or venous) by choosing a thoracic incision appropriate to the involved vessel. The physician examines the abnormal vessel and repairs it by clamping proximally and distally to the defect and sewing in synthetic graft material in order to correct the defect. The physician confirms vessel patency with Doppler probe or angiography prior to closing the wound. The physician leaves chest and, possibly, mediastinal drains in place.

Coding Tips

Establishing both inflow and outflow by any method is included. That portion of the operative arteriogram performed by the surgeon is also included. Angioscopy performed during therapeutic intervention should be reported in addition to the code for the primary procedure; see 35400. Any graft harvest is not reported separately. For repair of a thoracic aortic aneurysm, see 33858–33875. For repair of an innominate, subclavian aneurysm by thoracic incision, see 35021–35022. For direct repair of an intrathoracic blood vessel, see 35211–35216. For repair of an intrathoracic blood vessel with vein graft, see 35241–35246.

ICD-10-CM Diagnostic Codes

I77.2	Rupture of artery
I77.5	Necrosis of artery
I77.810	Thoracic aortic ectasia
I77.812	Thoracoabdominal aortic ectasia
I80.8	Phlebitis and thrombophlebitis of other sites
I87.1	Compression of vein
S25.01XA	Minor laceration of thoracic aorta, initial encounter
S25.02XA	Major laceration of thoracic aorta, initial encounter
S25.111A	Minor laceration of right innominate or subclavian artery, initial encounter ☑
S25.121A	Major laceration of right innominate or subclavian artery, initial encounter ☑
S25.191A	Other specified injury of right innominate or subclavian artery, initial encounter ☑
S25.21XA	Minor laceration of superior vena cava, initial encounter
S25.22XA	Major laceration of superior vena cava, initial encounter
S25.29XA	Other specified injury of superior vena cava, initial encounter
S25.311A	Minor laceration of right innominate or subclavian vein, initial encounter ☑
S25.321A	Major laceration of right innominate or subclavian vein, initial encounter ☑
S25.391A	Other specified injury of right innominate or subclavian vein, initial encounter ☑
S25.411A	Minor laceration of right pulmonary blood vessels, initial encounter ☑
S25.421A	Major laceration of right pulmonary blood vessels, initial encounter ☑
S25.491A	Other specified injury of right pulmonary blood vessels, initial encounter ☑
S25.511A	Laceration of intercostal blood vessels, right side, initial encounter ☑
S25.591A	Other specified injury of intercostal blood vessels, right side, initial encounter ☑
S35.11XA	Minor laceration of inferior vena cava, initial encounter
S35.12XA	Major laceration of inferior vena cava, initial encounter
S35.19XA	Other injury of inferior vena cava, initial encounter

AMA: **35271** 2019,Jul **35276** 2019,Jul; 2018,Jun

Relative Value Units/Medicare Edits

Non-Facility RVU	Work	PE	MP	Total
35271	24.58	10.43	5.86	40.87
35276	25.83	11.05	5.99	42.87
Facility RVU	**Work**	**PE**	**MP**	**Total**
35271	24.58	10.43	5.86	40.87
35276	25.83	11.05	5.99	42.87

	FUD	Status	MUE	Modifiers				IOM Reference
35271	90	A	2(3)	51	50	62*	80	None
35276	90	A	2(3)	51	50	62*	80	

* with documentation

35281

35281 Repair blood vessel with graft other than vein; intra-abdominal

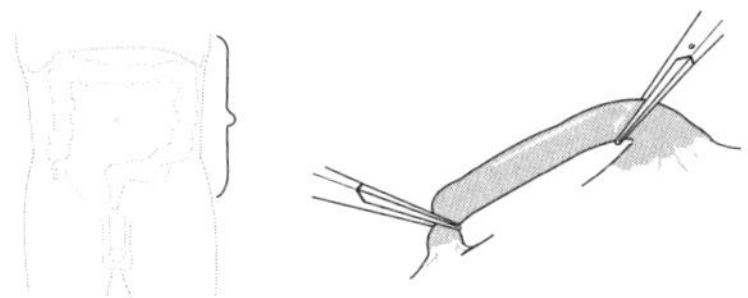

A defective vessel of the abdominal area, venous or arterial, is repaired using a graft other than vein

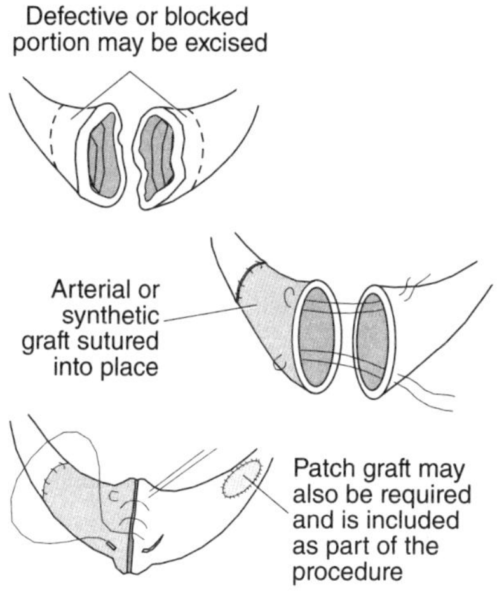

Explanation

The physician exposes the abnormal blood vessel (arterial or venous) by choosing an abdominal incision appropriate to the involved vessel. The physician examines the abnormal vessel and repairs it by clamping proximally and distally to the defect, and sewing in synthetic graft material in order to correct the defect. The physician confirms vessel patency with Doppler probe or angiography prior to closing the wound. The physician leaves surgical drains in place.

Coding Tips

Establishing both inflow and outflow by any method is included. That portion of the operative arteriogram performed by the surgeon is also included. Angioscopy performed during therapeutic intervention should be reported in addition to the code for the primary procedure; see 35400. Any graft harvest is not reported separately. For repair of an intra-abdominal aneurysm, see 35081–35132. For direct repair of an intra-abdominal blood vessel, see 35221. For repair of an intra-abdominal blood vessel with vein graft, see 35251.

ICD-10-CM Diagnostic Codes

I77.1	Stricture of artery
I77.2	Rupture of artery
I77.811	Abdominal aortic ectasia
I77.812	Thoracoabdominal aortic ectasia
I82.0	Budd-Chiari syndrome
K55.011	Focal (segmental) acute (reversible) ischemia of small intestine
K55.012	Diffuse acute (reversible) ischemia of small intestine
K55.021	Focal (segmental) acute infarction of small intestine
K55.022	Diffuse acute infarction of small intestine
K55.031	Focal (segmental) acute (reversible) ischemia of large intestine
K55.032	Diffuse acute (reversible) ischemia of large intestine

K55.041	Focal (segmental) acute infarction of large intestine
K55.042	Diffuse acute infarction of large intestine
S35.01XA	Minor laceration of abdominal aorta, initial encounter
S35.02XA	Major laceration of abdominal aorta, initial encounter
S35.09XA	Other injury of abdominal aorta, initial encounter
S35.211A	Minor laceration of celiac artery, initial encounter
S35.212A	Major laceration of celiac artery, initial encounter
S35.218A	Other injury of celiac artery, initial encounter
S35.221A	Minor laceration of superior mesenteric artery, initial encounter
S35.222A	Major laceration of superior mesenteric artery, initial encounter
S35.228A	Other injury of superior mesenteric artery, initial encounter
S35.231A	Minor laceration of inferior mesenteric artery, initial encounter
S35.232A	Major laceration of inferior mesenteric artery, initial encounter
S35.238A	Other injury of inferior mesenteric artery, initial encounter
S35.291A	Minor laceration of branches of celiac and mesenteric artery, initial encounter
S35.292A	Major laceration of branches of celiac and mesenteric artery, initial encounter
S35.298A	Other injury of branches of celiac and mesenteric artery, initial encounter
S35.311A	Laceration of portal vein, initial encounter
S35.318A	Other specified injury of portal vein, initial encounter
S35.321A	Laceration of splenic vein, initial encounter
S35.328A	Other specified injury of splenic vein, initial encounter
S35.331A	Laceration of superior mesenteric vein, initial encounter
S35.338A	Other specified injury of superior mesenteric vein, initial encounter
S35.341A	Laceration of inferior mesenteric vein, initial encounter
S35.348A	Other specified injury of inferior mesenteric vein, initial encounter
S35.411A	Laceration of right renal artery, initial encounter ☑
S35.414A	Laceration of right renal vein, initial encounter ☑
S35.491A	Other specified injury of right renal artery, initial encounter ☑
S35.494A	Other specified injury of right renal vein, initial encounter ☑
S35.511A	Injury of right iliac artery, initial encounter ☑
S35.514A	Injury of right iliac vein, initial encounter ☑
S35.531A	Injury of right uterine artery, initial encounter ☑
S35.534A	Injury of right uterine vein, initial encounter ☑
S35.59XA	Injury of other iliac blood vessels, initial encounter
S35.8X1A	Laceration of other blood vessels at abdomen, lower back and pelvis level, initial encounter

AMA: 35281 2019,Jul

Relative Value Units/Medicare Edits

Non-Facility RVU	Work	PE	MP	Total
35281	30.06	10.01	7.54	47.61
Facility RVU	**Work**	**PE**	**MP**	**Total**
35281	30.06	10.01	7.54	47.61

	FUD	Status	MUE	Modifiers				IOM Reference
35281	90	A	2(3)	51	50	62*	80	None

* with documentation

35286

35286 Repair blood vessel with graft other than vein; lower extremity

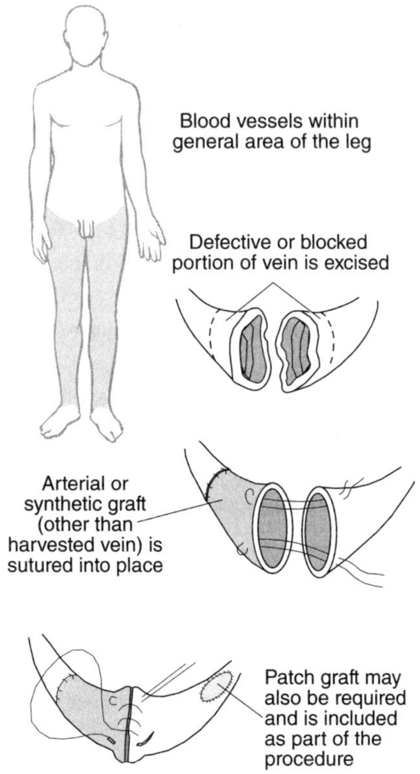

Explanation

The physician makes an incision in the skin of a lower extremity over the site of an injured blood vessel. The vessel is isolated and dissected from adjacent critical structures and vessel clamps are applied. If the defect is too extensive to repair directly, the physician repairs the injured vessel with a length of synthetic graft material. The clamps are removed and the skin incision is repaired with layered closure.

Coding Tips

Establishing both inflow and outflow by any method is included. That portion of the operative arteriogram performed by the surgeon is also included. Angioscopy performed during therapeutic intervention should be reported in addition to the code for the primary procedure, see 35400. Any graft harvest is not reported separately. For repair of an aneurysm, lower extremity, see 35141–35152. For direct repair of a blood vessel, lower extremity, see 35226. For repair of a blood vessel of lower extremity with vein graft, see 35256. For repair of a congenital arteriovenous fistula, see 35184. For repair of an acquired or traumatic arteriovenous blood fistula, see 35190.

ICD-10-CM Diagnostic Codes

I77.2	Rupture of artery
S75.021A	Major laceration of femoral artery, right leg, initial encounter ☑
S75.022A	Major laceration of femoral artery, left leg, initial encounter ☑
S75.221A	Major laceration of greater saphenous vein at hip and thigh level, right leg, initial encounter ☑
S75.222A	Major laceration of greater saphenous vein at hip and thigh level, left leg, initial encounter ☑
S85.011A	Laceration of popliteal artery, right leg, initial encounter ☑
S85.012A	Laceration of popliteal artery, left leg, initial encounter ☑

S85.141A Laceration of anterior tibial artery, right leg, initial encounter ☑
S85.142A Laceration of anterior tibial artery, left leg, initial encounter ☑
S85.171A Laceration of posterior tibial artery, right leg, initial encounter ☑
S85.172A Laceration of posterior tibial artery, left leg, initial encounter ☑
S85.211A Laceration of peroneal artery, right leg, initial encounter ☑
S85.212A Laceration of peroneal artery, left leg, initial encounter ☑
S85.311A Laceration of greater saphenous vein at lower leg level, right leg, initial encounter ☑
S85.312A Laceration of greater saphenous vein at lower leg level, left leg, initial encounter ☑
S85.411A Laceration of lesser saphenous vein at lower leg level, right leg, initial encounter ☑
S85.412A Laceration of lesser saphenous vein at lower leg level, left leg, initial encounter ☑
S85.511A Laceration of popliteal vein, right leg, initial encounter ☑
S85.512A Laceration of popliteal vein, left leg, initial encounter ☑
S85.811A Laceration of other blood vessels at lower leg level, right leg, initial encounter ☑
S85.812A Laceration of other blood vessels at lower leg level, left leg, initial encounter ☑
S95.011A Laceration of dorsal artery of right foot, initial encounter ☑
S95.012A Laceration of dorsal artery of left foot, initial encounter ☑
S95.211A Laceration of dorsal vein of right foot, initial encounter ☑
S95.212A Laceration of dorsal vein of left foot, initial encounter ☑
S95.811A Laceration of other blood vessels at ankle and foot level, right leg, initial encounter ☑
S95.812A Laceration of other blood vessels at ankle and foot level, left leg, initial encounter ☑

AMA: 35286 2020,Dec; 2019,Dec; 2019,Jul

Relative Value Units/Medicare Edits

Non-Facility RVU	Work	PE	MP	Total
35286	17.19	5.76	4.25	27.2
Facility RVU	**Work**	**PE**	**MP**	**Total**
35286	17.19	5.76	4.25	27.2

	FUD	Status	MUE	Modifiers				IOM Reference
35286	90	A	2(3)	51	50	62*	80	None

* with documentation

35301

35301 Thromboendarterectomy, including patch graft, if performed; carotid, vertebral, subclavian, by neck incision

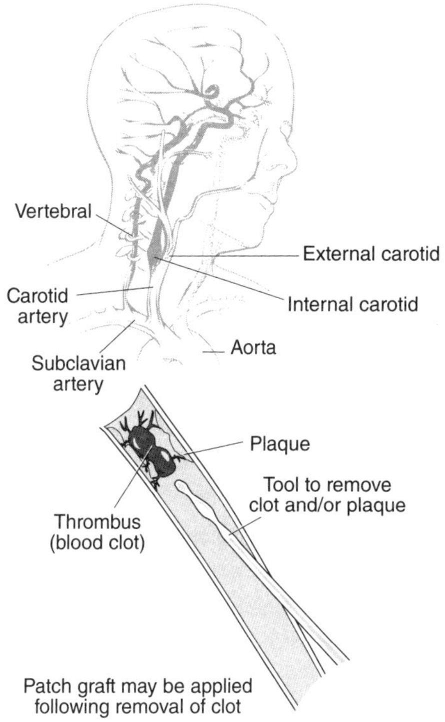

Explanation

The physician makes an incision in the skin of the neck over the site of plaque or abnormal lining of the carotid, vertebral, or subclavian artery. The vessel is isolated and dissected from adjacent critical structures and vessel clamps are applied. A temporary vascular shunt may be placed, bypassing the area and allowing blood supply to continue uninterrupted during the procedure. The vessel is incised. Using a blunt, spatula-like tool, the plaque and the vessel lining are separated from the artery and removed. The edge of the normal artery lining may be sutured to the artery wall to prevent separation when blood flow resumes. After the plaque and lining are removed, a patch graft may be applied and sutured to the vessel. This enlarges the diameter of the artery. The vessel clamps are removed and the skin incision is repaired with layered closure.

Coding Tips

Establishing both inflow and outflow by any method is included. That portion of the operative arteriogram performed by the surgeon is also included. Angioscopy performed during therapeutic intervention should be reported in addition to the code for the primary procedure, see 35400. Report 35390 in addition to 35301 for reoperation on the carotid artery involving repeat thromboendarterectomy more than one month after the original operation. Any graft harvest of saphenous or upper extremity vein is not reported separately. Do not report this procedure with codes for repair of an aneurysm (35001–35152) as aneurysm repair includes endarterectomy and treatment of associated occlusive disease.

ICD-10-CM Diagnostic Codes

G45.0 Vertebro-basilar artery syndrome
G45.1 Carotid artery syndrome (hemispheric)
G45.2 Multiple and bilateral precerebral artery syndromes

G45.3	Amaurosis fugax
G45.8	Other transient cerebral ischemic attacks and related syndromes
I63.011	Cerebral infarction due to thrombosis of right vertebral artery ☑
I63.012	Cerebral infarction due to thrombosis of left vertebral artery ☑
I63.013	Cerebral infarction due to thrombosis of bilateral vertebral arteries ☑
I63.031	Cerebral infarction due to thrombosis of right carotid artery ☑
I63.032	Cerebral infarction due to thrombosis of left carotid artery ☑
I63.033	Cerebral infarction due to thrombosis of bilateral carotid arteries ☑
I63.09	Cerebral infarction due to thrombosis of other precerebral artery
I63.111	Cerebral infarction due to embolism of right vertebral artery ☑
I63.112	Cerebral infarction due to embolism of left vertebral artery ☑
I63.113	Cerebral infarction due to embolism of bilateral vertebral arteries ☑
I63.131	Cerebral infarction due to embolism of right carotid artery ☑
I63.132	Cerebral infarction due to embolism of left carotid artery ☑
I63.133	Cerebral infarction due to embolism of bilateral carotid arteries ☑
I63.19	Cerebral infarction due to embolism of other precerebral artery
I65.01	Occlusion and stenosis of right vertebral artery ☑
I65.02	Occlusion and stenosis of left vertebral artery ☑
I65.03	Occlusion and stenosis of bilateral vertebral arteries ☑
I65.21	Occlusion and stenosis of right carotid artery ☑
I65.22	Occlusion and stenosis of left carotid artery ☑
I65.23	Occlusion and stenosis of bilateral carotid arteries ☑
I65.8	Occlusion and stenosis of other precerebral arteries
I67.81	Acute cerebrovascular insufficiency
I67.82	Cerebral ischemia
I67.841	Reversible cerebrovascular vasoconstriction syndrome
I67.848	Other cerebrovascular vasospasm and vasoconstriction
I67.858	Other hereditary cerebrovascular disease
I67.89	Other cerebrovascular disease
I73.89	Other specified peripheral vascular diseases
I76	Septic arterial embolism
I77.1	Stricture of artery

Relative Value Units/Medicare Edits

Non-Facility RVU	Work	PE	MP	Total
35301	21.16	6.59	5.35	33.1
Facility RVU	**Work**	**PE**	**MP**	**Total**
35301	21.16	6.59	5.35	33.1

	FUD	Status	MUE	Modifiers				IOM Reference
35301	90	A	2(3)	51	50	62*	80	None

* with documentation

Terms To Know

angioscopy. Visualization of capillary blood vessels with a microscope, or the inside of a blood vessel with a fiberoptic-equipped catheter.

35302-35304

35302	Thromboendarterectomy, including patch graft, if performed; superficial femoral artery
35303	popliteal artery
35304	tibioperoneal trunk artery

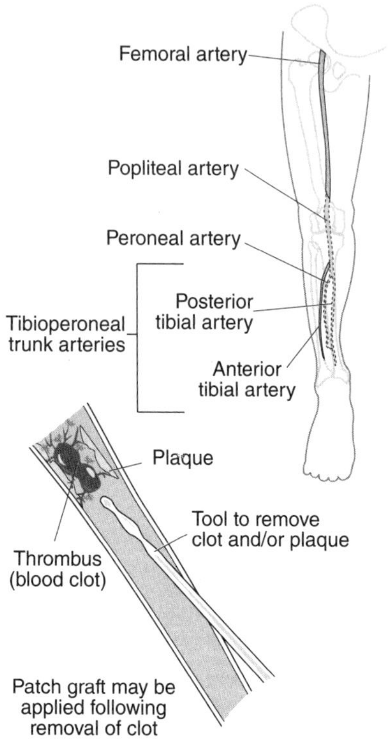

Explanation

The physician makes an incision in the skin of the leg over the site of a blood clot, plaque, or abnormal lining of the superficial femoral (35302), popliteal (35303), or tibioperoneal trunk (35304) arteries. The vessels are isolated and dissected from adjacent critical structures and vessel clamps are applied. The vessels are incised. Using a blunt, spatula-like tool, the plaque and the vessel lining are separated from the arteries and removed. The edge of the normal artery linings may be sutured to the artery walls to prevent separation when blood flow resumes. After the plaque and lining are removed, a patch graft may be applied and sutured to the vessels. This enlarges the diameter of the arteries. The vessel clamps are removed and the skin incision is repaired with layered closure.

Coding Tips

Establishing both inflow and outflow by any method is included. That portion of the operative arteriogram performed by the surgeon is also included. Angioscopy performed during therapeutic intervention should be reported in addition to the code for the primary procedure, see 35400. Any graft harvest of saphenous or upper extremity vein (35500) is not reported separately. Do not report 35302 or 35303 with 37225 or 37227 when the procedures are performed in the same vessel. Do not report 35304 with 37229, 37231, 37233, or 37235 when the procedures are performed in the same vessel.

ICD-10-CM Diagnostic Codes

D68.61	Antiphospholipid syndrome
I70.211	Atherosclerosis of native arteries of extremities with intermittent claudication, right leg A ☑

N Newborn: 0 P Pediatric: 0-17 M Maternity: 9-64 A Adult: 15-124 AMA: CPT Assist

I70.221	Atherosclerosis of native arteries of extremities with rest pain, right leg A ☑
I70.231	Atherosclerosis of native arteries of right leg with ulceration of thigh A ☑
I70.232	Atherosclerosis of native arteries of right leg with ulceration of calf A ☑
I70.233	Atherosclerosis of native arteries of right leg with ulceration of ankle A ☑
I70.234	Atherosclerosis of native arteries of right leg with ulceration of heel and midfoot A ☑
I70.235	Atherosclerosis of native arteries of right leg with ulceration of other part of foot A ☑
I70.261	Atherosclerosis of native arteries of extremities with gangrene, right leg A ☑
I70.291	Other atherosclerosis of native arteries of extremities, right leg A ☑
I70.461	Atherosclerosis of autologous vein bypass graft(s) of the extremities with gangrene, right leg A ☑
I70.561	Atherosclerosis of nonautologous biological bypass graft(s) of the extremities with gangrene, right leg A ☑
I70.661	Atherosclerosis of nonbiological bypass graft(s) of the extremities with gangrene, right leg A ☑
I70.761	Atherosclerosis of other type of bypass graft(s) of the extremities with gangrene, right leg A ☑
I72.4	Aneurysm of artery of lower extremity
I74.3	Embolism and thrombosis of arteries of the lower extremities
I75.021	Atheroembolism of right lower extremity ☑
I76	Septic arterial embolism
I77.1	Stricture of artery
I77.2	Rupture of artery
S75.021A	Major laceration of femoral artery, right leg, initial encounter ☑
S85.011A	Laceration of popliteal artery, right leg, initial encounter ☑
S85.141A	Laceration of anterior tibial artery, right leg, initial encounter ☑
S85.171A	Laceration of posterior tibial artery, right leg, initial encounter ☑
S85.181A	Other specified injury of posterior tibial artery, right leg, initial encounter ☑
S85.211A	Laceration of peroneal artery, right leg, initial encounter ☑

Relative Value Units/Medicare Edits

Non-Facility RVU	Work	PE	MP	Total
35302	21.35	6.1	5.28	32.73
35303	23.6	6.42	5.86	35.88
35304	24.6	6.62	6.13	37.35
Facility RVU	**Work**	**PE**	**MP**	**Total**
35302	21.35	6.1	5.28	32.73
35303	23.6	6.42	5.86	35.88
35304	24.6	6.62	6.13	37.35

	FUD	Status	MUE	Modifiers				IOM Reference
35302	90	A	1(2)	51	50	62*	80	None
35303	90	A	1(2)	51	50	62*	80	
35304	90	A	1(2)	51	50	62*	80	

* with documentation

35305-35306

35305 Thromboendarterectomy, including patch graft, if performed; tibial or peroneal artery, initial vessel

\+ **35306** each additional tibial or peroneal artery (List separately in addition to code for primary procedure)

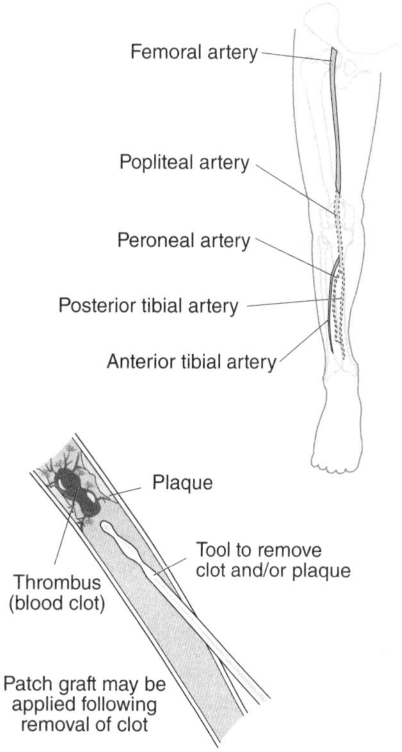

Explanation

A thromboendarterectomy is performed on a tibial or peroneal artery. The physician makes an incision in the skin over the site of plaque or abnormal lining of a tibial or peroneal artery. The vessel is isolated and dissected from adjacent critical structures and vessel clamps are applied. The vessel is incised. Using a blunt, spatula-like tool, the plaque and the vessel lining are separated from the artery and removed. The edge of the normal artery lining may be sutured to the artery wall to prevent separation when blood flow resumes. After the plaque and lining are removed, a patch graft may be applied and sutured to the vessel. This enlarges the diameter of the artery. The vessel clamps are removed, and the skin incision is repaired with layered closure. Report 35305 for thromboendarterectomy of the initial tibial or peroneal artery and 35306 for each additional tibial or peroneal artery.

Coding Tips

Report 35306 in addition to 35305. Establishing both inflow and outflow by any method is included. That portion of the operative arteriogram performed by the surgeon is also included. Angioscopy performed during therapeutic intervention should be reported in addition to the code for the primary procedure, see 35400. Any graft harvest of saphenous or upper extremity vein (35500) is not reported separately. Do not report 35305 or 35306 with transluminal peripheral atherectomy (37229, 37231, 37233, 37235) when performed in the same vessel.

ICD-10-CM Diagnostic Codes

I70.211	Atherosclerosis of native arteries of extremities with intermittent claudication, right leg A ☑

I70.221	Atherosclerosis of native arteries of extremities with rest pain, right leg [A] ☑
I70.231	Atherosclerosis of native arteries of right leg with ulceration of thigh [A] ☑
I70.232	Atherosclerosis of native arteries of right leg with ulceration of calf [A] ☑
I70.233	Atherosclerosis of native arteries of right leg with ulceration of ankle [A] ☑
I70.234	Atherosclerosis of native arteries of right leg with ulceration of heel and midfoot [A] ☑
I70.235	Atherosclerosis of native arteries of right leg with ulceration of other part of foot [A] ☑
I70.238	Atherosclerosis of native arteries of right leg with ulceration of other part of lower leg [A] ☑
I70.261	Atherosclerosis of native arteries of extremities with gangrene, right leg [A] ☑
I70.291	Other atherosclerosis of native arteries of extremities, right leg [A] ☑
I70.361	Atherosclerosis of unspecified type of bypass graft(s) of the extremities with gangrene, right leg [A] ☑
I70.461	Atherosclerosis of autologous vein bypass graft(s) of the extremities with gangrene, right leg [A] ☑
I70.561	Atherosclerosis of nonautologous biological bypass graft(s) of the extremities with gangrene, right leg [A] ☑
I70.661	Atherosclerosis of nonbiological bypass graft(s) of the extremities with gangrene, right leg [A] ☑
I70.761	Atherosclerosis of other type of bypass graft(s) of the extremities with gangrene, right leg [A] ☑
I72.4	Aneurysm of artery of lower extremity
I74.3	Embolism and thrombosis of arteries of the lower extremities
I75.021	Atheroembolism of right lower extremity ☑
I77.1	Stricture of artery
I77.2	Rupture of artery
I77.79	Dissection of other specified artery
S85.141A	Laceration of anterior tibial artery, right leg, initial encounter ☑
S85.171A	Laceration of posterior tibial artery, right leg, initial encounter ☑
S85.211A	Laceration of peroneal artery, right leg, initial encounter ☑

Relative Value Units/Medicare Edits

Non-Facility RVU	Work	PE	MP	Total
35305	23.6	6.45	5.88	35.93
35306	9.25	1.43	2.29	12.97
Facility RVU	**Work**	**PE**	**MP**	**Total**
35305	23.6	6.45	5.88	35.93
35306	9.25	1.43	2.29	12.97

	FUD	Status	MUE	Modifiers				IOM Reference
35305	90	A	1(2)	51	50	62*	80	None
35306	N/A	A	2(3)	N/A	N/A	62*	80	

* with documentation

35311

35311 Thromboendarterectomy, including patch graft, if performed; subclavian, innominate, by thoracic incision

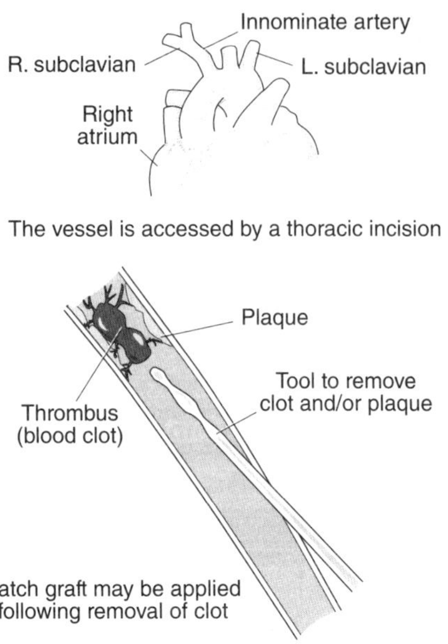

Explanation

The physician exposes the innominate or subclavian artery by median sternotomy or lateral thoracotomy. The physician clamps the aortic arch widely around the origin of the diseased artery and clamps the distal end of the diseased artery. After making a longitudinal incision in the diseased artery, the physician uses a spatula to remove the atherosclerotic material. The physician may tack (suture) down the inner layer of the artery with a few 6-0 sutures before closing the artery with suture. A patch graft may be used to enlarge the arterial lumen. The physician unclamps the aorta, as well as the distal arterial clamp, and closes the sternotomy or thoracotomy, leaving a chest tube in place.

Coding Tips

Establishing both inflow and outflow by any method is included. That portion of the operative arteriogram performed by the surgeon is also included. Angioscopy performed during therapeutic intervention should be reported in addition to the code for the primary procedure; see 35400. Any graft harvest is not reported separately. Do not report this procedure with codes for repair of an aneurysm (35001–35152) as aneurysm repair includes endarterectomy and treatment of associated occlusive disease. For innominate or subclavian embolectomy and/or thrombectomy, see 34051. For repair of a congenital arteriovenous fistula, see 35182. For repair of an acquired or traumatic arteriovenous fistula, see 35189.

ICD-10-CM Diagnostic Codes

G45.2	Multiple and bilateral precerebral artery syndromes
G45.8	Other transient cerebral ischemic attacks and related syndromes
G45.9	Transient cerebral ischemic attack, unspecified
G54.0	Brachial plexus disorders
I63.09	Cerebral infarction due to thrombosis of other precerebral artery
I63.19	Cerebral infarction due to embolism of other precerebral artery
I63.29	Cerebral infarction due to unspecified occlusion or stenosis of other precerebral arteries
I70.8	Atherosclerosis of other arteries [A]

I74.8 Embolism and thrombosis of other arteries

S25.191A Other specified injury of right innominate or subclavian artery, initial encounter ☑

S25.192A Other specified injury of left innominate or subclavian artery, initial encounter ☑

Relative Value Units/Medicare Edits

Non-Facility RVU	Work	PE	MP	Total
35311	28.6	10.32	6.62	45.54
Facility RVU	**Work**	**PE**	**MP**	**Total**
35311	28.6	10.32	6.62	45.54

	FUD	Status	MUE	Modifiers				IOM Reference
35311	90	A	1(2)	51	50	62*	80	None

* with documentation

Terms To Know

angioscopy. Visualization of capillary blood vessels with a microscope, or the inside of a blood vessel with a fiberoptic-equipped catheter.

arteriogram. Radiograph of arteries.

atherosclerosis. Buildup of yellowish plaques composed of cholesterol and lipoid material within the arteries.

embolism. Obstruction of a blood vessel resulting from a clot or foreign substance.

fistula. Abnormal tube-like passage between two body cavities or organs or from an organ to the outside surface.

graft. Tissue implant from another part of the body or another person.

thrombosis. Condition arising from the presence or formation of blood clots within a blood vessel that may cause vascular obstruction and insufficient oxygenation.

35321

35321 Thromboendarterectomy, including patch graft, if performed; axillary-brachial

Explanation

The physician makes an incision in the skin of the axilla or arm over the site of a blood clot, plaque, or abnormal lining of the axillary or brachial artery. The vessel is isolated and dissected from adjacent critical structures and vessel clamps are applied. The vessel is incised. Using a blunt, spatula-like tool, the plaque and the vessel lining are separated from the artery and removed. The edge of the normal artery lining may be sutured to the artery wall to prevent separation when blood flow resumes. After the plaque and lining are removed, a patch graft may be applied and sutured to the vessel. This enlarges the diameter of the artery. The vessel clamps are removed and the skin incision is repaired with layered closure.

Coding Tips

Establishing both inflow and outflow by any method is included. That portion of the operative arteriogram performed by the surgeon is also included. Angioscopy performed during therapeutic intervention should be reported in addition to the code for the primary procedure; see 35400. Any graft harvest is not reported separately. Do not report this procedure with codes for repair of an aneurysm (35001–35152) as aneurysm repair includes endarterectomy and treatment of associated occlusive disease. For axillary, brachial embolectomy and/or thrombectomy, see 34101. For repair of a congenital arteriovenous fistula, see 35184. For repair of an acquired or traumatic arteriovenous fistula, see 35190.

ICD-10-CM Diagnostic Codes

I70.92 Chronic total occlusion of artery of the extremities A

I74.2 Embolism and thrombosis of arteries of the upper extremities

I75.011 Atheroembolism of right upper extremity ☑

I75.012 Atheroembolism of left upper extremity ☑

I75.013 Atheroembolism of bilateral upper extremities ☑

I77.1 Stricture of artery

I77.2 Rupture of artery

Relative Value Units/Medicare Edits

Non-Facility RVU	Work	PE	MP	Total
35321	16.59	5.67	4.12	26.38
Facility RVU	**Work**	**PE**	**MP**	**Total**
35321	16.59	5.67	4.12	26.38

	FUD	Status	MUE	Modifiers				IOM Reference
35321	90	A	1(2)	51	50	62*	80	None

* with documentation

Terms To Know

angioscopy. Visualization of capillary blood vessels with a microscope, or the inside of a blood vessel with a fiberoptic-equipped catheter.

dissection. Separating by cutting tissue or body structures apart.

graft. Tissue implant from another part of the body or another person.

plaque. Accumulation of a soft sticky substance on the teeth largely composed of bacteria and its byproducts.

35331

35331 Thromboendarterectomy, including patch graft, if performed; abdominal aorta

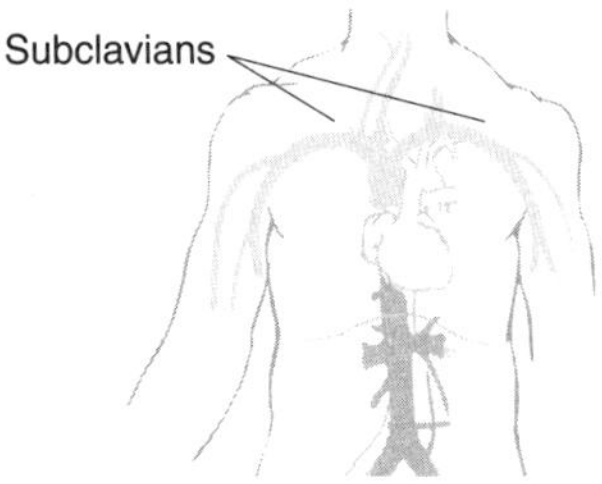

Abdominal aorta and select branches

A thromboendarterectomy is performed on the abdominal aorta

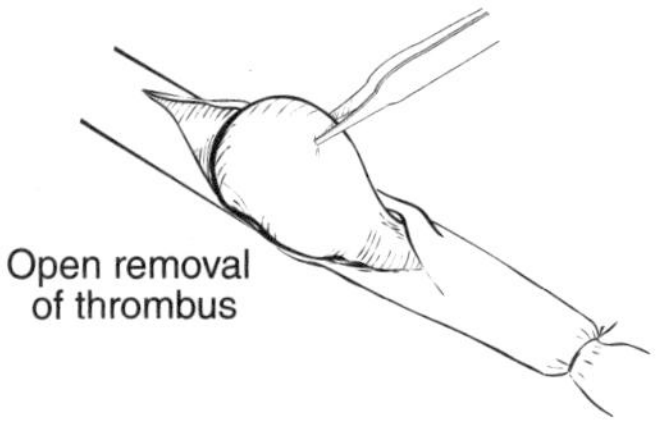

Patch graft may be applied following removal of clot

Explanation

The physician exposes the abdominal aorta using a transperitoneal approach, placing a long incision in the midabdomen. The transverse colon and small bowel are retracted to allow dissection and exposure of the aorta. The iliac arteries are exposed and control of blood flow is achieved with umbilical tape or rubber catheters placed proximal to the diseased area. The physician anticoagulates the patient and cross-clamps the iliac arteries and proximal aorta. A longitudinal incision down the affected portion of abdominal aorta is performed and a spatula is used to remove the atherosclerotic material. The inner layer of the aorta may be tacked down with small sutures. A patch graft may be applied and sutured to the vessel. The physician sutures the aorta closed and closes the retroperitoneum and abdominal wound, leaving drains in place.

Coding Tips

Establishing both inflow and outflow by any method is included. That portion of the operative arteriogram performed by the surgeon is also included. Angioscopy performed during therapeutic intervention should be reported in addition to the code for the primary procedure; see 35400. Any graft harvest is not reported separately. Do not report this procedure with codes for repair of aneurysm (35001–35152) as aneurysm repair includes endarterectomy and treatment of associated occlusive disease. For repair of a congenital arteriovenous fistula, see 35182. For repair of an acquired or traumatic arteriovenous fistula, see 35189.

ICD-10-CM Diagnostic Codes

I70.0	Atherosclerosis of aorta 🅰
I74.01	Saddle embolus of abdominal aorta
I74.09	Other arterial embolism and thrombosis of abdominal aorta
I76	Septic arterial embolism
I77.1	Stricture of artery
I77.89	Other specified disorders of arteries and arterioles

Relative Value Units/Medicare Edits

Non-Facility RVU	Work	PE	MP	Total
35331	27.72	7.97	6.91	42.6
Facility RVU	**Work**	**PE**	**MP**	**Total**
35331	27.72	7.97	6.91	42.6

	FUD	Status	MUE	Modifiers				IOM Reference
35331	90	A	1(2)	51	50	62*	80	None

* with documentation

Terms To Know

angioscopy. Visualization of capillary blood vessels with a microscope, or the inside of a blood vessel with a fiberoptic-equipped catheter.

arteriogram. Radiograph of arteries.

artery. Vessel through which oxygenated blood passes away from the heart to any part of the body.

atherosclerosis. Buildup of yellowish plaques composed of cholesterol and lipoid material within the arteries.

catheter. Flexible tube inserted into an area of the body for introducing or withdrawing fluid.

embolism. Obstruction of a blood vessel resulting from a clot or foreign substance.

incision. Act of cutting into tissue or an organ.

suture. Numerous stitching techniques employed in wound closure.

thrombosis. Condition arising from the presence or formation of blood clots within a blood vessel that may cause vascular obstruction and insufficient oxygenation.

35341

35341 Thromboendarterectomy, including patch graft, if performed; mesenteric, celiac, or renal

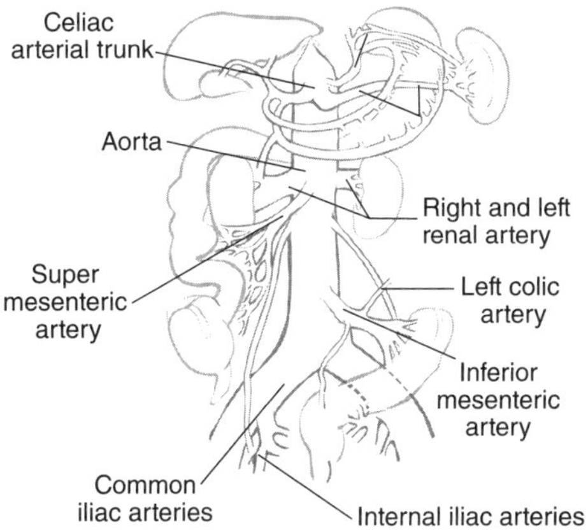

A thromboendarterectomy is performed on the mesenteric, celiac, and renal arteries

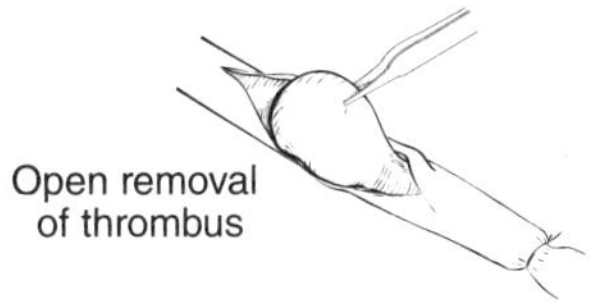

Patch graft may be applied following removal of clot

Explanation

The physician exposes the involved mesenteric, celiac, or renal artery using an abdominal incision, retracting and dissecting past large and small bowel. The aorta is clamped to isolate the involved vessel with a longitudinal incision placed down the affected vessel, and a spatula is used to remove the atherosclerotic material. If there is significant stenosis at the arterial takeoff, the aorta may be opened and the atherosclerotic material removed from within the aorta before suturing the aorta and diseased artery closed. A patch graft may be applied and sutured to the vessel An arteriography may be performed or a Doppler probe may be used to establish patency of the vessel, before closing the abdominal wound, leaving drains in place.

Coding Tips

Establishing both inflow and outflow by any method is included. That portion of the operative arteriogram performed by the surgeon is also included. Angioscopy performed during therapeutic intervention should be reported in addition to the code for the primary procedure; see 35400. Any graft harvest is not reported separately. Do not report this procedure with codes for repair of an aneurysm (35001–35152) as aneurysm repair includes endarterectomy and treatment of associated occlusive disease. For renal, celiac, mesenteric, or aortoiliac embolectomy and/or thrombectomy, by abdominal incision, see 34151. For repair of a congenital arteriovenous fistula, see 35182. For repair of an acquired or traumatic arteriovenous fistula, see 35189.

ICD-10-CM Diagnostic Codes

I70.1	Atherosclerosis of renal artery A
I70.8	Atherosclerosis of other arteries A
I77.1	Stricture of artery
I77.89	Other specified disorders of arteries and arterioles
Q27.1	Congenital renal artery stenosis
Q27.2	Other congenital malformations of renal artery
Q79.61	Classical Ehlers-Danlos syndrome
Q79.62	Hypermobile Ehlers-Danlos syndrome
Q79.63	Vascular Ehlers-Danlos syndrome

Relative Value Units/Medicare Edits

Non-Facility RVU	Work	PE	MP	Total
35341	26.21	7.93	6.49	40.63
Facility RVU	**Work**	**PE**	**MP**	**Total**
35341	26.21	7.93	6.49	40.63

	FUD	Status	MUE	Modifiers				IOM Reference
35341	90	A	3(3)	51	50	62*	80	None

* with documentation

Terms To Know

aneurysm. Circumscribed dilation or outpouching of an artery wall, often containing blood clots and connecting directly with the lumen of the artery.

angioscopy. Visualization of capillary blood vessels with a microscope, or the inside of a blood vessel with a fiberoptic-equipped catheter.

embolism. Obstruction of a blood vessel resulting from a clot or foreign substance.

endarterectomy. Removal of the thickened, endothelial lining of a diseased or damaged artery.

fistula. Abnormal tube-like passage between two body cavities or organs or from an organ to the outside surface.

35351

35351 Thromboendarterectomy, including patch graft, if performed; iliac

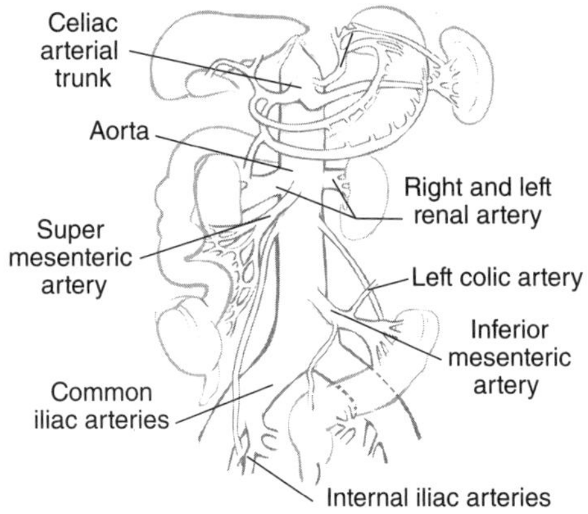

A thromboendarterectomy is performed on the iliac artery

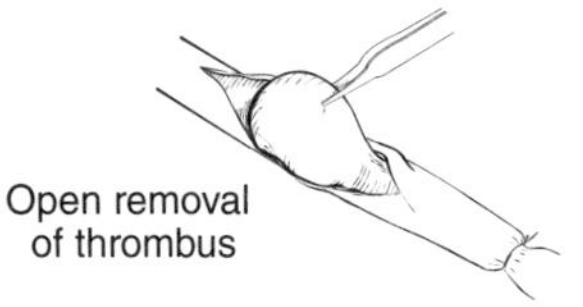

Patch graft may be applied following removal of clot

Explanation

The physician exposes the involved iliac artery using an abdominal incision, retracting and dissecting past large and small bowel. The aorta is clamped to isolate the involved vessel, with a longitudinal incision down the affected vessel, and a spatula is used to remove the atherosclerotic material. If there is significant stenosis at the arterial takeoff, the aorta may be opened and the atherosclerotic material removed before suturing the aorta and diseased artery closed. A patch graft may be applied and sutured to the vessel. The physician may perform arteriography or use a Doppler probe to establish patency of the vessel before closing the abdominal wound, leaving drains in place.

Coding Tips

Establishing both inflow and outflow by any method is included. That portion of the operative arteriogram performed by the surgeon is also included. Angioscopy performed during therapeutic intervention should be reported in addition to the code for the primary procedure, see 35400. Any graft harvest is not reported separately. Do not report this procedure with codes for repair of an aneurysm (35001–35152) as aneurysm repair includes endarterectomy and treatment of associated occlusive disease. For repair of a congenital arteriovenous fistula, see 35182. For repair of an acquired or traumatic arteriovenous fistula, see 35189.

ICD-10-CM Diagnostic Codes

I74.5	Embolism and thrombosis of iliac artery
I76	Septic arterial embolism
I77.1	Stricture of artery
I77.72	Dissection of iliac artery
I77.89	Other specified disorders of arteries and arterioles
S35.511A	Injury of right iliac artery, initial encounter ☑
S35.512A	Injury of left iliac artery, initial encounter ☑
S35.59XA	Injury of other iliac blood vessels, initial encounter

Relative Value Units/Medicare Edits

Non-Facility RVU	Work	PE	MP	Total
35351	24.61	6.91	6.12	37.64
Facility RVU	**Work**	**PE**	**MP**	**Total**
35351	24.61	6.91	6.12	37.64

	FUD	Status	MUE	Modifiers				IOM Reference
35351	90	A	1(3)	51	50	62*	80	None

* with documentation

Terms To Know

aneurysm. Circumscribed dilation or outpouching of an artery wall, often containing blood clots and connecting directly with the lumen of the artery.

angioscopy. Visualization of capillary blood vessels with a microscope, or the inside of a blood vessel with a fiberoptic-equipped catheter.

arteriogram. Radiograph of arteries.

atherosclerosis. Buildup of yellowish plaques composed of cholesterol and lipoid material within the arteries.

complication. Condition arising after the beginning of observation and treatment that modifies the course of the patient's illness or the medical care required, or an undesired result or misadventure in medical care.

digital subtraction angiography. Diagnostic imaging technique that applies computer technology to fluoroscopy for the purpose of visualizing the same vascular structures observable with conventional angiography.

embolism. Obstruction of a blood vessel resulting from a clot or foreign substance.

fistula. Abnormal tube-like passage between two body cavities or organs or from an organ to the outside surface.

graft. Tissue implant from another part of the body or another person.

harvest. Removal of cells or tissue from their native site to be used as a graft or transplant to another part of the donor's body or placed into another person.

patency. State of a tube-like structure or conduit being open and unobstructed.

stenosis. Narrowing or constriction of a passage.

N Newborn: 0 P Pediatric: 0-17 M Maternity: 9-64 A Adult: 15-124 AMA: CPT Assist

35355

35355 Thromboendarterectomy, including patch graft, if performed; iliofemoral

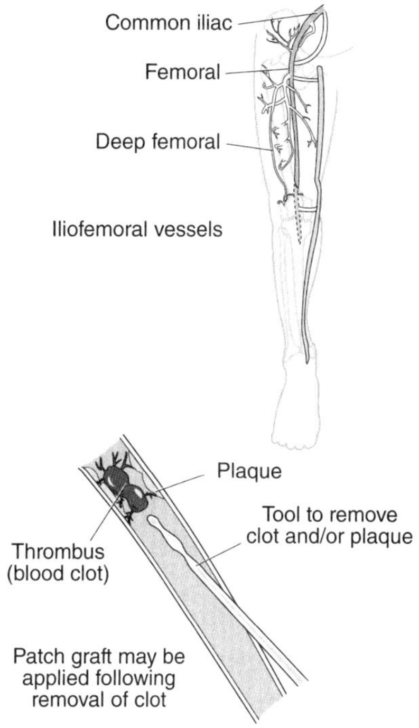

Explanation

The physician exposes the involved iliac artery using abdominal and femoral incisions, retracting and dissecting past large and small bowel. The femoral artery is exposed via a femoral incision. The aorta is clamped to isolate the involved vessel, a longitudinal incision is performed down the involved vessel, and a spatula is used to remove the atherosclerotic material. If there is significant stenosis at the arterial takeoff, the physician may open the aorta and remove the atherosclerotic material from within the aorta before suturing the aorta and diseased artery closed. A patch graft may be applied and sutured to the vessel. An arteriography may be performed or a Doppler probe may be used to establish patency of the vessel before closing the abdominal and femoral wounds, leaving drains in place.

Coding Tips

Establishing both inflow and outflow by any method is included. That portion of the operative arteriogram performed by the surgeon is also included. Angioscopy performed during therapeutic intervention should be reported in addition to the code for the primary procedure; see 35400. Any graft harvest is not reported separately. Do not report this procedure with codes for repair of an aneurysm (35001–35152) as aneurysm repair includes endarterectomy and treatment of associated occlusive disease.

ICD-10-CM Diagnostic Codes

D68.61 Antiphospholipid syndrome
I70.211 Atherosclerosis of native arteries of extremities with intermittent claudication, right leg A ☑
I70.221 Atherosclerosis of native arteries of extremities with rest pain, right leg A ☑
I70.231 Atherosclerosis of native arteries of right leg with ulceration of thigh A ☑
I70.232 Atherosclerosis of native arteries of right leg with ulceration of calf A ☑
I70.233 Atherosclerosis of native arteries of right leg with ulceration of ankle A ☑
I70.234 Atherosclerosis of native arteries of right leg with ulceration of heel and midfoot A ☑
I70.235 Atherosclerosis of native arteries of right leg with ulceration of other part of foot A ☑
I70.238 Atherosclerosis of native arteries of right leg with ulceration of other part of lower leg A ☑
I70.261 Atherosclerosis of native arteries of extremities with gangrene, right leg A ☑
I70.291 Other atherosclerosis of native arteries of extremities, right leg A ☑
I70.461 Atherosclerosis of autologous vein bypass graft(s) of the extremities with gangrene, right leg A ☑
I70.561 Atherosclerosis of nonautologous biological bypass graft(s) of the extremities with gangrene, right leg A ☑
I70.661 Atherosclerosis of nonbiological bypass graft(s) of the extremities with gangrene, right leg A ☑
I70.761 Atherosclerosis of other type of bypass graft(s) of the extremities with gangrene, right leg A ☑
I72.4 Aneurysm of artery of lower extremity
I74.3 Embolism and thrombosis of arteries of the lower extremities
I74.5 Embolism and thrombosis of iliac artery
I75.021 Atheroembolism of right lower extremity ☑
I76 Septic arterial embolism
I77.1 Stricture of artery
I77.72 Dissection of iliac artery
S35.511A Injury of right iliac artery, initial encounter ☑
S35.59XA Injury of other iliac blood vessels, initial encounter
S75.091A Other specified injury of femoral artery, right leg, initial encounter ☑

Relative Value Units/Medicare Edits

Non-Facility RVU	Work	PE	MP	Total
35355	19.86	5.34	4.91	30.11
Facility RVU	**Work**	**PE**	**MP**	**Total**
35355	19.86	5.34	4.91	30.11

	FUD	Status	MUE	Modifiers				IOM Reference
35355	90	A	1(2)	51	50	62*	80	None

* with documentation

35361

35361 Thromboendarterectomy, including patch graft, if performed; combined aortoiliac

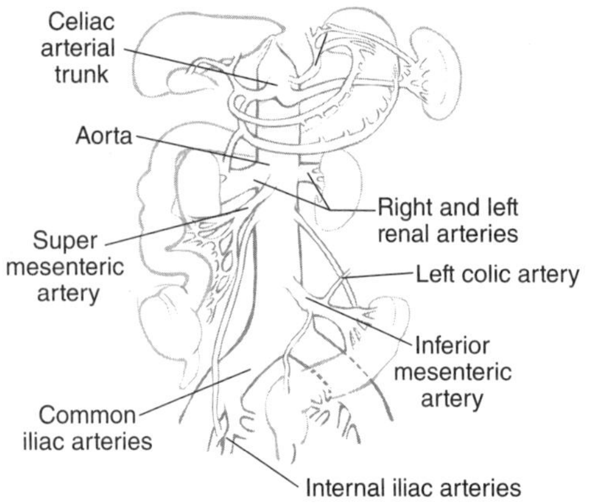

A thromboendarterectomy is performed on the combined aortoiliac artery

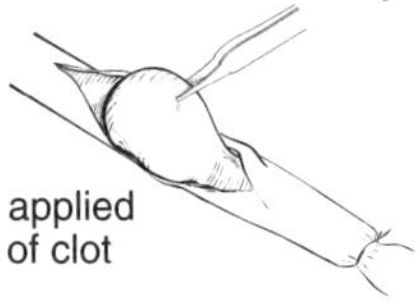
Patch graft may be applied following removal of clot

Explanation

The physician exposes the involved iliac artery using an abdominal incision, retracting and dissecting past large and small bowel. The proximal aorta is clamped above the diseased area, a longitudinal incision is performed down the distal aorta and affected iliac artery, and a spatula is utilized to remove the atherosclerotic material before suturing the aorta and iliac artery closed. A patch graft may be applied and sutured to the vessel. Arteriography or use of a Doppler probe may be necessary to establish patency of the vessel before closing the abdominal wound, leaving drains in place.

Coding Tips

Establishing both inflow and outflow by any method is included. That portion of the operative arteriogram performed by the surgeon is also included. Angioscopy performed during therapeutic intervention should be reported in addition to the code for the primary procedure; see 35400. Any graft harvest is not reported separately. Do not report this procedure with codes for repair of an aneurysm (35001–35152) as aneurysm repair includes endarterectomy and treatment of associated occlusive disease. For renal, celiac, mesenteric, or aortoiliac embolectomy and/or thrombectomy, by abdominal incision, see 34151. For repair of a congenital arteriovenous fistula, see 35182. For repair of an acquired or traumatic arteriovenous fistula, see 35189.

ICD-10-CM Diagnostic Codes

I70.0	Atherosclerosis of aorta 🅰
I74.01	Saddle embolus of abdominal aorta
I74.09	Other arterial embolism and thrombosis of abdominal aorta
I74.19	Embolism and thrombosis of other parts of aorta
I74.5	Embolism and thrombosis of iliac artery
I76	Septic arterial embolism
I77.1	Stricture of artery
I77.72	Dissection of iliac artery
I77.89	Other specified disorders of arteries and arterioles
S35.02XA	Major laceration of abdominal aorta, initial encounter
S35.511A	Injury of right iliac artery, initial encounter ☑
S35.512A	Injury of left iliac artery, initial encounter ☑

Relative Value Units/Medicare Edits

Non-Facility RVU	Work	PE	MP	Total
35361	30.24	6.81	7.55	44.6
Facility RVU	**Work**	**PE**	**MP**	**Total**
35361	30.24	6.81	7.55	44.6

	FUD	Status	MUE	Modifiers				IOM Reference
35361	90	A	1(2)	51	50	62*	80	None

* with documentation

Terms To Know

aneurysm. Circumscribed dilation or outpouching of an artery wall, often containing blood clots and connecting directly with the lumen of the artery.

angioscopy. Visualization of capillary blood vessels with a microscope, or the inside of a blood vessel with a fiberoptic-equipped catheter.

arteriogram. Radiograph of arteries.

atherosclerosis. Buildup of yellowish plaques composed of cholesterol and lipoid material within the arteries.

complication. Condition arising after the beginning of observation and treatment that modifies the course of the patient's illness or the medical care required, or an undesired result or misadventure in medical care.

embolism. Obstruction of a blood vessel resulting from a clot or foreign substance.

graft. Tissue implant from another part of the body or another person.

harvest. Removal of cells or tissue from their native site to be used as a graft or transplant to another part of the donor's body or placed into another person.

incision. Act of cutting into tissue or an organ.

patency. State of a tube-like structure or conduit being open and unobstructed.

proximal. Located closest to a specified reference point, usually the midline or trunk.

 🅽 Newborn: 0 🅿 Pediatric: 0-17 🅼 Maternity: 9-64 🅰 Adult: 15-124 AMA: CPT Assist

35363

35363 Thromboendarterectomy, including patch graft, if performed; combined aortoiliofemoral

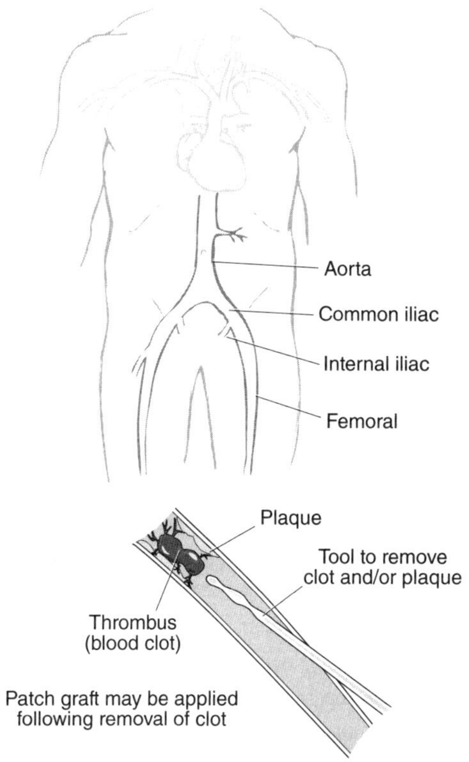

Explanation

The physician exposes the involved abdominal aorta and iliac artery using an abdominal incision, retracting and dissecting past large and small bowel. The involved femoral artery is exposed via a femoral incision and dissection. The proximal aorta is clamped above the diseased area, a longitudinal incision is performed down the distal aorta and affected iliac artery, and a spatula is used to remove the atherosclerotic material before suturing the aorta and iliac artery closed. A longitudinal incision is performed down the femoral artery and a spatula is used to remove any atherosclerotic material before sewing the femoral artery closed. A patch graft may be applied and sutured to the vessel. An arteriography or Doppler imaging may be performed to establish patency of the vessel. The physician closes the femoral and abdominal wounds, leaving drains in place.

Coding Tips

Establishing both inflow and outflow by any method is included. That portion of the operative arteriogram performed by the surgeon is also included. Angioscopy performed during therapeutic intervention should be reported in addition to the code for the primary procedure; see 35400. Any graft harvest is not reported separately. Do not report this procedure with codes for repair of aneurysm (35001–35152) as aneurysm repair includes endarterectomy and treatment of associated occlusive disease. For renal, celiac, mesentery, aortoiliac, embolectomy and/or thrombectomy, by abdominal incision, see 34151. For repair of a congenital arteriovenous fistula, see 35182. For repair of an acquired or traumatic arteriovenous fistula, see 35189.

ICD-10-CM Diagnostic Codes

D68.61 Antiphospholipid syndrome
I70.0 Atherosclerosis of aorta A
I70.211 Atherosclerosis of native arteries of extremities with intermittent claudication, right leg A ☑
I70.221 Atherosclerosis of native arteries of extremities with rest pain, right leg A ☑
I70.231 Atherosclerosis of native arteries of right leg with ulceration of thigh A ☑
I70.232 Atherosclerosis of native arteries of right leg with ulceration of calf A ☑
I70.233 Atherosclerosis of native arteries of right leg with ulceration of ankle A ☑
I70.234 Atherosclerosis of native arteries of right leg with ulceration of heel and midfoot A ☑
I70.235 Atherosclerosis of native arteries of right leg with ulceration of other part of foot A ☑
I70.238 Atherosclerosis of native arteries of right leg with ulceration of other part of lower leg A ☑
I70.261 Atherosclerosis of native arteries of extremities with gangrene, right leg A ☑
I70.291 Other atherosclerosis of native arteries of extremities, right leg A ☑
I70.461 Atherosclerosis of autologous vein bypass graft(s) of the extremities with gangrene, right leg A ☑
I70.561 Atherosclerosis of nonautologous biological bypass graft(s) of the extremities with gangrene, right leg A ☑
I70.661 Atherosclerosis of nonbiological bypass graft(s) of the extremities with gangrene, right leg A ☑
I74.01 Saddle embolus of abdominal aorta
I74.09 Other arterial embolism and thrombosis of abdominal aorta
I74.19 Embolism and thrombosis of other parts of aorta
I74.3 Embolism and thrombosis of arteries of the lower extremities
I74.5 Embolism and thrombosis of iliac artery
I75.021 Atheroembolism of right lower extremity ☑
I76 Septic arterial embolism
I77.1 Stricture of artery
I77.72 Dissection of iliac artery
S35.511A Injury of right iliac artery, initial encounter ☑
S35.59XA Injury of other iliac blood vessels, initial encounter
S75.091A Other specified injury of femoral artery, right leg, initial encounter ☑

Relative Value Units/Medicare Edits

Non-Facility RVU	Work	PE	MP	Total
35363	32.35	7.13	8.06	47.54
Facility RVU	**Work**	**PE**	**MP**	**Total**
35363	32.35	7.13	8.06	47.54

	FUD	Status	MUE	Modifiers				IOM Reference
35363	90	A	1(2)	51	50	62*	80	None

* with documentation

35371-35372

35371 Thromboendarterectomy, including patch graft, if performed; common femoral
35372 deep (profunda) femoral

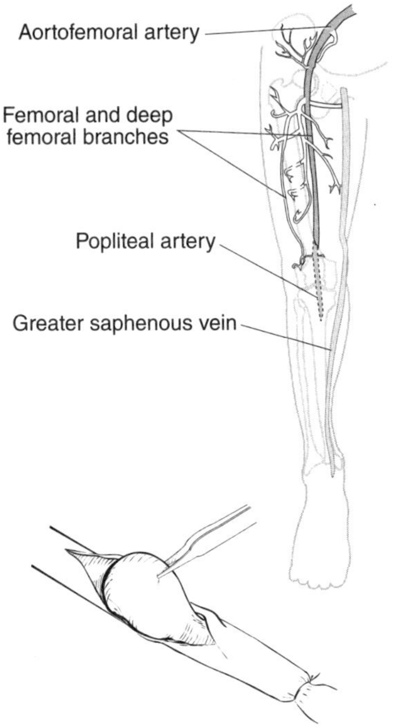

Explanation

The physician makes an incision in the skin over the leg at the site of a blood clot, plaque, or abnormal lining of the common femoral artery (35371) or the deep (profunda) femoral artery (35372). The vessel is isolated and dissected from adjacent critical structures and vessel clamps are applied. The vessel is incised. Using a blunt, spatula-like tool, the plaque and the vessel lining are separated from the artery and removed. The edge of the normal artery lining may be sutured to the artery wall to prevent separation when blood flow resumes. After the plaque and lining are removed, a patch graft may be applied and sutured to the vessel. This enlarges the diameter of the artery. The vessel clamps are removed and the skin incision is repaired with layered closure.

Coding Tips

Unless the procedure involves a significant length of the deep or superficial femoral artery, report only the common femoral procedure (35371). Establishing both inflow and outflow by any method is included. That portion of the operative arteriogram performed by the surgeon is also included. Angioscopy performed during therapeutic intervention should be reported in addition to the code for the primary procedure; see 35400. Any graft harvest is not reported separately. Do not report this procedure with codes for repair of an aneurysm (35001–35152) as aneurysm repair includes endarterectomy and treatment of associated occlusive disease. For femoropopliteal embolectomy and/or thrombectomy, see 34201. For repair of a congenital arteriovenous fistula, see 35184. For repair of an acquired or traumatic arteriovenous fistula, see 35190.

ICD-10-CM Diagnostic Codes

I70.211 Atherosclerosis of native arteries of extremities with intermittent claudication, right leg A ✓
I70.221 Atherosclerosis of native arteries of extremities with rest pain, right leg A ✓
I70.231 Atherosclerosis of native arteries of right leg with ulceration of thigh A ✓
I70.232 Atherosclerosis of native arteries of right leg with ulceration of calf A ✓
I70.233 Atherosclerosis of native arteries of right leg with ulceration of ankle A ✓
I70.234 Atherosclerosis of native arteries of right leg with ulceration of heel and midfoot A ✓
I70.235 Atherosclerosis of native arteries of right leg with ulceration of other part of foot A ✓
I70.238 Atherosclerosis of native arteries of right leg with ulceration of other part of lower leg A ✓
I70.261 Atherosclerosis of native arteries of extremities with gangrene, right leg A ✓
I70.291 Other atherosclerosis of native arteries of extremities, right leg A ✓
I70.461 Atherosclerosis of autologous vein bypass graft(s) of the extremities with gangrene, right leg A ✓
I70.561 Atherosclerosis of nonautologous biological bypass graft(s) of the extremities with gangrene, right leg A ✓
I70.661 Atherosclerosis of nonbiological bypass graft(s) of the extremities with gangrene, right leg A ✓
I70.761 Atherosclerosis of other type of bypass graft(s) of the extremities with gangrene, right leg A ✓
I70.92 Chronic total occlusion of artery of the extremities A
I74.3 Embolism and thrombosis of arteries of the lower extremities
I75.021 Atheroembolism of right lower extremity ✓
I76 Septic arterial embolism
I77.1 Stricture of artery

AMA: 35371 2020,Dec

Relative Value Units/Medicare Edits

Non-Facility RVU	Work	PE	MP	Total
35371	15.31	4.77	3.79	23.87
35372	18.58	5.42	4.6	28.6
Facility RVU	**Work**	**PE**	**MP**	**Total**
35371	15.31	4.77	3.79	23.87
35372	18.58	5.42	4.6	28.6

	FUD	Status	MUE	Modifiers				IOM Reference
35371	90	A	1(2)	51	50	62*	80	None
35372	90	A	1(2)	51	50	62*	80	

* with documentation

Terms To Know

embolism. Obstruction of a blood vessel resulting from a clot or foreign substance.

Arteries and Veins

N Newborn: 0 P Pediatric: 0-17 M Maternity: 9-64 A Adult: 15-124 AMA: CPT Assist

35390

\+ **35390** Reoperation, carotid, thromboendarterectomy, more than 1 month after original operation (List separately in addition to code for primary procedure)

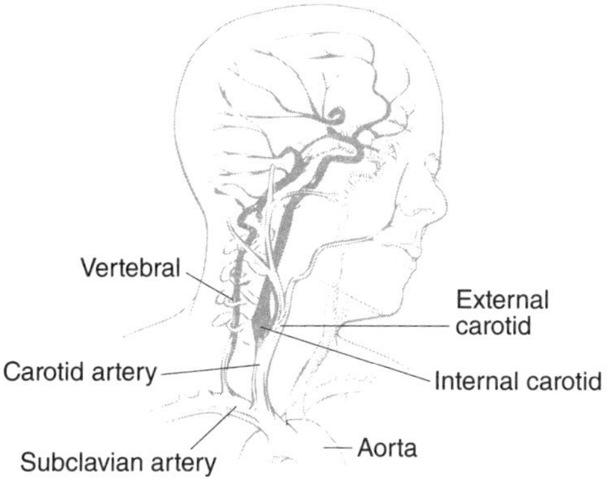

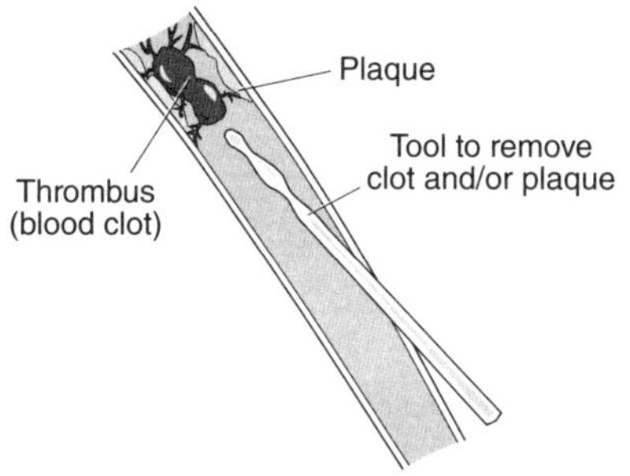

Explanation

The physician makes an incision in the skin of the neck over the site of plaque or abnormal lining of the carotid, vertebral, or subclavian artery. The vessel is isolated and dissected from adjacent critical structures, and vessel clamps are applied. A temporary vascular shunt may be placed, bypassing the area and allowing blood supply to continue uninterrupted during the procedure. The vessel is incised. Using a blunt, spatula-like tool, the plaque and the vessel lining are separated from the artery and removed. The edge of the normal artery lining may be sutured to the artery wall to prevent separation when blood flow resumes. After the plaque and lining are removed, a patch graft may be applied and sutured to the vessel. This enlarges the diameter of the artery. The vessel clamps are removed and the skin incision is repaired with layered closure.

Coding Tips

Report 35390 in addition to 35301 and for a repeat thromboendarterectomy on the carotid artery.

ICD-10-CM Diagnostic Codes

This/these CPT code(s) are add-on code(s). See the primary procedure code that this code is performed with for your ICD-10-CM code selections. Diagnostic code(s) would be the same as the actual procedure performed.

Relative Value Units/Medicare Edits

Non-Facility RVU	Work	PE	MP	Total
35390	3.19	0.66	0.78	4.63
Facility RVU	**Work**	**PE**	**MP**	**Total**
35390	3.19	0.66	0.78	4.63

	FUD	Status	MUE	Modifiers				IOM Reference
35390	N/A	A	1(3)	N/A	N/A	62*	80	None

* with documentation

Terms To Know

artery. Vessel through which oxygenated blood passes away from the heart to any part of the body.

atherosclerosis. Buildup of yellowish plaques composed of cholesterol and lipoid material within the arteries.

graft. Tissue implant from another part of the body or another person.

plaque. Accumulation of a soft sticky substance on the teeth largely composed of bacteria and its byproducts.

shunt. Surgically created passage between blood vessels or other natural passages, such as an arteriovenous anastomosis, to divert or bypass blood flow from the normal channel.

suture. Numerous stitching techniques employed in wound closure.

buried suture. Continuous or interrupted suture placed under the skin for a layered closure.

continuous suture. Running stitch with tension evenly distributed across a single strand to provide a leakproof closure line.

interrupted suture. Series of single stitches with tension isolated at each stitch, in which all stitches are not affected if one becomes loose, and the isolated sutures cannot act as a wick to transport an infection.

purse-string suture. Continuous suture placed around a tubular structure and tightened, to reduce or close the lumen.

retention suture. Secondary stitching that bridges the primary suture, providing support for the primary repair; a plastic or rubber bolster may be placed over the primary repair and under the retention sutures.

thrombus. Stationary blood clot inside a blood vessel.

35400

\+ **35400** Angioscopy (noncoronary vessels or grafts) during therapeutic intervention (List separately in addition to code for primary procedure)

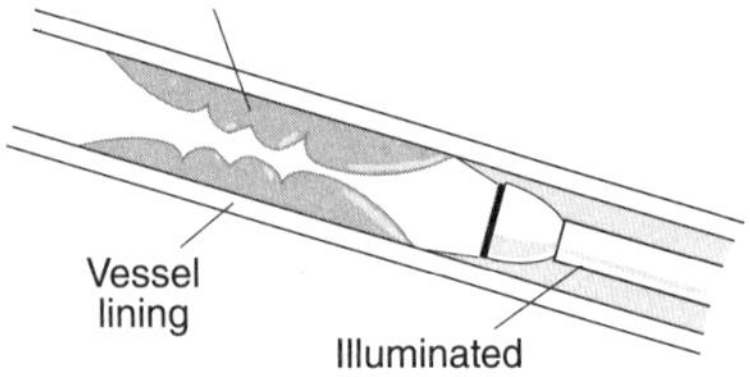

Explanation

The purpose of this procedure is to use an endoscope to look inside a blood vessel. The physician places an introducer sheath in the vessel to be examined, using percutaneous puncture or a cutdown technique. The physician places an angioscopy catheter through the introducer sheath into the vessel to be examined. The physician advances the angioscope through the vessel, clearing the view with injections of saline. Once the inside of the vessel has been examined, the angioscope and sheath are withdrawn. Vessel hemostasis is achieved using sutures or manual pressure.

Coding Tips

Fiberoptic intraoperative angioscopy provides three-dimensional endovascular visualization for assessment of vessels during revascularization procedures, such as endarterectomy and bypass.

ICD-10-CM Diagnostic Codes

This/these CPT code(s) are add-on code(s). See the primary procedure code that this code is performed with for your ICD-10-CM code selections.

Relative Value Units/Medicare Edits

Non-Facility RVU	Work	PE	MP	Total
35400	3.0	0.57	0.74	4.31
Facility RVU	**Work**	**PE**	**MP**	**Total**
35400	3.0	0.57	0.74	4.31

	FUD	Status	MUE	Modifiers				IOM Reference
35400	N/A	A	1(3)	N/A	N/A	62*	80*	None

* with documentation

Terms To Know

angioscopy. Visualization of capillary blood vessels with a microscope, or the inside of a blood vessel with a fiberoptic-equipped catheter.

bypass. Auxiliary or diverted route to maintain continuous flow.

catheter. Flexible tube inserted into an area of the body for introducing or withdrawing fluid.

35500

\+ **35500** Harvest of upper extremity vein, 1 segment, for lower extremity or coronary artery bypass procedure (List separately in addition to code for primary procedure)

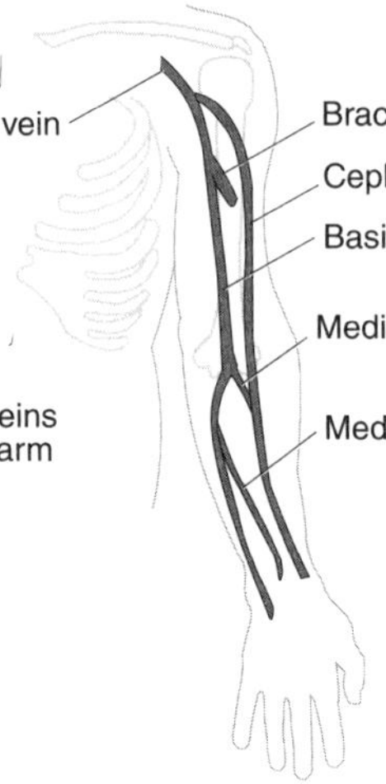

Explanation

The physician harvests a vein from an upper extremity (arm) to use for a planned bypass procedure on a lower extremity vessel (leg) or coronary artery. An incision is made over the site on the arm. Tissue is dissected to the vein. The portion of the vein to be removed is released from the surrounding structures, and is tied off above and below the portion of vein to be removed. The vein is removed. The wound is closed with layered sutures. The portion of vein removed is prepared for use in a separately reportable bypass graft procedure of a leg vessel or coronary artery.

Coding Tips

Report 35500 in addition to 33510–33536, 35556, 35566, 35570, 35571, and 35583–35587. For endoscopic harvest of veins for a coronary artery bypass procedure, see 33508. Note that 35500 reports harvest of a single vein segment. For harvest of more than one vein segment, see 35682 or 35683.

ICD-10-CM Diagnostic Codes

This/these CPT code(s) are add-on code(s). See the primary procedure code that this code is performed with for your ICD-10-CM code selections. Diagnostic code(s) would be the same as the actual procedure performed.

AMA: 35500 2021,Dec

Relative Value Units/Medicare Edits

Non-Facility RVU	Work	PE	MP	Total
35500	6.44	1.26	1.58	9.28
Facility RVU	**Work**	**PE**	**MP**	**Total**
35500	6.44	1.26	1.58	9.28

	FUD	Status	MUE	Modifiers				IOM Reference
35500	N/A	A	2(3)	N/A	N/A	62*	80	None

* with documentation

N Newborn: 0 P Pediatric: 0-17 M Maternity: 9-64 A Adult: 15-124 AMA: CPT Assist

35501

35501 Bypass graft, with vein; common carotid-ipsilateral internal carotid

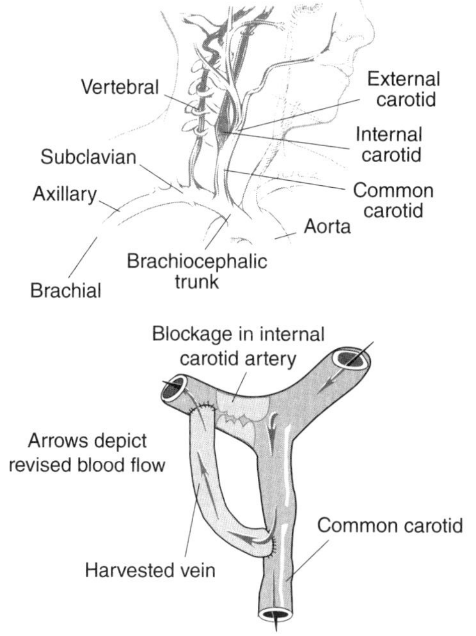

A portion of blocked internal carotid artery is bypassed

Explanation

The physician bypasses a blocked segment of common carotid artery to a segment of internal carotid artery on the same side of the neck. Through an incision in the skin of the neck in front of the sternocleidomastoid muscle, the physician isolates and dissects the common carotid artery, separating it from adjacent structures. After vessel clamps are affixed above and below the defect, the physician creates a bypass around the defective section of common carotid artery. The common carotid artery may be cut through below the damaged area and sutured to one end of the harvest vein (end-to-end), which is then sutured to the internal carotid artery beyond the affected area. As an alternative, the ends of the harvested vein are sutured into the side of the common carotid arterial wall and to the side of the internal carotid arterial wall (end-to-side). Either method results in a bypass of the damaged area. When the clamps are removed, the section of vein graft forms a new path through which blood can easily bypass the blocked area. The defective common carotid artery is not removed. After the graft is complete, the skin incision is repaired with layered closure.

Coding Tips

Establishing both inflow and outflow by any method is included. That portion of the operative arteriogram performed by the surgeon is also included. Angioscopy performed during therapeutic intervention should be reported in addition to the code for the primary procedure, see 35400. Harvesting of the saphenous vein graft is included in the description of the work for 35501 and should not be reported as a separate procedure. For harvesting of a femoropopliteal vein segment, use 35572 in addition to the bypass procedure. If a composite (combination of vein and synthetic graft) is used, report 35681 in addition to the code for the primary procedure.

ICD-10-CM Diagnostic Codes

G45.1	Carotid artery syndrome (hemispheric)
G45.3	Amaurosis fugax
G45.8	Other transient cerebral ischemic attacks and related syndromes
G45.9	Transient cerebral ischemic attack, unspecified
I63.031	Cerebral infarction due to thrombosis of right carotid artery ☑
I63.032	Cerebral infarction due to thrombosis of left carotid artery ☑
I63.131	Cerebral infarction due to embolism of right carotid artery ☑
I63.132	Cerebral infarction due to embolism of left carotid artery ☑
I63.81	Other cerebral infarction due to occlusion or stenosis of small artery
I63.89	Other cerebral infarction
I65.21	Occlusion and stenosis of right carotid artery ☑
I65.22	Occlusion and stenosis of left carotid artery ☑
I65.23	Occlusion and stenosis of bilateral carotid arteries ☑
I67.81	Acute cerebrovascular insufficiency
I67.82	Cerebral ischemia
I67.850	Cerebral autosomal dominant arteriopathy with subcortical infarcts and leukoencephalopathy
I67.858	Other hereditary cerebrovascular disease
I67.89	Other cerebrovascular disease
I72.0	Aneurysm of carotid artery
I77.1	Stricture of artery
I77.2	Rupture of artery
I77.71	Dissection of carotid artery
S15.011A	Minor laceration of right carotid artery, initial encounter ☑
S15.012A	Minor laceration of left carotid artery, initial encounter ☑
S15.021A	Major laceration of right carotid artery, initial encounter ☑
S15.022A	Major laceration of left carotid artery, initial encounter ☑
S15.091A	Other specified injury of right carotid artery, initial encounter ☑
S15.092A	Other specified injury of left carotid artery, initial encounter ☑
S15.8XXA	Injury of other specified blood vessels at neck level, initial encounter

Relative Value Units/Medicare Edits

Non-Facility RVU	Work	PE	MP	Total
35501	29.09	6.37	7.26	42.72
Facility RVU	**Work**	**PE**	**MP**	**Total**
35501	29.09	6.37	7.26	42.72

	FUD	Status	MUE	Modifiers				IOM Reference
35501	90	A	1(3)	51	50	62*	80	None

* with documentation

Arteries and Veins

35506

35506 Bypass graft, with vein; carotid-subclavian or subclavian-carotid

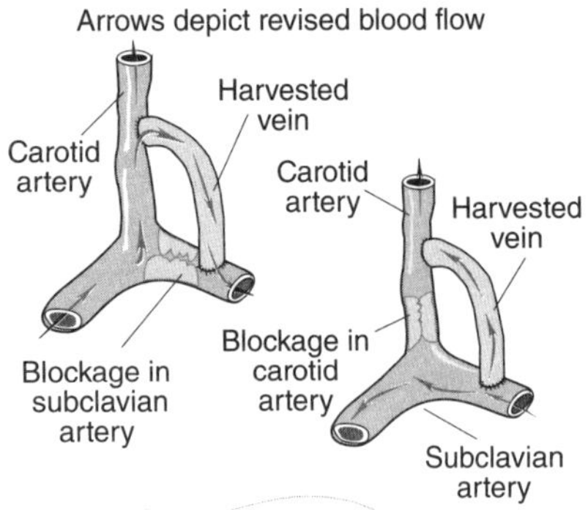

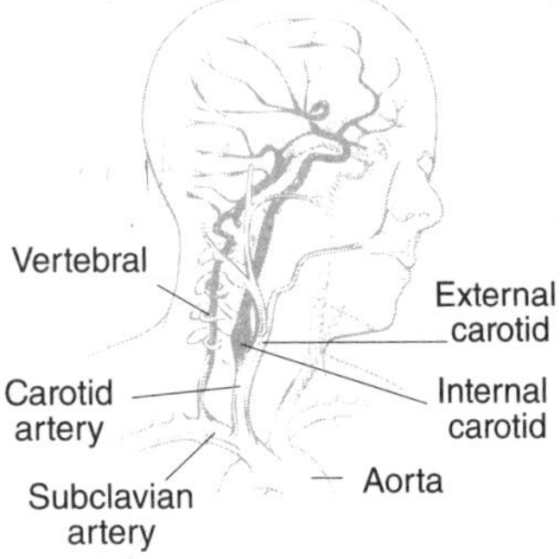

Explanation

The physician bypasses a segment of blocked common carotid or subclavian artery. Through an incision in the skin at the side of the neck, the physician isolates and dissects the subclavian and common carotid arteries, separating them from adjacent critical structures. In this procedure, a blocked common carotid arterial flow may be bypassed to the subclavian artery, or a blocked subclavian arterial flow may be bypassed to the common carotid artery. To create a bypass around a section of artery that is damaged or blocked, the physician uses a harvested vein and one of two methods of repair. After vessel clamps have been affixed above and below the damaged area, the graft is sewn to the side of the two arteries (end-to-side) or cut ends may be sewn (end-to-end). The graft is attached above the portion of blocked artery. The blocked portion of artery is not removed. When the clamps are removed in either case, the section of vein graft forms a new path through which blood can easily bypass the blocked area. After the graft is complete, the skin incision is repaired with layered closure.

Coding Tips

Establishing both inflow and outflow by any method is included. That portion of the operative arteriogram performed by the surgeon is also included. Angioscopy performed during therapeutic intervention should be reported in addition to the code for the primary procedure, see 35400. Harvesting of the saphenous vein graft is included in the description of the work for 35506 and should not be reported as a separate procedure. For harvesting of a femoropopliteal vein segment, use 35572 in addition to the bypass procedure. If a composite (combination of vein and synthetic graft) is used, report 35681 in addition to the code for the primary procedure. If synthetic graft material is used, see 35606.

ICD-10-CM Diagnostic Codes

G45.1	Carotid artery syndrome (hemispheric)
G45.2	Multiple and bilateral precerebral artery syndromes
G45.3	Amaurosis fugax
G45.8	Other transient cerebral ischemic attacks and related syndromes
G45.9	Transient cerebral ischemic attack, unspecified
I63.031	Cerebral infarction due to thrombosis of right carotid artery ☑
I63.032	Cerebral infarction due to thrombosis of left carotid artery ☑
I63.09	Cerebral infarction due to thrombosis of other precerebral artery
I63.131	Cerebral infarction due to embolism of right carotid artery ☑
I63.132	Cerebral infarction due to embolism of left carotid artery ☑
I63.19	Cerebral infarction due to embolism of other precerebral artery
I63.89	Other cerebral infarction
I65.21	Occlusion and stenosis of right carotid artery ☑
I65.22	Occlusion and stenosis of left carotid artery ☑
I65.23	Occlusion and stenosis of bilateral carotid arteries ☑
I65.8	Occlusion and stenosis of other precerebral arteries
I67.81	Acute cerebrovascular insufficiency
I67.82	Cerebral ischemia
I67.850	Cerebral autosomal dominant arteriopathy with subcortical infarcts and leukoencephalopathy
I67.858	Other hereditary cerebrovascular disease
I67.89	Other cerebrovascular disease
I77.1	Stricture of artery
I77.2	Rupture of artery
I77.79	Dissection of other specified artery
I77.89	Other specified disorders of arteries and arterioles
Q28.1	Other malformations of precerebral vessels
S15.011A	Minor laceration of right carotid artery, initial encounter ☑
S15.012A	Minor laceration of left carotid artery, initial encounter ☑
S15.021A	Major laceration of right carotid artery, initial encounter ☑
S15.022A	Major laceration of left carotid artery, initial encounter ☑
S15.091A	Other specified injury of right carotid artery, initial encounter ☑
S15.092A	Other specified injury of left carotid artery, initial encounter ☑
S25.191A	Other specified injury of right innominate or subclavian artery, initial encounter ☑
S25.192A	Other specified injury of left innominate or subclavian artery, initial encounter ☑

Relative Value Units/Medicare Edits

Non-Facility RVU	Work	PE	MP	Total
35506	25.33	5.67	6.3	37.3
Facility RVU	**Work**	**PE**	**MP**	**Total**
35506	25.33	5.67	6.3	37.3

	FUD	Status	MUE	Modifiers				IOM Reference
35506	90	A	1(3)	51	50	62*	80	None

* with documentation

Terms To Know

infarction. Area of necrosis in tissue, due to ischemia from lack of circulation, usually from a thrombus or an embolus.

ischemia. Deficiency in blood supply causing tissues to be deprived of oxygen, resulting from trauma, mechanical or functional constriction of blood vessels, or a physical obstruction.

35508

35508 Bypass graft, with vein; carotid-vertebral

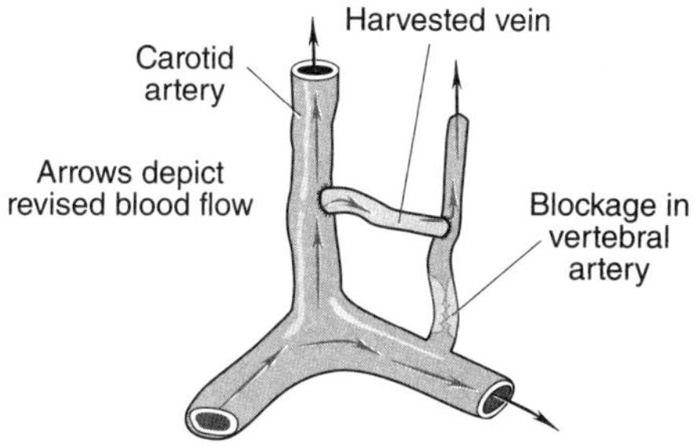

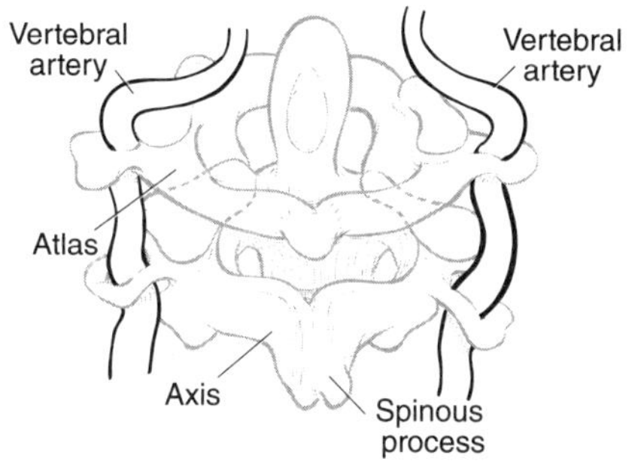

Posterior view of the first two vertebrae showing route of vertebral arteries

Explanation

Through an incision in the skin of the neck, the physician isolates and dissects the vertebral and carotid arteries, separating them from adjacent critical structures. The physician creates a bypass around a section of vertebral artery that is damaged or blocked, using a harvested vein and one of two methods of repair. After vessel clamps have been affixed above and below the damaged area, the graft is sewn to the side of the carotid artery and either sewn to the side of the vertebral artery beyond the affected area (end-to-side) or sewn over the cut end of the vertebral artery after dividing it beyond the affected area (end-to-end). The damaged or blocked section of the vertebral artery is not removed. When the clamps are removed, the section of vein graft forms a new path through which blood can easily bypass the blocked area. After the graft is complete, the skin incision is repaired with a layered closure.

Coding Tips

Establishing both inflow and outflow by any method is included. That portion of the operative arteriogram performed by the surgeon is also included. Angioscopy performed during therapeutic intervention should be reported in addition to the code for the primary procedure; see 35400. Harvesting of the saphenous vein graft is included in the description of the work for 35508 and should not be reported as a separate procedure. For harvesting of a femoropopliteal vein segment, use 35572 in addition to the bypass procedure. If a composite (combination of vein and synthetic graft) is used, report 35681 in addition to the code for the primary procedure. If synthetic graft material is used, see 35642.

ICD-10-CM Diagnostic Codes

G45.0	Vertebro-basilar artery syndrome
I63.011	Cerebral infarction due to thrombosis of right vertebral artery ☑
I63.012	Cerebral infarction due to thrombosis of left vertebral artery ☑
I63.013	Cerebral infarction due to thrombosis of bilateral vertebral arteries ☑
I63.033	Cerebral infarction due to thrombosis of bilateral carotid arteries ☑
I63.111	Cerebral infarction due to embolism of right vertebral artery ☑
I63.112	Cerebral infarction due to embolism of left vertebral artery ☑
I63.113	Cerebral infarction due to embolism of bilateral vertebral arteries ☑
I63.133	Cerebral infarction due to embolism of bilateral carotid arteries ☑
I65.01	Occlusion and stenosis of right vertebral artery ☑
I65.02	Occlusion and stenosis of left vertebral artery ☑
I65.03	Occlusion and stenosis of bilateral vertebral arteries ☑
I76	Septic arterial embolism
I77.1	Stricture of artery
I77.2	Rupture of artery
I77.74	Dissection of vertebral artery
I77.89	Other specified disorders of arteries and arterioles
S15.111A	Minor laceration of right vertebral artery, initial encounter ☑
S15.112A	Minor laceration of left vertebral artery, initial encounter ☑
S15.121A	Major laceration of right vertebral artery, initial encounter ☑
S15.122A	Major laceration of left vertebral artery, initial encounter ☑
S15.191A	Other specified injury of right vertebral artery, initial encounter ☑
S15.192A	Other specified injury of left vertebral artery, initial encounter ☑

Relative Value Units/Medicare Edits

Non-Facility RVU	Work	PE	MP	Total
35508	26.09	6.36	6.5	38.95
Facility RVU	**Work**	**PE**	**MP**	**Total**
35508	26.09	6.36	6.5	38.95

	FUD	Status	MUE	Modifiers				IOM Reference
35508	90	A	1(3)	51	50	62*	80	None

* with documentation

Terms To Know

arteriogram. Radiograph of arteries.

bypass graft. Surgically created alternative blood vessel used to reroute blood flow around an area of obstruction or disease.

ischemia. Deficiency in blood supply causing tissues to be deprived of oxygen, resulting from trauma, mechanical or functional constriction of blood vessels, or a physical obstruction.

35509

35509 Bypass graft, with vein; carotid-contralateral carotid

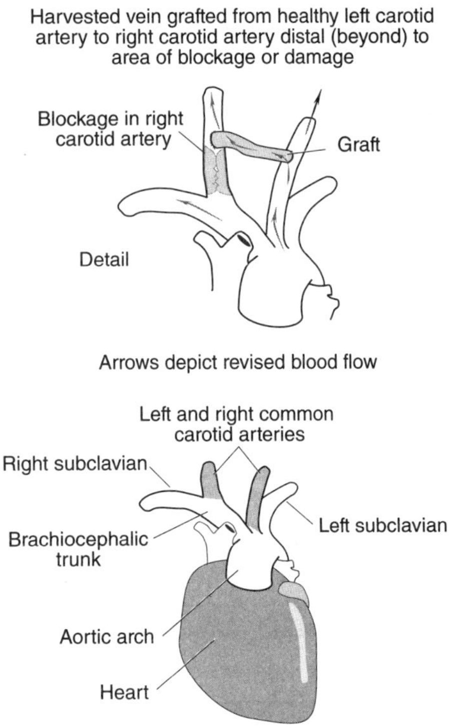

Explanation

The physician performs a vein bypass graft from one carotid to the contralateral carotid. Through incisions in the skin of the neck, the physician isolates and dissects the carotid arteries, separating them from adjacent critical structures. The physician creates a bypass around a section of carotid artery that is damaged or blocked, using a harvested vein and one of two methods of repair. After vessel clamps have been affixed above and below the damaged area, the ends of the vein graft are sutured into the side of the carotid arterial wall (end-to-side). In the second method, the carotid artery may be cut through above the damaged area and sutured to one end of a harvested vein, which is sutured to the side of the carotid artery on the opposite side of the neck (end-to-end). In either case, the blocked or damaged section of artery is not removed. When the clamps are removed, the section of vein graft forms a new path through which blood can easily bypass the blocked or damaged area. After the graft is complete, the skin incisions are repaired with layered closures.

Coding Tips

Establishing both inflow and outflow by any method is included. That portion of the operative arteriogram performed by the surgeon is also included. Angioscopy performed during therapeutic intervention should be reported in addition to the code for the primary procedure; see 35400. Harvesting of the saphenous vein graft is included in the description of the work for 35509 and should not be reported as a separate procedure. For harvesting of a femoropopliteal vein segment, use 35572 in addition to the bypass procedure. If a composite (combination of vein and synthetic graft) is used, report 35681 in addition to the code for the primary procedure.

ICD-10-CM Diagnostic Codes

G45.1	Carotid artery syndrome (hemispheric)
G45.3	Amaurosis fugax
G45.9	Transient cerebral ischemic attack, unspecified
I63.031	Cerebral infarction due to thrombosis of right carotid artery ☑
I63.032	Cerebral infarction due to thrombosis of left carotid artery ☑
I63.131	Cerebral infarction due to embolism of right carotid artery ☑
I63.132	Cerebral infarction due to embolism of left carotid artery ☑
I63.81	Other cerebral infarction due to occlusion or stenosis of small artery
I63.89	Other cerebral infarction
I65.21	Occlusion and stenosis of right carotid artery ☑
I65.22	Occlusion and stenosis of left carotid artery ☑
I65.23	Occlusion and stenosis of bilateral carotid arteries ☑
I67.81	Acute cerebrovascular insufficiency
I67.850	Cerebral autosomal dominant arteriopathy with subcortical infarcts and leukoencephalopathy
I67.858	Other hereditary cerebrovascular disease
I72.0	Aneurysm of carotid artery
I77.71	Dissection of carotid artery
S15.011A	Minor laceration of right carotid artery, initial encounter ☑
S15.012A	Minor laceration of left carotid artery, initial encounter ☑
S15.021A	Major laceration of right carotid artery, initial encounter ☑
S15.022A	Major laceration of left carotid artery, initial encounter ☑
S15.091A	Other specified injury of right carotid artery, initial encounter ☑
S15.092A	Other specified injury of left carotid artery, initial encounter ☑
S15.8XXA	Injury of other specified blood vessels at neck level, initial encounter

Relative Value Units/Medicare Edits

Non-Facility RVU	Work	PE	MP	Total
35509	28.09	6.24	6.98	41.31
Facility RVU	**Work**	**PE**	**MP**	**Total**
35509	28.09	6.24	6.98	41.31

	FUD	Status	MUE	Modifiers				IOM Reference
35509	90	A	1(3)	51	50	62*	80	None

* with documentation

35510

35510 Bypass graft, with vein; carotid-brachial

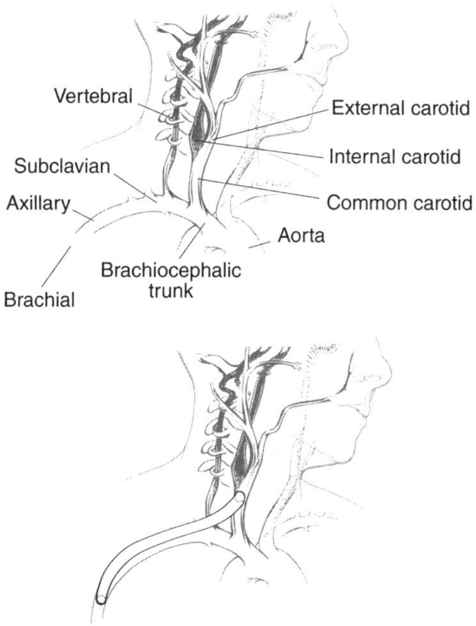

A vein graft from the carotid to the brachial artery is performed

Explanation

Through an incision in the skin at the side of the neck, the physician dissects down to the common carotid artery, separating soft tissue and adjacent critical structures. Soft tissue must be cleared for several centimeters. Dissection through the skin and soft tissue at the distal anastomosis site of this bypass graft is also done over the brachial artery in the arm. Next, a tunnel is made from the carotid through the axilla and down the arm to the brachial artery site. To create a bypass graft around the section of brachial artery that is damaged or blocked, the physician uses a harvested vein, usually the greater saphenous. After vascular clamps have been affixed above and below the anastomosis area on the carotid artery, the proximal arteriotomy is carried out and the harvested vein is sutured to the carotid artery. When this is completed and checked for hemorrhaging, the arterial clamps are removed. The vein graft is tunneled through the prepared space to the brachial artery and the distal arteriotomy and anastomosis are carried out in the same manner. The clamps are removed, additional sutures may be placed for complete hemostasis, and the patency of the graft is checked. The incisions are closed and the appropriate pulses are checked again before dressings are applied.

Coding Tips

Establishing both inflow and outflow by any method is included. That portion of the operative arteriogram performed by the surgeon is also included. Angioscopy performed during therapeutic intervention should be reported in addition to the code for the primary procedure; see 35400. Harvesting of the saphenous vein graft is included in the description of the work for 35510 and should not be reported as a separate procedure. For harvesting of a femoropopliteal vein segment, use 35572 in addition to the bypass procedure. If a composite (combination of vein and synthetic graft) is used, report 35681 in addition to the code for the primary procedure.

ICD-10-CM Diagnostic Codes

I70.92	Chronic total occlusion of artery of the extremities [A]
I74.2	Embolism and thrombosis of arteries of the upper extremities
I74.8	Embolism and thrombosis of other arteries
I75.011	Atheroembolism of right upper extremity ☑
I75.012	Atheroembolism of left upper extremity ☑
I75.013	Atheroembolism of bilateral upper extremities ☑
I77.1	Stricture of artery
I77.2	Rupture of artery
S45.111A	Laceration of brachial artery, right side, initial encounter ☑
S45.112A	Laceration of brachial artery, left side, initial encounter ☑
S45.191A	Other specified injury of brachial artery, right side, initial encounter ☑
S45.192A	Other specified injury of brachial artery, left side, initial encounter ☑

Relative Value Units/Medicare Edits

Non-Facility RVU	Work	PE	MP	Total
35510	24.39	5.55	6.08	36.02
Facility RVU	**Work**	**PE**	**MP**	**Total**
35510	24.39	5.55	6.08	36.02

	FUD	Status	MUE	Modifiers				IOM Reference
35510	90	A	1(3)	51	50	62*	80	None

* with documentation

Terms To Know

anastomosis. Surgically created connection between ducts, blood vessels, or bowel segments to allow flow from one to the other.

bypass graft. Surgically created alternative blood vessel used to reroute blood flow around an area of obstruction or disease.

dissection. Separating by cutting tissue or body structures apart.

hemostasis. Interruption of blood flow or the cessation or arrest of bleeding.

patency. State of a tube-like structure or conduit being open and unobstructed.

35511

35511 Bypass graft, with vein; subclavian-subclavian

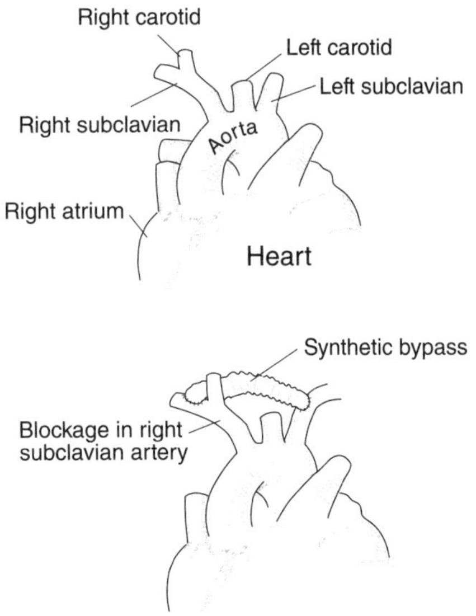

Harvested vein grafted from healthy left subclavian artery to right subclavian artery distal (beyond) area of blockage or damage

Explanation

Through incisions in the skin at the base of the neck, the physician isolates and dissects the subclavian arteries, separating them from adjacent critical structures. The physician creates a bypass around a section of subclavian artery that is damaged or blocked, using a harvested vein and one of two methods of repair after vessel clamps have been affixed above and below the defect. In the first method of repair the ends of the vein graft are sutured into the sides of the walls of the two subclavian arteries, resulting in a bypass of the damaged area. In the second method, the subclavian artery may be cut through beyond the damaged area and sutured to one end of a harvested vein, which is sutured to the subclavian artery on the opposite side of the neck. In either case, the blocked or damaged portion of the artery is not removed. When the clamps are removed, the section of vein graft forms a new path through which blood can easily bypass the blocked area. After the graft is complete, the skin incisions are repaired with a layered closure.

Coding Tips

Establishing both inflow and outflow by any method is included. That portion of the operative arteriogram performed by the surgeon is also included. Angioscopy performed during therapeutic intervention should be reported in addition to the code for the primary procedure; see 35400. Harvesting of the saphenous vein graft is included in the description of the work for 35511 and should not be reported as a separate procedure. For harvesting of a femoropopliteal vein segment, use 35572 in addition to the bypass procedure. If a composite (combination of vein and synthetic graft) is used, report 35681 in addition to the code for the primary procedure. If synthetic graft material is used, see 35612.

ICD-10-CM Diagnostic Codes

I74.2	Embolism and thrombosis of arteries of the upper extremities
I74.8	Embolism and thrombosis of other arteries
I75.011	Atheroembolism of right upper extremity ☑
I75.012	Atheroembolism of left upper extremity ☑
I75.013	Atheroembolism of bilateral upper extremities ☑
I77.1	Stricture of artery
I77.2	Rupture of artery
I77.5	Necrosis of artery
I77.79	Dissection of other specified artery
I77.89	Other specified disorders of arteries and arterioles
S25.111A	Minor laceration of right innominate or subclavian artery, initial encounter ☑
S25.112A	Minor laceration of left innominate or subclavian artery, initial encounter ☑
S25.121A	Major laceration of right innominate or subclavian artery, initial encounter ☑
S25.122A	Major laceration of left innominate or subclavian artery, initial encounter ☑
S25.191A	Other specified injury of right innominate or subclavian artery, initial encounter ☑
S25.192A	Other specified injury of left innominate or subclavian artery, initial encounter ☑

Relative Value Units/Medicare Edits

Non-Facility RVU	Work	PE	MP	Total
35511	22.2	5.09	5.53	32.82
Facility RVU	**Work**	**PE**	**MP**	**Total**
35511	22.2	5.09	5.53	32.82

	FUD	Status	MUE	Modifiers				IOM Reference
35511	90	A	1(3)	51	50	62*	80	None

* with documentation

Terms To Know

angioscopy. Visualization of capillary blood vessels with a microscope, or the inside of a blood vessel with a fiberoptic-equipped catheter.

ischemia. Deficiency in blood supply causing tissues to be deprived of oxygen, resulting from trauma, mechanical or functional constriction of blood vessels, or a physical obstruction.

35512

35512 Bypass graft, with vein; subclavian-brachial

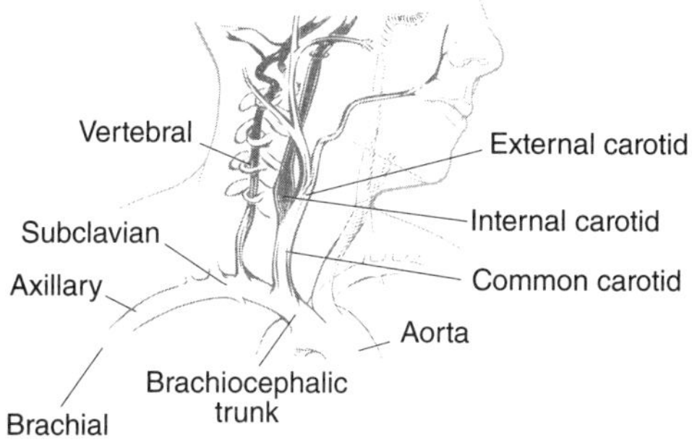

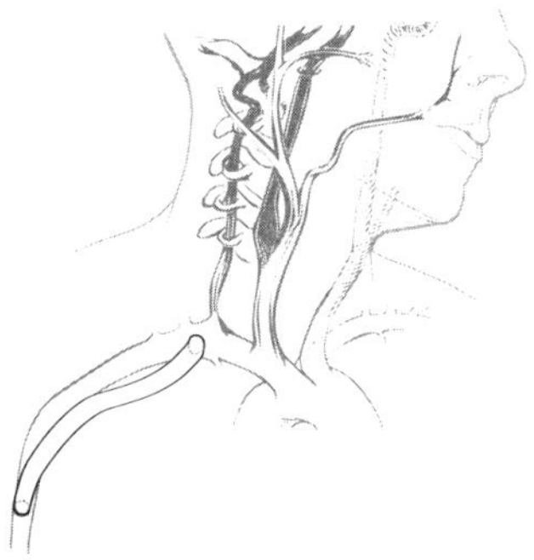

A vein graft from the subclavian to the brachial artery is performed

Explanation

Through an incision in the skin at the base of the neck, the physician dissects down to the subclavian artery just above the clavicle, separating soft tissue and adjacent critical structures. Soft tissue must be cleared for several centimeters. Dissection through the skin and soft tissue at the distal anastomosis site for this bypass graft is also done over the brachial artery in the arm. Next, a tunnel is made from the subclavian, under the clavicle, through the axilla, and down the arm to the brachial artery site. To create a bypass graft around the section of brachial artery that is damaged or blocked, the physician uses a harvested vein, usually the greater saphenous. After vascular clamps have been affixed above and below the anastomosis area on the subclavian artery, the proximal arteriotomy is carried out and the harvested vein is sutured to the subclavian artery. When this is completed and checked for hemorrhaging, the arterial clamps are removed. The vein graft is tunneled through the prepared space to the brachial artery and the distal arteriotomy and anastomosis are carried out in the same manner. The clamps are removed, additional sutures may be placed for complete hemostasis, and the patency of the graft is checked. The incisions are closed and the appropriate pulses are checked again before dressings are applied.

Coding Tips

Establishing both inflow and outflow by any method is included. That portion of the operative arteriogram performed by the surgeon is also included. Angioscopy performed during therapeutic intervention should be reported in addition to the code for the primary procedure; see 35400. Harvesting of the saphenous vein graft is included in the description of the work for 35512 and should not be reported as a separate procedure. For harvesting of a femoropopliteal vein segment, use 35572 in addition to the bypass procedure. If a composite (combination of vein and synthetic graft) is used, report 35681 in addition to the code for the primary procedure.

ICD-10-CM Diagnostic Codes

I72.1	Aneurysm of artery of upper extremity
I74.2	Embolism and thrombosis of arteries of the upper extremities
I74.8	Embolism and thrombosis of other arteries
I75.011	Atheroembolism of right upper extremity ☑
I75.012	Atheroembolism of left upper extremity ☑
I75.013	Atheroembolism of bilateral upper extremities ☑
I77.1	Stricture of artery
I77.2	Rupture of artery
I77.79	Dissection of other specified artery
I77.89	Other specified disorders of arteries and arterioles
S45.111A	Laceration of brachial artery, right side, initial encounter ☑
S45.112A	Laceration of brachial artery, left side, initial encounter ☑
S45.191A	Other specified injury of brachial artery, right side, initial encounter ☑
S45.192A	Other specified injury of brachial artery, left side, initial encounter ☑

Relative Value Units/Medicare Edits

Non-Facility RVU	Work	PE	MP	Total
35512	23.89	5.47	5.96	35.32
Facility RVU	Work	PE	MP	Total
35512	23.89	5.47	5.96	35.32

	FUD	Status	MUE	Modifiers				IOM Reference
35512	90	A	1(3)	51	50	62*	80	None

* with documentation

Terms To Know

anastomosis. Surgically created connection between ducts, blood vessels, or bowel segments to allow flow from one to the other.

arteriotomy. Incision into an artery.

axillary region. Area immediately surrounding the armpit.

vascular insufficiency. Inadequate blood flow and oxygenation.

Arteries and Veins

35515

35515 Bypass graft, with vein; subclavian-vertebral

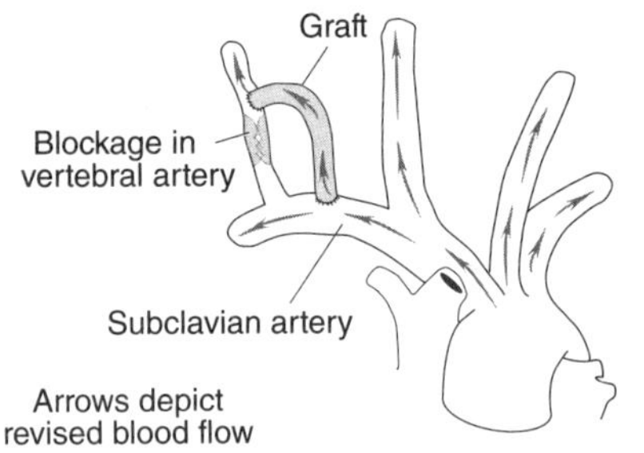

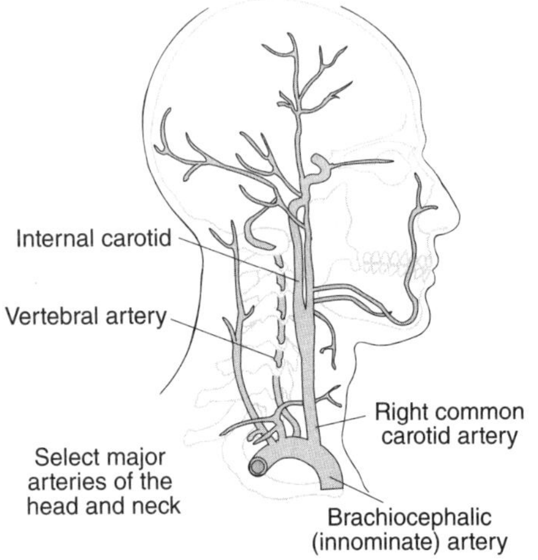

Explanation

Through an incision in the skin of the neck, the physician isolates and dissects the vertebral and subclavian arteries, separating them from adjacent critical structures. The physician creates a bypass around a section of vertebral artery that is damaged or blocked, using a harvested vein and one of two methods of repair. Once vessel clamps are affixed above and below the defect, the ends of the harvested vein are sutured into the sides of the subclavian and vertebral arterial walls resulting in a bypass of the damaged area (end-to-side). In the second method, the vertebral artery can be cut through above the damaged area and sutured to one end of a harvested vein (end-to-end). The remaining end is sutured to the subclavian artery. In either case, the blocked or damaged vertebral artery is not removed. When the clamps are removed, the section of vein graft forms a new path through which blood can easily bypass the blocked area. After the graft is complete, the skin incision is repaired with a layered closure.

Coding Tips

Establishing both inflow and outflow by any method is included. That portion of the operative arteriogram performed by the surgeon is also included. Angioscopy performed during therapeutic intervention should be reported in addition to the code for the primary procedure; see 35400. Harvesting of the saphenous vein graft is included in the description of the work for 35515 and should not be reported as a separate procedure. For harvesting of a femoropopliteal vein segment, use 35572 in addition to the bypass procedure. If a composite (combination of vein and synthetic graft) is used, report 35681 in addition to the code for the primary procedure.

ICD-10-CM Diagnostic Codes

G45.0	Vertebro-basilar artery syndrome
I63.011	Cerebral infarction due to thrombosis of right vertebral artery ☑
I63.012	Cerebral infarction due to thrombosis of left vertebral artery ☑
I63.111	Cerebral infarction due to embolism of right vertebral artery ☑
I63.112	Cerebral infarction due to embolism of left vertebral artery ☑
I65.01	Occlusion and stenosis of right vertebral artery ☑
I65.02	Occlusion and stenosis of left vertebral artery ☑
I65.03	Occlusion and stenosis of bilateral vertebral arteries ☑
I77.74	Dissection of vertebral artery
I77.89	Other specified disorders of arteries and arterioles
S15.111A	Minor laceration of right vertebral artery, initial encounter ☑
S15.112A	Minor laceration of left vertebral artery, initial encounter ☑
S15.121A	Major laceration of right vertebral artery, initial encounter ☑
S15.122A	Major laceration of left vertebral artery, initial encounter ☑
S15.191A	Other specified injury of right vertebral artery, initial encounter ☑
S15.192A	Other specified injury of left vertebral artery, initial encounter ☑

Relative Value Units/Medicare Edits

Non-Facility RVU	Work	PE	MP	Total
35515	26.09	6.36	6.5	38.95
Facility RVU	**Work**	**PE**	**MP**	**Total**
35515	26.09	6.36	6.5	38.95

	FUD	Status	MUE	Modifiers				IOM Reference
35515	90	A	1(3)	51	50	62*	80	None

* with documentation

Terms To Know

angioscopy. Visualization of capillary blood vessels with a microscope, or the inside of a blood vessel with a fiberoptic-equipped catheter.

graft. Tissue implant from another part of the body or another person.

ischemia. Deficiency in blood supply causing tissues to be deprived of oxygen, resulting from trauma, mechanical or functional constriction of blood vessels, or a physical obstruction.

occlusion. Constriction, closure, or blockage of a passage.

stenosis. Narrowing or constriction of a passage.

stricture. Narrowing of an anatomical structure.

N Newborn: 0 **P** Pediatric: 0-17 **M** Maternity: 9-64 **A** Adult: 15-124 **AMA: CPT Assist**

35516

35516 Bypass graft, with vein; subclavian-axillary

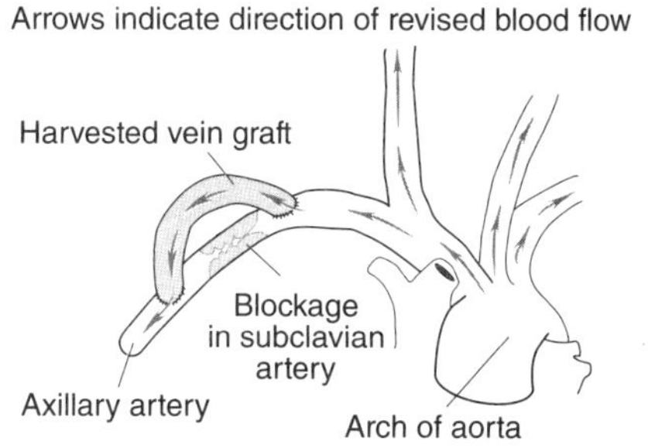

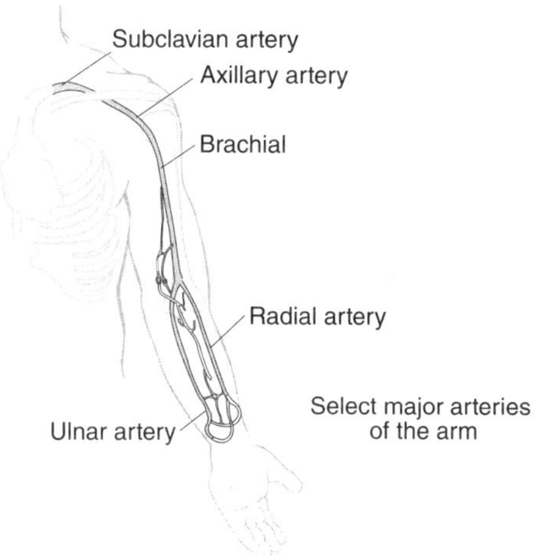

Explanation

Through an incision in the skin at the base of the neck and axilla, the physician isolates and dissects the subclavian and axillary arteries, separating them from adjacent critical structures. The physician creates a bypass around a section of subclavian artery that is damaged or blocked, using a harvested vein and one of two methods of repair. Once vessel clamps have been affixed above and below the defect, the ends of the harvested vein are sutured into the sides of the subclavian and axillary arterial walls resulting in a bypass of the damaged area (end-to-side). In the second method, the subclavian artery may be cut through before the damaged area and sutured to one end of a harvested vein, which is sutured to the axillary artery (end-to-end). The blocked or damaged portion of the subclavian artery is not removed. When the clamps are removed, the section of vein graft forms a new path through which blood can easily bypass the blocked area. After the graft is complete, the skin incisions are repaired with a layered closure.

Coding Tips

Establishing both inflow and outflow by any method is included. That portion of the operative arteriogram performed by the surgeon is also included. Angioscopy performed during therapeutic intervention should be reported in addition to the code for the primary procedure; see 35400. Harvesting of the saphenous vein graft is included in the description of the work for 35516 and should not be reported as a separate procedure. For harvesting of a femoropopliteal vein segment, use 35572 in addition to the bypass procedure. If a composite (combination of vein and synthetic graft) is used, report 35681 in addition to the code for the primary procedure. If synthetic graft material is used, see 35616.

ICD-10-CM Diagnostic Codes

G45.2	Multiple and bilateral precerebral artery syndromes
G45.8	Other transient cerebral ischemic attacks and related syndromes
I63.19	Cerebral infarction due to embolism of other precerebral artery
I63.29	Cerebral infarction due to unspecified occlusion or stenosis of other precerebral arteries
I63.89	Other cerebral infarction
I65.8	Occlusion and stenosis of other precerebral arteries
I67.850	Cerebral autosomal dominant arteriopathy with subcortical infarcts and leukoencephalopathy
I67.858	Other hereditary cerebrovascular disease
I70.92	Chronic total occlusion of artery of the extremities A
I74.2	Embolism and thrombosis of arteries of the upper extremities
I74.8	Embolism and thrombosis of other arteries
I75.011	Atheroembolism of right upper extremity ☑
I75.012	Atheroembolism of left upper extremity ☑
I75.013	Atheroembolism of bilateral upper extremities ☑
I77.1	Stricture of artery
I77.2	Rupture of artery
I77.5	Necrosis of artery
I77.79	Dissection of other specified artery
I77.89	Other specified disorders of arteries and arterioles
S15.8XXA	Injury of other specified blood vessels at neck level, initial encounter
S25.111A	Minor laceration of right innominate or subclavian artery, initial encounter ☑
S25.112A	Minor laceration of left innominate or subclavian artery, initial encounter ☑
S25.121A	Major laceration of right innominate or subclavian artery, initial encounter ☑
S25.122A	Major laceration of left innominate or subclavian artery, initial encounter ☑
S25.191A	Other specified injury of right innominate or subclavian artery, initial encounter ☑
S25.192A	Other specified injury of left innominate or subclavian artery, initial encounter ☑

Relative Value Units/Medicare Edits

Non-Facility RVU	Work	PE	MP	Total
35516	24.21	5.5	6.03	35.74
Facility RVU	**Work**	**PE**	**MP**	**Total**
35516	24.21	5.5	6.03	35.74

	FUD	Status	MUE	Modifiers				IOM Reference
35516	90	A	1(3)	51	50	62*	80	None

* with documentation

Terms To Know

bypass graft. Surgically created alternative blood vessel used to reroute blood flow around an area of obstruction or disease.

35518

35518 Bypass graft, with vein; axillary-axillary

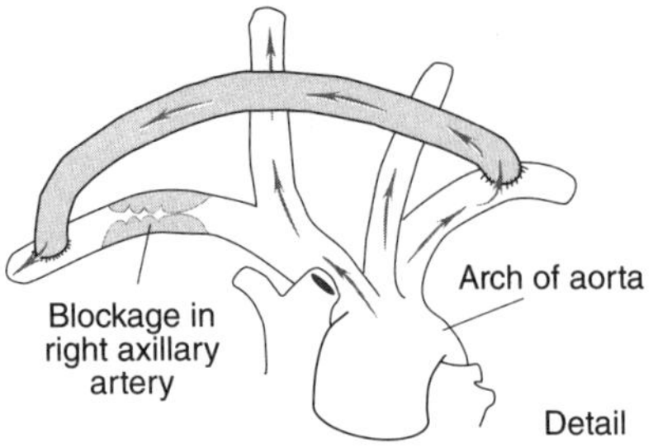

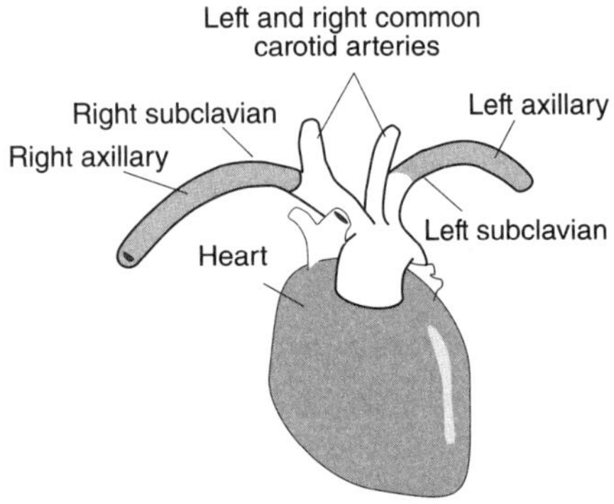

Explanation

The physician makes an incision in the skin of both axillae. The physician creates a bypass around the section of axillary artery that is damaged or blocked, using a harvested vein and one of two methods of repair. Once vessel clamps have been affixed above and below the defect, the ends of the harvested vein are sutured into the sides of the two axillary arterial walls, resulting in a bypass of the damaged area. In the second method, the axillary artery may be cut through beyond the damaged area and sutured to one end of a harvested vein, which is passed across the front of the chest under the skin and sutured to the side of the contralateral axillary artery. The blocked or damaged portion of the axillary artery is not removed. When the clamps are removed, the section of vein graft forms a new path through which blood can easily bypass the blocked area. After the graft is complete, the skin incisions are repaired with layered closures.

Coding Tips

Establishing both inflow and outflow by any method is included. That portion of the operative arteriogram performed by the surgeon is also included. Angioscopy performed during therapeutic intervention should be reported in addition to the code for the primary procedure; see 35400. Harvesting of the saphenous vein graft is included in the description of the work for 35518 and should not be reported as a separate procedure. For harvesting of a femoropopliteal vein segment, use 35572 in addition to the bypass procedure. If a composite (combination of vein and synthetic graft) is used, report 35681 in addition to the code for the primary procedure.

ICD-10-CM Diagnostic Codes

G45.2	Multiple and bilateral precerebral artery syndromes
I63.09	Cerebral infarction due to thrombosis of other precerebral artery
I63.19	Cerebral infarction due to embolism of other precerebral artery
I63.81	Other cerebral infarction due to occlusion or stenosis of small artery
I63.89	Other cerebral infarction
I65.8	Occlusion and stenosis of other precerebral arteries
I67.81	Acute cerebrovascular insufficiency
I67.850	Cerebral autosomal dominant arteriopathy with subcortical infarcts and leukoencephalopathy
I67.858	Other hereditary cerebrovascular disease
I74.8	Embolism and thrombosis of other arteries
I76	Septic arterial embolism
I77.1	Stricture of artery
I77.2	Rupture of artery
I77.5	Necrosis of artery
I77.79	Dissection of other specified artery
I77.89	Other specified disorders of arteries and arterioles
S15.8XXA	Injury of other specified blood vessels at neck level, initial encounter
S45.011A	Laceration of axillary artery, right side, initial encounter ☑
S45.012A	Laceration of axillary artery, left side, initial encounter ☑
S45.091A	Other specified injury of axillary artery, right side, initial encounter ☑
S45.092A	Other specified injury of axillary artery, left side, initial encounter ☑

Relative Value Units/Medicare Edits

Non-Facility RVU	Work	PE	MP	Total
35518	22.65	5.16	5.64	33.45
Facility RVU	**Work**	**PE**	**MP**	**Total**
35518	22.65	5.16	5.64	33.45

	FUD	Status	MUE	Modifiers				IOM Reference
35518	90	A	1(3)	51	50	62*	80	None

* with documentation

Terms To Know

angioscopy. Visualization of capillary blood vessels with a microscope, or the inside of a blood vessel with a fiberoptic-equipped catheter.

arteriogram. Radiograph of arteries.

atherosclerosis. Buildup of yellowish plaques composed of cholesterol and lipoid material within the arteries.

graft. Tissue implant from another part of the body or another person.

35521

35521 Bypass graft, with vein; axillary-femoral

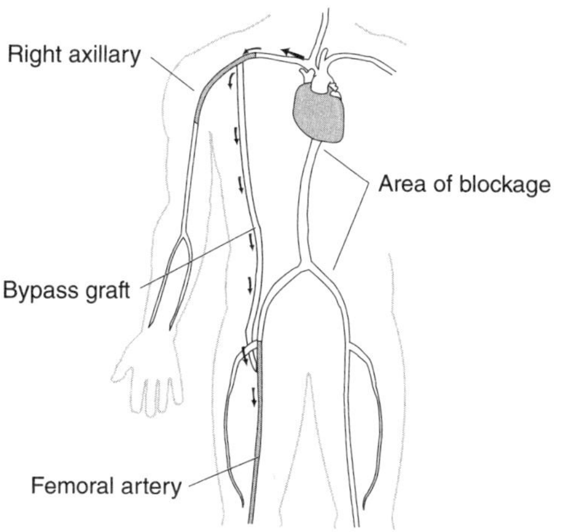

Explanation

The physician makes incisions in the skin of the axilla and upper thigh. The axillary and femoral arteries are isolated and dissected from adjacent critical structures. The physician creates a bypass around the section of damaged or blocked artery using a harvested vein and one of two methods of repair. Once vessel clamps have been affixed above and below the areas of anastomosis, the harvested vein is sutured to an incision in the side of the axillary artery and passed through a subcutaneous tunnel on the side of the body and to the upper thigh. The harvested vein is sutured to the femoral artery (common, deep, or superficial) in an end-to-side or end-to-end fashion. The blocked or damaged portion of artery is not removed. When the clamps are removed, the section of vein graft forms a new path through which blood can easily bypass the blocked area. After the graft is complete, the skin incisions are repaired with layered closures.

Coding Tips

Establishing both inflow and outflow by any method is included. That portion of the operative arteriogram performed by the surgeon is also included. Angioscopy performed during therapeutic intervention should be reported in addition to the code for the primary procedure; see 35400. Harvesting of the saphenous vein graft is included in the description of the work for 35521 and should not be reported as a separate procedure. For harvesting of a femoropopliteal vein segment, use 35572 in addition to the bypass procedure. If a composite (combination of vein and synthetic graft) is used, report 35681 in addition to the code for the primary procedure. If synthetic graft material is used, see 35621.

ICD-10-CM Diagnostic Codes

A52.02	Syphilitic aortitis
I70.0	Atherosclerosis of aorta A
I70.8	Atherosclerosis of other arteries A
I70.92	Chronic total occlusion of artery of the extremities A
I71.010	Dissection of ascending aorta
I71.011	Dissection of aortic arch
I71.012	Dissection of descending thoracic aorta
I71.02	Dissection of abdominal aorta
I71.03	Dissection of thoracoabdominal aorta
I73.89	Other specified peripheral vascular diseases
I73.9	Peripheral vascular disease, unspecified
I74.01	Saddle embolus of abdominal aorta
I74.09	Other arterial embolism and thrombosis of abdominal aorta
I74.19	Embolism and thrombosis of other parts of aorta
I74.5	Embolism and thrombosis of iliac artery
I76	Septic arterial embolism
I77.1	Stricture of artery
I77.3	Arterial fibromuscular dysplasia
I77.5	Necrosis of artery
I77.72	Dissection of iliac artery
I77.89	Other specified disorders of arteries and arterioles
Q25.21	Interruption of aortic arch
Q25.41	Absence and aplasia of aorta
Q25.42	Hypoplasia of aorta
Q25.43	Congenital aneurysm of aorta
Q25.44	Congenital dilation of aorta
Q25.45	Double aortic arch
Q25.46	Tortuous aortic arch
Q25.47	Right aortic arch
Q25.48	Anomalous origin of subclavian artery
Q25.8	Other congenital malformations of other great arteries
S25.01XA	Minor laceration of thoracic aorta, initial encounter
S25.02XA	Major laceration of thoracic aorta, initial encounter
S25.09XA	Other specified injury of thoracic aorta, initial encounter
S35.01XA	Minor laceration of abdominal aorta, initial encounter
S35.02XA	Major laceration of abdominal aorta, initial encounter
S35.09XA	Other injury of abdominal aorta, initial encounter
S35.511A	Injury of right iliac artery, initial encounter ☑
S35.512A	Injury of left iliac artery, initial encounter ☑
S35.59XA	Injury of other iliac blood vessels, initial encounter

Relative Value Units/Medicare Edits

Non-Facility RVU	Work	PE	MP	Total
35521	24.13	5.86	6.01	36.0
Facility RVU	**Work**	**PE**	**MP**	**Total**
35521	24.13	5.86	6.01	36.0

	FUD	Status	MUE	Modifiers				IOM Reference
35521	90	A	1(3)	51	50	62*	80	None

* with documentation

Terms To Know

aneurysm. Circumscribed dilation or outpouching of an artery wall, often containing blood clots and connecting directly with the lumen of the artery.

bypass graft. Surgically created alternative blood vessel used to reroute blood flow around an area of obstruction or disease.

35522

35522 Bypass graft, with vein; axillary-brachial

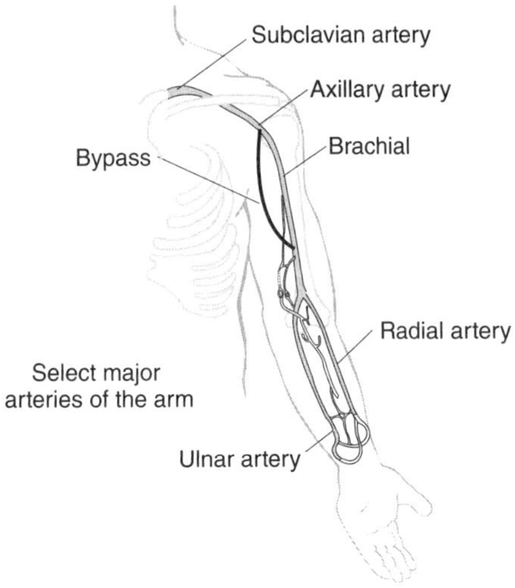

A bypass from the axillary artery to another site along the brachial artery is performed

Explanation

Through an incision in the skin of the chest wall, the physician dissects down to the axillary artery just below the clavicle, separating soft tissue and adjacent critical structures. Soft tissue must be cleared for several centimeters. Dissection through the skin and soft tissue at the distal anastomosis site for this bypass graft is also done over the brachial artery in the arm near the elbow. Next, a tunnel is made from the exposed axillary, through the axilla and down the arm to the brachial artery site. To create a bypass graft around the section of brachial artery that is damaged or blocked, the physician uses a harvested vein, usually the greater saphenous. After vascular clamps have been affixed above and below the anastomosis area on the axillary artery, the proximal arteriotomy is carried out and the harvested vein is sutured to the axillary artery. When this is completed and checked for hemorrhaging, the arterial clamps are removed. The vein graft is tunneled through the prepared space to the brachial artery and the distal arteriotomy and anastomosis are carried out in the same manner. The clamps are removed, additional sutures may be placed for complete hemostasis, and the patency of the graft is checked. The incisions are closed and the appropriate pulses are checked again before dressings are applied.

Coding Tips

Establishing both inflow and outflow by any method is included. That portion of the operative arteriogram performed by the surgeon is also included. Angioscopy performed during therapeutic intervention should be reported in addition to the code for the primary procedure; see 35400. Harvesting of the saphenous vein graft is included in the description of the work for 35522 and should not be reported as a separate procedure. For harvesting of a femoropopliteal vein segment, use 35572 in addition to the bypass procedure.

ICD-10-CM Diagnostic Codes

I70.92	Chronic total occlusion of artery of the extremities A
I72.1	Aneurysm of artery of upper extremity
I73.9	Peripheral vascular disease, unspecified
I74.2	Embolism and thrombosis of arteries of the upper extremities
I74.8	Embolism and thrombosis of other arteries
I75.011	Atheroembolism of right upper extremity ☑
I75.012	Atheroembolism of left upper extremity ☑
I75.013	Atheroembolism of bilateral upper extremities ☑
I77.1	Stricture of artery
I77.2	Rupture of artery
I77.5	Necrosis of artery
I77.89	Other specified disorders of arteries and arterioles
S45.111A	Laceration of brachial artery, right side, initial encounter ☑
S45.112A	Laceration of brachial artery, left side, initial encounter ☑
S45.191A	Other specified injury of brachial artery, right side, initial encounter ☑
S45.192A	Other specified injury of brachial artery, left side, initial encounter ☑

Relative Value Units/Medicare Edits

Non-Facility RVU	Work	PE	MP	Total
35522	23.15	5.35	5.76	34.26
Facility RVU	**Work**	**PE**	**MP**	**Total**
35522	23.15	5.35	5.76	34.26

	FUD	Status	MUE	Modifiers				IOM Reference
35522	90	A	1(3)	51	50	62*	80	None

* with documentation

Terms To Know

anastomosis. Surgically created connection between ducts, blood vessels, or bowel segments to allow flow from one to the other.

bypass graft. Surgically created alternative blood vessel used to reroute blood flow around an area of obstruction or disease.

35523

35523 Bypass graft, with vein; brachial-ulnar or -radial

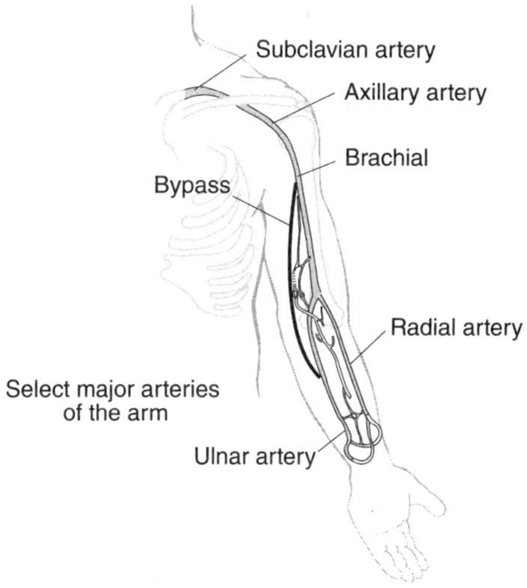

A bypass from the brachial artery to another site along the ulnar or radial artery

Explanation

The physician performs a brachial-ulnar or brachioradial bypass graft. Through an incision in the skin of the upper arm, the physician dissects down to the brachial artery at a site above the diseased or damaged portion of the artery. Soft tissue and adjacent critical structures are separated. Soft tissue must be cleared for several centimeters. Dissection through the skin and soft tissue at the distal anastomosis site for this bypass graft is also done over the radial or ulnar artery. A tunnel is made from the exposed proximal brachial site down the arm to the radial or ulnar artery site. To create a bypass graft around the section of the artery that is damaged or blocked, the physician uses a harvested vein, usually the greater saphenous. After vascular clamps have been affixed above and below the proximal anastomosis area on the brachial artery, arteriotomy is carried out and the harvested vein is sutured to the artery. When this is completed and checked for hemorrhaging, the arterial clamps are removed. The vein graft is tunneled through the prepared space to the distal site on the radial or ulnar artery and arteriotomy and anastomosis are carried out again in the same manner. The clamps are removed, additional sutures may be placed for complete hemostasis, and the patency of the graft is checked. The incisions are closed and the appropriate pulses are checked again before dressings are applied.

Coding Tips

Establishing both inflow and outflow by any method is included. That portion of the operative arteriogram performed by the surgeon is also included. Angioscopy performed during therapeutic intervention should be reported in addition to the code for the primary procedure, see 35400. Harvesting of the saphenous vein graft is included in the description of the work for 35523 and should not be reported as a separate procedure. For harvesting of a femoropopliteal vein segment, use 35572 in addition to the bypass procedure. If a composite (combination of vein and synthetic graft) is used, report 35681 in addition to the code for the primary procedure. For a bypass graft performed with synthetic conduit, see 37799. Do not report 33523 with 35206, 35500, 35525, or 36838.

ICD-10-CM Diagnostic Codes

I70.92	Chronic total occlusion of artery of the extremities A
I73.9	Peripheral vascular disease, unspecified
I74.2	Embolism and thrombosis of arteries of the upper extremities
I74.8	Embolism and thrombosis of other arteries
I75.011	Atheroembolism of right upper extremity ☑
I75.012	Atheroembolism of left upper extremity ☑
I75.013	Atheroembolism of bilateral upper extremities ☑
I77.1	Stricture of artery
I77.2	Rupture of artery
I77.5	Necrosis of artery
I77.89	Other specified disorders of arteries and arterioles
S45.111A	Laceration of brachial artery, right side, initial encounter ☑
S45.112A	Laceration of brachial artery, left side, initial encounter ☑
S45.191A	Other specified injury of brachial artery, right side, initial encounter ☑
S45.192A	Other specified injury of brachial artery, left side, initial encounter ☑
S55.011A	Laceration of ulnar artery at forearm level, right arm, initial encounter ☑
S55.012A	Laceration of ulnar artery at forearm level, left arm, initial encounter ☑
S55.091A	Other specified injury of ulnar artery at forearm level, right arm, initial encounter ☑
S55.092A	Other specified injury of ulnar artery at forearm level, left arm, initial encounter ☑
S55.111A	Laceration of radial artery at forearm level, right arm, initial encounter ☑
S55.112A	Laceration of radial artery at forearm level, left arm, initial encounter ☑
S55.191A	Other specified injury of radial artery at forearm level, right arm, initial encounter ☑
S55.192A	Other specified injury of radial artery at forearm level, left arm, initial encounter ☑

Relative Value Units/Medicare Edits

Non-Facility RVU	Work	PE	MP	Total
35523	24.13	5.91	6.01	36.05
Facility RVU	**Work**	**PE**	**MP**	**Total**
35523	24.13	5.91	6.01	36.05

	FUD	Status	MUE	Modifiers				IOM Reference
35523	90	A	1(3)	51	50	62*	80	None

* with documentation

Terms To Know

anastomosis. Surgically created connection between ducts, blood vessels, or bowel segments to allow flow from one to the other.

bypass graft. Surgically created alternative blood vessel used to reroute blood flow around an area of obstruction or disease.

35525

35525 Bypass graft, with vein; brachial-brachial

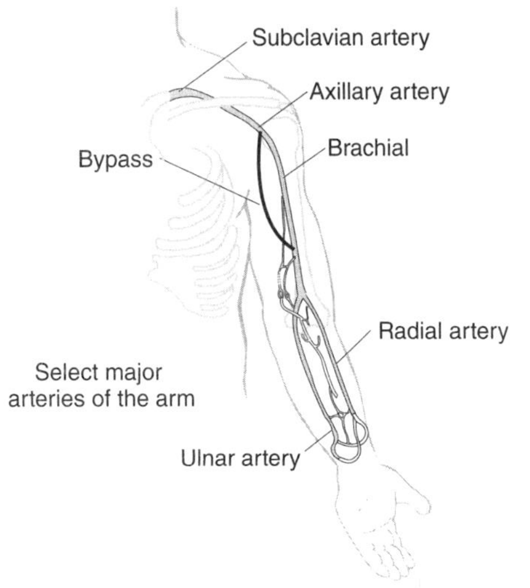

A bypass from the brachial artery to another site along the brachial artery is performed

Explanation

Through an incision in the skin of the upper arm, the physician dissects down to the brachial artery at a site above the diseased or damaged portion of the artery, usually in the mid to distal part, and separates soft tissue and adjacent critical structures. Soft tissue must be cleared for several centimeters. Dissection through the skin and soft tissue at the distal anastomosis site for this bypass graft is also done over the distal brachial artery in the arm, most often below the elbow. Next, a tunnel is made from the exposed proximal brachial site, down the arm to the distal brachial artery site. To create a bypass graft around the section of the artery that is damaged or blocked, the physician uses a harvested vein, usually the greater saphenous. After vascular clamps have been affixed above and below the proximal anastomosis area on the brachial artery, arteriotomy is carried out and the harvested vein is sutured to the brachial artery. When this is completed and checked for hemorrhaging, the arterial clamps are removed. The vein graft is tunneled through the prepared space to the distal site on the brachial artery and arteriotomy and anastomosis are carried out again in the same manner. The clamps are removed, additional sutures may be placed for complete hemostasis, and the patency of the graft is checked. The incisions are closed and the appropriate pulses are checked again before dressings are applied.

Coding Tips

Establishing both inflow and outflow by any method is included. That portion of the operative arteriogram performed by the surgeon is also included. Angioscopy performed during therapeutic intervention should be reported in addition to the code for the primary procedure; see 35400. Harvesting of the saphenous vein graft is included in the description of the work for 35525 and should not be reported as a separate procedure. To report harvesting of an upper extremity vein, use 35500 in addition to the bypass procedure. For harvesting of a femoropopliteal vein segment, use 35572 in addition to the bypass procedure.

ICD-10-CM Diagnostic Codes

I70.92	Chronic total occlusion of artery of the extremities 🅰
I73.9	Peripheral vascular disease, unspecified
I74.2	Embolism and thrombosis of arteries of the upper extremities
I74.8	Embolism and thrombosis of other arteries
I75.011	Atheroembolism of right upper extremity ☑
I75.012	Atheroembolism of left upper extremity ☑
I75.013	Atheroembolism of bilateral upper extremities ☑
I77.1	Stricture of artery
I77.2	Rupture of artery
I77.5	Necrosis of artery
I77.89	Other specified disorders of arteries and arterioles
S45.111A	Laceration of brachial artery, right side, initial encounter ☑
S45.112A	Laceration of brachial artery, left side, initial encounter ☑
S45.191A	Other specified injury of brachial artery, right side, initial encounter ☑
S45.192A	Other specified injury of brachial artery, left side, initial encounter ☑

Relative Value Units/Medicare Edits

Non-Facility RVU	Work	PE	MP	Total
35525	21.69	6.12	5.37	33.18
Facility RVU	**Work**	**PE**	**MP**	**Total**
35525	21.69	6.12	5.37	33.18

	FUD	Status	MUE	Modifiers				IOM Reference
35525	90	A	1(3)	51	50	62*	80	None

* with documentation

Terms To Know

bypass graft. Surgically created alternative blood vessel used to reroute blood flow around an area of obstruction or disease.

thrombosis. Condition arising from the presence or formation of blood clots within a blood vessel that may cause vascular obstruction and insufficient oxygenation.

35526

35526 Bypass graft, with vein; aortosubclavian, aortoinnominate, or aortocarotid

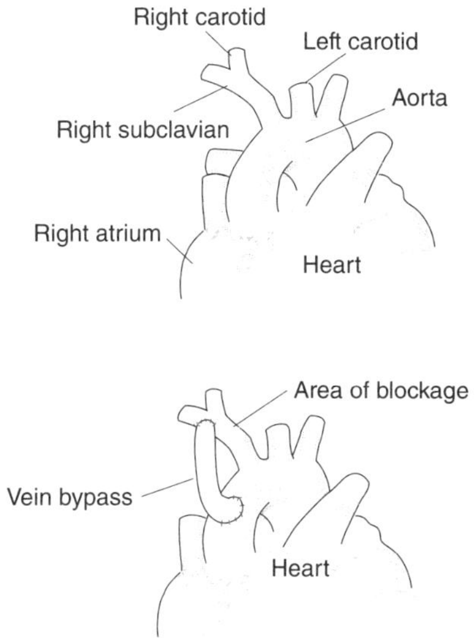

A vein graft is employed to bypass a blockage in the great arteries

Explanation

The physician exposes the aorta by median sternotomy and exposes the aortocarotid, aortoinnominate, or aortosubclavian artery extending this incision in the appropriate direction. The physician clamps the middle part of the right anterolateral aspect of the anterior ascending aorta with a J clamp. The physician makes a 2 cm to 3 cm longitudinal incision in the clamped portion of the aorta and sews the venous graft to the aortic incision. The physician clamps the vein and releases the aortic clamp to assess the anastomosis for leaks. The physician clamps the distal end of the diseased artery. The physician makes a longitudinal incision in the diseased artery, distal to the blockage, and sews the venous graft to the arterial incision. The physician may also use harvested vein to enlarge the arterial lumen (patch graft). The physician removes the clamp from the vein graft. The physician may perform arteriography or use a Doppler probe to establish patency of the graft. The physician closes the sternotomy or thoracotomy, leaving a chest tube in place.

Coding Tips

Establishing both inflow and outflow by any method is included. That portion of the operative arteriogram performed by the surgeon is also included. Angioscopy performed during therapeutic intervention should be reported in addition to the code for the primary procedure; see 35400. If synthetic graft material is used, see 35626. Harvesting of the saphenous vein graft is included in the description of the work for 35526 and should not be reported as a separate procedure. For harvesting of a femoropopliteal vein segment, use 35572 in addition to the bypass procedure. If a composite (combination of vein and synthetic graft) is used, report 35681 in addition to the code for the primary procedure.

ICD-10-CM Diagnostic Codes

G45.1	Carotid artery syndrome (hemispheric)
G45.2	Multiple and bilateral precerebral artery syndromes
G45.3	Amaurosis fugax
G45.8	Other transient cerebral ischemic attacks and related syndromes
I63.031	Cerebral infarction due to thrombosis of right carotid artery ☑
I63.09	Cerebral infarction due to thrombosis of other precerebral artery
I63.131	Cerebral infarction due to embolism of right carotid artery ☑
I63.19	Cerebral infarction due to embolism of other precerebral artery
I63.81	Other cerebral infarction due to occlusion or stenosis of small artery
I65.21	Occlusion and stenosis of right carotid artery ☑
I65.8	Occlusion and stenosis of other precerebral arteries
I67.81	Acute cerebrovascular insufficiency
I67.82	Cerebral ischemia
I67.850	Cerebral autosomal dominant arteriopathy with subcortical infarcts and leukoencephalopathy
I67.858	Other hereditary cerebrovascular disease
I70.92	Chronic total occlusion of artery of the extremities [A]
I74.2	Embolism and thrombosis of arteries of the upper extremities
I75.011	Atheroembolism of right upper extremity ☑
I77.1	Stricture of artery
I77.2	Rupture of artery
I77.71	Dissection of carotid artery
I77.79	Dissection of other specified artery
I77.89	Other specified disorders of arteries and arterioles
Q28.1	Other malformations of precerebral vessels
Q28.8	Other specified congenital malformations of circulatory system
S15.011A	Minor laceration of right carotid artery, initial encounter ☑
S15.021A	Major laceration of right carotid artery, initial encounter ☑
S15.091A	Other specified injury of right carotid artery, initial encounter ☑
S15.8XXA	Injury of other specified blood vessels at neck level, initial encounter
S25.111A	Minor laceration of right innominate or subclavian artery, initial encounter ☑
S25.121A	Major laceration of right innominate or subclavian artery, initial encounter ☑
S25.191A	Other specified injury of right innominate or subclavian artery, initial encounter ☑

Relative Value Units/Medicare Edits

Non-Facility RVU	Work	PE	MP	Total
35526	31.55	11.86	7.31	50.72
Facility RVU	**Work**	**PE**	**MP**	**Total**
35526	31.55	11.86	7.31	50.72

	FUD	Status	MUE	Modifiers				IOM Reference
35526	90	A	1(3)	51	50	62*	80	None

* with documentation

Terms To Know

anastomosis. Surgically created connection between ducts, blood vessels, or bowel segments to allow flow from one to the other.

sternotomy. Incision into the sternum, the bone that forms the front of the chest cavity and connects with the ribs.

thoracotomy. Surgical procedure for opening the chest wall in order to access the lungs, esophagus, trachea, aorta, heart, and diaphragm.

35531

35531 Bypass graft, with vein; aortoceliac or aortomesenteric

Schematic of an aortomesenteric bypass

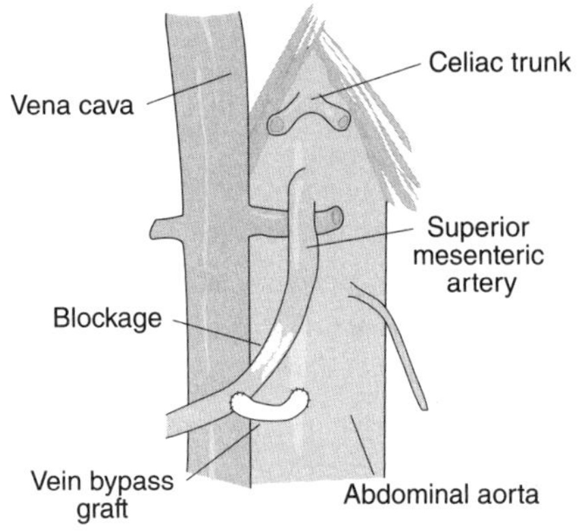

Bypass around blockage of an upper abdominal artery (celiac or mesentery)

Explanation

The physician exposes the involved aortomesenteric or aortoceliac artery using an upper midline abdominal incision, retracting and dissecting past large and small bowel. The physician exposes the distal thoracic aorta, administers heparin for anticoagulation, and clamps the aorta both proximal and distal to the celiac axis origin. The physician cuts out an elliptical disk of aortic wall from the anterior surface of the aorta. The physician exposes the involved vessel (aortomesenteric or aortoceliac artery) and divides it proximal to the occlusion, closing off the proximal stump with suture. The physician sews a venous graft from the clamped aorta to the nondiseased distal artery. The physician may use harvested vein to enlarge the arterial lumen (patch graft). The physician may perform arteriography or use a Doppler probe to establish patency of the graft. The physician closes the abdominal wound, leaving drains in place.

Coding Tips

Establishing both inflow and outflow by any method is included. That portion of the operative arteriogram performed by the surgeon is also included. Angioscopy performed during therapeutic intervention should be reported in addition to the code for the primary procedure; see 35400. Harvesting of the saphenous vein graft is included in the description of the work for 35531 and should not be reported as a separate procedure. For harvesting of a femoropopliteal vein segment, use 35572 in addition to the bypass procedure. If a composite (combination of vein and synthetic graft) is used, report 35681 in addition to the code for the primary procedure. If synthetic graft material is used, see 35631.

ICD-10-CM Diagnostic Codes

I70.8	Atherosclerosis of other arteries A
I75.89	Atheroembolism of other site
I77.1	Stricture of artery
I77.4	Celiac artery compression syndrome
I77.5	Necrosis of artery
I77.79	Dissection of other specified artery
I77.89	Other specified disorders of arteries and arterioles
K55.011	Focal (segmental) acute (reversible) ischemia of small intestine
K55.012	Diffuse acute (reversible) ischemia of small intestine
K55.021	Focal (segmental) acute infarction of small intestine
K55.022	Diffuse acute infarction of small intestine
K55.031	Focal (segmental) acute (reversible) ischemia of large intestine
K55.032	Diffuse acute (reversible) ischemia of large intestine
K55.041	Focal (segmental) acute infarction of large intestine
K55.042	Diffuse acute infarction of large intestine
K55.1	Chronic vascular disorders of intestine
K55.8	Other vascular disorders of intestine
S35.211A	Minor laceration of celiac artery, initial encounter
S35.212A	Major laceration of celiac artery, initial encounter
S35.218A	Other injury of celiac artery, initial encounter
S35.221A	Minor laceration of superior mesenteric artery, initial encounter
S35.222A	Major laceration of superior mesenteric artery, initial encounter
S35.228A	Other injury of superior mesenteric artery, initial encounter
S35.231A	Minor laceration of inferior mesenteric artery, initial encounter
S35.232A	Major laceration of inferior mesenteric artery, initial encounter
S35.238A	Other injury of inferior mesenteric artery, initial encounter
S35.291A	Minor laceration of branches of celiac and mesenteric artery, initial encounter
S35.292A	Major laceration of branches of celiac and mesenteric artery, initial encounter
S35.298A	Other injury of branches of celiac and mesenteric artery, initial encounter
S35.8X1A	Laceration of other blood vessels at abdomen, lower back and pelvis level, initial encounter
S35.8X8A	Other specified injury of other blood vessels at abdomen, lower back and pelvis level, initial encounter
T81.710A	Complication of mesenteric artery following a procedure, not elsewhere classified, initial encounter

Relative Value Units/Medicare Edits

Non-Facility RVU	Work	PE	MP	Total
35531	39.11	8.19	9.77	57.07
Facility RVU	**Work**	**PE**	**MP**	**Total**
35531	39.11	8.19	9.77	57.07

	FUD	Status	MUE	Modifiers				IOM Reference
35531	90	A	1(3)	51	50	62*	80	None

* with documentation

35533

35533 Bypass graft, with vein; axillary-femoral-femoral

Axillary-femoral-femoral bypass

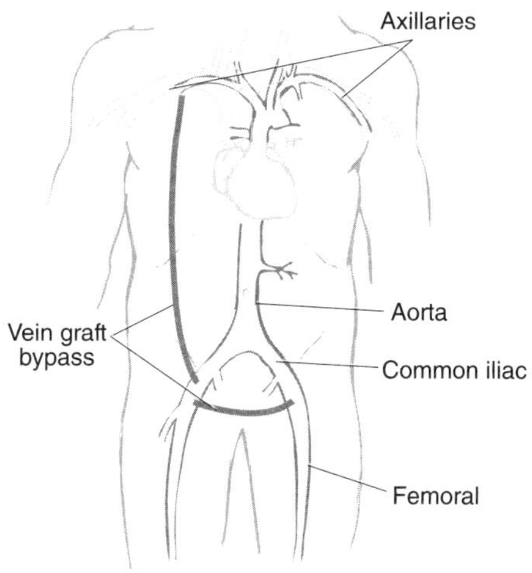

Explanation

Through incisions in the skin of the axilla and both upper thighs, the physician creates a bypass using a harvested vein around the section of diseased or damaged artery. Once vessel clamps have been affixed above and below the area of anastomosis, the harvested vein is sutured to the side of the axillary artery and passed through a subcutaneous tunnel to the upper thigh, where it is sutured end-to-end or end-to-side to the femoral artery. A second harvested vein is sutured end-to-side to the femoral artery or to the vein graft descending from the axilla where it joins the femoral artery, and is passed through another subcutaneous tunnel to the opposite thigh, where it is sutured end-to-end or end-to-side to the femoral artery. When the clamps are removed, the two grafted vein limbs form a new path through which blood can easily bypass the blocked area. The section of the blocked or damaged vessel is not removed. After the graft is complete, the incisions are repaired with layered closures.

Coding Tips

Establishing both inflow and outflow by any method is included. That portion of the operative arteriogram performed by the surgeon is also included. Angioscopy performed during therapeutic intervention should be reported in addition to the code for the primary procedure, see 35400. Harvesting of the saphenous vein graft is included in the description of the work for 35533 and should not be reported as a separate procedure. For harvesting of a femoropopliteal vein segment, use 35572 in addition to the bypass procedure. If a composite (combination of vein and synthetic graft) is used, report 35681 in addition to the code for the primary procedure. If synthetic graft material is used, see 35654.

ICD-10-CM Diagnostic Codes

A52.01	Syphilitic aneurysm of aorta
A52.02	Syphilitic aortitis
I70.0	Atherosclerosis of aorta A
I70.92	Chronic total occlusion of artery of the extremities A
I71.010	Dissection of ascending aorta
I71.011	Dissection of aortic arch
I71.012	Dissection of descending thoracic aorta
I71.02	Dissection of abdominal aorta
I71.03	Dissection of thoracoabdominal aorta
I72.2	Aneurysm of renal artery
I72.8	Aneurysm of other specified arteries
I73.89	Other specified peripheral vascular diseases
I74.01	Saddle embolus of abdominal aorta
I74.09	Other arterial embolism and thrombosis of abdominal aorta
I74.19	Embolism and thrombosis of other parts of aorta
I74.5	Embolism and thrombosis of iliac artery
I75.89	Atheroembolism of other site
I76	Septic arterial embolism
I77.1	Stricture of artery
I77.3	Arterial fibromuscular dysplasia
I77.4	Celiac artery compression syndrome
I77.5	Necrosis of artery
I77.72	Dissection of iliac artery
I77.73	Dissection of renal artery
I77.79	Dissection of other specified artery
I77.810	Thoracic aortic ectasia
I77.811	Abdominal aortic ectasia
I77.812	Thoracoabdominal aortic ectasia
I82.0	Budd-Chiari syndrome
K55.011	Focal (segmental) acute (reversible) ischemia of small intestine
K55.012	Diffuse acute (reversible) ischemia of small intestine
K55.021	Focal (segmental) acute infarction of small intestine
K55.022	Diffuse acute infarction of small intestine
K55.031	Focal (segmental) acute (reversible) ischemia of large intestine
K55.032	Diffuse acute (reversible) ischemia of large intestine
K55.041	Focal (segmental) acute infarction of large intestine
K55.042	Diffuse acute infarction of large intestine
K55.1	Chronic vascular disorders of intestine
K55.8	Other vascular disorders of intestine
N28.0	Ischemia and infarction of kidney
Q25.21	Interruption of aortic arch
Q25.41	Absence and aplasia of aorta
Q25.46	Tortuous aortic arch
Q25.47	Right aortic arch
Q25.48	Anomalous origin of subclavian artery
Q25.8	Other congenital malformations of other great arteries
Q27.1	Congenital renal artery stenosis
Q27.2	Other congenital malformations of renal artery
Q79.61	Classical Ehlers-Danlos syndrome
Q79.62	Hypermobile Ehlers-Danlos syndrome
Q79.63	Vascular Ehlers-Danlos syndrome
Q87.418	Marfan syndrome with other cardiovascular manifestations
S25.01XA	Minor laceration of thoracic aorta, initial encounter
S25.02XA	Major laceration of thoracic aorta, initial encounter
S25.09XA	Other specified injury of thoracic aorta, initial encounter
S25.811A	Laceration of other blood vessels of thorax, right side, initial encounter ☑
S25.812A	Laceration of other blood vessels of thorax, left side, initial encounter ☑
S25.891A	Other specified injury of other blood vessels of thorax, right side, initial encounter ☑

S25.892A	Other specified injury of other blood vessels of thorax, left side, initial encounter ☑
S35.01XA	Minor laceration of abdominal aorta, initial encounter
S35.02XA	Major laceration of abdominal aorta, initial encounter
S35.09XA	Other injury of abdominal aorta, initial encounter
S35.211A	Minor laceration of celiac artery, initial encounter
S35.212A	Major laceration of celiac artery, initial encounter
S35.218A	Other injury of celiac artery, initial encounter
S35.221A	Minor laceration of superior mesenteric artery, initial encounter
S35.222A	Major laceration of superior mesenteric artery, initial encounter
S35.228A	Other injury of superior mesenteric artery, initial encounter
S35.231A	Minor laceration of inferior mesenteric artery, initial encounter
S35.232A	Major laceration of inferior mesenteric artery, initial encounter
S35.238A	Other injury of inferior mesenteric artery, initial encounter
S35.291A	Minor laceration of branches of celiac and mesenteric artery, initial encounter
S35.292A	Major laceration of branches of celiac and mesenteric artery, initial encounter
S35.298A	Other injury of branches of celiac and mesenteric artery, initial encounter
S35.411A	Laceration of right renal artery, initial encounter ☑
S35.412A	Laceration of left renal artery, initial encounter ☑
S35.491A	Other specified injury of right renal artery, initial encounter ☑
S35.492A	Other specified injury of left renal artery, initial encounter ☑
S35.511A	Injury of right iliac artery, initial encounter ☑
S35.512A	Injury of left iliac artery, initial encounter ☑
S35.8X1A	Laceration of other blood vessels at abdomen, lower back and pelvis level, initial encounter
S35.8X8A	Other specified injury of other blood vessels at abdomen, lower back and pelvis level, initial encounter
T81.710A	Complication of mesenteric artery following a procedure, not elsewhere classified, initial encounter

Relative Value Units/Medicare Edits

Non-Facility RVU	Work	PE	MP	Total
35533	29.92	6.76	7.47	44.15
Facility RVU	**Work**	**PE**	**MP**	**Total**
35533	29.92	6.76	7.47	44.15

	FUD	Status	MUE	Modifiers				IOM Reference
35533	90	A	1(3)	51	50	62*	80	None

* with documentation

35535

35535 Bypass graft, with vein; hepatorenal

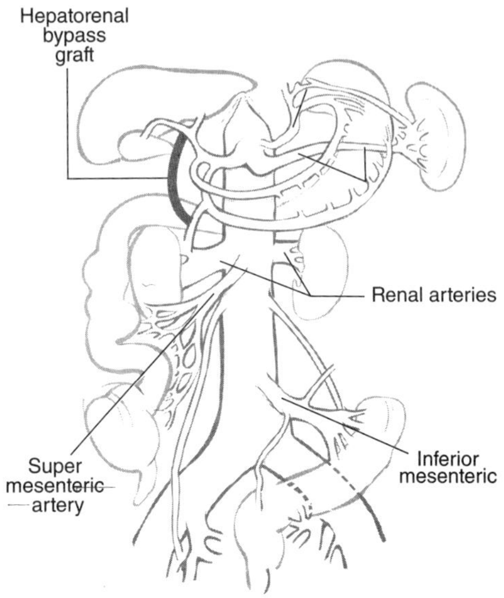

Vein bypass graft from the liver artery to one of the renal arteries

Explanation

The physician performs hepatorenal bypass graft. With the patient placed supine, a right subcostal (beneath the ribs) incision is made and extended through the subcutaneous tissue, fat, and muscle. The abdominal cavity is entered, the stomach is retracted, and the lesser omentum is entered. The physician locates the common hepatic, proper hepatic, and gastroduodenal arteries. These are dissected and encircled with Silastic vessel loops. After the physician mobilizes the right renal vein, the right renal artery is exposed, dissected, and encircled with Silastic vessel loops. The physician harvests a greater saphenous vein segment and forms a proximal end-to-end anastomosis to the common hepatic artery. Distal anastomosis is then performed with the renal artery in either a side-to-side or end-to-end fashion. Bleeding is controlled and Doppler or duplex is performed to verify revascularization. After the graft is complete, the incisions are repaired with layered closure.

Coding Tips

Angioscopy performed during therapeutic intervention should be reported in addition to the code for the primary procedure, see 35400. Harvesting of the saphenous vein graft is included in the description of the work for 35535 and should not be reported as a separate procedure. For harvesting of a femoropopliteal vein segment, use 35572 in addition to the bypass procedure. If a composite (combination of vein and synthetic graft) is used, report 35681 in addition to the code for the primary procedure. Do not report 35535 with 35221, 35251, 35281, 35500, 35536, 35560, 35631, or 35636.

ICD-10-CM Diagnostic Codes

I15.0	Renovascular hypertension
I15.1	Hypertension secondary to other renal disorders
I70.1	Atherosclerosis of renal artery [A]
I72.2	Aneurysm of renal artery
I75.81	Atheroembolism of kidney
I77.1	Stricture of artery
I77.3	Arterial fibromuscular dysplasia
I77.5	Necrosis of artery

I77.73	Dissection of renal artery
I77.89	Other specified disorders of arteries and arterioles
N26.2	Page kidney
N28.0	Ischemia and infarction of kidney
Q27.1	Congenital renal artery stenosis
Q27.2	Other congenital malformations of renal artery
Q27.34	Arteriovenous malformation of renal vessel
S35.411A	Laceration of right renal artery, initial encounter ☑
S35.412A	Laceration of left renal artery, initial encounter ☑
S35.491A	Other specified injury of right renal artery, initial encounter ☑
S35.492A	Other specified injury of left renal artery, initial encounter ☑
T81.711A	Complication of renal artery following a procedure, not elsewhere classified, initial encounter

Relative Value Units/Medicare Edits

Non-Facility RVU	Work	PE	MP	Total
35535	38.13	8.05	9.52	55.7
Facility RVU	**Work**	**PE**	**MP**	**Total**
35535	38.13	8.05	9.52	55.7

	FUD	Status	MUE	Modifiers				IOM Reference
35535	90	A	1(3)	51	50	62*	80	None

* with documentation

Terms To Know

atherosclerosis. Buildup of yellowish plaques composed of cholesterol and lipoid material within the arteries.

occlusion. Constriction, closure, or blockage of a passage.

stenosis. Narrowing or constriction of a passage.

35536

35536 Bypass graft, with vein; splenorenal

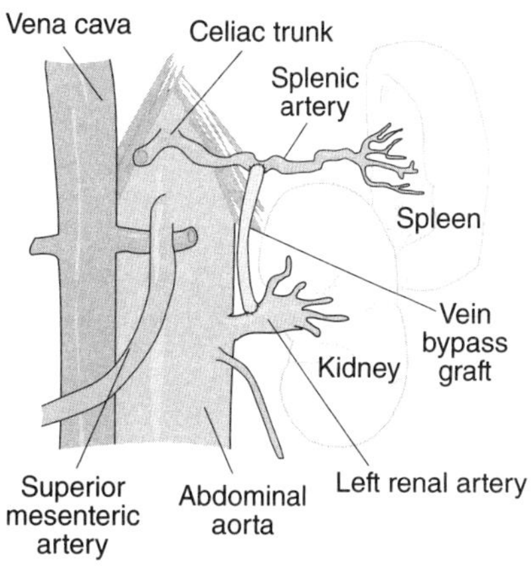

Explanation

The physician performs a bilateral subcostal incision from the right midrectus position extending into the left flank, and dissects past bowel and pancreas to expose the splenic vein. The physician exposes the splenic artery by careful dissection. The physician exposes the left renal artery by dissecting through the posterior parietal peritoneum, partially clamps it, and excises an ellipse of renal artery at its upper border. The physician performs end-to-side anastomosis of vein graft material from the splenic artery to the renal artery. The physician removes the clamps and assesses the anastomotic sites for leaks. The physician may perform Doppler studies or arteriography to establish patency of the graft. The physician closes the abdominal wound, leaving drains in place.

Coding Tips

Establishing both inflow and outflow by any method is included. That portion of the operative arteriogram performed by the surgeon is also included. Angioscopy performed during therapeutic intervention should be reported in addition to the code for the primary procedure; see 35400. Harvesting of the saphenous vein graft is included in the description of the work for 35536 and should not be reported as a separate procedure. For harvesting of a femoropopliteal vein segment, use 35572 in addition to the bypass procedure. If a composite (combination of vein and synthetic graft) is used, report 35681 in addition to the code for the primary procedure. If synthetic graft material is used, see 35636.

ICD-10-CM Diagnostic Codes

D73.5	Infarction of spleen
I70.1	Atherosclerosis of renal artery 🅰
I74.8	Embolism and thrombosis of other arteries
I75.81	Atheroembolism of kidney
I76	Septic arterial embolism
I77.1	Stricture of artery
I77.3	Arterial fibromuscular dysplasia
I77.5	Necrosis of artery
I77.73	Dissection of renal artery
I77.89	Other specified disorders of arteries and arterioles
N26.2	Page kidney

N28.0 Ischemia and infarction of kidney
Q27.1 Congenital renal artery stenosis
Q27.2 Other congenital malformations of renal artery
Q27.34 Arteriovenous malformation of renal vessel
S35.291A Minor laceration of branches of celiac and mesenteric artery, initial encounter
S35.292A Major laceration of branches of celiac and mesenteric artery, initial encounter
S35.298A Other injury of branches of celiac and mesenteric artery, initial encounter
S35.411A Laceration of right renal artery, initial encounter ☑
S35.412A Laceration of left renal artery, initial encounter ☑
S35.491A Other specified injury of right renal artery, initial encounter ☑
S35.492A Other specified injury of left renal artery, initial encounter ☑
S35.8X1A Laceration of other blood vessels at abdomen, lower back and pelvis level, initial encounter
S35.8X8A Other specified injury of other blood vessels at abdomen, lower back and pelvis level, initial encounter

Relative Value Units/Medicare Edits

Non-Facility RVU	Work	PE	MP	Total
35536	33.73	7.35	8.39	49.47
Facility RVU	**Work**	**PE**	**MP**	**Total**
35536	33.73	7.35	8.39	49.47

	FUD	Status	MUE	Modifiers				IOM Reference
35536	90	A	1(3)	51	50	62*	80	None

* with documentation

Terms To Know

anastomosis. Surgically created connection between ducts, blood vessels, or bowel segments to allow flow from one to the other.

atherosclerosis. Buildup of yellowish plaques composed of cholesterol and lipoid material within the arteries.

doppler. Ultrasonography used to augment two-dimensional images by registering velocity. When emitted sound waves reflect back off a moving object, the frequency of the reflected sound waves varies in relation to the speed of the moving object and may be used in many different procedures.

hyperplasia. Abnormal proliferation in the number of normal cells in regular tissue arrangement.

patency. State of a tube-like structure or conduit being open and unobstructed.

35537-35538

35537 Bypass graft, with vein; aortoiliac
35538 Bypass graft, with vein; aortobi-iliac

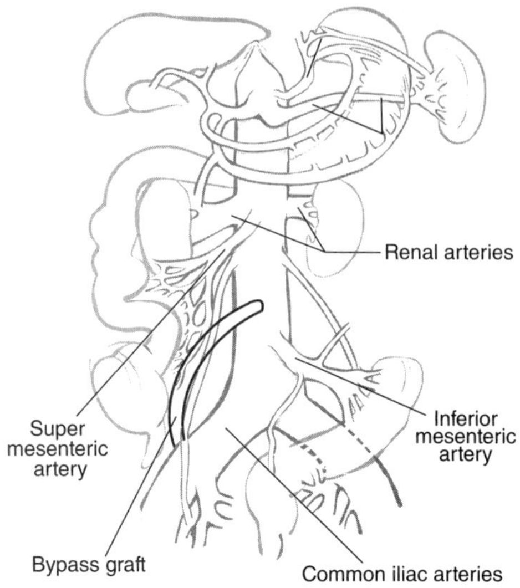

Bypass from the aorta to iliac artery

Explanation

The physician exposes the involved abdominal aorta and iliac arteries using an abdominal incision, retracting and dissecting past large and small bowel. The physician partially clamps the aorta above the diseased area and places a longitudinal incision down the clamped portion of the aorta. The physician sews in a (two) venous graft(s), clamps the graft(s), and removes the aortic clamp to assess the anastomosis(es) for leaks. The physician clamps the iliac artery(ies) distal to the stenosis and incises and attaches the distal venous graft to the iliac artery(ies). The physician may also use harvested vein to enlarge the aortic or arterial lumen (patch graft). The physician may perform arteriography or use a Doppler probe to establish patency of the graft. The physician closes the abdominal wound, leaving drains in place. A bypass graft to a single iliac artery is performed in 35537; both iliac arteries are bypassed in 35538.

Coding Tips

Establishing both inflow and outflow by any method is included. That portion of the operative arteriogram performed by the surgeon is also included. Angioscopy performed during therapeutic intervention should be reported in addition to the code for the primary procedure, see 35400. Harvesting of the saphenous vein graft is included in the description of the work for 35537 and 35538 and should not be reported as a separate procedure. For harvesting of a femoropopliteal vein segment, use 35572 in addition to the bypass procedure. If a composite (combination of vein and synthetic graft) is used, report 35681 in addition to the code for the primary procedure. Do not report 35537 or 35538 with each other. For a bypass graft performed with a synthetic graft, see 35637 or 35638.

ICD-10-CM Diagnostic Codes

A52.01 Syphilitic aneurysm of aorta
A52.02 Syphilitic aortitis
I70.0 Atherosclerosis of aorta 🅰
I71.02 Dissection of abdominal aorta
I73.89 Other specified peripheral vascular diseases

I73.9	Peripheral vascular disease, unspecified
I74.01	Saddle embolus of abdominal aorta
I74.09	Other arterial embolism and thrombosis of abdominal aorta
I74.19	Embolism and thrombosis of other parts of aorta
I74.5	Embolism and thrombosis of iliac artery
I75.89	Atheroembolism of other site
I76	Septic arterial embolism
I77.1	Stricture of artery
I77.3	Arterial fibromuscular dysplasia
I77.5	Necrosis of artery
I77.72	Dissection of iliac artery
I77.811	Abdominal aortic ectasia
I77.812	Thoracoabdominal aortic ectasia
I77.89	Other specified disorders of arteries and arterioles
Q25.21	Interruption of aortic arch
Q25.29	Other atresia of aorta
Q25.41	Absence and aplasia of aorta
Q25.42	Hypoplasia of aorta
Q25.43	Congenital aneurysm of aorta
Q25.44	Congenital dilation of aorta
Q25.45	Double aortic arch
Q25.46	Tortuous aortic arch
Q25.47	Right aortic arch
Q25.48	Anomalous origin of subclavian artery
Q25.49	Other congenital malformations of aorta
S35.01XA	Minor laceration of abdominal aorta, initial encounter
S35.02XA	Major laceration of abdominal aorta, initial encounter
S35.09XA	Other injury of abdominal aorta, initial encounter
S35.511A	Injury of right iliac artery, initial encounter ☑
S35.512A	Injury of left iliac artery, initial encounter ☑
S35.59XA	Injury of other iliac blood vessels, initial encounter
S35.8X1A	Laceration of other blood vessels at abdomen, lower back and pelvis level, initial encounter
S35.8X8A	Other specified injury of other blood vessels at abdomen, lower back and pelvis level, initial encounter

Relative Value Units/Medicare Edits

Non-Facility RVU	Work	PE	MP	Total
35537	41.88	8.65	10.47	61.0
35538	47.03	9.55	11.73	68.31
Facility RVU	**Work**	**PE**	**MP**	**Total**
35537	41.88	8.65	10.47	61.0
35538	47.03	9.55	11.73	68.31

	FUD	Status	MUE	Modifiers				IOM Reference
35537	90	A	1(3)	51	N/A	62*	80	None
35538	90	A	1(3)	51	N/A	62*	80	

* with documentation

35539-35540

35539 Bypass graft, with vein; aortofemoral
35540 aortobifemoral

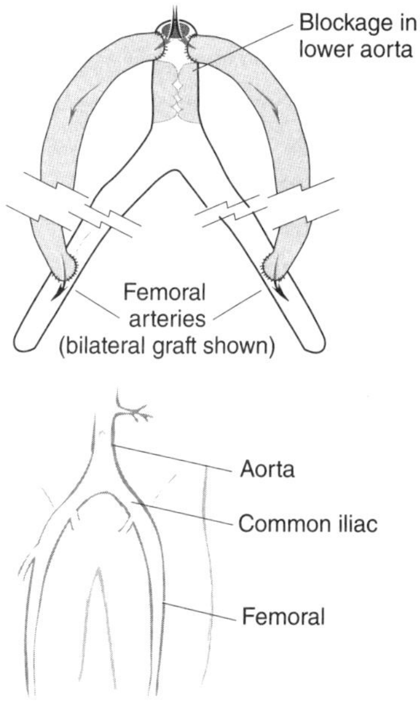

Explanation

The physician makes an incision in the skin of the abdomen over a section of damaged or blocked lower aorta. The artery is isolated and dissected. Through a separate skin incision in the upper thigh, the femoral artery is isolated and dissected from adjacent critical structures. The physician creates a bypass around the damaged or blocked lower aorta using a harvested vein. Once vessel clamps have been affixed above the defect, the lower aorta may be cut through or tied off with sutures above the damaged or blocked area and sutured to one end of the harvested vein in an end-to-end or side-to-side fashion. In 35539, the graft to one femoral artery is passed through a tunnel on the inside of the upper thigh and sutured to the femoral artery. In 35540, a bifemoral bypass is accomplished and a second harvested vein is placed in a similar fashion to the second side. When the clamps are removed, the two grafted vein limbs form a new path through which blood can easily bypass the blocked area. The blocked or damaged portion of artery is not removed. After the graft is complete, the skin incisions are repaired with layered closures.

Coding Tips

Establishing both inflow and outflow by any method is included. That portion of the operative arteriogram performed by the surgeon is also included. Angioscopy performed during therapeutic intervention should be reported in addition to the code for the primary procedure, see 35400. Harvesting of the saphenous vein graft is included in the description of the work for 35539 and 35540 and should not be reported as a separate procedure. For harvesting of a femoropopliteal vein segment, use 35572 in addition to the bypass procedure. If a composite (combination of vein and synthetic graft) is used, report 35681 in addition to the code for the primary procedure. Do not report 35539 or 35540 with each other. For a bypass graft performed with a synthetic graft, see 35646 or 35647.

ICD-10-CM Diagnostic Codes

A52.01	Syphilitic aneurysm of aorta
A52.02	Syphilitic aortitis
I70.0	Atherosclerosis of aorta 🅰

I71.02 Dissection of abdominal aorta
I73.89 Other specified peripheral vascular diseases
I73.9 Peripheral vascular disease, unspecified
I74.01 Saddle embolus of abdominal aorta
I74.09 Other arterial embolism and thrombosis of abdominal aorta
I74.19 Embolism and thrombosis of other parts of aorta
I74.5 Embolism and thrombosis of iliac artery
I75.89 Atheroembolism of other site
I76 Septic arterial embolism
I77.1 Stricture of artery
I77.3 Arterial fibromuscular dysplasia
I77.5 Necrosis of artery
I77.72 Dissection of iliac artery
I77.811 Abdominal aortic ectasia
I77.812 Thoracoabdominal aortic ectasia
I77.89 Other specified disorders of arteries and arterioles
I79.0 Aneurysm of aorta in diseases classified elsewhere
Q25.21 Interruption of aortic arch
Q25.29 Other atresia of aorta
Q25.41 Absence and aplasia of aorta
Q25.42 Hypoplasia of aorta
Q25.43 Congenital aneurysm of aorta
Q25.44 Congenital dilation of aorta
Q25.45 Double aortic arch
Q25.46 Tortuous aortic arch
Q25.47 Right aortic arch
Q25.48 Anomalous origin of subclavian artery
Q25.49 Other congenital malformations of aorta
S35.01XA Minor laceration of abdominal aorta, initial encounter
S35.02XA Major laceration of abdominal aorta, initial encounter
S35.09XA Other injury of abdominal aorta, initial encounter
S35.8X1A Laceration of other blood vessels at abdomen, lower back and pelvis level, initial encounter
S35.8X8A Other specified injury of other blood vessels at abdomen, lower back and pelvis level, initial encounter

Relative Value Units/Medicare Edits

Non-Facility RVU	Work	PE	MP	Total
35539	44.11	9.0	11.01	64.12
35540	49.33	9.8	12.31	71.44
Facility RVU	**Work**	**PE**	**MP**	**Total**
35539	44.11	9.0	11.01	64.12
35540	49.33	9.8	12.31	71.44

	FUD	Status	MUE	Modifiers				IOM Reference
35539	90	A	1(3)	51	50	62*	80	None
35540	90	A	1(3)	51	50	62*	N/A	

* with documentation

35556

35556 Bypass graft, with vein; femoral-popliteal

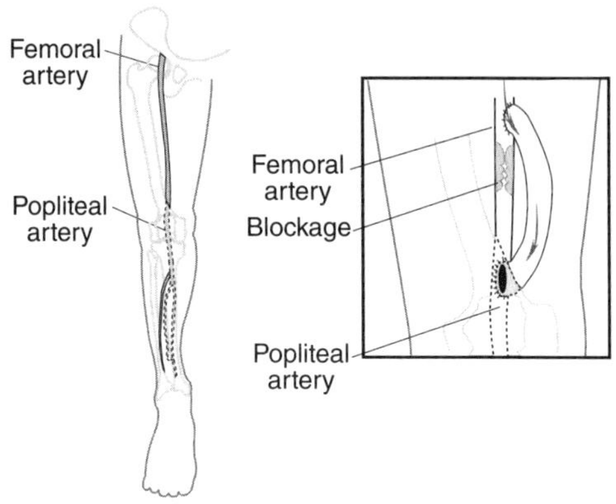

Explanation

Through incisions in the skin of the leg overlying the femoral and popliteal arteries, the physician isolates and dissects a section of artery that is damaged or blocked. The physician creates a bypass around the superficial femoral artery, using a harvested vein and one of two methods of repair. Once vessel clamps have been affixed above and below the defect, the superficial femoral artery may be cut through above the damaged or blocked area and sutured to one end of a harvested vein. The vein is passed through a tunnel down the thigh muscles and behind the knee and sutured to the popliteal artery. In the second method, the ends of the harvested vein are sutured into the side of the femoral and popliteal arterial walls, resulting in a bypass of the damaged area. When the clamps are removed, the section of vein forms a new path through which blood can easily bypass the blocked area. The blocked or damaged portion of artery is not removed. After the graft is complete, the skin incisions are repaired with layered closures.

Coding Tips

Establishing both inflow and outflow by any method is included. That portion of the operative arteriogram performed by the surgeon is also included. Angioscopy performed during therapeutic intervention should be reported in addition to the code for the primary procedure; see 35400. Harvesting of the saphenous vein graft is included in the description of the work for 35556 and should not be reported as a separate procedure. For harvesting of a femoropopliteal vein segment, use 35572 in addition to the bypass procedure. If a composite (combination of vein and synthetic graft) is used, report 35681 in addition to the code for the primary procedure. To report the harvesting and construction of an autogenous composite graft of two segments from two distant locations, report 35682 in addition to the bypass procedure. For autogenous composite of three or more segments from distant sites, see 35683. Report 35700 in addition to 35556 for reoperation more than one month after the original operation. If synthetic graft material is used, see 35656.

ICD-10-CM Diagnostic Codes

I70.211 Atherosclerosis of native arteries of extremities with intermittent claudication, right leg A ☑
I70.221 Atherosclerosis of native arteries of extremities with rest pain, right leg A ☑
I70.231 Atherosclerosis of native arteries of right leg with ulceration of thigh A ☑
I70.232 Atherosclerosis of native arteries of right leg with ulceration of calf A ☑

 N Newborn: 0 P Pediatric: 0-17 M Maternity: 9-64 A Adult: 15-124 AMA: CPT Assist

I70.233 Atherosclerosis of native arteries of right leg with ulceration of ankle A ☑
I70.234 Atherosclerosis of native arteries of right leg with ulceration of heel and midfoot A ☑
I70.235 Atherosclerosis of native arteries of right leg with ulceration of other part of foot A ☑
I70.238 Atherosclerosis of native arteries of right leg with ulceration of other part of lower leg A ☑
I70.261 Atherosclerosis of native arteries of extremities with gangrene, right leg A ☑
I70.291 Other atherosclerosis of native arteries of extremities, right leg A ☑
I70.461 Atherosclerosis of autologous vein bypass graft(s) of the extremities with gangrene, right leg A ☑
I70.511 Atherosclerosis of nonautologous biological bypass graft(s) of the extremities with intermittent claudication, right leg A ☑
I70.521 Atherosclerosis of nonautologous biological bypass graft(s) of the extremities with rest pain, right leg A ☑
I70.531 Atherosclerosis of nonautologous biological bypass graft(s) of the right leg with ulceration of thigh A ☑
I70.561 Atherosclerosis of nonautologous biological bypass graft(s) of the extremities with gangrene, right leg A ☑
I70.611 Atherosclerosis of nonbiological bypass graft(s) of the extremities with intermittent claudication, right leg A ☑
I70.621 Atherosclerosis of nonbiological bypass graft(s) of the extremities with rest pain, right leg A ☑
I70.631 Atherosclerosis of nonbiological bypass graft(s) of the right leg with ulceration of thigh A ☑
I70.661 Atherosclerosis of nonbiological bypass graft(s) of the extremities with gangrene, right leg A ☑
I70.92 Chronic total occlusion of artery of the extremities A
I72.4 Aneurysm of artery of lower extremity
I74.3 Embolism and thrombosis of arteries of the lower extremities
I75.021 Atheroembolism of right lower extremity ☑
I76 Septic arterial embolism
I77.1 Stricture of artery
I77.2 Rupture of artery
I77.5 Necrosis of artery
S75.011A Minor laceration of femoral artery, right leg, initial encounter ☑
S75.021A Major laceration of femoral artery, right leg, initial encounter ☑
S75.091A Other specified injury of femoral artery, right leg, initial encounter ☑

AMA: 35556 2021,Dec

Relative Value Units/Medicare Edits

Non-Facility RVU	Work	PE	MP	Total
35556	26.75	7.38	6.63	40.76
Facility RVU	**Work**	**PE**	**MP**	**Total**
35556	26.75	7.38	6.63	40.76

	FUD	Status	MUE	Modifiers				IOM Reference
35556	90	A	1(3)	51	50	62*	80	None

* with documentation

35558

35558 Bypass graft, with vein; femoral-femoral

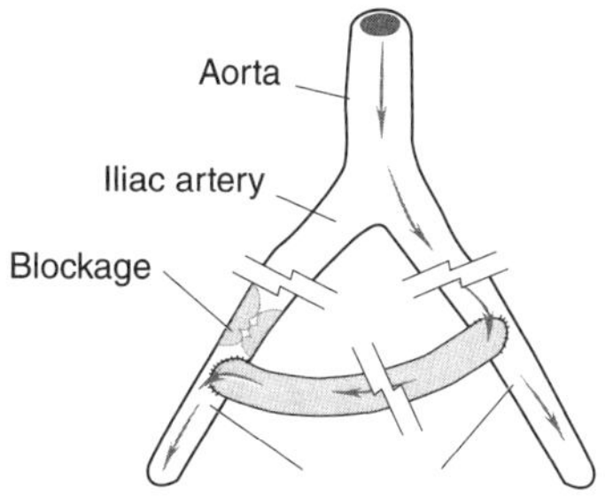

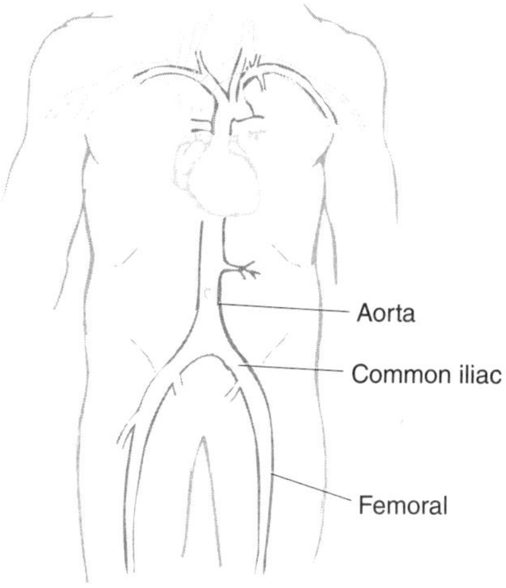

Explanation

Through incisions in the skin of the upper thighs, the physician isolates and dissects a section of the femoral arteries. The physician creates a bypass using a harvested vein. Once vessel clamps have been affixed above and below the area of anastomosis, the femoral artery may be cut through below the damaged area and sutured to one end of a harvested vein, which is sutured to the femoral artery in the opposite leg, resulting in a bypass of the damaged or blocked area. When the clamps are removed, the section of vein forms a new path through which blood can easily bypass the blocked area. The blocked or damaged portion of the artery is not removed. After the graft is complete, the skin incisions are repaired with layered closures.

Coding Tips

Establishing both inflow and outflow by any method is included. That portion of the operative arteriogram performed by the surgeon is also included. Angioscopy performed during therapeutic intervention should be reported in addition to the code for the primary procedure; see 35400. Harvesting of the saphenous vein graft is included in the description of the work for 35558 and should not be reported as a separate procedure. For harvesting of a femoropopliteal vein segment, use 35572 in addition to the bypass procedure. If a composite (combination of vein and synthetic graft) is used, report 35681 in addition to the code for the primary procedure. If synthetic graft material is used, see 35661.

ICD-10-CM Diagnostic Codes

I70.211 Atherosclerosis of native arteries of extremities with intermittent claudication, right leg A ☑
I70.221 Atherosclerosis of native arteries of extremities with rest pain, right leg A ☑

I70.231	Atherosclerosis of native arteries of right leg with ulceration of thigh A ☑
I70.232	Atherosclerosis of native arteries of right leg with ulceration of calf A ☑
I70.233	Atherosclerosis of native arteries of right leg with ulceration of ankle A ☑
I70.234	Atherosclerosis of native arteries of right leg with ulceration of heel and midfoot A ☑
I70.235	Atherosclerosis of native arteries of right leg with ulceration of other part of foot A ☑
I70.238	Atherosclerosis of native arteries of right leg with ulceration of other part of lower leg A ☑
I70.261	Atherosclerosis of native arteries of extremities with gangrene, right leg A ☑
I70.291	Other atherosclerosis of native arteries of extremities, right leg A ☑
I70.461	Atherosclerosis of autologous vein bypass graft(s) of the extremities with gangrene, right leg A ☑
I70.511	Atherosclerosis of nonautologous biological bypass graft(s) of the extremities with intermittent claudication, right leg A ☑
I70.521	Atherosclerosis of nonautologous biological bypass graft(s) of the extremities with rest pain, right leg A ☑
I70.531	Atherosclerosis of nonautologous biological bypass graft(s) of the right leg with ulceration of thigh A ☑
I70.561	Atherosclerosis of nonautologous biological bypass graft(s) of the extremities with gangrene, right leg A ☑
I70.611	Atherosclerosis of nonbiological bypass graft(s) of the extremities with intermittent claudication, right leg A ☑
I70.621	Atherosclerosis of nonbiological bypass graft(s) of the extremities with rest pain, right leg A ☑
I70.631	Atherosclerosis of nonbiological bypass graft(s) of the right leg with ulceration of thigh A ☑
I70.661	Atherosclerosis of nonbiological bypass graft(s) of the extremities with gangrene, right leg A ☑
I70.92	Chronic total occlusion of artery of the extremities A
I74.3	Embolism and thrombosis of arteries of the lower extremities
I75.021	Atheroembolism of right lower extremity ☑
I76	Septic arterial embolism
I77.1	Stricture of artery
I77.2	Rupture of artery
I77.5	Necrosis of artery
I77.89	Other specified disorders of arteries and arterioles
S75.011A	Minor laceration of femoral artery, right leg, initial encounter ☑
S75.021A	Major laceration of femoral artery, right leg, initial encounter ☑

Relative Value Units/Medicare Edits

Non-Facility RVU	Work	PE	MP	Total
35558	23.13	7.44	5.73	36.3
Facility RVU	**Work**	**PE**	**MP**	**Total**
35558	23.13	7.44	5.73	36.3

	FUD	Status	MUE	Modifiers				IOM Reference
35558	90	A	1(3)	51	50	62*	80	None

* with documentation

35560

35560 Bypass graft, with vein; aortorenal

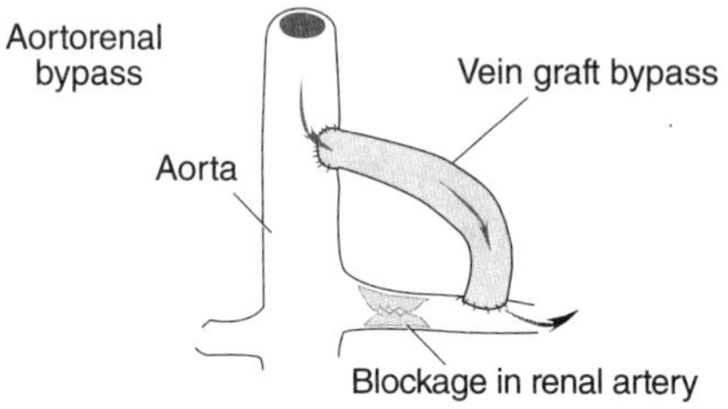

Surgical placement of a vein bypass graft from the aorta to the renal artery

Explanation

The physician exposes the involved abdominal aorta and renal artery using an abdominal incision, retracting and dissecting past large and small bowel. The aorta is partially clamped below the renal takeoff and a small longitudinal incision is performed down the clamped portion of the aorta. The venous graft is sutured and clamped and the aortic clamp is removed to assess the anastomosis for leaks. The renal artery is clamped distal to the stenosis and incised. The distal venous graft is attached to the distal renal artery. A harvested vein may be utilized to enlarge the renal arterial lumen (patch graft). The physician may perform arteriography or use a Doppler probe to establish patency of the graft. The abdominal wound is closed, leaving drains in place.

Coding Tips

Establishing both inflow and outflow by any method is included. That portion of the operative arteriogram performed by the surgeon is also included. Angioscopy performed during therapeutic intervention should be reported in addition to the code for the primary procedure; see 35400. Harvesting of the saphenous vein graft is included in the description of the work for 35560 and should not be reported as a separate procedure. For harvesting of a femoropopliteal vein segment, use 35572 in addition to the bypass procedure. If a composite (combination of vein and synthetic graft) is used, report 35681 in addition to the code for the primary procedure. If synthetic graft material is used, see 35631.

ICD-10-CM Diagnostic Codes

I15.0	Renovascular hypertension
I15.1	Hypertension secondary to other renal disorders
I70.1	Atherosclerosis of renal artery A
I72.2	Aneurysm of renal artery
I73.9	Peripheral vascular disease, unspecified
I75.81	Atheroembolism of kidney
I77.1	Stricture of artery
I77.3	Arterial fibromuscular dysplasia
I77.5	Necrosis of artery
I77.73	Dissection of renal artery
I77.89	Other specified disorders of arteries and arterioles
N26.2	Page kidney
N28.0	Ischemia and infarction of kidney
Q27.1	Congenital renal artery stenosis
Q27.2	Other congenital malformations of renal artery
Q27.34	Arteriovenous malformation of renal vessel
S35.411A	Laceration of right renal artery, initial encounter ☑

S35.412A Laceration of left renal artery, initial encounter ☑

S35.491A Other specified injury of right renal artery, initial encounter ☑

S35.492A Other specified injury of left renal artery, initial encounter ☑

T81.711A Complication of renal artery following a procedure, not elsewhere classified, initial encounter

Relative Value Units/Medicare Edits

Non-Facility RVU	Work	PE	MP	Total
35560	34.03	7.4	8.48	49.91
Facility RVU	**Work**	**PE**	**MP**	**Total**
35560	34.03	7.4	8.48	49.91

	FUD	Status	MUE	Modifiers				IOM Reference
35560	90	A	1(3)	51	50	62*	80	None

* with documentation

Terms To Know

angioscopy. Visualization of capillary blood vessels with a microscope, or the inside of a blood vessel with a fiberoptic-equipped catheter.

arteriogram. Radiograph of arteries.

atherosclerosis. Buildup of yellowish plaques composed of cholesterol and lipoid material within the arteries.

graft. Tissue implant from another part of the body or another person.

hyperplasia. Abnormal proliferation in the number of normal cells in regular tissue arrangement.

secondary. Second in order of occurrence or importance, or appearing during the course of another disease or condition.

35563

35563 Bypass graft, with vein; ilioiliac

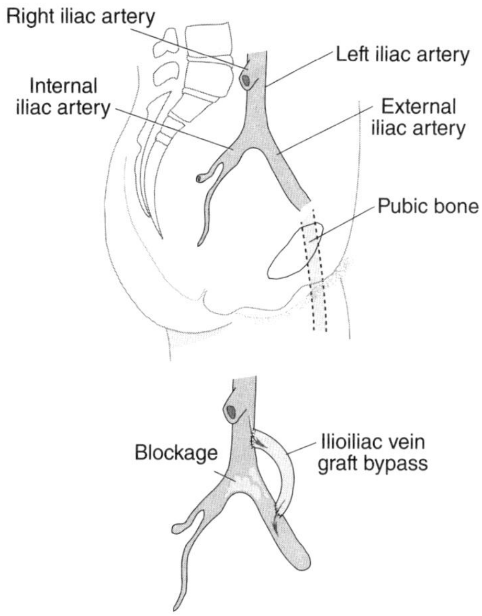

The end-to-side installment of a vein bypass graft from an iliac artery to another point on the iliac artery bypasses a blockage

Explanation

The physician exposes the iliac arteries using an abdominal incision, retracting and dissecting past large and small bowel. The patent (nondiseased) iliac artery is partially clamped and a longitudinal incision is performed down the clamped portion of the aorta. A venous graft is attached and clamped. The iliac clamp is removed to assess the anastomosis for leaks. The diseased iliac artery is clamped distal to the stenosis and a distal incision is performed. The distal venous graft is attached to the diseased iliac artery. A harvested vein may be used to enlarge the aortic or arterial lumen (patch graft). The physician may perform arteriography or use a Doppler probe to establish patency of the graft. The abdominal wound is closed, leaving drains in place.

Coding Tips

Establishing both inflow and outflow by any method is included. That portion of the operative arteriogram performed by the surgeon is also included. Angioscopy performed during therapeutic intervention should be reported in addition to the code for the primary procedure; see 35400. Harvesting of the saphenous vein graft is included in the description of the work for 35563 and should not be reported as a separate procedure. For harvesting of a femoropopliteal vein segment, use 35572 in addition to the bypass procedure. If a composite (combination of vein and synthetic graft) is used, report 35681 in addition to the code for the primary procedure. If synthetic graft material is used, see 35663.

ICD-10-CM Diagnostic Codes

I72.3 Aneurysm of iliac artery

I73.89 Other specified peripheral vascular diseases

I73.9 Peripheral vascular disease, unspecified

I74.5 Embolism and thrombosis of iliac artery

I76 Septic arterial embolism

I77.1 Stricture of artery

● New ▲ Revised + Add On ★ Telemedicine [Resequenced] ☑ Laterality

I77.5	Necrosis of artery
I77.72	Dissection of iliac artery
S35.511A	Injury of right iliac artery, initial encounter ☑
S35.512A	Injury of left iliac artery, initial encounter ☑
S35.59XA	Injury of other iliac blood vessels, initial encounter

Relative Value Units/Medicare Edits

Non-Facility RVU	Work	PE	MP	Total
35563	26.12	6.17	6.51	38.8
Facility RVU	**Work**	**PE**	**MP**	**Total**
35563	26.12	6.17	6.51	38.8

	FUD	Status	MUE	Modifiers				IOM Reference
35563	90	A	1(3)	51	50	62*	80	None

* with documentation

Terms To Know

anastomosis. Surgically created connection between ducts, blood vessels, or bowel segments to allow flow from one to the other.

aneurysm. Circumscribed dilation or outpouching of an artery wall, often containing blood clots and connecting directly with the lumen of the artery.

angioscopy. Visualization of capillary blood vessels with a microscope, or the inside of a blood vessel with a fiberoptic-equipped catheter.

arteriogram. Radiograph of arteries.

artery. Vessel through which oxygenated blood passes away from the heart to any part of the body.

atherosclerosis. Buildup of yellowish plaques composed of cholesterol and lipoid material within the arteries.

complication. Condition arising after the beginning of observation and treatment that modifies the course of the patient's illness or the medical care required, or an undesired result or misadventure in medical care.

embolism. Obstruction of a blood vessel resulting from a clot or foreign substance.

graft. Tissue implant from another part of the body or another person.

harvest. Removal of cells or tissue from their native site to be used as a graft or transplant to another part of the donor's body or placed into another person.

necrosis. Death of cells or tissue within a living organ or structure.

stricture. Narrowing of an anatomical structure.

thrombosis. Condition arising from the presence or formation of blood clots within a blood vessel that may cause vascular obstruction and insufficient oxygenation.

35565

35565 Bypass graft, with vein; iliofemoral

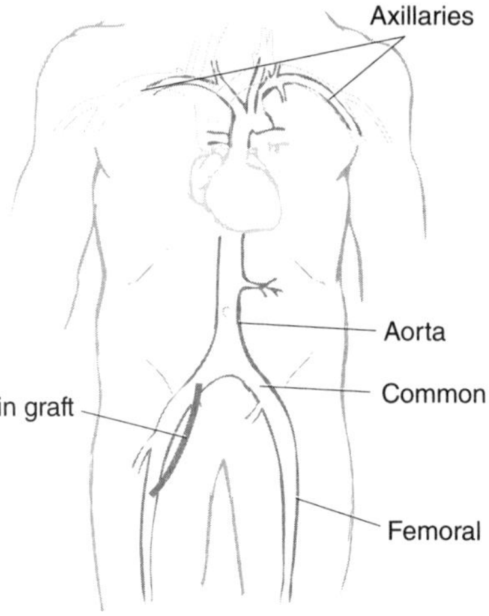

An iliofemoral bypass graft is performed

Explanation

Through incisions in the skin of the lower abdomen overlying the iliac artery and in the skin of the upper thigh overlying the femoral artery, the physician isolates and dissects a section of common iliac artery. The physician creates a bypass around the iliac artery, using a harvested vein and one of two methods of repair. Once vessel clamps have been affixed above and below the defect, the iliac artery may be cut or tied off with sutures above the damaged area and sutured to one end of a harvested vein. The graft is passed through a tunnel on the inside of the upper thigh and is sutured to the side of the femoral artery. In the second method, the end of the harvested vein is sutured to the side of the iliac artery. Either method results in a bypass of the damaged area. When the clamps are removed, the section of vein forms a new path through which blood can easily bypass the blocked area. After the graft is complete, the skin incisions are repaired with layered closures.

Coding Tips

Establishing both inflow and outflow by any method is included. That portion of the operative arteriogram performed by the surgeon is also included. Angioscopy performed during therapeutic intervention should be reported in addition to the code for the primary procedure; see 35400. Harvesting of the saphenous vein graft is included in the description of the work for 35565 and should not be reported as a separate procedure. To report harvesting of an upper extremity vein, use 35500 in addition to the bypass procedure. For harvesting of a femoropopliteal vein segment, use 35572 in addition to the bypass procedure. If a composite (combination of vein and synthetic graft) is used, report 35681 in addition to the code for the primary procedure. If synthetic graft material is used, see 35665.

ICD-10-CM Diagnostic Codes

I70.92	Chronic total occlusion of artery of the extremities 🅰
I73.89	Other specified peripheral vascular diseases
I74.3	Embolism and thrombosis of arteries of the lower extremities
I74.5	Embolism and thrombosis of iliac artery
I75.021	Atheroembolism of right lower extremity ☑
I75.022	Atheroembolism of left lower extremity ☑
I75.023	Atheroembolism of bilateral lower extremities ☑
I76	Septic arterial embolism

I77.1	Stricture of artery
I77.2	Rupture of artery
I77.5	Necrosis of artery
I77.72	Dissection of iliac artery
I77.89	Other specified disorders of arteries and arterioles
I79.8	Other disorders of arteries, arterioles and capillaries in diseases classified elsewhere
S35.511A	Injury of right iliac artery, initial encounter ☑
S35.512A	Injury of left iliac artery, initial encounter ☑
S35.59XA	Injury of other iliac blood vessels, initial encounter

Relative Value Units/Medicare Edits

Non-Facility RVU	Work	PE	MP	Total
35565	25.13	7.1	6.19	38.42
Facility RVU	**Work**	**PE**	**MP**	**Total**
35565	25.13	7.1	6.19	38.42

	FUD	Status	MUE	Modifiers				IOM Reference
35565	90	A	1(3)	51	50	62*	80	None

* with documentation

Terms To Know

bypass graft. Surgically created alternative blood vessel used to reroute blood flow around an area of obstruction or disease.

harvest. Removal of cells or tissue from their native site to be used as a graft or transplant to another part of the donor's body or placed into another person.

35566

35566 Bypass graft, with vein; femoral-anterior tibial, posterior tibial, peroneal artery or other distal vessels

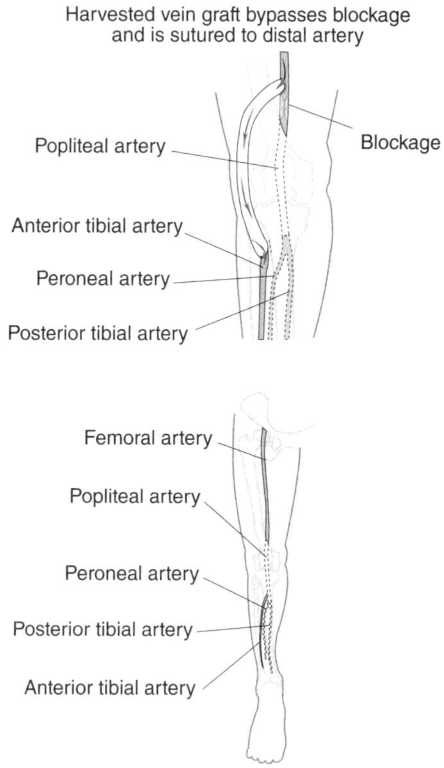

Explanation

Through incisions in the skin of the leg overlying the superficial femoral artery, the physician isolates and dissects sections of the femoral and anterior tibial, posterior tibial, or peroneal arteries. The physician creates a bypass around the affected artery using a harvested vein. Once vessel clamps have been affixed above and below the defect, the superficial femoral artery may be cut through above the damaged area and sutured to one end of a harvested vein, which is passed through an intramuscular tunnel and sutured to the anterior tibial, posterior tibial, peroneal, or other distal vessel. In the second method, the ends of the harvested vein are sutured to the side of the femoral artery and anterior tibial, posterior tibial, peroneal, or other distal vessel wall, resulting in a bypass of the damaged area. When the clamps are removed, the section of vein forms a new path through which blood can easily bypass the blocked area. The blocked or damaged portion of artery is left in place and not removed. After the graft is complete, the skin incisions are repaired with layered closures.

Coding Tips

Establishing both inflow and outflow by any method is included. That portion of the operative arteriogram performed by the surgeon is also included. Angioscopy performed during therapeutic intervention should be reported in addition to the code for the primary procedure; see 35400. Harvesting of the saphenous vein graft is included in the description of the work for 35566 and should not be reported as a separate procedure. For harvesting of a femoropopliteal vein segment, use 35572 in addition to the bypass procedure. To report harvesting of an upper extremity vein, use 35500 in addition to the bypass procedure. If a composite (combination of vein and synthetic graft) is used, report 35681 in addition to the code for the primary procedure. To report the harvesting and construction of an autogenous composite graft of two segments from two distant locations, report 35682 in addition to the bypass procedure. For autogenous composite of three or more segments from distant sites, see 35683. Report 35700 in addition to 35566 for reoperation more than one month after the original operation. If synthetic graft material is used, see 35666.

ICD-10-CM Diagnostic Codes

I70.211	Atherosclerosis of native arteries of extremities with intermittent claudication, right leg A ☑
I70.221	Atherosclerosis of native arteries of extremities with rest pain, right leg A ☑
I70.231	Atherosclerosis of native arteries of right leg with ulceration of thigh A ☑
I70.232	Atherosclerosis of native arteries of right leg with ulceration of calf A ☑
I70.233	Atherosclerosis of native arteries of right leg with ulceration of ankle A ☑
I70.234	Atherosclerosis of native arteries of right leg with ulceration of heel and midfoot A ☑
I70.261	Atherosclerosis of native arteries of extremities with gangrene, right leg A ☑
I70.461	Atherosclerosis of autologous vein bypass graft(s) of the extremities with gangrene, right leg A ☑
I70.511	Atherosclerosis of nonautologous biological bypass graft(s) of the extremities with intermittent claudication, right leg A ☑
I70.521	Atherosclerosis of nonautologous biological bypass graft(s) of the extremities with rest pain, right leg A ☑
I70.531	Atherosclerosis of nonautologous biological bypass graft(s) of the right leg with ulceration of thigh A ☑
I70.561	Atherosclerosis of nonautologous biological bypass graft(s) of the extremities with gangrene, right leg A ☑
I70.611	Atherosclerosis of nonbiological bypass graft(s) of the extremities with intermittent claudication, right leg A ☑
I70.621	Atherosclerosis of nonbiological bypass graft(s) of the extremities with rest pain, right leg A ☑
I70.631	Atherosclerosis of nonbiological bypass graft(s) of the right leg with ulceration of thigh A ☑
I70.661	Atherosclerosis of nonbiological bypass graft(s) of the extremities with gangrene, right leg A ☑
I70.92	Chronic total occlusion of artery of the extremities A
I75.021	Atheroembolism of right lower extremity ☑
I76	Septic arterial embolism
I77.1	Stricture of artery
I77.2	Rupture of artery
I77.5	Necrosis of artery

AMA: 35566 2021,Dec

Relative Value Units/Medicare Edits

Non-Facility RVU	Work	PE	MP	Total
35566	32.35	8.21	8.04	48.6
Facility RVU	**Work**	**PE**	**MP**	**Total**
35566	32.35	8.21	8.04	48.6

	FUD	Status	MUE	Modifiers				IOM Reference
35566	90	A	1(3)	51	50	62*	80	None

* with documentation

35570

35570 Bypass graft, with vein; tibial-tibial, peroneal-tibial, or tibial/peroneal trunk-tibial

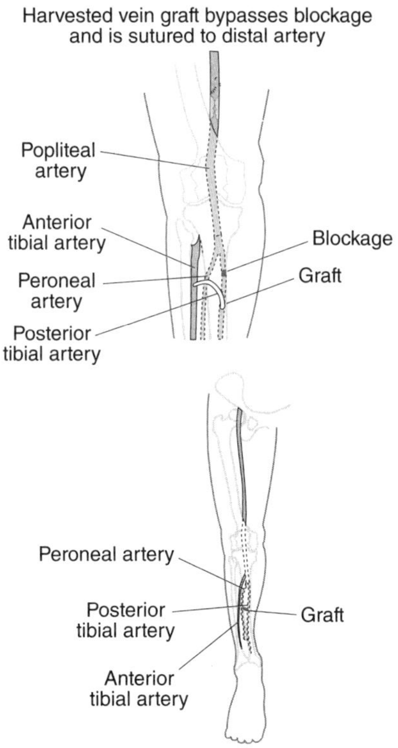

Explanation

The physician performs tibial-tibial, peroneal-tibial, or tibioperoneal trunk-tibial bypass graft. Through incisions in the skin of the leg overlying the affected tibial, peroneal, or tibioperoneal trunk artery, the physician isolates and dissects a section of arteries from adjacent critical structures. The physician creates a bypass around the affected artery using a harvested vein and one of two methods of repair. Once vessel clamps have been affixed above and below the defect, the artery may be cut through above the damaged area and sutured to one end of a harvested vein, which is sutured to the targeted tibial artery. In the second method, the ends of the harvested vein are sutured to the side of the bypassed artery and tibial vessel wall, resulting in a bypass of the damaged area. When the clamps are removed, the section of vein forms a new path through which blood can bypass the blocked area. The blocked or damaged portion of artery is left in place and not removed. After the graft is complete, the skin incisions are repaired with layered closures.

Coding Tips

Establishing both inflow and outflow by any method is included. That portion of the operative arteriogram performed by the surgeon is also included. Angioscopy performed during therapeutic intervention should be reported in addition to the code for the primary procedure, see 35400. Harvesting of the saphenous vein graft is included in the description of the work for 35570 and should not be reported as a separate procedure. For harvesting of a femoropopliteal vein segment, use 35572 in addition to the bypass procedure. If a composite (combination of vein and synthetic graft) is used, report 35681 in addition to the code for the primary procedure. Report 35700 in addition to 35570 for reoperation more than one month after the original operation. Do not report 35570 with 35256 or 35286.

ICD-10-CM Diagnostic Codes

I70.92	Chronic total occlusion of artery of the extremities 🅰
I73.89	Other specified peripheral vascular diseases
I74.3	Embolism and thrombosis of arteries of the lower extremities
I75.021	Atheroembolism of right lower extremity ☑
I75.022	Atheroembolism of left lower extremity ☑
I75.023	Atheroembolism of bilateral lower extremities ☑
I76	Septic arterial embolism
I77.1	Stricture of artery
I77.2	Rupture of artery
I77.5	Necrosis of artery
I77.89	Other specified disorders of arteries and arterioles
I79.8	Other disorders of arteries, arterioles and capillaries in diseases classified elsewhere
S85.141A	Laceration of anterior tibial artery, right leg, initial encounter ☑
S85.142A	Laceration of anterior tibial artery, left leg, initial encounter ☑
S85.151A	Other specified injury of anterior tibial artery, right leg, initial encounter ☑
S85.152A	Other specified injury of anterior tibial artery, left leg, initial encounter ☑
S85.171A	Laceration of posterior tibial artery, right leg, initial encounter ☑
S85.172A	Laceration of posterior tibial artery, left leg, initial encounter ☑
S85.181A	Other specified injury of posterior tibial artery, right leg, initial encounter ☑
S85.182A	Other specified injury of posterior tibial artery, left leg, initial encounter ☑
S85.211A	Laceration of peroneal artery, right leg, initial encounter ☑
S85.212A	Laceration of peroneal artery, left leg, initial encounter ☑
S85.291A	Other specified injury of peroneal artery, right leg, initial encounter ☑
S85.292A	Other specified injury of peroneal artery, left leg, initial encounter ☑
S85.811A	Laceration of other blood vessels at lower leg level, right leg, initial encounter ☑
S85.812A	Laceration of other blood vessels at lower leg level, left leg, initial encounter ☑
S85.891A	Other specified injury of other blood vessels at lower leg level, right leg, initial encounter ☑
S85.892A	Other specified injury of other blood vessels at lower leg level, left leg, initial encounter ☑

AMA: **35570** 2021,Dec

Relative Value Units/Medicare Edits

Non-Facility RVU	Work	PE	MP	Total
35570	29.15	6.75	7.28	43.18
Facility RVU	**Work**	**PE**	**MP**	**Total**
35570	29.15	6.75	7.28	43.18

	FUD	Status	MUE	Modifiers				IOM Reference
35570	90	A	1(3)	51	50	62*	80	None

* with documentation

35571

35571 Bypass graft, with vein; popliteal-tibial, -peroneal artery or other distal vessels

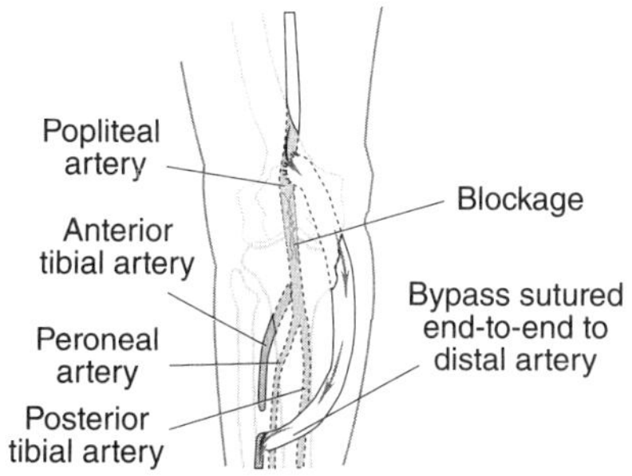

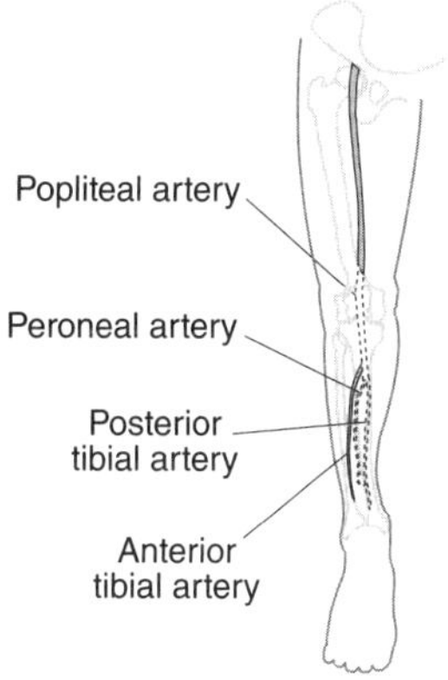

Explanation

Through incisions in the skin of the leg overlying the popliteal arteries, the physician isolates and dissects a section of arteries from adjacent critical structures. The physician creates a bypass around the artery, using a harvested vein and one of two methods of repair. Once vessel clamps have been affixed above and below the defect, the popliteal artery may be cut through above the damaged area and sutured to one end of a harvested vein, which is sutured to the tibial, peroneal, or other distal artery. In the second method, the ends of the harvested vein are sutured into the side of the popliteal and the tibial or peroneal arterial wall resulting in a bypass of the damaged area. When the clamps are removed, the section of vein forms a new path through which blood can easily bypass the blocked area. After the graft is complete, the incisions are repaired with layered closures.

Coding Tips

Establishing both inflow and outflow by any method is included. That portion of the operative arteriogram performed by the surgeon is also included. Angioscopy performed during therapeutic intervention should be reported in addition to the code for the primary procedure, see 35400. Harvesting of the saphenous vein graft is included in the description of the work for 35571 and should not be reported as a separate procedure. To report harvesting of an upper extremity vein, use 35500 in addition to the bypass procedure. For harvesting of a femoropopliteal vein segment, use 35572 in addition to the bypass procedure. If a composite (combination of vein and synthetic graft) is used, report 35681 in addition to the code for the primary procedure. To report the harvesting and construction of an autogenous composite graft of two segments from two distant locations, report 35682 in addition to the bypass procedure. For autogenous composite of three or more segments from distant sites, see 35683. Report 35700 in addition to 35571 for reoperation more than one month after the original operation. If synthetic graft material is used, see 35671.

ICD-10-CM Diagnostic Codes

I70.92	Chronic total occlusion of artery of the extremities 🅰
I73.89	Other specified peripheral vascular diseases
I74.3	Embolism and thrombosis of arteries of the lower extremities
I75.021	Atheroembolism of right lower extremity ☑
I76	Septic arterial embolism
I77.89	Other specified disorders of arteries and arterioles
I79.8	Other disorders of arteries, arterioles and capillaries in diseases classified elsewhere
S85.011A	Laceration of popliteal artery, right leg, initial encounter ☑
S85.012A	Laceration of popliteal artery, left leg, initial encounter ☑
S85.091A	Other specified injury of popliteal artery, right leg, initial encounter ☑
S85.141A	Laceration of anterior tibial artery, right leg, initial encounter ☑
S85.142A	Laceration of anterior tibial artery, left leg, initial encounter ☑
S85.151A	Other specified injury of anterior tibial artery, right leg, initial encounter ☑
S85.171A	Laceration of posterior tibial artery, right leg, initial encounter ☑
S85.172A	Laceration of posterior tibial artery, left leg, initial encounter ☑
S85.181A	Other specified injury of posterior tibial artery, right leg, initial encounter ☑
S85.211A	Laceration of peroneal artery, right leg, initial encounter ☑
S85.212A	Laceration of peroneal artery, left leg, initial encounter ☑
S85.291A	Other specified injury of peroneal artery, right leg, initial encounter ☑
S85.811A	Laceration of other blood vessels at lower leg level, right leg, initial encounter ☑
S85.812A	Laceration of other blood vessels at lower leg level, left leg, initial encounter ☑
S85.891A	Other specified injury of other blood vessels at lower leg level, right leg, initial encounter ☑

AMA: **35571** 2021,Dec

Relative Value Units/Medicare Edits

Non-Facility RVU	Work	PE	MP	Total
35571	25.52	6.87	6.34	38.73
Facility RVU	**Work**	**PE**	**MP**	**Total**
35571	25.52	6.87	6.34	38.73

	FUD	Status	MUE	Modifiers				IOM Reference
35571	90	A	1(3)	51	50	62*	80	None

* with documentation

35572

+ **35572** Harvest of femoropopliteal vein, 1 segment, for vascular reconstruction procedure (eg, aortic, vena caval, coronary, peripheral artery) (List separately in addition to code for primary procedure)

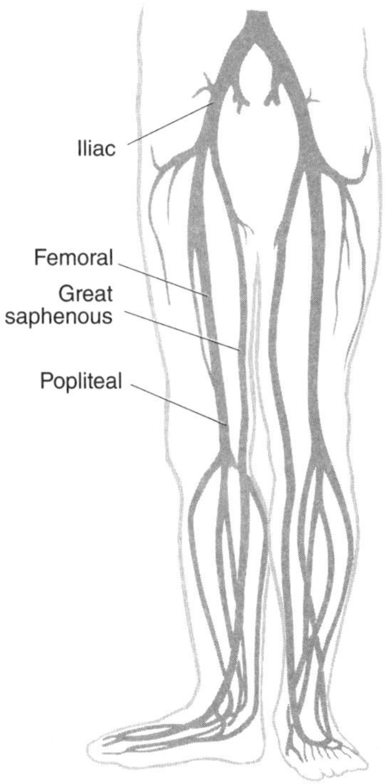

A single segment of femoropopliteal vein is harvested for a vascular reconstruction

Explanation

The physician harvests one segment of the femoropopliteal vein for a vascular reconstructive procedure. The leg is prepared circumferentially to make the leg accessible and provide optimal access. A single incision or multiple incisions can be made to harvest the vein. The vein is first located through an approximately 10 cm incision and dissected. The skin is cut over the course of the vein. If multiple incisions are made, the index finger is used to continue dissection along the anterior surface of the vein, with the incisions made about 2 to 4 cm from the last incision and the physician's finger underneath, or an external vein stripper is used with incisions made where the stripper meets resistance again. Branches of the vein are ligated. Dissection can begin at the proximal or distal end. The length of vein needed is estimated based on its intended purpose and the desired length is mobilized and divided at both ends. The vein is placed in a prepared solution of blood and saline at room temperature and prepared with diluted blood placed to flush the vein. A vascular device is applied, the vein is gently distended, and uncontrolled branches are closed. The vein is returned to the solution until used.

Coding Tips

Code 35572 should be reported twice when performed bilaterally. Do not report with modifier 50 per CPT guidelines. Medicare may still require the use of modifier 50. Report 35572 in addition to 33510–33516, 33517–33523, 33533–33536, 34502, 34520, 35001, 35002, 35011–35022, 35102, 35103, 35121–35152, 35231–35256, 35501–35587, and 35879–35907. For endoscopic vein harvest, see 33508.

ICD-10-CM Diagnostic Codes

This/these CPT code(s) are add-on code(s). See the primary procedure code that this code is performed with for your ICD-10-CM code selections. Diagnostic code(s) would be the same as the actual procedure performed.

AMA: 35572 2021,Dec

Relative Value Units/Medicare Edits

Non-Facility RVU	Work	PE	MP	Total
35572	6.81	1.53	1.67	10.01
Facility RVU	**Work**	**PE**	**MP**	**Total**
35572	6.81	1.53	1.67	10.01

	FUD	Status	MUE	Modifiers				IOM Reference
35572	N/A	A	2(3)	N/A	N/A	N/A	80	None

* with documentation

Terms To Know

anterior. Situated in the front area or toward the belly surface of the body; an anatomical reference point used to show the position and relationship of one body structure to another.

dissection. Separating by cutting tissue or body structures apart.

distal. *1)* Located farther away from a specified reference point or the trunk. *2)* Pertaining to the area farthest from the center of the body or the point of origin.

harvest. Removal of cells or tissue from their native site to be used as a graft or transplant to another part of the donor's body or placed into another person.

incision. Act of cutting into tissue or an organ.

ligate. To tie off a blood vessel or duct with a suture or a soft, thin wire (ligature wire).

proximal. Located closest to a specified reference point, usually the midline or trunk.

reconstruction. Recreating, restoring, or rebuilding a body part or organ.

vein. Vessel through which oxygen-depleted blood passes back to the heart.

35583

35583 In-situ vein bypass; femoral-popliteal

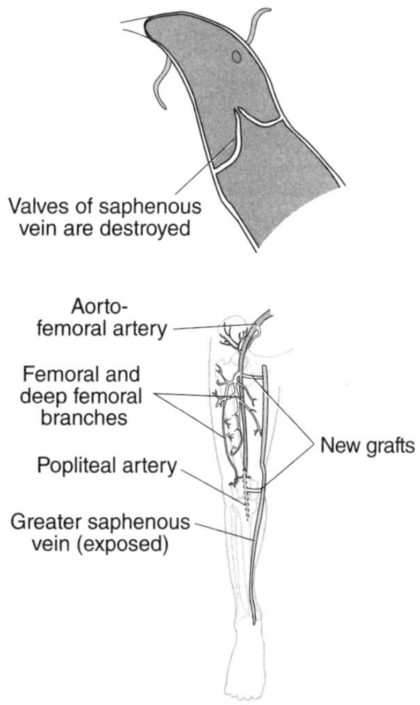

Saphenous vein is attached to femoral (at top) and popliteal arteries, converting it into a de facto artery

Explanation

Through an incision in the skin of the leg overlying the greater saphenous vein, the physician isolates and dissects the greater saphenous vein from adjacent critical structures from the upper thigh to the level of the knee. Vessel clamps are affixed above and below the site of the anastomosis to the femoral and popliteal arteries. All side branches of the saphenous vein are tied off. The vessel's valves are destroyed. The upper end of the saphenous vein is divided and sutured into the femoral artery either end-to-end or end-to-side. The lower end is divided and sutured into the popliteal artery either end-to-end or end-to-side. The clamps are removed, and blood flows backward toward the feet, as if the vein were an artery. When the procedure is complete, the skin incision is repaired with a layered closure.

Coding Tips

Establishing both inflow and outflow by any method is included. That portion of the operative arteriogram performed by the surgeon is also included. Angioscopy performed during therapeutic intervention should be reported in addition to the code for the primary procedure; see 35400. Harvesting of the saphenous vein graft is included in the description of the work for 35583 and should not be reported as a separate procedure. For harvesting of a femoropopliteal vein segment, use 35572 in addition to the bypass procedure. To report harvesting of an upper extremity vein, use 35500 in addition to the bypass procedure. Report 35700 in addition to 35583 for reoperation more than one month after the original operation. Aortobifemoral bypass using synthetic conduit and femoral-popliteal bypass with vein conduit in-situ should be reported with 35646 and 35583. Aorto(uni)femoral bypass with synthetic conduit and femoral popliteal bypass with vein conduit in-situ should be reported with 35647 and 35583. Aortofemoral bypass using vein conduit and femoral-popliteal bypass with vein conduit in-situ should be reported with 35539 and 35583.

ICD-10-CM Diagnostic Codes

I70.211 Atherosclerosis of native arteries of extremities with intermittent claudication, right leg A ✓
I70.221 Atherosclerosis of native arteries of extremities with rest pain, right leg A ✓
I70.231 Atherosclerosis of native arteries of right leg with ulceration of thigh A ✓
I70.232 Atherosclerosis of native arteries of right leg with ulceration of calf A ✓
I70.233 Atherosclerosis of native arteries of right leg with ulceration of ankle A ✓
I70.234 Atherosclerosis of native arteries of right leg with ulceration of heel and midfoot A ✓
I70.261 Atherosclerosis of native arteries of extremities with gangrene, right leg A ✓
I70.411 Atherosclerosis of autologous vein bypass graft(s) of the extremities with intermittent claudication, right leg A ✓
I70.421 Atherosclerosis of autologous vein bypass graft(s) of the extremities with rest pain, right leg A ✓
I70.431 Atherosclerosis of autologous vein bypass graft(s) of the right leg with ulceration of thigh A ✓
I70.432 Atherosclerosis of autologous vein bypass graft(s) of the right leg with ulceration of calf A ✓
I70.433 Atherosclerosis of autologous vein bypass graft(s) of the right leg with ulceration of ankle A ✓
I70.434 Atherosclerosis of autologous vein bypass graft(s) of the right leg with ulceration of heel and midfoot A ✓
I70.461 Atherosclerosis of autologous vein bypass graft(s) of the extremities with gangrene, right leg A ✓
I70.511 Atherosclerosis of nonautologous biological bypass graft(s) of the extremities with intermittent claudication, right leg A ✓
I70.521 Atherosclerosis of nonautologous biological bypass graft(s) of the extremities with rest pain, right leg A ✓
I70.531 Atherosclerosis of nonautologous biological bypass graft(s) of the right leg with ulceration of thigh A ✓
I70.532 Atherosclerosis of nonautologous biological bypass graft(s) of the right leg with ulceration of calf A ✓
I70.533 Atherosclerosis of nonautologous biological bypass graft(s) of the right leg with ulceration of ankle A ✓
I70.534 Atherosclerosis of nonautologous biological bypass graft(s) of the right leg with ulceration of heel and midfoot A ✓
I70.561 Atherosclerosis of nonautologous biological bypass graft(s) of the extremities with gangrene, right leg A ✓
I70.611 Atherosclerosis of nonbiological bypass graft(s) of the extremities with intermittent claudication, right leg A ✓
I70.621 Atherosclerosis of nonbiological bypass graft(s) of the extremities with rest pain, right leg A ✓
I70.631 Atherosclerosis of nonbiological bypass graft(s) of the right leg with ulceration of thigh A ✓
I70.632 Atherosclerosis of nonbiological bypass graft(s) of the right leg with ulceration of calf A ✓
I70.633 Atherosclerosis of nonbiological bypass graft(s) of the right leg with ulceration of ankle A ✓
I70.634 Atherosclerosis of nonbiological bypass graft(s) of the right leg with ulceration of heel and midfoot A ✓
I70.635 Atherosclerosis of nonbiological bypass graft(s) of the right leg with ulceration of other part of foot A ✓
I70.638 Atherosclerosis of nonbiological bypass graft(s) of the right leg with ulceration of other part of lower leg A ✓
I70.661 Atherosclerosis of nonbiological bypass graft(s) of the extremities with gangrene, right leg A ✓
I70.691 Other atherosclerosis of nonbiological bypass graft(s) of the extremities, right leg A ✓
I70.711 Atherosclerosis of other type of bypass graft(s) of the extremities with intermittent claudication, right leg A ✓
I70.721 Atherosclerosis of other type of bypass graft(s) of the extremities with rest pain, right leg A ✓
I70.731 Atherosclerosis of other type of bypass graft(s) of the right leg with ulceration of thigh A ✓
I70.732 Atherosclerosis of other type of bypass graft(s) of the right leg with ulceration of calf A ✓
I70.733 Atherosclerosis of other type of bypass graft(s) of the right leg with ulceration of ankle A ✓
I70.734 Atherosclerosis of other type of bypass graft(s) of the right leg with ulceration of heel and midfoot A ✓
I70.761 Atherosclerosis of other type of bypass graft(s) of the extremities with gangrene, right leg A ✓
I70.92 Chronic total occlusion of artery of the extremities A
I72.4 Aneurysm of artery of lower extremity
I74.3 Embolism and thrombosis of arteries of the lower extremities
I75.021 Atheroembolism of right lower extremity ✓
I76 Septic arterial embolism
I77.1 Stricture of artery
I77.2 Rupture of artery
I77.5 Necrosis of artery
I80.01 Phlebitis and thrombophlebitis of superficial vessels of right lower extremity ✓
I80.11 Phlebitis and thrombophlebitis of right femoral vein ✓
I80.221 Phlebitis and thrombophlebitis of right popliteal vein ✓
I80.231 Phlebitis and thrombophlebitis of right tibial vein ✓
I82.411 Acute embolism and thrombosis of right femoral vein ✓
I82.431 Acute embolism and thrombosis of right popliteal vein ✓
I82.441 Acute embolism and thrombosis of right tibial vein ✓
I82.511 Chronic embolism and thrombosis of right femoral vein ✓
I82.531 Chronic embolism and thrombosis of right popliteal vein ✓
I82.541 Chronic embolism and thrombosis of right tibial vein ✓

AMA: 35583 2021,Dec

Relative Value Units/Medicare Edits

Non-Facility RVU	Work	PE	MP	Total
35583	27.75	7.52	6.91	42.18
Facility RVU	**Work**	**PE**	**MP**	**Total**
35583	27.75	7.52	6.91	42.18

	FUD	Status	MUE	Modifiers				IOM Reference
35583	90	A	1(2)	51	50	62*	80	None

* with documentation

35585

35585 In-situ vein bypass; femoral-anterior tibial, posterior tibial, or peroneal artery

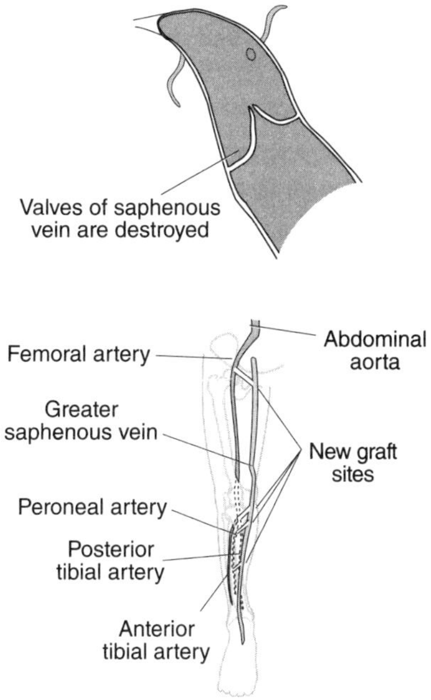

Saphenous vein is attached to femoral (at top) and one of the distal arteries at bottom, thus converting it into a de facto artery

Explanation

Through an incision in the skin of the leg overlying the greater saphenous vein, the physician isolates and dissects the greater saphenous vein from adjacent critical structures. Vessel clamps are affixed above and below the site of anastomosis in the femoral artery and the distal artery. All side branches of the Saphenous are tied off. The vessel's valves are destroyed. The upper end of the saphenous vein is divided and sutured end-to-end or end-to-side in the femoral artery above the blockage. The lower end is divided and sutured end-to-end or end-to-side to the anterior tibial, posterior tibial, or peroneal artery below the blockage. The clamps are removed, and blood flows backward toward the feet, as if the vein were an artery. When the procedure is complete, the skin incision is repaired with a layered closure.

Coding Tips

Establishing both inflow and outflow by any method is included. That portion of the operative arteriogram performed by the surgeon is also included. Angioscopy performed during therapeutic intervention should be reported in addition to the code for the primary procedure; see 35400. Harvesting of the saphenous vein graft is included in the description of the work for 35585 and should not be reported as a separate procedure. To report harvesting of an upper extremity vein, use 35500 in addition to the bypass procedure. For harvesting of a femoropopliteal vein segment, use 35572 in addition to the bypass procedure. If a composite (combination of vein and synthetic graft) is used, report 35681 in addition to the code for the primary procedure. To report the harvesting and construction of an autogenous composite graft of two segments from two distant locations, report 35682 in addition to the bypass procedure. For autogenous composite of three or more segments from distant sites, see 35683. Report 35700 in addition to 35585 for reoperation more than one month after the original operation.

ICD-10-CM Diagnostic Codes

I70.211	Atherosclerosis of native arteries of extremities with intermittent claudication, right leg A ☑
I70.221	Atherosclerosis of native arteries of extremities with rest pain, right leg A ☑
I70.231	Atherosclerosis of native arteries of right leg with ulceration of thigh A ☑
I70.232	Atherosclerosis of native arteries of right leg with ulceration of calf A ☑
I70.233	Atherosclerosis of native arteries of right leg with ulceration of ankle A ☑
I70.234	Atherosclerosis of native arteries of right leg with ulceration of heel and midfoot A ☑
I70.261	Atherosclerosis of native arteries of extremities with gangrene, right leg A ☑
I70.411	Atherosclerosis of autologous vein bypass graft(s) of the extremities with intermittent claudication, right leg A ☑
I70.421	Atherosclerosis of autologous vein bypass graft(s) of the extremities with rest pain, right leg A ☑
I70.431	Atherosclerosis of autologous vein bypass graft(s) of the right leg with ulceration of thigh A ☑
I70.432	Atherosclerosis of autologous vein bypass graft(s) of the right leg with ulceration of calf A ☑
I70.433	Atherosclerosis of autologous vein bypass graft(s) of the right leg with ulceration of ankle A ☑
I70.434	Atherosclerosis of autologous vein bypass graft(s) of the right leg with ulceration of heel and midfoot A ☑
I70.435	Atherosclerosis of autologous vein bypass graft(s) of the right leg with ulceration of other part of foot A ☑
I70.438	Atherosclerosis of autologous vein bypass graft(s) of the right leg with ulceration of other part of lower leg A ☑
I70.461	Atherosclerosis of autologous vein bypass graft(s) of the extremities with gangrene, right leg A ☑
I70.511	Atherosclerosis of nonautologous biological bypass graft(s) of the extremities with intermittent claudication, right leg A ☑
I70.521	Atherosclerosis of nonautologous biological bypass graft(s) of the extremities with rest pain, right leg A ☑
I70.531	Atherosclerosis of nonautologous biological bypass graft(s) of the right leg with ulceration of thigh A ☑
I70.532	Atherosclerosis of nonautologous biological bypass graft(s) of the right leg with ulceration of calf A ☑
I70.533	Atherosclerosis of nonautologous biological bypass graft(s) of the right leg with ulceration of ankle A ☑
I70.534	Atherosclerosis of nonautologous biological bypass graft(s) of the right leg with ulceration of heel and midfoot A ☑
I70.561	Atherosclerosis of nonautologous biological bypass graft(s) of the extremities with gangrene, right leg A ☑
I70.611	Atherosclerosis of nonbiological bypass graft(s) of the extremities with intermittent claudication, right leg A ☑
I70.621	Atherosclerosis of nonbiological bypass graft(s) of the extremities with rest pain, right leg A ☑
I70.631	Atherosclerosis of nonbiological bypass graft(s) of the right leg with ulceration of thigh A ☑
I70.632	Atherosclerosis of nonbiological bypass graft(s) of the right leg with ulceration of calf A ☑
I70.633	Atherosclerosis of nonbiological bypass graft(s) of the right leg with ulceration of ankle A ☑

 ● New ▲ Revised + Add On ★ Telemedicine [Resequenced] ☑ Laterality

I70.634	Atherosclerosis of nonbiological bypass graft(s) of the right leg with ulceration of heel and midfoot A ☑
I70.635	Atherosclerosis of nonbiological bypass graft(s) of the right leg with ulceration of other part of foot A ☑
I70.638	Atherosclerosis of nonbiological bypass graft(s) of the right leg with ulceration of other part of lower leg A ☑
I70.661	Atherosclerosis of nonbiological bypass graft(s) of the extremities with gangrene, right leg A ☑
I70.691	Other atherosclerosis of nonbiological bypass graft(s) of the extremities, right leg A ☑
I70.711	Atherosclerosis of other type of bypass graft(s) of the extremities with intermittent claudication, right leg A ☑
I70.721	Atherosclerosis of other type of bypass graft(s) of the extremities with rest pain, right leg A ☑
I70.731	Atherosclerosis of other type of bypass graft(s) of the right leg with ulceration of thigh A ☑
I70.732	Atherosclerosis of other type of bypass graft(s) of the right leg with ulceration of calf A ☑
I70.733	Atherosclerosis of other type of bypass graft(s) of the right leg with ulceration of ankle A ☑
I70.734	Atherosclerosis of other type of bypass graft(s) of the right leg with ulceration of heel and midfoot A ☑
I70.761	Atherosclerosis of other type of bypass graft(s) of the extremities with gangrene, right leg A ☑
I70.92	Chronic total occlusion of artery of the extremities A
I72.4	Aneurysm of artery of lower extremity
I74.3	Embolism and thrombosis of arteries of the lower extremities
I75.021	Atheroembolism of right lower extremity ☑
I76	Septic arterial embolism
I77.1	Stricture of artery
I77.2	Rupture of artery
I77.5	Necrosis of artery
I80.01	Phlebitis and thrombophlebitis of superficial vessels of right lower extremity ☑
I80.231	Phlebitis and thrombophlebitis of right tibial vein ☑
I82.411	Acute embolism and thrombosis of right femoral vein ☑
I82.441	Acute embolism and thrombosis of right tibial vein ☑
I82.491	Acute embolism and thrombosis of other specified deep vein of right lower extremity ☑
I82.511	Chronic embolism and thrombosis of right femoral vein ☑
I82.541	Chronic embolism and thrombosis of right tibial vein ☑

AMA: **35585** 2021,Dec

Relative Value Units/Medicare Edits

Non-Facility RVU	Work	PE	MP	Total
35585	32.35	8.43	8.06	48.84
Facility RVU	**Work**	**PE**	**MP**	**Total**
35585	32.35	8.43	8.06	48.84

	FUD	Status	MUE	Modifiers				IOM Reference
35585	90	A	2(3)	51	50	62*	80	None

* with documentation

35587

35587 In-situ vein bypass; popliteal-tibial, peroneal

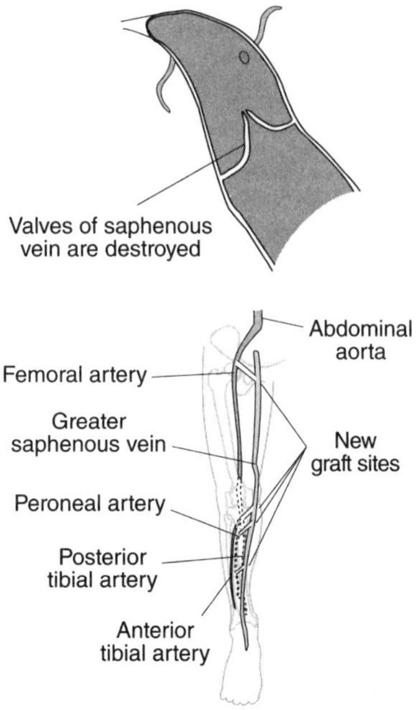

Saphenous vein is attached to the popliteal-tibial (at top) and the peroneal artery at bottom, thus converting the vein into a de facto artery

Explanation

Through an incision in the skin of the leg overlying the greater saphenous vein from the knee to the ankle, the physician isolates and dissects the greater saphenous vein from adjacent critical structures along its length. Vessel clamps are affixed above and below the site of anastomosis on the popliteal and peroneal arteries. All side branches of the saphenous vein are tied off. The vessel's valves are destroyed. The upper end of the saphenous vein is divided and sutured into the popliteal-tibial artery. The lower end is divided and sutured into the peroneal artery. The clamps are removed and blood flows backward through the vein toward the feet, as if it were an artery. When the procedure is complete, the incision is repaired with layered closure.

Coding Tips

Establishing both inflow and outflow by any method is included. That portion of the operative arteriogram performed by the surgeon is also included. Angioscopy performed during therapeutic intervention should be reported in addition to the code for the primary procedure; see 35400. Harvesting of the saphenous vein graft is included in the description of the work for 35587 and should not be reported as a separate procedure. To report harvesting of an upper extremity vein, use 35500 in addition to the bypass procedure. For harvesting of a femoropopliteal vein segment, use 35572 in addition to the bypass procedure. If a composite (combination of vein and synthetic graft) is used, report 35681 in addition to the code for the primary procedure. To report the harvesting and construction of an autogenous composite graft of two segments from two distant locations, report 35682 in addition to the bypass procedure. For autogenous composite of three or more segments from distant sites, see 35683. Report 35700 in addition to 35587 for reoperation more than one month after the original operation.

ICD-10-CM Diagnostic Codes

I70.211	Atherosclerosis of native arteries of extremities with intermittent claudication, right leg A ☑

I70.221 Atherosclerosis of native arteries of extremities with rest pain, right leg A ☑
I70.231 Atherosclerosis of native arteries of right leg with ulceration of thigh A ☑
I70.232 Atherosclerosis of native arteries of right leg with ulceration of calf A ☑
I70.233 Atherosclerosis of native arteries of right leg with ulceration of ankle A ☑
I70.234 Atherosclerosis of native arteries of right leg with ulceration of heel and midfoot A ☑
I70.235 Atherosclerosis of native arteries of right leg with ulceration of other part of foot A ☑
I70.238 Atherosclerosis of native arteries of right leg with ulceration of other part of lower leg A ☑
I70.261 Atherosclerosis of native arteries of extremities with gangrene, right leg A ☑
I70.92 Chronic total occlusion of artery of the extremities A
I74.3 Embolism and thrombosis of arteries of the lower extremities
I75.021 Atheroembolism of right lower extremity ☑
I76 Septic arterial embolism
I77.1 Stricture of artery
I77.2 Rupture of artery
I77.5 Necrosis of artery
I77.89 Other specified disorders of arteries and arterioles
I80.221 Phlebitis and thrombophlebitis of right popliteal vein ☑
I80.231 Phlebitis and thrombophlebitis of right tibial vein ☑
I80.291 Phlebitis and thrombophlebitis of other deep vessels of right lower extremity ☑
I82.531 Chronic embolism and thrombosis of right popliteal vein ☑
I82.541 Chronic embolism and thrombosis of right tibial vein ☑
I82.591 Chronic embolism and thrombosis of other specified deep vein of right lower extremity ☑

AMA: **35587** 2021,Dec

Relative Value Units/Medicare Edits

Non-Facility RVU	Work	PE	MP	Total
35587	26.21	6.31	6.53	39.05
Facility RVU	**Work**	**PE**	**MP**	**Total**
35587	26.21	6.31	6.53	39.05

	FUD	Status	MUE	Modifiers				IOM Reference
35587	90	A	1(3)	51	50	62*	80	None

* with documentation

35600

35600 Harvest of upper extremity artery, 1 segment, for coronary artery bypass procedure, open

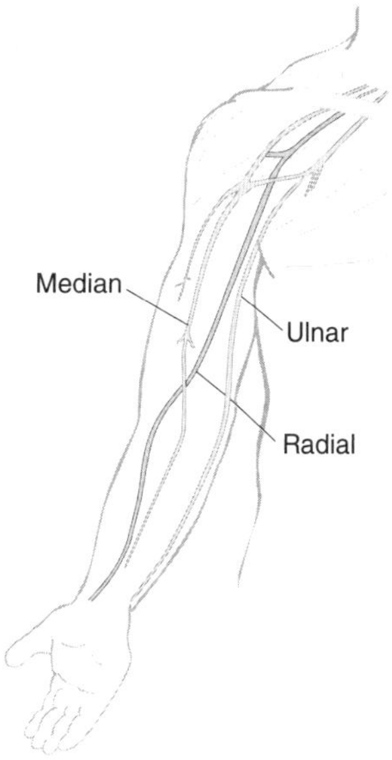

An upper extremity artery or segment is harvested for a coronary artery bypass procedure

Explanation

The physician harvests an artery from an upper extremity (arm) to use for a planned bypass procedure on a coronary artery using an open approach. An incision is made over the site on the arm. Tissue is dissected to the artery. The portion of the artery to be removed is released from the surrounding structures and is tied off above and below the portion of artery to be removed. The artery is removed and the wound closed with layered sutures. The portion of artery removed is prepared for use in the bypass graft.

Coding Tips

This is a unilateral procedure. If performed bilaterally, some payers require that the service be reported twice with modifier 50 appended to the second code while others require identification of the service only once with modifier 50 appended. Check with individual payers. Modifier 50 identifies a procedure performed identically on the opposite side of the body (mirror image). As exempt from modifier 51, 35600 has not been designated in CPT as an add-on service/procedure. However, codes identified as exempt from modifier 51 are not subject to multiple procedure rules. No reimbursement reduction or modifier 51 is applied. For endoscopic harvest of an upper extremity artery for coronary artery bypass, see 33509. Report 35600 in addition to 33533–33536.

ICD-10-CM Diagnostic Codes

I20.0 Unstable angina
I20.1 Angina pectoris with documented spasm
I20.81 Angina pectoris with coronary microvascular dysfunction
I21.01 ST elevation (STEMI) myocardial infarction involving left main coronary artery
I21.02 ST elevation (STEMI) myocardial infarction involving left anterior descending coronary artery
I21.09 ST elevation (STEMI) myocardial infarction involving other coronary artery of anterior wall

I21.11	ST elevation (STEMI) myocardial infarction involving right coronary artery
I21.19	ST elevation (STEMI) myocardial infarction involving other coronary artery of inferior wall
I21.21	ST elevation (STEMI) myocardial infarction involving left circumflex coronary artery
I21.29	ST elevation (STEMI) myocardial infarction involving other sites
I21.4	Non-ST elevation (NSTEMI) myocardial infarction
I21.A1	Myocardial infarction type 2
I21.B	Myocardial infarction with coronary microvascular dysfunction
I22.0	Subsequent ST elevation (STEMI) myocardial infarction of anterior wall
I22.1	Subsequent ST elevation (STEMI) myocardial infarction of inferior wall
I22.2	Subsequent non-ST elevation (NSTEMI) myocardial infarction
I22.8	Subsequent ST elevation (STEMI) myocardial infarction of other sites
I24.0	Acute coronary thrombosis not resulting in myocardial infarction
I24.89	Other forms of acute ischemic heart disease
I25.110	Atherosclerotic heart disease of native coronary artery with unstable angina pectoris A
I25.111	Atherosclerotic heart disease of native coronary artery with angina pectoris with documented spasm A
I25.112	Atherosclerotic heart disease of native coronary artery with refractory angina pectoris A
I25.118	Atherosclerotic heart disease of native coronary artery with other forms of angina pectoris A
I25.3	Aneurysm of heart
I25.41	Coronary artery aneurysm
I25.42	Coronary artery dissection
I25.5	Ischemic cardiomyopathy
I25.6	Silent myocardial ischemia
I25.710	Atherosclerosis of autologous vein coronary artery bypass graft(s) with unstable angina pectoris A
I25.711	Atherosclerosis of autologous vein coronary artery bypass graft(s) with angina pectoris with documented spasm A
I25.712	Atherosclerosis of autologous vein coronary artery bypass graft(s) with refractory angina pectoris A
I25.720	Atherosclerosis of autologous artery coronary artery bypass graft(s) with unstable angina pectoris A
I25.721	Atherosclerosis of autologous artery coronary artery bypass graft(s) with angina pectoris with documented spasm A
I25.722	Atherosclerosis of autologous artery coronary artery bypass graft(s) with refractory angina pectoris A
I25.730	Atherosclerosis of nonautologous biological coronary artery bypass graft(s) with unstable angina pectoris A
I25.731	Atherosclerosis of nonautologous biological coronary artery bypass graft(s) with angina pectoris with documented spasm A
I25.732	Atherosclerosis of nonautologous biological coronary artery bypass graft(s) with refractory angina pectoris A
I25.750	Atherosclerosis of native coronary artery of transplanted heart with unstable angina
I25.751	Atherosclerosis of native coronary artery of transplanted heart with angina pectoris with documented spasm
I25.752	Atherosclerosis of native coronary artery of transplanted heart with refractory angina pectoris A
I25.760	Atherosclerosis of bypass graft of coronary artery of transplanted heart with unstable angina A
I25.761	Atherosclerosis of bypass graft of coronary artery of transplanted heart with angina pectoris with documented spasm A
I25.762	Atherosclerosis of bypass graft of coronary artery of transplanted heart with refractory angina pectoris A
I25.790	Atherosclerosis of other coronary artery bypass graft(s) with unstable angina pectoris A
I25.791	Atherosclerosis of other coronary artery bypass graft(s) with angina pectoris with documented spasm A
I25.810	Atherosclerosis of coronary artery bypass graft(s) without angina pectoris A
I25.811	Atherosclerosis of native coronary artery of transplanted heart without angina pectoris
I25.812	Atherosclerosis of bypass graft of coronary artery of transplanted heart without angina pectoris A
I25.82	Chronic total occlusion of coronary artery
I25.83	Coronary atherosclerosis due to lipid rich plaque A
I25.84	Coronary atherosclerosis due to calcified coronary lesion
I50.1	Left ventricular failure, unspecified
I50.21	Acute systolic (congestive) heart failure
I50.22	Chronic systolic (congestive) heart failure
I50.23	Acute on chronic systolic (congestive) heart failure
I50.31	Acute diastolic (congestive) heart failure
I50.32	Chronic diastolic (congestive) heart failure
I50.33	Acute on chronic diastolic (congestive) heart failure
I50.41	Acute combined systolic (congestive) and diastolic (congestive) heart failure
I50.42	Chronic combined systolic (congestive) and diastolic (congestive) heart failure
I50.43	Acute on chronic combined systolic (congestive) and diastolic (congestive) heart failure
I50.811	Acute right heart failure
I50.812	Chronic right heart failure
I50.813	Acute on chronic right heart failure
I50.814	Right heart failure due to left heart failure
I50.82	Biventricular heart failure
I50.83	High output heart failure
I50.84	End stage heart failure
Q24.5	Malformation of coronary vessels
Q26.2	Total anomalous pulmonary venous connection

AMA: 35600 2021,Dec

Relative Value Units/Medicare Edits

Non-Facility RVU	Work	PE	MP	Total
35600	3.59	0.99	0.86	5.44
Facility RVU	**Work**	**PE**	**MP**	**Total**
35600	3.59	0.99	0.86	5.44

	FUD	Status	MUE	Modifiers				IOM Reference
35600	N/A	A	2(3)	N/A	N/A	62*	80	None

* with documentation

35601

35601 Bypass graft, with other than vein; common carotid-ipsilateral internal carotid

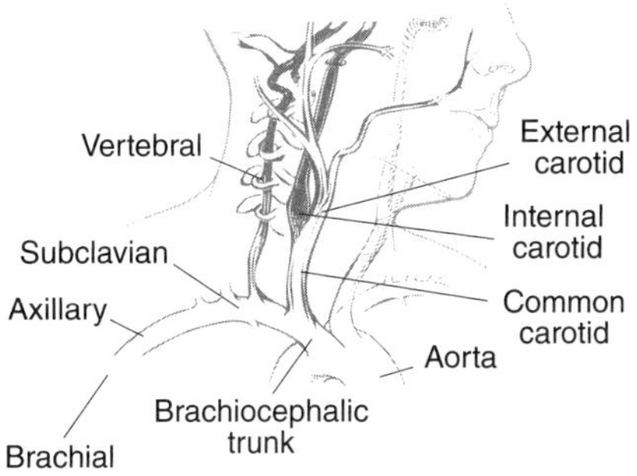

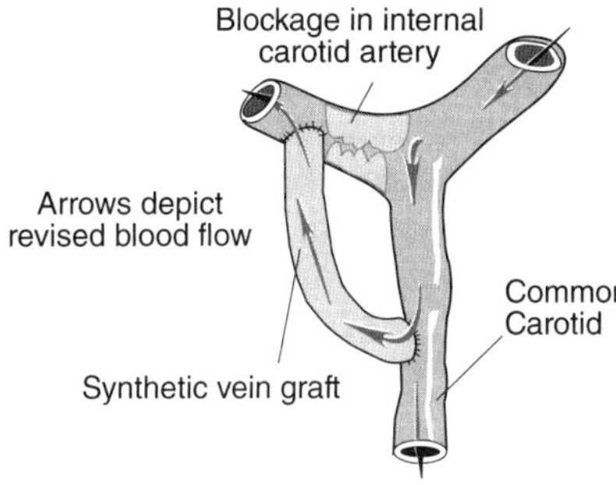

A portion of blocked internal carotid artery is bypassed

Explanation

Through an incision in the skin of the neck in front of the sternocleidomastoid muscle, the physician isolates and dissects the common carotid and internal carotid arteries, separating them from adjacent critical structures. The physician creates a bypass around the section of common carotid artery that is damaged or blocked, using a synthetic vein graft and one of two methods of repair involving the internal carotid artery on the same side of the neck. After vessel clamps have been affixed above and below the damaged area, the common carotid artery may be cut through below the damaged area and sutured to one end of the synthetic vein (end-to-end), which is sutured to the internal carotid artery beyond the affected area. In the second method, the ends of the synthetic vein are sutured into the side of the common carotid arterial wall and the internal carotid arterial wall (end-to-side). Either method results in a bypass of the damaged area. When the clamps are removed, the section of synthetic graft forms a new path through which blood can easily bypass the blocked area. The damaged or blocked carotid artery is not removed. After the graft is complete, the skin incision is repaired with layered closure.

Coding Tips

Establishing both inflow and outflow by any method is included. That portion of the operative arteriogram performed by the surgeon is also included. Angioscopy performed during therapeutic intervention should be reported in addition to the code for the primary procedure, see 35400. If a composite (combination of vein and synthetic graft) is used, report 35681 in addition to the code for the primary procedure. For open transcervical common carotid-common carotid bypass performed in addition to endovascular repair of the descending thoracic aorta, see 33891. For transposition and/or reimplantation of arteries, see 35691–35695.

ICD-10-CM Diagnostic Codes

G45.1	Carotid artery syndrome (hemispheric)
G45.8	Other transient cerebral ischemic attacks and related syndromes
G45.9	Transient cerebral ischemic attack, unspecified
I63.031	Cerebral infarction due to thrombosis of right carotid artery ☑
I63.032	Cerebral infarction due to thrombosis of left carotid artery ☑
I63.131	Cerebral infarction due to embolism of right carotid artery ☑
I63.132	Cerebral infarction due to embolism of left carotid artery ☑
I63.231	Cerebral infarction due to unspecified occlusion or stenosis of right carotid arteries ☑
I63.232	Cerebral infarction due to unspecified occlusion or stenosis of left carotid arteries ☑
I63.81	Other cerebral infarction due to occlusion or stenosis of small artery
I63.89	Other cerebral infarction
I65.21	Occlusion and stenosis of right carotid artery ☑
I65.22	Occlusion and stenosis of left carotid artery ☑
I65.23	Occlusion and stenosis of bilateral carotid arteries ☑
I67.81	Acute cerebrovascular insufficiency
I67.82	Cerebral ischemia
I67.850	Cerebral autosomal dominant arteriopathy with subcortical infarcts and leukoencephalopathy
I67.858	Other hereditary cerebrovascular disease
I67.89	Other cerebrovascular disease
I77.1	Stricture of artery
I77.2	Rupture of artery
I77.89	Other specified disorders of arteries and arterioles
S15.011A	Minor laceration of right carotid artery, initial encounter ☑
S15.012A	Minor laceration of left carotid artery, initial encounter ☑
S15.021A	Major laceration of right carotid artery, initial encounter ☑
S15.022A	Major laceration of left carotid artery, initial encounter ☑
S15.091A	Other specified injury of right carotid artery, initial encounter ☑
S15.092A	Other specified injury of left carotid artery, initial encounter ☑

Relative Value Units/Medicare Edits

Non-Facility RVU	Work	PE	MP	Total
35601	27.09	7.16	6.75	41.0
Facility RVU	**Work**	**PE**	**MP**	**Total**
35601	27.09	7.16	6.75	41.0

	FUD	Status	MUE	Modifiers				IOM Reference
35601	90	A	1(3)	51	50	62*	80	None

* with documentation

35606

35606 Bypass graft, with other than vein; carotid-subclavian

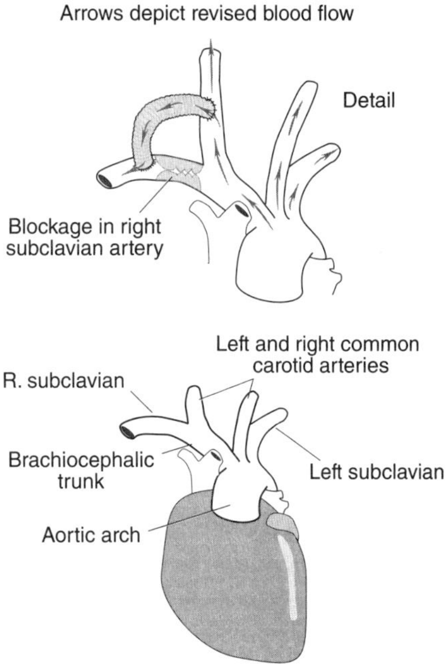

Synthetic material grafted from healthy left subclavian artery to right subclavian artery distal (beyond) to area of blockage or damage

Explanation

Through an incision in the skin at the side of the neck, the physician isolates and dissects the subclavian and carotid arteries, separating them from adjacent critical structures. To create a bypass around a section of subclavian artery that is damaged or blocked, the physician uses a synthetic vein and one of two methods of repair. After vessel clamps have been affixed above and below the damaged area, the graft is sewn to the side of the carotid artery and sewn to the side of the subclavian artery beyond the affected area (end-to-side) or sewn to the cut end of the subclavian artery after dividing it beyond the affected area (end-to-end). The damaged or blocked portion of the subclavian artery is not removed. When the clamps are removed in either case, the section of synthetic graft vein forms a new path through which blood can easily bypass the blocked area. After the graft is complete, the skin incision is repaired with a layered closure.

Coding Tips

Establishing both inflow and outflow by any method is included. That portion of the operative arteriogram performed by the surgeon is also included. Angioscopy performed during therapeutic intervention should be reported in addition to the code for the primary procedure; see 35400. If a composite (combination of vein and synthetic graft) is used, report 35681 in addition to the code for the primary procedure. For transposition and/or reimplantation of arteries, see 35691–35695. Do not report 35606 for open subclavian to carotid artery transposition performed with endovascular thoracic aneurysm repair; use 33889.

ICD-10-CM Diagnostic Codes

G45.2	Multiple and bilateral precerebral artery syndromes
G45.8	Other transient cerebral ischemic attacks and related syndromes
G45.9	Transient cerebral ischemic attack, unspecified
I63.09	Cerebral infarction due to thrombosis of other precerebral artery
I63.19	Cerebral infarction due to embolism of other precerebral artery
I63.29	Cerebral infarction due to unspecified occlusion or stenosis of other precerebral arteries
I63.81	Other cerebral infarction due to occlusion or stenosis of small artery
I63.89	Other cerebral infarction
I65.8	Occlusion and stenosis of other precerebral arteries
I67.81	Acute cerebrovascular insufficiency
I67.850	Cerebral autosomal dominant arteriopathy with subcortical infarcts and leukoencephalopathy
I67.858	Other hereditary cerebrovascular disease
I70.92	Chronic total occlusion of artery of the extremities [A]
I74.2	Embolism and thrombosis of arteries of the upper extremities
I74.8	Embolism and thrombosis of other arteries
I75.011	Atheroembolism of right upper extremity ☑
I75.012	Atheroembolism of left upper extremity ☑
I75.013	Atheroembolism of bilateral upper extremities ☑
I77.1	Stricture of artery
I77.2	Rupture of artery
I77.5	Necrosis of artery
I77.89	Other specified disorders of arteries and arterioles
S15.8XXA	Injury of other specified blood vessels at neck level, initial encounter
S25.111A	Minor laceration of right innominate or subclavian artery, initial encounter ☑
S25.112A	Minor laceration of left innominate or subclavian artery, initial encounter ☑
S25.121A	Major laceration of right innominate or subclavian artery, initial encounter ☑
S25.122A	Major laceration of left innominate or subclavian artery, initial encounter ☑
S25.191A	Other specified injury of right innominate or subclavian artery, initial encounter ☑
S25.192A	Other specified injury of left innominate or subclavian artery, initial encounter ☑

Relative Value Units/Medicare Edits

Non-Facility RVU	Work	PE	MP	Total
35606	22.46	6.42	5.57	34.45
Facility RVU	**Work**	**PE**	**MP**	**Total**
35606	22.46	6.42	5.57	34.45

	FUD	Status	MUE	Modifiers				IOM Reference
35606	90	A	1(3)	51	50	62*	80	None

* with documentation

Arteries and Veins

35612

35612 Bypass graft, with other than vein; subclavian-subclavian

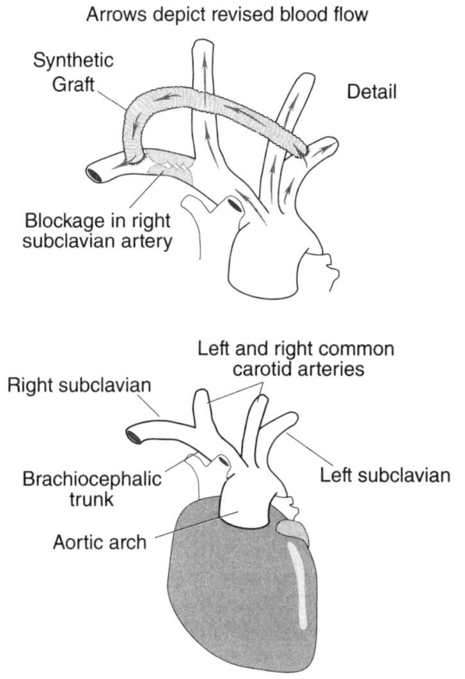

Synthetic material grafted from healthy left subclavian artery to right subclavian artery distal (beyond) to area of blockage or damage

Explanation

Through incisions in the skin at the base of the neck, the physician isolates and dissects the subclavian arteries, separating them from adjacent critical structures. The physician creates a bypass around a section of subclavian artery that is damaged or blocked, using a synthetic vein and one of two methods of repair. Once vessel clamps have been affixed above and below the defect, the ends of the synthetic vein graft are sutured into the sides of the walls of the two subclavian arteries, resulting in a bypass of the damaged area. In the second method, the subclavian artery may be cut through beyond the damaged area and sutured to one end of a synthetic vein, which is sutured to the subclavian artery on the opposite side of the neck. In either case, the blocked or damaged portion of the artery is not removed. When the clamps are removed, the section of synthetic vein graft forms a new path through which blood can easily bypass the blocked area. After the graft is complete, the skin incisions are repaired with a layered closure.

Coding Tips

Establishing both inflow and outflow by any method is included. That portion of the operative arteriogram performed by the surgeon is also included. Angioscopy performed during therapeutic intervention should be reported in addition to the code for the primary procedure, see 35400. For transposition and/or reimplantation of arteries, see 35691–35695.

ICD-10-CM Diagnostic Codes

G45.9	Transient cerebral ischemic attack, unspecified
I63.09	Cerebral infarction due to thrombosis of other precerebral artery
I63.19	Cerebral infarction due to embolism of other precerebral artery
I63.29	Cerebral infarction due to unspecified occlusion or stenosis of other precerebral arteries
I63.81	Other cerebral infarction due to occlusion or stenosis of small artery
I63.89	Other cerebral infarction
I65.8	Occlusion and stenosis of other precerebral arteries
I67.81	Acute cerebrovascular insufficiency
I67.850	Cerebral autosomal dominant arteriopathy with subcortical infarcts and leukoencephalopathy
I67.858	Other hereditary cerebrovascular disease
I70.92	Chronic total occlusion of artery of the extremities A
I74.2	Embolism and thrombosis of arteries of the upper extremities
I74.8	Embolism and thrombosis of other arteries
I75.011	Atheroembolism of right upper extremity ☑
I75.012	Atheroembolism of left upper extremity ☑
I75.013	Atheroembolism of bilateral upper extremities ☑
I77.1	Stricture of artery
I77.2	Rupture of artery
I77.5	Necrosis of artery
I77.89	Other specified disorders of arteries and arterioles
S15.8XXA	Injury of other specified blood vessels at neck level, initial encounter
S25.111A	Minor laceration of right innominate or subclavian artery, initial encounter ☑
S25.112A	Minor laceration of left innominate or subclavian artery, initial encounter ☑
S25.121A	Major laceration of right innominate or subclavian artery, initial encounter ☑
S25.122A	Major laceration of left innominate or subclavian artery, initial encounter ☑
S25.191A	Other specified injury of right innominate or subclavian artery, initial encounter ☑
S25.192A	Other specified injury of left innominate or subclavian artery, initial encounter ☑

Relative Value Units/Medicare Edits

Non-Facility RVU	Work	PE	MP	Total
35612	20.35	5.26	5.07	30.68
Facility RVU	**Work**	**PE**	**MP**	**Total**
35612	20.35	5.26	5.07	30.68

	FUD	Status	MUE	Modifiers				IOM Reference
35612	90	A	1(3)	51	50	62*	80	None

* with documentation

Terms To Know

angioscopy. Visualization of capillary blood vessels with a microscope, or the inside of a blood vessel with a fiberoptic-equipped catheter.

atherosclerosis. Buildup of yellowish plaques composed of cholesterol and lipoid material within the arteries.

infarction. Area of necrosis in tissue, due to ischemia from lack of circulation, usually from a thrombus or an embolus.

35616

35616 Bypass graft, with other than vein; subclavian-axillary

Arrows indicate direction of revised blood flow

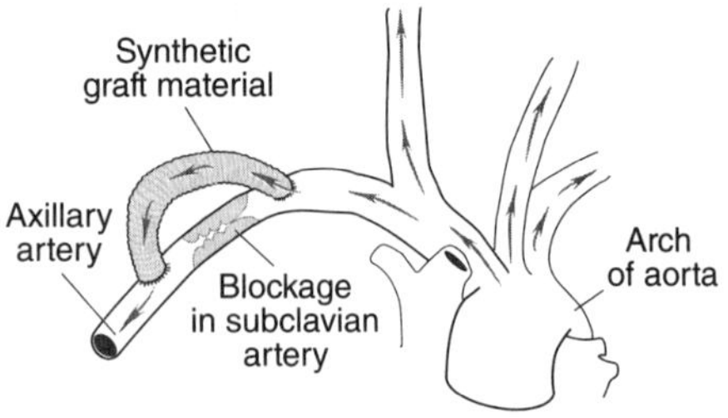

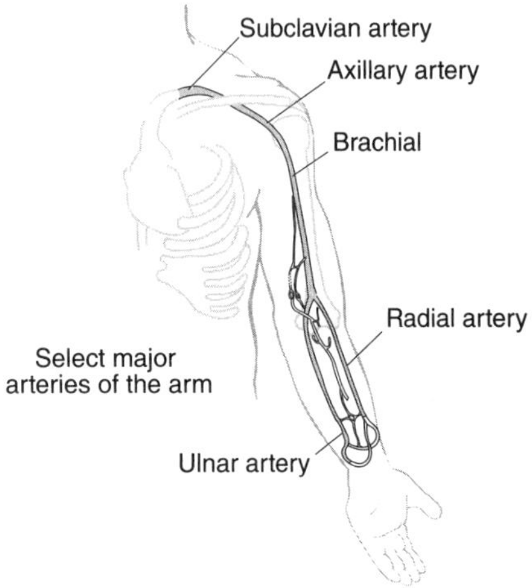

Explanation

Through an incision in the skin at the base of the neck and axilla, the physician isolates and dissects the subclavian and axillary arteries, separating them from adjacent critical structures. The physician creates a bypass around a section of subclavian artery that is damaged or blocked, using a synthetic vein and one of two methods of repair. Once vessel clamps have been affixed above and below the defect, the ends of the synthetic vein are sutured into the sides of the subclavian and axillary arterial walls resulting in a bypass of the damaged area (end-to-side). In the second method, the subclavian artery may be cut through before the damaged area and sutured to one end of a synthetic vein, which is then sutured to the axillary artery (end-to-end). The blocked or damaged portion of the subclavian artery is not removed. When the clamps are removed, the section of synthetic vein graft forms a new path through which blood can easily bypass the blocked area. After the graft is complete, the skin incisions are repaired with a layered closure.

Coding Tips

Establishing both inflow and outflow by any method is included. That portion of the operative arteriogram performed by the surgeon is also included. Angioscopy performed during therapeutic intervention should be reported in addition to the code for the primary procedure; see 35400. For transposition and/or reimplantation of arteries, see 35691–35695.

ICD-10-CM Diagnostic Codes

G45.8	Other transient cerebral ischemic attacks and related syndromes
G45.9	Transient cerebral ischemic attack, unspecified
I63.09	Cerebral infarction due to thrombosis of other precerebral artery
I63.19	Cerebral infarction due to embolism of other precerebral artery
I63.29	Cerebral infarction due to unspecified occlusion or stenosis of other precerebral arteries
I63.81	Other cerebral infarction due to occlusion or stenosis of small artery
I63.89	Other cerebral infarction
I65.8	Occlusion and stenosis of other precerebral arteries
I67.850	Cerebral autosomal dominant arteriopathy with subcortical infarcts and leukoencephalopathy
I67.858	Other hereditary cerebrovascular disease
I70.92	Chronic total occlusion of artery of the extremities [A]
I72.1	Aneurysm of artery of upper extremity
I74.2	Embolism and thrombosis of arteries of the upper extremities
I74.8	Embolism and thrombosis of other arteries
I75.011	Atheroembolism of right upper extremity ☑
I75.012	Atheroembolism of left upper extremity ☑
I75.013	Atheroembolism of bilateral upper extremities ☑
I77.1	Stricture of artery
I77.2	Rupture of artery
I77.5	Necrosis of artery
I77.89	Other specified disorders of arteries and arterioles
S15.8XXA	Injury of other specified blood vessels at neck level, initial encounter
S25.111A	Minor laceration of right innominate or subclavian artery, initial encounter ☑
S25.112A	Minor laceration of left innominate or subclavian artery, initial encounter ☑
S25.121A	Major laceration of right innominate or subclavian artery, initial encounter ☑
S25.122A	Major laceration of left innominate or subclavian artery, initial encounter ☑
S25.191A	Other specified injury of right innominate or subclavian artery, initial encounter ☑
S25.192A	Other specified injury of left innominate or subclavian artery, initial encounter ☑

Relative Value Units/Medicare Edits

Non-Facility RVU	Work	PE	MP	Total
35616	21.82	5.03	5.43	32.28
Facility RVU	**Work**	**PE**	**MP**	**Total**
35616	21.82	5.03	5.43	32.28

	FUD	Status	MUE	Modifiers				IOM Reference
35616	90	A	1(3)	51	50	62*	80	None

* with documentation

Terms To Know

angioscopy. Visualization of capillary blood vessels with a microscope, or the inside of a blood vessel with a fiberoptic-equipped catheter.

arteriogram. Radiograph of arteries.

atherosclerosis. Buildup of yellowish plaques composed of cholesterol and lipoid material within the arteries.

35621

35621 Bypass graft, with other than vein; axillary-femoral

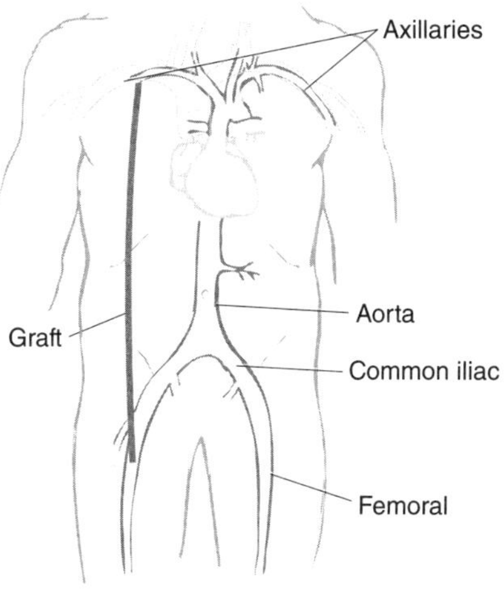

A graft other than vein is used in a bypass procedure from the axillary artery to the femoral artery

Explanation

The physician makes incisions in the skin of the axilla and upper thigh. The artery is isolated and dissected from adjacent critical structures. The physician creates a bypass around a section of artery that is damaged or blocked using a synthetic vein and one of two repair methods. Once vessel clamps have been affixed above and below the areas of anastomosis, the synthetic vein is sutured to an incision in the side of the axillary artery and passed through a subcutaneous tunnel on the side of the body and to the upper thigh. The synthetic vein is sutured to the femoral artery (common, deep, or superficial) in an end-to-side or end-to-end fashion. The blocked or damaged portion of the artery is not removed. When the clamps are removed, the section of synthetic vein graft forms a new path through which blood can easily bypass the blocked area. After the graft is complete, the skin incisions are repaired with layered closures.

Coding Tips

Establishing both inflow and outflow by any method is included. That portion of the operative arteriogram performed by the surgeon is also included. Angioscopy performed during therapeutic intervention should be reported in addition to the code for the primary procedure; see 35400.

ICD-10-CM Diagnostic Codes

A52.02 Syphilitic aortitis
I70.0 Atherosclerosis of aorta A
I70.8 Atherosclerosis of other arteries A
I70.92 Chronic total occlusion of artery of the extremities A
I71.010 Dissection of ascending aorta
I71.011 Dissection of aortic arch
I71.012 Dissection of descending thoracic aorta
I71.02 Dissection of abdominal aorta
I71.03 Dissection of thoracoabdominal aorta
I74.01 Saddle embolus of abdominal aorta
I74.09 Other arterial embolism and thrombosis of abdominal aorta
I74.19 Embolism and thrombosis of other parts of aorta
I74.5 Embolism and thrombosis of iliac artery
I76 Septic arterial embolism
I77.1 Stricture of artery
I77.3 Arterial fibromuscular dysplasia
I77.5 Necrosis of artery
I77.72 Dissection of iliac artery
K55.1 Chronic vascular disorders of intestine
K55.8 Other vascular disorders of intestine
Q25.21 Interruption of aortic arch
Q25.41 Absence and aplasia of aorta
Q25.46 Tortuous aortic arch
Q25.47 Right aortic arch
Q25.48 Anomalous origin of subclavian artery
Q25.8 Other congenital malformations of other great arteries
S25.01XA Minor laceration of thoracic aorta, initial encounter
S25.02XA Major laceration of thoracic aorta, initial encounter
S25.09XA Other specified injury of thoracic aorta, initial encounter
S25.811A Laceration of other blood vessels of thorax, right side, initial encounter ☑
S25.812A Laceration of other blood vessels of thorax, left side, initial encounter ☑
S25.891A Other specified injury of other blood vessels of thorax, right side, initial encounter ☑
S25.892A Other specified injury of other blood vessels of thorax, left side, initial encounter ☑
S35.01XA Minor laceration of abdominal aorta, initial encounter
S35.02XA Major laceration of abdominal aorta, initial encounter
S35.09XA Other injury of abdominal aorta, initial encounter
S35.511A Injury of right iliac artery, initial encounter ☑
S35.512A Injury of left iliac artery, initial encounter ☑
S35.59XA Injury of other iliac blood vessels, initial encounter
S35.8X1A Laceration of other blood vessels at abdomen, lower back and pelvis level, initial encounter
S35.8X8A Other specified injury of other blood vessels at abdomen, lower back and pelvis level, initial encounter

Relative Value Units/Medicare Edits

Non-Facility RVU	Work	PE	MP	Total
35621	21.03	5.87	5.2	32.1
Facility RVU	Work	PE	MP	Total
35621	21.03	5.87	5.2	32.1

	FUD	Status	MUE	Modifiers				IOM Reference
35621	90	A	1(3)	51	50	62*	80	None

* with documentation

Terms To Know

embolism. Obstruction of a blood vessel resulting from a clot or foreign substance.

thrombosis. Condition arising from the presence or formation of blood clots within a blood vessel that may cause vascular obstruction and insufficient oxygenation.

35623

35623 Bypass graft, with other than vein; axillary-popliteal or -tibial

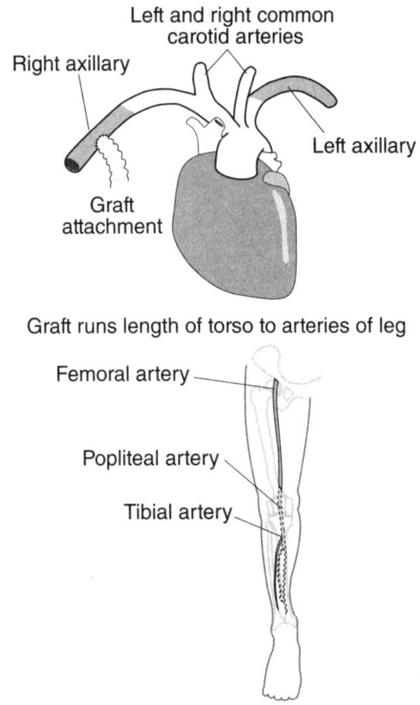

A bypass graft other than vein (synthetic) is surgically attached from the axillary artery to the popliteal or tibial artery of the leg

Explanation

The physician makes incisions in the skin of the axilla and behind the knee or in the lower leg. The artery is isolated and dissected from adjacent critical structures. The physician creates a bypass around a section of artery that is damaged or blocked using a synthetic vein and one of two repair methods. Once vessel clamps have been affixed above and below the areas of anastomosis, the synthetic vein is sutured to an incision in the side of the axillary artery and passed through a subcutaneous tunnel on the side of the body and behind the knee or upper thigh. The synthetic vein is sutured to the popliteal or tibial artery in an end-to-side or end-to-end fashion. The blocked or damaged portion of the artery is not removed. When the clamps are removed, the section of synthetic vein graft forms a new path through which blood can easily bypass the blocked area. After the graft is complete, the skin incisions are repaired with layered closures.

Coding Tips

Establishing both inflow and outflow by any method is included. That portion of the operative arteriogram performed by the surgeon is also included. Angioscopy performed during therapeutic intervention should be reported in addition to the code for the primary procedure; see 35400.

ICD-10-CM Diagnostic Codes

A52.02 Syphilitic aortitis
I70.0 Atherosclerosis of aorta [A]
I70.8 Atherosclerosis of other arteries [A]
I70.92 Chronic total occlusion of artery of the extremities [A]
I71.010 Dissection of ascending aorta
I71.011 Dissection of aortic arch
I71.012 Dissection of descending thoracic aorta
I71.02 Dissection of abdominal aorta
I71.03 Dissection of thoracoabdominal aorta
I74.01 Saddle embolus of abdominal aorta
I74.09 Other arterial embolism and thrombosis of abdominal aorta
I74.19 Embolism and thrombosis of other parts of aorta
I74.5 Embolism and thrombosis of iliac artery
I76 Septic arterial embolism
I77.1 Stricture of artery
I77.3 Arterial fibromuscular dysplasia
I77.5 Necrosis of artery
I77.72 Dissection of iliac artery
I77.89 Other specified disorders of arteries and arterioles
K55.8 Other vascular disorders of intestine
Q25.41 Absence and aplasia of aorta
Q25.46 Tortuous aortic arch
Q25.47 Right aortic arch
Q25.48 Anomalous origin of subclavian artery
Q25.8 Other congenital malformations of other great arteries
S25.01XA Minor laceration of thoracic aorta, initial encounter
S25.02XA Major laceration of thoracic aorta, initial encounter
S25.09XA Other specified injury of thoracic aorta, initial encounter
S25.811A Laceration of other blood vessels of thorax, right side, initial encounter ☑
S25.812A Laceration of other blood vessels of thorax, left side, initial encounter ☑
S25.891A Other specified injury of other blood vessels of thorax, right side, initial encounter ☑
S25.892A Other specified injury of other blood vessels of thorax, left side, initial encounter ☑
S35.01XA Minor laceration of abdominal aorta, initial encounter
S35.02XA Major laceration of abdominal aorta, initial encounter
S35.09XA Other injury of abdominal aorta, initial encounter
S35.511A Injury of right iliac artery, initial encounter ☑
S35.512A Injury of left iliac artery, initial encounter ☑
S35.59XA Injury of other iliac blood vessels, initial encounter
S35.8X1A Laceration of other blood vessels at abdomen, lower back and pelvis level, initial encounter
S35.8X8A Other specified injury of other blood vessels at abdomen, lower back and pelvis level, initial encounter

Relative Value Units/Medicare Edits

Non-Facility RVU	Work	PE	MP	Total
35623	25.92	6.14	6.45	38.51
Facility RVU	**Work**	**PE**	**MP**	**Total**
35623	25.92	6.14	6.45	38.51

	FUD	Status	MUE	Modifiers				IOM Reference
35623	90	A	1(3)	51	50	62*	80	None

* with documentation

35626

35626 Bypass graft, with other than vein; aortosubclavian, aortoinnominate, or aortocarotid

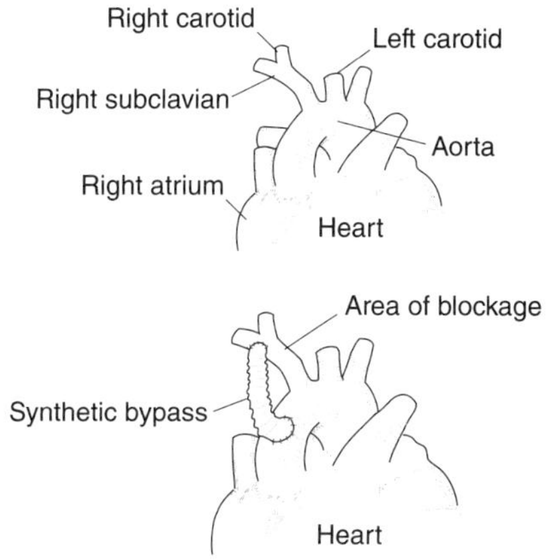

A graft other than vein (e.g., synthetic) is employed to bypass a blockage in the great arteries

Explanation

The physician exposes the aorta by median sternotomy and exposes the aortocarotid, aortoinnominate, or aortosubclavian artery, extending this incision in the appropriate direction. The physician clamps the middle part of the right anterolateral aspect of the anterior ascending aorta with a J clamp. The physician makes a 2 cm to 3 cm longitudinal incision in the clamped portion of the aorta and sews the arterial or synthetic graft to the aortic incision. The physician clamps the graft and releases the aortic clamp to assess the anastomosis for leaks. The physician clamps the distal end of the diseased artery. The physician makes a longitudinal incision in the diseased artery, distal to the blockage, and sews the graft to the arterial incision. The physician may also use graft material to enlarge the arterial lumen (patch graft). The physician removes the clamp from the graft. The physician may perform arteriography or use a Doppler probe to establish patency of the graft. The physician closes the sternotomy or thoracotomy, leaving a chest tube in place.

Coding Tips

Establishing both inflow and outflow by any method is included. That portion of the operative arteriogram performed by the surgeon is also included. Angioscopy performed during therapeutic intervention should be reported in addition to the code for the primary procedure, see 35400. For transposition and/or reimplantation of arteries, see 35691-35695.

ICD-10-CM Diagnostic Codes

G45.1 Carotid artery syndrome (hemispheric)
G45.2 Multiple and bilateral precerebral artery syndromes
G45.8 Other transient cerebral ischemic attacks and related syndromes
I63.031 Cerebral infarction due to thrombosis of right carotid artery ☑
I63.032 Cerebral infarction due to thrombosis of left carotid artery ☑
I63.131 Cerebral infarction due to embolism of right carotid artery ☑
I63.132 Cerebral infarction due to embolism of left carotid artery ☑
I63.19 Cerebral infarction due to embolism of other precerebral artery
I63.81 Other cerebral infarction due to occlusion or stenosis of small artery
I65.21 Occlusion and stenosis of right carotid artery ☑
I65.22 Occlusion and stenosis of left carotid artery ☑
I65.8 Occlusion and stenosis of other precerebral arteries
I67.81 Acute cerebrovascular insufficiency
I67.82 Cerebral ischemia
I67.850 Cerebral autosomal dominant arteriopathy with subcortical infarcts and leukoencephalopathy
I67.858 Other hereditary cerebrovascular disease
I67.89 Other cerebrovascular disease
I70.92 Chronic total occlusion of artery of the extremities [A]
I74.2 Embolism and thrombosis of arteries of the upper extremities
I75.011 Atheroembolism of right upper extremity ☑
I75.012 Atheroembolism of left upper extremity ☑
I77.1 Stricture of artery
I77.2 Rupture of artery
I77.71 Dissection of carotid artery
I77.76 Dissection of artery of upper extremity
I77.77 Dissection of artery of lower extremity
I77.79 Dissection of other specified artery
I77.89 Other specified disorders of arteries and arterioles
Q28.1 Other malformations of precerebral vessels
Q28.8 Other specified congenital malformations of circulatory system
S15.011A Minor laceration of right carotid artery, initial encounter ☑
S15.012A Minor laceration of left carotid artery, initial encounter ☑
S15.021A Major laceration of right carotid artery, initial encounter ☑
S15.022A Major laceration of left carotid artery, initial encounter ☑
S15.091A Other specified injury of right carotid artery, initial encounter ☑
S15.092A Other specified injury of left carotid artery, initial encounter ☑
S15.8XXA Injury of other specified blood vessels at neck level, initial encounter
S25.111A Minor laceration of right innominate or subclavian artery, initial encounter ☑
S25.112A Minor laceration of left innominate or subclavian artery, initial encounter ☑
S25.121A Major laceration of right innominate or subclavian artery, initial encounter ☑
S25.122A Major laceration of left innominate or subclavian artery, initial encounter ☑
S25.191A Other specified injury of right innominate or subclavian artery, initial encounter ☑
S25.192A Other specified injury of left innominate or subclavian artery, initial encounter ☑

Relative Value Units/Medicare Edits

Non-Facility RVU	Work	PE	MP	Total
35626	29.14	10.3	7.09	46.53
Facility RVU	**Work**	**PE**	**MP**	**Total**
35626	29.14	10.3	7.09	46.53

	FUD	Status	MUE	Modifiers				IOM Reference
35626	90	A	3(3)	51	50	62*	80	None

* with documentation

35631

35631 Bypass graft, with other than vein; aortoceliac, aortomesenteric, aortorenal

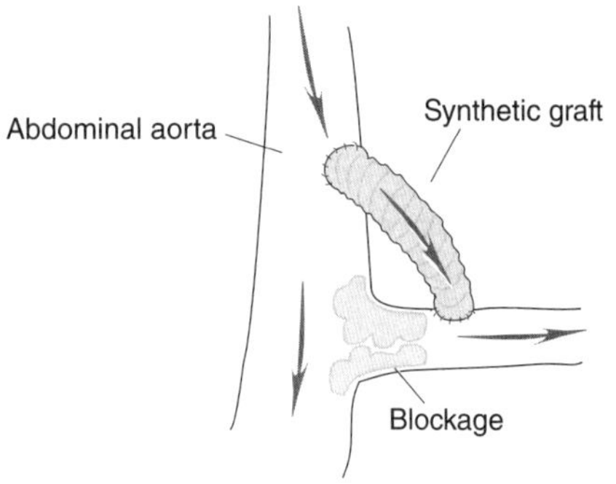

A bypass graft of material other than vein is surgically installed from the aorta to the celiac, mesenteric, or renal arteries. The graft is typically placed in an end-to-side fashion on both the aorta and the recipient vessel downstream from the blockage

Explanation

The physician exposes the involved aortomesenteric, aortoceliac, or aortorenal artery using an upper midline abdominal incision, retracting and dissecting past large and small bowel. The distal thoracic aorta is exposed, heparin is administered for anticoagulation, and the aorta is clamped both proximal and distal to the celiac axis origin. An elliptical disk of aortic wall is cut out from the anterior surface of the aorta. The involved vessel (aortomesenteric, aortoceliac, or aortorenal artery) is exposed and divided proximal to the occlusion, closing off the proximal stump with suture. A synthetic or arterial graft is sewn from the clamped aorta to the undiseased distal artery. Graft material may be utilized to enlarge the arterial lumen (patch graft). The physician may perform arteriography or use a Doppler probe to establish patency of the graft. The abdominal wound is closed, leaving drains in place.

Coding Tips

Establishing both inflow and outflow by any method is included. That portion of the operative arteriogram performed by the surgeon is also included. Angioscopy performed during therapeutic intervention should be reported in addition to the code for the primary procedure, see 35400.

ICD-10-CM Diagnostic Codes

I15.0	Renovascular hypertension
I16.0	Hypertensive urgency
I16.1	Hypertensive emergency
I70.1	Atherosclerosis of renal artery [A]
I75.81	Atheroembolism of kidney
I75.89	Atheroembolism of other site
I77.1	Stricture of artery
I77.3	Arterial fibromuscular dysplasia
I77.4	Celiac artery compression syndrome
I77.5	Necrosis of artery
I77.73	Dissection of renal artery
I77.79	Dissection of other specified artery
K55.011	Focal (segmental) acute (reversible) ischemia of small intestine
K55.012	Diffuse acute (reversible) ischemia of small intestine
K55.021	Focal (segmental) acute infarction of small intestine
K55.022	Diffuse acute infarction of small intestine
K55.031	Focal (segmental) acute (reversible) ischemia of large intestine
K55.032	Diffuse acute (reversible) ischemia of large intestine
K55.041	Focal (segmental) acute infarction of large intestine
K55.042	Diffuse acute infarction of large intestine
K55.1	Chronic vascular disorders of intestine
K55.8	Other vascular disorders of intestine
N26.2	Page kidney
N28.0	Ischemia and infarction of kidney
Q27.1	Congenital renal artery stenosis
Q27.2	Other congenital malformations of renal artery
Q27.34	Arteriovenous malformation of renal vessel
S35.212A	Major laceration of celiac artery, initial encounter
S35.218A	Other injury of celiac artery, initial encounter
S35.222A	Major laceration of superior mesenteric artery, initial encounter
S35.228A	Other injury of superior mesenteric artery, initial encounter
S35.232A	Major laceration of inferior mesenteric artery, initial encounter
S35.238A	Other injury of inferior mesenteric artery, initial encounter
S35.292A	Major laceration of branches of celiac and mesenteric artery, initial encounter
S35.298A	Other injury of branches of celiac and mesenteric artery, initial encounter
S35.411A	Laceration of right renal artery, initial encounter ☑
S35.412A	Laceration of left renal artery, initial encounter ☑
S35.491A	Other specified injury of right renal artery, initial encounter ☑
S35.492A	Other specified injury of left renal artery, initial encounter ☑
S35.8X1A	Laceration of other blood vessels at abdomen, lower back and pelvis level, initial encounter
T81.710A	Complication of mesenteric artery following a procedure, not elsewhere classified, initial encounter
T81.711A	Complication of renal artery following a procedure, not elsewhere classified, initial encounter

Relative Value Units/Medicare Edits

Non-Facility RVU	Work	PE	MP	Total
35631	36.03	9.31	8.88	54.22
Facility RVU	**Work**	**PE**	**MP**	**Total**
35631	36.03	9.31	8.88	54.22

	FUD	Status	MUE	Modifiers				IOM Reference
35631	90	A	4(3)	51	50	62*	80	None

* with documentation

35632-35634

35632 Bypass graft, with other than vein; ilio-celiac
35633 ilio-mesenteric
35634 iliorenal

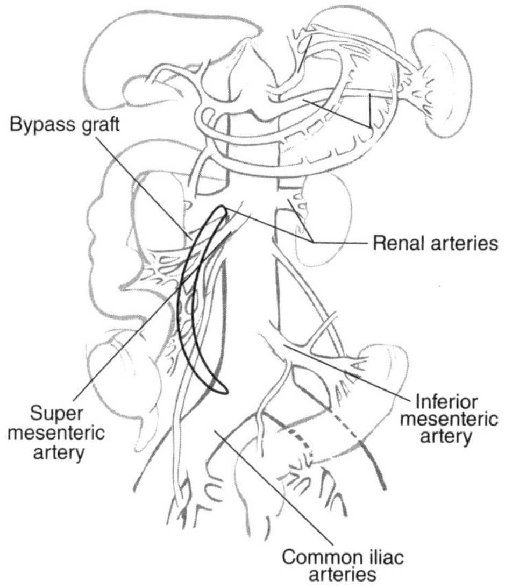

Bypass graft of a material other than vein is placed from the iliac artery to the celiac, mesenteric, or renal arteries

Explanation

The physician performs ilio-celiac (35632), ilio-mesenteric (35633), or iliorenal (35634) bypass using a synthetic graft. Through a midline abdominal incision, the physician retracts the intestines and exposes the common iliac artery and the involved vessel (celiac, mesenteric, or renal artery). The common iliac artery is clamped proximally and distally. The physician makes an oval incision on the anterolateral aspect of the common iliac artery, temporarily releases the distal clamp, and administers heparin for anticoagulation. A synthetic graft is attached to the common iliac artery at the site of the arteriotomy and sutured in place. An end-to-end anastomosis of the synthetic graft to the disease-free portion of the celiac, mesenteric, or renal artery is created. The physician may perform arteriography or Doppler to establish patency of the graft. The physician closes the abdominal wound, leaving drains in place.

Coding Tips

Do not report 35632 or 35633 with 35221, 35251, 35281, 35531, or 35631. Do not report 35634 with 35221, 35251, 35281, 35560, 35536, or 35631. Angioscopy performed during therapeutic intervention should be reported in addition to the code for the primary procedure, see 35400.

ICD-10-CM Diagnostic Codes

I15.0	Renovascular hypertension
I15.1	Hypertension secondary to other renal disorders
I70.1	Atherosclerosis of renal artery A
I70.8	Atherosclerosis of other arteries A
I74.5	Embolism and thrombosis of iliac artery
I75.81	Atheroembolism of kidney
I75.89	Atheroembolism of other site
I77.1	Stricture of artery
I77.3	Arterial fibromuscular dysplasia
I77.4	Celiac artery compression syndrome
I77.5	Necrosis of artery
I77.72	Dissection of iliac artery
I77.73	Dissection of renal artery
I77.79	Dissection of other specified artery
I77.89	Other specified disorders of arteries and arterioles
K55.011	Focal (segmental) acute (reversible) ischemia of small intestine
K55.012	Diffuse acute (reversible) ischemia of small intestine
K55.021	Focal (segmental) acute infarction of small intestine
K55.022	Diffuse acute infarction of small intestine
K55.031	Focal (segmental) acute (reversible) ischemia of large intestine
K55.032	Diffuse acute (reversible) ischemia of large intestine
K55.041	Focal (segmental) acute infarction of large intestine
K55.042	Diffuse acute infarction of large intestine
K55.1	Chronic vascular disorders of intestine
K55.8	Other vascular disorders of intestine
N26.2	Page kidney
N28.0	Ischemia and infarction of kidney
Q27.1	Congenital renal artery stenosis
S35.211A	Minor laceration of celiac artery, initial encounter
S35.212A	Major laceration of celiac artery, initial encounter
S35.218A	Other injury of celiac artery, initial encounter
S35.221A	Minor laceration of superior mesenteric artery, initial encounter
S35.222A	Major laceration of superior mesenteric artery, initial encounter
S35.228A	Other injury of superior mesenteric artery, initial encounter
S35.231A	Minor laceration of inferior mesenteric artery, initial encounter
S35.232A	Major laceration of inferior mesenteric artery, initial encounter
S35.238A	Other injury of inferior mesenteric artery, initial encounter
S35.291A	Minor laceration of branches of celiac and mesenteric artery, initial encounter
S35.292A	Major laceration of branches of celiac and mesenteric artery, initial encounter
S35.298A	Other injury of branches of celiac and mesenteric artery, initial encounter
S35.411A	Laceration of right renal artery, initial encounter ☑
S35.412A	Laceration of left renal artery, initial encounter ☑
S35.491A	Other specified injury of right renal artery, initial encounter ☑
S35.492A	Other specified injury of left renal artery, initial encounter ☑
S35.8X1A	Laceration of other blood vessels at abdomen, lower back and pelvis level, initial encounter
S35.8X8A	Other specified injury of other blood vessels at abdomen, lower back and pelvis level, initial encounter
T81.710A	Complication of mesenteric artery following a procedure, not elsewhere classified, initial encounter

Relative Value Units/Medicare Edits

Non-Facility RVU	Work	PE	MP	Total
35632	36.13	7.74	9.01	52.88
35633	39.11	9.14	9.75	58.0
35634	35.33	7.61	8.81	51.75
Facility RVU	**Work**	**PE**	**MP**	**Total**
35632	36.13	7.74	9.01	52.88
35633	39.11	9.14	9.75	58.0
35634	35.33	7.61	8.81	51.75

	FUD	Status	MUE	Modifiers				IOM Reference
35632	90	A	1(3)	51	50	62*	80	None
35633	90	A	1(3)	51	50	62*	80	
35634	90	A	1(3)	51	50	62*	80	

* with documentation

Terms To Know

bypass graft. Surgically created alternative blood vessel used to reroute blood flow around an area of obstruction or disease.

doppler. Ultrasonography used to augment two-dimensional images by registering velocity. When emitted sound waves reflect back off a moving object, the frequency of the reflected sound waves varies in relation to the speed of the moving object and may be used in many different procedures.

infarction. Area of necrosis in tissue, due to ischemia from lack of circulation, usually from a thrombus or an embolus.

ischemia. Deficiency in blood supply causing tissues to be deprived of oxygen, resulting from trauma, mechanical or functional constriction of blood vessels, or a physical obstruction.

necrosis. Death of cells or tissue within a living organ or structure.

35636

35636 Bypass graft, with other than vein; splenorenal (splenic to renal arterial anastomosis)

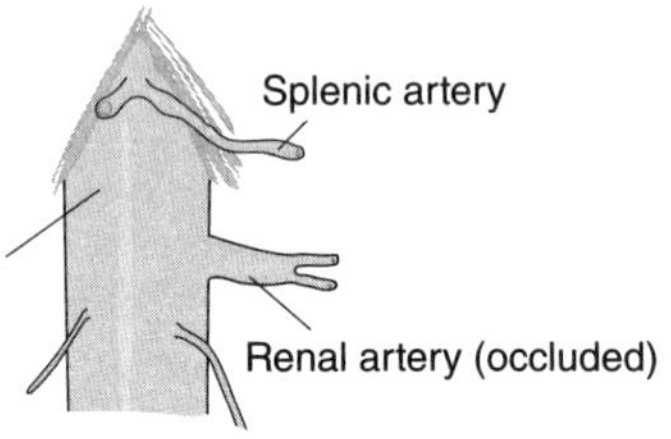

This procedure serves to bypass a diseased or occluded renal artery. The spleen remains perfused by a more distal splenic artery

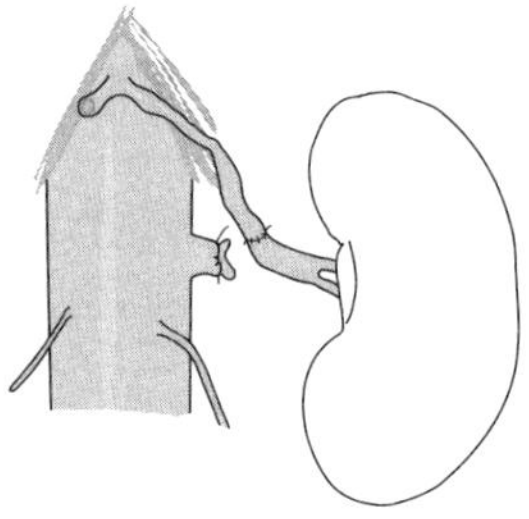

Renal artery is ligated and the splenic artery is anastomosed to remnant renal artery. This procedure is performed on the left kidney

Explanation

The physician performs a bilateral subcostal incision from the right midrectus position extending into the left flank, and dissects past bowel and pancreas to expose the splenic artery. The splenic artery is exposed by careful dissection. The left renal artery is exposed by dissecting through the posterior parietal peritoneum and partially clamped. An ellipse of renal artery is excised at its upper border. An end-to-side anastomosis of synthetic or arterial graft material from the splenic artery to the renal artery is performed. The clamps are removed and the anastomotic sites are assessed for leaks. The physician may perform Doppler studies or arteriography to establish patency of the graft. The abdominal wound is closed, leaving drains in place.

Coding Tips

Establishing both inflow and outflow by any method is included. That portion of the operative arteriogram performed by the surgeon is also included. Angioscopy performed during therapeutic intervention should be reported in addition to the code for the primary procedure; see 35400.

ICD-10-CM Diagnostic Codes

I15.0	Renovascular hypertension
I70.1	Atherosclerosis of renal artery A
I73.9	Peripheral vascular disease, unspecified
I74.8	Embolism and thrombosis of other arteries
I75.81	Atheroembolism of kidney
I76	Septic arterial embolism
I77.1	Stricture of artery
I77.3	Arterial fibromuscular dysplasia
I77.5	Necrosis of artery
I77.73	Dissection of renal artery
I77.89	Other specified disorders of arteries and arterioles

N26.2	Page kidney
N28.0	Ischemia and infarction of kidney
Q27.1	Congenital renal artery stenosis
Q27.2	Other congenital malformations of renal artery
Q27.34	Arteriovenous malformation of renal vessel
S35.411A	Laceration of right renal artery, initial encounter ☑
S35.412A	Laceration of left renal artery, initial encounter ☑
S35.491A	Other specified injury of right renal artery, initial encounter ☑
S35.492A	Other specified injury of left renal artery, initial encounter ☑
S35.8X1A	Laceration of other blood vessels at abdomen, lower back and pelvis level, initial encounter
S35.8X8A	Other specified injury of other blood vessels at abdomen, lower back and pelvis level, initial encounter

Relative Value Units/Medicare Edits

Non-Facility RVU	Work	PE	MP	Total
35636	31.75	7.04	7.91	46.7
Facility RVU	**Work**	**PE**	**MP**	**Total**
35636	31.75	7.04	7.91	46.7

	FUD	Status	MUE	Modifiers				IOM Reference
35636	90	A	1(3)	51	50	62*	80	None

* with documentation

Terms To Know

aneurysm. Circumscribed dilation or outpouching of an artery wall, often containing blood clots and connecting directly with the lumen of the artery.

angioscopy. Visualization of capillary blood vessels with a microscope, or the inside of a blood vessel with a fiberoptic-equipped catheter.

arteriogram. Radiograph of arteries.

hyperplasia. Abnormal proliferation in the number of normal cells in regular tissue arrangement.

35637-35638

35637 Bypass graft, with other than vein; aortoiliac
35638 aortobi-iliac

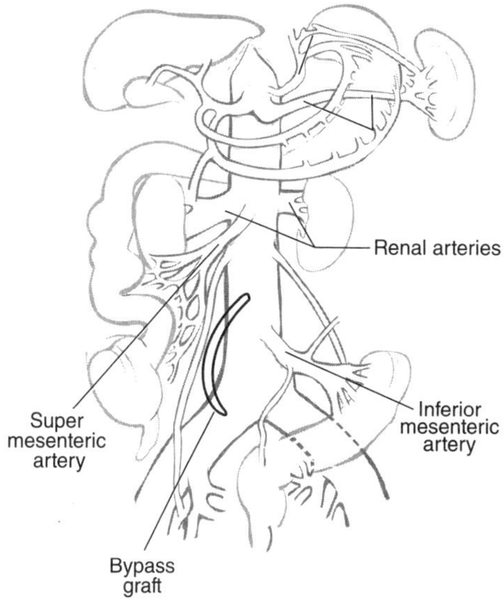

Bypass graft of a material other than vein extending from the aorta to iliac artery

Explanation

The physician makes an incision in the abdominal wall and separates the muscles to expose the internal organs, which are checked for any undetected disease. The aorta and iliac arteries are located and the obstruction is isolated by clamping the vessels. An artificial graft, commonly of polyester or polytetrafluoroethylene, is made ready. Synthetic grafts are preferred in aortoiliac bypass since they more closely match the luminal dimensions of the replaced arteries. The graft is sewn into place, with one end anastomosed to the aorta and the other end to the iliac artery. The clamps are removed, blood flows freely, and the anastomotic sites are assessed for leaks. The physician may perform Doppler studies or arteriography to establish patency of the graft. The abdominal wound is closed in layers. Report 35637 for an artificial bypass graft to a single iliac artery and 35638 when both iliac arteries are bypassed.

Coding Tips

Establishing both inflow and outflow by any method is included. That portion of the operative arteriogram performed by the surgeon is also included. Angioscopy performed during therapeutic intervention should be reported in addition to the code for the primary procedure, see 35400. Do not report 35637 with 35638 or 35646. Do not report 35638 with 35637 or 35646. For open placement of aorto-bi-iliac prosthesis following unsuccessful endovascular repair, see 34831.

ICD-10-CM Diagnostic Codes

A52.01	Syphilitic aneurysm of aorta
A52.02	Syphilitic aortitis
I70.0	Atherosclerosis of aorta A
I71.02	Dissection of abdominal aorta
I71.31	Pararenal abdominal aortic aneurysm, ruptured
I71.32	Juxtarenal abdominal aortic aneurysm, ruptured
I71.33	Infrarenal abdominal aortic aneurysm, ruptured
I71.41	Pararenal abdominal aortic aneurysm, without rupture

I71.42	Juxtarenal abdominal aortic aneurysm, without rupture
I71.43	Infrarenal abdominal aortic aneurysm, without rupture
I71.51	Supraceliac aneurysm of the thoracoabdominal aorta, ruptured
I71.52	Paravisceral aneurysm of the thoracoabdominal aorta, ruptured
I71.61	Supraceliac aneurysm of the thoracoabdominal aorta, without rupture
I71.62	Paravisceral aneurysm of the thoracoabdominal aorta, without rupture
I72.3	Aneurysm of iliac artery
I73.9	Peripheral vascular disease, unspecified
I74.01	Saddle embolus of abdominal aorta
I74.5	Embolism and thrombosis of iliac artery
I76	Septic arterial embolism
I77.1	Stricture of artery
I77.3	Arterial fibromuscular dysplasia
I77.5	Necrosis of artery
I77.72	Dissection of iliac artery
I77.811	Abdominal aortic ectasia
I77.812	Thoracoabdominal aortic ectasia
I77.89	Other specified disorders of arteries and arterioles
I79.0	Aneurysm of aorta in diseases classified elsewhere
Q25.21	Interruption of aortic arch
Q25.41	Absence and aplasia of aorta
Q25.42	Hypoplasia of aorta
Q25.43	Congenital aneurysm of aorta
Q25.44	Congenital dilation of aorta
Q25.45	Double aortic arch
Q25.46	Tortuous aortic arch
Q25.47	Right aortic arch
Q25.48	Anomalous origin of subclavian artery
S35.01XA	Minor laceration of abdominal aorta, initial encounter
S35.02XA	Major laceration of abdominal aorta, initial encounter
S35.09XA	Other injury of abdominal aorta, initial encounter
S35.511A	Injury of right iliac artery, initial encounter ☑
S35.512A	Injury of left iliac artery, initial encounter ☑
S35.59XA	Injury of other iliac blood vessels, initial encounter
S35.8X1A	Laceration of other blood vessels at abdomen, lower back and pelvis level, initial encounter
S35.8X8A	Other specified injury of other blood vessels at abdomen, lower back and pelvis level, initial encounter

Relative Value Units/Medicare Edits

Non-Facility RVU	Work	PE	MP	Total
35637	33.05	7.27	8.23	48.55
35638	33.6	8.82	8.33	50.75
Facility RVU	**Work**	**PE**	**MP**	**Total**
35637	33.05	7.27	8.23	48.55
35638	33.6	8.82	8.33	50.75

	FUD	Status	MUE	Modifiers				IOM Reference
35637	90	A	1(3)	51	N/A	62*	80	None
35638	90	A	1(3)	51	N/A	62*	80	

* with documentation

35642-35645

35642 Bypass graft, with other than vein; carotid-vertebral
35645 subclavian-vertebral

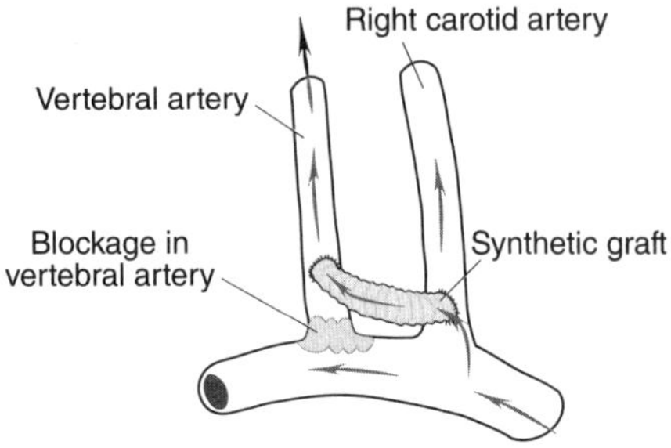

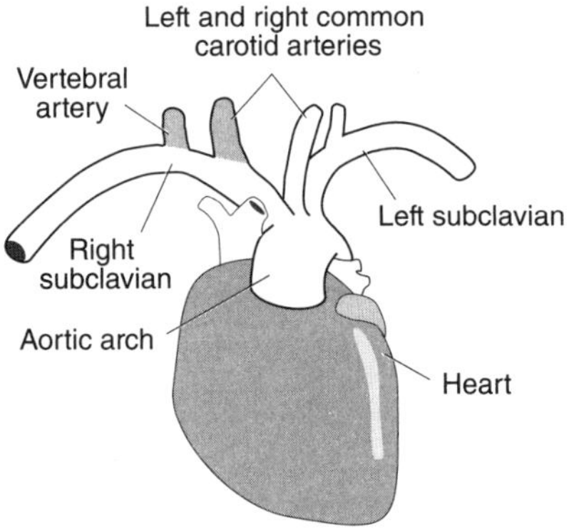

Explanation

Through an incision in the skin of the neck, the physician isolates and dissects the vertebral and carotid arteries, separating them from adjacent critical structures. The physician creates a bypass around a section of vertebral artery that is damaged or blocked, using a synthetic vein and one of two methods of repair. In 35642, after vessel clamps have been affixed above and below the damaged area, the synthetic graft is sewn to the side of the carotid artery and sewn to the side of the vertebral artery beyond the affected area (end-to-side) or sewn to the cut end of the vertebral artery after dividing it beyond the affected area (end-to-end). The damaged or blocked section of the vertebral artery is not removed. In 35645, the physician isolates and dissects the vertebral and subclavian arteries, separating them from adjacent critical structures. Once vessel clamps are affixed above and below the defect, the ends of the synthetic vein are sutured into the sides of the subclavian and vertebral arterial walls resulting in a bypass of the damaged area (end-to-side). In the second method, the vertebral artery can be cut through above the damaged area and sutured to one end of a synthetic vein (end-to-end). The remaining end is sutured to the subclavian artery. In either case, the blocked or damaged vertebral artery is not removed. For both procedures, when the clamps are removed, the section of synthetic vein graft forms a new path through which blood can easily bypass the blocked area. After the graft is complete, the skin incision is repaired with a layered closure.

Coding Tips

Establishing both inflow and outflow by any method is included. That portion of the operative arteriogram performed by the surgeon is also included. Angioscopy performed during therapeutic intervention should be reported in addition to the code for the primary procedure; see 35400. If a subclavian-vertebral bypass graft is performed with harvested vein, see 35515. If a carotid-vertebral bypass graft is performed with a harvested vein, see 35508.

ICD-10-CM Diagnostic Codes

G45.0	Vertebro-basilar artery syndrome
I63.011	Cerebral infarction due to thrombosis of right vertebral artery ☑
I63.012	Cerebral infarction due to thrombosis of left vertebral artery ☑
I63.013	Cerebral infarction due to thrombosis of bilateral vertebral arteries ☑
I63.033	Cerebral infarction due to thrombosis of bilateral carotid arteries ☑
I63.111	Cerebral infarction due to embolism of right vertebral artery ☑
I63.112	Cerebral infarction due to embolism of left vertebral artery ☑
I63.113	Cerebral infarction due to embolism of bilateral vertebral arteries ☑
I63.133	Cerebral infarction due to embolism of bilateral carotid arteries ☑
I65.01	Occlusion and stenosis of right vertebral artery ☑
I65.02	Occlusion and stenosis of left vertebral artery ☑
I65.03	Occlusion and stenosis of bilateral vertebral arteries ☑
I76	Septic arterial embolism
I77.1	Stricture of artery
I77.2	Rupture of artery
I77.74	Dissection of vertebral artery
I77.89	Other specified disorders of arteries and arterioles
S15.111A	Minor laceration of right vertebral artery, initial encounter ☑
S15.112A	Minor laceration of left vertebral artery, initial encounter ☑
S15.121A	Major laceration of right vertebral artery, initial encounter ☑
S15.122A	Major laceration of left vertebral artery, initial encounter ☑
S15.191A	Other specified injury of right vertebral artery, initial encounter ☑
S15.192A	Other specified injury of left vertebral artery, initial encounter ☑

Relative Value Units/Medicare Edits

Non-Facility RVU	Work	PE	MP	Total
35642	18.94	5.39	4.69	29.02
35645	18.43	4.79	4.58	27.8
Facility RVU	**Work**	**PE**	**MP**	**Total**
35642	18.94	5.39	4.69	29.02
35645	18.43	4.79	4.58	27.8

	FUD	Status	MUE	Modifiers				IOM Reference
35642	90	A	1(3)	51	50	62*	80	None
35645	90	A	1(3)	51	50	62*	80	

* with documentation

35646-35647

35646 Bypass graft, with other than vein; aortobifemoral
35647 aortofemoral

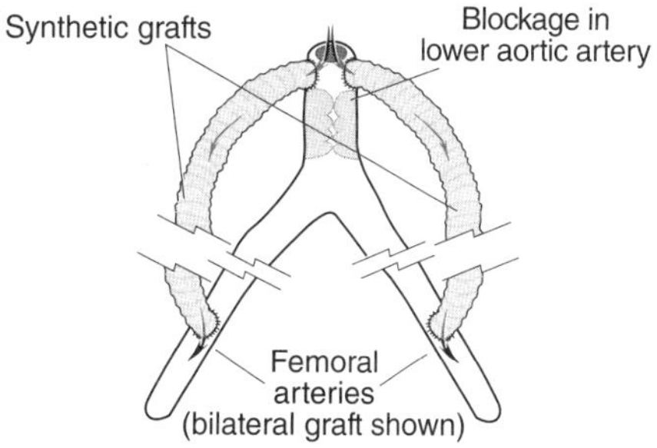

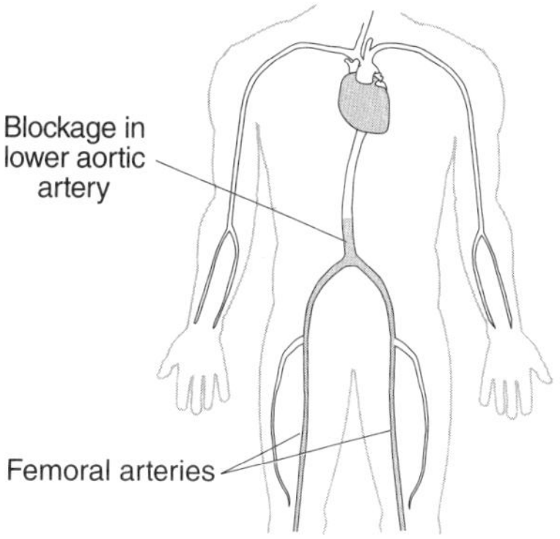

Explanation

The physician makes an incision in the skin of the abdomen over a section of damaged or blocked lower aorta. The artery is isolated and dissected. Through a separate skin incision in the upper thigh, the femoral artery is isolated and dissected from adjacent critical structures. The physician creates a bypass around the damage or blocked lower aorta using a synthetic vein. Once vessel clamps have been affixed above the defect, the lower aorta may be cut through or tied off with sutures above the damaged or blocked area and sutured to one end of the synthetic vein in an end-to-end or side-to-side fashion. The graft to one femoral artery is passed through a tunnel on the inside of the upper thigh and sutured to the femoral artery. A second synthetic vein is placed in a similar fashion to the second side. When the clamps are removed, the two grafted synthetic vein limbs form a new path through which blood can easily bypass the blocked area. The blocked or damaged portion of artery is not removed. After the graft is complete, the skin incisions are repaired with layered closure. Report 35646 when both femoral arteries are bypassed and 35647 when a single femoral artery is bypassed.

Coding Tips

Establishing inflow and outflow by any method is included. That portion of the operative arteriogram performed by the surgeon is also included. Angioscopy performed during therapeutic intervention should be reported in addition to the code for the primary procedure, see 35400. For bypass graft performed with vein graft, see 35540. When 35647 is performed with another separately identifiable procedure, the highest dollar value code is listed as the primary procedure and subsequent procedures are appended with modifier 51. For a bypass graft performed with a vein, see 35539. Do not report 35646 for open placement of aortobifemoral prosthesis following unsuccessful endovascular repair; use 34832.

Arteries and Veins

● New ▲ Revised + Add On ★ Telemedicine [Resequenced] ☑ Laterality

ICD-10-CM Diagnostic Codes

A52.01	Syphilitic aneurysm of aorta
A52.02	Syphilitic aortitis
I70.0	Atherosclerosis of aorta A
I71.02	Dissection of abdominal aorta
I71.31	Pararenal abdominal aortic aneurysm, ruptured
I71.32	Juxtarenal abdominal aortic aneurysm, ruptured
I71.33	Infrarenal abdominal aortic aneurysm, ruptured
I71.41	Pararenal abdominal aortic aneurysm, without rupture
I71.42	Juxtarenal abdominal aortic aneurysm, without rupture
I71.43	Infrarenal abdominal aortic aneurysm, without rupture
I73.89	Other specified peripheral vascular diseases
I73.9	Peripheral vascular disease, unspecified
I74.01	Saddle embolus of abdominal aorta
I74.09	Other arterial embolism and thrombosis of abdominal aorta
I74.19	Embolism and thrombosis of other parts of aorta
I74.5	Embolism and thrombosis of iliac artery
I75.89	Atheroembolism of other site
I76	Septic arterial embolism
I77.1	Stricture of artery
I77.3	Arterial fibromuscular dysplasia
I77.5	Necrosis of artery
I77.72	Dissection of iliac artery
I77.811	Abdominal aortic ectasia
I77.812	Thoracoabdominal aortic ectasia
I77.89	Other specified disorders of arteries and arterioles
I79.0	Aneurysm of aorta in diseases classified elsewhere
Q25.21	Interruption of aortic arch
Q25.29	Other atresia of aorta
Q25.41	Absence and aplasia of aorta
Q25.42	Hypoplasia of aorta
Q25.43	Congenital aneurysm of aorta
Q25.44	Congenital dilation of aorta
Q25.45	Double aortic arch
Q25.46	Tortuous aortic arch
Q25.47	Right aortic arch
Q25.48	Anomalous origin of subclavian artery
Q25.49	Other congenital malformations of aorta
S35.01XA	Minor laceration of abdominal aorta, initial encounter
S35.02XA	Major laceration of abdominal aorta, initial encounter
S35.09XA	Other injury of abdominal aorta, initial encounter
S35.8X1A	Laceration of other blood vessels at abdomen, lower back and pelvis level, initial encounter
S35.8X8A	Other specified injury of other blood vessels at abdomen, lower back and pelvis level, initial encounter

Relative Value Units/Medicare Edits

Non-Facility RVU	Work	PE	MP	Total
35646	32.98	8.73	8.17	49.88
35647	29.73	8.25	7.39	45.37
Facility RVU	**Work**	**PE**	**MP**	**Total**
35646	32.98	8.73	8.17	49.88
35647	29.73	8.25	7.39	45.37

	FUD	Status	MUE	Modifiers				IOM Reference
35646	90	A	1(3)	51	N/A	62*	80	None
35647	90	A	1(3)	51	50	62*	80	

* with documentation

Terms To Know

bypass graft. Surgically created alternative blood vessel used to reroute blood flow around an area of obstruction or disease.

embolism. Obstruction of a blood vessel resulting from a clot or foreign substance.

graft. Tissue implant from another part of the body or another person.

thrombosis. Condition arising from the presence or formation of blood clots within a blood vessel that may cause vascular obstruction and insufficient oxygenation.

35650

35650 Bypass graft, with other than vein; axillary-axillary

Arrows indicate direction of revised blood flow

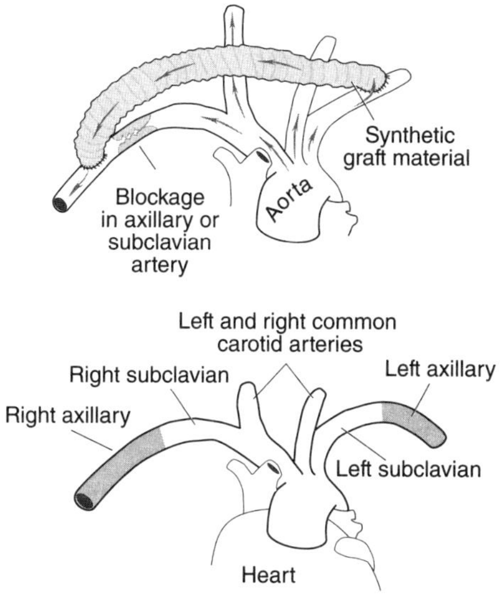

Explanation

The physician makes an incision in the skin of both axillae. The physician creates a bypass around a section of artery that is damaged or blocked, using a synthetic graft and one of two repair methods. Once vessel clamps have been affixed above and below the defect, the ends of the synthetic graft are sutured into the sides of the two axillary arterial walls, resulting in a bypass of the damaged area. In the second method, the axillary artery may be cut through beyond the damaged area and sutured to one end of a synthetic graft, which is passed across the front of the chest under the skin and sutured to the side of the contralateral axillary artery. The blocked or damaged portion of the axillary artery is not removed. When the clamps are removed, the section of synthetic vein graft forms a new path through which blood can easily bypass the blocked area. After the graft is complete, the skin incisions are repaired with layered closures.

Coding Tips

Establishing both inflow and outflow by any method is included. That portion of the operative arteriogram performed by the surgeon is also included. Angioscopy performed during therapeutic intervention should be reported in addition to the code for the primary procedure; see 35400. If a bypass graft is performed with harvested vein, see 35518.

ICD-10-CM Diagnostic Codes

G45.8	Other transient cerebral ischemic attacks and related syndromes
G45.9	Transient cerebral ischemic attack, unspecified
I63.19	Cerebral infarction due to embolism of other precerebral artery
I63.81	Other cerebral infarction due to occlusion or stenosis of small artery
I63.89	Other cerebral infarction
I67.81	Acute cerebrovascular insufficiency
I67.850	Cerebral autosomal dominant arteriopathy with subcortical infarcts and leukoencephalopathy
I67.858	Other hereditary cerebrovascular disease
I70.8	Atherosclerosis of other arteries [A]
I70.92	Chronic total occlusion of artery of the extremities [A]
I73.89	Other specified peripheral vascular diseases
I73.9	Peripheral vascular disease, unspecified
I74.2	Embolism and thrombosis of arteries of the upper extremities
I74.8	Embolism and thrombosis of other arteries
I75.011	Atheroembolism of right upper extremity ☑
I75.012	Atheroembolism of left upper extremity ☑
I75.013	Atheroembolism of bilateral upper extremities ☑
I76	Septic arterial embolism
I77.1	Stricture of artery
I77.2	Rupture of artery
I77.5	Necrosis of artery
I77.79	Dissection of other specified artery
I77.89	Other specified disorders of arteries and arterioles
S15.8XXA	Injury of other specified blood vessels at neck level, initial encounter
S25.111A	Minor laceration of right innominate or subclavian artery, initial encounter ☑
S25.112A	Minor laceration of left innominate or subclavian artery, initial encounter ☑
S25.121A	Major laceration of right innominate or subclavian artery, initial encounter ☑
S25.122A	Major laceration of left innominate or subclavian artery, initial encounter ☑
S25.191A	Other specified injury of right innominate or subclavian artery, initial encounter ☑
S25.192A	Other specified injury of left innominate or subclavian artery, initial encounter ☑
S45.011A	Laceration of axillary artery, right side, initial encounter ☑
S45.012A	Laceration of axillary artery, left side, initial encounter ☑
S45.091A	Other specified injury of axillary artery, right side, initial encounter ☑
S45.092A	Other specified injury of axillary artery, left side, initial encounter ☑

Relative Value Units/Medicare Edits

Non-Facility RVU	Work	PE	MP	Total
35650	20.16	4.77	5.01	29.94
Facility RVU	**Work**	**PE**	**MP**	**Total**
35650	20.16	4.77	5.01	29.94

	FUD	Status	MUE	Modifiers				IOM Reference
35650	90	A	1(3)	51	50	62*	80	None

* with documentation

Terms To Know

angioscopy. Visualization of capillary blood vessels with a microscope, or the inside of a blood vessel with a fiberoptic-equipped catheter.

arteriogram. Radiograph of arteries.

bypass. Auxiliary or diverted route to maintain continuous flow.

claudication. Lameness, pain, and weakness occurring in the arms or legs during exercise due to muscles not receiving the needed oxygen and nutrients.

35654

35654 Bypass graft, with other than vein; axillary-femoral-femoral

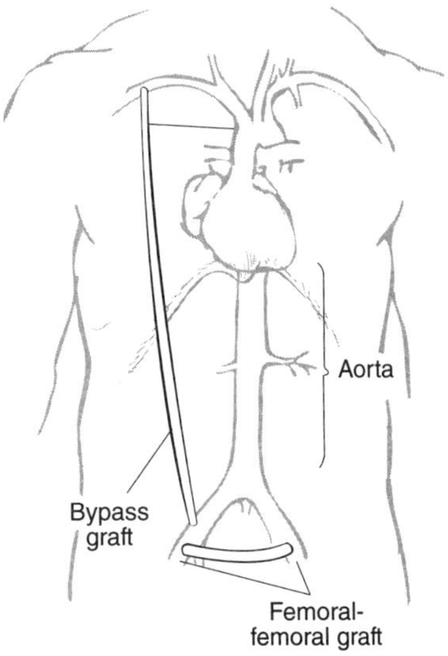

An axillary-femoral-femoral bypass graft is performed

Explanation

Through an incision in the skin of the axilla and both upper thighs, the physician creates a bypass around a section of lower aorta that is damaged or blocked, using a synthetic graft. Once vessel clamps have been affixed above and below the defect, the synthetic graft is sutured to the side of the axillary artery and passed through a subcutaneous tunnel to the upper thigh where it is sutured end-to-end or end-to-side to the femoral artery. A second synthetic graft is sutured end-to-side to the femoral artery and passed through another subcutaneous tunnel to the opposite thigh where it is sutured end-to-end or end-to-side to the femoral artery. The section of blocked artery is not removed. When the clamps are removed, the two synthetic grafted limbs form a new path through which blood can easily bypass the blocked area. After the graft is complete, the skin incisions are repaired with layered closures.

Coding Tips

Establishing both inflow and outflow by any method is included. That portion of the operative arteriogram performed by the surgeon is also included. Angioscopy performed during therapeutic intervention should be reported in addition to the code for the primary procedure, see 35400. If a bypass graft is performed with harvested vein, see 35533.

ICD-10-CM Diagnostic Codes

A52.02	Syphilitic aortitis
I70.0	Atherosclerosis of aorta A
I70.92	Chronic total occlusion of artery of the extremities A
I71.010	Dissection of ascending aorta
I71.011	Dissection of aortic arch
I71.012	Dissection of descending thoracic aorta
I71.02	Dissection of abdominal aorta
I71.03	Dissection of thoracoabdominal aorta
I74.01	Saddle embolus of abdominal aorta
I74.09	Other arterial embolism and thrombosis of abdominal aorta
I74.19	Embolism and thrombosis of other parts of aorta
I74.5	Embolism and thrombosis of iliac artery
I75.89	Atheroembolism of other site
I76	Septic arterial embolism
I77.1	Stricture of artery
I77.3	Arterial fibromuscular dysplasia
I77.5	Necrosis of artery
I77.72	Dissection of iliac artery
I77.73	Dissection of renal artery
I77.79	Dissection of other specified artery
I77.89	Other specified disorders of arteries and arterioles
Q25.41	Absence and aplasia of aorta
Q25.46	Tortuous aortic arch
Q25.47	Right aortic arch
Q25.48	Anomalous origin of subclavian artery
Q25.8	Other congenital malformations of other great arteries
Q27.1	Congenital renal artery stenosis
Q27.2	Other congenital malformations of renal artery
Q28.8	Other specified congenital malformations of circulatory system
Q79.61	Classical Ehlers-Danlos syndrome
Q79.62	Hypermobile Ehlers-Danlos syndrome
Q79.63	Vascular Ehlers-Danlos syndrome
Q87.418	Marfan syndrome with other cardiovascular manifestations
S25.01XA	Minor laceration of thoracic aorta, initial encounter
S25.02XA	Major laceration of thoracic aorta, initial encounter
S25.811A	Laceration of other blood vessels of thorax, right side, initial encounter ☑
S25.812A	Laceration of other blood vessels of thorax, left side, initial encounter ☑
S25.891A	Other specified injury of other blood vessels of thorax, right side, initial encounter ☑
S25.892A	Other specified injury of other blood vessels of thorax, left side, initial encounter ☑
S35.01XA	Minor laceration of abdominal aorta, initial encounter
S35.02XA	Major laceration of abdominal aorta, initial encounter
S35.8X1A	Laceration of other blood vessels at abdomen, lower back and pelvis level, initial encounter
T81.710A	Complication of mesenteric artery following a procedure, not elsewhere classified, initial encounter

Relative Value Units/Medicare Edits

Non-Facility RVU	Work	PE	MP	Total
35654	26.28	7.11	6.52	39.91
Facility RVU	**Work**	**PE**	**MP**	**Total**
35654	26.28	7.11	6.52	39.91

	FUD	Status	MUE	Modifiers				IOM Reference
35654	90	A	1(3)	51	N/A	62*	80	None

* with documentation

35656

35656 Bypass graft, with other than vein; femoral-popliteal

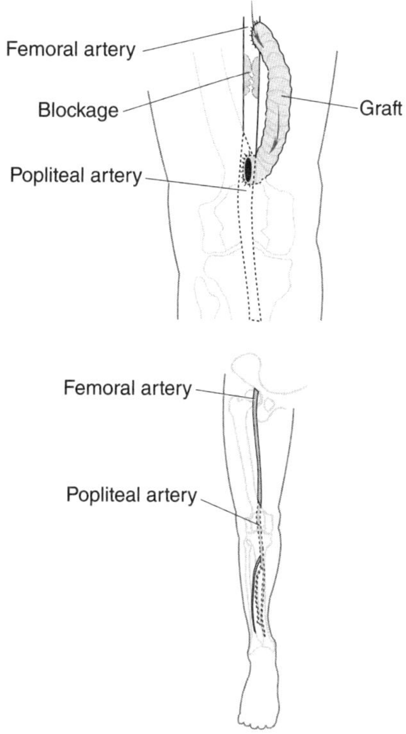

Explanation

Through incisions in the skin of the leg overlying the femoral and popliteal arteries, the physician isolates and dissects a section of artery that is damaged or blocked. The physician creates a bypass around the superficial femoral artery, using a synthetic vein and one of two methods of repair. Once vessel clamps have been affixed above and below the defect, the superficial femoral artery may be cut through above the damaged or blocked area and sutured to one end of a synthetic vein, which is passed through a tunnel down the thigh muscles to behind the knee and sutured to the popliteal artery. In the second method, the ends of the synthetic vein are sutured into the side of the femoral and popliteal arterial walls, resulting in a bypass of the damaged area. When the clamps are removed, the section of synthetic vein forms a new path through which blood can easily bypass the blocked area. The blocked or damaged portion of artery is not removed. After the graft is complete, the skin incisions are repaired with layered closures.

Coding Tips

Establishing both inflow and outflow by any method is included. That portion of the operative arteriogram performed by the surgeon is also included. Angioscopy performed during therapeutic intervention should be reported in addition to the code for the primary procedure, see 35400. Report 35700 in addition to 35656 for reoperation more than one month after the original operation. If in-situ vein bypass is performed, see 35583.

ICD-10-CM Diagnostic Codes

I70.211 Atherosclerosis of native arteries of extremities with intermittent claudication, right leg A ☑

I70.221 Atherosclerosis of native arteries of extremities with rest pain, right leg A ☑

I70.231 Atherosclerosis of native arteries of right leg with ulceration of thigh A ☑

I70.232 Atherosclerosis of native arteries of right leg with ulceration of calf A ☑

I70.233 Atherosclerosis of native arteries of right leg with ulceration of ankle A ☑

I70.234 Atherosclerosis of native arteries of right leg with ulceration of heel and midfoot A ☑

I70.235 Atherosclerosis of native arteries of right leg with ulceration of other part of foot A ☑

I70.261 Atherosclerosis of native arteries of extremities with gangrene, right leg A ☑

I70.291 Other atherosclerosis of native arteries of extremities, right leg A ☑

I70.461 Atherosclerosis of autologous vein bypass graft(s) of the extremities with gangrene, right leg A ☑

I70.511 Atherosclerosis of nonautologous biological bypass graft(s) of the extremities with intermittent claudication, right leg A ☑

I70.521 Atherosclerosis of nonautologous biological bypass graft(s) of the extremities with rest pain, right leg A ☑

I70.531 Atherosclerosis of nonautologous biological bypass graft(s) of the right leg with ulceration of thigh A ☑

I70.561 Atherosclerosis of nonautologous biological bypass graft(s) of the extremities with gangrene, right leg A ☑

I70.611 Atherosclerosis of nonbiological bypass graft(s) of the extremities with intermittent claudication, right leg A ☑

I70.621 Atherosclerosis of nonbiological bypass graft(s) of the extremities with rest pain, right leg A ☑

I70.631 Atherosclerosis of nonbiological bypass graft(s) of the right leg with ulceration of thigh A ☑

I70.661 Atherosclerosis of nonbiological bypass graft(s) of the extremities with gangrene, right leg A ☑

I70.92 Chronic total occlusion of artery of the extremities A

I74.3 Embolism and thrombosis of arteries of the lower extremities

I75.021 Atheroembolism of right lower extremity ☑

I76 Septic arterial embolism

I77.1 Stricture of artery

I77.2 Rupture of artery

I77.5 Necrosis of artery

S75.011A Minor laceration of femoral artery, right leg, initial encounter ☑

S75.021A Major laceration of femoral artery, right leg, initial encounter ☑

S75.091A Other specified injury of femoral artery, right leg, initial encounter ☑

Relative Value Units/Medicare Edits

Non-Facility RVU	Work	PE	MP	Total
35656	20.47	5.85	5.08	31.4
Facility RVU	**Work**	**PE**	**MP**	**Total**
35656	20.47	5.85	5.08	31.4

	FUD	Status	MUE	Modifiers				IOM Reference
35656	90	A	1(3)	51	50	62*	80	None

* with documentation

35661

35661 Bypass graft, with other than vein; femoral-femoral

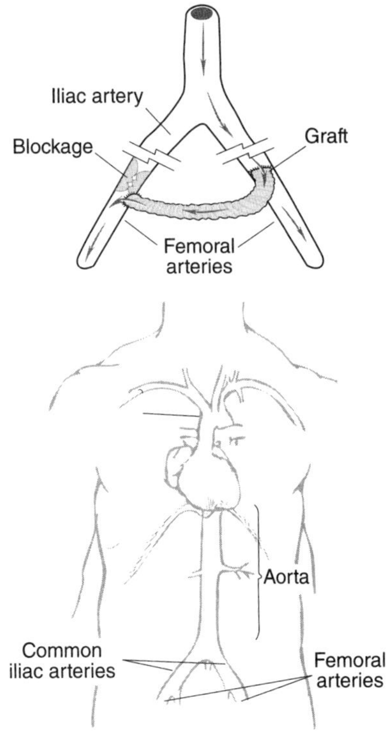

Explanation

Through incisions in the skin of the upper thighs, the physician isolates and dissects a section of the femoral arteries. The physician creates a bypass using a synthetic vein. Once vessel clamps have been affixed above and below the area of anastomosis, the femoral artery may be cut through below the damaged area and sutured to one end of a synthetic vein, which is sutured to the femoral artery in the opposite leg, resulting in a bypass of the damaged or blocked area. When the clamps are removed, the section of synthetic vein forms a new path through which blood can easily bypass the blocked area. The blocked or damaged portion of the artery is not removed. After the graft is complete, the skin incisions are repaired with layered closures.

Coding Tips

Establishing both inflow and outflow by any method is included. That portion of the operative arteriogram performed by the surgeon is also included. Angioscopy performed during therapeutic intervention should be reported in addition to the code for the primary procedure; see 35400. If a bypass graft is performed with harvested vein, see 35558.

ICD-10-CM Diagnostic Codes

I70.211 Atherosclerosis of native arteries of extremities with intermittent claudication, right leg A ☑

I70.221 Atherosclerosis of native arteries of extremities with rest pain, right leg A ☑

I70.231 Atherosclerosis of native arteries of right leg with ulceration of thigh A ☑

I70.232 Atherosclerosis of native arteries of right leg with ulceration of calf A ☑

I70.233 Atherosclerosis of native arteries of right leg with ulceration of ankle A ☑

I70.234 Atherosclerosis of native arteries of right leg with ulceration of heel and midfoot A ☑

I70.261 Atherosclerosis of native arteries of extremities with gangrene, right leg A ☑

I70.291 Other atherosclerosis of native arteries of extremities, right leg A ☑

I70.461 Atherosclerosis of autologous vein bypass graft(s) of the extremities with gangrene, right leg A ☑

I70.511 Atherosclerosis of nonautologous biological bypass graft(s) of the extremities with intermittent claudication, right leg A ☑

I70.521 Atherosclerosis of nonautologous biological bypass graft(s) of the extremities with rest pain, right leg A ☑

I70.531 Atherosclerosis of nonautologous biological bypass graft(s) of the right leg with ulceration of thigh A ☑

I70.561 Atherosclerosis of nonautologous biological bypass graft(s) of the extremities with gangrene, right leg A ☑

I70.611 Atherosclerosis of nonbiological bypass graft(s) of the extremities with intermittent claudication, right leg A ☑

I70.621 Atherosclerosis of nonbiological bypass graft(s) of the extremities with rest pain, right leg A ☑

I70.631 Atherosclerosis of nonbiological bypass graft(s) of the right leg with ulceration of thigh A ☑

I70.661 Atherosclerosis of nonbiological bypass graft(s) of the extremities with gangrene, right leg A ☑

I70.92 Chronic total occlusion of artery of the extremities A

I74.3 Embolism and thrombosis of arteries of the lower extremities

I75.021 Atheroembolism of right lower extremity ☑

I76 Septic arterial embolism

I77.1 Stricture of artery

I77.2 Rupture of artery

I77.5 Necrosis of artery

S75.011A Minor laceration of femoral artery, right leg, initial encounter ☑

S75.021A Major laceration of femoral artery, right leg, initial encounter ☑

S75.091A Other specified injury of femoral artery, right leg, initial encounter ☑

Relative Value Units/Medicare Edits

Non-Facility RVU	Work	PE	MP	Total
35661	20.35	6.32	5.04	31.71
Facility RVU	**Work**	**PE**	**MP**	**Total**
35661	20.35	6.32	5.04	31.71

	FUD	Status	MUE	Modifiers				IOM Reference
35661	90	A	1(3)	51	50	62*	80	None

* with documentation

35663

35663 Bypass graft, with other than vein; ilioiliac

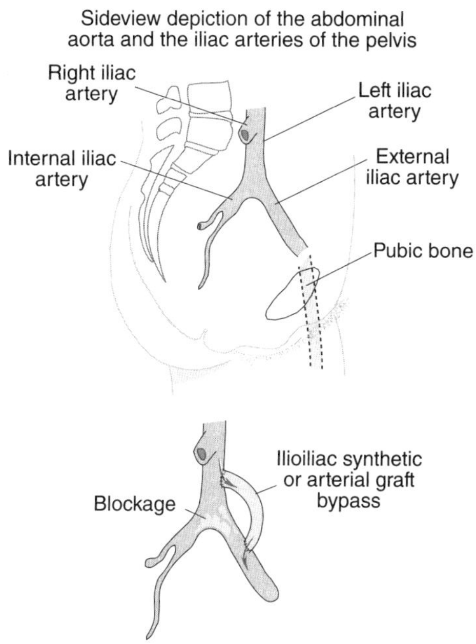

Explanation

The physician exposes the iliac arteries using an abdominal incision, retracting and dissecting past large and small bowel. The patent (nondiseased) iliac artery is partially clamped and a longitudinal incision is performed down the clamped portion of the aorta. A synthetic or arterial graft is sewn in, the graft is clamped, and the iliac clamp is removed to assess patency of the anastomosis. The diseased iliac artery is clamped distal to the stenosis, a distal incision is performed, and the distal graft is attached to the diseased iliac artery. Graft material may be utilized to enlarge the aortic or arterial lumen (patch graft). The physician may perform arteriography or use a Doppler probe to establish patency of the graft. The abdominal wound is closed, leaving drains in place.

Coding Tips

Establishing both inflow and outflow by any method is included. That portion of the operative arteriogram performed by the surgeon is also included. Angioscopy performed during therapeutic intervention should be reported in addition to the code for the primary procedure; see 35400. If a bypass graft is performed with harvested vein, see 35563.

ICD-10-CM Diagnostic Codes

I73.89	Other specified peripheral vascular diseases
I73.9	Peripheral vascular disease, unspecified
I74.5	Embolism and thrombosis of iliac artery
I76	Septic arterial embolism
I77.1	Stricture of artery
I77.5	Necrosis of artery
I77.72	Dissection of iliac artery
S35.511A	Injury of right iliac artery, initial encounter ☑
S35.512A	Injury of left iliac artery, initial encounter ☑
S35.59XA	Injury of other iliac blood vessels, initial encounter

Relative Value Units/Medicare Edits

Non-Facility RVU	Work	PE	MP	Total
35663	23.93	5.83	5.97	35.73
Facility RVU	**Work**	**PE**	**MP**	**Total**
35663	23.93	5.83	5.97	35.73

	FUD	Status	MUE	Modifiers				IOM Reference
35663	90	A	1(3)	51	50	62*	80	None

* with documentation

Terms To Know

anastomosis. Surgically created connection between ducts, blood vessels, or bowel segments to allow flow from one to the other.

angioscopy. Visualization of capillary blood vessels with a microscope, or the inside of a blood vessel with a fiberoptic-equipped catheter.

arteriogram. Radiograph of arteries.

artery. Vessel through which oxygenated blood passes away from the heart to any part of the body.

atherosclerosis. Buildup of yellowish plaques composed of cholesterol and lipoid material within the arteries.

bypass. Auxiliary or diverted route to maintain continuous flow.

complication. Condition arising after the beginning of observation and treatment that modifies the course of the patient's illness or the medical care required, or an undesired result or misadventure in medical care.

distal. *1)* Located farther away from a specified reference point or the trunk. *2)* Pertaining to the area farthest from the center of the body or the point of origin.

graft. Tissue implant from another part of the body or another person.

harvest. Removal of cells or tissue from their native site to be used as a graft or transplant to another part of the donor's body or placed into another person.

shunt. Surgically created passage between blood vessels or other natural passages, such as an arteriovenous anastomosis, to divert or bypass blood flow from the normal channel.

stenosis. Narrowing or constriction of a passage.

stricture. Narrowing of an anatomical structure.

35665

35665 Bypass graft, with other than vein; iliofemoral

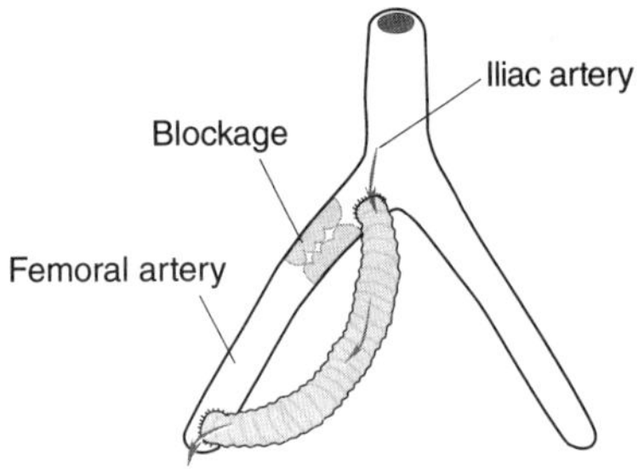

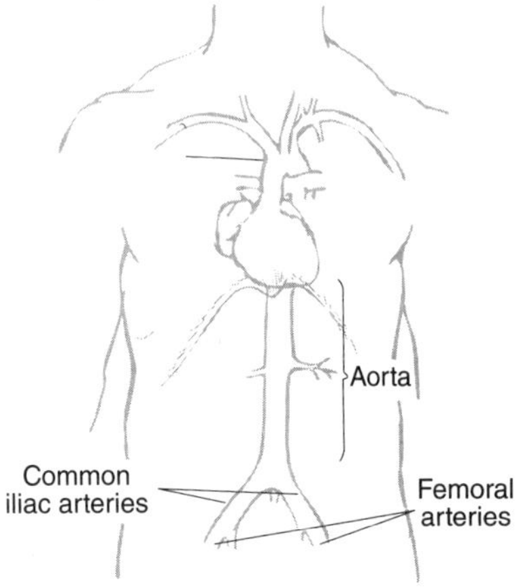

Explanation

Through incisions in the skin of the lower abdomen overlying the iliac artery, and in the skin of the upper thigh overlying the femoral artery, the physician isolates and dissects a section of common iliac artery. The physician creates a bypass around the iliac artery, using a synthetic vein and one of two methods of repair. Once vessel clamps have been affixed above and below the defect, the iliac artery may be cut or tied off with sutures above the damaged area and sutured to one end of a synthetic vein. The graft is passed through a tunnel on the inside of the upper thigh and is sutured to the side of the femoral artery. In the second method, the end of the synthetic vein is sutured to the side of the iliac artery. Either method results in a bypass of the damaged area. When the clamps are removed, the section of synthetic vein forms a new path through which blood can easily bypass the blocked area. After the graft is complete, the skin incisions are repaired with layered closures.

Coding Tips

Establishing both inflow and outflow by any method is included. That portion of the operative arteriogram performed by the surgeon is also included. Angioscopy performed during therapeutic intervention should be reported in addition to the code for the primary procedure; see 35400. If a bypass graft is performed with harvested vein, see 35565.

ICD-10-CM Diagnostic Codes

I70.92	Chronic total occlusion of artery of the extremities A
I72.3	Aneurysm of iliac artery
I72.4	Aneurysm of artery of lower extremity
I73.89	Other specified peripheral vascular diseases
I74.3	Embolism and thrombosis of arteries of the lower extremities
I74.5	Embolism and thrombosis of iliac artery
I75.021	Atheroembolism of right lower extremity ☑
I75.022	Atheroembolism of left lower extremity ☑
I75.023	Atheroembolism of bilateral lower extremities ☑
I76	Septic arterial embolism
I77.1	Stricture of artery
I77.2	Rupture of artery
I77.5	Necrosis of artery
I77.72	Dissection of iliac artery
I77.89	Other specified disorders of arteries and arterioles
I79.8	Other disorders of arteries, arterioles and capillaries in diseases classified elsewhere
M79.604	Pain in right leg ☑
M79.605	Pain in left leg ☑
M79.651	Pain in right thigh ☑
M79.652	Pain in left thigh ☑
S35.511A	Injury of right iliac artery, initial encounter ☑
S35.512A	Injury of left iliac artery, initial encounter ☑
S35.59XA	Injury of other iliac blood vessels, initial encounter
S35.8X1A	Laceration of other blood vessels at abdomen, lower back and pelvis level, initial encounter
S35.8X8A	Other specified injury of other blood vessels at abdomen, lower back and pelvis level, initial encounter

Relative Value Units/Medicare Edits

Non-Facility RVU	Work	PE	MP	Total
35665	22.35	6.55	5.48	34.38
Facility RVU	**Work**	**PE**	**MP**	**Total**
35665	22.35	6.55	5.48	34.38

	FUD	Status	MUE	Modifiers				IOM Reference
35665	90	A	1(3)	51	50	62*	80	None

* with documentation

35666

35666 Bypass graft, with other than vein; femoral-anterior tibial, posterior tibial, or peroneal artery

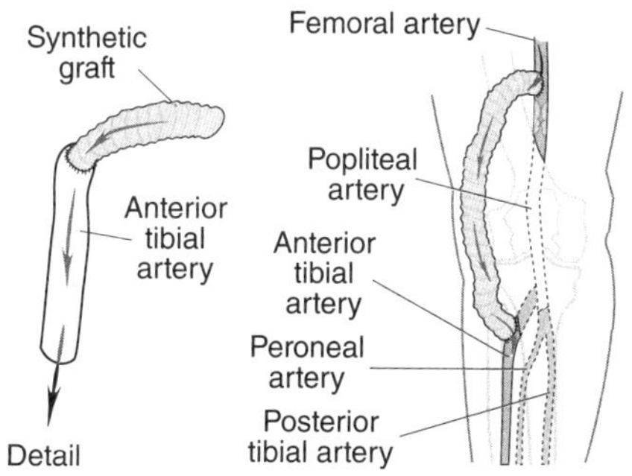

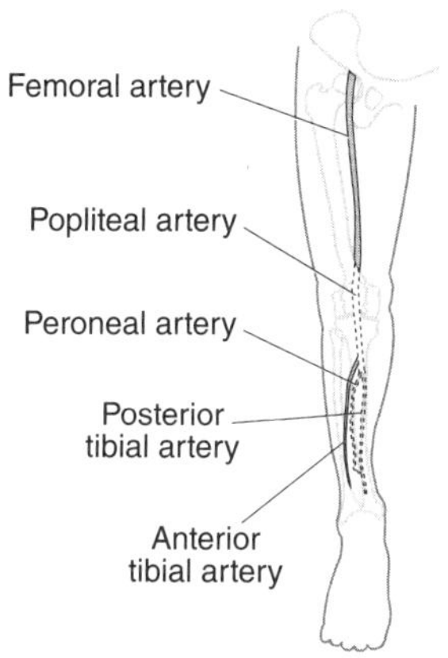

Explanation

Through incisions in the skin of the leg overlying the superficial femoral artery, the physician isolates and dissects sections of the femoral and anterior tibial, posterior tibial or peroneal arteries. The physician creates a bypass around the affected artery using a synthetic vein. Once vessel clamps have been affixed above and below the defect, the superficial femoral artery may be cut through above the damaged area and sutured to one end of a synthetic vein, which is passed through an intramuscular tunnel and sutured to the anterior tibial, posterior tibial, peroneal, or other distal vessel. In the second method, the ends of the synthetic vein are sutured to the side of the femoral artery and anterior tibial, posterior tibial, peroneal, or other distal vessel wall, resulting in a bypass of the damaged area. When the clamps are removed, the section of synthetic vein forms a new path through which blood can easily bypass the blocked area. The blocked or damaged portion of artery is left in place and not removed. After the graft is complete, the skin incisions are repaired with layered closures.

Coding Tips

Establishing both inflow and outflow by any method is included. That portion of the operative arteriogram performed by the surgeon is also included. Angioscopy performed during therapeutic intervention should be reported in addition to the code for the primary procedure; see 35400. Report 35700 in addition to 35666 for reoperation more than one month after the original operation. If a bypass graft is performed with a harvested vein, see 35566. If an in-situ vein bypass is performed, see 35585.

ICD-10-CM Diagnostic Codes

I70.211 Atherosclerosis of native arteries of extremities with intermittent claudication, right leg A ☑
I70.221 Atherosclerosis of native arteries of extremities with rest pain, right leg A ☑
I70.231 Atherosclerosis of native arteries of right leg with ulceration of thigh A ☑
I70.232 Atherosclerosis of native arteries of right leg with ulceration of calf A ☑
I70.233 Atherosclerosis of native arteries of right leg with ulceration of ankle A ☑
I70.234 Atherosclerosis of native arteries of right leg with ulceration of heel and midfoot A ☑
I70.235 Atherosclerosis of native arteries of right leg with ulceration of other part of foot A ☑
I70.238 Atherosclerosis of native arteries of right leg with ulceration of other part of lower leg A ☑
I70.261 Atherosclerosis of native arteries of extremities with gangrene, right leg A ☑
I70.461 Atherosclerosis of autologous vein bypass graft(s) of the extremities with gangrene, right leg A ☑
I70.511 Atherosclerosis of nonautologous biological bypass graft(s) of the extremities with intermittent claudication, right leg A ☑
I70.521 Atherosclerosis of nonautologous biological bypass graft(s) of the extremities with rest pain, right leg A ☑
I70.531 Atherosclerosis of nonautologous biological bypass graft(s) of the right leg with ulceration of thigh A ☑
I70.561 Atherosclerosis of nonautologous biological bypass graft(s) of the extremities with gangrene, right leg A ☑
I70.611 Atherosclerosis of nonbiological bypass graft(s) of the extremities with intermittent claudication, right leg A ☑
I70.621 Atherosclerosis of nonbiological bypass graft(s) of the extremities with rest pain, right leg A ☑
I70.631 Atherosclerosis of nonbiological bypass graft(s) of the right leg with ulceration of thigh A ☑
I70.661 Atherosclerosis of nonbiological bypass graft(s) of the extremities with gangrene, right leg A ☑
I70.92 Chronic total occlusion of artery of the extremities A
I72.4 Aneurysm of artery of lower extremity
I74.3 Embolism and thrombosis of arteries of the lower extremities
I75.021 Atheroembolism of right lower extremity ☑
I76 Septic arterial embolism
I77.1 Stricture of artery
I77.2 Rupture of artery
I77.5 Necrosis of artery
S75.021A Major laceration of femoral artery, right leg, initial encounter ☑

Relative Value Units/Medicare Edits

Non-Facility RVU	Work	PE	MP	Total
35666	23.66	8.17	5.88	37.71
Facility RVU	**Work**	**PE**	**MP**	**Total**
35666	23.66	8.17	5.88	37.71

	FUD	Status	MUE	Modifiers				IOM Reference
35666	90	A	2(3)	51	50	62*	80	None

* with documentation

● New ▲ Revised + Add On ★ Telemedicine [Resequenced] ☑ Laterality

35671

35671 Bypass graft, with other than vein; popliteal-tibial or -peroneal artery

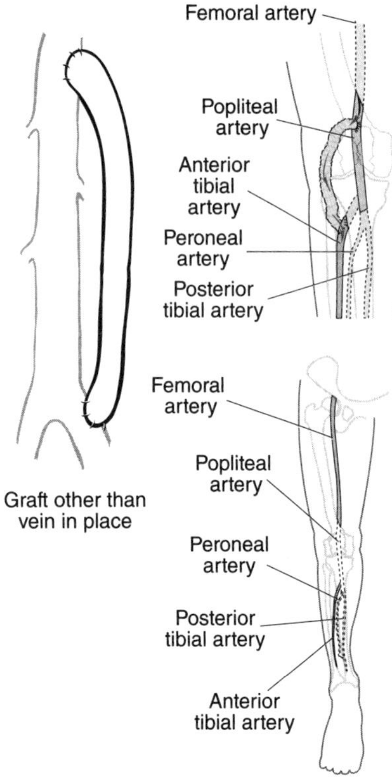

Explanation

Through incisions in the skin of the leg overlying the popliteal arteries, the physician isolates and dissects a section of artery from adjacent critical structures. The physician creates a bypass around the artery, using a synthetic vein and one of two methods of repair. Once vessel clamps have been affixed above and below the defect, the popliteal artery may be cut through above the damaged area and sutured to one end of a synthetic vein, which is sutured to the tibial, peroneal, or other distal artery. In the second method, the ends of the synthetic vein are sutured into the side of the popliteal and the tibial or peroneal arterial wall resulting in a bypass of the damaged area. When the clamps are removed, the section of synthetic vein forms a new path through which blood can easily bypass the blocked area. After the graft is complete, the incision is repaired with layered closures.

Coding Tips

Establishing both inflow and outflow by any method is included. That portion of the operative arteriogram performed by the surgeon is also included. Angioscopy performed during therapeutic intervention should be reported in addition to the code for the primary procedure; see 35400. Report 35700 in addition to 35671 for reoperation more than one month after the original operation. If a bypass graft is performed with a harvested vein, see 35571. If an in-situ vein bypass is performed, see 35587.

ICD-10-CM Diagnostic Codes

I70.92	Chronic total occlusion of artery of the extremities 🅰
I73.89	Other specified peripheral vascular diseases
I73.9	Peripheral vascular disease, unspecified
I74.3	Embolism and thrombosis of arteries of the lower extremities
I75.021	Atheroembolism of right lower extremity ☑
I75.022	Atheroembolism of left lower extremity ☑
I75.023	Atheroembolism of bilateral lower extremities ☑
I76	Septic arterial embolism
I77.89	Other specified disorders of arteries and arterioles
I79.8	Other disorders of arteries, arterioles and capillaries in diseases classified elsewhere
S85.011A	Laceration of popliteal artery, right leg, initial encounter ☑
S85.012A	Laceration of popliteal artery, left leg, initial encounter ☑
S85.091A	Other specified injury of popliteal artery, right leg, initial encounter ☑
S85.092A	Other specified injury of popliteal artery, left leg, initial encounter ☑
S85.141A	Laceration of anterior tibial artery, right leg, initial encounter ☑
S85.142A	Laceration of anterior tibial artery, left leg, initial encounter ☑
S85.151A	Other specified injury of anterior tibial artery, right leg, initial encounter ☑
S85.152A	Other specified injury of anterior tibial artery, left leg, initial encounter ☑
S85.171A	Laceration of posterior tibial artery, right leg, initial encounter ☑
S85.172A	Laceration of posterior tibial artery, left leg, initial encounter ☑
S85.181A	Other specified injury of posterior tibial artery, right leg, initial encounter ☑
S85.182A	Other specified injury of posterior tibial artery, left leg, initial encounter ☑
S85.211A	Laceration of peroneal artery, right leg, initial encounter ☑
S85.212A	Laceration of peroneal artery, left leg, initial encounter ☑
S85.291A	Other specified injury of peroneal artery, right leg, initial encounter ☑
S85.292A	Other specified injury of peroneal artery, left leg, initial encounter ☑
S85.811A	Laceration of other blood vessels at lower leg level, right leg, initial encounter ☑
S85.812A	Laceration of other blood vessels at lower leg level, left leg, initial encounter ☑
S85.891A	Other specified injury of other blood vessels at lower leg level, right leg, initial encounter ☑
S85.892A	Other specified injury of other blood vessels at lower leg level, left leg, initial encounter ☑

Relative Value Units/Medicare Edits

Non-Facility RVU	Work	PE	MP	Total
35671	20.77	7.28	5.15	33.2
Facility RVU	**Work**	**PE**	**MP**	**Total**
35671	20.77	7.28	5.15	33.2

	FUD	Status	MUE	Modifiers				IOM Reference
35671	90	A	2(3)	51	50	62*	80	None

* with documentation

35681-35683

+ 35681 Bypass graft; composite, prosthetic and vein (List separately in addition to code for primary procedure)

+ 35682 autogenous composite, 2 segments of veins from 2 locations (List separately in addition to code for primary procedure)

+ 35683 autogenous composite, 3 or more segments of vein from 2 or more locations (List separately in addition to code for primary procedure)

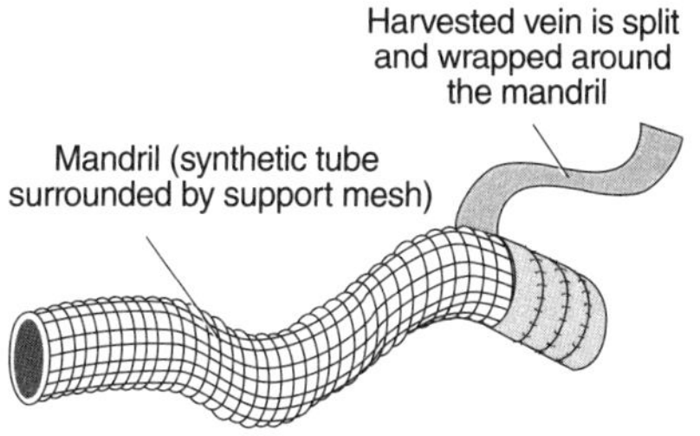

The vein material is harvested from a site distant from the site of the primary procedure

Explanation

In 35681 the physician constructs a composite graft from donor and synthetic materials. One common composite would involve the reconfiguring of a harvested vein into a length of larger diameter graft material. The harvested vein would be split lengthwise and wrapped in a spiral and sutured around a larger diameter mandrill. This length of composite graft would be used to complete the primary procedure. In 35682 a graft is constructed using tissue acquired from two veins at separate locations in the patient's body for the transplantation. In 35683 a graft is constructed using three or more segments of vein from two or more locations in the patient's body. In all three procedures veins are harvested by making an incision over the site where the vein will be removed. Tissues are dissected down to the vein and the vein is released from surrounding tissues. The vein is tied off above and below the area of vein that is to be removed. The vein is removed. The wound is closed with layered sutures. The portion of vein(s) removed is prepared for use in a separately reportable bypass graft procedure.

Coding Tips

Report 35682 and 35683 in addition to 35556, 35566, 35570, 35571, and 35583–35587. Codes 35682–35683 should be reported only when two or more vein segments are harvested from a site distant to the site of the arterial bypass graft. Do not report 35681 with 35682 or 35683; do not report 35682 with 35681 or 35683; do not report 35683 with 35681 or 35682. For harvest of a single upper extremity vein segment for lower extremity bypass, see 35500.

ICD-10-CM Diagnostic Codes

This/these CPT code(s) are add-on code(s). See the primary procedure code that this code is performed with for your ICD-10-CM code selections.

AMA: **35682** 2021,Dec **35683** 2021,Dec

Relative Value Units/Medicare Edits

Non-Facility RVU	Work	PE	MP	Total
35681	1.6	0.33	0.4	2.33
35682	7.19	1.32	1.78	10.29
35683	8.49	1.32	2.11	11.92
Facility RVU	**Work**	**PE**	**MP**	**Total**
35681	1.6	0.33	0.4	2.33
35682	7.19	1.32	1.78	10.29
35683	8.49	1.32	2.11	11.92

	FUD	Status	MUE	Modifiers				IOM Reference
35681	N/A	A	1(3)	N/A	N/A	62*	80	None
35682	N/A	A	1(2)	N/A	N/A	62*	80*	
35683	N/A	A	1(2)	N/A	N/A	62*	80*	

* with documentation

Terms To Know

atherosclerosis. Buildup of yellowish plaques composed of cholesterol and lipoid material within the arteries.

autogenous transplant. Tissue, such as bone, that is harvested from the patient and used for transplantation back into the same patient.

bypass graft. Surgically created alternative blood vessel used to reroute blood flow around an area of obstruction or disease.

dissection. Separating by cutting tissue or body structures apart.

graft. Tissue implant from another part of the body or another person.

harvest. Removal of cells or tissue from their native site to be used as a graft or transplant to another part of the donor's body or placed into another person.

incision. Act of cutting into tissue or an organ.

prosthesis. Man-made substitute for a missing body part.

transplantation. Grafting or movement of an organ or tissue from one site or person to another.

venous. Relating to the veins.

35685

+ **35685** Placement of vein patch or cuff at distal anastomosis of bypass graft, synthetic conduit (List separately in addition to code for primary procedure)

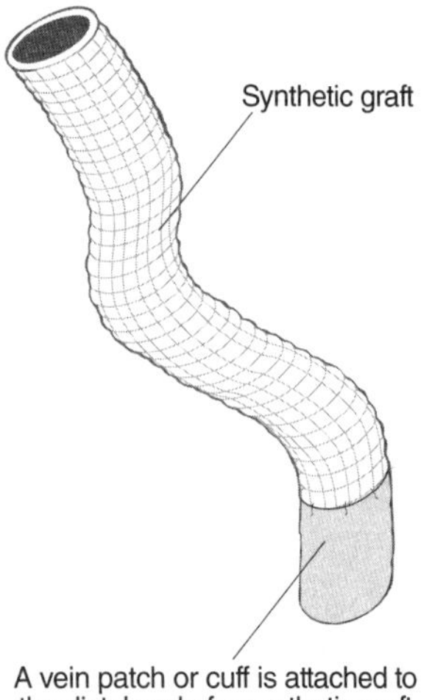

Explanation

The physician places a vein patch or cuff at a distal arterial anastomosis site during a bypass graft, synthetic conduit procedure of the lower extremity. The physician harvests the vein to be used for the vein patch from a previously chosen site. The vein patch is positioned and anastomosed between the distal portion of the synthetic vein graft and the native artery, end-to-end or side-to-end. The physician returns to the bypass graft surgery having performed this additional procedure.

Coding Tips

Report 35685 in addition to 35656, 35666, or 35671.

ICD-10-CM Diagnostic Codes

This/these CPT code(s) are add-on code(s). See the primary procedure code that this code is performed with for your ICD-10-CM code selections. Diagnostic code(s) would be the same as the actual procedure performed.

AMA: 35685 2018,Jun

Relative Value Units/Medicare Edits

Non-Facility RVU	Work	PE	MP	Total
35685	4.04	0.71	1.02	5.77
Facility RVU	**Work**	**PE**	**MP**	**Total**
35685	4.04	0.71	1.02	5.77

	FUD	Status	MUE	Modifiers				IOM Reference
35685	N/A	A	2(3)	N/A	N/A	62*	80	None

* with documentation

35686

+ **35686** Creation of distal arteriovenous fistula during lower extremity bypass surgery (non-hemodialysis) (List separately in addition to code for primary procedure)

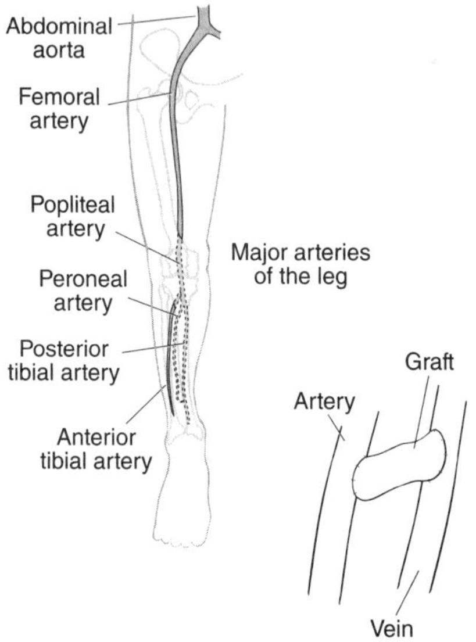

Explanation

The physician creates a fistula between an artery and vein during a lower extremity bypass procedure. The physician harvests the vein to be used for creation of the fistula from a previously chosen site. The vein is anastomosed between the tibial or peroneal artery and a vein at or beyond the distal bypass anastomosis site. The physician returns to the bypass graft surgery having performed this adjuvant (additional) procedure.

Coding Tips

Report 35686 in addition to 35556, 35566, 35570, 35571, 35583–35587, 35623, 35656, 35666, or 35671.

ICD-10-CM Diagnostic Codes

This/these CPT code(s) are add-on code(s). See the primary procedure code that this code is performed with for your ICD-10-CM code selections. Diagnostic code(s) would be the same as the actual procedure performed.

Relative Value Units/Medicare Edits

Non-Facility RVU	Work	PE	MP	Total
35686	3.34	0.52	0.82	4.68
Facility RVU	**Work**	**PE**	**MP**	**Total**
35686	3.34	0.52	0.82	4.68

	FUD	Status	MUE	Modifiers				IOM Reference
35686	N/A	A	1(3)	N/A	N/A	62*	80	None

* with documentation

35691

35691 Transposition and/or reimplantation; vertebral to carotid artery

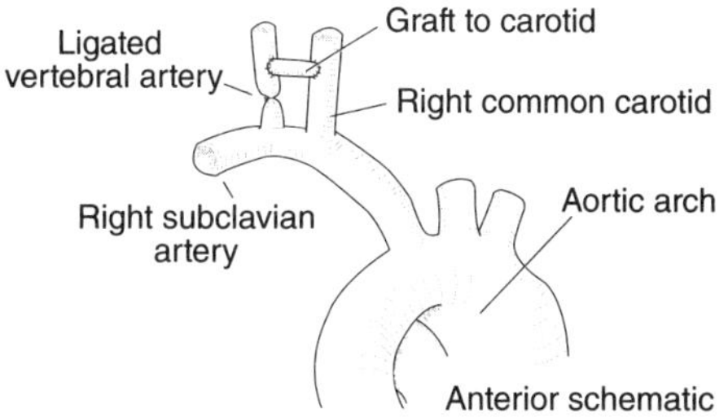

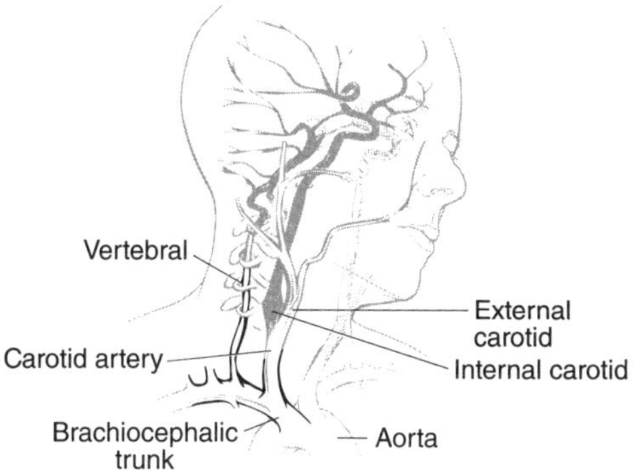

Explanation

The physician performs a supraclavicular incision and exposes the vertebral and carotid arteries by careful dissection. The adventitia of the chosen translocation site in the posterolateral wall of the common carotid artery is cleared. The physician anticoagulates the patient with heparin and divides the vertebral artery above the stenotic area. The proximal vertebral stump is ligated with sutures and a small arteriotomy in the common carotid arterial wall with an aortic punch is performed. The vertebral artery is attached using an end-to-side anastomosis to the carotid artery. The physician may perform arteriography or use a Doppler probe to establish patency of the graft. The supraclavicular wound is closed, leaving a drain in place.

Coding Tips

Establishing both inflow and outflow by any method is included. That portion of the operative arteriogram performed by the surgeon is also included. Angioscopy performed during therapeutic intervention should be reported in addition to the code for the primary procedure, see 35400.

ICD-10-CM Diagnostic Codes

G45.0	Vertebro-basilar artery syndrome
I63.011	Cerebral infarction due to thrombosis of right vertebral artery ☑
I63.012	Cerebral infarction due to thrombosis of left vertebral artery ☑
I63.013	Cerebral infarction due to thrombosis of bilateral vertebral arteries ☑
I63.033	Cerebral infarction due to thrombosis of bilateral carotid arteries ☑
I63.111	Cerebral infarction due to embolism of right vertebral artery ☑
I63.112	Cerebral infarction due to embolism of left vertebral artery ☑
I63.113	Cerebral infarction due to embolism of bilateral vertebral arteries ☑
I65.01	Occlusion and stenosis of right vertebral artery ☑
I65.02	Occlusion and stenosis of left vertebral artery ☑
I65.03	Occlusion and stenosis of bilateral vertebral arteries ☑
I76	Septic arterial embolism
I77.1	Stricture of artery
I77.2	Rupture of artery
I77.74	Dissection of vertebral artery
I77.89	Other specified disorders of arteries and arterioles
S15.111A	Minor laceration of right vertebral artery, initial encounter ☑
S15.112A	Minor laceration of left vertebral artery, initial encounter ☑
S15.121A	Major laceration of right vertebral artery, initial encounter ☑
S15.122A	Major laceration of left vertebral artery, initial encounter ☑
S15.191A	Other specified injury of right vertebral artery, initial encounter ☑
S15.192A	Other specified injury of left vertebral artery, initial encounter ☑

Relative Value Units/Medicare Edits

Non-Facility RVU	Work	PE	MP	Total
35691	18.41	4.78	4.57	27.76
Facility RVU	**Work**	**PE**	**MP**	**Total**
35691	18.41	4.78	4.57	27.76

	FUD	Status	MUE	Modifiers				IOM Reference
35691	90	A	1(3)	51	50	62*	80	None

* with documentation

Terms To Know

adventitia. Outermost layer of connective tissue covering an organ or other tissue.

Arteries and Veins

35693

35693 Transposition and/or reimplantation; vertebral to subclavian artery

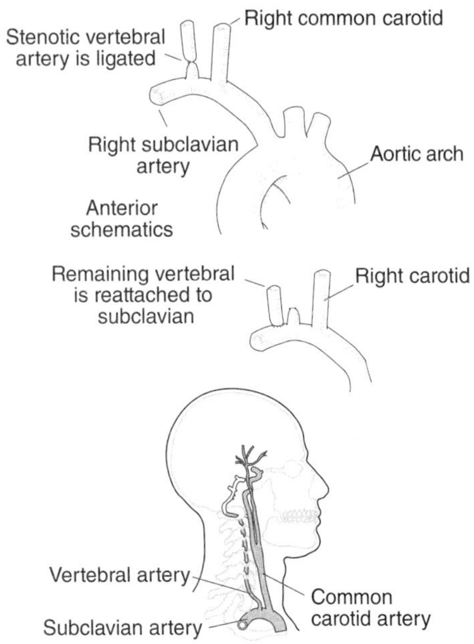

Explanation

The physician performs a supraclavicular incision and exposes the vertebral and subclavian arteries by careful dissection. The adventitia of the chosen translocation site in the subclavian artery lateral to the thyrocervical trunk is cleared. The physician anticoagulates the patient with heparin and divides the vertebral artery above the stenotic area. The proximal vertebral stump is ligated with sutures and a small arteriotomy is made in the subclavian artery wall with an aortic punch. The vertebral artery is attached using an end-to-side anastomosis to the subclavian artery. The physician may perform arteriography or use a Doppler probe to establish patency of the graft. The supraclavicular wound is closed, leaving a drain in place.

Coding Tips

Establishing both inflow and outflow by any method is included. That portion of the operative arteriogram performed by the surgeon is also included. Angioscopy performed during therapeutic intervention should be reported in addition to the code for the primary procedure, see 35400.

ICD-10-CM Diagnostic Codes

G45.0 Vertebro-basilar artery syndrome
I63.011 Cerebral infarction due to thrombosis of right vertebral artery ☑
I63.012 Cerebral infarction due to thrombosis of left vertebral artery ☑
I63.013 Cerebral infarction due to thrombosis of bilateral vertebral arteries ☑
I63.033 Cerebral infarction due to thrombosis of bilateral carotid arteries ☑
I63.111 Cerebral infarction due to embolism of right vertebral artery ☑
I63.112 Cerebral infarction due to embolism of left vertebral artery ☑
I63.113 Cerebral infarction due to embolism of bilateral vertebral arteries ☑
I63.89 Other cerebral infarction
I65.01 Occlusion and stenosis of right vertebral artery ☑
I65.02 Occlusion and stenosis of left vertebral artery ☑
I65.03 Occlusion and stenosis of bilateral vertebral arteries ☑
I76 Septic arterial embolism
I77.1 Stricture of artery
I77.2 Rupture of artery
I77.74 Dissection of vertebral artery
I77.89 Other specified disorders of arteries and arterioles
S15.111A Minor laceration of right vertebral artery, initial encounter ☑
S15.112A Minor laceration of left vertebral artery, initial encounter ☑
S15.121A Major laceration of right vertebral artery, initial encounter ☑
S15.122A Major laceration of left vertebral artery, initial encounter ☑
S15.191A Other specified injury of right vertebral artery, initial encounter ☑
S15.192A Other specified injury of left vertebral artery, initial encounter ☑

Relative Value Units/Medicare Edits

Non-Facility RVU	Work	PE	MP	Total
35693	15.73	4.98	3.91	24.62
Facility RVU	**Work**	**PE**	**MP**	**Total**
35693	15.73	4.98	3.91	24.62

	FUD	Status	MUE	Modifiers				IOM Reference
35693	90	A	1(3)	51	50	62*	80	None

* with documentation

Terms To Know

transposition. Removal or exchange from one side to another; change of position from one place to another.

35694

35694 Transposition and/or reimplantation; subclavian to carotid artery

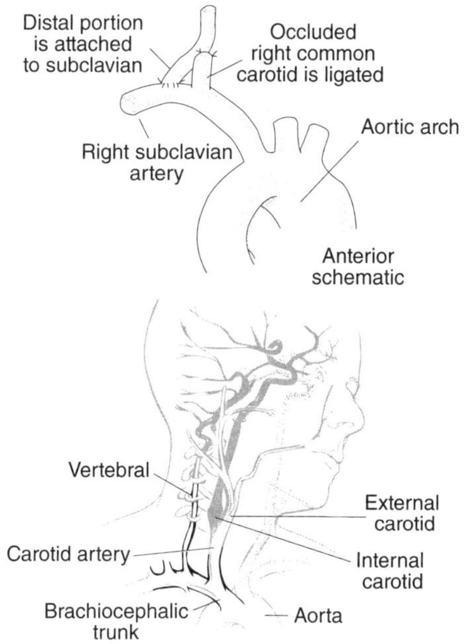

Explanation

The physician performs a supraclavicular incision and exposes the carotid and subclavian arteries by careful dissection. The adventitia of the chosen translocation site in the posterolateral wall of the common carotid artery is cleared. The physician anticoagulates the patient's blood with heparin and divides the subclavian artery distal to the stenotic area. The proximal subclavian stump is ligated with sutures and a small arteriotomy in the common carotid artery wall is performed with an aortic punch. The subclavian artery is attached using an end-to-side anastomosis to the carotid artery. The physician may perform arteriography or use a Doppler probe to establish patency of the graft. The supraclavicular wound is closed, leaving a drain in place.

Coding Tips

Establishing both inflow and outflow by any method is included. That portion of the operative arteriogram performed by the surgeon is also included. Angioscopy performed during therapeutic intervention should be reported in addition to the code for the primary procedure; see 35400. For an open subclavian to carotid artery transposition performed in conjunction with an endovascular repair of the descending aorta, see 33889. For a bypass graft completed with a harvested vein, subclavian to carotid, see 35506.

ICD-10-CM Diagnostic Codes

I63.09	Cerebral infarction due to thrombosis of other precerebral artery
I63.19	Cerebral infarction due to embolism of other precerebral artery
I65.8	Occlusion and stenosis of other precerebral arteries
I76	Septic arterial embolism
I77.1	Stricture of artery
I77.2	Rupture of artery
I77.75	Dissection of other precerebral arteries
S25.121A	Major laceration of right innominate or subclavian artery, initial encounter ☑
S25.122A	Major laceration of left innominate or subclavian artery, initial encounter ☑

Relative Value Units/Medicare Edits

Non-Facility RVU	Work	PE	MP	Total
35694	19.28	4.92	4.79	28.99
Facility RVU	**Work**	**PE**	**MP**	**Total**
35694	19.28	4.92	4.79	28.99

	FUD	Status	MUE	Modifiers				IOM Reference
35694	90	A	1(3)	51	50	62*	80	None

* with documentation

Terms To Know

adventitia. Outermost layer of connective tissue covering an organ or other tissue.

amaurosis fugax. Carotid artery plaque that breaks free and moves to the retinal artery causing decreased blood to the retina and temporary loss of vision. Frequently occurs prior to a stroke.

anastomosis. Surgically created connection between ducts, blood vessels, or bowel segments to allow flow from one to the other.

infarction. Area of necrosis in tissue, due to ischemia from lack of circulation, usually from a thrombus or an embolus.

 ● New ▲ Revised + Add On ★ Telemedicine [Resequenced] ☑ Laterality

35695

35695 Transposition and/or reimplantation; carotid to subclavian artery

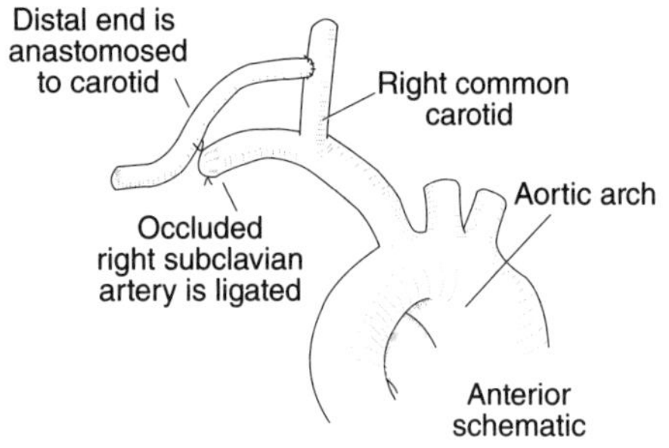

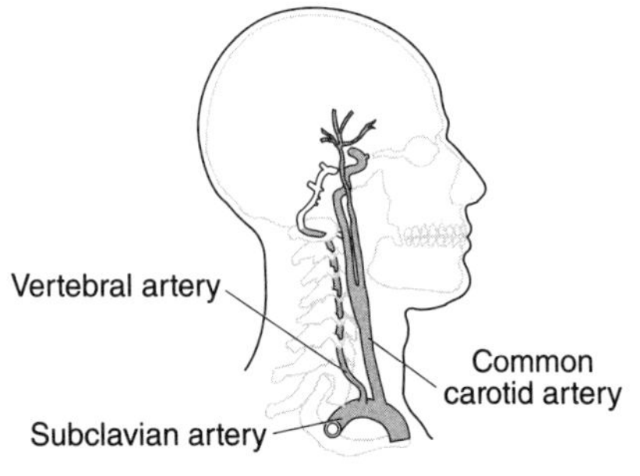

Explanation

The physician performs a supraclavicular incision and exposes the carotid and subclavian arteries by careful dissection. The adventitia of the chosen translocation site in the subclavian artery lateral to the thyrocervical trunk is cleared. The physician anticoagulates the patient's blood with heparin and divides the carotid artery above the stenotic area. The proximal carotid stump is ligated with sutures and a small arteriotomy in the subclavian artery wall is made with an aortic punch. The carotid artery is attached using an end-to-side anastomosis to the subclavian artery. The physician may perform arteriography or use a Doppler probe to establish patency of the graft. The supraclavicular wound is closed, leaving a drain in place.

Coding Tips

Establishing both inflow and outflow by any method is included. That portion of the operative arteriogram performed by the surgeon is also included. Angioscopy performed during therapeutic intervention should be reported in addition to the code for the primary procedure; see 35400. For a bypass graft completed with a harvested vein, carotid to subclavian, see 35506. For a synthetic bypass graft, carotid to subclavian, see 35606.

ICD-10-CM Diagnostic Codes

G45.1	Carotid artery syndrome (hemispheric)
I63.031	Cerebral infarction due to thrombosis of right carotid artery ☑
I63.032	Cerebral infarction due to thrombosis of left carotid artery ☑
I63.033	Cerebral infarction due to thrombosis of bilateral carotid arteries ☑
I63.131	Cerebral infarction due to embolism of right carotid artery ☑
I63.132	Cerebral infarction due to embolism of left carotid artery ☑
I63.133	Cerebral infarction due to embolism of bilateral carotid arteries ☑
I65.21	Occlusion and stenosis of right carotid artery ☑
I65.22	Occlusion and stenosis of left carotid artery ☑
I65.23	Occlusion and stenosis of bilateral carotid arteries ☑
I77.1	Stricture of artery
I77.2	Rupture of artery
I77.5	Necrosis of artery
I77.71	Dissection of carotid artery
S15.011A	Minor laceration of right carotid artery, initial encounter ☑
S15.012A	Minor laceration of left carotid artery, initial encounter ☑
S15.021A	Major laceration of right carotid artery, initial encounter ☑
S15.022A	Major laceration of left carotid artery, initial encounter ☑
S15.091A	Other specified injury of right carotid artery, initial encounter ☑
S15.092A	Other specified injury of left carotid artery, initial encounter ☑

Relative Value Units/Medicare Edits

Non-Facility RVU	Work	PE	MP	Total
35695	20.06	5.04	4.98	30.08
Facility RVU	**Work**	**PE**	**MP**	**Total**
35695	20.06	5.04	4.98	30.08

	FUD	Status	MUE	Modifiers				IOM Reference
35695	90	A	1(3)	51	50	62*	80	None

* with documentation

Terms To Know

adventitia. Outermost layer of connective tissue covering an organ or other tissue.

anastomosis. Surgically created connection between ducts, blood vessels, or bowel segments to allow flow from one to the other.

angioscopy. Visualization of capillary blood vessels with a microscope, or the inside of a blood vessel with a fiberoptic-equipped catheter.

ligate. To tie off a blood vessel or duct with a suture or a soft, thin wire (ligature wire).

35697

\+ **35697** Reimplantation, visceral artery to infrarenal aortic prosthesis, each artery (List separately in addition to code for primary procedure)

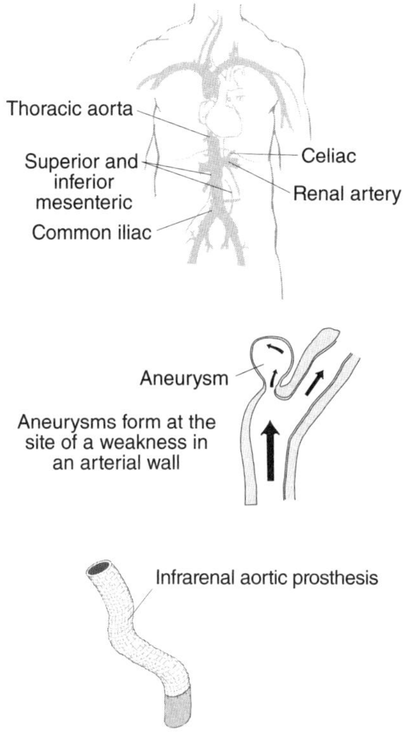

Explanation

A reimplantation of a visceral artery to an infrarenal aortic prosthesis, each artery, is done in addition to the primary procedure of an open aortic aneurysm repair (35081). This surgery is performed when a visceral artery, such as the inferior mesenteric, has been determined not to supply sufficient blood flow to vital organs, after repair of the aortic aneurysm. After the aortic prosthesis has been placed and blood flow is re-established through the aorta, the physician dissects soft tissue from around the origin of the visceral artery in the aorta where it exits. A small button-shaped patch of aortic tissue is removed from this site. Next, a clamp is placed on the aortic prosthesis at the intended site for reimplantation and a hole is cut the size of the button patch, which is anastomosed to the recipient hole in the prosthesis. The suturing is tested by removing the clamps and placing any additional sutures for complete hemostasis.

Coding Tips

Report 35697 in addition to the code for the aortic aneurysm repair (35081–35092). Do not report 35697 with 33877.

ICD-10-CM Diagnostic Codes

This/these CPT code(s) are add-on code(s). See the primary procedure code that this code is performed with for your ICD-10-CM code selections.

Relative Value Units/Medicare Edits

Non-Facility RVU	Work	PE	MP	Total
35697	3.0	0.53	0.74	4.27
Facility RVU	**Work**	**PE**	**MP**	**Total**
35697	3.0	0.53	0.74	4.27

	FUD	Status	MUE	Modifiers				IOM Reference
35697	N/A	A	2(3)	N/A	N/A	62	80	None

* with documentation

Terms To Know

anastomosis. Surgically created connection between ducts, blood vessels, or bowel segments to allow flow from one to the other.

aneurysm. Circumscribed dilation or outpouching of an artery wall, often containing blood clots and connecting directly with the lumen of the artery.

clamp. Tool used to grip, compress, join, or fasten body parts.

dissection. Separating by cutting tissue or body structures apart.

hemostasis. Interruption of blood flow or the cessation or arrest of bleeding.

prosthesis. Man-made substitute for a missing body part.

reimplant. Reinsert or reattach tissue.

suture. Numerous stitching techniques employed in wound closure.

35700

\+ **35700** Reoperation, femoral-popliteal or femoral (popliteal)-anterior tibial, posterior tibial, peroneal artery, or other distal vessels, more than 1 month after original operation (List separately in addition to code for primary procedure)

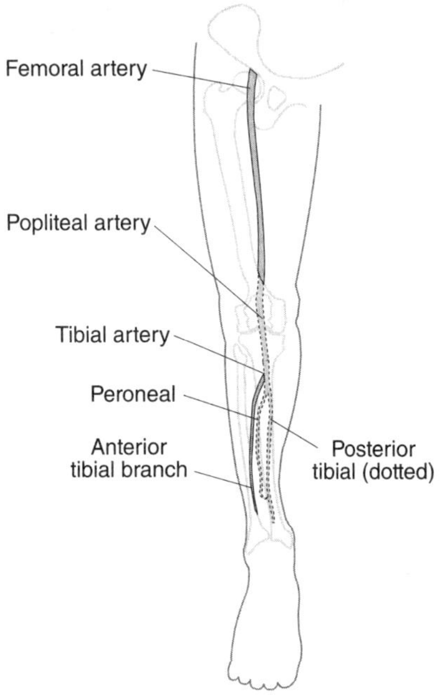

Original grafts may require replacement or patency testing with balloon catheter

Explanation

This code is only used with other codes to identify the reoperation aspect of this procedure, which usually requires more effort when performed again. Through incisions in the skin of the leg, overlying the affected artery, the physician isolates the graft. The physician makes an incision in the proximal portion of the graft and passes a Fogarty balloon catheter through the graft to clear and straighten it. If an arteriograph indicates the graft must be replaced, the physician makes a second incision distal to the inguinal incision, releases the graft, and places vein clamps above and below the stricture. The physician replaces the graft by suturing the ends of a new graft to the side of the arteries to form a bypass of the damaged area. The clamps are removed. After the stricture is controlled or the graft is otherwise complete, the incisions are repaired with layered closures.

Coding Tips

Report 35700 in addition to 35556, 35566, 35570, 35571, 35583, 35585, 35587, 35656, 35666, and 35671. This code is used instead of modifier 22.

ICD-10-CM Diagnostic Codes

This/these CPT code(s) are add-on code(s). See the primary procedure code that this code is performed with for your ICD-10-CM code selections. Diagnostic code(s) would be the same as the actual procedure performed.

Relative Value Units/Medicare Edits

Non-Facility RVU	Work	PE	MP	Total
35700	3.08	0.58	0.76	4.42
Facility RVU	**Work**	**PE**	**MP**	**Total**
35700	3.08	0.58	0.76	4.42

	FUD	Status	MUE	Modifiers				IOM Reference
35700	N/A	A	2(3)	N/A	N/A	62*	80	None

* with documentation

Terms To Know

anterior. Situated in the front area or toward the belly surface of the body; an anatomical reference point used to show the position and relationship of one body structure to another.

artery. Vessel through which oxygenated blood passes away from the heart to any part of the body.

bypass. Auxiliary or diverted route to maintain continuous flow.

catheter. Flexible tube inserted into an area of the body for introducing or withdrawing fluid.

distal. *1)* Located farther away from a specified reference point or the trunk. *2)* Pertaining to the area farthest from the center of the body or the point of origin.

graft. Tissue implant from another part of the body or another person.

incision. Act of cutting into tissue or an organ.

proximal. Located closest to a specified reference point, usually the midline or trunk.

suture. Numerous stitching techniques employed in wound closure.

35701-35703

35701 Exploration not followed by surgical repair, artery; neck (eg, carotid, subclavian)

35702 upper extremity (eg, axillary, brachial, radial, ulnar)

35703 lower extremity (eg, common femoral, deep femoral, superficial femoral, popliteal, tibial, peroneal)

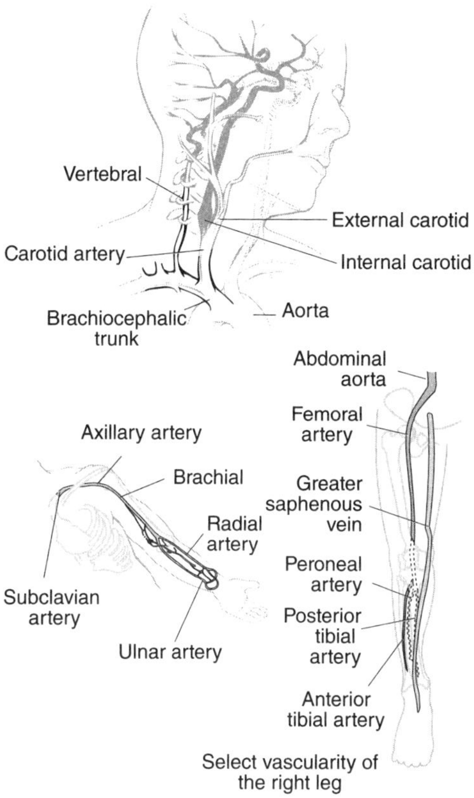

Explanation

Through an incision in the skin overlying the targeted artery, the physician dissects around surrounding structures as necessary to access the artery, freeing it so it can be examined. The artery is released from any surrounding scar tissue that may be compressing it. Finding no perforations or other signs of injury, the physician repairs the skin incision with a layered closure. Report 35701 for exploration of arteries of the neck (e.g., carotid or subclavian); 35702 for those of the upper extremity (e.g., axillary, brachial, radial, or ulnar); and 35703 for those of the lower extremity (e.g., common, deep, or superficial femoral, peroneal, popliteal, or tibial).

Coding Tips

Additional surgical procedures may only be reported if the artery exploration is performed through a separate incision. If the carotid artery is examined through the same incision used for a procedure performed during the same operative session, the exploration is not reported. If the carotid artery is examined and a defect is discovered and repaired, report the repair, not the exploration. Do not report 35702-35703 with 35206, 35207, 35236, 35256, 35266, 35286, or 35860 in the same extremity. For vascular exploration of the chest not followed by surgical repair, see 32100; of the abdomen, see 49000. For an exploration for postoperative hemorrhage, thrombosis, or infection of the neck, see 35800. For excision of an infected graft of the neck, see 35901. For exploration for postoperative hemorrhage, thrombosis, or infection, see 35860. If the procedure is completed through an operating microscope, report 69990 in addition to the primary procedure. However, head gear (e.g., loupes or binoculars) is considered an integral part of this procedure.

ICD-10-CM Diagnostic Codes

G45.1	Carotid artery syndrome (hemispheric)
G45.3	Amaurosis fugax
G45.8	Other transient cerebral ischemic attacks and related syndromes
G45.9	Transient cerebral ischemic attack, unspecified
I63.031	Cerebral infarction due to thrombosis of right carotid artery ☑
I63.131	Cerebral infarction due to embolism of right carotid artery ☑
I63.231	Cerebral infarction due to unspecified occlusion or stenosis of right carotid arteries ☑
I63.81	Other cerebral infarction due to occlusion or stenosis of small artery
I63.89	Other cerebral infarction
I65.21	Occlusion and stenosis of right carotid artery ☑
I67.81	Acute cerebrovascular insufficiency
I67.82	Cerebral ischemia
I67.850	Cerebral autosomal dominant arteriopathy with subcortical infarcts and leukoencephalopathy
I67.858	Other hereditary cerebrovascular disease
I70.92	Chronic total occlusion of artery of the extremities A
I73.89	Other specified peripheral vascular diseases
I74.2	Embolism and thrombosis of arteries of the upper extremities
I74.3	Embolism and thrombosis of arteries of the lower extremities
I75.011	Atheroembolism of right upper extremity ☑
I76	Septic arterial embolism
I77.1	Stricture of artery
I77.2	Rupture of artery
I77.71	Dissection of carotid artery
I77.76	Dissection of artery of upper extremity
I77.77	Dissection of artery of lower extremity
I77.89	Other specified disorders of arteries and arterioles
I79.8	Other disorders of arteries, arterioles and capillaries in diseases classified elsewhere
S15.011A	Minor laceration of right carotid artery, initial encounter ☑
S15.021A	Major laceration of right carotid artery, initial encounter ☑
S15.091A	Other specified injury of right carotid artery, initial encounter ☑
S15.8XXA	Injury of other specified blood vessels at neck level, initial encounter
S17.8XXA	Crushing injury of other specified parts of neck, initial encounter
S45.011A	Laceration of axillary artery, right side, initial encounter ☑
S45.091A	Other specified injury of axillary artery, right side, initial encounter ☑
S45.111A	Laceration of brachial artery, right side, initial encounter ☑
S45.191A	Other specified injury of brachial artery, right side, initial encounter ☑
S55.011A	Laceration of ulnar artery at forearm level, right arm, initial encounter ☑
S55.091A	Other specified injury of ulnar artery at forearm level, right arm, initial encounter ☑
S55.111A	Laceration of radial artery at forearm level, right arm, initial encounter ☑
S55.191A	Other specified injury of radial artery at forearm level, right arm, initial encounter ☑
S65.011A	Laceration of ulnar artery at wrist and hand level of right arm, initial encounter ☑

Arteries and Veins

S65.091A	Other specified injury of ulnar artery at wrist and hand level of right arm, initial encounter ☑
S65.111A	Laceration of radial artery at wrist and hand level of right arm, initial encounter ☑
S65.191A	Other specified injury of radial artery at wrist and hand level of right arm, initial encounter ☑
S75.001A	Unspecified injury of femoral artery, right leg, initial encounter ☑
S75.011A	Minor laceration of femoral artery, right leg, initial encounter ☑
S75.021A	Major laceration of femoral artery, right leg, initial encounter ☑
S75.091A	Other specified injury of femoral artery, right leg, initial encounter ☑
S85.011A	Laceration of popliteal artery, right leg, initial encounter ☑
S85.091A	Other specified injury of popliteal artery, right leg, initial encounter ☑
S85.111A	Laceration of unspecified tibial artery, right leg, initial encounter ☑
S85.121A	Other specified injury of unspecified tibial artery, right leg, initial encounter ☑
S85.141A	Laceration of anterior tibial artery, right leg, initial encounter ☑
S85.151A	Other specified injury of anterior tibial artery, right leg, initial encounter ☑
S85.171A	Laceration of posterior tibial artery, right leg, initial encounter ☑
S85.181A	Other specified injury of posterior tibial artery, right leg, initial encounter ☑
S85.211A	Laceration of peroneal artery, right leg, initial encounter ☑
S85.291A	Other specified injury of peroneal artery, right leg, initial encounter ☑

AMA: 35701 2019,Dec **35702** 2019,Dec **35703** 2019,Dec

Relative Value Units/Medicare Edits

Non-Facility RVU	Work	PE	MP	Total
35701	7.5	4.22	1.29	13.01
35702	7.12	3.31	1.67	12.1
35703	7.5	2.95	1.79	12.24
Facility RVU	**Work**	**PE**	**MP**	**Total**
35701	7.5	4.22	1.29	13.01
35702	7.12	3.31	1.67	12.1
35703	7.5	2.95	1.79	12.24

	FUD	Status	MUE	Modifiers				IOM Reference
35701	90	A	1(2)	51	50	62*	80	None
35702	90	A	2(2)	51	50	62*	80	
35703	90	A	2(2)	51	50	62*	80	

* with documentation

Terms To Know

dissect. Cut apart or separate tissue for surgical purposes or for visual or microscopic study.

stenosis. Narrowing or constriction of a passage.

35800

35800 Exploration for postoperative hemorrhage, thrombosis or infection; neck

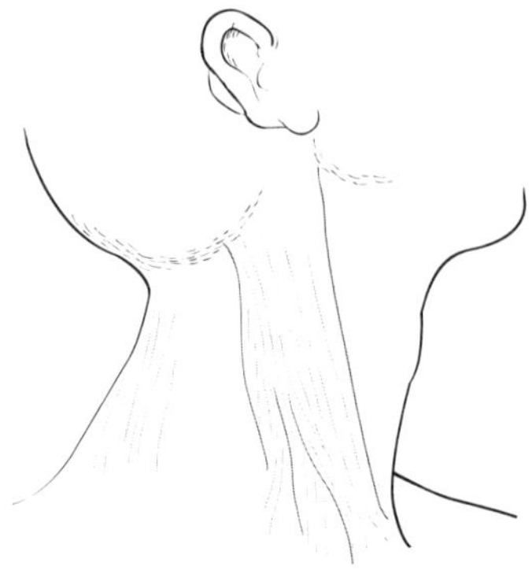

The physician makes an incision in the neck to explore a suspect vessel or to determine where blood loss, clot, or infection is coming from in an attempt to resolve postsurgical complication

Explanation

Through an incision in the neck over the affected area, the physician isolates the vessel and explores it for postoperative complications such as hemorrhage, thrombosis, or infection. The physician dissects any adjacent critical structures as necessary to access the vessel. The complication is identified and corrected. A hemorrhage is controlled by ligation or suture repair of the artery. Thrombosis requires opening of the artery and the removal of the clot. Any infection is drained, and sometimes a temporary tube is placed so the infection can continue to drain. The physician sutures the skin incision with a layered closure once the postsurgical complication has been treated.

Coding Tips

This code is used to report exploration for postoperative hemorrhage, thrombosis, or infection complications of veins and arteries of the neck only, including correction of the problem. For exploration of a vessel (not followed by surgical repair), of the carotid, or for exploration of other vessels of the neck when no other procedure is performed, see 35701. For thrombectomy of an arterial or a venous graft, see 35875–35876. For excision of an infected graft of the neck, see 35901.

ICD-10-CM Diagnostic Codes

G97.51	Postprocedural hemorrhage of a nervous system organ or structure following a nervous system procedure
G97.52	Postprocedural hemorrhage of a nervous system organ or structure following other procedure
G97.61	Postprocedural hematoma of a nervous system organ or structure following a nervous system procedure
G97.62	Postprocedural hematoma of a nervous system organ or structure following other procedure
G97.63	Postprocedural seroma of a nervous system organ or structure following a nervous system procedure
G97.64	Postprocedural seroma of a nervous system organ or structure following other procedure
G97.82	Other postprocedural complications and disorders of nervous system
I77.2	Rupture of artery
I77.71	Dissection of carotid artery

I97.89	Other postprocedural complications and disorders of the circulatory system, not elsewhere classified
T79.2XXA	Traumatic secondary and recurrent hemorrhage and seroma, initial encounter
T79.8XXA	Other early complications of trauma, initial encounter
T80.211A	Bloodstream infection due to central venous catheter, initial encounter
T80.212A	Local infection due to central venous catheter, initial encounter
T80.218A	Other infection due to central venous catheter, initial encounter
T80.29XA	Infection following other infusion, transfusion and therapeutic injection, initial encounter
T81.31XA	Disruption of external operation (surgical) wound, not elsewhere classified, initial encounter
T81.328A	Disruption or dehiscence of closure of other specified internal operation (surgical) wound, initial encounter
T81.42XA	Infection following a procedure, deep incisional surgical site, initial encounter
T81.43XA	Infection following a procedure, organ and space surgical site, initial encounter
T81.44XA	Sepsis following a procedure, initial encounter
T81.49XA	Infection following a procedure, other surgical site, initial encounter
T81.718A	Complication of other artery following a procedure, not elsewhere classified, initial encounter
T81.72XA	Complication of vein following a procedure, not elsewhere classified, initial encounter
T82.311A	Breakdown (mechanical) of carotid arterial graft (bypass), initial encounter
T82.318A	Breakdown (mechanical) of other vascular grafts, initial encounter
T82.321A	Displacement of carotid arterial graft (bypass), initial encounter
T82.328A	Displacement of other vascular grafts, initial encounter
T82.331A	Leakage of carotid arterial graft (bypass), initial encounter
T82.338A	Leakage of other vascular grafts, initial encounter
T82.391A	Other mechanical complication of carotid arterial graft (bypass), initial encounter
T82.398A	Other mechanical complication of other vascular grafts, initial encounter
T82.518A	Breakdown (mechanical) of other cardiac and vascular devices and implants, initial encounter
T82.528A	Displacement of other cardiac and vascular devices and implants, initial encounter
T82.538A	Leakage of other cardiac and vascular devices and implants, initial encounter
T82.598A	Other mechanical complication of other cardiac and vascular devices and implants, initial encounter
T82.7XXA	Infection and inflammatory reaction due to other cardiac and vascular devices, implants and grafts, initial encounter
T82.818A	Embolism due to vascular prosthetic devices, implants and grafts, initial encounter
T82.828A	Fibrosis due to vascular prosthetic devices, implants and grafts, initial encounter
T82.838A	Hemorrhage due to vascular prosthetic devices, implants and grafts, initial encounter
T82.848A	Pain due to vascular prosthetic devices, implants and grafts, initial encounter
T82.858A	Stenosis of other vascular prosthetic devices, implants and grafts, initial encounter
T82.868A	Thrombosis due to vascular prosthetic devices, implants and grafts, initial encounter
T82.898A	Other specified complication of vascular prosthetic devices, implants and grafts, initial encounter
T88.8XXA	Other specified complications of surgical and medical care, not elsewhere classified, initial encounter

AMA: 35800 2019,Dec

Relative Value Units/Medicare Edits

Non-Facility RVU	Work	PE	MP	Total
35800	12.0	7.52	2.34	21.86
Facility RVU	**Work**	**PE**	**MP**	**Total**
35800	12.0	7.52	2.34	21.86

	FUD	Status	MUE	Modifiers				IOM Reference
35800	90	A	2(3)	51	N/A	62*	80	None

* with documentation

Terms To Know

cautery. Destruction or burning of tissue by means of a hot instrument, an electric current, or a caustic chemical, such as silver nitrate.

complication. Condition arising after the beginning of observation and treatment that modifies the course of the patient's illness or the medical care required, or an undesired result or misadventure in medical care.

exploration. Examination for diagnostic purposes.

hemorrhage. Internal or external bleeding with loss of significant amounts of blood.

infection. Presence of microorganisms in body tissues that may result in cellular damage.

thrombosis. Condition arising from the presence or formation of blood clots within a blood vessel that may cause vascular obstruction and insufficient oxygenation.

35820

35820 Exploration for postoperative hemorrhage, thrombosis or infection; chest

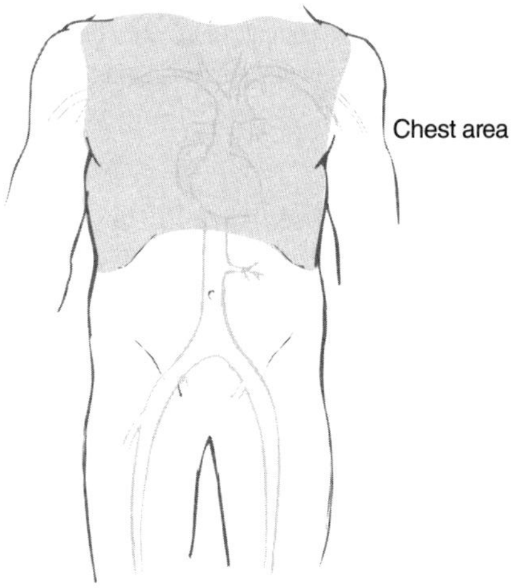

A surgical exploration is performed in the chest cavity to find and identify postoperative hemorrhage, thrombosis (clotting), or infection

Explanation

The physician reopens the original incision site and inspects the operative area for active bleeding, hematoma, thrombus, and exudate. The physician removes or debrides any observed hematoma, thrombus, and infected tissues. The physician looks for and corrects any active bleeding sites using electrocautery or ligation of bleeding vessels. The physician may leave an infected wound open, but generally closes the incision, leaving drains and chest tubes in place.

Coding Tips

This code is used to report exploration for postoperative hemorrhage, thrombosis, or infection complications of veins and arteries of the chest only, including correction of the problem. This procedure may be performed during the postoperative global period of the initial procedure. To indicate that this is an unplanned return to the operating/procedure room by the same physician, append modifier 78. For thrombectomy of an arterial or a venous graft, see 35875–35876. For excision of an infected graft of the thorax, see 35905.

ICD-10-CM Diagnostic Codes

I26.90	Septic pulmonary embolism without acute cor pulmonale
I26.99	Other pulmonary embolism without acute cor pulmonale
I97.610	Postprocedural hemorrhage of a circulatory system organ or structure following a cardiac catheterization
I97.611	Postprocedural hemorrhage of a circulatory system organ or structure following cardiac bypass
I97.618	Postprocedural hemorrhage of a circulatory system organ or structure following other circulatory system procedure
I97.620	Postprocedural hemorrhage of a circulatory system organ or structure following other procedure
I97.621	Postprocedural hematoma of a circulatory system organ or structure following other procedure
I97.622	Postprocedural seroma of a circulatory system organ or structure following other procedure
I97.630	Postprocedural hematoma of a circulatory system organ or structure following a cardiac catheterization
I97.631	Postprocedural hematoma of a circulatory system organ or structure following cardiac bypass
I97.638	Postprocedural hematoma of a circulatory system organ or structure following other circulatory system procedure
I97.648	Postprocedural seroma of a circulatory system organ or structure following other circulatory system procedure
I97.89	Other postprocedural complications and disorders of the circulatory system, not elsewhere classified
J94.2	Hemothorax
J94.8	Other specified pleural conditions
J95.830	Postprocedural hemorrhage of a respiratory system organ or structure following a respiratory system procedure
J95.831	Postprocedural hemorrhage of a respiratory system organ or structure following other procedure
J95.860	Postprocedural hematoma of a respiratory system organ or structure following a respiratory system procedure
J95.861	Postprocedural hematoma of a respiratory system organ or structure following other procedure
J95.862	Postprocedural seroma of a respiratory system organ or structure following a respiratory system procedure
J95.863	Postprocedural seroma of a respiratory system organ or structure following other procedure
K68.11	Postprocedural retroperitoneal abscess
T80.0XXA	Air embolism following infusion, transfusion and therapeutic injection, initial encounter
T80.211A	Bloodstream infection due to central venous catheter, initial encounter
T80.212A	Local infection due to central venous catheter, initial encounter
T80.218A	Other infection due to central venous catheter, initial encounter
T80.29XA	Infection following other infusion, transfusion and therapeutic injection, initial encounter
T81.11XA	Postprocedural cardiogenic shock, initial encounter
T81.41XA	Infection following a procedure, superficial incisional surgical site, initial encounter
T81.42XA	Infection following a procedure, deep incisional surgical site, initial encounter
T81.43XA	Infection following a procedure, organ and space surgical site, initial encounter
T81.44XA	Sepsis following a procedure, initial encounter
T81.49XA	Infection following a procedure, other surgical site, initial encounter
T81.718A	Complication of other artery following a procedure, not elsewhere classified, initial encounter
T81.72XA	Complication of vein following a procedure, not elsewhere classified, initial encounter
T82.310A	Breakdown (mechanical) of aortic (bifurcation) graft (replacement), initial encounter
T82.318A	Breakdown (mechanical) of other vascular grafts, initial encounter
T82.320A	Displacement of aortic (bifurcation) graft (replacement), initial encounter
T82.328A	Displacement of other vascular grafts, initial encounter
T82.330A	Leakage of aortic (bifurcation) graft (replacement), initial encounter
T82.338A	Leakage of other vascular grafts, initial encounter

T82.390A	Other mechanical complication of aortic (bifurcation) graft (replacement), initial encounter
T82.398A	Other mechanical complication of other vascular grafts, initial encounter
T82.518A	Breakdown (mechanical) of other cardiac and vascular devices and implants, initial encounter
T82.528A	Displacement of other cardiac and vascular devices and implants, initial encounter
T82.538A	Leakage of other cardiac and vascular devices and implants, initial encounter
T82.598A	Other mechanical complication of other cardiac and vascular devices and implants, initial encounter
T82.7XXA	Infection and inflammatory reaction due to other cardiac and vascular devices, implants and grafts, initial encounter
T82.817A	Embolism due to cardiac prosthetic devices, implants and grafts, initial encounter
T82.818A	Embolism due to vascular prosthetic devices, implants and grafts, initial encounter
T82.828A	Fibrosis due to vascular prosthetic devices, implants and grafts, initial encounter
T82.838A	Hemorrhage due to vascular prosthetic devices, implants and grafts, initial encounter
T82.848A	Pain due to vascular prosthetic devices, implants and grafts, initial encounter
T82.858A	Stenosis of other vascular prosthetic devices, implants and grafts, initial encounter
T82.868A	Thrombosis due to vascular prosthetic devices, implants and grafts, initial encounter
T82.898A	Other specified complication of vascular prosthetic devices, implants and grafts, initial encounter
T88.8XXA	Other specified complications of surgical and medical care, not elsewhere classified, initial encounter

AMA: 35820 2024,Oct; 2024,May

Relative Value Units/Medicare Edits

Non-Facility RVU	Work	PE	MP	Total
35820	36.89	13.51	8.81	59.21
Facility RVU	**Work**	**PE**	**MP**	**Total**
35820	36.89	13.51	8.81	59.21

	FUD	Status	MUE	Modifiers				IOM Reference
35820	90	A	2(3)	51	N/A	62*	80	None

* with documentation

Terms To Know

complication. Condition arising after the beginning of observation and treatment that modifies the course of the patient's illness or the medical care required, or an undesired result or misadventure in medical care.

debridement. Removal of dead or contaminated tissue and foreign matter from a wound.

electrocautery. Division or cutting of tissue using high-frequency electrical current to produce heat, which destroys cells.

hematoma. Tumor-like collection of blood in some part of the body caused by a break in a blood vessel wall, usually as a result of trauma.

35840

35840 Exploration for postoperative hemorrhage, thrombosis or infection; abdomen

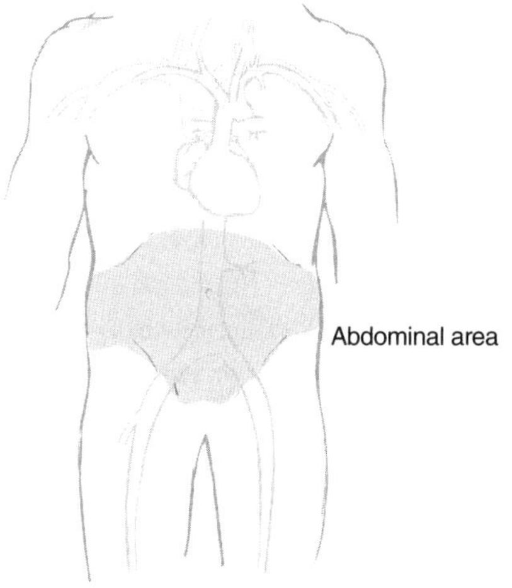

A surgical exploration is performed in the abdominal cavity to find and identify postoperative hemorrhage, thrombosis (clotting), or infection

Explanation

The physician reopens the original incision site and inspects the operative area for active bleeding, hematoma, thrombus, and exudate. The physician removes or debrides any observed hematoma, thrombus, and infected tissues. The physician looks for and corrects any active bleeding sites using electrocautery or ligation of bleeding vessels. The physician may leave an infected wound open, but generally closes the incision, leaving drains in place.

Coding Tips

This code is used to report exploration for postoperative hemorrhage, thrombosis, or infection complications of veins and arteries of the abdomen only, including correction of the problem. For thrombectomy of arterial or venous graft, see 35875–35876. For an excision of an infected graft of the abdomen, see 35907.

ICD-10-CM Diagnostic Codes

D78.21	Postprocedural hemorrhage of the spleen following a procedure on the spleen
D78.22	Postprocedural hemorrhage of the spleen following other procedure
D78.31	Postprocedural hematoma of the spleen following a procedure on the spleen
D78.32	Postprocedural hematoma of the spleen following other procedure
D78.33	Postprocedural seroma of the spleen following a procedure on the spleen
D78.34	Postprocedural seroma of the spleen following other procedure
I77.2	Rupture of artery
K68.11	Postprocedural retroperitoneal abscess
K91.840	Postprocedural hemorrhage of a digestive system organ or structure following a digestive system procedure
K91.841	Postprocedural hemorrhage of a digestive system organ or structure following other procedure

● New ▲ Revised + Add On ★ Telemedicine [Resequenced] ☑ Laterality

K91.870 Postprocedural hematoma of a digestive system organ or structure following a digestive system procedure

K91.871 Postprocedural hematoma of a digestive system organ or structure following other procedure

K91.872 Postprocedural seroma of a digestive system organ or structure following a digestive system procedure

K91.873 Postprocedural seroma of a digestive system organ or structure following other procedure

K91.89 Other postprocedural complications and disorders of digestive system

N99.0 Postprocedural (acute) (chronic) kidney failure

N99.520 Hemorrhage of incontinent external stoma of urinary tract

N99.521 Infection of incontinent external stoma of urinary tract

N99.522 Malfunction of incontinent external stoma of urinary tract

N99.523 Herniation of incontinent stoma of urinary tract

N99.524 Stenosis of incontinent stoma of urinary tract

N99.528 Other complication of incontinent external stoma of urinary tract

N99.530 Hemorrhage of continent stoma of urinary tract

N99.531 Infection of continent stoma of urinary tract

N99.532 Malfunction of continent stoma of urinary tract

N99.533 Herniation of continent stoma of urinary tract

N99.534 Stenosis of continent stoma of urinary tract

N99.538 Other complication of continent stoma of urinary tract

N99.820 Postprocedural hemorrhage of a genitourinary system organ or structure following a genitourinary system procedure

N99.821 Postprocedural hemorrhage of a genitourinary system organ or structure following other procedure

N99.840 Postprocedural hematoma of a genitourinary system organ or structure following a genitourinary system procedure

N99.841 Postprocedural hematoma of a genitourinary system organ or structure following other procedure

N99.842 Postprocedural seroma of a genitourinary system organ or structure following a genitourinary system procedure

N99.843 Postprocedural seroma of a genitourinary system organ or structure following other procedure

N99.89 Other postprocedural complications and disorders of genitourinary system

T81.31XA Disruption of external operation (surgical) wound, not elsewhere classified, initial encounter

T81.321A Disruption or dehiscence of closure of internal operation (surgical) wound of abdominal wall muscle or fascia, initial encounter

T81.328A Disruption or dehiscence of closure of other specified internal operation (surgical) wound, initial encounter

T81.41XA Infection following a procedure, superficial incisional surgical site, initial encounter

T81.42XA Infection following a procedure, deep incisional surgical site, initial encounter

T81.43XA Infection following a procedure, organ and space surgical site, initial encounter

T81.44XA Sepsis following a procedure, initial encounter

T81.49XA Infection following a procedure, other surgical site, initial encounter

T81.710A Complication of mesenteric artery following a procedure, not elsewhere classified, initial encounter

T81.711A Complication of renal artery following a procedure, not elsewhere classified, initial encounter

T81.718A Complication of other artery following a procedure, not elsewhere classified, initial encounter

T81.72XA Complication of vein following a procedure, not elsewhere classified, initial encounter

T82.7XXA Infection and inflammatory reaction due to other cardiac and vascular devices, implants and grafts, initial encounter

T82.818A Embolism due to vascular prosthetic devices, implants and grafts, initial encounter

T82.828A Fibrosis due to vascular prosthetic devices, implants and grafts, initial encounter

T82.838A Hemorrhage due to vascular prosthetic devices, implants and grafts, initial encounter

T82.848A Pain due to vascular prosthetic devices, implants and grafts, initial encounter

T82.856A Stenosis of peripheral vascular stent, initial encounter

T82.858A Stenosis of other vascular prosthetic devices, implants and grafts, initial encounter

T82.868A Thrombosis due to vascular prosthetic devices, implants and grafts, initial encounter

T82.898A Other specified complication of vascular prosthetic devices, implants and grafts, initial encounter

T88.8XXA Other specified complications of surgical and medical care, not elsewhere classified, initial encounter

Relative Value Units/Medicare Edits

Non-Facility RVU	Work	PE	MP	Total
35840	20.75	10.41	5.04	36.2
Facility RVU	**Work**	**PE**	**MP**	**Total**
35840	20.75	10.41	5.04	36.2

	FUD	Status	MUE	Modifiers				IOM Reference
35840	90	A	2(3)	51	N/A	62*	80	None

* with documentation

Terms To Know

cautery. Destruction or burning of tissue by means of a hot instrument, an electric current, or a caustic chemical, such as silver nitrate.

exudate. Fluid or other material, such as debris from cells, that has escaped blood vessel circulation and is deposited in or on tissues and usually occurs due to inflammation.

hematoma. Tumor-like collection of blood in some part of the body caused by a break in a blood vessel wall, usually as a result of trauma.

seroma. Swelling caused by the collection of serum, or clear fluid, in the tissues.

35860

35860 Exploration for postoperative hemorrhage, thrombosis or infection; extremity

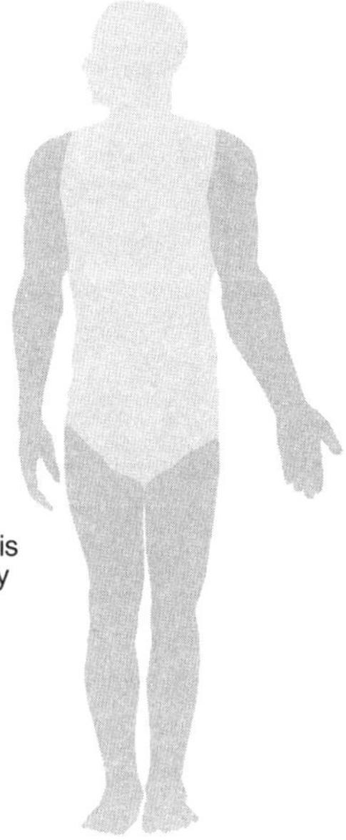

Explanation

Through an incision in the extremity over the affected area, the physician isolates the vessel and explores it for postoperative complications such as hemorrhage, thrombosis, or infection. The physician dissects any adjacent critical structures as necessary to access the vessel. The complication is identified and corrected. A hemorrhage is controlled by ligation or suture repair of the artery. Thrombosis requires opening of the artery and the removal of the clot. Any infection is drained, and sometimes a temporary tube is placed so the infection can continue to drain. The physician sutures the skin incision with a layered closure once the postsurgical complication has been treated.

Coding Tips

This code is used to report exploration for postoperative hemorrhage, thrombosis, and infection complications of veins and arteries of an extremity only, including correction of the problem. For exploration of a vessel of the extremity (not followed by surgical repair) when no other procedure is performed, see 35702 and 35703. For thrombectomy of an arterial or a venous graft, see 35875–35876. For an excision of an infected graft of the extremity, see 35903.

ICD-10-CM Diagnostic Codes

I77.2	Rupture of artery
L76.21	Postprocedural hemorrhage of skin and subcutaneous tissue following a dermatologic procedure
L76.22	Postprocedural hemorrhage of skin and subcutaneous tissue following other procedure
L76.31	Postprocedural hematoma of skin and subcutaneous tissue following a dermatologic procedure
L76.32	Postprocedural hematoma of skin and subcutaneous tissue following other procedure
L76.33	Postprocedural seroma of skin and subcutaneous tissue following a dermatologic procedure
L76.34	Postprocedural seroma of skin and subcutaneous tissue following other procedure
M96.830	Postprocedural hemorrhage of a musculoskeletal structure following a musculoskeletal system procedure
M96.831	Postprocedural hemorrhage of a musculoskeletal structure following other procedure
M96.841	Postprocedural hematoma of a musculoskeletal structure following other procedure
M96.842	Postprocedural seroma of a musculoskeletal structure following a musculoskeletal system procedure
M96.843	Postprocedural seroma of a musculoskeletal structure following other procedure
T81.31XA	Disruption of external operation (surgical) wound, not elsewhere classified, initial encounter
T81.328A	Disruption or dehiscence of closure of other specified internal operation (surgical) wound, initial encounter
T81.33XA	Disruption of traumatic injury wound repair, initial encounter
T81.41XA	Infection following a procedure, superficial incisional surgical site, initial encounter
T81.42XA	Infection following a procedure, deep incisional surgical site, initial encounter
T81.43XA	Infection following a procedure, organ and space surgical site, initial encounter
T81.44XA	Sepsis following a procedure, initial encounter
T81.49XA	Infection following a procedure, other surgical site, initial encounter
T81.718A	Complication of other artery following a procedure, not elsewhere classified, initial encounter
T81.72XA	Complication of vein following a procedure, not elsewhere classified, initial encounter
T82.312A	Breakdown (mechanical) of femoral arterial graft (bypass), initial encounter
T82.318A	Breakdown (mechanical) of other vascular grafts, initial encounter
T82.322A	Displacement of femoral arterial graft (bypass), initial encounter
T82.328A	Displacement of other vascular grafts, initial encounter
T82.332A	Leakage of femoral arterial graft (bypass), initial encounter
T82.338A	Leakage of other vascular grafts, initial encounter
T82.392A	Other mechanical complication of femoral arterial graft (bypass), initial encounter
T82.398A	Other mechanical complication of other vascular grafts, initial encounter
T82.7XXA	Infection and inflammatory reaction due to other cardiac and vascular devices, implants and grafts, initial encounter
T82.818A	Embolism due to vascular prosthetic devices, implants and grafts, initial encounter
T82.828A	Fibrosis due to vascular prosthetic devices, implants and grafts, initial encounter
T82.838A	Hemorrhage due to vascular prosthetic devices, implants and grafts, initial encounter
T82.848A	Pain due to vascular prosthetic devices, implants and grafts, initial encounter
T82.856A	Stenosis of peripheral vascular stent, initial encounter
T82.858A	Stenosis of other vascular prosthetic devices, implants and grafts, initial encounter
T82.868A	Thrombosis due to vascular prosthetic devices, implants and grafts, initial encounter

● New ▲ Revised + Add On ★ Telemedicine [Resequenced] ☑ Laterality

T82.898A Other specified complication of vascular prosthetic devices, implants and grafts, initial encounter

T88.8XXA Other specified complications of surgical and medical care, not elsewhere classified, initial encounter

AMA: 35860 2019,Dec

Relative Value Units/Medicare Edits

Non-Facility RVU	Work	PE	MP	Total
35860	15.25	5.83	3.72	24.8
Facility RVU	Work	PE	MP	Total
35860	15.25	5.83	3.72	24.8

	FUD	Status	MUE	Modifiers				IOM Reference
35860	90	A	2(3)	51	N/A	62*	80	None

* with documentation

Terms To Know

complication. Condition arising after the beginning of observation and treatment that modifies the course of the patient's illness or the medical care required, or an undesired result or misadventure in medical care.

embolism. Obstruction of a blood vessel resulting from a clot or foreign substance.

excision. Surgical removal of an organ or tissue.

hemorrhage. Internal or external bleeding with loss of significant amounts of blood.

infection. Presence of microorganisms in body tissues that may result in cellular damage.

seroma. Swelling caused by the collection of serum, or clear fluid, in the tissues.

thrombosis. Condition arising from the presence or formation of blood clots within a blood vessel that may cause vascular obstruction and insufficient oxygenation.

35870

35870 Repair of graft-enteric fistula

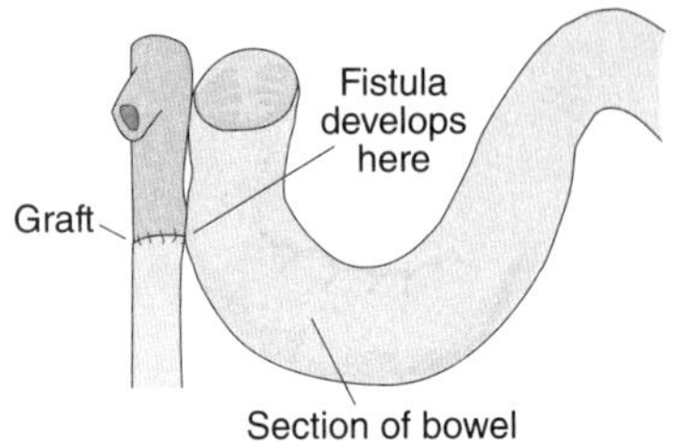

Explanation

The physician opens the abdomen under antibiotic cover and exposes the graft-enteric fistula site by careful dissection (most often aortic/Dacron anastomosis with a fistulous connection to the duodenum). The fistula is disconnected and the enteric defect is repaired using two layers of suture. The vascular prosthesis is examined and removed with an appropriate new bypass graft sewn in if there is obvious graft infection. If there is no obvious infection, the graft is repaired with local sutures. The wound is closed, leaving drains in place.

Coding Tips

When 35870 is performed with another separately identifiable procedure, the highest dollar value code is listed as the primary procedure, and subsequent procedures are appended with modifier 51. For arteriovenous fistula repairs, see 35180–35190.

ICD-10-CM Diagnostic Codes

I77.2 Rupture of artery

T82.818A Embolism due to vascular prosthetic devices, implants and grafts, initial encounter

T82.828A Fibrosis due to vascular prosthetic devices, implants and grafts, initial encounter

T82.838A Hemorrhage due to vascular prosthetic devices, implants and grafts, initial encounter

T82.848A Pain due to vascular prosthetic devices, implants and grafts, initial encounter

T82.858A Stenosis of other vascular prosthetic devices, implants and grafts, initial encounter

T82.868A Thrombosis due to vascular prosthetic devices, implants and grafts, initial encounter

T82.898A Other specified complication of vascular prosthetic devices, implants and grafts, initial encounter

Relative Value Units/Medicare Edits

Non-Facility RVU	Work	PE	MP	Total
35870	24.5	5.98	6.1	36.58
Facility RVU	**Work**	**PE**	**MP**	**Total**
35870	24.5	5.98	6.1	36.58

	FUD	Status	MUE	Modifiers				IOM Reference
35870	90	A	1(3)	51	N/A	62*	80	None

* with documentation

Terms To Know

anastomosis. Surgically created connection between ducts, blood vessels, or bowel segments to allow flow from one to the other.

bypass. Auxiliary or diverted route to maintain continuous flow.

complication. Condition arising after the beginning of observation and treatment that modifies the course of the patient's illness or the medical care required, or an undesired result or misadventure in medical care.

fistula. Abnormal tube-like passage between two body cavities or organs or from an organ to the outside surface.

graft. Tissue implant from another part of the body or another person.

infection. Presence of microorganisms in body tissues that may result in cellular damage.

prosthesis. Man-made substitute for a missing body part.

rupture. Tearing or breaking open of tissue.

suture. Numerous stitching techniques employed in wound closure.

buried suture. Continuous or interrupted suture placed under the skin for a layered closure.

continuous suture. Running stitch with tension evenly distributed across a single strand to provide a leakproof closure line.

interrupted suture. Series of single stitches with tension isolated at each stitch, in which all stitches are not affected if one becomes loose, and the isolated sutures cannot act as a wick to transport an infection.

purse-string suture. Continuous suture placed around a tubular structure and tightened, to reduce or close the lumen.

retention suture. Secondary stitching that bridges the primary suture, providing support for the primary repair; a plastic or rubber bolster may be placed over the primary repair and under the retention sutures.

35875-35876

35875 Thrombectomy of arterial or venous graft (other than hemodialysis graft or fistula);

35876 with revision of arterial or venous graft

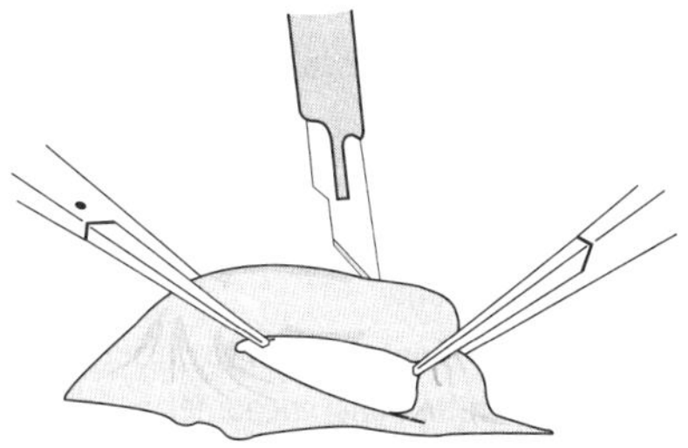

An arterial or venous thrombus is isolated and dissected from graft

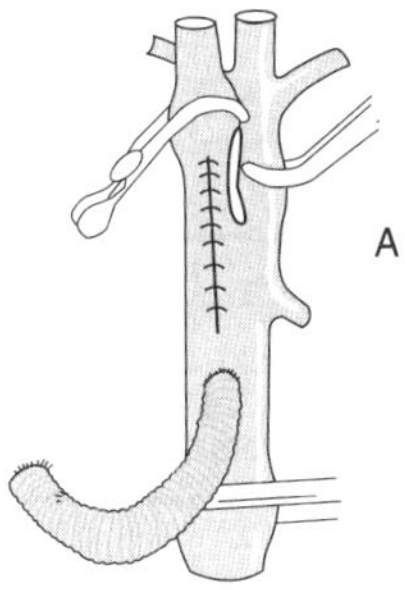

A new graft is placed

Explanation

Through an incision in the skin overlying the arterial or venous graft, the physician isolates the site of the thrombus. The physician dissects any muscle, overlying vessel, and/or adjacent critical structures to access the graft. To excise the thrombus from the graft, the blood vessel is clamped above and below the thrombus, an incision is made into the vessel or graft and the thrombus is removed. The graft or vessel is sutured at the site of the thrombectomy and the clamps are removed. To remove the thrombus with a catheter, the physician makes an incision in the vessel above or below the graft and threads the catheter past the thrombus. A balloon or tool at the tip of the catheter is inflated or extended. The physician withdraws the catheter, repeating as necessary, to capture and retrieve all of the thrombus. The blood vessel is repaired with sutures. After either procedure, the skin incision is repaired with a layered closure. In 35876, the thrombotic graft is removed, the graft site is repaired with sutures, and, avoiding the repair site, a new graft is sutured into place on the vessel. The skin incision is repaired with a layered closure.

Coding Tips

Establishing both inflow and outflow by any method is included. That portion of the operative arteriogram performed by the surgeon is also included. Angioscopy performed during therapeutic intervention should be reported in addition to the code for the primary procedure, see 35400. For thrombectomy of a hemodialysis graft or fistula, see 36831 and 36833. For initial placement of a bypass graft using a vein, see 35501–35571. For an initial in-situ vein graft placement, see 35583–35587. For an initial placement of a bypass graft other than vein, see 35601–35681. For excision of an infected graft, see 35901–35907.

ICD-10-CM Diagnostic Codes

T82.818A Embolism due to vascular prosthetic devices, implants and grafts, initial encounter

T82.828A Fibrosis due to vascular prosthetic devices, implants and grafts, initial encounter

T82.848A Pain due to vascular prosthetic devices, implants and grafts, initial encounter

T82.856A Stenosis of peripheral vascular stent, initial encounter

T82.858A Stenosis of other vascular prosthetic devices, implants and grafts, initial encounter

T82.868A Thrombosis due to vascular prosthetic devices, implants and grafts, initial encounter

T82.898A Other specified complication of vascular prosthetic devices, implants and grafts, initial encounter

Relative Value Units/Medicare Edits

Non-Facility RVU	Work	PE	MP	Total
35875	10.72	4.0	2.65	17.37
35876	17.82	5.41	4.38	27.61
Facility RVU	**Work**	**PE**	**MP**	**Total**
35875	10.72	4.0	2.65	17.37
35876	17.82	5.41	4.38	27.61

	FUD	Status	MUE	Modifiers				IOM Reference
35875	90	A	2(3)	51	N/A	62*	N/A	None
35876	90	A	2(3)	51	N/A	62*	80	

* with documentation

Terms To Know

catheter. Flexible tube inserted into an area of the body for introducing or withdrawing fluid.

complication. Condition arising after the beginning of observation and treatment that modifies the course of the patient's illness or the medical care required, or an undesired result or misadventure in medical care.

dissect. Cut apart or separate tissue for surgical purposes or for visual or microscopic study.

fistula. Abnormal tube-like passage between two body cavities or organs or from an organ to the outside surface.

graft. Tissue implant from another part of the body or another person.

in situ. Located in the natural position or contained within the origin site, not spread into neighboring tissue.

incision. Act of cutting into tissue or an organ.

thrombectomy. Removal of a clot (thrombus) from a blood vessel utilizing various methods.

thrombus. Stationary blood clot inside a blood vessel.

35879-35881

35879 Revision, lower extremity arterial bypass, without thrombectomy, open; with vein patch angioplasty

35881 with segmental vein interposition

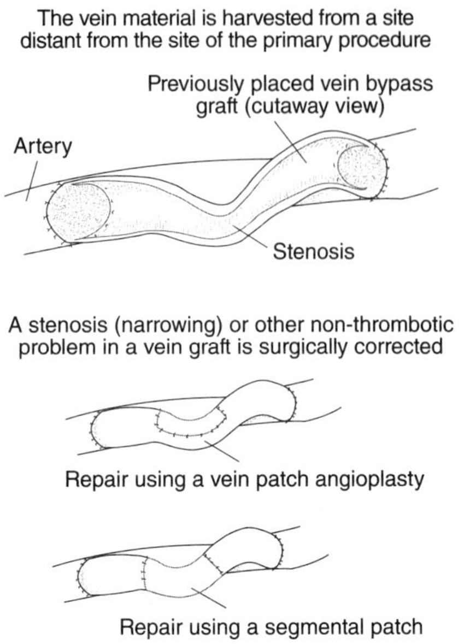

Explanation

The physician revises a lower extremity arterial bypass with vein-patch angioplasty or segmental vein interposition. A previous lower-extremity arterial bypass graft requires open revision due to graft-threatening stenosis. The physician makes an incision in a lower extremity over the site of a previous arterial bypass graft. Dissection is carried down to the graft. In 35879, angioplasty of the stenosed area is performed by excising the area of stenosis and using a patch of vein to close the created wound. In 35881, a segment of vein is excised from another area. The area of stenosis is excised and the vein segment is positioned between the two ends of the graft and anastomosed in an end to end fashion. A thrombectomy is not performed. The wound is closed with layered sutures.

Coding Tips

Codes 35879 and 35881 should be used to report open revision of stenotic arterial bypass grafts when the stenosis is such that it threatens the viability of the previously constructed arterial graft. For thrombectomy with revision of any non-coronary arterial or venous graft (except hemodialysis graft or fistula), including those of the lower extremity, report 35876. For direct repair (other than for fistula) of a lower extremity blood vessel (with or without patch angioplasty), see 35226. For repair of a lower extremity blood vessel using a vein graft, see 35256. For fistula repair of a lower extremity, see 35184 or 35190. For the revision of a femoral anastomosis of a synthetic arterial bypass graft, see 35883 and 35884. For excision of an infected graft, see 35901–35907 and the appropriate revascularization code.

ICD-10-CM Diagnostic Codes

I70.411 Atherosclerosis of autologous vein bypass graft(s) of the extremities with intermittent claudication, right leg A ✓

I70.421 Atherosclerosis of autologous vein bypass graft(s) of the extremities with rest pain, right leg A ✓

I70.431 Atherosclerosis of autologous vein bypass graft(s) of the right leg with ulceration of thigh A ✓

I70.432 Atherosclerosis of autologous vein bypass graft(s) of the right leg with ulceration of calf A ☑

I70.433 Atherosclerosis of autologous vein bypass graft(s) of the right leg with ulceration of ankle A ☑

I70.434 Atherosclerosis of autologous vein bypass graft(s) of the right leg with ulceration of heel and midfoot A ☑

I70.461 Atherosclerosis of autologous vein bypass graft(s) of the extremities with gangrene, right leg A ☑

I70.491 Other atherosclerosis of autologous vein bypass graft(s) of the extremities, right leg A ☑

I70.511 Atherosclerosis of nonautologous biological bypass graft(s) of the extremities with intermittent claudication, right leg A ☑

I70.521 Atherosclerosis of nonautologous biological bypass graft(s) of the extremities with rest pain, right leg A ☑

I70.531 Atherosclerosis of nonautologous biological bypass graft(s) of the right leg with ulceration of thigh A ☑

I70.532 Atherosclerosis of nonautologous biological bypass graft(s) of the right leg with ulceration of calf A ☑

I70.533 Atherosclerosis of nonautologous biological bypass graft(s) of the right leg with ulceration of ankle A ☑

I70.534 Atherosclerosis of nonautologous biological bypass graft(s) of the right leg with ulceration of heel and midfoot A ☑

I70.561 Atherosclerosis of nonautologous biological bypass graft(s) of the extremities with gangrene, right leg A ☑

I70.611 Atherosclerosis of nonbiological bypass graft(s) of the extremities with intermittent claudication, right leg A ☑

I70.621 Atherosclerosis of nonbiological bypass graft(s) of the extremities with rest pain, right leg A ☑

I70.631 Atherosclerosis of nonbiological bypass graft(s) of the right leg with ulceration of thigh A ☑

I70.632 Atherosclerosis of nonbiological bypass graft(s) of the right leg with ulceration of calf A ☑

I70.633 Atherosclerosis of nonbiological bypass graft(s) of the right leg with ulceration of ankle A ☑

I70.634 Atherosclerosis of nonbiological bypass graft(s) of the right leg with ulceration of heel and midfoot A ☑

I70.661 Atherosclerosis of nonbiological bypass graft(s) of the extremities with gangrene, right leg A ☑

Relative Value Units/Medicare Edits

Non-Facility RVU	Work	PE	MP	Total
35879	17.41	5.24	4.34	26.99
35881	19.35	6.03	4.79	30.17
Facility RVU	**Work**	**PE**	**MP**	**Total**
35879	17.41	5.24	4.34	26.99
35881	19.35	6.03	4.79	30.17

	FUD	Status	MUE	Modifiers				IOM Reference
35879	90	A	2(3)	51	50	62*	80	None
35881	90	A	1(3)	51	50	62*	80	

* with documentation

35883-35884

35883 Revision, femoral anastomosis of synthetic arterial bypass graft in groin, open; with nonautogenous patch graft (eg, polyester, ePTFE, bovine pericardium)

35884 Revision, femoral anastomosis of synthetic arterial bypass graft in groin, open; with autogenous vein patch graft

A revision of a femoral bypass in the groin is performed due to formation of an anastomotic aneurysm

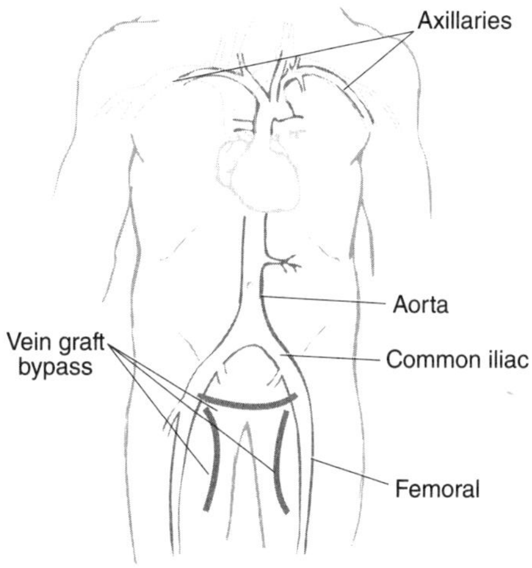

The aneurysm is excised and a patch graft applied

Explanation

The physician performs open revision of the femoral anastomosis of a synthetic arterial bypass graft in the groin using a nonautogenous patch graft such as bovine pericardium, polyester, or expanded polytetrafluoroethylene (ePTFE) in 35883 or an autogenous vein patch graft in 35884. This procedure is performed due to formation of an anastomotic aneurysm in the femoral artery, which occurs due to a defect in the anastomosis. The physician makes an incision in the skin of the upper thigh to isolate and dissect the anastomotic aneurysm. An arteriotomy is performed and the aneurysm is excised. A patch graft is placed and the skin incision repaired.

Coding Tips

These are unilateral procedures. If performed bilaterally, some payers require that the service be reported twice with modifier 50 appended to the second code, while others require identification of the service only once with modifier 50 appended. Check with individual payers. Modifier 50 identifies a procedure performed identically on the opposite side of the body (mirror image). Do not report 35883 or 35884 with 35700, 35875, or 35876. Do not report these codes with each other.

ICD-10-CM Diagnostic Codes

T81.41XA Infection following a procedure, superficial incisional surgical site, initial encounter

T81.42XA Infection following a procedure, deep incisional surgical site, initial encounter

T81.43XA Infection following a procedure, organ and space surgical site, initial encounter

T81.44XA Sepsis following a procedure, initial encounter

T81.49XA Infection following a procedure, other surgical site, initial encounter

T81.718A Complication of other artery following a procedure, not elsewhere classified, initial encounter

T82.7XXA	Infection and inflammatory reaction due to other cardiac and vascular devices, implants and grafts, initial encounter
T82.818A	Embolism due to vascular prosthetic devices, implants and grafts, initial encounter
T82.828A	Fibrosis due to vascular prosthetic devices, implants and grafts, initial encounter
T82.838A	Hemorrhage due to vascular prosthetic devices, implants and grafts, initial encounter
T82.848A	Pain due to vascular prosthetic devices, implants and grafts, initial encounter
T82.856A	Stenosis of peripheral vascular stent, initial encounter
T82.858A	Stenosis of other vascular prosthetic devices, implants and grafts, initial encounter
T82.868A	Thrombosis due to vascular prosthetic devices, implants and grafts, initial encounter
T82.898A	Other specified complication of vascular prosthetic devices, implants and grafts, initial encounter

Relative Value Units/Medicare Edits

Non-Facility RVU	Work	PE	MP	Total
35883	23.15	6.11	5.74	35.0
35884	24.65	5.5	6.14	36.29
Facility RVU	**Work**	**PE**	**MP**	**Total**
35883	23.15	6.11	5.74	35.0
35884	24.65	5.5	6.14	36.29

	FUD	Status	MUE	Modifiers				IOM Reference
35883	90	A	1(3)	51	50	62*	80	None
35884	90	A	1(3)	51	50	62*	80	

* with documentation

Terms To Know

anastomosis. Surgically created connection between ducts, blood vessels, or bowel segments to allow flow from one to the other.

aneurysm. Circumscribed dilation or outpouching of an artery wall, often containing blood clots and connecting directly with the lumen of the artery.

arteriotomy. Incision into an artery.

autograft. Any tissue harvested from one anatomical site of a person and grafted to another anatomical site of the same person. Most commonly, blood vessels, skin, tendons, fascia, and bone are used as autografts.

graft. Tissue implant from another part of the body or another person.

pericardium. Thin and slippery case in which the heart lies that is lined with fluid so that the heart is free to pulse and move as it beats.

35901

35901 Excision of infected graft; neck

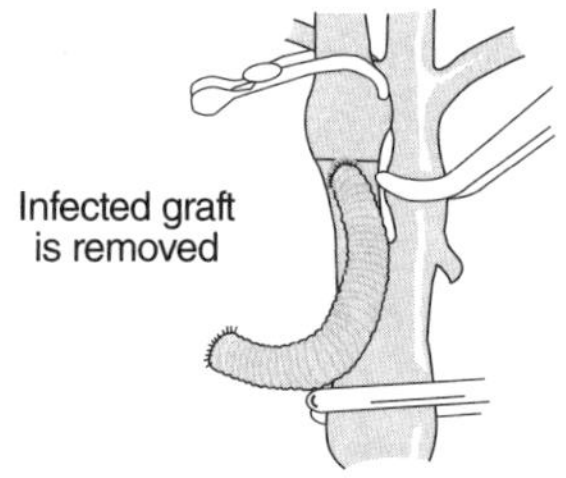

The physician removes an infected graft from the neck and repairs the blood vessel

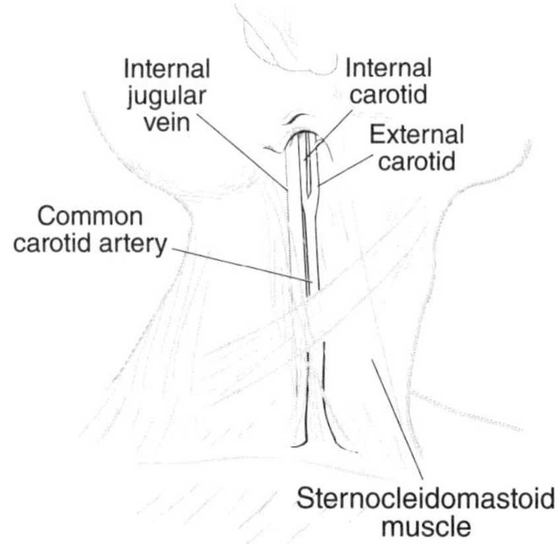

Explanation

Through an incision in the skin of the neck overlying the graft, the physician dissects around any muscle, vessels, or other structures to access the graft site. The physician dissects around the vessel, and applies vessel clamps above and below the graft. The physician excises above and below the existing infected graft. The blood vessel is repaired with sutures. A catheter may be left in place to help drain infection. The skin is loosely closed. If the excised graft is replaced with a new graft, report the appropriate revascularization code.

Coding Tips

Establishing both inflow and outflow by any method is included. That portion of the operative arteriogram performed by the surgeon is also included. Angioscopy performed during therapeutic intervention should be reported in addition to the code for the primary procedure; see 35400. For a thrombectomy of an arterial or venous graft, see 35875–35876. For an initial placement of a bypass graft using a vein, see 35501–35571. For an initial placement of a bypass graft other than vein, see 35601–35681.

ICD-10-CM Diagnostic Codes

T82.7XXA Infection and inflammatory reaction due to other cardiac and vascular devices, implants and grafts, initial encounter

AMA: 35901 2018,Aug

Relative Value Units/Medicare Edits

Non-Facility RVU	Work	PE	MP	Total
35901	8.38	3.61	2.08	14.07
Facility RVU	**Work**	**PE**	**MP**	**Total**
35901	8.38	3.61	2.08	14.07

	FUD	Status	MUE	Modifiers				IOM Reference
35901	90	A	1(3)	51	N/A	62*	80	None

* with documentation

Terms To Know

angioscopy. Visualization of capillary blood vessels with a microscope, or the inside of a blood vessel with a fiberoptic-equipped catheter.

arteriogram. Radiograph of arteries.

catheter. Flexible tube inserted into an area of the body for introducing or withdrawing fluid.

complication. Condition arising after the beginning of observation and treatment that modifies the course of the patient's illness or the medical care required, or an undesired result or misadventure in medical care.

excision. Surgical removal of an organ or tissue.

graft. Tissue implant from another part of the body or another person.

incision. Act of cutting into tissue or an organ.

infection. Presence of microorganisms in body tissues that may result in cellular damage.

revascularization. Restoration of blood flow and oxygen supply to a body part. This may apply to an extremity, the heart, or penis.

suture. Numerous stitching techniques employed in wound closure.

35903

35903 Excision of infected graft; extremity

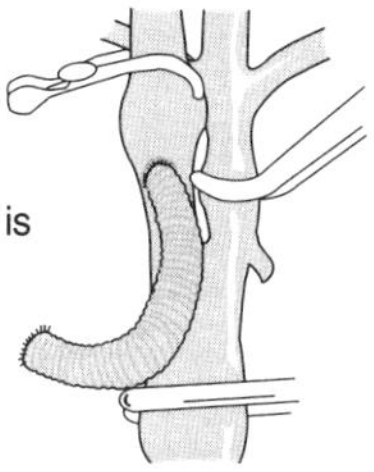

The physician removes an infected graft from an extremity and repairs the blood vessel

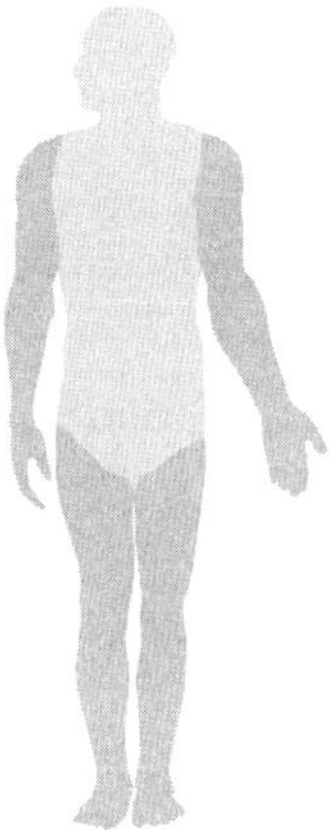

Explanation

Through an incision in the skin of the extremity overlying the graft, the physician dissects around any muscle, vessels or other structures to access the graft site. The physician dissects around the vessel, and applies vessel clamps above and below the graft. The physician excises above and below the existing infected graft. The blood vessel is repaired with sutures. A catheter may be left in place to help drain infection. The skin is loosely closed. If the excised graft is replaced with a new graft, report the appropriate revascularization code.

Coding Tips

Establishing both inflow and outflow by any method is included. That portion of the operative arteriogram performed by the surgeon is also included. Angioscopy performed during therapeutic intervention should be reported in addition to the code for the primary procedure, see 35400. For a thrombectomy of an arterial or venous graft, see 35875–35876. For an initial placement of a bypass graft using a vein, see 35501–35571. For an initial in-situ vein graft placement, see 35583–35587. For an initial placement of a bypass graft other than vein, see 35601–35681.

ICD-10-CM Diagnostic Codes

T81.41XA	Infection following a procedure, superficial incisional surgical site, initial encounter
T81.42XA	Infection following a procedure, deep incisional surgical site, initial encounter
T81.43XA	Infection following a procedure, organ and space surgical site, initial encounter
T81.44XA	Sepsis following a procedure, initial encounter
T81.49XA	Infection following a procedure, other surgical site, initial encounter

T82.7XXA Infection and inflammatory reaction due to other cardiac and vascular devices, implants and grafts, initial encounter

T88.8XXA Other specified complications of surgical and medical care, not elsewhere classified, initial encounter

AMA: 35903 2018,Aug

Relative Value Units/Medicare Edits

Non-Facility RVU	Work	PE	MP	Total
35903	9.53	4.75	2.36	16.64
Facility RVU	**Work**	**PE**	**MP**	**Total**
35903	9.53	4.75	2.36	16.64

	FUD	Status	MUE	Modifiers				IOM Reference
35903	90	A	2(3)	51	N/A	62*	80	None

* with documentation

Terms To Know

catheter. Flexible tube inserted into an area of the body for introducing or withdrawing fluid.

complication. Condition arising after the beginning of observation and treatment that modifies the course of the patient's illness or the medical care required, or an undesired result or misadventure in medical care.

excision. Surgical removal of an organ or tissue.

graft. Tissue implant from another part of the body or another person.

incision. Act of cutting into tissue or an organ.

infection. Presence of microorganisms in body tissues that may result in cellular damage.

suture. Numerous stitching techniques employed in wound closure.

buried suture. Continuous or interrupted suture placed under the skin for a layered closure.

continuous suture. Running stitch with tension evenly distributed across a single strand to provide a leakproof closure line.

interrupted suture. Series of single stitches with tension isolated at each stitch, in which all stitches are not affected if one becomes loose, and the isolated sutures cannot act as a wick to transport an infection.

purse-string suture. Continuous suture placed around a tubular structure and tightened, to reduce or close the lumen.

retention suture. Secondary stitching that bridges the primary suture, providing support for the primary repair; a plastic or rubber bolster may be placed over the primary repair and under the retention sutures.

35905

35905 Excision of infected graft; thorax

Explanation

Through an incision in the skin of the thorax overlying the graft, the physician dissects around any muscle, vessels or other structures to access the graft site. The physician dissects around the vessel, and applies vessel clamps above and below the graft. The physician excises above and below the existing infected graft. The blood vessel is repaired with sutures. A catheter may be left in place to help drain infection. The skin is loosely closed. If the excised graft is replaced with a new graft, report the appropriate revascularization code.

Coding Tips

Establishing both inflow and outflow by any method is included. That portion of the operative arteriogram performed by the surgeon is also included. Angioscopy performed during therapeutic intervention should be reported in addition to the code for the primary procedure; see 35400. For a thrombectomy of an arterial or a venous graft, see 35875–35876. For an initial placement of a bypass graft using a vein, see 35501–35571. For an initial placement of a bypass graft other than vein, see 35601–35681.

ICD-10-CM Diagnostic Codes

T82.7XXA Infection and inflammatory reaction due to other cardiac and vascular devices, implants and grafts, initial encounter

AMA: 35905 2018,Aug

Relative Value Units/Medicare Edits

Non-Facility RVU	Work	PE	MP	Total
35905	33.52	7.32	8.35	49.19
Facility RVU	**Work**	**PE**	**MP**	**Total**
35905	33.52	7.32	8.35	49.19

	FUD	Status	MUE	Modifiers				IOM Reference
35905	90	A	1(3)	51	N/A	62*	80	None

* with documentation

Terms To Know

angiography. Radiographic imaging of the arteries.

angioscopy. Visualization of capillary blood vessels with a microscope, or the inside of a blood vessel with a fiberoptic-equipped catheter.

excision. Surgical removal of an organ or tissue.

graft. Tissue implant from another part of the body or another person.

infection. Presence of microorganisms in body tissues that may result in cellular damage.

revascularize. Restoring blood flow or blood supply to a body part.

35907

35907 Excision of infected graft; abdomen

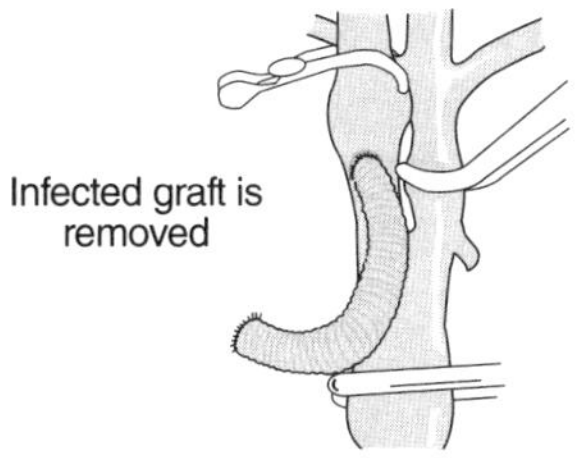

The physician removes an infected graft from the abdomen and repairs the blood vessel

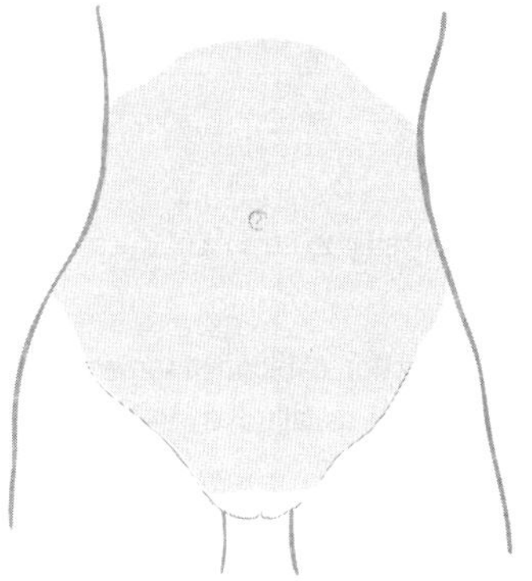

Explanation

Through an incision in the skin of the abdomen overlying the graft, the physician dissects around any muscle, vessels or other structures to access the graft site. The physician dissects around the vessel, and applies vessel clamps above and below the graft. The physician excises above and below the existing infected graft. The blood vessel is repaired with sutures. A catheter may be left in place to help drain infection. The skin is loosely closed. If the excised graft is replaced with a new graft, report the appropriate revascularization code.

Coding Tips

Establishing both inflow and outflow by any method is included. That portion of the operative arteriogram performed by the surgeon is also included. Angioscopy performed during therapeutic intervention should be reported in addition to the code for the primary procedure, see 35400. For a thrombectomy of an arterial or a venous graft, see 35875–35876. For an initial placement of a bypass graft using a vein, see 35501–35571. For an initial in-situ vein graft placement, see 35583–35587. For an initial placement of a bypass graft other than vein, see 35601–35681.

ICD-10-CM Diagnostic Codes

T81.44XA Sepsis following a procedure, initial encounter

T82.7XXA Infection and inflammatory reaction due to other cardiac and vascular devices, implants and grafts, initial encounter

T82.898A Other specified complication of vascular prosthetic devices, implants and grafts, initial encounter

AMA: 35907 2018,Aug

Relative Value Units/Medicare Edits

Non-Facility RVU	Work	PE	MP	Total
35907	37.27	9.32	9.29	55.88
Facility RVU	**Work**	**PE**	**MP**	**Total**
35907	37.27	9.32	9.29	55.88

	FUD	Status	MUE	Modifiers				IOM Reference
35907	90	A	1(3)	51	N/A	62*	80	None

* with documentation

Terms To Know

catheter. Flexible tube inserted into an area of the body for introducing or withdrawing fluid.

complication. Condition arising after the beginning of observation and treatment that modifies the course of the patient's illness or the medical care required, or an undesired result or misadventure in medical care.

excision. Surgical removal of an organ or tissue.

graft. Tissue implant from another part of the body or another person.

incision. Act of cutting into tissue or an organ.

infection. Presence of microorganisms in body tissues that may result in cellular damage.

suture. Numerous stitching techniques employed in wound closure.

buried suture. Continuous or interrupted suture placed under the skin for a layered closure.

continuous suture. Running stitch with tension evenly distributed across a single strand to provide a leakproof closure line.

interrupted suture. Series of single stitches with tension isolated at each stitch, in which all stitches are not affected if one becomes loose, and the isolated sutures cannot act as a wick to transport an infection.

purse-string suture. Continuous suture placed around a tubular structure and tightened, to reduce or close the lumen.

retention suture. Secondary stitching that bridges the primary suture, providing support for the primary repair; a plastic or rubber bolster may be placed over the primary repair and under the retention sutures.

36000-36005

36000 Introduction of needle or intracatheter, vein

36002 Injection procedures (eg, thrombin) for percutaneous treatment of extremity pseudoaneurysm

36005 Injection procedure for extremity venography (including introduction of needle or intracatheter)

Explanation

In 36000, the provider places a needle or a catheter through a puncture in the skin and into a peripheral vein. In 36002, the physician or other qualified health care provider injects a pseudoaneurysm, which is a pulsatile hematoma with a fibrous capsule that maintains persistent communication with the adjacent vessel. The vessel wall does not heal and blood flows back and forth between the vessel and hematoma during the cardiac cycle. Under ultrasound control, the physician advances a 22-gauge needle into the lumen of the pseudoaneurysm and injects thrombin to cause thrombosis of the pseudoaneurysm. In 36005, an opaque substance is injected through the catheter for venography. Once the procedure is complete, the catheter is removed and pressure is applied to stop bleeding at the injection site.

Coding Tips

Report 36005 if the catheter is inserted for a venography and 36000 if the catheter is inserted for another purpose. These codes are often incorrectly used to report placement of a routine IV. These codes include local anesthesia, introduction of needles or catheter, injection of contrast material with or without automatic power injection, and/or necessary pre- and postinjection care. See CPT notes for additional guidelines. Supplies (catheters, drugs, and contrast media) are not included in the listed service for the injection procedures. For imaging guidance performed in addition to 36002, see 76942, 77002, 77012, or 77021. For ultrasound guided compression repair of pseudoaneurysms, see 76936. Do not report 36002 for vascular sealant of an arteriotomy site. For radiological supervision and interpretation performed in addition to 36005, see 75820 and 75822. For cardiac catheterizations and injection procedures performed in addition to cardiac catheterization, see 93452–93461, 93563–93569, and 93573–93575. Do not report 36005 with 36836 or 36837.

ICD-10-CM Diagnostic Codes

The application of this code is too broad to adequately present ICD-10-CM diagnostic code links here. Refer to your ICD-10-CM book.

AMA: 36000 2022,Jan; 2018,Mar **36002** 2023,Jan; 2018,Mar **36005** 2023,Mar; 2022,Oct; 2018,Mar

Relative Value Units/Medicare Edits

Non-Facility RVU	Work	PE	MP	Total
36000	0.18	0.73	0.02	0.93
36002	1.96	2.32	0.31	4.59
36005	0.95	6.37	0.16	7.48
Facility RVU	**Work**	**PE**	**MP**	**Total**
36000	0.18	0.07	0.02	0.27
36002	1.96	0.79	0.31	3.06
36005	0.95	0.28	0.16	1.39

	FUD	Status	MUE	Modifiers				IOM Reference
36000	N/A	B	4(3)	N/A	N/A	N/A	N/A	None
36002	0	A	2(3)	51	50	N/A	N/A	
36005	0	A	2(3)	51	50	N/A	80*	

* with documentation

Terms To Know

catheter. Flexible tube inserted into an area of the body for introducing or withdrawing fluid.

hematoma. Tumor-like collection of blood in some part of the body caused by a break in a blood vessel wall, usually as a result of trauma.

percutaneous. Through the skin.

pseudoaneurysm. False aneurysm produced by a dilated vessel wall, or a ruptured blood vessel that has formed a clot that pulsates, mimicking a true aneurysm.

supervision and interpretation. Radiology services that usually contain an invasive component and are reported by the radiologist for supervision of the procedure and the personnel involved with performing the examination, reading the film, and preparing the written report.

thrombosis. Condition arising from the presence or formation of blood clots within a blood vessel that may cause vascular obstruction and insufficient oxygenation.

ultrasound. Imaging using ultra-high sound frequency bounced off body structures.

vein. Vessel through which oxygen-depleted blood passes back to the heart.

venography. Radiographic study of the veins.

36010

36010 Introduction of catheter, superior or inferior vena cava

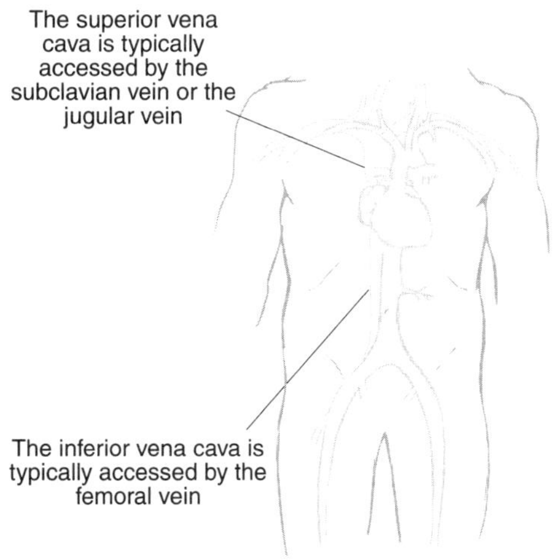

Explanation

The physician punctures a distal vein (typically antecubital, internal jugular, subclavian, or femoral) with a large needle and passes a guidewire via the needle into the punctured vein. The physician removes the needle while leaving the guidewire in place, and enlarges the skin opening slightly with a blade. The physician may slide an introducer sheath over the guidewire into the venous lumen, or may slide the catheter directly into the venous lumen without using an introducer sheath. If using an introducer sheath, the physician inserts the catheter into the vein through an O-ring in the introducer sheath (this prevents blood from leaking around the catheter) into the superior or inferior vena cava. The physician may check the catheter position with fluoroscope or with an x-ray.

Coding Tips

When medically necessary, report moderate (conscious) sedation provided by the performing physician with 99151-99153. When provided by another physician, report 99155-99157. Listed services for injection procedures include necessary local anesthesia, introduction of needles or catheter, injection of contrast material with or without automatic power injection, and/or necessary pre- and postinjection care specifically related to the injection procedure. Supplies (catheters, drugs, and contrast media) are not included in the listed service for the injection procedures. For radiology supervision and interpretation, see 75825–75827. For introduction of catheter, right heart or main pulmonary artery, see 36013; aorta, see 36200. For other cardiac catheterizations and injection procedures performed in addition to cardiac catheterization, see 93452–93461 and 93563–93568.

ICD-10-CM Diagnostic Codes

I26.01	Septic pulmonary embolism with acute cor pulmonale
I26.09	Other pulmonary embolism with acute cor pulmonale
I26.90	Septic pulmonary embolism without acute cor pulmonale
I26.99	Other pulmonary embolism without acute cor pulmonale
I27.0	Primary pulmonary hypertension
I27.20	Pulmonary hypertension, unspecified
I27.21	Secondary pulmonary arterial hypertension
I27.22	Pulmonary hypertension due to left heart disease
I27.23	Pulmonary hypertension due to lung diseases and hypoxia
I27.24	Chronic thromboembolic pulmonary hypertension
I27.29	Other secondary pulmonary hypertension
I27.82	Chronic pulmonary embolism
I27.83	Eisenmenger's syndrome
I27.89	Other specified pulmonary heart diseases
I80.11	Phlebitis and thrombophlebitis of right femoral vein ☑
I80.12	Phlebitis and thrombophlebitis of left femoral vein ☑
I80.13	Phlebitis and thrombophlebitis of femoral vein, bilateral ☑
I82.210	Acute embolism and thrombosis of superior vena cava
I82.211	Chronic embolism and thrombosis of superior vena cava
I82.220	Acute embolism and thrombosis of inferior vena cava
I82.221	Chronic embolism and thrombosis of inferior vena cava
I82.3	Embolism and thrombosis of renal vein
I82.411	Acute embolism and thrombosis of right femoral vein ☑
I82.412	Acute embolism and thrombosis of left femoral vein ☑
I82.413	Acute embolism and thrombosis of femoral vein, bilateral ☑
I82.511	Chronic embolism and thrombosis of right femoral vein ☑
I82.512	Chronic embolism and thrombosis of left femoral vein ☑
I82.513	Chronic embolism and thrombosis of femoral vein, bilateral ☑
I87.1	Compression of vein
I87.8	Other specified disorders of veins
N18.4	Chronic kidney disease, stage 4 (severe)
N18.5	Chronic kidney disease, stage 5
N18.6	End stage renal disease

AMA: 36010 2018,Oct

Relative Value Units/Medicare Edits

Non-Facility RVU	Work	PE	MP	Total
36010	2.18	13.32	0.4	15.9
Facility RVU	**Work**	**PE**	**MP**	**Total**
36010	2.18	0.59	0.4	3.17

	FUD	Status	MUE	Modifiers				IOM Reference
36010	N/A	A	2(3)	51	50	N/A	N/A	None

* with documentation

Terms To Know

catheter. Flexible tube inserted into an area of the body for introducing or withdrawing fluid.

fluoroscopy. Radiology technique that allows visual examination of part of the body or a function of an organ using a device that projects an x-ray image on a fluorescent screen.

guidewire. Flexible metal instrument designed to lead another instrument in its proper course.

36011-36012

36011 Selective catheter placement, venous system; first order branch (eg, renal vein, jugular vein)

36012 second order, or more selective, branch (eg, left adrenal vein, petrosal sinus)

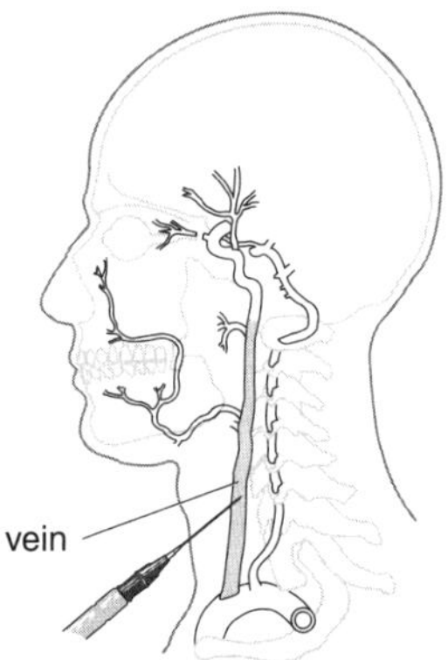

Explanation

Through a puncture through the skin, the physician passes a needle into the vein and threads a guidewire through the needle into the vein. The needle is removed and the wire is passed to the desired location in the venous system. A catheter follows the wire into the selected point in the vein and the wire is removed. A first order branch from the vena cava (36011) is any initial vessel draining directly into the vena cava (e.g., renal vein or jugular vein). A second order branch of the vena cava (36012) is any vein draining into a first order branch (e.g., left adrenal, petrosal sinus). Contrast material for venography is injected into the catheter that has traveled to an area upstream of the site under investigation. Once the procedure is complete, the catheter is removed, and pressure applied to stop bleeding at the injection site.

Coding Tips

These codes include local anesthesia, introduction of needles or catheter, injection of contrast material with or without automatic power injection, and/or necessary pre- and postinjection care specifically related to the injection performed by the physician. Supplies (catheters, drugs, and contrast media) are not included in the listed service for the injection procedures. For chemotherapy of malignant disease, see 96401–96549. For an injection procedure in addition to cardiac catheterization, see 93452–93461 and 93563–93568. For radiological supervision and interpretation of the venography, see 75820–75891. Named or unnamed venous branches beyond a second-order branch should be reported with 36012.

ICD-10-CM Diagnostic Codes

I15.0	Renovascular hypertension
I15.1	Hypertension secondary to other renal disorders
I16.0	Hypertensive urgency
I16.1	Hypertensive emergency
I82.3	Embolism and thrombosis of renal vein
I82.C11	Acute embolism and thrombosis of right internal jugular vein ☑
I82.C12	Acute embolism and thrombosis of left internal jugular vein ☑
I82.C13	Acute embolism and thrombosis of internal jugular vein, bilateral ☑
I82.C21	Chronic embolism and thrombosis of right internal jugular vein ☑
I82.C22	Chronic embolism and thrombosis of left internal jugular vein ☑
I82.C23	Chronic embolism and thrombosis of internal jugular vein, bilateral ☑
I87.1	Compression of vein
I87.2	Venous insufficiency (chronic) (peripheral)
I87.8	Other specified disorders of veins

AMA: 36011 2018,Oct **36012** 2018,Oct

Relative Value Units/Medicare Edits

Non-Facility RVU	Work	PE	MP	Total
36011	3.14	19.86	0.52	23.52
36012	3.51	20.48	0.57	24.56
Facility RVU	**Work**	**PE**	**MP**	**Total**
36011	3.14	0.89	0.52	4.55
36012	3.51	0.99	0.57	5.07

	FUD	Status	MUE	Modifiers				IOM Reference
36011	N/A	A	4(3)	51	50	N/A	N/A	None
36012	N/A	A	4(3)	51	50	N/A	N/A	

* with documentation

Terms To Know

catheter. Flexible tube inserted into an area of the body for introducing or withdrawing fluid.

contrast material. Radiopaque substance placed into the body to enable a system or body structure to be visualized, such as nonionic and low osmolar contrast media (LOCM), ionic and high osmolar contrast media (HOCM), barium, and gadolinium.

guidewire. Flexible metal instrument designed to lead another instrument in its proper course.

implantable venous access device. Catheter implanted for continuous access to the venous system for long-term parenteral feeding or for the administration of fluids or medications.

vein. Vessel through which oxygen-depleted blood passes back to the heart.

vena cava. Main venous trunk that empties into the right atrium from both the lower and upper regions, beginning at the junction of the common iliac veins inferiorly and the two brachiocephalic veins superiorly.

venography. Radiographic study of the veins.

36013

36013 Introduction of catheter, right heart or main pulmonary artery

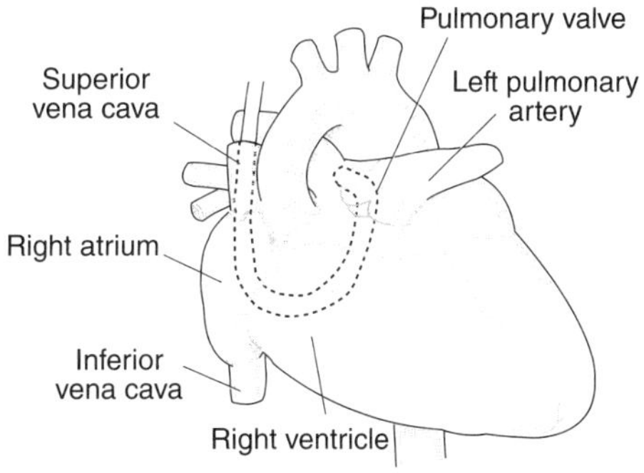

Introduction of a catheter into the right side of the heart or into the main pulmonary artery

Explanation

The physician punctures a distal vein (typically antecubital, internal jugular, subclavian, or femoral) with a large needle and passes a guidewire via the needle into the punctured vein. The physician removes the needle while leaving the guidewire in place, and enlarges the skin opening slightly with a blade. The physician slides an introducer sheath over the guidewire into the venous lumen. The physician inserts the catheter into the vein through an O-ring in the introducer sheath (this prevents blood from leaking around the catheter) and advances the catheter into the right heart or main pulmonary artery, using fluoroscopic guidance or while measuring pressures through the catheter lumen to ensure that the catheter tip is in the desired place. The physician may use the catheter to inject contrast material to perform venography or pulmonary arteriography.

Coding Tips

Listed services for injection procedures include necessary local anesthesia, introduction of needles or catheter, injection of contrast material with or without automatic power injection, and/or necessary pre- and postinjection care specifically related to the injection procedure. Catheters, drugs, and contrast media are not included in the listed service for the injection procedures. For radiology supervision and interpretation, see 75741–75746. For introduction of catheter, superior or inferior vena cava, see 36010; aorta, see 36200. For other cardiac catheterizations and injection procedures in addition to cardiac catheterization, see 93452–93461 and 93563–93568.

ICD-10-CM Diagnostic Codes

I05.0	Rheumatic mitral stenosis
I05.1	Rheumatic mitral insufficiency
I05.2	Rheumatic mitral stenosis with insufficiency
I05.8	Other rheumatic mitral valve diseases
I08.0	Rheumatic disorders of both mitral and aortic valves
I08.1	Rheumatic disorders of both mitral and tricuspid valves
I08.2	Rheumatic disorders of both aortic and tricuspid valves
I08.3	Combined rheumatic disorders of mitral, aortic and tricuspid valves
I08.8	Other rheumatic multiple valve diseases
I25.3	Aneurysm of heart
I25.89	Other forms of chronic ischemic heart disease
I27.0	Primary pulmonary hypertension
I27.21	Secondary pulmonary arterial hypertension
I27.22	Pulmonary hypertension due to left heart disease
I27.23	Pulmonary hypertension due to lung diseases and hypoxia
I27.24	Chronic thromboembolic pulmonary hypertension
I27.29	Other secondary pulmonary hypertension
I27.82	Chronic pulmonary embolism
I27.83	Eisenmenger's syndrome
I27.89	Other specified pulmonary heart diseases
I28.0	Arteriovenous fistula of pulmonary vessels
I28.1	Aneurysm of pulmonary artery
I28.8	Other diseases of pulmonary vessels
I34.0	Nonrheumatic mitral (valve) insufficiency
I34.1	Nonrheumatic mitral (valve) prolapse
I34.2	Nonrheumatic mitral (valve) stenosis
I37.0	Nonrheumatic pulmonary valve stenosis
I37.1	Nonrheumatic pulmonary valve insufficiency
I37.2	Nonrheumatic pulmonary valve stenosis with insufficiency
I37.8	Other nonrheumatic pulmonary valve disorders
I42.0	Dilated cardiomyopathy
I42.1	Obstructive hypertrophic cardiomyopathy
I42.2	Other hypertrophic cardiomyopathy
I42.5	Other restrictive cardiomyopathy
I42.6	Alcoholic cardiomyopathy
I42.7	Cardiomyopathy due to drug and external agent
I42.8	Other cardiomyopathies
I50.1	Left ventricular failure, unspecified
I50.21	Acute systolic (congestive) heart failure
I50.22	Chronic systolic (congestive) heart failure
I50.23	Acute on chronic systolic (congestive) heart failure
I50.31	Acute diastolic (congestive) heart failure
I50.32	Chronic diastolic (congestive) heart failure
I50.33	Acute on chronic diastolic (congestive) heart failure
I50.41	Acute combined systolic (congestive) and diastolic (congestive) heart failure
I50.42	Chronic combined systolic (congestive) and diastolic (congestive) heart failure
I50.43	Acute on chronic combined systolic (congestive) and diastolic (congestive) heart failure
I50.811	Acute right heart failure
I50.812	Chronic right heart failure
I50.813	Acute on chronic right heart failure
I50.814	Right heart failure due to left heart failure
I50.82	Biventricular heart failure
I50.83	High output heart failure
I50.84	End stage heart failure
J81.0	Acute pulmonary edema
J81.1	Chronic pulmonary edema
Q21.0	Ventricular septal defect
Q21.11	Secundum atrial septal defect
Q21.12	Patent foramen ovale
Q21.13	Coronary sinus atrial septal defect
Q21.14	Superior sinus venosus atrial septal defect
Q21.15	Inferior sinus venosus atrial septal defect
Q21.3	Tetralogy of Fallot

Q21.4	Aortopulmonary septal defect
Q21.8	Other congenital malformations of cardiac septa
Q22.0	Pulmonary valve atresia
Q22.1	Congenital pulmonary valve stenosis
Q22.2	Congenital pulmonary valve insufficiency
Q22.3	Other congenital malformations of pulmonary valve
Q22.4	Congenital tricuspid stenosis
Q22.5	Ebstein's anomaly
Q22.6	Hypoplastic right heart syndrome
Q22.8	Other congenital malformations of tricuspid valve
Q23.0	Congenital stenosis of aortic valve
Q23.1	Congenital insufficiency of aortic valve
Q23.2	Congenital mitral stenosis
Q23.3	Congenital mitral insufficiency
Q23.4	Hypoplastic left heart syndrome
Q24.3	Pulmonary infundibular stenosis
Q24.8	Other specified congenital malformations of heart
R57.0	Cardiogenic shock

AMA: 36013 2019,Jun

Relative Value Units/Medicare Edits

Non-Facility RVU	Work	PE	MP	Total
36013	2.52	20.12	0.35	22.99
Facility RVU	**Work**	**PE**	**MP**	**Total**
36013	2.52	0.8	0.35	3.67

	FUD	Status	MUE	Modifiers				IOM Reference
36013	N/A	A	2(3)	51	N/A	N/A	N/A	None

* with documentation

Terms To Know

implantable venous access device. Catheter implanted for continuous access to the venous system for long-term parenteral feeding or for the administration of fluids or medications.

tetralogy of Fallot. Specific combination of congenital cardiac defects: obstruction of the right ventricular outflow tract with pulmonary stenosis, interventricular septal defect, malposition of the aorta, overriding the interventricular septum and receiving blood from both the venous and arterial systems, and enlargement of the right ventricle.

ventricular septal defect. Congenital cardiac anomaly resulting in a continual opening in the septum between the ventricles that, in severe cases, causes oxygenated blood to flow back into the lungs, resulting in pulmonary hypertension.

36014-36015

36014 Selective catheter placement, left or right pulmonary artery

36015 Selective catheter placement, segmental or subsegmental pulmonary artery

Introduction through to the right pulmonary artery shown

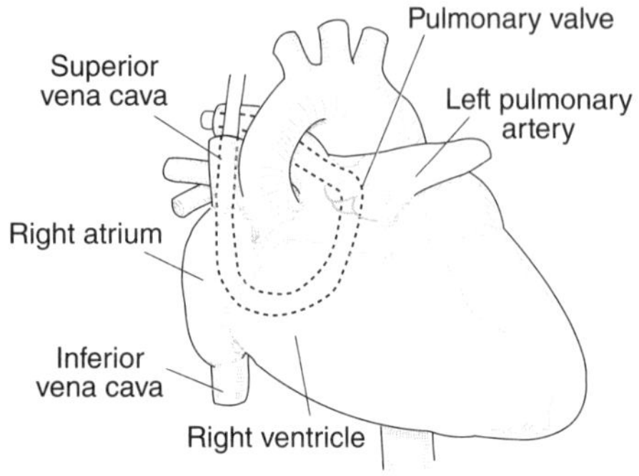

Explanation

The physician punctures a distal vein (typically antecubital, internal jugular, subclavian, or femoral) with a large needle and passes a guidewire via the needle into the punctured vein. The physician removes the needle while leaving the guidewire in place, and enlarges the skin opening slightly with a blade. The physician slides an introducer sheath over the guidewire into the venous lumen. The physician inserts the catheter into the vein through an O-ring in the introducer sheath (this prevents blood from leaking around the catheter) and advances the catheter into one of the main pulmonary arteries (right or left) in 36014 or into one of the segmental or subsegmental pulmonary arteries in 36015, using fluoroscopic guidance and possibly measuring pressures through the catheter lumen to ensure that the catheter tip is in the desired place. The physician may use the catheter to inject contrast material to perform venography or pulmonary arteriography.

Coding Tips

Placement of a CVP line and/or a Swan-Ganz catheter may be reported separately when placed at a different site than the intra-pulmonary catheter for 36014. For an insertion of a flow directed catheter (e.g., Swan-Ganz), see 93503. Listed services for injection procedures include necessary local anesthesia, introduction of needles or catheter, injection of contrast material with or without automatic power injection, and/or necessary pre- and post-injection care specifically related to the injection procedure. Supplies (catheters, drugs, and contrast media) are not included in the listed service for the injection procedures. For venous catheterization for selective organ blood sampling, see 36500. For cardiac catheterizations, injection procedures in addition to cardiac catheterization, see 93452–93461 and 93563–93568.

ICD-10-CM Diagnostic Codes

C34.01	Malignant neoplasm of right main bronchus ☑
C34.02	Malignant neoplasm of left main bronchus ☑
C34.11	Malignant neoplasm of upper lobe, right bronchus or lung ☑
C34.12	Malignant neoplasm of upper lobe, left bronchus or lung ☑
C34.2	Malignant neoplasm of middle lobe, bronchus or lung
C34.31	Malignant neoplasm of lower lobe, right bronchus or lung ☑
C34.32	Malignant neoplasm of lower lobe, left bronchus or lung ☑
C34.81	Malignant neoplasm of overlapping sites of right bronchus and lung ☑

C34.82 Malignant neoplasm of overlapping sites of left bronchus and lung ☑
I26.01 Septic pulmonary embolism with acute cor pulmonale
I26.02 Saddle embolus of pulmonary artery with acute cor pulmonale
I26.09 Other pulmonary embolism with acute cor pulmonale
I26.90 Septic pulmonary embolism without acute cor pulmonale
I26.92 Saddle embolus of pulmonary artery without acute cor pulmonale
I26.93 Single subsegmental thrombotic pulmonary embolism without acute cor pulmonale
I26.94 Multiple subsegmental thrombotic pulmonary emboli without acute cor pulmonale
I26.99 Other pulmonary embolism without acute cor pulmonale
I27.0 Primary pulmonary hypertension
I27.21 Secondary pulmonary arterial hypertension
I27.22 Pulmonary hypertension due to left heart disease
I27.23 Pulmonary hypertension due to lung diseases and hypoxia
I27.24 Chronic thromboembolic pulmonary hypertension
I27.29 Other secondary pulmonary hypertension
I27.82 Chronic pulmonary embolism
I27.83 Eisenmenger's syndrome
I27.89 Other specified pulmonary heart diseases
I28.0 Arteriovenous fistula of pulmonary vessels
I28.1 Aneurysm of pulmonary artery
I28.8 Other diseases of pulmonary vessels
I31.4 Cardiac tamponade
I42.0 Dilated cardiomyopathy
I50.1 Left ventricular failure, unspecified
I50.21 Acute systolic (congestive) heart failure
I50.22 Chronic systolic (congestive) heart failure
I50.23 Acute on chronic systolic (congestive) heart failure
I50.31 Acute diastolic (congestive) heart failure
I50.32 Chronic diastolic (congestive) heart failure
I50.33 Acute on chronic diastolic (congestive) heart failure
I50.41 Acute combined systolic (congestive) and diastolic (congestive) heart failure
I50.42 Chronic combined systolic (congestive) and diastolic (congestive) heart failure
I50.43 Acute on chronic combined systolic (congestive) and diastolic (congestive) heart failure
I50.811 Acute right heart failure
I50.812 Chronic right heart failure
I50.813 Acute on chronic right heart failure
I50.814 Right heart failure due to left heart failure
I50.82 Biventricular heart failure
I50.83 High output heart failure
I50.84 End stage heart failure
J44.0 Chronic obstructive pulmonary disease with (acute) lower respiratory infection
J44.1 Chronic obstructive pulmonary disease with (acute) exacerbation
J44.81 Bronchiolitis obliterans and bronchiolitis obliterans syndrome
J4A.0 Restrictive allograft syndrome
J4A.8 Other chronic lung allograft dysfunction
J81.0 Acute pulmonary edema
J81.1 Chronic pulmonary edema
J90 Pleural effusion, not elsewhere classified
J91.0 Malignant pleural effusion
J91.8 Pleural effusion in other conditions classified elsewhere
J98.11 Atelectasis
J98.19 Other pulmonary collapse

AMA: 36014 2019,Jun; 2018,Oct **36015** 2019,Jun; 2018,Oct

Relative Value Units/Medicare Edits

Non-Facility RVU	Work	PE	MP	Total
36014	3.02	19.6	0.48	23.1
36015	3.51	20.86	0.44	24.81

Facility RVU	Work	PE	MP	Total
36014	3.02	0.91	0.48	4.41
36015	3.51	1.04	0.44	4.99

	FUD	Status	MUE	Modifiers				IOM Reference
36014	N/A	A	2(3)	51	50	N/A	N/A	None
36015	N/A	A	4(3)	51	50	N/A	N/A	

* with documentation

Terms To Know

catheter. Flexible tube inserted into an area of the body for introducing or withdrawing fluid.

contrast material. Radiopaque substance placed into the body to enable a system or body structure to be visualized, such as nonionic and low osmolar contrast media (LOCM), ionic and high osmolar contrast media (HOCM), barium, and gadolinium.

distal. *1)* Located farther away from a specified reference point or the trunk. *2)* Pertaining to the area farthest from the center of the body or the point of origin.

guidewire. Flexible metal instrument designed to lead another instrument in its proper course.

introducer. Instrument, such as a catheter, needle, or tube, through which another instrument or device is introduced into the body.

36100

36100 Introduction of needle or intracatheter, carotid or vertebral artery

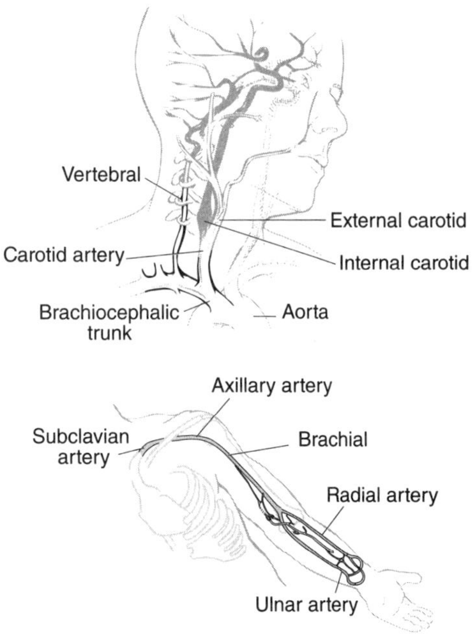

Explanation

Through the skin of the neck, the physician inserts a needle into the carotid or vertebral artery. A guidewire is threaded through the needle into the artery and the needle is removed. A catheter follows the wire into the artery. The wire is removed. Contrast material is injected through the catheter into the artery for arteriography. Once the procedure is complete, the catheter is removed and pressure is applied to the puncture site to stop bleeding.

Coding Tips

Note that 36100 is a unilateral procedure. If performed bilaterally, some payers require that the service be reported twice with modifier 50 appended to the second code, while others require identification of the service only once with modifier 50 appended. Check with individual payers. Modifier 50 identifies a procedure performed identically on the opposite side of the body (mirror image). These codes include local anesthesia, introduction of needles or catheter, injection of contrast material with or without automatic power injection, and/or necessary pre- and postinjection care specifically related to the injection. Supplies (catheters, drugs, and contrast media) are not included in the listed service. For introduction of a needle or intracatheter, vein, see 36000; extremity artery, see 36140; and aortic translumbar, see 36160.

ICD-10-CM Diagnostic Codes

G45.0 Vertebro-basilar artery syndrome
G45.1 Carotid artery syndrome (hemispheric)
G45.8 Other transient cerebral ischemic attacks and related syndromes
G45.9 Transient cerebral ischemic attack, unspecified
I63.011 Cerebral infarction due to thrombosis of right vertebral artery ☑
I63.012 Cerebral infarction due to thrombosis of left vertebral artery ☑
I63.013 Cerebral infarction due to thrombosis of bilateral vertebral arteries ☑
I63.031 Cerebral infarction due to thrombosis of right carotid artery ☑
I63.032 Cerebral infarction due to thrombosis of left carotid artery ☑
I63.033 Cerebral infarction due to thrombosis of bilateral carotid arteries ☑
I63.111 Cerebral infarction due to embolism of right vertebral artery ☑
I63.112 Cerebral infarction due to embolism of left vertebral artery ☑
I63.113 Cerebral infarction due to embolism of bilateral vertebral arteries ☑
I63.131 Cerebral infarction due to embolism of right carotid artery ☑
I63.132 Cerebral infarction due to embolism of left carotid artery ☑
I63.133 Cerebral infarction due to embolism of bilateral carotid arteries ☑
I63.89 Other cerebral infarction
I65.01 Occlusion and stenosis of right vertebral artery ☑
I65.02 Occlusion and stenosis of left vertebral artery ☑
I65.03 Occlusion and stenosis of bilateral vertebral arteries ☑
I65.21 Occlusion and stenosis of right carotid artery ☑
I65.22 Occlusion and stenosis of left carotid artery ☑
I65.23 Occlusion and stenosis of bilateral carotid arteries ☑
I67.81 Acute cerebrovascular insufficiency
I67.82 Cerebral ischemia
I67.850 Cerebral autosomal dominant arteriopathy with subcortical infarcts and leukoencephalopathy
I67.858 Other hereditary cerebrovascular disease
I72.0 Aneurysm of carotid artery
I76 Septic arterial embolism
I77.1 Stricture of artery
I77.2 Rupture of artery
I77.71 Dissection of carotid artery
I77.74 Dissection of vertebral artery

Relative Value Units/Medicare Edits

Non-Facility RVU	Work	PE	MP	Total
36100	3.02	12.06	0.73	15.81
Facility RVU	**Work**	**PE**	**MP**	**Total**
36100	3.02	0.7	0.73	4.45

	FUD	Status	MUE	Modifiers				IOM Reference
36100	N/A	A	2(3)	51	50	N/A	N/A	None

* with documentation

Terms To Know

aortic arch. Thoracic aorta, ascending/arch.

arteriogram. Radiograph of arteries.

catheter. Flexible tube inserted into an area of the body for introducing or withdrawing fluid.

contrast material. Radiopaque substance placed into the body to enable a system or body structure to be visualized, such as nonionic and low osmolar contrast media (LOCM), ionic and high osmolar contrast media (HOCM), barium, and gadolinium.

guidewire. Flexible metal instrument designed to lead another instrument in its proper course.

36140

36140 Introduction of needle or intracatheter, upper or lower extremity artery

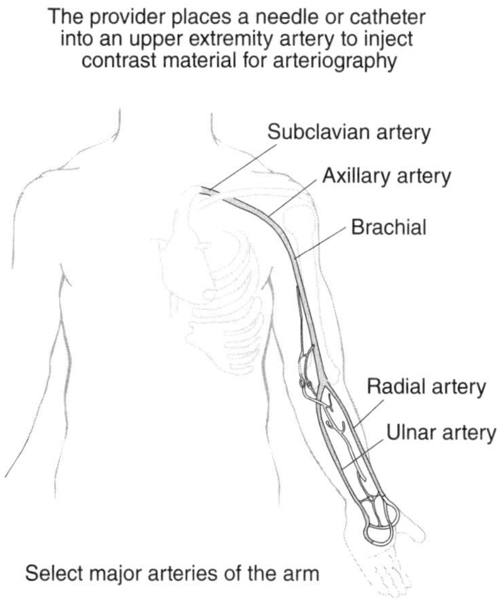

Explanation

Through a puncture in the skin over an upper or lower extremity artery, the physician injects a needle into the artery and threads a guidewire through it. The needle is removed. A catheter follows the wire into the artery and the wire is removed. Contrast material for arteriography is injected into the catheter placed upstream of the site under investigation. Once the procedure is complete, the catheter is removed and pressure is applied to stop bleeding at the injection site.

Coding Tips

When medically necessary, report moderate (conscious) sedation provided by the performing physician with 99151-99153. When provided by another physician, report 99155-99157. Note that 36140 includes local anesthesia, introduction of needles or catheter, injection of contrast material with or without automatic power injection, and/or necessary pre- and postinjection care specifically related to the injection. Supplies (catheters, drugs, and contrast media) are not included in this procedure. For introduction of a needle or an intracatheter, vein, see 36000. Chemotherapy codes are reported in addition to intracatheter placements. For an injection procedure in addition to cardiac catheterization, see 93452–93461 and 93563–93568. For radiological supervision and interpretation, see 75710 or 75716. For insertion of an arteriovenous cannula, see 36810–36821. Do not report 36140 with 36836 or 36837.

ICD-10-CM Diagnostic Codes

I70.211 Atherosclerosis of native arteries of extremities with intermittent claudication, right leg A ☑
I70.218 Atherosclerosis of native arteries of extremities with intermittent claudication, other extremity A
I70.221 Atherosclerosis of native arteries of extremities with rest pain, right leg A ☑
I70.228 Atherosclerosis of native arteries of extremities with rest pain, other extremity A
I70.231 Atherosclerosis of native arteries of right leg with ulceration of thigh A ☑
I70.232 Atherosclerosis of native arteries of right leg with ulceration of calf A ☑
I70.233 Atherosclerosis of native arteries of right leg with ulceration of ankle A ☑
I70.234 Atherosclerosis of native arteries of right leg with ulceration of heel and midfoot A ☑
I70.261 Atherosclerosis of native arteries of extremities with gangrene, right leg A ☑
I70.268 Atherosclerosis of native arteries of extremities with gangrene, other extremity A
I70.411 Atherosclerosis of autologous vein bypass graft(s) of the extremities with intermittent claudication, right leg A ☑
I70.418 Atherosclerosis of autologous vein bypass graft(s) of the extremities with intermittent claudication, other extremity A
I70.421 Atherosclerosis of autologous vein bypass graft(s) of the extremities with rest pain, right leg A ☑
I70.428 Atherosclerosis of autologous vein bypass graft(s) of the extremities with rest pain, other extremity A
I70.431 Atherosclerosis of autologous vein bypass graft(s) of the right leg with ulceration of thigh A ☑
I70.432 Atherosclerosis of autologous vein bypass graft(s) of the right leg with ulceration of calf A ☑
I70.433 Atherosclerosis of autologous vein bypass graft(s) of the right leg with ulceration of ankle A ☑
I70.434 Atherosclerosis of autologous vein bypass graft(s) of the right leg with ulceration of heel and midfoot A ☑
I70.435 Atherosclerosis of autologous vein bypass graft(s) of the right leg with ulceration of other part of foot A ☑
I70.438 Atherosclerosis of autologous vein bypass graft(s) of the right leg with ulceration of other part of lower leg A ☑
I70.461 Atherosclerosis of autologous vein bypass graft(s) of the extremities with gangrene, right leg A ☑
I70.468 Atherosclerosis of autologous vein bypass graft(s) of the extremities with gangrene, other extremity A
I70.491 Other atherosclerosis of autologous vein bypass graft(s) of the extremities, right leg A ☑
I70.498 Other atherosclerosis of autologous vein bypass graft(s) of the extremities, other extremity A
I70.511 Atherosclerosis of nonautologous biological bypass graft(s) of the extremities with intermittent claudication, right leg A ☑
I70.521 Atherosclerosis of nonautologous biological bypass graft(s) of the extremities with rest pain, right leg A ☑
I70.528 Atherosclerosis of nonautologous biological bypass graft(s) of the extremities with rest pain, other extremity A
I70.531 Atherosclerosis of nonautologous biological bypass graft(s) of the right leg with ulceration of thigh A ☑
I70.532 Atherosclerosis of nonautologous biological bypass graft(s) of the right leg with ulceration of calf A ☑
I70.533 Atherosclerosis of nonautologous biological bypass graft(s) of the right leg with ulceration of ankle A ☑
I70.534 Atherosclerosis of nonautologous biological bypass graft(s) of the right leg with ulceration of heel and midfoot A ☑
I70.535 Atherosclerosis of nonautologous biological bypass graft(s) of the right leg with ulceration of other part of foot A ☑
I70.538 Atherosclerosis of nonautologous biological bypass graft(s) of the right leg with ulceration of other part of lower leg A ☑

 ● New ▲ Revised + Add On ★ Telemedicine [Resequenced] ☑ Laterality

I70.561 Atherosclerosis of nonautologous biological bypass graft(s) of the extremities with gangrene, right leg A ☑

I70.568 Atherosclerosis of nonautologous biological bypass graft(s) of the extremities with gangrene, other extremity A

I70.591 Other atherosclerosis of nonautologous biological bypass graft(s) of the extremities, right leg A ☑

I70.598 Other atherosclerosis of nonautologous biological bypass graft(s) of the extremities, other extremity A

I70.611 Atherosclerosis of nonbiological bypass graft(s) of the extremities with intermittent claudication, right leg A ☑

I70.618 Atherosclerosis of nonbiological bypass graft(s) of the extremities with intermittent claudication, other extremity A

I70.621 Atherosclerosis of nonbiological bypass graft(s) of the extremities with rest pain, right leg A ☑

I70.628 Atherosclerosis of nonbiological bypass graft(s) of the extremities with rest pain, other extremity A

I70.631 Atherosclerosis of nonbiological bypass graft(s) of the right leg with ulceration of thigh A ☑

I70.632 Atherosclerosis of nonbiological bypass graft(s) of the right leg with ulceration of calf A ☑

I70.633 Atherosclerosis of nonbiological bypass graft(s) of the right leg with ulceration of ankle A ☑

I70.634 Atherosclerosis of nonbiological bypass graft(s) of the right leg with ulceration of heel and midfoot A ☑

I70.635 Atherosclerosis of nonbiological bypass graft(s) of the right leg with ulceration of other part of foot A ☑

I70.638 Atherosclerosis of nonbiological bypass graft(s) of the right leg with ulceration of other part of lower leg A ☑

I70.661 Atherosclerosis of nonbiological bypass graft(s) of the extremities with gangrene, right leg A ☑

I70.668 Atherosclerosis of nonbiological bypass graft(s) of the extremities with gangrene, other extremity A

I70.691 Other atherosclerosis of nonbiological bypass graft(s) of the extremities, right leg A ☑

I70.698 Other atherosclerosis of nonbiological bypass graft(s) of the extremities, other extremity A

I70.711 Atherosclerosis of other type of bypass graft(s) of the extremities with intermittent claudication, right leg A ☑

I70.718 Atherosclerosis of other type of bypass graft(s) of the extremities with intermittent claudication, other extremity A

I70.721 Atherosclerosis of other type of bypass graft(s) of the extremities with rest pain, right leg A ☑

I70.728 Atherosclerosis of other type of bypass graft(s) of the extremities with rest pain, other extremity A

I70.731 Atherosclerosis of other type of bypass graft(s) of the right leg with ulceration of thigh A ☑

I70.732 Atherosclerosis of other type of bypass graft(s) of the right leg with ulceration of calf A ☑

I70.733 Atherosclerosis of other type of bypass graft(s) of the right leg with ulceration of ankle A ☑

I70.734 Atherosclerosis of other type of bypass graft(s) of the right leg with ulceration of heel and midfoot A ☑

I70.761 Atherosclerosis of other type of bypass graft(s) of the extremities with gangrene, right leg A ☑

I70.768 Atherosclerosis of other type of bypass graft(s) of the extremities with gangrene, other extremity A

I70.791 Other atherosclerosis of other type of bypass graft(s) of the extremities, right leg A ☑

I70.798 Other atherosclerosis of other type of bypass graft(s) of the extremities, other extremity A

I70.92 Chronic total occlusion of artery of the extremities A

I74.2 Embolism and thrombosis of arteries of the upper extremities

I74.3 Embolism and thrombosis of arteries of the lower extremities

I75.011 Atheroembolism of right upper extremity ☑

I75.021 Atheroembolism of right lower extremity ☑

I77.1 Stricture of artery

I77.2 Rupture of artery

AMA: 36140 2023,Mar; 2022,Oct

Relative Value Units/Medicare Edits

Non-Facility RVU	Work	PE	MP	Total
36140	1.76	12.97	0.36	15.09
Facility RVU	**Work**	**PE**	**MP**	**Total**
36140	1.76	0.48	0.36	2.6

	FUD	Status	MUE	Modifiers				IOM Reference
36140	N/A	A	3(3)	51	N/A	N/A	N/A	None

* with documentation

Terms To Know

arteriography. Radiologic study of an artery upon injection of dye.

catheter. Flexible tube inserted into an area of the body for introducing or withdrawing fluid.

36160

36160 Introduction of needle or intracatheter, aortic, translumbar

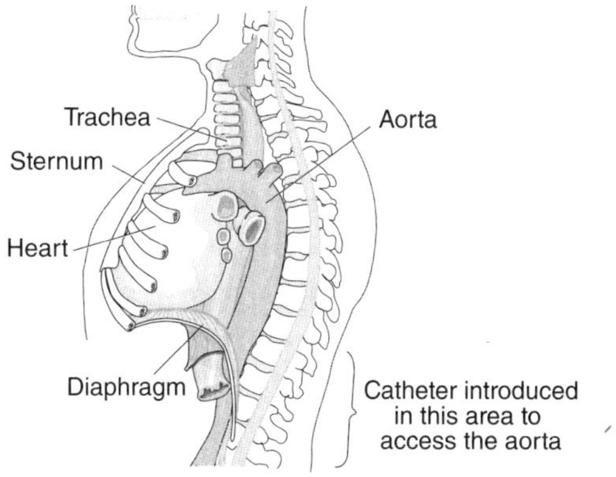

Explanation

The physician punctures the left lumbar area, typically just above a rib, to direct a large needle into the aorta. When pulsatile red blood is obtained through the needle, indicating successful aortic puncture, the physician passes a guidewire via the needle into the punctured aorta. The physician removes the needle while leaving the guidewire in place, and enlarges the skin opening slightly with a blade. The physician slides a catheter over the guidewire into the aortic lumen and secures the catheter in place with suture.

Coding Tips

This code includes local anesthesia, introduction of needles or catheter, injection of contrast material with or without automatic power injection, and/or necessary pre- and postinjection care specifically related to the injection. Other catheters, drugs, and contrast media are not included in the listed service. For introduction of needle or intracatheter, vein, see 36000; carotid or vertebral artery, see 36100; extremity artery, see 36140; chemotherapy of a malignant disease, see 96401–96549; an injection procedure in addition to cardiac catheterization, see 93452–93461 and 93563–93568.

ICD-10-CM Diagnostic Codes

A52.01	Syphilitic aneurysm of aorta
A52.02	Syphilitic aortitis
I70.0	Atherosclerosis of aorta Ⓐ
I71.02	Dissection of abdominal aorta
I71.03	Dissection of thoracoabdominal aorta
I71.11	Aneurysm of the ascending aorta, ruptured
I71.12	Aneurysm of the aortic arch, ruptured
I71.13	Aneurysm of the descending thoracic aorta, ruptured
I71.21	Aneurysm of the ascending aorta, without rupture
I71.22	Aneurysm of the aortic arch, without rupture
I71.23	Aneurysm of the descending thoracic aorta, without rupture
I71.51	Supraceliac aneurysm of the thoracoabdominal aorta, ruptured
I71.52	Paravisceral aneurysm of the thoracoabdominal aorta, ruptured
I71.61	Supraceliac aneurysm of the thoracoabdominal aorta, without rupture
I71.62	Paravisceral aneurysm of the thoracoabdominal aorta, without rupture
I74.01	Saddle embolus of abdominal aorta
I74.09	Other arterial embolism and thrombosis of abdominal aorta
I74.11	Embolism and thrombosis of thoracic aorta
I74.19	Embolism and thrombosis of other parts of aorta
I76	Septic arterial embolism
I77.1	Stricture of artery
I77.2	Rupture of artery
I77.3	Arterial fibromuscular dysplasia
I77.5	Necrosis of artery
I77.810	Thoracic aortic ectasia
I77.811	Abdominal aortic ectasia
I77.812	Thoracoabdominal aortic ectasia
I77.89	Other specified disorders of arteries and arterioles
I79.0	Aneurysm of aorta in diseases classified elsewhere
I79.1	Aortitis in diseases classified elsewhere
I79.8	Other disorders of arteries, arterioles and capillaries in diseases classified elsewhere

Relative Value Units/Medicare Edits

Non-Facility RVU	Work	PE	MP	Total
36160	2.52	13.41	0.35	16.28
Facility RVU	**Work**	**PE**	**MP**	**Total**
36160	2.52	0.72	0.35	3.59

	FUD	Status	MUE	Modifiers				IOM Reference
36160	N/A	A	2(3)	51	N/A	N/A	N/A	None

* with documentation

Terms To Know

aneurysm. Circumscribed dilation or outpouching of an artery wall, often containing blood clots and connecting directly with the lumen of the artery.

atherosclerosis. Buildup of yellowish plaques composed of cholesterol and lipoid material within the arteries.

catheter. Flexible tube inserted into an area of the body for introducing or withdrawing fluid.

guidewire. Flexible metal instrument designed to lead another instrument in its proper course.

lumen. Space inside an intestine, artery, vein, duct, or tube.

retrograde. Moving against the usual direction of flow.

rupture. Tearing or breaking open of tissue.

stricture. Narrowing of an anatomical structure.

36200

36200 Introduction of catheter, aorta

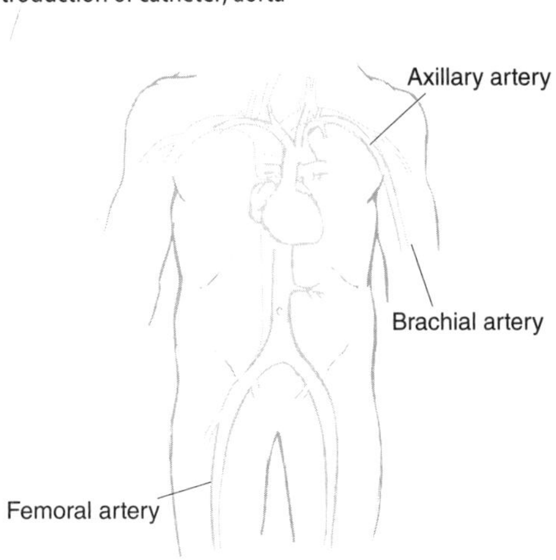

Explanation

The physician punctures a distal artery (typically femoral, brachial, radial, or axillary) with a large needle and passes a guidewire via the needle into the punctured artery. The physician removes the needle while leaving the guidewire in place, and enlarges the skin opening slightly with a blade. The physician slides an introducer sheath over the guidewire into the arterial lumen. The physician inserts a catheter into the artery through an O-ring in the introducer sheath (this prevents blood from leaking around the catheter) and advances the catheter into the aorta. The physician may use the catheter to inject contrast material to perform aortography, measure aortic pressures, or to administer medication.

Coding Tips

When medically necessary, report moderate (conscious) sedation provided by the performing physician with 99151-99153. When provided by another physician, report 99155-99157. Listed services for injection procedures include necessary local anesthesia, introduction of needles or catheter, injection of contrast material with or without automatic power injection, and/or necessary pre- and postinjection care specifically related to the injection procedure. Catheters, drugs, and contrast media are not included in the listed service for the injection procedures. For introduction of a catheter, superior or inferior vena cava, see 36010; for right heart or main artery, see 36013. For other cardiac catheterizations, injection procedures in addition to cardiac catheterization, see 93452–93461 and 93563–93568. For nonselective angiography of the extracranial carotid, cerebral vessels, and cervicocerebral arch, see 36221.

ICD-10-CM Diagnostic Codes

A52.01	Syphilitic aneurysm of aorta
A52.02	Syphilitic aortitis
I70.0	Atherosclerosis of aorta [A]
I70.211	Atherosclerosis of native arteries of extremities with intermittent claudication, right leg [A] ✓
I70.212	Atherosclerosis of native arteries of extremities with intermittent claudication, left leg [A] ✓
I70.221	Atherosclerosis of native arteries of extremities with rest pain, right leg [A] ✓
I70.222	Atherosclerosis of native arteries of extremities with rest pain, left leg [A] ✓
I74.01	Saddle embolus of abdominal aorta
I74.09	Other arterial embolism and thrombosis of abdominal aorta
I74.11	Embolism and thrombosis of thoracic aorta
I74.19	Embolism and thrombosis of other parts of aorta
I76	Septic arterial embolism
I77.1	Stricture of artery
I77.2	Rupture of artery
I77.3	Arterial fibromuscular dysplasia
I77.5	Necrosis of artery
I77.810	Thoracic aortic ectasia
I77.811	Abdominal aortic ectasia
I77.812	Thoracoabdominal aortic ectasia
I77.89	Other specified disorders of arteries and arterioles
I79.0	Aneurysm of aorta in diseases classified elsewhere
I79.1	Aortitis in diseases classified elsewhere
I79.8	Other disorders of arteries, arterioles and capillaries in diseases classified elsewhere

AMA: 36200 2023,Jun; 2021,Dec; 2021,Jul; 2018,Oct

Relative Value Units/Medicare Edits

Non-Facility RVU	Work	PE	MP	Total
36200	2.77	14.09	0.61	17.47
Facility RVU	**Work**	**PE**	**MP**	**Total**
36200	2.77	0.69	0.61	4.07

	FUD	Status	MUE	Modifiers				IOM Reference
36200	0	A	2(3)	51	50	N/A	N/A	None

* with documentation

Terms To Know

contrast material. Radiopaque substance placed into the body to enable a system or body structure to be visualized, such as nonionic and low osmolar contrast media (LOCM), ionic and high osmolar contrast media (HOCM), barium, and gadolinium.

embolism. Obstruction of a blood vessel resulting from a clot or foreign substance.

guidewire. Flexible metal instrument designed to lead another instrument in its proper course.

sheath. Covering enclosing an organ or part.

thrombus. Stationary blood clot inside a blood vessel.

36215-36216

36215 Selective catheter placement, arterial system; each first order thoracic or brachiocephalic branch, within a vascular family

36216 initial second order thoracic or brachiocephalic branch, within a vascular family

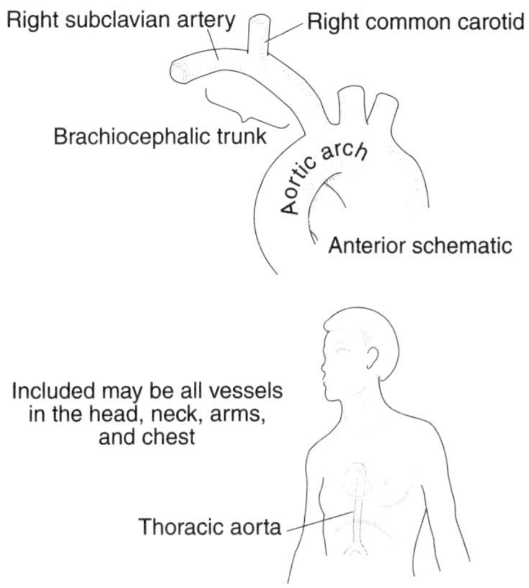

Explanation

The physician passes a needle into the skin into an extremity artery, usually in the upper thigh. A guidewire is threaded through the needle into the vessel. The needle is removed. The wire is threaded into the aorta and up to the thoracic aorta where it is manipulated into a branch off the aortic arch. A catheter follows the wire into a first order thoracic or brachiocephalic artery. The wire is removed. The catheter may pass through the first order vessel into a second order thoracic or brachiocephalic artery. Contrast material for arteriography is injected into the catheter that has been guided to an area upstream of the site under investigation. In 36215, the catheter remains in a first order artery. In 36216, the catheter travels further to a second order artery. Upon completion, the catheter is removed, and pressure applied to stop bleeding at the puncture site.

Coding Tips

These codes include introduction of needles or catheters, injection of contrast material with or without automatic power injection, and/or necessary pre- and postinjection care specifically related to the injection. Supplies (catheters, drugs, and contrast media) are not included in the listed service. Code the highest order vessel cannulated, but not any lesser order vessels cannulated in the approach. Report 36218 for each additional second order, third order, and more selective order vessel cannulated in the same vascular family. Right and left vessels belong to different vascular families; code separate catheterizations when performed. For radiological supervision and interpretation, see 75710. For catheter placement for coronary angiography, see 93454–93461. Do not report 36215-36216 with 36836 or 36837.

ICD-10-CM Diagnostic Codes

C34.01	Malignant neoplasm of right main bronchus ☑
C34.11	Malignant neoplasm of upper lobe, right bronchus or lung ☑
C34.2	Malignant neoplasm of middle lobe, bronchus or lung
C34.31	Malignant neoplasm of lower lobe, right bronchus or lung ☑
C34.81	Malignant neoplasm of overlapping sites of right bronchus and lung ☑
G45.0	Vertebro-basilar artery syndrome
G45.1	Carotid artery syndrome (hemispheric)
G45.2	Multiple and bilateral precerebral artery syndromes
G45.3	Amaurosis fugax
G90.01	Carotid sinus syncope
I05.0	Rheumatic mitral stenosis
I05.1	Rheumatic mitral insufficiency
I05.2	Rheumatic mitral stenosis with insufficiency
I05.8	Other rheumatic mitral valve diseases
I06.0	Rheumatic aortic stenosis
I06.1	Rheumatic aortic insufficiency
I06.2	Rheumatic aortic stenosis with insufficiency
I07.0	Rheumatic tricuspid stenosis
I07.1	Rheumatic tricuspid insufficiency
I07.2	Rheumatic tricuspid stenosis and insufficiency
I08.0	Rheumatic disorders of both mitral and aortic valves
I08.1	Rheumatic disorders of both mitral and tricuspid valves
I08.2	Rheumatic disorders of both aortic and tricuspid valves
I08.3	Combined rheumatic disorders of mitral, aortic and tricuspid valves
I25.3	Aneurysm of heart
I26.01	Septic pulmonary embolism with acute cor pulmonale
I26.02	Saddle embolus of pulmonary artery with acute cor pulmonale
I26.09	Other pulmonary embolism with acute cor pulmonale
I26.90	Septic pulmonary embolism without acute cor pulmonale
I26.92	Saddle embolus of pulmonary artery without acute cor pulmonale
I27.0	Primary pulmonary hypertension
I27.21	Secondary pulmonary arterial hypertension
I27.22	Pulmonary hypertension due to left heart disease
I27.23	Pulmonary hypertension due to lung diseases and hypoxia
I27.24	Chronic thromboembolic pulmonary hypertension
I27.29	Other secondary pulmonary hypertension
I27.82	Chronic pulmonary embolism
I27.83	Eisenmenger's syndrome
I28.0	Arteriovenous fistula of pulmonary vessels
I28.1	Aneurysm of pulmonary artery
I31.4	Cardiac tamponade
I34.0	Nonrheumatic mitral (valve) insufficiency
I34.1	Nonrheumatic mitral (valve) prolapse
I34.2	Nonrheumatic mitral (valve) stenosis
I35.0	Nonrheumatic aortic (valve) stenosis
I35.1	Nonrheumatic aortic (valve) insufficiency
I35.2	Nonrheumatic aortic (valve) stenosis with insufficiency
I37.0	Nonrheumatic pulmonary valve stenosis
I37.1	Nonrheumatic pulmonary valve insufficiency
I37.2	Nonrheumatic pulmonary valve stenosis with insufficiency
I42.0	Dilated cardiomyopathy
I42.1	Obstructive hypertrophic cardiomyopathy
I42.6	Alcoholic cardiomyopathy
I42.7	Cardiomyopathy due to drug and external agent
I50.21	Acute systolic (congestive) heart failure
I50.22	Chronic systolic (congestive) heart failure
I50.23	Acute on chronic systolic (congestive) heart failure

I50.31	Acute diastolic (congestive) heart failure
I50.32	Chronic diastolic (congestive) heart failure
I50.33	Acute on chronic diastolic (congestive) heart failure
I50.41	Acute combined systolic (congestive) and diastolic (congestive) heart failure
I50.42	Chronic combined systolic (congestive) and diastolic (congestive) heart failure
I50.43	Acute on chronic combined systolic (congestive) and diastolic (congestive) heart failure
I50.811	Acute right heart failure
I50.812	Chronic right heart failure
I50.813	Acute on chronic right heart failure
I50.814	Right heart failure due to left heart failure
I50.82	Biventricular heart failure
I50.83	High output heart failure
I50.84	End stage heart failure
I63.011	Cerebral infarction due to thrombosis of right vertebral artery ☑
I63.02	Cerebral infarction due to thrombosis of basilar artery
I63.031	Cerebral infarction due to thrombosis of right carotid artery ☑
I63.111	Cerebral infarction due to embolism of right vertebral artery ☑
I63.12	Cerebral infarction due to embolism of basilar artery
I63.131	Cerebral infarction due to embolism of right carotid artery ☑
I65.01	Occlusion and stenosis of right vertebral artery ☑
I65.1	Occlusion and stenosis of basilar artery
I65.21	Occlusion and stenosis of right carotid artery ☑
I67.81	Acute cerebrovascular insufficiency
I67.82	Cerebral ischemia
I67.841	Reversible cerebrovascular vasoconstriction syndrome
I67.850	Cerebral autosomal dominant arteriopathy with subcortical infarcts and leukoencephalopathy
I70.0	Atherosclerosis of aorta A
I70.8	Atherosclerosis of other arteries A
I70.92	Chronic total occlusion of artery of the extremities A
I71.03	Dissection of thoracoabdominal aorta
I72.0	Aneurysm of carotid artery
I72.1	Aneurysm of artery of upper extremity
I72.5	Aneurysm of other precerebral arteries
I72.6	Aneurysm of vertebral artery
I74.19	Embolism and thrombosis of other parts of aorta
I74.2	Embolism and thrombosis of arteries of the upper extremities
I75.011	Atheroembolism of right upper extremity ☑
I76	Septic arterial embolism
I77.1	Stricture of artery
I77.2	Rupture of artery
I77.3	Arterial fibromuscular dysplasia
I77.5	Necrosis of artery
I77.71	Dissection of carotid artery
I77.74	Dissection of vertebral artery
I77.75	Dissection of other precerebral arteries
I77.76	Dissection of artery of upper extremity
I77.77	Dissection of artery of lower extremity
I77.810	Thoracic aortic ectasia
I77.812	Thoracoabdominal aortic ectasia
J44.0	Chronic obstructive pulmonary disease with (acute) lower respiratory infection
J44.1	Chronic obstructive pulmonary disease with (acute) exacerbation
J81.0	Acute pulmonary edema
J81.1	Chronic pulmonary edema
J98.11	Atelectasis
Q21.0	Ventricular septal defect
Q21.3	Tetralogy of Fallot
Q21.4	Aortopulmonary septal defect
Q22.5	Ebstein's anomaly
Q22.6	Hypoplastic right heart syndrome
Q23.0	Congenital stenosis of aortic valve
Q23.1	Congenital insufficiency of aortic valve
Q23.2	Congenital mitral stenosis
Q23.3	Congenital mitral insufficiency
R57.0	Cardiogenic shock

AMA: 36215 2023,Oct; 2023,Mar; 2022,Oct; 2021,Jul; 2018,Oct **36216** 2023,Oct; 2023,Mar; 2022,Oct; 2020,Sep; 2018,Oct

Relative Value Units/Medicare Edits

Non-Facility RVU	Work	PE	MP	Total
36215	4.17	25.75	0.6	30.52
36216	5.27	25.1	1.09	31.46
Facility RVU	**Work**	**PE**	**MP**	**Total**
36215	4.17	1.44	0.6	6.21
36216	5.27	1.61	1.09	7.97

	FUD	Status	MUE	Modifiers				IOM Reference
36215	0	A	6(3)	51	N/A	N/A	N/A	None
36216	0	A	4(3)	51	N/A	N/A	N/A	

* with documentation

Terms To Know

aortic arch. Thoracic aorta, ascending/arch.

first order. First vessel in the arterial or venous system that branches off the main vessel and supplies additional branches within the same vascular family.

second order catheter placement. Catheter manipulation into a vessel that branches off the aorta. May be noted in the record as a second branch or second family placement.

36217-36218

36217 Selective catheter placement, arterial system; initial third order or more selective thoracic or brachiocephalic branch, within a vascular family

+ **36218** additional second order, third order, and beyond, thoracic or brachiocephalic branch, within a vascular family (List in addition to code for initial second or third order vessel as appropriate)

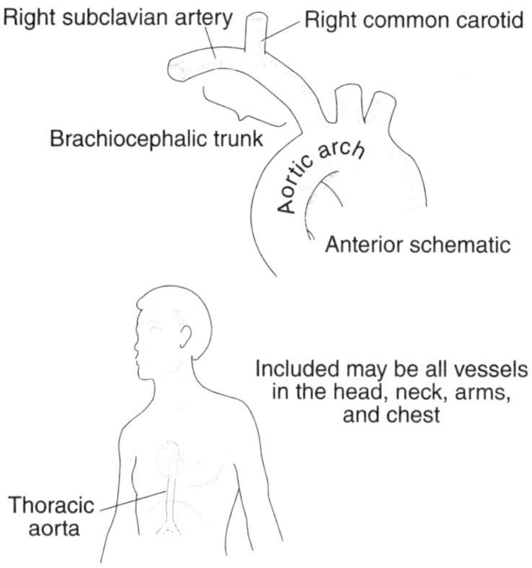

Explanation

The physician punctures the skin and underlying artery with a needle and threads a guidance wire through the needle into the artery. The needle is removed. The guidewire is manipulated into the specific artery. A catheter follows the wire into a first order thoracic or brachiocephalic artery. The catheter passes through the first order vessel into the second order thoracic or brachiocephalic artery. The catheter continues to a third order vessel. Contrast material for arteriography is injected into the catheter that has been guided to the site under investigation. Once the procedure is complete, the catheter is removed and pressure is applied to stop bleeding at the injection site. Report 36218 for an additional second order, third order, and beyond, thoracic or brachiocephalic branch, within a vascular family.

Coding Tips

These codes include introduction of needles or catheter, injection of contrast material with or without automatic power injection, and/or necessary pre- and postinjection care specifically related to the injection. Supplies (catheters, drugs, and contrast media) are not included in the listed service. Code the highest order vessel cannulated, but not any lesser order vessels cannulated in the approach. Report 36218 for each additional second order, third order, and more selective order vessel cannulated in the same vascular family. Right and left vessels belong to different vascular families; therefore, code separate catheterizations when performed. Report 36218 in addition to 36216, 36217, 36225, and 36226. Do not report 36218 when performing diagnostic angiography of extracranial and intracranial cervicocerebral vessels. Named or unnamed arterial branches beyond a third-order arterial branch should be reported with 36218 or 36248, as appropriate. For angiography, see 36222–36228 and 75600–75774. Transcatheter therapy is reported using 37200, 37211, 37213, 37214, 37236–37239, 37241–37244, 61624, and 61626. For angiography of the coronary artery, arterial conduit, or venous bypass graft performed at the same time as cardiac catheterizations, see 93454-93461, 93564, or 93593-93597. For angiography of the internal mammary artery without concomitant heart catheterization, see 36216 or 36217. Do not report 36217-36218 with 36836 or 36837.

ICD-10-CM Diagnostic Codes

C34.01	Malignant neoplasm of right main bronchus ☑
C34.11	Malignant neoplasm of upper lobe, right bronchus or lung ☑
C34.2	Malignant neoplasm of middle lobe, bronchus or lung
C34.31	Malignant neoplasm of lower lobe, right bronchus or lung ☑
C34.81	Malignant neoplasm of overlapping sites of right bronchus and lung ☑
G45.0	Vertebro-basilar artery syndrome
G45.1	Carotid artery syndrome (hemispheric)
G45.2	Multiple and bilateral precerebral artery syndromes
G45.3	Amaurosis fugax
G90.01	Carotid sinus syncope
I05.0	Rheumatic mitral stenosis
I05.1	Rheumatic mitral insufficiency
I05.2	Rheumatic mitral stenosis with insufficiency
I05.8	Other rheumatic mitral valve diseases
I06.0	Rheumatic aortic stenosis
I06.1	Rheumatic aortic insufficiency
I06.2	Rheumatic aortic stenosis with insufficiency
I07.0	Rheumatic tricuspid stenosis
I07.1	Rheumatic tricuspid insufficiency
I07.2	Rheumatic tricuspid stenosis and insufficiency
I08.0	Rheumatic disorders of both mitral and aortic valves
I08.1	Rheumatic disorders of both mitral and tricuspid valves
I08.2	Rheumatic disorders of both aortic and tricuspid valves
I08.3	Combined rheumatic disorders of mitral, aortic and tricuspid valves
I25.3	Aneurysm of heart
I26.01	Septic pulmonary embolism with acute cor pulmonale
I26.02	Saddle embolus of pulmonary artery with acute cor pulmonale
I26.09	Other pulmonary embolism with acute cor pulmonale
I26.90	Septic pulmonary embolism without acute cor pulmonale
I26.92	Saddle embolus of pulmonary artery without acute cor pulmonale
I27.0	Primary pulmonary hypertension
I27.21	Secondary pulmonary arterial hypertension
I27.22	Pulmonary hypertension due to left heart disease
I27.23	Pulmonary hypertension due to lung diseases and hypoxia
I27.24	Chronic thromboembolic pulmonary hypertension
I27.29	Other secondary pulmonary hypertension
I27.82	Chronic pulmonary embolism
I27.83	Eisenmenger's syndrome
I28.0	Arteriovenous fistula of pulmonary vessels
I28.1	Aneurysm of pulmonary artery
I31.4	Cardiac tamponade
I34.0	Nonrheumatic mitral (valve) insufficiency
I34.1	Nonrheumatic mitral (valve) prolapse
I34.2	Nonrheumatic mitral (valve) stenosis
I35.0	Nonrheumatic aortic (valve) stenosis
I35.1	Nonrheumatic aortic (valve) insufficiency
I35.2	Nonrheumatic aortic (valve) stenosis with insufficiency

I37.0 Nonrheumatic pulmonary valve stenosis
I37.1 Nonrheumatic pulmonary valve insufficiency
I37.2 Nonrheumatic pulmonary valve stenosis with insufficiency
I42.0 Dilated cardiomyopathy
I42.1 Obstructive hypertrophic cardiomyopathy
I42.6 Alcoholic cardiomyopathy
I42.7 Cardiomyopathy due to drug and external agent
I50.21 Acute systolic (congestive) heart failure
I50.22 Chronic systolic (congestive) heart failure
I50.23 Acute on chronic systolic (congestive) heart failure
I50.31 Acute diastolic (congestive) heart failure
I50.32 Chronic diastolic (congestive) heart failure
I50.33 Acute on chronic diastolic (congestive) heart failure
I50.41 Acute combined systolic (congestive) and diastolic (congestive) heart failure
I50.42 Chronic combined systolic (congestive) and diastolic (congestive) heart failure
I50.43 Acute on chronic combined systolic (congestive) and diastolic (congestive) heart failure
I50.811 Acute right heart failure
I50.812 Chronic right heart failure
I50.813 Acute on chronic right heart failure
I50.814 Right heart failure due to left heart failure
I50.82 Biventricular heart failure
I50.83 High output heart failure
I50.84 End stage heart failure
I63.011 Cerebral infarction due to thrombosis of right vertebral artery ☑
I63.02 Cerebral infarction due to thrombosis of basilar artery
I63.031 Cerebral infarction due to thrombosis of right carotid artery ☑
I63.111 Cerebral infarction due to embolism of right vertebral artery ☑
I63.12 Cerebral infarction due to embolism of basilar artery
I63.131 Cerebral infarction due to embolism of right carotid artery ☑
I65.01 Occlusion and stenosis of right vertebral artery ☑
I65.1 Occlusion and stenosis of basilar artery
I65.21 Occlusion and stenosis of right carotid artery ☑
I67.81 Acute cerebrovascular insufficiency
I67.82 Cerebral ischemia
I67.841 Reversible cerebrovascular vasoconstriction syndrome
I67.850 Cerebral autosomal dominant arteriopathy with subcortical infarcts and leukoencephalopathy
I70.0 Atherosclerosis of aorta A
I70.8 Atherosclerosis of other arteries A
I70.92 Chronic total occlusion of artery of the extremities A
I71.03 Dissection of thoracoabdominal aorta
I72.0 Aneurysm of carotid artery
I72.1 Aneurysm of artery of upper extremity
I72.5 Aneurysm of other precerebral arteries
I72.6 Aneurysm of vertebral artery
I74.19 Embolism and thrombosis of other parts of aorta
I74.2 Embolism and thrombosis of arteries of the upper extremities
I75.011 Atheroembolism of right upper extremity ☑
I76 Septic arterial embolism
I77.1 Stricture of artery
I77.2 Rupture of artery
I77.3 Arterial fibromuscular dysplasia
I77.5 Necrosis of artery
I77.71 Dissection of carotid artery
I77.74 Dissection of vertebral artery
I77.75 Dissection of other precerebral arteries
I77.76 Dissection of artery of upper extremity
I77.77 Dissection of artery of lower extremity
I77.810 Thoracic aortic ectasia
I77.812 Thoracoabdominal aortic ectasia
J44.0 Chronic obstructive pulmonary disease with (acute) lower respiratory infection
J44.1 Chronic obstructive pulmonary disease with (acute) exacerbation
J81.0 Acute pulmonary edema
J81.1 Chronic pulmonary edema
J98.11 Atelectasis
Q21.0 Ventricular septal defect
Q21.3 Tetralogy of Fallot
Q21.4 Aortopulmonary septal defect
Q22.5 Ebstein's anomaly
Q22.6 Hypoplastic right heart syndrome
Q23.0 Congenital stenosis of aortic valve
Q23.1 Congenital insufficiency of aortic valve
Q23.2 Congenital mitral stenosis
Q23.3 Congenital mitral insufficiency
R57.0 Cardiogenic shock

AMA: 36217 2023,Mar; 2022,Oct; 2020,Sep; 2018,Oct **36218** 2023,Mar; 2022,Oct; 2020,Sep; 2018,Oct

Relative Value Units/Medicare Edits

Non-Facility RVU	Work	PE	MP	Total
36217	6.29	45.72	1.46	53.47
36218	1.01	5.0	0.21	6.22
Facility RVU	**Work**	**PE**	**MP**	**Total**
36217	6.29	2.03	1.46	9.78
36218	1.01	0.32	0.21	1.54

	FUD	Status	MUE	Modifiers				IOM Reference
36217	0	A	2(3)	51	N/A	N/A	N/A	None
36218	N/A	A	6(3)	N/A	N/A	N/A	N/A	

* with documentation

36221

36221 Non-selective catheter placement, thoracic aorta, with angiography of the extracranial carotid, vertebral, and/or intracranial vessels, unilateral or bilateral, and all associated radiological supervision and interpretation, includes angiography of the cervicocerebral arch, when performed

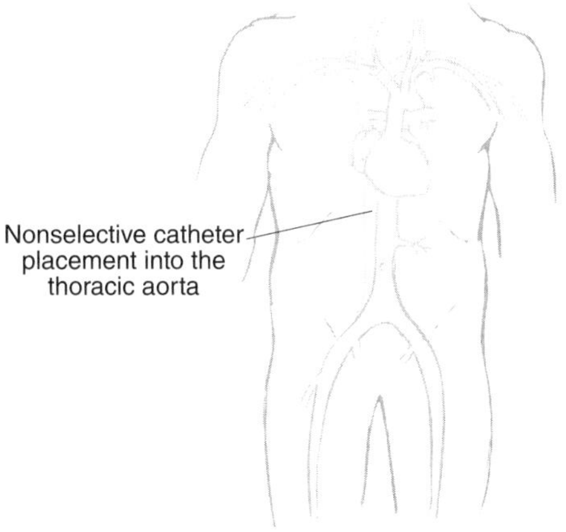

Explanation

The physician punctures a distal artery (typically femoral, brachial, radial, or axillary) with a large needle and passes a guidewire via the needle into the punctured artery. The needle is removed while leaving the guidewire in place, and the skin opening is enlarged slightly with a blade. An introducer sheath is inserted over the guidewire and into the arterial lumen. A catheter is introduced into the artery through an O-ring in the introducer sheath, which prevents blood from leaking around the catheter, and advanced into the thoracic aorta. The physician injects contrast material to perform angiography of the cervicocerebral arch, the extracranial carotid, and the vertebral and/or other intracranial vessels, unilaterally or bilaterally. Upon completion, the catheter is removed and pressure is applied to stop bleeding at the access site.

Coding Tips

When medically necessary, report moderate (conscious) sedation provided by the performing physician with 99151-99153. When provided by another physician, report 99155-99157. This code includes access of the vessel, placement of the catheter(s), injection(s) of the contrast, fluoroscopy, radiologic supervision and interpretation, and closure of the arteriotomy by pressure or by application of an arterial closure device. Diagnostic angiography may be followed by interventional procedures at the same operative session, and may be reported separately using appropriate coding guidelines. Do not report 36221 with 36222–36226. Do not report with the transcatheter placement of an intravascular stent of the common carotid or innominate artery on the same side (37217). For 3D rendering, see 76376–76377. For ultrasound guidance for vascular access, see 76937.

ICD-10-CM Diagnostic Codes

C70.0	Malignant neoplasm of cerebral meninges
C71.0	Malignant neoplasm of cerebrum, except lobes and ventricles
C71.1	Malignant neoplasm of frontal lobe
C71.2	Malignant neoplasm of temporal lobe
C71.3	Malignant neoplasm of parietal lobe
C71.4	Malignant neoplasm of occipital lobe
C71.5	Malignant neoplasm of cerebral ventricle
C71.6	Malignant neoplasm of cerebellum
C71.7	Malignant neoplasm of brain stem
C75.1	Malignant neoplasm of pituitary gland
C75.2	Malignant neoplasm of craniopharyngeal duct
C75.4	Malignant neoplasm of carotid body
C76.0	Malignant neoplasm of head, face and neck
C79.31	Secondary malignant neoplasm of brain
C79.32	Secondary malignant neoplasm of cerebral meninges
D18.02	Hemangioma of intracranial structures
I60.01	Nontraumatic subarachnoid hemorrhage from right carotid siphon and bifurcation ☑
I60.11	Nontraumatic subarachnoid hemorrhage from right middle cerebral artery ☑
I60.4	Nontraumatic subarachnoid hemorrhage from basilar artery
I60.51	Nontraumatic subarachnoid hemorrhage from right vertebral artery ☑
I63.311	Cerebral infarction due to thrombosis of right middle cerebral artery ☑
I63.321	Cerebral infarction due to thrombosis of right anterior cerebral artery ☑
I63.331	Cerebral infarction due to thrombosis of right posterior cerebral artery ☑
I63.341	Cerebral infarction due to thrombosis of right cerebellar artery ☑
I63.411	Cerebral infarction due to embolism of right middle cerebral artery ☑
I63.421	Cerebral infarction due to embolism of right anterior cerebral artery ☑
I63.431	Cerebral infarction due to embolism of right posterior cerebral artery ☑
I63.441	Cerebral infarction due to embolism of right cerebellar artery ☑
I65.01	Occlusion and stenosis of right vertebral artery ☑
I65.1	Occlusion and stenosis of basilar artery
I65.21	Occlusion and stenosis of right carotid artery ☑
I66.01	Occlusion and stenosis of right middle cerebral artery ☑
I66.11	Occlusion and stenosis of right anterior cerebral artery ☑
I66.21	Occlusion and stenosis of right posterior cerebral artery ☑
I66.3	Occlusion and stenosis of cerebellar arteries
I67.0	Dissection of cerebral arteries, nonruptured
I67.1	Cerebral aneurysm, nonruptured
I67.2	Cerebral atherosclerosis [A]
I67.81	Acute cerebrovascular insufficiency
I67.82	Cerebral ischemia
I67.841	Reversible cerebrovascular vasoconstriction syndrome
I72.0	Aneurysm of carotid artery
I72.6	Aneurysm of vertebral artery
I76	Septic arterial embolism
I77.1	Stricture of artery
I77.2	Rupture of artery
I77.71	Dissection of carotid artery
I77.74	Dissection of vertebral artery
I97.820	Postprocedural cerebrovascular infarction following cardiac surgery
I97.821	Postprocedural cerebrovascular infarction following other surgery
Q28.2	Arteriovenous malformation of cerebral vessels

S15.011A Minor laceration of right carotid artery, initial encounter ☑
S15.021A Major laceration of right carotid artery, initial encounter ☑
S15.111A Minor laceration of right vertebral artery, initial encounter ☑
S15.121A Major laceration of right vertebral artery, initial encounter ☑

AMA: 36221 2021,Dec; 2018,Oct

Relative Value Units/Medicare Edits

Non-Facility RVU	Work	PE	MP	Total
36221	3.92	24.32	0.88	29.12
Facility RVU	**Work**	**PE**	**MP**	**Total**
36221	3.92	1.05	0.88	5.85

	FUD	Status	MUE	Modifiers				IOM Reference
36221	0	A	1(3)	51	N/A	N/A	N/A	None

* with documentation

Terms To Know

angiography. Radiographic imaging of the arteries. Imaging may be performed to study the vasculature of any given organ, body system, or area of circulation such as the brain, heart, chest, kidneys, limbs, gastrointestinal tract, aorta, and pulmonary circulation to visualize the formation and the function of the blood vessels to detect problems such as a blockage or stricture. A catheter is inserted through an accessible blood vessel and the artery is injected with a radiopaque contrast material after which x-rays are taken.

nonselective placement. Insertion of a large needle with passage of a guidewire via the needle into the punctured vein or artery. The needle is removed leaving the guidewire and catheter in place. In direct punctures to peripheral veins or arteries, the catheter is not manipulated further after the initial stick is secured. Regardless of the site of the puncture, catheterization of the aorta or of the vena cava is considered nonselective placement.

36222-36223

36222 Selective catheter placement, common carotid or innominate artery, unilateral, any approach, with angiography of the ipsilateral extracranial carotid circulation and all associated radiological supervision and interpretation, includes angiography of the cervicocerebral arch, when performed

36223 Selective catheter placement, common carotid or innominate artery, unilateral, any approach, with angiography of the ipsilateral intracranial carotid circulation and all associated radiological supervision and interpretation, includes angiography of the extracranial carotid and cervicocerebral arch, when performed

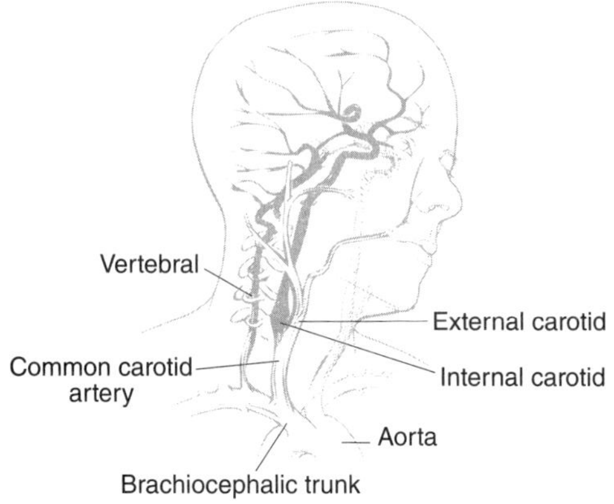

Selective catheter is placed in the common carotid artery

Explanation

The physician passes a needle through the skin and into an extremity artery, usually in the upper thigh. A guidewire is threaded through the needle into the vessel. The needle is removed. The wire is threaded into the aorta and up to the thoracic aorta where it is manipulated into a branch off the aortic arch. A catheter follows the wire into the common carotid or innominate artery on one side. The wire is removed. Contrast material is injected into the catheter for arteriography. Report 36222 when angiography of the ipsilateral extracranial carotid circulation is also included. In 36223, angiography of the ipsilateral extracranial and intracranial carotid circulation is performed. Angiography of the cervicocerebral arch may also be performed. Upon completion, the catheter is removed and pressure is applied to stop bleeding at the access site.

Coding Tips

When medically necessary, report moderate (conscious) sedation provided by the performing physician with 99151-99153. When provided by another physician, report 99155-99157. These procedures include access of the vessel, placement of the catheter(s), injection(s) of the contrast, fluoroscopy, radiologic supervision and interpretation, and closure of the arteriotomy by pressure or by application of an arterial closure device. Diagnostic angiography may be followed by interventional procedures at the same operative session, and may be reported separately using appropriate coding guidelines. These are unilateral procedures. If performed bilaterally, some payers require that the service be reported twice with modifier 50 appended to the second code while others require identification of the service only once with modifier 50 appended. Check with individual payers. Modifier 50 identifies a procedure performed identically on the opposite side of the body (mirror image). Do not report 36222–36224 together to report ipsilateral angiography. Report the single code that represents the most complex service, with 36224 being the most complex and 36222 being the least complex. For 3D rendering, see

76376–76377. For ultrasound guidance for vascular access, see 76937. Do not report 36222 or 36223 with 37215, 37216, 37218 for the treated carotid artery. Do not report 36222 or 36223 with the transcatheter placement of an intravascular stent of the common carotid or innominate artery on the same side (37217).

ICD-10-CM Diagnostic Codes

G45.0	Vertebro-basilar artery syndrome
G45.1	Carotid artery syndrome (hemispheric)
G45.2	Multiple and bilateral precerebral artery syndromes
G45.3	Amaurosis fugax
I60.01	Nontraumatic subarachnoid hemorrhage from right carotid siphon and bifurcation ☑
I60.8	Other nontraumatic subarachnoid hemorrhage
I61.8	Other nontraumatic intracerebral hemorrhage
I63.011	Cerebral infarction due to thrombosis of right vertebral artery ☑
I63.031	Cerebral infarction due to thrombosis of right carotid artery ☑
I63.111	Cerebral infarction due to embolism of right vertebral artery ☑
I63.131	Cerebral infarction due to embolism of right carotid artery ☑
I63.19	Cerebral infarction due to embolism of other precerebral artery
I63.311	Cerebral infarction due to thrombosis of right middle cerebral artery ☑
I63.321	Cerebral infarction due to thrombosis of right anterior cerebral artery ☑
I63.333	Cerebral infarction due to thrombosis of bilateral posterior cerebral arteries ☑
I63.343	Cerebral infarction due to thrombosis of bilateral cerebellar arteries ☑
I63.411	Cerebral infarction due to embolism of right middle cerebral artery ☑
I63.421	Cerebral infarction due to embolism of right anterior cerebral artery ☑
I63.433	Cerebral infarction due to embolism of bilateral posterior cerebral arteries ☑
I63.443	Cerebral infarction due to embolism of bilateral cerebellar arteries ☑
I65.01	Occlusion and stenosis of right vertebral artery ☑
I65.1	Occlusion and stenosis of basilar artery
I65.21	Occlusion and stenosis of right carotid artery ☑
I65.8	Occlusion and stenosis of other precerebral arteries
I67.1	Cerebral aneurysm, nonruptured
I67.2	Cerebral atherosclerosis [A]
I67.81	Acute cerebrovascular insufficiency
I67.82	Cerebral ischemia
I67.841	Reversible cerebrovascular vasoconstriction syndrome
I67.848	Other cerebrovascular vasospasm and vasoconstriction
I67.89	Other cerebrovascular disease
I72.0	Aneurysm of carotid artery
I72.8	Aneurysm of other specified arteries
I76	Septic arterial embolism
I77.1	Stricture of artery
I77.2	Rupture of artery
I77.71	Dissection of carotid artery
I77.74	Dissection of vertebral artery
I77.79	Dissection of other specified artery
I77.89	Other specified disorders of arteries and arterioles
I97.820	Postprocedural cerebrovascular infarction following cardiac surgery
I97.821	Postprocedural cerebrovascular infarction following other surgery
Q28.1	Other malformations of precerebral vessels
Q28.8	Other specified congenital malformations of circulatory system
S09.0XXA	Injury of blood vessels of head, not elsewhere classified, initial encounter
S15.011A	Minor laceration of right carotid artery, initial encounter ☑
S15.021A	Major laceration of right carotid artery, initial encounter ☑
S15.091A	Other specified injury of right carotid artery, initial encounter ☑
S15.111A	Minor laceration of right vertebral artery, initial encounter ☑
S15.121A	Major laceration of right vertebral artery, initial encounter ☑
S15.191A	Other specified injury of right vertebral artery, initial encounter ☑
S15.8XXA	Injury of other specified blood vessels at neck level, initial encounter
S25.111A	Minor laceration of right innominate or subclavian artery, initial encounter ☑
S25.121A	Major laceration of right innominate or subclavian artery, initial encounter ☑
S25.191A	Other specified injury of right innominate or subclavian artery, initial encounter ☑

AMA: 36222 2020,Sep; 2018,Oct **36223** 2020,Sep; 2018,Oct

Relative Value Units/Medicare Edits

Non-Facility RVU	Work	PE	MP	Total
36222	5.28	29.93	1.3	36.51
36223	5.75	42.24	1.64	49.63
Facility RVU	**Work**	**PE**	**MP**	**Total**
36222	5.28	1.84	1.3	8.42
36223	5.75	2.34	1.64	9.73

	FUD	Status	MUE	Modifiers				IOM Reference
36222	0	A	1(3)	51	50	N/A	N/A	None
36223	0	A	1(3)	51	50	N/A	N/A	

* with documentation

Terms To Know

angiography. Radiographic imaging of the arteries.

guidewire. Flexible metal instrument designed to lead another instrument in its proper course.

ipsilateral. Located on, or affecting, the same side of the body, usually as it relates to a bilateral body part.

selective placement. Introduction and manipulation of a catheter or guidewire within a vascular tree or family into a specified target area that is identified and monitored by radiographic imaging in order to carry out a diagnostic or therapeutic procedure.

36224

36224 Selective catheter placement, internal carotid artery, unilateral, with angiography of the ipsilateral intracranial carotid circulation and all associated radiological supervision and interpretation, includes angiography of the extracranial carotid and cervicocerebral arch, when performed

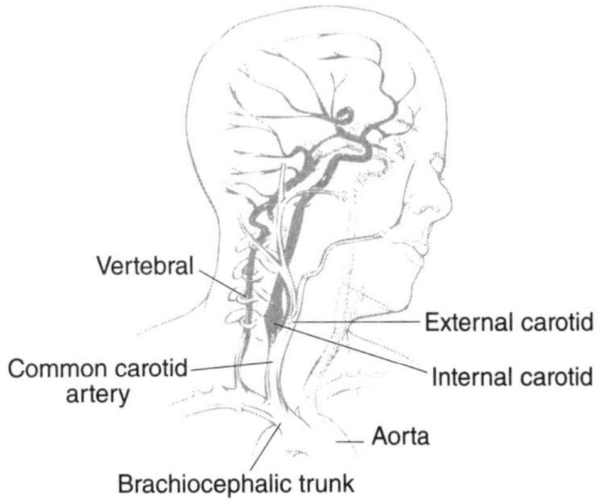

Selective catheter is placed in the internal carotid artery

Explanation

The physician passes a needle through the skin and into an extremity artery, usually in the upper thigh. A guidewire is threaded through the needle into the vessel. The needle is removed. The wire is threaded into the aorta and up to the thoracic aorta where it is manipulated into a branch off the aortic arch. A catheter follows the wire into the internal carotid artery on one side. The wire is removed. Contrast material is injected into the catheter for arteriography, including the intracranial carotid circulation. Angiography of the ipsilateral extracranial carotid circulation and the cervicocerebral arch may also be performed. Upon completion, the catheter is removed and pressure is applied to stop bleeding at the access site.

Coding Tips

When medically necessary, report moderate (conscious) sedation provided by the performing physician with 99151-99153. When provided by another physician, report 99155-99157. This code includes access of the vessel, placement of the catheter(s), injection(s) of the contrast, fluoroscopy, radiologic supervision and interpretation, and closure of the arteriotomy by pressure or by application of an arterial closure device. Diagnostic angiography may be followed by interventional procedures at the same operative session, and may be reported separately using appropriate coding guidelines. Do not report 36222–36224 together to report ipsilateral angiography. Do not report 36224 with 37215, 37216, or 37218 for the treated carotid artery. Do not report these codes with transcatheter placement of an intravascular stent of the common carotid or innominate artery on the same side (37217). Report the single code that represents the most complex service, with 36224 being the most complex and 36222 being the least complex. For 3D rendering, see 76376–76377. For ultrasound guidance for vascular access, see 76937.

ICD-10-CM Diagnostic Codes

G45.1 Carotid artery syndrome (hemispheric)
G45.3 Amaurosis fugax
I60.01 Nontraumatic subarachnoid hemorrhage from right carotid siphon and bifurcation ☑
I63.031 Cerebral infarction due to thrombosis of right carotid artery ☑
I63.131 Cerebral infarction due to embolism of right carotid artery ☑
I63.311 Cerebral infarction due to thrombosis of right middle cerebral artery ☑
I63.321 Cerebral infarction due to thrombosis of right anterior cerebral artery ☑
I63.411 Cerebral infarction due to embolism of right middle cerebral artery ☑
I63.421 Cerebral infarction due to embolism of right anterior cerebral artery ☑
I65.21 Occlusion and stenosis of right carotid artery ☑
I66.01 Occlusion and stenosis of right middle cerebral artery ☑
I66.11 Occlusion and stenosis of right anterior cerebral artery ☑
I67.1 Cerebral aneurysm, nonruptured
I67.2 Cerebral atherosclerosis [A]
I67.81 Acute cerebrovascular insufficiency
I67.82 Cerebral ischemia
I67.841 Reversible cerebrovascular vasoconstriction syndrome
I67.848 Other cerebrovascular vasospasm and vasoconstriction
I72.0 Aneurysm of carotid artery
I76 Septic arterial embolism
I77.1 Stricture of artery
I77.71 Dissection of carotid artery
I97.820 Postprocedural cerebrovascular infarction following cardiac surgery
I97.821 Postprocedural cerebrovascular infarction following other surgery
S15.011A Minor laceration of right carotid artery, initial encounter ☑
S15.021A Major laceration of right carotid artery, initial encounter ☑
S15.091A Other specified injury of right carotid artery, initial encounter ☑

AMA: 36224 2020,Sep; 2018,Oct

Relative Value Units/Medicare Edits

Non-Facility RVU	Work	PE	MP	Total
36224	6.25	53.12	1.91	61.28
Facility RVU	**Work**	**PE**	**MP**	**Total**
36224	6.25	2.77	1.91	10.93

	FUD	Status	MUE	Modifiers				IOM Reference
36224	0	A	1(3)	51	50	N/A	N/A	None

* with documentation

36225

36225 Selective catheter placement, subclavian or innominate artery, unilateral, with angiography of the ipsilateral vertebral circulation and all associated radiological supervision and interpretation, includes angiography of the cervicocerebral arch, when performed

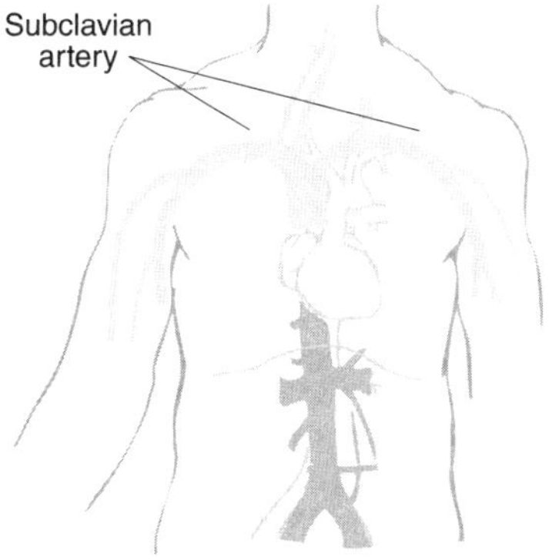

Selective catheter is placed in the subclavian artery

Explanation

The physician passes a needle through the skin and into an extremity artery. A guidewire is threaded through the needle into the vessel. The needle is removed. The wire is threaded into the thoracic aorta where it is manipulated into a branch off the aortic arch. A catheter follows the wire into the subclavian or innominate artery on one side. The wire is removed. Contrast material is injected into the catheter for arteriography, including the ipsilateral vertebral circulation. Angiography of the cervicocerebral arch may also be performed. Upon completion, the catheter is removed and pressure is applied to stop bleeding at the access site.

Coding Tips

When medically necessary, report moderate (conscious) sedation provided by the performing physician with 99151-99153. When provided by another physician, report 99155-99157. This code includes access of the vessel, placement of the catheter(s), injection(s) of the contrast, fluoroscopy, radiologic supervision and interpretation, and closure of the arteriotomy by pressure or by application of an arterial closure device. Diagnostic angiography may be followed by interventional procedures at the same operative session and may be reported separately using appropriate coding guidelines. Do not report 36225 and 36226 together to report ipsilateral angiography. Report the single code that represents the most complex service, with 36226 being the most complex. Do not report 36225 with transcatheter placement of an intravascular stent of the common carotid or innominate artery on the same side (37217). For 3D rendering, see 76376–76377. For ultrasound guidance for vascular access, see 76937.

ICD-10-CM Diagnostic Codes

G45.0	Vertebro-basilar artery syndrome
G45.1	Carotid artery syndrome (hemispheric)
G45.2	Multiple and bilateral precerebral artery syndromes
G45.3	Amaurosis fugax
G45.8	Other transient cerebral ischemic attacks and related syndromes
I60.01	Nontraumatic subarachnoid hemorrhage from right carotid siphon and bifurcation ☑
I60.4	Nontraumatic subarachnoid hemorrhage from basilar artery
I60.51	Nontraumatic subarachnoid hemorrhage from right vertebral artery ☑
I60.6	Nontraumatic subarachnoid hemorrhage from other intracranial arteries
I60.8	Other nontraumatic subarachnoid hemorrhage
I61.8	Other nontraumatic intracerebral hemorrhage
I63.011	Cerebral infarction due to thrombosis of right vertebral artery ☑
I63.031	Cerebral infarction due to thrombosis of right carotid artery ☑
I63.09	Cerebral infarction due to thrombosis of other precerebral artery
I63.111	Cerebral infarction due to embolism of right vertebral artery ☑
I63.131	Cerebral infarction due to embolism of right carotid artery ☑
I63.19	Cerebral infarction due to embolism of other precerebral artery
I63.311	Cerebral infarction due to thrombosis of right middle cerebral artery ☑
I63.321	Cerebral infarction due to thrombosis of right anterior cerebral artery ☑
I63.331	Cerebral infarction due to thrombosis of right posterior cerebral artery ☑
I63.341	Cerebral infarction due to thrombosis of right cerebellar artery ☑
I63.411	Cerebral infarction due to embolism of right middle cerebral artery ☑
I63.421	Cerebral infarction due to embolism of right anterior cerebral artery ☑
I63.431	Cerebral infarction due to embolism of right posterior cerebral artery ☑
I63.441	Cerebral infarction due to embolism of right cerebellar artery ☑
I63.81	Other cerebral infarction due to occlusion or stenosis of small artery
I63.89	Other cerebral infarction
I65.01	Occlusion and stenosis of right vertebral artery ☑
I65.03	Occlusion and stenosis of bilateral vertebral arteries ☑
I65.1	Occlusion and stenosis of basilar artery
I65.21	Occlusion and stenosis of right carotid artery ☑
I65.23	Occlusion and stenosis of bilateral carotid arteries ☑
I65.8	Occlusion and stenosis of other precerebral arteries
I67.1	Cerebral aneurysm, nonruptured
I67.2	Cerebral atherosclerosis A
I67.81	Acute cerebrovascular insufficiency
I67.82	Cerebral ischemia
I67.841	Reversible cerebrovascular vasoconstriction syndrome
I67.848	Other cerebrovascular vasospasm and vasoconstriction
I67.850	Cerebral autosomal dominant arteriopathy with subcortical infarcts and leukoencephalopathy
I67.858	Other hereditary cerebrovascular disease
I67.89	Other cerebrovascular disease
I72.0	Aneurysm of carotid artery
I72.6	Aneurysm of vertebral artery
I72.8	Aneurysm of other specified arteries
I76	Septic arterial embolism
I77.1	Stricture of artery
I77.2	Rupture of artery
I77.71	Dissection of carotid artery
I77.74	Dissection of vertebral artery
I77.79	Dissection of other specified artery

I97.820	Postprocedural cerebrovascular infarction following cardiac surgery
I97.821	Postprocedural cerebrovascular infarction following other surgery
S09.0XXA	Injury of blood vessels of head, not elsewhere classified, initial encounter
S15.011A	Minor laceration of right carotid artery, initial encounter ☑
S15.021A	Major laceration of right carotid artery, initial encounter ☑
S15.091A	Other specified injury of right carotid artery, initial encounter ☑
S15.111A	Minor laceration of right vertebral artery, initial encounter ☑
S15.121A	Major laceration of right vertebral artery, initial encounter ☑
S15.191A	Other specified injury of right vertebral artery, initial encounter ☑
S25.111A	Minor laceration of right innominate or subclavian artery, initial encounter ☑
S25.121A	Major laceration of right innominate or subclavian artery, initial encounter ☑

AMA: 36225 2020,Sep; 2018,Oct

Relative Value Units/Medicare Edits

Non-Facility RVU	Work	PE	MP	Total
36225	5.75	39.76	1.63	47.14
Facility RVU	**Work**	**PE**	**MP**	**Total**
36225	5.75	2.27	1.63	9.65

	FUD	Status	MUE	Modifiers				IOM Reference
36225	0	A	1(3)	51	50	N/A	N/A	None

* with documentation

36226

36226 Selective catheter placement, vertebral artery, unilateral, with angiography of the ipsilateral vertebral circulation and all associated radiological supervision and interpretation, includes angiography of the cervicocerebral arch, when performed

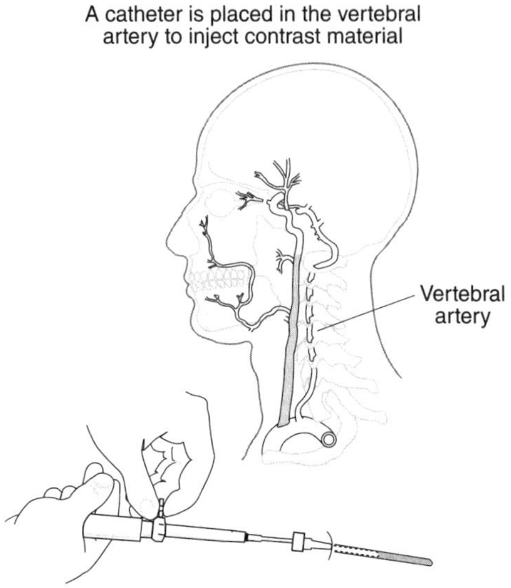

Explanation

The physician passes a needle through the skin and into an extremity artery. A guidewire is threaded through the needle into the vessel. The needle is removed. The wire is threaded into the thoracic aorta where it is manipulated into a branch off the aortic arch. A catheter follows the wire into the vertebral artery on one side. The wire is removed. Contrast material is injected into the catheter for arteriography, including the ipsilateral vertebral circulation. Angiography of the cervicocerebral arch may also be performed. Upon completion, the catheter is removed and pressure is applied to stop bleeding at the access site.

Coding Tips

When medically necessary, report moderate (conscious) sedation provided by the performing physician with 99151-99153. When provided by another physician, report 99155-99157. This code includes access of the vessel, placement of the catheter(s), injection(s) of the contrast, fluoroscopy, radiologic supervision and interpretation, and closure of the arteriotomy by pressure or by application of an arterial closure device. Diagnostic angiography may be followed by interventional procedures at the same operative session and may be reported separately using appropriate coding guidelines. Do not report 36226 with transcatheter placement of an intravascular stent of the common carotid or innominate artery on the same side (37217). Do not report 36225 and 36226 together to report ipsilateral angiography. Report the single code that represents the most complex service, with 36226 being the most complex. For 3D rendering, see 76376–76377. For ultrasound guidance for vascular access, see 76937.

ICD-10-CM Diagnostic Codes

I60.4	Nontraumatic subarachnoid hemorrhage from basilar artery
I60.51	Nontraumatic subarachnoid hemorrhage from right vertebral artery ☑

I60.8	Other nontraumatic subarachnoid hemorrhage
I61.8	Other nontraumatic intracerebral hemorrhage
I63.011	Cerebral infarction due to thrombosis of right vertebral artery ☑
I63.111	Cerebral infarction due to embolism of right vertebral artery ☑
I63.333	Cerebral infarction due to thrombosis of bilateral posterior cerebral arteries ☑
I63.343	Cerebral infarction due to thrombosis of bilateral cerebellar arteries ☑
I63.433	Cerebral infarction due to embolism of bilateral posterior cerebral arteries ☑
I63.443	Cerebral infarction due to embolism of bilateral cerebellar arteries ☑
I63.89	Other cerebral infarction
I65.01	Occlusion and stenosis of right vertebral artery ☑
I65.1	Occlusion and stenosis of basilar artery
I67.1	Cerebral aneurysm, nonruptured
I67.2	Cerebral atherosclerosis [A]
I67.81	Acute cerebrovascular insufficiency
I67.82	Cerebral ischemia
I67.841	Reversible cerebrovascular vasoconstriction syndrome
I67.848	Other cerebrovascular vasospasm and vasoconstriction
I67.850	Cerebral autosomal dominant arteriopathy with subcortical infarcts and leukoencephalopathy
I67.858	Other hereditary cerebrovascular disease
I67.89	Other cerebrovascular disease
I77.74	Dissection of vertebral artery
I97.820	Postprocedural cerebrovascular infarction following cardiac surgery
I97.821	Postprocedural cerebrovascular infarction following other surgery
S15.111A	Minor laceration of right vertebral artery, initial encounter ☑
S15.121A	Major laceration of right vertebral artery, initial encounter ☑
S15.191A	Other specified injury of right vertebral artery, initial encounter ☑

AMA: 36226 2020,Sep; 2018,Oct

Relative Value Units/Medicare Edits

Non-Facility RVU	Work	PE	MP	Total
36226	6.25	51.58	1.88	59.71
Facility RVU	**Work**	**PE**	**MP**	**Total**
36226	6.25	2.73	1.88	10.86

	FUD	Status	MUE	Modifiers				IOM Reference
36226	0	A	1(3)	51	50	N/A	N/A	None

* with documentation

36227-36228

+ **36227** Selective catheter placement, external carotid artery, unilateral, with angiography of the ipsilateral external carotid circulation and all associated radiological supervision and interpretation (List separately in addition to code for primary procedure)
+ **36228** Selective catheter placement, each intracranial branch of the internal carotid or vertebral arteries, unilateral, with angiography of the selected vessel circulation and all associated radiological supervision and interpretation (eg, middle cerebral artery, posterior inferior cerebellar artery) (List separately in addition to code for primary procedure)

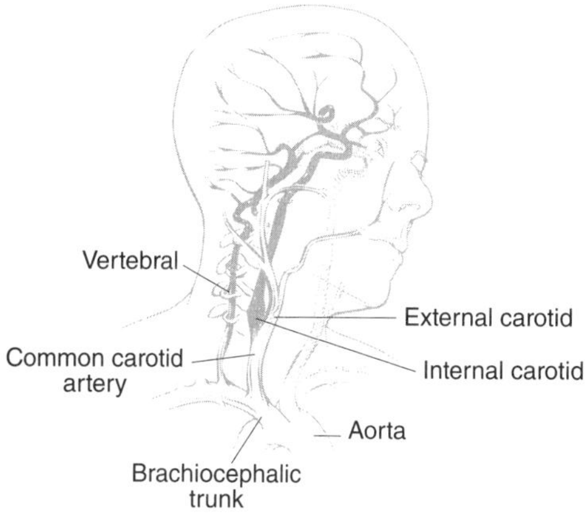

Explanation

In 36227, during selective angiography of the common carotid, internal carotid, or innominate artery, the physician also manipulates the catheter to the external carotid artery. Contrast material is injected into the catheter for arteriography, including the ipsilateral external carotid circulation. In 36228, during selective angiography of the internal carotid or vertebral artery, the physician further manipulates the catheter into additional intracranial branches of the artery, such as the middle cerebral or posterior inferior cerebellar arteries. Contrast material is injected into the catheter for arteriography, including the selected vessels circulation.

Coding Tips

When medically necessary, report moderate (conscious) sedation provided by the performing physician with 99151-99153. When provided by another physician, report 99155-99157. These codes include accessing the vessel, catheter placement(s), injection(s) of contrast, fluoroscopy, and radiological supervision and interpretation. Although it includes any additional second or third order selective catheter placements in the affected vessels, 36228 cannot be reported more than twice per side at the same operative session. Report 36227 in addition to 36222-36224. Report 36228 in addition to 36223-36226. Codes 36227 and 36228 should be reported twice when performed bilaterally. Do not report with modifier 50 per CPT guidelines. Medicare may still require the use of modifier 50. Do not report these codes with transcatheter placement of an intravascular stent of the common carotid or innominate artery on the same side (37217).

ICD-10-CM Diagnostic Codes

This/these CPT code(s) are add-on code(s). See the primary procedure code that this code is performed with for your ICD-10-CM code selections. Diagnostic code(s) would be the same as the actual procedure performed.

AMA: 36227 2020,Sep; 2018,Oct **36228** 2020,Sep; 2018,Oct

Relative Value Units/Medicare Edits

Non-Facility RVU	Work	PE	MP	Total
36227	2.09	4.56	0.63	7.28
36228	4.25	32.9	1.36	38.51
Facility RVU	**Work**	**PE**	**MP**	**Total**
36227	2.09	0.86	0.63	3.58
36228	4.25	1.77	1.36	7.38

	FUD	Status	MUE	Modifiers				IOM Reference
36227	N/A	A	1(3)	N/A	50	N/A	N/A	None
36228	N/A	A	2(3)	N/A	50	N/A	N/A	

* with documentation

Terms To Know

angiography. Radiographic imaging of the arteries. Imaging may be performed to study the vasculature of any given organ, body system, or area of circulation such as the brain, heart, chest, kidneys, limbs, gastrointestinal tract, aorta, and pulmonary circulation to visualize the formation and the function of the blood vessels to detect problems such as a blockage or stricture. A catheter is inserted through an accessible blood vessel and the artery is injected with a radiopaque contrast material after which x-rays are taken.

catheter. Flexible tube inserted into an area of the body for introducing or withdrawing fluid.

cerebellum. Portion of the brain in the rear cranial fossa behind the brain stem responsible for movement coordination.

contrast material. Any internally administered substance that has a different opacity from soft tissue on radiography or computed tomograph; includes barium, used to opacify parts of the gastrointestinal tract; water-soluble iodinated compounds, used to opacify blood vessels or the genitourinary tract; may refer to air occurring naturally or introduced into the body; also, paramagnetic substances used in magnetic resonance imaging. Substances may also be documented as contrast agent or contrast medium.

selective placement. Introduction and manipulation of a catheter or guidewire within a vascular tree or family into a specified target area that is identified and monitored by radiographic imaging in order to carry out a diagnostic or therapeutic procedure.

36245-36248

36245 Selective catheter placement, arterial system; each first order abdominal, pelvic, or lower extremity artery branch, within a vascular family

36246 initial second order abdominal, pelvic, or lower extremity artery branch, within a vascular family

36247 initial third order or more selective abdominal, pelvic, or lower extremity artery branch, within a vascular family

\+ **36248** additional second order, third order, and beyond, abdominal, pelvic, or lower extremity artery branch, within a vascular family (List in addition to code for initial second or third order vessel as appropriate)

Selective catheter placement, arterial system

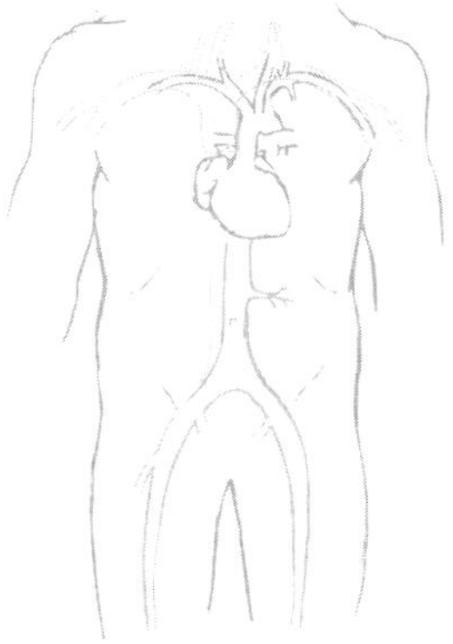

Explanation

The physician inserts a needle through the skin and into an underlying artery, usually a lower extremity artery, and threads a guidewire through the needle and into the artery. The needle is removed. The wire is threaded into the specific vessel. A catheter follows the wire into the artery branch. The wire is removed. Contrast material for arteriography is injected into the catheter that has been guided to the site under investigation. In 36245, the catheter remains in a first order artery. In 36246, the catheter travels to a second order artery. In 36247, the catheter placement is in the initial third order or more selective abdominal, pelvic, or lower extremity artery branch, within a vascular family. Report 36248 for any additional second order, third order and beyond, abdominal, pelvic, or lower extremity artery branch, within a vascular family. Once the procedure is complete, the catheter is removed, and pressure is applied to stop bleeding at the injection site.

Coding Tips

When medically necessary, report moderate (conscious) sedation provided by the performing physician with 99151-99153. When provided by another physician, report 99155-99157. These codes include introduction of needles or a catheter, injection of contrast material with or without automatic power injection, and/or necessary pre- and postinjection care specifically related to the injection. Supplies (catheters, drugs, and contrast media) are not included in the listed service. Report only the highest order vessel cannulated in each vascular family, but not any lesser order vessels cannulated in the approach. Report 36248 for each additional second order, third order, and more selective order vessel cannulated in the same vascular family. Report 36248 in addition to 36246 and 36247. Do not report 36245–36248 with 36836 or 36837. Right and left vessels belong to different vascular families; therefore, code separate catheterizations when performed.

ICD-10-CM Diagnostic Codes

The application of this code is too broad to adequately present ICD-10-CM diagnostic code links here. Refer to your ICD-10-CM book.

AMA: 36245 2023,Mar; 2022,Oct; 2020,Sep; 2018,Oct **36246** 2023,Mar; 2022,Oct; 2020,Sep; 2018,Oct **36247** 2023,Mar; 2022,Oct; 2020,Sep; 2018,Oct **36248** 2022,Oct; 2020,Sep; 2018,Oct

Relative Value Units/Medicare Edits

Non-Facility RVU	Work	PE	MP	Total
36245	4.65	31.02	0.83	36.5
36246	5.02	18.52	1.04	24.58
36247	6.04	34.69	1.03	41.76
36248	1.01	2.3	0.12	3.43
Facility RVU	**Work**	**PE**	**MP**	**Total**
36245	4.65	1.4	0.83	6.88
36246	5.02	1.32	1.04	7.38
36247	6.04	1.62	1.03	8.69
36248	1.01	0.27	0.12	1.4

	FUD	Status	MUE	Modifiers				IOM Reference
36245	N/A	A	6(3)	51	50	N/A	N/A	None
36246	0	A	4(3)	51	50	N/A	N/A	
36247	0	A	3(3)	51	50	N/A	N/A	
36248	N/A	A	6(3)	N/A	N/A	N/A	N/A	

* with documentation

Terms To Know

artery. Vessel through which oxygenated blood passes away from the heart to any part of the body.

catheter. Flexible tube inserted into an area of the body for introducing or withdrawing fluid.

contrast material. Radiopaque substance placed into the body to enable a system or body structure to be visualized, such as nonionic and low osmolar contrast media (LOCM), ionic and high osmolar contrast media (HOCM), barium, and gadolinium.

first order. First vessel in the arterial or venous system that branches off the main vessel and supplies additional branches within the same vascular family.

guidewire. Flexible metal instrument designed to lead another instrument in its proper course.

second order catheter placement. Catheter manipulation into a vessel that branches off the aorta. May be noted in the record as a second branch or second family placement.

third order catheter placement. Catheter placement (manipulation) into the third or greater vessel that branches off the aorta. May be noted in the record as an additional order catheterization or a third branch placement.

36251-36252

36251 Selective catheter placement (first-order), main renal artery and any accessory renal artery(s) for renal angiography, including arterial puncture and catheter placement(s), fluoroscopy, contrast injection(s), image postprocessing, permanent recording of images, and radiological supervision and interpretation, including pressure gradient measurements when performed, and flush aortogram when performed; unilateral

36252 bilateral

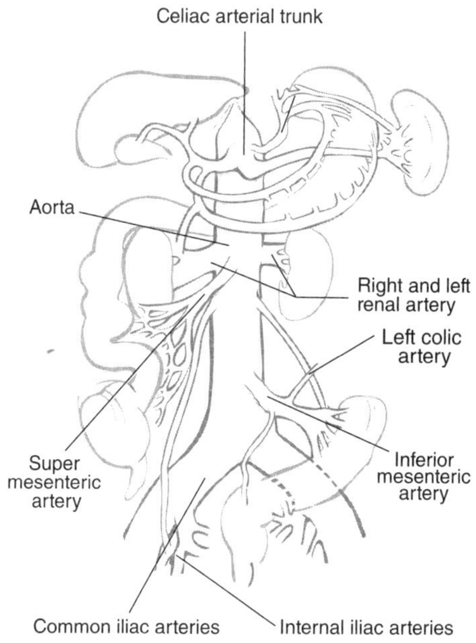

Explanation

The physician inserts a needle through the skin and into an underlying artery, usually a lower extremity artery, and threads a guidewire through the needle and into the artery. The needle is removed. The wire is threaded into the main renal artery and any accessory renal arteries, first order (branch) only. A catheter follows the wire into the arteries. The wire is removed. Contrast material for arteriography is injected into the catheter. Images are taken, the catheter is removed, and pressure applied to stop bleeding at the injection site. These codes include image postprocessing, permanent recording of images, and radiological supervision and interpretation (e.g., pressure gradient measurements and flush aortogram). Report 36251 for a unilateral procedure and 36252 for a bilateral procedure.

Coding Tips

When medically necessary, report moderate (conscious) sedation provided by the performing physician with 99151-99153. When provided by another physician, report 99155-99157. These codes include introduction of needles or a catheter, injection of contrast material, fluoroscopic guidance, image postprocessing and permanent recording, radiological supervision and interpretation with or without pressure gradient measurement, and flush aortogram. Do not report closure device placement at the vascular access site separately. Do not report 36253 with 36251 when the procedure is performed on the same kidney. Do not report these codes with 0338T or 0339T.

ICD-10-CM Diagnostic Codes

C64.1	Malignant neoplasm of right kidney, except renal pelvis ☑
C65.1	Malignant neoplasm of right renal pelvis ☑

C79.01	Secondary malignant neoplasm of right kidney and renal pelvis ☑
D09.19	Carcinoma in situ of other urinary organs
D30.01	Benign neoplasm of right kidney ☑
D30.11	Benign neoplasm of right renal pelvis ☑
D41.01	Neoplasm of uncertain behavior of right kidney ☑
D41.11	Neoplasm of uncertain behavior of right renal pelvis ☑
D41.21	Neoplasm of uncertain behavior of right ureter ☑
I15.0	Renovascular hypertension
I15.1	Hypertension secondary to other renal disorders
I70.1	Atherosclerosis of renal artery [A]
I72.2	Aneurysm of renal artery
I75.81	Atheroembolism of kidney
I77.73	Dissection of renal artery
N17.0	Acute kidney failure with tubular necrosis
N17.1	Acute kidney failure with acute cortical necrosis
N17.2	Acute kidney failure with medullary necrosis
N17.8	Other acute kidney failure
N26.1	Atrophy of kidney (terminal)
N26.2	Page kidney
N27.0	Small kidney, unilateral
N27.1	Small kidney, bilateral
N28.0	Ischemia and infarction of kidney
N28.82	Megaloureter
Q27.1	Congenital renal artery stenosis
Q27.2	Other congenital malformations of renal artery
S35.411A	Laceration of right renal artery, Initial encounter ☑
S35.491A	Other specified injury of right renal artery, initial encounter ☑
S37.011A	Minor contusion of right kidney, initial encounter ☑
S37.021A	Major contusion of right kidney, initial encounter ☑
S37.061A	Major laceration of right kidney, initial encounter ☑
S37.091A	Other injury of right kidney, initial encounter ☑

AMA: **36251** 2020,Sep; 2018,Oct **36252** 2020,Sep; 2018,Oct

Relative Value Units/Medicare Edits

Non-Facility RVU	Work	PE	MP	Total
36251	5.1	31.81	0.92	37.83
36252	6.74	32.81	1.49	41.04
Facility RVU	**Work**	**PE**	**MP**	**Total**
36251	5.1	1.44	0.92	7.46
36252	6.74	2.2	1.49	10.43

	FUD	Status	MUE	Modifiers				IOM Reference
36251	0	A	1(3)	51	N/A	N/A	N/A	None
36252	0	A	1(3)	51	N/A	N/A	N/A	

* with documentation

36253-36254

36253 Superselective catheter placement (one or more second order or higher renal artery branches) renal artery and any accessory renal artery(s) for renal angiography, including arterial puncture, catheterization, fluoroscopy, contrast injection(s), image postprocessing, permanent recording of images, and radiological supervision and interpretation, including pressure gradient measurements when performed, and flush aortogram when performed; unilateral

36254 bilateral

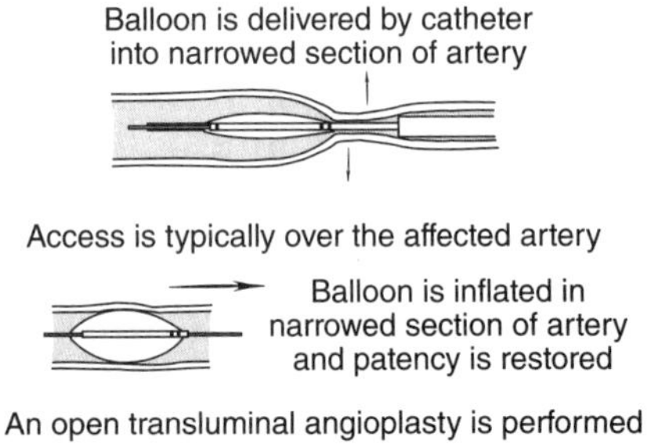

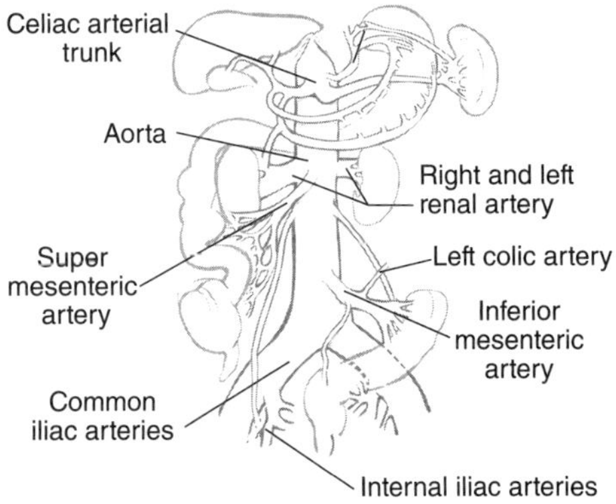

Explanation

A superselective catheterization is performed on one or more of the second order (branch) or higher of the renal artery branches. Superselective catheterization is needed for extremely small vessels or vessels that have sharp angles when branching to another order. The physician inserts a needle through the skin and into an underlying artery, usually a lower extremity artery, and threads a guidewire through the needle and into the artery. The needle is removed. The wire is threaded into the targeted artery and any accessory renal arteries of the second order or higher. A super fine and small catheter follows the wire into the arteries. The wire is removed. Contrast material for arteriography is injected into the catheter. Images are taken, the catheter is removed, and pressure is applied to stop bleeding at the injection site. These codes include image postprocessing, permanent recording of images, and radiological supervision and interpretation (e.g., pressure gradient measurements and flush aortogram). Report 36253 for a unilateral procedure and 36254 for a bilateral procedure.

Coding Tips

When medically necessary, report moderate (conscious) sedation provided by the performing physician with 99151-99153. When provided by another physician, report 99155-99157. These codes include needle or catheter placement, injection of contrast material, fluoroscopic guidance, image postprocessing and permanent storage of images, radiologic supervision and interpretation with or without pressure gradient measurements, and flush aortogram. Do not report closure device placement at the vascular access site separately. Do not report 36253 with 36251 when the procedure is performed on the same kidney. Do not report 36254 with 36252. Do not report these codes with 0338T or 0339T.

ICD-10-CM Diagnostic Codes

C64.1 Malignant neoplasm of right kidney, except renal pelvis ☑
C65.1 Malignant neoplasm of right renal pelvis ☑
C79.01 Secondary malignant neoplasm of right kidney and renal pelvis ☑
D30.01 Benign neoplasm of right kidney ☑
D30.11 Benign neoplasm of right renal pelvis ☑
D41.01 Neoplasm of uncertain behavior of right kidney ☑
D41.11 Neoplasm of uncertain behavior of right renal pelvis ☑
D41.21 Neoplasm of uncertain behavior of right ureter ☑
I15.0 Renovascular hypertension
I15.1 Hypertension secondary to other renal disorders
I70.1 Atherosclerosis of renal artery A
I72.2 Aneurysm of renal artery
I75.81 Atheroembolism of kidney
I77.73 Dissection of renal artery
N17.0 Acute kidney failure with tubular necrosis
N17.1 Acute kidney failure with acute cortical necrosis
N17.2 Acute kidney failure with medullary necrosis
N17.8 Other acute kidney failure
N26.1 Atrophy of kidney (terminal)
N26.2 Page kidney
N27.0 Small kidney, unilateral
N27.1 Small kidney, bilateral
N28.0 Ischemia and infarction of kidney
N28.82 Megaloureter
Q27.1 Congenital renal artery stenosis
Q27.2 Other congenital malformations of renal artery
S35.411A Laceration of right renal artery, initial encounter ☑
S35.491A Other specified injury of right renal artery, initial encounter ☑
S37.011A Minor contusion of right kidney, initial encounter ☑
S37.021A Major contusion of right kidney, initial encounter ☑
S37.061A Major laceration of right kidney, initial encounter ☑
S37.091A Other injury of right kidney, initial encounter ☑

AMA: 36253 2020,Sep; 2018,Oct **36254** 2020,Sep; 2018,Oct

Relative Value Units/Medicare Edits

Non-Facility RVU	Work	PE	MP	Total
36253	7.3	50.84	0.88	59.02
36254	7.9	48.55	1.72	58.17
Facility RVU	**Work**	**PE**	**MP**	**Total**
36253	7.3	2.11	0.88	10.29
36254	7.9	2.54	1.72	12.16

	FUD	Status	MUE	Modifiers				IOM Reference
36253	0	A	1(3)	51	N/A	N/A	N/A	None
36254	0	A	1(3)	51	N/A	N/A	N/A	

* with documentation

36260

36260 Insertion of implantable intra-arterial infusion pump (eg, for chemotherapy of liver)

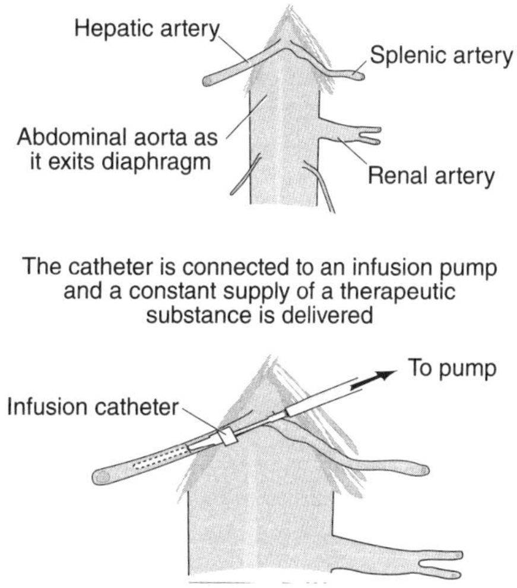

Explanation

The physician performs an upper abdominal incision and exposes the hepatic artery. The physician punctures the hepatic artery with a large needle and passes a guidewire via the needle into the punctured artery. The physician removes the needle while leaving the guidewire in place. The physician slides the infusion catheter over the guidewire into the arterial lumen. The physician secures the catheter with suture and closes the abdominal wound around the proximal end of the infusion catheter. The physician may use the catheter to administer chemotherapeutic medication.

Coding Tips

For removal of an intra-arterial infusion pump, see 36262. Supplies used when providing this procedure may be reported with C1772. Check with the specific payer to determine coverage. For revision of an implanted intra-arterial infusion pump, see 36261.

ICD-10-CM Diagnostic Codes

C22.0 Liver cell carcinoma
C22.1 Intrahepatic bile duct carcinoma
C22.2 Hepatoblastoma
C22.3 Angiosarcoma of liver
C22.4 Other sarcomas of liver
C22.7 Other specified carcinomas of liver
C78.7 Secondary malignant neoplasm of liver and intrahepatic bile duct
C7B.02 Secondary carcinoid tumors of liver
D01.5 Carcinoma in situ of liver, gallbladder and bile ducts
D01.7 Carcinoma in situ of other specified digestive organs
D37.6 Neoplasm of uncertain behavior of liver, gallbladder and bile ducts

Associated HCPCS Codes

C1772 Infusion pump, programmable (implantable)

Relative Value Units/Medicare Edits

Non-Facility RVU	Work	PE	MP	Total
36260	9.91	7.33	2.55	19.79
Facility RVU	**Work**	**PE**	**MP**	**Total**
36260	9.91	7.33	2.55	19.79

	FUD	Status	MUE	Modifiers				IOM Reference
36260	90	A	1(2)	51	N/A	N/A	N/A	None

* with documentation

Terms To Know

artery. Vessel through which oxygenated blood passes away from the heart to any part of the body.

carcinoma in situ. Malignancy that arises from the cells of the vessel, gland, or organ of origin that remains confined to that site or has not invaded neighboring tissue.

catheter. Flexible tube inserted into an area of the body for introducing or withdrawing fluid.

in situ. Located in the natural position or contained within the origin site, not spread into neighboring tissue.

malignant. Any condition tending to progress toward death, specifically an invasive tumor with a loss of cellular differentiation that has the ability to spread or metastasize to other body areas.

proximal. Located closest to a specified reference point, usually the midline or trunk.

36261

36261 Revision of implanted intra-arterial infusion pump

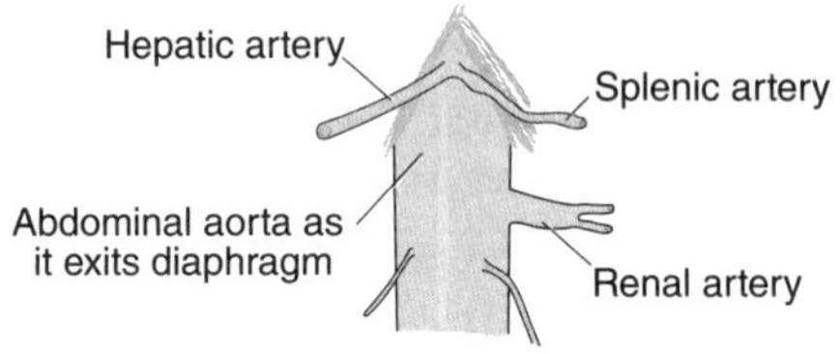

The catheter is connected to an infusion pump and a constant supply of a therapeutic substance is delivered

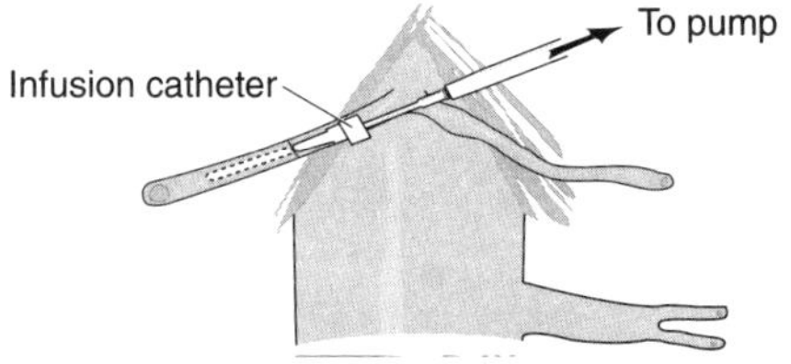

Explanation

The physician performs an upper abdominal incision and exposes the hepatic artery, locating the previously implanted infusion catheter. The physician may unkink the catheter or replace it over a wire. The physician secures the catheter with suture and closes the abdominal wound around the proximal end of the infusion catheter. The physician may use the catheter to administer chemotherapeutic medication.

Coding Tips

Supplies used when providing this procedure may be reported with the appropriate HCPCS Level II code. Check with the specific payer to determine coverage. For insertion of an implantable intra-arterial infusion pump, see 36260. For removal of an implanted intra-arterial infusion pump, see 36262.

ICD-10-CM Diagnostic Codes

C22.0	Liver cell carcinoma
C22.1	Intrahepatic bile duct carcinoma
C22.2	Hepatoblastoma
C22.3	Angiosarcoma of liver
C22.4	Other sarcomas of liver
C22.7	Other specified carcinomas of liver
C78.7	Secondary malignant neoplasm of liver and intrahepatic bile duct
C7B.02	Secondary carcinoid tumors of liver
D01.5	Carcinoma in situ of liver, gallbladder and bile ducts
D01.7	Carcinoma in situ of other specified digestive organs
D37.6	Neoplasm of uncertain behavior of liver, gallbladder and bile ducts
Z45.2	Encounter for adjustment and management of vascular access device
Z95.828	Presence of other vascular implants and grafts

Relative Value Units/Medicare Edits

Non-Facility RVU	Work	PE	MP	Total
36261	5.63	5.38	1.46	12.47
Facility RVU	**Work**	**PE**	**MP**	**Total**
36261	5.63	5.38	1.46	12.47

	FUD	Status	MUE	Modifiers				IOM Reference
36261	90	A	1(2)	51	N/A	N/A	80	None

* with documentation

Terms To Know

catheter. Flexible tube inserted into an area of the body for introducing or withdrawing fluid.

complication. Condition arising after the beginning of observation and treatment that modifies the course of the patient's illness or the medical care required, or an undesired result or misadventure in medical care.

infection. Presence of microorganisms in body tissues that may result in cellular damage.

proximal. Located closest to a specified reference point, usually the midline or trunk.

suture. Numerous stitching techniques employed in wound closure.

buried suture. Continuous or interrupted suture placed under the skin for a layered closure.

continuous suture. Running stitch with tension evenly distributed across a single strand to provide a leakproof closure line.

interrupted suture. Series of single stitches with tension isolated at each stitch, in which all stitches are not affected if one becomes loose, and the isolated sutures cannot act as a wick to transport an infection.

purse-string suture. Continuous suture placed around a tubular structure and tightened, to reduce or close the lumen.

retention suture. Secondary stitching that bridges the primary suture, providing support for the primary repair; a plastic or rubber bolster may be placed over the primary repair and under the retention sutures.

36262

36262 Removal of implanted intra-arterial infusion pump

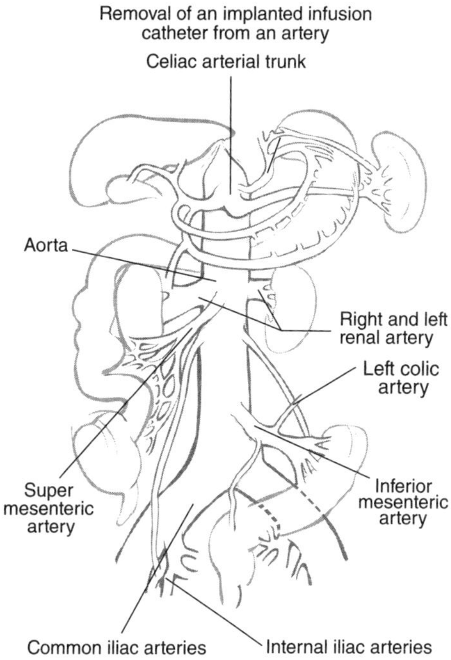

Explanation

The physician performs an upper abdominal incision and exposes the hepatic artery while dissecting free the previously implanted infusion catheter. The physician removes the catheter, and may repair the arteriotomy with suture. The physician closes the abdominal wound, and may leave a drain in place.

Coding Tips

For insertion of an implantable intra-arterial infusion pump, see 36260. For revision of an implanted intra-arterial infusion pump, see 36261.

ICD-10-CM Diagnostic Codes

T82.514A	Breakdown (mechanical) of infusion catheter, initial encounter
T82.518A	Breakdown (mechanical) of other cardiac and vascular devices and implants, initial encounter
T82.524A	Displacement of infusion catheter, initial encounter
T82.528A	Displacement of other cardiac and vascular devices and implants, initial encounter
T82.534A	Leakage of infusion catheter, initial encounter
T82.538A	Leakage of other cardiac and vascular devices and implants, initial encounter
T82.594A	Other mechanical complication of infusion catheter, initial encounter
T82.598A	Other mechanical complication of other cardiac and vascular devices and implants, initial encounter
T82.7XXA	Infection and inflammatory reaction due to other cardiac and vascular devices, implants and grafts, initial encounter
T82.818A	Embolism due to vascular prosthetic devices, implants and grafts, initial encounter
T82.828A	Fibrosis due to vascular prosthetic devices, implants and grafts, initial encounter
T82.838A	Hemorrhage due to vascular prosthetic devices, implants and grafts, initial encounter

T82.848A Pain due to vascular prosthetic devices, implants and grafts, initial encounter

T82.858A Stenosis of other vascular prosthetic devices, implants and grafts, initial encounter

T82.868A Thrombosis due to vascular prosthetic devices, implants and grafts, initial encounter

T82.898A Other specified complication of vascular prosthetic devices, implants and grafts, initial encounter

Z45.2 Encounter for adjustment and management of vascular access device

Z95.828 Presence of other vascular implants and grafts

Relative Value Units/Medicare Edits

Non-Facility RVU	Work	PE	MP	Total
36262	4.11	4.36	1.07	9.54
Facility RVU	**Work**	**PE**	**MP**	**Total**
36262	4.11	4.36	1.07	9.54

	FUD	Status	MUE	Modifiers				IOM Reference
36262	90	A	1(2)	51	N/A	N/A	N/A	None

* with documentation

Terms To Know

arteriotomy. Incision into an artery.

catheter. Flexible tube inserted into an area of the body for introducing or withdrawing fluid.

complication. Condition arising after the beginning of observation and treatment that modifies the course of the patient's illness or the medical care required, or an undesired result or misadventure in medical care.

incision. Act of cutting into tissue or an organ.

infection. Presence of microorganisms in body tissues that may result in cellular damage.

malignant. Any condition tending to progress toward death, specifically an invasive tumor with a loss of cellular differentiation that has the ability to spread or metastasize to other body areas.

36468

36468 Injection(s) of sclerosant for spider veins (telangiectasia), limb or trunk

A solution is injected directly into the tiny distended veins in the arms, legs, or body trunk causing the walls of the vein to close

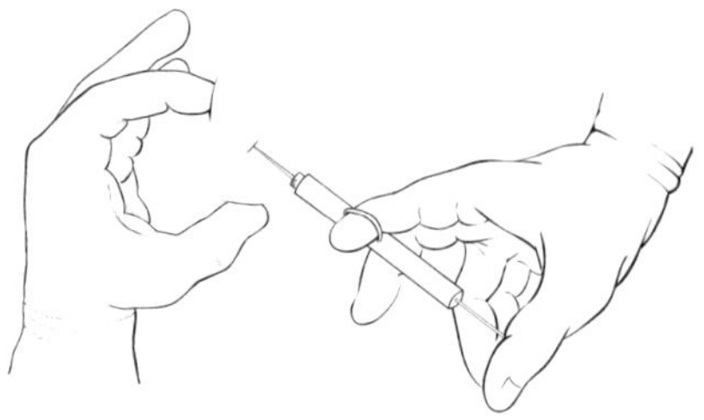

Explanation

The physician inserts a tiny needle through the skin and directly into the tiny, distended veins in the arm, leg, or trunk. A sclerosant for telangiectasias (spider veins) is injected into these veins. The solution causes the walls of the veins to become inflamed, collapse, and stick together so the veins close.

Coding Tips

This code should only be reported once per extremity. Do not report 36468 with 37241 for the same surgical field. Because this procedure usually is not done out of medical necessity, the patient may be responsible for charges. Verify with the insurance carrier for coverage. For ultrasound guidance performed with 36468, see 76942. Do not report 36468 with 29520, 29530, 29540, 29550, 29580, 29581, or 29584 for the same extremity. For treatment of larger varicose veins in the leg, with sclerosing solutions, see 36470–36471. For removal of a varicose vein/vein cluster, see 37785.

ICD-10-CM Diagnostic Codes

I78.0 Hereditary hemorrhagic telangiectasia

I78.8 Other diseases of capillaries

I78.9 Disease of capillaries, unspecified

I79.8 Other disorders of arteries, arterioles and capillaries in diseases classified elsewhere

Z41.1 Encounter for cosmetic surgery

AMA: **36468** 2018,Mar

Relative Value Units/Medicare Edits

Non-Facility RVU	Work	PE	MP	Total
36468	0.0	0.0	0.0	0.0
Facility RVU	**Work**	**PE**	**MP**	**Total**
36468	0.0	0.0	0.0	0.0

	FUD	Status	MUE	Modifiers				IOM Reference
36468	0	R	2(3)	51	N/A	N/A	80*	None

* with documentation

36470-36471

36470 Injection of sclerosant; single incompetent vein (other than telangiectasia)

36471 multiple incompetent veins (other than telangiectasia), same leg

A solution is injected directly into the tiny distended veins in the leg causing the walls of the vein to close

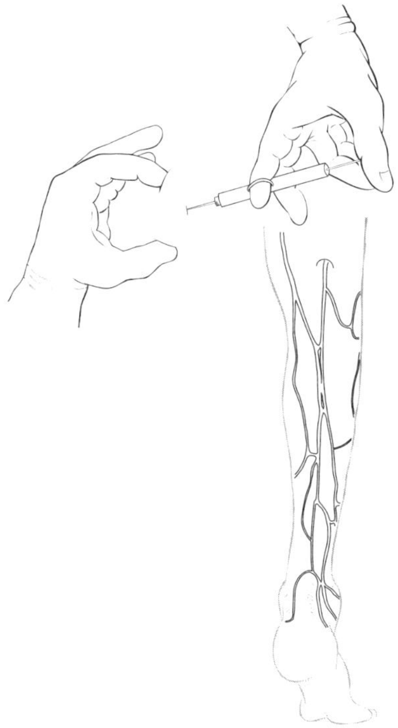

Explanation

The physician inserts a tiny needle through the skin and injects sclerosant into a single, incompetent vein, other than telangiectasias (spider veins), of the leg. The patient stands while the sclerosant injection is given. The leg is elevated and wrapped in an elastic dressing. The solution causes the walls of the veins to become inflamed, collapse, and stick together so the veins close. Report 36471 for injection of sclerosant into multiple incompetent veins, other than telangiectasias, of the same leg.

Coding Tips

Note that 36471 is a unilateral procedure. If performed bilaterally, some payers require that the service be reported twice with modifier 50 appended to the second code, while others require identification of the service only once with modifier 50 appended. Check with individual payers. Modifier 50 identifies a procedure performed identically on the opposite side of the body (mirror image). For ultrasound guidance performed with 36470-36471, see 76942. Do not report these codes with 29520, 29530, 29540, 29550, 29580, 29581, or 29584 for the same extremity. Do not report these codes with 37241 for the same surgical field. Do not report 36471 more than once per extremity. If extremity truncal vein injection of noncompounded foam sclerosant with ultrasound guided compression maneuvers to guide dispersion of the injectate is performed, see 36465-36466. For injections of spider veins (telangiectasia) of the arm, limb, or trunk, see 36468. Because this procedure usually is not done out of medical necessity, the patient may be responsible for charges. Verify with the insurance carrier for coverage.

ICD-10-CM Diagnostic Codes

I83.011 Varicose veins of right lower extremity with ulcer of thigh [A] ☑

I83.012 Varicose veins of right lower extremity with ulcer of calf [A] ☑

I83.013 Varicose veins of right lower extremity with ulcer of ankle [A] ☑

I83.014 Varicose veins of right lower extremity with ulcer of heel and midfoot [A] ☑

I83.015 Varicose veins of right lower extremity with ulcer other part of foot [A] ☑

I83.018 Varicose veins of right lower extremity with ulcer other part of lower leg [A] ☑

I83.11 Varicose veins of right lower extremity with inflammation [A] ☑

I83.211 Varicose veins of right lower extremity with both ulcer of thigh and inflammation [A] ☑

I83.212 Varicose veins of right lower extremity with both ulcer of calf and inflammation [A] ☑

I83.213 Varicose veins of right lower extremity with both ulcer of ankle and inflammation [A] ☑

I83.214 Varicose veins of right lower extremity with both ulcer of heel and midfoot and inflammation [A] ☑

I83.215 Varicose veins of right lower extremity with both ulcer other part of foot and inflammation [A] ☑

I83.218 Varicose veins of right lower extremity with both ulcer of other part of lower extremity and inflammation [A] ☑

I83.811 Varicose veins of right lower extremity with pain [A] ☑

I83.891 Varicose veins of right lower extremity with other complications [A] ☑

I83.91 Asymptomatic varicose veins of right lower extremity [A] ☑

AMA: 36470 2018,Dec; 2018,Mar **36471** 2018,Dec

Relative Value Units/Medicare Edits

Non-Facility RVU	Work	PE	MP	Total
36470	0.75	2.56	0.15	3.46
36471	1.5	4.19	0.3	5.99
Facility RVU	**Work**	**PE**	**MP**	**Total**
36470	0.75	0.22	0.15	1.12
36471	1.5	0.43	0.3	2.23

	FUD	Status	MUE	Modifiers				IOM Reference
36470	0	A	1(2)	51	50	N/A	N/A	None
36471	0	A	1(2)	51	50	N/A	N/A	

* with documentation

Terms To Know

sclerose. To become hard or firm and indurated from increased formation of connective tissue or disease.

ulcer. Open sore or excavating lesion of skin or the tissue on the surface of an organ from the sloughing of chronically inflamed and necrosing tissue.

varicose vein. Abnormal, permanently distended or stretched vein.

[36465, 36466]

36465 Injection of non-compounded foam sclerosant with ultrasound compression maneuvers to guide dispersion of the injectate, inclusive of all imaging guidance and monitoring; single incompetent extremity truncal vein (eg, great saphenous vein, accessory saphenous vein)

36466 Injection of non-compounded foam sclerosant with ultrasound compression maneuvers to guide dispersion of the injectate, inclusive of all imaging guidance and monitoring; multiple incompetent truncal veins (eg, great saphenous vein, accessory saphenous vein), same leg

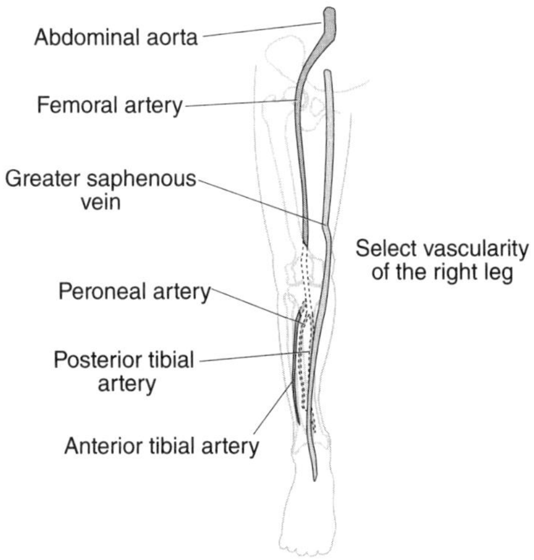

Explanation

The physician performs ultrasound guided foam sclerotherapy (UGFS) of varicose veins. UGFS is a minimally invasive and relatively safe treatment of restricted amounts of small varicose veins. In UGFS, a non-compounded foam sclerosant is injected into an extremity truncal vein (e.g., great saphenous vein, accessory saphenous vein) using ultrasound-guided compression of the junction of the central vein (saphenofemoral junction or saphenopopliteal junction) to limit the dispersion of the injectate. The physician creates a detailed outline or mapping of the veins in the lower legs to identify all vein abnormalities along with additional nearby structures to include deep veins and arteries via duplex ultrasound examination. Once completed, the patient is placed in the supine position and the leg being treated is exposed. The physician guides the needle into the vein using ultrasonic guidance and injects a non-compounded foam. Foam volumes vary from 1 mL to 16 mL per treatment. The injected vein collapses and is eventually absorbed by the body. The physician may need to repeat the injection process a number of times along the vein in order to completely target the incompetent truncal vein. Report 36465 for injection of a non-compounded foam sclerosant into a single incompetent extremity truncal vein and 36466 for multiple incompetent truncal veins of the same leg.

Coding Tips

When these procedures are performed in the office, all supplies and equipment are included. Codes may be reported only once per extremity per day. Application of compression bandages and/or stockings is included and may not be reported separately. Do not report 36465 or 36466 with 29520, 29530, 29540, 29550, 29580, 29581, or 29584 for the same extremity. Do not report 36465 or 36466 with 37241 when performed in the same surgical field. For a truncal vein injection in an extremity using compounded foam sclerosants or injection of a sclerosant into an incompetent vein without compression maneuvers to guide dispersion of the injectate, see 36470 and 36471. For endovenous ablation therapy of incompetent veins by transcatheter delivery of a chemical adhesive, see 36482 or 36483. For vascular embolization and occlusion procedures, see 37241-37244.

ICD-10-CM Diagnostic Codes

I78.0	Hereditary hemorrhagic telangiectasia
I82.491	Acute embolism and thrombosis of other specified deep vein of right lower extremity ☑
I82.591	Chronic embolism and thrombosis of other specified deep vein of right lower extremity ☑
I82.811	Embolism and thrombosis of superficial veins of right lower extremity ☑
I83.011	Varicose veins of right lower extremity with ulcer of thigh A ☑
I83.012	Varicose veins of right lower extremity with ulcer of calf A ☑
I83.013	Varicose veins of right lower extremity with ulcer of ankle A ☑
I83.014	Varicose veins of right lower extremity with ulcer of heel and midfoot A ☑
I83.015	Varicose veins of right lower extremity with ulcer other part of foot A ☑
I83.018	Varicose veins of right lower extremity with ulcer other part of lower leg A ☑
I83.11	Varicose veins of right lower extremity with inflammation A ☑
I83.211	Varicose veins of right lower extremity with both ulcer of thigh and inflammation A ☑
I83.212	Varicose veins of right lower extremity with both ulcer of calf and inflammation A ☑
I83.213	Varicose veins of right lower extremity with both ulcer of ankle and inflammation A ☑
I83.214	Varicose veins of right lower extremity with both ulcer of heel and midfoot and inflammation A ☑
I83.215	Varicose veins of right lower extremity with both ulcer other part of foot and inflammation A ☑
I83.218	Varicose veins of right lower extremity with both ulcer of other part of lower extremity and inflammation A ☑
I83.811	Varicose veins of right lower extremity with pain A ☑
I83.891	Varicose veins of right lower extremity with other complications A ☑
I83.91	Asymptomatic varicose veins of right lower extremity A ☑
I87.2	Venous insufficiency (chronic) (peripheral)

AMA: 36465 2019,Feb; 2018,Dec; 2018,Mar **36466** 2019,Feb; 2018,Dec; 2018,Mar

Relative Value Units/Medicare Edits

Non-Facility RVU	Work	PE	MP	Total
36465	2.35	35.41	0.46	38.22
36466	3.0	36.76	0.59	40.35
Facility RVU	**Work**	**PE**	**MP**	**Total**
36465	2.35	0.68	0.46	3.49
36466	3.0	0.86	0.59	4.45

	FUD	Status	MUE	Modifiers				IOM Reference
36465	0	A	1(2)	51	50	N/A	N/A	None
36466	0	A	1(2)	51	50	N/A	N/A	

* with documentation

36473-36474

36473 Endovenous ablation therapy of incompetent vein, extremity, inclusive of all imaging guidance and monitoring, percutaneous, mechanochemical; first vein treated

\+ **36474** subsequent vein(s) treated in a single extremity, each through separate access sites (List separately in addition to code for primary procedure)

Incompetent veins are treated with endovenous ablation including imaging guidance and monitoring

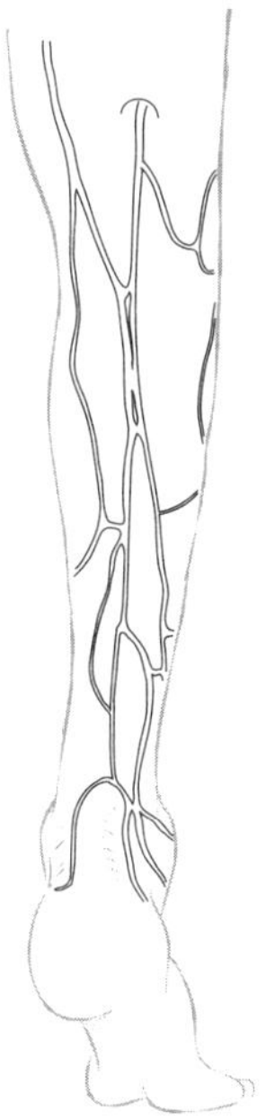

Explanation

The physician uses endovenous ablation therapy to treat venous incompetence in an extremity vein. Mechanochemical endovenous ablation (MOCA) uses a rotating wire in conjunction with an infused sclerosing agent to damage the wall of the vein. The most common site of treatment is the greater saphenous vein. The procedure includes any imaging guidance and monitoring. The leg is prepared and draped and a local anesthetic is applied to the puncture site. A needle is inserted into the access site. A guidewire is placed into the vessel using ultrasound guidance. An introducer sheath is placed over the guidewire and the guidewire is removed. A wire catheter system is introduced and the tip is advanced to the site of the venous incompetence under ultrasound guidance. The wire catheter system is connected to a handle with a motor that provides the rotation to the wire. The system is started for about 10 seconds to create vasospasm and slowly withdrawn with continuous infusion of sclerosing agent. The ablation catheter and introducer sheath are removed and pressure is applied to the puncture site. A compression stocking is applied for the immediate 24 hours and replaced daily for the following two weeks. Report 36473 for the initial vein treated and 36474 for subsequent veins treated in the same extremity via different access sites.

Coding Tips

When these procedures are performed in an office setting, required supplies and equipment are included and may not be reported separately. Codes may be reported only once per extremity per day. Application of compression bandages and/or stockings are included, when performed, and may not be reported separately. Report 36474 in addition to 36473. Report 36474 for subsequent veins treated in the same extremity; it may only be reported once per extremity. Do not report 36473 or 36474 with 36000-36005, 36410, 36425, 36475-36479, 37241, 75894, 76000, 76937, 76942, 76998, 77022, 93970, or 93971 for the same surgical field. Do not report these codes with 29520, 29530, 29540, 29550, 29580, 29581, or 29584 for the same extremity. For injection of an adhesive via catheter, see 37799.

ICD-10-CM Diagnostic Codes

I83.011	Varicose veins of right lower extremity with ulcer of thigh A ☑
I83.012	Varicose veins of right lower extremity with ulcer of calf A ☑
I83.013	Varicose veins of right lower extremity with ulcer of ankle A ☑
I83.014	Varicose veins of right lower extremity with ulcer of heel and midfoot A ☑
I83.015	Varicose veins of right lower extremity with ulcer other part of foot A ☑
I83.018	Varicose veins of right lower extremity with ulcer other part of lower leg A ☑
I83.11	Varicose veins of right lower extremity with inflammation A ☑
I83.211	Varicose veins of right lower extremity with both ulcer of thigh and inflammation A ☑
I83.212	Varicose veins of right lower extremity with both ulcer of calf and inflammation A ☑
I83.213	Varicose veins of right lower extremity with both ulcer of ankle and inflammation A ☑
I83.214	Varicose veins of right lower extremity with both ulcer of heel and midfoot and inflammation A ☑
I83.215	Varicose veins of right lower extremity with both ulcer other part of foot and inflammation A ☑
I83.218	Varicose veins of right lower extremity with both ulcer of other part of lower extremity and inflammation A ☑
I83.811	Varicose veins of right lower extremity with pain A ☑
I83.891	Varicose veins of right lower extremity with other complications A ☑
I83.91	Asymptomatic varicose veins of right lower extremity A ☑
I86.8	Varicose veins of other specified sites A

AMA: **36473** 2019,Feb; 2018,Mar **36474** 2019,Feb; 2018,Mar

Relative Value Units/Medicare Edits

Non-Facility RVU	Work	PE	MP	Total
36473	3.5	31.4	0.74	35.64
36474	1.75	5.38	0.34	7.47
Facility RVU	**Work**	**PE**	**MP**	**Total**
36473	3.5	1.08	0.74	5.32
36474	1.75	0.51	0.34	2.6

	FUD	Status	MUE	Modifiers				IOM Reference
36473	0	A	1(3)	51	50	N/A	N/A	None
36474	N/A	A	1(3)	N/A	50	N/A	N/A	

* with documentation

36475-36476

36475 Endovenous ablation therapy of incompetent vein, extremity, inclusive of all imaging guidance and monitoring, percutaneous, radiofrequency; first vein treated

\+ **36476** subsequent vein(s) treated in a single extremity, each through separate access sites (List separately in addition to code for primary procedure)

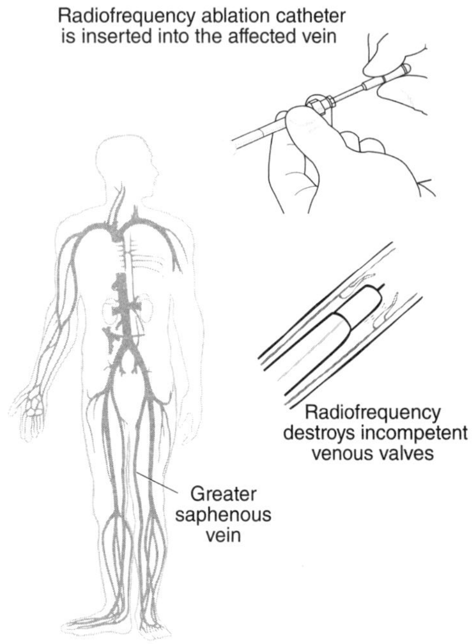

Radiofrequency endovenous ablation therapy is performed on a site in an extremity

Explanation

The physician uses percutaneous, radiofrequency, endovenous ablation therapy to treat venous incompetence in an extremity vein. Radiofrequency energy is used to heat and seal the vein closed. The most common site of treatment is the greater saphenous vein. The procedure includes any imaging guidance and monitoring. The leg is prepared and draped and a local anesthetic is applied to the puncture site. A needle is inserted into the access site. A guidewire is placed into the vessel using ultrasound guidance. An introducer sheath is placed over the guidewire and the guidewire is removed. The radiofrequency ablation catheter system is introduced and the tip is advanced to the site of the venous incompetence under ultrasound guidance. A local anesthetic agent is injected into the tissues surrounding the vein within its fascial sheath along the course of the vein. Ultrasonography is used to position the catheter tip at the level of the terminal valve and the catheter electrodes are deployed. The electrodes should be just distal to the valve cusps of the terminal valve. Radiofrequency energy is applied until the thermocouple temperature rises to 80° to 85°C and remains at this temperature for 10 to 15 seconds. Once this temperature is reached, the catheter tip is slowly withdrawn until it reaches the introducer sheath in the distal vein. The ablation catheter and introducer sheath are removed and pressure is applied to the puncture site. Report 36475 for the first vein treated in a single extremity and 36476 for each additional vein treated through a separate access site in the same extremity.

Coding Tips

When these procedures are performed in an office setting, required supplies and equipment are included and may not be reported separately. Application of compression bandages and/or stockings are included, when performed, and may not be reported separately. Report 36476 for subsequent veins treated in the same extremity; it may only be reported once per extremity. Report 36476 in addition to 36475. Do not report 36475 or 36476 with 36000–36005, 36410, 36425, 36478, 36479, 36482, 36483, 37241–37244, 75894, 76000, 76937, 76942, 76998, 77022, 93970, or 93971 in the same surgical field. Do not report 36468 with 29520, 29530, 29540, 29550, 29580, 29581, or 29584 for the same extremity.

ICD-10-CM Diagnostic Codes

I83.011 Varicose veins of right lower extremity with ulcer of thigh A ✓

I83.012 Varicose veins of right lower extremity with ulcer of calf A ✓

I83.013 Varicose veins of right lower extremity with ulcer of ankle A ✓

I83.014 Varicose veins of right lower extremity with ulcer of heel and midfoot A ✓

I83.015 Varicose veins of right lower extremity with ulcer other part of foot A ✓

I83.018 Varicose veins of right lower extremity with ulcer other part of lower leg A ✓

I83.11 Varicose veins of right lower extremity with inflammation A ✓

I83.211 Varicose veins of right lower extremity with both ulcer of thigh and inflammation A ✓

I83.212 Varicose veins of right lower extremity with both ulcer of calf and inflammation A ✓

I83.213 Varicose veins of right lower extremity with both ulcer of ankle and inflammation A ✓

I83.214 Varicose veins of right lower extremity with both ulcer of heel and midfoot and inflammation A ✓

I83.215 Varicose veins of right lower extremity with both ulcer other part of foot and inflammation A ✓

I83.218 Varicose veins of right lower extremity with both ulcer of other part of lower extremity and inflammation A ✓

I83.811 Varicose veins of right lower extremity with pain A ✓

I83.891 Varicose veins of right lower extremity with other complications A ✓

I83.91 Asymptomatic varicose veins of right lower extremity A ✓

I86.8 Varicose veins of other specified sites A

AMA: 36475 2024,Jan; 2018,Mar **36476** 2018,Mar

Relative Value Units/Medicare Edits

Non-Facility RVU	Work	PE	MP	Total
36475	5.3	25.26	1.15	31.71
36476	2.65	5.14	0.56	8.35
Facility RVU	**Work**	**PE**	**MP**	**Total**
36475	5.3	1.7	1.15	8.15
36476	2.65	0.69	0.56	3.9

	FUD	Status	MUE	Modifiers				IOM Reference
36475	0	A	1(3)	51	50	N/A	N/A	None
36476	N/A	A	2(3)	N/A	50	N/A	N/A	

* with documentation

36478-36479

36478 Endovenous ablation therapy of incompetent vein, extremity, inclusive of all imaging guidance and monitoring, percutaneous, laser; first vein treated

\+ **36479** subsequent vein(s) treated in a single extremity, each through separate access sites (List separately in addition to code for primary procedure)

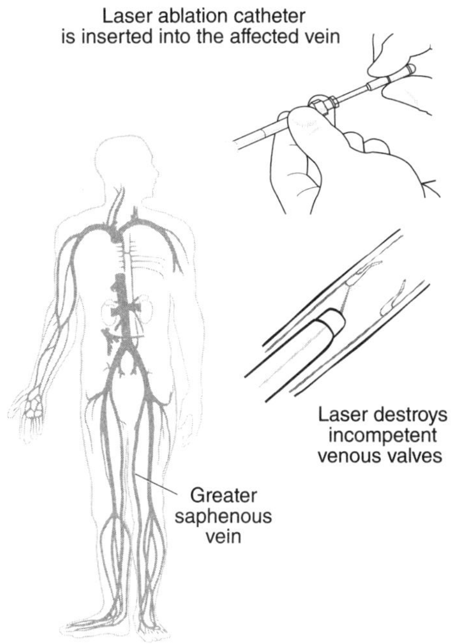

Laser endovenous ablation therapy is performed on a site in an extremity

Explanation

The physician uses percutaneous, laser, endovenous ablation therapy to treat venous incompetence in an extremity vein. Laser energy is used to heat the vein and seal the vein closed. The most common site of treatment is the greater saphenous vein. The procedure includes any imaging guidance and monitoring. The leg is prepared and draped and a local anesthetic is applied to the puncture site. A needle is inserted into the access site. A guidewire is placed into the vessel using ultrasound guidance. An introducer sheath is placed over the guidewire and the guidewire is removed. The laser ablation catheter system is introduced and the tip is advanced to the site of the venous incompetence under ultrasound guidance. A local anesthetic agent is injected into the tissues surrounding the vein within its fascial sheath. The anesthetic is injected along the course of the vein. Ultrasonography is used to position the catheter tip at the level of the terminal valve and laser energy is applied via a laser fiber along the length of the vein as the catheter is slowly withdrawn. When the laser catheter tip reaches the introducer sheath in the distal vein, the laser energy is terminated. The ablation catheter and introducer sheath are removed and pressure is applied at the puncture site. Report 36478 for the first vein treated in a single extremity and 36479 for each additional vein treated through a separate access site in the same extremity.

Coding Tips

When these procedures are performed in an office setting, required supplies and equipment are included and may not be reported separately. Application of compression bandages and/or stockings are included, when performed, and may not be reported separately. Report 36479 for subsequent veins treated in the same extremity; it may only be reported once per extremity. Report 36479 in addition to 36478. Do not report 36478 or 36479 with 36000–36005, 36410, 36425, 36475, 36476, 36482, 36483, 37241, 75894, 76000, 76937, 76942, 76998, 77022, 93970, or 93971 in the same surgical field. Do not report 36468 with 29520, 29530, 29540, 29550, 29580, 29581, or 29584 for the same extremity.

ICD-10-CM Diagnostic Codes

I83.011	Varicose veins of right lower extremity with ulcer of thigh A ☑
I83.012	Varicose veins of right lower extremity with ulcer of calf A ☑
I83.013	Varicose veins of right lower extremity with ulcer of ankle A ☑
I83.014	Varicose veins of right lower extremity with ulcer of heel and midfoot A ☑
I83.015	Varicose veins of right lower extremity with ulcer other part of foot A ☑
I83.018	Varicose veins of right lower extremity with ulcer other part of lower leg A ☑
I83.11	Varicose veins of right lower extremity with inflammation A ☑
I83.211	Varicose veins of right lower extremity with both ulcer of thigh and inflammation A ☑
I83.212	Varicose veins of right lower extremity with both ulcer of calf and inflammation A ☑
I83.213	Varicose veins of right lower extremity with both ulcer of ankle and inflammation A ☑
I83.214	Varicose veins of right lower extremity with both ulcer of heel and midfoot and inflammation A ☑
I83.215	Varicose veins of right lower extremity with both ulcer other part of foot and inflammation A ☑
I83.218	Varicose veins of right lower extremity with both ulcer of other part of lower extremity and inflammation A ☑
I83.811	Varicose veins of right lower extremity with pain A ☑
I83.891	Varicose veins of right lower extremity with other complications A ☑
I83.91	Asymptomatic varicose veins of right lower extremity A ☑
I86.8	Varicose veins of other specified sites A

AMA: **36478** 2020,May; 2018,Mar **36479** 2020,May; 2018,Mar

Relative Value Units/Medicare Edits

Non-Facility RVU	Work	PE	MP	Total
36478	5.3	22.57	1.09	28.96
36479	2.65	5.78	0.55	8.98
Facility RVU	**Work**	**PE**	**MP**	**Total**
36478	5.3	1.76	1.09	8.15
36479	2.65	0.78	0.55	3.98

	FUD	Status	MUE	Modifiers				IOM Reference
36478	0	A	1(3)	51	50	N/A	N/A	None
36479	N/A	A	2(3)	N/A	50	N/A	N/A	

* with documentation

[36482, 36483]

36482 Endovenous ablation therapy of incompetent vein, extremity, by transcatheter delivery of a chemical adhesive (eg, cyanoacrylate) remote from the access site, inclusive of all imaging guidance and monitoring, percutaneous; first vein treated

\+ **36483** Endovenous ablation therapy of incompetent vein, extremity, by transcatheter delivery of a chemical adhesive (eg, cyanoacrylate) remote from the access site, inclusive of all imaging guidance and monitoring, percutaneous; subsequent vein(s) treated in a single extremity, each through separate access sites (List separately in addition to code for primary procedure)

Incompetent veins treated with chemical adhesive

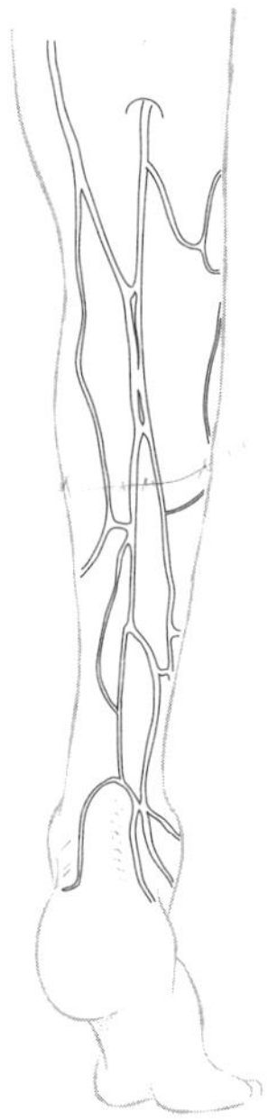

Explanation

The physician creates a detailed outline or mapping of the veins in the lower legs to identify all vein abnormalities, along with additional nearby structures to include deep veins and arteries, via duplex ultrasound examination. The patient is placed in the supine position and the leg being treated is exposed. A local anesthetic is administered. Through a small incision, the physician uses a needle to position an intravenous catheter the length of the incompetent vein. A chemical adhesive, such as cyanoacrylate, is injected through the catheter via a special type of applicator and into the vein under imaging guidance. A small amount of the chemical adhesive is injected approximately every 3 cm along the vein causing sclerosis or a hardening of the vein. To minimize dispersing of the chemical adhesive, ultrasound compression of the outflow vein is often included in these procedures. Imaging guidance and monitoring are included in these procedures. Report 36482 for the first vein treated and 36483 for subsequent veins treated in a single extremity, each through separate access sites.

Coding Tips

When these procedures are performed in the office, all supplies and equipment are included. Codes may be reported only once per extremity per day. Application of compression bandages and/or stockings is included and may not be reported separately. Report 36483 in addition to 36482. Report 36483 only once per extremity. Do not report 36482 or 36483 with 36000, 36002, 36005, 36410, 36425, 36475, 36476, 36478, 36479, 37241, 75894, 76000, 76937, 76942, 76998, 77022, 93970, or 93971 when performed in the same surgical field. Do not report 36468 with 29520, 29530, 29540, 29550, 29580, 29581, or 29584 for the same extremity.

ICD-10-CM Diagnostic Codes

I82.491	Acute embolism and thrombosis of other specified deep vein of right lower extremity ☑
I82.591	Chronic embolism and thrombosis of other specified deep vein of right lower extremity ☑
I82.811	Embolism and thrombosis of superficial veins of right lower extremity ☑
I83.011	Varicose veins of right lower extremity with ulcer of thigh A ☑
I83.012	Varicose veins of right lower extremity with ulcer of calf A ☑
I83.013	Varicose veins of right lower extremity with ulcer of ankle A ☑
I83.014	Varicose veins of right lower extremity with ulcer of heel and midfoot A ☑
I83.015	Varicose veins of right lower extremity with ulcer other part of foot A ☑
I83.018	Varicose veins of right lower extremity with ulcer other part of lower leg A ☑
I83.11	Varicose veins of right lower extremity with inflammation A ☑
I83.211	Varicose veins of right lower extremity with both ulcer of thigh and inflammation A ☑
I83.212	Varicose veins of right lower extremity with both ulcer of calf and inflammation A ☑
I83.213	Varicose veins of right lower extremity with both ulcer of ankle and inflammation A ☑
I83.214	Varicose veins of right lower extremity with both ulcer of heel and midfoot and inflammation A ☑
I83.215	Varicose veins of right lower extremity with both ulcer other part of foot and inflammation A ☑
I83.218	Varicose veins of right lower extremity with both ulcer of other part of lower extremity and inflammation A ☑
I83.811	Varicose veins of right lower extremity with pain A ☑
I83.891	Varicose veins of right lower extremity with other complications A ☑
I83.91	Asymptomatic varicose veins of right lower extremity A ☑
I87.2	Venous insufficiency (chronic) (peripheral)

AMA: 36482 2019,Feb; 2018,Mar **36483** 2019,Feb; 2018,Mar

Relative Value Units/Medicare Edits

Non-Facility RVU	Work	PE	MP	Total
36482	3.5	45.05	0.72	49.27
36483	1.75	1.95	0.39	4.09
Facility RVU	**Work**	**PE**	**MP**	**Total**
36482	3.5	1.04	0.72	5.26
36483	1.75	0.45	0.39	2.59

	FUD	Status	MUE	Modifiers				IOM Reference
36482	0	A	1(3)	51	50	N/A	N/A	None
36483	N/A	A	2(3)	N/A	50	N/A	N/A	

* with documentation

36500

36500 Venous catheterization for selective organ blood sampling

Explanation

The physician inserts a needle through the skin and into a peripheral vein. A guidewire is threaded through the needle into the vessel. The needle is removed. The wire is manipulated into the vein draining from the organ to be sampled. The catheter follows the guidewire into the vein. Once the catheter has been placed, the guidewire is removed and the blood sample obtained. The catheter is removed and pressure is applied to the puncture site to stop the flow of blood.

Coding Tips

This procedure does not include laboratory analysis. If a specimen is transported to an outside laboratory, report 99000 for handling or conveyance. For catheterization in the superior or inferior vena cava, see 36010. For radiological supervision and interpretation, see 75893.

ICD-10-CM Diagnostic Codes

C25.0	Malignant neoplasm of head of pancreas
C25.1	Malignant neoplasm of body of pancreas
C25.2	Malignant neoplasm of tail of pancreas
C25.3	Malignant neoplasm of pancreatic duct
C25.4	Malignant neoplasm of endocrine pancreas
C25.7	Malignant neoplasm of other parts of pancreas
C25.8	Malignant neoplasm of overlapping sites of pancreas
C56.1	Malignant neoplasm of right ovary ☑
C56.2	Malignant neoplasm of left ovary ☑
C56.3	Malignant neoplasm of bilateral ovaries ☑
C74.01	Malignant neoplasm of cortex of right adrenal gland ☑
C74.02	Malignant neoplasm of cortex of left adrenal gland ☑
C75.0	Malignant neoplasm of parathyroid gland
C79.61	Secondary malignant neoplasm of right ovary ☑
C79.62	Secondary malignant neoplasm of left ovary ☑
C79.63	Secondary malignant neoplasm of bilateral ovaries ☑
D13.6	Benign neoplasm of pancreas
D13.7	Benign neoplasm of endocrine pancreas
D27.0	Benign neoplasm of right ovary ☑
D27.1	Benign neoplasm of left ovary ☑
D35.01	Benign neoplasm of right adrenal gland ☑
D35.02	Benign neoplasm of left adrenal gland ☑
D35.1	Benign neoplasm of parathyroid gland
D35.2	Benign neoplasm of pituitary gland
D37.8	Neoplasm of uncertain behavior of other specified digestive organs
D44.2	Neoplasm of uncertain behavior of parathyroid gland
D44.3	Neoplasm of uncertain behavior of pituitary gland
D44.4	Neoplasm of uncertain behavior of craniopharyngeal duct
E21.0	Primary hyperparathyroidism
E21.1	Secondary hyperparathyroidism, not elsewhere classified
E21.2	Other hyperparathyroidism
E22.0	Acromegaly and pituitary gigantism
E22.8	Other hyperfunction of pituitary gland
E24.0	Pituitary-dependent Cushing's disease
E24.2	Drug-induced Cushing's syndrome
E24.3	Ectopic ACTH syndrome
E24.4	Alcohol-induced pseudo-Cushing's syndrome
E24.8	Other Cushing's syndrome
E26.01	Conn's syndrome
E26.02	Glucocorticoid-remediable aldosteronism
E26.09	Other primary hyperaldosteronism
E26.1	Secondary hyperaldosteronism
E26.89	Other hyperaldosteronism
E28.1	Androgen excess
E28.2	Polycystic ovarian syndrome

Relative Value Units/Medicare Edits

Non-Facility RVU	Work	PE	MP	Total
36500	3.51	1.15	0.67	5.33
Facility RVU	**Work**	**PE**	**MP**	**Total**
36500	3.51	1.15	0.67	5.33

	FUD	Status	MUE	Modifiers				IOM Reference
36500	0	A	4(3)	51	N/A	N/A	N/A	None

* with documentation

Terms To Know

cannula. Tube inserted into a blood vessel, duct, or body cavity to facilitate passage.

catheter. Flexible tube inserted into an area of the body for introducing or withdrawing fluid.

guidewire. Flexible metal instrument designed to lead another instrument in its proper course.

peripheral. Outside of a structure or organ.

puncture. Creating a hole.

specimen. Tissue cells or sample of fluid taken for analysis, pathologic examination, and diagnosis.

supervision and interpretation. Radiology services that usually contain an invasive component and are reported by the radiologist for supervision of the procedure and the personnel involved with performing the examination, reading the film, and preparing the written report.

vena cava. Main venous trunk that empties into the right atrium from both the lower and upper regions, beginning at the junction of the common iliac veins inferiorly and the two brachiocephalic veins superiorly.

venous. Relating to the veins.

36511-36513

36511 Therapeutic apheresis; for white blood cells
36512 for red blood cells
36513 for platelets

Explanation

Therapeutic apheresis is the removal of some specific circulating blood component, cells or plasma solute, that is directly responsible for a disease process. Cells and plasma components may also be mobilized from other tissue storage during apheresis, such as from the spleen and lymph nodes, for enhanced clearance of the undesired element. The patient is prepared much the same as giving a regular blood donation. Whole blood is drawn out of one arm and into an instrument called a separator, which uses a microprocessing technique to draw the blood, anticoagulate it, and separate the component to be removed by centrifugal spinning, filtration, or column adsorption with the help of computerized calibration. The cells to be removed are collected while the remainder of the blood is recombined and returned to the patient through a tube and needle in the other arm. Report 36511 for white blood cell isolation and removal (leukapheresis or lymphocytapheresis), 36512 for red blood cell removal, and 36513 for removal of platelets.

Coding Tips

Use 36512 for automated red cell exchange. Do not report 36513 for donor platelet collections; only report this code for treatment of the patient when platelets are removed using apheresis. For therapeutic plasma pheresis, see 36514. For therapeutic apheresis with extracorporeal immunoadsorption or selective adsorption or filtration with plasma reinfusion, see 36516. For manual red cell exchange, see 36450, 36455, or 36456.

ICD-10-CM Diagnostic Codes

The application of this code is too broad to adequately present ICD-10-CM diagnostic code links here. Refer to your ICD-10-CM book.

AMA: 36512 2021,Oct

Relative Value Units/Medicare Edits

Non-Facility RVU	Work	PE	MP	Total
36511	2.0	1.15	0.13	3.28
36512	2.0	1.0	0.12	3.12
36513	2.0	0.94	0.19	3.13
Facility RVU	**Work**	**PE**	**MP**	**Total**
36511	2.0	1.15	0.13	3.28
36512	2.0	1.0	0.12	3.12
36513	2.0	0.94	0.19	3.13

	FUD	Status	MUE	Modifiers				IOM Reference
36511	0	A	1(3)	51	N/A	N/A	N/A	None
36512	0	A	1(3)	51	N/A	N/A	N/A	
36513	0	A	1(3)	51	N/A	N/A	N/A	

* with documentation

36514-36516

36514 Therapeutic apheresis; for plasma pheresis
36516 with extracorporeal immunoadsorption, selective adsorption or selective filtration and plasma reinfusion

Explanation

Therapeutic apheresis is the removal of specific circulating blood components, cells, or plasma solute that is directly responsible for a disease process. Cells and plasma components may also be mobilized from other tissue storage during apheresis, such as from the spleen and lymph nodes, for enhanced clearance of the undesired element. The patient is prepared much the same as giving a regular blood donation. Whole blood is drawn out of one arm and into an instrument called a separator, which uses a microprocessing technique to draw the blood, anticoagulate it, and separate the component to be removed by centrifugal spinning, filtration, or column adsorption with the help of computerized calibration. Plasmapheresis, reported with 36514, is the isolation of the plasma from the blood. Plasma exchange isolates, discards, and replaces the plasma with a substitute fluid, like albumin. Plasma exchange is nonspecific since the plasma is discarded on the basis that toxins and antibodies accumulate in the plasma. The best method requires treating a disorder by removing the offending abnormal plasma component selectively. Report 36516 for extracorporeal immunoadsorption, selective adsorption, or selective filtration, such as dextran sulfate cellulose columns, to selectively remove low-density lipoproteins with plasma reinfusion.

Coding Tips

For therapeutic apheresis for white blood cells, see 36511; red blood cells, see 36512; and platelets, see 36513. For professional supervision only for 36516, append modifier 26.

ICD-10-CM Diagnostic Codes

B60.01	Babesiosis due to Babesia microti
B60.02	Babesiosis due to Babesia duncani
B60.03	Babesiosis due to Babesia divergens
D57.03	Hb-SS disease with cerebral vascular involvement
D57.213	Sickle-cell/Hb-C disease with cerebral vascular involvement
D57.218	Sickle-cell/Hb-C disease with crisis with other specified complication
D57.813	Other sickle-cell disorders with cerebral vascular involvement
D59.11	Warm autoimmune hemolytic anemia
D59.12	Cold autoimmune hemolytic anemia
D59.13	Mixed type autoimmune hemolytic anemia
D59.31	Infection-associated hemolytic-uremic syndrome
D59.32	Hereditary hemolytic-uremic syndrome
D68.01	Von Willebrand disease, type 1
D68.020	Von Willebrand disease, type 2A
D68.03	Von Willebrand disease, type 3
D68.04	Acquired von Willebrand disease
M05.211	Rheumatoid vasculitis with rheumatoid arthritis of right shoulder ☑
M05.221	Rheumatoid vasculitis with rheumatoid arthritis of right elbow ☑
M05.231	Rheumatoid vasculitis with rheumatoid arthritis of right wrist ☑
M05.241	Rheumatoid vasculitis with rheumatoid arthritis of right hand ☑
M05.251	Rheumatoid vasculitis with rheumatoid arthritis of right hip ☑
M05.261	Rheumatoid vasculitis with rheumatoid arthritis of right knee ☑

M05.271	Rheumatoid vasculitis with rheumatoid arthritis of right ankle and foot ☑
M05.311	Rheumatoid heart disease with rheumatoid arthritis of right shoulder ☑
M05.321	Rheumatoid heart disease with rheumatoid arthritis of right elbow ☑
M05.331	Rheumatoid heart disease with rheumatoid arthritis of right wrist ☑
M05.341	Rheumatoid heart disease with rheumatoid arthritis of right hand ☑
M05.351	Rheumatoid heart disease with rheumatoid arthritis of right hip ☑
M05.361	Rheumatoid heart disease with rheumatoid arthritis of right knee ☑
M05.371	Rheumatoid heart disease with rheumatoid arthritis of right ankle and foot ☑
M31.11	Hematopoietic stem cell transplantation-associated thrombotic microangiopathy [HSCT-TMA]
M31.19	Other thrombotic microangiopathy
N18.31	Chronic kidney disease, stage 3a
N18.32	Chronic kidney disease, stage 3b
T80.310A	ABO incompatibility with acute hemolytic transfusion reaction, initial encounter
T80.311A	ABO incompatibility with delayed hemolytic transfusion reaction, initial encounter
T86.01	Bone marrow transplant rejection
T86.02	Bone marrow transplant failure
T86.03	Bone marrow transplant infection

AMA: 36514 2018,May

Relative Value Units/Medicare Edits

Non-Facility RVU	Work	PE	MP	Total
36514	1.81	17.98	0.15	19.94
36516	1.56	51.39	0.31	53.26
Facility RVU	**Work**	**PE**	**MP**	**Total**
36514	1.81	0.79	0.15	2.75
36516	1.56	0.67	0.31	2.54

	FUD	Status	MUE	Modifiers				IOM Reference
36514	0	A	1(3)	51	N/A	N/A	N/A	None
36516	0	A	1(3)	51	N/A	N/A	N/A	

* with documentation

36555-36556

36555 Insertion of non-tunneled centrally inserted central venous catheter; younger than 5 years of age

36556 age 5 years or older

A non-tunneled centrally inserted CVC is inserted

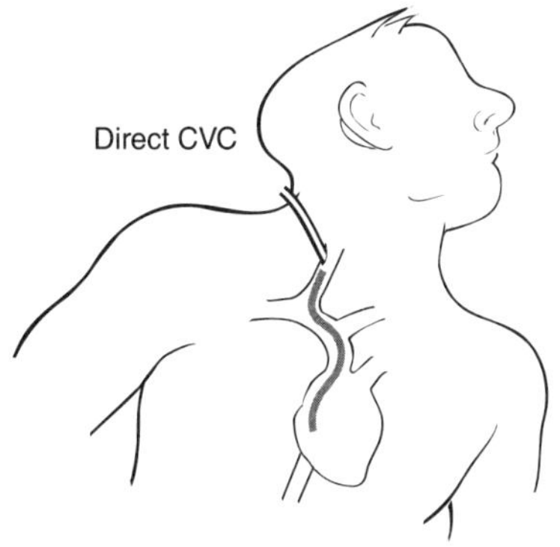

Explanation

A central venous access device (CVAD) or catheter is one in which the tip terminates in the subclavian, brachiocephalic, or iliac vein; the superior or inferior vena cava; or the right atrium. A centrally inserted CVAD has an entry site in the inferior vena cava or the jugular, subclavian, or femoral vein. For insertion of a non-tunneled, centrally inserted CVAD, the site over the access vein (e.g., subclavian, jugular) is injected with local anesthesia and punctured with a needle. A guidewire is inserted. The central venous catheter is placed over the guidewire. Ultrasound guidance may be used to gain venous access and/or fluoroscopy to check the positioning of the catheter tip. The catheter is secured into position and dressed. Non-tunneled catheters are percutaneously inserted for short term (five to seven days) use; to infuse medications, fluids, blood products, and parenteral nutrition; and to take blood draws. Report 36555 for insertion for children younger than 5 years of age and 36556 for a patient 5 years of age or older.

Coding Tips

When medically necessary, report moderate (conscious) sedation provided by the performing physician with 99151-99153. When provided by another physician, report 99155-99157. If imaging guidance is used, either for obtaining access to the venous access site or for manipulating the catheter into its final end position, see 76937 or 77001. For central venous catheter without a subcutaneous port or pump inserted peripherally in patients younger than 5 years old, see 36568. For central venous catheter without a subcutaneous port or pump inserted peripherally in patients older than age 5, see 36569.

ICD-10-CM Diagnostic Codes

The application of this code is too broad to adequately present ICD-10-CM diagnostic code links here. Refer to your ICD-10-CM book.

AMA: 36555 2023,Sep; 2019,May; 2018,Nov **36556** 2023,Sep; 2019,May; 2018,Nov

Relative Value Units/Medicare Edits

Non-Facility RVU	Work	PE	MP	Total
36555	1.93	3.51	0.16	5.6
36556	1.75	4.37	0.23	6.35
Facility RVU	**Work**	**PE**	**MP**	**Total**
36555	1.93	0.39	0.16	2.48
36556	1.75	0.51	0.23	2.49

	FUD	Status	MUE	Modifiers				IOM Reference
36555	0	A	2(3)	N/A	N/A	N/A	N/A	None
36556	0	A	2(3)	N/A	N/A	N/A	N/A	

* with documentation

Terms To Know

catheter. Flexible tube inserted into an area of the body for introducing or withdrawing fluid.

fluoroscopy. Radiology technique that allows visual examination of part of the body or a function of an organ using a device that projects an x-ray image on a fluorescent screen.

guidewire. Flexible metal instrument designed to lead another instrument in its proper course.

infusion. Introduction of a therapeutic fluid, other than blood, into the bloodstream.

insertion. Placement or implantation into a body part.

jugular vein. Two pairs of veins on either side of the neck that open into the subclavian, sending blood from the head and neck to the heart.

parenteral nutrition. Nutrients provided subcutaneously, intravenously, intramuscularly, or intradermally for patients during the postoperative period and in other conditions, such as shock, coma, and renal failure.

vena cava. Main venous trunk that empties into the right atrium from both the lower and upper regions, beginning at the junction of the common iliac veins inferiorly and the two brachiocephalic veins superiorly.

36557-36558

36557 Insertion of tunneled centrally inserted central venous catheter, without subcutaneous port or pump; younger than 5 years of age

36558 age 5 years or older

A tunneled centrally inserted CVC is inserted

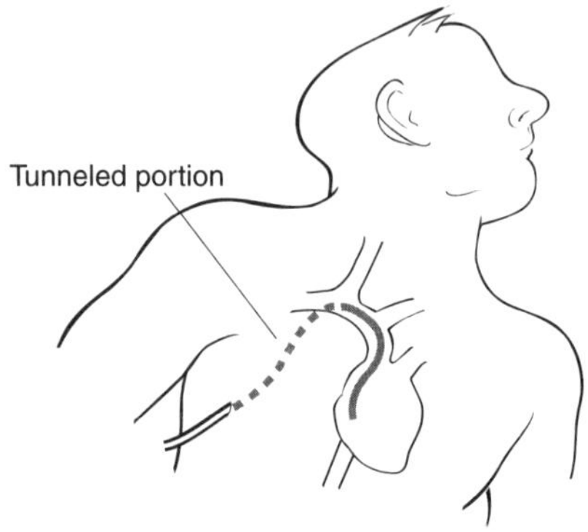

Explanation

A central venous access device (CVAD) or catheter is one in which the tip terminates in the subclavian, brachiocephalic, or iliac vein; the superior or inferior vena cava; or the right atrium. A centrally inserted CVAD has an entry site in the inferior vena cava or the jugular, subclavian, or femoral vein. A tunneled catheter has an entrance site at a distance from its entrance into the vascular system; they are "tunneled" through the skin and subcutaneous tissue to a great vein. For insertion of a tunneled, centrally inserted CVAD, without subcutaneous port or pump, standard preparations are made and the site over the access vein (e.g., subclavian, jugular) is injected with local anesthesia and punctured with a needle or accessed by cutdown approach. A guidewire is inserted. A subcutaneous tunnel is created using a blunt pair of forceps or sharp tunneling tools, over the clavicle from the anterior chest wall to the venotomy site, which is dilated to the right size. The catheter is passed through this tunnel over the guidewire and into the target vein. Ultrasound guidance may be used to gain venous access and/or fluoroscopy to check the positioning of the catheter tip. The catheter is secured into position and any incisions are sutured. Report 36557 for insertion for children younger than 5 years of age and 36558 for a patient 5 years of age or older.

Coding Tips

When medically necessary, report moderate (conscious) sedation provided by the performing physician with 99151-99153. When provided by another physician, report 99155-99157. If imaging guidance is used, either for obtaining access to the venous access site or for manipulating the catheter into its final end position, see 76937 or 77001. For central venous catheter with a port inserted peripherally on patients age 5 years or older, see 36571.

ICD-10-CM Diagnostic Codes

The application of this code is too broad to adequately present ICD-10-CM diagnostic code links here. Refer to your ICD-10-CM book.

AMA: **36557** 2018,Nov **36558** 2018,Nov

Relative Value Units/Medicare Edits

Non-Facility RVU	Work	PE	MP	Total
36557	4.89	28.0	1.25	34.14
36558	4.59	19.07	0.64	24.3
Facility RVU	**Work**	**PE**	**MP**	**Total**
36557	4.89	3.46	1.25	9.6
36558	4.59	2.4	0.64	7.63

	FUD	Status	MUE	Modifiers				IOM Reference
36557	10	A	2(3)	51	50	N/A	80*	None
36558	10	A	2(3)	51	50	N/A	80*	

* with documentation

Terms To Know

anterior. Situated in the front area or toward the belly surface of the body.

catheter. Flexible tube inserted into an area of the body for introducing or withdrawing fluid.

cutdown. Small, incised opening in the skin to expose a blood vessel, especially over a vein (venous cutdown) to allow venipuncture and permit a needle or cannula to be inserted for the withdrawal of blood or administration of fluids.

forceps. Tool used for grasping or compressing tissue.

guidewire. Flexible metal instrument designed to lead another instrument in its proper course.

jugular vein. Two pairs of veins on either side of the neck that open into the subclavian, sending blood from the head and neck to the heart.

vascular. Pertaining to blood vessels.

venotomy. Incision or puncture of a vein.

36560-36563

36560 Insertion of tunneled centrally inserted central venous access device, with subcutaneous port; younger than 5 years of age

36561 age 5 years or older

36563 Insertion of tunneled centrally inserted central venous access device with subcutaneous pump

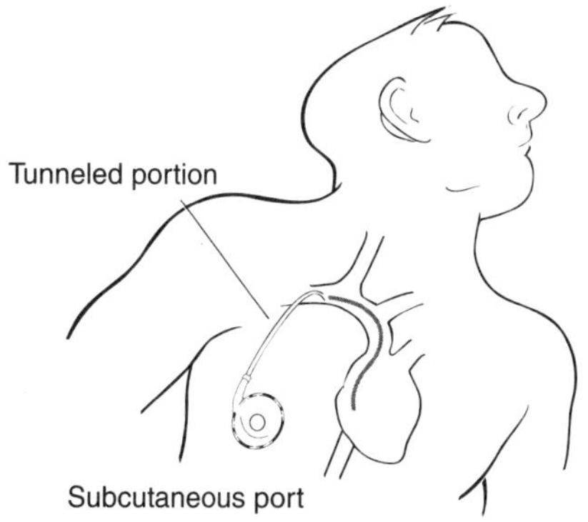

Explanation

For insertion of a tunneled, centrally inserted CVAD, with subcutaneous port/pump, the site over the access vein (e.g., subclavian, jugular) is injected with local anesthesia and punctured with a needle or accessed by cutdown approach. A guidewire is inserted. A subcutaneous tunnel is created using a blunt pair of forceps or sharp tunneling tools, over the clavicle, from the anterior chest wall to the venotomy site, which is dilated to the right size. The catheter is passed through this tunnel over the guidewire and into the target vein. The subcutaneous pocket for the port/pump is created with an incision through the skin overlying the second rib, a few centimeters from the midline. Blunt dissection and cautery are used to create the pocket in the chest wall and the port/pump is placed. The catheter is connected to the port/pump and checked by injection. Ultrasound guidance may be used to gain venous access and/or fluoroscopy to check the positioning of the catheter tip. The catheter and port/pump are secured into position and any incisions are sutured. Report 36560 for insertion with a port for children younger than 5 years of age and 36561 for a patient 5 years of age or older. Report 36563 for insertion with a pump.

Coding Tips

When medically necessary, report moderate (conscious) sedation provided by the performing physician with 99151-99153. When provided by another physician, report 99155-99157. If imaging guidance is used, either for obtaining access to the venous access site or for manipulating the catheter into its final end position, see 76937 or 77001. For a peripherally inserted central venous access device with subcutaneous port, younger than 5 years of age, see 36570; 5 years or older, see 36571.

ICD-10-CM Diagnostic Codes

The application of this code is too broad to adequately present ICD-10-CM diagnostic code links here. Refer to your ICD-10-CM book.

AMA: 36560 2018,Nov **36561** 2022,Jan; 2018,Nov

Relative Value Units/Medicare Edits

Non-Facility RVU	Work	PE	MP	Total
36560	6.04	28.84	1.55	36.43
36561	5.79	21.99	0.96	28.74
36563	5.99	25.09	1.23	32.31
Facility RVU	**Work**	**PE**	**MP**	**Total**
36560	6.04	3.88	1.55	11.47
36561	5.79	3.06	0.96	9.81
36563	5.99	3.5	1.23	10.72

	FUD	Status	MUE	Modifiers				IOM Reference
36560	10	A	2(3)	51	50	N/A	80*	None
36561	10	A	2(3)	51	50	N/A	80*	
36563	10	A	1(3)	51	N/A	N/A	80*	

* with documentation

Terms To Know

guidewire. Flexible metal instrument designed to lead another instrument in its proper course.

injection. Forcing a liquid substance into a body part such as a joint or muscle.

puncture. Creating a hole.

subcutaneous. Below the skin.

36565-36566

36565 Insertion of tunneled centrally inserted central venous access device, requiring 2 catheters via 2 separate venous access sites; without subcutaneous port or pump (eg, Tesio type catheter)

36566 with subcutaneous port(s)

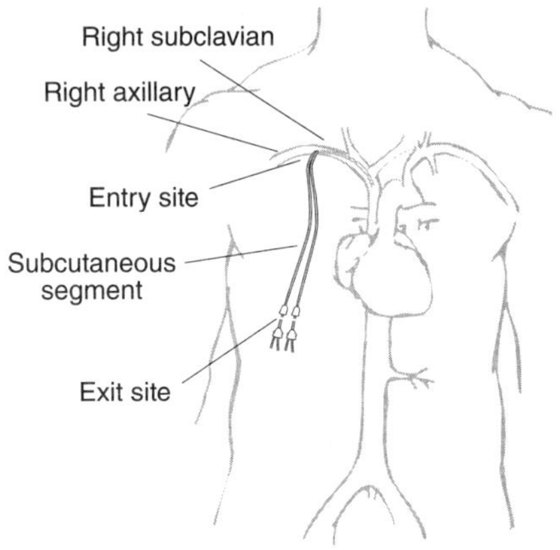

Tesio type catheters are double lumen devices. They are typically inserted into the superior vena cava and positioned before tunneling to an exit site or connecting to a subcutaneous port

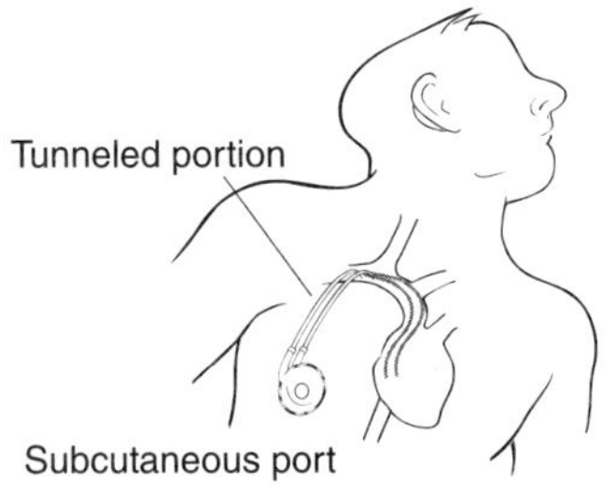

Explanation

For insertion of a tunneled, centrally inserted CVAD, requiring two catheters via two separate venous access sites, the sites of access (e.g., subclavian, jugular vein) for each catheter are injected with local anesthesia and two punctures are made with a needle or cutdown approach. Guidewires are inserted. Two subcutaneous tunnels are created using a blunt pair of forceps or sharp tunneling tools, over the clavicle, from the anterior chest wall to the venotomy sites, which are dilated to the right size. The catheters are each passed through their tunnel, over the guidewires, and into their venotomy sites. Ultrasound guidance may be used to gain venous access and/or fluoroscopy to check the positioning of the catheter tip. In 36565, the catheters are secured into position and any incisions are sutured. In 36566, two subcutaneous pockets for the ports are created with incisions through the skin in the chest wall, a few centimeters from the midline. Blunt dissection and cautery are used to create the pockets in the chest wall and the ports are placed. The catheters are connected to their respective ports and checked by injection. The catheters and ports are secured into position and any incisions are sutured.

Coding Tips

When medically necessary, report moderate (conscious) sedation provided by the performing physician with 99151-99153. When provided by another physician, report 99155-99157. If imaging guidance is used, either for obtaining access to the venous access site or for manipulating the catheter into its final end position, see 76937 or 77001.

ICD-10-CM Diagnostic Codes

The application of this code is too broad to adequately present ICD-10-CM diagnostic code links here. Refer to your ICD-10-CM book.

Relative Value Units/Medicare Edits

Non-Facility RVU	Work	PE	MP	Total
36565	5.79	17.45	1.25	24.49
36566	6.29	116.56	1.12	123.97
Facility RVU	**Work**	**PE**	**MP**	**Total**
36565	5.79	2.94	1.25	9.98
36566	6.29	3.14	1.12	10.55

	FUD	Status	MUE	Modifiers				IOM Reference
36565	10	A	1(3)	51	50	N/A	80*	None
36566	10	A	1(3)	51	50	N/A	80*	

* with documentation

Terms To Know

fluoroscopy. Radiology technique that allows visual examination of part of the body or a function of an organ using a device that projects an x-ray image on a fluorescent screen.

guidewire. Flexible metal instrument designed to lead another instrument in its proper course.

injection. Forcing a liquid substance into a body part such as a joint or muscle.

moderate sedation. Medically controlled state of depressed consciousness, with or without analgesia, while maintaining the patient's airway, protective reflexes, and ability to respond to stimulation or verbal commands.

puncture. Creating a hole.

subcutaneous. Below the skin.

vena cava. Main venous trunk that empties into the right atrium from both the lower and upper regions, beginning at the junction of the common iliac veins inferiorly and the two brachiocephalic veins superiorly.

venotomy. Incision or puncture of a vein.

36568-36569 [36572, 36573]

36568 Insertion of peripherally inserted central venous catheter (PICC), without subcutaneous port or pump, without imaging guidance; younger than 5 years of age

36569 age 5 years or older

36572 Insertion of peripherally inserted central venous catheter (PICC), without subcutaneous port or pump, including all imaging guidance, image documentation, and all associated radiological supervision and interpretation required to perform the insertion; younger than 5 years of age

36573 Insertion of peripherally inserted central venous catheter (PICC), without subcutaneous port or pump, including all imaging guidance, image documentation, and all associated radiological supervision and interpretation required to perform the insertion; age 5 years or older

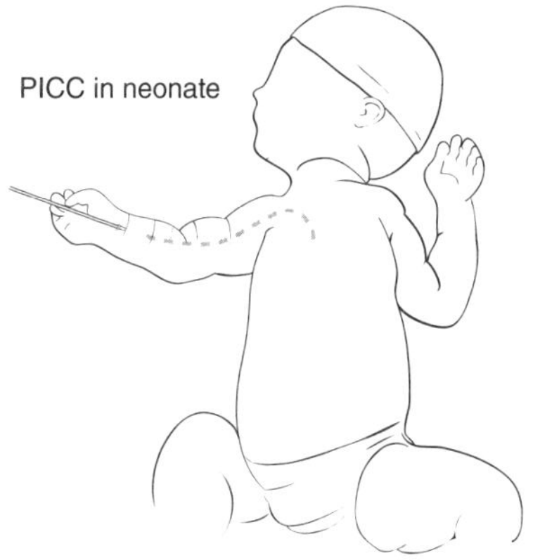

A central venous catheter is inserted from a periphery

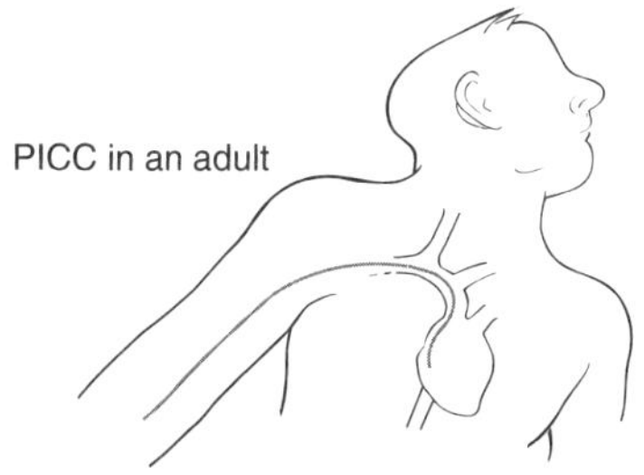

Explanation

A central venous access device or catheter is one in which the tip terminates in the subclavian, brachiocephalic, or iliac vein; the superior or inferior vena cava; or the right atrium. A peripherally inserted central venous catheter (PICC) has an entry site in the basilic or cephalic vein in the arm and is threaded into the superior vena cava above the right atrium. PICC lines are used for antibiotic therapy, chemotherapy, total parenteral nutrition, lab work, pain medications, blood transfusions, and hydration the same as a central line. For insertion of a (non-tunneled) peripherally inserted central venous catheter, without subcutaneous port or pump, the access vein (basilic or cephalic) is injected with local anesthesia and punctured with a needle. A guidewire is inserted. The central venous catheter is placed over the guidewire. The catheter is secured into position and dressed. Report 36568 for insertion of a PICC, without imaging, for children younger than 5 years of age; for a patient 5 years of age or older, report 36569. Report 36572 for insertion of a PICC, with imaging, for children younger than 5 years age; for a patient 5 years of age or older, report 36573.

Coding Tips

When medically necessary, report moderate (conscious) sedation provided by the performing physician with 99151-99153. When provided by another physician, report 99155-99157. Do not report 36568, 36569, 36572, or 36573 with 76937 or 77001. Do not report 36572 or 36573 with 71045-71048 as these services include confirming the catheter tip location. Report 36572 or 36573 for non-tunneled central venous catheter placement. If confirmation of catheter tip placement is not performed by the provider inserting the PICC line, append modifier 52 to 36572 or 36573. For midline catheter placement, see 36400, 36405, 36406, and 36410.

ICD-10-CM Diagnostic Codes

The application of this code is too broad to adequately present ICD-10-CM diagnostic code links here. Refer to your ICD-10-CM book.

AMA: **36568** 2019,May; 2019,Mar **36569** 2019,May; 2019,Mar **36572** 2019,May; 2019,Mar **36573** 2019,May; 2019,Mar

Relative Value Units/Medicare Edits

Non-Facility RVU	Work	PE	MP	Total
36568	2.11	0.34	0.25	2.7
36569	1.9	0.6	0.29	2.79
36572	1.82	8.97	0.23	11.02
36573	1.7	9.39	0.17	11.26
Facility RVU	**Work**	**PE**	**MP**	**Total**
36568	2.11	0.34	0.25	2.7
36569	1.9	0.6	0.29	2.79
36572	1.82	0.33	0.23	2.38
36573	1.7	0.57	0.17	2.44

	FUD	Status	MUE	Modifiers				IOM Reference
36568	0	A	2(3)	N/A	N/A	N/A	N/A	None
36569	0	A	2(3)	N/A	N/A	N/A	N/A	
36572	0	A	1(3)	N/A	N/A	N/A	N/A	
36573	0	A	1(3)	N/A	N/A	N/A	N/A	

* with documentation

Terms To Know

guidewire. Flexible metal instrument designed to lead another instrument in its proper course.

injection. Forcing a liquid substance into a body part such as a joint or muscle.

subcutaneous. Below the skin.

ultrasound. Imaging using ultra-high sound frequency bounced off body structures.

vena cava. Main venous trunk that empties into the right atrium from both the lower and upper regions, beginning at the junction of the common iliac veins inferiorly and the two brachiocephalic veins superiorly.

36570-36571

36570 Insertion of peripherally inserted central venous access device, with subcutaneous port; younger than 5 years of age

36571 age 5 years or older

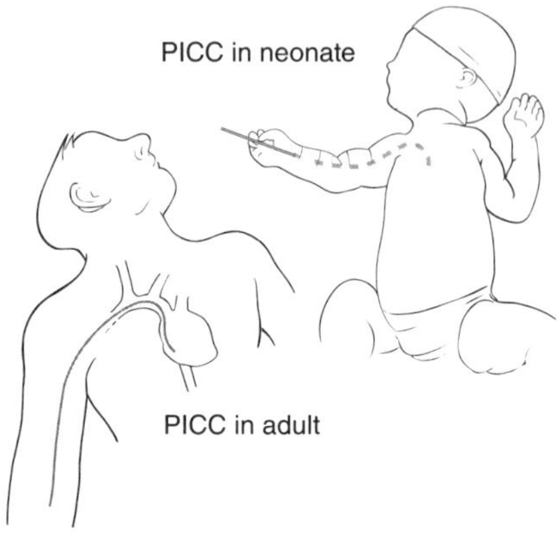

A central venous catheter is inserted from a periphery, with use of a subcutaneous port

Explanation

A central venous access device or catheter is one in which the tip terminates in the subclavian, brachiocephalic, or iliac vein; the superior or inferior vena cava; or the right atrium. A peripherally inserted central venous catheter (PICC) has an entry site in the basilic or cephalic vein in the arm and is threaded into the superior vena cava above the right atrium. PICC lines are used for antibiotic therapy, chemotherapy, total parenteral nutrition, lab work, pain medications, blood transfusions, and hydration the same as a central line. For insertion of a peripherally inserted central venous catheter with a subcutaneous port, the site over the access vein (basilic or cephalic) is injected with local anesthesia and punctured with a needle. A guidewire is inserted. The central venous catheter is placed over the guidewire and fed through the vein in the arm into the superior vena cava. The port may be placed in the chest in a subcutaneous pocket created through an incision in the chest wall, or placed in the arm through a small incision just above or halfway between the elbow crease and the shoulder on the inside of the arm. The port is attached to the catheter and checked. Ultrasound guidance may be used to gain venous access and/or fluoroscopy to check the positioning of the catheter tip. The catheter and port are secured into position and incisions are closed and dressed. Report 36570 for insertion for children younger than 5 years of age and 36571 for a patient 5 years of age or older.

Coding Tips

When medically necessary, report moderate (conscious) sedation provided by the performing physician with 99151-99153. When provided by another physician, report 99155-99157. If imaging guidance is used, either for obtaining access to the venous access site or for manipulating the catheter into its final end position, see 76937 or 77001. For insertion of a tunneled, centrally inserted central venous access device with subcutaneous port for patients younger than 5 years of age, see 36560; 5 years of age or older, see 36561.

ICD-10-CM Diagnostic Codes

The application of this code is too broad to adequately present ICD-10-CM diagnostic code links here. Refer to your ICD-10-CM book.

AMA: **36570** 2019,Mar **36571** 2019,Mar

Relative Value Units/Medicare Edits

Non-Facility RVU	Work	PE	MP	Total
36570	5.11	36.42	1.31	42.84
36571	5.09	30.77	1.06	36.92
Facility RVU	**Work**	**PE**	**MP**	**Total**
36570	5.11	3.54	1.31	9.96
36571	5.09	3.14	1.06	9.29

	FUD	Status	MUE	Modifiers				IOM Reference
36570	10	A	2(3)	51	50	N/A	80*	None
36571	10	A	2(3)	51	50	N/A	80*	

* with documentation

Terms To Know

chemotherapy. Treatment of disease, especially cancerous conditions, using chemical agents.

fluoroscopy. Radiology technique that allows visual examination of part of the body or a function of an organ using a device that projects an x-ray image on a fluorescent screen.

guidewire. Flexible metal instrument designed to lead another instrument in its proper course.

incision. Act of cutting into tissue or an organ.

injection. Forcing a liquid substance into a body part such as a joint or muscle.

insertion. Placement or implantation into a body part.

parenteral nutrition. Nutrients provided subcutaneously, intravenously, intramuscularly, or intradermally for patients during the postoperative period and in other conditions, such as shock, coma, and renal failure.

36575-36576

36575 Repair of tunneled or non-tunneled central venous access catheter, without subcutaneous port or pump, central or peripheral insertion site

36576 Repair of central venous access device, with subcutaneous port or pump, central or peripheral insertion site

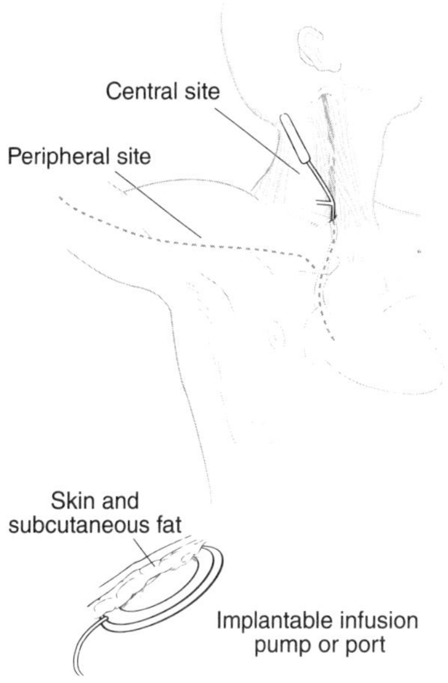

A CVA catheter or device, central or peripheral access, is repaired

Explanation

Code 36575 reports repair of a central venous access device (CVAD) that has external catheters with the access ports outside the body, and no subcutaneous ports or pumps, whether centrally or peripherally inserted, tunneled or non-tunneled. The repair is done on the catheter that is placed without any replacement of components. A Hickman catheter is an example of a tunneled CVAD with an external port. Code 36576 reports repair of a central venous access device (CVAD) that has an internal access port/pump in a subcutaneous pocket that is connected to the catheter, whether centrally or peripherally inserted. The repair is done on the device as it is placed within the patient, without any replacement of components, catheter or subcutaneous port/pump.

Coding Tips

When medically necessary, report moderate (conscious) sedation provided by the performing physician with 99151-99153. When provided by another physician, report 99155-99157. If imaging guidance is used, either for obtaining access to the venous access site or for manipulating the catheter into its final end position, see 76937 or 77001. For mechanical removal of pericatheter obstructive material, see 36595. For mechanical removal of intracatheter obstructive material, see 36596.

ICD-10-CM Diagnostic Codes

T82.41XA Breakdown (mechanical) of vascular dialysis catheter, initial encounter

T82.42XA Displacement of vascular dialysis catheter, initial encounter

T82.43XA Leakage of vascular dialysis catheter, initial encounter

T82.49XA Other complication of vascular dialysis catheter, initial encounter

T82.514A Breakdown (mechanical) of infusion catheter, initial encounter

T82.524A	Displacement of infusion catheter, initial encounter
T82.534A	Leakage of infusion catheter, initial encounter
T82.594A	Other mechanical complication of infusion catheter, initial encounter
T82.598A	Other mechanical complication of other cardiac and vascular devices and implants, initial encounter
T82.898A	Other specified complication of vascular prosthetic devices, implants and grafts, initial encounter
Z45.2	Encounter for adjustment and management of vascular access device

Relative Value Units/Medicare Edits

Non-Facility RVU	Work	PE	MP	Total
36575	0.67	3.54	0.07	4.28
36576	2.99	6.66	0.57	10.22
Facility RVU	**Work**	**PE**	**MP**	**Total**
36575	0.67	0.24	0.07	0.98
36576	2.99	1.87	0.57	5.43

	FUD	Status	MUE	Modifiers				IOM Reference
36575	0	A	2(3)	51	N/A	N/A	80*	None
36576	10	A	2(3)	51	N/A	N/A	80*	

* with documentation

Terms To Know

anesthesia. Loss of feeling or sensation, usually induced to permit the performance of surgery or other painful procedures.

Hickman catheter. Central venous catheter used for long-term delivery of medications, such as antibiotics, nutritional substances, or chemotherapeutic agents.

moderate sedation. Medically controlled state of depressed consciousness, with or without analgesia, while maintaining the patient's airway, protective reflexes, and ability to respond to stimulation or verbal commands.

peripheral. Outside of a structure or organ.

subcutaneous. Below the skin.

36578

36578 Replacement, catheter only, of central venous access device, with subcutaneous port or pump, central or peripheral insertion site

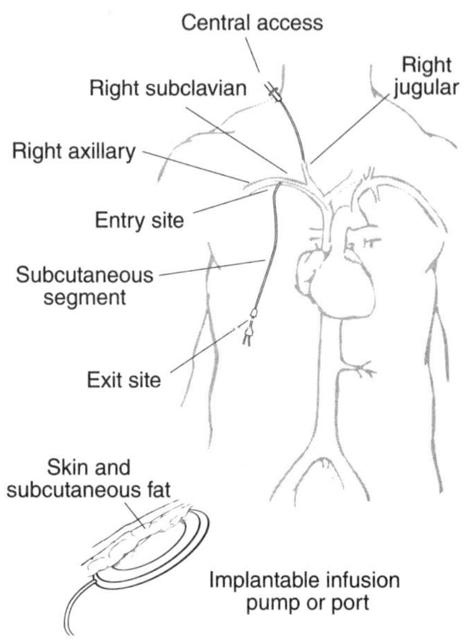

The catheter alone is replaced in a CVA device, with subcutaneous port or pump, central or peripheral access site

Explanation

The catheter only of a central venous access device with a subcutaneous port or pump is replaced, whether centrally or peripherally inserted. Local anesthesia is given and the subcutaneous pocket over the port is incised. The catheter is disconnected. A guidewire is placed through the existing catheter, which is removed over the guidewire. A new central venous catheter of correct length is placed into position and connected to the port/pump device that has not been removed or replaced. The connection with the new catheter is checked, as well as the catheter and port secured, and the wound is dressed.

Coding Tips

When medically necessary, report moderate (conscious) sedation provided by the performing physician with 99151-99153. When provided by another physician, report 99155-99157. For complete replacement of an entire device through the same venous access, see 36582 or 36583. If imaging guidance is used, either for obtaining access to the venous access site or for manipulating the catheter into its final end position, see 76937 or 77001.

ICD-10-CM Diagnostic Codes

T80.211A	Bloodstream infection due to central venous catheter, initial encounter
T80.212A	Local infection due to central venous catheter, initial encounter
T80.218A	Other infection due to central venous catheter, initial encounter
T82.41XA	Breakdown (mechanical) of vascular dialysis catheter, initial encounter
T82.42XA	Displacement of vascular dialysis catheter, initial encounter
T82.43XA	Leakage of vascular dialysis catheter, initial encounter
T82.49XA	Other complication of vascular dialysis catheter, initial encounter
T82.514A	Breakdown (mechanical) of infusion catheter, initial encounter
T82.524A	Displacement of infusion catheter, initial encounter
T82.534A	Leakage of infusion catheter, initial encounter

T82.594A	Other mechanical complication of infusion catheter, initial encounter
T82.598A	Other mechanical complication of other cardiac and vascular devices and implants, initial encounter
T82.7XXA	Infection and inflammatory reaction due to other cardiac and vascular devices, implants and grafts, initial encounter
T82.818A	Embolism due to vascular prosthetic devices, implants and grafts, initial encounter
T82.828A	Fibrosis due to vascular prosthetic devices, implants and grafts, initial encounter
T82.838A	Hemorrhage due to vascular prosthetic devices, implants and grafts, initial encounter
T82.848A	Pain due to vascular prosthetic devices, implants and grafts, initial encounter
T82.858A	Stenosis of other vascular prosthetic devices, implants and grafts, initial encounter
T82.868A	Thrombosis due to vascular prosthetic devices, implants and grafts, initial encounter
T82.898A	Other specified complication of vascular prosthetic devices, implants and grafts, initial encounter
Z45.2	Encounter for adjustment and management of vascular access device

Relative Value Units/Medicare Edits

Non-Facility RVU	Work	PE	MP	Total
36578	3.29	8.79	0.66	12.74
Facility RVU	**Work**	**PE**	**MP**	**Total**
36578	3.29	2.09	0.66	6.04

	FUD	Status	MUE	Modifiers				IOM Reference
36578	10	A	2(3)	51	N/A	N/A	80*	None

* with documentation

Terms To Know

anesthesia. Loss of feeling or sensation, usually induced to permit the performance of surgery or other painful procedures.

catheter. Flexible tube inserted into an area of the body for introducing or withdrawing fluid.

complication. Condition arising after the beginning of observation and treatment that modifies the course of the patient's illness or the medical care required, or an undesired result or misadventure in medical care.

guidewire. Flexible metal instrument designed to lead another instrument in its proper course.

36580-36581

36580 Replacement, complete, of a non-tunneled centrally inserted central venous catheter, without subcutaneous port or pump, through same venous access

36581 Replacement, complete, of a tunneled centrally inserted central venous catheter, without subcutaneous port or pump, through same venous access

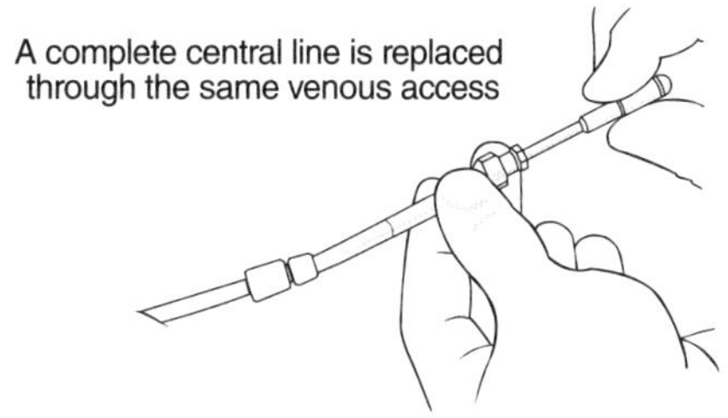

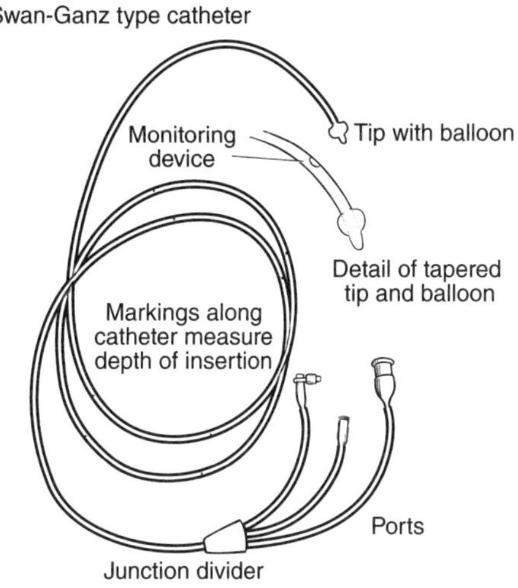

Explanation

In 36580, a non-tunneled, centrally inserted central venous catheter, without subcutaneous port or pump, is replaced through the same venous access site. Local anesthesia is given. In 36581, sutures securing the cuff of the indwelling catheter are freed from the skin. A guidewire is first passed through the existing central line catheter and the catheter is removed. A new central venous catheter is placed back into position over the guidewire, secured into position, and the wound dressed.

Coding Tips

When medically necessary, report moderate (conscious) sedation provided by the performing physician with 99151-99153. When provided by another physician, report 99155-99157. If imaging guidance is used for obtaining access to the venous access site or for manipulating the replacement catheter into its final end position, see 76937 or 77001. For replacement of a multicatheter device placed at separate venous access sites, use the appropriate code and indicate a frequency of two in the units column. If a venous access device is removed and a new one placed at a different access site, do not report 36580 or 36581; use the appropriate codes for the removal of the old device (if a removal code exists) and the insertion of the new device.

ICD-10-CM Diagnostic Codes

T80.211A	Bloodstream infection due to central venous catheter, initial encounter
T80.212A	Local infection due to central venous catheter, initial encounter

T80.218A Other infection due to central venous catheter, initial encounter

T82.41XA Breakdown (mechanical) of vascular dialysis catheter, initial encounter

T82.42XA Displacement of vascular dialysis catheter, initial encounter

T82.43XA Leakage of vascular dialysis catheter, initial encounter

T82.49XA Other complication of vascular dialysis catheter, initial encounter

T82.514A Breakdown (mechanical) of infusion catheter, initial encounter

T82.524A Displacement of infusion catheter, initial encounter

T82.534A Leakage of infusion catheter, initial encounter

T82.594A Other mechanical complication of infusion catheter, initial encounter

T82.598A Other mechanical complication of other cardiac and vascular devices and implants, initial encounter

T82.7XXA Infection and inflammatory reaction due to other cardiac and vascular devices, implants and grafts, initial encounter

T82.818A Embolism due to vascular prosthetic devices, implants and grafts, initial encounter

T82.828A Fibrosis due to vascular prosthetic devices, implants and grafts, initial encounter

T82.838A Hemorrhage due to vascular prosthetic devices, implants and grafts, initial encounter

T82.848A Pain due to vascular prosthetic devices, implants and grafts, initial encounter

T82.858A Stenosis of other vascular prosthetic devices, implants and grafts, initial encounter

T82.868A Thrombosis due to vascular prosthetic devices, implants and grafts, initial encounter

T82.898A Other specified complication of vascular prosthetic devices, implants and grafts, initial encounter

Z45.2 Encounter for adjustment and management of vascular access device

AMA: **36581** 2023,Jul

Relative Value Units/Medicare Edits

Non-Facility RVU	Work	PE	MP	Total
36580	1.31	4.1	0.17	5.58
36581	3.23	19.14	0.42	22.79
Facility RVU	**Work**	**PE**	**MP**	**Total**
36580	1.31	0.43	0.17	1.91
36581	3.23	1.73	0.42	5.38

	FUD	Status	MUE	Modifiers				IOM Reference
36580	0	A	2(3)	N/A	N/A	N/A	N/A	None
36581	10	A	2(3)	51	N/A	N/A	80*	

* with documentation

Terms To Know

catheter. Flexible tube inserted into an area of the body for introducing or withdrawing fluid.

guidewire. Flexible metal instrument designed to lead another instrument in its proper course.

36582-36583

36582 Replacement, complete, of a tunneled centrally inserted central venous access device, with subcutaneous port, through same venous access

36583 Replacement, complete, of a tunneled centrally inserted central venous access device, with subcutaneous pump, through same venous access

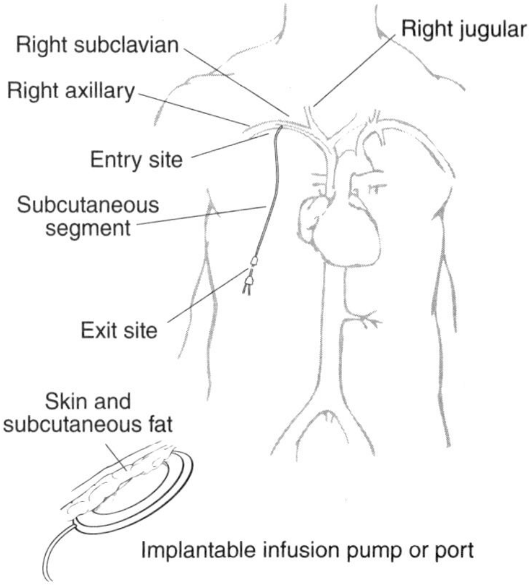

A complete replacement is performed for a tunneled CVA device, with subcutaneous port or pump, through the same venous access

Explanation

A tunneled, centrally inserted central venous catheter, along with a subcutaneous port (36582) or pump (36583) device is replaced. Local anesthesia is given and the subcutaneous pocket over the port/pump device is incised. The pump/port is dissected free and tested. The catheter is disconnected and the pump/port device is removed from its pocket. A guidewire is placed over the existing catheter, which is removed, and a new central venous catheter is threaded into position over the guidewire. A new pump/port device is inserted into the subcutaneous pocket and the catheter is connected. The connection is checked with an injection. The new pump/port is secured into the pocket, incisions are closed, and the wound is dressed.

Coding Tips

When medically necessary, report moderate (conscious) sedation provided by the performing physician with 99151-99153. When provided by another physician, report 99155-99157. If imaging guidance is used, either for obtaining access to the venous access site or for manipulating the catheter into its final end position, see 76937 or 77001. Supplies used when providing this procedure may be reported with HCPCS Level II code C1751. Check with the specific payer to determine coverage.

ICD-10-CM Diagnostic Codes

T80.211A Bloodstream infection due to central venous catheter, initial encounter

T80.212A Local infection due to central venous catheter, initial encounter

T80.218A Other infection due to central venous catheter, initial encounter

T82.41XA Breakdown (mechanical) of vascular dialysis catheter, initial encounter

T82.42XA Displacement of vascular dialysis catheter, initial encounter

T82.43XA Leakage of vascular dialysis catheter, initial encounter

T82.49XA Other complication of vascular dialysis catheter, initial encounter
T82.514A Breakdown (mechanical) of infusion catheter, initial encounter
T82.524A Displacement of infusion catheter, initial encounter
T82.534A Leakage of infusion catheter, initial encounter
T82.594A Other mechanical complication of infusion catheter, initial encounter
T82.598A Other mechanical complication of other cardiac and vascular devices and implants, initial encounter
T82.7XXA Infection and inflammatory reaction due to other cardiac and vascular devices, implants and grafts, initial encounter
T82.818A Embolism due to vascular prosthetic devices, implants and grafts, initial encounter
T82.828A Fibrosis due to vascular prosthetic devices, implants and grafts, initial encounter
T82.838A Hemorrhage due to vascular prosthetic devices, implants and grafts, initial encounter
T82.848A Pain due to vascular prosthetic devices, implants and grafts, initial encounter
T82.858A Stenosis of other vascular prosthetic devices, implants and grafts, initial encounter
T82.868A Thrombosis due to vascular prosthetic devices, implants and grafts, initial encounter
T82.898A Other specified complication of vascular prosthetic devices, implants and grafts, initial encounter
Z45.2 Encounter for adjustment and management of vascular access device

Relative Value Units/Medicare Edits

Non-Facility RVU	Work	PE	MP	Total
36582	4.99	19.87	0.86	25.72
36583	5.04	27.54	1.29	33.87
Facility RVU	**Work**	**PE**	**MP**	**Total**
36582	4.99	2.63	0.86	8.48
36583	5.04	3.51	1.29	9.84

	FUD	Status	MUE	Modifiers				IOM Reference
36582	10	A	2(3)	51	N/A	N/A	80*	None
36583	10	A	2(3)	51	N/A	N/A	80*	

* with documentation

Terms To Know

anesthesia. Loss of feeling or sensation, usually induced to permit the performance of surgery or other painful procedures.

catheter. Flexible tube inserted into an area of the body for introducing or withdrawing fluid.

complication. Condition arising after the beginning of observation and treatment that modifies the course of the patient's illness or the medical care required, or an undesired result or misadventure in medical care.

36584-36585

36584 Replacement, complete, of a peripherally inserted central venous catheter (PICC), without subcutaneous port or pump, through same venous access, including all imaging guidance, image documentation, and all associated radiological supervision and interpretation required to perform the replacement

36585 Replacement, complete, of a peripherally inserted central venous access device, with subcutaneous port, through same venous access

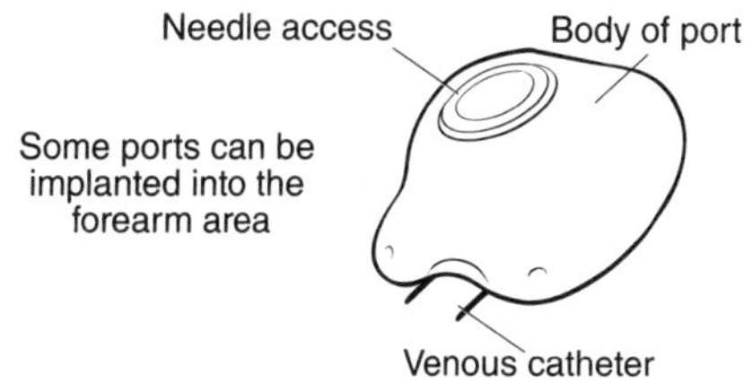

A PICC system is replaced in its entirety. The replacement is accomplished through the same venous access as the previous catheter previous catheter system

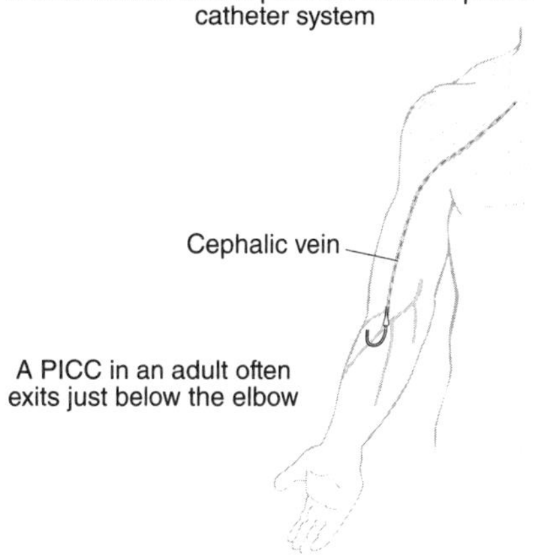

Explanation

In 36584, a peripherally inserted central venous catheter (PICC), without subcutaneous port or pump, is replaced through the same venous access site. Local anesthesia is given and the sutures securing the cuff of the catheter with external port are freed from the skin and it is partially withdrawn. This service includes all imaging guidance and documentation, as well as the supervision and interpretation. In 36585, a peripherally inserted central venous catheter (PICC), along with a subcutaneous port, is replaced through the same venous access site. Local anesthesia is given, the skin over the subcutaneous pocket is incised, and the port is dissected free. In both cases, a sheath is placed over the nonfunctioning catheter and it is completely withdrawn. A guidewire is inserted into the access site through the sheath and advanced. A new catheter of correct length is placed over the guidewire and the sheath and guidewire are removed. The catheter is fastened in position and the wound is dressed.

Coding Tips

Complete replacement, also referred to as complete exchange, involves removal of the entire device via the same access site. When medically necessary, report moderate (conscious) sedation provided by the performing physician with 99151-99153. When provided by another physician, report 99155-99157. Imaging guidance is included in 36584 and is not reported separately. If confirmation of catheter tip placement is not performed by the provider inserting the PICC line, append modifier 52 to 36584. For replacement of a peripherally inserted central venous catheter without subcutaneous port or pump, through the same venous access, without imaging guidance, see 37799. Do not report 36584 with 76937 or 77001.

ICD-10-CM Diagnostic Codes

T80.211A	Bloodstream infection due to central venous catheter, initial encounter
T80.212A	Local infection due to central venous catheter, initial encounter
T80.218A	Other infection due to central venous catheter, initial encounter
T82.41XA	Breakdown (mechanical) of vascular dialysis catheter, initial encounter
T82.42XA	Displacement of vascular dialysis catheter, initial encounter
T82.43XA	Leakage of vascular dialysis catheter, initial encounter
T82.49XA	Other complication of vascular dialysis catheter, initial encounter
T82.514A	Breakdown (mechanical) of infusion catheter, initial encounter
T82.524A	Displacement of infusion catheter, initial encounter
T82.534A	Leakage of infusion catheter, initial encounter
T82.594A	Other mechanical complication of infusion catheter, initial encounter
T82.598A	Other mechanical complication of other cardiac and vascular devices and implants, initial encounter
T82.7XXA	Infection and inflammatory reaction due to other cardiac and vascular devices, implants and grafts, initial encounter
T82.818A	Embolism due to vascular prosthetic devices, implants and grafts, initial encounter
T82.828A	Fibrosis due to vascular prosthetic devices, implants and grafts, initial encounter
T82.838A	Hemorrhage due to vascular prosthetic devices, implants and grafts, initial encounter
T82.848A	Pain due to vascular prosthetic devices, implants and grafts, initial encounter
T82.858A	Stenosis of other vascular prosthetic devices, implants and grafts, initial encounter
T82.868A	Thrombosis due to vascular prosthetic devices, implants and grafts, initial encounter
T82.898A	Other specified complication of vascular prosthetic devices, implants and grafts, initial encounter
Z45.2	Encounter for adjustment and management of vascular access device

AMA: 36584 2019,May; 2019,Mar

Relative Value Units/Medicare Edits

Non-Facility RVU	Work	PE	MP	Total
36584	1.2	8.25	0.12	9.57
36585	4.59	28.26	0.69	33.54
Facility RVU	**Work**	**PE**	**MP**	**Total**
36584	1.2	0.39	0.12	1.71
36585	4.59	2.97	0.69	8.25

	FUD	Status	MUE	Modifiers				IOM Reference
36584	0	A	2(3)	N/A	N/A	N/A	N/A	None
36585	10	A	2(3)	51	N/A	N/A	80*	

* with documentation

36589-36590

36589 Removal of tunneled central venous catheter, without subcutaneous port or pump

36590 Removal of tunneled central venous access device, with subcutaneous port or pump, central or peripheral insertion

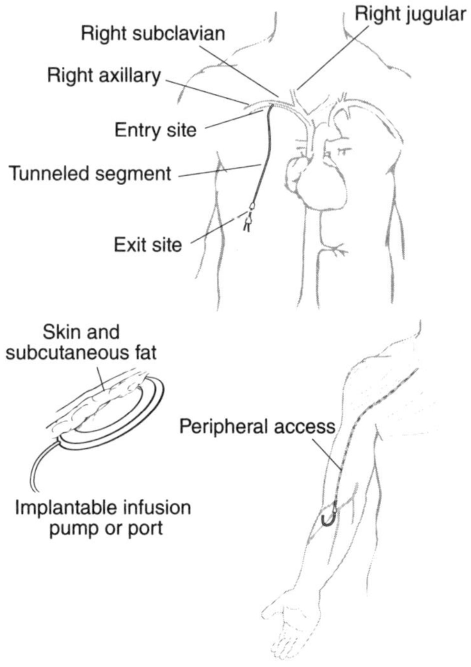

Explanation

In 36589, a tunneled central venous catheter without subcutaneous port or pump is removed. Local anesthesia is given and the sutures securing the cuff of the tunneled catheter's external port are freed from the skin. In 36590, a tunneled central venous access device, both catheter and subcutaneous port or pump, is removed. Local anesthesia is given and the subcutaneous pocket over the port/pump device is incised and the pump/port is dissected free. The catheter is disconnected and the pump/port device is removed from its pocket. In both cases, a guidewire is placed over the existing catheter, which is withdrawn over the guidewire, and the guidewire is removed. The incisions are closed and the wound is dressed.

Coding Tips

When medically necessary, report moderate (conscious) sedation provided by the performing physician with 99151-99153. When provided by another physician, report 99155-99157. Do not report 36589 or 36590 for removal of non-tunneled central venous catheters. If imaging guidance is used, either for obtaining access to the venous access site or for manipulating the catheter into its final end position, see 76937 or 77001.

ICD-10-CM Diagnostic Codes

T80.211A	Bloodstream infection due to central venous catheter, initial encounter
T80.212A	Local infection due to central venous catheter, initial encounter
T80.218A	Other infection due to central venous catheter, initial encounter
T82.41XA	Breakdown (mechanical) of vascular dialysis catheter, initial encounter
T82.42XA	Displacement of vascular dialysis catheter, initial encounter
T82.43XA	Leakage of vascular dialysis catheter, initial encounter
T82.49XA	Other complication of vascular dialysis catheter, initial encounter

T82.514A Breakdown (mechanical) of infusion catheter, initial encounter
T82.524A Displacement of infusion catheter, initial encounter
T82.534A Leakage of infusion catheter, initial encounter
T82.594A Other mechanical complication of infusion catheter, initial encounter
T82.598A Other mechanical complication of other cardiac and vascular devices and implants, initial encounter
T82.7XXA Infection and inflammatory reaction due to other cardiac and vascular devices, implants and grafts, initial encounter
T82.818A Embolism due to vascular prosthetic devices, implants and grafts, initial encounter
T82.828A Fibrosis due to vascular prosthetic devices, implants and grafts, initial encounter
T82.838A Hemorrhage due to vascular prosthetic devices, implants and grafts, initial encounter
T82.848A Pain due to vascular prosthetic devices, implants and grafts, initial encounter
T82.858A Stenosis of other vascular prosthetic devices, implants and grafts, initial encounter
T82.868A Thrombosis due to vascular prosthetic devices, implants and grafts, initial encounter
T82.898A Other specified complication of vascular prosthetic devices, implants and grafts, initial encounter
Z45.2 Encounter for adjustment and management of vascular access device

Relative Value Units/Medicare Edits

Non-Facility RVU	Work	PE	MP	Total
36589	2.28	2.29	0.34	4.91
36590	3.1	3.0	0.54	6.64
Facility RVU	**Work**	**PE**	**MP**	**Total**
36589	2.28	1.41	0.34	4.03
36590	3.1	1.98	0.54	5.62

	FUD	Status	MUE	Modifiers				IOM Reference
36589	10	A	2(3)	51	N/A	N/A	80*	None
36590	10	A	2(3)	51	N/A	N/A	80*	

* with documentation

36591

36591 Collection of blood specimen from a completely implantable venous access device

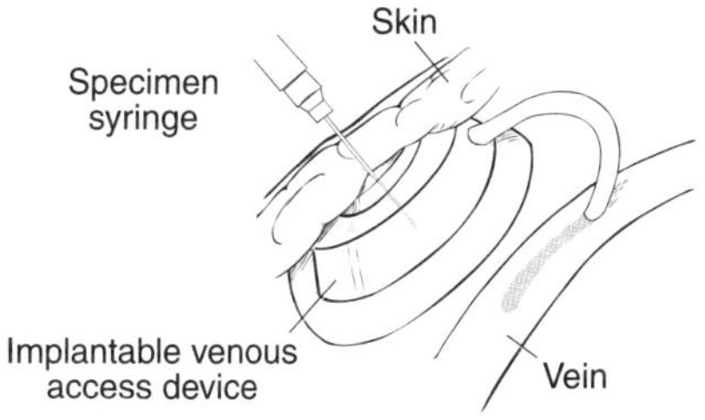

A blood specimen is collected from a partially or completely implantable venous access device

Explanation

The physician obtains a blood specimen from a previously placed, completely implantable venous access device. Completely implanted devices are those that have access through a subcutaneous port (e.g., Port-A-Cath, Infusaport). An implantable access device requires a percutaneous noncoring needle to accomplish the blood draw. The skin is cleansed with alcohol or iodine solution. The needle is placed into the port. Heparin is withdrawn. A second needle is inserted and the blood specimen obtained. The port is flushed with heparin solution.

Coding Tips

This service may only be reported in addition to laboratory services. To report collection of venous blood by venipuncture, see 36415. Medicare and some payers may require HCPCS Level II code G0471 to report this service when provided in a federally qualified health center (FQHC). To report collection of capillary blood, see 36416. Code 36591 is included in the codes for critical care services 99291–99292. Surgical trays, A4550, are not separately reimbursed by Medicare; however, other third-party payers may cover them. Check with the specific payer to determine coverage.

ICD-10-CM Diagnostic Codes

The application of this code is too broad to adequately present ICD-10-CM diagnostic code links here. Refer to your ICD-10-CM book.

AMA: 36591 2022,Jan; 2019,Aug

Relative Value Units/Medicare Edits

Non-Facility RVU	Work	PE	MP	Total
36591	0.0	0.82	0.01	0.83
Facility RVU	**Work**	**PE**	**MP**	**Total**
36591	0.0	0.82	0.01	0.83

	FUD	Status	MUE	Modifiers				IOM Reference
36591	N/A	T	2(3)	N/A	N/A	N/A	80*	None

* with documentation

36592

36592 Collection of blood specimen using established central or peripheral catheter, venous, not otherwise specified

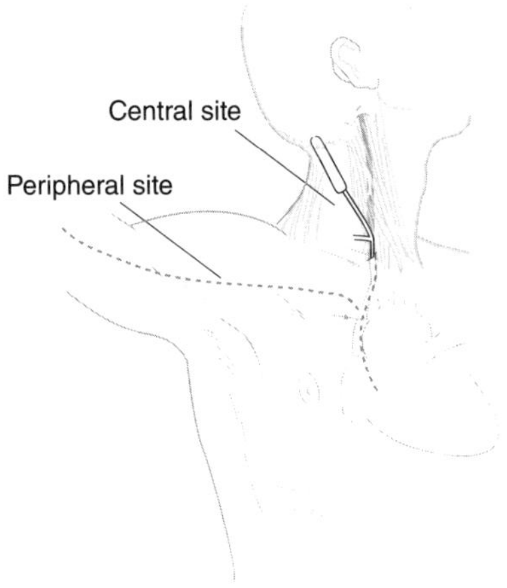

Blood specimen is collected from established catheter

Explanation

The physician obtains a blood specimen from an established central venous or peripheral venous catheter. A central venous catheter (CVC) is one that is inserted through the skin into central veins, such as the femoral, internal jugular, or subclavian veins. Peripheral catheters include those inserted in the arm veins (basilic or cephalic), such as a PICC line, saline lock, or heparin lock. In order to clear the catheter of any material that could contaminate the sample and affect the test results, a specific volume of infusing fluid and blood must be discarded before a blood specimen is obtained; this volume will vary depending on the type of catheter utilized. With a central venous catheter, a three-way stopcock is attached to the catheter's hub and two syringes attached to the stopcock. Using one syringe, the catheter is flushed with normal saline. A specific amount of blood is aspirated into the same syringe used for the saline flush and discarded. The blood sample is then withdrawn using the other syringe and placed into an appropriate tube for laboratory analysis. If using a peripheral venous catheter, a specific amount of blood is also aspirated and discarded before the blood sample is drawn.

Coding Tips

This service may only be reported in addition to laboratory services. To report blood collection from an established arterial catheter, see 37799.

ICD-10-CM Diagnostic Codes

The application of this code is too broad to adequately present ICD-10-CM diagnostic code links here. Refer to your ICD-10-CM book.

Relative Value Units/Medicare Edits

Non-Facility RVU	Work	PE	MP	Total
36592	0.0	0.89	0.01	0.9
Facility RVU	**Work**	**PE**	**MP**	**Total**
36592	0.0	0.89	0.01	0.9

	FUD	Status	MUE	Modifiers				IOM Reference
36592	N/A	T	1(3)	N/A	N/A	N/A	80*	None

* with documentation

36593

36593 Declotting by thrombolytic agent of implanted vascular access device or catheter

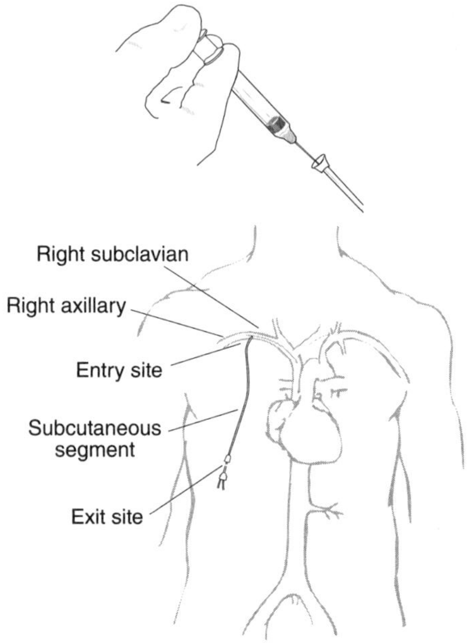

A thrombolytic agent is used to declot a catheter or implanted vascular access device

Explanation

To remove a clot from an implanted vascular access device or catheter, the physician injects a thrombolytic agent (e.g., Streptokinase) into the catheter to dissolve the clot. The patient is observed for any abnormal signs of bleeding.

Coding Tips

When 36593 is performed with another separately identifiable procedure, the highest dollar value code is listed as the primary procedure and subsequent procedures are appended with modifier 51. Supplies used when providing this procedure may be reported with HCPCS Level II code J2995. Check with the specific payer to determine coverage.

ICD-10-CM Diagnostic Codes

T82.818A	Embolism due to vascular prosthetic devices, implants and grafts, initial encounter
T82.848A	Pain due to vascular prosthetic devices, implants and grafts, initial encounter
T82.856A	Stenosis of peripheral vascular stent, initial encounter
T82.858A	Stenosis of other vascular prosthetic devices, implants and grafts, initial encounter
T82.868A	Thrombosis due to vascular prosthetic devices, implants and grafts, initial encounter
T82.898A	Other specified complication of vascular prosthetic devices, implants and grafts, initial encounter

Relative Value Units/Medicare Edits

Non-Facility RVU	Work	PE	MP	Total
36593	0.0	1.02	0.02	1.04
Facility RVU	**Work**	**PE**	**MP**	**Total**
36593	0.0	1.02	0.02	1.04

	FUD	Status	MUE	Modifiers				IOM Reference
36593	N/A	A	2(3)	N/A	N/A	N/A	80*	None

* with documentation

Terms To Know

catheter. Flexible tube inserted into an area of the body for introducing or withdrawing fluid.

complication. Condition arising after the beginning of observation and treatment that modifies the course of the patient's illness or the medical care required, or an undesired result or misadventure in medical care.

embolism. Obstruction of a blood vessel resulting from a clot or foreign substance.

implantable venous access device. Catheter implanted for continuous access to the venous system for long-term parenteral feeding or for the administration of fluids or medications.

stenosis. Narrowing or constriction of a passage.

thrombolytic agent. Drugs or other substances used to dissolve blood clots in blood vessels or in tubes that have been placed into the body.

thrombosis. Condition arising from the presence or formation of blood clots within a blood vessel that may cause vascular obstruction and insufficient oxygenation.

36595

36595 Mechanical removal of pericatheter obstructive material (eg, fibrin sheath) from central venous device via separate venous access

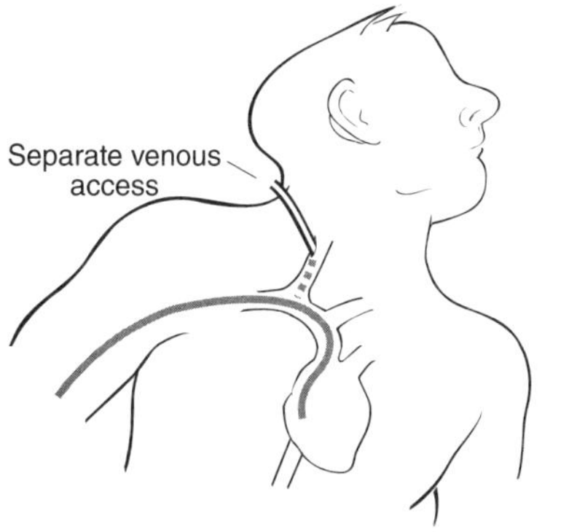

A CVC that has become obstructed is addressed mechanically via a second venous access site. The obstructive matter is on the exterior of the catheter lumen

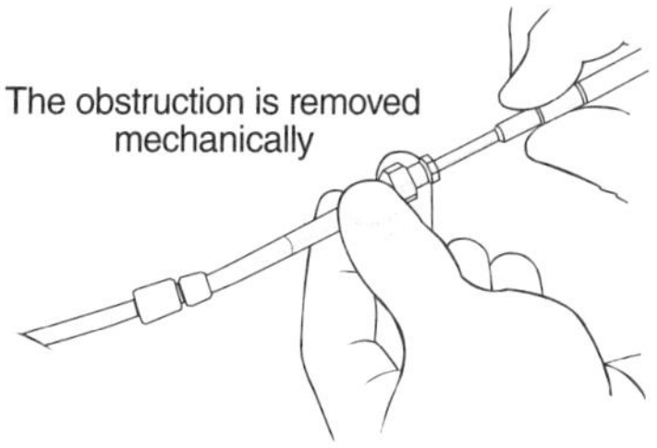

Explanation

Pericatheter obstructive material such as a fibrin sheath is removed from around a central venous device via separate venous access. Central venous catheters often fail because of the accumulation of an obstructing thrombus or fibrin sheath around the tip of the catheter. The catheter is first checked that it can aspirate and flush forward. The pericatheter material is identified by contrast material injection. Generally, a right femoral vein access is used. A guidewire followed by an angiographic catheter are advanced into the superior vena cava and exchanged for a loop snare with its catheter, which are advanced cephalad along the length of the central venous catheter beyond the ports. The loop snare is tightly closed about the central venous catheter to encircle it and slowly pulled down and off the tip of the catheter, stripping off the pericatheter obstructive material. This is repeated a few times and the catheter is rechecked for infusion and injection ability of the ports. A contrast study is done again to identify any fibrin and the process may be repeated until the fibrin sheath is completely removed.

Coding Tips

Do not report 36593 in addition to 36595. For venous catheterization, see 36010–36012. For radiological supervision and interpretation, see 75901.

ICD-10-CM Diagnostic Codes

T82.49XA Other complication of vascular dialysis catheter, initial encounter

T82.594A Other mechanical complication of infusion catheter, initial encounter

T82.598A Other mechanical complication of other cardiac and vascular devices and implants, initial encounter

T82.818A Embolism due to vascular prosthetic devices, implants and grafts, initial encounter

T82.828A Fibrosis due to vascular prosthetic devices, implants and grafts, initial encounter

T82.856A	Stenosis of peripheral vascular stent, initial encounter
T82.858A	Stenosis of other vascular prosthetic devices, implants and grafts, initial encounter
T82.868A	Thrombosis due to vascular prosthetic devices, implants and grafts, initial encounter
T82.898A	Other specified complication of vascular prosthetic devices, implants and grafts, initial encounter
Z45.2	Encounter for adjustment and management of vascular access device

Relative Value Units/Medicare Edits

Non-Facility RVU	Work	PE	MP	Total
36595	3.59	13.47	0.42	17.48
Facility RVU	Work	PE	MP	Total
36595	3.59	1.28	0.42	5.29

	FUD	Status	MUE	Modifiers				IOM Reference
36595	0	A	2(3)	51	N/A	N/A	N/A	None

* with documentation

Terms To Know

aspiration. Drawing fluid out by suction.

cephalad. Toward the head.

fibrin. Main fibrous composition of blood clots.

guidewire. Flexible metal instrument designed to lead another instrument in its proper course.

infection. Presence of microorganisms in body tissues that may result in cellular damage.

infusion. Introduction of a therapeutic fluid, other than blood, into the bloodstream.

injection. Forcing a liquid substance into a body part such as a joint or muscle.

snare. Wire used as a loop to excise a polyp or lesion.

thrombus. Stationary blood clot inside a blood vessel.

vena cava. Main venous trunk that empties into the right atrium from both the lower and upper regions, beginning at the junction of the common iliac veins inferiorly and the two brachiocephalic veins superiorly.

36596

36596 Mechanical removal of intraluminal (intracatheter) obstructive material from central venous device through device lumen

Explanation

Intraluminal obstructive material, such as a thrombus or fibrin sheath, is removed from inside a central venous device through the lumen of the device. This does not require a separate access incision. The central venous catheter is first checked that it can aspirate and flush forward. The obstructing material is disrupted and removed mechanically by using an angioplasty balloon or other catheter introduced into the central venous catheter through its entry site on the skin. The catheter is checked for unimpeded, restored flow and the process may be repeated until the central venous catheter is cleared.

Coding Tips

Do not report 36593 in addition to 36596. For venous catheterization, see 36010–36012. For radiological supervision and interpretation, see 75902.

ICD-10-CM Diagnostic Codes

T82.49XA	Other complication of vascular dialysis catheter, initial encounter
T82.594A	Other mechanical complication of infusion catheter, initial encounter
T82.598A	Other mechanical complication of other cardiac and vascular devices and implants, initial encounter
T82.818A	Embolism due to vascular prosthetic devices, implants and grafts, initial encounter
T82.828A	Fibrosis due to vascular prosthetic devices, implants and grafts, initial encounter
T82.858A	Stenosis of other vascular prosthetic devices, implants and grafts, initial encounter
T82.868A	Thrombosis due to vascular prosthetic devices, implants and grafts, initial encounter
T82.898A	Other specified complication of vascular prosthetic devices, implants and grafts, initial encounter
Z45.2	Encounter for adjustment and management of vascular access device

Relative Value Units/Medicare Edits

Non-Facility RVU	Work	PE	MP	Total
36596	0.75	2.58	0.11	3.44
Facility RVU	Work	PE	MP	Total
36596	0.75	0.47	0.11	1.33

	FUD	Status	MUE	Modifiers				IOM Reference
36596	0	A	2(3)	51	N/A	N/A	N/A	None

* with documentation

Terms To Know

complication. Condition arising after the beginning of observation and treatment that modifies the course of the patient's illness or the medical care required, or an undesired result or misadventure in medical care.

incision. Act of cutting into tissue or an organ.

lumen. Space inside an intestine, artery, vein, duct, or tube.

thrombus. Stationary blood clot inside a blood vessel.

36597

36597 Repositioning of previously placed central venous catheter under fluoroscopic guidance

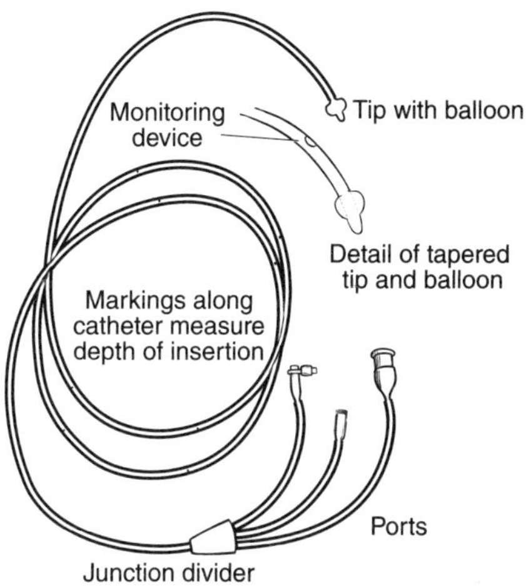

A central venous catheter is repositioned using fluoroscopic guidance, a type of live-image radiology

Explanation

A previously placed central venous catheter needs to be repositioned. It is possible for a catheter position to change significantly after the procedure is completed. Catheter position change and tip migration occur most often with subclavian venous access in women and obese patients, because the soft tissues of the chest wall move inferiorly with standing and often cause the catheter to get pulled back. When a catheter tip is incorrectly placed, it can increase the risks of thrombosis, fibrin sheath formation, perforation of the vein, and even arrhythmias. Fluoroscopy is used to check the positioning of the catheter tip and guide it to its correct position. Local anesthesia is given, and the sutures securing the cuff of the catheter may be freed from the skin. The catheter is partially withdrawn, and a sheath may be placed over the catheter at the existing venous access site. A guidewire is inserted through the catheter and advanced. The central venous catheter is maneuvered back into correct position and monitored with fluoroscopy to view correct placement of the tip.

Coding Tips

For fluoroscopic guidance, see 76000.

ICD-10-CM Diagnostic Codes

T82.41XA	Breakdown (mechanical) of vascular dialysis catheter, initial encounter
T82.42XA	Displacement of vascular dialysis catheter, initial encounter
T82.43XA	Leakage of vascular dialysis catheter, initial encounter
T82.49XA	Other complication of vascular dialysis catheter, initial encounter
T82.514A	Breakdown (mechanical) of infusion catheter, initial encounter
T82.524A	Displacement of infusion catheter, initial encounter
T82.534A	Leakage of infusion catheter, initial encounter
T82.594A	Other mechanical complication of infusion catheter, initial encounter
T82.598A	Other mechanical complication of other cardiac and vascular devices and implants, initial encounter
T82.898A	Other specified complication of vascular prosthetic devices, implants and grafts, initial encounter
Z45.2	Encounter for adjustment and management of vascular access device
Z45.89	Encounter for adjustment and management of other implanted devices
Z46.89	Encounter for fitting and adjustment of other specified devices

Relative Value Units/Medicare Edits

Non-Facility RVU	Work	PE	MP	Total
36597	1.21	1.93	0.15	3.29
Facility RVU	**Work**	**PE**	**MP**	**Total**
36597	1.21	0.4	0.15	1.76

	FUD	Status	MUE	Modifiers				IOM Reference
36597	0	A	2(3)	51	N/A	N/A	N/A	None

* with documentation

Terms To Know

arrhythmias. Heart disorder of rhythm or rate, due to an electrical conduction system malfunction.

catheter. Flexible tube inserted into an area of the body for introducing or withdrawing fluid.

fluoroscopy. Radiology technique that allows visual examination of part of the body or a function of an organ using a device that projects an x-ray image on a fluorescent screen.

guidewire. Flexible metal instrument designed to lead another instrument in its proper course.

introducer. Instrument, such as a catheter, needle, or tube, through which another instrument or device is introduced into the body.

soft tissue. Nonepithelial tissues outside of the skeleton that includes subcutaneous adipose tissue, fibrous tissue, fascia, muscles, blood and lymph vessels, and peripheral nervous system tissue.

thrombosis. Condition arising from the presence or formation of blood clots within a blood vessel that may cause vascular obstruction and insufficient oxygenation.

36598

36598 Contrast injection(s) for radiologic evaluation of existing central venous access device, including fluoroscopy, image documentation and report

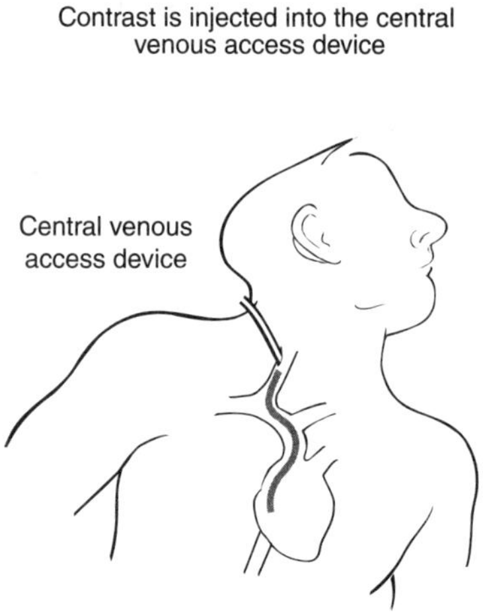

Explanation

A previously placed central venous access device is evaluated for complications that may be interfering with its proper functioning or the ability to draw blood from the catheter. Complications may include the presence of a fibrin sheath around the end of the catheter, migration of the catheter tip, patency of the tubing, kinking, fracture, or leaks. A small amount of contrast agent is injected into the catheter and the central venous access device is examined under fluoroscopy as the flow is evaluated. Images are documented and a radiological report is prepared.

Coding Tips

Fluoroscopic guidance is included in 36598. Do not report 36598 with 76000. Do not report mechanical removal of pericatheter obstructive material separately (36595). Do not report mechanical removal of intraluminal (intracatheter) obstructive material separately (36596). For complete diagnostic studies (venography), see 75820, 75825, and 75827.

ICD-10-CM Diagnostic Codes

T80.211A	Bloodstream infection due to central venous catheter, initial encounter
T80.212A	Local infection due to central venous catheter, initial encounter
T82.41XA	Breakdown (mechanical) of vascular dialysis catheter, initial encounter
T82.42XA	Displacement of vascular dialysis catheter, initial encounter
T82.43XA	Leakage of vascular dialysis catheter, initial encounter
T82.514A	Breakdown (mechanical) of infusion catheter, initial encounter
T82.524A	Displacement of infusion catheter, initial encounter
T82.534A	Leakage of infusion catheter, initial encounter
T82.594A	Other mechanical complication of infusion catheter, initial encounter
T82.598A	Other mechanical complication of other cardiac and vascular devices and implants, initial encounter
T82.7XXA	Infection and inflammatory reaction due to other cardiac and vascular devices, implants and grafts, initial encounter
T82.818A	Embolism due to vascular prosthetic devices, implants and grafts, initial encounter
T82.828A	Fibrosis due to vascular prosthetic devices, implants and grafts, initial encounter
T82.838A	Hemorrhage due to vascular prosthetic devices, implants and grafts, initial encounter
T82.848A	Pain due to vascular prosthetic devices, implants and grafts, initial encounter
T82.858A	Stenosis of other vascular prosthetic devices, implants and grafts, initial encounter
T82.868A	Thrombosis due to vascular prosthetic devices, implants and grafts, initial encounter
T82.898A	Other specified complication of vascular prosthetic devices, implants and grafts, initial encounter
Z45.2	Encounter for adjustment and management of vascular access device

Relative Value Units/Medicare Edits

Non-Facility RVU	Work	PE	MP	Total
36598	0.74	2.74	0.07	3.55
Facility RVU	**Work**	**PE**	**MP**	**Total**
36598	0.74	0.23	0.07	1.04

	FUD	Status	MUE	Modifiers				IOM Reference
36598	0	T	2(3)	51	50	N/A	80*	None

* with documentation

Terms To Know

central venous access device. Catheter or other device introduced through a large vein, such as the subclavian or femoral vein, terminating in the superior or inferior vena cava or the right atrium and used to measure venous pressure or administer medication or fluids.

contrast material. Radiopaque substance placed into the body to enable a system or body structure to be visualized, such as nonionic and low osmolar contrast media (LOCM), ionic and high osmolar contrast media (HOCM), barium, and gadolinium.

embolism. Obstruction of a blood vessel resulting from a clot or foreign substance.

fluoroscopy. Radiology technique that allows visual examination of part of the body or a function of an organ using a device that projects an x-ray image on a fluorescent screen.

injection. Forcing a liquid substance into a body part such as a joint or muscle.

stenosis. Narrowing or constriction of a passage.

36600

36600 Arterial puncture, withdrawal of blood for diagnosis

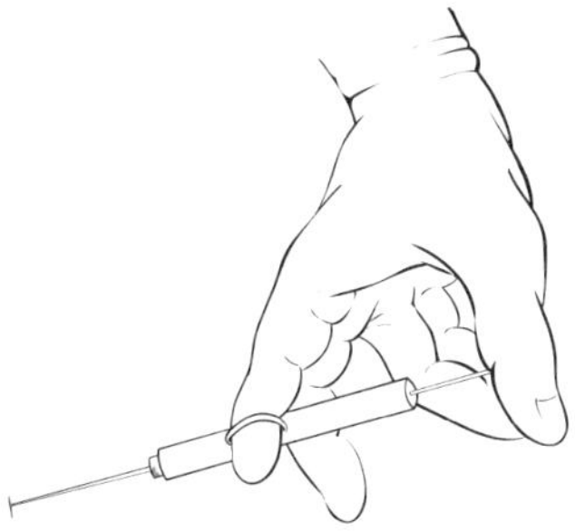

Any artery is punctured by a needle to withdraw blood for testing

Explanation

The physician inserts a needle through the skin and punctures the artery to withdraw blood for testing. No catheter is left in the artery. Pressure is applied to the puncture site to stop the flow of blood.

Coding Tips

Report 36600 only once when multiple tests are performed on the same arterial blood draw. This procedure does not include laboratory analysis. If specimen is transported to an outside laboratory, report 99000 for handling or conveyance. This service is included in the codes for critical care services including 99291-99292 and 99468-99476.

ICD-10-CM Diagnostic Codes

The application of this code is too broad to adequately present ICD-10-CM diagnostic code links here. Refer to your ICD-10-CM book.

AMA: 36600 2022,Jan; 2019,Aug

Relative Value Units/Medicare Edits

Non-Facility RVU	Work	PE	MP	Total
36600	0.32	0.48	0.02	0.82
Facility RVU	**Work**	**PE**	**MP**	**Total**
36600	0.32	0.1	0.02	0.44

	FUD	Status	MUE	Modifiers				IOM Reference
36600	N/A	A	4(3)	51	N/A	N/A	N/A	None

* with documentation

36620-36640

36620 Arterial catheterization or cannulation for sampling, monitoring or transfusion (separate procedure); percutaneous

36625 cutdown

36640 Arterial catheterization for prolonged infusion therapy (chemotherapy), cutdown

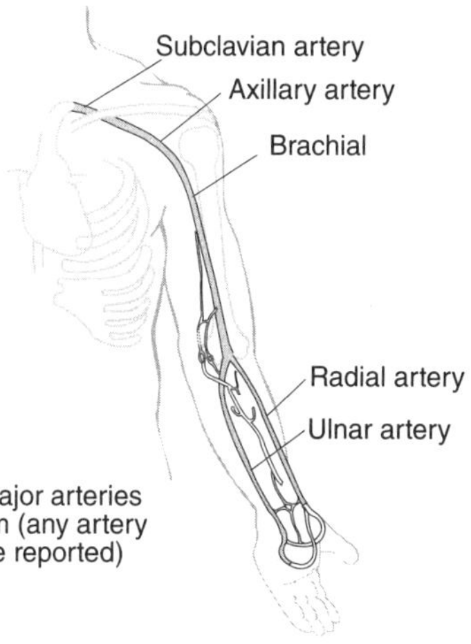

An artery is percutaneously catheterized or cannulized for sampling, monitoring, or for transfusion

Explanation

The physician accesses, in most cases, the ulnar or radial artery to insert a cannula, or tube-shaped portal. In 36620, the physician inserts a needle through the skin to puncture the artery, and then inserts a cannula. In 36625, the physician makes an incision in the skin overlying the artery and dissects the surrounding tissue to access it. The artery is sometimes nicked with a thin-bladed scalpel before the physician inserts the cannula. This cannula acts as a portal for sampling, monitoring or transfusion. Once the procedure is complete, the cannula is removed. In an open procedure, the opening in the artery may be sutured and the incision repaired with a layered closure. Pressure is applied to the puncture if a percutaneous approach is used. In 36640, the physician accesses the artery supplying the area to be treated. To insert a cannula, or tube-shaped portal for prolonged infusion therapy, the physician makes an incision above the artery and dissects the surrounding tissue to access it. The artery is sometimes nicked with a thin-bladed scalpel before the physician inserts the catheter. The catheter may be advanced to a site immediately upstream of the site to be treated. This catheter acts as a portal for the infusion of chemotherapy drugs and will remain in place until chemotherapy is completed. The catheter is removed, the hole in the artery is repaired, and the incision is repaired with a layered closure.

Coding Tips

Codes 36620 and 36625, separate procedures by definition, are usually a component of a more complex service and are not identified separately. When performed alone or with other unrelated procedures/services, they may be reported. If performed alone, list the code; if performed with other procedures/services, list the code and append modifier 59 or an X{EPSU} modifier. Code 36620 is included in critical care codes 99468–99476. These codes include only the insertion of the catheter. For transfusion via venous access, see 36430–36460. For occlusion therapy via arterial catheterization, see 75894. For chemotherapy administration, see 96420–96425.

ICD-10-CM Diagnostic Codes

The application of this code is too broad to adequately present ICD-10-CM diagnostic code links here. Refer to your ICD-10-CM book.

Relative Value Units/Medicare Edits

Non-Facility RVU	Work	PE	MP	Total
36620	1.0	0.21	0.09	1.3
36625	2.11	0.66	0.33	3.1
36640	2.1	1.24	0.16	3.5
Facility RVU	**Work**	**PE**	**MP**	**Total**
36620	1.0	0.21	0.09	1.3
36625	2.11	0.66	0.33	3.1
36640	2.1	1.24	0.16	3.5

	FUD	Status	MUE	Modifiers				IOM Reference
36620	0	A	3(3)	N/A	N/A	N/A	N/A	None
36625	0	A	2(3)	N/A	N/A	N/A	N/A	
36640	0	A	1(3)	51	N/A	N/A	N/A	

* with documentation

Terms To Know

artery. Vessel through which oxygenated blood passes away from the heart to any part of the body.

cannula. Tube inserted into a blood vessel, duct, or body cavity to facilitate passage.

chemotherapy. Treatment of disease, especially cancerous conditions, using chemical agents.

incision. Act of cutting into tissue or an organ.

infusion. Introduction of a therapeutic fluid, other than blood, into the bloodstream.

percutaneous. Through the skin.

suture. Numerous stitching techniques employed in wound closure.

transfusion. Process of transferring whole blood or blood components from one person, the donor, to another person, the recipient, or the process of taking liquid from one vessel and putting it into another.

36680

36680 Placement of needle for intraosseous infusion

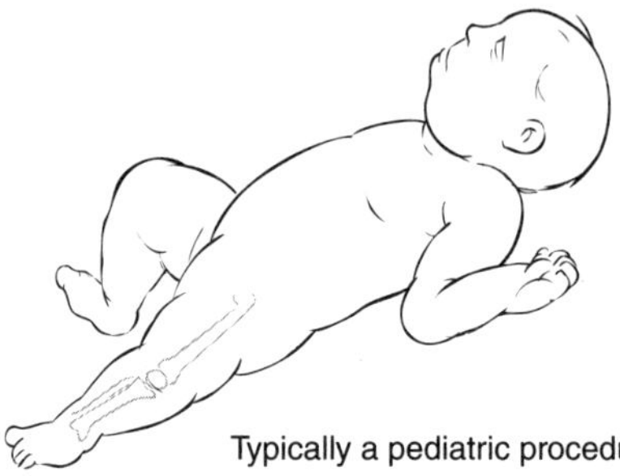

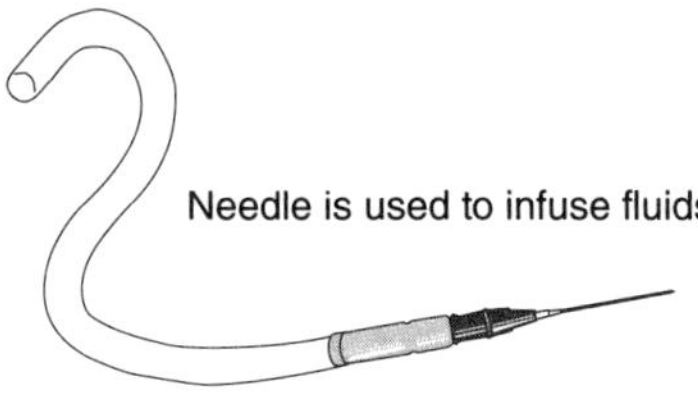

Explanation

The physician inserts a hollow needle through the skin and through the muscle tissue to puncture the bone marrow cavity, usually in the tibia or femur, of a patient whose vessels otherwise seem inaccessible. This needle is used as a method of infusing fluids into the blood vessels in the bone marrow.

Coding Tips

This is typically a pediatric procedure for severe dehydration. When 36680 is performed with another distinct or independent procedure, in which the procedures are not normally performed on the same day, and another modifier does not apply (e.g., modifier 51), the highest dollar value code is listed as the primary procedure and subsequent procedures are appended with modifier 59 or an X{EPSU} modifier. For IV infusion for hydration, see 96360–96361. For IV infusion for therapy/diagnosis, administered by physician or under direct supervision of a physician, see 96365–96368.

ICD-10-CM Diagnostic Codes

E66.01	Morbid (severe) obesity due to excess calories
E66.09	Other obesity due to excess calories
E66.1	Drug-induced obesity
E66.2	Morbid (severe) obesity with alveolar hypoventilation
E66.811	Obesity, class 1
E66.812	Obesity, class 2
E66.813	Obesity, class 3
E86.0	Dehydration
E86.1	Hypovolemia
G40.001	Localization-related (focal) (partial) idiopathic epilepsy and epileptic syndromes with seizures of localized onset, not intractable, with status epilepticus
G40.011	Localization-related (focal) (partial) idiopathic epilepsy and epileptic syndromes with seizures of localized onset, intractable, with status epilepticus

G40.101 Localization-related (focal) (partial) symptomatic epilepsy and epileptic syndromes with simple partial seizures, not intractable, with status epilepticus
G40.111 Localization-related (focal) (partial) symptomatic epilepsy and epileptic syndromes with simple partial seizures, intractable, with status epilepticus
G40.201 Localization-related (focal) (partial) symptomatic epilepsy and epileptic syndromes with complex partial seizures, not intractable, with status epilepticus
G40.211 Localization-related (focal) (partial) symptomatic epilepsy and epileptic syndromes with complex partial seizures, intractable, with status epilepticus
G40.301 Generalized idiopathic epilepsy and epileptic syndromes, not intractable, with status epilepticus
G40.311 Generalized idiopathic epilepsy and epileptic syndromes, intractable, with status epilepticus
G40.401 Other generalized epilepsy and epileptic syndromes, not intractable, with status epilepticus
G40.411 Other generalized epilepsy and epileptic syndromes, intractable, with status epilepticus
G40.501 Epileptic seizures related to external causes, not intractable, with status epilepticus
G40.801 Other epilepsy, not intractable, with status epilepticus
G40.803 Other epilepsy, intractable, with status epilepticus
G40.811 Lennox-Gastaut syndrome, not intractable, with status epilepticus
G40.813 Lennox-Gastaut syndrome, intractable, with status epilepticus
G40.821 Epileptic spasms, not intractable, with status epilepticus
G40.823 Epileptic spasms, intractable, with status epilepticus
G40.89 Other seizures
G40.A01 Absence epileptic syndrome, not intractable, with status epilepticus
G40.A11 Absence epileptic syndrome, intractable, with status epilepticus
G40.B01 Juvenile myoclonic epilepsy, not intractable, with status epilepticus
G40.B11 Juvenile myoclonic epilepsy, intractable, with status epilepticus
P28.5 Respiratory failure of newborn N
P28.81 Respiratory arrest of newborn N
P29.81 Cardiac arrest of newborn N
P29.89 Other cardiovascular disorders originating in the perinatal period N
R09.2 Respiratory arrest
R57.1 Hypovolemic shock

Relative Value Units/Medicare Edits

Non-Facility RVU	Work	PE	MP	Total
36680	1.2	0.35	0.22	1.77
Facility RVU	**Work**	**PE**	**MP**	**Total**
36680	1.2	0.35	0.22	1.77

	FUD	Status	MUE	Modifiers				IOM Reference
36680	0	A	1(3)	51	N/A	N/A	80*	None

* with documentation

36800

36800 Insertion of cannula for hemodialysis, other purpose (separate procedure); vein to vein

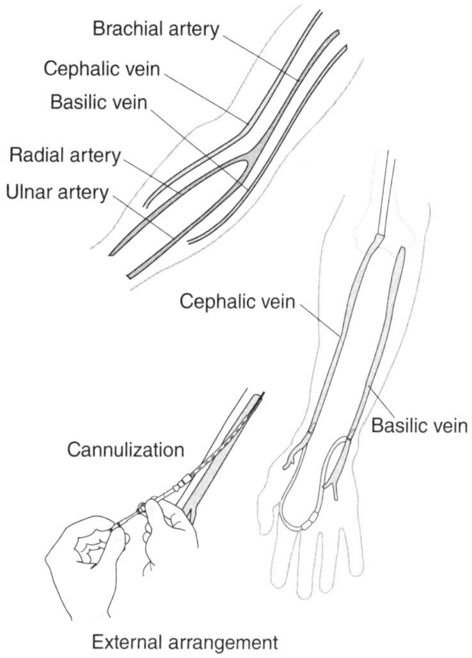

Vein-to-vein cannulization is established, usually for dialysis

Explanation

The physician isolates two veins, usually in the nondominant forearm, and inserts a needle through the skin and into each vessel. A guidance wire may be threaded through the needle into each vessel. The needle is removed. An end of a single cannula is inserted into each puncture, and any guidance wire removed. The cannula remains external, and may be left in place for several days. (This hemodialysis cannula is used to remove blood from the vein, route it through the dialysis machine, then reinfuse it.)

Coding Tips

This separate procedure by definition is usually a component of a more complex service and is not identified separately. When performed alone or with other unrelated procedures/services, it may be reported. If performed alone, list the code; if performed with other procedures/services, list the code and append modifier 59 or X{EPSU}. This type of hemodialysis cannula is infrequently used; verify this is the correct code by obtaining a copy of the cannula label from the medical record. This code includes venipuncture when performed by the physician. If the hemodialysis procedure is done intraoperatively and is a standard and necessary part of the main procedure during the same surgical session, the cannula insertion should not be reported separately.

ICD-10-CM Diagnostic Codes

D59.31 Infection-associated hemolytic-uremic syndrome
D59.32 Hereditary hemolytic-uremic syndrome
E87.21 Acute metabolic acidosis
E87.22 Chronic metabolic acidosis
E87.5 Hyperkalemia
I12.0 Hypertensive chronic kidney disease with stage 5 chronic kidney disease or end stage renal disease

I12.9	Hypertensive chronic kidney disease with stage 1 through stage 4 chronic kidney disease, or unspecified chronic kidney disease
I13.0	Hypertensive heart and chronic kidney disease with heart failure and stage 1 through stage 4 chronic kidney disease, or unspecified chronic kidney disease
I13.10	Hypertensive heart and chronic kidney disease without heart failure, with stage 1 through stage 4 chronic kidney disease, or unspecified chronic kidney disease
I13.11	Hypertensive heart and chronic kidney disease without heart failure, with stage 5 chronic kidney disease, or end stage renal disease
I13.2	Hypertensive heart and chronic kidney disease with heart failure and with stage 5 chronic kidney disease, or end stage renal disease
I16.0	Hypertensive urgency
I16.1	Hypertensive emergency
I82.3	Embolism and thrombosis of renal vein
M35.04	Sjögren syndrome with tubulo-interstitial nephropathy
M35.0A	Sjögren syndrome with glomerular disease
N00.0	Acute nephritic syndrome with minor glomerular abnormality
N00.1	Acute nephritic syndrome with focal and segmental glomerular lesions
N00.2	Acute nephritic syndrome with diffuse membranous glomerulonephritis
N00.3	Acute nephritic syndrome with diffuse mesangial proliferative glomerulonephritis
N00.4	Acute nephritic syndrome with diffuse endocapillary proliferative glomerulonephritis
N00.5	Acute nephritic syndrome with diffuse mesangiocapillary glomerulonephritis
N00.6	Acute nephritic syndrome with dense deposit disease
N00.7	Acute nephritic syndrome with diffuse crescentic glomerulonephritis
N00.A	Acute nephritic syndrome with C3 glomerulonephritis
N01.0	Rapidly progressive nephritic syndrome with minor glomerular abnormality
N01.1	Rapidly progressive nephritic syndrome with focal and segmental glomerular lesions
N01.2	Rapidly progressive nephritic syndrome with diffuse membranous glomerulonephritis
N01.3	Rapidly progressive nephritic syndrome with diffuse mesangial proliferative glomerulonephritis
N01.4	Rapidly progressive nephritic syndrome with diffuse endocapillary proliferative glomerulonephritis
N01.5	Rapidly progressive nephritic syndrome with diffuse mesangiocapillary glomerulonephritis
N01.6	Rapidly progressive nephritic syndrome with dense deposit disease
N01.7	Rapidly progressive nephritic syndrome with diffuse crescentic glomerulonephritis
N01.A	Rapidly progressive nephritic syndrome with C3 glomerulonephritis
N03.0	Chronic nephritic syndrome with minor glomerular abnormality
N03.1	Chronic nephritic syndrome with focal and segmental glomerular lesions
N03.2	Chronic nephritic syndrome with diffuse membranous glomerulonephritis
N03.3	Chronic nephritic syndrome with diffuse mesangial proliferative glomerulonephritis
N03.4	Chronic nephritic syndrome with diffuse endocapillary proliferative glomerulonephritis
N03.5	Chronic nephritic syndrome with diffuse mesangiocapillary glomerulonephritis
N03.6	Chronic nephritic syndrome with dense deposit disease
N03.7	Chronic nephritic syndrome with diffuse crescentic glomerulonephritis
N03.A	Chronic nephritic syndrome with C3 glomerulonephritis
N04.0	Nephrotic syndrome with minor glomerular abnormality
N04.1	Nephrotic syndrome with focal and segmental glomerular lesions
N04.21	Primary membranous nephropathy with nephrotic syndrome
N04.3	Nephrotic syndrome with diffuse mesangial proliferative glomerulonephritis
N04.4	Nephrotic syndrome with diffuse endocapillary proliferative glomerulonephritis
N04.5	Nephrotic syndrome with diffuse mesangiocapillary glomerulonephritis
N04.6	Nephrotic syndrome with dense deposit disease
N04.7	Nephrotic syndrome with diffuse crescentic glomerulonephritis
N04.A	Nephrotic syndrome with C3 glomerulonephritis
N08	Glomerular disorders in diseases classified elsewhere
N10	Acute pyelonephritis
N11.0	Nonobstructive reflux-associated chronic pyelonephritis
N11.1	Chronic obstructive pyelonephritis
N12	Tubulo-interstitial nephritis, not specified as acute or chronic
N15.8	Other specified renal tubulo-interstitial diseases
N16	Renal tubulo-interstitial disorders in diseases classified elsewhere
N17.0	Acute kidney failure with tubular necrosis
N17.1	Acute kidney failure with acute cortical necrosis
N17.2	Acute kidney failure with medullary necrosis
N17.8	Other acute kidney failure
N18.31	Chronic kidney disease, stage 3a
N18.32	Chronic kidney disease, stage 3b
N18.4	Chronic kidney disease, stage 4 (severe)
N18.5	Chronic kidney disease, stage 5
N18.6	End stage renal disease

AMA: 36800 2023,Mar; 2022,Oct

Relative Value Units/Medicare Edits

Non-Facility RVU	Work	PE	MP	Total
36800	2.43	0.84	0.29	3.56
Facility RVU	**Work**	**PE**	**MP**	**Total**
36800	2.43	0.84	0.29	3.56

	FUD	Status	MUE	Modifiers				IOM Reference
36800	0	A	1(3)	51	N/A	N/A	N/A	None

* with documentation

36810

36810 Insertion of cannula for hemodialysis, other purpose (separate procedure); arteriovenous, external (Scribner type)

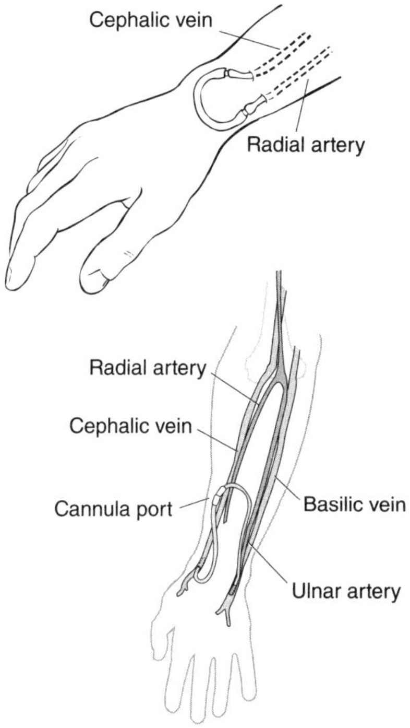

One end of the cannula is inserted into the artery and the other end is inserted into the vein to create a portal for hemodialysis

Explanation

The physician isolates an artery and a vein, usually in the nondominant forearm, and inserts a needle through the skin and into each vessel. A guidewire may be threaded through the needle into each vessel. The needle is removed. An end of a single cannula is inserted into each puncture, and any guidance wire removed. The Scribner cannula remains external, and may be left in place for several days. (This hemodialysis cannula is used to remove blood from the vessel, route it through the dialysis machine, then reinfuse it.)

Coding Tips

This separate procedure by definition is usually a component of a more complex service and is not identified separately. When performed alone or with other unrelated procedures/services, it may be reported. If performed alone, list the code; if performed with other procedures/services, list the code and append modifier 59 or an X{EPSU} modifier. This type of hemodialysis cannula is infrequently used; verify this is the correct code by obtaining a copy of the cannula label from the medical record. This code includes venipuncture when performed by the physician. If the hemodialysis procedure is done intraoperatively and is a standard and necessary part of the main procedure during the same surgical session, the cannula insertion should not be reported separately.

ICD-10-CM Diagnostic Codes

D59.31	Infection-associated hemolytic-uremic syndrome
D59.32	Hereditary hemolytic-uremic syndrome
E87.21	Acute metabolic acidosis
E87.22	Chronic metabolic acidosis
E87.5	Hyperkalemia
I12.0	Hypertensive chronic kidney disease with stage 5 chronic kidney disease or end stage renal disease
I12.9	Hypertensive chronic kidney disease with stage 1 through stage 4 chronic kidney disease, or unspecified chronic kidney disease
I13.0	Hypertensive heart and chronic kidney disease with heart failure and stage 1 through stage 4 chronic kidney disease, or unspecified chronic kidney disease
I13.10	Hypertensive heart and chronic kidney disease without heart failure, with stage 1 through stage 4 chronic kidney disease, or unspecified chronic kidney disease
I13.11	Hypertensive heart and chronic kidney disease without heart failure, with stage 5 chronic kidney disease, or end stage renal disease
I13.2	Hypertensive heart and chronic kidney disease with heart failure and with stage 5 chronic kidney disease, or end stage renal disease
I16.0	Hypertensive urgency
I16.1	Hypertensive emergency
I82.3	Embolism and thrombosis of renal vein
M35.04	Sjögren syndrome with tubulo-interstitial nephropathy
M35.0A	Sjögren syndrome with glomerular disease
N00.0	Acute nephritic syndrome with minor glomerular abnormality
N00.1	Acute nephritic syndrome with focal and segmental glomerular lesions
N00.2	Acute nephritic syndrome with diffuse membranous glomerulonephritis
N00.3	Acute nephritic syndrome with diffuse mesangial proliferative glomerulonephritis
N00.4	Acute nephritic syndrome with diffuse endocapillary proliferative glomerulonephritis
N00.5	Acute nephritic syndrome with diffuse mesangiocapillary glomerulonephritis
N00.6	Acute nephritic syndrome with dense deposit disease
N00.7	Acute nephritic syndrome with diffuse crescentic glomerulonephritis
N00.A	Acute nephritic syndrome with C3 glomerulonephritis
N01.0	Rapidly progressive nephritic syndrome with minor glomerular abnormality
N01.1	Rapidly progressive nephritic syndrome with focal and segmental glomerular lesions
N01.2	Rapidly progressive nephritic syndrome with diffuse membranous glomerulonephritis
N01.3	Rapidly progressive nephritic syndrome with diffuse mesangial proliferative glomerulonephritis
N01.4	Rapidly progressive nephritic syndrome with diffuse endocapillary proliferative glomerulonephritis
N01.5	Rapidly progressive nephritic syndrome with diffuse mesangiocapillary glomerulonephritis
N01.6	Rapidly progressive nephritic syndrome with dense deposit disease
N01.7	Rapidly progressive nephritic syndrome with diffuse crescentic glomerulonephritis
N01.A	Rapidly progressive nephritic syndrome with C3 glomerulonephritis
N03.0	Chronic nephritic syndrome with minor glomerular abnormality
N03.1	Chronic nephritic syndrome with focal and segmental glomerular lesions

N03.2 Chronic nephritic syndrome with diffuse membranous glomerulonephritis
N03.3 Chronic nephritic syndrome with diffuse mesangial proliferative glomerulonephritis
N03.4 Chronic nephritic syndrome with diffuse endocapillary proliferative glomerulonephritis
N03.5 Chronic nephritic syndrome with diffuse mesangiocapillary glomerulonephritis
N03.6 Chronic nephritic syndrome with dense deposit disease
N03.7 Chronic nephritic syndrome with diffuse crescentic glomerulonephritis
N03.A Chronic nephritic syndrome with C3 glomerulonephritis
N04.0 Nephrotic syndrome with minor glomerular abnormality
N04.1 Nephrotic syndrome with focal and segmental glomerular lesions
N04.21 Primary membranous nephropathy with nephrotic syndrome
N04.3 Nephrotic syndrome with diffuse mesangial proliferative glomerulonephritis
N04.4 Nephrotic syndrome with diffuse endocapillary proliferative glomerulonephritis
N04.5 Nephrotic syndrome with diffuse mesangiocapillary glomerulonephritis
N04.6 Nephrotic syndrome with dense deposit disease
N04.7 Nephrotic syndrome with diffuse crescentic glomerulonephritis
N08 Glomerular disorders in diseases classified elsewhere
N10 Acute pyelonephritis
N11.0 Nonobstructive reflux-associated chronic pyelonephritis
N11.1 Chronic obstructive pyelonephritis
N12 Tubulo-interstitial nephritis, not specified as acute or chronic
N15.8 Other specified renal tubulo-interstitial diseases
N16 Renal tubulo-interstitial disorders in diseases classified elsewhere
N17.0 Acute kidney failure with tubular necrosis
N17.1 Acute kidney failure with acute cortical necrosis
N17.2 Acute kidney failure with medullary necrosis
N17.8 Other acute kidney failure
N18.31 Chronic kidney disease, stage 3a
N18.32 Chronic kidney disease, stage 3b
N18.4 Chronic kidney disease, stage 4 (severe)
N18.5 Chronic kidney disease, stage 5
N18.6 End stage renal disease

AMA: **36810** 2023,Mar; 2022,Oct

Relative Value Units/Medicare Edits

Non-Facility RVU	Work	PE	MP	Total
36810	3.96	1.82	0.41	6.19
Facility RVU	**Work**	**PE**	**MP**	**Total**
36810	3.96	1.82	0.41	6.19

	FUD	Status	MUE	Modifiers				IOM Reference
36810	0	A	1(3)	51	N/A	N/A	N/A	None

* with documentation

36815

36815 Insertion of cannula for hemodialysis, other purpose (separate procedure); arteriovenous, external revision, or closure

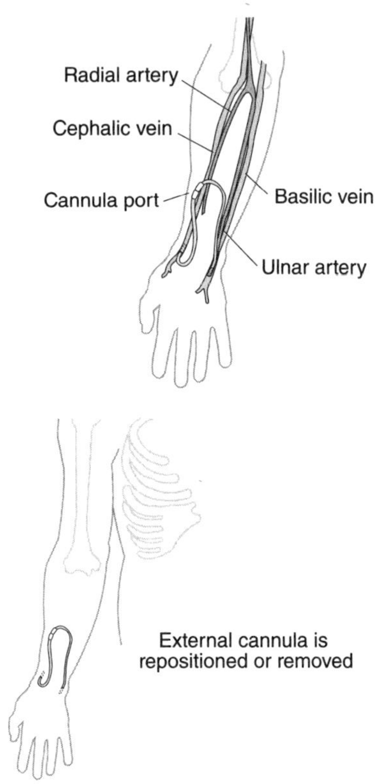

Explanation

The physician repositions an external cannula or removes it. The cannula forms a ready connection between the artery and vein or vein and vein for hemodialysis or another purpose. Closure of the insertion site is performed using sutures on the vessels or skin as necessary.

Coding Tips

This separate procedure by definition is usually a component of a more complex service and is not identified separately. When performed alone or with other unrelated procedures/services, it may be reported. If performed alone, list the code; if performed with other procedures/services, list the code and append modifier 59 or an X{EPSU} modifier. This type of hemodialysis cannula is infrequently used; verify this is the correct code by obtaining a copy of the cannula label from the medical record. This code includes venipuncture when performed by the physician. If the hemodialysis procedure is done intraoperatively and is a standard and necessary part of the main procedure during the same surgical session, the cannula insertion should not be reported separately.

ICD-10-CM Diagnostic Codes

D59.31 Infection-associated hemolytic-uremic syndrome
D59.32 Hereditary hemolytic-uremic syndrome
E87.21 Acute metabolic acidosis
E87.22 Chronic metabolic acidosis
E87.5 Hyperkalemia
I12.0 Hypertensive chronic kidney disease with stage 5 chronic kidney disease or end stage renal disease

I12.9	Hypertensive chronic kidney disease with stage 1 through stage 4 chronic kidney disease, or unspecified chronic kidney disease
I13.0	Hypertensive heart and chronic kidney disease with heart failure and stage 1 through stage 4 chronic kidney disease, or unspecified chronic kidney disease
I13.10	Hypertensive heart and chronic kidney disease without heart failure, with stage 1 through stage 4 chronic kidney disease, or unspecified chronic kidney disease
I13.11	Hypertensive heart and chronic kidney disease without heart failure, with stage 5 chronic kidney disease, or end stage renal disease
I13.2	Hypertensive heart and chronic kidney disease with heart failure and with stage 5 chronic kidney disease, or end stage renal disease
I16.0	Hypertensive urgency
I16.1	Hypertensive emergency
I82.3	Embolism and thrombosis of renal vein
M35.04	Sjögren syndrome with tubulo-interstitial nephropathy
M35.0A	Sjögren syndrome with glomerular disease
N00.0	Acute nephritic syndrome with minor glomerular abnormality
N00.1	Acute nephritic syndrome with focal and segmental glomerular lesions
N00.2	Acute nephritic syndrome with diffuse membranous glomerulonephritis
N00.3	Acute nephritic syndrome with diffuse mesangial proliferative glomerulonephritis
N00.4	Acute nephritic syndrome with diffuse endocapillary proliferative glomerulonephritis
N00.5	Acute nephritic syndrome with diffuse mesangiocapillary glomerulonephritis
N00.6	Acute nephritic syndrome with dense deposit disease
N00.7	Acute nephritic syndrome with diffuse crescentic glomerulonephritis
N00.A	Acute nephritic syndrome with C3 glomerulonephritis
N01.0	Rapidly progressive nephritic syndrome with minor glomerular abnormality
N01.1	Rapidly progressive nephritic syndrome with focal and segmental glomerular lesions
N01.2	Rapidly progressive nephritic syndrome with diffuse membranous glomerulonephritis
N01.3	Rapidly progressive nephritic syndrome with diffuse mesangial proliferative glomerulonephritis
N01.4	Rapidly progressive nephritic syndrome with diffuse endocapillary proliferative glomerulonephritis
N01.5	Rapidly progressive nephritic syndrome with diffuse mesangiocapillary glomerulonephritis
N01.6	Rapidly progressive nephritic syndrome with dense deposit disease
N01.7	Rapidly progressive nephritic syndrome with diffuse crescentic glomerulonephritis
N01.A	Rapidly progressive nephritic syndrome with C3 glomerulonephritis
N03.0	Chronic nephritic syndrome with minor glomerular abnormality
N03.1	Chronic nephritic syndrome with focal and segmental glomerular lesions
N03.2	Chronic nephritic syndrome with diffuse membranous glomerulonephritis
N03.3	Chronic nephritic syndrome with diffuse mesangial proliferative glomerulonephritis
N03.4	Chronic nephritic syndrome with diffuse endocapillary proliferative glomerulonephritis
N03.5	Chronic nephritic syndrome with diffuse mesangiocapillary glomerulonephritis
N03.6	Chronic nephritic syndrome with dense deposit disease
N03.7	Chronic nephritic syndrome with diffuse crescentic glomerulonephritis
N03.A	Chronic nephritic syndrome with C3 glomerulonephritis
N04.0	Nephrotic syndrome with minor glomerular abnormality
N04.1	Nephrotic syndrome with focal and segmental glomerular lesions
N04.21	Primary membranous nephropathy with nephrotic syndrome
N04.3	Nephrotic syndrome with diffuse mesangial proliferative glomerulonephritis
N04.4	Nephrotic syndrome with diffuse endocapillary proliferative glomerulonephritis
N04.5	Nephrotic syndrome with diffuse mesangiocapillary glomerulonephritis
N04.6	Nephrotic syndrome with dense deposit disease
N04.7	Nephrotic syndrome with diffuse crescentic glomerulonephritis
N04.A	Nephrotic syndrome with C3 glomerulonephritis
N10	Acute pyelonephritis
N11.0	Nonobstructive reflux-associated chronic pyelonephritis
N11.1	Chronic obstructive pyelonephritis
N17.0	Acute kidney failure with tubular necrosis
N17.1	Acute kidney failure with acute cortical necrosis
N17.2	Acute kidney failure with medullary necrosis
N18.31	Chronic kidney disease, stage 3a
N18.32	Chronic kidney disease, stage 3b
N18.4	Chronic kidney disease, stage 4 (severe)
N18.5	Chronic kidney disease, stage 5
N18.6	End stage renal disease

AMA: 36815 2023,Mar; 2022,Oct

Relative Value Units/Medicare Edits

Non-Facility RVU	Work	PE	MP	Total
36815	2.62	0.71	0.64	3.97
Facility RVU	**Work**	**PE**	**MP**	**Total**
36815	2.62	0.71	0.64	3.97

	FUD	Status	MUE	Modifiers				IOM Reference
36815	0	A	1(3)	51	N/A	N/A	N/A	None

* with documentation

Terms To Know

cannulation. Insertion of a flexible length of hollow tubing into a blood vessel, duct, or body cavity, usually for extracorporeal circulation or chemotherapy infusion to a particular region of the body.

nephrotic syndrome. Condition where levels of albumin in the blood and urine are far below the norm.

36818

36818 Arteriovenous anastomosis, open; by upper arm cephalic vein transposition

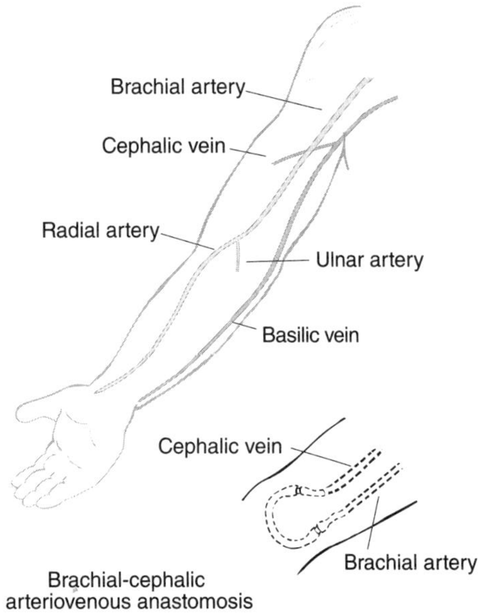

Explanation

A vascular surgeon creates a connection between an artery and a vein for a vascular access site in patients with end stage renal disease that require hemodialysis. The surgeon dissects down to the cephalic vein on the medial side of the upper arm and mobilizes the vein. A subcutaneous tunnel on the anterior side of the arm is created, and the mobilized cephalic vein is transposed to this tunnel and anastomosed to the brachial artery.

Coding Tips

This is a unilateral procedure. If performed bilaterally, some payers require that the service be reported twice with modifier 50 appended to the second code, while others require identification of the service only once with modifier 50 appended. Check with individual payers. Modifier 50 identifies a procedure performed identically on the opposite side of the body (mirror image). Do not report 36818 with 36819, 36820, 36821, or 36830 during a unilateral upper extremity procedure. For bilateral, upper extremity, open arteriovenous anastomosis performed at the same operative session, use modifier 50 or 59 as appropriate. When central dialysis segment angioplasty is performed with 36818–36833, see 36907. When central dialysis segment stent placement is performed with 36818–36833, see 36908.

ICD-10-CM Diagnostic Codes

D59.31	Infection-associated hemolytic-uremic syndrome
D59.32	Hereditary hemolytic-uremic syndrome
I12.0	Hypertensive chronic kidney disease with stage 5 chronic kidney disease or end stage renal disease
I13.0	Hypertensive heart and chronic kidney disease with heart failure and stage 1 through stage 4 chronic kidney disease, or unspecified chronic kidney disease
I13.11	Hypertensive heart and chronic kidney disease without heart failure, with stage 5 chronic kidney disease, or end stage renal disease
I13.2	Hypertensive heart and chronic kidney disease with heart failure and with stage 5 chronic kidney disease, or end stage renal disease
I16.0	Hypertensive urgency
I16.1	Hypertensive emergency
M35.04	Sjögren syndrome with tubulo-interstitial nephropathy
M35.0A	Sjögren syndrome with glomerular disease
N00.0	Acute nephritic syndrome with minor glomerular abnormality
N00.1	Acute nephritic syndrome with focal and segmental glomerular lesions
N00.2	Acute nephritic syndrome with diffuse membranous glomerulonephritis
N00.3	Acute nephritic syndrome with diffuse mesangial proliferative glomerulonephritis
N00.4	Acute nephritic syndrome with diffuse endocapillary proliferative glomerulonephritis
N00.5	Acute nephritic syndrome with diffuse mesangiocapillary glomerulonephritis
N00.6	Acute nephritic syndrome with dense deposit disease
N00.7	Acute nephritic syndrome with diffuse crescentic glomerulonephritis
N00.A	Acute nephritic syndrome with C3 glomerulonephritis
N01.0	Rapidly progressive nephritic syndrome with minor glomerular abnormality
N01.1	Rapidly progressive nephritic syndrome with focal and segmental glomerular lesions
N01.2	Rapidly progressive nephritic syndrome with diffuse membranous glomerulonephritis
N01.3	Rapidly progressive nephritic syndrome with diffuse mesangial proliferative glomerulonephritis
N01.4	Rapidly progressive nephritic syndrome with diffuse endocapillary proliferative glomerulonephritis
N01.5	Rapidly progressive nephritic syndrome with diffuse mesangiocapillary glomerulonephritis
N01.6	Rapidly progressive nephritic syndrome with dense deposit disease
N01.7	Rapidly progressive nephritic syndrome with diffuse crescentic glomerulonephritis
N01.A	Rapidly progressive nephritic syndrome with C3 glomerulonephritis
N03.0	Chronic nephritic syndrome with minor glomerular abnormality
N03.1	Chronic nephritic syndrome with focal and segmental glomerular lesions
N03.2	Chronic nephritic syndrome with diffuse membranous glomerulonephritis
N03.3	Chronic nephritic syndrome with diffuse mesangial proliferative glomerulonephritis
N03.4	Chronic nephritic syndrome with diffuse endocapillary proliferative glomerulonephritis
N03.5	Chronic nephritic syndrome with diffuse mesangiocapillary glomerulonephritis
N03.6	Chronic nephritic syndrome with dense deposit disease
N03.7	Chronic nephritic syndrome with diffuse crescentic glomerulonephritis
N03.A	Chronic nephritic syndrome with C3 glomerulonephritis
N04.0	Nephrotic syndrome with minor glomerular abnormality
N04.1	Nephrotic syndrome with focal and segmental glomerular lesions
N04.21	Primary membranous nephropathy with nephrotic syndrome

N04.3	Nephrotic syndrome with diffuse mesangial proliferative glomerulonephritis
N04.4	Nephrotic syndrome with diffuse endocapillary proliferative glomerulonephritis
N04.5	Nephrotic syndrome with diffuse mesangiocapillary glomerulonephritis
N04.6	Nephrotic syndrome with dense deposit disease
N04.7	Nephrotic syndrome with diffuse crescentic glomerulonephritis
N04.A	Nephrotic syndrome with C3 glomerulonephritis
N07.0	Hereditary nephropathy, not elsewhere classified with minor glomerular abnormality
N07.1	Hereditary nephropathy, not elsewhere classified with focal and segmental glomerular lesions
N07.2	Hereditary nephropathy, not elsewhere classified with diffuse membranous glomerulonephritis
N07.3	Hereditary nephropathy, not elsewhere classified with diffuse mesangial proliferative glomerulonephritis
N07.4	Hereditary nephropathy, not elsewhere classified with diffuse endocapillary proliferative glomerulonephritis
N07.5	Hereditary nephropathy, not elsewhere classified with diffuse mesangiocapillary glomerulonephritis
N07.6	Hereditary nephropathy, not elsewhere classified with dense deposit disease
N07.7	Hereditary nephropathy, not elsewhere classified with diffuse crescentic glomerulonephritis
N07.A	Hereditary nephropathy, not elsewhere classified with C3 glomerulonephritis
N11.0	Nonobstructive reflux-associated chronic pyelonephritis
N11.1	Chronic obstructive pyelonephritis
N12	Tubulo-interstitial nephritis, not specified as acute or chronic
N16	Renal tubulo-interstitial disorders in diseases classified elsewhere
N17.0	Acute kidney failure with tubular necrosis
N17.1	Acute kidney failure with acute cortical necrosis
N17.2	Acute kidney failure with medullary necrosis
N18.31	Chronic kidney disease, stage 3a
N18.32	Chronic kidney disease, stage 3b
N18.4	Chronic kidney disease, stage 4 (severe)
N18.5	Chronic kidney disease, stage 5
N18.6	End stage renal disease

AMA: 36818 2023,Mar; 2022,Oct

Relative Value Units/Medicare Edits

Non-Facility RVU	Work	PE	MP	Total
36818	12.39	4.82	3.05	20.26
Facility RVU	**Work**	**PE**	**MP**	**Total**
36818	12.39	4.82	3.05	20.26

	FUD	Status	MUE	Modifiers				IOM Reference
36818	90	A	1(3)	51	N/A	62*	80	None

* with documentation

36819

36819 Arteriovenous anastomosis, open; by upper arm basilic vein transposition

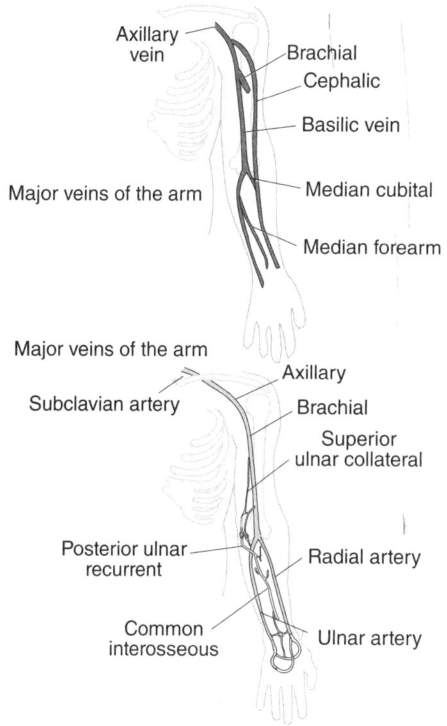

The basilic vein is transposed in an open arteriovenous anastomosis

Explanation

A vascular surgeon creates a connection between an artery and a vein for a vascular access site in patients with end-stage renal disease that require hemodialysis. The surgeon dissects down to the basilic vein on the medial side of the upper arm and mobilizes the vein. A subcutaneous tunnel on the anterior side of the arm is created and the mobilized basilic vein is transposed to this tunnel and anastomosed to the brachial artery.

Coding Tips

This is a unilateral procedure. If performed bilaterally, some payers require that the service be reported twice with modifier 50 appended to the second code, while others require identification of the service only once with modifier 50 appended. Check with individual payers. Modifier 50 identifies a procedure performed identically on the opposite side of the body (mirror image). Do not report 36819 with 36818, 36820, 36821, or 36830 during a unilateral upper extremity procedure. For bilateral, upper extremity, open arteriovenous anastomoses performed at the same operative session, use modifier 50 or 59 as appropriate. When central dialysis segment angioplasty is performed with 36818-36833, use 36907. When central dialysis segment stent placement is performed with 36818-36833, use 36908.

ICD-10-CM Diagnostic Codes

D59.31	Infection-associated hemolytic-uremic syndrome
D59.32	Hereditary hemolytic-uremic syndrome
E87.21	Acute metabolic acidosis
E87.22	Chronic metabolic acidosis
I12.0	Hypertensive chronic kidney disease with stage 5 chronic kidney disease or end stage renal disease

I13.0	Hypertensive heart and chronic kidney disease with heart failure and stage 1 through stage 4 chronic kidney disease, or unspecified chronic kidney disease
I13.11	Hypertensive heart and chronic kidney disease without heart failure, with stage 5 chronic kidney disease, or end stage renal disease
I13.2	Hypertensive heart and chronic kidney disease with heart failure and with stage 5 chronic kidney disease, or end stage renal disease
I16.0	Hypertensive urgency
I16.1	Hypertensive emergency
I82.3	Embolism and thrombosis of renal vein
M35.04	Sjögren syndrome with tubulo-interstitial nephropathy
M35.0A	Sjögren syndrome with glomerular disease
N00.0	Acute nephritic syndrome with minor glomerular abnormality
N00.1	Acute nephritic syndrome with focal and segmental glomerular lesions
N00.2	Acute nephritic syndrome with diffuse membranous glomerulonephritis
N00.3	Acute nephritic syndrome with diffuse mesangial proliferative glomerulonephritis
N00.4	Acute nephritic syndrome with diffuse endocapillary proliferative glomerulonephritis
N00.5	Acute nephritic syndrome with diffuse mesangiocapillary glomerulonephritis
N00.6	Acute nephritic syndrome with dense deposit disease
N00.7	Acute nephritic syndrome with diffuse crescentic glomerulonephritis
N00.8	Acute nephritic syndrome with other morphologic changes
N00.A	Acute nephritic syndrome with C3 glomerulonephritis
N01.0	Rapidly progressive nephritic syndrome with minor glomerular abnormality
N01.1	Rapidly progressive nephritic syndrome with focal and segmental glomerular lesions
N01.2	Rapidly progressive nephritic syndrome with diffuse membranous glomerulonephritis
N01.3	Rapidly progressive nephritic syndrome with diffuse mesangial proliferative glomerulonephritis
N01.4	Rapidly progressive nephritic syndrome with diffuse endocapillary proliferative glomerulonephritis
N01.5	Rapidly progressive nephritic syndrome with diffuse mesangiocapillary glomerulonephritis
N01.6	Rapidly progressive nephritic syndrome with dense deposit disease
N01.7	Rapidly progressive nephritic syndrome with diffuse crescentic glomerulonephritis
N01.8	Rapidly progressive nephritic syndrome with other morphologic changes
N01.A	Rapidly progressive nephritic syndrome with C3 glomerulonephritis
N03.0	Chronic nephritic syndrome with minor glomerular abnormality
N03.1	Chronic nephritic syndrome with focal and segmental glomerular lesions
N03.2	Chronic nephritic syndrome with diffuse membranous glomerulonephritis
N03.3	Chronic nephritic syndrome with diffuse mesangial proliferative glomerulonephritis
N03.4	Chronic nephritic syndrome with diffuse endocapillary proliferative glomerulonephritis
N03.5	Chronic nephritic syndrome with diffuse mesangiocapillary glomerulonephritis
N03.6	Chronic nephritic syndrome with dense deposit disease
N03.7	Chronic nephritic syndrome with diffuse crescentic glomerulonephritis
N03.8	Chronic nephritic syndrome with other morphologic changes
N03.A	Chronic nephritic syndrome with C3 glomerulonephritis
N04.0	Nephrotic syndrome with minor glomerular abnormality
N04.1	Nephrotic syndrome with focal and segmental glomerular lesions
N04.21	Primary membranous nephropathy with nephrotic syndrome
N04.3	Nephrotic syndrome with diffuse mesangial proliferative glomerulonephritis
N04.4	Nephrotic syndrome with diffuse endocapillary proliferative glomerulonephritis
N04.5	Nephrotic syndrome with diffuse mesangiocapillary glomerulonephritis
N04.6	Nephrotic syndrome with dense deposit disease
N04.7	Nephrotic syndrome with diffuse crescentic glomerulonephritis
N04.8	Nephrotic syndrome with other morphologic changes
N04.A	Nephrotic syndrome with C3 glomerulonephritis
N07.0	Hereditary nephropathy, not elsewhere classified with minor glomerular abnormality
N07.1	Hereditary nephropathy, not elsewhere classified with focal and segmental glomerular lesions
N07.2	Hereditary nephropathy, not elsewhere classified with diffuse membranous glomerulonephritis
N07.3	Hereditary nephropathy, not elsewhere classified with diffuse mesangial proliferative glomerulonephritis
N07.4	Hereditary nephropathy, not elsewhere classified with diffuse endocapillary proliferative glomerulonephritis
N07.5	Hereditary nephropathy, not elsewhere classified with diffuse mesangiocapillary glomerulonephritis
N07.6	Hereditary nephropathy, not elsewhere classified with dense deposit disease
N07.7	Hereditary nephropathy, not elsewhere classified with diffuse crescentic glomerulonephritis
N07.8	Hereditary nephropathy, not elsewhere classified with other morphologic lesions
N07.A	Hereditary nephropathy, not elsewhere classified with C3 glomerulonephritis
N08	Glomerular disorders in diseases classified elsewhere
N10	Acute pyelonephritis
N11.0	Nonobstructive reflux-associated chronic pyelonephritis
N11.1	Chronic obstructive pyelonephritis
N11.8	Other chronic tubulo-interstitial nephritis
N12	Tubulo-interstitial nephritis, not specified as acute or chronic
N15.8	Other specified renal tubulo-interstitial diseases
N16	Renal tubulo-interstitial disorders in diseases classified elsewhere
N17.0	Acute kidney failure with tubular necrosis
N17.1	Acute kidney failure with acute cortical necrosis
N17.2	Acute kidney failure with medullary necrosis

N17.8	Other acute kidney failure
N18.31	Chronic kidney disease, stage 3a
N18.32	Chronic kidney disease, stage 3b
N18.4	Chronic kidney disease, stage 4 (severe)
N18.5	Chronic kidney disease, stage 5
N18.6	End stage renal disease

AMA: 36819 2023,Mar

Relative Value Units/Medicare Edits

Non-Facility RVU	Work	PE	MP	Total
36819	13.29	4.85	3.31	21.45
Facility RVU	**Work**	**PE**	**MP**	**Total**
36819	13.29	4.85	3.31	21.45

	FUD	Status	MUE	Modifiers				IOM Reference
36819	90	A	1(3)	51	N/A	62*	80	None

* with documentation

Terms To Know

anastomosis. Surgically created connection between ducts, blood vessels, or bowel segments to allow flow from one to the other.

arteriovenous fistula. Connecting passage between an artery and a vein.

end-stage renal disease. Chronic, advanced kidney disease requiring renal dialysis or a kidney transplant to prevent imminent death.

hemodialysis. Cleansing of wastes and contaminating elements from the blood by virtue of different diffusion rates through a semipermeable membrane, which separates blood from a filtration solution that diffuses other elements out of the blood.

transposition. Removal or exchange from one side to another; change of position from one place to another.

36820

36820 Arteriovenous anastomosis, open; by forearm vein transposition

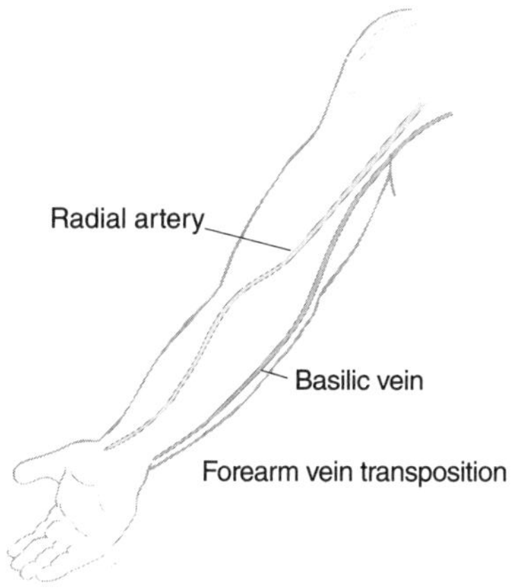

Explanation

The physician creates a connection between an artery or vein, using a forearm vein in the arm-inverted end to end. The physician dissects down to the vein and artery. The subfascial plane is identified and elevated laterally to the flexor carpi radialis (FCR) and medially to the brachioradialis (BR). The plane between the BR and FCR is dissected and the perforating vessels are identified and cauterized. The pedicle is followed to the antecubital fossa. The tourniquet is released, and the vessels are further cleaned of their adventitia under loupe visualization. Using microvascular techniques, a suture for the arterial anastomosis is performed and closure is completed. Suction drains are placed in the neck. If a Doppler is to be used for postoperative assessment, a suture is placed to mark the pedicle site. A splint is fabricated and secured to the arm with an elastic bandage.

Coding Tips

When this procedure is performed on the upper arm, basilic vein, see 36819; on the upper arm cephalic vein, see 36818. For insertion of a cannula for hemodialysis, other purpose (separate procedure), see 36800–36815. When central dialysis segment angioplasty is performed with 36818-36833, use 36907. When central dialysis segment stent placement is performed with 36818-36833, use 36908.

ICD-10-CM Diagnostic Codes

D59.31	Infection-associated hemolytic-uremic syndrome
D59.32	Hereditary hemolytic-uremic syndrome
I12.0	Hypertensive chronic kidney disease with stage 5 chronic kidney disease or end stage renal disease
I13.0	Hypertensive heart and chronic kidney disease with heart failure and stage 1 through stage 4 chronic kidney disease, or unspecified chronic kidney disease
I13.11	Hypertensive heart and chronic kidney disease without heart failure, with stage 5 chronic kidney disease, or end stage renal disease
I13.2	Hypertensive heart and chronic kidney disease with heart failure and with stage 5 chronic kidney disease, or end stage renal disease
I16.0	Hypertensive urgency
I16.1	Hypertensive emergency
I82.3	Embolism and thrombosis of renal vein
M35.04	Sjögren syndrome with tubulo-interstitial nephropathy

M35.0A Sjögren syndrome with glomerular disease
N00.0 Acute nephritic syndrome with minor glomerular abnormality
N00.1 Acute nephritic syndrome with focal and segmental glomerular lesions
N00.2 Acute nephritic syndrome with diffuse membranous glomerulonephritis
N00.3 Acute nephritic syndrome with diffuse mesangial proliferative glomerulonephritis
N00.4 Acute nephritic syndrome with diffuse endocapillary proliferative glomerulonephritis
N00.5 Acute nephritic syndrome with diffuse mesangiocapillary glomerulonephritis
N00.6 Acute nephritic syndrome with dense deposit disease
N00.7 Acute nephritic syndrome with diffuse crescentic glomerulonephritis
N00.A Acute nephritic syndrome with C3 glomerulonephritis
N01.0 Rapidly progressive nephritic syndrome with minor glomerular abnormality
N01.1 Rapidly progressive nephritic syndrome with focal and segmental glomerular lesions
N01.2 Rapidly progressive nephritic syndrome with diffuse membranous glomerulonephritis
N01.3 Rapidly progressive nephritic syndrome with diffuse mesangial proliferative glomerulonephritis
N01.4 Rapidly progressive nephritic syndrome with diffuse endocapillary proliferative glomerulonephritis
N01.5 Rapidly progressive nephritic syndrome with diffuse mesangiocapillary glomerulonephritis
N01.6 Rapidly progressive nephritic syndrome with dense deposit disease
N01.7 Rapidly progressive nephritic syndrome with diffuse crescentic glomerulonephritis
N01.A Rapidly progressive nephritic syndrome with C3 glomerulonephritis
N03.0 Chronic nephritic syndrome with minor glomerular abnormality
N03.1 Chronic nephritic syndrome with focal and segmental glomerular lesions
N03.2 Chronic nephritic syndrome with diffuse membranous glomerulonephritis
N03.3 Chronic nephritic syndrome with diffuse mesangial proliferative glomerulonephritis
N03.4 Chronic nephritic syndrome with diffuse endocapillary proliferative glomerulonephritis
N03.5 Chronic nephritic syndrome with diffuse mesangiocapillary glomerulonephritis
N03.6 Chronic nephritic syndrome with dense deposit disease
N03.7 Chronic nephritic syndrome with diffuse crescentic glomerulonephritis
N03.A Chronic nephritic syndrome with C3 glomerulonephritis
N04.0 Nephrotic syndrome with minor glomerular abnormality
N04.1 Nephrotic syndrome with focal and segmental glomerular lesions
N04.21 Primary membranous nephropathy with nephrotic syndrome
N04.3 Nephrotic syndrome with diffuse mesangial proliferative glomerulonephritis
N04.4 Nephrotic syndrome with diffuse endocapillary proliferative glomerulonephritis
N04.5 Nephrotic syndrome with diffuse mesangiocapillary glomerulonephritis
N04.6 Nephrotic syndrome with dense deposit disease
N04.7 Nephrotic syndrome with diffuse crescentic glomerulonephritis
N04.A Nephrotic syndrome with C3 glomerulonephritis
N07.0 Hereditary nephropathy, not elsewhere classified with minor glomerular abnormality
N07.1 Hereditary nephropathy, not elsewhere classified with focal and segmental glomerular lesions
N07.2 Hereditary nephropathy, not elsewhere classified with diffuse membranous glomerulonephritis
N07.3 Hereditary nephropathy, not elsewhere classified with diffuse mesangial proliferative glomerulonephritis
N07.4 Hereditary nephropathy, not elsewhere classified with diffuse endocapillary proliferative glomerulonephritis
N07.5 Hereditary nephropathy, not elsewhere classified with diffuse mesangiocapillary glomerulonephritis
N07.6 Hereditary nephropathy, not elsewhere classified with dense deposit disease
N07.7 Hereditary nephropathy, not elsewhere classified with diffuse crescentic glomerulonephritis
N07.A Hereditary nephropathy, not elsewhere classified with C3 glomerulonephritis
N11.0 Nonobstructive reflux-associated chronic pyelonephritis
N11.1 Chronic obstructive pyelonephritis
N11.8 Other chronic tubulo-interstitial nephritis
N12 Tubulo-interstitial nephritis, not specified as acute or chronic
N15.8 Other specified renal tubulo-interstitial diseases
N16 Renal tubulo-interstitial disorders in diseases classified elsewhere
N17.0 Acute kidney failure with tubular necrosis
N17.1 Acute kidney failure with acute cortical necrosis
N17.2 Acute kidney failure with medullary necrosis
N18.31 Chronic kidney disease, stage 3a
N18.32 Chronic kidney disease, stage 3b
N18.4 Chronic kidney disease, stage 4 (severe)
N18.5 Chronic kidney disease, stage 5
N18.6 End stage renal disease

AMA: 36820 2023,Mar; 2022,Oct

Relative Value Units/Medicare Edits

Non-Facility RVU	Work	PE	MP	Total
36820	13.07	5.04	3.23	21.34
Facility RVU	**Work**	**PE**	**MP**	**Total**
36820	13.07	5.04	3.23	21.34

	FUD	Status	MUE	Modifiers				IOM Reference
36820	90	A	1(3)	51	50	62*	80	None

* with documentation

36821

36821 Arteriovenous anastomosis, open; direct, any site (eg, Cimino type) (separate procedure)

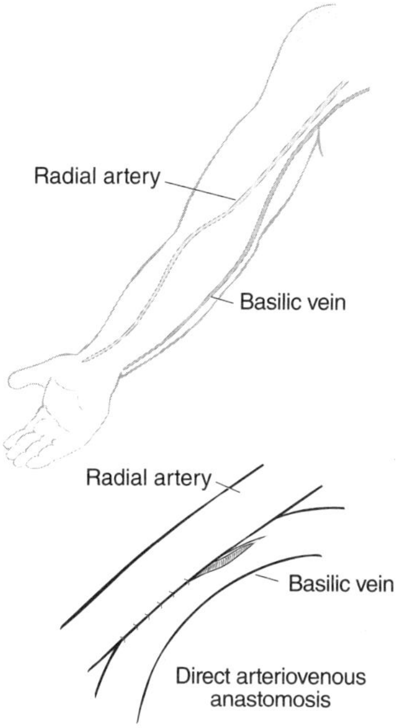

Explanation

Through an incision, usually in the skin over an artery in the nondominant wrist or antecubital fossa, the physician isolates a desired section of artery and neighboring vein. Vessel clamps are placed on the vein and adjacent artery. The vein is dissected free, divided, and the downstream portion of the vein is sutured to an opening created in the adjacent artery, usually in an end-to-side fashion, allowing blood to flow both down the artery and into the vein. Large branches of the vein may be tied off to cause flow down a single vein. The skin incision is repaired with a layered closure. This arteriovenous anastomosis will allow an increased blood flow through the vein, usually for hemodialysis.

Coding Tips

This separate procedure by definition is usually a component of a more complex service and is not identified separately. When performed alone or with other unrelated procedures/services, it may be reported. If performed alone, list the code; if performed with other procedures/services, list the code and append modifier 59 or an X{EPSU} modifier. For insertion of cannula for hemodialysis, other purpose (separate procedure), see 36800–36815. When central dialysis segment angioplasty is performed with 36818-36833, use 36907. When central dialysis segment stent placement is performed with 36818-36833, use 36908.

ICD-10-CM Diagnostic Codes

D59.31	Infection-associated hemolytic-uremic syndrome
D59.32	Hereditary hemolytic-uremic syndrome
E87.21	Acute metabolic acidosis
E87.22	Chronic metabolic acidosis
E87.5	Hyperkalemia
I12.0	Hypertensive chronic kidney disease with stage 5 chronic kidney disease or end stage renal disease
I13.0	Hypertensive heart and chronic kidney disease with heart failure and stage 1 through stage 4 chronic kidney disease, or unspecified chronic kidney disease
I13.11	Hypertensive heart and chronic kidney disease without heart failure, with stage 5 chronic kidney disease, or end stage renal disease
I13.2	Hypertensive heart and chronic kidney disease with heart failure and with stage 5 chronic kidney disease, or end stage renal disease
I16.0	Hypertensive urgency
I16.1	Hypertensive emergency
I82.3	Embolism and thrombosis of renal vein
M35.04	Sjögren syndrome with tubulo-interstitial nephropathy
M35.0A	Sjögren syndrome with glomerular disease
N00.0	Acute nephritic syndrome with minor glomerular abnormality
N00.1	Acute nephritic syndrome with focal and segmental glomerular lesions
N00.2	Acute nephritic syndrome with diffuse membranous glomerulonephritis
N00.3	Acute nephritic syndrome with diffuse mesangial proliferative glomerulonephritis
N00.4	Acute nephritic syndrome with diffuse endocapillary proliferative glomerulonephritis
N00.5	Acute nephritic syndrome with diffuse mesangiocapillary glomerulonephritis
N00.6	Acute nephritic syndrome with dense deposit disease
N00.7	Acute nephritic syndrome with diffuse crescentic glomerulonephritis
N00.8	Acute nephritic syndrome with other morphologic changes
N00.A	Acute nephritic syndrome with C3 glomerulonephritis
N01.0	Rapidly progressive nephritic syndrome with minor glomerular abnormality
N01.1	Rapidly progressive nephritic syndrome with focal and segmental glomerular lesions
N01.2	Rapidly progressive nephritic syndrome with diffuse membranous glomerulonephritis
N01.3	Rapidly progressive nephritic syndrome with diffuse mesangial proliferative glomerulonephritis
N01.4	Rapidly progressive nephritic syndrome with diffuse endocapillary proliferative glomerulonephritis
N01.5	Rapidly progressive nephritic syndrome with diffuse mesangiocapillary glomerulonephritis
N01.6	Rapidly progressive nephritic syndrome with dense deposit disease
N01.7	Rapidly progressive nephritic syndrome with diffuse crescentic glomerulonephritis
N01.8	Rapidly progressive nephritic syndrome with other morphologic changes
N01.A	Rapidly progressive nephritic syndrome with C3 glomerulonephritis
N03.0	Chronic nephritic syndrome with minor glomerular abnormality
N03.1	Chronic nephritic syndrome with focal and segmental glomerular lesions
N03.2	Chronic nephritic syndrome with diffuse membranous glomerulonephritis

N03.3 Chronic nephritic syndrome with diffuse mesangial proliferative glomerulonephritis
N03.4 Chronic nephritic syndrome with diffuse endocapillary proliferative glomerulonephritis
N03.5 Chronic nephritic syndrome with diffuse mesangiocapillary glomerulonephritis
N03.6 Chronic nephritic syndrome with dense deposit disease
N03.7 Chronic nephritic syndrome with diffuse crescentic glomerulonephritis
N03.8 Chronic nephritic syndrome with other morphologic changes
N03.A Chronic nephritic syndrome with C3 glomerulonephritis
N04.0 Nephrotic syndrome with minor glomerular abnormality
N04.1 Nephrotic syndrome with focal and segmental glomerular lesions
N04.21 Primary membranous nephropathy with nephrotic syndrome
N04.3 Nephrotic syndrome with diffuse mesangial proliferative glomerulonephritis
N04.4 Nephrotic syndrome with diffuse endocapillary proliferative glomerulonephritis
N04.5 Nephrotic syndrome with diffuse mesangiocapillary glomerulonephritis
N04.6 Nephrotic syndrome with dense deposit disease
N04.7 Nephrotic syndrome with diffuse crescentic glomerulonephritis
N04.8 Nephrotic syndrome with other morphologic changes
N04.A Nephrotic syndrome with C3 glomerulonephritis
N07.0 Hereditary nephropathy, not elsewhere classified with minor glomerular abnormality
N07.1 Hereditary nephropathy, not elsewhere classified with focal and segmental glomerular lesions
N07.2 Hereditary nephropathy, not elsewhere classified with diffuse membranous glomerulonephritis
N07.3 Hereditary nephropathy, not elsewhere classified with diffuse mesangial proliferative glomerulonephritis
N07.4 Hereditary nephropathy, not elsewhere classified with diffuse endocapillary proliferative glomerulonephritis
N07.5 Hereditary nephropathy, not elsewhere classified with diffuse mesangiocapillary glomerulonephritis
N07.6 Hereditary nephropathy, not elsewhere classified with dense deposit disease
N07.7 Hereditary nephropathy, not elsewhere classified with diffuse crescentic glomerulonephritis
N07.8 Hereditary nephropathy, not elsewhere classified with other morphologic lesions
N07.A Hereditary nephropathy, not elsewhere classified with C3 glomerulonephritis
N08 Glomerular disorders in diseases classified elsewhere
N10 Acute pyelonephritis
N11.0 Nonobstructive reflux-associated chronic pyelonephritis
N11.1 Chronic obstructive pyelonephritis
N11.8 Other chronic tubulo-interstitial nephritis
N12 Tubulo-interstitial nephritis, not specified as acute or chronic
N15.8 Other specified renal tubulo-interstitial diseases
N16 Renal tubulo-interstitial disorders in diseases classified elsewhere
N17.0 Acute kidney failure with tubular necrosis
N17.1 Acute kidney failure with acute cortical necrosis
N17.2 Acute kidney failure with medullary necrosis
N17.8 Other acute kidney failure
N18.31 Chronic kidney disease, stage 3a
N18.32 Chronic kidney disease, stage 3b
N18.4 Chronic kidney disease, stage 4 (severe)
N18.5 Chronic kidney disease, stage 5
N18.6 End stage renal disease

AMA: 36821 2023,Mar; 2022,Oct

Relative Value Units/Medicare Edits

Non-Facility RVU	Work	PE	MP	Total
36821	11.9	4.56	2.93	19.39
Facility RVU	**Work**	**PE**	**MP**	**Total**
36821	11.9	4.56	2.93	19.39

	FUD	Status	MUE	Modifiers				IOM Reference
36821	90	A	2(3)	51	N/A	62*	80	None

* with documentation

Terms To Know

anastomosis. Surgically created connection between ducts, blood vessels, or bowel segments to allow flow from one to the other.

arteriovenous fistula. Connecting passage between an artery and a vein.

end-stage renal disease. Chronic, advanced kidney disease requiring renal dialysis or a kidney transplant to prevent imminent death.

hemodialysis. Cleansing of wastes and contaminating elements from the blood by virtue of different diffusion rates through a semipermeable membrane, which separates blood from a filtration solution that diffuses other elements out of the blood.

transposition. Removal or exchange from one side to another; change of position from one place to another.

36825-36830

36825 Creation of arteriovenous fistula by other than direct arteriovenous anastomosis (separate procedure); autogenous graft
36830 nonautogenous graft (eg, biological collagen, thermoplastic graft)

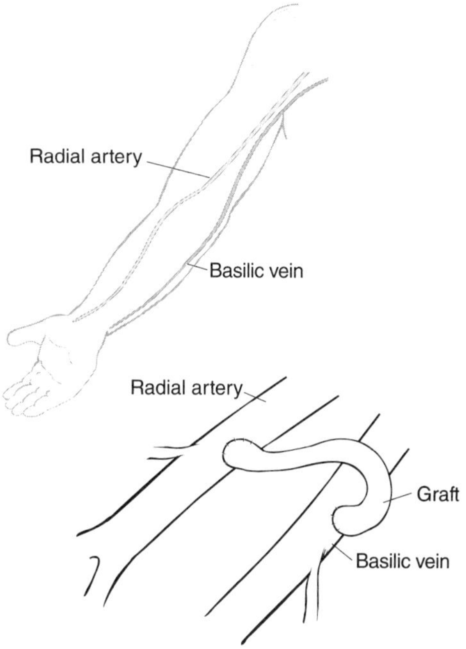

Explanation

The physician creates an arteriovenous fistula by other than direct anastomosis. The physician makes an incision in the skin over an artery and vein, and the vein and artery are dissected free. A vessel clamp is affixed to each. A length of harvested vein from the patient is used for an autogenous graft in 36825 and is sutured to the incised artery and vein, usually in an end-to-side fashion. The graft is passed in a superficial subcutaneous tunnel that is created bluntly and connects the arterial and venous sites. The clamps are removed, allowing the blood to flow through the graft, creating an arteriovenous fistula. The skin incision is repaired with a layered closure. Report 36830 if a nonautogenous graft, such as biological collagen or a thermoplastic graft, is used.

Coding Tips

These separate procedures by definition are usually a component of a more complex service and are not identified separately. When performed alone or with other unrelated procedures/services, they may be reported. If performed alone, list the code; if performed with other procedures/services, list the code and append modifier 59 or an X{EPSU} modifier. For direct arteriovenous anastomosis, see 36821. When central dialysis segment angioplasty is performed with 36818-36833, use 36907. When central dialysis segment stent placement is performed with 36818-36833, use 36908.

ICD-10-CM Diagnostic Codes

D59.31	Infection-associated hemolytic-uremic syndrome
D59.32	Hereditary hemolytic-uremic syndrome
E87.21	Acute metabolic acidosis
E87.22	Chronic metabolic acidosis
E87.5	Hyperkalemia
I12.0	Hypertensive chronic kidney disease with stage 5 chronic kidney disease or end stage renal disease
I13.0	Hypertensive heart and chronic kidney disease with heart failure and stage 1 through stage 4 chronic kidney disease, or unspecified chronic kidney disease
I13.10	Hypertensive heart and chronic kidney disease without heart failure, with stage 1 through stage 4 chronic kidney disease, or unspecified chronic kidney disease
I13.11	Hypertensive heart and chronic kidney disease without heart failure, with stage 5 chronic kidney disease, or end stage renal disease
I13.2	Hypertensive heart and chronic kidney disease with heart failure and with stage 5 chronic kidney disease, or end stage renal disease
I16.0	Hypertensive urgency
I16.1	Hypertensive emergency
I82.3	Embolism and thrombosis of renal vein
M35.04	Sjögren syndrome with tubulo-interstitial nephropathy
M35.0A	Sjögren syndrome with glomerular disease
N00.0	Acute nephritic syndrome with minor glomerular abnormality
N00.1	Acute nephritic syndrome with focal and segmental glomerular lesions
N00.2	Acute nephritic syndrome with diffuse membranous glomerulonephritis
N00.3	Acute nephritic syndrome with diffuse mesangial proliferative glomerulonephritis
N00.4	Acute nephritic syndrome with diffuse endocapillary proliferative glomerulonephritis
N00.5	Acute nephritic syndrome with diffuse mesangiocapillary glomerulonephritis
N00.6	Acute nephritic syndrome with dense deposit disease
N00.7	Acute nephritic syndrome with diffuse crescentic glomerulonephritis
N00.8	Acute nephritic syndrome with other morphologic changes
N00.A	Acute nephritic syndrome with C3 glomerulonephritis
N01.0	Rapidly progressive nephritic syndrome with minor glomerular abnormality
N01.1	Rapidly progressive nephritic syndrome with focal and segmental glomerular lesions
N01.2	Rapidly progressive nephritic syndrome with diffuse membranous glomerulonephritis
N01.3	Rapidly progressive nephritic syndrome with diffuse mesangial proliferative glomerulonephritis
N01.4	Rapidly progressive nephritic syndrome with diffuse endocapillary proliferative glomerulonephritis
N01.5	Rapidly progressive nephritic syndrome with diffuse mesangiocapillary glomerulonephritis
N01.6	Rapidly progressive nephritic syndrome with dense deposit disease
N01.7	Rapidly progressive nephritic syndrome with diffuse crescentic glomerulonephritis
N01.8	Rapidly progressive nephritic syndrome with other morphologic changes
N01.A	Rapidly progressive nephritic syndrome with C3 glomerulonephritis
N03.0	Chronic nephritic syndrome with minor glomerular abnormality
N03.1	Chronic nephritic syndrome with focal and segmental glomerular lesions

N03.2	Chronic nephritic syndrome with diffuse membranous glomerulonephritis
N03.3	Chronic nephritic syndrome with diffuse mesangial proliferative glomerulonephritis
N03.4	Chronic nephritic syndrome with diffuse endocapillary proliferative glomerulonephritis
N03.5	Chronic nephritic syndrome with diffuse mesangiocapillary glomerulonephritis
N03.6	Chronic nephritic syndrome with dense deposit disease
N03.7	Chronic nephritic syndrome with diffuse crescentic glomerulonephritis
N03.8	Chronic nephritic syndrome with other morphologic changes
N03.A	Chronic nephritic syndrome with C3 glomerulonephritis
N04.0	Nephrotic syndrome with minor glomerular abnormality
N04.1	Nephrotic syndrome with focal and segmental glomerular lesions
N04.21	Primary membranous nephropathy with nephrotic syndrome
N04.22	Secondary membranous nephropathy with nephrotic syndrome
N04.3	Nephrotic syndrome with diffuse mesangial proliferative glomerulonephritis
N04.4	Nephrotic syndrome with diffuse endocapillary proliferative glomerulonephritis
N04.5	Nephrotic syndrome with diffuse mesangiocapillary glomerulonephritis
N04.6	Nephrotic syndrome with dense deposit disease
N04.7	Nephrotic syndrome with diffuse crescentic glomerulonephritis
N04.8	Nephrotic syndrome with other morphologic changes
N04.A	Nephrotic syndrome with C3 glomerulonephritis
N07.0	Hereditary nephropathy, not elsewhere classified with minor glomerular abnormality
N07.1	Hereditary nephropathy, not elsewhere classified with focal and segmental glomerular lesions
N07.2	Hereditary nephropathy, not elsewhere classified with diffuse membranous glomerulonephritis
N07.3	Hereditary nephropathy, not elsewhere classified with diffuse mesangial proliferative glomerulonephritis
N07.4	Hereditary nephropathy, not elsewhere classified with diffuse endocapillary proliferative glomerulonephritis
N07.5	Hereditary nephropathy, not elsewhere classified with diffuse mesangiocapillary glomerulonephritis
N07.6	Hereditary nephropathy, not elsewhere classified with dense deposit disease
N07.7	Hereditary nephropathy, not elsewhere classified with diffuse crescentic glomerulonephritis
N07.8	Hereditary nephropathy, not elsewhere classified with other morphologic lesions
N07.A	Hereditary nephropathy, not elsewhere classified with C3 glomerulonephritis
N08	Glomerular disorders in diseases classified elsewhere
N10	Acute pyelonephritis
N11.0	Nonobstructive reflux-associated chronic pyelonephritis
N11.1	Chronic obstructive pyelonephritis
N11.8	Other chronic tubulo-interstitial nephritis
N12	Tubulo-interstitial nephritis, not specified as acute or chronic
N15.8	Other specified renal tubulo-interstitial diseases
N16	Renal tubulo-interstitial disorders in diseases classified elsewhere
N17.0	Acute kidney failure with tubular necrosis
N17.1	Acute kidney failure with acute cortical necrosis
N17.2	Acute kidney failure with medullary necrosis
N17.8	Other acute kidney failure
N18.31	Chronic kidney disease, stage 3a
N18.32	Chronic kidney disease, stage 3b
N18.4	Chronic kidney disease, stage 4 (severe)
N18.5	Chronic kidney disease, stage 5
N18.6	End stage renal disease

AMA: **36830** 2023,Nov

Relative Value Units/Medicare Edits

Non-Facility RVU	Work	PE	MP	Total
36825	14.17	5.62	3.53	23.32
36830	12.03	4.58	2.97	19.58
Facility RVU	**Work**	**PE**	**MP**	**Total**
36825	14.17	5.62	3.53	23.32
36830	12.03	4.58	2.97	19.58

	FUD	Status	MUE	Modifiers				IOM Reference
36825	90	A	1(3)	51	N/A	62*	80	None
36830	90	A	2(3)	51	N/A	62*	80	

* with documentation

Terms To Know

anastomosis. Surgically created connection between ducts, blood vessels, or bowel segments to allow flow from one to the other.

arteriovenous fistula. Connecting passage between an artery and a vein.

nonautogenous. Derived from a source other than the same individual or recipient (e.g., cells, tissue, blood vessels, and other organs donated from another human).

36831

36831 Thrombectomy, open, arteriovenous fistula without revision, autogenous or nonautogenous dialysis graft (separate procedure)

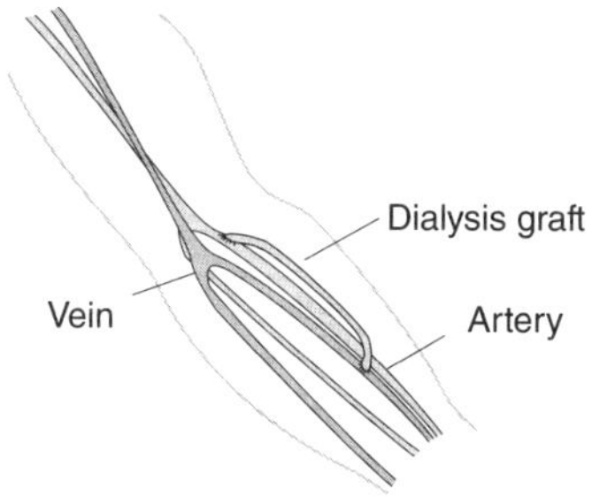

A previously placed dialysis graft, autogenous or nonautogenous, has developed a thrombus

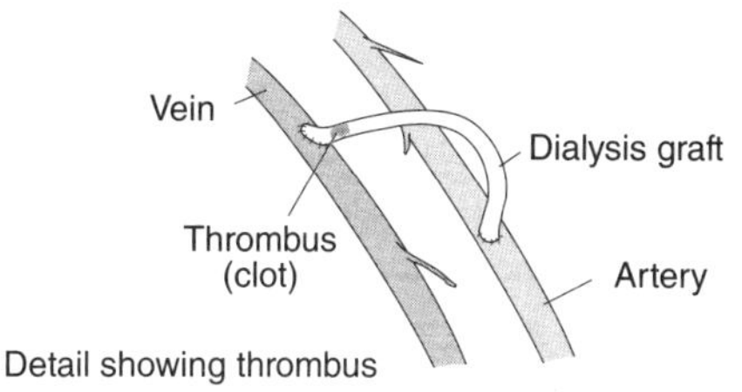

Explanation

The physician removes a blood clot from a surgically created connection between an artery and a vein (arteriovenous fistula). The procedure involves making an incision over the site of an existing fistula. The fistula is isolated and dissected free. Vessel clamps are affixed above and below the fistula. The blood clot is removed, the clamps are taken off, and the incision is repaired by layered sutures. The procedure may involve a vein acquired from the patient or the construction of a synthetic graft.

Coding Tips

This separate procedure by definition is usually a component of a more complex service and is not identified separately. When performed alone or with other unrelated procedures/services, it may be reported. If performed alone, list the code; if performed with other procedures/services, list the code and append modifier 59 of an X{EPSU} modifier. Use this procedure for thrombectomy associated with reduced flow. If a vein is acquired from the patient or the construction of a synthetic graft is performed, it may be reported with a separate code. For cannula declotting, see 36860–36861. For thrombectomy with revision of an arteriovenous fistula, see 36833. When central dialysis segment angioplasty is performed with 36818-36833, use 36907. When central dialysis segment stent placement is performed with 36818-36833, use 36908.

ICD-10-CM Diagnostic Codes

T82.818A Embolism due to vascular prosthetic devices, implants and grafts, initial encounter

T82.828A Fibrosis due to vascular prosthetic devices, implants and grafts, initial encounter

T82.848A Pain due to vascular prosthetic devices, implants and grafts, initial encounter

T82.856A Stenosis of peripheral vascular stent, initial encounter

T82.858A Stenosis of other vascular prosthetic devices, implants and grafts, initial encounter

T82.868A Thrombosis due to vascular prosthetic devices, implants and grafts, initial encounter

T82.898A Other specified complication of vascular prosthetic devices, implants and grafts, initial encounter

Relative Value Units/Medicare Edits

Non-Facility RVU	Work	PE	MP	Total
36831	11.0	4.41	2.73	18.14
Facility RVU	**Work**	**PE**	**MP**	**Total**
36831	11.0	4.41	2.73	18.14

	FUD	Status	MUE	Modifiers				IOM Reference
36831	90	A	1(3)	51	N/A	62*	80	None

* with documentation

Terms To Know

chronic. Persistent, continuing, or recurring.

complication. Condition arising after the beginning of observation and treatment that modifies the course of the patient's illness or the medical care required, or an undesired result or misadventure in medical care.

fistula. Abnormal tube-like passage between two body cavities or organs or from an organ to the outside surface.

graft. Tissue implant from another part of the body or another person.

incision. Act of cutting into tissue or an organ.

renal failure. Inability of a kidney to eliminate metabolites and retain electrolytes at a normal level.

thrombus. Stationary blood clot inside a blood vessel.

36832-36833

36832 Revision, open, arteriovenous fistula; without thrombectomy, autogenous or nonautogenous dialysis graft (separate procedure)

36833 with thrombectomy, autogenous or nonautogenous dialysis graft (separate procedure)

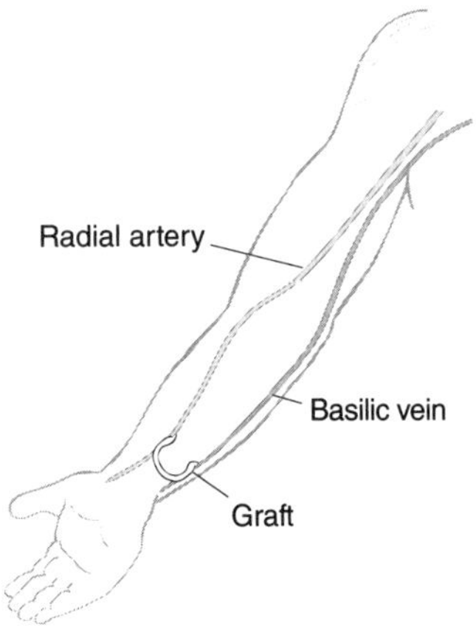

Explanation

In 36832, the physician makes an incision at the site of an already existing artificial fistula between an artery and a vein. The fistula is dissected free. Vessel clamps are affixed above and below the fistula, which is incised. Revisions are made to the fistula at its juncture to the vein and/or artery and may require creating a new anastomosis with a graft obtained from a separate site or created with synthetic material. After the repair has been made, the fistula is sutured, the clamps removed, and the skin incision repaired with a layered closure. Report 36833 when the physician removes a blood clot at the fistula site in addition to revising the existing arteriovenous fistula.

Coding Tips

These codes should be reported only for open revision of an arteriovenous fistula. These separate procedures by definition are usually a component of a more complex service and are not identified separately. When performed alone or with other unrelated procedures/services, they may be reported. If performed alone, list the code; if performed with other procedures/services, list the code and append modifier 59 or an X{EPSU} modifier. For cannula declotting, see 36860–36861. For open thrombectomy without revision of an arteriovenous fistula, see 36831. When central dialysis segment angioplasty is performed with 36818-36833, use 36907. When central dialysis segment stent placement is performed with 36818-36833, use 36908. When percutaneous thrombectomy is performed within the dialysis circuit, see 36904-36906. Do not report 36832 or 36833 with 36901-36906 for revision of the dialysis circuit.

ICD-10-CM Diagnostic Codes

T82.318A	Breakdown (mechanical) of other vascular grafts, initial encounter
T82.328A	Displacement of other vascular grafts, initial encounter
T82.338A	Leakage of other vascular grafts, initial encounter
T82.398A	Other mechanical complication of other vascular grafts, initial encounter
T82.510A	Breakdown (mechanical) of surgically created arteriovenous fistula, initial encounter
T82.518A	Breakdown (mechanical) of other cardiac and vascular devices and implants, initial encounter
T82.520A	Displacement of surgically created arteriovenous fistula, initial encounter
T82.528A	Displacement of other cardiac and vascular devices and implants, initial encounter
T82.530A	Leakage of surgically created arteriovenous fistula, initial encounter
T82.538A	Leakage of other cardiac and vascular devices and implants, initial encounter
T82.590A	Other mechanical complication of surgically created arteriovenous fistula, initial encounter
T82.598A	Other mechanical complication of other cardiac and vascular devices and implants, initial encounter
T82.7XXA	Infection and inflammatory reaction due to other cardiac and vascular devices, implants and grafts, initial encounter
T82.818A	Embolism due to vascular prosthetic devices, implants and grafts, initial encounter
T82.828A	Fibrosis due to vascular prosthetic devices, implants and grafts, initial encounter
T82.838A	Hemorrhage due to vascular prosthetic devices, implants and grafts, initial encounter
T82.848A	Pain due to vascular prosthetic devices, implants and grafts, initial encounter
T82.856A	Stenosis of peripheral vascular stent, initial encounter
T82.858A	Stenosis of other vascular prosthetic devices, implants and grafts, initial encounter
T82.868A	Thrombosis due to vascular prosthetic devices, implants and grafts, initial encounter
T82.898A	Other specified complication of vascular prosthetic devices, implants and grafts, initial encounter
Z45.89	Encounter for adjustment and management of other implanted devices
Z46.89	Encounter for fitting and adjustment of other specified devices

AMA: **36832** 2022,May

Relative Value Units/Medicare Edits

Non-Facility RVU	Work	PE	MP	Total
36832	13.5	5.39	3.34	22.23
36833	14.5	5.61	3.6	23.71
Facility RVU	**Work**	**PE**	**MP**	**Total**
36832	13.5	5.39	3.34	22.23
36833	14.5	5.61	3.6	23.71

	FUD	Status	MUE	Modifiers				IOM Reference
36832	90	A	2(3)	51	N/A	62*	80	None
36833	90	A	1(3)	51	N/A	62*	80	

* with documentation

Arteries and Veins

[36836, 36837]

36836 Percutaneous arteriovenous fistula creation, upper extremity, single access of both the peripheral artery and peripheral vein, including fistula maturation procedures (eg, transluminal balloon angioplasty, coil embolization) when performed, including all vascular access, imaging guidance and radiologic supervision and interpretation

36837 Percutaneous arteriovenous fistula creation, upper extremity, separate access sites of the peripheral artery and peripheral vein, including fistula maturation procedures (eg, transluminal balloon angioplasty, coil embolization) when performed, including all vascular access, imaging guidance and radiologic supervision and interpretation

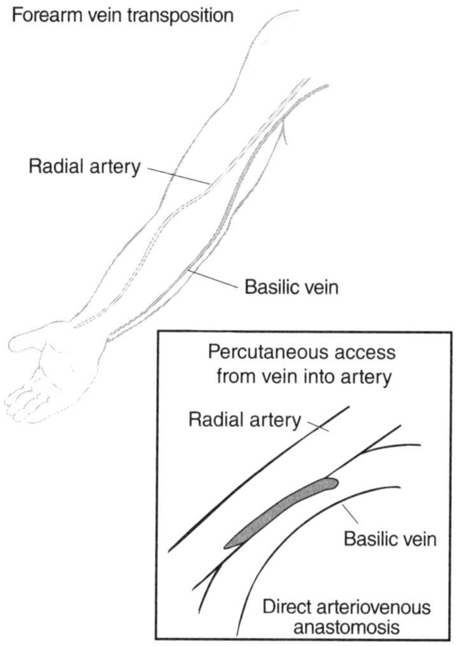

Explanation

The physician creates an arteriovenous (AV) fistula, which is a surgically created connection between an artery and a vein, in an upper extremity using a minimally invasive, catheter-based percutaneous approach. The procedure is typically performed by a vascular specialist and is created for long-term dialysis access. Conscious sedation, regional anesthesia, or local anesthesia may be used. Code 36836 is reported for the creation of an AV fistula via a single access site for the arteriovenous puncture, along with thermal energy. In one technique, the cubital vein is accessed using a standard micropuncture needle and wire. Using ultrasound guidance, the access needle is advanced intravenously into the perforating vein and into the proximal radial artery. A guidewire is positioned through the vein into the radial artery followed by a sheath, which allows the device to be inserted into the artery. The access needle is withdrawn, and a 6-F sheath is advanced over the guidewire into the artery. The device catheter is placed through the sheath and the walls of the artery and vein are engaged. The catheter is activated, creating a fistula via a low-power direct current. The device and sheath are removed, and hemostasis is accomplished with pressure. A Doppler study may be performed to confirm fistula flow and measure brachial artery flow volume, and balloon angioplasty may be performed immediately following fistula creation to quickly increase blood flow in the fistula. In an alternate method (36837), separate access sites are employed, and the AV fistula is created using magnetic-guided arterial and venous catheters along with radiofrequency (RF) energy. Most commonly, the brachial vein is accessed using a standard micropuncture needle and wire. The guidewire is advanced intravenously, under imaging guidance, through the brachial vein into the ulnar vein, and a dilator and sheath are placed. The brachial artery is accessed, also under imaging guidance, using a standard micropuncture needle and wire. The guidewire is advanced intravenously into the ulnar artery, and a dilator and sheath are placed. A magnetic catheter is inserted into the artery and a second magnetic catheter is inserted into the vein. The magnets draw the artery and vein together. Once alignment is confirmed, an RF cutting electrode is deployed in the venous catheter, which aligns with a ceramic backstop in the arterial catheter. The electrode is energized, and a channel is created between the vein and artery. The catheters are removed, and the accessed brachial vein is embolized with a coil to force blood into the superficial veins for dialysis. All prosthetic materials are removed, and hemostasis is accomplished with pressure. A fistulogram is performed to confirm fistula flow. In either procedure, the patient must have vessels that are more than 2 mm in diameter and have less than 2 mm of separation between the artery and vein at the site of fistula creation. These codes include all fistula maturation procedures such as coil embolization or transluminal balloon angioplasty if performed, and include all vascular access, imaging guidance, and any radiologic supervision/interpretation.

Coding Tips

When medically necessary, report moderate (conscious) sedation provided by the performing physician with 99151-99153. When provided by another physician, report 99155-99157. Vascular access, angiography, blood flow redirection, imaging guidance, and radiological supervision and interpretation are included in 36836 and 36837 and are not reported separately. Do not report 36836 or 36837 with 36005, 36140, 36215–36218, 36245–36247, 36901–36909, 37236, 37238, 37241, 37242, 37246, 37248, 37252, 75710, 75716, 75820, 75822, 75894, 75898, 76937, or 77001. Do not report 36836 with 36837. For open approach creation of an arteriovenous fistula, see 36800, 36810, 36815, 36818, 36819, 36820, or 36821. For percutaneous arteriovenous fistula creation for any location other that an upper extremity, see 37799.

ICD-10-CM Diagnostic Codes

D59.31	Infection-associated hemolytic-uremic syndrome
D59.32	Hereditary hemolytic-uremic syndrome
E87.5	Hyperkalemia
I12.0	Hypertensive chronic kidney disease with stage 5 chronic kidney disease or end stage renal disease
I13.11	Hypertensive heart and chronic kidney disease without heart failure, with stage 5 chronic kidney disease, or end stage renal disease
I13.2	Hypertensive heart and chronic kidney disease with heart failure and with stage 5 chronic kidney disease, or end stage renal disease
N00.0	Acute nephritic syndrome with minor glomerular abnormality
N00.1	Acute nephritic syndrome with focal and segmental glomerular lesions
N00.2	Acute nephritic syndrome with diffuse membranous glomerulonephritis
N00.3	Acute nephritic syndrome with diffuse mesangial proliferative glomerulonephritis
N00.4	Acute nephritic syndrome with diffuse endocapillary proliferative glomerulonephritis
N00.5	Acute nephritic syndrome with diffuse mesangiocapillary glomerulonephritis
N00.6	Acute nephritic syndrome with dense deposit disease
N00.7	Acute nephritic syndrome with diffuse crescentic glomerulonephritis

N01.0	Rapidly progressive nephritic syndrome with minor glomerular abnormality
N01.1	Rapidly progressive nephritic syndrome with focal and segmental glomerular lesions
N01.2	Rapidly progressive nephritic syndrome with diffuse membranous glomerulonephritis
N01.3	Rapidly progressive nephritic syndrome with diffuse mesangial proliferative glomerulonephritis
N01.4	Rapidly progressive nephritic syndrome with diffuse endocapillary proliferative glomerulonephritis
N01.5	Rapidly progressive nephritic syndrome with diffuse mesangiocapillary glomerulonephritis
N01.6	Rapidly progressive nephritic syndrome with dense deposit disease
N01.7	Rapidly progressive nephritic syndrome with diffuse crescentic glomerulonephritis
N01.A	Rapidly progressive nephritic syndrome with C3 glomerulonephritis
N03.0	Chronic nephritic syndrome with minor glomerular abnormality
N03.1	Chronic nephritic syndrome with focal and segmental glomerular lesions
N03.2	Chronic nephritic syndrome with diffuse membranous glomerulonephritis
N03.3	Chronic nephritic syndrome with diffuse mesangial proliferative glomerulonephritis
N03.4	Chronic nephritic syndrome with diffuse endocapillary proliferative glomerulonephritis
N03.5	Chronic nephritic syndrome with diffuse mesangiocapillary glomerulonephritis
N03.6	Chronic nephritic syndrome with dense deposit disease
N03.7	Chronic nephritic syndrome with diffuse crescentic glomerulonephritis
N03.A	Chronic nephritic syndrome with C3 glomerulonephritis
N04.0	Nephrotic syndrome with minor glomerular abnormality
N04.1	Nephrotic syndrome with focal and segmental glomerular lesions
N04.21	Primary membranous nephropathy with nephrotic syndrome
N04.22	Secondary membranous nephropathy with nephrotic syndrome
N04.3	Nephrotic syndrome with diffuse mesangial proliferative glomerulonephritis
N04.4	Nephrotic syndrome with diffuse endocapillary proliferative glomerulonephritis
N04.5	Nephrotic syndrome with diffuse mesangiocapillary glomerulonephritis
N04.6	Nephrotic syndrome with dense deposit disease
N04.7	Nephrotic syndrome with diffuse crescentic glomerulonephritis
N04.A	Nephrotic syndrome with C3 glomerulonephritis
N11.1	Chronic obstructive pyelonephritis
N11.8	Other chronic tubulo-interstitial nephritis
N12	Tubulo-interstitial nephritis, not specified as acute or chronic
N16	Renal tubulo-interstitial disorders in diseases classified elsewhere
N17.0	Acute kidney failure with tubular necrosis
N17.1	Acute kidney failure with acute cortical necrosis
N17.2	Acute kidney failure with medullary necrosis
N18.4	Chronic kidney disease, stage 4 (severe)
N18.5	Chronic kidney disease, stage 5
N18.6	End stage renal disease
Z99.2	Dependence on renal dialysis

AMA: 36836 2023,Mar; 2022,Oct **36837** 2023,Mar; 2022,Oct

Relative Value Units/Medicare Edits

Non-Facility RVU	Work	PE	MP	Total
36836	7.2	232.31	1.01	240.52
36837	9.3	275.61	1.37	286.28
Facility RVU	**Work**	**PE**	**MP**	**Total**
36836	7.2	2.19	1.01	10.4
36837	9.3	2.78	1.37	13.45

	FUD	Status	MUE	Modifiers				IOM Reference
36836	0	A	1(2)	51	N/A	62*	80	None
36837	0	A	1(2)	51	N/A	62*	80	

* with documentation

Terms To Know

fistula. Abnormal tube-like passage between two body cavities or organs or from an organ to the outside surface.

hemodialysis. Cleansing of wastes and contaminating elements from the blood by virtue of different diffusion rates through a semipermeable membrane, which separates blood from a filtration solution that diffuses other elements out of the blood.

percutaneous. Through the skin.

36835

36835 Insertion of Thomas shunt (separate procedure)

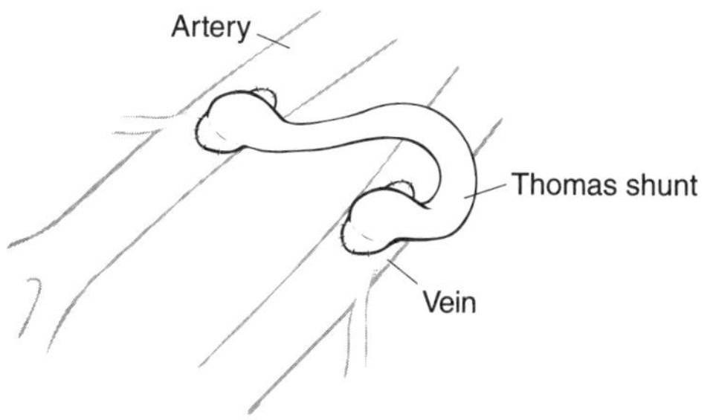

The Thomas shunt is a specialized synthetic graft and is typically used for infant and pediatric patients

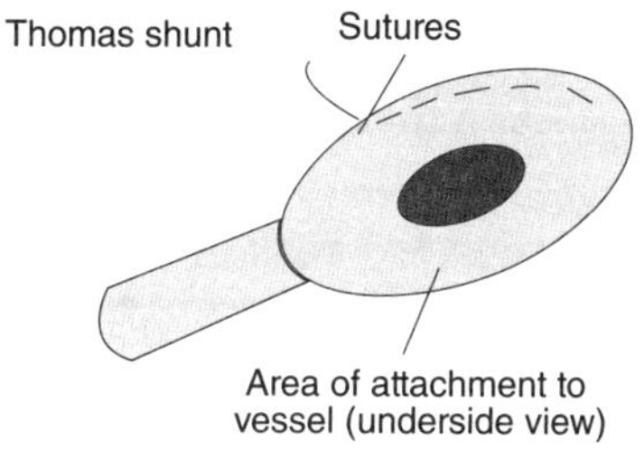

Explanation

Through an incision in the skin overlying a large vein or artery of a child, the physician dissects the vessel that will receive a synthetic shunt. The vessel may be clamped. The vessel is nicked, and a needle threads a guidance wire into the vein or artery. The shunt follows, and the wire is removed. The physician sutures the synthetic shunt either end-to-end, or end-to-side, to the vein or artery. The shunt is most often used for access in hemodialysis.

Coding Tips

This separate procedure by definition is usually a component of a more complex service and is not identified separately. When performed alone or with other unrelated procedures/services, it may be reported. If performed alone, list the code; if performed with other procedures/services, list the code and append modifier 59 or an X{EPSU} modifier. This type of shunt is infrequently used; verify this is the correct code by obtaining a copy of the shunt label from the medical record. This code includes venipuncture performed by the physician. Supplies used when providing this procedure may be reported with C1750. Check with the specific payer to determine coverage.

ICD-10-CM Diagnostic Codes

D59.31	Infection-associated hemolytic-uremic syndrome
D59.32	Hereditary hemolytic-uremic syndrome
E87.21	Acute metabolic acidosis
E87.22	Chronic metabolic acidosis
E87.5	Hyperkalemia
I12.0	Hypertensive chronic kidney disease with stage 5 chronic kidney disease or end stage renal disease
I13.0	Hypertensive heart and chronic kidney disease with heart failure and stage 1 through stage 4 chronic kidney disease, or unspecified chronic kidney disease
I13.10	Hypertensive heart and chronic kidney disease without heart failure, with stage 1 through stage 4 chronic kidney disease, or unspecified chronic kidney disease
I13.11	Hypertensive heart and chronic kidney disease without heart failure, with stage 5 chronic kidney disease, or end stage renal disease
I13.2	Hypertensive heart and chronic kidney disease with heart failure and with stage 5 chronic kidney disease, or end stage renal disease
I16.0	Hypertensive urgency
I16.1	Hypertensive emergency
I82.3	Embolism and thrombosis of renal vein
M35.04	Sjögren syndrome with tubulo-interstitial nephropathy
M35.0A	Sjögren syndrome with glomerular disease
N00.0	Acute nephritic syndrome with minor glomerular abnormality
N00.1	Acute nephritic syndrome with focal and segmental glomerular lesions
N00.2	Acute nephritic syndrome with diffuse membranous glomerulonephritis
N00.3	Acute nephritic syndrome with diffuse mesangial proliferative glomerulonephritis
N00.4	Acute nephritic syndrome with diffuse endocapillary proliferative glomerulonephritis
N00.5	Acute nephritic syndrome with diffuse mesangiocapillary glomerulonephritis
N00.6	Acute nephritic syndrome with dense deposit disease
N00.7	Acute nephritic syndrome with diffuse crescentic glomerulonephritis
N00.A	Acute nephritic syndrome with C3 glomerulonephritis
N01.0	Rapidly progressive nephritic syndrome with minor glomerular abnormality
N01.1	Rapidly progressive nephritic syndrome with focal and segmental glomerular lesions
N01.2	Rapidly progressive nephritic syndrome with diffuse membranous glomerulonephritis
N01.3	Rapidly progressive nephritic syndrome with diffuse mesangial proliferative glomerulonephritis
N01.4	Rapidly progressive nephritic syndrome with diffuse endocapillary proliferative glomerulonephritis
N01.5	Rapidly progressive nephritic syndrome with diffuse mesangiocapillary glomerulonephritis
N01.6	Rapidly progressive nephritic syndrome with dense deposit disease
N01.7	Rapidly progressive nephritic syndrome with diffuse crescentic glomerulonephritis
N01.A	Rapidly progressive nephritic syndrome with C3 glomerulonephritis
N03.0	Chronic nephritic syndrome with minor glomerular abnormality
N03.1	Chronic nephritic syndrome with focal and segmental glomerular lesions
N03.2	Chronic nephritic syndrome with diffuse membranous glomerulonephritis
N03.3	Chronic nephritic syndrome with diffuse mesangial proliferative glomerulonephritis
N03.4	Chronic nephritic syndrome with diffuse endocapillary proliferative glomerulonephritis

N03.5	Chronic nephritic syndrome with diffuse mesangiocapillary glomerulonephritis
N03.6	Chronic nephritic syndrome with dense deposit disease
N03.7	Chronic nephritic syndrome with diffuse crescentic glomerulonephritis
N03.A	Chronic nephritic syndrome with C3 glomerulonephritis
N04.0	Nephrotic syndrome with minor glomerular abnormality
N04.1	Nephrotic syndrome with focal and segmental glomerular lesions
N04.21	Primary membranous nephropathy with nephrotic syndrome
N04.22	Secondary membranous nephropathy with nephrotic syndrome
N04.3	Nephrotic syndrome with diffuse mesangial proliferative glomerulonephritis
N04.4	Nephrotic syndrome with diffuse endocapillary proliferative glomerulonephritis
N04.5	Nephrotic syndrome with diffuse mesangiocapillary glomerulonephritis
N04.6	Nephrotic syndrome with dense deposit disease
N04.7	Nephrotic syndrome with diffuse crescentic glomerulonephritis
N04.A	Nephrotic syndrome with C3 glomerulonephritis
N10	Acute pyelonephritis
N11.0	Nonobstructive reflux-associated chronic pyelonephritis
N11.1	Chronic obstructive pyelonephritis
N17.0	Acute kidney failure with tubular necrosis
N17.1	Acute kidney failure with acute cortical necrosis
N17.2	Acute kidney failure with medullary necrosis
N18.31	Chronic kidney disease, stage 3a
N18.32	Chronic kidney disease, stage 3b
N18.4	Chronic kidney disease, stage 4 (severe)
N18.5	Chronic kidney disease, stage 5
N18.6	End stage renal disease
T80.211A	Bloodstream infection due to central venous catheter, initial encounter
T80.212A	Local infection due to central venous catheter, initial encounter
T82.318A	Breakdown (mechanical) of other vascular grafts, initial encounter
T82.41XA	Breakdown (mechanical) of vascular dialysis catheter, initial encounter
T82.42XA	Displacement of vascular dialysis catheter, initial encounter
T82.43XA	Leakage of vascular dialysis catheter, initial encounter
T82.510A	Breakdown (mechanical) of surgically created arteriovenous fistula, initial encounter
T82.514A	Breakdown (mechanical) of infusion catheter, initial encounter
T82.518A	Breakdown (mechanical) of other cardiac and vascular devices and implants, initial encounter
T82.520A	Displacement of surgically created arteriovenous fistula, initial encounter
T82.524A	Displacement of infusion catheter, initial encounter
T82.528A	Displacement of other cardiac and vascular devices and implants, initial encounter
T82.530A	Leakage of surgically created arteriovenous fistula, initial encounter
T82.534A	Leakage of infusion catheter, initial encounter
T82.538A	Leakage of other cardiac and vascular devices and implants, initial encounter
T82.7XXA	Infection and inflammatory reaction due to other cardiac and vascular devices, implants and grafts, initial encounter
T82.818A	Embolism due to vascular prosthetic devices, implants and grafts, initial encounter
T82.828A	Fibrosis due to vascular prosthetic devices, implants and grafts, initial encounter
T82.838A	Hemorrhage due to vascular prosthetic devices, implants and grafts, initial encounter
T82.848A	Pain due to vascular prosthetic devices, implants and grafts, initial encounter
T82.856A	Stenosis of peripheral vascular stent, initial encounter
T82.858A	Stenosis of other vascular prosthetic devices, implants and grafts, initial encounter
T82.868A	Thrombosis due to vascular prosthetic devices, implants and grafts, initial encounter

Relative Value Units/Medicare Edits

Non-Facility RVU	Work	PE	MP	Total
36835	7.51	5.06	1.84	14.41
Facility RVU	**Work**	**PE**	**MP**	**Total**
36835	7.51	5.06	1.84	14.41

	FUD	Status	MUE	Modifiers				IOM Reference
36835	90	A	1(3)	51	N/A	N/A	N/A	None

* with documentation

Terms To Know

artery. Vessel through which oxygenated blood passes away from the heart to any part of the body.

guidewire. Flexible metal instrument designed to lead another instrument in its proper course.

hemodialysis. Cleansing of wastes and contaminating elements from the blood by virtue of different diffusion rates through a semipermeable membrane, which separates blood from a filtration solution that diffuses other elements out of the blood.

vein. Vessel through which oxygen-depleted blood passes back to the heart.

36838

36838 Distal revascularization and interval ligation (DRIL), upper extremity hemodialysis access (steal syndrome)

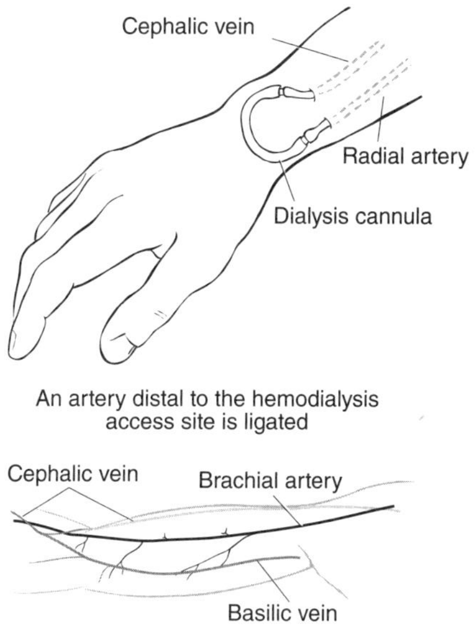

An artery distal to the hemodialysis access site is ligated

Explanation

A DRIL procedure, distal revascularization and interval ligation, is done to treat Steal syndrome occurring in patients with a permanent indwelling access site in the arm for hemodialysis. In Steal syndrome, the hand becomes cold and painful, due to ischemia because the hemodialysis access is taking the arm's blood supply. The DRIL procedure restores blood flow to the hand and preserves the access site. It is a two-step procedure. The surgeon first creates a bypass graft around the access site, using a harvested vein conduit, usually the greater saphenous. An incision is made in the upper arm for the proximal anastomosis, which is placed above the dialysis access site, nearer to the axilla. Soft tissue is dissected to expose the brachial artery. An incision is also made lower in the arm for the site of the distal anastomosis, which is placed below the dialysis access site, down in the forearm. A tunnel is created from one site to the other and the graft is completed using the harvested vein. This is the revascularization portion of the procedure and allows a good flow of blood around the access site. The second part of the procedure is the ligation. The brachial artery is tied off at a point between the dialysis access and the distal anastomosis site of the bypass graft. Now the arterial blood flow being pumped from the heart runs through the bypass, supplying the hand with oxygen before entering the access site. The incisions are closed and pulses are checked for good perfusion before applying dressings.

Coding Tips

Do not report 36838 with 35512, 35522, 35523, 36832, 37607, or 37618.

ICD-10-CM Diagnostic Codes

T80.211A Bloodstream infection due to central venous catheter, initial encounter
T80.212A Local infection due to central venous catheter, initial encounter
T82.318A Breakdown (mechanical) of other vascular grafts, initial encounter
T82.328A Displacement of other vascular grafts, initial encounter
T82.338A Leakage of other vascular grafts, initial encounter
T82.41XA Breakdown (mechanical) of vascular dialysis catheter, initial encounter
T82.42XA Displacement of vascular dialysis catheter, initial encounter
T82.43XA Leakage of vascular dialysis catheter, initial encounter
T82.510A Breakdown (mechanical) of surgically created arteriovenous fistula, initial encounter
T82.514A Breakdown (mechanical) of infusion catheter, initial encounter
T82.518A Breakdown (mechanical) of other cardiac and vascular devices and implants, initial encounter
T82.520A Displacement of surgically created arteriovenous fistula, initial encounter
T82.524A Displacement of infusion catheter, initial encounter
T82.528A Displacement of other cardiac and vascular devices and implants, initial encounter
T82.530A Leakage of surgically created arteriovenous fistula, initial encounter
T82.534A Leakage of infusion catheter, initial encounter
T82.538A Leakage of other cardiac and vascular devices and implants, initial encounter
T82.7XXA Infection and inflammatory reaction due to other cardiac and vascular devices, implants and grafts, initial encounter
T82.818A Embolism due to vascular prosthetic devices, implants and grafts, initial encounter
T82.828A Fibrosis due to vascular prosthetic devices, implants and grafts, initial encounter
T82.838A Hemorrhage due to vascular prosthetic devices, implants and grafts, initial encounter
T82.848A Pain due to vascular prosthetic devices, implants and grafts, initial encounter
T82.856A Stenosis of peripheral vascular stent, initial encounter
T82.858A Stenosis of other vascular prosthetic devices, implants and grafts, initial encounter
T82.868A Thrombosis due to vascular prosthetic devices, implants and grafts, initial encounter
Z45.89 Encounter for adjustment and management of other implanted devices

Relative Value Units/Medicare Edits

Non-Facility RVU	Work	PE	MP	Total
36838	21.69	6.31	5.4	33.4
Facility RVU	**Work**	**PE**	**MP**	**Total**
36838	21.69	6.31	5.4	33.4

	FUD	Status	MUE	Modifiers				IOM Reference
36838	90	A	1(3)	51	50	62*	80	None

* with documentation

36860-36861

36860 External cannula declotting (separate procedure); without balloon catheter

36861 with balloon catheter

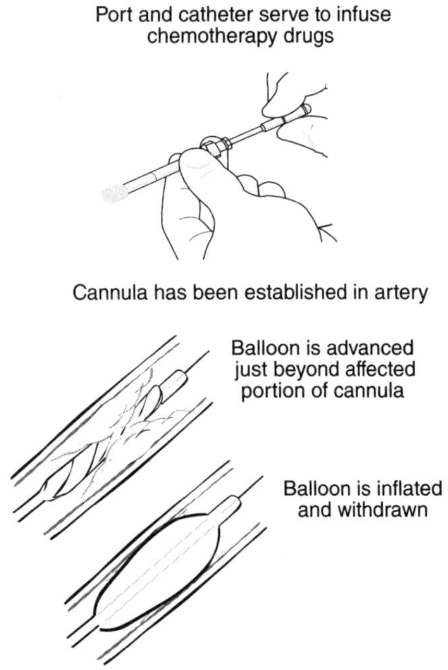

Explanation

To remove a blood clot lodged in a previously placed cannula, the physician may inject a solution containing enzymes into the cannula to dissolve the clot (in 36860) or the physician may, after injecting a solution containing enzymes, insert a balloon catheter (in 36861) into the cannula to retrieve a clot there. The balloon is inserted and inflated beyond the clot. The catheter is slowly pulled out, capturing and retrieving the clot. Once the clot is dissolved or retrieved, the catheter is removed and the cannula is left in place.

Coding Tips

These separate procedures by definition are usually a component of a more complex service and are not identified separately. When performed alone or with other unrelated procedures/services, they may be reported. If performed alone, list the code; if performed with other procedures/services, list the code and append modifier 59 or an X{EPSU} modifier. If imaging guidance is performed with 36861, see 76000.

ICD-10-CM Diagnostic Codes

T82.49XA	Other complication of vascular dialysis catheter, initial encounter
T82.594A	Other mechanical complication of infusion catheter, initial encounter
T82.818A	Embolism due to vascular prosthetic devices, implants and grafts, initial encounter
T82.828A	Fibrosis due to vascular prosthetic devices, implants and grafts, initial encounter
T82.848A	Pain due to vascular prosthetic devices, implants and grafts, initial encounter
T82.856A	Stenosis of peripheral vascular stent, initial encounter
T82.858A	Stenosis of other vascular prosthetic devices, implants and grafts, initial encounter
T82.868A	Thrombosis due to vascular prosthetic devices, implants and grafts, initial encounter
T82.898A	Other specified complication of vascular prosthetic devices, implants and grafts, initial encounter

Relative Value Units/Medicare Edits

Non-Facility RVU	Work	PE	MP	Total
36860	2.01	4.45	0.51	6.97
36861	2.52	0.93	0.64	4.09
Facility RVU	**Work**	**PE**	**MP**	**Total**
36860	2.01	0.74	0.51	3.26
36861	2.52	0.93	0.64	4.09

	FUD	Status	MUE	Modifiers				IOM Reference
36860	0	A	2(3)	51	N/A	N/A	N/A	None
36861	0	A	2(3)	51	N/A	N/A	N/A	

* with documentation

Terms To Know

cannula. Tube inserted into a blood vessel, duct, or body cavity to facilitate passage.

catheter. Flexible tube inserted into an area of the body for introducing or withdrawing fluid.

complication. Condition arising after the beginning of observation and treatment that modifies the course of the patient's illness or the medical care required, or an undesired result or misadventure in medical care.

embolism. Obstruction of a blood vessel resulting from a clot or foreign substance.

thrombosis. Condition arising from the presence or formation of blood clots within a blood vessel that may cause vascular obstruction and insufficient oxygenation.

36901-36903

36901 Introduction of needle(s) and/or catheter(s), dialysis circuit, with diagnostic angiography of the dialysis circuit, including all direct puncture(s) and catheter placement(s), injection(s) of contrast, all necessary imaging from the arterial anastomosis and adjacent artery through entire venous outflow including the inferior or superior vena cava, fluoroscopic guidance, radiological supervision and interpretation and image documentation and report;

36902 with transluminal balloon angioplasty, peripheral dialysis segment, including all imaging and radiological supervision and interpretation necessary to perform the angioplasty

36903 with transcatheter placement of intravascular stent(s), peripheral dialysis segment, including all imaging and radiological supervision and interpretation necessary to perform the stenting, and all angioplasty within the peripheral dialysis segment

Major arteries of the arm

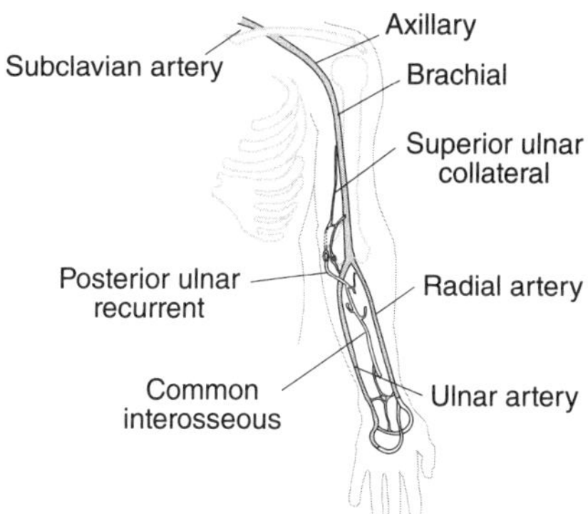

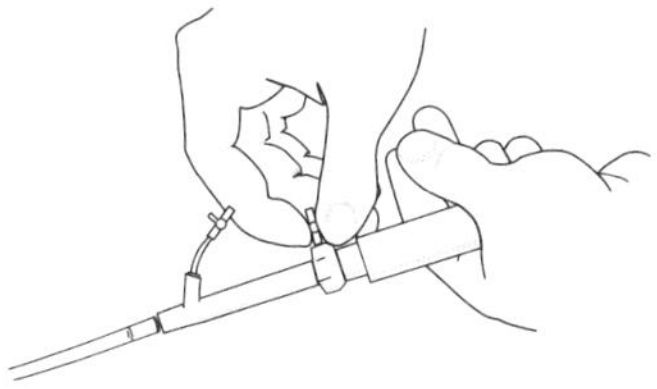

Needles or catheter are inserted into the dialysis circuit for diagnostic angiography

Explanation

The physician inserts a needle or catheter into a dialysis circuit via a puncture in the skin overlying the circuit of a dialysis patient. The catheter is guided into the circuit and vessel to an area upstream of the site under investigation, and contrast material is injected into it. Report 36901 for the initial access, including shunt access, contrast injections, and all fluoroscopic imaging deemed necessary from the arterial anastomosis and adjacent artery through the entire venous outflow (inferior and superior vena cava included). In 36902, a catheter with a balloon attached is inserted into the peripheral dialysis segment and fed into the narrowed portion where its balloon may be inflated several times in order to stretch the diameter, allowing a more normal flow of blood through the area. In 36903, a catheter with a stent-transporting tip is threaded over the guidewire into the peripheral dialysis segment and the wire is extracted. The catheter travels to the point where the vessel needs additional support. The compressed stent is passed from the catheter into the vessel, where it deploys, expanding to support the vessel walls. Once the procedure is complete, the catheter is removed and pressure is applied over the puncture site.

Coding Tips

Direct access, imaging of the dialysis circuit, catheter manipulation, catheter advancement to the vena cava for imaging, all dialysis circuit punctures, and venous side branches communicating with the dialysis circuit that require catheterization are included in 36901. If ultrasound guidance is required to safely puncture the dialysis circuit for evaluation, it may be reported separately, see 76937. Report 36902 once per encounter for all angioplasty services performed in the peripheral segment of the circuit. Report 36903 once per encounter regardless of the number of stents placed in the peripheral segment. Selective catheterization of the proximal artery is not inherent to the work of 36901-36903; code 36215 may be reported separately. Do not report 36215 for catheter tip placement near the arterial anastomosis of the AV access as it is inherent to the work of 36901-36903. Do not report 36901 with 36833, 36836, 36837, 36902–36906. Do not report 36902 with 36833, 36836, 36837, or 36903–36906. Do not report 36903 with 36833, 36836, 36837, or 36904–36906. Do not report 36901, 36902, or 36903 more than once per session.

ICD-10-CM Diagnostic Codes

T82.510A	Breakdown (mechanical) of surgically created arteriovenous fistula, initial encounter
T82.511A	Breakdown (mechanical) of surgically created arteriovenous shunt, initial encounter
T82.520A	Displacement of surgically created arteriovenous fistula, initial encounter
T82.521A	Displacement of surgically created arteriovenous shunt, initial encounter
T82.530A	Leakage of surgically created arteriovenous fistula, initial encounter
T82.531A	Leakage of surgically created arteriovenous shunt, initial encounter
T82.590A	Other mechanical complication of surgically created arteriovenous fistula, initial encounter
T82.591A	Other mechanical complication of surgically created arteriovenous shunt, initial encounter
T82.7XXA	Infection and inflammatory reaction due to other cardiac and vascular devices, implants and grafts, initial encounter
T82.818A	Embolism due to vascular prosthetic devices, implants and grafts, initial encounter
T82.828A	Fibrosis due to vascular prosthetic devices, implants and grafts, initial encounter
T82.838A	Hemorrhage due to vascular prosthetic devices, implants and grafts, initial encounter
T82.848A	Pain due to vascular prosthetic devices, implants and grafts, initial encounter
T82.856A	Stenosis of peripheral vascular stent, initial encounter
T82.858A	Stenosis of other vascular prosthetic devices, implants and grafts, initial encounter
T82.868A	Thrombosis due to vascular prosthetic devices, implants and grafts, initial encounter
T82.898A	Other specified complication of vascular prosthetic devices, implants and grafts, initial encounter

AMA: **36901** 2023,Mar; 2022,Oct; 2021,Jul **36902** 2023,Mar; 2022,Oct; 2021,Jul **36903** 2023,Mar; 2022,Oct; 2021,Jul

Relative Value Units/Medicare Edits

Non-Facility RVU	Work	PE	MP	Total
36901	3.36	16.92	0.51	20.79
36902	4.83	29.98	0.72	35.53
36903	6.39	117.09	1.03	124.51

Facility RVU	Work	PE	MP	Total
36901	3.36	1.03	0.51	4.9
36902	4.83	1.44	0.72	6.99
36903	6.39	1.77	1.03	9.19

	FUD	Status	MUE	Modifiers				IOM Reference
36901	0	A	1(3)	51	N/A	N/A	N/A	None
36902	0	A	1(3)	51	N/A	N/A	N/A	
36903	0	A	1(3)	51	N/A	N/A	N/A	

* with documentation

Terms To Know

anastomosis. Surgically created connection between ducts, blood vessels, or bowel segments to allow flow from one to the other.

angiography. Radiographic imaging of the arteries. Imaging may be performed to study the vasculature of any given organ, body system, or area of circulation such as the brain, heart, chest, kidneys, limbs, gastrointestinal tract, aorta, and pulmonary circulation to visualize the formation and the function of the blood vessels to detect problems such as a blockage or stricture. A catheter is inserted through an accessible blood vessel and the artery is injected with a radiopaque contrast material after which x-rays are taken.

stent. Tube to provide support in a body cavity or lumen.

transcatheter. Procedure or treatment performed via a catheter.

transluminal balloon angioplasty. Balloon-tipped catheter is placed within a narrowed artery or vein and the balloon is inflated to stretch the vessel to a larger diameter for increased blood flow.

36904-36906

36904 Percutaneous transluminal mechanical thrombectomy and/or infusion for thrombolysis, dialysis circuit, any method, including all imaging and radiological supervision and interpretation, diagnostic angiography, fluoroscopic guidance, catheter placement(s), and intraprocedural pharmacological thrombolytic injection(s);

36905 with transluminal balloon angioplasty, peripheral dialysis segment, including all imaging and radiological supervision and interpretation necessary to perform the angioplasty

36906 with transcatheter placement of intravascular stent(s), peripheral dialysis segment, including all imaging and radiological supervision and interpretation necessary to perform the stenting, and all angioplasty within the peripheral dialysis circuit

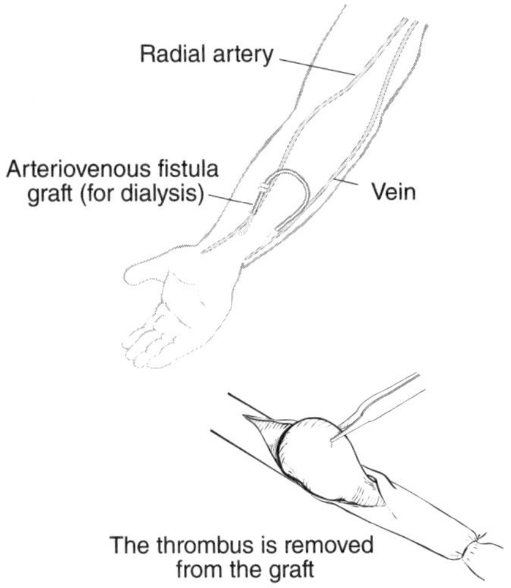

A thrombus (clot) is removed percutaneously from the dialysis circuit

Explanation

The physician treats the dialysis circuit occlusion with mechanical thrombectomy and/or thrombolysis infusion. The devices used for mechanical thrombectomy include those that fragment the thrombus with or without removal of the clot, as well as those that come into contact with the vessel wall. The dialysis circuit is cannulated to gain access and 5,000 units of heparin are administered. Angiography is performed to confirm the occluded segment. A hydrophilic wire is passed across the occlusion, followed by passing of the device over a stiff exchange length wire. The distal and proximal balloons are inflated in the segment on either side of a treatment zone containing infusion to isolate the treatment zone and to sustain the fluid concentration that is infused. One milligram of tissue plasminogen activator (TPA) is infused into the treatment zone. A thrombectomy device is run at 4,000 rpm for five minutes. After the proximal balloon is deflated, small clots are removed via the integral aspiration port to prevent embolization. Thrombolysis infusion may be performed with a catheter threaded over the wire for pharmaceutical administration directly within the thrombosis. When the procedure is complete, the instruments are removed, and pressure is applied over the puncture site to stop the bleeding. This procedure is reported with 36904 and includes imaging guidance, diagnostic angiography, catheter placement, and intraprocedural pharmacological thrombolytic injections. Report 36905 when the peripheral dialysis segment is treated with balloon angioplasty. A catheter with a balloon attached is inserted into the segment and fed into the narrowed portion, where its balloon may be inflated several times to stretch the diameter allowing a more normal flow of blood through the area. Report 36906 when the peripheral dialysis segment is treated with an intravascular stent. A catheter with a stent-transporting tip is threaded over the guidewire into the vessel and the wire is extracted. The catheter travels to the point where the vessel needs additional support. The compressed stent is passed from the catheter into the vessel, where it deploys, expanding to support the vessel walls. Once the procedure is complete, the catheter is removed, and pressure is applied over the puncture site.

Coding Tips

Diagnostic angiography, fluoroscopy, all manipulation required to remove a thrombus, and catheter placements are included in 36904. Report 36905 once per encounter for all angioplasty services performed in the peripheral segment of the circuit. Do not report 36904 with 36836 or 36837. Do not report 36905 with 36836, 36837, or 36904. Do not report 36906 with 36836, 36837, or 39601–36905. Report 36904, 36905, and 36906 only once per operative session. For transluminal balloon angioplasty, see 36907. For transcatheter placement of intravascular stents within the central vein of the dialysis circuit, see 36908. Selective catheterization of the proximal artery is not inherent to the work of 36904-36906; code 36215 may be reported separately. Do not report 36215 for catheter tip placement near the arterial anastomosis of the AV access as it is inherent to the work of 36904-36906.

ICD-10-CM Diagnostic Codes

T82.328A	Displacement of other vascular grafts, initial encounter
T82.338A	Leakage of other vascular grafts, initial encounter
T82.398A	Other mechanical complication of other vascular grafts, initial encounter
T82.41XA	Breakdown (mechanical) of vascular dialysis catheter, initial encounter
T82.42XA	Displacement of vascular dialysis catheter, initial encounter
T82.43XA	Leakage of vascular dialysis catheter, initial encounter
T82.49XA	Other complication of vascular dialysis catheter, initial encounter
T82.510A	Breakdown (mechanical) of surgically created arteriovenous fistula, initial encounter
T82.511A	Breakdown (mechanical) of surgically created arteriovenous shunt, initial encounter
T82.520A	Displacement of surgically created arteriovenous fistula, initial encounter
T82.521A	Displacement of surgically created arteriovenous shunt, initial encounter
T82.530A	Leakage of surgically created arteriovenous fistula, initial encounter
T82.531A	Leakage of surgically created arteriovenous shunt, initial encounter
T82.590A	Other mechanical complication of surgically created arteriovenous fistula, initial encounter
T82.591A	Other mechanical complication of surgically created arteriovenous shunt, initial encounter
T82.818A	Embolism due to vascular prosthetic devices, implants and grafts, initial encounter
T82.828A	Fibrosis due to vascular prosthetic devices, implants and grafts, initial encounter
T82.838A	Hemorrhage due to vascular prosthetic devices, implants and grafts, initial encounter
T82.848A	Pain due to vascular prosthetic devices, implants and grafts, initial encounter
T82.856A	Stenosis of peripheral vascular stent, initial encounter
T82.858A	Stenosis of other vascular prosthetic devices, implants and grafts, initial encounter
T82.868A	Thrombosis due to vascular prosthetic devices, implants and grafts, initial encounter
T82.898A	Other specified complication of vascular prosthetic devices, implants and grafts, initial encounter

AMA: **36904** 2023,Mar; 2022,Oct; 2022,Jun; 2021,Jul **36905** 2023,Mar; 2022,Oct; 2022,Jun; 2021,Jul **36906** 2023,Mar; 2022,Oct; 2022,Jun; 2021,Jul

Relative Value Units/Medicare Edits

Non-Facility RVU	Work	PE	MP	Total
36904	7.5	44.54	1.12	53.16
36905	9.0	56.61	1.24	66.85
36906	10.42	146.54	1.51	158.47
Facility RVU	**Work**	**PE**	**MP**	**Total**
36904	7.5	2.1	1.12	10.72
36905	9.0	2.63	1.24	12.87
36906	10.42	2.93	1.51	14.86

	FUD	Status	MUE	Modifiers				IOM Reference
36904	0	A	1(3)	51	N/A	62*	N/A	None
36905	0	A	1(3)	51	N/A	62*	N/A	
36906	0	A	1(3)	51	N/A	62*	N/A	

* with documentation

Terms To Know

cannulation. Insertion of a flexible length of hollow tubing into a blood vessel, duct, or body cavity, usually for extracorporeal circulation or chemotherapy infusion to a particular region of the body.

thrombectomy. Removal of a clot (thrombus) from a blood vessel utilizing various methods.

thrombolysis. Chemical process of dissolving or breaking down a blood clot by inducing a complex chain of events involving the action of plasminogen to solubilize fibrin clots and degrade fibrinogen.

transluminal balloon angioplasty. Balloon-tipped catheter is placed within a narrowed artery or vein and the balloon is inflated to stretch the vessel to a larger diameter for increased blood flow.

36907-36908

+ **36907** Transluminal balloon angioplasty, central dialysis segment, performed through dialysis circuit, including all imaging and radiological supervision and interpretation required to perform the angioplasty (List separately in addition to code for primary procedure)
+ **36908** Transcatheter placement of intravascular stent(s), central dialysis segment, performed through dialysis circuit, including all imaging and radiological supervision and interpretation required to perform the stenting, and all angioplasty in the central dialysis segment (List separately in addition to code for primary procedure)

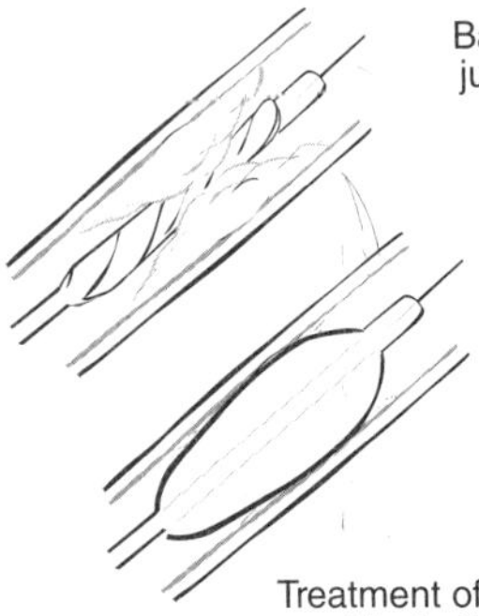

Treatment of the central dialysis segment by balloon angioplasty or stent

Explanation

The physician inserts a needle or catheter into a dialysis circuit via a puncture in the skin. The catheter is guided into the circuit to an area upstream of the investigation site and contrast material is injected. In 36907, a catheter with a balloon attached is inserted into the central dialysis segment and fed into the narrowed portion, where its balloon may be inflated several times in order to stretch the diameter, allowing a more normal blood flow through the area. In 36908, a catheter with a stent-transporting tip is threaded over the guidewire into the central dialysis segment and the wire is extracted. The catheter travels to the point where the vessel needs additional support. The compressed stent is passed from the catheter out into the vessel, where it deploys, expanding to support the vessel walls. Once the procedure is complete, the catheter is removed and pressure is applied over the puncture site. All imaging and radiological supervision and interpretation is included.

Coding Tips

Report 36907 and 36908 in addition to 36818-36833 or 36901-36906. Report 36907 once for all angioplasty performed within the central dialysis segment. Report 36908 once per encounter for all stenting performed within the central dialysis segment. Report 36908 once per encounter regardless of the number of stents placed or lesions treated. Do not report 36907 with 36836, 36837, or 36908. Do not report 36908 with 36836, 36837, or 36907.

ICD-10-CM Diagnostic Codes

This/these CPT code(s) are add-on code(s). See the primary procedure code that this code is performed with for your ICD-10-CM code selections. Diagnostic code(s) would be the same as the actual procedure performed.

AMA: 36907 2023,Mar; 2022,Oct; 2021,Jul **36908** 2023,Mar; 2022,Oct; 2021,Jul

Relative Value Units/Medicare Edits

Non-Facility RVU	Work	PE	MP	Total
36907	3.0	13.88	0.45	17.33
36908	4.25	36.57	0.71	41.53
Facility RVU	**Work**	**PE**	**MP**	**Total**
36907	3.0	0.8	0.45	4.25
36908	4.25	1.07	0.71	6.03

	FUD	Status	MUE	Modifiers				IOM Reference
36907	N/A	A	1(3)	N/A	N/A	N/A	N/A	None
36908	N/A	A	1(3)	N/A	N/A	N/A	N/A	

* with documentation

Terms To Know

angioplasty. Reconstruction or repair of a diseased or damaged blood vessel.

dialysis. Artificial filtering of the blood to remove contaminating waste elements and restore normal balance.

guidewire. Flexible metal instrument designed to lead another instrument in its proper course.

stent. Tube to provide support in a body cavity or lumen.

supervision and interpretation. Radiology services that usually contain an invasive component and are reported by the radiologist for supervision of the procedure and the personnel involved with performing the examination, reading the film, and preparing the written report.

36909

\+ **36909** Dialysis circuit permanent vascular embolization or occlusion (including main circuit or any accessory veins), endovascular, including all imaging and radiological supervision and interpretation necessary to complete the intervention (List separately in addition to code for primary procedure)

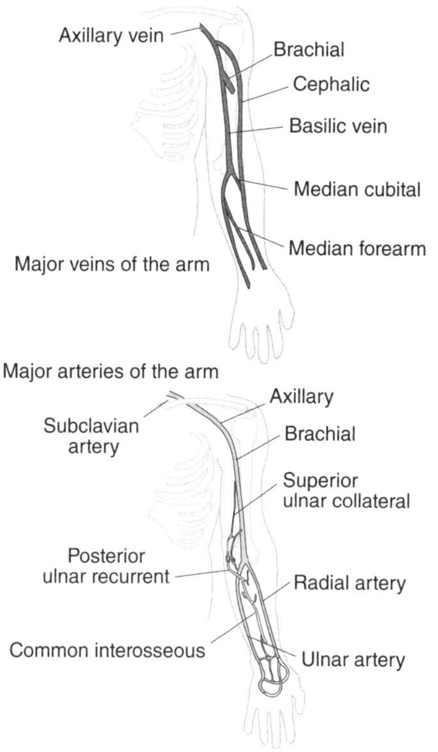

Endovascular embolization or occlusion of dialysis circuit

Explanation

The physician performs embolization or occlusion of a dialysis circuit (main circuit or any accessory vein) due to complications or to assist in circuit maturity and/or patency. A needle is inserted through the skin and into a blood vessel. A guidewire is threaded through the needle into the vessel. The needle is removed. A catheter is threaded into the vessel and the wire is extracted. The catheter travels to the appropriate blood vessel and beads, coils, or another vessel-blocking device are released. The beads or other device block the vessel. The catheter is removed and pressure is applied over the puncture site to stop bleeding.

Coding Tips

Report 36909 in addition to 36901-36906. Report 36909 once per encounter/day for all permanent vascular occlusions within the circuit. For open ligation/occlusion of dialysis access, see 37607. Do not report 36909 with 36836 or 36837.

ICD-10-CM Diagnostic Codes

This/these CPT code(s) are add-on code(s). See the primary procedure code that this code is performed with for your ICD-10-CM code selections. Diagnostic code(s) would be the same as the actual procedure performed.

AMA: 36909 2023,Mar; 2022,Oct; 2022,Jun; 2021,Jul

Relative Value Units/Medicare Edits

Non-Facility RVU	Work	PE	MP	Total
36909	4.12	50.75	0.67	55.54
Facility RVU	**Work**	**PE**	**MP**	**Total**
36909	4.12	1.06	0.67	5.85

	FUD	Status	MUE	Modifiers				IOM Reference
36909	N/A	A	1(3)	N/A	N/A	N/A	N/A	None

* with documentation

Terms To Know

catheter. Flexible tube inserted into an area of the body for introducing or withdrawing fluid.

embolization. Placement of a clotting agent, such as a coil, plastic particles, gel, foam, etc., into an area of hemorrhage to stop the bleeding or to block blood flow to a problem area, such as an aneurysm or a tumor.

hemodialysis. Cleansing of wastes and contaminating elements from the blood by virtue of different diffusion rates through a semipermeable membrane, which separates blood from a filtration solution that diffuses other elements out of the blood.

occlusion. Constriction, closure, or blockage of a passage.

patency. State of a tube-like structure or conduit being open and unobstructed.

37140

37140 Venous anastomosis, open; portocaval

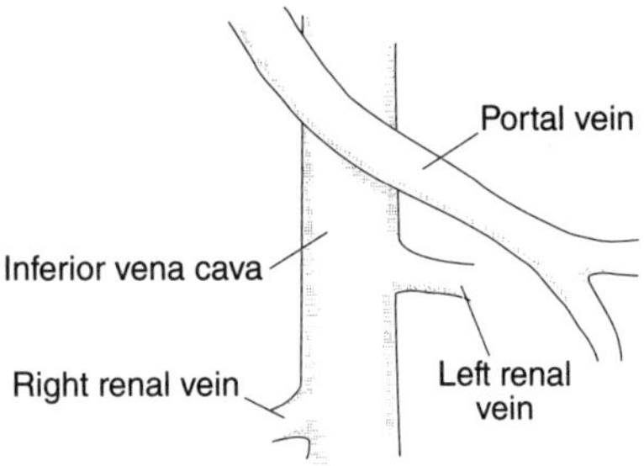

Schematic of portocaval anatomy

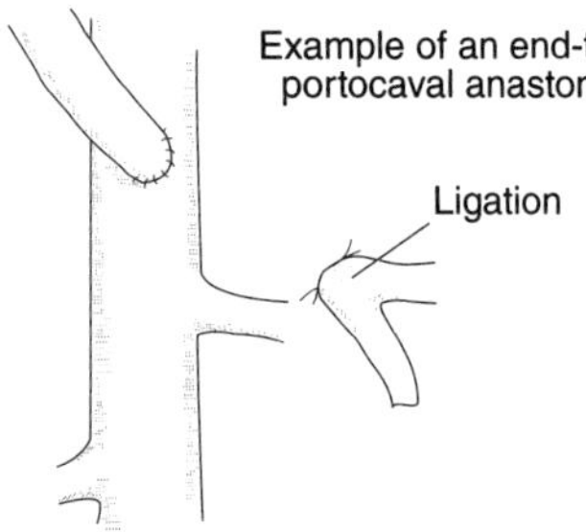

Explanation

The physician performs portocaval venous anastomosis. The physician places a long right thoracoabdominal incision and exposes the liver. The physician exposes the inferior vena cava and portal vein through careful dissection. The physician places a plastic sling around the portal vein and ties it closed, just proximal to its bifurcation. The physician clamps and divides the portal vein. The physician applies a partial exclusion vascular clamp to the front of the vena cava and removes a small oval of tissue from the vena cava to allow end-to-side anastomosis of portal vein to the inferior vena cava. The physician removes the clamps and checks for appropriate flow without anastomotic leakage. The physician closes the incision, leaving a chest tube in place (but no abdominal drains, as this may lead to protein loss from postoperative drainage of ascites).

Coding Tips

When 37140 is performed with another separately identifiable procedure, the highest dollar value code is listed as the primary procedure and subsequent procedures are appended with modifier 51. For a percutaneous procedure, see 37182. For a peritoneal-venous shunt, see 49425. For venous anastomosis, renoportal, see 37145.

ICD-10-CM Diagnostic Codes

I81	Portal vein thrombosis
I82.0	Budd-Chiari syndrome
I85.11	Secondary esophageal varices with bleeding
I87.1	Compression of vein
K70.0	Alcoholic fatty liver A
K70.30	Alcoholic cirrhosis of liver without ascites A
K70.31	Alcoholic cirrhosis of liver with ascites A
K74.69	Other cirrhosis of liver
K75.1	Phlebitis of portal vein
K76.0	Fatty (change of) liver, not elsewhere classified
K76.1	Chronic passive congestion of liver
K76.3	Infarction of liver
K76.5	Hepatic veno-occlusive disease
K76.6	Portal hypertension
K76.89	Other specified diseases of liver

Relative Value Units/Medicare Edits

Non-Facility RVU	Work	PE	MP	Total
37140	40.0	18.97	10.33	69.3
Facility RVU	**Work**	**PE**	**MP**	**Total**
37140	40.0	18.97	10.33	69.3

	FUD	Status	MUE	Modifiers				IOM Reference
37140	90	A	1(2)	51	N/A	62*	N/A	None

* with documentation

Terms To Know

anastomosis. Surgically created connection between ducts, blood vessels, or bowel segments to allow flow from one to the other.

bifurcated. Having two branches or divisions, such as the left pulmonary veins that split off from the left atrium to carry oxygenated blood away from the heart.

Budd-Chiari syndrome. Thrombus or other obstruction of the hepatic vein, with an enlarged liver, intractable ascites, portal hypertension, and the growth of extensive collateral vessels.

dissection. Separating by cutting tissue or body structures apart.

hypertension. Abnormally increased pressure, usually referring to arterial pressure, exceeding an acceptable range.

incision. Act of cutting into tissue or an organ.

portal hypertension. Abnormally high blood pressure in the portal vein.

shunt. Surgically created passage between blood vessels or other natural passages, such as an arteriovenous anastomosis, to divert or bypass blood flow from the normal channel.

thrombosis. Condition arising from the presence or formation of blood clots within a blood vessel that may cause vascular obstruction and insufficient oxygenation.

thrombus. Stationary blood clot inside a blood vessel.

varices. Enlarged, dilated, or twisted turning veins.

 N Newborn: 0 P Pediatric: 0-17 M Maternity: 9-64 A Adult: 15-124 AMA: CPT Assist

37145

37145 Venous anastomosis, open; renoportal

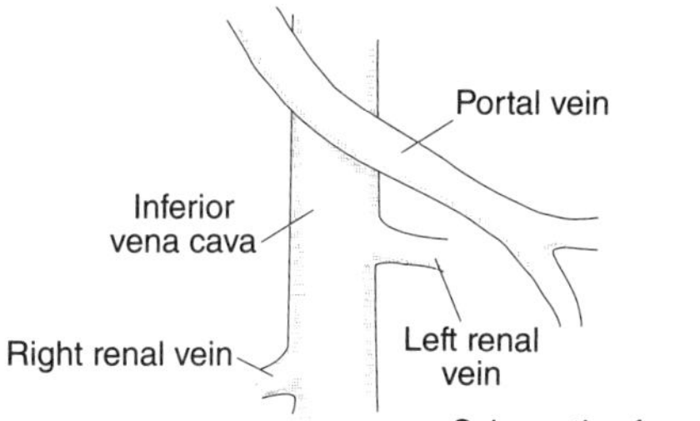

Schematic of portocaval anatomy

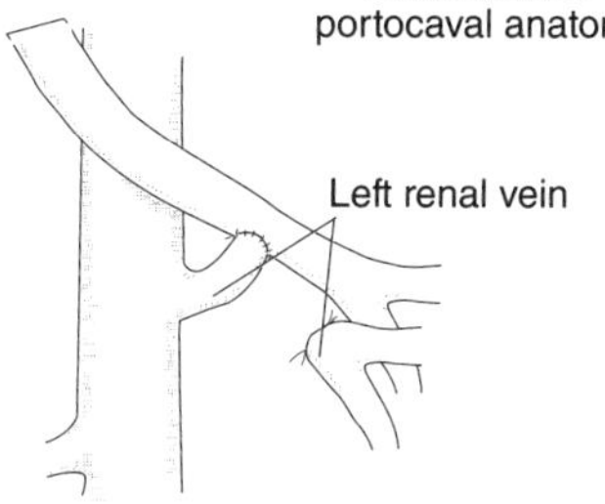

Example of a renoportal anastomosis

Explanation

The physician performs an abdominal incision and exposes the left renal vein and inferior vena cava. The physician transects the left renal vein and attaches it to the portal circulation by sewing the vena caval end to the portal vein, the superior mesenteric vein, or the splenic vein. Alternatively, the physician may divide the portal vein and attach its splanchnic end to the end of the transected renal vein. The physician assesses patency of the anastomosis and may measure venous pressures before closing the abdomen.

Coding Tips

When 37145 is performed with another separately identifiable procedure, the highest dollar value code is listed as the primary procedure, and subsequent procedures are appended with modifier 51. For venous anastomosis, portocaval, see 37140.

ICD-10-CM Diagnostic Codes

I81	Portal vein thrombosis
I82.0	Budd-Chiari syndrome
I82.3	Embolism and thrombosis of renal vein
I85.11	Secondary esophageal varices with bleeding
N28.0	Ischemia and infarction of kidney
Q27.34	Arteriovenous malformation of renal vessel
S35.414A	Laceration of right renal vein, initial encounter ☑
S35.494A	Other specified injury of right renal vein, initial encounter ☑

Relative Value Units/Medicare Edits

Non-Facility RVU	Work	PE	MP	Total
37145	37.0	17.75	9.56	64.31
Facility RVU	**Work**	**PE**	**MP**	**Total**
37145	37.0	17.75	9.56	64.31

	FUD	Status	MUE	Modifiers				IOM Reference
37145	90	A	1(3)	51	N/A	N/A	80	None

* with documentation

37160

37160 Venous anastomosis, open; caval-mesenteric

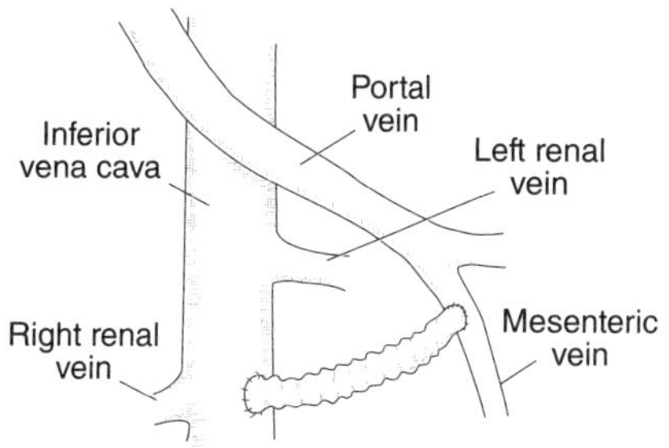

Example of a synthetic side-to-side caval-mesenteric anastomosis

This shunting procedure is designed to reduce pressure in the portal system and as therapy for esophagogastric varices

Explanation

The physician performs an upper midline vertical abdominal incision and retracts the transverse colon in a cephalad direction. The physician exposes the anterior surface of the inferior vena cava and frees the posterior surface of the superior mesenteric vein after careful dissection through the root of the transverse mesocolon. The physician isolates a long segment of the superior mesenteric vein with ties and partially occludes the inferior vena cava. The physician removes an ellipse of tissue from the inferior vena cava and performs and end-to-side anastomosis of Dacron graft to the inferior vena cava. The physician occludes the superior mesenteric vein, cuts an ellipse from its anterior surface, and sews the end of the Dacron graft to the side of the superior mesenteric vein. The physician assesses patency of the anastomosis and may measure venous pressures before closing the abdomen.

Coding Tips

When 37160 is performed with another separately identifiable procedure, the highest dollar value code is listed as the primary procedure, and subsequent procedures are appended with modifier 51. For venous anastomosis, portocaval, see 37140. For venous anastomosis, renoportal, see 37145.

ICD-10-CM Diagnostic Codes

I81	Portal vein thrombosis
I82.890	Acute embolism and thrombosis of other specified veins
I82.891	Chronic embolism and thrombosis of other specified veins
I85.11	Secondary esophageal varices with bleeding
I87.1	Compression of vein
K70.0	Alcoholic fatty liver 🅰
K70.30	Alcoholic cirrhosis of liver without ascites 🅰
K70.31	Alcoholic cirrhosis of liver with ascites 🅰
K74.60	Unspecified cirrhosis of liver
K74.69	Other cirrhosis of liver
K76.0	Fatty (change of) liver, not elsewhere classified
K76.1	Chronic passive congestion of liver
K76.3	Infarction of liver
K76.5	Hepatic veno-occlusive disease
K76.6	Portal hypertension
K76.89	Other specified diseases of liver
K76.9	Liver disease, unspecified
R16.0	Hepatomegaly, not elsewhere classified

R16.2 Hepatomegaly with splenomegaly, not elsewhere classified

Relative Value Units/Medicare Edits

Non-Facility RVU	Work	PE	MP	Total
37160	38.0	18.24	9.81	66.05
Facility RVU	**Work**	**PE**	**MP**	**Total**
37160	38.0	18.24	9.81	66.05

	FUD	Status	MUE	Modifiers				IOM Reference
37160	90	A	1(3)	51	N/A	62*	80	None

* with documentation

Terms To Know

acute. Sudden, severe. Documentation and reporting of an acute condition is important to establishing medical necessity.

anastomosis. Surgically created connection between ducts, blood vessels, or bowel segments to allow flow from one to the other.

cephalad. Toward the head.

chronic. Persistent, continuing, or recurring.

dissection. Separating by cutting tissue or body structures apart.

embolism. Obstruction of a blood vessel resulting from a clot or foreign substance.

graft. Tissue implant from another part of the body or another person.

incision. Act of cutting into tissue or an organ.

patency. State of a tube-like structure or conduit being open and unobstructed.

shunt. Surgically created passage between blood vessels or other natural passages, such as an arteriovenous anastomosis, to divert or bypass blood flow from the normal channel.

vascular insufficiency. Inadequate blood flow and oxygenation.

37184-37185

37184 Primary percutaneous transluminal mechanical thrombectomy, noncoronary, non-intracranial, arterial or arterial bypass graft, including fluoroscopic guidance and intraprocedural pharmacological thrombolytic injection(s); initial vessel

\+ **37185** second and all subsequent vessel(s) within the same vascular family (List separately in addition to code for primary mechanical thrombectomy procedure)

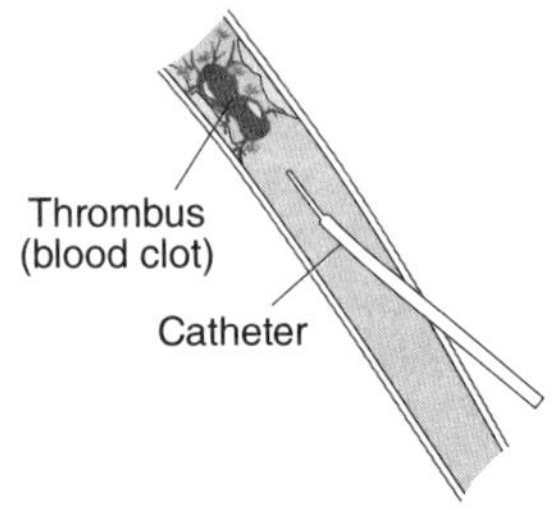

A transluminal device removes a blood clot from an artery or artery graft other than from the heart

Explanation

The physician treats an acute noncoronary, nonintracranial arterial occlusion with a combination of thrombolytic drugs and percutaneous mechanical thrombectomy. The devices used for mechanical thrombectomy include those that fragment the thrombus with or without removal of the clot, as well as those that come into contact with the wall of the vessel. For the procedure using the Trellis device, the artery is cannulated to gain access and 5,000 units of heparin are administered. Angiography is performed to confirm the occluded arteries. A hydrophilic wire is passed across the occlusion, followed by passing of the Trellis device over a stiff exchange length wire. The distal and proximal balloons are inflated in the artery on either side of a treatment zone containing infusion to isolate the treatment zone and to sustain the fluid concentration that is infused. One milligram of tissue plasminogen activator (TPA) is infused into the treatment zone. The Turbo Trellis is run at 4,000 rpm for five minutes. After the proximal balloon is deflated, small clots are removed via the integral aspiration port to prevent embolization. Fluoroscopic guidance services and injections administered during the course of the procedure are included in the service. Separately reportable procedures include other percutaneous interventions such as stent placement and diagnostic studies. Report 37184 for the first vessel and 37185 for the second and subsequent vessels in the same vascular family.

Coding Tips

Do not report 37184 with 61645, 76000 or 96374. Do not report 37185 with 76000 or 96375. Do not report 37185 with 61645 when treating the same vascular territory. Codes 37184 and 37185 should not be used to report mechanical thrombectomy performed to remove short segments of thrombus or embolus discovered during other percutaneous interventional procedures, see 37186.

ICD-10-CM Diagnostic Codes

I26.01 Septic pulmonary embolism with acute cor pulmonale
I26.02 Saddle embolus of pulmonary artery with acute cor pulmonale
I26.90 Septic pulmonary embolism without acute cor pulmonale
I26.92 Saddle embolus of pulmonary artery without acute cor pulmonale
I26.93 Single subsegmental thrombotic pulmonary embolism without acute cor pulmonale

 N Newborn: 0 P Pediatric: 0-17 M Maternity: 9-64 A Adult: 15-124 AMA: CPT Assist

I26.94	Multiple subsegmental thrombotic pulmonary emboli without acute cor pulmonale
I72.8	Aneurysm of other specified arteries
I73.89	Other specified peripheral vascular diseases
I74.01	Saddle embolus of abdominal aorta
I74.09	Other arterial embolism and thrombosis of abdominal aorta
I74.11	Embolism and thrombosis of thoracic aorta
I74.19	Embolism and thrombosis of other parts of aorta
I74.2	Embolism and thrombosis of arteries of the upper extremities
I74.3	Embolism and thrombosis of arteries of the lower extremities
I74.5	Embolism and thrombosis of iliac artery
I74.8	Embolism and thrombosis of other arteries
I75.011	Atheroembolism of right upper extremity ☑
I75.012	Atheroembolism of left upper extremity ☑
I75.013	Atheroembolism of bilateral upper extremities ☑
I75.021	Atheroembolism of right lower extremity ☑
I75.022	Atheroembolism of left lower extremity ☑
I75.023	Atheroembolism of bilateral lower extremities ☑
I75.81	Atheroembolism of kidney
I75.89	Atheroembolism of other site
I76	Septic arterial embolism
K55.011	Focal (segmental) acute (reversible) ischemia of small intestine
K55.012	Diffuse acute (reversible) ischemia of small intestine
K55.021	Focal (segmental) acute infarction of small intestine
K55.022	Diffuse acute infarction of small intestine
K55.031	Focal (segmental) acute (reversible) ischemia of large intestine
K55.032	Diffuse acute (reversible) ischemia of large intestine
K55.041	Focal (segmental) acute infarction of large intestine
K55.042	Diffuse acute infarction of large intestine
K55.1	Chronic vascular disorders of intestine
K55.8	Other vascular disorders of intestine
N28.0	Ischemia and infarction of kidney
T82.818A	Embolism due to vascular prosthetic devices, implants and grafts, initial encounter
T82.868A	Thrombosis due to vascular prosthetic devices, implants and grafts, initial encounter

AMA: 37184 2023,Jan; 2022,Jun; 2019,Sep **37185** 2023,Jan; 2022,Jun; 2019,Sep

Relative Value Units/Medicare Edits

Non-Facility RVU	Work	PE	MP	Total
37184	8.41	40.27	1.57	50.25
37185	3.28	10.04	0.63	13.95
Facility RVU	**Work**	**PE**	**MP**	**Total**
37184	8.41	2.57	1.57	12.55
37185	3.28	0.83	0.63	4.74

	FUD	Status	MUE	Modifiers				IOM Reference
37184	0	A	1(2)	51	50	62	N/A	None
37185	N/A	A	2(3)	N/A	N/A	62	N/A	

* with documentation

37186

\+ **37186** Secondary percutaneous transluminal thrombectomy (eg, nonprimary mechanical, snare basket, suction technique), noncoronary, non-intracranial, arterial or arterial bypass graft, including fluoroscopic guidance and intraprocedural pharmacological thrombolytic injections, provided in conjunction with another percutaneous intervention other than primary mechanical thrombectomy (List separately in addition to code for primary procedure)

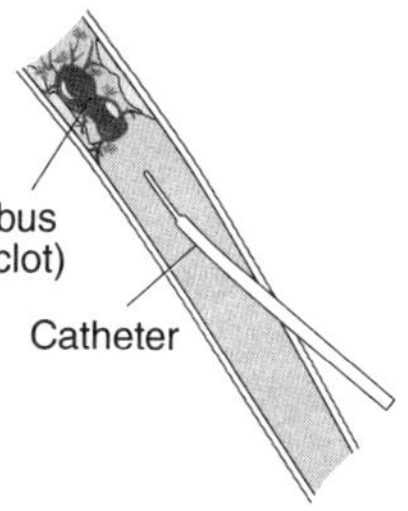

Secondary percutaneous transluminal thrombectomy occurs prior to, or after, the primary procedure

Explanation

The physician performs a secondary thrombectomy of a noncoronary, non-intracranial arterial occlusion. Prior to or after a percutaneous intervention is performed, such as balloon angioplasty or placement of a stent, the transcatheter removal of small sections of the thrombus or embolism is performed using suction, a snare basket, or a mechanical thrombectomy device under fluoroscopic guidance. Thrombolytic injections may also be used during the procedure.

Coding Tips

When medically necessary, report moderate (conscious) sedation provided by the performing physician with 99151-99153. When provided by another physician, report 99155-99157. Do not report 37186 with 76000 or 96375. Do not report 37186 with 61645 when treating the same vascular territory.

ICD-10-CM Diagnostic Codes

This/these CPT code(s) are add-on code(s). See the primary procedure code that this code is performed with for your ICD-10-CM code selections.

AMA: 37186 2022,Jun; 2019,Sep

Relative Value Units/Medicare Edits

Non-Facility RVU	Work	PE	MP	Total
37186	4.92	28.9	1.01	34.83
Facility RVU	**Work**	**PE**	**MP**	**Total**
37186	4.92	1.17	1.01	7.1

	FUD	Status	MUE	Modifiers				IOM Reference
37186	N/A	A	2(3)	N/A	N/A	62	N/A	None

* with documentation

37187-37188

37187 Percutaneous transluminal mechanical thrombectomy, vein(s), including intraprocedural pharmacological thrombolytic injections and fluoroscopic guidance

37188 Percutaneous transluminal mechanical thrombectomy, vein(s), including intraprocedural pharmacological thrombolytic injections and fluoroscopic guidance, repeat treatment on subsequent day during course of thrombolytic therapy

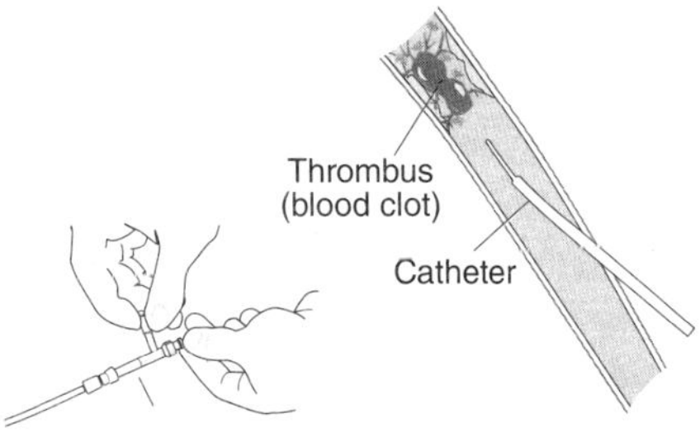

Explanation

The physician performs a percutaneous transluminal mechanical venous thrombectomy. A catheter sheath is inserted through a small incision in the vein, most commonly a groin incision in the femoral vein or an incision below the knee in the popliteal vein. Contrast is injected through the sheath and a separately reportable venography is performed to visualize the area of the vein being treated. Fluoroscopic guidance may be used. A guidewire is inserted through the sheath and advanced past the clot. A catheter is passed over the wire to the blocked area. A device at the tip of the catheter, a mechanical tool or a high-velocity liquid jet, is used to break the clot. A thrombolytic agent may be injected. When the procedure is completed, all instruments are removed and a compression bandage is applied. Report 37187 for the initial treatment. Report 37188 for repeat treatment on a subsequent day during the course of thrombolytic therapy.

Coding Tips

When medically necessary, report moderate (conscious) sedation provided by the performing physician with 99151-99153. When provided by another physician, report 99155-99157. Do not report 37187 or 37188 with 76000 or 96375. Supplies used when providing this procedure may be reported with A4300. Check with the specific payer to determine coverage.

ICD-10-CM Diagnostic Codes

I80.01 Phlebitis and thrombophlebitis of superficial vessels of right lower extremity ☑
I80.11 Phlebitis and thrombophlebitis of right femoral vein ☑
I80.211 Phlebitis and thrombophlebitis of right iliac vein ☑
I80.221 Phlebitis and thrombophlebitis of right popliteal vein ☑
I80.231 Phlebitis and thrombophlebitis of right tibial vein ☑
I80.291 Phlebitis and thrombophlebitis of other deep vessels of right lower extremity ☑
I82.0 Budd-Chiari syndrome
I82.1 Thrombophlebitis migrans
I82.210 Acute embolism and thrombosis of superior vena cava
I82.211 Chronic embolism and thrombosis of superior vena cava
I82.220 Acute embolism and thrombosis of inferior vena cava
I82.221 Chronic embolism and thrombosis of inferior vena cava
I82.290 Acute embolism and thrombosis of other thoracic veins
I82.291 Chronic embolism and thrombosis of other thoracic veins
I82.3 Embolism and thrombosis of renal vein
I82.411 Acute embolism and thrombosis of right femoral vein ☑
I82.421 Acute embolism and thrombosis of right iliac vein ☑
I82.431 Acute embolism and thrombosis of right popliteal vein ☑
I82.441 Acute embolism and thrombosis of right tibial vein ☑
I82.491 Acute embolism and thrombosis of other specified deep vein of right lower extremity ☑
I82.511 Chronic embolism and thrombosis of right femoral vein ☑
I82.521 Chronic embolism and thrombosis of right iliac vein ☑
I82.531 Chronic embolism and thrombosis of right popliteal vein ☑
I82.541 Chronic embolism and thrombosis of right tibial vein ☑
I82.591 Chronic embolism and thrombosis of other specified deep vein of right lower extremity ☑
I82.611 Acute embolism and thrombosis of superficial veins of right upper extremity ☑
I82.621 Acute embolism and thrombosis of deep veins of right upper extremity ☑
I82.711 Chronic embolism and thrombosis of superficial veins of right upper extremity ☑
I82.721 Chronic embolism and thrombosis of deep veins of right upper extremity ☑
I82.811 Embolism and thrombosis of superficial veins of right lower extremity ☑
I82.A11 Acute embolism and thrombosis of right axillary vein ☑
I82.A21 Chronic embolism and thrombosis of right axillary vein ☑
I82.B11 Acute embolism and thrombosis of right subclavian vein ☑
I82.B21 Chronic embolism and thrombosis of right subclavian vein ☑
I82.C11 Acute embolism and thrombosis of right internal jugular vein ☑
I82.C21 Chronic embolism and thrombosis of right internal jugular vein ☑

AMA: **37187** 2023,May; 2022,Jun **37188** 2023,May; 2022,Jun

Relative Value Units/Medicare Edits

Non-Facility RVU	Work	PE	MP	Total
37187	7.78	40.62	1.27	49.67
37188	5.46	36.12	0.97	42.55
Facility RVU	**Work**	**PE**	**MP**	**Total**
37187	7.78	2.4	1.27	11.45
37188	5.46	1.76	0.97	8.19

	FUD	Status	MUE	Modifiers				IOM Reference
37187	0	A	1(3)	51	50	62	N/A	None
37188	0	A	1(3)	N/A	50	62	N/A	

* with documentation

Terms To Know

Budd-Chiari syndrome. Thrombus or other obstruction of the hepatic vein, with an enlarged liver, intractable ascites, portal hypertension, and the growth of extensive collateral vessels.

embolism. Obstruction of a blood vessel resulting from a clot or foreign substance.

37191-37193

37191 Insertion of intravascular vena cava filter, endovascular approach including vascular access, vessel selection, and radiological supervision and interpretation, intraprocedural roadmapping, and imaging guidance (ultrasound and fluoroscopy), when performed

37192 Repositioning of intravascular vena cava filter, endovascular approach including vascular access, vessel selection, and radiological supervision and interpretation, intraprocedural roadmapping, and imaging guidance (ultrasound and fluoroscopy), when performed

37193 Retrieval (removal) of intravascular vena cava filter, endovascular approach including vascular access, vessel selection, and radiological supervision and interpretation, intraprocedural roadmapping, and imaging guidance (ultrasound and fluoroscopy), when performed

Select major vessels

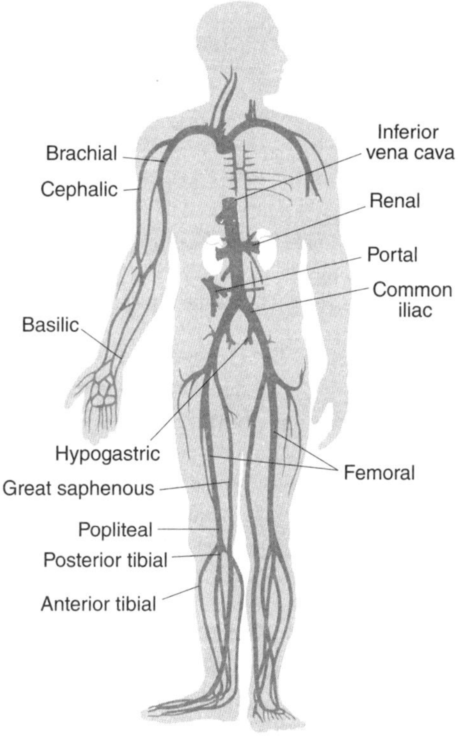

Explanation

An inferior vena cava (IVC) filter is placed most commonly for refractory deep vein thrombosis and pulmonary embolism or when anticoagulation is contraindicated. In 37191, the physician places a needle in the femoral (or internal jugular) vein, advances a guidewire through the needle, removes the needle over the wire, and advances an introducer sheath over the wire into the femoral vein. The physician advances the filter through the introducer sheath into the inferior vena cava under fluoroscopic guidance. The physician removes the introducer sheath and compresses the femoral vein manually until hemostasis is achieved. Report 37192 for the repositioning of an already placed filter utilizing an endovascular approach and associated radiologic guidance when applicable. In 37193, the physician utilizes the same approach to remove the filter.

Coding Tips

When medically necessary, report moderate (conscious) sedation provided by the performing physician with 99151-99153. When provided by another physician, report 99155-99157. These codes include access and vessel selection, radiological supervision and interpretation, roadmapping, and imaging guidance by ultrasound and/or fluoroscopy. For open surgical interruption of the inferior vena cava through laparotomy or retroperitoneal exposure, see 37619. Do not report 37192 with 37191. Do not report 37193 with 37197.

ICD-10-CM Diagnostic Codes

I26.01	Septic pulmonary embolism with acute cor pulmonale
I26.09	Other pulmonary embolism with acute cor pulmonale
I26.90	Septic pulmonary embolism without acute cor pulmonale
I26.99	Other pulmonary embolism without acute cor pulmonale
I27.82	Chronic pulmonary embolism
I82.220	Acute embolism and thrombosis of inferior vena cava
I82.221	Chronic embolism and thrombosis of inferior vena cava
I82.290	Acute embolism and thrombosis of other thoracic veins
I82.291	Chronic embolism and thrombosis of other thoracic veins
I82.3	Embolism and thrombosis of renal vein
I82.411	Acute embolism and thrombosis of right femoral vein ☑
I82.412	Acute embolism and thrombosis of left femoral vein ☑
I82.413	Acute embolism and thrombosis of femoral vein, bilateral ☑
I82.421	Acute embolism and thrombosis of right iliac vein ☑
I82.422	Acute embolism and thrombosis of left iliac vein ☑
I82.423	Acute embolism and thrombosis of iliac vein, bilateral ☑
I82.431	Acute embolism and thrombosis of right popliteal vein ☑
I82.432	Acute embolism and thrombosis of left popliteal vein ☑
I82.433	Acute embolism and thrombosis of popliteal vein, bilateral ☑
I82.441	Acute embolism and thrombosis of right tibial vein ☑
I82.442	Acute embolism and thrombosis of left tibial vein ☑
I82.443	Acute embolism and thrombosis of tibial vein, bilateral ☑
I82.491	Acute embolism and thrombosis of other specified deep vein of right lower extremity ☑
I82.492	Acute embolism and thrombosis of other specified deep vein of left lower extremity ☑
I82.493	Acute embolism and thrombosis of other specified deep vein of lower extremity, bilateral ☑
I82.511	Chronic embolism and thrombosis of right femoral vein ☑
I82.512	Chronic embolism and thrombosis of left femoral vein ☑
I82.513	Chronic embolism and thrombosis of femoral vein, bilateral ☑
I82.521	Chronic embolism and thrombosis of right iliac vein ☑
I82.522	Chronic embolism and thrombosis of left iliac vein ☑
I82.523	Chronic embolism and thrombosis of iliac vein, bilateral ☑
I82.531	Chronic embolism and thrombosis of right popliteal vein ☑
I82.532	Chronic embolism and thrombosis of left popliteal vein ☑
I82.533	Chronic embolism and thrombosis of popliteal vein, bilateral ☑
I82.541	Chronic embolism and thrombosis of right tibial vein ☑
I82.542	Chronic embolism and thrombosis of left tibial vein ☑
I82.543	Chronic embolism and thrombosis of tibial vein, bilateral ☑
I82.591	Chronic embolism and thrombosis of other specified deep vein of right lower extremity ☑
I82.592	Chronic embolism and thrombosis of other specified deep vein of left lower extremity ☑
I82.593	Chronic embolism and thrombosis of other specified deep vein of lower extremity, bilateral ☑
I82.811	Embolism and thrombosis of superficial veins of right lower extremity ☑

I82.812 Embolism and thrombosis of superficial veins of left lower extremity ☑

I82.813 Embolism and thrombosis of superficial veins of lower extremities, bilateral ☑

T82.515A Breakdown (mechanical) of umbrella device, initial encounter

T82.518A Breakdown (mechanical) of other cardiac and vascular devices and implants, initial encounter

T82.525A Displacement of umbrella device, initial encounter

T82.528A Displacement of other cardiac and vascular devices and implants, initial encounter

T82.535A Leakage of umbrella device, initial encounter

T82.538A Leakage of other cardiac and vascular devices and implants, initial encounter

T82.595A Other mechanical complication of umbrella device, initial encounter

T82.598A Other mechanical complication of other cardiac and vascular devices and implants, initial encounter

T82.7XXA Infection and inflammatory reaction due to other cardiac and vascular devices, implants and grafts, initial encounter

T82.818A Embolism due to vascular prosthetic devices, implants and grafts, initial encounter

T82.828A Fibrosis due to vascular prosthetic devices, implants and grafts, initial encounter

T82.848A Pain due to vascular prosthetic devices, implants and grafts, initial encounter

T82.858A Stenosis of other vascular prosthetic devices, implants and grafts, initial encounter

T82.868A Thrombosis due to vascular prosthetic devices, implants and grafts, initial encounter

T82.898A Other specified complication of vascular prosthetic devices, implants and grafts, initial encounter

Relative Value Units/Medicare Edits

Non-Facility RVU	Work	PE	MP	Total
37191	4.46	54.11	0.63	59.2
37192	7.1	28.86	1.75	37.71
37193	7.1	35.84	1.06	44.0
Facility RVU	**Work**	**PE**	**MP**	**Total**
37191	4.46	1.33	0.63	6.42
37192	7.1	1.2	1.75	10.05
37193	7.1	1.93	1.06	10.09

	FUD	Status	MUE	Modifiers				IOM Reference
37191	0	A	1(3)	51	N/A	N/A	N/A	None
37192	0	A	1(3)	51	N/A	N/A	N/A	
37193	0	A	1(3)	51	N/A	N/A	N/A	

* with documentation

37195

37195 Thrombolysis, cerebral, by intravenous infusion

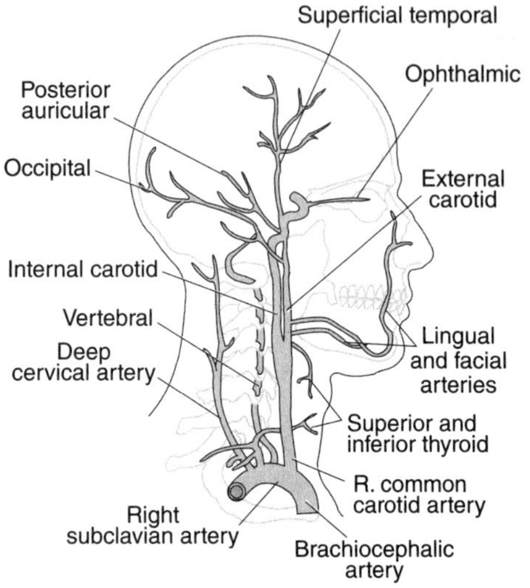

Explanation

The physician remedies a stroke-causing blood clot obstructing blood flow to the brain. The physician infuses a thrombolytic ("clot-busting") drug through an intravenous catheter to help dissolve the clot and restore normal blood flow to the brain.

Coding Tips

This code should only be reported when the physician personally administers the medication. If a nurse administers the medication in the emergency department, the ordering physician should not report 37195 but may report an E/M code if all criteria for a specific code are met. For transcatheter therapy, infusion for thrombolysis other than coronary (or cerebral), see 37211-37214. For thrombolysis of the coronary vessels, see 92975 and 92977.

ICD-10-CM Diagnostic Codes

G45.8 Other transient cerebral ischemic attacks and related syndromes

G45.9 Transient cerebral ischemic attack, unspecified

G46.0 Middle cerebral artery syndrome

G46.1 Anterior cerebral artery syndrome

G46.2 Posterior cerebral artery syndrome

I63.311 Cerebral infarction due to thrombosis of right middle cerebral artery ☑

I63.312 Cerebral infarction due to thrombosis of left middle cerebral artery ☑

I63.321 Cerebral infarction due to thrombosis of right anterior cerebral artery ☑

I63.322 Cerebral infarction due to thrombosis of left anterior cerebral artery ☑

I63.331 Cerebral infarction due to thrombosis of right posterior cerebral artery ☑

I63.332 Cerebral infarction due to thrombosis of left posterior cerebral artery ☑

I63.39 Cerebral infarction due to thrombosis of other cerebral artery

I63.411 Cerebral infarction due to embolism of right middle cerebral artery ☑

Arteries and Veins

I63.412	Cerebral infarction due to embolism of left middle cerebral artery ☑
I63.421	Cerebral infarction due to embolism of right anterior cerebral artery ☑
I63.422	Cerebral infarction due to embolism of left anterior cerebral artery ☑
I63.431	Cerebral infarction due to embolism of right posterior cerebral artery ☑
I63.432	Cerebral infarction due to embolism of left posterior cerebral artery ☑
I63.6	Cerebral infarction due to cerebral venous thrombosis, nonpyogenic
I63.81	Other cerebral infarction due to occlusion or stenosis of small artery
I63.89	Other cerebral infarction
I66.01	Occlusion and stenosis of right middle cerebral artery ☑
I66.02	Occlusion and stenosis of left middle cerebral artery ☑
I66.03	Occlusion and stenosis of bilateral middle cerebral arteries ☑
I66.11	Occlusion and stenosis of right anterior cerebral artery ☑
I66.12	Occlusion and stenosis of left anterior cerebral artery ☑
I66.13	Occlusion and stenosis of bilateral anterior cerebral arteries ☑
I66.21	Occlusion and stenosis of right posterior cerebral artery ☑
I66.22	Occlusion and stenosis of left posterior cerebral artery ☑
I66.23	Occlusion and stenosis of bilateral posterior cerebral arteries ☑
I66.8	Occlusion and stenosis of other cerebral arteries
I67.848	Other cerebrovascular vasospasm and vasoconstriction
I67.850	Cerebral autosomal dominant arteriopathy with subcortical infarcts and leukoencephalopathy
I67.858	Other hereditary cerebrovascular disease
I97.810	Intraoperative cerebrovascular infarction during cardiac surgery
I97.811	Intraoperative cerebrovascular infarction during other surgery
I97.820	Postprocedural cerebrovascular infarction following cardiac surgery
I97.821	Postprocedural cerebrovascular infarction following other surgery

AMA: **37195** 2020,Jan

Relative Value Units/Medicare Edits

Non-Facility RVU	Work	PE	MP	Total
37195	0.0	0.0	0.0	0.0
Facility RVU	**Work**	**PE**	**MP**	**Total**
37195	0.0	0.0	0.0	0.0

	FUD	Status	MUE	Modifiers				IOM Reference
37195	N/A	C	1(3)	N/A	N/A	N/A	80*	None

* with documentation

Terms To Know

infarction. Area of necrosis in tissue, due to ischemia from lack of circulation, usually from a thrombus or an embolus.

thrombolysis. Chemical process of dissolving or breaking down a blood clot by inducing a complex chain of events involving the action of plasminogen to solubilize fibrin clots and degrade fibrinogen.

37197

37197 Transcatheter retrieval, percutaneous, of intravascular foreign body (eg, fractured venous or arterial catheter), includes radiological supervision and interpretation, and imaging guidance (ultrasound or fluoroscopy), when performed

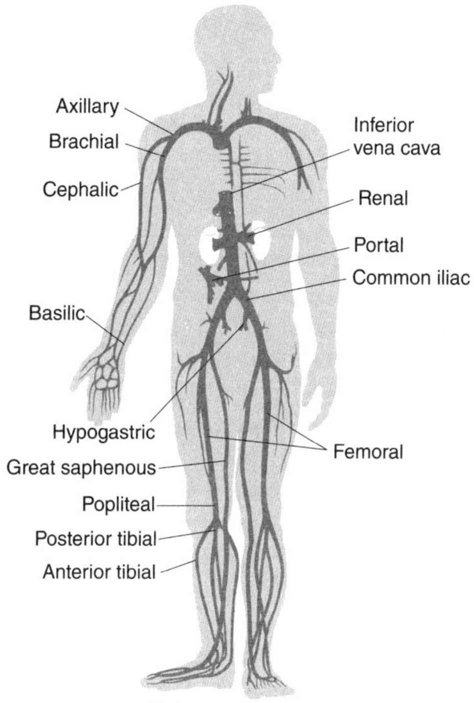

Select major veins

Explanation

The physician places a needle into a blood vessel. A guidewire is threaded through the needle into the vessel and the needle is removed. A catheter is threaded into the vessel and the wire is extracted. The catheter, equipped with a grasping instrument, travels to the site of the foreign body typically using imaging guidance. The instrument grasps the foreign body, typically a fractured catheter, and retrieves it. The catheter is removed and pressure is applied over the puncture site to stop the bleeding.

Coding Tips

When medically necessary, report moderate (conscious) sedation provided by the performing physician with 99151-99153. When provided by another physician, report 99155-99157. For percutaneous retrieval of a vena cava filter, see 37193. For transcatheter removal of a permanent leadless pacemaker, see 33275.

ICD-10-CM Diagnostic Codes

T81.510A	Adhesions due to foreign body accidentally left in body following surgical operation, initial encounter
T81.511A	Adhesions due to foreign body accidentally left in body following infusion or transfusion, initial encounter
T81.512A	Adhesions due to foreign body accidentally left in body following kidney dialysis, initial encounter
T81.513A	Adhesions due to foreign body accidentally left in body following injection or immunization, initial encounter
T81.515A	Adhesions due to foreign body accidentally left in body following heart catheterization, initial encounter

T81.517A Adhesions due to foreign body accidentally left in body following removal of catheter or packing, initial encounter

T81.518A Adhesions due to foreign body accidentally left in body following other procedure, initial encounter

T81.520A Obstruction due to foreign body accidentally left in body following surgical operation, initial encounter

T81.521A Obstruction due to foreign body accidentally left in body following infusion or transfusion, initial encounter

T81.522A Obstruction due to foreign body accidentally left in body following kidney dialysis, initial encounter

T81.523A Obstruction due to foreign body accidentally left in body following injection or immunization, initial encounter

T81.525A Obstruction due to foreign body accidentally left in body following heart catheterization, initial encounter

T81.527A Obstruction due to foreign body accidentally left in body following removal of catheter or packing, initial encounter

T81.528A Obstruction due to foreign body accidentally left in body following other procedure, initial encounter

T81.530A Perforation due to foreign body accidentally left in body following surgical operation, initial encounter

T81.531A Perforation due to foreign body accidentally left in body following infusion or transfusion, initial encounter

T81.532A Perforation due to foreign body accidentally left in body following kidney dialysis, initial encounter

T81.533A Perforation due to foreign body accidentally left in body following injection or immunization, initial encounter

T81.535A Perforation due to foreign body accidentally left in body following heart catheterization, initial encounter

T81.537A Perforation due to foreign body accidentally left in body following removal of catheter or packing, initial encounter

T81.538A Perforation due to foreign body accidentally left in body following other procedure, initial encounter

T81.590A Other complications of foreign body accidentally left in body following surgical operation, initial encounter

T81.591A Other complications of foreign body accidentally left in body following infusion or transfusion, initial encounter

T81.592A Other complications of foreign body accidentally left in body following kidney dialysis, initial encounter

T81.593A Other complications of foreign body accidentally left in body following injection or immunization, initial encounter

T81.595A Other complications of foreign body accidentally left in body following heart catheterization, initial encounter

T81.597A Other complications of foreign body accidentally left in body following removal of catheter or packing, initial encounter

T81.598A Other complications of foreign body accidentally left in body following other procedure, initial encounter

T82.310A Breakdown (mechanical) of aortic (bifurcation) graft (replacement), initial encounter

T82.311A Breakdown (mechanical) of carotid arterial graft (bypass), initial encounter

T82.312A Breakdown (mechanical) of femoral arterial graft (bypass), initial encounter

T82.318A Breakdown (mechanical) of other vascular grafts, initial encounter

T82.390A Other mechanical complication of aortic (bifurcation) graft (replacement), initial encounter

T82.391A Other mechanical complication of carotid arterial graft (bypass), initial encounter

T82.392A Other mechanical complication of femoral arterial graft (bypass), initial encounter

T82.398A Other mechanical complication of other vascular grafts, initial encounter

T82.41XA Breakdown (mechanical) of vascular dialysis catheter, initial encounter

T82.49XA Other complication of vascular dialysis catheter, initial encounter

T82.513A Breakdown (mechanical) of balloon (counterpulsation) device, initial encounter

T82.514A Breakdown (mechanical) of infusion catheter, initial encounter

T82.515A Breakdown (mechanical) of umbrella device, initial encounter

T82.518A Breakdown (mechanical) of other cardiac and vascular devices and implants, initial encounter

T82.593A Other mechanical complication of balloon (counterpulsation) device, initial encounter

T82.594A Other mechanical complication of infusion catheter, initial encounter

T82.595A Other mechanical complication of umbrella device, initial encounter

T82.598A Other mechanical complication of other cardiac and vascular devices and implants, initial encounter

T82.898A Other specified complication of vascular prosthetic devices, implants and grafts, initial encounter

AMA: 37197 2021,Dec

Relative Value Units/Medicare Edits

Non-Facility RVU	Work	PE	MP	Total
37197	6.04	38.89	1.01	45.94
Facility RVU	**Work**	**PE**	**MP**	**Total**
37197	6.04	1.71	1.01	8.76

	FUD	Status	MUE	Modifiers				IOM Reference
37197	0	A	2(3)	51	N/A	N/A	N/A	None

* with documentation

Arteries and Veins

37200

37200 Transcatheter biopsy

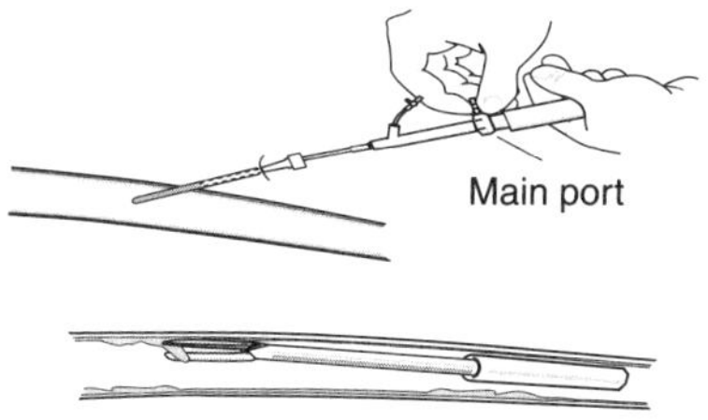

A biopsy instrument extracts tissue from vessel wall for biopsy

Explanation

A needle is inserted through the skin and into a blood vessel, and a guidewire is threaded through the needle into the vessel. The needle is removed. A catheter is threaded into the vessel, and the wire extracted. The catheter equipped with a biopsy instrument travels to the area to be sampled. The instrument extracts for biopsy tissue affixed to the vessel wall. Pressure is applied over the puncture site to stop bleeding after the catheter is removed. This procedure may also be performed through a skin incision with direct exposure of the access vessel.

Coding Tips

When 37200 is performed with another separately identifiable procedure, the highest dollar value code is listed as the primary procedure, and subsequent procedures are appended with modifier 51. For radiological supervision and interpretation, see 75970.

ICD-10-CM Diagnostic Codes

The application of this code is too broad to adequately present ICD-10-CM diagnostic code links here. Refer to your ICD-10-CM book.

Relative Value Units/Medicare Edits

Non-Facility RVU	Work	PE	MP	Total
37200	4.55	1.21	0.47	6.23
Facility RVU	**Work**	**PE**	**MP**	**Total**
37200	4.55	1.21	0.47	6.23

	FUD	Status	MUE	Modifiers				IOM Reference
37200	0	A	2(3)	51	N/A	N/A	N/A	None

* with documentation

Terms To Know

biopsy. Tissue or fluid removed for diagnostic purposes through analysis of the cells in the biopsy material.

catheter. Flexible tube inserted into an area of the body for introducing or withdrawing fluid.

guidewire. Flexible metal instrument designed to lead another instrument in its proper course.

incision. Act of cutting into tissue or an organ.

37211-37214

37211 Transcatheter therapy, arterial infusion for thrombolysis other than coronary or intracranial, any method, including radiological supervision and interpretation, initial treatment day

37212 Transcatheter therapy, venous infusion for thrombolysis, any method, including radiological supervision and interpretation, initial treatment day

37213 Transcatheter therapy, arterial or venous infusion for thrombolysis other than coronary, any method, including radiological supervision and interpretation, continued treatment on subsequent day during course of thrombolytic therapy, including follow-up catheter contrast injection, position change, or exchange, when performed;

37214 cessation of thrombolysis including removal of catheter and vessel closure by any method

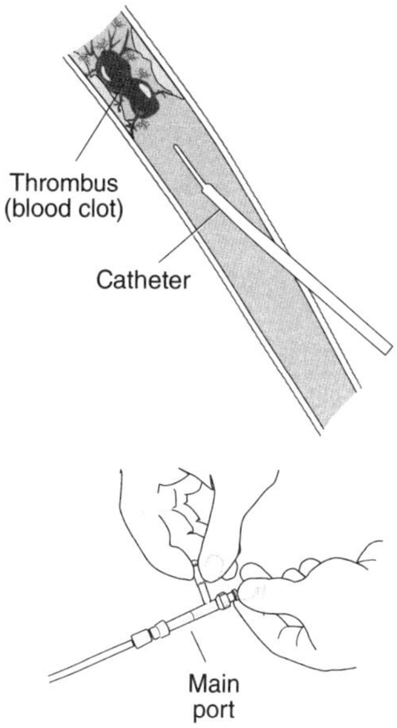

Thrombolysis is performed using intra-arterial or intravenous infusion

Explanation

Transcatheter thrombolysis infusion is most commonly used to treat symptomatic inferior vena cava thrombosis that is responding poorly to the routine anticoagulation regimen or symptomatic iliofemoral or femoropopliteal deep vein thrombosis (DVT) in patients with a low risk of bleeding. A diagnostic arteriography or venography is performed to pinpoint the extent of the thrombosis. The physician places a needle into the blood vessel. A guidewire is threaded through the needle to the site of the clot using fluoroscopic guidance and the needle is removed. An infusion catheter is threaded to the site and the wire is extracted. A thrombolytic pharmaceutical is administered directly to the thrombosis. During the infusion, the patient is on bed rest with frequent monitoring. Once the thrombosis has dissipated satisfactorily, the infusion is stopped and the catheter removed. Pressure is applied over the puncture site to stop the bleeding. Report 37211 for the first day of arterial transcatheter therapy; 37212 for the first day of venous transcatheter therapy; 37213 for each subsequent day of arterial or venous therapy, including follow-up catheter contrast injection, position change, or exchange, if applicable; and 37214 for the last day the thrombolysis is administered, including removal of the catheter and closure of the access site. These codes are not for use when thrombolysis is performed on coronary or intracranial arteries.

● New ▲ Revised + Add On ★ Telemedicine [Resequenced] ☑ Laterality

Coding Tips

When medically necessary, report moderate (conscious) sedation provided by the performing physician with 99151-99153. When provided by another physician, report 99155-99157. Codes 37211–37214 are resequenced codes and will not display in numeric order. These are unilateral procedures. If performed bilaterally, some payers require that the service be reported twice with modifier 50 appended to the second code while others require identification of the service only once with modifier 50 appended. Check with individual payers. Modifier 50 identifies a procedure performed identically on the opposite side of the body (mirror image). Catheter placement, diagnostic studies, and any other percutaneous interventions performed are separately reportable. Fluoroscopic guidance and radiological supervision and interpretation are included in 37211–37214. These codes should only be reported once per treatment day. For ultrasound guidance for vascular access, see 76937. For declotting of an implanted vascular access device or catheter by thrombolytic agent, see 36593. For mechanical thrombectomy and/or thrombolysis infusion performed on an intracranial artery, see 61645.

ICD-10-CM Diagnostic Codes

G45.2	Multiple and bilateral precerebral artery syndromes
I26.01	Septic pulmonary embolism with acute cor pulmonale
I26.02	Saddle embolus of pulmonary artery with acute cor pulmonale
I26.90	Septic pulmonary embolism without acute cor pulmonale
I26.92	Saddle embolus of pulmonary artery without acute cor pulmonale
I26.93	Single subsegmental thrombotic pulmonary embolism without acute cor pulmonale
I26.94	Multiple subsegmental thrombotic pulmonary emboli without acute cor pulmonale
I63.011	Cerebral infarction due to thrombosis of right vertebral artery ☑
I63.02	Cerebral infarction due to thrombosis of basilar artery
I63.031	Cerebral infarction due to thrombosis of right carotid artery ☑
I63.111	Cerebral infarction due to embolism of right vertebral artery ☑
I63.12	Cerebral infarction due to embolism of basilar artery
I63.131	Cerebral infarction due to embolism of right carotid artery ☑
I63.6	Cerebral infarction due to cerebral venous thrombosis, nonpyogenic
I65.01	Occlusion and stenosis of right vertebral artery ☑
I65.1	Occlusion and stenosis of basilar artery
I65.21	Occlusion and stenosis of right carotid artery ☑
I72.6	Aneurysm of vertebral artery
I74.01	Saddle embolus of abdominal aorta
I74.11	Embolism and thrombosis of thoracic aorta
I74.2	Embolism and thrombosis of arteries of the upper extremities
I74.3	Embolism and thrombosis of arteries of the lower extremities
I74.5	Embolism and thrombosis of iliac artery
I75.011	Atheroembolism of right upper extremity ☑
I75.021	Atheroembolism of right lower extremity ☑
I75.81	Atheroembolism of kidney
I76	Septic arterial embolism
I80.211	Phlebitis and thrombophlebitis of right iliac vein ☑
I80.221	Phlebitis and thrombophlebitis of right popliteal vein ☑
I80.231	Phlebitis and thrombophlebitis of right tibial vein ☑
I81	Portal vein thrombosis
I82.0	Budd-Chiari syndrome
I82.1	Thrombophlebitis migrans
I82.210	Acute embolism and thrombosis of superior vena cava
I82.211	Chronic embolism and thrombosis of superior vena cava
I82.220	Acute embolism and thrombosis of inferior vena cava
I82.221	Chronic embolism and thrombosis of inferior vena cava
I82.3	Embolism and thrombosis of renal vein
I82.411	Acute embolism and thrombosis of right femoral vein ☑
I82.421	Acute embolism and thrombosis of right iliac vein ☑
I82.431	Acute embolism and thrombosis of right popliteal vein ☑
I82.441	Acute embolism and thrombosis of right tibial vein ☑
I82.511	Chronic embolism and thrombosis of right femoral vein ☑
I82.521	Chronic embolism and thrombosis of right iliac vein ☑
I82.531	Chronic embolism and thrombosis of right popliteal vein ☑
I82.541	Chronic embolism and thrombosis of right tibial vein ☑
I82.611	Acute embolism and thrombosis of superficial veins of right upper extremity ☑
I82.621	Acute embolism and thrombosis of deep veins of right upper extremity ☑
I82.711	Chronic embolism and thrombosis of superficial veins of right upper extremity ☑
I82.721	Chronic embolism and thrombosis of deep veins of right upper extremity ☑
I82.811	Embolism and thrombosis of superficial veins of right lower extremity ☑
I82.A11	Acute embolism and thrombosis of right axillary vein ☑
I82.A21	Chronic embolism and thrombosis of right axillary vein ☑
I82.B11	Acute embolism and thrombosis of right subclavian vein ☑
I82.B21	Chronic embolism and thrombosis of right subclavian vein ☑
I82.C11	Acute embolism and thrombosis of right internal jugular vein ☑
I82.C21	Chronic embolism and thrombosis of right internal jugular vein ☑
K55.011	Focal (segmental) acute (reversible) ischemia of small intestine
K55.012	Diffuse acute (reversible) ischemia of small intestine
K55.021	Focal (segmental) acute infarction of small intestine
K55.022	Diffuse acute infarction of small intestine
K55.031	Focal (segmental) acute (reversible) ischemia of large intestine
K55.032	Diffuse acute (reversible) ischemia of large intestine
K55.041	Focal (segmental) acute infarction of large intestine
K55.042	Diffuse acute infarction of large intestine
K55.1	Chronic vascular disorders of intestine
N28.0	Ischemia and infarction of kidney
T82.818A	Embolism due to vascular prosthetic devices, implants and grafts, initial encounter
T82.868A	Thrombosis due to vascular prosthetic devices, implants and grafts, initial encounter

AMA: 37211 2022,Jun; 2019,Sep **37212** 2022,Jun; 2019,Sep **37213** 2022,Jun; 2019,Sep **37214** 2022,Jun; 2019,Sep

Relative Value Units/Medicare Edits

Non-Facility RVU	Work	PE	MP	Total
37211	7.75	2.06	1.47	11.28
37212	6.81	1.84	1.18	9.83
37213	4.75	1.16	0.81	6.72
37214	2.49	0.61	0.45	3.55
Facility RVU	**Work**	**PE**	**MP**	**Total**
37211	7.75	2.06	1.47	11.28
37212	6.81	1.84	1.18	9.83
37213	4.75	1.16	0.81	6.72
37214	2.49	0.61	0.45	3.55

	FUD	Status	MUE	Modifiers				IOM Reference
37211	0	A	1(2)	51	50	N/A	N/A	None
37212	0	A	1(2)	51	50	N/A	N/A	
37213	0	A	1(2)	51	N/A	N/A	N/A	
37214	0	A	1(2)	51	N/A	N/A	N/A	

* with documentation

Terms To Know

artery. Vessel through which oxygenated blood passes away from the heart to any part of the body.

infusion. Introduction of a therapeutic fluid, other than blood, into the bloodstream.

thrombolysis. Chemical process of dissolving or breaking down a blood clot by inducing a complex chain of events involving the action of plasminogen to solubilize fibrin clots and degrade fibrinogen.

transcatheter therapy. Therapeutic procedure or treatment performed via a catheter as opposed to open access.

vein. Vessel through which oxygen-depleted blood passes back to the heart.

37215-37216

37215 Transcatheter placement of intravascular stent(s), cervical carotid artery, open or percutaneous, including angioplasty, when performed, and radiological supervision and interpretation; with distal embolic protection

37216 without distal embolic protection

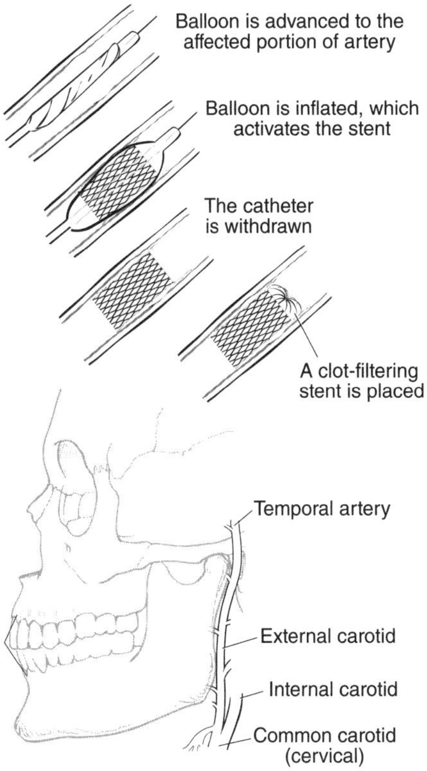

Explanation

The physician places an intravascular stent via open or percutaneous approach through a catheter into the cervical carotid artery. The open procedure is carried out by making an incision exposing the cervical carotid artery and creating an arteriotomy. In the percutaneous approach, a needle is inserted through the skin into the access blood vessel, usually the brachial or femoral artery. A guidewire is threaded through the needle into the cervical carotid artery and the needle is removed. Long sheaths or guiding catheters are advanced into the stenosed cervical carotid artery. A filter protection device may be inserted distal to the stenosis to capture emboli. After filter opening, predilation of the stenosis with angioplasty balloons may be performed. A catheter with a stent-transporting tip is threaded over the guidewire into the vessel and the wire is extracted. The catheter travels to the point where the vessel needs additional support. The compressed stent is passed from the catheter out into the vessel, where it deploys, expanding to support the vessel walls. The catheter is removed and pressure is applied over the puncture site. Report 37215 when stenting is performed with a filter protection device (distal embolic protection) and 37216 when stenting is performed without a filter protection device. The procedures include radiologic supervision and interpretation, as well as angioplasty, when performed.

Coding Tips

When medically necessary, report moderate (conscious) sedation provided by the performing physician with 99151-99153. When provided by another physician, report 99155-99157. These procedures include all ipsilateral selective carotid catheterization; all diagnostic imaging for ipsilateral, cervical, and cerebral carotid arteriography; and all related radiological supervision and interpretation. When ipsilateral carotid arteriogram (including imaging and selective catheterization) confirms the need for carotid stenting, 37215 and 37216 are inclusive of these services. If carotid stenting is not indicated, then the appropriate codes for carotid catheterization and imaging should be reported in lieu of 37215 and 37216. Do not report 37215 or 37216 with 36222–36224 for the carotid artery being treated. For transcatheter placement of an extracranial vertebral artery stent(s), see Category III codes 0075T–0076T. For percutaneous transcatheter placement of intravascular stents other than coronary, carotid, or vertebral, see 37236–37239. Supplies used when providing this procedure may be reported with HCPCS Level II code C1884 or C1886. Check with the specific payer to determine coverage.

ICD-10-CM Diagnostic Codes

G45.1	Carotid artery syndrome (hemispheric)
G45.8	Other transient cerebral ischemic attacks and related syndromes
I63.031	Cerebral infarction due to thrombosis of right carotid artery ☑
I63.131	Cerebral infarction due to embolism of right carotid artery ☑
I63.81	Other cerebral infarction due to occlusion or stenosis of small artery
I63.89	Other cerebral infarction
I65.21	Occlusion and stenosis of right carotid artery ☑
I67.81	Acute cerebrovascular insufficiency
I67.82	Cerebral ischemia
I67.848	Other cerebrovascular vasospasm and vasoconstriction
I67.850	Cerebral autosomal dominant arteriopathy with subcortical infarcts and leukoencephalopathy
I67.858	Other hereditary cerebrovascular disease
I67.89	Other cerebrovascular disease
I72.0	Aneurysm of carotid artery
I76	Septic arterial embolism
I77.1	Stricture of artery
I77.3	Arterial fibromuscular dysplasia
I77.89	Other specified disorders of arteries and arterioles

Relative Value Units/Medicare Edits

Non-Facility RVU	Work	PE	MP	Total
37215	17.75	6.71	4.58	29.04
37216	17.98	9.37	1.83	29.18
Facility RVU	**Work**	**PE**	**MP**	**Total**
37215	17.75	6.71	4.58	29.04
37216	17.98	9.37	1.83	29.18

	FUD	Status	MUE	Modifiers				IOM Reference
37215	90	R	1(2)	51	50	N/A	80*	None
37216	90	N	0(3)	N/A	N/A	N/A	N/A	

* with documentation

37217

37217 Transcatheter placement of intravascular stent(s), intrathoracic common carotid artery or innominate artery by retrograde treatment, open ipsilateral cervical carotid artery exposure, including angioplasty, when performed, and radiological supervision and interpretation

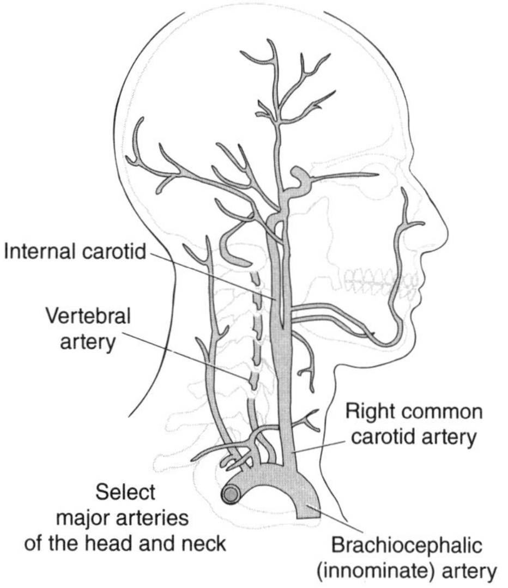

Intravascular stents are placed into the common carotid or innominate artery

Explanation

Placing stents into the intrathoracic common carotid artery or innominate artery via a catheter is a less invasive alternative to open endarterectomy. The procedure is carried out by making an incision exposing the cervical carotid artery and creating an arteriotomy. A catheter is inserted through the artery and threaded to the target. A stent delivery system, which may also include an embolic capturing device, is loaded into a delivery pod and advanced to the blocked or narrowed artery through the catheter. The embolic protection device is deployed first, distal to the lesion so that any emboli are collected as the blood passes through the device. The stent is advanced out of the pod until it expands to open the narrowing. The instruments are removed. The artery and overlying tissues are closed. The procedure includes radiologic supervision and interpretation, as well as angioplasty, when performed.

Coding Tips

This procedure includes all open vessel exposure and vascular access closure, access to and selective catheterization of the vessel being treated, traversing of the lesion, supervision and interpretation of radiology services that are related to the intervention when applicable including imaging performed to document completion of the intervention, and standard closure by suture of the arteriotomy site. None of these services can be reported separately. Carotid artery revascularization services, such as 33891, 35301, 35509–35510, 35601, and 35606, may be reported separately when performed during the same session. Do not report 37217 with 35201, 36221–36227, 37246, or 37247 when ipsilateral services are performed. For percutaneous or open transcatheter placement of an intravascular cervical carotid artery stent, see 37215–37216. For transcatheter placement of an intracranial stent, see 61635. For percutaneous or open transcatheter placement of an extracranial vertebral artery stent(s), see 0075T–0076T. For percutaneous or open antegrade transcatheter placement of innominate and/or intrathoracic carotid artery stent(s), see 37218.

ICD-10-CM Diagnostic Codes

G45.1	Carotid artery syndrome (hemispheric)
G45.9	Transient cerebral ischemic attack, unspecified
I63.031	Cerebral infarction due to thrombosis of right carotid artery ☑
I63.032	Cerebral infarction due to thrombosis of left carotid artery ☑
I63.131	Cerebral infarction due to embolism of right carotid artery ☑
I63.132	Cerebral infarction due to embolism of left carotid artery ☑
I63.231	Cerebral infarction due to unspecified occlusion or stenosis of right carotid arteries ☑
I63.232	Cerebral infarction due to unspecified occlusion or stenosis of left carotid arteries ☑
I63.81	Other cerebral infarction due to occlusion or stenosis of small artery
I63.89	Other cerebral infarction
I65.21	Occlusion and stenosis of right carotid artery ☑
I65.22	Occlusion and stenosis of left carotid artery ☑
I65.23	Occlusion and stenosis of bilateral carotid arteries ☑
I65.8	Occlusion and stenosis of other precerebral arteries
I67.81	Acute cerebrovascular insufficiency
I67.82	Cerebral ischemia
I67.848	Other cerebrovascular vasospasm and vasoconstriction
I67.850	Cerebral autosomal dominant arteriopathy with subcortical infarcts and leukoencephalopathy
I67.858	Other hereditary cerebrovascular disease
I67.89	Other cerebrovascular disease
I72.0	Aneurysm of carotid artery
I76	Septic arterial embolism
I77.1	Stricture of artery
I77.3	Arterial fibromuscular dysplasia
I77.71	Dissection of carotid artery
I77.89	Other specified disorders of arteries and arterioles

Relative Value Units/Medicare Edits

Non-Facility RVU	Work	PE	MP	Total
37217	20.38	6.22	4.98	31.58
Facility RVU	**Work**	**PE**	**MP**	**Total**
37217	20.38	6.22	4.98	31.58

	FUD	Status	MUE	Modifiers				IOM Reference
37217	90	A	1(2)	51	50	N/A	80*	None

* with documentation

Terms To Know

stent. Tube to provide support in a body cavity or lumen.

transcatheter. Procedure or treatment performed via a catheter.

37218

37218 Transcatheter placement of intravascular stent(s), intrathoracic common carotid artery or innominate artery, open or percutaneous antegrade approach, including angioplasty, when performed, and radiological supervision and interpretation

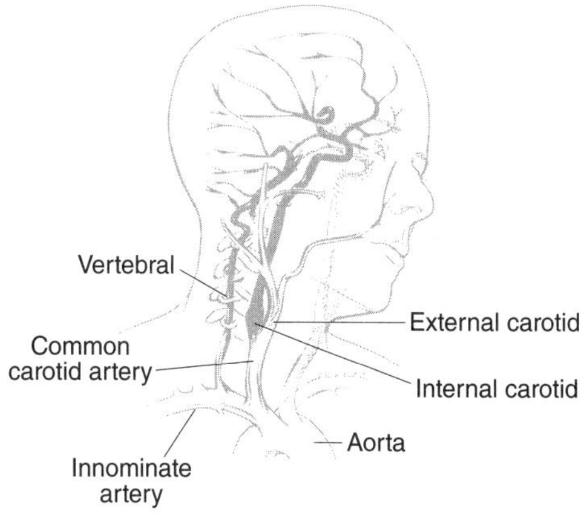

Explanation

The physician places an intravascular stent via open or percutaneous antegrade approach through a catheter into the intrathoracic common carotid artery or innominate artery. A catheter is inserted through the artery and threaded to the target. A stent delivery system, which may also include an embolic capturing device, is loaded into a delivery pod and advanced to the blocked or narrowed artery through the catheter. The embolic protection device is deployed first, distal to the lesion, so that any emboli are collected as the blood passes through the device. The stent is advanced out of the pod until it expands to open the narrowing. The instruments are removed. The artery and overlying tissues are closed. The procedure includes radiologic supervision and interpretation, as well as angioplasty, when performed.

Coding Tips

When medically necessary, report moderate (conscious) sedation provided by the performing physician with 99151-99153. When provided by another physician, report 99155-99157. This code includes all ipsilateral, extracranial, intrathoracic, selective innominate, and carotid catheterization, imaging for stent deployment, and radiological supervision and interpretation. Report this code when arteriogram determines the need for the stent; however, if stenting is not medically necessary, see codes for selective catheterization and imaging. For percutaneous or open transcatheter placement of intravascular cervical carotid artery stent, see 37215 and 37216. For percutaneous or open transcatheter placement of an extracranial vertebral artery stent, see 0075T and 0076T. For transcatheter placement of an intracranial stent, see 61635. Do not report 37218 with 36222-36224.

ICD-10-CM Diagnostic Codes

G45.1	Carotid artery syndrome (hemispheric)
G45.9	Transient cerebral ischemic attack, unspecified
I63.031	Cerebral infarction due to thrombosis of right carotid artery ☑
I63.032	Cerebral infarction due to thrombosis of left carotid artery ☑
I63.131	Cerebral infarction due to embolism of right carotid artery ☑
I63.132	Cerebral infarction due to embolism of left carotid artery ☑
I63.231	Cerebral infarction due to unspecified occlusion or stenosis of right carotid arteries ☑
I63.232	Cerebral infarction due to unspecified occlusion or stenosis of left carotid arteries ☑

I63.81	Other cerebral infarction due to occlusion or stenosis of small artery
I63.89	Other cerebral infarction
I65.21	Occlusion and stenosis of right carotid artery ☑
I65.22	Occlusion and stenosis of left carotid artery ☑
I65.23	Occlusion and stenosis of bilateral carotid arteries ☑
I65.8	Occlusion and stenosis of other precerebral arteries
I67.81	Acute cerebrovascular insufficiency
I67.82	Cerebral ischemia
I67.848	Other cerebrovascular vasospasm and vasoconstriction
I67.850	Cerebral autosomal dominant arteriopathy with subcortical infarcts and leukoencephalopathy
I67.858	Other hereditary cerebrovascular disease
I67.89	Other cerebrovascular disease
I72.0	Aneurysm of carotid artery
I76	Septic arterial embolism
I77.1	Stricture of artery
I77.3	Arterial fibromuscular dysplasia
I77.71	Dissection of carotid artery
I77.89	Other specified disorders of arteries and arterioles

Relative Value Units/Medicare Edits

Non-Facility RVU	Work	PE	MP	Total
37218	14.75	6.0	3.55	24.3
Facility RVU	**Work**	**PE**	**MP**	**Total**
37218	14.75	6.0	3.55	24.3

	FUD	Status	MUE	Modifiers				IOM Reference
37218	90	A	1(2)	51	50	N/A	80*	None

* with documentation

Terms To Know

arteriography. Radiologic study of an artery upon injection of dye.

ipsilateral. Located on, or affecting, the same side of the body, usually as it relates to a bilateral body part.

37220-37223

37220 Revascularization, endovascular, open or percutaneous, iliac artery, unilateral, initial vessel; with transluminal angioplasty

37221 with transluminal stent placement(s), includes angioplasty within the same vessel, when performed

\+ **37222** Revascularization, endovascular, open or percutaneous, iliac artery, each additional ipsilateral iliac vessel; with transluminal angioplasty (List separately in addition to code for primary procedure)

\+ **37223** with transluminal stent placement(s), includes angioplasty within the same vessel, when performed (List separately in addition to code for primary procedure)

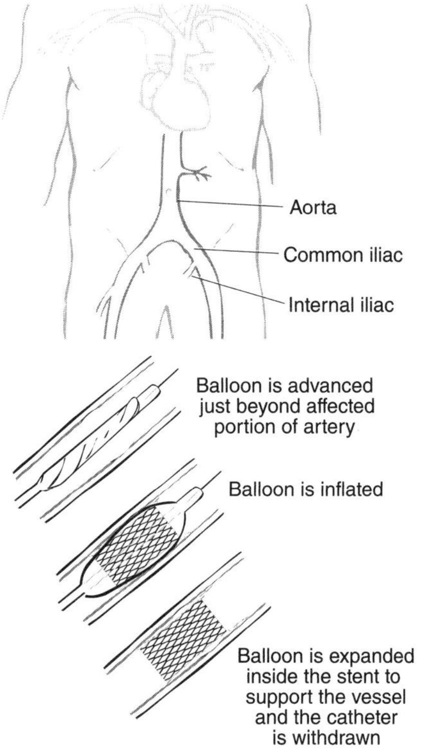

Explanation

The physician treats an iliac artery occlusion or stenosis by endovascular revascularization (restoration of blood supply) in 37220. Access is gained using a small open incision or a percutaneous sheath. Typically, a femoral approach under local anesthesia is used. After sheath placement, intra-arterial heparin is administered. Using a retrograde approach and under angiographic guidance, the occlusion is crossed using a catheter and guidewire. The balloon catheter is inflated in order to dilate the vessel to a larger diameter. Report 37220 for revascularization of the initial vessel and 37222 for each additional vessel on the same side (ipsilateral). Report 37221 if stent placement follows; angioplasty within the same vessel is included in this code. Following dilation and stent deployment, an angiogram is performed to assure appropriate placement and to evaluate the final result. Report 37223 for each additional ipsilateral vessel into which a stent is placed.

Coding Tips

When medically necessary, report moderate (conscious) sedation provided by the performing physician with 99151-99153. When provided by another physician, report 99155-99157. There are up to three vessels within the iliac region that can be treated within the same surgical session; report 37220 or

37221 for the initial vessel treated within one leg and 37222 and 37223 for other vessels when treated. Codes 37222–37223 are specific to additional vessels treated, not separate lesions within the same vessel. These procedures include accessing and selective catheterization of the vessel, traversing the lesion, radiological supervision and interpretation related to the vessel, embolic protection if utilized, closure of the arteriotomy, and imaging related to the completion of the procedure. Report 37220-37223 in addition to 34701-34711, 34718, or 34845-34848 when performed outside the treatment area of the endograft.

ICD-10-CM Diagnostic Codes

I70.211	Atherosclerosis of native arteries of extremities with intermittent claudication, right leg A ☑
I70.221	Atherosclerosis of native arteries of extremities with rest pain, right leg A ☑
I70.231	Atherosclerosis of native arteries of right leg with ulceration of thigh A ☑
I70.232	Atherosclerosis of native arteries of right leg with ulceration of calf A ☑
I70.233	Atherosclerosis of native arteries of right leg with ulceration of ankle A ☑
I72.3	Aneurysm of iliac artery
I74.5	Embolism and thrombosis of iliac artery
I76	Septic arterial embolism
I77.1	Stricture of artery
I77.2	Rupture of artery
I77.3	Arterial fibromuscular dysplasia
I77.5	Necrosis of artery
I77.72	Dissection of iliac artery
S35.511A	Injury of right iliac artery, initial encounter ☑
S35.59XA	Injury of other iliac blood vessels, initial encounter

AMA: 37220 2020,Jul; 2019,Jun **37221** 2020,Jul; 2019,Jun **37222** 2020,Jul; 2019,Jun **37223** 2020,Jul; 2019,Jun

Relative Value Units/Medicare Edits

Non-Facility RVU	Work	PE	MP	Total
37220	7.9	64.01	1.74	73.65
37221	9.75	78.45	2.21	90.41
37222	3.73	13.64	0.81	18.18
37223	4.25	32.06	0.98	37.29
Facility RVU	**Work**	**PE**	**MP**	**Total**
37220	7.9	2.0	1.74	11.64
37221	9.75	2.38	2.21	14.34
37222	3.73	0.84	0.81	5.38
37223	4.25	0.93	0.98	6.16

	FUD	Status	MUE	Modifiers				IOM Reference
37220	0	A	1(2)	51	50	N/A	N/A	None
37221	0	A	1(2)	51	50	N/A	80*	
37222	N/A	A	2(3)	N/A	50	N/A	80*	
37223	N/A	A	2(3)	N/A	50	N/A	80*	

* with documentation

37224-37227

37224 Revascularization, endovascular, open or percutaneous, femoral, popliteal artery(s), unilateral; with transluminal angioplasty

37225 with atherectomy, includes angioplasty within the same vessel, when performed

37226 with transluminal stent placement(s), includes angioplasty within the same vessel, when performed

37227 with transluminal stent placement(s) and atherectomy, includes angioplasty within the same vessel, when performed

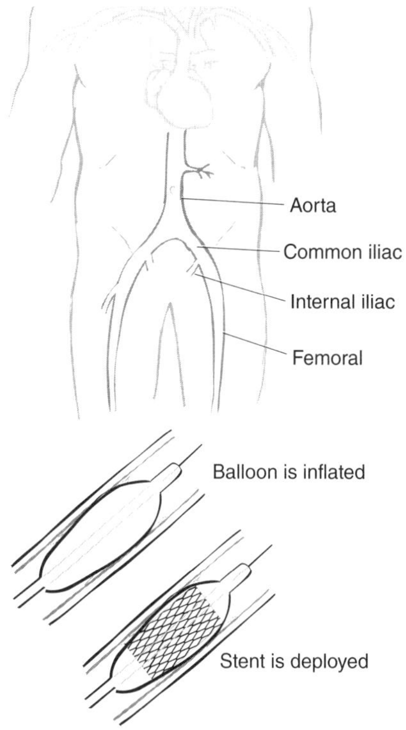

Explanation

The physician treats occlusive disease of a unilateral femoral or popliteal artery by endovascular revascularization (restoration of blood supply) using angioplasty in 37224. Access is gained using a femoral cutdown incision or a percutaneous sheath. Under local anesthesia, the physician accesses the femoral artery. After sheath or needle placement, intra-arterial heparin may be administered. A guidewire is inserted into the artery, followed by a catheter with an attached balloon. The catheter is advanced through the arterial system and into the narrowed portion of the targeted artery. There, the balloon is inflated in order to dilate the vessel to a larger diameter; several inflations may be necessary to achieve maximal results. The physician withdraws the deflated catheter and applies pressure to the puncture site to staunch the bleeding or closes the arteriotomy with suture. In 37225, the physician also performs atherectomy. The physician slides a guidewire through the atherectomy catheter or device, and inserts the guidewire/atherectomy catheter combination through the introducer sheath. The atherectomy device is fluoroscopically positioned at the site of the stenosis. The physician activates the device to remove the stenotic tissue and rechecks the diameter of the lesion by angiography. Several passes with the atherectomy device may be required. The physician removes the atherectomy catheter, guidewire, and introducer sheath. In 37226, the physician places one or more transluminal stents percutaneously using a guidewire or by incision. A catheter with a stent-transporting tip is threaded into the vessel. The catheter travels to the point where the vessel needs additional support, and the compressed stent is passed from the catheter into the vessel, where it deploys and expands to support the vessel walls. The catheter is removed. Pressure is applied over the percutaneous puncture site or, if performed via open approach, the vessel may be repaired and the skin incision closed by sutures. Angioplasty within the same vessel is included in 37226. Report 37227 if the physician performs both stent placement and atherectomy.

Coding Tips

When medically necessary, report moderate (conscious) sedation provided by the performing physician with 99151-99153. When provided by another physician, report 99155-99157. These procedures include accessing and selective catheterization of the vessel, traversing the lesion, radiological supervision and interpretation related to the vessel, embolic protection if utilized, closure of the arteriotomy, and imaging related to the completion of the procedure. These codes pertain to open and/or percutaneous access. There is only one vessel within the femoral/popliteal region that can be treated within the same surgical session. A single code is reported based on the specific procedures performed in this area, including the common, deep, and superficial femoral arteries and the popliteal artery. Do not report these codes in addition to 0505T, when performed in the femoral-popliteal. Supplies used when providing 37224 or 37226 may be reported with HCPCS Level II code C2623. Check with the specific payer to determine coverage.

ICD-10-CM Diagnostic Codes

I70.211 Atherosclerosis of native arteries of extremities with intermittent claudication, right leg A ☑

I70.221 Atherosclerosis of native arteries of extremities with rest pain, right leg A ☑

I70.231 Atherosclerosis of native arteries of right leg with ulceration of thigh A ☑

I70.232 Atherosclerosis of native arteries of right leg with ulceration of calf A ☑

I70.233 Atherosclerosis of native arteries of right leg with ulceration of ankle A ☑

I70.241 Atherosclerosis of native arteries of left leg with ulceration of thigh A ☑

I70.242 Atherosclerosis of native arteries of left leg with ulceration of calf A ☑

I70.243 Atherosclerosis of native arteries of left leg with ulceration of ankle A ☑

I70.244 Atherosclerosis of native arteries of left leg with ulceration of heel and midfoot A ☑

I70.261 Atherosclerosis of native arteries of extremities with gangrene, right leg A ☑

I70.511 Atherosclerosis of nonautologous biological bypass graft(s) of the extremities with intermittent claudication, right leg A ☑

I70.512 Atherosclerosis of nonautologous biological bypass graft(s) of the extremities with intermittent claudication, left leg A ☑

I70.521 Atherosclerosis of nonautologous biological bypass graft(s) of the extremities with rest pain, right leg A ☑

I70.531 Atherosclerosis of nonautologous biological bypass graft(s) of the right leg with ulceration of thigh A ☑

I70.532 Atherosclerosis of nonautologous biological bypass graft(s) of the right leg with ulceration of calf A ☑

I70.533 Atherosclerosis of nonautologous biological bypass graft(s) of the right leg with ulceration of ankle A ☑

I70.534 Atherosclerosis of nonautologous biological bypass graft(s) of the right leg with ulceration of heel and midfoot A ☑

I70.562 Atherosclerosis of nonautologous biological bypass graft(s) of the extremities with gangrene, left leg A ☑

I70.611 Atherosclerosis of nonbiological bypass graft(s) of the extremities with intermittent claudication, right leg A ☑

I70.621 Atherosclerosis of nonbiological bypass graft(s) of the extremities with rest pain, right leg A ☑

I70.631 Atherosclerosis of nonbiological bypass graft(s) of the right leg with ulceration of thigh A ☑

I70.632 Atherosclerosis of nonbiological bypass graft(s) of the right leg with ulceration of calf A ☑

I70.633 Atherosclerosis of nonbiological bypass graft(s) of the right leg with ulceration of ankle A ☑

I70.634 Atherosclerosis of nonbiological bypass graft(s) of the right leg with ulceration of heel and midfoot A ☑

I70.92 Chronic total occlusion of artery of the extremities A

I72.4 Aneurysm of artery of lower extremity

I74.3 Embolism and thrombosis of arteries of the lower extremities

I76 Septic arterial embolism

I77.1 Stricture of artery

I77.2 Rupture of artery

I77.3 Arterial fibromuscular dysplasia

I77.5 Necrosis of artery

AMA: 37224 2020,Jul; 2019,Jun **37225** 2020,Jul; 2019,Jun **37226** 2023,Dec; 2020,Jul; 2019,Jun **37227** 2020,Jul; 2019,Jun

Relative Value Units/Medicare Edits

Non-Facility RVU	Work	PE	MP	Total
37224	8.75	74.88	1.99	85.62
37225	11.75	242.41	2.54	256.7
37226	10.24	225.21	2.33	237.78
37227	14.25	310.48	3.07	327.8
Facility RVU	**Work**	**PE**	**MP**	**Total**
37224	8.75	2.2	1.99	12.94
37225	11.75	3.12	2.54	17.41
37226	10.24	2.52	2.33	15.09
37227	14.25	3.51	3.07	20.83

	FUD	Status	MUE	Modifiers				IOM Reference
37224	0	A	1(2)	51	50	N/A	80*	None
37225	0	A	1(2)	51	50	N/A	80*	
37226	0	A	1(2)	51	50	N/A	80*	
37227	0	A	1(2)	51	50	N/A	80*	

* with documentation

37228-37231

37228 Revascularization, endovascular, open or percutaneous, tibial, peroneal artery, unilateral, initial vessel; with transluminal angioplasty

37229 with atherectomy, includes angioplasty within the same vessel, when performed

37230 with transluminal stent placement(s), includes angioplasty within the same vessel, when performed

37231 Revascularization, endovascular, open or percutaneous, tibial, peroneal artery, unilateral, initial vessel; with transluminal stent placement(s) and atherectomy, includes angioplasty within the same vessel, when performed

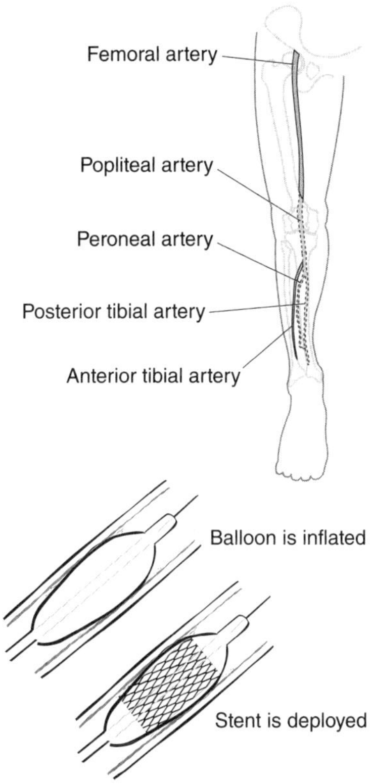

Explanation

The physician treats occlusive disease of a unilateral tibial or peroneal artery by endovascular revascularization (restoration of blood supply) using angioplasty in 37228. Access is gained using a femoral cutdown incision or a percutaneous sheath. Under local anesthesia, the physician accesses the femoral artery. After sheath or needle placement, intra-arterial heparin may be administered. A guidewire is inserted into the artery, followed by a catheter with an attached balloon. The catheter is advanced through the arterial system and into the narrowed portion of the targeted artery. There, the balloon is inflated in order to dilate the vessel to a larger diameter; several inflations may be necessary to achieve maximal results. The physician withdraws the deflated catheter and applies pressure to the puncture site to staunch the bleeding or closes the arteriotomy with suture. In 37229, the physician also performs atherectomy. The physician slides a guidewire through the atherectomy catheter or device, and inserts the guidewire/atherectomy catheter combination through the introducer sheath. The atherectomy device is fluoroscopically positioned at the site of the stenosis. The physician activates the device to remove the stenotic tissue and then rechecks the diameter of the lesion by angiography. Several passes with the atherectomy device may be required. The physician removes the atherectomy catheter, guidewire, and introducer sheath. In 37230, the physician places one or more transluminal stents percutaneously using a guidewire or by incision. A catheter with a stent-transporting tip is threaded into the vessel. The catheter travels to the point where the vessel needs additional support, and the compressed stent is passed from the catheter into the vessel, where it deploys and expands to support the vessel walls. The catheter is removed. Pressure is applied over the percutaneous puncture site or, if performed via open approach, the vessel may be repaired and the skin incision closed by sutures. Angioplasty within the same vessel is included in 37230. Report 37231 if the physician performs both stent placement and atherectomy.

Coding Tips

When medically necessary, report moderate (conscious) sedation provided by the performing physician with 99151-99153. When provided by another physician, report 99155-99157. These procedures include accessing and selective catheterization of the vessel, traversing the lesion, radiological supervision and interpretation related to the vessel, embolic protection if utilized, closure of the arteriotomy, and imaging related to the completion of the procedure. These codes pertain to open and/or percutaneous access. There are up to three vessels within the tibial/peroneal region that can be treated within the same surgical session. Report 37227, 37228, 37229, or 37230 for the initial vessel treated within one leg. Report add-on codes 37232–37235 for other vessels when treated.

ICD-10-CM Diagnostic Codes

I70.211	Atherosclerosis of native arteries of extremities with intermittent claudication, right leg A ☑
I70.221	Atherosclerosis of native arteries of extremities with rest pain, right leg A ☑
I70.231	Atherosclerosis of native arteries of right leg with ulceration of thigh A ☑
I70.232	Atherosclerosis of native arteries of right leg with ulceration of calf A ☑
I70.233	Atherosclerosis of native arteries of right leg with ulceration of ankle A ☑
I70.261	Atherosclerosis of native arteries of extremities with gangrene, right leg A ☑
I70.511	Atherosclerosis of nonautologous biological bypass graft(s) of the extremities with intermittent claudication, right leg A ☑
I70.521	Atherosclerosis of nonautologous biological bypass graft(s) of the extremities with rest pain, right leg A ☑
I70.531	Atherosclerosis of nonautologous biological bypass graft(s) of the right leg with ulceration of thigh A ☑
I70.532	Atherosclerosis of nonautologous biological bypass graft(s) of the right leg with ulceration of calf A ☑
I70.533	Atherosclerosis of nonautologous biological bypass graft(s) of the right leg with ulceration of ankle A ☑
I70.534	Atherosclerosis of nonautologous biological bypass graft(s) of the right leg with ulceration of heel and midfoot A ☑
I70.535	Atherosclerosis of nonautologous biological bypass graft(s) of the right leg with ulceration of other part of foot A ☑
I70.611	Atherosclerosis of nonbiological bypass graft(s) of the extremities with intermittent claudication, right leg A ☑
I70.621	Atherosclerosis of nonbiological bypass graft(s) of the extremities with rest pain, right leg A ☑
I70.631	Atherosclerosis of nonbiological bypass graft(s) of the right leg with ulceration of thigh A ☑
I70.632	Atherosclerosis of nonbiological bypass graft(s) of the right leg with ulceration of calf A ☑

I70.633	Atherosclerosis of nonbiological bypass graft(s) of the right leg with ulceration of ankle A ☑
I70.634	Atherosclerosis of nonbiological bypass graft(s) of the right leg with ulceration of heel and midfoot A ☑
I70.635	Atherosclerosis of nonbiological bypass graft(s) of the right leg with ulceration of other part of foot A ☑
I70.92	Chronic total occlusion of artery of the extremities A
I72.4	Aneurysm of artery of lower extremity
I74.3	Embolism and thrombosis of arteries of the lower extremities
I75.022	Atheroembolism of left lower extremity ☑
I76	Septic arterial embolism
I77.1	Stricture of artery
I77.2	Rupture of artery
I77.3	Arterial fibromuscular dysplasia
I77.5	Necrosis of artery

AMA: **37228** 2020,Jul; 2019,Jun **37229** 2020,Jul; 2019,Jun **37230** 2020,Jul; 2019,Jun **37231** 2020,Jul; 2019,Jun

Relative Value Units/Medicare Edits

Non-Facility RVU	Work	PE	MP	Total
37228	10.75	108.2	2.38	121.33
37229	13.8	244.6	2.79	261.19
37230	13.55	245.1	2.96	261.61
37231	14.75	327.96	2.68	345.39
Facility RVU	**Work**	**PE**	**MP**	**Total**
37228	10.75	2.6	2.38	15.73
37229	13.8	3.56	2.79	20.15
37230	13.55	3.65	2.96	20.16
37231	14.75	3.92	2.68	21.35

	FUD	Status	MUE	Modifiers				IOM Reference
37228	0	A	1(2)	51	50	N/A	80*	None
37229	0	A	1(2)	51	50	N/A	80*	
37230	0	A	1(2)	51	50	N/A	80*	
37231	0	A	1(2)	51	50	N/A	80*	

* with documentation

37232-37235

+ **37232** Revascularization, endovascular, open or percutaneous, tibial/peroneal artery, unilateral, each additional vessel; with transluminal angioplasty (List separately in addition to code for primary procedure)
+ **37233** with atherectomy, includes angioplasty within the same vessel, when performed (List separately in addition to code for primary procedure)
+ **37234** with transluminal stent placement(s), includes angioplasty within the same vessel, when performed (List separately in addition to code for primary procedure)
+ **37235** with transluminal stent placement(s) and atherectomy, includes angioplasty within the same vessel, when performed (List separately in addition to code for primary procedure)

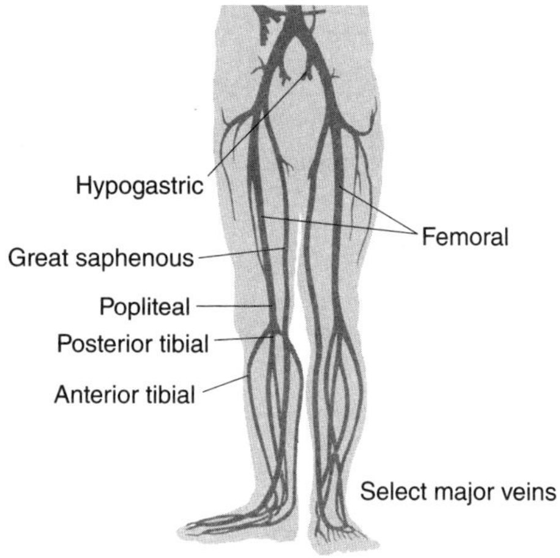

Explanation

The physician treats occlusive disease of unilateral tibial or peroneal arteries by endovascular revascularization (restoration of blood supply) using angioplasty. Access is gained using a femoral cutdown incision or a percutaneous sheath. Under local anesthesia, the physician accesses the femoral artery. After sheath or needle placement, intra-arterial heparin may be administered. A guidewire is inserted into the artery, followed by a catheter with an attached balloon. The catheter is advanced through the arterial system and into the narrowed portion of the targeted artery. The balloon is inflated in order to dilate the vessel to a larger diameter; several inflations may be necessary to achieve maximal results. The physician withdraws the deflated catheter and applies pressure to the puncture site to staunch the bleeding or closes the arteriotomy with suture. In some cases, the physician also performs atherectomy. The physician slides a guidewire through the atherectomy catheter or device and inserts the guidewire/atherectomy catheter combination through the introducer sheath. The atherectomy device is fluoroscopically positioned at the site of the stenosis. The physician activates the device to remove the stenotic tissue and rechecks the diameter of the lesion by angiography. Several passes with the atherectomy device may be required. The physician removes the atherectomy catheter, guidewire, and introducer sheath. In other cases, the physician places one or more transluminal stents percutaneously using a guidewire or by incision. A catheter with a stent-transporting tip is threaded into the vessel. The catheter travels to the point where the vessel needs additional support, and the compressed stent is passed from the catheter into the vessel, where it deploys and expands to support the vessel walls. The catheter is removed. Pressure is applied over the percutaneous puncture site or, if performed via open approach, the vessel may be repaired and the skin incision closed by sutures. Angioplasty within the same vessel is included in the codes for this procedure.

Coding Tips

When medically necessary, report moderate (conscious) sedation provided by the performing physician with 99151-99153. When provided by another physician, report 99155-99157. These procedures include accessing and selective catheterization of the vessel, traversing the lesion, radiological supervision and interpretation related to the vessel, embolic protection if utilized, closure of the arteriotomy, and imaging related to the completion of the procedure. These codes pertain to open and/or percutaneous access. These codes are based on the degree of progression where a code with more intensive procedures includes less intensive procedures (i.e., angioplasty, stent placement, atherectomy). Stent placement includes angioplasty when performed by the physician. Report 37232 with applicable codes in range 37228-37231 for each additional vessel. Report 37233 with 37229 and 37231 for each additional vessel. Report 37234 with 37229, 37230, and 37231 for each additional vessel. Report 37235 with 37231 when the physician performs both stent placement and atherectomy on more than one vessel. There are up to three vessels within the tibial/peroneal region that can be treated within the same surgical session. Report 37227-37230 for the initial vessel treated within one leg. Report add-on codes 37232–37235 for other vessels when treated.

ICD-10-CM Diagnostic Codes

I70.211	Atherosclerosis of native arteries of extremities with intermittent claudication, right leg A ☑
I70.221	Atherosclerosis of native arteries of extremities with rest pain, right leg A ☑
I70.231	Atherosclerosis of native arteries of right leg with ulceration of thigh A ☑
I70.232	Atherosclerosis of native arteries of right leg with ulceration of calf A ☑
I70.233	Atherosclerosis of native arteries of right leg with ulceration of ankle A ☑
I70.234	Atherosclerosis of native arteries of right leg with ulceration of heel and midfoot A ☑
I70.235	Atherosclerosis of native arteries of right leg with ulceration of other part of foot A ☑
I70.261	Atherosclerosis of native arteries of extremities with gangrene, right leg A ☑
I70.511	Atherosclerosis of nonautologous biological bypass graft(s) of the extremities with intermittent claudication, right leg A ☑
I70.521	Atherosclerosis of nonautologous biological bypass graft(s) of the extremities with rest pain, right leg A ☑
I70.531	Atherosclerosis of nonautologous biological bypass graft(s) of the right leg with ulceration of thigh A ☑
I70.532	Atherosclerosis of nonautologous biological bypass graft(s) of the right leg with ulceration of calf A ☑
I70.533	Atherosclerosis of nonautologous biological bypass graft(s) of the right leg with ulceration of ankle A ☑
I70.534	Atherosclerosis of nonautologous biological bypass graft(s) of the right leg with ulceration of heel and midfoot A ☑
I70.535	Atherosclerosis of nonautologous biological bypass graft(s) of the right leg with ulceration of other part of foot A ☑
I70.561	Atherosclerosis of nonautologous biological bypass graft(s) of the extremities with gangrene, right leg A ☑
I70.621	Atherosclerosis of nonbiological bypass graft(s) of the extremities with rest pain, right leg A ☑
I70.631	Atherosclerosis of nonbiological bypass graft(s) of the right leg with ulceration of thigh A ☑
I70.632	Atherosclerosis of nonbiological bypass graft(s) of the right leg with ulceration of calf A ☑
I70.633	Atherosclerosis of nonbiological bypass graft(s) of the right leg with ulceration of ankle A ☑
I70.634	Atherosclerosis of nonbiological bypass graft(s) of the right leg with ulceration of heel and midfoot A ☑
I70.635	Atherosclerosis of nonbiological bypass graft(s) of the right leg with ulceration of other part of foot A ☑
I70.661	Atherosclerosis of nonbiological bypass graft(s) of the extremities with gangrene, right leg A ☑
I70.92	Chronic total occlusion of artery of the extremities A
I74.3	Embolism and thrombosis of arteries of the lower extremities
I76	Septic arterial embolism
I77.1	Stricture of artery
I77.3	Arterial fibromuscular dysplasia
I77.5	Necrosis of artery

AMA: **37232** 2020,Jul; 2019,Jun **37233** 2020,Jul; 2019,Jun **37234** 2020,Jul; 2019,Jun **37235** 2020,Jul; 2019,Jun

Relative Value Units/Medicare Edits

Non-Facility RVU	Work	PE	MP	Total
37232	4.0	19.32	0.82	24.14
37233	6.5	23.26	1.25	31.01
37234	5.5	100.0	1.18	106.68
37235	7.8	106.97	1.1	115.87
Facility RVU	**Work**	**PE**	**MP**	**Total**
37232	4.0	0.97	0.82	5.79
37233	6.5	1.61	1.25	9.36
37234	5.5	1.5	1.18	8.18
37235	7.8	1.79	1.1	10.69

	FUD	Status	MUE	Modifiers				IOM Reference
37232	N/A	A	2(3)	N/A	50	N/A	80*	None
37233	N/A	A	2(3)	N/A	50	N/A	80*	
37234	N/A	A	2(3)	N/A	50	N/A	80*	
37235	N/A	A	2(3)	N/A	50	N/A	80*	

* with documentation

[37246, 37247]

37246 Transluminal balloon angioplasty (except lower extremity artery(ies) for occlusive disease, intracranial, coronary, pulmonary, or dialysis circuit), open or percutaneous, including all imaging and radiological supervision and interpretation necessary to perform the angioplasty within the same artery; initial artery

\+ **37247** Transluminal balloon angioplasty (except lower extremity artery(ies) for occlusive disease, intracranial, coronary, pulmonary, or dialysis circuit), open or percutaneous, including all imaging and radiological supervision and interpretation necessary to perform the angioplasty within the same artery; each additional artery (List separately in addition to code for primary procedure)

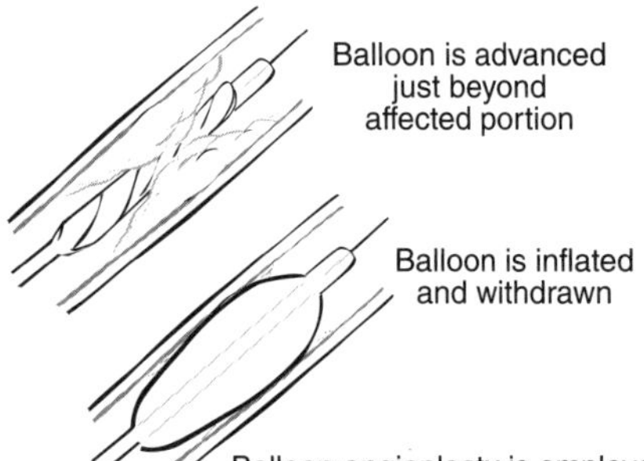

Balloon angioplasty is employed to treat occlusive disease

Explanation

Transluminal balloon angioplasty is performed by open or percutaneous approach (except lower limb arterial occlusion, intracranial, coronary, pulmonary, or dialysis circuit). In an open procedure, the physician makes an incision in the skin overlying the vessel. The vessel is dissected from adjacent critical structures, and vessel clamps are applied. The physician may nick the vessel to create an opening into which a catheter with a balloon attached is inserted into the vessel and threaded. The catheter is fed into the narrowed portion of the vessel, where its balloon is inflated in the narrowed area. The blood vessel is stretched to a larger diameter, allowing a more normal outflow of blood through the area. Several inflations may be performed along the narrowed area. The catheter is slowly withdrawn after deflation. Occasionally, the opening in the vessel is repaired with sutures. In a percutaneous approach, the physician isolates the vessel and inserts a large needle through the skin and into the vessel. A guidewire is threaded through the needle into the vessel. The needle is removed. A catheter with a balloon attached follows the wire into the vessel. The wire is removed. The catheter is fed through the vascular system and into the narrowed portion of the affected vessel and the balloon is inflated. The blood vessel is stretched to a larger diameter, allowing a more normal outflow of blood through the area. Several inflations may be performed along the narrowed area. The catheter is slowly withdrawn after deflation. Pressure is applied to the puncture site to stop the bleeding after the catheter is removed. These codes include all radiological imaging within the same artery. Report 37246 for the initial artery treated and 37247 for each additional artery.

Coding Tips

Report 37247 in addition to 37246. Radiological supervision and interpretation and imaging used to record the completion of the intervention are included in these codes. Do not report these codes with 37215-37218 or 37220-37237 during the same operative encounter in the same artery. Do not report these codes with 34841-34848 for angioplasty for insertion of bare metal/covered stent into the visceral branches within the endoprosthesis target zone. Do not report 37246-37247 with 36836 or 36837.

ICD-10-CM Diagnostic Codes

I70.1	Atherosclerosis of renal artery A
I70.8	Atherosclerosis of other arteries A
I74.8	Embolism and thrombosis of other arteries
I75.81	Atheroembolism of kidney
I77.1	Stricture of artery
I77.3	Arterial fibromuscular dysplasia
I77.4	Celiac artery compression syndrome
I77.89	Other specified disorders of arteries and arterioles
K55.011	Focal (segmental) acute (reversible) ischemia of small intestine
K55.012	Diffuse acute (reversible) ischemia of small intestine
K55.021	Focal (segmental) acute infarction of small intestine
K55.022	Diffuse acute infarction of small intestine
K55.031	Focal (segmental) acute (reversible) ischemia of large intestine
K55.032	Diffuse acute (reversible) ischemia of large intestine
K55.041	Focal (segmental) acute infarction of large intestine
K55.042	Diffuse acute infarction of large intestine
K55.1	Chronic vascular disorders of intestine
K55.8	Other vascular disorders of intestine
N28.0	Ischemia and infarction of kidney
Q27.1	Congenital renal artery stenosis
Q27.2	Other congenital malformations of renal artery

AMA: 37246 2023,Jun; 2023,May; 2023,Mar; 2022,Oct; 2021,Dec **37247** 2022,Oct

Relative Value Units/Medicare Edits

Non-Facility RVU	Work	PE	MP	Total
37246	7.0	45.02	1.31	53.33
37247	3.5	13.16	0.68	17.34
Facility RVU	**Work**	**PE**	**MP**	**Total**
37246	7.0	1.83	1.31	10.14
37247	3.5	0.87	0.68	5.05

	FUD	Status	MUE	Modifiers				IOM Reference
37246	0	A	1(2)	51	50	N/A	N/A	None
37247	N/A	A	2(3)	N/A	50	N/A	N/A	

* with documentation

Terms To Know

hypertension. Abnormally increased pressure, usually referring to arterial pressure, exceeding an acceptable range.

ischemia. Deficiency in blood supply causing tissues to be deprived of oxygen, resulting from trauma, mechanical or functional constriction of blood vessels, or a physical obstruction.

occlusion. Constriction, closure, or blockage of a passage.

transluminal balloon angioplasty. Balloon-tipped catheter is placed within a narrowed artery or vein and the balloon is inflated to stretch the vessel to a larger diameter for increased blood flow.

[37248, 37249]

37248 Transluminal balloon angioplasty (except dialysis circuit), open or percutaneous, including all imaging and radiological supervision and interpretation necessary to perform the angioplasty within the same vein; initial vein

\+ **37249** Transluminal balloon angioplasty (except dialysis circuit), open or percutaneous, including all imaging and radiological supervision and interpretation necessary to perform the angioplasty within the same vein; each additional vein (List separately in addition to code for primary procedure)

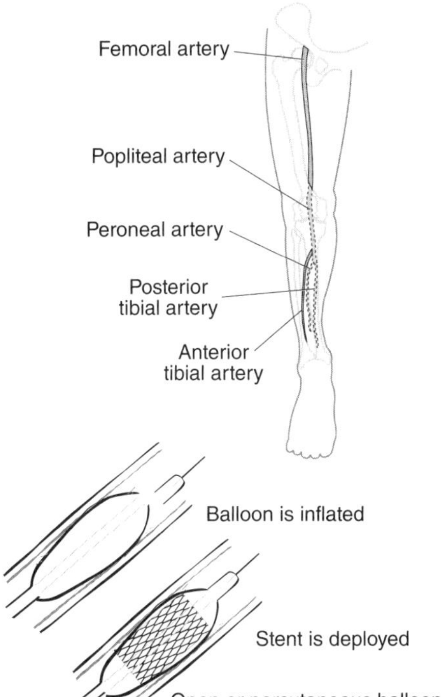

Open or percutaneous balloon angioplasty including imaging

Explanation

Transluminal balloon angioplasty is performed by open or percutaneous approach (except dialysis circuit). In an open procedure, the physician makes an incision in the skin overlying the vessel. The vessel is dissected from adjacent critical structures and vessel clamps are applied. The physician may nick the vessel to create an opening into which a catheter with a balloon attached is inserted into the vessel and threaded. The catheter is fed into the narrowed portion of the vessel, where its balloon is inflated in the narrowed area. The blood vessel is stretched to a larger diameter, allowing a more normal outflow of blood through the area. Several inflations may be performed along the narrowed area. The catheter is slowly withdrawn after deflation. Occasionally, the opening in the vessel is repaired with sutures. In a percutaneous approach, the physician isolates the vessel and inserts a large needle through the skin and into the vessel. A guidewire is threaded through the needle into the vessel. The needle is removed. A catheter with a balloon attached follows the wire into the vessel. The wire is removed. The catheter is fed through the vascular system and into the narrowed portion of the affected vessel and the balloon is inflated. The blood vessel is stretched to a larger diameter, allowing a more normal outflow of blood through the area. Several inflations may be performed along the narrowed area. The catheter is slowly withdrawn after deflation. Pressure is applied to the puncture site to stop the bleeding after the catheter is removed. These codes include all radiological imaging within the same vein. Report 37248 for the initial vein treated and 37249 for each additional vein.

Coding Tips

Report 37249 in addition to 37248. Radiological supervision and interpretation and imaging used to record the completion of the intervention are included in these codes. Do not report 37248 or 37249 with 37238 or 37239 during the same operative encounter in the same vein. Intravascular ultrasound may be reported separately, see 37252 and 37253. Do not report these codes in addition to 0505T when performed in the femoral-popliteal. Do not report these codes in addition to 0620T when performed in the tibial-peroneal. Do not report these codes with 36836 or 36837. For balloon angioplasty performed through the dialysis circuit, see 36902-36908. For transluminal balloon angioplasty in aorta/visceral artery during fenestrated endovascular repair, see 34841-34848; in the iliac, femoral, popliteal, or tibial/peroneal artery due to occlusive disease, see 37220-37235; in an intracranial artery, see 61630 or 61635.

ICD-10-CM Diagnostic Codes

The application of this code is too broad to adequately present ICD-10-CM diagnostic code links here. Refer to your ICD-10-CM book.

AMA: **37248** 2023,Nov; 2023,May; 2023,Mar; 2022,Oct **37249** 2022,Oct

Relative Value Units/Medicare Edits

Non-Facility RVU	Work	PE	MP	Total
37248	6.0	32.86	0.91	39.77
37249	2.97	9.51	0.53	13.01
Facility RVU	**Work**	**PE**	**MP**	**Total**
37248	6.0	1.74	0.91	8.65
37249	2.97	0.74	0.53	4.24

	FUD	Status	MUE	Modifiers				IOM Reference
37248	0	A	1(2)	51	50	N/A	N/A	None
37249	N/A	A	3(3)	N/A	50	N/A	N/A	

* with documentation

Arteries and Veins

37236-37237

37236 Transcatheter placement of an intravascular stent(s) (except lower extremity artery(s) for occlusive disease, cervical carotid, extracranial vertebral or intrathoracic carotid, intracranial, or coronary), open or percutaneous, including radiological supervision and interpretation and including all angioplasty within the same vessel, when performed; initial artery

\+ **37237** each additional artery (List separately in addition to code for primary procedure)

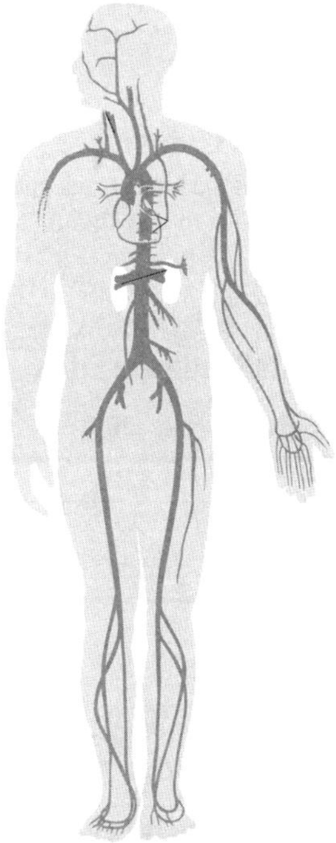

Map of major arteries

Explanation

The physician places one or more intravascular stents through a catheter into an artery other than a coronary, cervical or intrathoracic carotid, extracranial vertebral, iliac, intracranial, or lower extremity artery. The procedure may be performed via a percutaneous or an open approach. In the percutaneous approach, a guidewire is threaded through the needle into the blood vessel and the needle is removed. In the open approach, the physician makes an incision in the skin overlying the vessel to be catheterized. The vessel is dissected and nicked with a small blade. After the approach, a catheter with a stent-transporting tip is threaded over the guidewire into the vessel and the wire is extracted. The catheter travels to the point where the vessel needs additional support. The compressed stent is passed from the catheter out into the vessel, where it deploys, expanding to support the vessel walls. The catheter is removed and pressure is applied over the puncture site or layered closure is performed. Report 37236 for stents placed in the initial artery and 37237 for each additional artery where a stent is placed. These procedures include radiologic supervision and interpretation, as well as angioplasty, when performed.

Coding Tips

When medically necessary, report moderate (conscious) sedation provided by the performing physician with 99151-99153. When provided by another physician, report 99155-99157. Report 37237 in addition to 37236. These codes include all balloon angioplasty procedures performed in the treated vessel including pre- and postdilation, treatment of lesions outside of the stented segment but within the same vessel, and use of a smaller or larger balloon to achieve the same therapeutic result. Angioplasty performed in vessels other than the one being reported with this code can be reported separately. Selective and/or nonselective catheterization is reported separately in addition to 37236–37237. These codes include supervision and interpretation of radiology services related to the intervention, as well as imaging to document completion of the intervention. Also included are closure of the arteriotomy via pressure and application of an arterial closure device or standard closure of the puncture site by suture. Extensive repairs or replacement of the artery may be reported separately, see 35226 or 35286. Ultrasound guidance for vascular access (76937) may be reported separately, as well as intravascular ultrasound (37252–37253). If a stent is being deployed for the purpose of serving as a lattice work for embolization coils, use the embolization code and not the stent deployment code. Do not report 37236–37237 with 34841–34848 for bare metal or covered stents placed into the visceral branches within the endoprosthesis target zone. Do not report these codes with 36836 or 36837. For transcatheter placement of intravascular stent in the intracranial vessels, see 61635. For stent placement in iliac, femoral, popliteal, or tibial/peroneal artery for occlusive disease, see 37221, 37223, 37226, 37227, 37230, 37231, 37234, and 37235. For open or percutaneous antegrade transcatheter placement of intrathoracic carotid/innominate artery stent, see 37218. For open or percutaneous transcatheter placement of extracranial vertebral artery stent, see 0075T and 0076T. For placement of stent at arterial anastomosis of the dialysis circuit, see 36903 or 36906.

ICD-10-CM Diagnostic Codes

A52.01	Syphilitic aneurysm of aorta
I15.0	Renovascular hypertension
I70.0	Atherosclerosis of aorta A
I70.1	Atherosclerosis of renal artery A
I70.218	Atherosclerosis of native arteries of extremities with intermittent claudication, other extremity A
I70.228	Atherosclerosis of native arteries of extremities with rest pain, other extremity A
I70.25	Atherosclerosis of native arteries of other extremities with ulceration A
I70.268	Atherosclerosis of native arteries of extremities with gangrene, other extremity A
I70.92	Chronic total occlusion of artery of the extremities A
I71.02	Dissection of abdominal aorta
I71.03	Dissection of thoracoabdominal aorta
I72.1	Aneurysm of artery of upper extremity
I74.01	Saddle embolus of abdominal aorta
I74.2	Embolism and thrombosis of arteries of the upper extremities
I74.5	Embolism and thrombosis of iliac artery
I75.011	Atheroembolism of right upper extremity ☑
I75.012	Atheroembolism of left upper extremity ☑
I75.81	Atheroembolism of kidney
I77.1	Stricture of artery
I77.3	Arterial fibromuscular dysplasia
I77.72	Dissection of iliac artery
I77.73	Dissection of renal artery
K55.011	Focal (segmental) acute (reversible) ischemia of small intestine
K55.012	Diffuse acute (reversible) ischemia of small intestine
K55.021	Focal (segmental) acute infarction of small intestine
K55.022	Diffuse acute infarction of small intestine
K55.031	Focal (segmental) acute (reversible) ischemia of large intestine

K55.032 Diffuse acute (reversible) ischemia of large intestine
K55.041 Focal (segmental) acute infarction of large intestine
K55.042 Diffuse acute infarction of large intestine
K55.1 Chronic vascular disorders of intestine
Q25.21 Interruption of aortic arch
Q25.29 Other atresia of aorta
Q25.3 Supravalvular aortic stenosis
Q25.41 Absence and aplasia of aorta
Q25.42 Hypoplasia of aorta
Q25.43 Congenital aneurysm of aorta
Q25.44 Congenital dilation of aorta
Q25.45 Double aortic arch
Q25.46 Tortuous aortic arch
Q25.47 Right aortic arch
Q25.48 Anomalous origin of subclavian artery
Q25.5 Atresia of pulmonary artery
Q25.71 Coarctation of pulmonary artery
Q27.1 Congenital renal artery stenosis
Q27.34 Arteriovenous malformation of renal vessel

AMA: 37236 2023,Jun; 2023,May; 2023,Mar; 2022,Oct; 2021,Dec **37237** 2023,May

Relative Value Units/Medicare Edits

Non-Facility RVU	Work	PE	MP	Total
37236	8.75	70.03	1.91	80.69
37237	4.25	32.73	0.96	37.94
Facility RVU	**Work**	**PE**	**MP**	**Total**
37236	8.75	2.18	1.91	12.84
37237	4.25	0.94	0.96	6.15

	FUD	Status	MUE	Modifiers				IOM Reference
37236	0	A	1(2)	51	50	N/A	80*	None
37237	N/A	A	2(3)	N/A	50	N/A	80*	

* with documentation

37238-37239

37238 Transcatheter placement of an intravascular stent(s), open or percutaneous, including radiological supervision and interpretation and including angioplasty within the same vessel, when performed; initial vein

\+ **37239** each additional vein (List separately in addition to code for primary procedure)

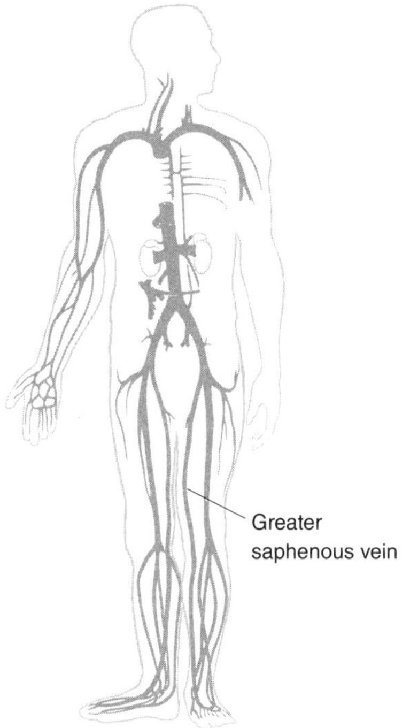

Map of major veins

Explanation

The physician places one or more intravascular stents through a catheter into a vein. The procedure may be performed via a percutaneous or an open approach. In the percutaneous approach, a guidewire is threaded through the needle into the blood vessel and the needle is removed. In the open approach, the physician makes an incision in the skin overlying the vessel to be catheterized. The vessel is dissected and nicked with a small blade. After the approach, a catheter with a stent-transporting tip is threaded over the guidewire into the vessel and the wire is extracted. The catheter travels to the point where the vessel needs additional support. The compressed stent is passed from the catheter out into the vessel, where it deploys, expanding to support the vessel walls. The catheter is removed and pressure is applied over the puncture site or layered closure is performed. Report 37238 for stents placed in the initial vein and 37239 for each additional vein where a stent is placed.

Coding Tips

When medically necessary, report moderate (conscious) sedation provided by the performing physician with 99151-99153. When provided by another physician, report 99155-99157. Report 37239 in addition to 37238. These codes include all balloon angioplasty procedures performed in the treated vessel, including pre- and postdilation, treatment of lesions outside of the stented segment but within the same vessel, and use of a smaller or larger balloon to achieve the same therapeutic result. Angioplasty performed in vessels other than the one being reported with this code can be reported separately. Selective and/or nonselective catheterization is reported separately in addition to 37238–37239. These codes include supervision and interpretation of radiology services related to the intervention, as well as imaging to document completion of the intervention. Also included is closure of the arteriotomy via pressure and application of an arterial closure device or standard closure of the puncture site by suture. Extensive repairs or replacement of the artery may be reported separately, see 35226 or 35286. Ultrasound guidance for vascular access (76937) may be reported separately, as well as intravascular ultrasound (37252–37253). If a stent is being deployed for the purpose of serving as a lattice work for embolization coils, use the embolization code and not the stent deployment code. Do not report these codes in addition to 0505T, when performed in the femoral-popliteal. Do not report these codes in addition to 0620T, when performed in the tibial-peroneal. Do not report these codes with 36836 or 36837. For transcatheter placement of an intravascular stent in the intracranial vessels, see 61635. For stent placement in iliac, femoral, popliteal, or tibial/peroneal artery for occlusive disease, see 37221, 37223, 37226, 37227, 37230, 37231, 37234, and 37235; for cervical carotid, see 37215-37216; for intracoronary, see 92928, 92929, 92933, 92934, 92937, 92938, 92941, 92943, and 92944; for open retrograde intrathoracic common carotid or innominate vessels, see 37217. For open or percutaneous antegrade transcatheter placement of an intrathoracic carotid/innominate artery stent, see 37218. For open or percutaneous transcatheter placement of an extracranial vertebral artery stent, see 0075T and 0076T. For placement of a stent within the peripheral segment of dialysis segment, see 36903 or 36906. For transcatheter placement of an intravascular stent within the central dialysis segment performed through the dialysis segment, see 36908.

ICD-10-CM Diagnostic Codes

I80.11 Phlebitis and thrombophlebitis of right femoral vein ☑
I80.12 Phlebitis and thrombophlebitis of left femoral vein ☑
I80.211 Phlebitis and thrombophlebitis of right iliac vein ☑
I80.212 Phlebitis and thrombophlebitis of left iliac vein ☑
I80.221 Phlebitis and thrombophlebitis of right popliteal vein ☑
I80.222 Phlebitis and thrombophlebitis of left popliteal vein ☑
I80.231 Phlebitis and thrombophlebitis of right tibial vein ☑
I80.232 Phlebitis and thrombophlebitis of left tibial vein ☑
I80.241 Phlebitis and thrombophlebitis of right peroneal vein ☑
I81 Portal vein thrombosis
I82.210 Acute embolism and thrombosis of superior vena cava
I82.220 Acute embolism and thrombosis of inferior vena cava
I82.221 Chronic embolism and thrombosis of inferior vena cava
I82.411 Acute embolism and thrombosis of right femoral vein ☑
I82.412 Acute embolism and thrombosis of left femoral vein ☑
I82.421 Acute embolism and thrombosis of right iliac vein ☑
I82.422 Acute embolism and thrombosis of left iliac vein ☑
I82.451 Acute embolism and thrombosis of right peroneal vein ☑
I82.511 Chronic embolism and thrombosis of right femoral vein ☑
I82.512 Chronic embolism and thrombosis of left femoral vein ☑
I82.521 Chronic embolism and thrombosis of right iliac vein ☑
I82.522 Chronic embolism and thrombosis of left iliac vein ☑
I82.621 Acute embolism and thrombosis of deep veins of right upper extremity ☑
I82.622 Acute embolism and thrombosis of deep veins of left upper extremity ☑
I82.721 Chronic embolism and thrombosis of deep veins of right upper extremity ☑
I82.722 Chronic embolism and thrombosis of deep veins of left upper extremity ☑
I82.A11 Acute embolism and thrombosis of right axillary vein ☑
I82.A12 Acute embolism and thrombosis of left axillary vein ☑
I82.B11 Acute embolism and thrombosis of right subclavian vein ☑
I82.B12 Acute embolism and thrombosis of left subclavian vein ☑
I87.001 Postthrombotic syndrome without complications of right lower extremity ☑
I87.002 Postthrombotic syndrome without complications of left lower extremity ☑
I87.091 Postthrombotic syndrome with other complications of right lower extremity ☑
I87.092 Postthrombotic syndrome with other complications of left lower extremity ☑
I87.1 Compression of vein
Q26.0 Congenital stenosis of vena cava
Q26.1 Persistent left superior vena cava

AMA: **37238** 2023,May; 2023,Mar; 2022,Oct

Relative Value Units/Medicare Edits

Non-Facility RVU	Work	PE	MP	Total
37238	6.04	94.05	1.2	101.29
37239	2.97	47.05	0.59	50.61
Facility RVU	**Work**	**PE**	**MP**	**Total**
37238	6.04	1.7	1.2	8.94
37239	2.97	0.82	0.59	4.38

	FUD	Status	MUE	Modifiers				IOM Reference
37238	0	A	1(2)	51	50	N/A	80*	None
37239	N/A	A	2(3)	N/A	50	N/A	80*	

* with documentation

Terms To Know

catheter. Flexible tube inserted into an area of the body for introducing or withdrawing fluid.

guidewire. Flexible metal instrument designed to lead another instrument in its proper course.

stent. Tube to provide support in a body cavity or lumen.

37241-37242

37241 Vascular embolization or occlusion, inclusive of all radiological supervision and interpretation, intraprocedural roadmapping, and imaging guidance necessary to complete the intervention; venous, other than hemorrhage (eg, congenital or acquired venous malformations, venous and capillary hemangiomas, varices, varicoceles)

37242 arterial, other than hemorrhage or tumor (eg, congenital or acquired arterial malformations, arteriovenous malformations, arteriovenous fistulas, aneurysms, pseudoaneurysms)

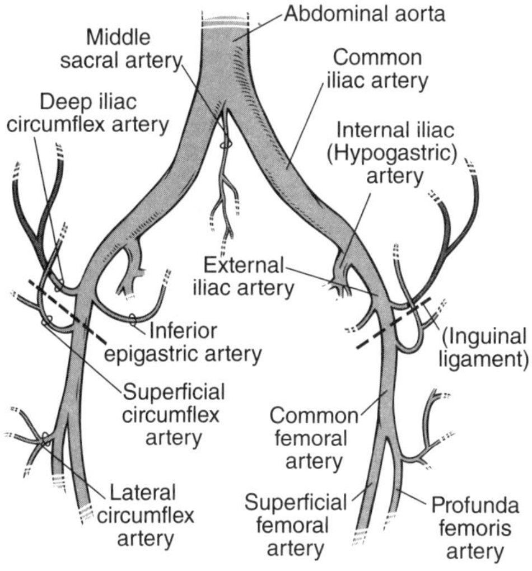

Pelvic arterial anatomy

Explanation

Embolization or occlusion of a blood vessel is performed. A needle is inserted through the skin and into a blood vessel. A guidewire is threaded through the needle into the vessel. The needle is removed. A catheter is threaded into the vessel and the wire is extracted. The catheter travels to the appropriate blood vessel and beads, coils, or another vessel-blocking device are released. The beads or other device block the vessel. The catheter is removed and pressure is applied over the puncture site to stop bleeding. Report 37241 for occlusion of a vein for any condition other than hemorrhage. Report 37242 when the occlusion is of an artery to treat a condition other than hemorrhage or tumor.

Coding Tips

When medically necessary, report moderate (conscious) sedation provided by the performing physician with 99151-99153. When provided by another physician, report 99155-99157. Only one embolization code should be reported for each surgical field, including the entire area directly involved in and immediately surrounding the procedure. If an intravascular stent is deployed for the purpose of providing a lattice work for embolization coils, report the embolization codes. The code representing the immediate cause for the embolization should be used. Diagnostic angiography and catheter placement may be reported separately. Report with an appropriate modifier. Do not report 37241 for treatment of incompetent veins. Do not report 37241 with 36465, 36466, 36468, 36470, 36471, 36473-36479, 75894, or 75898 in the same surgical field. Do not report 37242 with 75894 or 75898 in the same surgical field. Do not report these codes with 36836 or 36837. For sclerosis of veins or endovenous ablation of incompetent extremity veins, see 36468–36479. For percutaneous treatment of an extremity pseudoaneurysms, see 36002. For permanent endovascular embolization or occlusion within the dialysis circuit, see 36909.

ICD-10-CM Diagnostic Codes

D18.01	Hemangioma of skin and subcutaneous tissue
D18.02	Hemangioma of intracranial structures
D18.03	Hemangioma of intra-abdominal structures
I28.0	Arteriovenous fistula of pulmonary vessels
I28.1	Aneurysm of pulmonary artery
I71.11	Aneurysm of the ascending aorta, ruptured
I71.12	Aneurysm of the aortic arch, ruptured
I71.13	Aneurysm of the descending thoracic aorta, ruptured
I71.21	Aneurysm of the ascending aorta, without rupture
I71.22	Aneurysm of the aortic arch, without rupture
I71.23	Aneurysm of the descending thoracic aorta, without rupture
I71.31	Pararenal abdominal aortic aneurysm, ruptured
I71.32	Juxtarenal abdominal aortic aneurysm, ruptured
I71.33	Infrarenal abdominal aortic aneurysm, ruptured
I71.41	Pararenal abdominal aortic aneurysm, without rupture
I71.42	Juxtarenal abdominal aortic aneurysm, without rupture
I71.43	Infrarenal abdominal aortic aneurysm, without rupture
I71.51	Supraceliac aneurysm of the thoracoabdominal aorta, ruptured
I71.52	Paravisceral aneurysm of the thoracoabdominal aorta, ruptured
I71.61	Supraceliac aneurysm of the thoracoabdominal aorta, without rupture
I71.62	Paravisceral aneurysm of the thoracoabdominal aorta, without rupture
I72.0	Aneurysm of carotid artery
I72.1	Aneurysm of artery of upper extremity
I72.2	Aneurysm of renal artery
I72.3	Aneurysm of iliac artery
I72.4	Aneurysm of artery of lower extremity
I72.6	Aneurysm of vertebral artery
I77.0	Arteriovenous fistula, acquired
I83.011	Varicose veins of right lower extremity with ulcer of thigh A ☑
I83.012	Varicose veins of right lower extremity with ulcer of calf A ☑
I83.013	Varicose veins of right lower extremity with ulcer of ankle A ☑
I83.014	Varicose veins of right lower extremity with ulcer of heel and midfoot A ☑
I83.018	Varicose veins of right lower extremity with ulcer other part of lower leg A ☑
I83.11	Varicose veins of right lower extremity with inflammation A ☑
I83.211	Varicose veins of right lower extremity with both ulcer of thigh and inflammation A ☑
I83.212	Varicose veins of right lower extremity with both ulcer of calf and inflammation A ☑
I83.213	Varicose veins of right lower extremity with both ulcer of ankle and inflammation A ☑
I83.214	Varicose veins of right lower extremity with both ulcer of heel and midfoot and inflammation A ☑
I83.811	Varicose veins of right lower extremity with pain A ☑
I83.813	Varicose veins of bilateral lower extremities with pain A ☑
I83.891	Varicose veins of right lower extremity with other complications A ☑
I83.92	Asymptomatic varicose veins of left lower extremity A ☑
I85.00	Esophageal varices without bleeding
I85.01	Esophageal varices with bleeding

I85.10	Secondary esophageal varices without bleeding
I85.11	Secondary esophageal varices with bleeding
I86.0	Sublingual varices
I86.1	Scrotal varices
I86.2	Pelvic varices
I86.3	Vulval varices
I86.4	Gastric varices
Q24.5	Malformation of coronary vessels
Q25.0	Patent ductus arteriosus
Q25.1	Coarctation of aorta
Q25.21	Interruption of aortic arch
Q25.3	Supravalvular aortic stenosis
Q25.41	Absence and aplasia of aorta
Q25.42	Hypoplasia of aorta
Q25.43	Congenital aneurysm of aorta
Q25.44	Congenital dilation of aorta
Q25.45	Double aortic arch
Q25.46	Tortuous aortic arch
Q25.47	Right aortic arch
Q25.48	Anomalous origin of subclavian artery
Q25.5	Atresia of pulmonary artery
Q25.6	Stenosis of pulmonary artery
Q25.71	Coarctation of pulmonary artery
Q25.72	Congenital pulmonary arteriovenous malformation
Q26.0	Congenital stenosis of vena cava
Q26.1	Persistent left superior vena cava
Q26.2	Total anomalous pulmonary venous connection
Q26.3	Partial anomalous pulmonary venous connection
Q26.5	Anomalous portal venous connection
Q27.31	Arteriovenous malformation of vessel of upper limb
Q27.32	Arteriovenous malformation of vessel of lower limb
Q27.33	Arteriovenous malformation of digestive system vessel
Q27.34	Arteriovenous malformation of renal vessel
Q28.0	Arteriovenous malformation of precerebral vessels
Q28.2	Arteriovenous malformation of cerebral vessels

AMA: 37241 2024,May; 2023,Mar; 2022,Oct; 2019,Sep; 2018,Jul; 2018,Mar
37242 2024,May; 2023,Mar; 2022,Oct; 2019,Sep; 2018,Jul; 2018,Mar

Relative Value Units/Medicare Edits

Non-Facility RVU	Work	PE	MP	Total
37241	8.75	125.62	1.29	135.66
37242	9.8	196.01	1.54	207.35
Facility RVU	**Work**	**PE**	**MP**	**Total**
37241	8.75	2.39	1.29	12.43
37242	9.8	2.5	1.54	13.84

	FUD	Status	MUE	Modifiers				IOM Reference
37241	0	A	2(3)	51	N/A	N/A	N/A	None
37242	0	A	2(3)	51	N/A	N/A	N/A	

* with documentation

37243

37243 Vascular embolization or occlusion, inclusive of all radiological supervision and interpretation, intraprocedural roadmapping, and imaging guidance necessary to complete the intervention; for tumors, organ ischemia, or infarction

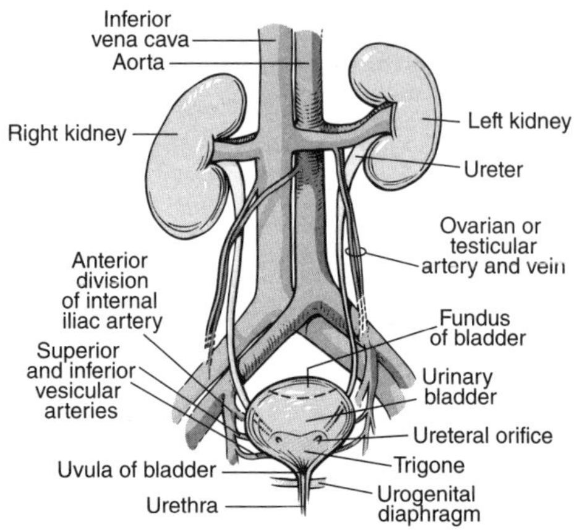

Embolization or occlusion for tumors, organ ischemia, or infarction

Explanation

Embolization or occlusion of an artery is performed to treat tumors or organ infarction/ischemia. A needle is inserted through the skin and into the artery. A guidewire is threaded through the needle and the needle is removed. A catheter is threaded into the vessel over the guidewire and the wire is extracted. The catheter travels to the appropriate site and beads, coils, or another vessel-blocking device are released. The beads or other device block the artery that supplies the tumor or that portion of the organ with blood. The catheter is removed and pressure is applied over the puncture site to stop bleeding.

Coding Tips

When medically necessary, report moderate (conscious) sedation provided by the performing physician with 99151-99153. When provided by another physician, report 99155-99157. Only one embolization code should be reported for each surgical field, including the entire area directly involved in and immediately surrounding the procedure. If chemotherapy or radioisotopes are used with the embolization procedure, additional codes such as 79445 or 96420 may be reported. The code representing the immediate cause for the embolization should be used. Diagnostic angiography and catheter placement may be reported separately. Report with an appropriate modifier. Do not report 37243 with 75894 or 75898 in the same surgical field.

ICD-10-CM Diagnostic Codes

C22.0	Liver cell carcinoma
C23	Malignant neoplasm of gallbladder
C24.0	Malignant neoplasm of extrahepatic bile duct
C24.1	Malignant neoplasm of ampulla of Vater
C41.0	Malignant neoplasm of bones of skull and face
C41.1	Malignant neoplasm of mandible
C41.2	Malignant neoplasm of vertebral column
C41.3	Malignant neoplasm of ribs, sternum and clavicle
C41.4	Malignant neoplasm of pelvic bones, sacrum and coccyx
C64.1	Malignant neoplasm of right kidney, except renal pelvis ☑
C65.1	Malignant neoplasm of right renal pelvis ☑

C71.0 Malignant neoplasm of cerebrum, except lobes and ventricles
C71.1 Malignant neoplasm of frontal lobe
C71.2 Malignant neoplasm of temporal lobe
C71.3 Malignant neoplasm of parietal lobe
C71.4 Malignant neoplasm of occipital lobe
C71.5 Malignant neoplasm of cerebral ventricle
C71.6 Malignant neoplasm of cerebellum
C71.7 Malignant neoplasm of brain stem
C72.0 Malignant neoplasm of spinal cord
C76.0 Malignant neoplasm of head, face and neck
D16.01 Benign neoplasm of scapula and long bones of right upper limb ☑
D16.11 Benign neoplasm of short bones of right upper limb ☑
D16.12 Benign neoplasm of short bones of left upper limb ☑
D18.02 Hemangioma of intracranial structures
D25.0 Submucous leiomyoma of uterus
D25.1 Intramural leiomyoma of uterus
D25.2 Subserosal leiomyoma of uterus
D32.0 Benign neoplasm of cerebral meninges
D32.1 Benign neoplasm of spinal meninges
D36.11 Benign neoplasm of peripheral nerves and autonomic nervous system of face, head, and neck
D36.12 Benign neoplasm of peripheral nerves and autonomic nervous system, upper limb, including shoulder
D36.13 Benign neoplasm of peripheral nerves and autonomic nervous system of lower limb, including hip
D36.14 Benign neoplasm of peripheral nerves and autonomic nervous system of thorax
D36.15 Benign neoplasm of peripheral nerves and autonomic nervous system of abdomen
D36.16 Benign neoplasm of peripheral nerves and autonomic nervous system of pelvis
D48.110 Desmoid tumor of head and neck
D48.111 Desmoid tumor of chest wall
D48.112 Desmoid tumor, intrathoracic
D48.113 Desmoid tumor of abdominal wall
D48.114 Desmoid tumor, intraabdominal
D48.115 Desmoid tumor of upper extremity and shoulder girdle
D48.116 Desmoid tumor of lower extremity and pelvic girdle
D48.117 Desmoid tumor of back

AMA: 37243 2024,May; 2019,Sep; 2018,Jul; 2018,Mar

Relative Value Units/Medicare Edits

Non-Facility RVU	Work	PE	MP	Total
37243	11.74	238.3	1.23	251.27
Facility RVU	**Work**	**PE**	**MP**	**Total**
37243	11.74	3.29	1.23	16.26

	FUD	Status	MUE	Modifiers				IOM Reference
37243	0	A	1(3)	51	N/A	N/A	N/A	None

* with documentation

37244

37244 Vascular embolization or occlusion, inclusive of all radiological supervision and interpretation, intraprocedural roadmapping, and imaging guidance necessary to complete the intervention; for arterial or venous hemorrhage or lymphatic extravasation

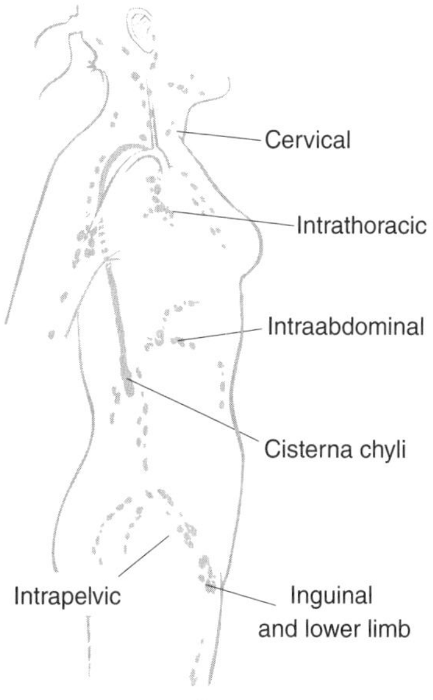

Lymphatic system

Explanation

Embolization or occlusion of a blood vessel is performed to treat hemorrhage. A needle is inserted through the skin and into a blood vessel. A guidewire is threaded through the needle and the needle is removed. A catheter is threaded into the vessel over the guidewire and the wire is extracted. The catheter travels to the appropriate site and beads, coils, or another vessel-blocking device are released. The beads or other device block the vessel. The catheter is removed and pressure is applied over the puncture site to stop the bleeding.

Coding Tips

When medically necessary, report moderate (conscious) sedation provided by the performing physician with 99151-99153. When provided by another physician, report 99155-99157. Only one embolization code should be reported for each surgical field, including the entire area directly involved in and immediately surrounding the procedure. The code representing the immediate cause for the embolization should be used. Diagnostic angiography and catheter placement may be reported separately. Report with an appropriate modifier. Do not report 37244 with 75894 or 75898 in the same surgical field. For embolization procedures of the head and neck, see 61626 or 61710.

ICD-10-CM Diagnostic Codes

I61.0 Nontraumatic intracerebral hemorrhage in hemisphere, subcortical
I61.1 Nontraumatic intracerebral hemorrhage in hemisphere, cortical
I61.3 Nontraumatic intracerebral hemorrhage in brain stem
I61.4 Nontraumatic intracerebral hemorrhage in cerebellum
I61.5 Nontraumatic intracerebral hemorrhage, intraventricular
I62.01 Nontraumatic acute subdural hemorrhage
I62.02 Nontraumatic subacute subdural hemorrhage
I62.03 Nontraumatic chronic subdural hemorrhage

 ● New ▲ Revised + Add On ★ Telemedicine [Resequenced] ☑ Laterality

I62.1 Nontraumatic extradural hemorrhage
N99.820 Postprocedural hemorrhage of a genitourinary system organ or structure following a genitourinary system procedure
O72.0 Third-stage hemorrhage M
O72.2 Delayed and secondary postpartum hemorrhage M
O72.3 Postpartum coagulation defects M
R04.0 Epistaxis
R04.2 Hemoptysis
S15.011A Minor laceration of right carotid artery, initial encounter ☑
S15.012A Minor laceration of left carotid artery, initial encounter ☑
S15.021A Major laceration of right carotid artery, initial encounter ☑
S15.022A Major laceration of left carotid artery, initial encounter ☑
S15.111A Minor laceration of right vertebral artery, initial encounter ☑
S15.112A Minor laceration of left vertebral artery, initial encounter ☑
S15.121A Major laceration of right vertebral artery, initial encounter ☑
S15.122A Major laceration of left vertebral artery, initial encounter ☑
S25.01XA Minor laceration of thoracic aorta, initial encounter
S25.02XA Major laceration of thoracic aorta, initial encounter
S25.411A Minor laceration of right pulmonary blood vessels, initial encounter ☑
S25.412A Minor laceration of left pulmonary blood vessels, initial encounter ☑
S25.421A Major laceration of right pulmonary blood vessels, initial encounter ☑
S25.422A Major laceration of left pulmonary blood vessels, initial encounter ☑
S25.511A Laceration of intercostal blood vessels, right side, initial encounter ☑
S25.512A Laceration of intercostal blood vessels, left side, initial encounter ☑
S35.01XA Minor laceration of abdominal aorta, initial encounter
S35.02XA Major laceration of abdominal aorta, initial encounter
S35.11XA Minor laceration of inferior vena cava, initial encounter
S35.12XA Major laceration of inferior vena cava, initial encounter
S45.011A Laceration of axillary artery, right side, initial encounter ☑
S45.012A Laceration of axillary artery, left side, initial encounter ☑

AMA: **37244** 2024,May; 2019,Sep; 2018,Jul; 2018,Mar

Relative Value Units/Medicare Edits

Non-Facility RVU	Work	PE	MP	Total
37244	13.75	176.7	1.5	191.95
Facility RVU	**Work**	**PE**	**MP**	**Total**
37244	13.75	3.92	1.5	19.17

	FUD	Status	MUE	Modifiers				IOM Reference
37244	0	A	2(3)	51	N/A	N/A	N/A	None

* with documentation

Terms To Know

embolization. Placement of a clotting agent, such as a coil, plastic particles, gel, foam, etc., into an area of hemorrhage to stop the bleeding or to block blood flow to a problem area, such as an aneurysm or a tumor.

37252-37253

\+ **37252** Intravascular ultrasound (noncoronary vessel) during diagnostic evaluation and/or therapeutic intervention, including radiological supervision and interpretation; initial noncoronary vessel (List separately in addition to code for primary procedure)

\+ **37253** each additional noncoronary vessel (List separately in addition to code for primary procedure)

Explanation

Intravascular ultrasound may be used during diagnostic evaluation of the noncoronary artery or vein. It may also be used before and after a therapeutic intervention upon a noncoronary artery or vein to assess patency and integrity of the vessel. A needle is inserted through the skin and into a blood vessel. A guidewire is threaded through the needle into a noncoronary blood vessel. The needle is removed. An intravascular ultrasound catheter is placed over the guidewire. The ultrasound catheter is used to obtain images from inside the vessel to assess area and extent of disease prior to interventional therapy, as well as adequacy of therapy after interventional therapy. Report 37252 for the initial noncoronary vessel. In 37253, the physician advances the ultrasound catheter into additional noncoronary vessels to assess patency and structure. The catheter and guidewire are removed and pressure is applied over the puncture site to stop bleeding. These codes include radiological supervision and interpretation.

Coding Tips

When medically necessary, report moderate (conscious) sedation provided by the performing physician with 99151-99153. When provided by another physician, report 99155-99157. Use 37253 in addition to 37252. Intravascular ultrasound services include all transducer manipulations within the specific vessel being examined, before and after therapeutic intervention. Report 37252 one time, in addition to the primary code, for a lesion that extends into multiple vessels. Catheterization may be reported separately, see 36005–36248. Do not report 37252–37253 with 36836, 36837, 37191–37193, or 37197. These codes may be reported with an extensive number of primary procedures ranging from 33361-34848, 36010-37249, 61623, 75600-77001, and 0075T-0338T. Refer to the CPT manual for details.

ICD-10-CM Diagnostic Codes

This/these CPT code(s) are add-on code(s). See the primary procedure code that this code is performed with for your ICD-10-CM code selections.

AMA: **37252** 2023,Mar; 2023,Feb; 2022,Oct; 2021,Jun; 2019,Nov **37253** 2023,Feb; 2021,Jun; 2019,Nov

Relative Value Units/Medicare Edits

Non-Facility RVU	Work	PE	MP	Total
37252	1.8	25.7	0.35	27.85
37253	1.44	3.41	0.27	5.12
Facility RVU	**Work**	**PE**	**MP**	**Total**
37252	1.8	0.44	0.35	2.59
37253	1.44	0.35	0.27	2.06

	FUD	Status	MUE	Modifiers				IOM Reference
37252	N/A	A	1(2)	N/A	N/A	62*	80*	None
37253	N/A	A	5(3)	N/A	N/A	62*	80*	

* with documentation

 N Newborn: 0 P Pediatric: 0-17 M Maternity: 9-64 A Adult: 15-124 AMA: CPT Assist

37500

37500 Vascular endoscopy, surgical, with ligation of perforator veins, subfascial (SEPS)

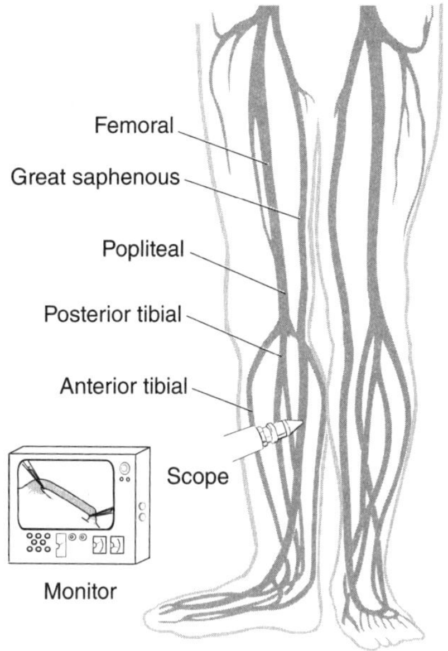

Incompetent perforator veins are treated endoscopically in the subfascial plane of the lower leg. The veins are typically ligated or transected

Explanation

Subfascial endoscopic perforator surgery (SEPS) is performed as a minimally invasive way to treat patients with chronic venous insufficiency (CVI) of the lower extremities. Incompetent calf perforator veins are ligated in this procedure. Perforator veins are an irregular group of veins growing as tributaries of the greater saphenous vein, which connect between it and other veins in the lower leg. They are considered incompetent when the direction of blood flow within the perforator vein changes upon applying distal pressure. SEP is carried out under regional or general anesthesia. A rollover tourniquet technique is used to exsanguinate the leg and a single stab incision is made over the medial aspect of the calf through which the operating telescope is inserted. The subfascial plane is created with blunt dissection and maintained open by insufflating with carbon dioxide gas at low pressure. The perforators are identified and ligated, or transected, with a 5 mm ultrasonic scalpel. Patients may be given elastic stockings to wear for the next two weeks.

Coding Tips

This is a unilateral procedure. If performed bilaterally, some payers require that the service be reported twice with modifier 50 appended to the second code, while others require identification of the service only once with modifier 50 appended. Check with individual payers. Modifier 50 identifies a procedure performed identically on the opposite side of the body (mirror image). For other treatment of long and/or short saphenous veins, see 37700–37735 and 37780. For open radical ligation of perforators (Linton type), with or without a skin graft, see 37760. For injection of a sclerosing solution, spider veins (telangiectasia), see 36468. For injection of a sclerosing solution for larger veins, see 36470–36471.

ICD-10-CM Diagnostic Codes

I83.011 Varicose veins of right lower extremity with ulcer of thigh A ☑
I83.012 Varicose veins of right lower extremity with ulcer of calf A ☑
I83.013 Varicose veins of right lower extremity with ulcer of ankle A ☑
I83.014 Varicose veins of right lower extremity with ulcer of heel and midfoot A ☑
I83.015 Varicose veins of right lower extremity with ulcer other part of foot A ☑
I83.018 Varicose veins of right lower extremity with ulcer other part of lower leg A ☑
I83.11 Varicose veins of right lower extremity with inflammation A ☑
I83.211 Varicose veins of right lower extremity with both ulcer of thigh and inflammation A ☑
I83.212 Varicose veins of right lower extremity with both ulcer of calf and inflammation A ☑
I83.213 Varicose veins of right lower extremity with both ulcer of ankle and inflammation A ☑
I83.214 Varicose veins of right lower extremity with both ulcer of heel and midfoot and inflammation A ☑
I83.215 Varicose veins of right lower extremity with both ulcer other part of foot and inflammation A ☑
I83.218 Varicose veins of right lower extremity with both ulcer of other part of lower extremity and inflammation A ☑
I83.811 Varicose veins of right lower extremity with pain A ☑
I83.891 Varicose veins of right lower extremity with other complications A ☑
I87.1 Compression of vein
I87.2 Venous insufficiency (chronic) (peripheral)

AMA: **37500** 2021,Dec

Relative Value Units/Medicare Edits

Non-Facility RVU	Work	PE	MP	Total
37500	11.67	4.01	2.89	18.57
Facility RVU	**Work**	**PE**	**MP**	**Total**
37500	11.67	4.01	2.89	18.57

	FUD	Status	MUE	Modifiers				IOM Reference
37500	90	A	1(3)	51	50	62*	N/A	None

* with documentation

Terms To Know

incompetent. Inability of a valve or structure to perform its normal function.

subfascial. Beneath the band of fibrous tissue that lies deep to the skin, encloses muscles, and separates their layers.

ulcer. Open sore or excavating lesion of skin or the tissue on the surface of an organ from the sloughing of chronically inflamed and necrosing tissue.

varicose vein. Abnormal, permanently distended or stretched vein.

37565

37565 Ligation, internal jugular vein

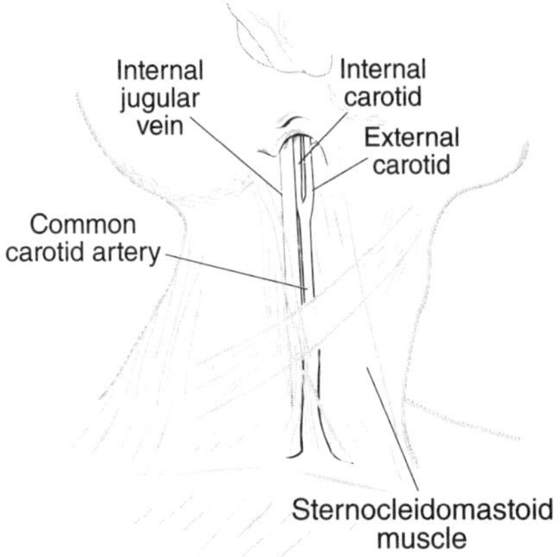

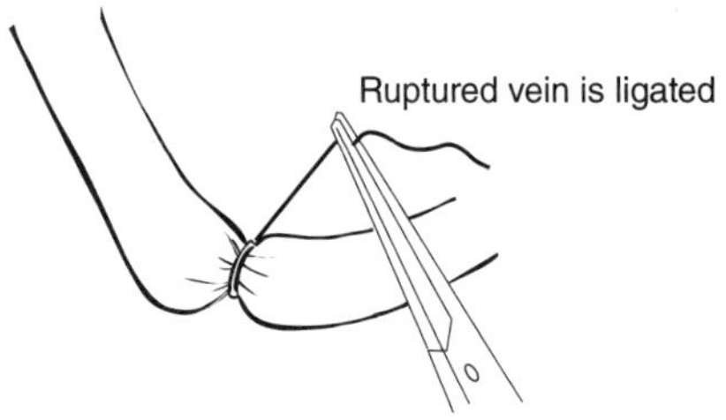

Explanation

Through an incision in the skin at side of neck in front of the sternocleidomastoid muscle, the physician isolates and dissects the internal jugular vein, separating it from critical structures. Using a vascular clip or ligature, the blood flow is reduced and the vein is ligated. Once the vein has been tied off, the skin incision is repaired with a layered closure.

Coding Tips

For ligation of the internal or common carotid artery, see 37605 and 37606.

ICD-10-CM Diagnostic Codes

G97.31 Intraoperative hemorrhage and hematoma of a nervous system organ or structure complicating a nervous system procedure

G97.48 Accidental puncture and laceration of other nervous system organ or structure during a nervous system procedure

G97.51 Postprocedural hemorrhage of a nervous system organ or structure following a nervous system procedure

G97.61 Postprocedural hematoma of a nervous system organ or structure following a nervous system procedure

G97.63 Postprocedural seroma of a nervous system organ or structure following a nervous system procedure

H93.11 Tinnitus, right ear ☑

H93.A1 Pulsatile tinnitus, right ear ☑

I82.C11 Acute embolism and thrombosis of right internal jugular vein ☑

I82.C12 Acute embolism and thrombosis of left internal jugular vein ☑

I82.C13 Acute embolism and thrombosis of internal jugular vein, bilateral ☑

I82.C21 Chronic embolism and thrombosis of right internal jugular vein ☑

I82.C22 Chronic embolism and thrombosis of left internal jugular vein ☑

I82.C23 Chronic embolism and thrombosis of internal jugular vein, bilateral ☑

R58 Hemorrhage, not elsewhere classified

S11.81XA Laceration without foreign body of other specified part of neck, initial encounter

S11.82XA Laceration with foreign body of other specified part of neck, initial encounter

S11.83XA Puncture wound without foreign body of other specified part of neck, initial encounter

S11.84XA Puncture wound with foreign body of other specified part of neck, initial encounter

S11.85XA Open bite of other specified part of neck, initial encounter

S11.89XA Other open wound of other specified part of neck, initial encounter

S15.311A Minor laceration of right internal jugular vein, initial encounter ☑

S15.312A Minor laceration of left internal jugular vein, initial encounter ☑

S15.321A Major laceration of right internal jugular vein, initial encounter ☑

S15.322A Major laceration of left internal jugular vein, initial encounter ☑

S15.391A Other specified injury of right internal jugular vein, initial encounter ☑

S15.392A Other specified injury of left internal jugular vein, initial encounter ☑

S16.2XXA Laceration of muscle, fascia and tendon at neck level, initial encounter

Relative Value Units/Medicare Edits

Non-Facility RVU	Work	PE	MP	Total
37565	12.05	7.24	2.44	21.73
Facility RVU	**Work**	**PE**	**MP**	**Total**
37565	12.05	7.24	2.44	21.73

	FUD	Status	MUE	Modifiers				IOM Reference
37565	90	A	1(2)	51	50	62*	80*	None

* with documentation

Terms To Know

dissect. Cut apart or separate tissue for surgical purposes or for visual or microscopic study.

embolism. Obstruction of a blood vessel resulting from a clot or foreign substance.

hemorrhage syndrome. Fulminating meningococcal septicemia occurring in children younger than 10 years of age with vomiting, cyanosis, diarrhea, purpura, convulsions, circulatory collapse, meningitis, and hemorrhaging into adrenal glands.

ligation. Tying off a blood vessel or duct with a suture or a soft, thin wire.

seroma. Swelling caused by the collection of serum, or clear fluid, in the tissues.

37600

37600 Ligation; external carotid artery

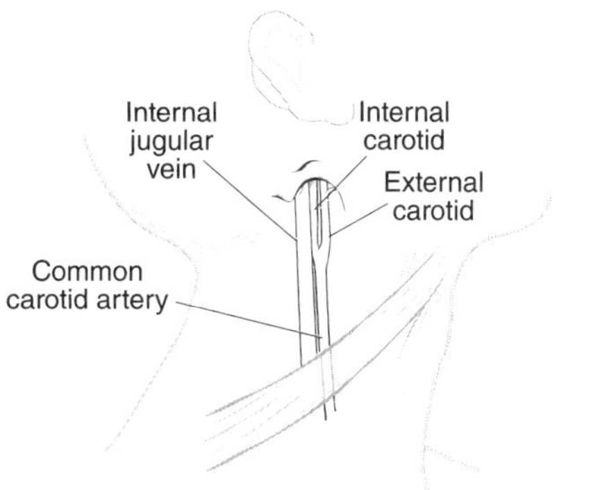

Deep dissection showing bifurcation of carotid arteries

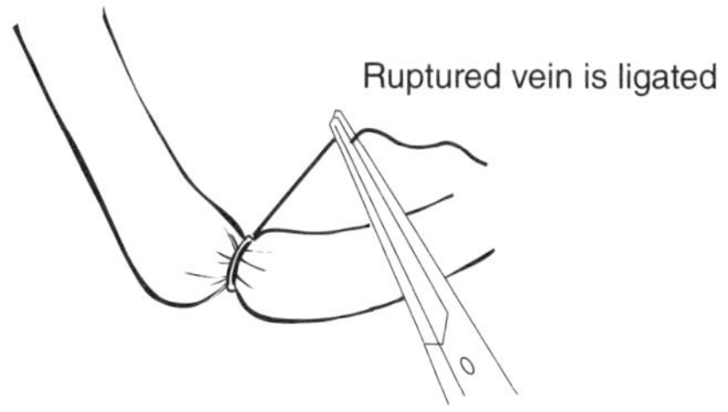

Explanation

Through an incision in the skin at the side of the neck in front of the sternocleidomastoid muscle, the physician isolates and dissects the external carotid artery, separating it from critical structures. Using a vascular clip or ligature, the blood flow is reduced and the artery is ligated. Once the artery has been tied off, the skin incision is repaired with a layered closure.

Coding Tips

Angioscopy during therapeutic intervention is listed separately, see 35400. For ligation of the internal or common carotid artery, see 37605 or 37606.

ICD-10-CM Diagnostic Codes

S15.011A Minor laceration of right carotid artery, initial encounter ☑
S15.012A Minor laceration of left carotid artery, initial encounter ☑
S15.021A Major laceration of right carotid artery, initial encounter ☑
S15.022A Major laceration of left carotid artery, initial encounter ☑
S15.091A Other specified injury of right carotid artery, initial encounter ☑
S15.092A Other specified injury of left carotid artery, initial encounter ☑

Relative Value Units/Medicare Edits

Non-Facility RVU	Work	PE	MP	Total
37600	12.42	7.8	2.13	22.35
Facility RVU	**Work**	**PE**	**MP**	**Total**
37600	12.42	7.8	2.13	22.35

	FUD	Status	MUE	Modifiers				IOM Reference
37600	90	A	1(3)	51	N/A	62*	80	None

* with documentation

37605-37606

37605 Ligation; internal or common carotid artery
37606 internal or common carotid artery, with gradual occlusion, as with Selverstone or Crutchfield clamp

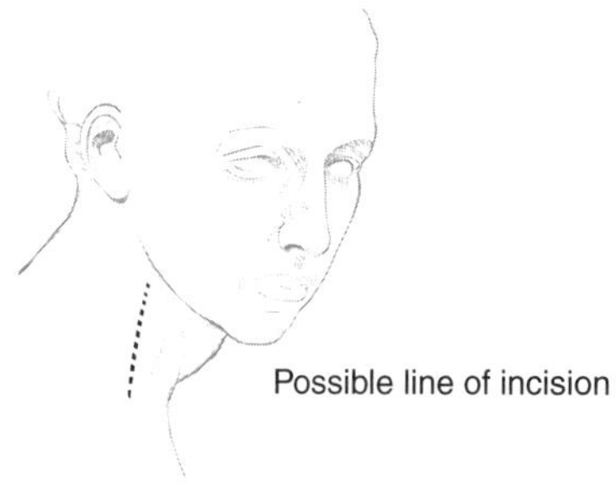

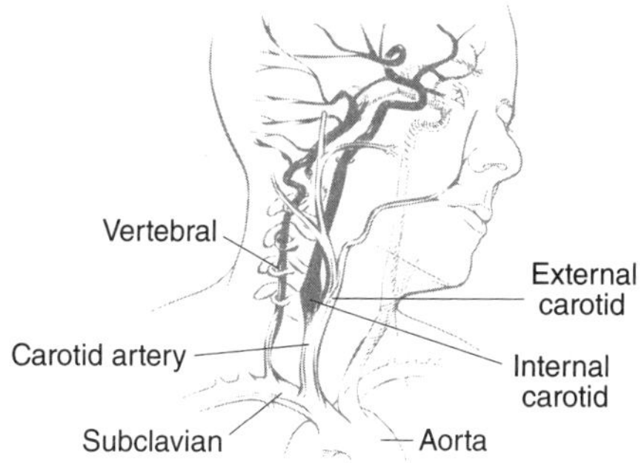

Explanation

Through an incision in the skin at the side of the neck, the physician isolates and dissects the internal or common carotid artery, separating it from critical structures. After vessel clamps have been affixed above and below the injured or affected artery, the physician sutures the artery to permanently stop the flow of blood through it (37605). The physician may apply a gradual occluding clamp (37606) to assess the effect of a ligation prior to complete occlusion (37605). Once the artery has been ligated or the occluding clamp has been placed, the vessel clamp is removed and the skin incision is repaired with a layered closure.

Coding Tips

Angioscopy during therapeutic intervention is listed separately, see 35400. Neurologic monitoring of the patient is normally a function of the anesthesiologist or neurologist. This code includes any neurologic monitoring performed by the physician. For ligation of the external carotid artery, see 37600. For ligation treatment of intracranial aneurysm, see 61703. For transcatheter permanent arterial occlusion or embolization, see 61624 and 61626. For temporary endovascular arterial balloon occlusion, see 61623.

ICD-10-CM Diagnostic Codes

S11.81XA Laceration without foreign body of other specified part of neck, initial encounter
S11.82XA Laceration with foreign body of other specified part of neck, initial encounter
S11.83XA Puncture wound without foreign body of other specified part of neck, initial encounter
S11.84XA Puncture wound with foreign body of other specified part of neck, initial encounter
S11.85XA Open bite of other specified part of neck, initial encounter
S11.89XA Other open wound of other specified part of neck, initial encounter

S15.011A	Minor laceration of right carotid artery, initial encounter ☑
S15.012A	Minor laceration of left carotid artery, initial encounter ☑
S15.021A	Major laceration of right carotid artery, initial encounter ☑
S15.022A	Major laceration of left carotid artery, initial encounter ☑
S15.091A	Other specified injury of right carotid artery, initial encounter ☑
S15.092A	Other specified injury of left carotid artery, initial encounter ☑
S16.2XXA	Laceration of muscle, fascia and tendon at neck level, initial encounter

Relative Value Units/Medicare Edits

Non-Facility RVU	Work	PE	MP	Total
37605	14.28	3.87	3.56	21.71
37606	8.81	9.9	3.67	22.38
Facility RVU	**Work**	**PE**	**MP**	**Total**
37605	14.28	3.87	3.56	21.71
37606	8.81	9.9	3.67	22.38

	FUD	Status	MUE	Modifiers				IOM Reference
37605	90	A	1(3)	51	N/A	62*	80	None
37606	90	A	1(3)	51	N/A	N/A	80	

* with documentation

Terms To Know

dissect. Cut apart or separate tissue for surgical purposes or for visual or microscopic study.

ligation. Tying off a blood vessel or duct with a suture or a soft, thin wire.

occlusion. Constriction, closure, or blockage of a passage.

37607

37607 Ligation or banding of angioaccess arteriovenous fistula

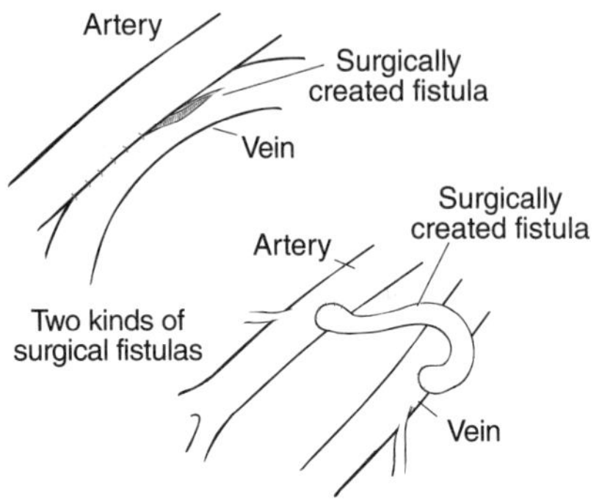

An arteriovenous fistula that occurs at the site of an access is ligated or banded

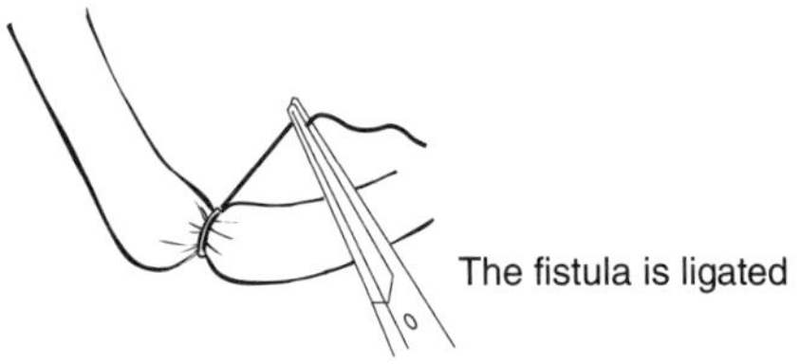

Explanation

The physician exposes a surgically created arteriovenous fistula by careful dissection. The physician isolates the fistula with ties or clamps. The physician may tie the arteriovenous fistula off completely (ligation) with suture, or the physician may partially obstruct (banding) the lumen of the fistula with a broader band in order to reduce flow. The physician closes the skin incision.

Coding Tips

This code is used to report ligation or banding of a surgically created arteriovenous fistula. It should not be used to report repair of traumatic or congenital arteriovenous fistulas. For repair of traumatic or congenital arteriovenous fistulas, see 35180–35190. For creation of an arteriovenous fistula by other than direct arteriovenous anastomosis, see 36825–36830.

ICD-10-CM Diagnostic Codes

T82.318A	Breakdown (mechanical) of other vascular grafts, initial encounter
T82.338A	Leakage of other vascular grafts, initial encounter
T82.398A	Other mechanical complication of other vascular grafts, initial encounter
T82.510A	Breakdown (mechanical) of surgically created arteriovenous fistula, initial encounter
T82.518A	Breakdown (mechanical) of other cardiac and vascular devices and implants, initial encounter
T82.530A	Leakage of surgically created arteriovenous fistula, initial encounter
T82.538A	Leakage of other cardiac and vascular devices and implants, initial encounter
T82.590A	Other mechanical complication of surgically created arteriovenous fistula, initial encounter
T82.598A	Other mechanical complication of other cardiac and vascular devices and implants, initial encounter
T82.7XXA	Infection and inflammatory reaction due to other cardiac and vascular devices, implants and grafts, initial encounter

T82.818A	Embolism due to vascular prosthetic devices, implants and grafts, initial encounter
T82.828A	Fibrosis due to vascular prosthetic devices, implants and grafts, initial encounter
T82.838A	Hemorrhage due to vascular prosthetic devices, implants and grafts, initial encounter
T82.858A	Stenosis of other vascular prosthetic devices, implants and grafts, initial encounter
T82.868A	Thrombosis due to vascular prosthetic devices, implants and grafts, initial encounter
T82.898A	Other specified complication of vascular prosthetic devices, implants and grafts, initial encounter
T82.9XXA	Unspecified complication of cardiac and vascular prosthetic device, implant and graft, initial encounter
Z45.2	Encounter for adjustment and management of vascular access device
Z45.89	Encounter for adjustment and management of other implanted devices
Z46.89	Encounter for fitting and adjustment of other specified devices

AMA: 37607 2022,May

Relative Value Units/Medicare Edits

Non-Facility RVU	Work	PE	MP	Total
37607	6.25	3.32	1.5	11.07
Facility RVU	**Work**	**PE**	**MP**	**Total**
37607	6.25	3.32	1.5	11.07

	FUD	Status	MUE	Modifiers				IOM Reference
37607	90	A	1(3)	51	N/A	62*	N/A	None

* with documentation

Terms To Know

anastomosis. Surgically created connection between ducts, blood vessels, or bowel segments to allow flow from one to the other.

clamp. Tool used to grip, compress, join, or fasten body parts.

complication. Condition arising after the beginning of observation and treatment that modifies the course of the patient's illness or the medical care required, or an undesired result or misadventure in medical care.

dissection. Separating by cutting tissue or body structures apart.

fistula. Abnormal tube-like passage between two body cavities or organs or from an organ to the outside surface.

incision. Act of cutting into tissue or an organ.

revision. Reordering or rearrangement of tissue to suit a particular need or function.

37609

37609 Ligation or biopsy, temporal artery

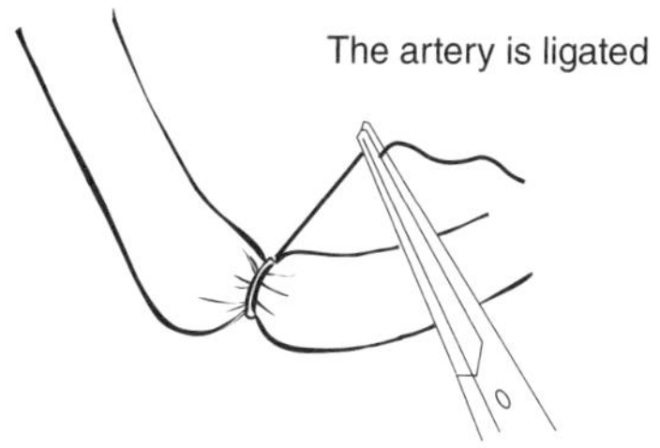

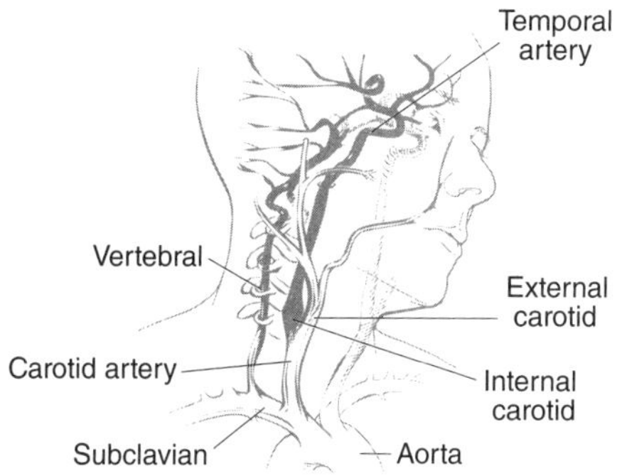

Explanation

Through an incision in the skin in front of the ear, the physician isolates and dissects the temporal artery, separating it from critical structures. Using a vascular clip or ligature, the artery is ligated or tissue samples are taken for biopsy. Once the artery has been tied off, the skin incision is repaired with a layered closure.

Coding Tips

Angioscopy during therapeutic intervention is listed separately, see 35400. For ligation of the external, internal, or common carotid artery, see 37600–37606.

ICD-10-CM Diagnostic Codes

G44.1	Vascular headache, not elsewhere classified
I77.2	Rupture of artery
M31.5	Giant cell arteritis with polymyalgia rheumatica
M31.6	Other giant cell arteritis
M35.0B	Sjögren syndrome with vasculitis
R58	Hemorrhage, not elsewhere classified

Relative Value Units/Medicare Edits

Non-Facility RVU	Work	PE	MP	Total
37609	3.05	5.64	0.64	9.33
Facility RVU	**Work**	**PE**	**MP**	**Total**
37609	3.05	2.42	0.64	6.11

	FUD	Status	MUE	Modifiers				IOM Reference
37609	10	A	1(2)	51	50	N/A	N/A	None

* with documentation

37615

37615 Ligation, major artery (eg, post-traumatic, rupture); neck

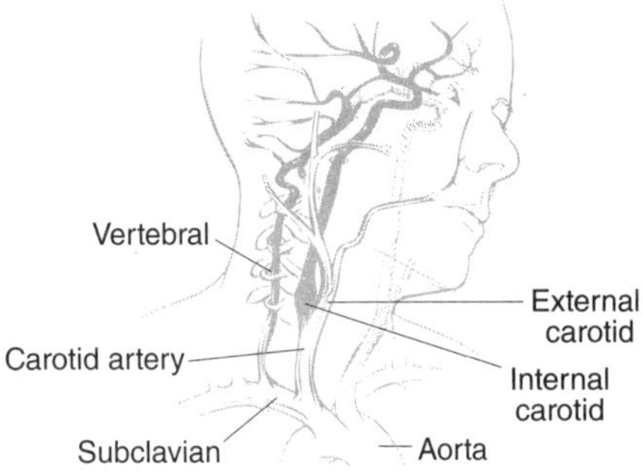

A major artery of the neck is ligated

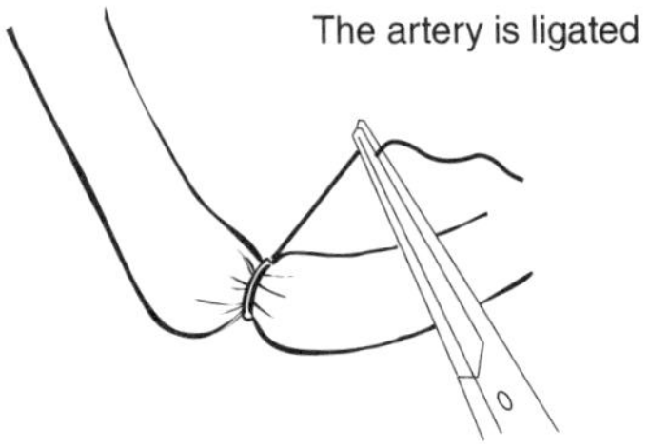

Explanation

Through an incision in the skin in the side of the neck, usually in front of the sternocleidomastoid muscle, the physician isolates and dissects the ruptured or otherwise traumatized vessel, separating it from critical structures. Using a vascular clip or ligature, the vessel is ligated with sutures. Once the vessel has been tied off, the skin incision is repaired with a layered closure.

Coding Tips

Angioscopy during therapeutic intervention is listed separately, see 35400. For ligation, major artery (e.g., post-traumatic, rupture), chest, see 37616; abdomen, see 37617; extremity, see 37618. For ligation of the external, internal, or common carotid artery for reasons other than trauma, see 37600–37606. If an artery is ligated in the course of dissecting another structure, or if a vessel is accidentally injured during dissection, requiring ligation, the procedure is not reported separately.

ICD-10-CM Diagnostic Codes

S11.81XA Laceration without foreign body of other specified part of neck, initial encounter
S11.82XA Laceration with foreign body of other specified part of neck, initial encounter
S11.83XA Puncture wound without foreign body of other specified part of neck, initial encounter
S11.84XA Puncture wound with foreign body of other specified part of neck, initial encounter
S11.85XA Open bite of other specified part of neck, initial encounter
S11.89XA Other open wound of other specified part of neck, initial encounter
S15.111A Minor laceration of right vertebral artery, initial encounter ☑
S15.112A Minor laceration of left vertebral artery, initial encounter ☑
S15.121A Major laceration of right vertebral artery, initial encounter ☑
S15.122A Major laceration of left vertebral artery, initial encounter ☑
S15.191A Other specified injury of right vertebral artery, initial encounter ☑
S15.192A Other specified injury of left vertebral artery, initial encounter ☑
S15.8XXA Injury of other specified blood vessels at neck level, initial encounter

Relative Value Units/Medicare Edits

Non-Facility RVU	Work	PE	MP	Total
37615	7.8	6.11	1.54	15.45
Facility RVU	**Work**	**PE**	**MP**	**Total**
37615	7.8	6.11	1.54	15.45

	FUD	Status	MUE	Modifiers				IOM Reference
37615	90	A	2(3)	51	N/A	62*	80	None

* with documentation

Terms To Know

angioscopy. Visualization of capillary blood vessels with a microscope, or the inside of a blood vessel with a fiberoptic-equipped catheter.

complication. Condition arising after the beginning of observation and treatment that modifies the course of the patient's illness or the medical care required, or an undesired result or misadventure in medical care.

hematoma. Tumor-like collection of blood in some part of the body caused by a break in a blood vessel wall, usually as a result of trauma.

ligation. Tying off a blood vessel or duct with a suture or a soft, thin wire.

seroma. Swelling caused by the collection of serum, or clear fluid, in the tissues.

37616

37616 Ligation, major artery (eg, post-traumatic, rupture); chest

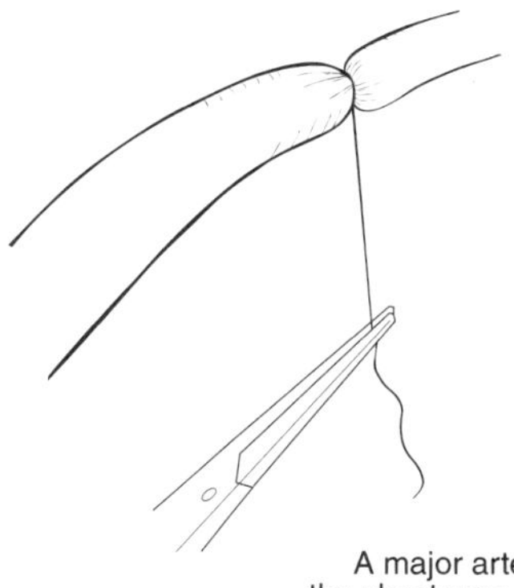

A major artery of the chest area is ligated

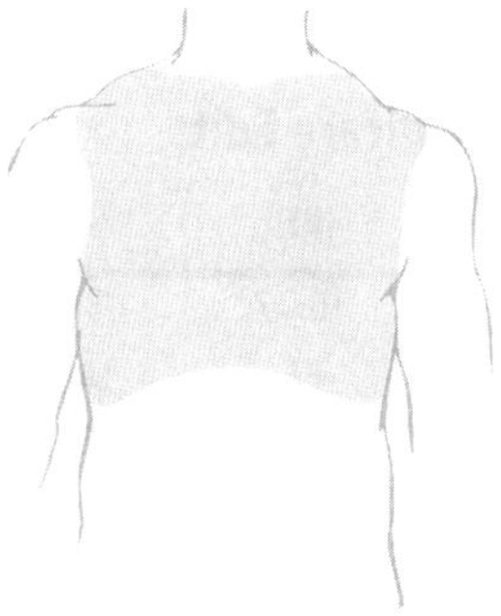

Explanation

The physician performs an incision of the chest wall (thoracotomy or median sternotomy) to best expose the involved artery. The physician identifies the injured artery and quickly clamps it to reduce blood loss. The physician then ties off the artery completely (ligation), proximal and distal to the site of injury. The physician closes the chest, leaving chest tubes in place.

Coding Tips

Angioscopy during therapeutic intervention is listed separately, see 35400. For ligation, major artery (e.g., posttraumatic, rupture) of the neck, see 37615; abdomen, see 37617; extremity, see 37618. If an artery is ligated in the course of dissecting another structure, or if a vessel is accidentally injured during dissection, requiring ligation, it is not reported separately.

ICD-10-CM Diagnostic Codes

S21.121A Laceration with foreign body of right front wall of thorax without penetration into thoracic cavity, initial encounter

S21.122A Laceration with foreign body of left front wall of thorax without penetration into thoracic cavity, initial encounter

S21.141A Puncture wound with foreign body of right front wall of thorax without penetration into thoracic cavity, initial encounter

S21.142A Puncture wound with foreign body of left front wall of thorax without penetration into thoracic cavity, initial encounter

S25.01XA Minor laceration of thoracic aorta, initial encounter

S25.02XA Major laceration of thoracic aorta, initial encounter

S25.09XA Other specified injury of thoracic aorta, initial encounter

S25.411A Minor laceration of right pulmonary blood vessels, initial encounter ☑

S25.412A Minor laceration of left pulmonary blood vessels, initial encounter ☑

S25.421A Major laceration of right pulmonary blood vessels, initial encounter ☑

S25.422A Major laceration of left pulmonary blood vessels, initial encounter ☑

S25.491A Other specified injury of right pulmonary blood vessels, initial encounter ☑

S25.492A Other specified injury of left pulmonary blood vessels, initial encounter ☑

S25.511A Laceration of intercostal blood vessels, right side, initial encounter ☑

S25.512A Laceration of intercostal blood vessels, left side, initial encounter ☑

S25.591A Other specified injury of intercostal blood vessels, right side, initial encounter ☑

S25.592A Other specified injury of intercostal blood vessels, left side, initial encounter ☑

S25.811A Laceration of other blood vessels of thorax, right side, initial encounter ☑

S25.812A Laceration of other blood vessels of thorax, left side, initial encounter ☑

S25.891A Other specified injury of other blood vessels of thorax, right side, initial encounter ☑

S25.892A Other specified injury of other blood vessels of thorax, left side, initial encounter ☑

Relative Value Units/Medicare Edits

Non-Facility RVU	Work	PE	MP	Total
37616	18.97	9.9	4.63	33.5
Facility RVU	**Work**	**PE**	**MP**	**Total**
37616	18.97	9.9	4.63	33.5

	FUD	Status	MUE	Modifiers				IOM Reference
37616	90	A	1(3)	51	N/A	62*	80	None

* with documentation

Terms To Know

angioscopy. Visualization of capillary blood vessels with a microscope, or the inside of a blood vessel with a fiberoptic-equipped catheter.

distal. *1)* Located farther away from a specified reference point or the trunk. *2)* Pertaining to the area farthest from the center of the body or the point of origin.

hemorrhage syndrome. Fulminating meningococcal septicemia occurring in children younger than 10 years of age with vomiting, cyanosis, diarrhea, purpura, convulsions, circulatory collapse, meningitis, and hemorrhaging into adrenal glands.

ligation. Tying off a blood vessel or duct with a suture or a soft, thin wire.

proximal. Located closest to a specified reference point, usually the midline or trunk.

sternotomy. Incision into the sternum, the bone that forms the front of the chest cavity and connects with the ribs.

thoracotomy. Surgical procedure for opening the chest wall in order to access the lungs, esophagus, trachea, aorta, heart, and diaphragm.

37617

37617 Ligation, major artery (eg, post-traumatic, rupture); abdomen

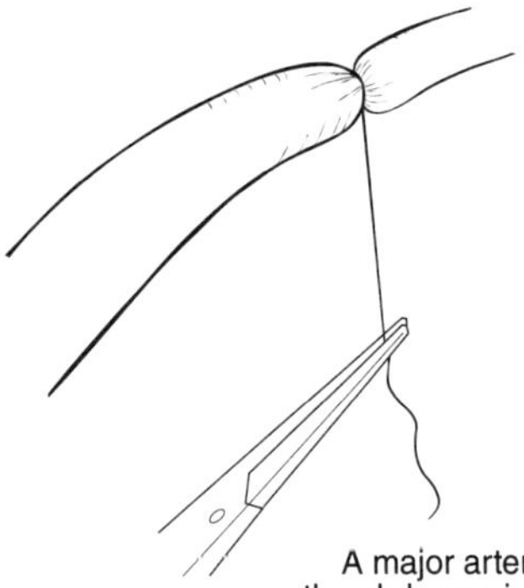

A major artery of the abdomen is ligated

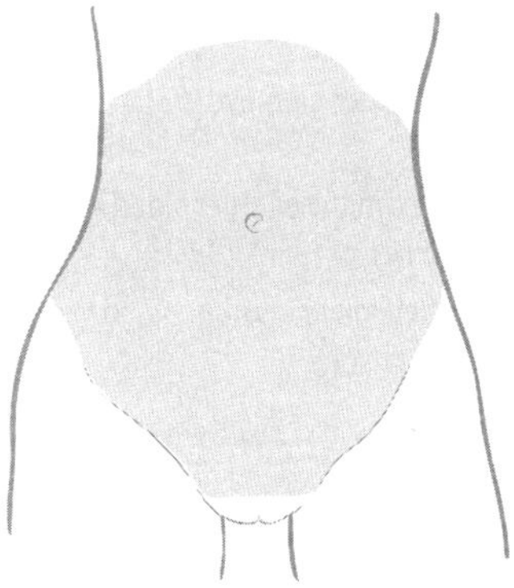

Explanation

The physician performs an abdominal incision to best expose the involved artery. The physician identifies the injured artery and quickly clamps it to reduce blood loss. The physician ties off the artery completely (ligation), proximal and distal to the site of injury. The physician closes the abdomen, leaving drains in place.

Coding Tips

Angioscopy during therapeutic intervention is listed separately, see 35400. For ligation, major artery (e.g., post-traumatic, rupture) of the neck, see 37615; chest, see 37616; extremity, see 37618. If an artery is ligated in the course of dissecting another structure, or if a vessel is accidentally injured during dissection, requiring ligation, it is not reported separately.

ICD-10-CM Diagnostic Codes

S35.01XA Minor laceration of abdominal aorta, initial encounter
S35.02XA Major laceration of abdominal aorta, initial encounter
S35.09XA Other injury of abdominal aorta, initial encounter
S35.211A Minor laceration of celiac artery, initial encounter
S35.212A Major laceration of celiac artery, initial encounter
S35.218A Other injury of celiac artery, initial encounter
S35.221A Minor laceration of superior mesenteric artery, initial encounter
S35.222A Major laceration of superior mesenteric artery, initial encounter
S35.228A Other injury of superior mesenteric artery, initial encounter
S35.231A Minor laceration of inferior mesenteric artery, initial encounter
S35.232A Major laceration of inferior mesenteric artery, initial encounter
S35.238A Other injury of inferior mesenteric artery, initial encounter
S35.291A Minor laceration of branches of celiac and mesenteric artery, initial encounter
S35.292A Major laceration of branches of celiac and mesenteric artery, initial encounter
S35.298A Other injury of branches of celiac and mesenteric artery, initial encounter
S35.411A Laceration of right renal artery, initial encounter ☑
S35.412A Laceration of left renal artery, initial encounter ☑
S35.491A Other specified injury of right renal artery, initial encounter ☑
S35.492A Other specified injury of left renal artery, initial encounter ☑
S35.511A Injury of right iliac artery, initial encounter ☑
S35.512A Injury of left iliac artery, initial encounter ☑
S35.59XA Injury of other iliac blood vessels, initial encounter
S35.8X1A Laceration of other blood vessels at abdomen, lower back and pelvis level, initial encounter
S35.8X8A Other specified injury of other blood vessels at abdomen, lower back and pelvis level, initial encounter

Relative Value Units/Medicare Edits

Non-Facility RVU	Work	PE	MP	Total
37617	23.79	10.05	5.47	39.31
Facility RVU	**Work**	**PE**	**MP**	**Total**
37617	23.79	10.05	5.47	39.31

	FUD	Status	MUE	Modifiers				IOM Reference
37617	90	A	3(3)	51	N/A	62*	80	None

* with documentation

Terms To Know

aneurysm. Circumscribed dilation or outpouching of an artery wall, often containing blood clots and connecting directly with the lumen of the artery.

angioscopy. Visualization of capillary blood vessels with a microscope, or the inside of a blood vessel with a fiberoptic-equipped catheter.

dissection. Separating by cutting tissue or body structures apart.

distal. *1)* Located farther away from a specified reference point or the trunk. *2)* Pertaining to the area farthest from the center of the body or the point of origin.

hematoma. Tumor-like collection of blood in some part of the body caused by a break in a blood vessel wall, usually as a result of trauma.

ligation. Tying off a blood vessel or duct with a suture or a soft, thin wire.

proximal. Located closest to a specified reference point, usually the midline or trunk.

37618

37618 Ligation, major artery (eg, post-traumatic, rupture); extremity

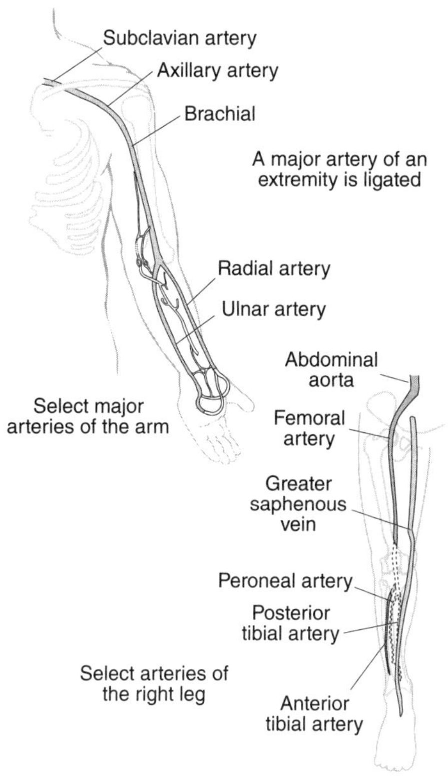

Explanation

Through an incision in the skin of an extremity, usually over the damaged or traumatized vessel, the physician isolates and dissects the vessel, separating it from critical structures. Using a vascular clip or ligature, the vessel is ligated with sutures or vascular clips. Once the vessel has been tied off, the skin incision is repaired with a layered closure.

Coding Tips

Angioscopy during therapeutic intervention is listed separately, see 35400. For ligation, major artery (e.g., post-traumatic, rupture) of the neck, see 37615; chest, see 37616; abdomen, see 37617. If an artery is ligated in the course of dissecting another structure, or if a vessel is accidentally injured during dissection, requiring ligation, it is not reported separately.

ICD-10-CM Diagnostic Codes

S45.011A Laceration of axillary artery, right side, initial encounter ☑
S45.091A Other specified injury of axillary artery, right side, initial encounter ☑
S45.111A Laceration of brachial artery, right side, initial encounter ☑
S45.191A Other specified injury of brachial artery, right side, initial encounter ☑
S45.811A Laceration of other specified blood vessels at shoulder and upper arm level, right arm, initial encounter ☑
S55.011A Laceration of ulnar artery at forearm level, right arm, initial encounter ☑
S55.091A Other specified injury of ulnar artery at forearm level, right arm, initial encounter ☑
S55.111A Laceration of radial artery at forearm level, right arm, initial encounter ☑
S55.191A Other specified injury of radial artery at forearm level, right arm, initial encounter ☑
S55.811A Laceration of other blood vessels at forearm level, right arm, initial encounter ☑
S55.891A Other specified injury of other blood vessels at forearm level, right arm, initial encounter ☑
S65.011A Laceration of ulnar artery at wrist and hand level of right arm, initial encounter ☑
S65.091A Other specified injury of ulnar artery at wrist and hand level of right arm, initial encounter ☑
S65.111A Laceration of radial artery at wrist and hand level of right arm, initial encounter ☑
S65.191A Other specified injury of radial artery at wrist and hand level of right arm, initial encounter ☑
S65.811A Laceration of other blood vessels at wrist and hand level of right arm, initial encounter ☑
S75.011A Minor laceration of femoral artery, right leg, initial encounter ☑
S75.021A Major laceration of femoral artery, right leg, initial encounter ☑
S75.091A Other specified injury of femoral artery, right leg, initial encounter ☑
S75.811A Laceration of other blood vessels at hip and thigh level, right leg, initial encounter ☑
S85.011A Laceration of popliteal artery, right leg, initial encounter ☑
S85.091A Other specified injury of popliteal artery, right leg, initial encounter ☑
S85.141A Laceration of anterior tibial artery, right leg, initial encounter ☑
S85.151A Other specified injury of anterior tibial artery, right leg, initial encounter ☑
S85.171A Laceration of posterior tibial artery, right leg, initial encounter ☑
S85.181A Other specified injury of posterior tibial artery, right leg, initial encounter ☑
S85.211A Laceration of peroneal artery, right leg, initial encounter ☑
S85.291A Other specified injury of peroneal artery, right leg, initial encounter ☑
S85.811A Laceration of other blood vessels at lower leg level, right leg, initial encounter ☑
S95.011A Laceration of dorsal artery of right foot, initial encounter ☑
S95.091A Other specified injury of dorsal artery of right foot, initial encounter ☑
S95.111A Laceration of plantar artery of right foot, initial encounter ☑
S95.191A Other specified injury of plantar artery of right foot, initial encounter ☑

Relative Value Units/Medicare Edits

Non-Facility RVU	Work	PE	MP	Total
37618	6.03	4.26	1.44	11.73
Facility RVU	**Work**	**PE**	**MP**	**Total**
37618	6.03	4.26	1.44	11.73

	FUD	Status	MUE	Modifiers				IOM Reference
37618	90	A	2(3)	51	N/A	62*	80	None

* with documentation

37619

37619 Ligation of inferior vena cava

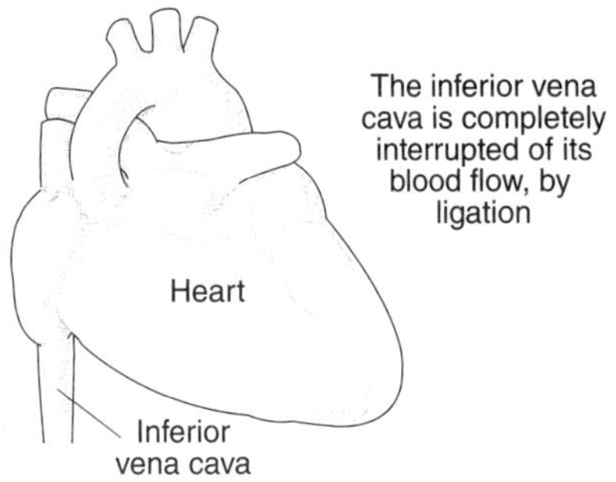

The inferior vena cava (or IVC) is the major return vessel of the lower body. It extends from the right atrium of the heart down to the bifurcation of the iliac veins

Explanation

The physician performs an upper midline abdominal incision and dissects to expose the inferior vena cava. The physician interrupts vena caval flow by tying the cava off with suture or clipping it. The physician closes the abdomen, leaving drains in place.

Coding Tips

For endovascular placement of an intravascular filter, see 37191. For phleborrhaphy and arteriorrhaphy, see 35201–35286.

ICD-10-CM Diagnostic Codes

I26.01	Septic pulmonary embolism with acute cor pulmonale
I26.90	Septic pulmonary embolism without acute cor pulmonale
I27.82	Chronic pulmonary embolism
I82.220	Acute embolism and thrombosis of inferior vena cava
I82.221	Chronic embolism and thrombosis of inferior vena cava
I82.3	Embolism and thrombosis of renal vein
I82.411	Acute embolism and thrombosis of right femoral vein ☑
I82.421	Acute embolism and thrombosis of right iliac vein ☑
I82.431	Acute embolism and thrombosis of right popliteal vein ☑
I82.441	Acute embolism and thrombosis of right tibial vein ☑
I82.511	Chronic embolism and thrombosis of right femoral vein ☑
I82.521	Chronic embolism and thrombosis of right iliac vein ☑
I82.531	Chronic embolism and thrombosis of right popliteal vein ☑
I82.541	Chronic embolism and thrombosis of right tibial vein ☑
I82.811	Embolism and thrombosis of superficial veins of right lower extremity ☑
O86.81	Puerperal septic thrombophlebitis M
O87.1	Deep phlebothrombosis in the puerperium M
S35.11XA	Minor laceration of inferior vena cava, initial encounter
S35.12XA	Major laceration of inferior vena cava, initial encounter
S35.19XA	Other injury of inferior vena cava, initial encounter

Relative Value Units/Medicare Edits

Non-Facility RVU	Work	PE	MP	Total
37619	30.0	13.78	7.73	51.51
Facility RVU	**Work**	**PE**	**MP**	**Total**
37619	30.0	13.78	7.73	51.51

	FUD	Status	MUE	Modifiers				IOM Reference
37619	90	A	1(2)	51	N/A	N/A	80	None

* with documentation

Terms To Know

bifurcation. Point of division into two separate branches or structures, such as the site where the trachea divides into the right and left main bronchi or the common carotid artery becomes the external and internal carotid arteries. For diagnostic purposes, a bifurcation is a congenital anomaly that results in an imperfect closure of an organ or other anatomical structure, such as the ureter, renal pelvis, hard or soft palate, lip, etc.

dissection. Separating by cutting tissue or body structures apart.

drain. Device that creates a channel to allow fluid from a cavity, wound, or infected area to exit the body.

embolism. Obstruction of a blood vessel resulting from a clot or foreign substance.

intravascular. Within a blood vessel.

ligation. Tying off a blood vessel or duct with a suture or a soft, thin wire.

phlebo-. Relating to the vein.

suture. Numerous stitching techniques employed in wound closure.

thrombosis. Condition arising from the presence or formation of blood clots within a blood vessel that may cause vascular obstruction and insufficient oxygenation.

vena cava. Main venous trunk that empties into the right atrium from both the lower and upper regions, beginning at the junction of the common iliac veins inferiorly and the two brachiocephalic veins superiorly.

37650

37650 Ligation of femoral vein

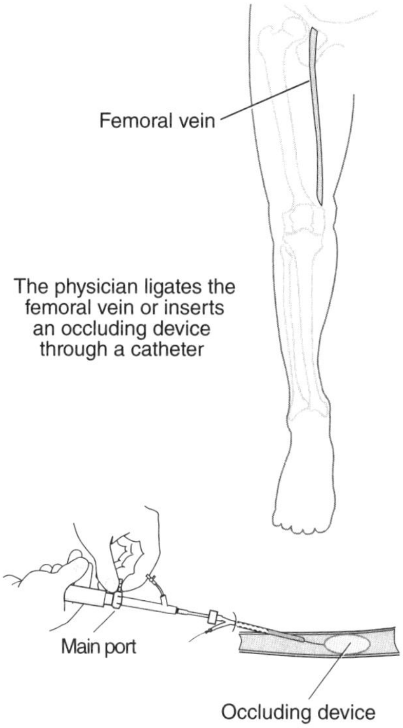

Explanation

Through a small incision in the skin of the upper leg overlying the femoral vein, the physician isolates and dissects the femoral vein from other critical structures. After affixing vessel clamps, the physician either ligates the vein or inserts a catheter into the femoral vein. A guidewire may be inserted prior to the catheter, then removed. Through the catheter, the physician places an occluding device (one that blocks blood flow) in the vein. The catheter is removed and the skin incision is repaired with a layered closure.

Coding Tips

This is a unilateral procedure. If performed bilaterally, some payers require that the service be reported twice with modifier 50 appended to the second code, while others require identification of the service only once with modifier 50 appended. Check with individual payers. Modifier 50 identifies a procedure performed identically on the opposite side of the body (mirror image). For femoral vein repair, see 35226, 36256, or 35286. For ligation of the common iliac vein, see 37660.

ICD-10-CM Diagnostic Codes

- I26.01 Septic pulmonary embolism with acute cor pulmonale
- I26.09 Other pulmonary embolism with acute cor pulmonale
- I26.90 Septic pulmonary embolism without acute cor pulmonale
- I26.99 Other pulmonary embolism without acute cor pulmonale
- I27.82 Chronic pulmonary embolism
- I80.11 Phlebitis and thrombophlebitis of right femoral vein ☑
- I82.411 Acute embolism and thrombosis of right femoral vein ☑
- I82.511 Chronic embolism and thrombosis of right femoral vein ☑
- I83.011 Varicose veins of right lower extremity with ulcer of thigh A ☑
- I83.012 Varicose veins of right lower extremity with ulcer of calf A ☑
- I83.013 Varicose veins of right lower extremity with ulcer of ankle A ☑
- I83.014 Varicose veins of right lower extremity with ulcer of heel and midfoot A ☑
- I83.015 Varicose veins of right lower extremity with ulcer other part of foot A ☑
- I83.018 Varicose veins of right lower extremity with ulcer other part of lower leg A ☑
- I83.11 Varicose veins of right lower extremity with inflammation A ☑
- I83.211 Varicose veins of right lower extremity with both ulcer of thigh and inflammation A ☑
- I83.212 Varicose veins of right lower extremity with both ulcer of calf and inflammation A ☑
- I83.213 Varicose veins of right lower extremity with both ulcer of ankle and inflammation A ☑
- I83.214 Varicose veins of right lower extremity with both ulcer of heel and midfoot and inflammation A ☑
- I83.215 Varicose veins of right lower extremity with both ulcer other part of foot and inflammation A ☑
- I83.218 Varicose veins of right lower extremity with both ulcer of other part of lower extremity and inflammation A ☑
- I83.811 Varicose veins of right lower extremity with pain A ☑
- I83.891 Varicose veins of right lower extremity with other complications A ☑
- I83.91 Asymptomatic varicose veins of right lower extremity A ☑
- I87.001 Postthrombotic syndrome without complications of right lower extremity ☑
- I87.011 Postthrombotic syndrome with ulcer of right lower extremity ☑
- I87.021 Postthrombotic syndrome with inflammation of right lower extremity ☑
- I87.031 Postthrombotic syndrome with ulcer and inflammation of right lower extremity ☑
- I87.091 Postthrombotic syndrome with other complications of right lower extremity ☑
- I87.2 Venous insufficiency (chronic) (peripheral)
- S75.111A Minor laceration of femoral vein at hip and thigh level, right leg, initial encounter ☑
- S75.121A Major laceration of femoral vein at hip and thigh level, right leg, initial encounter ☑

Relative Value Units/Medicare Edits

Non-Facility RVU	Work	PE	MP	Total
37650	8.49	2.96	2.11	13.56
Facility RVU	**Work**	**PE**	**MP**	**Total**
37650	8.49	2.96	2.11	13.56

	FUD	Status	MUE	Modifiers				IOM Reference
37650	90	A	1(2)	51	50	62*	N/A	None

* with documentation

37660

37660 Ligation of common iliac vein

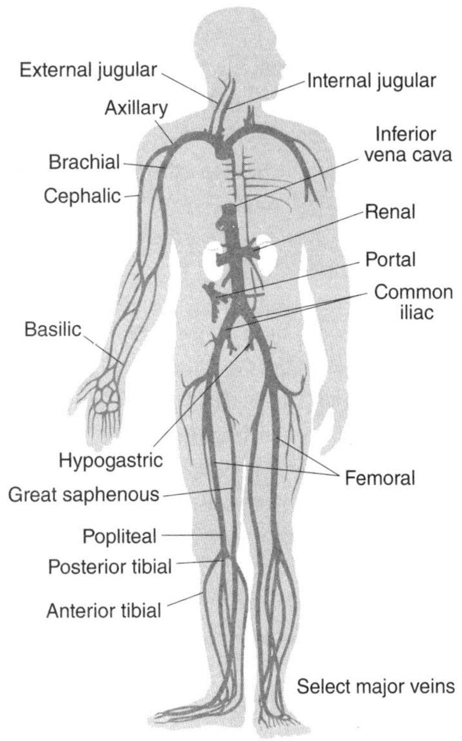

Explanation

The physician performs a lower midline abdominal incision and dissects to expose the common iliac vein. The physician interrupts common iliac venous flow by tying the common iliac vein off with suture. The physician closes the abdomen, leaving drains in place.

Coding Tips

This is a unilateral procedure. If performed bilaterally, some payers require that the service be reported twice with modifier 50 appended to the second code, while others require identification of the service only once with modifier 50 appended. Check with individual payers. Modifier 50 identifies a procedure performed identically on the opposite side of the body (mirror image).

ICD-10-CM Diagnostic Codes

I80.211 Phlebitis and thrombophlebitis of right iliac vein ☑
I80.212 Phlebitis and thrombophlebitis of left iliac vein ☑
I80.213 Phlebitis and thrombophlebitis of iliac vein, bilateral ☑
I82.421 Acute embolism and thrombosis of right iliac vein ☑
I82.422 Acute embolism and thrombosis of left iliac vein ☑
I82.423 Acute embolism and thrombosis of iliac vein, bilateral ☑
I82.521 Chronic embolism and thrombosis of right iliac vein ☑
I82.522 Chronic embolism and thrombosis of left iliac vein ☑
I82.523 Chronic embolism and thrombosis of iliac vein, bilateral ☑
K91.71 Accidental puncture and laceration of a digestive system organ or structure during a digestive system procedure
K91.72 Accidental puncture and laceration of a digestive system organ or structure during other procedure
K91.840 Postprocedural hemorrhage of a digestive system organ or structure following a digestive system procedure
K91.841 Postprocedural hemorrhage of a digestive system organ or structure following other procedure
K91.870 Postprocedural hematoma of a digestive system organ or structure following a digestive system procedure
K91.871 Postprocedural hematoma of a digestive system organ or structure following other procedure
K91.872 Postprocedural seroma of a digestive system organ or structure following a digestive system procedure
K91.873 Postprocedural seroma of a digestive system organ or structure following other procedure
M96.810 Intraoperative hemorrhage and hematoma of a musculoskeletal structure complicating a musculoskeletal system procedure
M96.811 Intraoperative hemorrhage and hematoma of a musculoskeletal structure complicating other procedure
M96.820 Accidental puncture and laceration of a musculoskeletal structure during a musculoskeletal system procedure
M96.821 Accidental puncture and laceration of a musculoskeletal structure during other procedure
S35.514A Injury of right iliac vein, initial encounter ☑
S35.515A Injury of left iliac vein, initial encounter ☑

Relative Value Units/Medicare Edits

Non-Facility RVU	Work	PE	MP	Total
37660	22.28	11.31	5.73	39.32
Facility RVU	**Work**	**PE**	**MP**	**Total**
37660	22.28	11.31	5.73	39.32

	FUD	Status	MUE	Modifiers				IOM Reference
37660	90	A	1(2)	51	50	62*	80	None

* with documentation

Terms To Know

aneurysm. Circumscribed dilation or outpouching of an artery wall, often containing blood clots and connecting directly with the lumen of the artery.

embolism. Obstruction of a blood vessel resulting from a clot or foreign substance.

hematoma. Tumor-like collection of blood in some part of the body caused by a break in a blood vessel wall, usually as a result of trauma.

37700

37700 Ligation and division of long saphenous vein at saphenofemoral junction, or distal interruptions

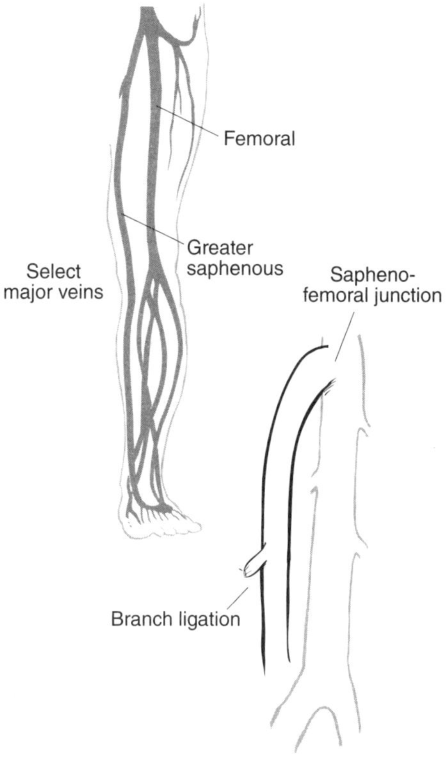

Explanation

Through multiple small incisions in the skin of the upper thigh and along the femoral vein or its branches lower in the thigh, the physician isolates and separates the saphenous vein at the point it joins the femoral vein or at several points farther down the leg. The physician affixes vessel clamps and ligates sections of the saphenous vein along the leg as necessary. Once the ligations are completed, each skin incision is repaired with a layered closure.

Coding Tips

This is a unilateral procedure. If performed bilaterally, some payers require that the service be reported twice with modifier 50 appended to the second code, while others require identification of the service only once with modifier 50 appended. Check with individual payers. Modifier 50 identifies a procedure performed identically on the opposite side of the body (mirror image). Do not report 37700 with 37718 or 37722. For injection of a sclerosing solution, spider veins (telangiectasia), see 36468. For injection of a sclerosing solution for larger veins, see 36470–36471.

ICD-10-CM Diagnostic Codes

- I80.01 Phlebitis and thrombophlebitis of superficial vessels of right lower extremity ☑
- I80.11 Phlebitis and thrombophlebitis of right femoral vein ☑
- I80.291 Phlebitis and thrombophlebitis of other deep vessels of right lower extremity ☑
- I83.011 Varicose veins of right lower extremity with ulcer of thigh A ☑
- I83.012 Varicose veins of right lower extremity with ulcer of calf A ☑
- I83.013 Varicose veins of right lower extremity with ulcer of ankle A ☑
- I83.014 Varicose veins of right lower extremity with ulcer of heel and midfoot A ☑
- I83.015 Varicose veins of right lower extremity with ulcer other part of foot A ☑
- I83.018 Varicose veins of right lower extremity with ulcer other part of lower leg A ☑
- I83.11 Varicose veins of right lower extremity with inflammation A ☑
- I83.211 Varicose veins of right lower extremity with both ulcer of thigh and inflammation A ☑
- I83.212 Varicose veins of right lower extremity with both ulcer of calf and inflammation A ☑
- I83.213 Varicose veins of right lower extremity with both ulcer of ankle and inflammation A ☑
- I83.214 Varicose veins of right lower extremity with both ulcer of heel and midfoot and inflammation A ☑
- I83.215 Varicose veins of right lower extremity with both ulcer other part of foot and inflammation A ☑
- I83.218 Varicose veins of right lower extremity with both ulcer of other part of lower extremity and inflammation A ☑
- I83.811 Varicose veins of right lower extremity with pain A ☑
- I83.891 Varicose veins of right lower extremity with other complications A ☑
- I83.91 Asymptomatic varicose veins of right lower extremity A ☑
- I87.2 Venous insufficiency (chronic) (peripheral)

AMA: **37700** 2018,Mar

Relative Value Units/Medicare Edits

Non-Facility RVU	Work	PE	MP	Total
37700	3.82	2.49	0.95	7.26
Facility RVU	**Work**	**PE**	**MP**	**Total**
37700	3.82	2.49	0.95	7.26

	FUD	Status	MUE	Modifiers				IOM Reference
37700	90	A	1(2)	51	50	N/A	N/A	None

* with documentation

37718-37722

37718 Ligation, division, and stripping, short saphenous vein
37722 Ligation, division, and stripping, long (greater) saphenous veins from saphenofemoral junction to knee or below

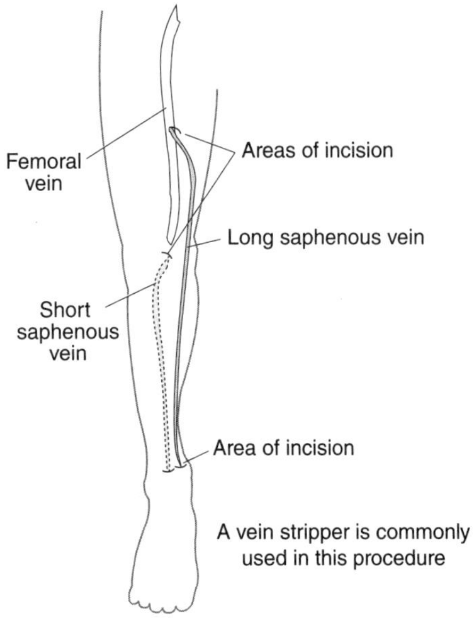

Explanation

The physician makes a skin incision in the upper thigh or upper leg exposing the short saphenous vein (37718) or the long saphenous veins (37722). Additional skin incisions are made at the knee and the ankle and along the leg as necessary. A long wire is threaded through the length of the vein and brought out at the ankle. The vein is tied to the end of the wire and the wire is pulled out along with the vein. Once the vein has been removed, the skin incisions are repaired with layered closures. The leg is wrapped with an elastic pressure dressing postoperatively.

Coding Tips

These are unilateral procedures. If performed bilaterally, some payers require that the service be reported twice with modifier 50 appended to the second code, while others require identification of the service only once with modifier 50 appended. Check with individual payers. Modifier 50 identifies a procedure performed identically on the opposite side of the body (mirror image). Ligation, division, and stripping of the greater saphenous vein are reported with 37722; for the short saphenous vein, report 37718. Do not report 37718 with 37735 or 37780. Do not report 37722 with 37700 or 37735.

ICD-10-CM Diagnostic Codes

I80.01 Phlebitis and thrombophlebitis of superficial vessels of right lower extremity ☑
I80.11 Phlebitis and thrombophlebitis of right femoral vein ☑
I80.291 Phlebitis and thrombophlebitis of other deep vessels of right lower extremity ☑
I83.011 Varicose veins of right lower extremity with ulcer of thigh A ☑
I83.012 Varicose veins of right lower extremity with ulcer of calf A ☑
I83.013 Varicose veins of right lower extremity with ulcer of ankle A ☑
I83.014 Varicose veins of right lower extremity with ulcer of heel and midfoot A ☑
I83.015 Varicose veins of right lower extremity with ulcer other part of foot A ☑
I83.018 Varicose veins of right lower extremity with ulcer other part of lower leg A ☑
I83.11 Varicose veins of right lower extremity with inflammation A ☑
I83.211 Varicose veins of right lower extremity with both ulcer of thigh and inflammation A ☑
I83.212 Varicose veins of right lower extremity with both ulcer of calf and inflammation A ☑
I83.213 Varicose veins of right lower extremity with both ulcer of ankle and inflammation A ☑
I83.214 Varicose veins of right lower extremity with both ulcer of heel and midfoot and inflammation A ☑
I83.215 Varicose veins of right lower extremity with both ulcer other part of foot and inflammation A ☑
I83.218 Varicose veins of right lower extremity with both ulcer of other part of lower extremity and inflammation A ☑
I83.811 Varicose veins of right lower extremity with pain A ☑
I83.891 Varicose veins of right lower extremity with other complications A ☑
I83.91 Asymptomatic varicose veins of right lower extremity A ☑
I87.2 Venous insufficiency (chronic) (peripheral)

AMA: 37718 2018,Mar **37722** 2018,Mar

Relative Value Units/Medicare Edits

Non-Facility RVU	Work	PE	MP	Total
37718	7.13	2.72	1.76	11.61
37722	8.16	3.44	2.03	13.63
Facility RVU	**Work**	**PE**	**MP**	**Total**
37718	7.13	2.72	1.76	11.61
37722	8.16	3.44	2.03	13.63

	FUD	Status	MUE	Modifiers				IOM Reference
37718	90	A	1(2)	51	50	62*	N/A	None
37722	90	A	1(2)	51	50	62*	N/A	

* with documentation

37735

37735 Ligation and division and complete stripping of long or short saphenous veins with radical excision of ulcer and skin graft and/or interruption of communicating veins of lower leg, with excision of deep fascia

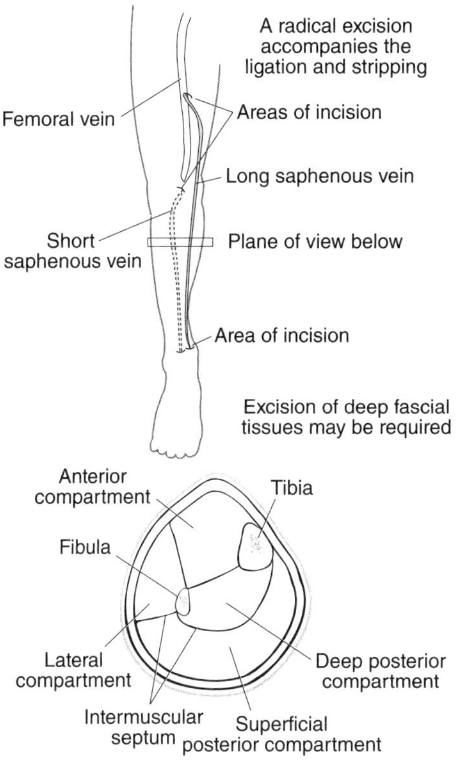

Explanation

The physician makes a skin incision in the upper thigh and the upper leg exposing the long and short saphenous veins. Additional skin incisions are made at the ankle and along the leg as necessary. A long wire is passed through the length of the vein and brought out at the ankle. Each vein is tied to the end of the wire and the vein is pulled out along with the wire. The physician uses a scalpel to remove the skin ulcer from the leg. The ulcer site is covered with a piece of skin that has been shaved from another part of the patient's body. Veins that connect superficial veins with deep veins may be tied off. The tough, fibrous envelope containing the muscle of the leg is split and removed at points where the superficial and deep veins connect. The skin incisions are repaired with layered closures. The leg is wrapped with an elastic pressure dressing postoperatively.

Coding Tips

This is a unilateral procedure. If performed bilaterally, some payers require that the service be reported twice with modifier 50 appended to the second code, while others require identification of the service only once with modifier 50 appended. Check with individual payers. Modifier 50 identifies a procedure performed identically on the opposite side of the body (mirror image). This code includes any debridement performed by the physician. For ligation and division and complete stripping of saphenous veins without excision of ulcer, skin grafting, or interruption of communicating veins, see 37700–37722. Do not report 37735 with 37700, 37718, 37722, or 37780. For injection of a sclerosing solution, spider veins (telangiectasia), see 36468. For injection of a sclerosing solution for larger veins, see 36470–36471.

ICD-10-CM Diagnostic Codes

I83.011	Varicose veins of right lower extremity with ulcer of thigh [A] ☑
I83.012	Varicose veins of right lower extremity with ulcer of calf [A] ☑
I83.013	Varicose veins of right lower extremity with ulcer of ankle [A] ☑
I83.014	Varicose veins of right lower extremity with ulcer of heel and midfoot [A] ☑
I83.015	Varicose veins of right lower extremity with ulcer other part of foot [A] ☑
I83.11	Varicose veins of right lower extremity with inflammation [A] ☑
I83.211	Varicose veins of right lower extremity with both ulcer of thigh and inflammation [A] ☑
I83.212	Varicose veins of right lower extremity with both ulcer of calf and inflammation [A] ☑
I83.213	Varicose veins of right lower extremity with both ulcer of ankle and inflammation [A] ☑
I83.214	Varicose veins of right lower extremity with both ulcer of heel and midfoot and inflammation [A] ☑
I83.811	Varicose veins of right lower extremity with pain [A] ☑
I83.891	Varicose veins of right lower extremity with other complications [A] ☑
I83.91	Asymptomatic varicose veins of right lower extremity [A] ☑
I87.2	Venous insufficiency (chronic) (peripheral)
L97.111	Non-pressure chronic ulcer of right thigh limited to breakdown of skin ☑
L97.112	Non-pressure chronic ulcer of right thigh with fat layer exposed ☑
L97.113	Non-pressure chronic ulcer of right thigh with necrosis of muscle ☑
L97.114	Non-pressure chronic ulcer of right thigh with necrosis of bone ☑
L97.115	Non-pressure chronic ulcer of right thigh with muscle involvement without evidence of necrosis ☑
L97.116	Non-pressure chronic ulcer of right thigh with bone involvement without evidence of necrosis ☑
L97.211	Non-pressure chronic ulcer of right calf limited to breakdown of skin ☑
L97.212	Non-pressure chronic ulcer of right calf with fat layer exposed ☑
L97.213	Non-pressure chronic ulcer of right calf with necrosis of muscle ☑
L97.214	Non-pressure chronic ulcer of right calf with necrosis of bone ☑
L97.215	Non-pressure chronic ulcer of right calf with muscle involvement without evidence of necrosis ☑
L97.216	Non-pressure chronic ulcer of right calf with bone involvement without evidence of necrosis ☑
L97.311	Non-pressure chronic ulcer of right ankle limited to breakdown of skin ☑
L97.312	Non-pressure chronic ulcer of right ankle with fat layer exposed ☑
L97.313	Non-pressure chronic ulcer of right ankle with necrosis of muscle ☑
L97.314	Non-pressure chronic ulcer of right ankle with necrosis of bone ☑
L97.315	Non-pressure chronic ulcer of right ankle with muscle involvement without evidence of necrosis ☑
L97.316	Non-pressure chronic ulcer of right ankle with bone involvement without evidence of necrosis ☑
L97.411	Non-pressure chronic ulcer of right heel and midfoot limited to breakdown of skin ☑

L97.412 Non-pressure chronic ulcer of right heel and midfoot with fat layer exposed ☑
L97.413 Non-pressure chronic ulcer of right heel and midfoot with necrosis of muscle ☑
L97.414 Non-pressure chronic ulcer of right heel and midfoot with necrosis of bone ☑
L97.415 Non-pressure chronic ulcer of right heel and midfoot with muscle involvement without evidence of necrosis ☑
L97.416 Non-pressure chronic ulcer of right heel and midfoot with bone involvement without evidence of necrosis ☑
L97.525 Non-pressure chronic ulcer of other part of left foot with muscle involvement without evidence of necrosis ☑
L97.526 Non-pressure chronic ulcer of other part of left foot with bone involvement without evidence of necrosis ☑
L97.825 Non-pressure chronic ulcer of other part of left lower leg with muscle involvement without evidence of necrosis ☑
L97.826 Non-pressure chronic ulcer of other part of left lower leg with bone involvement without evidence of necrosis ☑

AMA: **37735** 2018,Mar

Relative Value Units/Medicare Edits

Non-Facility RVU	Work	PE	MP	Total
37735	10.9	3.56	2.71	17.17
Facility RVU	**Work**	**PE**	**MP**	**Total**
37735	10.9	3.56	2.71	17.17

	FUD	Status	MUE	Modifiers				IOM Reference
37735	90	A	1(2)	51	50	62*	N/A	None

* with documentation

Terms To Know

debridement. Removal of dead or contaminated tissue and foreign matter from a wound.

fascia. Fibrous sheet or band of tissue that envelops organs, muscles, and groupings of muscles.

graft. Tissue implant from another part of the body or another person.

inflammation. Cytologic and chemical reactions that occur in affected blood vessels and adjacent tissues in response to injury or abnormal stimulation from a physical, chemical, or biologic agent.

ligation. Tying off a blood vessel or duct with a suture or a soft, thin wire.

radical. Extensive surgery.

ulcer. Open sore or excavating lesion of skin or the tissue on the surface of an organ from the sloughing of chronically inflamed and necrosing tissue.

varicose vein. Abnormal, permanently distended or stretched vein.

37760-37761

37760 Ligation of perforator veins, subfascial, radical (Linton type), including skin graft, when performed, open,1 leg

37761 Ligation of perforator vein(s), subfascial, open, including ultrasound guidance, when performed, 1 leg

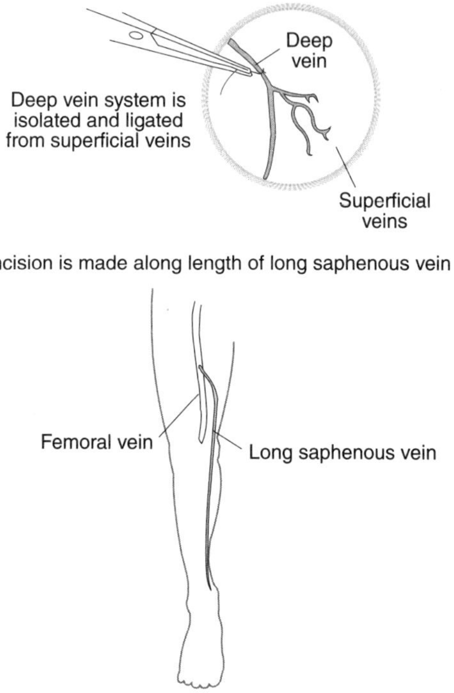

Explanation

The physician performs a radical (Linton type) subfascial ligation (tying) of the perforator veins in 37760 and an open subfascial perforator vein ligation in 37761. Through incisions along the course of the saphenous vein, the veins connecting the deep and superficial veins of the leg are isolated. They are ligated, isolating the two systems along the course of the leg. The incisions may be sutured or covered with skin grafts taken from another part of the patient's body. Code 37760 includes skin grafts, when performed, and code 37761 includes the use of ultrasonic guidance, when performed. Both codes report a procedure involving one leg.

Coding Tips

These are unilateral procedures. If performed bilaterally, some payers require the service be reported twice with modifier 50 appended to the second code, while others require identification of the service only once with modifier 50 appended. Check with individual payers. Modifier 50 identifies a procedure performed identically on the opposite side of the body (mirror image). This code includes any skin graft the physician may perform. For endoscopic ligation of perforator veins, subfascial (SEPS), see 37500. For other treatment of long and/or short saphenous veins, see 37700–37735 and 37780. For injection of a sclerosing solution, spider veins (telangiectasia), see 36468. For injection of a sclerosing solution for larger veins, see 36470–36471. For 37760–37761 codes 76937, 76942, 76998, and 93971 are not separately reportable.

ICD-10-CM Diagnostic Codes

I83.011 Varicose veins of right lower extremity with ulcer of thigh A ☑
I83.012 Varicose veins of right lower extremity with ulcer of calf A ☑
I83.013 Varicose veins of right lower extremity with ulcer of ankle A ☑

I83.014 Varicose veins of right lower extremity with ulcer of heel and midfoot A ☑

I83.015 Varicose veins of right lower extremity with ulcer other part of foot A ☑

I83.018 Varicose veins of right lower extremity with ulcer other part of lower leg A ☑

I83.11 Varicose veins of right lower extremity with inflammation A ☑

I83.211 Varicose veins of right lower extremity with both ulcer of thigh and inflammation A ☑

I83.212 Varicose veins of right lower extremity with both ulcer of calf and inflammation A ☑

I83.213 Varicose veins of right lower extremity with both ulcer of ankle and inflammation A ☑

I83.214 Varicose veins of right lower extremity with both ulcer of heel and midfoot and inflammation A ☑

I83.215 Varicose veins of right lower extremity with both ulcer other part of foot and inflammation A ☑

I83.218 Varicose veins of right lower extremity with both ulcer of other part of lower extremity and inflammation A ☑

I83.811 Varicose veins of right lower extremity with pain A ☑

I83.891 Varicose veins of right lower extremity with other complications A ☑

I83.91 Asymptomatic varicose veins of right lower extremity A ☑

AMA: **37760** 2023,Jan; 2018,Mar **37761** 2023,Jan; 2018,Mar

Relative Value Units/Medicare Edits

Non-Facility RVU	Work	PE	MP	Total
37760	10.78	3.54	2.68	17.0
37761	9.13	4.55	2.22	15.9
Facility RVU	**Work**	**PE**	**MP**	**Total**
37760	10.78	3.54	2.68	17.0
37761	9.13	4.55	2.22	15.9

	FUD	Status	MUE	Modifiers				IOM Reference
37760	90	A	1(2)	51	50	62*	N/A	None
37761	90	A	1(2)	51	50	62*	80	

* with documentation

Terms To Know

ligation. Tying off a blood vessel or duct with a suture or a soft, thin wire.

sclerose. To become hard or firm and indurated from increased formation of connective tissue or disease.

ulcer. Open sore or excavating lesion of skin or the tissue on the surface of an organ from the sloughing of chronically inflamed and necrosing tissue.

37765-37766

37765 Stab phlebectomy of varicose veins, 1 extremity; 10-20 stab incisions

37766 more than 20 incisions

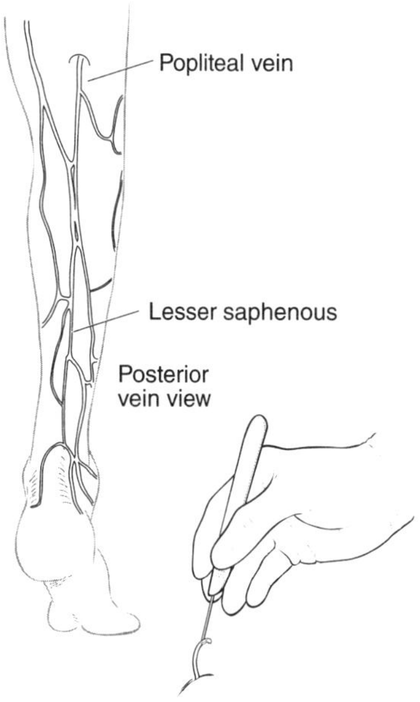

Stab incisions are made over the varicose vein and a hooked device retrieves the section of vein

Explanation

Stab phlebectomy for varicose veins is an ambulatory procedure that permits removal of nearly any incompetent vein below the saphenofemoral and saphenopopliteal junction. The varicose veins are identified with an indelible marking pen while the patient is standing. The patient is placed supine for further marking. Diluted lidocaine is injected into the tissues in large volumes until the perivenous tissues are engorged and distended with the anesthetic. Regional nerve blocks may be used for extensive areas. Tiny stab incisions are made with a scalpel or 18-gauge needle. The varicose vein is dissected with the phlebectomy hook. The vein is undermined along its course, all fibroadipose attachments to the vein are freed, and the vein is grasped with the hook and removed with mosquito forceps. Hemostasis is achieved by applying local compression to the veins already removed. The varicose vein is progressively extracted from one stab incision to the next. No skin closure is needed. Bandages are applied. Large pads are placed along the site of vein removal and covered with an inelastic bandage, followed by a second bandage of highly elastic material. Report 37765 when 10 to 20 stab incisions are made and 37766 when more than 20 are reported.

Coding Tips

For open ligation of subfascial or radical perforator veins, see 37760; for endoscopic ligation of perforator veins, subfascial (SEPS), see 37500. If a stab phlebectomy is performed with less than 10 incisions, see 37799.

ICD-10-CM Diagnostic Codes

I83.011 Varicose veins of right lower extremity with ulcer of thigh A ☑

I83.012 Varicose veins of right lower extremity with ulcer of calf A ☑

I83.013 Varicose veins of right lower extremity with ulcer of ankle A ☑

I83.014 Varicose veins of right lower extremity with ulcer of heel and midfoot A ☑

I83.015 Varicose veins of right lower extremity with ulcer other part of foot A ☑

I83.018 Varicose veins of right lower extremity with ulcer other part of lower leg A ☑

I83.11 Varicose veins of right lower extremity with inflammation A ☑

I83.211 Varicose veins of right lower extremity with both ulcer of thigh and inflammation A ☑

I83.212 Varicose veins of right lower extremity with both ulcer of calf and inflammation A ☑

I83.213 Varicose veins of right lower extremity with both ulcer of ankle and inflammation A ☑

I83.214 Varicose veins of right lower extremity with both ulcer of heel and midfoot and inflammation A ☑

I83.215 Varicose veins of right lower extremity with both ulcer other part of foot and inflammation A ☑

I83.218 Varicose veins of right lower extremity with both ulcer of other part of lower extremity and inflammation A ☑

I83.811 Varicose veins of right lower extremity with pain A ☑

I83.891 Varicose veins of right lower extremity with other complications A ☑

I83.91 Asymptomatic varicose veins of right lower extremity A ☑

AMA: **37765** 2018,Mar **37766** 2018,Mar

Relative Value Units/Medicare Edits

Non-Facility RVU	Work	PE	MP	Total
37765	4.8	6.66	1.09	12.55
37766	6.0	7.41	1.35	14.76
Facility RVU	**Work**	**PE**	**MP**	**Total**
37765	4.8	2.09	1.09	7.98
37766	6.0	2.43	1.35	9.78

	FUD	Status	MUE	Modifiers				IOM Reference
37765	10	A	1(2)	51	50	62*	N/A	None
37766	10	A	1(2)	51	50	62*	N/A	

* with documentation

Terms To Know

forceps. Tool used for grasping or compressing tissue.

hemostasis. Interruption of blood flow or the cessation or arrest of bleeding.

incision. Act of cutting into tissue or an organ.

supine. Lying on the back.

ulcer. Open sore or excavating lesion of skin or the tissue on the surface of an organ from the sloughing of chronically inflamed and necrosing tissue.

varicose vein. Abnormal, permanently distended or stretched vein.

37780

37780 Ligation and division of short saphenous vein at saphenopopliteal junction (separate procedure)

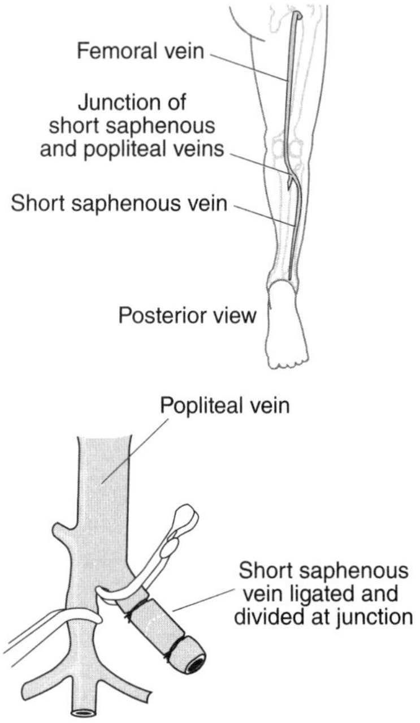

Explanation

The physician makes an incision in the skin overlying the short saphenous vein at its junction with the saphenopopliteal vein at the knee. The vessels are dissected and ties are placed around the short saphenous vein which is divided between the ties. Once the ties are in place and the vein has been divided, the skin incision is repaired with a layered closure.

Coding Tips

This separate procedure by definition is usually a component of a more complex service and is not identified separately. When performed alone or with other unrelated procedures/services, it may be reported. If performed alone, list the code; if performed with other procedures/services, list the code and append modifier 59 or an X{EPSU} modifier. This is a unilateral procedure. If performed bilaterally, some payers require that the service be reported twice with modifier 50 appended to the second code, while others require identification of the service only once with modifier 50 appended. Check with individual payers. Modifier 50 identifies a procedure performed identically on the opposite side of the body (mirror image). For other treatment of long or short saphenous veins, see 37700–37735. For injection of a sclerosing solution, spider veins (telangiectasia), see 36468. For injection of a sclerosing solution for larger veins, see 36470–36471.

ICD-10-CM Diagnostic Codes

I80.221 Phlebitis and thrombophlebitis of right popliteal vein ☑

I80.291 Phlebitis and thrombophlebitis of other deep vessels of right lower extremity ☑

I83.011 Varicose veins of right lower extremity with ulcer of thigh A ☑

I83.012 Varicose veins of right lower extremity with ulcer of calf A ☑

I83.013 Varicose veins of right lower extremity with ulcer of ankle A ☑

I83.014 Varicose veins of right lower extremity with ulcer of heel and midfoot A ☑

I83.015 Varicose veins of right lower extremity with ulcer other part of foot [A] ☑
I83.018 Varicose veins of right lower extremity with ulcer other part of lower leg [A] ☑
I83.11 Varicose veins of right lower extremity with inflammation [A] ☑
I83.211 Varicose veins of right lower extremity with both ulcer of thigh and inflammation [A] ☑
I83.212 Varicose veins of right lower extremity with both ulcer of calf and inflammation [A] ☑
I83.213 Varicose veins of right lower extremity with both ulcer of ankle and inflammation [A] ☑
I83.214 Varicose veins of right lower extremity with both ulcer of heel and midfoot and inflammation [A] ☑
I83.215 Varicose veins of right lower extremity with both ulcer other part of foot and inflammation [A] ☑
I83.218 Varicose veins of right lower extremity with both ulcer of other part of lower extremity and inflammation [A] ☑
I83.811 Varicose veins of right lower extremity with pain [A] ☑
I83.891 Varicose veins of right lower extremity with other complications [A] ☑
I83.91 Asymptomatic varicose veins of right lower extremity [A] ☑
I87.2 Venous insufficiency (chronic) (peripheral)

Relative Value Units/Medicare Edits

Non-Facility RVU	Work	PE	MP	Total
37780	3.93	2.1	0.98	7.01
Facility RVU	**Work**	**PE**	**MP**	**Total**
37780	3.93	2.1	0.98	7.01

	FUD	Status	MUE	Modifiers				IOM Reference
37780	90	A	1(2)	51	50	62*	N/A	None

* with documentation

Terms To Know

dissect. Cut apart or separate tissue for surgical purposes or for visual or microscopic study.

ligation. Tying off a blood vessel or duct with a suture or a soft, thin wire.

varicose vein. Abnormal, permanently distended or stretched vein.

37785

37785 Ligation, division, and/or excision of varicose vein cluster(s), 1 leg

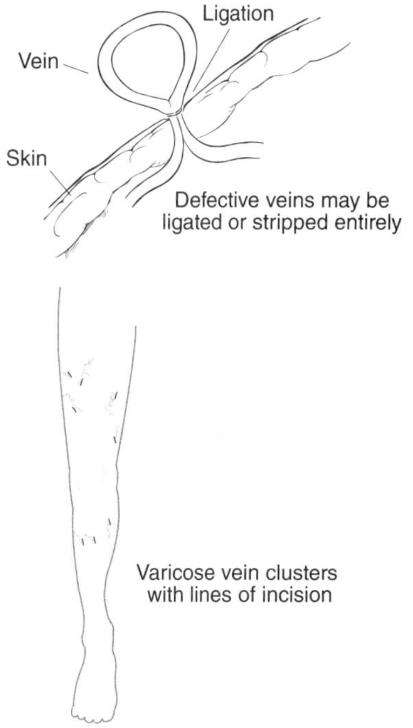

Explanation

The physician ligates, divides, and/or excises varicose vein cluster(s) in one leg. The physician makes small incisions in the skin over localized areas of superficial varicose veins along the leg. These veins are isolated and dissected free of neighboring tissue, tied with sutures and divided, or stripped out bluntly. Pressure is applied over the site to stop bleeding. All incisions are repaired with a layered closure. The legs are wrapped in an elastic pressure dressing postoperatively.

Coding Tips

This is a unilateral procedure. If performed bilaterally, some payers require that the service be reported twice with modifier 50 appended to the second code, while others require identification of the service only once with modifier 50 appended. Check with individual payers. Modifier 50 identifies a procedure performed identically on the opposite side of the body (mirror image). For initial treatment of varicose veins, see 37700–37780. For injection of a sclerosing solution, spider veins (telangiectasia), see 36468. For injection of a sclerosing solution for larger veins, see 36470–36471.

ICD-10-CM Diagnostic Codes

I83.011 Varicose veins of right lower extremity with ulcer of thigh [A] ☑
I83.012 Varicose veins of right lower extremity with ulcer of calf [A] ☑
I83.013 Varicose veins of right lower extremity with ulcer of ankle [A] ☑
I83.014 Varicose veins of right lower extremity with ulcer of heel and midfoot [A] ☑
I83.015 Varicose veins of right lower extremity with ulcer other part of foot [A] ☑
I83.018 Varicose veins of right lower extremity with ulcer other part of lower leg [A] ☑
I83.021 Varicose veins of left lower extremity with ulcer of thigh [A] ☑
I83.022 Varicose veins of left lower extremity with ulcer of calf [A] ☑
I83.023 Varicose veins of left lower extremity with ulcer of ankle [A] ☑

I83.024 Varicose veins of left lower extremity with ulcer of heel and midfoot [A] ☑

I83.025 Varicose veins of left lower extremity with ulcer other part of foot [A] ☑

I83.028 Varicose veins of left lower extremity with ulcer other part of lower leg [A] ☑

I83.11 Varicose veins of right lower extremity with inflammation [A] ☑

I83.12 Varicose veins of left lower extremity with inflammation [A] ☑

I83.211 Varicose veins of right lower extremity with both ulcer of thigh and inflammation [A] ☑

I83.212 Varicose veins of right lower extremity with both ulcer of calf and inflammation [A] ☑

I83.213 Varicose veins of right lower extremity with both ulcer of ankle and inflammation [A] ☑

I83.214 Varicose veins of right lower extremity with both ulcer of heel and midfoot and inflammation [A] ☑

I83.215 Varicose veins of right lower extremity with both ulcer other part of foot and inflammation [A] ☑

I83.218 Varicose veins of right lower extremity with both ulcer of other part of lower extremity and inflammation [A] ☑

I83.221 Varicose veins of left lower extremity with both ulcer of thigh and inflammation [A] ☑

I83.222 Varicose veins of left lower extremity with both ulcer of calf and inflammation [A] ☑

I83.223 Varicose veins of left lower extremity with both ulcer of ankle and inflammation [A] ☑

I83.224 Varicose veins of left lower extremity with both ulcer of heel and midfoot and inflammation [A] ☑

I83.225 Varicose veins of left lower extremity with both ulcer other part of foot and inflammation [A] ☑

I83.228 Varicose veins of left lower extremity with both ulcer of other part of lower extremity and inflammation [A] ☑

I83.811 Varicose veins of right lower extremity with pain [A] ☑

I83.812 Varicose veins of left lower extremity with pain [A] ☑

I83.813 Varicose veins of bilateral lower extremities with pain [A] ☑

I83.891 Varicose veins of right lower extremity with other complications [A] ☑

I83.892 Varicose veins of left lower extremity with other complications [A] ☑

I83.893 Varicose veins of bilateral lower extremities with other complications [A] ☑

I83.91 Asymptomatic varicose veins of right lower extremity [A] ☑

I83.92 Asymptomatic varicose veins of left lower extremity [A] ☑

I83.93 Asymptomatic varicose veins of bilateral lower extremities [A] ☑

Relative Value Units/Medicare Edits

Non-Facility RVU	Work	PE	MP	Total
37785	3.93	5.55	0.97	10.45
Facility RVU	**Work**	**PE**	**MP**	**Total**
37785	3.93	2.68	0.97	7.58

	FUD	Status	MUE	Modifiers				IOM Reference
37785	90	A	1(2)	51	50	N/A	N/A	None

* with documentation

38300-38305

38300 Drainage of lymph node abscess or lymphadenitis; simple
38305 extensive

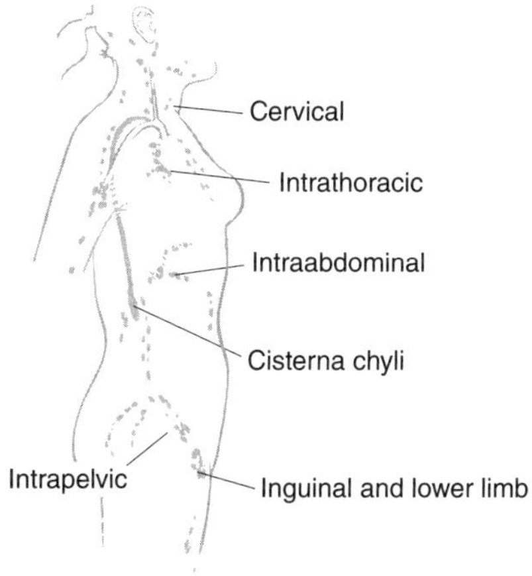

Explanation

The physician performs this procedure to drain inflamed lymph nodes. The physician makes an incision over the affected lymph node and the abscess or infection is drained. The wound is irrigated and closed with sutures or Steri-strips. Report 38305 if the procedure is extensive.

Coding Tips

These are bilateral procedures and as such are reported once even if the procedure is performed on both sides. When 38300 or 38305 is performed with another separately identifiable procedure, the highest dollar value code is listed as the primary procedure and subsequent procedures are appended with modifier 51. For injection for sentinel node identification, see 38792. For imaging guidance, see 76942, 77012, and 77021. For fine needle aspiration, see 10021 For fine needle aspiration, see 10004-10012 and 10021.

ICD-10-CM Diagnostic Codes

A18.2	Tuberculous peripheral lymphadenopathy
A51.49	Other secondary syphilitic conditions
I88.0	Nonspecific mesenteric lymphadenitis
I88.1	Chronic lymphadenitis, except mesenteric
I88.8	Other nonspecific lymphadenitis
I89.8	Other specified noninfective disorders of lymphatic vessels and lymph nodes
L04.0	Acute lymphadenitis of face, head and neck
L04.1	Acute lymphadenitis of trunk
L04.2	Acute lymphadenitis of upper limb
L04.3	Acute lymphadenitis of lower limb
L04.8	Acute lymphadenitis of other sites
R59.0	Localized enlarged lymph nodes
R59.1	Generalized enlarged lymph nodes

Relative Value Units/Medicare Edits

Non-Facility RVU	Work	PE	MP	Total
38300	2.36	7.23	0.6	10.19
38305	6.68	6.6	1.72	15.0
Facility RVU	**Work**	**PE**	**MP**	**Total**
38300	2.36	3.4	0.6	6.36
38305	6.68	6.6	1.72	15.0

	FUD	Status	MUE	Modifiers				IOM Reference
38300	10	A	1(3)	51	N/A	N/A	N/A	None
38305	90	A	1(3)	51	N/A	N/A	N/A	

* with documentation

Terms To Know

abscess. Circumscribed collection of pus resulting from bacteria, frequently associated with swelling and other signs of inflammation.

infection. Presence of microorganisms in body tissues that may result in cellular damage.

irrigate. Washing out, lavage.

lymph nodes. Bean-shaped structures along the lymphatic vessels that intercept and destroy foreign materials in the tissue and bloodstream.

lymphadenitis. Inflammation or enlargement of the lymph nodes.

38381

38381 Suture and/or ligation of thoracic duct; thoracic approach

The thoracic duct is a major drainage channel of the lymphatic system. It enters near the junction of the left internal jugular and subclavian veins

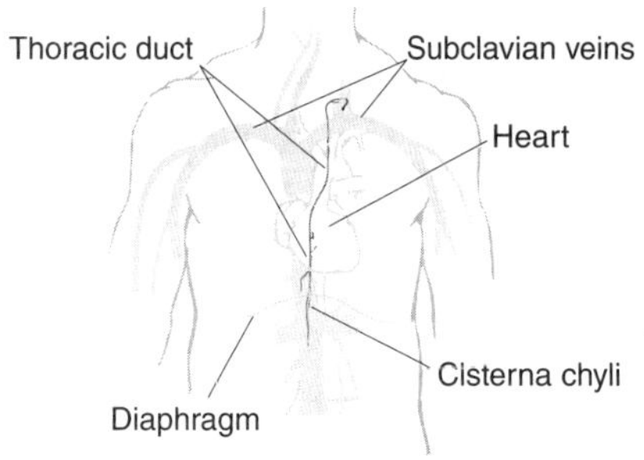

The thoracic duct is accessed by a thoracic incision and is ligated or sutured

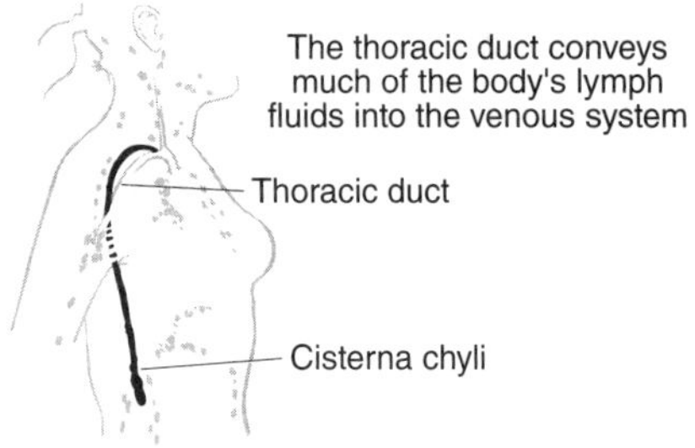

Explanation

The thoracic duct is sutured or ligated. The thoracic duct is a tubular structure, approximately 2 to 3 mm in diameter, that originates in the cisterna chyli, which lies above the second lumbar vertebral body. It ascends on the right, anterior to the vertebral bodies, entering the chest through the aortic hiatus. At the fourth or fifth thoracic vertebra, it crosses to the left and empties into the left jugulosubclavian venous junction. Tears or injury can occur in any segment (cervical, thoracic, abdominal) and the approach is dependent on the site of the leak. An incision is made in the left neck, right or left chest, or abdomen. The involved compartment is drained of all effluent and the leak identified. The duct is ligated a few centimeters below the leak and also a few centimeters above it. Dry gauze is placed at the site of the leak to ensure that the ligation has completely sealed the leak. When it has been determined that the leak is completely sealed, the gauze is removed and glue or other sealant is applied to the area. If the leak is repaired by thoracotomy, chest tubes are placed. Incisions are closed. Report 38381 for a thoracic approach.

Coding Tips

When 38381 is performed with another separately identifiable procedure, the highest dollar value code is listed as the primary procedure, and subsequent procedures are appended with modifier 51.

ICD-10-CM Diagnostic Codes

I89.8	Other specified noninfective disorders of lymphatic vessels and lymph nodes
S27.898A	Other injury of other specified intrathoracic organs, initial encounter

Relative Value Units/Medicare Edits

Non-Facility RVU	Work	PE	MP	Total
38381	13.38	7.32	3.28	23.98
Facility RVU	**Work**	**PE**	**MP**	**Total**
38381	13.38	7.32	3.28	23.98

	FUD	Status	MUE	Modifiers				IOM Reference
38381	90	A	1(2)	51	N/A	62*	80	None

* with documentation

Terms To Know

closure. Repairing an incision or wound by suture or other means.

dissect. Cut apart or separate tissue for surgical purposes or for visual or microscopic study.

fistula. Abnormal tube-like passage between two body cavities or organs or from an organ to the outside surface.

incision. Act of cutting into tissue or an organ.

ligation. Tying off a blood vessel or duct with a suture or a soft, thin wire.

lymphadenitis. Inflammation or enlargement of the lymph nodes.

lymphangitis. Inflammation of the lymph channels most often caused by *Streptococcus*.

lymphoma. Tumors occurring in the lymphoid tissues that are most commonly malignant.

malignant. Any condition tending to progress toward death, specifically an invasive tumor with a loss of cellular differentiation that has the ability to spread or metastasize to other body areas.

secondary. Second in order of occurrence or importance, or appearing during the course of another disease or condition.

suture. Numerous stitching techniques employed in wound closure.

38746

+ **38746** Thoracic lymphadenectomy by thoracotomy, mediastinal and regional lymphadenectomy (List separately in addition to code for primary procedure)

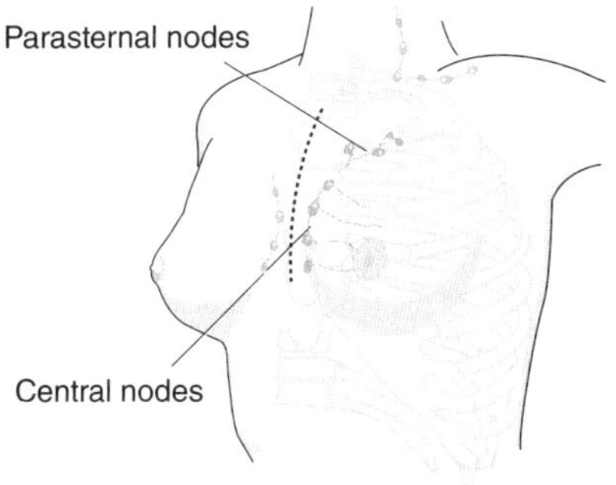

Typical access incision for thoracic lymphadenectomy

Explanation

The physician performs a regional and mediastinal lymphadenectomy via an open approach. Using a scalpel, the surgeon makes a long incision around the side of the chest between two of the ribs. The incision is carried through all of the tissue layers into the chest cavity. Rib spreaders are inserted into the wound and the ribs are spread apart exposing the lung, the heart, and other structures. Alternately, the chest cavity can be opened and the operation performed through a vertical incision in the center of the chest through the sternum. The skin incision is carried down to the sternum bone and a saw is used to split the sternum. With the sternum split in half, the chest is entered by spreading the sternum apart with a set of rib spreaders. Lymph nodes near the lungs, around the heart, and behind the trachea are removed. The area is irrigated and the retractors are removed. If applicable, the sternotomy is repaired using wires to bring the two halves of the sternum together, and the operative wound is closed by sutures or staples.

Coding Tips

Report 38746 in addition to 21601, 31760, 31766, 31786, 32096-32200, 32220-32320, 32440-32491, 32503-32505, 33025, 33030, 33050-33130, 39200-39220, 39560, 39561, 43101, 43112, 43117, 43118, 43122, 43123, 43351, 60270, or 60505. For thoracoscopic mediastinal and regional lymphadenectomy, see 32674.

ICD-10-CM Diagnostic Codes

This/these CPT code(s) are add-on code(s). See the primary procedure code that this code is performed with for your ICD-10-CM code selections. Diagnostic code(s) would be the same as the actual procedure performed.

AMA: 38746 2019,Feb

Relative Value Units/Medicare Edits

Non-Facility RVU	Work	PE	MP	Total
38746	4.12	1.16	1.01	6.29
Facility RVU	**Work**	**PE**	**MP**	**Total**
38746	4.12	1.16	1.01	6.29

	FUD	Status	MUE	Modifiers				IOM Reference
38746	N/A	A	1(2)	N/A	N/A	62*	80	None

* with documentation

39000-39010

39000 Mediastinotomy with exploration, drainage, removal of foreign body, or biopsy; cervical approach

39010 transthoracic approach, including either transthoracic or median sternotomy

The mediastinum describes tissues and organs bounded by lungs, spinal column, and sternum. Exploration, drainage, or removal of a foreign body or a biopsy is performed

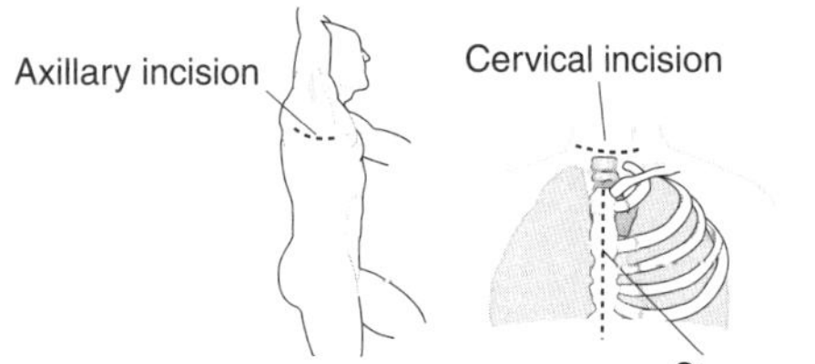

A sternal (median sternotomy) or axillary incision is employed

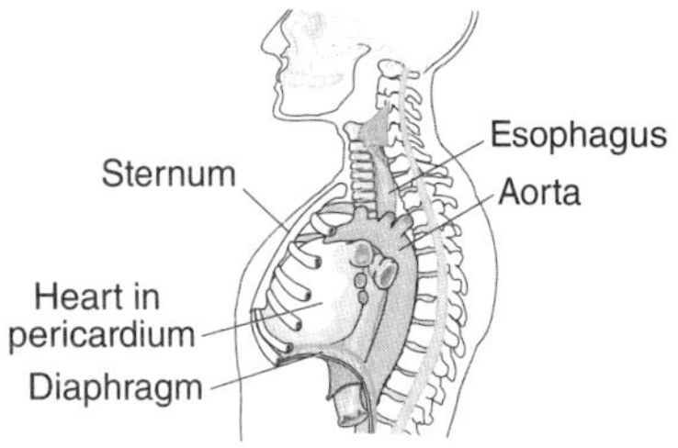

The heart, pericardium, bases of great vessels, trachea, bronchi, esophagus, thymus, thoracic lymph nodes, thoracic duct, and phrenic and vagus nerves are all part of the mediastinum

Explanation

The physician makes an incision low in the front of the neck, pulling back the sternomastoid muscles and the cranial vessels to the side and drawing the trachea and thyroid to the center. The space behind the esophagus is exposed. The foreign body is removed, biopsy of any abnormal mass performed, and Penrose drains are placed. The incision is closed with sutures or staples. Report 39010 if using a transthoracic approach.

Coding Tips

When 39000 or 39010 is performed with another separately identifiable procedure, the highest dollar value code is listed as the primary procedure and subsequent procedures are appended with modifier 51. Do not report 39010 with 33955, 33956, 33963, or 33964. For mediastinoscopy, with or without biopsy, see 39401. For video-assisted thoracic surgery (VATS) pericardial biopsy, see 32604.

ICD-10-CM Diagnostic Codes

A15.4	Tuberculosis of intrathoracic lymph nodes
C33	Malignant neoplasm of trachea
C34.01	Malignant neoplasm of right main bronchus ☑
C34.02	Malignant neoplasm of left main bronchus ☑
C34.11	Malignant neoplasm of upper lobe, right bronchus or lung ☑
C34.12	Malignant neoplasm of upper lobe, left bronchus or lung ☑
C34.2	Malignant neoplasm of middle lobe, bronchus or lung
C34.31	Malignant neoplasm of lower lobe, right bronchus or lung ☑
C34.32	Malignant neoplasm of lower lobe, left bronchus or lung ☑
C34.81	Malignant neoplasm of overlapping sites of right bronchus and lung ☑
C34.82	Malignant neoplasm of overlapping sites of left bronchus and lung ☑
C37	Malignant neoplasm of thymus
C38.0	Malignant neoplasm of heart
C38.1	Malignant neoplasm of anterior mediastinum
C38.2	Malignant neoplasm of posterior mediastinum
C38.8	Malignant neoplasm of overlapping sites of heart, mediastinum and pleura
C45.0	Mesothelioma of pleura
C77.1	Secondary and unspecified malignant neoplasm of intrathoracic lymph nodes
C78.01	Secondary malignant neoplasm of right lung ☑
C78.02	Secondary malignant neoplasm of left lung ☑
C78.1	Secondary malignant neoplasm of mediastinum
C78.2	Secondary malignant neoplasm of pleura
C7A.090	Malignant carcinoid tumor of the bronchus and lung
C7A.091	Malignant carcinoid tumor of the thymus
C81.02	Nodular lymphocyte predominant Hodgkin lymphoma, intrathoracic lymph nodes
C81.12	Nodular sclerosis Hodgkin lymphoma, intrathoracic lymph nodes
C81.22	Mixed cellularity Hodgkin lymphoma, intrathoracic lymph nodes
C81.32	Lymphocyte depleted Hodgkin lymphoma, intrathoracic lymph nodes
C81.42	Lymphocyte-rich Hodgkin lymphoma, intrathoracic lymph nodes
C81.72	Other Hodgkin lymphoma, intrathoracic lymph nodes
C82.02	Follicular lymphoma grade I, intrathoracic lymph nodes
C82.12	Follicular lymphoma grade II, intrathoracic lymph nodes
C82.32	Follicular lymphoma grade IIIa, intrathoracic lymph nodes
C82.52	Diffuse follicle center lymphoma, intrathoracic lymph nodes
C82.62	Cutaneous follicle center lymphoma, intrathoracic lymph nodes
C82.82	Other types of follicular lymphoma, intrathoracic lymph nodes
C83.02	Small cell B-cell lymphoma, intrathoracic lymph nodes
C83.12	Mantle cell lymphoma, intrathoracic lymph nodes
C83.32	Diffuse large B-cell lymphoma, intrathoracic lymph nodes
C83.52	Lymphoblastic (diffuse) lymphoma, intrathoracic lymph nodes
C83.72	Burkitt lymphoma, intrathoracic lymph nodes
C84.02	Mycosis fungoides, intrathoracic lymph nodes
C84.12	Sezary disease, intrathoracic lymph nodes
C84.Z2	Other mature T/NK-cell lymphomas, intrathoracic lymph nodes
C85.22	Mediastinal (thymic) large B-cell lymphoma, intrathoracic lymph nodes
C85.82	Other specified types of non-Hodgkin lymphoma, intrathoracic lymph nodes
D02.1	Carcinoma in situ of trachea
D02.21	Carcinoma in situ of right bronchus and lung ☑
D02.22	Carcinoma in situ of left bronchus and lung ☑
D02.3	Carcinoma in situ of other parts of respiratory system
D14.2	Benign neoplasm of trachea
D14.31	Benign neoplasm of right bronchus and lung ☑
D14.32	Benign neoplasm of left bronchus and lung ☑
D15.0	Benign neoplasm of thymus
D15.2	Benign neoplasm of mediastinum
D19.0	Benign neoplasm of mesothelial tissue of pleura
D38.1	Neoplasm of uncertain behavior of trachea, bronchus and lung

D38.2	Neoplasm of uncertain behavior of pleura
D38.3	Neoplasm of uncertain behavior of mediastinum
D38.4	Neoplasm of uncertain behavior of thymus
D3A.090	Benign carcinoid tumor of the bronchus and lung
D3A.091	Benign carcinoid tumor of the thymus
J85.3	Abscess of mediastinum
J86.0	Pyothorax with fistula
J91.0	Malignant pleural effusion
J98.51	Mediastinitis
J98.59	Other diseases of mediastinum, not elsewhere classified
S21.321A	Laceration with foreign body of right front wall of thorax with penetration into thoracic cavity, initial encounter
S21.322A	Laceration with foreign body of left front wall of thorax with penetration into thoracic cavity, initial encounter
S21.341A	Puncture wound with foreign body of right front wall of thorax with penetration into thoracic cavity, initial encounter
S21.342A	Puncture wound with foreign body of left front wall of thorax with penetration into thoracic cavity, initial encounter
S21.421A	Laceration with foreign body of right back wall of thorax with penetration into thoracic cavity, initial encounter
S21.422A	Laceration with foreign body of left back wall of thorax with penetration into thoracic cavity, initial encounter
S21.441A	Puncture wound with foreign body of right back wall of thorax with penetration into thoracic cavity, initial encounter
S21.442A	Puncture wound with foreign body of left back wall of thorax with penetration into thoracic cavity, initial encounter

AMA: 39000 2021,Apr **39010** 2021,Apr

Relative Value Units/Medicare Edits

Non-Facility RVU	Work	PE	MP	Total
39000	7.57	5.88	1.7	15.15
39010	13.19	7.1	3.18	23.47
Facility RVU	**Work**	**PE**	**MP**	**Total**
39000	7.57	5.88	1.7	15.15
39010	13.19	7.1	3.18	23.47

	FUD	Status	MUE	Modifiers				IOM Reference
39000	90	A	1(2)	51	N/A	62*	80	None
39010	90	A	1(2)	51	N/A	62*	80	

* with documentation

Terms To Know

abscess. Circumscribed collection of pus resulting from bacteria, frequently associated with swelling and other signs of inflammation.

hemorrhage syndrome. Fulminating meningococcal septicemia occurring in children younger than 10 years of age with vomiting, cyanosis, diarrhea, purpura, convulsions, circulatory collapse, meningitis, and hemorrhaging into adrenal glands.

39200

39200 Resection of mediastinal cyst

The mediastinum is the mass of tissues and organs bounded by lungs, spinal column, and sternum

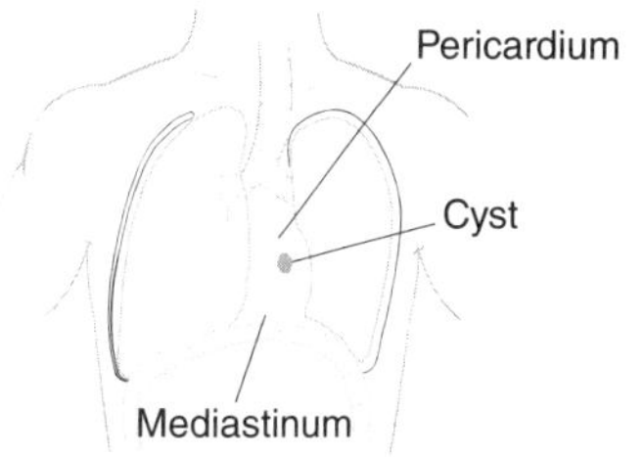

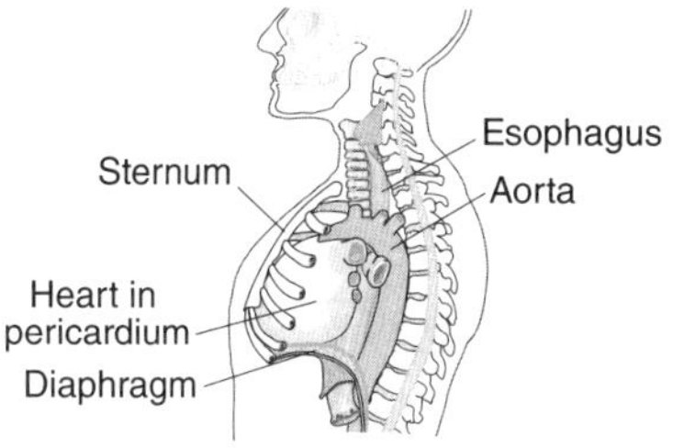

The heart, pericardium, bases of great vessels, trachea, bronchi, esophagus, thymus, thoracic lymph nodes, thoracic duct, and phrenic and vagus nerves are all part of the mediastinum

Explanation

The physician makes an incision from in front of the axilla just below the nipple line. The incision extends below the tip of the shoulder blade and ascends to halfway between the spinal column and the shoulder blade. The physician exposes the rib cage, retracting muscles. A rib spreader is used to ease access to the thoracic cavity. The cyst is located and removed. The rib spreader is removed, and the wound is closed with sutures or staples.

Coding Tips

This procedure may also be performed endoscopically. For thoracoscopic (endoscopic) excision of a mediastinal cyst, tumor, or mass, see 32662. For mediastinotomy with exploration, drainage, removal of foreign body, or biopsy, thoracic approach, see 39010; cervical approach, see 39000.

ICD-10-CM Diagnostic Codes

Q34.1	Congenital cyst of mediastinum

Relative Value Units/Medicare Edits

Non-Facility RVU	Work	PE	MP	Total
39200	15.09	6.99	3.72	25.8
Facility RVU	**Work**	**PE**	**MP**	**Total**
39200	15.09	6.99	3.72	25.8

	FUD	Status	MUE	Modifiers				IOM Reference
39200	90	A	1(2)	51	N/A	62*	80	None

* with documentation

39220

39220 Resection of mediastinal tumor

The mediastinum is the mass of tissues and organs bounded by lungs, spinal column, and sternum

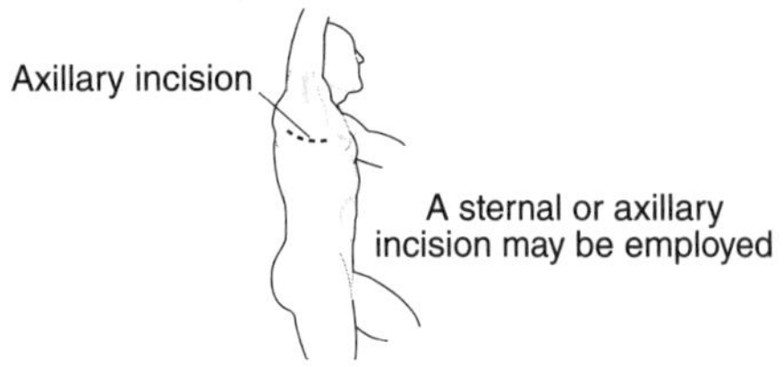

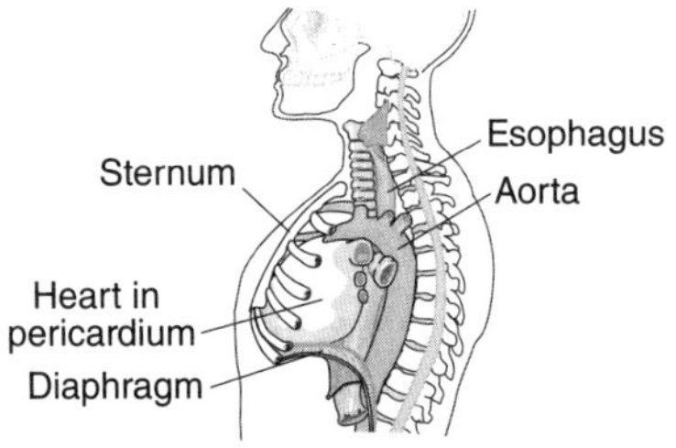

The heart, pericardium, bases of great vessels, trachea, bronchi, esophagus, thymus, thoracic lymph nodes, thoracic duct, and phrenic and vagus nerves are all part of the mediastinum

Explanation

The physician makes an incision from in front of the axilla just below the nipple line. The incision extends below the tip of the shoulder blade and ascends to halfway between the spinal column and the shoulder blade. The physician exposes the rib cage by cutting through the muscles. The chest cavity is entered between the ribs by using a rib spreader. The tumor is located and dissected from the surrounding tissue. The wound is closed using sutures or staples.

Coding Tips

This procedure may be performed endoscopically. For thoracoscopic (endoscopic) resection of a mediastinal cyst, tumor, or mass, see 32662. For mediastinotomy with exploration, drainage, removal of foreign body, or biopsy, thoracic approach, see 39010; cervical approach, see 39000. For resection of a mediastinal cyst, see 39200.

ICD-10-CM Diagnostic Codes

C38.1	Malignant neoplasm of anterior mediastinum
C38.2	Malignant neoplasm of posterior mediastinum
C38.3	Malignant neoplasm of mediastinum, part unspecified
C38.8	Malignant neoplasm of overlapping sites of heart, mediastinum and pleura
D15.2	Benign neoplasm of mediastinum
D38.3	Neoplasm of uncertain behavior of mediastinum

Relative Value Units/Medicare Edits

Non-Facility RVU	Work	PE	MP	Total
39220	19.55	9.69	4.47	33.71
Facility RVU	**Work**	**PE**	**MP**	**Total**
39220	19.55	9.69	4.47	33.71

	FUD	Status	MUE	Modifiers				IOM Reference
39220	90	A	1(2)	51	N/A	62*	80	None

* with documentation

Terms To Know

axillary. Area under the arm.

benign. Mild or nonmalignant in nature.

biopsy. Tissue or fluid removed for diagnostic purposes through analysis of the cells in the biopsy material.

dissect. Cut apart or separate tissue for surgical purposes or for visual or microscopic study.

excision. Surgical removal of an organ or tissue.

incision. Act of cutting into tissue or an organ.

malignant. Any condition tending to progress toward death, specifically an invasive tumor with a loss of cellular differentiation that has the ability to spread or metastasize to other body areas.

manubrium. Sternum.

mediastinotomy. Incision into the mediastinum for purposes of exploration, foreign body removal, drainage, or biopsy.

mediastinum. Collection of organs and tissues that separate the pleural sacs. Located between the sternum and spine above the diaphragm, it contains the heart and great vessels, trachea and bronchi, esophagus, thymus, lymph nodes, and nerves.

neoplasm. New abnormal growth, tumor.

tumor. Pathological swelling or enlargement; a neoplastic growth of uncontrolled, abnormal multiplication of cells.

39401-39402

39401 Mediastinoscopy; includes biopsy(ies) of mediastinal mass (eg, lymphoma), when performed

39402 with lymph node biopsy(ies) (eg, lung cancer staging)

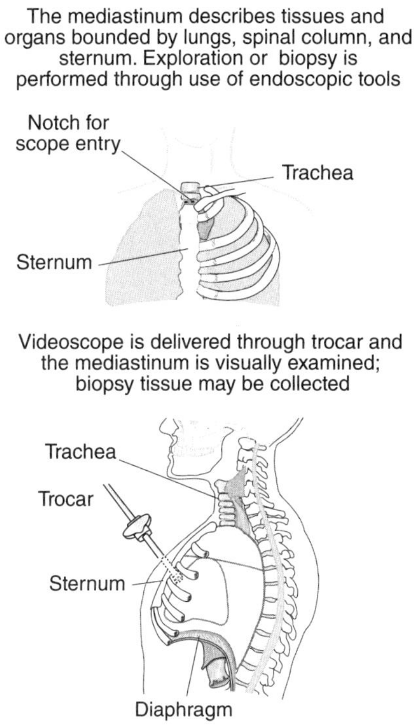

Explanation

The physician performs a mediastinoscopy. The physician makes a small incision in the notch above the sternum. The mediastinoscope is inserted and explorations are carried out between the trachea and the major vessels. The mediastinal lymph nodes, thymus, and thyroid are visualized and a biopsy(ies) may be performed through the mediastinoscope during the procedure. The scope is removed and the incision is closed with sutures or Steri-strips. Report 39401 for biopsy of a mediastinal mass. Report 39402 for a biopsy of the lymph nodes.

Coding Tips

For thoracoscopy, diagnostic, lungs, pericardial sac, mediastinal and pleural space without biopsy, see 32601; pericardial sac with biopsy, see 32604; and mediastinal space with biopsy, see 32606. For thoracoscopy, surgical with excision of mediastinal cyst, tumor, or mass, see 32662. For mediastinotomy with exploration, drainage, removal of foreign body, or biopsy, thoracic approach, see 39010; cervical approach, see 39000. For resection of a mediastinal cyst, see 39200. For resection of a mediastinal tumor, see 39220.

ICD-10-CM Diagnostic Codes

A15.4	Tuberculosis of intrathoracic lymph nodes
A15.8	Other respiratory tuberculosis
C33	Malignant neoplasm of trachea
C34.01	Malignant neoplasm of right main bronchus ☑
C34.02	Malignant neoplasm of left main bronchus ☑
C34.11	Malignant neoplasm of upper lobe, right bronchus or lung ☑
C34.12	Malignant neoplasm of upper lobe, left bronchus or lung ☑
C34.2	Malignant neoplasm of middle lobe, bronchus or lung
C34.31	Malignant neoplasm of lower lobe, right bronchus or lung ☑
C34.32	Malignant neoplasm of lower lobe, left bronchus or lung ☑
C34.81	Malignant neoplasm of overlapping sites of right bronchus and lung ☑
C34.82	Malignant neoplasm of overlapping sites of left bronchus and lung ☑
C37	Malignant neoplasm of thymus
C38.1	Malignant neoplasm of anterior mediastinum
C38.2	Malignant neoplasm of posterior mediastinum
C38.4	Malignant neoplasm of pleura
C38.8	Malignant neoplasm of overlapping sites of heart, mediastinum and pleura
C45.0	Mesothelioma of pleura
C78.01	Secondary malignant neoplasm of right lung ☑
C78.02	Secondary malignant neoplasm of left lung ☑
C78.1	Secondary malignant neoplasm of mediastinum
C78.2	Secondary malignant neoplasm of pleura
C7A.090	Malignant carcinoid tumor of the bronchus and lung
C7A.091	Malignant carcinoid tumor of the thymus
C81.02	Nodular lymphocyte predominant Hodgkin lymphoma, intrathoracic lymph nodes
C81.12	Nodular sclerosis Hodgkin lymphoma, intrathoracic lymph nodes
C81.22	Mixed cellularity Hodgkin lymphoma, intrathoracic lymph nodes
C81.42	Lymphocyte-rich Hodgkin lymphoma, intrathoracic lymph nodes
C82.02	Follicular lymphoma grade I, intrathoracic lymph nodes
C82.12	Follicular lymphoma grade II, intrathoracic lymph nodes
C82.32	Follicular lymphoma grade IIIa, intrathoracic lymph nodes
C82.42	Follicular lymphoma grade IIIb, intrathoracic lymph nodes
C82.52	Diffuse follicle center lymphoma, intrathoracic lymph nodes
C82.62	Cutaneous follicle center lymphoma, intrathoracic lymph nodes
C82.82	Other types of follicular lymphoma, intrathoracic lymph nodes
C83.02	Small cell B-cell lymphoma, intrathoracic lymph nodes
C83.32	Diffuse large B-cell lymphoma, intrathoracic lymph nodes
C83.52	Lymphoblastic (diffuse) lymphoma, intrathoracic lymph nodes
C83.72	Burkitt lymphoma, intrathoracic lymph nodes
C83.82	Other non-follicular lymphoma, intrathoracic lymph nodes
C84.02	Mycosis fungoides, intrathoracic lymph nodes
C84.12	Sezary disease, intrathoracic lymph nodes
C84.Z2	Other mature T/NK-cell lymphomas, intrathoracic lymph nodes
C85.22	Mediastinal (thymic) large B-cell lymphoma, intrathoracic lymph nodes
C85.82	Other specified types of non-Hodgkin lymphoma, intrathoracic lymph nodes
C96.Z	Other specified malignant neoplasms of lymphoid, hematopoietic and related tissue
D02.1	Carcinoma in situ of trachea
D02.21	Carcinoma in situ of right bronchus and lung ☑
D02.22	Carcinoma in situ of left bronchus and lung ☑
D02.3	Carcinoma in situ of other parts of respiratory system
D14.2	Benign neoplasm of trachea
D14.31	Benign neoplasm of right bronchus and lung ☑
D14.32	Benign neoplasm of left bronchus and lung ☑
D15.0	Benign neoplasm of thymus
D15.2	Benign neoplasm of mediastinum

D19.0	Benign neoplasm of mesothelial tissue of pleura
D38.1	Neoplasm of uncertain behavior of trachea, bronchus and lung
D38.2	Neoplasm of uncertain behavior of pleura
D38.3	Neoplasm of uncertain behavior of mediastinum
D38.4	Neoplasm of uncertain behavior of thymus
D3A.090	Benign carcinoid tumor of the bronchus and lung
D3A.091	Benign carcinoid tumor of the thymus
D86.0	Sarcoidosis of lung
D86.1	Sarcoidosis of lymph nodes
D86.2	Sarcoidosis of lung with sarcoidosis of lymph nodes
E32.8	Other diseases of thymus
J91.0	Malignant pleural effusion
J98.51	Mediastinitis
R22.2	Localized swelling, mass and lump, trunk
R59.0	Localized enlarged lymph nodes
R59.1	Generalized enlarged lymph nodes

Relative Value Units/Medicare Edits

Non-Facility RVU	Work	PE	MP	Total
39401	5.44	2.38	1.29	9.11
39402	7.25	2.88	1.76	11.89
Facility RVU	**Work**	**PE**	**MP**	**Total**
39401	5.44	2.38	1.29	9.11
39402	7.25	2.88	1.76	11.89

	FUD	Status	MUE	Modifiers				IOM Reference
39401	0	A	1(3)	51	N/A	N/A	N/A	None
39402	0	A	1(3)	51	N/A	N/A	N/A	

* with documentation

Terms To Know

pleura. One of the two membranes that surround the lungs. The visceral pleura encases the lung and the parietal pleura lines the inner chest walls.

thymus. Lymphoid organ located in the front of the upper mediastinum, composed of two symmetrical pyramid-shaped lobes, that is the site where T-lymphocytes are produced.

thyroid. Endocrine gland located in the front of the lower neck composed of two lobes on either side of the trachea, responsible for secreting and storing the thyroid hormones that regulate metabolism.

trachea. Tube descending from the larynx and branching into the right and left main bronchi.

tuberculosis. Bacterial infection that typically spreads by inhalation of an airborne agent that usually attacks the lungs, but may also affect other organs.

49425-49427

49425 Insertion of peritoneal-venous shunt
49426 Revision of peritoneal-venous shunt
49427 Injection procedure (eg, contrast media) for evaluation of previously placed peritoneal-venous shunt

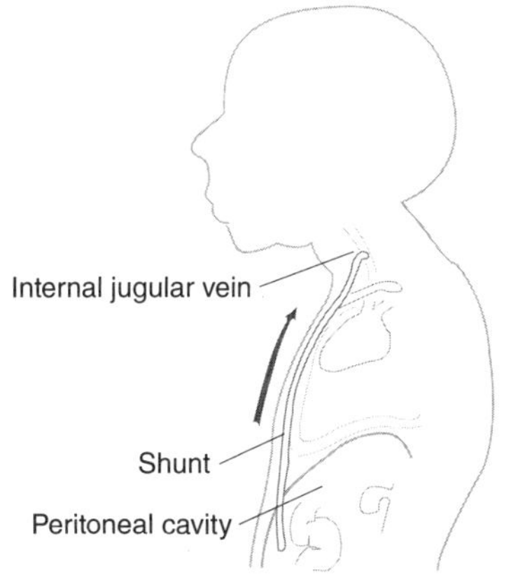

A shunt is prepared and inserted, revised, or injection performed to evaluate shunt function from the peritoneal cavity to a major vein

Explanation

In 49425, the physician places a peritoneal-venous shunt. The physician makes a small lateral upper abdominal incision. Dissection is carried through the abdominal wall layers, the peritoneum is entered, and the peritoneal end of the catheter is inserted into the peritoneal cavity and sutured into place. A subcutaneous tunnel is created from the abdominal incision up to the neck and the catheter is pulled through the tunnel into the neck. A counter incision is made in the neck over the internal jugular vein and the venous end of the catheter is inserted into the jugular vein. The incisions are closed. In 49426, the peritoneal-venous shunt is revised. The physician may remove the shunt by incisions over the venous and peritoneal insertion sites with a subcutaneous tunnel created from the abdominal incision up to the neck where the catheter is pulled through the tunnel into the neck. A counter incision is made in the neck over the internal jugular vein and the venous end of the catheter is inserted into the jugular vein. Alternately, the physician may make an incision over the dysfunctional end of the shunt and replace that portion of the shunt and insert it back into the peritoneal cavity or jugular vein. In 49427, the physician injects contrast material through the skin into the reservoir of a peritoneal-venous shunt. Radiography is used to visualize the flow of contrast through the shunt into the peritoneal and venous ends for evaluation.

Coding Tips

For shunt patency test, see 78291. For radiological supervision and interpretation of an injection procedure performed to evaluate previously placed peritoneal-venous shunt, see 75809 or 78291.

ICD-10-CM Diagnostic Codes

K70.11	Alcoholic hepatitis with ascites A
K70.31	Alcoholic cirrhosis of liver with ascites A
K71.51	Toxic liver disease with chronic active hepatitis with ascites
R18.0	Malignant ascites
R18.8	Other ascites
T85.618A	Breakdown (mechanical) of other specified internal prosthetic devices, implants and grafts, initial encounter
T85.628A	Displacement of other specified internal prosthetic devices, implants and grafts, initial encounter
T85.638A	Leakage of other specified internal prosthetic devices, implants and grafts, initial encounter
T85.698A	Other mechanical complication of other specified internal prosthetic devices, implants and grafts, initial encounter
T85.79XA	Infection and inflammatory reaction due to other internal prosthetic devices, implants and grafts, initial encounter
T85.818A	Embolism due to other internal prosthetic devices, implants and grafts, initial encounter
T85.828A	Fibrosis due to other internal prosthetic devices, implants and grafts, initial encounter
T85.838A	Hemorrhage due to other internal prosthetic devices, implants and grafts, initial encounter
T85.848A	Pain due to other internal prosthetic devices, implants and grafts, initial encounter
T85.858A	Stenosis due to other internal prosthetic devices, implants and grafts, initial encounter
T85.868A	Thrombosis due to other internal prosthetic devices, implants and grafts, initial encounter
T85.898A	Other specified complication of other internal prosthetic devices, implants and grafts, initial encounter
Z45.89	Encounter for adjustment and management of other implanted devices

Relative Value Units/Medicare Edits

Non-Facility RVU	Work	PE	MP	Total
49425	12.22	8.17	3.15	23.54
49426	10.41	7.14	2.68	20.23
49427	0.89	0.14	0.11	1.14
Facility RVU	**Work**	**PE**	**MP**	**Total**
49425	12.22	8.17	3.15	23.54
49426	10.41	7.14	2.68	20.23
49427	0.89	0.14	0.11	1.14

	FUD	Status	MUE	Modifiers				IOM Reference
49425	90	A	1(2)	51	N/A	62*	80	None
49426	90	A	1(3)	51	N/A	N/A	N/A	
49427	0	A	1(3)	51	N/A	N/A	80*	

* with documentation

Terms To Know

patency. State of a tube-like structure or conduit being open and unobstructed.

peritoneum. Strong, continuous membrane that forms the lining of the abdominal and pelvic cavity. The parietal peritoneum, or outer layer, is attached to the abdominopelvic walls and the visceral peritoneum, or inner layer, surrounds the organs inside the abdominal cavity.

shunt. Surgically created passage between blood vessels or other natural passages, such as an arteriovenous anastomosis, to divert or bypass blood flow from the normal channel.

49428-49429

49428 Ligation of peritoneal-venous shunt
49429 Removal of peritoneal-venous shunt

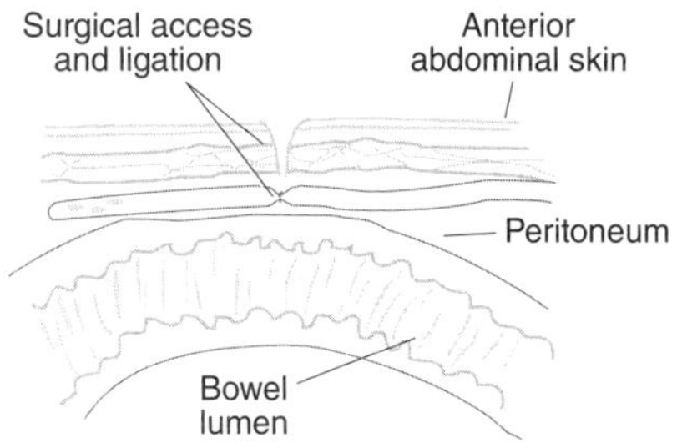

Access is usually by incising the skin over the percutaneous tunnel. This measure is often the simplest way to close off the shunt and assess the body's ability to absorb the excess fluids

Explanation

In 49428, the physician performs ligation of a previously placed peritoneo-venous shunt. The physician makes an incision over the path of the shunt. The shunt tubing under the incision is isolated and ligated with sutures. The incision is closed. In 49429, the physician performs removal of a peritoneal venous shunt. An incision is made over the abdominal insertion site of the shunt. The shunt is dissected from surrounding scar tissue and removed from the abdominal cavity. The fascia and peritoneum of the abdominal insertion site is closed. Usually, the venous end of the catheter can be removed by placing traction on the shunt through the abdominal incision and pulling it through the subcutaneous tunnel. If necessary, a second incision is made over the venous insertion site and the catheter removed from the jugular vein. The incisions are closed.

Coding Tips

For revision of peritoneal-venous shunt, see 49426. For an injection procedure for evaluation of a previously placed peritoneal-venous shunt, see 49427.

ICD-10-CM Diagnostic Codes

K68.11	Postprocedural retroperitoneal abscess
R18.0	Malignant ascites
R18.8	Other ascites
R50.82	Postprocedural fever
T81.41XA	Infection following a procedure, superficial incisional surgical site, initial encounter
T81.42XA	Infection following a procedure, deep incisional surgical site, initial encounter
T81.43XA	Infection following a procedure, organ and space surgical site, initial encounter
T81.44XA	Sepsis following a procedure, initial encounter
T81.49XA	Infection following a procedure, other surgical site, initial encounter
T82.818A	Embolism due to vascular prosthetic devices, implants and grafts, initial encounter
T82.828A	Fibrosis due to vascular prosthetic devices, implants and grafts, initial encounter
T82.838A	Hemorrhage due to vascular prosthetic devices, implants and grafts, initial encounter
T82.848A	Pain due to vascular prosthetic devices, implants and grafts, initial encounter
T82.856A	Stenosis of peripheral vascular stent, initial encounter
T82.858A	Stenosis of other vascular prosthetic devices, implants and grafts, initial encounter
T82.868A	Thrombosis due to vascular prosthetic devices, implants and grafts, initial encounter
T82.898A	Other specified complication of vascular prosthetic devices, implants and grafts, initial encounter
Z45.2	Encounter for adjustment and management of vascular access device

Relative Value Units/Medicare Edits

Non-Facility RVU	Work	PE	MP	Total
49428	6.87	4.34	1.76	12.97
49429	7.44	4.41	1.9	13.75
Facility RVU	**Work**	**PE**	**MP**	**Total**
49428	6.87	4.34	1.76	12.97
49429	7.44	4.41	1.9	13.75

	FUD	Status	MUE	Modifiers				IOM Reference
49428	10	A	1(2)	51	N/A	N/A	N/A	None
49429	10	A	1(2)	51	N/A	N/A	N/A	

* with documentation

Terms To Know

complication. Condition arising after the beginning of observation and treatment that modifies the course of the patient's illness or the medical care required, or an undesired result or misadventure in medical care.

dissection. Separating by cutting tissue or body structures apart.

fascia. Fibrous sheet or band of tissue that envelops organs, muscles, and groupings of muscles.

ligation. Tying off a blood vessel or duct with a suture or a soft, thin wire.

peritoneal cavity. Space between the lining of the abdominal wall, or parietal peritoneum, and the surface layer of the abdominal organs, or visceral peritoneum. It contains a thin, watery fluid that keeps the peritoneal surfaces moist.

peritoneum. Strong, continuous membrane that forms the lining of the abdominal and pelvic cavity. The parietal peritoneum, or outer layer, is attached to the abdominopelvic walls and the visceral peritoneum, or inner layer, surrounds the organs inside the abdominal cavity.

peritonitis. Inflammation and infection within the peritoneal cavity, the space between the membrane lining the abdominopelvic walls and covering the internal organs.

shunt. Surgically created passage between blood vessels or other natural passages, such as an arteriovenous anastomosis, to divert or bypass blood flow from the normal channel.

49435

\+ **49435** Insertion of subcutaneous extension to intraperitoneal cannula or catheter with remote chest exit site (List separately in addition to code for primary procedure)

The catheter is extended and exits the chest

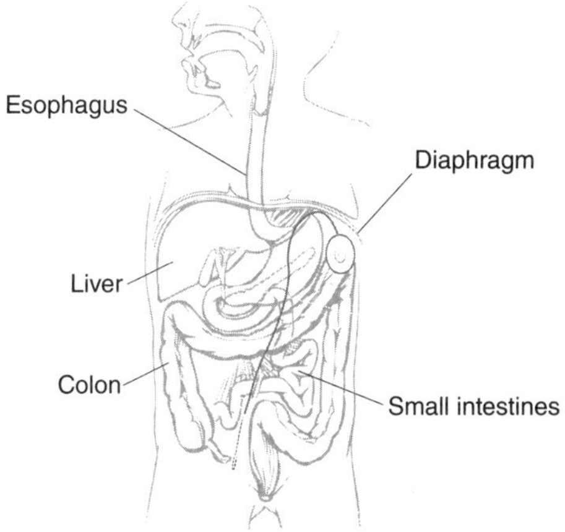

Explanation

A permanent, subcutaneous intraperitoneal catheter is lengthened with an extension and brought to the surface of the skin during the primary procedure in which a catheter/cannula is established. In the primary procedure, the physician makes a small abdominal incision, opens the peritoneum, and establishes the cannula. In 49435, the physician fits an extension to the cannula and tunnels subcutaneously to accommodate the extension. The physician makes a separate incision in the chest as an exit site for the extension. The extension is brought out through the skin and may be attached to the drug delivery system. The operative incision is closed.

Coding Tips

Report 49435 in addition to 49324 or 49421.

ICD-10-CM Diagnostic Codes

This/these CPT code(s) are add-on code(s). See the primary procedure code that this code is performed with for your ICD-10-CM code selections. Diagnostic code(s) would be the same as the actual procedure performed.

Relative Value Units/Medicare Edits

Non-Facility RVU	Work	PE	MP	Total
49435	2.25	0.68	0.56	3.49
Facility RVU	**Work**	**PE**	**MP**	**Total**
49435	2.25	0.68	0.56	3.49

	FUD	Status	MUE	Modifiers				IOM Reference
49435	N/A	A	1(2)	N/A	N/A	62*	80	None

* with documentation

49436

49436 Delayed creation of exit site from embedded subcutaneous segment of intraperitoneal cannula or catheter

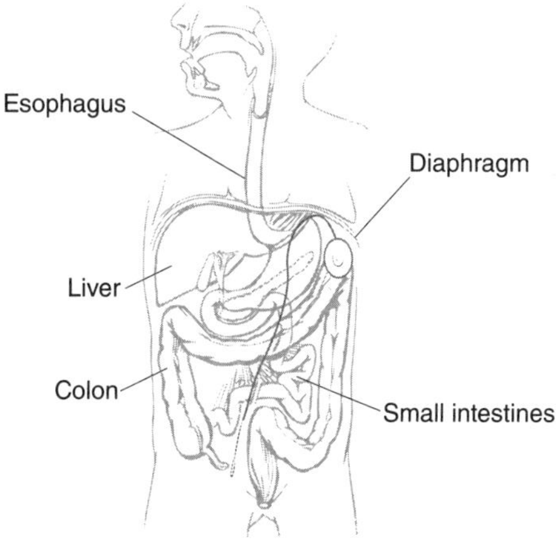

An exit site for the intraperitoneal catheter is created in a subsequent operative session

Explanation

A previously implanted, permanent subcutaneous intraperitoneal catheter is brought to the surface of the skin. The physician makes a small abdominal incision, opens the peritoneum, and locates the end of the existing intraperitoneal cannula. An extension may be fitted to the existing cannula. The physician makes a separate incision as an exit site for the cannula. The cannula is brought out through the skin and may be attached to the drug delivery system. The operative incision is closed.

Coding Tips

For laparoscopic insertion of intraperitoneal cannula or catheter, see 49324. For revision of previously placed intraperitoneal cannula or catheter with removal of intraluminal obstructive material if performed, see 49325; with omentectomy, see 49326. For insertion of subcutaneous extension at time of laparoscopic placement of intraperitoneal catheter, see 49435.

ICD-10-CM Diagnostic Codes

K68.11 Postprocedural retroperitoneal abscess
T81.41XA Infection following a procedure, superficial incisional surgical site, initial encounter
T81.42XA Infection following a procedure, deep incisional surgical site, initial encounter
T81.43XA Infection following a procedure, organ and space surgical site, initial encounter
T81.44XA Sepsis following a procedure, initial encounter
T81.49XA Infection following a procedure, other surgical site, initial encounter
T82.818A Embolism due to vascular prosthetic devices, implants and grafts, initial encounter
T82.828A Fibrosis due to vascular prosthetic devices, implants and grafts, initial encounter
T82.838A Hemorrhage due to vascular prosthetic devices, implants and grafts, initial encounter
T82.848A Pain due to vascular prosthetic devices, implants and grafts, initial encounter

T82.858A	Stenosis of other vascular prosthetic devices, implants and grafts, initial encounter
T82.868A	Thrombosis due to vascular prosthetic devices, implants and grafts, initial encounter
T82.898A	Other specified complication of vascular prosthetic devices, implants and grafts, initial encounter

Relative Value Units/Medicare Edits

Non-Facility RVU	Work	PE	MP	Total
49436	2.72	12.67	0.69	16.08
Facility RVU	**Work**	**PE**	**MP**	**Total**
49436	2.72	2.2	0.69	5.61

	FUD	Status	MUE	Modifiers				IOM Reference
49436	10	A	1(2)	51	N/A	62*	80	None

* with documentation

Terms To Know

cannula. Tube inserted into a blood vessel, duct, or body cavity to facilitate passage.

catheter. Flexible tube inserted into an area of the body for introducing or withdrawing fluid.

peritoneal cavity. Space between the lining of the abdominal wall, or parietal peritoneum, and the surface layer of the abdominal organs, or visceral peritoneum. It contains a thin, watery fluid that keeps the peritoneal surfaces moist.

subcutaneous. Below the skin.

49904-49906

49904 Omental flap, extra-abdominal (eg, for reconstruction of sternal and chest wall defects)

\+ **49905** Omental flap, intra-abdominal (List separately in addition to code for primary procedure)

49906 Free omental flap with microvascular anastomosis

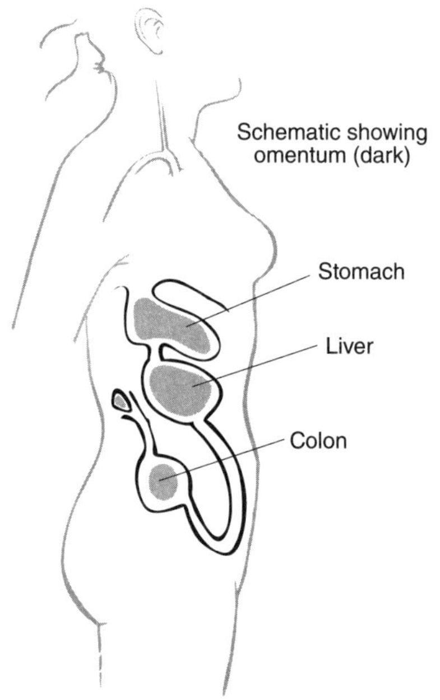

A flap of omentum is used in an extra-abdominal repair, such as of the chest wall

Explanation

The physician mobilizes an omental flap for reconstruction of a defect. The surgical recipient site of the flap is prepared. An upper abdominal transverse or midline incision is made. A laparotomy and manual exploration of the abdominal cavity is done first and the omentum and transverse colon are delivered from the cavity. The omentum is dissected from the transverse colon from left to right and small vessels are ligated. When completely separated from the transverse colon, the omentum is dissected from the stomach with careful clamping, division, and ligation of vessels. The omentum is fully mobilized and pedicled on the right or left gastroepiploic vessel, depending on the purpose. More incisions and tunneling may be necessary to bring the flap into its new location to fill a defect. The flap may be used as a pedicled transposition flap or a free microvascular transfer flap. Report 49904 when the flap is transpositioned to repair an extra-abdominal defect, such as chest wounds after radiation and mastectomy or lower extremity trauma wounds. Report 49905 when the omental flap is repositioned to repair a defect intra-abdominally. Report 49906 when the omentum is used as a free vascularized transfer flap to repair defects such as hemifacial atrophy. Microvascular anastomosis is performed to maintain blood flow to the omental flap. The abdominal incision is closed. If a separate split-thickness skin graft is required for omental coverage, it is done immediately and applied directly over the omentum and a dressing is applied.

Coding Tips

Report 49905 separately in addition to the primary procedure. Do not report 69990 in addition to 49906 as the operating microscope is considered an inclusive component of the surgery.

ICD-10-CM Diagnostic Codes

S21.111A Laceration without foreign body of right front wall of thorax without penetration into thoracic cavity, initial encounter

S21.112A Laceration without foreign body of left front wall of thorax without penetration into thoracic cavity, initial encounter

S21.121A Laceration with foreign body of right front wall of thorax without penetration into thoracic cavity, initial encounter

S21.122A Laceration with foreign body of left front wall of thorax without penetration into thoracic cavity, initial encounter

S21.131A Puncture wound without foreign body of right front wall of thorax without penetration into thoracic cavity, initial encounter

S21.132A Puncture wound without foreign body of left front wall of thorax without penetration into thoracic cavity, initial encounter

S21.141A Puncture wound with foreign body of right front wall of thorax without penetration into thoracic cavity, initial encounter

S21.142A Puncture wound with foreign body of left front wall of thorax without penetration into thoracic cavity, initial encounter

S21.151A Open bite of right front wall of thorax without penetration into thoracic cavity, initial encounter

S21.152A Open bite of left front wall of thorax without penetration into thoracic cavity, initial encounter

S28.1XXA Traumatic amputation (partial) of part of thorax, except breast, initial encounter

S29.021A Laceration of muscle and tendon of front wall of thorax, initial encounter

S31.112A Laceration without foreign body of abdominal wall, epigastric region without penetration into peritoneal cavity, initial encounter

S31.115A Laceration without foreign body of abdominal wall, periumbilic region without penetration into peritoneal cavity, initial encounter

S31.120A Laceration of abdominal wall with foreign body, right upper quadrant without penetration into peritoneal cavity, initial encounter ☑

S31.121A Laceration of abdominal wall with foreign body, left upper quadrant without penetration into peritoneal cavity, initial encounter ☑

S31.122A Laceration of abdominal wall with foreign body, epigastric region without penetration into peritoneal cavity, initial encounter

S31.123A Laceration of abdominal wall with foreign body, right lower quadrant without penetration into peritoneal cavity, initial encounter ☑

S31.124A Laceration of abdominal wall with foreign body, left lower quadrant without penetration into peritoneal cavity, initial encounter ☑

S31.125A Laceration of abdominal wall with foreign body, periumbilic region without penetration into peritoneal cavity, initial encounter

S31.131A Puncture wound of abdominal wall without foreign body, left upper quadrant without penetration into peritoneal cavity, initial encounter ☑

S31.132A Puncture wound of abdominal wall without foreign body, epigastric region without penetration into peritoneal cavity, initial encounter

S31.133A Puncture wound of abdominal wall without foreign body, right lower quadrant without penetration into peritoneal cavity, initial encounter ☑

S31.134A Puncture wound of abdominal wall without foreign body, left lower quadrant without penetration into peritoneal cavity, initial encounter ☑

S31.135A Puncture wound of abdominal wall without foreign body, periumbilic region without penetration into peritoneal cavity, initial encounter

S31.140A Puncture wound of abdominal wall with foreign body, right upper quadrant without penetration into peritoneal cavity, initial encounter ☑

S31.141A Puncture wound of abdominal wall with foreign body, left upper quadrant without penetration into peritoneal cavity, initial encounter ☑

S31.143A Puncture wound of abdominal wall with foreign body, right lower quadrant without penetration into peritoneal cavity, initial encounter ☑

S31.144A Puncture wound of abdominal wall with foreign body, left lower quadrant without penetration into peritoneal cavity, initial encounter ☑

S31.150A Open bite of abdominal wall, right upper quadrant without penetration into peritoneal cavity, initial encounter ☑

S31.151A Open bite of abdominal wall, left upper quadrant without penetration into peritoneal cavity, initial encounter ☑

S31.152A Open bite of abdominal wall, epigastric region without penetration into peritoneal cavity, initial encounter

S31.153A Open bite of abdominal wall, right lower quadrant without penetration into peritoneal cavity, initial encounter ☑

S31.154A Open bite of abdominal wall, left lower quadrant without penetration into peritoneal cavity, initial encounter ☑

S31.155A Open bite of abdominal wall, periumbilic region without penetration into peritoneal cavity, initial encounter

T21.31XA Burn of third degree of chest wall, initial encounter

T21.71XA Corrosion of third degree of chest wall, initial encounter

AMA: 49905 2020,Feb **49906** 2019,Dec

Relative Value Units/Medicare Edits

Non-Facility RVU	Work	PE	MP	Total
49904	22.35	14.38	4.97	41.7
49905	6.54	2.42	1.51	10.47
49906	0.0	0.0	0.0	0.0
Facility RVU	**Work**	**PE**	**MP**	**Total**
49904	22.35	14.38	4.97	41.7
49905	6.54	2.42	1.51	10.47
49906	0.0	0.0	0.0	0.0

	FUD	Status	MUE	Modifiers				IOM Reference
49904	90	A	1(3)	51	N/A	62*	N/A	None
49905	N/A	A	1(3)	N/A	N/A	62	80	
49906	90	C	1(3)	51	N/A	62*	N/A	

* with documentation

60270

60270 Thyroidectomy, including substernal thyroid; sternal split or transthoracic approach

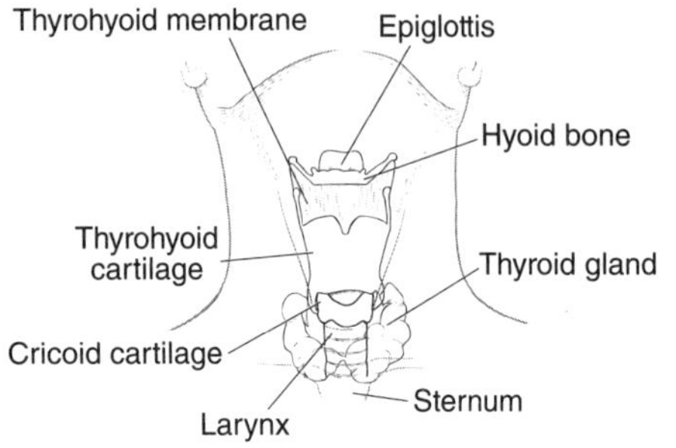

The thyroid gland is removed, including portions that occur below the sternum

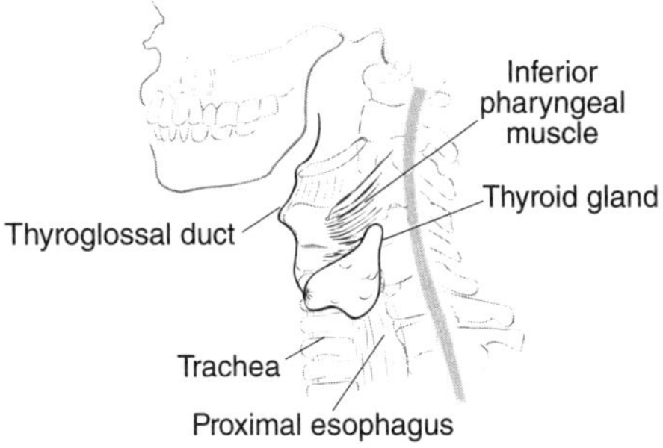

Explanation

The physician removes the thyroid, including the substernal thyroid gland. The physician exposes the thyroid via sternal split or transthoracic approach. The platysmas is divided and the strap muscles separated in the midline. The thyroid gland is mobilized and the superior and inferior thyroid vessels are ligated. The parathyroid glands are preserved and the thyroid is resected free of the trachea and removed. Any substernal thyroid is bluntly dissected. Upper sternal incision may be necessary for complete excision of substernal thyroid. The platysmas and skin are closed.

Coding Tips

The approach is considered inherent to the procedure and should not be reported separately.

ICD-10-CM Diagnostic Codes

C73	Malignant neoplasm of thyroid gland
C79.89	Secondary malignant neoplasm of other specified sites
D09.3	Carcinoma in situ of thyroid and other endocrine glands
D09.8	Carcinoma in situ of other specified sites
D34	Benign neoplasm of thyroid gland
D44.0	Neoplasm of uncertain behavior of thyroid gland
E01.0	Iodine-deficiency related diffuse (endemic) goiter
E04.0	Nontoxic diffuse goiter
E04.1	Nontoxic single thyroid nodule
E04.2	Nontoxic multinodular goiter
E04.8	Other specified nontoxic goiter
E05.00	Thyrotoxicosis with diffuse goiter without thyrotoxic crisis or storm
E05.01	Thyrotoxicosis with diffuse goiter with thyrotoxic crisis or storm
E05.10	Thyrotoxicosis with toxic single thyroid nodule without thyrotoxic crisis or storm
E05.11	Thyrotoxicosis with toxic single thyroid nodule with thyrotoxic crisis or storm
E05.20	Thyrotoxicosis with toxic multinodular goiter without thyrotoxic crisis or storm
E05.21	Thyrotoxicosis with toxic multinodular goiter with thyrotoxic crisis or storm
E05.30	Thyrotoxicosis from ectopic thyroid tissue without thyrotoxic crisis or storm

Relative Value Units/Medicare Edits

Non-Facility RVU	Work	PE	MP	Total
60270	23.2	13.0	4.68	40.88
Facility RVU	**Work**	**PE**	**MP**	**Total**
60270	23.2	13.0	4.68	40.88

	FUD	Status	MUE	Modifiers				IOM Reference
60270	90	A	1(2)	51	N/A	62*	80	None

* with documentation

Terms To Know

dissection. Separating by cutting tissue or body structures apart.

excision. Surgical removal of an organ or tissue.

goiter. Abnormal enlargement of the thyroid gland commonly caused by a deficiency of dietary iodine.

incision. Act of cutting into tissue or an organ.

ligate. To tie off a blood vessel or duct with a suture or a soft, thin wire (ligature wire).

lymphoma. Tumors occurring in the lymphoid tissues that are most commonly malignant.

malignant. Any condition tending to progress toward death, specifically an invasive tumor with a loss of cellular differentiation that has the ability to spread or metastasize to other body areas.

60505

60505 Parathyroidectomy or exploration of parathyroid(s); with mediastinal exploration, sternal split or transthoracic approach

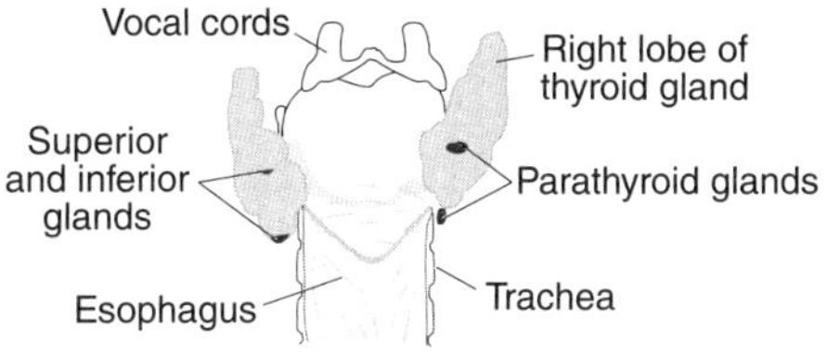

Posterior view of parathyroid glands

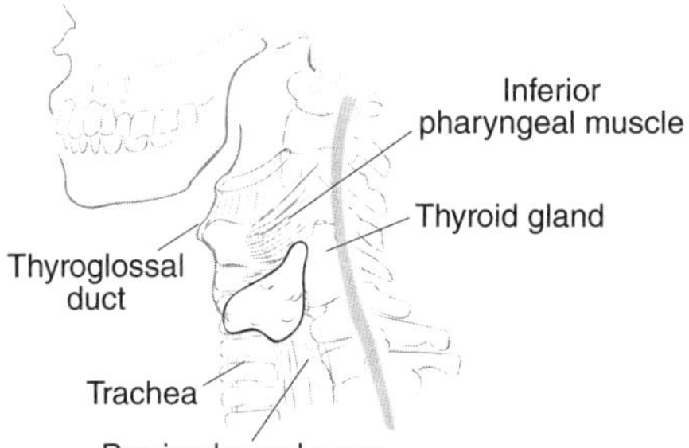

Parathyroid glands are removed or merely explored and biopsied. Usually four glands occur (two per thyroid lobe)

Explanation

The physician removes or explores the parathyroids, glands adjacent to the thyroids with mediastinal exploration, sternal split or transthoracic approach. The physician exposes the thyroid via a sternal split or transthoracic approach. The parathyroid glands are identified and tissue is excised for separately reportable pathological examination. The mediastinum is explored. The parathyroid may be removed; usually a port remains following excision. The platysmas and skin are closed.

Coding Tips

The approach is considered inherent to the procedure and should not be reported separately.

ICD-10-CM Diagnostic Codes

C75.0	Malignant neoplasm of parathyroid gland
D35.1	Benign neoplasm of parathyroid gland
D44.2	Neoplasm of uncertain behavior of parathyroid gland
E20.0	Idiopathic hypoparathyroidism
E20.1	Pseudohypoparathyroidism
E20.810	Autosomal dominant hypocalcemia
E20.812	Autoimmune hypoparathyroidism
E20.818	Other specified hypoparathyroidism due to impaired parathyroid hormone secretion
E20.89	Other specified hypoparathyroidism
E20.9	Hypoparathyroidism, unspecified
E21.0	Primary hyperparathyroidism
E21.1	Secondary hyperparathyroidism, not elsewhere classified
E21.2	Other hyperparathyroidism
E83.51	Hypocalcemia
E83.52	Hypercalcemia

Relative Value Units/Medicare Edits

Non-Facility RVU	Work	PE	MP	Total
60505	23.06	14.48	4.56	42.1
Facility RVU	**Work**	**PE**	**MP**	**Total**
60505	23.06	14.48	4.56	42.1

	FUD	Status	MUE	Modifiers				IOM Reference
60505	90	A	1(3)	51	N/A	62*	80	None

* with documentation

Terms To Know

benign. Mild or nonmalignant in nature.

carcinoma in situ. Malignancy that arises from the cells of the vessel, gland, or organ of origin that remains confined to that site or has not invaded neighboring tissue.

excision. Surgical removal of an organ or tissue.

exploration. Examination for diagnostic purposes.

malignant. Any condition tending to progress toward death, specifically an invasive tumor with a loss of cellular differentiation that has the ability to spread or metastasize to other body areas.

mediastinum. Collection of organs and tissues that separate the pleural sacs. Located between the sternum and spine above the diaphragm, it contains the heart and great vessels, trachea and bronchi, esophagus, thymus, lymph nodes, and nerves.

platysma. Muscle originating from the neck region attached to the mandible that opens the jaw.

secondary. Second in order of occurrence or importance, or appearing during the course of another disease or condition.

60521-60522

60521 Thymectomy, partial or total; sternal split or transthoracic approach, without radical mediastinal dissection (separate procedure)

60522 sternal split or transthoracic approach, with radical mediastinal dissection (separate procedure)

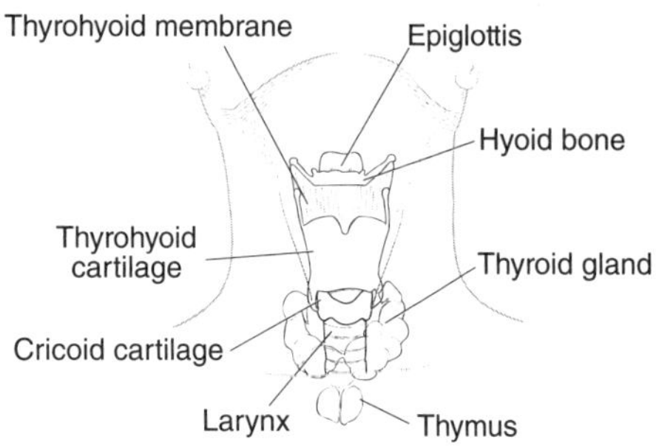

The thymus is removed, either partially or in total

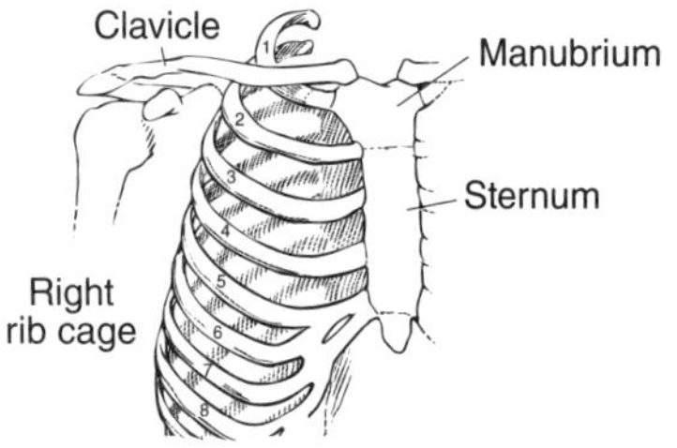

Explanation

The physician removes part or all of the thymus gland. The physician exposes the thymus via a sternal split or transthoracic approach. The sternum is retracted and strap muscles separated. The superior lobe of the thymus is separated from the inferior aspect of the thyroid. The blood supply to the thymus is divided and the thymus is dissected free from the pericardium and removed. In 60522, the mediastinum is dissected. In both procedures, the incision is closed.

Coding Tips

Note that 60521 and 60522, separate procedures by definition, are usually components of a more complex service and are not identified separately. When performed alone or with other unrelated procedures/services, they may be reported. If performed alone, list the code; if performed with other procedures/services, list the code and append modifier 59 or an X{EPSU} modifier. The approach is considered inherent to the procedure and should not be reported separately. For thoracoscopic video-assisted thoracic surgery (VATS), thymectomy, see 32673.

ICD-10-CM Diagnostic Codes

C37	Malignant neoplasm of thymus
C7A.091	Malignant carcinoid tumor of the thymus
D15.0	Benign neoplasm of thymus
D38.4	Neoplasm of uncertain behavior of thymus
D3A.091	Benign carcinoid tumor of the thymus
G70.01	Myasthenia gravis with (acute) exacerbation

Relative Value Units/Medicare Edits

Non-Facility RVU	Work	PE	MP	Total
60521	19.18	9.64	4.61	33.43
60522	23.48	11.24	5.74	40.46
Facility RVU	**Work**	**PE**	**MP**	**Total**
60521	19.18	9.64	4.61	33.43
60522	23.48	11.24	5.74	40.46

	FUD	Status	MUE	Modifiers				IOM Reference
60521	90	A	1(2)	51	N/A	62*	80	None
60522	90	A	1(2)	51	N/A	62*	80	

* with documentation

Terms To Know

anomaly. Irregularity in the structure or position of an organ or tissue.

benign. Mild or nonmalignant in nature.

congenital. Present at birth, occurring through heredity or an influence during gestation up to the moment of birth.

dissection. Separating by cutting tissue or body structures apart.

excision. Surgical removal of an organ or tissue.

incision. Act of cutting into tissue or an organ.

malignant. Any condition tending to progress toward death, specifically an invasive tumor with a loss of cellular differentiation that has the ability to spread or metastasize to other body areas.

pericardium. Thin and slippery case in which the heart lies that is lined with fluid so that the heart is free to pulse and move as it beats.

secondary. Second in order of occurrence or importance, or appearing during the course of another disease or condition.

60600-60605

60600 Excision of carotid body tumor; without excision of carotid artery
60605 with excision of carotid artery

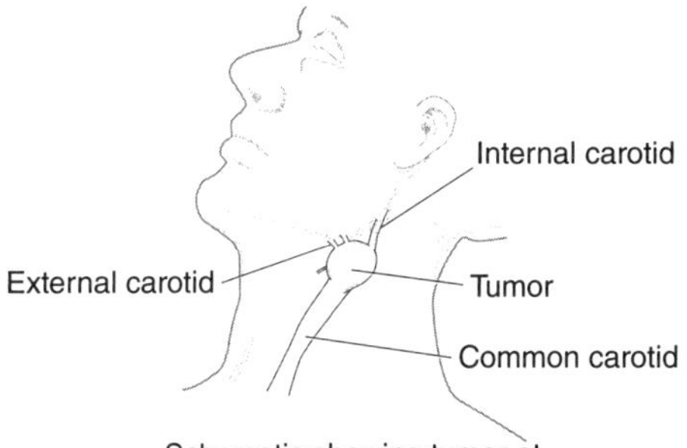

Schematic showing tumor at bifurcation of carotid artery

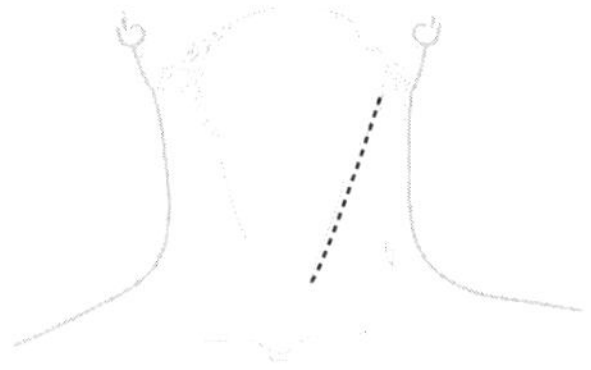
Typical incision to access the carotid body

Explanation

This physician removes a tumor from a small epithelioid structure (carotid body) just above the bifurcation of the carotid. The physician exposes the carotid body via an incision anterior to the sternocleidomastoid. After dissection down to the carotid sheath, the vein is retracted and the carotid bifurcation exposed. The blood supply to the tumor is ligated and the tumor resected. The incision is closed. Report 60605 if the carotid body tumor excision is performed with excision of the carotid artery.

Coding Tips

When 60600 or 60605 is performed with another separately identifiable procedure, the highest dollar value code is listed as the primary procedure, and subsequent procedures are appended with modifier 51.

ICD-10-CM Diagnostic Codes

C75.4	Malignant neoplasm of carotid body
D35.5	Benign neoplasm of carotid body

Relative Value Units/Medicare Edits

Non-Facility RVU	Work	PE	MP	Total
60600	25.09	9.72	5.84	40.65
60605	31.96	8.4	7.96	48.32
Facility RVU	**Work**	**PE**	**MP**	**Total**
60600	25.09	9.72	5.84	40.65
60605	31.96	8.4	7.96	48.32

	FUD	Status	MUE	Modifiers				IOM Reference
60600	90	A	1(3)	51	N/A	62*	80	None
60605	90	A	1(3)	51	N/A	62*	80	

* with documentation

64415-64416

64415 Injection(s), anesthetic agent(s) and/or steroid; brachial plexus, including imaging guidance, when performed

64416 brachial plexus, continuous infusion by catheter (including catheter placement), including imaging guidance, when performed

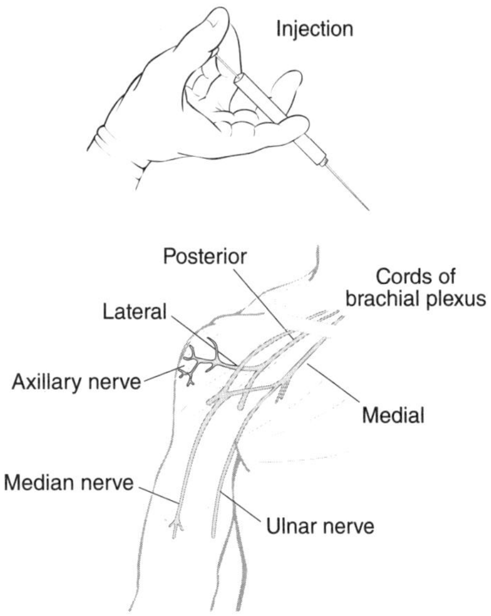

An anesthetic agent is injected to block the brachial plexus, a group of nerves serving the arm and upper thorax

Explanation

The physician injects one or more anesthetic agents and/or steroids near the brachial plexus to relieve pain and inflammation in 64415. The physician draws a local anesthetic and/or steroid into a syringe and injects it into a targeted area near the brachial plexus, approached in one of several locations: interscalene, superior trunk, supraclavicular, infraclavicular, or axillary. In 64416, continuous infusion of local anesthetic and/or steroid through a catheter is done to provide a nerve block lasting longer than the block effect achieved through a single injection. An indwelling catheter is placed and positioned to provide anesthesia to the brachial plexus. An infusion pump is connected to the catheter to supply a continuous flow of infused agent at a set rate. The infusion system may be used for regional surgical anesthesia when general anesthesia is not required and for postoperative pain management. Catheter placement is included in 64416 and is not reported separately. Imaging guidance and any contrast injection, when performed, is included in both codes.

Coding Tips

These are unilateral procedures. If performed bilaterally, some payers require that the service be reported twice with modifier 50 appended to the second code while others require identification of the service only once with modifier 50 appended. Check with individual payers. Supplies used when providing this procedure may be reported with the appropriate HCPCS Level II code. Check with the specific payer to determine coverage. Imaging guidance and localization may be reported separately. For anesthesia by injection performed by a different provider, see 01991 and 01992. Do not report 64415 or 64416 with 76942, 77002, or 77003. Do not report 64416 with 01996.

ICD-10-CM Diagnostic Codes

G54.0 Brachial plexus disorders
G56.41 Causalgia of right upper limb ☑
G56.42 Causalgia of left upper limb ☑
G56.43 Causalgia of bilateral upper limbs ☑
G90.511 Complex regional pain syndrome I of right upper limb ☑
G90.512 Complex regional pain syndrome I of left upper limb ☑
G90.513 Complex regional pain syndrome I of upper limb, bilateral ☑
M12.511 Traumatic arthropathy, right shoulder ☑
M12.512 Traumatic arthropathy, left shoulder ☑
M25.511 Pain in right shoulder ☑
M25.512 Pain in left shoulder ☑
M25.521 Pain in right elbow ☑
M25.522 Pain in left elbow ☑
M25.541 Pain in joints of right hand ☑
M25.542 Pain in joints of left hand ☑
M50.13 Cervical disc disorder with radiculopathy, cervicothoracic region
M54.12 Radiculopathy, cervical region
M54.13 Radiculopathy, cervicothoracic region
M54.2 Cervicalgia
M79.11 Myalgia of mastication muscle
M79.12 Myalgia of auxiliary muscles, head and neck
M79.18 Myalgia, other site
M79.601 Pain in right arm ☑
M79.602 Pain in left arm ☑
M79.621 Pain in right upper arm ☑
M79.622 Pain in left upper arm ☑
M79.631 Pain in right forearm ☑
M79.632 Pain in left forearm ☑
M79.641 Pain in right hand ☑
M79.642 Pain in left hand ☑
M79.644 Pain in right finger(s) ☑
M79.645 Pain in left finger(s) ☑
M79.7 Fibromyalgia
S13.4XXA Sprain of ligaments of cervical spine, initial encounter
S13.8XXA Sprain of joints and ligaments of other parts of neck, initial encounter
S16.1XXA Strain of muscle, fascia and tendon at neck level, initial encounter
S43.421A Sprain of right rotator cuff capsule, initial encounter ☑
S43.422A Sprain of left rotator cuff capsule, initial encounter ☑

AMA: **64415** 2023,Jan; 2022,Dec; 2022,Jul; 2021,Feb **64416** 2023,Jan; 2022,Dec; 2022,Jul; 2021,Feb

Relative Value Units/Medicare Edits

Non-Facility RVU	Work	PE	MP	Total
64415	1.5	2.39	0.13	4.02
64416	1.8	0.33	0.15	2.28
Facility RVU	**Work**	**PE**	**MP**	**Total**
64415	1.5	0.43	0.13	2.06
64416	1.8	0.33	0.15	2.28

	FUD	Status	MUE	Modifiers				IOM Reference
64415	0	A	1(3)	51	50	N/A	N/A	None
64416	0	A	1(2)	51	50	N/A	N/A	

* with documentation

92950

92950 Cardiopulmonary resuscitation (eg, in cardiac arrest)

Explanation

Cardiopulmonary arrest occurs when the patient's heart and lungs suddenly stop. In a clinical setting, cardiopulmonary resuscitation, the attempt at restarting the heart and lungs, is usually directed by a physician or another health care provider who is certified in Advanced Cardiac Life Support (ACLS). The patient's lungs are ventilated by mouth-to-mouth breathing or by a bag and mask. The patient's circulation is assisted using external chest compression. An electronic defibrillator may be used to shock the heart into restarting. Medications used to restart the heart include epinephrine and lidocaine.

Coding Tips

See also critical care services, 99291–99292, and neonatal and pediatric critical care services, 99468–99476. For critical care services provided during transport of a pediatric patient, see 99466–99467. For resuscitation services provided in the delivery or birthing room, see 99465.

ICD-10-CM Diagnostic Codes

I46.2	Cardiac arrest due to underlying cardiac condition
I46.8	Cardiac arrest due to other underlying condition
J80	Acute respiratory distress syndrome
J95.1	Acute pulmonary insufficiency following thoracic surgery
J95.2	Acute pulmonary insufficiency following nonthoracic surgery
J95.3	Chronic pulmonary insufficiency following surgery
J95.821	Acute postprocedural respiratory failure
J95.822	Acute and chronic postprocedural respiratory failure
J96.01	Acute respiratory failure with hypoxia
J96.02	Acute respiratory failure with hypercapnia
J96.21	Acute and chronic respiratory failure with hypoxia
J96.22	Acute and chronic respiratory failure with hypercapnia
P29.81	Cardiac arrest of newborn N
R06.03	Acute respiratory distress

Relative Value Units/Medicare Edits

Non-Facility RVU	Work	PE	MP	Total
92950	4.0	5.31	0.4	9.71
Facility RVU	**Work**	**PE**	**MP**	**Total**
92950	4.0	1.01	0.4	5.41

	FUD	Status	MUE	Modifiers				IOM Reference
92950	0	A	2(3)	N/A	N/A	N/A	80*	None

* with documentation

Terms To Know

cardiac arrest. Sudden, unexpected cessation of cardiac action, including absence of heart sounds and/or blood pressure.

respiratory distress syndrome. Premature neonates with respiratory distress and associated with reduced amounts of lung surfactant. Frequently fatal.

92953

92953 Temporary transcutaneous pacing

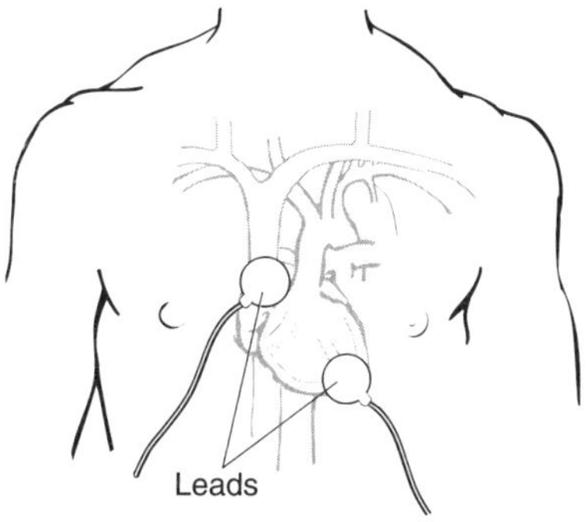

The heart is paced using transcutaneous leads (skin mounted)

Explanation

A temporary pacemaker is placed on the patient's heart to regulate heartbeats considered dangerously irregular. The physician applies electrodes to the chest wall. The electrodes give small electronic shocks through the chest to pace the heart as controlled by the physician.

Coding Tips

When medically necessary, report moderate (conscious) sedation provided by the performing physician with 99151-99153. When provided by another physician, report 99155-99157. When temporary pacing is done under physician direction from a remote location (e.g., hospital to ambulance or rescue personnel outside the hospital), report 99288 and not 92953. Temporary transcutaneous pacing is considered a component of critical care services. Do not report 92953 with 99291 or 99292. For temporary transvenous pacing, see 33210 and 33211.

ICD-10-CM Diagnostic Codes

I44.1	Atrioventricular block, second degree
I44.2	Atrioventricular block, complete
I45.2	Bifascicular block
I45.3	Trifascicular block
I49.5	Sick sinus syndrome
R00.1	Bradycardia, unspecified

AMA: 92953 2022,Dec; 2022,Jun; 2022,Jan; 2019,Aug

Relative Value Units/Medicare Edits

Non-Facility RVU	Work	PE	MP	Total
92953	0.01	0.01	0.01	0.03
Facility RVU	**Work**	**PE**	**MP**	**Total**
92953	0.01	0.01	0.01	0.03

	FUD	Status	MUE	Modifiers				IOM Reference
92953	0	A	2(3)	N/A	N/A	N/A	80*	None

* with documentation

Medicine

92960-92961

92960 Cardioversion, elective, electrical conversion of arrhythmia; external
92961 internal (separate procedure)

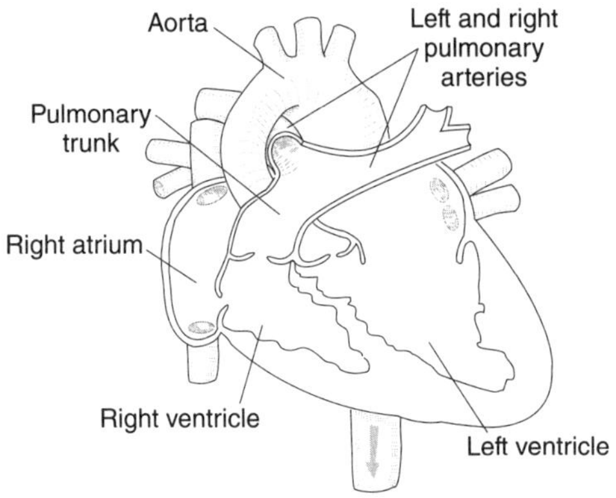

Explanation

The physician may administer an electronic shock to the patient's chest to regulate heartbeats considered dangerously irregular. The physician uses a defibrillator machine and places two paddles on the patient's chest and/or back. A measured electric shock is delivered through the chest to the heart to convert the heartbeat to a regular rhythm. Report 92960 for external cardioversion and 92961 when the procedure is performed internally.

Coding Tips

When medically necessary, report moderate (conscious) sedation provided by the performing physician with 99151-99153. When provided by another physician report 99155-99157. Note that 92961, a separate procedure by definition, is usually a component of a more complex service and is not identified separately. When performed alone or with other unrelated procedures/services, it may be reported. If performed alone, list the code; if performed with other procedures/services, list the code and append modifier 59 or an X{EPSU} modifier. Do not report 92961 with 93282-93284, 93287, 93289, 93295, 93296, 93618-93624, 93631, 93640-96342, 93650, 93653-93657, or 93662.

ICD-10-CM Diagnostic Codes

I44.0	Atrioventricular block, first degree
I44.1	Atrioventricular block, second degree
I44.2	Atrioventricular block, complete
I44.30	Unspecified atrioventricular block
I44.39	Other atrioventricular block
I44.4	Left anterior fascicular block
I44.5	Left posterior fascicular block
I44.69	Other fascicular block
I45.0	Right fascicular block
I45.19	Other right bundle-branch block
I45.2	Bifascicular block
I45.3	Trifascicular block
I45.4	Nonspecific intraventricular block
I45.5	Other specified heart block
I45.6	Pre-excitation syndrome
I45.81	Long QT syndrome
I45.89	Other specified conduction disorders
I47.0	Re-entry ventricular arrhythmia
I47.11	Inappropriate sinus tachycardia, so stated
I47.19	Other supraventricular tachycardia
I47.21	Torsades de pointes
I47.29	Other ventricular tachycardia
I48.0	Paroxysmal atrial fibrillation
I48.11	Longstanding persistent atrial fibrillation
I48.19	Other persistent atrial fibrillation
I48.21	Permanent atrial fibrillation
I48.3	Typical atrial flutter
I48.4	Atypical atrial flutter
I49.01	Ventricular fibrillation
I49.02	Ventricular flutter
I49.1	Atrial premature depolarization
I49.2	Junctional premature depolarization
I49.3	Ventricular premature depolarization
I49.49	Other premature depolarization
I49.5	Sick sinus syndrome
I49.8	Other specified cardiac arrhythmias

AMA: **92960** 2024,Jul

Relative Value Units/Medicare Edits

Non-Facility RVU	Work	PE	MP	Total
92960	2.0	2.44	0.15	4.59
92961	4.34	1.86	0.96	7.16
Facility RVU	**Work**	**PE**	**MP**	**Total**
92960	2.0	1.03	0.15	3.18
92961	4.34	1.86	0.96	7.16

	FUD	Status	MUE	Modifiers				IOM Reference
92960	0	A	2(3)	N/A	N/A	N/A	80*	None
92961	0	A	1(3)	N/A	N/A	N/A	N/A	

* with documentation

Terms To Know

anomalous atrioventricular excitation. Pre-excitation associated with paroxysmal tachycardia or atrial fibrillation with a short P-R interval on EKG and an early delta wave. The normal conduction pathway is bypassed.

arrhythmias. Heart disorder of rhythm or rate, due to an electrical conduction system malfunction.

atrioventricular block. Condition in which there is a disturbance of electrical conduction, such as a delay, intermittence, or absence in the transmission of an impulse from the atria to the ventricles and categorized according to degree of severity.

supraventricular tachycardia. Rapid beating of the heart, usually pertains to more than 100 beats per minute and can be as high as 250 beats per minute. SVT is caused by abnormal electrical impulses originating at the AV node or above it in the atria (upper chambers) of the heart.

 N Newborn: 0 P Pediatric: 0-17 M Maternity: 9-64 A Adult: 15-124 AMA: CPT Assist

92970-92971

92970 Cardioassist-method of circulatory assist; internal
92971 external

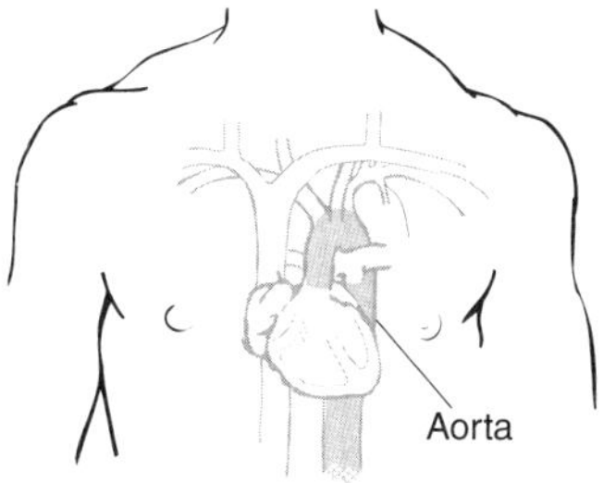

Internal circulatory assist involves accessing the aorta by catheter or cannula and inserting a blood flow assist device

External circulatory assist trousers

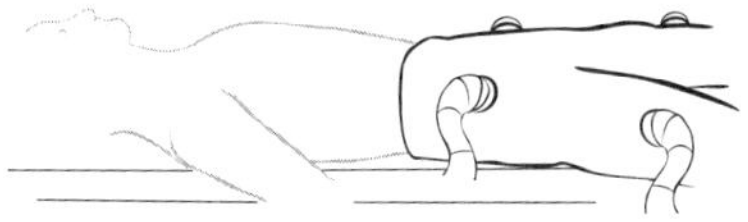

The trousers are rhythmically inflated and deflated, from the toes proximally toward the heart. The action improves venous return while reducing cardiac workload

Explanation

In 92970, in internal circulatory assist, the femoral artery is cannulated and a catheter with balloon or another device is inserted into the aorta. Various devices may be used to assist circulation. This code should be reported for the internal insertion of such a device but should not be used to report intra-aortic balloon pump (IABP) or implantation of ventricular assist devices that are reported elsewhere. In 92971, devices are placed at the outside of the body to assist circulation. One example of external circulatory assist is Military Anti-Shock Trousers (MAST), which apply counterpressure around the legs and abdomen. The artificial peripheral resistance helps coronary perfusion. In a related procedure, pressure cuffs are used to assist circulation. The patient is placed on a treatment table where their lower extremities are wrapped in a series of three compressive air cuffs, which inflate and deflate in synchronization with the patient's cardiac cycle. During diastole the three sets of air cuffs are inflated sequentially (distal to proximal) compressing the vascular beds within the muscles of the calves, lower thighs, and upper thighs. This action results in an increase in diastolic pressure, generation of retrograde arterial blood flow, and an increase in venous return. The cuffs are deflated simultaneously just prior to systole, which produces a rapid drop in vascular impedance, a decrease in ventricular workload, and an increase in cardiac output. The augmented diastolic pressure and retrograde aortic flow appear to improve myocardial perfusion, while systolic unloading appears to reduce cardiac workload and oxygen requirements. The increased venous return coupled with enhanced systolic flow appears to increase cardiac output.

Coding Tips

For balloon atrial-septostomy, see 33741. For placement of catheters for use in circulatory assist devices such as an intra-aortic balloon pump, see 33970.

ICD-10-CM Diagnostic Codes

I11.0 Hypertensive heart disease with heart failure
I13.2 Hypertensive heart and chronic kidney disease with heart failure and with stage 5 chronic kidney disease, or end stage renal disease
I16.0 Hypertensive urgency
I16.1 Hypertensive emergency
I50.21 Acute systolic (congestive) heart failure
I50.22 Chronic systolic (congestive) heart failure
I50.23 Acute on chronic systolic (congestive) heart failure
I50.31 Acute diastolic (congestive) heart failure
I50.32 Chronic diastolic (congestive) heart failure
I50.33 Acute on chronic diastolic (congestive) heart failure
I50.41 Acute combined systolic (congestive) and diastolic (congestive) heart failure
I50.42 Chronic combined systolic (congestive) and diastolic (congestive) heart failure
I50.43 Acute on chronic combined systolic (congestive) and diastolic (congestive) heart failure
I50.811 Acute right heart failure
I50.812 Chronic right heart failure
I50.813 Acute on chronic right heart failure
I50.814 Right heart failure due to left heart failure
I50.82 Biventricular heart failure
I50.83 High output heart failure
I50.84 End stage heart failure
I97.110 Postprocedural cardiac insufficiency following cardiac surgery
I97.111 Postprocedural cardiac insufficiency following other surgery
I97.120 Postprocedural cardiac arrest following cardiac surgery
I97.121 Postprocedural cardiac arrest following other surgery
I97.130 Postprocedural heart failure following cardiac surgery
I97.131 Postprocedural heart failure following other surgery
I97.710 Intraoperative cardiac arrest during cardiac surgery
I97.711 Intraoperative cardiac arrest during other surgery
R57.0 Cardiogenic shock

Relative Value Units/Medicare Edits

Non-Facility RVU	Work	PE	MP	Total
92970	3.51	1.2	0.8	5.51
92971	1.77	0.76	0.4	2.93
Facility RVU	**Work**	**PE**	**MP**	**Total**
92970	3.51	1.2	0.8	5.51
92971	1.77	0.76	0.4	2.93

	FUD	Status	MUE	Modifiers				IOM Reference
92970	0	A	1(3)	N/A	N/A	N/A	80*	None
92971	0	A	1(3)	N/A	N/A	N/A	80*	

* with documentation

92986-92990

92986 Percutaneous balloon valvuloplasty; aortic valve
92987 mitral valve
92990 pulmonary valve

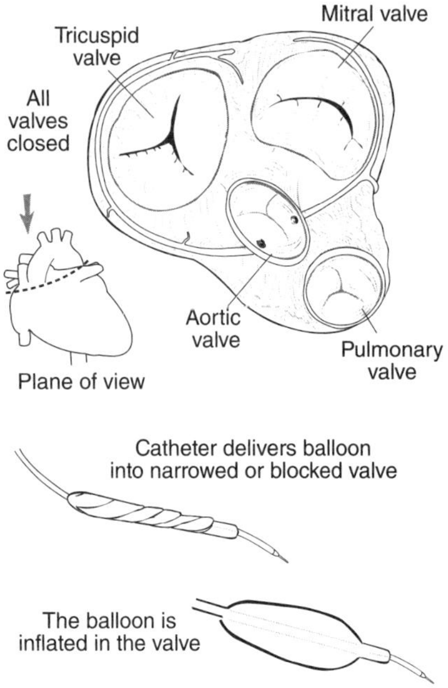

Explanation

The physician performs a percutaneous valvuloplasty. The physician makes a small incision in the arm or leg. Two catheters are placed: a central venous catheter and a second catheter threaded up to the heart. The physician inflates a balloon at the tip of the second catheter to open the blocked valve. The catheters are removed. Pressure is placed over the incision for 20 to 30 minutes to stem bleeding. The patient is observed for a period afterward. Report 92986 if the procedure is performed on the aortic valve; 92987 if the procedure is performed on the mitral valve; and 92990 if the procedure is performed on the pulmonary valve.

Coding Tips

When medically necessary, report moderate (conscious) sedation provided by the performing physician with 99151-99153. When provided by another physician, report 99155-99157. For open mitral valvuloplasty, see 33425-33427. For closed heart valvuloplasty, see 33471. For atrial septectomy or septostomy, transvenous method, balloon or blade, see 33741.

ICD-10-CM Diagnostic Codes

I05.0	Rheumatic mitral stenosis
I05.1	Rheumatic mitral insufficiency
I05.2	Rheumatic mitral stenosis with insufficiency
I05.8	Other rheumatic mitral valve diseases
I06.0	Rheumatic aortic stenosis
I06.1	Rheumatic aortic insufficiency
I06.2	Rheumatic aortic stenosis with insufficiency
I06.8	Other rheumatic aortic valve diseases
I08.0	Rheumatic disorders of both mitral and aortic valves
I08.8	Other rheumatic multiple valve diseases
I09.89	Other specified rheumatic heart diseases
I34.0	Nonrheumatic mitral (valve) insufficiency
I34.1	Nonrheumatic mitral (valve) prolapse
I34.2	Nonrheumatic mitral (valve) stenosis
I34.81	Nonrheumatic mitral (valve) annulus calcification
I34.89	Other nonrheumatic mitral valve disorders
I35.0	Nonrheumatic aortic (valve) stenosis
I35.1	Nonrheumatic aortic (valve) insufficiency
I35.2	Nonrheumatic aortic (valve) stenosis with insufficiency
I35.8	Other nonrheumatic aortic valve disorders
I37.0	Nonrheumatic pulmonary valve stenosis
I37.1	Nonrheumatic pulmonary valve insufficiency
I37.2	Nonrheumatic pulmonary valve stenosis with insufficiency
I37.8	Other nonrheumatic pulmonary valve disorders
Q22.1	Congenital pulmonary valve stenosis
Q23.1	Congenital insufficiency of aortic valve
Q23.3	Congenital mitral insufficiency

AMA: 92990 2024,Aug

Relative Value Units/Medicare Edits

Non-Facility RVU	Work	PE	MP	Total
92986	22.6	11.22	5.16	38.98
92987	23.38	11.49	5.3	40.17
92990	18.27	9.68	4.22	32.17
Facility RVU	**Work**	**PE**	**MP**	**Total**
92986	22.6	11.22	5.16	38.98
92987	23.38	11.49	5.3	40.17
92990	18.27	9.68	4.22	32.17

	FUD	Status	MUE	Modifiers				IOM Reference
92986	90	A	1(2)	51	N/A	N/A	80*	None
92987	90	A	1(2)	51	N/A	N/A	80*	
92990	90	A	1(2)	51	N/A	N/A	80*	

* with documentation

Terms To Know

aortic insufficiency. Malfunction of the aortic valve resulting in backflow of blood into the ventricle.

aortic valve. Heart valve, comprising three cusps, that divides the left ventricle and the aorta.

balloon catheter. Any catheter equipped with an inflatable balloon at the end to hold it in place in a body cavity or to be used for dilation of a vessel lumen.

mitral valve. Valve with two cusps that is between the left atrium and left ventricle of the heart.

pulmonary valve. Valve with three cusps between the right ventricle and the pulmonary artery.

valvuloplasty. Surgical repair of a valve.

 N Newborn: 0 P Pediatric: 0-17 M Maternity: 9-64 A Adult: 15-124 AMA: CPT Assist

92997-92998

92997 Percutaneous transluminal pulmonary artery balloon angioplasty; single vessel

+ **92998** each additional vessel (List separately in addition to code for primary procedure)

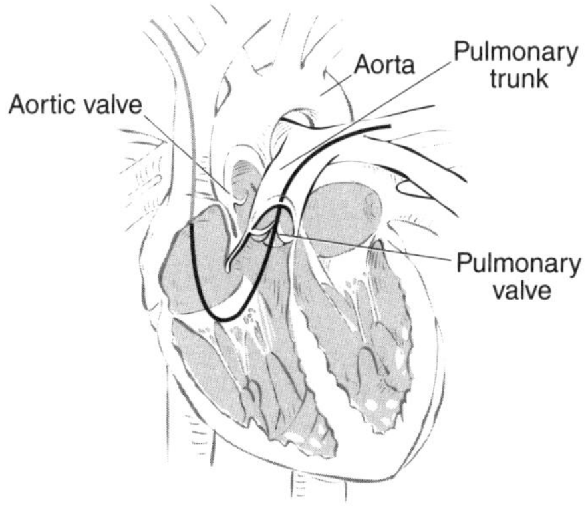

A pulmonary artery is approached transluminally by percutaneous entry. Balloon angioplasty is performed

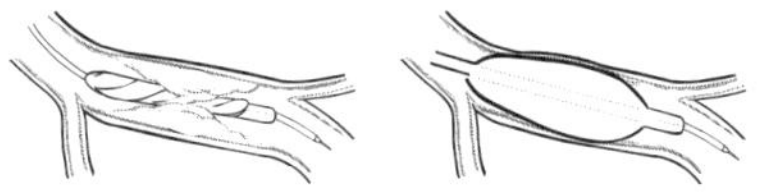

Explanation

The purpose of this procedure is to use a balloon to expand a narrowed pulmonary artery. The physician places an introducer sheath in the femoral vein, using percutaneous puncture. The physician places an angioplasty catheter through the introducer sheath into the femoral vein and advances it under fluoroscopic guidance to the right ventricle and out into the main pulmonary artery. The physician advances the angioplasty balloon into the narrowed pulmonary artery, using injections of x-ray contrast material to guide the way. In 92998, following single vessel percutaneous transluminal pulmonary artery balloon angioplasty, the physician redirects the balloon angioplasty catheter to an additional pulmonary artery. The physician may change to a different sized balloon catheter if the additional pulmonary artery is of a different size. For both procedures, the physician inflates the balloon to expand the pulmonary artery, sometimes using several balloon inflations. The physician removes the catheter and sheath from the femoral vein. Pressure is placed on the wound for 20 to 30 minutes to stem bleeding.

Coding Tips

Report 75741 or 75743 for the radiological supervision and interpretation, when appropriate. If intravascular ultrasound is used, report 37252-37253.

ICD-10-CM Diagnostic Codes

I26.01	Septic pulmonary embolism with acute cor pulmonale
I26.02	Saddle embolus of pulmonary artery with acute cor pulmonale
I26.09	Other pulmonary embolism with acute cor pulmonale
I26.90	Septic pulmonary embolism without acute cor pulmonale
I26.92	Saddle embolus of pulmonary artery without acute cor pulmonale
I26.93	Single subsegmental thrombotic pulmonary embolism without acute cor pulmonale
I26.94	Multiple subsegmental thrombotic pulmonary emboli without acute cor pulmonale
I26.99	Other pulmonary embolism without acute cor pulmonale
I28.8	Other diseases of pulmonary vessels
Q21.3	Tetralogy of Fallot
Q24.3	Pulmonary infundibular stenosis
Q25.5	Atresia of pulmonary artery
Q25.6	Stenosis of pulmonary artery
Q25.71	Coarctation of pulmonary artery
Q25.72	Congenital pulmonary arteriovenous malformation
Q25.79	Other congenital malformations of pulmonary artery

AMA: **92997** 2023,Jun; 2023,May **92998** 2023,Jun; 2023,May

Relative Value Units/Medicare Edits

Non-Facility RVU	Work	PE	MP	Total
92997	11.98	4.22	2.33	18.53
92998	5.99	2.01	1.3	9.3
Facility RVU	**Work**	**PE**	**MP**	**Total**
92997	11.98	4.22	2.33	18.53
92998	5.99	2.01	1.3	9.3

	FUD	Status	MUE	Modifiers				IOM Reference
92997	0	A	1(2)	51	N/A	N/A	80*	None
92998	N/A	A	7(3)	N/A	N/A	N/A	80*	

* with documentation

Terms To Know

embolism. Obstruction of a blood vessel resulting from a clot or foreign substance.

fluoroscopy. Radiology technique that allows visual examination of part of the body or a function of an organ using a device that projects an x-ray image on a fluorescent screen.

infarction. Area of necrosis in tissue, due to ischemia from lack of circulation, usually from a thrombus or an embolus.

percutaneous. Through the skin.

transluminal balloon angioplasty. Balloon-tipped catheter is placed within a narrowed artery or vein and the balloon is inflated to stretch the vessel to a larger diameter for increased blood flow.

[92920, 92921]

92920 Percutaneous transluminal coronary angioplasty; single major coronary artery or branch

\+ **92921** Percutaneous transluminal coronary angioplasty; each additional branch of a major coronary artery (List separately in addition to code for primary procedure)

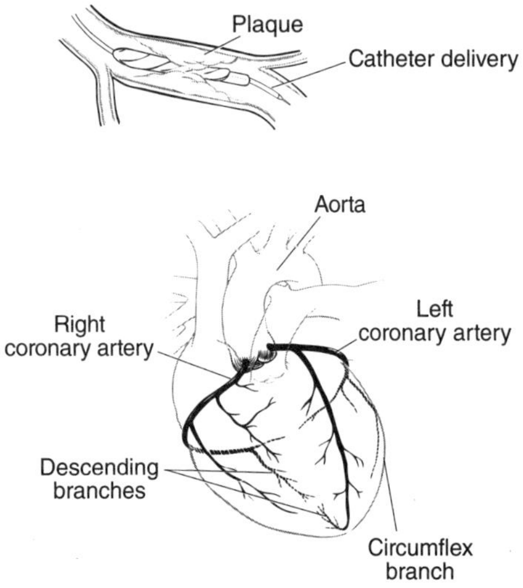

Percutaneous angioplasty of one or more major coronary arteries

Explanation

The physician makes a small incision in the arm or leg to access the artery for placement of two catheters. A central venous catheter is inserted through the femoral or brachial artery and a second catheter with a balloon tip is threaded up to the heart and into an obstructed native coronary artery. The physician inflates the balloon at the tip of the second catheter to flatten plaque obstructing the artery against the walls of the coronary artery. If sufficient results are not obtained after the first inflation, the physician may reinflate the balloon for a longer period of time or at greater pressure. The catheters are removed. Pressure is placed over the incision for 20 to 30 minutes to stop bleeding. Report 92920 for each angioplasty performed on a single major coronary artery or branch. Report 92921 for each additional branch of the major coronary artery treated during percutaneous coronary intervention.

Coding Tips

When medically necessary, report moderate (conscious) sedation provided by the performing physician with 99151-99153. When provided by another physician, report 99155-99157. Report 92921 in addition to 92920, 92924, 92928, 92933, 92937, 92941, or 92943. Do not report 92920 with 0913T. For percutaneous transcatheter therapeutic drug delivery by intracoronary drug-delivery balloon, see 0913T-0914T. Diagnostic coronary angiography performed at the time of the procedure may be reported in certain instances, such as when no prior catheter-based angiography study has been performed or a significant change in the patient's condition has occurred since the time of a prior study. Diagnostic coronary angiography services reported at the same surgical session as a percutaneous revascularization service may be reported separately. Only one base code from the percutaneous coronary intervention (PCI) codes should be reported for revascularization of a major coronary artery and its branches or revascularization of a bypass graft. The PCI base codes are 92920, 92924, 92928, 92933, 92937, 92941, and 92943, and the most intensive service for the target vessel should be selected. Services performed on additional branches should be reported using the add-on codes throughout the section. See CPT section guidelines for details on hierarchy and examples. Medicare and some other payers may require HCPCS Level II codes C9600–C9601 be reported for these services if drug eluting stents are used.

ICD-10-CM Diagnostic Codes

I20.0	Unstable angina
I20.81	Angina pectoris with coronary microvascular dysfunction
I21.01	ST elevation (STEMI) myocardial infarction involving left main coronary artery
I21.02	ST elevation (STEMI) myocardial infarction involving left anterior descending coronary artery
I21.09	ST elevation (STEMI) myocardial infarction involving other coronary artery of anterior wall
I21.11	ST elevation (STEMI) myocardial infarction involving right coronary artery
I21.19	ST elevation (STEMI) myocardial infarction involving other coronary artery of inferior wall
I21.21	ST elevation (STEMI) myocardial infarction involving left circumflex coronary artery
I21.29	ST elevation (STEMI) myocardial infarction involving other sites
I21.4	Non-ST elevation (NSTEMI) myocardial infarction
I21.A1	Myocardial infarction type 2
I21.B	Myocardial infarction with coronary microvascular dysfunction
I22.0	Subsequent ST elevation (STEMI) myocardial infarction of anterior wall
I22.1	Subsequent ST elevation (STEMI) myocardial infarction of inferior wall
I22.2	Subsequent non-ST elevation (NSTEMI) myocardial infarction
I22.8	Subsequent ST elevation (STEMI) myocardial infarction of other sites
I24.0	Acute coronary thrombosis not resulting in myocardial infarction
I24.1	Dressler's syndrome
I24.89	Other forms of acute ischemic heart disease
I25.110	Atherosclerotic heart disease of native coronary artery with unstable angina pectoris A
I25.111	Atherosclerotic heart disease of native coronary artery with angina pectoris with documented spasm A
I25.112	Atherosclerotic heart disease of native coronary artery with refractory angina pectoris A
I25.118	Atherosclerotic heart disease of native coronary artery with other forms of angina pectoris A
I25.2	Old myocardial infarction
I25.3	Aneurysm of heart
I25.41	Coronary artery aneurysm
I25.42	Coronary artery dissection
I25.5	Ischemic cardiomyopathy
I25.6	Silent myocardial ischemia
I25.710	Atherosclerosis of autologous vein coronary artery bypass graft(s) with unstable angina pectoris A
I25.711	Atherosclerosis of autologous vein coronary artery bypass graft(s) with angina pectoris with documented spasm A
I25.718	Atherosclerosis of autologous vein coronary artery bypass graft(s) with other forms of angina pectoris A
I25.720	Atherosclerosis of autologous artery coronary artery bypass graft(s) with unstable angina pectoris A

I25.721 Atherosclerosis of autologous artery coronary artery bypass graft(s) with angina pectoris with documented spasm [A]

I25.728 Atherosclerosis of autologous artery coronary artery bypass graft(s) with other forms of angina pectoris [A]

I25.730 Atherosclerosis of nonautologous biological coronary artery bypass graft(s) with unstable angina pectoris [A]

I25.731 Atherosclerosis of nonautologous biological coronary artery bypass graft(s) with angina pectoris with documented spasm [A]

I25.738 Atherosclerosis of nonautologous biological coronary artery bypass graft(s) with other forms of angina pectoris [A]

I25.750 Atherosclerosis of native coronary artery of transplanted heart with unstable angina

I25.760 Atherosclerosis of bypass graft of coronary artery of transplanted heart with unstable angina [A]

I25.761 Atherosclerosis of bypass graft of coronary artery of transplanted heart with angina pectoris with documented spasm [A]

I25.768 Atherosclerosis of bypass graft of coronary artery of transplanted heart with other forms of angina pectoris [A]

I25.790 Atherosclerosis of other coronary artery bypass graft(s) with unstable angina pectoris [A]

I25.791 Atherosclerosis of other coronary artery bypass graft(s) with angina pectoris with documented spasm [A]

I25.798 Atherosclerosis of other coronary artery bypass graft(s) with other forms of angina pectoris [A]

I25.810 Atherosclerosis of coronary artery bypass graft(s) without angina pectoris [A]

I25.812 Atherosclerosis of bypass graft of coronary artery of transplanted heart without angina pectoris [A]

I25.82 Chronic total occlusion of coronary artery

I25.84 Coronary atherosclerosis due to calcified coronary lesion

I25.89 Other forms of chronic ischemic heart disease

R57.0 Cardiogenic shock

R94.31 Abnormal electrocardiogram [ECG] [EKG]

T82.211A Breakdown (mechanical) of coronary artery bypass graft, initial encounter

T82.212A Displacement of coronary artery bypass graft, initial encounter

T82.213A Leakage of coronary artery bypass graft, initial encounter

T82.218A Other mechanical complication of coronary artery bypass graft, initial encounter

T82.818A Embolism due to vascular prosthetic devices, implants and grafts, initial encounter

T82.828A Fibrosis due to vascular prosthetic devices, implants and grafts, initial encounter

T82.838A Hemorrhage due to vascular prosthetic devices, implants and grafts, initial encounter

T82.848A Pain due to vascular prosthetic devices, implants and grafts, initial encounter

T82.858A Stenosis of other vascular prosthetic devices, implants and grafts, initial encounter

T82.868A Thrombosis due to vascular prosthetic devices, implants and grafts, initial encounter

T82.898A Other specified complication of vascular prosthetic devices, implants and grafts, initial encounter

AMA: 92920 2024,Jun

Relative Value Units/Medicare Edits

Non-Facility RVU	Work	PE	MP	Total
92920	9.85	3.37	2.23	15.45
92921	0.0	0.0	0.0	0.0
Facility RVU	**Work**	**PE**	**MP**	**Total**
92920	9.85	3.37	2.23	15.45
92921	0.0	0.0	0.0	0.0

	FUD	Status	MUE	Modifiers				IOM Reference
92920	0	A	3(3)	51	N/A	N/A	80*	None
92921	N/A	B	6(2)	N/A	N/A	N/A	N/A	

* with documentation

Terms To Know

angiography. Radiographic imaging of the arteries.

angioplasty. Reconstruction or repair of a diseased or damaged blood vessel.

angioplasty balloon. Balloon-tipped medical device used to clear the blockage of an artery. After insertion into the clogged artery, the balloon is inflated to expand a narrowing arterial section.

revascularization. Restoration of blood flow and oxygen supply to a body part. This may apply to an extremity, the heart, or penis.

[92924, 92925]

92924 Percutaneous transluminal coronary atherectomy, with coronary angioplasty when performed; single major coronary artery or branch

\+ **92925** Percutaneous transluminal coronary atherectomy, with coronary angioplasty when performed; each additional branch of a major coronary artery (List separately in addition to code for primary procedure)

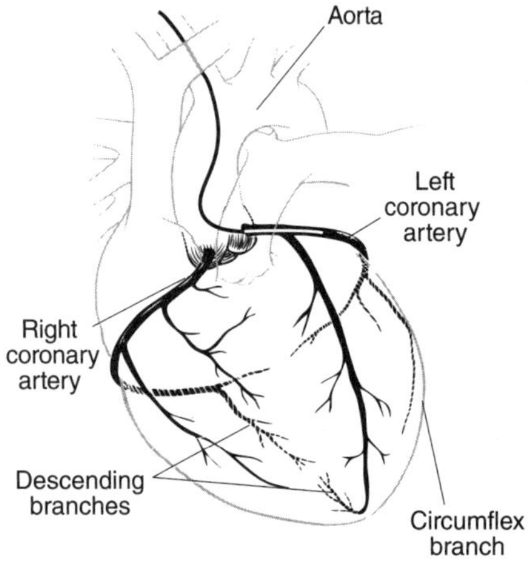

A coronary artery is approached transluminally by a percutaneous entry. Atherosclerotic deposits in the vessel are removed, mechanically or by other methods

Explanation

The physician removes the atherosclerotic plaque blocking a native coronary artery. The physician makes a small incision in the arm or leg to access the artery for placement of two catheters. A central venous catheter is inserted through the femoral or brachial artery and a second catheter threaded up to the coronary artery blockage. The plaque is removed using a rotary cutter introduced through a catheter under radiographic guidance. The blockage may also require subsequent inflation of the balloon on the tip of the second catheter to flatten any remaining plaque. The catheters are removed. Pressure is placed over the incision for 20 to 30 minutes to stop bleeding. Report 92924 for each atherectomy performed on a single major coronary artery or branch. Report 92925 for each additional branch of the major coronary artery treated during percutaneous coronary intervention.

Coding Tips

When medically necessary, report moderate (conscious) sedation provided by the performing physician with 99151-99153. When provided by another physician, report 99155-99157. Report 92925 in addition to 92924, 92928, 92933, 92937, 92941, or 92943. Do not report 92924 with 0913T. For percutaneous transcatheter therapeutic drug delivery by intracoronary drug-delivery balloon, see 0913T-0914T. Diagnostic coronary angiography performed at the time of the procedure may be reported in certain instances, such as when no prior catheter-based angiography study has been performed or a significant change in the patient's condition has occurred since the time of a prior study. Diagnostic coronary angiography services reported at the same surgical session as a percutaneous revascularization service may be reported separately. Only one base code from the percutaneous coronary intervention (PCI) codes should be reported for revascularization of a major coronary artery and its branches or revascularization of a bypass graft. The PCI base codes are 92920, 92924, 92928, 92933, 92937, 92941, and 92943, and the most intensive service for the target vessel should be selected. Services performed on additional branches should be reported using the add-on codes throughout the section. See CPT section guidelines for details on hierarchy and examples. Medicare and some other payers may require HCPCS Level II codes C9602–C9603 be reported for these services if drug eluting stents are used.

ICD-10-CM Diagnostic Codes

I20.0	Unstable angina
I20.81	Angina pectoris with coronary microvascular dysfunction
I21.01	ST elevation (STEMI) myocardial infarction involving left main coronary artery
I21.02	ST elevation (STEMI) myocardial infarction involving left anterior descending coronary artery
I21.09	ST elevation (STEMI) myocardial infarction involving other coronary artery of anterior wall
I21.11	ST elevation (STEMI) myocardial infarction involving right coronary artery
I21.19	ST elevation (STEMI) myocardial infarction involving other coronary artery of inferior wall
I21.21	ST elevation (STEMI) myocardial infarction involving left circumflex coronary artery
I21.29	ST elevation (STEMI) myocardial infarction involving other sites
I21.4	Non-ST elevation (NSTEMI) myocardial infarction
I21.B	Myocardial infarction with coronary microvascular dysfunction
I22.0	Subsequent ST elevation (STEMI) myocardial infarction of anterior wall
I22.1	Subsequent ST elevation (STEMI) myocardial infarction of inferior wall
I22.2	Subsequent non-ST elevation (NSTEMI) myocardial infarction
I22.8	Subsequent ST elevation (STEMI) myocardial infarction of other sites
I24.0	Acute coronary thrombosis not resulting in myocardial infarction
I24.1	Dressler's syndrome
I24.89	Other forms of acute ischemic heart disease
I25.10	Atherosclerotic heart disease of native coronary artery without angina pectoris A
I25.110	Atherosclerotic heart disease of native coronary artery with unstable angina pectoris A
I25.111	Atherosclerotic heart disease of native coronary artery with angina pectoris with documented spasm A
I25.112	Atherosclerotic heart disease of native coronary artery with refractory angina pectoris A
I25.118	Atherosclerotic heart disease of native coronary artery with other forms of angina pectoris A
I25.2	Old myocardial infarction
I25.3	Aneurysm of heart
I25.41	Coronary artery aneurysm
I25.42	Coronary artery dissection
I25.5	Ischemic cardiomyopathy
I25.6	Silent myocardial ischemia
I25.750	Atherosclerosis of native coronary artery of transplanted heart with unstable angina
I25.82	Chronic total occlusion of coronary artery
I25.84	Coronary atherosclerosis due to calcified coronary lesion
I25.89	Other forms of chronic ischemic heart disease
I25.9	Chronic ischemic heart disease, unspecified
R57.0	Cardiogenic shock

R94.31 Abnormal electrocardiogram [ECG] [EKG]

T82.211A Breakdown (mechanical) of coronary artery bypass graft, initial encounter

T82.212A Displacement of coronary artery bypass graft, initial encounter

T82.213A Leakage of coronary artery bypass graft, initial encounter

T82.218A Other mechanical complication of coronary artery bypass graft, initial encounter

T82.818A Embolism due to vascular prosthetic devices, implants and grafts, initial encounter

T82.828A Fibrosis due to vascular prosthetic devices, implants and grafts, initial encounter

T82.838A Hemorrhage due to vascular prosthetic devices, implants and grafts, initial encounter

T82.848A Pain due to vascular prosthetic devices, implants and grafts, initial encounter

T82.858A Stenosis of other vascular prosthetic devices, implants and grafts, initial encounter

T82.868A Thrombosis due to vascular prosthetic devices, implants and grafts, initial encounter

T82.898A Other specified complication of vascular prosthetic devices, implants and grafts, initial encounter

AMA: 92924 2024,Jun

Relative Value Units/Medicare Edits

Non-Facility RVU	Work	PE	MP	Total
92924	11.74	4.02	2.67	18.43
92925	0.0	0.0	0.0	0.0
Facility RVU	**Work**	**PE**	**MP**	**Total**
92924	11.74	4.02	2.67	18.43
92925	0.0	0.0	0.0	0.0

	FUD	Status	MUE	Modifiers				IOM Reference
92924	0	A	2(3)	51	N/A	N/A	80*	None
92925	N/A	B	6(2)	N/A	N/A	N/A	N/A	

* with documentation

Terms To Know

angiography. Radiographic imaging of the arteries.

angioplasty balloon. Balloon-tipped medical device used to clear the blockage of an artery. After insertion into the clogged artery, the balloon is inflated to expand a narrowing arterial section.

percutaneous transluminal coronary angioplasty. Procedure used to treat coronary artery obstruction. A balloon catheter is placed in the affected artery and the balloon is inflated to flatten the plaque against the wall of the artery and open the obstruction.

plaque. Accumulation of a soft sticky substance on the teeth largely composed of bacteria and its byproducts.

stent. Tube to provide support in a body cavity or lumen.

[92928, 92929]

92928 Percutaneous transcatheter placement of intracoronary stent(s), with coronary angioplasty when performed; single major coronary artery or branch

\+ **92929** Percutaneous transcatheter placement of intracoronary stent(s), with coronary angioplasty when performed; each additional branch of a major coronary artery (List separately in addition to code for primary procedure)

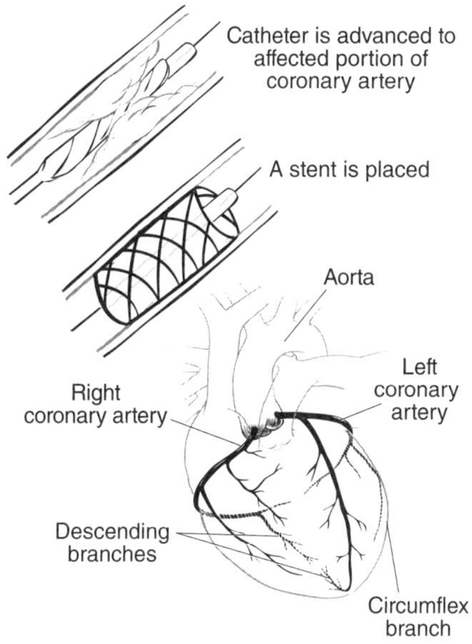

Explanation

A stent is used to hold open a blocked or collapsed native artery in the heart. The physician makes a small incision in the arm or leg to access the artery for placement of two catheters. A central venous catheter is inserted through the femoral or brachial artery and a second catheter is threaded up to the affected coronary artery. An obstruction may be treated first by inflating a balloon at the tip of the second catheter (PTCA) to flatten the obstruction. A stent is introduced through a catheter, placed under radiographic guidance, and expanded to fit the lumen of the artery by inflating the balloon on the second catheter. The catheters are removed. Pressure is placed over the incision for 20 to 30 minutes to stop the bleeding. Report 92928 for each stent placement performed on a single major coronary artery or branch. Report 92929 for each additional branch of the major coronary artery stented during percutaneous coronary intervention.

Coding Tips

When medically necessary, report moderate (conscious) sedation provided by the performing physician with 99151-99153. When provided by another physician, report 99155-99157. Report 92929 in addition to 92928, 92933, 92937, 92941, or 92943. Do not report 92928 with 0913T. For percutaneous transcatheter therapeutic drug delivery by intracoronary drug-delivery balloon, see 0913T-0914T. Diagnostic coronary angiography performed at the time of the procedure may be reported in certain instances, such as when no prior catheter-based angiography study has been performed or a significant change in the patient's condition has occurred since the time of a prior study. Diagnostic coronary angiography services reported at a different surgical session as a percutaneous revascularization service may be reported separately. Only one base code from the percutaneous coronary intervention (PCI) codes should be reported for revascularization of a major coronary artery and its branches or revascularization of a bypass graft. The PCI base codes are 92920,

92924, 92928, 92933, 92937, 92941, and 92943, and the most intensive service for the target vessel should be selected. Services performed on additional branches should be reported using the add-on codes throughout the section. See CPT section guidelines for details on hierarchy and examples.

ICD-10-CM Diagnostic Codes

I20.0	Unstable angina
I20.81	Angina pectoris with coronary microvascular dysfunction
I21.01	ST elevation (STEMI) myocardial infarction involving left main coronary artery
I21.02	ST elevation (STEMI) myocardial infarction involving left anterior descending coronary artery
I21.09	ST elevation (STEMI) myocardial infarction involving other coronary artery of anterior wall
I21.11	ST elevation (STEMI) myocardial infarction involving right coronary artery
I21.19	ST elevation (STEMI) myocardial infarction involving other coronary artery of inferior wall
I21.21	ST elevation (STEMI) myocardial infarction involving left circumflex coronary artery
I21.29	ST elevation (STEMI) myocardial infarction involving other sites
I21.4	Non-ST elevation (NSTEMI) myocardial infarction
I21.A1	Myocardial infarction type 2
I21.B	Myocardial infarction with coronary microvascular dysfunction
I22.0	Subsequent ST elevation (STEMI) myocardial infarction of anterior wall
I22.1	Subsequent ST elevation (STEMI) myocardial infarction of inferior wall
I22.2	Subsequent non-ST elevation (NSTEMI) myocardial infarction
I22.8	Subsequent ST elevation (STEMI) myocardial infarction of other sites
I24.0	Acute coronary thrombosis not resulting in myocardial infarction
I24.1	Dressler's syndrome
I24.89	Other forms of acute ischemic heart disease
I25.10	Atherosclerotic heart disease of native coronary artery without angina pectoris [A]
I25.110	Atherosclerotic heart disease of native coronary artery with unstable angina pectoris [A]
I25.111	Atherosclerotic heart disease of native coronary artery with angina pectoris with documented spasm [A]
I25.112	Atherosclerotic heart disease of native coronary artery with refractory angina pectoris [A]
I25.118	Atherosclerotic heart disease of native coronary artery with other forms of angina pectoris [A]
I25.119	Atherosclerotic heart disease of native coronary artery with unspecified angina pectoris [A]
I25.2	Old myocardial infarction
I25.3	Aneurysm of heart
I25.41	Coronary artery aneurysm
I25.42	Coronary artery dissection
I25.5	Ischemic cardiomyopathy
I25.6	Silent myocardial ischemia
I25.750	Atherosclerosis of native coronary artery of transplanted heart with unstable angina
I25.82	Chronic total occlusion of coronary artery
I25.84	Coronary atherosclerosis due to calcified coronary lesion
I25.89	Other forms of chronic ischemic heart disease
I25.9	Chronic ischemic heart disease, unspecified
R57.0	Cardiogenic shock
R94.31	Abnormal electrocardiogram [ECG] [EKG]
T82.211A	Breakdown (mechanical) of coronary artery bypass graft, initial encounter
T82.212A	Displacement of coronary artery bypass graft, initial encounter
T82.213A	Leakage of coronary artery bypass graft, initial encounter
T82.218A	Other mechanical complication of coronary artery bypass graft, initial encounter
T82.818A	Embolism due to vascular prosthetic devices, implants and grafts, initial encounter
T82.828A	Fibrosis due to vascular prosthetic devices, implants and grafts, initial encounter
T82.838A	Hemorrhage due to vascular prosthetic devices, implants and grafts, initial encounter
T82.848A	Pain due to vascular prosthetic devices, implants and grafts, initial encounter
T82.858A	Stenosis of other vascular prosthetic devices, implants and grafts, initial encounter
T82.868A	Thrombosis due to vascular prosthetic devices, implants and grafts, initial encounter
T82.898A	Other specified complication of vascular prosthetic devices, implants and grafts, initial encounter

AMA: 92928 2024,Jun

Relative Value Units/Medicare Edits

Non-Facility RVU	Work	PE	MP	Total
92928	10.96	3.75	2.48	17.19
92929	0.0	0.0	0.0	0.0
Facility RVU	**Work**	**PE**	**MP**	**Total**
92928	10.96	3.75	2.48	17.19
92929	0.0	0.0	0.0	0.0

	FUD	Status	MUE	Modifiers				IOM Reference
92928	0	A	3(3)	51	N/A	N/A	80*	None
92929	N/A	B	2(3)	N/A	N/A	N/A	N/A	

* with documentation

Terms To Know

percutaneous transluminal coronary angioplasty. Procedure used to treat coronary artery obstruction. A balloon catheter is placed in the affected artery and the balloon is inflated to flatten the plaque against the wall of the artery and open the obstruction.

revascularization. Restoration of blood flow and oxygen supply to a body part. This may apply to an extremity, the heart, or penis.

[92933, 92934]

92933 Percutaneous transluminal coronary atherectomy, with intracoronary stent, with coronary angioplasty when performed; single major coronary artery or branch

\+ **92934** Percutaneous transluminal coronary atherectomy, with intracoronary stent, with coronary angioplasty when performed; each additional branch of a major coronary artery (List separately in addition to code for primary procedure)

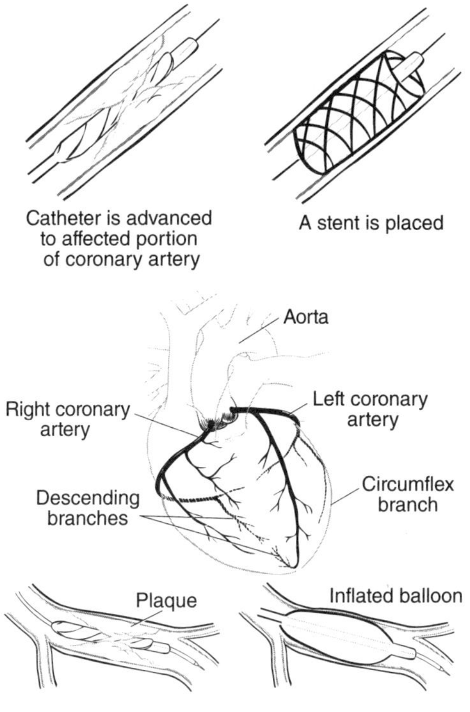

A balloon may be inflated or other intravascular therapy may accompany the procedure

Explanation

A stent is used to hold open a blocked native coronary artery. The physician makes a small incision in the arm or leg to access the artery for placement of two catheters. A central venous catheter is inserted through the femoral or brachial artery and a second catheter is threaded up to the affected coronary artery. Any obstruction is treated first by using a rotary cutter (atherectomy) to flatten or remove the obstruction. The obstruction may also be treated by inflating a balloon at the tip of the second catheter (PTCA). A stent is introduced through a catheter, placed under radiographic guidance, and expanded to fit the lumen of the artery by inflating the balloon on the second catheter. The catheters are removed. Pressure is placed over the incision for 20 to 30 minutes to stop the bleeding. Report 92933 for each atherectomy with stent placement performed on a single major coronary artery or branch. Report 92934 for each additional branch of the major coronary artery treated with atherectomy and stent during percutaneous coronary intervention.

Coding Tips

When medically necessary, report moderate (conscious) sedation provided by the performing physician with 99151-99153. When provided by another physician, report 99155-99157. Report 92934 in addition to 92933, 92937, 92941, or 92943. Do not report 92933 with 0913T. For percutaneous transcatheter therapeutic drug delivery by intracoronary drug-delivery balloon, see 0913T-0914T. Diagnostic coronary angiography performed at the time of the procedure may be reported in certain instances, such as when no prior catheter-based angiography study has been performed or a significant change in the patient's condition has occurred since the time of a prior study. Diagnostic coronary angiography services reported at the same surgical session as a percutaneous revascularization service may be reported separately. Only one base code from the percutaneous coronary intervention (PCI) codes should be reported for revascularization of a major coronary artery and its branches or revascularization of a bypass graft. The PCI base codes are 92920, 92924, 92928, 92933, 92937, 92941, and 92943, and the most intensive service for the target vessel should be selected. Services performed on additional branches should be reported using the add-on codes throughout the section. See CPT section guidelines for details on hierarchy and examples.

ICD-10-CM Diagnostic Codes

I20.0	Unstable angina
I20.81	Angina pectoris with coronary microvascular dysfunction
I21.01	ST elevation (STEMI) myocardial infarction involving left main coronary artery
I21.02	ST elevation (STEMI) myocardial infarction involving left anterior descending coronary artery
I21.09	ST elevation (STEMI) myocardial infarction involving other coronary artery of anterior wall
I21.11	ST elevation (STEMI) myocardial infarction involving right coronary artery
I21.19	ST elevation (STEMI) myocardial infarction involving other coronary artery of inferior wall
I21.21	ST elevation (STEMI) myocardial infarction involving left circumflex coronary artery
I21.29	ST elevation (STEMI) myocardial infarction involving other sites
I21.4	Non-ST elevation (NSTEMI) myocardial infarction
I21.A1	Myocardial infarction type 2
I21.B	Myocardial infarction with coronary microvascular dysfunction
I22.0	Subsequent ST elevation (STEMI) myocardial infarction of anterior wall
I22.1	Subsequent ST elevation (STEMI) myocardial infarction of inferior wall
I22.2	Subsequent non-ST elevation (NSTEMI) myocardial infarction
I22.8	Subsequent ST elevation (STEMI) myocardial infarction of other sites
I24.0	Acute coronary thrombosis not resulting in myocardial infarction
I24.1	Dressler's syndrome
I24.89	Other forms of acute ischemic heart disease
I25.10	Atherosclerotic heart disease of native coronary artery without angina pectoris A
I25.110	Atherosclerotic heart disease of native coronary artery with unstable angina pectoris A
I25.111	Atherosclerotic heart disease of native coronary artery with angina pectoris with documented spasm A
I25.112	Atherosclerotic heart disease of native coronary artery with refractory angina pectoris A
I25.118	Atherosclerotic heart disease of native coronary artery with other forms of angina pectoris A
I25.119	Atherosclerotic heart disease of native coronary artery with unspecified angina pectoris A
I25.2	Old myocardial infarction
I25.3	Aneurysm of heart
I25.41	Coronary artery aneurysm
I25.42	Coronary artery dissection

I25.5 Ischemic cardiomyopathy
I25.6 Silent myocardial ischemia
I25.750 Atherosclerosis of native coronary artery of transplanted heart with unstable angina
I25.82 Chronic total occlusion of coronary artery
I25.84 Coronary atherosclerosis due to calcified coronary lesion
I25.89 Other forms of chronic ischemic heart disease
I25.9 Chronic ischemic heart disease, unspecified
R57.0 Cardiogenic shock
R94.31 Abnormal electrocardiogram [ECG] [EKG]
T82.211A Breakdown (mechanical) of coronary artery bypass graft, initial encounter
T82.212A Displacement of coronary artery bypass graft, initial encounter
T82.213A Leakage of coronary artery bypass graft, initial encounter
T82.218A Other mechanical complication of coronary artery bypass graft, initial encounter
T82.818A Embolism due to vascular prosthetic devices, implants and grafts, initial encounter
T82.828A Fibrosis due to vascular prosthetic devices, implants and grafts, initial encounter
T82.838A Hemorrhage due to vascular prosthetic devices, implants and grafts, initial encounter
T82.848A Pain due to vascular prosthetic devices, implants and grafts, initial encounter
T82.858A Stenosis of other vascular prosthetic devices, implants and grafts, initial encounter
T82.868A Thrombosis due to vascular prosthetic devices, implants and grafts, initial encounter
T82.898A Other specified complication of vascular prosthetic devices, implants and grafts, initial encounter

AMA: 92933 2024,Jun; 2023,Nov **92934** 2023,Nov

Relative Value Units/Medicare Edits

Non-Facility RVU	Work	PE	MP	Total
92933	12.29	4.2	2.79	19.28
92934	0.0	0.0	0.0	0.0
Facility RVU	**Work**	**PE**	**MP**	**Total**
92933	12.29	4.2	2.79	19.28
92934	0.0	0.0	0.0	0.0

	FUD	Status	MUE	Modifiers				IOM Reference
92933	0	A	2(3)	51	N/A	N/A	80*	None
92934	N/A	B	2(3)	N/A	N/A	N/A	N/A	

* with documentation

Terms To Know

atherectomy. Surgical removal of arterial plaque from inside an artery. The procedure may be performed percutaneously, using a special catheter with a high-speed burr at the tip to bore through the sclerotic deposits, or transluminally by open incision.

revascularization. Restoration of blood flow and oxygen supply to a body part. This may apply to an extremity, the heart, or penis.

[92937, 92938]

92937 Percutaneous transluminal revascularization of or through coronary artery bypass graft (internal mammary, free arterial, venous), any combination of intracoronary stent, atherectomy and angioplasty, including distal protection when performed; single vessel

+ **92938** Percutaneous transluminal revascularization of or through coronary artery bypass graft (internal mammary, free arterial, venous), any combination of intracoronary stent, atherectomy and angioplasty, including distal protection when performed; each additional branch subtended by the bypass graft (List separately in addition to code for primary procedure)

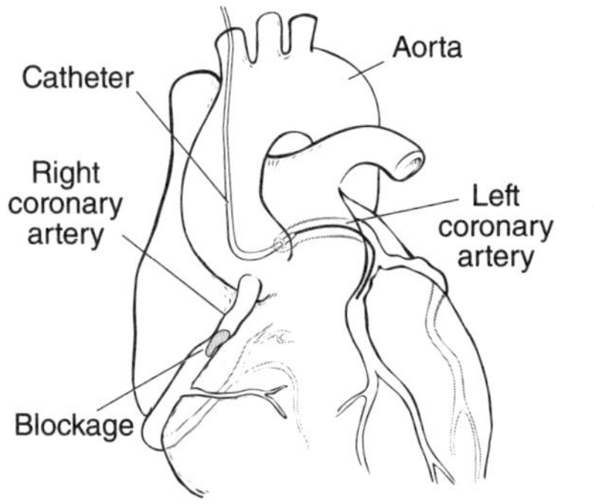

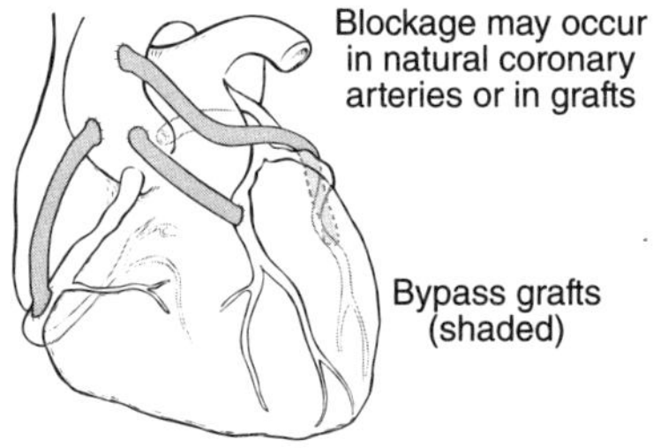

Explanation

The use of one or any combination of angioplasty, atherectomy, or stent placement is performed to restore a blocked coronary artery bypass graft (CABG). The physician makes a small incision in the arm or leg to access the artery for placement of two catheters. A central venous catheter is inserted through the femoral or brachial artery and a second catheter is threaded up to the affected graft. The obstruction may be treated by using a rotary cutter (atherectomy) to flatten or remove the obstruction, inflating a balloon at the tip of the second catheter (PTCA), or introducing a stent that is expanded to fit the lumen of the artery. The catheters are removed. Pressure is placed over the incision for 20 to 30 minutes to stop the bleeding. Report 92937 for treatment of the first CABG. Report 92938 for each additional graft treated.

Coding Tips

When medically necessary, report moderate (conscious) sedation provided by the performing physician with 99151-99153. When provided by another physician, report 99155-99157. Report 92938 in addition to 92937. Do not report 92937 with 0913T. For percutaneous transcatheter therapeutic drug delivery by intracoronary drug-delivery balloon, see 0913T-0914T. Diagnostic coronary angiography performed at the time of the procedure may be reported in certain instances, such as when no prior catheter-based angiography study has been performed or a significant change in the patient's condition has occurred since the time of a prior study. Diagnostic coronary angiography services reported at the same surgical session as a percutaneous revascularization service may be reported separately. Only one base code from the percutaneous coronary intervention (PCI) codes should be reported for revascularization of a major coronary artery and its branches or revascularization of a bypass graft. The PCI base codes are 92920, 92924, 92928, 92933, 92937, 92941, and 92943, and the most intensive service for the target vessel should be selected. Services performed on additional branches should be reported using the add-on codes throughout the section. See CPT section guidelines for details on hierarchy and examples. Medicare and some other payers may require HCPCS Level II codes C9604–C9605 be reported for these services if drug eluting stents are used.

ICD-10-CM Diagnostic Codes

I20.0	Unstable angina
I20.81	Angina pectoris with coronary microvascular dysfunction
I21.01	ST elevation (STEMI) myocardial infarction involving left main coronary artery
I21.02	ST elevation (STEMI) myocardial infarction involving left anterior descending coronary artery
I21.11	ST elevation (STEMI) myocardial infarction involving right coronary artery
I21.21	ST elevation (STEMI) myocardial infarction involving left circumflex coronary artery
I21.4	Non-ST elevation (NSTEMI) myocardial infarction
I21.A1	Myocardial infarction type 2
I21.B	Myocardial infarction with coronary microvascular dysfunction
I22.0	Subsequent ST elevation (STEMI) myocardial infarction of anterior wall
I22.1	Subsequent ST elevation (STEMI) myocardial infarction of inferior wall
I22.2	Subsequent non-ST elevation (NSTEMI) myocardial infarction
I24.0	Acute coronary thrombosis not resulting in myocardial infarction
I24.1	Dressler's syndrome
I24.89	Other forms of acute ischemic heart disease
I25.10	Atherosclerotic heart disease of native coronary artery without angina pectoris A
I25.110	Atherosclerotic heart disease of native coronary artery with unstable angina pectoris A
I25.111	Atherosclerotic heart disease of native coronary artery with angina pectoris with documented spasm A
I25.112	Atherosclerotic heart disease of native coronary artery with refractory angina pectoris A
I25.2	Old myocardial infarction
I25.3	Aneurysm of heart
I25.41	Coronary artery aneurysm
I25.42	Coronary artery dissection
I25.5	Ischemic cardiomyopathy
I25.6	Silent myocardial ischemia
I25.710	Atherosclerosis of autologous vein coronary artery bypass graft(s) with unstable angina pectoris A
I25.711	Atherosclerosis of autologous vein coronary artery bypass graft(s) with angina pectoris with documented spasm A
I25.720	Atherosclerosis of autologous artery coronary artery bypass graft(s) with unstable angina pectoris A
I25.721	Atherosclerosis of autologous artery coronary artery bypass graft(s) with angina pectoris with documented spasm A
I25.730	Atherosclerosis of nonautologous biological coronary artery bypass graft(s) with unstable angina pectoris A
I25.731	Atherosclerosis of nonautologous biological coronary artery bypass graft(s) with angina pectoris with documented spasm A
I25.750	Atherosclerosis of native coronary artery of transplanted heart with unstable angina
I25.760	Atherosclerosis of bypass graft of coronary artery of transplanted heart with unstable angina A
I25.761	Atherosclerosis of bypass graft of coronary artery of transplanted heart with angina pectoris with documented spasm A
I25.810	Atherosclerosis of coronary artery bypass graft(s) without angina pectoris A
I25.812	Atherosclerosis of bypass graft of coronary artery of transplanted heart without angina pectoris A
I25.82	Chronic total occlusion of coronary artery
I25.84	Coronary atherosclerosis due to calcified coronary lesion
R57.0	Cardiogenic shock
R94.31	Abnormal electrocardiogram [ECG] [EKG]
T82.211A	Breakdown (mechanical) of coronary artery bypass graft, initial encounter
T82.212A	Displacement of coronary artery bypass graft, initial encounter
T82.213A	Leakage of coronary artery bypass graft, initial encounter
T82.218A	Other mechanical complication of coronary artery bypass graft, initial encounter
T82.818A	Embolism due to vascular prosthetic devices, implants and grafts, initial encounter
T82.828A	Fibrosis due to vascular prosthetic devices, implants and grafts, initial encounter
T82.838A	Hemorrhage due to vascular prosthetic devices, implants and grafts, initial encounter
T82.848A	Pain due to vascular prosthetic devices, implants and grafts, initial encounter
T82.858A	Stenosis of other vascular prosthetic devices, implants and grafts, initial encounter
T82.868A	Thrombosis due to vascular prosthetic devices, implants and grafts, initial encounter

AMA: **92937** 2024,Jun

Relative Value Units/Medicare Edits

Non-Facility RVU	Work	PE	MP	Total
92937	10.95	3.75	2.49	17.19
92938	0.0	0.0	0.0	0.0
Facility RVU	**Work**	**PE**	**MP**	**Total**
92937	10.95	3.75	2.49	17.19
92938	0.0	0.0	0.0	0.0

	FUD	Status	MUE	Modifiers				IOM Reference
92937	0	A	2(3)	51	N/A	N/A	80*	None
92938	N/A	B	2(3)	N/A	N/A	N/A	N/A	

* with documentation

[92941]

92941 Percutaneous transluminal revascularization of acute total/subtotal occlusion during acute myocardial infarction, coronary artery or coronary artery bypass graft, any combination of intracoronary stent, atherectomy and angioplasty, including aspiration thrombectomy when performed, single vessel

Revascularization of occlusion in native or bypass coronary artery

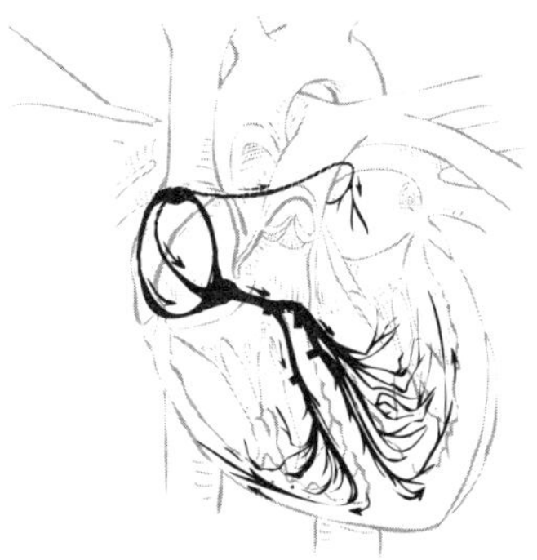

Explanation

The use of one or any combination of angioplasty, atherectomy, or stent placement is performed to restore an acutely blocked coronary artery bypass graft (CABG) or native coronary artery during an acute myocardial infarction. The physician makes a small incision in the arm or leg to access the artery for placement of two catheters. A central venous catheter is inserted through the femoral or brachial artery and a second catheter is threaded up to the affected vessel or graft. The obstruction may be treated by using a rotary cutter (atherectomy) to flatten or remove the obstruction, inflating a balloon at the tip of the second catheter (PTCA), or introducing a stent that is expanded to fit the lumen of the artery. The catheters are removed. Pressure is placed over the incision for 20 to 30 minutes to stop the bleeding.

Coding Tips

When medically necessary, report moderate (conscious) sedation provided by the performing physician with 99151-99153. When provided by another physician, report 99155-99157. Diagnostic coronary angiography performed at the time of the procedure may be reported in certain instances, such as when no prior catheter-based angiography study has been performed or a significant change in the patient's condition has occurred since the time of a prior study. Diagnostic coronary angiography services reported at the same surgical session as a percutaneous revascularization service may be reported separately. Only one base code from the percutaneous coronary intervention (PCI) codes should be reported for revascularization of a major coronary artery and its branches or revascularization of a bypass graft. The PCI base codes are 92920, 92924, 92928, 92933, 92937, 92941, and 92943, and the most intensive service for the target vessel should be selected. Services performed on additional branches should be reported using the add-on codes throughout the section. See CPT section guidelines for details on hierarchy and examples. Do not report 92941 with 0913T for intervention in the same major coronary artery or the same bypass graft. Code 92941 reports a single vessel. For additional vessels treated, see 92920–92938, 92943, 92944, 0913T, or 0914T. For transcatheter intra-arterial hyperoxemic reperfusion/supersaturated oxygen therapy (SSO2), see 0659T. Medicare and some other payers may require HCPCS Level II code C9606 be reported for this service if drug eluting stents are used.

ICD-10-CM Diagnostic Codes

I20.0	Unstable angina
I20.81	Angina pectoris with coronary microvascular dysfunction
I21.01	ST elevation (STEMI) myocardial infarction involving left main coronary artery
I21.02	ST elevation (STEMI) myocardial infarction involving left anterior descending coronary artery
I21.09	ST elevation (STEMI) myocardial infarction involving other coronary artery of anterior wall
I21.11	ST elevation (STEMI) myocardial infarction involving right coronary artery
I21.19	ST elevation (STEMI) myocardial infarction involving other coronary artery of inferior wall
I21.21	ST elevation (STEMI) myocardial infarction involving left circumflex coronary artery
I21.29	ST elevation (STEMI) myocardial infarction involving other sites
I21.4	Non-ST elevation (NSTEMI) myocardial infarction
I21.A1	Myocardial infarction type 2
I21.B	Myocardial infarction with coronary microvascular dysfunction
I22.0	Subsequent ST elevation (STEMI) myocardial infarction of anterior wall
I22.1	Subsequent ST elevation (STEMI) myocardial infarction of inferior wall
I22.2	Subsequent non-ST elevation (NSTEMI) myocardial infarction
I22.8	Subsequent ST elevation (STEMI) myocardial infarction of other sites
I24.0	Acute coronary thrombosis not resulting in myocardial infarction
I24.89	Other forms of acute ischemic heart disease
I25.10	Atherosclerotic heart disease of native coronary artery without angina pectoris A
I25.110	Atherosclerotic heart disease of native coronary artery with unstable angina pectoris A
I25.111	Atherosclerotic heart disease of native coronary artery with angina pectoris with documented spasm A
I25.112	Atherosclerotic heart disease of native coronary artery with refractory angina pectoris A
I25.5	Ischemic cardiomyopathy
I25.6	Silent myocardial ischemia
I25.710	Atherosclerosis of autologous vein coronary artery bypass graft(s) with unstable angina pectoris A
I25.711	Atherosclerosis of autologous vein coronary artery bypass graft(s) with angina pectoris with documented spasm A
I25.718	Atherosclerosis of autologous vein coronary artery bypass graft(s) with other forms of angina pectoris A
I25.720	Atherosclerosis of autologous artery coronary artery bypass graft(s) with unstable angina pectoris A
I25.721	Atherosclerosis of autologous artery coronary artery bypass graft(s) with angina pectoris with documented spasm A
I25.728	Atherosclerosis of autologous artery coronary artery bypass graft(s) with other forms of angina pectoris A
I25.730	Atherosclerosis of nonautologous biological coronary artery bypass graft(s) with unstable angina pectoris A
I25.731	Atherosclerosis of nonautologous biological coronary artery bypass graft(s) with angina pectoris with documented spasm A
I25.738	Atherosclerosis of nonautologous biological coronary artery bypass graft(s) with other forms of angina pectoris A
I25.750	Atherosclerosis of native coronary artery of transplanted heart with unstable angina

I25.760	Atherosclerosis of bypass graft of coronary artery of transplanted heart with unstable angina A
I25.761	Atherosclerosis of bypass graft of coronary artery of transplanted heart with angina pectoris with documented spasm A
I25.768	Atherosclerosis of bypass graft of coronary artery of transplanted heart with other forms of angina pectoris A
I25.790	Atherosclerosis of other coronary artery bypass graft(s) with unstable angina pectoris A
I25.791	Atherosclerosis of other coronary artery bypass graft(s) with angina pectoris with documented spasm A
I25.798	Atherosclerosis of other coronary artery bypass graft(s) with other forms of angina pectoris A
I25.810	Atherosclerosis of coronary artery bypass graft(s) without angina pectoris A
I25.812	Atherosclerosis of bypass graft of coronary artery of transplanted heart without angina pectoris A
I25.82	Chronic total occlusion of coronary artery
I25.84	Coronary atherosclerosis due to calcified coronary lesion
I25.89	Other forms of chronic ischemic heart disease
T82.818A	Embolism due to vascular prosthetic devices, implants and grafts, initial encounter
T82.828A	Fibrosis due to vascular prosthetic devices, implants and grafts, initial encounter
T82.838A	Hemorrhage due to vascular prosthetic devices, implants and grafts, initial encounter
T82.848A	Pain due to vascular prosthetic devices, implants and grafts, initial encounter
T82.858A	Stenosis of other vascular prosthetic devices, implants and grafts, initial encounter
T82.868A	Thrombosis due to vascular prosthetic devices, implants and grafts, initial encounter
T82.898A	Other specified complication of vascular prosthetic devices, implants and grafts, initial encounter

AMA: 92941 2024,Jun; 2020,Jul

Relative Value Units/Medicare Edits

Non-Facility RVU	Work	PE	MP	Total
92941	12.31	4.21	2.78	19.3
Facility RVU	**Work**	**PE**	**MP**	**Total**
92941	12.31	4.21	2.78	19.3

	FUD	Status	MUE	Modifiers				IOM Reference
92941	0	A	1(3)	51	N/A	N/A	80*	None

* with documentation

Terms To Know

atherectomy. Surgical removal of arterial plaque from inside an artery. The procedure may be performed percutaneously, using a special catheter with a high-speed burr at the tip to bore through the sclerotic deposits, or transluminally by open incision.

revascularization. Restoration of blood flow and oxygen supply to a body part. This may apply to an extremity, the heart, or penis.

[92943, 92944]

92943 Percutaneous transluminal revascularization of chronic total occlusion, coronary artery, coronary artery branch, or coronary artery bypass graft, any combination of intracoronary stent, atherectomy and angioplasty; single vessel

\+ **92944** Percutaneous transluminal revascularization of chronic total occlusion, coronary artery, coronary artery branch, or coronary artery bypass graft, any combination of intracoronary stent, atherectomy and angioplasty; each additional coronary artery, coronary artery branch, or bypass graft (List separately in addition to code for primary procedure)

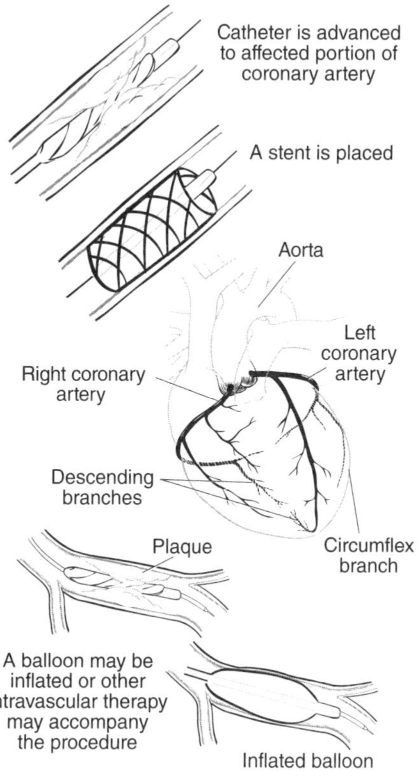

Explanation

The use of one or any combination of angioplasty, atherectomy, or stent placement is performed to restore a chronic totally blocked coronary artery bypass graft (CABG) or native coronary artery. The physician makes a small incision in the arm or leg to access the artery for placement of two catheters. A central venous catheter is inserted through the femoral or brachial artery and a second catheter is threaded up to the affected vessel or graft. The obstruction may be treated by using a rotary cutter (atherectomy) to flatten or remove the obstruction, inflating a balloon at the tip of the second catheter (PTCA), or introducing a stent that is expanded to fit the lumen of the artery. The catheters are removed. Pressure is placed over the incision for 20 to 30 minutes to stop the bleeding. Report 92943 for the treatment of the first native artery or CABG. Report 92944 for each additional graft or vessel treated.

Coding Tips

When medically necessary, report moderate (conscious) sedation provided by the performing physician with 99151-99153. When provided by another physician, report 99155-99157. Report 92944 in addition to 92924, 92928, 92933, 92937, 92941, and 92943. Do not report 92943 with 0913T. For percutaneous transcatheter therapeutic drug delivery by intracoronary drug-delivery balloon, see 0913T-0914T. Diagnostic coronary angiography performed at the time of the procedure may be reported in certain instances, such as when no prior catheter-based angiography study has been performed or a significant change in the patient's condition has occurred since the time of a prior study. Diagnostic coronary angiography services reported at the same surgical session as a percutaneous revascularization service may be reported separately. Only one base code from the percutaneous coronary intervention (PCI) codes should be reported for revascularization of a major coronary artery and its branches or revascularization of a bypass graft. The PCI base codes are 92920, 92924, 92928, 92933, 92937, 92941, and 92943, and the most intensive service for the target vessel should be selected. Services performed on additional branches should be reported using the add-on codes throughout the section. See CPT section guidelines for details on hierarchy and examples. For transcatheter placement of a radiation delivery device for coronary intravascular brachytherapy, see 92974. For intravascular application of a radioelement, see 77770–77772. Medicare and some other payers may require HCPCS Level II codes C9607–C9608 be reported for these services if drug eluting stents are used.

ICD-10-CM Diagnostic Codes

I25.110 Atherosclerotic heart disease of native coronary artery with unstable angina pectoris A

I25.111 Atherosclerotic heart disease of native coronary artery with angina pectoris with documented spasm A

I25.112 Atherosclerotic heart disease of native coronary artery with refractory angina pectoris A

I25.118 Atherosclerotic heart disease of native coronary artery with other forms of angina pectoris A

I25.5 Ischemic cardiomyopathy

I25.6 Silent myocardial ischemia

I25.710 Atherosclerosis of autologous vein coronary artery bypass graft(s) with unstable angina pectoris A

I25.711 Atherosclerosis of autologous vein coronary artery bypass graft(s) with angina pectoris with documented spasm A

I25.718 Atherosclerosis of autologous vein coronary artery bypass graft(s) with other forms of angina pectoris A

I25.720 Atherosclerosis of autologous artery coronary artery bypass graft(s) with unstable angina pectoris A

I25.721 Atherosclerosis of autologous artery coronary artery bypass graft(s) with angina pectoris with documented spasm A

I25.728 Atherosclerosis of autologous artery coronary artery bypass graft(s) with other forms of angina pectoris A

I25.730 Atherosclerosis of nonautologous biological coronary artery bypass graft(s) with unstable angina pectoris A

I25.731 Atherosclerosis of nonautologous biological coronary artery bypass graft(s) with angina pectoris with documented spasm A

I25.738 Atherosclerosis of nonautologous biological coronary artery bypass graft(s) with other forms of angina pectoris A

I25.760 Atherosclerosis of bypass graft of coronary artery of transplanted heart with unstable angina A

I25.761 Atherosclerosis of bypass graft of coronary artery of transplanted heart with angina pectoris with documented spasm A

I25.768 Atherosclerosis of bypass graft of coronary artery of transplanted heart with other forms of angina pectoris A

I25.790 Atherosclerosis of other coronary artery bypass graft(s) with unstable angina pectoris A

I25.791 Atherosclerosis of other coronary artery bypass graft(s) with angina pectoris with documented spasm A

I25.798 Atherosclerosis of other coronary artery bypass graft(s) with other forms of angina pectoris A

I25.810 Atherosclerosis of coronary artery bypass graft(s) without angina pectoris A

I25.812 Atherosclerosis of bypass graft of coronary artery of transplanted heart without angina pectoris A

I25.82 Chronic total occlusion of coronary artery

I25.84 Coronary atherosclerosis due to calcified coronary lesion

I25.89 Other forms of chronic ischemic heart disease

AMA: 92943 2024,Jun

Relative Value Units/Medicare Edits

Non-Facility RVU	Work	PE	MP	Total
92943	12.31	4.2	2.79	19.3
92944	0.0	0.0	0.0	0.0
Facility RVU	**Work**	**PE**	**MP**	**Total**
92943	12.31	4.2	2.79	19.3
92944	0.0	0.0	0.0	0.0

	FUD	Status	MUE	Modifiers				IOM Reference
92943	0	A	2(3)	51	N/A	N/A	80*	None
92944	N/A	B	2(3)	N/A	N/A	N/A	N/A	

* with documentation

Terms To Know

atherectomy. Surgical removal of arterial plaque from inside an artery. The procedure may be performed percutaneously, using a special catheter with a high-speed burr at the tip to bore through the sclerotic deposits, or transluminally by open incision.

bypass graft. Surgically created alternative blood vessel used to reroute blood flow around an area of obstruction or disease.

revascularization. Restoration of blood flow and oxygen supply to a body part. This may apply to an extremity, the heart, or penis.

[92972]

+ **92972** Percutaneous transluminal coronary lithotripsy (List separately in addition to code for primary procedure)

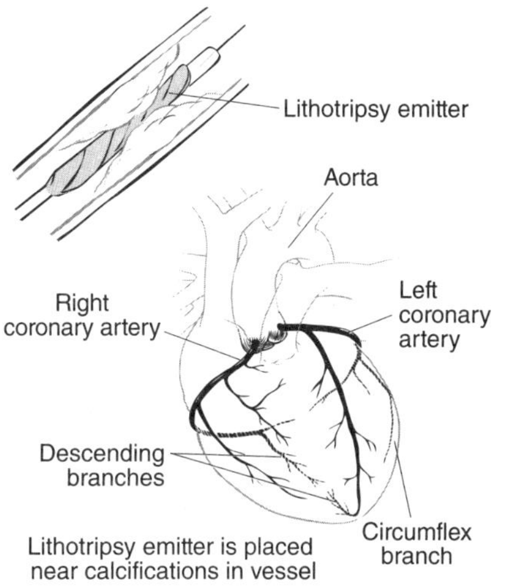

Explanation

The physician treats coronary artery calcification, which is known to hinder other percutaneous coronary interventions, with percutaneous transluminal coronary lithotripsy. This procedure is performed in conjunction with other percutaneous transluminal or transcatheter coronary procedures (angioplasty, atherectomy, stent placement, revascularization of bypass graft or occlusion, or thrombolysis). Following femoral or radial access and using a proprietary intravascular lithotripsy (IVL) device, the physician advances the coronary catheter to the target lesion. An integrated balloon is inflated with fluid at a low pressure to contact the arterial wall. IVL is then activated, creating a small bubble within the catheter balloon that rapidly expands and collapses, resulting in shockwaves that travel through the innermost layer of the vessel wall, where it cracks the calcium by creating microfractures.

Coding Tips

Report 92972 in addition to 92920, 92924, 92928, 92933, 92937, 92941, 92943, or 92975.

ICD-10-CM Diagnostic Codes

This/these CPT code(s) are add-on code(s). See the primary procedure code that this code is performed with for your ICD-10-CM code selections.

AMA: 92972 2024,Jun

Relative Value Units/Medicare Edits

Non-Facility RVU	Work	PE	MP	Total
92972	2.97	1.06	0.25	4.28
Facility RVU	**Work**	**PE**	**MP**	**Total**
92972	2.97	1.06	0.25	4.28

	FUD	Status	MUE	Modifiers				IOM Reference
92972	N/A	A	3(3)	N/A	N/A	N/A	N/A	None

* with documentation

[92973]

+ **92973** Percutaneous transluminal coronary thrombectomy mechanical (List separately in addition to code for primary procedure)

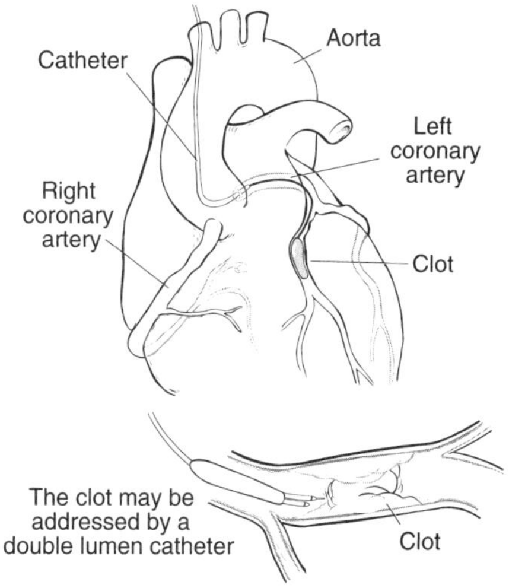

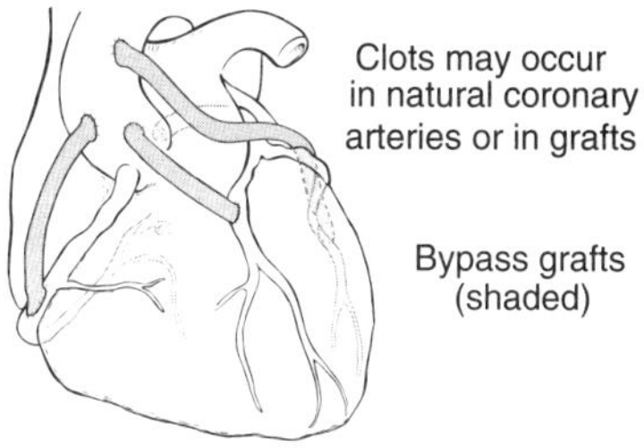

Explanation

The physician percutaneously removes a blood clot from a native or grafted coronary artery. A double lumen catheter is passed to the area of the clot. A high-pressure saline stream (via a pump) is introduced through a lumen that has multiple jet orifices located at the distal tip. The low-pressure zone created by the jets causes the clot to break up into small pieces and be pushed through the catheter with a force that drives debris from the thrombus through the other lumen (exhaust) and out of the body. The procedure is useful to clear fatty and degenerated arteries and to modify plaques in preparation for more definitive treatment with adjunctive balloon angioplasty or stenting.

Coding Tips

When medically necessary, report moderate (conscious) sedation provided by the performing physician with 99151-99153. When provided by another physician, report 99155-99157. Report 92973 in addition to 92920, 92924, 92928, 92933, 92937, 92941, 92943, 92975, 93454–93461, 93563, or 93564. Do not report 92973 with 0913T for intervention in the same major coronary artery or the same bypass graft. For intravascular radioelement application, see 77770–77772.

ICD-10-CM Diagnostic Codes

This/these CPT code(s) are add-on code(s). See the primary procedure code that this code is performed with for your ICD-10-CM code selections. Diagnostic code(s) would be the same as the actual procedure performed.

AMA: 92973 2024,Jun; 2020,Jul

Relative Value Units/Medicare Edits

Non-Facility RVU	Work	PE	MP	Total
92973	3.28	1.13	0.74	5.15
Facility RVU	**Work**	**PE**	**MP**	**Total**
92973	3.28	1.13	0.74	5.15

	FUD	Status	MUE	Modifiers				IOM Reference
92973	N/A	A	2(3)	N/A	N/A	N/A	80*	None

* with documentation

Terms To Know

catheterization. Use or insertion of a tubular device into a duct, blood vessel, hollow organ, or body cavity for injecting or withdrawing fluids for diagnostic or therapeutic purposes.

lumen. Space inside an intestine, artery, vein, duct, or tube.

moderate sedation. Medically controlled state of depressed consciousness, with or without analgesia, while maintaining the patient's airway, protective reflexes, and ability to respond to stimulation or verbal commands.

thrombectomy. Removal of a clot (thrombus) from a blood vessel utilizing various methods.

[92974]

\+ **92974** Transcatheter placement of radiation delivery device for subsequent coronary intravascular brachytherapy (List separately in addition to code for primary procedure)

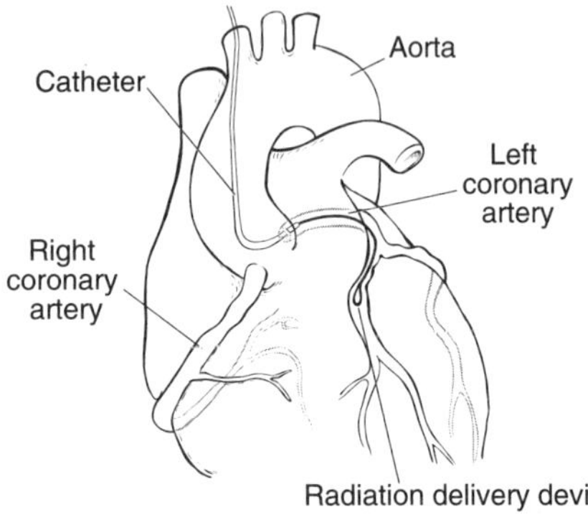

A radiation delivery device is introduced transcatheterally into a coronary artery

Explanation

Using an X-ray machine in a cardiac catheterization laboratory, the physician places the delivery catheter in the coronary artery at the site of the in-stent restenosis (reblockage in the artery). The transfer delivery device is connected to the delivery catheter; the transfer delivery device is used to deliver the radioactive seeds to the location. There are various methods for transcatheter placement, but commonly the methods involve the use of a guiding catheter. The radioactive seeds are positioned at the location for an appropriate length of time to administer radiation to the artery. At the completion of the radiation treatment, the radioactive seeds are returned to the transfer device.

Coding Tips

When medically necessary, report moderate (conscious) sedation provided by the performing physician with 99151-99153. When provided by another physician, report 99155-99157. Report 92974 in addition to 92920, 92924, 92928, 92933, 92937, 92941, 92943, and 93454–93461. For intravascular radioelement application, see 77770–77772.

ICD-10-CM Diagnostic Codes

This/these CPT code(s) are add-on code(s). See the primary procedure code that this code is performed with for your ICD-10-CM code selections. Diagnostic code(s) would be the same as the actual procedure performed.

Relative Value Units/Medicare Edits

Non-Facility RVU	Work	PE	MP	Total
92974	3.0	1.04	0.68	4.72
Facility RVU	**Work**	**PE**	**MP**	**Total**
92974	3.0	1.04	0.68	4.72

	FUD	Status	MUE	Modifiers				IOM Reference
92974	N/A	A	1(3)	N/A	N/A	N/A	80*	None

* with documentation

Medicine

[92975, 92977]

92975 Thrombolysis, coronary; by intracoronary infusion, including selective coronary angiography

92977 Thrombolysis, coronary; by intravenous infusion

Explanation

In 92975, the physician places a hollow catheter in the aorta from the arm or leg via a small incision. Using fluoroscopic guidance, the physician advances the catheter tip to the coronary artery to be treated and confirms the presence of thrombus (blood clot) in the artery by injecting contrast material through the catheter into the artery. In 92977, a catheter equipped with an infusion tip is threaded into the vessel. The physician infuses a thrombolytic agent (e.g., urokinase) into the affected artery in order to dissolve the thrombus. The physician may perform contrast injections to assess the size and extent of the thrombus after infusion of the thrombolytic agent. The catheter is removed from the patient's body. Pressure is placed over the incision to stem bleeding. The patient is observed for a period afterward.

Coding Tips

When medically necessary, report moderate (conscious) sedation provided by the performing physician with 99151-99153. When provided by another physician, report 99155-99157. For thrombolysis of vessels other than coronary, see 37211–37214. For cerebral thrombolysis, see 37195.

ICD-10-CM Diagnostic Codes

I21.01 ST elevation (STEMI) myocardial infarction involving left main coronary artery
I21.02 ST elevation (STEMI) myocardial infarction involving left anterior descending coronary artery
I21.09 ST elevation (STEMI) myocardial infarction involving other coronary artery of anterior wall
I21.11 ST elevation (STEMI) myocardial infarction involving right coronary artery
I21.19 ST elevation (STEMI) myocardial infarction involving other coronary artery of inferior wall
I21.21 ST elevation (STEMI) myocardial infarction involving left circumflex coronary artery
I21.29 ST elevation (STEMI) myocardial infarction involving other sites
I21.4 Non-ST elevation (NSTEMI) myocardial infarction
I21.A1 Myocardial infarction type 2
I21.B Myocardial infarction with coronary microvascular dysfunction
I22.0 Subsequent ST elevation (STEMI) myocardial infarction of anterior wall
I22.1 Subsequent ST elevation (STEMI) myocardial infarction of inferior wall
I22.2 Subsequent non-ST elevation (NSTEMI) myocardial infarction
I22.8 Subsequent ST elevation (STEMI) myocardial infarction of other sites
I24.0 Acute coronary thrombosis not resulting in myocardial infarction
I25.110 Atherosclerotic heart disease of native coronary artery with unstable angina pectoris A
I25.111 Atherosclerotic heart disease of native coronary artery with angina pectoris with documented spasm A
I25.112 Atherosclerotic heart disease of native coronary artery with refractory angina pectoris A
I25.118 Atherosclerotic heart disease of native coronary artery with other forms of angina pectoris A
I25.710 Atherosclerosis of autologous vein coronary artery bypass graft(s) with unstable angina pectoris A
I25.711 Atherosclerosis of autologous vein coronary artery bypass graft(s) with angina pectoris with documented spasm A
I25.718 Atherosclerosis of autologous vein coronary artery bypass graft(s) with other forms of angina pectoris A
I25.720 Atherosclerosis of autologous artery coronary artery bypass graft(s) with unstable angina pectoris A
I25.721 Atherosclerosis of autologous artery coronary artery bypass graft(s) with angina pectoris with documented spasm A
I25.728 Atherosclerosis of autologous artery coronary artery bypass graft(s) with other forms of angina pectoris A
I25.730 Atherosclerosis of nonautologous biological coronary artery bypass graft(s) with unstable angina pectoris A
I25.731 Atherosclerosis of nonautologous biological coronary artery bypass graft(s) with angina pectoris with documented spasm A
I25.738 Atherosclerosis of nonautologous biological coronary artery bypass graft(s) with other forms of angina pectoris A
I25.760 Atherosclerosis of bypass graft of coronary artery of transplanted heart with unstable angina A
I25.761 Atherosclerosis of bypass graft of coronary artery of transplanted heart with angina pectoris with documented spasm A
I25.768 Atherosclerosis of bypass graft of coronary artery of transplanted heart with other forms of angina pectoris A
I25.790 Atherosclerosis of other coronary artery bypass graft(s) with unstable angina pectoris A
I25.791 Atherosclerosis of other coronary artery bypass graft(s) with angina pectoris with documented spasm A
I25.798 Atherosclerosis of other coronary artery bypass graft(s) with other forms of angina pectoris A
I25.82 Chronic total occlusion of coronary artery

AMA: **92975** 2024,Jun

Relative Value Units/Medicare Edits

Non-Facility RVU	Work	PE	MP	Total
92975	6.99	2.38	1.61	10.98
92977	0.0	1.52	0.14	1.66
Facility RVU	**Work**	**PE**	**MP**	**Total**
92975	6.99	2.38	1.61	10.98
92977	0.0	1.52	0.14	1.66

	FUD	Status	MUE	Modifiers				IOM Reference
92975	0	A	1(3)	51	N/A	N/A	80*	None
92977	N/A	A	1(3)	N/A	N/A	N/A	80*	

* with documentation

Terms To Know

selective placement. Introduction and manipulation of a catheter or guidewire within a vascular tree or family into a specified target area that is identified and monitored by radiographic imaging in order to carry out a diagnostic or therapeutic procedure.

thrombolytic agent. Drugs or other substances used to dissolve blood clots in blood vessels or in tubes that have been placed into the body.

Medicine

[92978, 92979]

+ **92978** Endoluminal imaging of coronary vessel or graft using intravascular ultrasound (IVUS) or optical coherence tomography (OCT) during diagnostic evaluation and/or therapeutic intervention including imaging supervision, interpretation and report; initial vessel (List separately in addition to code for primary procedure)
+ **92979** Endoluminal imaging of coronary vessel or graft using intravascular ultrasound (IVUS) or optical coherence tomography (OCT) during diagnostic evaluation and/or therapeutic intervention including imaging supervision, interpretation and report; each additional vessel (List separately in addition to code for primary procedure)

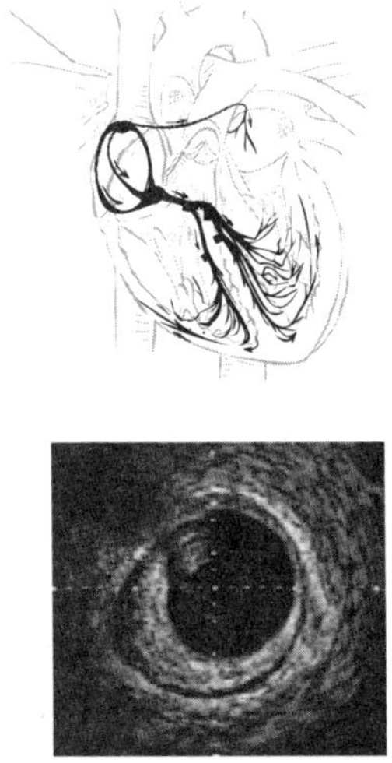

An intravascular ultrasound is used during a diagnostic study of a coronary vessel or coronary artery graft

Explanation

Intravascular ultrasound (IVUS) or optical coherence tomography (OCT) may be used for endoluminal imaging during diagnostic evaluation of a coronary vessel or graft. It may also be used before and after a therapeutic intervention on a coronary vessel or graft to assess patency and integrity of the vessel or graft. A needle is inserted through the skin and into a blood vessel. A guidewire is threaded through the needle into a coronary blood vessel or graft. The needle is removed. An intravascular ultrasound catheter is placed over the guidewire. The ultrasound probe is used to obtain images from inside the vessel to assess area and extent of disease prior to interventional therapy, as well as adequacy of therapy after interventional therapy. The ultrasound probe provides a two-dimensional, cross-sectional view of the vessel or graft as the probe is advanced and withdrawn along the area of interest. When the ultrasound examination is complete, the catheter is removed. OCT utilizes light instead of sound to provide cross-sectional images in high resolution within the lumen. Report 92978 for the initial vessel or graft. In 92979, the physician advances the ultrasound catheter into additional vessels or grafts to assess patency and structure. The catheter and guidewire are removed and pressure is applied over the puncture site to stop bleeding.

Coding Tips

When medically necessary, report moderate (conscious) sedation provided by the performing physician with 99151-99153. When provided by another physician, report 99155-99157. Report 92978 in addition to 92920, 92924, 92928, 92933, 92937, 92941, 92943, 92975, 93454–93461, 93563, and 93564. Use 92979 in addition to 92978. Transducer manipulation and repositioning within the specific vessel being examined both before and after therapeutic intervention is considered integral to the intravascular ultrasound service and should not be reported separately. Report 92978 once per encounter and 92979 once per additional vessel. Do not report 92978 with 0913T or 0914T for intervention in the same major coronary artery or the same bypass graft.

ICD-10-CM Diagnostic Codes

This/these CPT code(s) are add-on code(s). See the primary procedure code that this code is performed with for your ICD-10-CM code selections. Diagnostic code(s) would be the same as the actual procedure performed.

Relative Value Units/Medicare Edits

Non-Facility RVU	Work	PE	MP	Total
92978	0.0	0.0	0.0	0.0
92979	0.0	0.0	0.0	0.0
Facility RVU	**Work**	**PE**	**MP**	**Total**
92978	0.0	0.0	0.0	0.0
92979	0.0	0.0	0.0	0.0

	FUD	Status	MUE	Modifiers				IOM Reference
92978	N/A	C	1(3)	N/A	N/A	N/A	80*	None
92979	N/A	C	2(3)	N/A	N/A	N/A	80*	

* with documentation

Terms To Know

diagnostic procedures. Procedure performed on a patient to obtain information to assess the medical condition of the patient or to identify a disease and to determine the nature and severity of an illness or injury.

intravascular. Within a blood vessel.

therapeutic procedure. Manner of effecting change through the application of clinical skills and/or services that attempt to improve function.

ultrasound. Imaging using ultra-high sound frequency bounced off body structures.

[93150, 93151, 93152, 93153]

93150 Therapy activation of implanted phrenic nerve stimulator system, including all interrogation and programming

93151 Interrogation and programming (minimum one parameter) of implanted phrenic nerve stimulator system

93152 Interrogation and programming of implanted phrenic nerve stimulator system during polysomnography

93153 Interrogation without programming of implanted phrenic nerve stimulator system

Explanation

Following a specified period (typically one month to permit lead maturation and healing) after the patient undergoes insertion of a phrenic nerve stimulator system for the treatment of moderate to severe central sleep apnea, therapy initiation is undertaken. The system consists of a pulse generator much like a pacemaker, a stimulation electrode, and, when appropriate, a sensing electrode. Respiration sensing is accomplished by the electrodes determining the patient's position at rest/activity to allow for programming of applicable delivery times. This unit assists stable breathing by preventing episodes of apnea followed by rapid breathing. During activation, the device is programmed to automatically begin when the patient is at rest during normal hours of sleep, in a sleeping position, and after lead impedance is measured. Individualized settings, such as therapy start/stop times and stimulation parameters, are determined by testing performed in the office, interviews with the patient about sleep habits, and monitoring the patient's response to overnight stimulation if necessary. Report 93150 for therapy activation of the phrenic nerve stimulator system; this includes all interrogation and programming. Report 93151 for interrogation and programming of at least one parameter of the system; 93152 when interrogation and programming is performed during polysomnography; and 93153 when interrogation of the system is performed without programming.

Coding Tips

Do not report 93150 with 33276–33281 or 93151–93153. Do not report 93151 with 93150, 93152, or 93153. For interrogation without programming of an implanted phrenic nerve stimulator system, see 93153. Do not report 93152 with 33276, 93150, 93151, or 93153. For polysomnography, see 95808, 95810, 95811, 95782, or 95783. Do not report 93153 with 33276 or 93150–93152.

ICD-10-CM Diagnostic Codes

Z45.42	Encounter for adjustment and management of neurostimulator
Z96.82	Presence of neurostimulator

AMA: 93150 2024,Apr **93151** 2024,Apr **93152** 2024,Apr **93153** 2024,Apr

Relative Value Units/Medicare Edits

Non-Facility RVU	Work	PE	MP	Total
93150	0.85	2.08	0.06	2.99
93151	0.8	1.75	0.06	2.61
93152	1.82	2.77	0.13	4.72
93153	0.43	1.08	0.04	1.55
Facility RVU	**Work**	**PE**	**MP**	**Total**
93150	0.85	0.35	0.06	1.26
93151	0.8	0.33	0.06	1.19
93152	1.82	0.83	0.13	2.78
93153	0.43	0.17	0.04	0.64

	FUD	Status	MUE	Modifiers				IOM Reference
93150	N/A	A	1(2)	N/A	N/A	N/A	80*	None
93151	N/A	A	1(2)	N/A	N/A	N/A	80*	
93152	N/A	A	1(2)	N/A	N/A	N/A	80*	
93153	N/A	A	1(2)	N/A	N/A	N/A	80*	

* with documentation

Terms To Know

phrenic nerves. Two nerves that arise mainly from the fourth cervical nerve, providing motor nerve function to a side of the diaphragm, and serve in the breathing function. The right nerve plays a role in liver function.

polysomnography. Test involving monitoring of respiratory, cardiac, muscle, brain, and ocular function during sleep.

93355

93355 Echocardiography, transesophageal (TEE) for guidance of a transcatheter intracardiac or great vessel(s) structural intervention(s) (eg,TAVR, transcatheter pulmonary valve replacement, mitral valve repair, paravalvular regurgitation repair, left atrial appendage occlusion/closure, ventricular septal defect closure) (peri-and intra-procedural), real-time image acquisition and documentation, guidance with quantitative measurements, probe manipulation, interpretation, and report, including diagnostic transesophageal echocardiography and, when performed, administration of ultrasound contrast, Doppler, color flow, and 3D

Anatomy

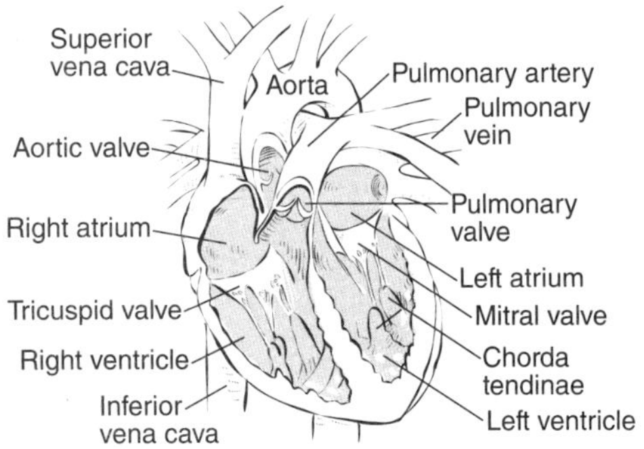

Explanation

Transesophageal echocardiography (TEE) is an invasive technique whereby the transducer is placed at the tip of an endoscope and introduced into the patient's esophagus as guidance for procedures performed on intracardiac or other great vessels and structures. The transducer sends sound waves to the heart and collects the echoes that bounce back. These echoes become high-quality moving pictures that show up on a computer screen. TEE provides high-quality, real-time images of the beating heart and mediastinal structures. This code reports the guidance during the procedure(s), as well as measurements of the surrounding structures. It includes probe navigation, image acquisition, and physician's interpretation and report. Diagnostic TEE is included and contrast administration, Doppler, color flow, and 3D images, when performed, are also included.

Coding Tips

Report this code when performed during transcatheter intracardiac therapy. It is reported only one time per interventional procedure and only by a provider not performing the intervention. For placement of a transesophageal probe by a different provider, see 93313. Do not report 93355 with 76376, 76377, 93312–93318, 93320, 93321, or 93325.

ICD-10-CM Diagnostic Codes

I05.0	Rheumatic mitral stenosis
I05.1	Rheumatic mitral insufficiency
I05.2	Rheumatic mitral stenosis with insufficiency
I05.8	Other rheumatic mitral valve diseases
I06.0	Rheumatic aortic stenosis
I06.1	Rheumatic aortic insufficiency
I06.2	Rheumatic aortic stenosis with insufficiency
I08.0	Rheumatic disorders of both mitral and aortic valves
I08.8	Other rheumatic multiple valve diseases
I34.0	Nonrheumatic mitral (valve) insufficiency
I34.1	Nonrheumatic mitral (valve) prolapse
I34.2	Nonrheumatic mitral (valve) stenosis
I34.81	Nonrheumatic mitral (valve) annulus calcification
I34.89	Other nonrheumatic mitral valve disorders
I35.0	Nonrheumatic aortic (valve) stenosis
I35.1	Nonrheumatic aortic (valve) insufficiency
I35.2	Nonrheumatic aortic (valve) stenosis with insufficiency
I35.8	Other nonrheumatic aortic valve disorders
I36.0	Nonrheumatic tricuspid (valve) stenosis
I36.1	Nonrheumatic tricuspid (valve) insufficiency
I36.2	Nonrheumatic tricuspid (valve) stenosis with insufficiency
I36.8	Other nonrheumatic tricuspid valve disorders
I37.0	Nonrheumatic pulmonary valve stenosis
I37.1	Nonrheumatic pulmonary valve insufficiency
I37.2	Nonrheumatic pulmonary valve stenosis with insufficiency
I37.8	Other nonrheumatic pulmonary valve disorders
Q21.0	Ventricular septal defect
Q21.3	Tetralogy of Fallot
Q21.4	Aortopulmonary septal defect
Q21.8	Other congenital malformations of cardiac septa
Q22.0	Pulmonary valve atresia
Q22.1	Congenital pulmonary valve stenosis
Q22.3	Other congenital malformations of pulmonary valve
Q22.4	Congenital tricuspid stenosis
Q22.6	Hypoplastic right heart syndrome
Q22.8	Other congenital malformations of tricuspid valve
Q23.0	Congenital stenosis of aortic valve
Q23.1	Congenital insufficiency of aortic valve
Q23.2	Congenital mitral stenosis
Q23.3	Congenital mitral insufficiency
Q23.81	Bicuspid aortic valve
Q23.82	Congenital mitral valve cleft leaflet
Q23.88	Other congenital malformations of aortic and mitral valves
Q24.8	Other specified congenital malformations of heart
T82.01XA	Breakdown (mechanical) of heart valve prosthesis, initial encounter
T82.02XA	Displacement of heart valve prosthesis, initial encounter
T82.03XA	Leakage of heart valve prosthesis, initial encounter
T82.09XA	Other mechanical complication of heart valve prosthesis, initial encounter
T82.6XXA	Infection and inflammatory reaction due to cardiac valve prosthesis, initial encounter

AMA: **93355** 2022,Jul

Relative Value Units/Medicare Edits

Non-Facility RVU	Work	PE	MP	Total
93355	4.66	1.59	0.33	6.58
Facility RVU	**Work**	**PE**	**MP**	**Total**
93355	4.66	1.59	0.33	6.58

	FUD	Status	MUE	Modifiers				IOM Reference
93355	N/A	A	1(3)	N/A	N/A	N/A	80*	None

* with documentation

93451

93451 Right heart catheterization including measurement(s) of oxygen saturation and cardiac output, when performed

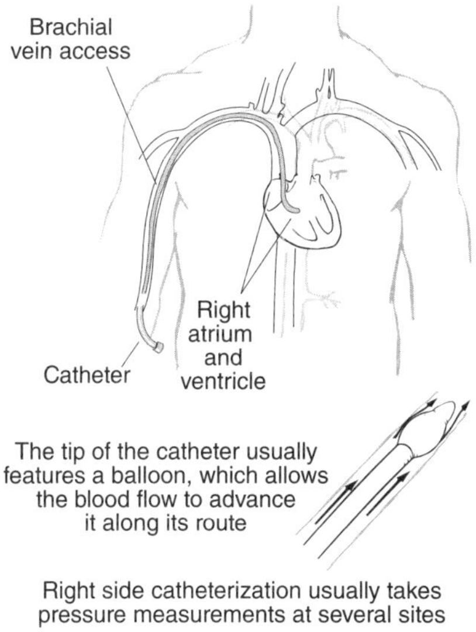

Explanation

The physician threads a catheter to the heart, most frequently through an introducing sheath placed percutaneously into the femoral vein. However, the physician may elect to use the subclavian, internal jugular, or antecubital vein instead. The catheter is threaded into the right atrium, through the tricuspid valve into the right ventricle, and across the pulmonary valve into the pulmonary arteries. ECG monitoring for the entirety of the procedure is included, as are intracardiac or intravascular pressure recordings, cardiac output and oxygen saturation measurements, and final evaluation and procedure report. This code applies to catheterizing the heart's right side only.

Coding Tips

When medically necessary, report moderate (conscious) sedation provided by the performing physician with 99151-99153. When provided by another physician, report 99155-99157. Right heart catheterization includes placement of the catheter into the right-side heart chambers or structures (right atrium, right ventricle, pulmonary artery, and wedge), specimen collection for blood gas measurements, and cardiac output measurements. For right heart catheterization performed in addition to other cardiac catheterizations, see 93453, 93456, 93457, 93460, or 93461. For placement of a flow directed catheter (Swan-Ganz) for hemodynamic monitoring not performed in addition to other cardiac catheterization procedures, see 93503. Report right ventricular or right atrial angiogram (93566) in addition to right heart catheterization when performed. This procedure includes introduction, positioning, and repositioning (when utilized) of the catheter within the vessel; recording of intracardiac and/or intravascular pressure; and final report evaluation. Additionally, all roadmapping angiography for catheter placement, as well as injections and imaging, are included. Report separately contrast injections and imaging that is separately indicated within a specific CPT code. Do not separately report contrast injections to view the access site when placing a closure device or the placement of the closure device at the vessel access site. Do not report 93451 with 33289, 93453, 93456, 93457, 93460, 93461, 0613T, or 0632T. Code 93451 may be reported in addition to 33274 and 33275 only if the catheterization is performed for reasons distinct from the leadless pacemaker procedure. Do not report 93451 with 33418, 0345T, 0483T, 0484T, 0544T, 0545T, or 0643T for diagnostic right catheterization intrinsic to the valve repair or annulus reconstruction. For right heart catheterization to evaluate congenital heart defects, see 93593, 93594, and 93596-93598.

ICD-10-CM Diagnostic Codes

I05.0	Rheumatic mitral stenosis
I05.1	Rheumatic mitral insufficiency
I05.2	Rheumatic mitral stenosis with insufficiency
I05.8	Other rheumatic mitral valve diseases
I06.0	Rheumatic aortic stenosis
I06.1	Rheumatic aortic insufficiency
I06.2	Rheumatic aortic stenosis with insufficiency
I06.8	Other rheumatic aortic valve diseases
I07.0	Rheumatic tricuspid stenosis
I07.1	Rheumatic tricuspid insufficiency
I07.2	Rheumatic tricuspid stenosis and insufficiency
I07.8	Other rheumatic tricuspid valve diseases
I08.0	Rheumatic disorders of both mitral and aortic valves
I08.1	Rheumatic disorders of both mitral and tricuspid valves
I08.2	Rheumatic disorders of both aortic and tricuspid valves
I08.3	Combined rheumatic disorders of mitral, aortic and tricuspid valves
I08.8	Other rheumatic multiple valve diseases
I09.81	Rheumatic heart failure
I09.89	Other specified rheumatic heart diseases
I21.01	ST elevation (STEMI) myocardial infarction involving left main coronary artery
I21.02	ST elevation (STEMI) myocardial infarction involving left anterior descending coronary artery
I21.09	ST elevation (STEMI) myocardial infarction involving other coronary artery of anterior wall
I21.11	ST elevation (STEMI) myocardial infarction involving right coronary artery
I21.19	ST elevation (STEMI) myocardial infarction involving other coronary artery of inferior wall
I21.21	ST elevation (STEMI) myocardial infarction involving left circumflex coronary artery
I21.29	ST elevation (STEMI) myocardial infarction involving other sites
I21.4	Non-ST elevation (NSTEMI) myocardial infarction
I21.A1	Myocardial infarction type 2
I21.B	Myocardial infarction with coronary microvascular dysfunction
I22.0	Subsequent ST elevation (STEMI) myocardial infarction of anterior wall
I22.1	Subsequent ST elevation (STEMI) myocardial infarction of inferior wall
I22.2	Subsequent non-ST elevation (NSTEMI) myocardial infarction
I22.8	Subsequent ST elevation (STEMI) myocardial infarction of other sites
I23.0	Hemopericardium as current complication following acute myocardial infarction A
I23.1	Atrial septal defect as current complication following acute myocardial infarction A
I23.2	Ventricular septal defect as current complication following acute myocardial infarction A
I25.3	Aneurysm of heart
I25.5	Ischemic cardiomyopathy

Medicine

I25.89	Other forms of chronic ischemic heart disease
I26.01	Septic pulmonary embolism with acute cor pulmonale
I26.02	Saddle embolus of pulmonary artery with acute cor pulmonale
I26.09	Other pulmonary embolism with acute cor pulmonale
I26.90	Septic pulmonary embolism without acute cor pulmonale
I26.92	Saddle embolus of pulmonary artery without acute cor pulmonale
I26.93	Single subsegmental thrombotic pulmonary embolism without acute cor pulmonale
I26.94	Multiple subsegmental thrombotic pulmonary emboli without acute cor pulmonale
I26.99	Other pulmonary embolism without acute cor pulmonale
I27.0	Primary pulmonary hypertension
I27.21	Secondary pulmonary arterial hypertension
I27.22	Pulmonary hypertension due to left heart disease
I27.23	Pulmonary hypertension due to lung diseases and hypoxia
I27.24	Chronic thromboembolic pulmonary hypertension
I27.29	Other secondary pulmonary hypertension
I27.81	Cor pulmonale (chronic)
I27.83	Eisenmenger's syndrome
I34.0	Nonrheumatic mitral (valve) insufficiency
I34.1	Nonrheumatic mitral (valve) prolapse
I34.2	Nonrheumatic mitral (valve) stenosis
I34.81	Nonrheumatic mitral (valve) annulus calcification
I34.89	Other nonrheumatic mitral valve disorders
I35.0	Nonrheumatic aortic (valve) stenosis
I35.1	Nonrheumatic aortic (valve) insufficiency
I35.2	Nonrheumatic aortic (valve) stenosis with insufficiency
I35.8	Other nonrheumatic aortic valve disorders
I36.0	Nonrheumatic tricuspid (valve) stenosis
I36.1	Nonrheumatic tricuspid (valve) insufficiency
I36.2	Nonrheumatic tricuspid (valve) stenosis with insufficiency
I36.8	Other nonrheumatic tricuspid valve disorders
I37.0	Nonrheumatic pulmonary valve stenosis
I37.1	Nonrheumatic pulmonary valve insufficiency
I37.2	Nonrheumatic pulmonary valve stenosis with insufficiency
I37.8	Other nonrheumatic pulmonary valve disorders
I38	Endocarditis, valve unspecified
I39	Endocarditis and heart valve disorders in diseases classified elsewhere
I40.0	Infective myocarditis
I40.1	Isolated myocarditis
I40.8	Other acute myocarditis
I42.0	Dilated cardiomyopathy
I42.1	Obstructive hypertrophic cardiomyopathy
I42.2	Other hypertrophic cardiomyopathy
I42.3	Endomyocardial (eosinophilic) disease
I42.4	Endocardial fibroelastosis
I42.5	Other restrictive cardiomyopathy
I42.6	Alcoholic cardiomyopathy
I42.7	Cardiomyopathy due to drug and external agent
I42.8	Other cardiomyopathies
I43	Cardiomyopathy in diseases classified elsewhere
I46.2	Cardiac arrest due to underlying cardiac condition
I46.8	Cardiac arrest due to other underlying condition
I50.1	Left ventricular failure, unspecified
I50.21	Acute systolic (congestive) heart failure
I50.22	Chronic systolic (congestive) heart failure
I50.23	Acute on chronic systolic (congestive) heart failure
I50.31	Acute diastolic (congestive) heart failure
I50.32	Chronic diastolic (congestive) heart failure
I50.33	Acute on chronic diastolic (congestive) heart failure
I50.41	Acute combined systolic (congestive) and diastolic (congestive) heart failure
I50.42	Chronic combined systolic (congestive) and diastolic (congestive) heart failure
I50.43	Acute on chronic combined systolic (congestive) and diastolic (congestive) heart failure
I50.811	Acute right heart failure
I50.812	Chronic right heart failure
I50.813	Acute on chronic right heart failure
I50.814	Right heart failure due to left heart failure
I50.82	Biventricular heart failure
I50.83	High output heart failure
I50.84	End stage heart failure
I50.9	Heart failure, unspecified
I51.0	Cardiac septal defect, acquired A
R57.0	Cardiogenic shock
R57.1	Hypovolemic shock
R57.8	Other shock

AMA: **93451** 2024,Mar; 2023,Jun; 2023,May; 2022,Jul; 2019,Jun; 2019,Apr; 2019,Mar; 2018,Dec

Relative Value Units/Medicare Edits

Non-Facility RVU	Work	PE	MP	Total
93451	2.47	22.57	0.46	25.5
Facility RVU	**Work**	**PE**	**MP**	**Total**
93451	2.47	22.57	0.46	25.5

	FUD	Status	MUE	Modifiers				IOM Reference
93451	0	A	1(3)	51	N/A	N/A	80*	None

* with documentation

Terms To Know

cardiac output. Measurement of the volume of blood ejected by the heart ventricle that is usually measured by a catheter with an opening in the right atrium and pulmonary artery.

catheterization. Use or insertion of a tubular device into a duct, blood vessel, hollow organ, or body cavity for injecting or withdrawing fluids for diagnostic or therapeutic purposes.

93452

93452 Left heart catheterization including intraprocedural injection(s) for left ventriculography, imaging supervision and interpretation, when performed

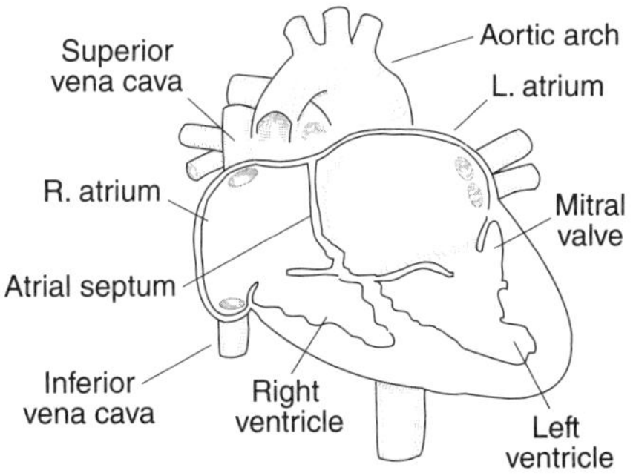

Left heart is catheterized

Explanation

The physician threads a catheter to the heart, most frequently through an introducing sheath placed percutaneously into the femoral, brachial, or axillary artery using retrograde technique. Using this technique, the catheter passes through the aortic valve into the left ventricle. Intracardiac and intravascular pressures are recorded. Left ventricular injections may be performed for left ventriculography; the physician injects dye through a previously placed catheter threaded through a central line into the left ventricle or atrium to evaluate function with fluoroscopy. Imaging supervision and interpretation, when performed, are included in this code, as is any required repositioning of catheters.

Coding Tips

When medically necessary, report moderate (conscious) sedation provided by the performing physician with 99151-99153. When provided by another physician, report 99155-99157. This procedure includes placement of the catheter into the left-side heart chambers or structures (left ventricle, left atrium) and left ventricular injection when utilized. Intraprocedural injections for left ventricular/atrial angiogram and imaging supervision and interpretation are also included. Do not report 93503 in addition to other diagnostic cardiac cath codes. When left heart catheterization is performed via transapical puncture into the left ventricle or transseptal puncture into the septum, report 93462 in addition to 93452, 93453, 93458–93461, 93653, and 93654. This procedure includes introduction, positioning, and repositioning (when utilized) of the catheter within the vessel; recording of intracardiac and/or intravascular pressure; and final report evaluation. All roadmapping angiography for catheter placement, as well as injections and imaging, are also included. Report separately contrast injections and imaging that is separately indicated within a specific CPT code. Do not separately report contrast injections to view the access site when placing a closure device or the placement of the closure device at the vessel access site. Do not report 93452 with 93453, 93458–93461, 93565, 0408T-0411T, or 0414T-0415T. Do not report 93452 with 33418, 0345T, 0483T, 0484T, 0544T, 0545T, or 0643T for diagnostic left catheterization intrinsic to the valve repair or annulus reconstruction. For left heart catheterization to evaluate congenital heart defects, see 93565 and 93595-93597.

ICD-10-CM Diagnostic Codes

C38.0	Malignant neoplasm of heart
D15.1	Benign neoplasm of heart
I05.0	Rheumatic mitral stenosis
I05.1	Rheumatic mitral insufficiency
I06.0	Rheumatic aortic stenosis
I06.1	Rheumatic aortic insufficiency
I07.0	Rheumatic tricuspid stenosis
I07.1	Rheumatic tricuspid insufficiency
I09.81	Rheumatic heart failure
I20.0	Unstable angina
I20.1	Angina pectoris with documented spasm
I20.81	Angina pectoris with coronary microvascular dysfunction
I21.01	ST elevation (STEMI) myocardial infarction involving left main coronary artery
I21.02	ST elevation (STEMI) myocardial infarction involving left anterior descending coronary artery
I21.11	ST elevation (STEMI) myocardial infarction involving right coronary artery
I21.21	ST elevation (STEMI) myocardial infarction involving left circumflex coronary artery
I21.4	Non-ST elevation (NSTEMI) myocardial infarction
I21.A1	Myocardial infarction type 2
I21.B	Myocardial infarction with coronary microvascular dysfunction
I22.0	Subsequent ST elevation (STEMI) myocardial infarction of anterior wall
I22.1	Subsequent ST elevation (STEMI) myocardial infarction of inferior wall
I22.2	Subsequent non-ST elevation (NSTEMI) myocardial infarction
I23.1	Atrial septal defect as current complication following acute myocardial infarction A
I23.2	Ventricular septal defect as current complication following acute myocardial infarction A
I23.3	Rupture of cardiac wall without hemopericardium as current complication following acute myocardial infarction A
I23.7	Postinfarction angina A
I24.0	Acute coronary thrombosis not resulting in myocardial infarction
I24.1	Dressler's syndrome
I25.10	Atherosclerotic heart disease of native coronary artery without angina pectoris A
I25.110	Atherosclerotic heart disease of native coronary artery with unstable angina pectoris A
I25.111	Atherosclerotic heart disease of native coronary artery with angina pectoris with documented spasm A
I25.112	Atherosclerotic heart disease of native coronary artery with refractory angina pectoris A
I25.2	Old myocardial infarction
I25.3	Aneurysm of heart
I25.41	Coronary artery aneurysm
I25.5	Ischemic cardiomyopathy
I25.6	Silent myocardial ischemia
I25.710	Atherosclerosis of autologous vein coronary artery bypass graft(s) with unstable angina pectoris A
I25.711	Atherosclerosis of autologous vein coronary artery bypass graft(s) with angina pectoris with documented spasm A
I25.712	Atherosclerosis of autologous vein coronary artery bypass graft(s) with refractory angina pectoris A
I25.720	Atherosclerosis of autologous artery coronary artery bypass graft(s) with unstable angina pectoris A

I25.721 Atherosclerosis of autologous artery coronary artery bypass graft(s) with angina pectoris with documented spasm A
I25.722 Atherosclerosis of autologous artery coronary artery bypass graft(s) with refractory angina pectoris A
I25.730 Atherosclerosis of nonautologous biological coronary artery bypass graft(s) with unstable angina pectoris A
I25.731 Atherosclerosis of nonautologous biological coronary artery bypass graft(s) with angina pectoris with documented spasm A
I25.732 Atherosclerosis of nonautologous biological coronary artery bypass graft(s) with refractory angina pectoris A
I25.750 Atherosclerosis of native coronary artery of transplanted heart with unstable angina
I25.751 Atherosclerosis of native coronary artery of transplanted heart with angina pectoris with documented spasm
I25.752 Atherosclerosis of native coronary artery of transplanted heart with refractory angina pectoris A
I25.760 Atherosclerosis of bypass graft of coronary artery of transplanted heart with unstable angina A
I25.761 Atherosclerosis of bypass graft of coronary artery of transplanted heart with angina pectoris with documented spasm A
I25.762 Atherosclerosis of bypass graft of coronary artery of transplanted heart with refractory angina pectoris A
I25.810 Atherosclerosis of coronary artery bypass graft(s) without angina pectoris A
I25.812 Atherosclerosis of bypass graft of coronary artery of transplanted heart without angina pectoris A
I25.82 Chronic total occlusion of coronary artery
I25.84 Coronary atherosclerosis due to calcified coronary lesion
I27.0 Primary pulmonary hypertension
I27.23 Pulmonary hypertension due to lung diseases and hypoxia
I27.24 Chronic thromboembolic pulmonary hypertension
I27.81 Cor pulmonale (chronic)
I27.83 Eisenmenger's syndrome
I34.1 Nonrheumatic mitral (valve) prolapse
I34.2 Nonrheumatic mitral (valve) stenosis
I35.0 Nonrheumatic aortic (valve) stenosis
I35.1 Nonrheumatic aortic (valve) insufficiency
I36.0 Nonrheumatic tricuspid (valve) stenosis
I36.1 Nonrheumatic tricuspid (valve) insufficiency
I37.0 Nonrheumatic pulmonary valve stenosis
I37.1 Nonrheumatic pulmonary valve insufficiency
I46.2 Cardiac arrest due to underlying cardiac condition
I50.21 Acute systolic (congestive) heart failure
I50.22 Chronic systolic (congestive) heart failure
I50.23 Acute on chronic systolic (congestive) heart failure
I50.31 Acute diastolic (congestive) heart failure
I50.32 Chronic diastolic (congestive) heart failure
I50.33 Acute on chronic diastolic (congestive) heart failure
I50.811 Acute right heart failure
I50.812 Chronic right heart failure
I50.813 Acute on chronic right heart failure
I50.814 Right heart failure due to left heart failure
I50.82 Biventricular heart failure
I50.83 High output heart failure
I50.84 End stage heart failure
R57.0 Cardiogenic shock
R57.1 Hypovolemic shock
T80.0XXA Air embolism following infusion, transfusion and therapeutic injection, initial encounter
T82.817A Embolism due to cardiac prosthetic devices, implants and grafts, initial encounter
T82.818A Embolism due to vascular prosthetic devices, implants and grafts, initial encounter

AMA: **93452** 2023,Jun

Relative Value Units/Medicare Edits

Non-Facility RVU	Work	PE	MP	Total
93452	4.5	21.12	0.9	26.52
Facility RVU	**Work**	**PE**	**MP**	**Total**
93452	4.5	21.12	0.9	26.52

	FUD	Status	MUE	Modifiers				IOM Reference
93452	0	A	1(3)	51	N/A	N/A	80*	None

* with documentation

Terms To Know

angiogram. Radiographic image of the arteries. Imaging may be performed to study the vasculature of any given organ, body system, or area of circulation such as the brain, heart, chest, kidneys, limbs, gastrointestinal tract, aorta, and pulmonary circulation to visualize the formation and the function of the blood vessels to detect problems such as a blockage or stricture.

aortic valve. Heart valve, comprising three cusps, that divides the left ventricle and the aorta.

fluoroscopy. Radiology technique that allows visual examination of part of the body or a function of an organ using a device that projects an x-ray image on a fluorescent screen.

supervision and interpretation. Radiology services that usually contain an invasive component and are reported by the radiologist for supervision of the procedure and the personnel involved with performing the examination, reading the film, and preparing the written report.

ventriculogram. Interventional procedure that demonstrates the contractility of the cardiac ventricles by serial recording of the distribution of intravenously injected radionuclide or that of radiographic contrast medium injected through an intracardiac catheter.

93453

93453 Combined right and left heart catheterization including intraprocedural injection(s) for left ventriculography, imaging supervision and interpretation, when performed

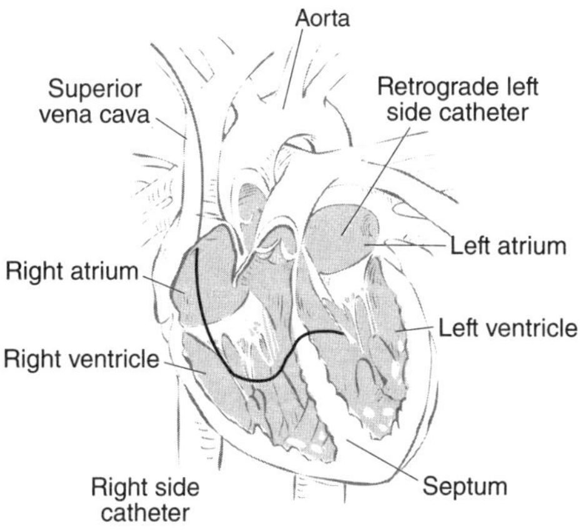

Both sides of the heart are catheterized

Explanation

This procedure is performed to evaluate both right and left heart function. To accomplish right heart catheterization, the physician threads a catheter through an introducing sheath placed percutaneously into the femoral, subclavian, internal jugular, or antecubital vein. The catheter is threaded into the right atrium, through the tricuspid valve into the right ventricle, and across the pulmonary valve into the pulmonary arteries. Left heart catheterization is also performed, in this case using retrograde technique. The catheter is inserted through an introducing sheath placed percutaneously into the femoral, brachial, or axillary artery. The catheter is passed through the aortic valve into the left ventricle. Intracardiac and intravascular pressures are recorded. Left ventricular injections may be performed for left ventriculography; the physician injects dye through a previously placed catheter threaded through a central line into the left ventricle or atrium to evaluate function with fluoroscopy. Imaging supervision and interpretation, when performed, are included in this code, as is any required repositioning of catheters.

Coding Tips

When medically necessary, report moderate (conscious) sedation provided by the performing physician with 99151-99153. When provided by another physician, report 99155-99157. Right heart catheterization includes placement of the catheter into the right-side heart chambers or structures (right atrium, right ventricle, pulmonary artery, and wedge), specimen collection for blood gas measurements, and cardiac output measurements. For right heart catheterization performed in addition to other cardiac catheterizations, see 93453, 93456, 93457, 93460, or 93461. When placement of a flow directed catheter (Swan-Ganz) for hemodynamic monitoring is not performed in addition to other cardiac catheterization procedures, see 93503. Report right ventricular or right atrial angiogram (93566) in addition to right heart catheterization when performed. Left heart catheterization includes placement of the catheter into the left-side heart chambers or structures (left ventricle, left atrium) and left ventricular injection when utilized. Intraprocedural injections for left ventricular/atrial angiogram and imaging supervision and interpretation are also included. Do not report 93503 in addition to other diagnostic cardiac cath codes. This procedure includes introduction, positioning, and repositioning (when utilized) of the catheter within the vessel; recording of intracardiac and/or intravascular pressure; and final report evaluation. All roadmapping angiography for catheter placement, as well as injections and imaging, are also included. Report separately contrast injections and imaging that are separately indicated within a specific CPT code. Do not separately report contrast injections to view the access site when placing a closure device or the placement of the closure device at the vessel access site. Do not report 93453 with 93451, 93452, 93456–93461, 93565, 0408T-0411T, or 0414T-0415T. Do not report 93453 with 33418, 0345T, 0483T, 0484T, 0544T, 0545T, or 0643T for diagnostic left and right catheterization intrinsic to the valve repair or annulus reconstruction. Code 93453 may be reported in addition to 33274 and 33275 only if the catheterization is performed for reasons distinct from the leadless pacemaker procedure.

ICD-10-CM Diagnostic Codes

C38.0	Malignant neoplasm of heart
I05.0	Rheumatic mitral stenosis
I05.1	Rheumatic mitral insufficiency
I06.0	Rheumatic aortic stenosis
I06.1	Rheumatic aortic insufficiency
I07.0	Rheumatic tricuspid stenosis
I07.1	Rheumatic tricuspid insufficiency
I09.81	Rheumatic heart failure
I20.0	Unstable angina
I20.1	Angina pectoris with documented spasm
I20.81	Angina pectoris with coronary microvascular dysfunction
I21.01	ST elevation (STEMI) myocardial infarction involving left main coronary artery
I21.02	ST elevation (STEMI) myocardial infarction involving left anterior descending coronary artery
I21.21	ST elevation (STEMI) myocardial infarction involving left circumflex coronary artery
I21.4	Non-ST elevation (NSTEMI) myocardial infarction
I21.A1	Myocardial infarction type 2
I21.B	Myocardial infarction with coronary microvascular dysfunction
I22.0	Subsequent ST elevation (STEMI) myocardial infarction of anterior wall
I22.1	Subsequent ST elevation (STEMI) myocardial infarction of inferior wall
I22.2	Subsequent non-ST elevation (NSTEMI) myocardial infarction
I23.0	Hemopericardium as current complication following acute myocardial infarction A
I23.1	Atrial septal defect as current complication following acute myocardial infarction A
I23.2	Ventricular septal defect as current complication following acute myocardial infarction A
I23.3	Rupture of cardiac wall without hemopericardium as current complication following acute myocardial infarction A
I23.7	Postinfarction angina A
I24.0	Acute coronary thrombosis not resulting in myocardial infarction
I24.1	Dressler's syndrome
I25.110	Atherosclerotic heart disease of native coronary artery with unstable angina pectoris A
I25.111	Atherosclerotic heart disease of native coronary artery with angina pectoris with documented spasm A
I25.112	Atherosclerotic heart disease of native coronary artery with refractory angina pectoris A
I25.2	Old myocardial infarction

I25.3 Aneurysm of heart
I25.41 Coronary artery aneurysm
I25.5 Ischemic cardiomyopathy
I25.6 Silent myocardial ischemia
I25.710 Atherosclerosis of autologous vein coronary artery bypass graft(s) with unstable angina pectoris [A]
I25.711 Atherosclerosis of autologous vein coronary artery bypass graft(s) with angina pectoris with documented spasm [A]
I25.82 Chronic total occlusion of coronary artery
I25.84 Coronary atherosclerosis due to calcified coronary lesion
I26.01 Septic pulmonary embolism with acute cor pulmonale
I26.02 Saddle embolus of pulmonary artery with acute cor pulmonale
I26.90 Septic pulmonary embolism without acute cor pulmonale
I26.92 Saddle embolus of pulmonary artery without acute cor pulmonale
I27.0 Primary pulmonary hypertension
I27.21 Secondary pulmonary arterial hypertension
I27.24 Chronic thromboembolic pulmonary hypertension
I27.81 Cor pulmonale (chronic)
I27.83 Eisenmenger's syndrome
I34.0 Nonrheumatic mitral (valve) insufficiency
I34.1 Nonrheumatic mitral (valve) prolapse
I34.2 Nonrheumatic mitral (valve) stenosis
I34.81 Nonrheumatic mitral (valve) annulus calcification
I34.89 Other nonrheumatic mitral valve disorders
I35.0 Nonrheumatic aortic (valve) stenosis
I35.1 Nonrheumatic aortic (valve) insufficiency
I36.0 Nonrheumatic tricuspid (valve) stenosis
I36.1 Nonrheumatic tricuspid (valve) insufficiency
I37.0 Nonrheumatic pulmonary valve stenosis
I37.1 Nonrheumatic pulmonary valve insufficiency
I40.0 Infective myocarditis
I40.1 Isolated myocarditis
I42.0 Dilated cardiomyopathy
I42.1 Obstructive hypertrophic cardiomyopathy
I42.3 Endomyocardial (eosinophilic) disease
I42.4 Endocardial fibroelastosis
I42.6 Alcoholic cardiomyopathy
I50.23 Acute on chronic systolic (congestive) heart failure
I50.33 Acute on chronic diastolic (congestive) heart failure
I50.813 Acute on chronic right heart failure
I50.814 Right heart failure due to left heart failure
I50.82 Biventricular heart failure
I50.83 High output heart failure
I50.84 End stage heart failure
I51.0 Cardiac septal defect, acquired [A]
R57.0 Cardiogenic shock
R57.1 Hypovolemic shock
T80.0XXA Air embolism following infusion, transfusion and therapeutic injection, initial encounter
T82.817A Embolism due to cardiac prosthetic devices, implants and grafts, initial encounter
T82.818A Embolism due to vascular prosthetic devices, implants and grafts, initial encounter

AMA: **93453** 2024,Mar; 2023,Jun; 2023,May; 2022,Jul; 2019,Jun; 2019,Apr; 2019,Mar

Relative Value Units/Medicare Edits

Non-Facility RVU	Work	PE	MP	Total
93453	5.99	26.66	1.19	33.84
Facility RVU	**Work**	**PE**	**MP**	**Total**
93453	5.99	26.66	1.19	33.84

	FUD	Status	MUE	Modifiers				IOM Reference
93453	0	A	1(3)	51	N/A	N/A	80*	None

* with documentation

Terms To Know

catheterization. Use or insertion of a tubular device into a duct, blood vessel, hollow organ, or body cavity for injecting or withdrawing fluids for diagnostic or therapeutic purposes.

left heart. Area of the heart consisting of the left atrium and left ventricle.

retrograde. Moving against the usual direction of flow.

right heart. Areas of the right heart, including the right atrium and right ventricle.

 [N] Newborn: 0 [P] Pediatric: 0-17 [M] Maternity: 9-64 [A] Adult: 15-124 AMA: CPT Assist

93454

93454 Catheter placement in coronary artery(s) for coronary angiography, including intraprocedural injection(s) for coronary angiography, imaging supervision and interpretation;

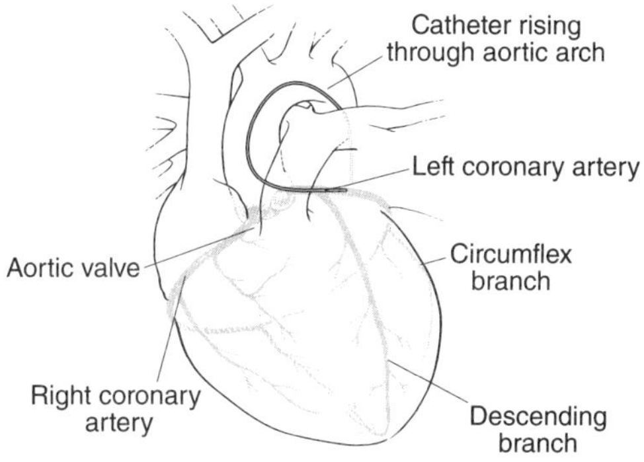

The catheter may enter the coronary grafts, but does not cross the aortic valve into the left ventricle

Explanation

The physician performs a catheter placement in one or more coronary arteries for coronary angiography, without concomitant left heart catheterization. The physician places an introducer sheath in an artery, typically the femoral artery, using percutaneous puncture. The physician advances an angiography catheter through the introducer sheath into the ascending aorta and advances it, under fluoroscopic guidance, to the opening of the coronary artery. The physician injects radiopaque contrast material through the catheter into the vessel while recording a cineangiogram. The physician removes the catheter and sheath from the femoral artery. Pressure is placed on the wound for 20 to 30 minutes to stem bleeding. This code includes imaging supervision and interpretation, as well as any required repositioning of catheters.

Coding Tips

When medically necessary, report moderate (conscious) sedation provided by the performing physician with 99151-99153. When provided by another physician, report 99155-99157. This procedure includes placement of the catheter into the coronary arteries involving selective placement of the native coronary artery origin in order to perform coronary angiogram. Codes 93454–93461, for other than congenital conditions, include intraprocedural injection and imaging when performing coronary angiogram. For right ventricle/atrium angiograms performed in addition to cardiac catheterization (93451–93461), report 93566. For aortography, see 93567. For pulmonary angiogram, see 93568. Do not report 93454 with 33418, 0345T, 0483T, 0484T, 0544T, 0545T, or 0643T for coronary angiography intrinsic to the valve repair or annulus reconstruction.

ICD-10-CM Diagnostic Codes

I20.0	Unstable angina
I20.1	Angina pectoris with documented spasm
I20.2	Refractory angina pectoris
I20.81	Angina pectoris with coronary microvascular dysfunction
I20.89	Other forms of angina pectoris
I21.01	ST elevation (STEMI) myocardial infarction involving left main coronary artery
I21.02	ST elevation (STEMI) myocardial infarction involving left anterior descending coronary artery
I21.09	ST elevation (STEMI) myocardial infarction involving other coronary artery of anterior wall
I21.11	ST elevation (STEMI) myocardial infarction involving right coronary artery
I21.19	ST elevation (STEMI) myocardial infarction involving other coronary artery of inferior wall
I21.21	ST elevation (STEMI) myocardial infarction involving left circumflex coronary artery
I21.29	ST elevation (STEMI) myocardial infarction involving other sites
I21.4	Non-ST elevation (NSTEMI) myocardial infarction
I21.A1	Myocardial infarction type 2
I21.B	Myocardial infarction with coronary microvascular dysfunction
I22.0	Subsequent ST elevation (STEMI) myocardial infarction of anterior wall
I22.1	Subsequent ST elevation (STEMI) myocardial infarction of inferior wall
I22.2	Subsequent non-ST elevation (NSTEMI) myocardial infarction
I22.8	Subsequent ST elevation (STEMI) myocardial infarction of other sites
I24.0	Acute coronary thrombosis not resulting in myocardial infarction
I24.89	Other forms of acute ischemic heart disease
I25.10	Atherosclerotic heart disease of native coronary artery without angina pectoris A
I25.110	Atherosclerotic heart disease of native coronary artery with unstable angina pectoris A
I25.111	Atherosclerotic heart disease of native coronary artery with angina pectoris with documented spasm A
I25.112	Atherosclerotic heart disease of native coronary artery with refractory angina pectoris A
I25.118	Atherosclerotic heart disease of native coronary artery with other forms of angina pectoris A
I25.3	Aneurysm of heart
I25.41	Coronary artery aneurysm
I25.5	Ischemic cardiomyopathy
I25.6	Silent myocardial ischemia
I25.752	Atherosclerosis of native coronary artery of transplanted heart with refractory angina pectoris A
I25.82	Chronic total occlusion of coronary artery
I25.84	Coronary atherosclerosis due to calcified coronary lesion
I25.89	Other forms of chronic ischemic heart disease
I42.0	Dilated cardiomyopathy
I42.1	Obstructive hypertrophic cardiomyopathy
I42.2	Other hypertrophic cardiomyopathy
I42.8	Other cardiomyopathies
I43	Cardiomyopathy in diseases classified elsewhere
I50.1	Left ventricular failure, unspecified
I50.21	Acute systolic (congestive) heart failure
I50.22	Chronic systolic (congestive) heart failure
I50.23	Acute on chronic systolic (congestive) heart failure
I50.31	Acute diastolic (congestive) heart failure
I50.32	Chronic diastolic (congestive) heart failure
I50.33	Acute on chronic diastolic (congestive) heart failure
I50.41	Acute combined systolic (congestive) and diastolic (congestive) heart failure
I50.42	Chronic combined systolic (congestive) and diastolic (congestive) heart failure

Medicine

● New ▲ Revised + Add On ★ Telemedicine [Resequenced] ☑ Laterality

I50.43	Acute on chronic combined systolic (congestive) and diastolic (congestive) heart failure
I50.811	Acute right heart failure
I50.812	Chronic right heart failure
I50.813	Acute on chronic right heart failure
I50.814	Right heart failure due to left heart failure
I50.82	Biventricular heart failure
I50.83	High output heart failure
I50.84	End stage heart failure
I51.7	Cardiomegaly

AMA: **93454** 2023,Jun

Relative Value Units/Medicare Edits

Non-Facility RVU	Work	PE	MP	Total
93454	4.54	21.29	0.91	26.74
Facility RVU	**Work**	**PE**	**MP**	**Total**
93454	4.54	21.29	0.91	26.74

	FUD	Status	MUE	Modifiers				IOM Reference
93454	0	A	1(3)	51	N/A	N/A	80*	None

* with documentation

Terms To Know

angiogram. Radiographic image of the arteries. Imaging may be performed to study the vasculature of any given organ, body system, or area of circulation such as the brain, heart, chest, kidneys, limbs, gastrointestinal tract, aorta, and pulmonary circulation to visualize the formation and the function of the blood vessels to detect problems such as a blockage or stricture.

catheterization. Use or insertion of a tubular device into a duct, blood vessel, hollow organ, or body cavity for injecting or withdrawing fluids for diagnostic or therapeutic purposes.

concomitant. Occurring at the same time, accompanying.

congenital. Present at birth, occurring through heredity or an influence during gestation up to the moment of birth.

radiopaque dye. Medium injected into the body that is impenetrable by x-rays.

supervision and interpretation. Radiology services that usually contain an invasive component and are reported by the radiologist for supervision of the procedure and the personnel involved with performing the examination, reading the film, and preparing the written report.

93455

93455 Catheter placement in coronary artery(s) for coronary angiography, including intraprocedural injection(s) for coronary angiography, imaging supervision and interpretation; with catheter placement(s) in bypass graft(s) (internal mammary, free arterial, venous grafts) including intraprocedural injection(s) for bypass graft angiography

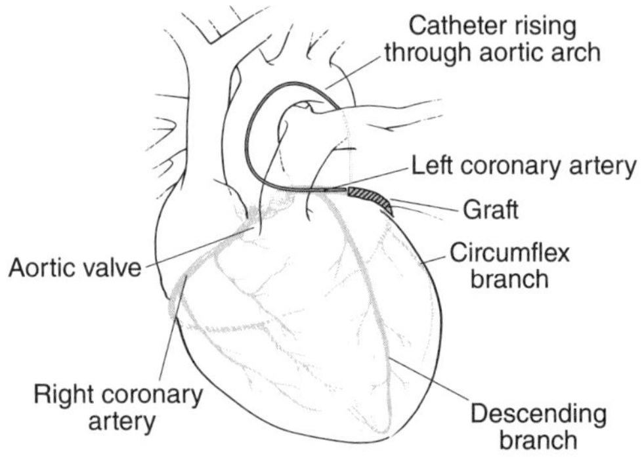

The catheter may enter the coronary grafts, but does not cross the aortic valve into the left ventricle

Explanation

The physician performs a catheter placement in one or more coronary arteries and bypass grafts (i.e., internal mammary, free arterial venous grafts) for coronary and bypass graft angiography, without concomitant left heart catheterization. The physician places an introducer sheath in an artery, typically the femoral artery, using percutaneous puncture. The physician advances an angiography catheter through the introducer sheath into the ascending aorta and advances it, under fluoroscopic guidance, to the opening of the coronary artery or the bypass graft. The physician injects radiopaque contrast material through the catheter into the vessel while recording a cineangiogram. The physician removes the catheter and sheath from the femoral artery. Pressure is placed on the wound for 20 to 30 minutes to stem bleeding. This code includes imaging supervision and interpretation, as well as any required repositioning of catheters.

Coding Tips

When medically necessary, report moderate (conscious) sedation provided by the performing physician with 99151-99153. When provided by another physician, report 99155-99157. This procedure includes placement of the catheter into the coronary arteries involving selective placement of the native coronary artery origin to perform coronary angiogram. Codes 93454–93461, for other than congenital conditions, include intraprocedural injection and imaging when performing coronary angiogram. These procedures (93455, 93457, 93459, 93461) include intraprocedural injections and imaging supervision and interpretation for bypass graft angiogram. Do not report 93563–93565 with 93452–93461. Do not report 93455 with 33418, 0345T, 0483T, 0484T, 0544T, 0545T, or 0643T for coronary angiography intrinsic to the valve repair or annulus reconstruction. Placement of the catheter in bypass grafts (venous, internal mammary, free arterial graft) involves selective placement of the graft origin for bypass angiogram and is most often performed in addition to coronary angiogram of native vessels.

ICD-10-CM Diagnostic Codes

I20.0	Unstable angina
I20.1	Angina pectoris with documented spasm
I20.2	Refractory angina pectoris
I20.81	Angina pectoris with coronary microvascular dysfunction

I21.01 ST elevation (STEMI) myocardial infarction involving left main coronary artery
I21.02 ST elevation (STEMI) myocardial infarction involving left anterior descending coronary artery
I21.11 ST elevation (STEMI) myocardial infarction involving right coronary artery
I21.21 ST elevation (STEMI) myocardial infarction involving left circumflex coronary artery
I21.4 Non-ST elevation (NSTEMI) myocardial infarction
I21.A1 Myocardial infarction type 2
I21.B Myocardial infarction with coronary microvascular dysfunction
I22.0 Subsequent ST elevation (STEMI) myocardial infarction of anterior wall
I22.1 Subsequent ST elevation (STEMI) myocardial infarction of inferior wall
I22.2 Subsequent non-ST elevation (NSTEMI) myocardial infarction
I24.0 Acute coronary thrombosis not resulting in myocardial infarction
I25.10 Atherosclerotic heart disease of native coronary artery without angina pectoris A
I25.110 Atherosclerotic heart disease of native coronary artery with unstable angina pectoris A
I25.111 Atherosclerotic heart disease of native coronary artery with angina pectoris with documented spasm A
I25.112 Atherosclerotic heart disease of native coronary artery with refractory angina pectoris A
I25.3 Aneurysm of heart
I25.41 Coronary artery aneurysm
I25.5 Ischemic cardiomyopathy
I25.6 Silent myocardial ischemia
I25.710 Atherosclerosis of autologous vein coronary artery bypass graft(s) with unstable angina pectoris A
I25.711 Atherosclerosis of autologous vein coronary artery bypass graft(s) with angina pectoris with documented spasm A
I25.712 Atherosclerosis of autologous vein coronary artery bypass graft(s) with refractory angina pectoris A
I25.720 Atherosclerosis of autologous artery coronary artery bypass graft(s) with unstable angina pectoris A
I25.721 Atherosclerosis of autologous artery coronary artery bypass graft(s) with angina pectoris with documented spasm A
I25.722 Atherosclerosis of autologous artery coronary artery bypass graft(s) with refractory angina pectoris A
I25.730 Atherosclerosis of nonautologous biological coronary artery bypass graft(s) with unstable angina pectoris A
I25.731 Atherosclerosis of nonautologous biological coronary artery bypass graft(s) with angina pectoris with documented spasm A
I25.732 Atherosclerosis of nonautologous biological coronary artery bypass graft(s) with refractory angina pectoris A
I25.750 Atherosclerosis of native coronary artery of transplanted heart with unstable angina
I25.751 Atherosclerosis of native coronary artery of transplanted heart with angina pectoris with documented spasm
I25.752 Atherosclerosis of native coronary artery of transplanted heart with refractory angina pectoris A
I25.760 Atherosclerosis of bypass graft of coronary artery of transplanted heart with unstable angina A
I25.761 Atherosclerosis of bypass graft of coronary artery of transplanted heart with angina pectoris with documented spasm A
I25.762 Atherosclerosis of bypass graft of coronary artery of transplanted heart with refractory angina pectoris A
I25.790 Atherosclerosis of other coronary artery bypass graft(s) with unstable angina pectoris A
I25.791 Atherosclerosis of other coronary artery bypass graft(s) with angina pectoris with documented spasm A
I25.810 Atherosclerosis of coronary artery bypass graft(s) without angina pectoris A
I25.812 Atherosclerosis of bypass graft of coronary artery of transplanted heart without angina pectoris A
I25.82 Chronic total occlusion of coronary artery
I25.84 Coronary atherosclerosis due to calcified coronary lesion
I25.89 Other forms of chronic ischemic heart disease
I42.0 Dilated cardiomyopathy
I42.1 Obstructive hypertrophic cardiomyopathy
I42.2 Other hypertrophic cardiomyopathy
I43 Cardiomyopathy in diseases classified elsewhere
I50.1 Left ventricular failure, unspecified
I50.21 Acute systolic (congestive) heart failure
I50.22 Chronic systolic (congestive) heart failure
I50.23 Acute on chronic systolic (congestive) heart failure
I50.31 Acute diastolic (congestive) heart failure
I50.32 Chronic diastolic (congestive) heart failure
I50.33 Acute on chronic diastolic (congestive) heart failure
I50.41 Acute combined systolic (congestive) and diastolic (congestive) heart failure
I50.42 Chronic combined systolic (congestive) and diastolic (congestive) heart failure
I50.43 Acute on chronic combined systolic (congestive) and diastolic (congestive) heart failure
I50.811 Acute right heart failure
I50.812 Chronic right heart failure
I50.813 Acute on chronic right heart failure
I50.814 Right heart failure due to left heart failure
I50.82 Biventricular heart failure
I50.83 High output heart failure
I50.84 End stage heart failure
I51.7 Cardiomegaly

AMA: 93455 2023,Jun

Relative Value Units/Medicare Edits

Non-Facility RVU	Work	PE	MP	Total
93455	5.29	23.44	1.06	29.79
Facility RVU	**Work**	**PE**	**MP**	**Total**
93455	5.29	23.44	1.06	29.79

	FUD	Status	MUE	Modifiers				IOM Reference
93455	0	A	1(3)	51	N/A	N/A	80*	None

* with documentation

93456-93457

93456 Catheter placement in coronary artery(s) for coronary angiography, including intraprocedural injection(s) for coronary angiography, imaging supervision and interpretation; with right heart catheterization

93457 with catheter placement(s) in bypass graft(s) (internal mammary, free arterial, venous grafts) including intraprocedural injection(s) for bypass graft angiography and right heart catheterization

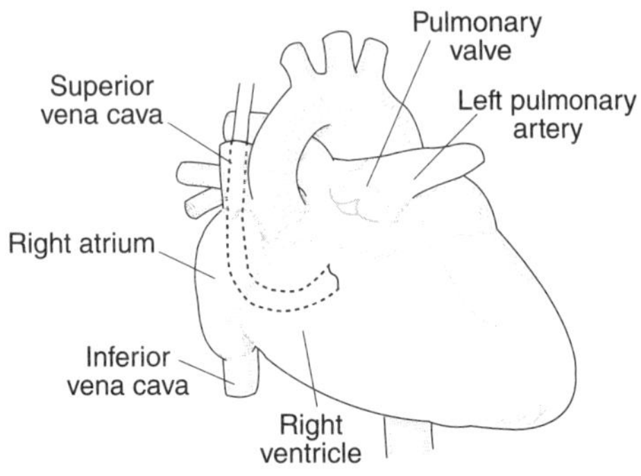

Introduction of a catheter into the right side of the heart

Explanation

The physician performs a catheter placement in one or more coronary arteries for coronary angiography, without concomitant left heart catheterization. The physician places an introducer sheath in an artery, typically the femoral artery, using percutaneous puncture. The physician advances an angiography catheter through the introducer sheath into the ascending aorta and advances it, under fluoroscopic guidance, to the opening of the coronary artery. The physician injects radiopaque contrast material through the catheter into the vessel while recording a cineangiogram. The physician removes the catheter and sheath from the femoral artery. Pressure is placed on the wound for 20 to 30 minutes to stem bleeding. These codes include imaging supervision and interpretation, as well as any required repositioning of catheters. Code 93456 includes right heart catheterization, in which the catheter is threaded into the right atrium, through the tricuspid valve into the right ventricle, and across the pulmonary valve into the pulmonary arteries. Code 93457 includes catheter placement in one or more bypass grafts for angiography, in addition to the right heart catheterization. Intracardiac or intravascular pressure recordings are included in these codes, as are cardiac output and oxygen saturation measurements, and final evaluation and procedure report.

Coding Tips

When medically necessary, report moderate (conscious) sedation provided by the performing physician with 99151-99153. When provided by another physician, report 99155-99157. These procedures include placement of the catheter into the coronary arteries involving selective placement of the native coronary artery origin in order to perform coronary angiogram. Codes 93454–93461, other than congenital conditions, include intraprocedural injection and imaging when performing coronary angiogram. Right heart catheterization includes placement of the catheter into the right-side heart chambers or structures (right atrium, right ventricle, pulmonary artery, and wedge), specimen collection for blood gas measurements, and cardiac output measurements. Report right ventricular or right atrial angiogram (93566) in addition to right heart catheterization when performed. Procedures 93455, 93457, 93459, and 93461 include intraprocedural injections and imaging supervision and interpretation for bypass graft angiogram. Placement of the catheter in bypass grafts (venous, internal mammary, free arterial graft) involves selective placement of the graft origin for bypass angiogram and is most often performed in addition to coronary angiogram of native vessels. For pharmacologic administration in addition to a cardiac catheterization procedure for re-evaluating hemodynamic measurements and responses, report 93463 with 93451–93453 and 93456–93461. These codes may be reported in addition to 33274 and 33275 only if the catheterization is performed for reasons distinct from the leadless pacemaker procedure. Do not report 93563–93565 with 93452–93461. Do not report 93456 or 93457 with 33418, 0345T, 0483T, 0484T, 0544T, 0545T, or 0643T for diagnostic coronary angiography or right heart catheterization intrinsic to the valve repair or annulus reconstruction.

ICD-10-CM Diagnostic Codes

C38.0	Malignant neoplasm of heart
I05.0	Rheumatic mitral stenosis
I05.1	Rheumatic mitral insufficiency
I06.0	Rheumatic aortic stenosis
I06.1	Rheumatic aortic insufficiency
I07.0	Rheumatic tricuspid stenosis
I07.1	Rheumatic tricuspid insufficiency
I09.81	Rheumatic heart failure
I20.0	Unstable angina
I20.2	Refractory angina pectoris
I20.81	Angina pectoris with coronary microvascular dysfunction
I21.01	ST elevation (STEMI) myocardial infarction involving left main coronary artery
I21.02	ST elevation (STEMI) myocardial infarction involving left anterior descending coronary artery
I21.21	ST elevation (STEMI) myocardial infarction involving left circumflex coronary artery
I21.4	Non-ST elevation (NSTEMI) myocardial infarction
I21.A1	Myocardial infarction type 2
I21.B	Myocardial infarction with coronary microvascular dysfunction
I22.0	Subsequent ST elevation (STEMI) myocardial infarction of anterior wall
I22.1	Subsequent ST elevation (STEMI) myocardial infarction of inferior wall
I22.2	Subsequent non-ST elevation (NSTEMI) myocardial infarction
I23.7	Postinfarction angina A
I24.0	Acute coronary thrombosis not resulting in myocardial infarction
I24.1	Dressler's syndrome
I25.10	Atherosclerotic heart disease of native coronary artery without angina pectoris A
I25.110	Atherosclerotic heart disease of native coronary artery with unstable angina pectoris A
I25.111	Atherosclerotic heart disease of native coronary artery with angina pectoris with documented spasm A
I25.112	Atherosclerotic heart disease of native coronary artery with refractory angina pectoris A
I25.3	Aneurysm of heart
I25.41	Coronary artery aneurysm
I25.5	Ischemic cardiomyopathy
I25.6	Silent myocardial ischemia
I25.82	Chronic total occlusion of coronary artery
I25.84	Coronary atherosclerosis due to calcified coronary lesion
I26.01	Septic pulmonary embolism with acute cor pulmonale

 N Newborn: 0 P Pediatric: 0-17 M Maternity: 9-64 A Adult: 15-124 AMA: CPT Assist

I26.02	Saddle embolus of pulmonary artery with acute cor pulmonale
I26.90	Septic pulmonary embolism without acute cor pulmonale
I26.92	Saddle embolus of pulmonary artery without acute cor pulmonale
I26.93	Single subsegmental thrombotic pulmonary embolism without acute cor pulmonale
I26.94	Multiple subsegmental thrombotic pulmonary emboli without acute cor pulmonale
I27.0	Primary pulmonary hypertension
I27.21	Secondary pulmonary arterial hypertension
I27.22	Pulmonary hypertension due to left heart disease
I27.23	Pulmonary hypertension due to lung diseases and hypoxia
I27.24	Chronic thromboembolic pulmonary hypertension
I27.81	Cor pulmonale (chronic)
I27.83	Eisenmenger's syndrome
I34.0	Nonrheumatic mitral (valve) insufficiency
I34.1	Nonrheumatic mitral (valve) prolapse
I34.2	Nonrheumatic mitral (valve) stenosis
I35.0	Nonrheumatic aortic (valve) stenosis
I35.1	Nonrheumatic aortic (valve) insufficiency
I36.0	Nonrheumatic tricuspid (valve) stenosis
I36.1	Nonrheumatic tricuspid (valve) insufficiency
I37.0	Nonrheumatic pulmonary valve stenosis
I37.1	Nonrheumatic pulmonary valve insufficiency
I40.0	Infective myocarditis
I40.1	Isolated myocarditis
I42.0	Dilated cardiomyopathy
I42.1	Obstructive hypertrophic cardiomyopathy
I42.3	Endomyocardial (eosinophilic) disease
I42.4	Endocardial fibroelastosis
I42.6	Alcoholic cardiomyopathy
I50.23	Acute on chronic systolic (congestive) heart failure
I50.33	Acute on chronic diastolic (congestive) heart failure
I50.813	Acute on chronic right heart failure
I50.814	Right heart failure due to left heart failure
I50.82	Biventricular heart failure
I50.83	High output heart failure
I50.84	End stage heart failure
I51.7	Cardiomegaly
R57.0	Cardiogenic shock
R57.1	Hypovolemic shock

AMA: 93456 2024,Mar; 2023,Jun; 2023,May; 2022,Jul; 2019,Jun; 2019,Apr; 2019,Mar **93457** 2023,Jun; 2023,May; 2022,Jul; 2019,Jun; 2019,Apr; 2019,Mar

Relative Value Units/Medicare Edits

Non-Facility RVU	Work	PE	MP	Total
93456	5.9	26.19	1.18	33.27
93457	6.64	28.31	1.31	36.26
Facility RVU	**Work**	**PE**	**MP**	**Total**
93456	5.9	26.19	1.18	33.27
93457	6.64	28.31	1.31	36.26

	FUD	Status	MUE	Modifiers				IOM Reference
93456	0	A	1(3)	51	N/A	N/A	80*	None
93457	0	A	1(3)	51	N/A	N/A	80*	

* with documentation

Terms To Know

angiography. Radiographic imaging of the arteries.

catheterization. Use or insertion of a tubular device into a duct, blood vessel, hollow organ, or body cavity for injecting or withdrawing fluids for diagnostic or therapeutic purposes.

cor pulmonale. Heart-lung disease appearing in identifiable forms as chronic or acute. The chronic form of this heart-lung disease is marked by dilation and hypertrophy failure of the right ventricle due to a disease that has affected the function of the lungs, excluding congenital or left heart diseases and is also called chronic cardiopulmonary disease. The acute form is an overload of the right ventricle from a rapid onset of pulmonary hypertension, usually arising from a pulmonary embolism.

myocardial infarction. Obstruction of circulation to the heart, resulting in necrosis.

myocardial infarction type 2. Often referred to as due to demand ischemia, myocardial infarction (MI) type 2 refers to an MI due to ischemia and necrosis resulting from an oxygen imbalance to the heart. This mismatch between oxygen decreased supply and increased demand is caused by conditions other than coronary artery disease such as vasospasm, embolism, anemia, hypertension, hypotension, or arrhythmias.

rheumatic heart failure. Decreased cardiac output, edema, and hypertension due to rheumatic heart disease.

rheumatic mitral stenosis. Narrowing of the mitral valve between the left atrium and left ventricle due to rheumatic fever. Symptoms include shortness of breath during or after exercise, fatigue, palpitations, chest discomfort, and swelling of feet or legs.

93458-93459

93458 Catheter placement in coronary artery(s) for coronary angiography, including intraprocedural injection(s) for coronary angiography, imaging supervision and interpretation; with left heart catheterization including intraprocedural injection(s) for left ventriculography, when performed

93459 with left heart catheterization including intraprocedural injection(s) for left ventriculography, when performed, catheter placement(s) in bypass graft(s) (internal mammary, free arterial, venous grafts) with bypass graft angiography

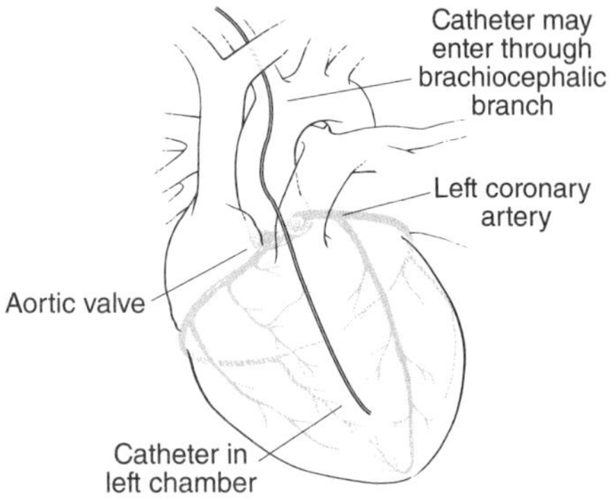

The catheter crosses the aortic valve and enters the left ventricle of the heart

Explanation

The physician places a catheter into one or more coronary arteries for coronary angiography. The physician threads a catheter to the heart, most frequently through an introducing sheath placed percutaneously into the femoral, brachial, or axillary artery using retrograde technique. The catheter passes through the aortic valve into the left ventricle. Intracardiac and intravascular pressures are recorded. Left ventricular injections may be performed for left ventriculography; the physician injects dye through a previously placed catheter threaded through a central line into the left ventricle or atrium to evaluate function with fluoroscopy. Code 93459 includes catheter placement in one or more bypass grafts with bypass graft angiography. The physician removes the catheter and sheath from the femoral artery. Pressure is placed on the wound for 20 to 30 minutes to stem bleeding. These codes include imaging supervision and interpretation, as well as any required repositioning of catheters.

Coding Tips

When medically necessary, report moderate (conscious) sedation provided by the performing physician with 99151-99153. When provided by another physician, report 99155-99157. These procedures include placement of the catheter into the coronary arteries involving selective placement of the native coronary artery origin in order to perform coronary angiogram. Codes 93454–93461, for other than congenital conditions, include intraprocedural injection and imaging when performing coronary angiogram. These procedures include placement of the catheter into the left-side heart chambers or structures (left ventricle, left atrium) and left ventricular injection when utilized. Intraprocedural injections for left ventricular/atrial angiogram and imaging supervision and interpretation are also included. Do not report 93503 in addition to other diagnostic cardiac cath codes. For left heart catheterization that is performed via transapical puncture into the left ventricle or transseptal puncture into the septum, report 93462 in addition to 93452, 93453, 93458–93461, 93653, and 93654. Right heart catheterization includes placement of the catheter into the right-side heart chambers or structures (right atrium, right ventricle, pulmonary artery, and wedge), specimen collection for blood gas measurements, and cardiac output measurements. Report right ventricular or right atrial angiogram (93566) in addition to right heart catheterization when performed. Procedures 93455, 93457, 93459, and 93461 include intraprocedural injections and imaging supervision and interpretation for bypass graft angiogram. Do not report 93563–93565 with 93452–93461. Placement of the catheter in bypass grafts (venous, internal mammary, free arterial graft) involves selective placement of the graft origin for bypass angiogram and is most often performed in addition to coronary angiogram of native vessels. For pharmacologic administration in addition to a cardiac catheterization procedure for re-evaluating hemodynamic measurements and responses, report 93463 in addition to 93451–93453 and 93456–93461. Do not report these codes with 0408T-0411T or 0414T-0415T. Do not report 93458 or 93459 with 33418, 0345T, 0483T, 0484T, 0544T, 0545T, or 0643T for diagnostic coronary angiography or left heart catheterization intrinsic to the valve repair or annulus reconstruction.

ICD-10-CM Diagnostic Codes

C38.0	Malignant neoplasm of heart
I05.0	Rheumatic mitral stenosis
I05.1	Rheumatic mitral insufficiency
I06.0	Rheumatic aortic stenosis
I06.1	Rheumatic aortic insufficiency
I07.0	Rheumatic tricuspid stenosis
I07.1	Rheumatic tricuspid insufficiency
I09.81	Rheumatic heart failure
I20.0	Unstable angina
I20.1	Angina pectoris with documented spasm
I20.2	Refractory angina pectoris
I20.81	Angina pectoris with coronary microvascular dysfunction
I21.01	ST elevation (STEMI) myocardial infarction involving left main coronary artery
I21.02	ST elevation (STEMI) myocardial infarction involving left anterior descending coronary artery
I21.09	ST elevation (STEMI) myocardial infarction involving other coronary artery of anterior wall
I21.11	ST elevation (STEMI) myocardial infarction involving right coronary artery
I21.19	ST elevation (STEMI) myocardial infarction involving other coronary artery of inferior wall
I21.21	ST elevation (STEMI) myocardial infarction involving left circumflex coronary artery
I21.4	Non-ST elevation (NSTEMI) myocardial infarction
I21.A1	Myocardial infarction type 2
I21.B	Myocardial infarction with coronary microvascular dysfunction
I22.0	Subsequent ST elevation (STEMI) myocardial infarction of anterior wall
I22.1	Subsequent ST elevation (STEMI) myocardial infarction of inferior wall
I22.2	Subsequent non-ST elevation (NSTEMI) myocardial infarction
I23.7	Postinfarction angina A
I24.0	Acute coronary thrombosis not resulting in myocardial infarction
I24.1	Dressler's syndrome
I24.89	Other forms of acute ischemic heart disease
I25.10	Atherosclerotic heart disease of native coronary artery without angina pectoris A
I25.110	Atherosclerotic heart disease of native coronary artery with unstable angina pectoris A

I25.111	Atherosclerotic heart disease of native coronary artery with angina pectoris with documented spasm A
I25.112	Atherosclerotic heart disease of native coronary artery with refractory angina pectoris A
I25.118	Atherosclerotic heart disease of native coronary artery with other forms of angina pectoris A
I25.2	Old myocardial infarction
I25.3	Aneurysm of heart
I25.41	Coronary artery aneurysm
I25.5	Ischemic cardiomyopathy
I25.6	Silent myocardial ischemia
I25.82	Chronic total occlusion of coronary artery
I25.84	Coronary atherosclerosis due to calcified coronary lesion
I26.01	Septic pulmonary embolism with acute cor pulmonale
I26.02	Saddle embolus of pulmonary artery with acute cor pulmonale
I26.90	Septic pulmonary embolism without acute cor pulmonale
I26.92	Saddle embolus of pulmonary artery without acute cor pulmonale
I27.0	Primary pulmonary hypertension
I27.81	Cor pulmonale (chronic)
I27.83	Eisenmenger's syndrome
I34.0	Nonrheumatic mitral (valve) insufficiency
I34.1	Nonrheumatic mitral (valve) prolapse
I34.2	Nonrheumatic mitral (valve) stenosis
I34.81	Nonrheumatic mitral (valve) annulus calcification
I34.89	Other nonrheumatic mitral valve disorders
I35.0	Nonrheumatic aortic (valve) stenosis
I35.1	Nonrheumatic aortic (valve) insufficiency
I35.2	Nonrheumatic aortic (valve) stenosis with insufficiency
I36.0	Nonrheumatic tricuspid (valve) stenosis
I36.1	Nonrheumatic tricuspid (valve) insufficiency
I37.0	Nonrheumatic pulmonary valve stenosis
I37.1	Nonrheumatic pulmonary valve insufficiency
I42.0	Dilated cardiomyopathy
I42.1	Obstructive hypertrophic cardiomyopathy
I50.23	Acute on chronic systolic (congestive) heart failure
I50.33	Acute on chronic diastolic (congestive) heart failure
I50.43	Acute on chronic combined systolic (congestive) and diastolic (congestive) heart failure
I50.813	Acute on chronic right heart failure
I50.814	Right heart failure due to left heart failure
I50.82	Biventricular heart failure
I50.83	High output heart failure
I50.84	End stage heart failure
I51.7	Cardiomegaly
R57.0	Cardiogenic shock
R57.1	Hypovolemic shock
T80.0XXA	Air embolism following infusion, transfusion and therapeutic injection, initial encounter
T82.817A	Embolism due to cardiac prosthetic devices, implants and grafts, initial encounter
T82.818A	Embolism due to vascular prosthetic devices, implants and grafts, initial encounter

AMA: **93458** 2023,Jun **93459** 2023,Jun

Relative Value Units/Medicare Edits

Non-Facility RVU	Work	PE	MP	Total
93458	5.6	24.04	1.12	30.76
93459	6.35	25.47	1.27	33.09
Facility RVU	**Work**	**PE**	**MP**	**Total**
93458	5.6	24.04	1.12	30.76
93459	6.35	25.47	1.27	33.09

	FUD	Status	MUE	Modifiers				IOM Reference
93458	0	A	1(3)	51	N/A	N/A	80*	None
93459	0	A	1(3)	51	N/A	N/A	80*	

* with documentation

Terms To Know

bypass graft. Surgically created alternative blood vessel used to reroute blood flow around an area of obstruction or disease.

fluoroscopy. Radiology technique that allows visual examination of part of the body or a function of an organ using a device that projects an x-ray image on a fluorescent screen.

ventriculogram. Interventional procedure that demonstrates the contractility of the cardiac ventricles by serial recording of the distribution of intravenously injected radionuclide or that of radiographic contrast medium injected through an intracardiac catheter.

93460-93461

93460 Catheter placement in coronary artery(s) for coronary angiography, including intraprocedural injection(s) for coronary angiography, imaging supervision and interpretation; with right and left heart catheterization including intraprocedural injection(s) for left ventriculography, when performed

93461 with right and left heart catheterization including intraprocedural injection(s) for left ventriculography, when performed, catheter placement(s) in bypass graft(s) (internal mammary, free arterial, venous grafts) with bypass graft angiography

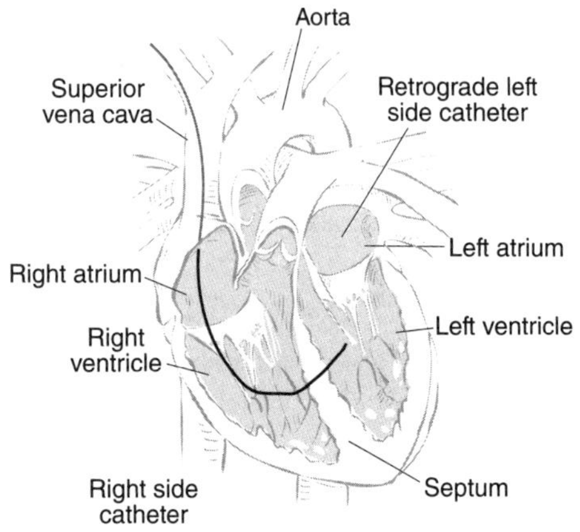

Both sides of the heart are catheterized with left ventriculogram

Explanation

The physician places a catheter in one or more coronary arteries for coronary angiography. In 93460, right and left heart function is evaluated. To accomplish right heart catheterization, the physician threads a catheter through an introducing sheath placed percutaneously into the femoral, subclavian, internal jugular, or antecubital vein. The catheter is threaded into the right atrium, through the tricuspid valve into the right ventricle, and across the pulmonary valve into the pulmonary arteries. Left heart catheterization is also performed, in this case using retrograde technique. The catheter is inserted through an introducing sheath placed percutaneously into the femoral, brachial, or axillary artery. The catheter is passed through the aortic valve into the left ventricle. Intracardiac and intravascular pressures are recorded. Left ventricular injections may be performed for left ventriculography; the physician injects dye through a previously placed catheter threaded through a central line into the left ventricle or atrium to evaluate function with fluoroscopy. Code 93461 includes catheter placement in one or more bypass grafts for angiography. The physician removes the catheter and sheath from the femoral artery. Pressure is placed on the wound for 20 to 30 minutes to stem bleeding. These codes include imaging supervision and interpretation, as well as any required repositioning of catheters.

Coding Tips

When medically necessary, report moderate (conscious) sedation provided by the performing physician with 99151-99153. When provided by another physician, report 99155-99157. These procedures include placement of the catheter into the coronary arteries involving selective placement of the native coronary artery origin in order to perform coronary angiogram. Codes 93454–93461, for other than congenital conditions, include intraprocedural injection and imaging when performing coronary angiogram. Right heart catheterization includes placement of the catheter into the right-side heart chambers or structures (right atrium, right ventricle, pulmonary artery, and wedge), specimen collection for blood gas measurements, and cardiac output measurements. Report right ventricular or right atrial angiogram (93566) in addition to right heart catheterization when performed. These procedures include placement of the catheter into the left-side heart chambers or structures (left ventricle, left atrium) and left ventricular injection when utilized. Intraprocedural injections for left ventricular/atrial angiogram and imaging supervision and interpretation are also included. For left heart catheterization performed via transapical puncture into the left ventricle or transseptal puncture into the septum, report 93462 with 93452, 93453, 93458–93461, 93653, and 93654. Procedures 93455, 93457, 93459, and 93461 include intraprocedural injections and imaging supervision and interpretation for bypass graft angiogram. Placement of the catheter in bypass grafts (venous, internal mammary, free arterial graft) involves selective placement of the graft origin for bypass angiogram and is most often performed in addition to coronary angiogram of native vessels. For pharmacologic administration in addition to a cardiac catheterization procedure for re-evaluating hemodynamic measurements and responses, report 93463 with 93451–93453 and 93456–93461. These codes may be reported in addition to 33274 and 33275 only if the catheterization is performed for reasons distinct from the leadless pacemaker procedure. Do not report 93563–93565 with 93452–93461, 0408T-0411T, or 0414T-0415T. Do not report 93460 or 93461 with 33418, 0345T, 0483T, 0484T, 0544T, 0545T, or 0643T for diagnostic coronary angiography or left and right heart catheterization intrinsic to the valve repair or annulus reconstruction.

ICD-10-CM Diagnostic Codes

C38.0	Malignant neoplasm of heart
I05.0	Rheumatic mitral stenosis
I05.1	Rheumatic mitral insufficiency
I06.0	Rheumatic aortic stenosis
I06.1	Rheumatic aortic insufficiency
I07.0	Rheumatic tricuspid stenosis
I07.1	Rheumatic tricuspid insufficiency
I08.3	Combined rheumatic disorders of mitral, aortic and tricuspid valves
I09.81	Rheumatic heart failure
I20.0	Unstable angina
I20.1	Angina pectoris with documented spasm
I20.2	Refractory angina pectoris
I20.81	Angina pectoris with coronary microvascular dysfunction
I21.01	ST elevation (STEMI) myocardial infarction involving left main coronary artery
I21.02	ST elevation (STEMI) myocardial infarction involving left anterior descending coronary artery
I21.09	ST elevation (STEMI) myocardial infarction involving other coronary artery of anterior wall
I21.11	ST elevation (STEMI) myocardial infarction involving right coronary artery
I21.19	ST elevation (STEMI) myocardial infarction involving other coronary artery of inferior wall
I21.21	ST elevation (STEMI) myocardial infarction involving left circumflex coronary artery
I21.4	Non-ST elevation (NSTEMI) myocardial infarction
I21.A1	Myocardial infarction type 2
I21.B	Myocardial infarction with coronary microvascular dysfunction
I22.0	Subsequent ST elevation (STEMI) myocardial infarction of anterior wall
I22.1	Subsequent ST elevation (STEMI) myocardial infarction of inferior wall

I22.2 Subsequent non-ST elevation (NSTEMI) myocardial infarction
I23.0 Hemopericardium as current complication following acute myocardial infarction A
I23.1 Atrial septal defect as current complication following acute myocardial infarction A
I23.2 Ventricular septal defect as current complication following acute myocardial infarction A
I23.3 Rupture of cardiac wall without hemopericardium as current complication following acute myocardial infarction A
I23.7 Postinfarction angina A
I24.0 Acute coronary thrombosis not resulting in myocardial infarction
I24.1 Dressler's syndrome
I25.10 Atherosclerotic heart disease of native coronary artery without angina pectoris A
I25.110 Atherosclerotic heart disease of native coronary artery with unstable angina pectoris A
I25.111 Atherosclerotic heart disease of native coronary artery with angina pectoris with documented spasm A
I25.112 Atherosclerotic heart disease of native coronary artery with refractory angina pectoris A
I25.2 Old myocardial infarction
I25.3 Aneurysm of heart
I25.41 Coronary artery aneurysm
I25.5 Ischemic cardiomyopathy
I25.6 Silent myocardial ischemia
I25.82 Chronic total occlusion of coronary artery
I25.84 Coronary atherosclerosis due to calcified coronary lesion
I26.01 Septic pulmonary embolism with acute cor pulmonale
I26.02 Saddle embolus of pulmonary artery with acute cor pulmonale
I26.90 Septic pulmonary embolism without acute cor pulmonale
I26.92 Saddle embolus of pulmonary artery without acute cor pulmonale
I27.0 Primary pulmonary hypertension
I27.81 Cor pulmonale (chronic)
I27.83 Eisenmenger's syndrome
I34.0 Nonrheumatic mitral (valve) insufficiency
I34.1 Nonrheumatic mitral (valve) prolapse
I34.2 Nonrheumatic mitral (valve) stenosis
I34.81 Nonrheumatic mitral (valve) annulus calcification
I34.89 Other nonrheumatic mitral valve disorders
I35.0 Nonrheumatic aortic (valve) stenosis
I35.1 Nonrheumatic aortic (valve) insufficiency
I35.2 Nonrheumatic aortic (valve) stenosis with insufficiency
I36.0 Nonrheumatic tricuspid (valve) stenosis
I36.1 Nonrheumatic tricuspid (valve) insufficiency
I37.0 Nonrheumatic pulmonary valve stenosis
I37.1 Nonrheumatic pulmonary valve insufficiency
I40.0 Infective myocarditis
I40.1 Isolated myocarditis
I42.0 Dilated cardiomyopathy
I42.1 Obstructive hypertrophic cardiomyopathy
I42.3 Endomyocardial (eosinophilic) disease
I42.4 Endocardial fibroelastosis
I42.6 Alcoholic cardiomyopathy
I50.23 Acute on chronic systolic (congestive) heart failure
I50.33 Acute on chronic diastolic (congestive) heart failure
I50.813 Acute on chronic right heart failure
I50.814 Right heart failure due to left heart failure
I50.82 Biventricular heart failure
I50.83 High output heart failure
I50.84 End stage heart failure
I51.7 Cardiomegaly
R57.0 Cardiogenic shock
R57.1 Hypovolemic shock
T80.0XXA Air embolism following infusion, transfusion and therapeutic injection, initial encounter
T82.817A Embolism due to cardiac prosthetic devices, implants and grafts, initial encounter
T82.818A Embolism due to vascular prosthetic devices, implants and grafts, initial encounter

AMA: 93460 2023,Jun; 2023,May; 2022,Jul; 2019,Jun; 2019,Apr; 2019,Mar **93461** 2024,Mar; 2023,Jun; 2023,May; 2022,Jul; 2019,Jun; 2019,Apr; 2019,Mar

Relative Value Units/Medicare Edits

Non-Facility RVU	Work	PE	MP	Total
93460	7.1	28.21	1.4	36.71
93461	7.85	31.09	1.56	40.5
Facility RVU	**Work**	**PE**	**MP**	**Total**
93460	7.1	28.21	1.4	36.71
93461	7.85	31.09	1.56	40.5

	FUD	Status	MUE	Modifiers				IOM Reference
93460	0	A	1(3)	51	N/A	N/A	80*	None
93461	0	A	1(3)	51	N/A	N/A	80*	

* with documentation

Terms To Know

angiogram. Radiographic image of the arteries. Imaging may be performed to study the vasculature of any given organ, body system, or area of circulation such as the brain, heart, chest, kidneys, limbs, gastrointestinal tract, aorta, and pulmonary circulation to visualize the formation and the function of the blood vessels to detect problems such as a blockage or stricture.

supervision and interpretation. Radiology services that usually contain an invasive component and are reported by the radiologist for supervision of the procedure and the personnel involved with performing the examination, reading the film, and preparing the written report.

93462

\+ **93462** Left heart catheterization by transseptal puncture through intact septum or by transapical puncture (List separately in addition to code for primary procedure)

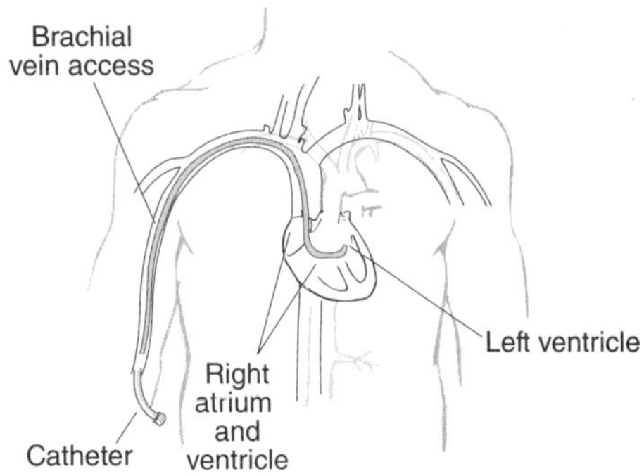

Explanation

Transseptal catheterization involves passing a catheter from the right femoral vein into the right atrium. The interatrial wall or septum is punctured and the catheter is passed into the left atrium or left ventricle. When the left atrium is accessed, the catheter may be further advanced through the mitral valve and into the left ventricle. The transapical or direct left ventricular puncture involves using a large bore needle to puncture the chest wall directly into the left ventricular cavity. These methods are used when the patient has had valve replacement and the left heart cannot be accessed any other way.

Coding Tips

When medically necessary, report moderate (conscious) sedation provided by the performing physician with 99151-99153. When provided by another physician, report 99155-99157. This procedure includes placement of the catheter into the left-side heart chambers or structures (left ventricle, left atrium) and left ventricular injection when utilized. Intraprocedural injections for left ventricular/atrial angiogram and imaging supervision and interpretation are also included. Report 93462 in addition to 33477, 33741, 33745, 93452, 93453, 93458–93461, 93582, 93595-93597, 93653, and 93654. For transseptal or transapical puncture performed for percutaneous transcatheter closure of ventricular septal defect, see 93581. Do not report 93462 with 93656. Do not report 93462 with 33418, 0345T, or 0544T unless transapical puncture is performed.

ICD-10-CM Diagnostic Codes

This/these CPT code(s) are add-on code(s). See the primary procedure code that this code is performed with for your ICD-10-CM code selections. Diagnostic code(s) would be the same as the actual procedure performed.

AMA: **93462** 2024,Mar; 2021,Dec; 2020,Nov

Relative Value Units/Medicare Edits

Non-Facility RVU	Work	PE	MP	Total
93462	3.73	1.48	0.85	6.06
Facility RVU	**Work**	**PE**	**MP**	**Total**
93462	3.73	1.48	0.85	6.06

	FUD	Status	MUE	Modifiers				IOM Reference
93462	N/A	A	1(3)	N/A	N/A	N/A	80*	None

* with documentation

93463

\+ **93463** Pharmacologic agent administration (eg, inhaled nitric oxide, intravenous infusion of nitroprusside, dobutamine, milrinone, or other agent) including assessing hemodynamic measurements before, during, after and repeat pharmacologic agent administration, when performed (List separately in addition to code for primary procedure)

Explanation

The physician administers a pharmacologic agent to invoke stress on coronary vessels in order to measure blood flow through and around the heart. This produces the same result as physical exercise. Arteries become enlarged as the body increases physical activity that requires more oxygen. When plaque is present within a vessel, it does not allow for this enlargement. This slows the ability of the oxygenated blood to reach the necessary organs, which can lead to ischemia.

Coding Tips

When medically necessary, report moderate (conscious) sedation provided by the performing physician with 99151-99153. When provided by another physician, report 99155-99157. Report 93463 in addition to 33477, 93451–93453, 93456–93461, 93580–93582, and 93593–93597. For pharmacologic administration in addition to a cardiac catheterization procedure for re-evaluating hemodynamic measurements and responses, report 93463 with 93451–93453 and 93456–93461. Do not report 93463 for intracoronary administration of pharmacologic administration with percutaneous coronary procedures, intracoronary assessment of pressures, flow and resistance, or intracoronary imaging procedures. Do not report 93463 with 92920–92944, 92975, or 92977.

ICD-10-CM Diagnostic Codes

This/these CPT code(s) are add-on code(s). See the primary procedure code that this code is performed with for your ICD-10-CM code selections. Diagnostic code(s) would be the same as the actual procedure performed.

AMA: **93463** 2023,Jun

Relative Value Units/Medicare Edits

Non-Facility RVU	Work	PE	MP	Total
93463	2.0	0.7	0.16	2.86
Facility RVU	**Work**	**PE**	**MP**	**Total**
93463	2.0	0.7	0.16	2.86

	FUD	Status	MUE	Modifiers				IOM Reference
93463	N/A	A	1(3)	N/A	N/A	N/A	80*	None

* with documentation

Terms To Know

ischemia. Deficiency in blood supply causing tissues to be deprived of oxygen, resulting from trauma, mechanical or functional constriction of blood vessels, or a physical obstruction.

pharmacological agent. Drug used to produce a chemical effect.

Medicine

93464

+ **93464** Physiologic exercise study (eg, bicycle or arm ergometry) including assessing hemodynamic measurements before and after (List separately in addition to code for primary procedure)

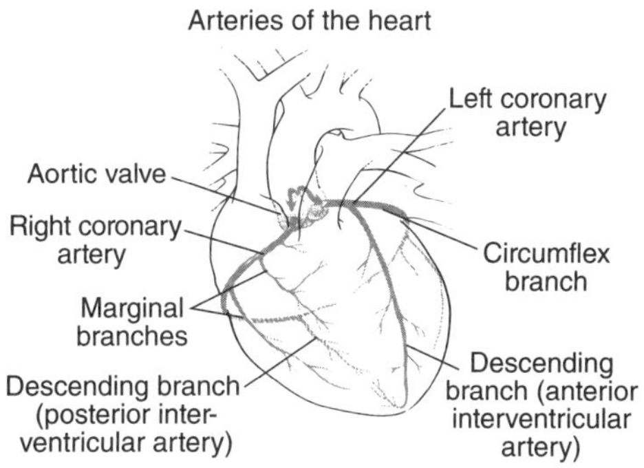

Explanation

The physician monitors a patient during physiologic exercise (e.g., stationary bicycle) to measure blood flow through and around the heart. During periods of exercise, the arteries become enlarged to allow increased blood flow to supply greater levels of oxygen to the necessary vessels and organs. When plaque is present within a vessel, it does not allow for this enlargement. The oxygenated blood's ability to reach the necessary organs is decreased, which can lead to ischemia. This study is often conducted when narrowing of a coronary artery is discovered during a cardiac catheter procedure.

Coding Tips

When medically necessary, report moderate (conscious) sedation provided by the performing physician with 99151-99153. When provided by another physician, report 99155-99157. This code is reported only one time per [redacted]theterization procedure. Report 93464 in addition to 33477, 93451–93453, [redacted]61, and 93593–93597. For pharmacologic agent administration, [redacted] His recording, see 93600.

[redacted]

This/the[redacted]rimary procedure code that this code is perfo[redacted]tions. Diagnostic code(s) would be the same as the actual p[redacted]

Relative Value Units/Medicare Edits

Non-Facility RVU	Work	PE	MP	Total
93464	1.8	4.61	0.12	6.53
Facility RVU	**Work**	**PE**	**MP**	**Total**
93464	1.8	4.61	0.12	6.53

	FUD	Status	MUE	Modifiers				IOM Reference
93464	N/A	A	1(3)	N/A	N/A	N/A	80*	None

* with documentation

93503

93503 Insertion and placement of flow directed catheter (eg, Swan-Ganz) for monitoring purposes

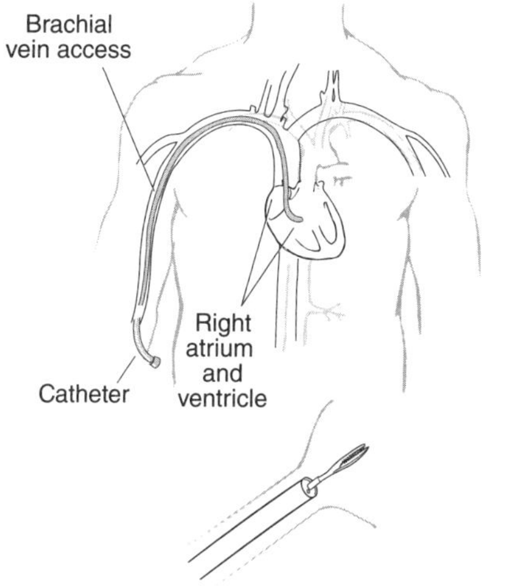

A biopsy tome is inserted through the catheter and several tiny tissue samples are collected from the walls of the heart

Explanation

The physician threads a catheter to the right heart through a central intravenous line often inserted up the femoral vein to take blood samples, pressure and electrical recordings, and/or other tests. This code applies to the insertion of a flow directed catheter, such as the Swan-Ganz device, used for measuring pressure and related parameters.

Coding Tips

Do not report 93503 with 0632T. For subsequent monitoring, see 99418.

ICD-10-CM Diagnostic Codes

I05.0	Rheumatic mitral stenosis
I05.1	Rheumatic mitral insufficiency
I05.2	Rheumatic mitral stenosis with insufficiency
I05.8	Other rheumatic mitral valve diseases
I06.0	Rheumatic aortic stenosis
I06.1	Rheumatic aortic insufficiency
I06.2	Rheumatic aortic stenosis with insufficiency
I06.8	Other rheumatic aortic valve diseases
I07.0	Rheumatic tricuspid stenosis
I07.1	Rheumatic tricuspid insufficiency
I07.2	Rheumatic tricuspid stenosis and insufficiency
I07.8	Other rheumatic tricuspid valve diseases
I08.0	Rheumatic disorders of both mitral and aortic valves
I08.1	Rheumatic disorders of both mitral and tricuspid valves
I08.2	Rheumatic disorders of both aortic and tricuspid valves
I08.3	Combined rheumatic disorders of mitral, aortic and tricuspid valves
I08.8	Other rheumatic multiple valve diseases
I09.0	Rheumatic myocarditis
I09.81	Rheumatic heart failure
I09.89	Other specified rheumatic heart diseases

I20.0	Unstable angina
I21.01	ST elevation (STEMI) myocardial infarction involving left main coronary artery
I21.02	ST elevation (STEMI) myocardial infarction involving left anterior descending coronary artery
I21.09	ST elevation (STEMI) myocardial infarction involving other coronary artery of anterior wall
I21.11	ST elevation (STEMI) myocardial infarction involving right coronary artery
I21.19	ST elevation (STEMI) myocardial infarction involving other coronary artery of inferior wall
I21.21	ST elevation (STEMI) myocardial infarction involving left circumflex coronary artery
I21.29	ST elevation (STEMI) myocardial infarction involving other sites
I21.4	Non-ST elevation (NSTEMI) myocardial infarction
I21.A1	Myocardial infarction type 2
I21.B	Myocardial infarction with coronary microvascular dysfunction
I22.0	Subsequent ST elevation (STEMI) myocardial infarction of anterior wall
I22.1	Subsequent ST elevation (STEMI) myocardial infarction of inferior wall
I22.2	Subsequent non-ST elevation (NSTEMI) myocardial infarction
I22.8	Subsequent ST elevation (STEMI) myocardial infarction of other sites
I25.10	Atherosclerotic heart disease of native coronary artery without angina pectoris A
I25.110	Atherosclerotic heart disease of native coronary artery with unstable angina pectoris A
I25.710	Atherosclerosis of autologous vein coronary artery bypass graft(s) with unstable angina pectoris A
I25.720	Atherosclerosis of autologous artery coronary artery bypass graft(s) with unstable angina pectoris A
I25.730	Atherosclerosis of nonautologous biological coronary artery bypass graft(s) with unstable angina pectoris A
I25.750	Atherosclerosis of native coronary artery of transplanted heart with unstable angina
I25.760	Atherosclerosis of bypass graft of coronary artery of transplanted heart with unstable angina A
I25.790	Atherosclerosis of other coronary artery bypass graft(s) with unstable angina pectoris A
I26.01	Septic pulmonary embolism with acute cor pulmonale
I26.02	Saddle embolus of pulmonary artery with acute cor pulmonale
I26.09	Other pulmonary embolism with acute cor pulmonale
I26.90	Septic pulmonary embolism without acute cor pulmonale
I26.92	Saddle embolus of pulmonary artery without acute cor pulmonale
I26.99	Other pulmonary embolism without acute cor pulmonale
I27.0	Primary pulmonary hypertension
I27.21	Secondary pulmonary arterial hypertension
I27.22	Pulmonary hypertension due to left heart disease
I27.23	Pulmonary hypertension due to lung diseases and hypoxia
I27.24	Chronic thromboembolic pulmonary hypertension
I27.29	Other secondary pulmonary hypertension
I27.81	Cor pulmonale (chronic)
I27.82	Chronic pulmonary embolism
I27.83	Eisenmenger's syndrome
I27.89	Other specified pulmonary heart diseases
I31.4	Cardiac tamponade
I34.0	Nonrheumatic mitral (valve) insufficiency
I34.1	Nonrheumatic mitral (valve) prolapse
I34.2	Nonrheumatic mitral (valve) stenosis
I34.81	Nonrheumatic mitral (valve) annulus calcification
I34.89	Other nonrheumatic mitral valve disorders
I35.0	Nonrheumatic aortic (valve) stenosis
I35.1	Nonrheumatic aortic (valve) insufficiency
I35.2	Nonrheumatic aortic (valve) stenosis with insufficiency
I35.8	Other nonrheumatic aortic valve disorders
I36.0	Nonrheumatic tricuspid (valve) stenosis
I36.1	Nonrheumatic tricuspid (valve) insufficiency
I36.2	Nonrheumatic tricuspid (valve) stenosis with insufficiency
I36.8	Other nonrheumatic tricuspid valve disorders
I37.0	Nonrheumatic pulmonary valve stenosis
I37.1	Nonrheumatic pulmonary valve insufficiency
I37.2	Nonrheumatic pulmonary valve stenosis with insufficiency
I37.8	Other nonrheumatic pulmonary valve disorders
I39	Endocarditis and heart valve disorders in diseases classified elsewhere
I40.0	Infective myocarditis
I40.1	Isolated myocarditis
I40.8	Other acute myocarditis
I41	Myocarditis in diseases classified elsewhere
I46.2	Cardiac arrest due to underlying cardiac condition
I46.8	Cardiac arrest due to other underlying condition
I50.1	Left ventricular failure, unspecified
I50.21	Acute systolic (congestive) heart failure
I50.22	Chronic systolic (congestive) heart [redacted]
I50.23	Acute on chronic syst[redacted]
I50.31	Acute dias[redacted]
I50.32	Ch[redacted]
I50.33	[redacted] heart failure
I5[redacted]	[redacted] systolic (congestive) and diastolic (congestive) heart failure
I50.42	Chronic combined systolic (congestive) and diastolic (congestive) heart failure
I50.43	Acute on chronic combined systolic (congestive) and diastolic (congestive) heart failure
I50.811	Acute right heart failure
I50.812	Chronic right heart failure
I50.813	Acute on chronic right heart failure
I50.814	Right heart failure due to left heart failure
I50.82	Biventricular heart failure
I50.83	High output heart failure
I50.84	End stage heart failure
I97.110	Postprocedural cardiac insufficiency following cardiac surgery
I97.111	Postprocedural cardiac insufficiency following other surgery
I97.120	Postprocedural cardiac arrest following cardiac surgery
I97.121	Postprocedural cardiac arrest following other surgery
I97.130	Postprocedural heart failure following cardiac surgery

I97.131	Postprocedural heart failure following other surgery
I97.190	Other postprocedural cardiac functional disturbances following cardiac surgery
I97.191	Other postprocedural cardiac functional disturbances following other surgery
J81.0	Acute pulmonary edema
J81.1	Chronic pulmonary edema
M32.11	Endocarditis in systemic lupus erythematosus
N17.0	Acute kidney failure with tubular necrosis
N17.1	Acute kidney failure with acute cortical necrosis
N17.2	Acute kidney failure with medullary necrosis
N17.8	Other acute kidney failure
P29.81	Cardiac arrest of newborn N
R57.0	Cardiogenic shock
R57.1	Hypovolemic shock
R57.8	Other shock
R65.21	Severe sepsis with septic shock
T86.22	Heart transplant failure
T86.23	Heart transplant infection
T86.31	Heart-lung transplant rejection
T86.32	Heart-lung transplant failure
T86.33	Heart-lung transplant infection
T86.39	Other complications of heart-lung transplant

AMA: 93503 2023,May; 2022,Jul

Relative Value Units/Medicare Edits

Non-Facility RVU	Work	PE	MP	Total
93503	2.0	0.39	0.18	2.57
Facility RVU	**Work**	**PE**	**MP**	**Total**
93503	2.0	0.39	0.18	2.57

	FUD	Status	MUE	Modifiers				IOM Reference
93503	0	A	2(3)	N/A	N/A	N/A	80*	None

* with documentation

93505

93505 Endomyocardial biopsy

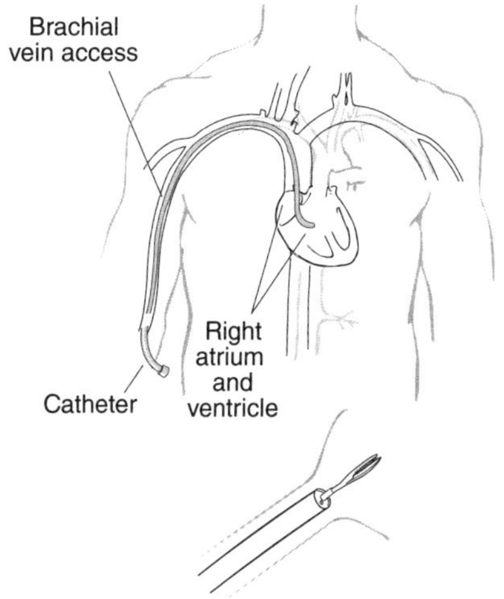

A biopsy tome is inserted through the catheter and several tiny tissue samples are collected from the walls of the heart

Explanation

The physician threads a catheter to the heart through a central intravenous line often inserted up the femoral vein to take tissue samples of the heart's septum.

Coding Tips

When medically necessary, report moderate (conscious) sedation provided by the performing physician with 99151-99153. When provided by another physician report 99155-99157. This code includes all biopsy specimens obtained from one or more endomyocardial sites. Report 76932 in addition to 93505 when ultrasonic guidance is used to obtain the biopsy. For transcatheter placement of a radiation delivery device in coronary intravascular brachytherapy, see 92974. For application of intravascular radioelements, see 77770–77772.

ICD-10-CM Diagnostic Codes

A18.84	Tuberculosis of heart
A52.03	Syphilitic endocarditis
B37.6	Candidal endocarditis
C38.0	Malignant neoplasm of heart
C79.89	Secondary malignant neoplasm of other specified sites
D15.1	Benign neoplasm of heart
D48.7	Neoplasm of uncertain behavior of other specified sites
D49.89	Neoplasm of unspecified behavior of other specified sites
I01.1	Acute rheumatic endocarditis
I25.2	Old myocardial infarction
I25.3	Aneurysm of heart
I33.0	Acute and subacute infective endocarditis
I40.0	Infective myocarditis
I40.1	Isolated myocarditis
I40.8	Other acute myocarditis
I41	Myocarditis in diseases classified elsewhere
I42.0	Dilated cardiomyopathy
I42.1	Obstructive hypertrophic cardiomyopathy

I42.2	Other hypertrophic cardiomyopathy
I42.3	Endomyocardial (eosinophilic) disease
I42.7	Cardiomyopathy due to drug and external agent
I42.8	Other cardiomyopathies
M32.11	Endocarditis in systemic lupus erythematosus
T86.21	Heart transplant rejection
T86.22	Heart transplant failure
T86.31	Heart-lung transplant rejection
T86.32	Heart-lung transplant failure

AMA: **93505** 2023,May

Relative Value Units/Medicare Edits

Non-Facility RVU	Work	PE	MP	Total
93505	4.12	14.21	0.79	19.12
Facility RVU	**Work**	**PE**	**MP**	**Total**
93505	4.12	14.21	0.79	19.12

	FUD	Status	MUE	Modifiers				IOM Reference
93505	0	A	1(2)	51	N/A	N/A	80*	None

* with documentation

Terms To Know

biopsy. Tissue or fluid removed for diagnostic purposes through analysis of the cells in the biopsy material.

catheterization. Use or insertion of a tubular device into a duct, blood vessel, hollow organ, or body cavity for injecting or withdrawing fluids for diagnostic or therapeutic purposes.

diagnostic procedures. Procedure performed on a patient to obtain information to assess the medical condition of the patient or to identify a disease and to determine the nature and severity of an illness or injury.

fluoroscopy. Radiology technique that allows visual examination of part of the body or a function of an organ using a device that projects an x-ray image on a fluorescent screen.

intravascular. Within a blood vessel.

moderate sedation. Medically controlled state of depressed consciousness, with or without analgesia, while maintaining the patient's airway, protective reflexes, and ability to respond to stimulation or verbal commands.

septum. Anatomical partition or dividing wall.

ultrasound. Imaging using ultra-high sound frequency bounced off body structures.

93563

\+ **93563** Injection procedure during cardiac catheterization including imaging supervision, interpretation, and report; for selective coronary angiography during congenital heart catheterization (List separately in addition to code for primary procedure)

Explanation

The physician injects dye into the coronary arteries to evaluate function during congenital heart catheterization procedures. Any required repositioning of catheters or use of automatic power injectors is included in this procedure, as is imaging supervision, interpretation, and report.

Coding Tips

When medically necessary, report moderate (conscious) sedation provided by the performing physician with 99151-99153. When provided by another physician, report 99155-99157. Report 93563 in addition to 33741, 33745, 93582, and 93593–93597. This procedure includes any radiological supervision, interpretation, and report. Contrast administration performed during cardiac catheterization for congenital conditions is reported separately with 93563–93568. Injection procedures for right ventricular, right atrial, aortic, or pulmonary angiogram performed with cardiac catheterizations are reported separately with 93566–93568. Report 93567 for supravalvular ascending aortogram done at the same session as cardiac catheterization. Report 93568 with right heart catheterization codes when done at the same session as a pulmonary angiogram. Injection procedures do not include catheter placement when applicable; however, repositioning of the catheter and automatic power injections should not be reported separately. Do not report 93563–93565 with 93452–93461. Do not report 93563 with 33418, 0345T, 0483T, 0484T, 0544T, or 0545T for coronary angiography intrinsic to the valve repair or annulus reconstruction.

ICD-10-CM Diagnostic Codes

This/these CPT code(s) are add-on code(s). See the primary procedure code that this code is performed with for your ICD-10-CM code selections.

AMA: **93563** 2024,Apr; 2023,Dec; 2023,Jun; 2023,May; 2021,Dec

Relative Value Units/Medicare Edits

Non-Facility RVU	Work	PE	MP	Total
93563	1.0	0.35	0.16	1.51
Facility RVU	**Work**	**PE**	**MP**	**Total**
93563	1.0	0.35	0.16	1.51

	FUD	Status	MUE	Modifiers				IOM Reference
93563	N/A	A	1(3)	N/A	N/A	N/A	80*	None

* with documentation

Terms To Know

aortography. Radiographic visualization of the aorta and its branches by injecting contrast medium through percutaneous puncture or catheterization technique.

congenital anomaly. Abnormality that is present at birth that may be the result of genetic factors, teratogens, or other conditions that affect the fetus in utero. The abnormalities may be readily apparent at birth or may remain undiscovered until some point after birth.

93564

\+ **93564** Injection procedure during cardiac catheterization including imaging supervision, interpretation, and report; for selective opacification of aortocoronary venous or arterial bypass graft(s) (eg, aortocoronary saphenous vein, free radial artery, or free mammary artery graft) to one or more coronary arteries and in situ arterial conduits (eg, internal mammary), whether native or used for bypass to one or more coronary arteries during congenital heart catheterization, when performed (List separately in addition to code for primary procedure)

Explanation

The physician injects dye into the coronary arteries to evaluate function during congenital heart catheterization procedures. This code is used when the physician chooses to visualize a specific aortocoronary vessel bypass graft that communicates with other coronary arteries or conduits. Any required repositioning of catheters or use of automatic power injectors is included in this procedure, as is imaging supervision, interpretation, and report.

Coding Tips

When medically necessary, report moderate (conscious) sedation provided by the performing physician with 99151-99153. When provided by another physician, report 99155-99157. Report 93564 in addition to 93582 and 93593–93597. This procedure includes any radiological supervision, interpretation, and report. Contrast administration performed during cardiac catheterization for congenital conditions is reported separately with 93563–93568. Report 93567 for supravalvular ascending aortogram done at the same session as cardiac catheterization. Injection procedures do not include catheter placement when applicable; however, repositioning of the catheter and automatic power injections should not be reported separately. Do not report 93564 with 93452–93461. Do not report 93564 with 33418, 0345T, 0483T, 0484T, 0544T, or 0545T for coronary angiography intrinsic to the valve repair or annulus reconstruction.

ICD-10-CM Diagnostic Codes

This/these CPT code(s) are add-on code(s). See the primary procedure code that this code is performed with for your ICD-10-CM code selections.

AMA: 93564 2024,Apr; 2023,Jun; 2021,Dec

Relative Value Units/Medicare Edits

Non-Facility RVU	Work	PE	MP	Total
93564	1.03	0.35	0.24	1.62
Facility RVU	**Work**	**PE**	**MP**	**Total**
93564	1.03	0.35	0.24	1.62

	FUD	Status	MUE	Modifiers				IOM Reference
93564	N/A	A	1(3)	N/A	N/A	N/A	80*	None

* with documentation

Terms To Know

aortography. Radiographic visualization of the aorta and its branches by injecting contrast medium through percutaneous puncture or catheterization technique.

bypass graft. Surgically created alternative blood vessel used to reroute blood flow around an area of obstruction or disease.

93565-93566

\+ **93565** Injection procedure during cardiac catheterization including imaging supervision, interpretation, and report; for selective left ventricular or left atrial angiography (List separately in addition to code for primary procedure)

\+ **93566** Injection procedure during cardiac catheterization including imaging supervision, interpretation, and report; for selective right ventricular or right atrial angiography (List separately in addition to code for primary procedure)

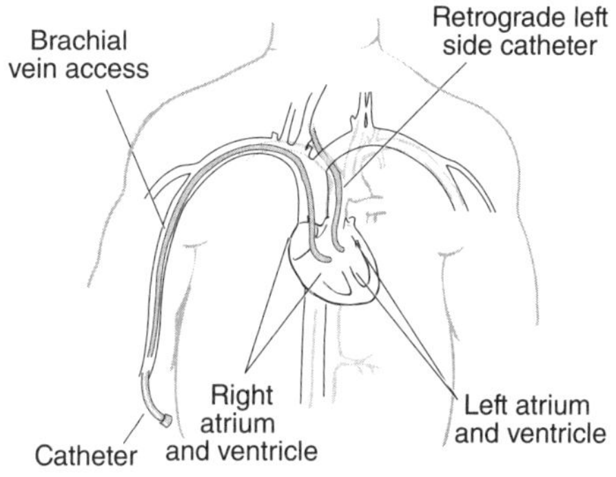

Catheters are placed into the right or left side of the heart

Explanation

The physician injects dye into the coronary arteries to evaluate function during heart catheterization procedures. Code 93565 is specific to the visualization of the left atrium or ventricle during catheterization procedures for congenital anomalies, while 93566 reports that associated with the right atrium or ventricle and may be associated with catheterization procedures for congenital or noncongenital indications. These codes do not report the introduction of catheters, but do include any required repositioning of catheters or use of automatic power injectors, as well as radiological supervision, interpretation, and report.

Coding Tips

When medically necessary, report moderate (conscious) sedation provided by the performing physician with 99151-99153. When provided by another physician, report 99155-99157. Report 93565 in addition to 33741, 33745, 93582, and 93593–93597. Report 93566 in addition to 33741, 33745, 93451, 93453, 93456, 93457, 93460, 93461, 93582, and 93593–93597. These procedures include any radiological supervision, interpretation, and report. Contrast administration performed during cardiac catheterization for congenital conditions is reported separately with 93563–93568. Injection procedures for right ventricular, right atrial, aortic, or pulmonary angiogram performed with cardiac catheterizations are reported separately with 93566–93568. For right ventricular or right atrial angiogram performed during the same session as a cardiac catheterization, report 93566 in addition to the applicable catheterization codes: 93451, 93453, 93456, 93457, 93460, or 93461. Injection procedures do not include catheter placement when applicable; however, repositioning of the catheter and automatic power injections should not be reported separately. Do not report 93565 with 93452–93461. Do not report 93566 with 33274 or 33275 for right ventriculography performed with leadless pacemaker insertion or removal. Do not report 93566 with 0545T for right ventricular or right atrial angiography intrinsic to annulus reconstruction.

ICD-10-CM Diagnostic Codes

This/these CPT code(s) are add-on code(s). See the primary procedure code that this code is performed with for your ICD-10-CM code selections. Diagnostic code(s) would be the same as the actual procedure performed.

AMA: **93565** 2024,Apr; 2023,Dec; 2023,Jun; 2021,Dec **93566** 2024,Apr; 2024,Mar; 2023,Dec; 2023,Jun; 2022,Jul; 2021,Dec; 2019,Mar

Relative Value Units/Medicare Edits

Non-Facility RVU	Work	PE	MP	Total
93565	0.5	0.17	0.12	0.79
93566	0.5	0.17	0.09	0.76
Facility RVU	**Work**	**PE**	**MP**	**Total**
93565	0.5	0.17	0.12	0.79
93566	0.5	0.17	0.09	0.76

	FUD	Status	MUE	Modifiers				IOM Reference
93565	N/A	A	1(3)	N/A	N/A	N/A	80*	None
93566	N/A	A	1(3)	N/A	N/A	N/A	80*	

* with documentation

Terms To Know

angiogram. Radiographic image of the arteries. Imaging may be performed to study the vasculature of any given organ, body system, or area of circulation such as the brain, heart, chest, kidneys, limbs, gastrointestinal tract, aorta, and pulmonary circulation to visualize the formation and the function of the blood vessels to detect problems such as a blockage or stricture.

catheterization. Use or insertion of a tubular device into a duct, blood vessel, hollow organ, or body cavity for injecting or withdrawing fluids for diagnostic or therapeutic purposes.

contrast material. Any internally administered substance that has a different opacity from soft tissue on radiography or computed tomograph; includes barium, used to opacify parts of the gastrointestinal tract; water-soluble iodinated compounds, used to opacify blood vessels or the genitourinary tract; may refer to air occurring naturally or introduced into the body; also, paramagnetic substances used in magnetic resonance imaging. Substances may also be documented as contrast agent or contrast medium.

supervision and interpretation. Radiology services that usually contain an invasive component and are reported by the radiologist for supervision of the procedure and the personnel involved with performing the examination, reading the film, and preparing the written report.

93567

\+ **93567** Injection procedure during cardiac catheterization including imaging supervision, interpretation, and report; for supravalvular aortography (List separately in addition to code for primary procedure)

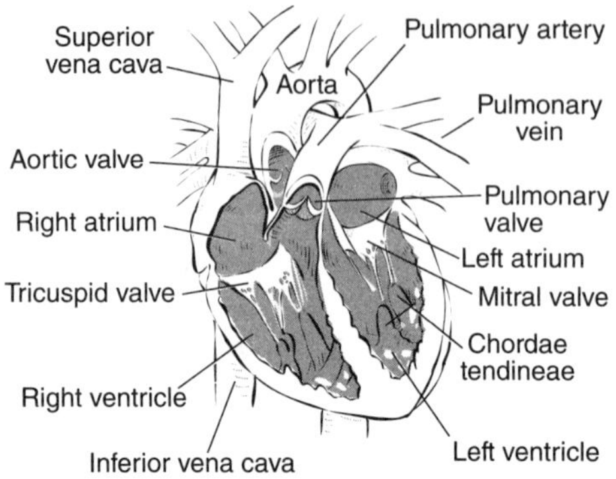

Injection for supravalvular aortography or pulmonary angiography

Explanation

In conjunction with congenital or noncongenital heart catheterization procedures, the physician injects dye into an area of interest to perform an aortogram. Code 93567 is specific to supravalvular ascending aortography, or the visualization of the valves just above the aorta and its branches. The physician repositions the previously placed catheter and attaches it to a power injector, making sure that air is removed from the tubing. After the catheter is positioned (using fluoroscopic guidance to confirm placement) power injection is performed to fill the aorta. Arterial pressures, electrocardiogram, and oxygen saturation are continuously monitored throughout the procedure. Upon injection completion, the injector is detached from the catheter. Note that 93567 does not report the introduction of catheters but does include any required repositioning of catheters or the use of automatic power injectors, as well as radiological supervision, interpretation, and report.

Coding Tips

When medically necessary, report moderate (conscious) sedation provided by the performing physician with 99151-99153. When provided by another physician, report 99155-99157. Report 93567 in addition to 33741, 33745, 93451–93461, and 93593–93597. This procedure includes any radiological supervision, interpretation, and report. Contrast administration performed during cardiac catheterization for congenital conditions is reported separately with 93563–93568. Injection procedures for right ventricular, right atrial, aortic, or pulmonary angiogram performed with cardiac catheterizations are reported separately with 93567–93568. Report 93567 for supravalvular ascending aortogram done at the same session as cardiac catheterization. Injection procedures do not include catheter placement when applicable; however, repositioning of the catheter and automatic power injections should not be reported separately. For non-supravalvular aortography or abdominal aortography performed at the time of cardiac catheterization, see 36221 and 75600–75630.

ICD-10-CM Diagnostic Codes

This/these CPT code(s) are add-on code(s). See the primary procedure code that this code is performed with for your ICD-10-CM code selections. Diagnostic code(s) would be the same as the actual procedure performed.

AMA: **93567** 2024,Apr; 2023,Dec; 2023,Jun; 2021,Dec

Relative Value Units/Medicare Edits

Non-Facility RVU	Work	PE	MP	Total
93567	0.7	0.24	0.16	1.1
Facility RVU	**Work**	**PE**	**MP**	**Total**
93567	0.7	0.24	0.16	1.1

	FUD	Status	MUE	Modifiers				IOM Reference
93567	N/A	A	1(3)	N/A	N/A	N/A	80*	None

* with documentation

Terms To Know

aortography. Radiographic visualization of the aorta and its branches by injecting contrast medium through percutaneous puncture or catheterization technique.

congenital. Present at birth, occurring through heredity or an influence during gestation up to the moment of birth.

contrast material. Any internally administered substance that has a different opacity from soft tissue on radiography or computed tomograph; includes barium, used to opacify parts of the gastrointestinal tract; water-soluble iodinated compounds, used to opacify blood vessels or the genitourinary tract; may refer to air occurring naturally or introduced into the body; also, paramagnetic substances used in magnetic resonance imaging. Substances may also be documented as contrast agent or contrast medium.

supra. Above.

valve. Fold or membrane within a body canal or passageway that prevents backflow of fluids running through it.

93568-93569 [93573, 93574, 93575]

\+ **93568** Injection procedure during cardiac catheterization including imaging supervision, interpretation, and report; for nonselective pulmonary arterial angiography (List separately in addition to code for primary procedure)

\+ **93569** Injection procedure during cardiac catheterization including imaging supervision, interpretation, and report; for selective pulmonary arterial angiography, unilateral (List separately in addition to code for primary procedure)

\+ **93573** Injection procedure during cardiac catheterization including imaging supervision, interpretation, and report; for selective pulmonary arterial angiography, bilateral (List separately in addition to code for primary procedure)

\+ **93574** Injection procedure during cardiac catheterization including imaging supervision, interpretation, and report; for selective pulmonary venous angiography of each distinct pulmonary vein during cardiac catheterization (List separately in addition to code for primary procedure)

\+ **93575** Injection procedure during cardiac catheterization including imaging supervision, interpretation, and report; for selective pulmonary angiography of major aortopulmonary collateral arteries (MAPCAs) arising off the aorta or its systemic branches, during cardiac catheterization for congenital heart defects, each distinct vessel (List separately in addition to code for primary procedure)

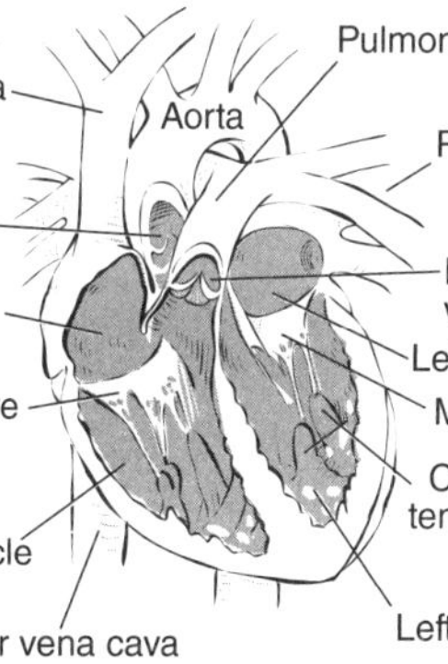

Injection during cardiac catheterization for arterial or venous angiography

Explanation

The physician injects dye into the pulmonary arteries to evaluate function during congenital or noncongenital heart catheterization procedures. Code 93568 is specific to nonselective pulmonary arterial angiography, in which the catheter remains in the vessel originally punctured or advances only to the aorta, at which point dye is injected for visualization of the pulmonary arteries. The physician repositions the previously placed catheter and attaches it to a power injector, making sure that air is removed from the tubing. After the catheter is positioned (using fluoroscopic guidance to confirm placement), power injection is performed to fill the aorta. Arterial pressures, electrocardiogram, and oxygen saturation are continuously monitored throughout the procedure. Upon injection completion, the injector is detached from the catheter. Codes 93569 and 93573 are specific to selective pulmonary arterial angiography, in which the catheter is advanced from the original vessel punctured or from an artery that branches off the aorta. Report 93569 for unilateral visualization of pulmonary arteries in the left or right lung, and

Medicine

93573 for bilateral visualization of the pulmonary arteries in both the left and right lungs. Report 93574 for selective pulmonary venous angiography of each distinct pulmonary vein during cardiac catheterization and 93575 for selective pulmonary angiography of major aortopulmonary collateral arteries (MAPCAs) arising off the aorta or its systemic branches during cardiac catheterization for congenital heart defects (each distinct vessel). These codes include radiological supervision, interpretation, and report.

Coding Tips

When medically necessary, report moderate (conscious) sedation provided by the performing physician with 99151-99153. When provided by another physician, report 99155-99157. Report 93568, 93569, and 93573–93575 in addition to 33361–33366, 33418, 33419, 33477, 33741, 33745, 33894, 33895, 33900–33904, 37187, 37188, 37236–37238, 37246, 37248, 92997, 92998, 93451, 93453, 93456, 93457, 93460, 93461, 93580–93583, and 93593–93597. Report 93569 and 93573–93575 in addition to 93505. These procedures include any radiological supervision, interpretation, and report. Contrast administration performed during cardiac catheterization for congenital conditions is reported separately with 93563–93568. Injection procedures for right ventricular, right atrial, aortic, or pulmonary angiogram performed with cardiac catheterizations are reported separately with 93567–93568. Report 93568 with right heart catheterization codes when done at the same session as a pulmonary angiogram. Injection procedures do not include catheter placement when applicable; however, repositioning of the catheter and automatic power injections should not be reported separately. Do not report 93568 with 33289 or 0632T. Selective introduction and positioning of angiographic catheter, injection, and radiologic supervision and interpretation are included with 93569 and 93573–93575 and should not be reported separately.

ICD-10-CM Diagnostic Codes

This/these CPT code(s) are add-on code(s). See the primary procedure code that this code is performed with for your ICD-10-CM code selections. Diagnostic code(s) would be the same as the actual procedure performed.

AMA: **93568** 2024,Apr; 2024,Feb; 2023,Dec; 2023,Jun; 2023,May; 2021,Dec; 2019,Jun; 2019,Apr **93569** 2024,Apr; 2024,Feb; 2023,Dec; 2023,May **93573** 2024,Apr; 2024,Feb; 2023,Dec; 2023,May **93574** 2024,Apr; 2024,Feb; 2023,Dec; 2023,May **93575** 2024,Apr; 2024,Feb; 2023,Dec; 2023,May

Relative Value Units/Medicare Edits

Non-Facility RVU	Work	PE	MP	Total
93568	0.88	0.3	0.18	1.36
93569	0.78	0.27	0.06	1.11
93573	1.3	0.45	0.09	1.84
93574	1.44	0.5	0.11	2.05
93575	1.92	0.66	0.14	2.72
Facility RVU	**Work**	**PE**	**MP**	**Total**
93568	0.88	0.3	0.18	1.36
93569	0.78	0.27	0.06	1.11
93573	1.3	0.45	0.09	1.84
93574	1.44	0.5	0.11	2.05
93575	1.92	0.66	0.14	2.72

	FUD	Status	MUE	Modifiers				IOM Reference
93568	N/A	A	1(3)	N/A	N/A	N/A	80*	None
93569	N/A	A	1(2)	N/A	N/A	N/A	80*	
93573	N/A	A	1(2)	N/A	N/A	N/A	80*	
93574	N/A	A	4(2)	N/A	N/A	N/A	80*	
93575	N/A	A	4(3)	N/A	N/A	N/A	80*	

* with documentation

Terms To Know

angiography. Radiographic imaging of the arteries.

catheterization. Use or insertion of a tubular device into a duct, blood vessel, hollow organ, or body cavity for injecting or withdrawing fluids for diagnostic or therapeutic purposes.

congenital. Present at birth, occurring through heredity or an influence during gestation up to the moment of birth.

93571-93572

\+ **93571** Intravascular Doppler velocity and/or pressure derived coronary flow reserve measurement (coronary vessel or graft) during coronary angiography including pharmacologically induced stress; initial vessel (List separately in addition to code for primary procedure)

\+ **93572** each additional vessel (List separately in addition to code for primary procedure)

Explanation

The physician measures intravascular Doppler velocity and/or pressure derived fractional flow reserve (FFR) or coronary flow reserve (CFR) during a coronary angiography to determine the hemodynamic significance of a lesion. A guidewire is passed through the coronary vessel or graft, and the baseline flow is measured distal to the lesion. Pharmacologic stress is induced with a bolus or infusion of a radiopharmaceutical agent such as adenosine; velocity blood flow measurements are taken and/or the FFR or CFR is calculated. The guidewire is repositioned in an unaffected artery and measurements are repeated for comparison. Report 93571 for Doppler measurements of the initial vessel; this is an add-on code to be reported with the appropriate primary procedure for the coronary or bypass graft diagnostic or interventional service. Report 93572 for each additional vessel.

Coding Tips

When medically necessary, report moderate (conscious) sedation provided by the performing physician with 99151-99153. When provided by another physician, report 99155-99157. Report 93571 in addition to 92920, 92924, 92928, 92933, 92937, 92941, 92943, 92975, 93454-93461, 93563, 93564, 93593–93597, and 0913T. Use 93572 in addition to 93571. Do not report 93571 or 93572 in addition to 0523T. Any required manipulation or repositioning of the Doppler transducer within the specific vessel being examined is included and should not be reported separately.

ICD-10-CM Diagnostic Codes

This/these CPT code(s) are add-on code(s). See the primary procedure code that this code is performed with for your ICD-10-CM code selections. Diagnostic code(s) would be the same as the actual procedure performed.

AMA: **93571** 2024,Mar

Relative Value Units/Medicare Edits

Non-Facility RVU	Work	PE	MP	Total
93571	0.0	0.0	0.0	0.0
93572	0.0	0.0	0.0	0.0
Facility RVU	**Work**	**PE**	**MP**	**Total**
93571	0.0	0.0	0.0	0.0
93572	0.0	0.0	0.0	0.0

	FUD	Status	MUE	Modifiers				IOM Reference
93571	N/A	C	1(3)	N/A	N/A	N/A	80*	None
93572	N/A	C	2(3)	N/A	N/A	N/A	80*	

* with documentation

Terms To Know

doppler. Ultrasonography used to augment two-dimensional images by registering velocity. When emitted sound waves reflect back off a moving object, the frequency of the reflected sound waves varies in relation to the speed of the moving object and may be used in many different procedures.

93580

93580 Percutaneous transcatheter closure of congenital interatrial communication (ie, Fontan fenestration, atrial septal defect) with implant

Atrial septal defects are small holes in the wall between the left and right atria. This can result in a right-to-left or left-to-right shunt

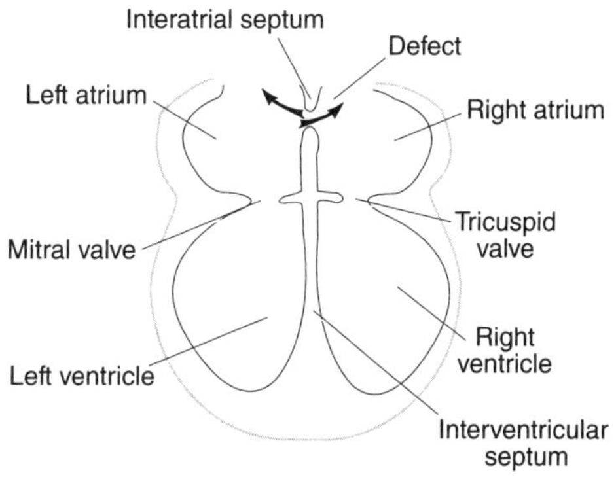

Posterior schematic showing atrial septal defect

Explanation

A congenital atrial septal defect is closed percutaneously by catheter. This procedure may be performed on infants or adults, usually under moderate sedation. After heparinization in induced, a combined right and left heart catheterization is first undertaken through the existing septal opening. Contrast material is injected for atrial and ventricular angiograms to map the anatomy. Using a specialized catheter, the atrial defect is crossed from the right atrium into the left. The catheter is threaded into the upper left pulmonary vein. A guidewire is inserted, the catheter is removed, and a balloon is threaded over the guidewire into position across the defect and inflated with low pressure. The "stretched" diameter of the defect is measured. Testing is carried out to ensure that the repair will remain hemodynamically stable by occluding the defect temporarily with the balloon while taking right-side pressures and saturation measurements. A dilator and sheath holding the device are advanced over the guidewire and positioned in the left atrium. Positioning is checked using echocardiography or fluoroscopy before releasing the device. The implant is deployed across the atrial opening and positioning is checked again. Any leaks, abnormal placement, or an improperly sized device may require removal of the implant and placement of a second device. The catheters and guidewires are removed.

Coding Tips

This procedure includes a right heart catheterization and injection of contrast for atrial and ventricular angiograms. Do not report 93580 with 93451–93453, 93456–93461, 93565–93566, or 93593–93598. For echocardiographic services performed with 93580, see 93303–93317 and 93662 as appropriate.

ICD-10-CM Diagnostic Codes

Q21.11	Secundum atrial septal defect
Q21.12	Patent foramen ovale
Q21.13	Coronary sinus atrial septal defect
Q21.14	Superior sinus venosus atrial septal defect
Q21.15	Inferior sinus venosus atrial septal defect
Q21.19	Other specified atrial septal defect
Q21.21	Partial atrioventricular septal defect
Q21.22	Transitional atrioventricular septal defect

Q21.23 Complete atrioventricular septal defect

AMA: **93580** 2023,May

Relative Value Units/Medicare Edits

Non-Facility RVU	Work	PE	MP	Total
93580	17.97	6.51	4.04	28.52
Facility RVU	**Work**	**PE**	**MP**	**Total**
93580	17.97	6.51	4.04	28.52

	FUD	Status	MUE	Modifiers				IOM Reference
93580	0	A	1(3)	51	N/A	N/A	80*	None

* with documentation

Terms To Know

angiography. Radiographic imaging of the arteries. Imaging may be performed to study the vasculature of any given organ, body system, or area of circulation such as the brain, heart, chest, kidneys, limbs, gastrointestinal tract, aorta, and pulmonary circulation to visualize the formation and the function of the blood vessels to detect problems such as a blockage or stricture. A catheter is inserted through an accessible blood vessel and the artery is injected with a radiopaque contrast material after which x-rays are taken.

anomaly. Irregularity in the structure or position of an organ or tissue.

atria. Two upper chambers of the heart. The left and right atria are divided by the septum, a muscular wall.

catheterization. Use or insertion of a tubular device into a duct, blood vessel, hollow organ, or body cavity for injecting or withdrawing fluids for diagnostic or therapeutic purposes.

congenital. Present at birth, occurring through heredity or an influence during gestation up to the moment of birth.

fluoroscopy. Radiology technique that allows visual examination of part of the body or a function of an organ using a device that projects an x-ray image on a fluorescent screen.

implant. Material or device inserted or placed within the body for therapeutic, reconstructive, or diagnostic purposes.

septum. Anatomical partition or dividing wall.

93581

93581 Percutaneous transcatheter closure of a congenital ventricular septal defect with implant

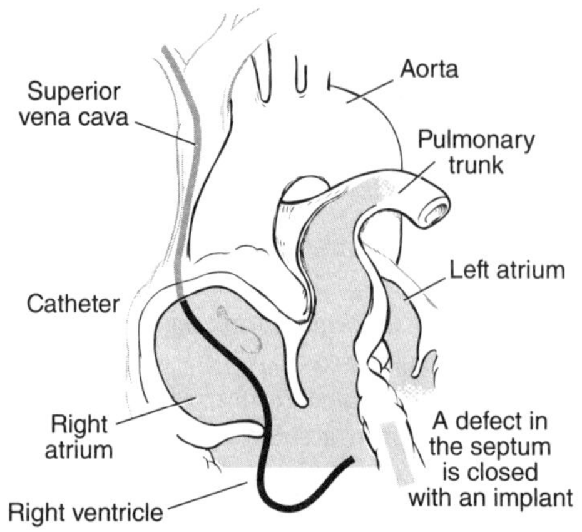

A ventricular septal defect (VSD) is addressed transcatheterally inserted percutaneously. Closure is accomplished using an implant

Explanation

A congenital ventricular septal defect is closed percutaneously by catheter. The patient is given local anesthesia and the femoral artery and vein are cannulated. A guidewire and catheter are inserted and advanced through the ventricular septum, into the right ventricle, and across the tricuspid valve into the right atrium. A separate venous sheath is placed in the jugular vein to allow passage of a snare catheter. The snare is advanced into the atrium and grasps the free wire or catheter that was threaded through the ventricular septal defect. This provides a through-and-through from the femoral vein to the ventricular septal defect and out the jugular. The jugular end is used to pass a dilator and sheath over the defect for the positioning of the occlusive device into the left ventricle. The sheath must be in the exact position with its tip in the left ventricle for delivery of the occlusive device. If necessary, traction is used at the opposite end to secure the sheath as the dilator is removed. If the sheath is displaced during removal of the dilator, the dilator is reinserted for correct positioning. Once the sheath is in place and the dilator removed, the delivery catheter loaded with an occlusive device is advanced to the center of the right atrium. The device is advanced out of the delivery catheter and into the tip of the sheath. It is gently advanced so that the distal legs are in the left ventricle and the center of the device is in the defect. A slight withdrawing of the sheath causes the distal legs to open within the left ventricle. Further withdrawal of the sheath allows the proximal legs to open in the right ventricle. The occlusion is confirmed with angiography and the delivery system and catheters are removed.

Coding Tips

This procedure includes a right heart catheterization and injection of contrast for atrial and ventricular angiograms. Do not report 93581 with 93451–93453, 93456–93461, 93565–93566, or 93593–93598. For echocardiographic services performed in addition to 93581, see 93303–93317 and 93662 as appropriate.

ICD-10-CM Diagnostic Codes

Q21.0 Ventricular septal defect

AMA: **93581** 2023,May

Relative Value Units/Medicare Edits

Non-Facility RVU	Work	PE	MP	Total
93581	24.39	8.67	5.64	38.7
Facility RVU	**Work**	**PE**	**MP**	**Total**
93581	24.39	8.67	5.64	38.7

	FUD	Status	MUE	Modifiers				IOM Reference
93581	0	A	1(3)	51	N/A	N/A	80*	None

* with documentation

Terms To Know

cannulation. Insertion of a flexible length of hollow tubing into a blood vessel, duct, or body cavity, usually for extracorporeal circulation or chemotherapy infusion to a particular region of the body.

congenital. Present at birth, occurring through heredity or an influence during gestation up to the moment of birth.

distal. *1)* Located farther away from a specified reference point or the trunk. *2)* Pertaining to the area farthest from the center of the body or the point of origin.

guidewire. Flexible metal instrument designed to lead another instrument in its proper course.

percutaneous. Through the skin.

proximal. Located closest to a specified reference point, usually the midline or trunk.

septum. Anatomical partition or dividing wall.

snare. Wire used as a loop to excise a polyp or lesion.

ventricular septal defect. Congenital cardiac anomaly resulting in a continual opening in the septum between the ventricles that, in severe cases, causes oxygenated blood to flow back into the lungs, resulting in pulmonary hypertension.

93582

93582 Percutaneous transcatheter closure of patent ductus arteriosus

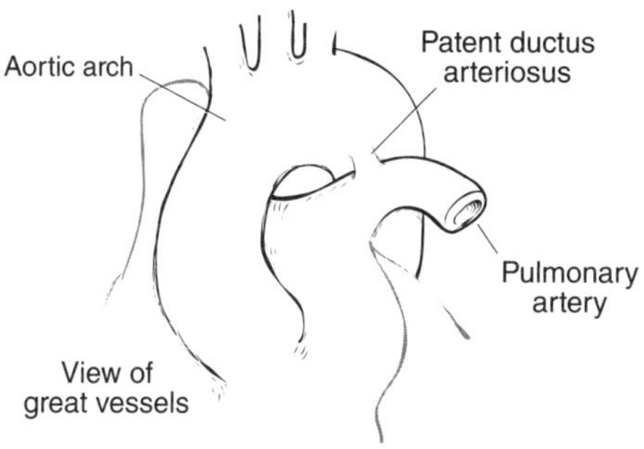

The ductus arteriosus is the natural shunt that bypasses lung circulation in the prenatal phase

Explanation

A patent ductus arteriosus (PDA) is closed using a transcatheter technique. A small incision is made in an extremity artery (usually the femoral artery). The physician threads a catheter through the arteries and heart to the PDA. A coil or other occlusion device is deployed into the PDA via the catheter. An angiography may be performed to check for patency of the closure device. The catheter is removed and the incision is closed.

Coding Tips

When medically necessary, report moderate (conscious) sedation provided by the performing physician with 99151-99153. When provided by another physician, report 99155-99157. This procedure includes catheter placement in the aorta, congenital right and left heart catheterization, as well as aortic arch angiography, if performed, and they may not be reported separately. Do not report 93582 with 36013, 36014, 36200, 75600, 75605, 93451, 93453, 93456–93461, 93567, or 93593–93598. For other cardiac angiography performed, see 93563–93566 or 93568. For left heart catheterization by transseptal puncture through intact septum or by transapical puncture, see 93462. For repair of patent ductus arteriosus by ligation, see 33820, 33822, or 33824. For intracardiac echocardiography services performed during the procedure, see 93662. Other echocardiographic procedures provided by another individual are reported with 93315–99317. For other cardiac angiographic procedures performed at the time of PDA closure, see 93563–93566, 93568, 93569, and 93573–93575.

ICD-10-CM Diagnostic Codes

Q25.0 Patent ductus arteriosus

AMA: 93582 2023,May; 2019,Apr

Relative Value Units/Medicare Edits

Non-Facility RVU	Work	PE	MP	Total
93582	12.31	4.18	2.83	19.32
Facility RVU	**Work**	**PE**	**MP**	**Total**
93582	12.31	4.18	2.83	19.32

	FUD	Status	MUE	Modifiers				IOM Reference
93582	0	A	1(2)	51	N/A	N/A	80*	None

* with documentation

93583

93583 Percutaneous transcatheter septal reduction therapy (eg, alcohol septal ablation) including temporary pacemaker insertion when performed

Explanation

Septal reduction therapy, also known as alcohol septal ablation (ASA), is performed to decrease the size of the cardiac septal muscle in patients with hypertrophic cardiomyopathy. A small incision is made in an extremity artery (usually the femoral artery). A catheter is threaded through the arteries to the heart and a coronary angiography is performed to locate the first septal perforator branch of the left anterior descending (LAD) artery. A balloon is inflated within the perforator and contrast is injected to ensure no flow back into the LAD. A slow injection of absolute alcohol is performed until a partial initial response is rendered. The balloon is deflated and an additional coronary angiogram is performed to ensure patency of the LAD. The catheters are removed and the incision is closed.

Coding Tips

When medically necessary, report moderate (conscious) sedation provided by the performing physician with 99151-99153. When provided by another physician, report 99155-99157. This procedure includes insertion of a temporary pacemaker and left heart catheterization. It also includes left anterior descending coronary angiography for the purpose of guiding the intervention. Diagnostic cardiac catheterization (93451, 93454–93457, 93563, 93564, 93566–93569, 93573–93575, 93593, 93594, 93598) may only be reported separately when no prior catheter-based study of the treatment area is available, the prior studies are inadequate, or the patient's condition has changed significantly enough to warrant the additional study. Do not report 93583 with 33210, 93452, 93453, 93458–93461, 93565, or 93595–93597. Do not report 93463 for the injection of alcohol for the procedure. For intracardiac echocardiography services performed during the procedure, see 93662.

ICD-10-CM Diagnostic Codes

I42.1	Obstructive hypertrophic cardiomyopathy
I42.2	Other hypertrophic cardiomyopathy
Q24.8	Other specified congenital malformations of heart

AMA: 93583 2023,May; 2019,Apr

Relative Value Units/Medicare Edits

Non-Facility RVU	Work	PE	MP	Total
93583	13.75	4.77	3.16	21.68
Facility RVU	**Work**	**PE**	**MP**	**Total**
93583	13.75	4.77	3.16	21.68

	FUD	Status	MUE	Modifiers				IOM Reference
93583	0	A	1(2)	51	N/A	N/A	80*	None

* with documentation

Terms To Know

cardiomyopathy. General term used to describe a number of conditions of the heart muscle.

congenital. Present at birth, occurring through heredity or an influence during gestation up to the moment of birth.

septum. Anatomical partition or dividing wall.

93590-93592

93590 Percutaneous transcatheter closure of paravalvular leak; initial occlusion device, mitral valve

93591 initial occlusion device, aortic valve

\+ **93592** each additional occlusion device (List separately in addition to code for primary procedure)

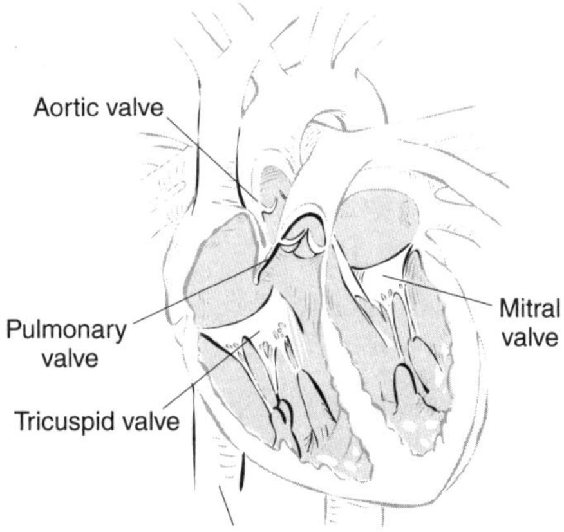

Paravalvular leak is repaired with an occlusion device

Explanation

Percutaneous transcatheter closure of a paravalvular leak (PVL) in the mitral or aortic valve can be achieved by antegrade or retrograde approach. A transesophageal echocardiogram (TEE) for a mitral valve leak or a transthoracic echocardiogram (TTE) for an aortic leak was performed within the previous six months, earlier if the patient was symptomatic. A retrograde transfemoral approach is performed utilizing a catheter and guidewire. Upon crossing the leak, the wire is removed and a stiff wire is inserted along with the device delivery system consisting of a guide catheter or sheath. The wire is removed allowing for advancement and deployment of an occlusion device. In cases where support becomes an issue, a transseptal access and snare may be employed to establish a rail. This entails the snaring of the initial wire within the left atrium or the formation of an apical ventricular rail by left ventricular puncture with the wire crossing the apex. In mitral PVL, if this approach does not achieve the desired results, an antegrade transseptal approach may be used. Upon completion of the procedure for 93590, TEE should indicate fluent leaflets, clear pulmonary veins, and if anterior leak, clear mitral valve. In 93591, the physician must evaluate that the coronary ostia is not covered and leaflets are fluent. For both procedures, the device deployed is dependent upon the defect size. Many closure devices are currently used in these procedures, such as embolization coils, double-umbrella devices, occluders, and plugs approved for other specific defects and may be suitable in most cases. However for PVLs they are limited by size, shape, specific characteristics, and features of delivery system. Report 93592 for each additional occlusion device.

Coding Tips

Report 93592 in addition to 93590 and 93591. Percutaneous access, fluoroscopy, angiography, placement of the access sheath, maneuvering the delivery system to the leak, device deployment, and positioning and repositioning the closure device are included in 93590 and 93591. Additional diagnostic cardiac catheterization procedures unrelated to the PVL closure may be reported separately. Do not report 93590 or 93591 with 93462 for transseptal puncture but do report transapical puncture (93462) with 93590 or 93591. Diagnostic catheterization and diagnostic coronary angiography codes may be reported in addition to 93590 or 93591 in cases where a previous examination is not available or the anatomic visualization is poor quality, there has been a clinical change in the patient's condition since the previous examination, or complications arise during the procedure requiring the additional study.

ICD-10-CM Diagnostic Codes

T82.03XA Leakage of heart valve prosthesis, initial encounter

T82.09XA Other mechanical complication of heart valve prosthesis, initial encounter

T82.223A Leakage of biological heart valve graft, initial encounter

T82.228A Other mechanical complication of biological heart valve graft, initial encounter

Relative Value Units/Medicare Edits

Non-Facility RVU	Work	PE	MP	Total
93590	21.7	7.8	1.76	31.26
93591	17.97	6.39	1.34	25.7
93592	8.0	2.72	0.54	11.26
Facility RVU	**Work**	**PE**	**MP**	**Total**
93590	21.7	7.8	1.76	31.26
93591	17.97	6.39	1.34	25.7
93592	8.0	2.72	0.54	11.26

	FUD	Status	MUE	Modifiers				IOM Reference
93590	0	A	1(2)	51	N/A	62*	80	None
93591	0	A	1(2)	51	N/A	62	80*	
93592	N/A	A	2(3)	N/A	N/A	62*	80	

* with documentation

Terms To Know

embolization. Placement of a clotting agent, such as a coil, plastic particles, gel, foam, etc., into an area of hemorrhage to stop the bleeding or to block blood flow to a problem area, such as an aneurysm or a tumor.

occlusion. Constriction, closure, or blockage of a passage.

retrograde. Moving against the usual direction of flow.

transcatheter. Procedure or treatment performed via a catheter.

transesophageal echocardiography. Guidance of a small probe into the esophagus under sedation to closely evaluate the heart and blood vessels within the chest.

93593-93594

93593 Right heart catheterization for congenital heart defect(s) including imaging guidance by the proceduralist to advance the catheter to the target zone; normal native connections

93594 Right heart catheterization for congenital heart defect(s) including imaging guidance by the proceduralist to advance the catheter to the target zone; abnormal native connections

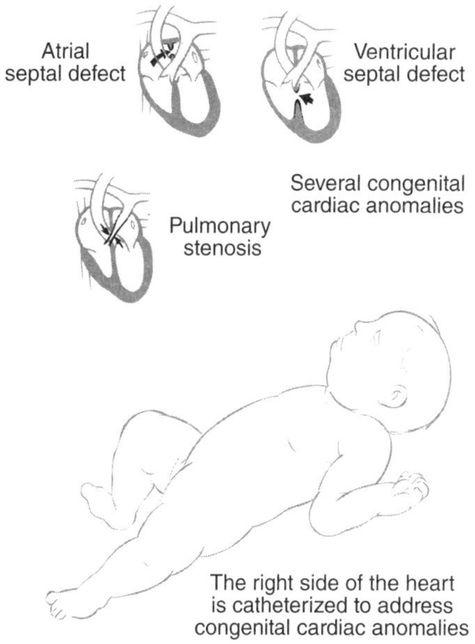

Explanation

The physician performs a right heart catheterization for congenital cardiac anomalies (regardless of patient's age). The physician investigates congenital cardiac anomalies by measuring pressures, taking blood samples for oximetry, and/or injecting contrast to assess chamber size and function. The physician places an introducer sheath in a vein (typically, the femoral vein) using percutaneous puncture. The physician places a lumen catheter through the introducer sheath into the femoral vein and advances it, under fluoroscopic guidance, to the heart chamber receiving venous circulation. The physician may use the fluid-filled catheter to record intracardiac pressures, withdraw blood samples, or inject radiopaque contrast material. The physician removes the catheter and sheath from the femoral vein. Pressure is placed on the wound for 20 to 30 minutes to stem bleeding. Report 93593 for a procedure performed on a patient with normal native connections (those in which the blood flow pathway follows the expected course through the right and left heart chambers and great vessels) and 93594 for a patient whose native connections are abnormal (those that exist when the blood flow pathway through the heart and great vessels follows alternative connections).

Coding Tips

Code selection for right heart catheterization for congenital heart defects is based on whether the patient's native anatomic connections from the great veins to the atria, atria to the ventricles, and ventricles to the great arteries are normal or abnormal. Normal native connection exists when the path of blood flow follows the typical course through the right and left heart chambers and great vessels. Abnormal native connection exists when the path of blood flow follows an alternative course through the heart and great vessels due to altered connections. These codes include obtaining blood samples for blood gas measurement, Fick cardiac output measurements, and catheter placement in one of more of the following: right atrium, right ventricle, pulmonary artery, and pulmonary wedge. These codes include fluoroscopy and ultrasound guidance for vascular access and catheter placement for hemodynamic evaluation when performed by the same clinician. In congenital heart disease, the subpulmonic ventricle may be a morphologic left ventricle and the subpulmonic atrium may be a morphologic left atrium; in either case, both structures are considered part of the right heart catheterization and left heart catheterization would not be reported separately. Thermodilution cardiac output assessment is not inherent in right heart catheterization for congenital cardiac anomalies and may be reported separately, see 93598. For right ventricular or right atrial angiography, see 93566. For insertion and placement of flow directed catheter for monitoring purposes when not performed along with other catheterization services, see 93503. For pharmacologic agent administration or physiological exercise study with cardiac catheterization, see 93463 or 93464. For contrast injections during cardiac catheterization for congenital heart defects, see 93563–93569, 93573–93575, and 93584–93588.

ICD-10-CM Diagnostic Codes

Q20.0	Common arterial trunk
Q20.1	Double outlet right ventricle
Q20.3	Discordant ventriculoarterial connection
Q20.4	Double inlet ventricle
Q20.5	Discordant atrioventricular connection
Q20.6	Isomerism of atrial appendages
Q20.8	Other congenital malformations of cardiac chambers and connections
Q21.0	Ventricular septal defect
Q21.11	Secundum atrial septal defect
Q21.12	Patent foramen ovale
Q21.13	Coronary sinus atrial septal defect
Q21.14	Superior sinus venosus atrial septal defect
Q21.15	Inferior sinus venosus atrial septal defect
Q21.21	Partial atrioventricular septal defect
Q21.22	Transitional atrioventricular septal defect
Q21.23	Complete atrioventricular septal defect
Q21.3	Tetralogy of Fallot
Q21.4	Aortopulmonary septal defect
Q22.0	Pulmonary valve atresia
Q22.1	Congenital pulmonary valve stenosis
Q22.2	Congenital pulmonary valve insufficiency
Q22.3	Other congenital malformations of pulmonary valve
Q22.4	Congenital tricuspid stenosis
Q22.5	Ebstein's anomaly
Q22.6	Hypoplastic right heart syndrome
Q23.0	Congenital stenosis of aortic valve
Q23.1	Congenital insufficiency of aortic valve
Q23.2	Congenital mitral stenosis
Q23.3	Congenital mitral insufficiency
Q23.81	Bicuspid aortic valve
Q23.82	Congenital mitral valve cleft leaflet
Q23.88	Other congenital malformations of aortic and mitral valves
Q24.0	Dextrocardia
Q24.1	Levocardia
Q24.2	Cor triatriatum
Q24.3	Pulmonary infundibular stenosis
Q24.4	Congenital subaortic stenosis
Q24.5	Malformation of coronary vessels
Q24.6	Congenital heart block
Q24.8	Other specified congenital malformations of heart
Q25.0	Patent ductus arteriosus
Q25.1	Coarctation of aorta
Q25.21	Interruption of aortic arch
Q25.29	Other atresia of aorta
Q25.3	Supravalvular aortic stenosis
Q25.41	Absence and aplasia of aorta
Q25.42	Hypoplasia of aorta
Q25.43	Congenital aneurysm of aorta
Q25.44	Congenital dilation of aorta
Q25.45	Double aortic arch
Q25.46	Tortuous aortic arch
Q25.47	Right aortic arch
Q25.48	Anomalous origin of subclavian artery
Q25.49	Other congenital malformations of aorta
Q25.5	Atresia of pulmonary artery
Q25.6	Stenosis of pulmonary artery
Q25.71	Coarctation of pulmonary artery
Q25.72	Congenital pulmonary arteriovenous malformation
Q25.79	Other congenital malformations of pulmonary artery
Q26.0	Congenital stenosis of vena cava
Q26.1	Persistent left superior vena cava
Q26.2	Total anomalous pulmonary venous connection
Q26.3	Partial anomalous pulmonary venous connection

AMA: 93593 2024,Apr; 2023,Jun; 2023,May; 2022,Jul; 2022,Apr; 2021,Dec
93594 2024,Apr; 2023,Jun; 2023,May; 2022,Jul; 2022,Apr; 2021,Dec

Relative Value Units/Medicare Edits

Non-Facility RVU	Work	PE	MP	Total
93593	0.0	0.0	0.0	0.0
93594	0.0	0.0	0.0	0.0
Facility RVU	**Work**	**PE**	**MP**	**Total**
93593	0.0	0.0	0.0	0.0
93594	0.0	0.0	0.0	0.0

	FUD	Status	MUE	Modifiers				IOM Reference
93593	0	C	1(3)	51	N/A	N/A	80*	None
93594	0	C	1(3)	51	N/A	N/A	80*	

* with documentation

Terms To Know

anomaly. Irregularity in the structure or position of an organ or tissue.

congenital. Present at birth, occurring through heredity or an influence during gestation up to the moment of birth.

tetralogy of Fallot. Specific combination of congenital cardiac defects: obstruction of the right ventricular outflow tract with pulmonary stenosis, interventricular septal defect, malposition of the aorta, overriding the interventricular septum and receiving blood from both the venous and arterial systems, and enlargement of the right ventricle.

93595

93595 Left heart catheterization for congenital heart defect(s) including imaging guidance by the proceduralist to advance the catheter to the target zone, normal or abnormal native connections

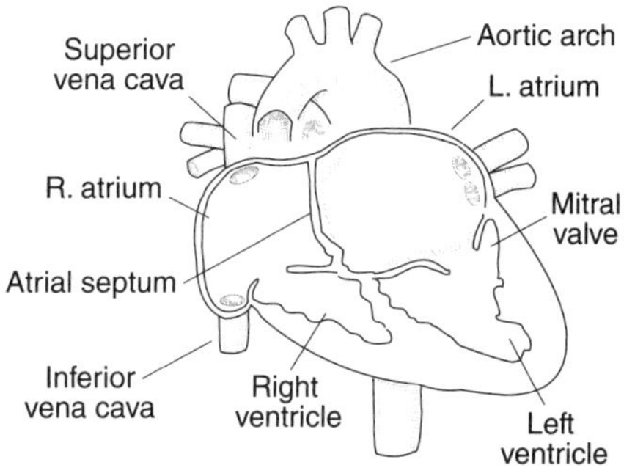

Left heart is catheterized

Explanation

The physician performs a left heart catheterization to evaluate a congenital heart defect. A catheter is threaded to the heart, most frequently through an introducing sheath placed percutaneously into the femoral, brachial, or axillary artery using retrograde technique. Using this technique, the catheter progresses through either normal or abnormal connections into the left ventricle or left atrium. Intracardiac and intravascular pressures are recorded. Left ventriculography or left atrial angiography may be performed and is reported separately; the physician injects dye through a previously placed catheter threaded through a central line into the left ventricle or atrium to evaluate function with fluoroscopy. Imaging guidance used to advance the catheter to the targeted area is included in this code.

Coding Tips

This code includes obtaining blood samples for blood gas measurement, Fick cardiac output measurements, and catheter placement in one of more of the following: right atrium, right ventricle, pulmonary artery, and pulmonary wedge. This code includes fluoroscopy and ultrasound guidance for vascular access and catheter placement for hemodynamic evaluation when performed by the same clinician. Thermodilution cardiac output assessment is not inherent in right heart catheterization for congenital cardiac anomalies and may be reported separately, see 93598. For left ventriculography, left atrial angiography, or angiography of morphologic left ventricle or morphologic left atrium performed during cardiac catheterization for congenital heart defects, see 93565. For insertion and placement of flow directed catheter for monitoring purposes when not performed along with other catheterization services, see 93503. To report left heart catheterization performed using transapical puncture of the left ventricle or transseptal puncture on an intact septum, report 93462 with 93595. For pharmacologic agent administration or physiological exercise study with cardiac catheterization, see 93463 or 93464. For contrast injections during cardiac catheterization for congenital heart defects, see 93563–93569, 93573–93575, and 93584–93588.

ICD-10-CM Diagnostic Codes

Q20.0	Common arterial trunk
Q20.2	Double outlet left ventricle
Q20.3	Discordant ventriculoarterial connection
Q20.4	Double inlet ventricle
Q20.5	Discordant atrioventricular connection
Q20.6	Isomerism of atrial appendages
Q20.8	Other congenital malformations of cardiac chambers and connections
Q21.0	Ventricular septal defect
Q21.11	Secundum atrial septal defect
Q21.12	Patent foramen ovale
Q21.13	Coronary sinus atrial septal defect
Q21.14	Superior sinus venosus atrial septal defect
Q21.15	Inferior sinus venosus atrial septal defect
Q21.21	Partial atrioventricular septal defect
Q21.22	Transitional atrioventricular septal defect
Q21.23	Complete atrioventricular septal defect
Q21.3	Tetralogy of Fallot
Q21.4	Aortopulmonary septal defect
Q22.0	Pulmonary valve atresia
Q22.1	Congenital pulmonary valve stenosis
Q22.2	Congenital pulmonary valve insufficiency
Q22.3	Other congenital malformations of pulmonary valve
Q22.4	Congenital tricuspid stenosis
Q22.5	Ebstein's anomaly
Q23.0	Congenital stenosis of aortic valve
Q23.1	Congenital insufficiency of aortic valve
Q23.2	Congenital mitral stenosis
Q23.3	Congenital mitral insufficiency
Q23.4	Hypoplastic left heart syndrome
Q23.81	Bicuspid aortic valve
Q23.82	Congenital mitral valve cleft leaflet
Q23.88	Other congenital malformations of aortic and mitral valves
Q24.0	Dextrocardia
Q24.1	Levocardia
Q24.2	Cor triatriatum
Q24.3	Pulmonary infundibular stenosis
Q24.4	Congenital subaortic stenosis
Q24.5	Malformation of coronary vessels
Q24.6	Congenital heart block
Q24.8	Other specified congenital malformations of heart
Q25.0	Patent ductus arteriosus
Q25.1	Coarctation of aorta
Q25.21	Interruption of aortic arch
Q25.29	Other atresia of aorta
Q25.3	Supravalvular aortic stenosis
Q25.41	Absence and aplasia of aorta
Q25.42	Hypoplasia of aorta
Q25.43	Congenital aneurysm of aorta
Q25.44	Congenital dilation of aorta
Q25.45	Double aortic arch
Q25.46	Tortuous aortic arch
Q25.47	Right aortic arch
Q25.48	Anomalous origin of subclavian artery
Q25.49	Other congenital malformations of aorta
Q25.5	Atresia of pulmonary artery
Q25.6	Stenosis of pulmonary artery
Q25.71	Coarctation of pulmonary artery

Q25.72	Congenital pulmonary arteriovenous malformation
Q25.79	Other congenital malformations of pulmonary artery
Q26.0	Congenital stenosis of vena cava
Q26.1	Persistent left superior vena cava
Q26.2	Total anomalous pulmonary venous connection
Q26.3	Partial anomalous pulmonary venous connection

AMA: **93595** 2023,Jun; 2023,May; 2022,Apr; 2021,Dec

Relative Value Units/Medicare Edits

Non-Facility RVU	Work	PE	MP	Total
93595	0.0	0.0	0.0	0.0
Facility RVU	**Work**	**PE**	**MP**	**Total**
93595	0.0	0.0	0.0	0.0

	FUD	Status	MUE	Modifiers				IOM Reference
93595	0	C	1(3)	51	N/A	N/A	80*	None

* with documentation

Terms To Know

congenital. Present at birth, occurring through heredity or an influence during gestation up to the moment of birth.

Ebstein's anomaly. Malformation of the tricuspid valve characterized by septal and posterior leaflets attaching to the wall of the right ventricle. Ebstein's anomaly causes the right ventricle to fuse with the atrium into a large right atrium and a small ventricle and leads to heart failure and abnormal cardiac rhythm.

ventriculogram. Interventional procedure that demonstrates the contractility of the cardiac ventricles by serial recording of the distribution of intravenously injected radionuclide or that of radiographic contrast medium injected through an intracardiac catheter.

93596-93597

93596 Right and left heart catheterization for congenital heart defect(s) including imaging guidance by the proceduralist to advance the catheter to the target zone(s); normal native connections

93597 Right and left heart catheterization for congenital heart defect(s) including imaging guidance by the proceduralist to advance the catheter to the target zone(s); abnormal native connections

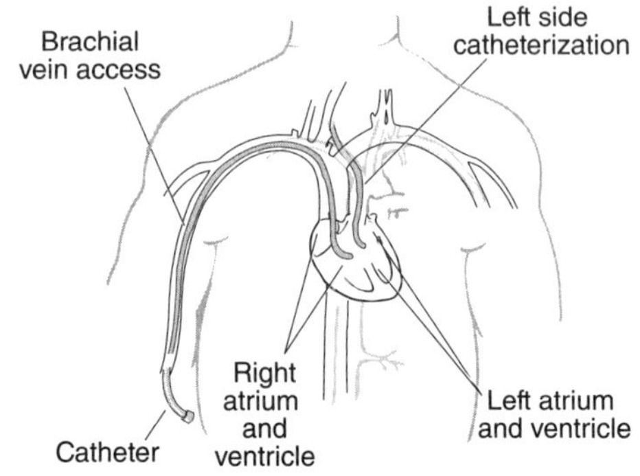

A combined right side catheterization and left side catheterization is performed to address congenital cardiac anomalies

Explanation

The physician performs combined right and left heart catheterization to investigate congenital cardiac anomalies. The physician places an introducer sheath in a vein (typically, the femoral vein) using percutaneous puncture. The physician places a lumen catheter through the introducer sheath into the femoral vein and advances it, under fluoroscopic guidance, to the heart chamber receiving venous circulation. The physician places an introducer sheath in an artery (typically, the femoral artery) using percutaneous puncture. The physician places a lumen catheter through the introducer sheath into the femoral artery and advances it, under fluoroscopic guidance, through the aorta to the heart chamber providing arterial circulation. The physician may use the fluid filled catheters to record intracardiac pressures, withdraw blood samples, or inject radiopaque contrast material. The physician removes the catheters and sheaths from the femoral vessels. Pressure is placed on the wound for 20 to 30 minutes to stem bleeding. Report 93596 for a procedure performed on a patient with normal native connections (those in which the blood flow pathway follows the expected course through the right and left heart chambers and great vessels) and 93597 for a patient whose native connections are abnormal (those that exist when the blood flow pathway through the heart and great vessels follows alternative connections).

Coding Tips

Code selection for right and left heart catheterization for congenital heart defects is based on whether the patient's native anatomic connections from the great veins to the atria, atria to the ventricles, and ventricles to the great arteries are normal or abnormal. Normal native connection exists when the path of blood flow follows the typical course through the right and left heart chambers and great vessels. Abnormal native connection exists when the path of blood flow follows an alternative course through the heart and great vessels due to altered connections. These codes include obtaining blood samples for blood gas measurement, Fick cardiac output measurements, and catheter placement in one of more of the following: right atrium, right ventricle, pulmonary artery, and pulmonary wedge. These codes include fluoroscopy and ultrasound guidance for vascular access and catheter placement for hemodynamic evaluation when performed by the same clinician. Thermodilution cardiac output assessment is not inherent in right heart catheterization for congenital cardiac anomalies and may be reported separately, see 93598. For left ventriculography, left atrial angiography, or angiography of morphologic left ventricle or morphologic left atrium performed during cardiac catheterization for congenital heart defects, see 93565. For insertion and placement of a flow directed catheter for monitoring purposes when not performed along with other catheterization services, see 93503. To report left heart catheterization performed using transapical puncture of the left ventricle or transseptal puncture on an intact septum, report 93462 with 93596 or 93597. For pharmacologic agent administration or physiological exercise study with cardiac catheterization, see 93463 or 93464. For contrast injections during cardiac catheterization for congenital heart defects, see 93563–93569, 93573–93575, and 93584–93588.

ICD-10-CM Diagnostic Codes

Q20.0	Common arterial trunk
Q20.1	Double outlet right ventricle
Q20.2	Double outlet left ventricle
Q20.3	Discordant ventriculoarterial connection
Q20.4	Double inlet ventricle
Q20.5	Discordant atrioventricular connection
Q20.6	Isomerism of atrial appendages
Q20.8	Other congenital malformations of cardiac chambers and connections
Q21.0	Ventricular septal defect
Q21.11	Secundum atrial septal defect
Q21.12	Patent foramen ovale
Q21.13	Coronary sinus atrial septal defect
Q21.14	Superior sinus venosus atrial septal defect
Q21.15	Inferior sinus venosus atrial septal defect
Q21.21	Partial atrioventricular septal defect
Q21.22	Transitional atrioventricular septal defect
Q21.23	Complete atrioventricular septal defect
Q21.3	Tetralogy of Fallot
Q21.4	Aortopulmonary septal defect
Q22.0	Pulmonary valve atresia
Q22.1	Congenital pulmonary valve stenosis
Q22.2	Congenital pulmonary valve insufficiency
Q22.3	Other congenital malformations of pulmonary valve
Q22.4	Congenital tricuspid stenosis
Q22.5	Ebstein's anomaly
Q22.6	Hypoplastic right heart syndrome
Q23.0	Congenital stenosis of aortic valve
Q23.1	Congenital insufficiency of aortic valve
Q23.2	Congenital mitral stenosis
Q23.3	Congenital mitral insufficiency
Q23.4	Hypoplastic left heart syndrome
Q23.81	Bicuspid aortic valve
Q23.82	Congenital mitral valve cleft leaflet
Q23.88	Other congenital malformations of aortic and mitral valves
Q24.0	Dextrocardia
Q24.1	Levocardia
Q24.2	Cor triatriatum
Q24.3	Pulmonary infundibular stenosis
Q24.4	Congenital subaortic stenosis
Q24.5	Malformation of coronary vessels
Q24.6	Congenital heart block
Q24.8	Other specified congenital malformations of heart
Q25.0	Patent ductus arteriosus
Q25.1	Coarctation of aorta
Q25.21	Interruption of aortic arch
Q25.29	Other atresia of aorta
Q25.3	Supravalvular aortic stenosis
Q25.41	Absence and aplasia of aorta
Q25.42	Hypoplasia of aorta
Q25.43	Congenital aneurysm of aorta
Q25.44	Congenital dilation of aorta
Q25.45	Double aortic arch
Q25.46	Tortuous aortic arch
Q25.47	Right aortic arch
Q25.48	Anomalous origin of subclavian artery
Q25.49	Other congenital malformations of aorta
Q25.5	Atresia of pulmonary artery
Q25.6	Stenosis of pulmonary artery
Q25.71	Coarctation of pulmonary artery
Q25.72	Congenital pulmonary arteriovenous malformation
Q25.79	Other congenital malformations of pulmonary artery
Q26.0	Congenital stenosis of vena cava
Q26.1	Persistent left superior vena cava
Q26.2	Total anomalous pulmonary venous connection
Q26.3	Partial anomalous pulmonary venous connection

AMA: 93596 2024,Apr; 2023,Jun; 2023,May; 2022,Jul; 2022,Apr; 2021,Dec
93597 2024,Apr; 2023,Jun; 2023,May; 2022,Jul; 2022,Apr; 2021,Dec

Relative Value Units/Medicare Edits

Non-Facility RVU	Work	PE	MP	Total
93596	0.0	0.0	0.0	0.0
93597	0.0	0.0	0.0	0.0
Facility RVU	**Work**	**PE**	**MP**	**Total**
93596	0.0	0.0	0.0	0.0
93597	0.0	0.0	0.0	0.0

	FUD	Status	MUE	Modifiers				IOM Reference
93596	0	C	1(3)	51	N/A	N/A	80*	None
93597	0	C	1(3)	51	N/A	N/A	80*	

* with documentation

Terms To Know

atresia. Congenital closure or absence of a tubular organ or an opening to the body surface.

coarctation of aorta. Localized deformation of the aortic media that causes a severe constriction of the vessel, resulting in high blood pressure in the arms and low pressure in the legs. This condition must be treated to prevent a cerebrovascular accident, endocarditis, congestive heart failure, or rupture of the aorta.

stenosis. Narrowing or constriction of a passage.

[93584, 93585, 93586, 93587, 93588]

+ **93584** Venography for congenital heart defect(s), including catheter placement, and radiological supervision and interpretation; anomalous or persistent superior vena cava when it exists as a second contralateral superior vena cava, with native drainage to heart (List separately in addition to code for primary procedure)
+ **93585** Venography for congenital heart defect(s), including catheter placement, and radiological supervision and interpretation; azygos/hemiazygos venous system (List separately in addition to code for primary procedure)
+ **93586** Venography for congenital heart defect(s), including catheter placement, and radiological supervision and interpretation; coronary sinus (List separately in addition to code for primary procedure)
+ **93587** Venography for congenital heart defect(s), including catheter placement, and radiological supervision and interpretation; venovenous collaterals originating at or above the heart (eg, from innominate vein) (List separately in addition to code for primary procedure)
+ **93588** Venography for congenital heart defect(s), including catheter placement, and radiological supervision and interpretation; venovenous collaterals originating below the heart (eg, from the inferior vena cava) (List separately in addition to code for primary procedure)

Explanation

The physician performs a venography during a separately reportable procedure to evaluate abnormalities of cardiac anatomy related to an existing congenital heart defect. Venography involves injection of a contrast dye into the venous system to visualize blood flow. An intravenous (IV) line is inserted and guided through a blood vessel, usually in the arm or hand. Contrast material is injected through the catheter into the targeted venous system. As the contrast dye circulates, real-time x-ray images (fluoroscopy) are continuously captured. Acquired images are analyzed to evaluate the area of the congenital heart defect for anatomical abnormalities. The catheter is removed, and pressure is applied to the insertion site to minimize bleeding. Report 93584 for venography involving an anomalous or persistent superior vena cava when it exists as a second contralateral superior vena cava, with native drainage to the heart; 93585 for the azygos/hemiazygos venous system; 93586 for the coronary sinus; 93587 for the venovenous collaterals originating at or above the heart, such as from the innominate vein; and 93588 for the venovenous collaterals originating below the heart, such as from the inferior vena cava. Catheter placement and radiological supervision and interpretation are included in these codes. These are add-on codes and are reported in addition to the primary procedure.

Coding Tips

These codes represent separately identifiable services and may be reported with one another, when appropriate. For angiography of other noncoronary and nonpulmonary arteries and veins performed as a distinct service, see radiology and vascular injection procedures under the cardiovascular section. Selective catheter placement for anomalous congenital venous structures is not included in standard congenital cardiac catheterization. Therefore, these codes include selective catheter in the specific venous structure being imaged as well as venography and radiologic supervision and interpretation with report. Report these codes only once per session. Report 93584–93588 with 93593, 93594, 93596, or 93597.

ICD-10-CM Diagnostic Codes

This/these CPT code(s) are add-on code(s). See the primary procedure code that this code is performed with for your ICD-10-CM code selections.

AMA: **93584** 2024,Apr **93585** 2024,Apr **93586** 2024,Apr **93587** 2024,Apr **93588** 2024,Apr

Relative Value Units/Medicare Edits

Non-Facility RVU	Work	PE	MP	Total
93584	1.2	0.43	0.1	1.73
93585	1.13	0.4	0.1	1.63
93586	1.43	0.51	0.12	2.06
93587	2.11	0.75	0.18	3.04
93588	2.13	0.76	0.18	3.07
Facility RVU	**Work**	**PE**	**MP**	**Total**
93584	1.2	0.43	0.1	1.73
93585	1.13	0.4	0.1	1.63
93586	1.43	0.51	0.12	2.06
93587	2.11	0.75	0.18	3.04
93588	2.13	0.76	0.18	3.07

	FUD	Status	MUE	Modifiers				IOM Reference
93584	N/A	A	1(2)	N/A	N/A	N/A	80*	None
93585	N/A	A	1(2)	N/A	N/A	N/A	80*	
93586	N/A	A	1(2)	N/A	N/A	N/A	80*	
93587	N/A	A	1(2)	N/A	N/A	N/A	80*	
93588	N/A	A	1(2)	N/A	N/A	N/A	80*	

* with documentation

93598

\+ **93598** Cardiac output measurement(s), thermodilution or other indicator dilution method, performed during cardiac catheterization for the evaluation of congenital heart defects (List separately in addition to code for primary procedure)

Explanation

Indicator dilution studies use a technique based on the principle that the volume of a fluid within a container can be determined by adding a known quantity of an indicator to the fluid and measuring the concentration of the indicator after it has completely mixed with the fluid. A time-concentration curve arises and the area of the inscribed curve is calculated. The physician threads a catheter through a central line leading to the heart and dye, such as nontoxic, water-soluble indocyanine green, or a thermal indicator, usually iced saline, is injected. In the thermodilution method, cardiac output is measured by a computer using an equation that incorporates body temperature, injection volume and temperature, time, and other calculated ratios over a denominator of the integral of the change in blood temperature during the cold injection, reflected by the area of the inscribed curve. This procedure is performed during a cardiac catheterization for the evaluation of congenital heart defects.

Coding Tips

Report 93598 in addition to 93593-93597. Do not report 93598 with 93451-93461. For pharmacologic agent administered during cardiac catheterization, see 93463. For physiological exercise study with cardiac catheterization, see 93464. For injections during cardiac catheterization, see 93563–93569, 93573–93575, and 93584–93588.

ICD-10-CM Diagnostic Codes

This/these CPT code(s) are add-on code(s). See the primary procedure code that this code is performed with for your ICD-10-CM code selections. Diagnostic code(s) would be the same as the actual procedure performed.

AMA: **93598** 2023,Jun; 2023,May; 2022,Dec; 2022,Jun; 2022,Apr; 2022,Jan

Relative Value Units/Medicare Edits

Non-Facility RVU	Work	PE	MP	Total
93598	0.0	0.0	0.0	0.0
Facility RVU	**Work**	**PE**	**MP**	**Total**
93598	0.0	0.0	0.0	0.0

	FUD	Status	MUE	Modifiers				IOM Reference
93598	N/A	C	1(2)	N/A	N/A	N/A	80*	None

* with documentation

Terms To Know

catheterization. Use or insertion of a tubular device into a duct, blood vessel, hollow organ, or body cavity for injecting or withdrawing fluids for diagnostic or therapeutic purposes.

congenital. Present at birth, occurring through heredity or an influence during gestation up to the moment of birth.

93600

93600 Bundle of His recording

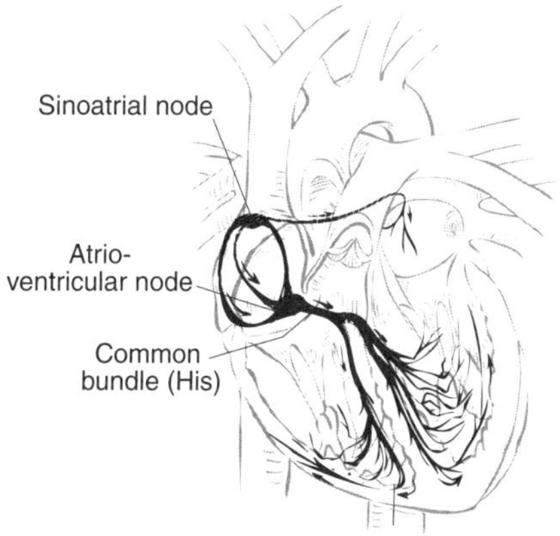

Conduction system of the heart

The His bundle is recorded, typically from the right atria

Explanation

The physician places a venous sheath, usually in a femoral vein, using standard techniques. The physician advances an electrical catheter through the venous sheath and into the right heart under fluoroscopic guidance. The physician attaches the catheter to an electrical recording device to allow depiction of the intracardiac electrograms obtained from electrodes on the catheter tip. The physician moves the catheter tip to the bundle of His, on the anteroseptal tricuspid annulus, and obtains recordings. Alternatively, the physician may obtain similar recordings by placing a catheter into the left ventricular outflow tract via the aorta.

Coding Tips

As exempt from modifier 51, 93600 has not been designated in CPT as an add-on service/procedure. However, codes identified as exempt from modifier 51 are not subject to multiple procedure rules. No reimbursement reduction or modifier 51 is applied. Do not report 93600 with 93619, 93620, 93653, 93654, or 93656. Procedure 93600 has both a technical and professional component. To report only the professional component, append modifier 26. To report only the technical component, append modifier TC. To report the complete procedure (i.e., both the professional and technical components), submit without a modifier. Fluoroscopic guidance is included in electrophysiological procedures and should not be reported separately. Procedure 93600 reports bundle of His recording only. For comprehensive electrophysiologic evaluation with bundle of His recording, see 93619–92622.

ICD-10-CM Diagnostic Codes

I44.0	Atrioventricular block, first degree
I44.1	Atrioventricular block, second degree
I44.2	Atrioventricular block, complete
I44.39	Other atrioventricular block
I44.4	Left anterior fascicular block
I44.5	Left posterior fascicular block
I44.69	Other fascicular block
I45.0	Right fascicular block
I45.19	Other right bundle-branch block
I45.2	Bifascicular block
I45.3	Trifascicular block

I45.4	Nonspecific intraventricular block
I45.5	Other specified heart block
I45.6	Pre-excitation syndrome
I45.89	Other specified conduction disorders
I46.2	Cardiac arrest due to underlying cardiac condition
I46.8	Cardiac arrest due to other underlying condition
I47.0	Re-entry ventricular arrhythmia
I47.11	Inappropriate sinus tachycardia, so stated
I47.21	Torsades de pointes
I47.29	Other ventricular tachycardia
I48.0	Paroxysmal atrial fibrillation
I48.11	Longstanding persistent atrial fibrillation
I48.19	Other persistent atrial fibrillation
I48.21	Permanent atrial fibrillation
I48.3	Typical atrial flutter
I48.4	Atypical atrial flutter
I49.01	Ventricular fibrillation
I49.02	Ventricular flutter
I49.1	Atrial premature depolarization
I49.2	Junctional premature depolarization
I49.3	Ventricular premature depolarization
I49.49	Other premature depolarization
I49.5	Sick sinus syndrome
I49.8	Other specified cardiac arrhythmias

AMA: **93600** 2021,Dec

Relative Value Units/Medicare Edits

Non-Facility RVU	Work	PE	MP	Total
93600	0.0	0.0	0.0	0.0
Facility RVU	**Work**	**PE**	**MP**	**Total**
93600	0.0	0.0	0.0	0.0

	FUD	Status	MUE	Modifiers				IOM Reference
93600	0	C	1(3)	N/A	N/A	N/A	80*	None

* with documentation

93602

93602 Intra-atrial recording

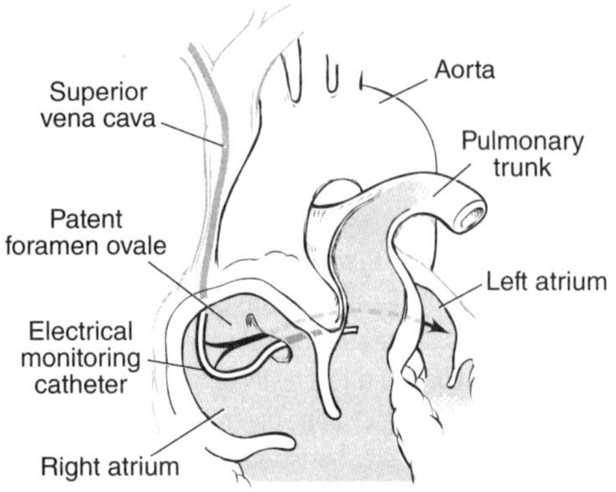

Intraatrial recordings are made. The monitor may be placed in the right atria or the left atria by retrograde approach. The septum may be probed from either side, as well

Explanation

The physician places a venous sheath, usually in a femoral vein, using standard techniques. The physician advances an electrical catheter through the venous sheath and into the right heart under fluoroscopic guidance. The physician attaches the catheter to an electrical recording device to allow depiction of the intracardiac electrograms obtained from electrodes on the catheter tip. The physician moves the catheter tip to the right atrium and obtains recordings. The physician may obtain left atrial recordings by crossing the interatrial septum. Alternatively, the physician may obtain left atrial recordings by placing an arterial catheter into the aorta and crossing both the aortic and mitral valves in a retrograde fashion.

Coding Tips

As exempt from modifier 51, 93602 has not been designated in CPT as an add-on service/procedure. However, codes identified as exempt from modifier 51 are not subject to multiple procedure rules. No reimbursement reduction or modifier 51 is applied. Do not report 93602 with 93619, 93620, 93653, 93654, or 93656. Procedure 93602 has both a technical and professional component. To report only the professional component, append modifier 26. To report only the technical component, append modifier TC. To report the complete procedure (i.e., both the professional and technical components), submit without a modifier. Fluoroscopic guidance is included in electrophysiological procedures and should not be reported separately. Procedure 93602 reports intra-atrial recording only. For comprehensive electrophysiologic evaluation including intra-atrial recording, see 93619–92622.

ICD-10-CM Diagnostic Codes

I44.0	Atrioventricular block, first degree
I44.1	Atrioventricular block, second degree
I44.2	Atrioventricular block, complete
I44.39	Other atrioventricular block
I45.5	Other specified heart block
I45.6	Pre-excitation syndrome
I45.89	Other specified conduction disorders
I48.0	Paroxysmal atrial fibrillation
I48.11	Longstanding persistent atrial fibrillation
I48.19	Other persistent atrial fibrillation

I48.21	Permanent atrial fibrillation
I48.3	Typical atrial flutter
I48.4	Atypical atrial flutter
I49.1	Atrial premature depolarization
I49.5	Sick sinus syndrome
I49.8	Other specified cardiac arrhythmias

AMA: **93602** 2021,Dec

Relative Value Units/Medicare Edits

Non-Facility RVU	Work	PE	MP	Total
93602	0.0	0.0	0.0	0.0
Facility RVU	**Work**	**PE**	**MP**	**Total**
93602	0.0	0.0	0.0	0.0

	FUD	Status	MUE	Modifiers				IOM Reference
93602	0	C	1(3)	N/A	N/A	N/A	80*	None

* with documentation

Terms To Know

fluoroscopy. Radiology technique that allows visual examination of part of the body or a function of an organ using a device that projects an x-ray image on a fluorescent screen.

retrograde. Moving against the usual direction of flow.

93603

93603 Right ventricular recording

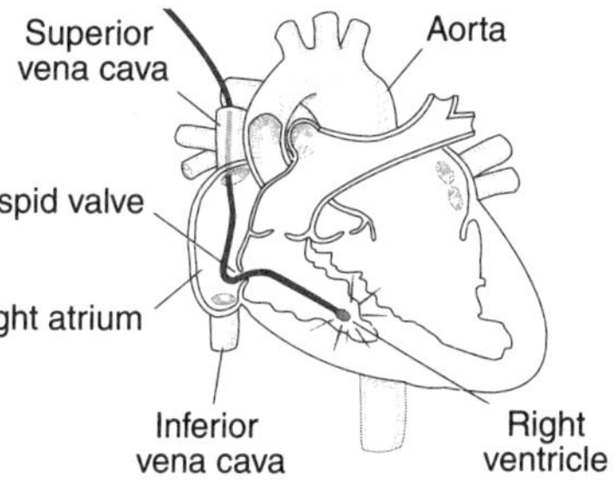

Recordings are collected from the right ventricle

Explanation

The physician places a venous sheath, usually in a femoral vein, using standard techniques. The physician advances an electrical catheter through the venous sheath and into the right heart under fluoroscopic guidance. The physician attaches the catheter to an electrical recording device to allow depiction of the intracardiac electrograms obtained from electrodes on the catheter tip. The physician moves the catheter tip to the right ventricle and obtains recordings.

Coding Tips

As exempt from modifier 51, 93603 has not been designated in CPT as an add-on service/procedure. However, codes identified as exempt from modifier 51 are not subject to multiple procedure rules. No reimbursement reduction or modifier 51 is applied. Do not report 93603 with 93619, 93620, 93653, 93654, or 93656. Procedure 93603 has both a technical and professional component. To report only the professional component, append modifier 26. To report only the technical component, append modifier TC. To report the complete procedure (i.e., both the professional and technical components), submit without a modifier. Fluoroscopic guidance is included in electrophysiological procedures and should not be reported separately. Procedure 93603 reports right ventricular recording only. For comprehensive electrophysiologic evaluation including right ventricular recording, see 93619–92622.

ICD-10-CM Diagnostic Codes

I42.8	Other cardiomyopathies
I44.0	Atrioventricular block, first degree
I44.1	Atrioventricular block, second degree
I44.2	Atrioventricular block, complete
I44.30	Unspecified atrioventricular block
I44.39	Other atrioventricular block
I45.4	Nonspecific intraventricular block
I45.5	Other specified heart block
I45.6	Pre-excitation syndrome
I45.89	Other specified conduction disorders
I45.9	Conduction disorder, unspecified
I47.0	Re-entry ventricular arrhythmia
I47.11	Inappropriate sinus tachycardia, so stated
I47.21	Torsades de pointes
I47.29	Other ventricular tachycardia
I49.01	Ventricular fibrillation

I49.02 Ventricular flutter
I49.3 Ventricular premature depolarization

AMA: 93603 2021,Dec

Relative Value Units/Medicare Edits

Non-Facility RVU	Work	PE	MP	Total
93603	0.0	0.0	0.0	0.0
Facility RVU	**Work**	**PE**	**MP**	**Total**
93603	0.0	0.0	0.0	0.0

	FUD	Status	MUE	Modifiers				IOM Reference
93603	0	C	1(3)	N/A	N/A	N/A	80*	None

* with documentation

Terms To Know

atrioventricular block. Condition in which there is a disturbance of electrical conduction, such as a delay, intermittence, or absence in the transmission of an impulse from the atria to the ventricles and categorized according to degree of severity.

electrode. Electric terminal specialized for a particular electrochemical reaction that acts as a medium between a body surface and another instrument, commonly termed a lead.

fluoroscopy. Radiology technique that allows visual examination of part of the body or a function of an organ using a device that projects an x-ray image on a fluorescent screen.

sheath. Covering enclosing an organ or part.

93609

+ **93609** Intraventricular and/or intra-atrial mapping of tachycardia site(s) with catheter manipulation to record from multiple sites to identify origin of tachycardia (List separately in addition to code for primary procedure)

Explanation

The physician places an appropriate arterial or venous sheath, usually femoral, to allow access to the chamber to be mapped. The physician advances an electrical catheter through the sheath and into the appropriate chamber under fluoroscopic guidance. The physician attaches the catheter to an electrical recording device to allow depiction of the intracardiac electrograms obtained from electrodes on the catheter tip. The physician moves the catheter tip throughout the chamber to be mapped and obtains recordings. The physician compares activation times from different sites in order to identify the origin of the tachycardia.

Coding Tips

When medically necessary, report moderate (conscious) sedation provided by the performing physician with 99151-99153. When provided by another physician, report 99155-99157. Report 93609 in addition to 93620, 93653, or 93656. Only one mapping procedure may be reported with a comprehensive electrophysiologic evaluation (93620) or intracardiac catheter ablation (93653). Three-dimensional mapping (93613) is the higher valued service and should be reported instead of 93609 when both are performed. Do not report 93609 with 93613 or 93654. Procedure 93609 has both a technical and professional component. To report only the professional component, append modifier 26. To report only the technical component, append modifier TC. To report the complete procedure (i.e., both the professional and technical components), submit without a modifier. Fluoroscopic guidance is included in electrophysiological procedures and should not be reported separately. Intraventricular and/or intra-atrial mapping is not included in comprehensive electrophysiologic evaluation, see 93620–92622.

ICD-10-CM Diagnostic Codes

This/these CPT code(s) are add-on code(s). See the primary procedure code that this code is performed with for your ICD-10-CM code selections. Diagnostic code(s) would be the same as the actual procedure performed.

AMA: 93609 2023,Oct; 2023,May; 2021,Dec

Relative Value Units/Medicare Edits

Non-Facility RVU	Work	PE	MP	Total
93609	0.0	0.0	0.0	0.0
Facility RVU	**Work**	**PE**	**MP**	**Total**
93609	0.0	0.0	0.0	0.0

	FUD	Status	MUE	Modifiers				IOM Reference
93609	N/A	C	1(3)	N/A	N/A	N/A	80*	None

* with documentation

Terms To Know

tachycardia. Excessively rapid beating action of the heart, defined as more than 100 beats per minute for an adult, that is usually defined by its origin (atrial or ventricular) and whether the onset and cessation occurs in sudden attacks (paroxysmal) or in a slow pattern (nonparoxysmal).

93610

93610 Intra-atrial pacing

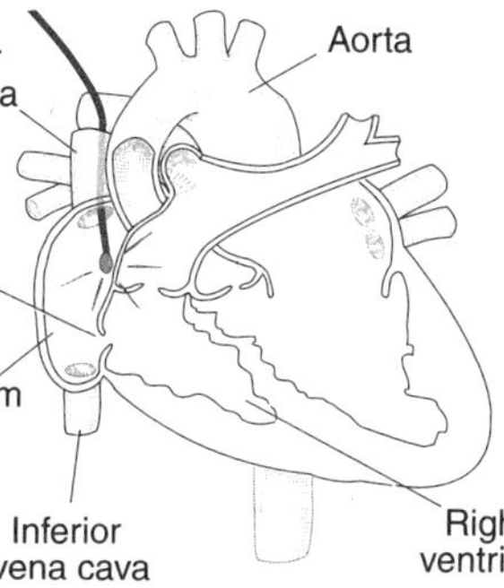

Schematic of right atrial pacing

Explanation

The physician places a venous sheath, usually in a femoral vein, using standard techniques. The physician advances an electrical catheter through the venous sheath and into the right heart under fluoroscopic guidance. The physician attaches the catheter to an electrical pacing device to allow transmission of pacing impulses through the catheter to the right atrium. The physician may pace the left atrium by placing the catheter in the coronary sinus or by crossing the interatrial septum. Alternatively, the physician may pace the left atrium by placing an arterial catheter into the aorta and crossing both the aortic and mitral valves in a retrograde fashion.

Coding Tips

As exempt from modifier 51, 93610 has not been designated in CPT as an add-on service/procedure. However, codes identified as exempt from modifier 51 are not subject to multiple procedure rules. No reimbursement reduction or modifier 51 is applied. Procedure 93610 has both a technical and professional component. To report only the professional component, append modifier 26. To report only the technical component, append modifier TC. To report the complete procedure (i.e., both the professional and technical components), submit without a modifier. Fluoroscopic guidance is included in electrophysiological procedures and should not be reported separately. Do not report 93610 with 93619, 93620, 93653, 93654, or 93656. Procedure 93610 reports intra-atrial pacing only. For comprehensive electrophysiologic evaluation including intra-atrial pacing, see 93619–92622.

ICD-10-CM Diagnostic Codes

I44.0	Atrioventricular block, first degree
I44.1	Atrioventricular block, second degree
I44.2	Atrioventricular block, complete
I44.39	Other atrioventricular block
I48.0	Paroxysmal atrial fibrillation
I48.11	Longstanding persistent atrial fibrillation
I48.19	Other persistent atrial fibrillation
I48.21	Permanent atrial fibrillation
I48.3	Typical atrial flutter
I48.4	Atypical atrial flutter
I49.1	Atrial premature depolarization
I49.5	Sick sinus syndrome

AMA: 93610 2021,Dec

Relative Value Units/Medicare Edits

Non-Facility RVU	Work	PE	MP	Total
93610	0.0	0.0	0.0	0.0
Facility RVU	**Work**	**PE**	**MP**	**Total**
93610	0.0	0.0	0.0	0.0

	FUD	Status	MUE	Modifiers				IOM Reference
93610	0	C	1(3)	N/A	N/A	N/A	80*	None

* with documentation

Terms To Know

arrhythmia. Irregular heartbeat.

fibrillation. Spontaneous contraction of individual muscle fibers.

sick sinus syndrome. Range of electrophysiological abnormalities of the heart including sinus bradycardia, sinus arrest, sinus node exit block, chronic atrial fibrillation, and bradycardia-tachycardia syndrome. Most often found in older patients with a history of heart disease, it is distinguished by delayed or failed conduction between the sinus node and atria, due to inadequate sinus node pacemaking or conduction disturbances.

tachycardia. Excessively rapid beating action of the heart, defined as more than 100 beats per minute for an adult, that is usually defined by its origin (atrial or ventricular) and whether the onset and cessation occurs in sudden attacks (paroxysmal) or in a slow pattern (nonparoxysmal).

93612

93612 Intraventricular pacing

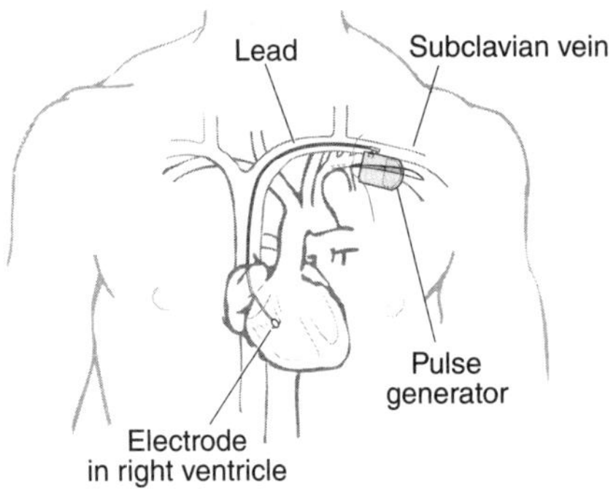

A ventricle of the heart is paced by an electrode positioned within the ventricle. Either left or right ventricle may be addressed according to the description

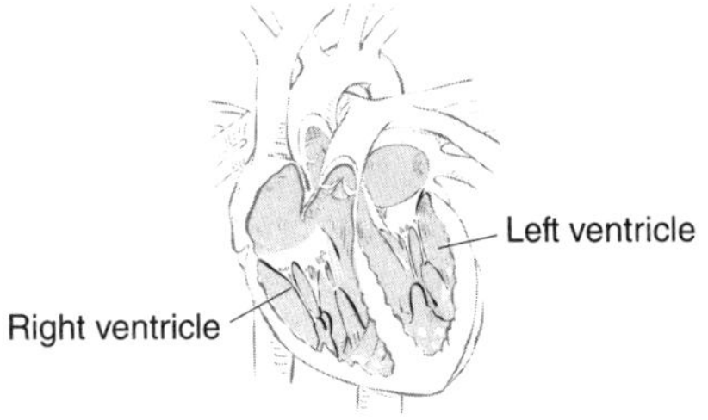

Explanation

The physician places a venous sheath using standard techniques. The physician advances an electrical catheter through the venous sheath and into the right ventricle under fluoroscopic guidance. The physician attaches the catheter to an electrical pacing device to allow transmission of pacing impulses through the catheter to the right ventricle. Alternatively, the physician may pace the left ventricle by placing the catheter in the right atrium, crossing the intra-atrial septum and mitral valve. Finally, the physician may pace the left ventricle by advancing a catheter through an arterial sheath, via the aorta, across the aortic valve into the left ventricle.

Coding Tips

As exempt from modifier 51, 93612 has not been designated in CPT as an add-on service/procedure. However, codes identified as exempt from modifier 51 are not subject to multiple procedure rules. No reimbursement reduction or modifier 51 is applied. Procedure 93612 has both a technical and professional component. To report only the professional component, append modifier 26. To report only the technical component, append modifier TC. To report the complete procedure (i.e., both the professional and technical components), submit without a modifier. Fluoroscopic guidance is included in electrophysiological procedures and should not be reported separately. Do not report 93612 with 93619, 93620–93622, 93653, 93654, or 93656. Procedure 93612 reports intraventricular pacing only. For comprehensive electrophysiologic evaluation including intraventricular pacing, see 93619–92622.

ICD-10-CM Diagnostic Codes

I44.0	Atrioventricular block, first degree
I44.1	Atrioventricular block, second degree
I44.2	Atrioventricular block, complete
I44.39	Other atrioventricular block
I44.4	Left anterior fascicular block
I44.5	Left posterior fascicular block
I44.69	Other fascicular block
I45.0	Right fascicular block
I45.19	Other right bundle-branch block
I45.2	Bifascicular block
I45.3	Trifascicular block
I45.4	Nonspecific intraventricular block
I47.0	Re-entry ventricular arrhythmia
I47.11	Inappropriate sinus tachycardia, so stated
I47.21	Torsades de pointes
I47.29	Other ventricular tachycardia
I49.01	Ventricular fibrillation
I49.02	Ventricular flutter
I49.3	Ventricular premature depolarization

AMA: **93612** 2021,Dec

Relative Value Units/Medicare Edits

Non-Facility RVU	Work	PE	MP	Total
93612	0.0	0.0	0.0	0.0
Facility RVU	**Work**	**PE**	**MP**	**Total**
93612	0.0	0.0	0.0	0.0

	FUD	Status	MUE	Modifiers				IOM Reference
93612	0	C	1(3)	N/A	N/A	N/A	80*	None

* with documentation

93613

\+ **93613** Intracardiac electrophysiologic 3-dimensional mapping (List separately in addition to code for primary procedure)

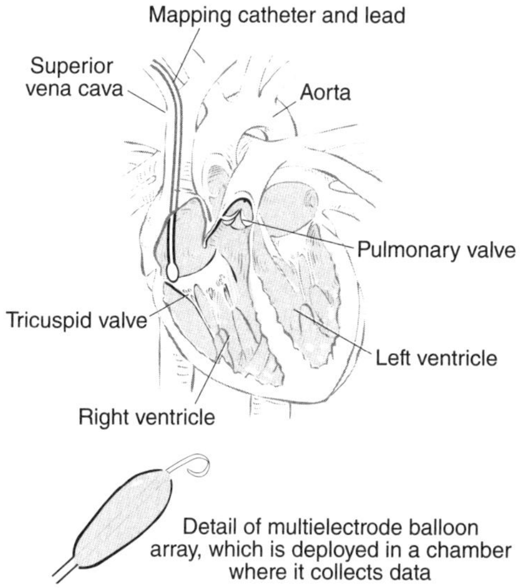

The heart is mapped by an intracardiac electrophysiologic sensor. The study yields three-dimensional views of the area under investigation

Explanation

Electrophysiologic studies use electric stimulation and monitoring in the diagnosis of conduction abnormalities that predispose patients to bradyarrhythmias and to determine a patient's chance of developing ventricular and supraventricular tachyarrhythmias. The physician inserts an electrode catheter percutaneously into the right subclavian vein and, under fluoroscopic guidance, positions the electrode catheter at the right ventricular apex, both for recording and stimulating the right atrium and the right ventricle. For mapping, additional electrode catheters are inserted percutaneously from the right femoral artery and advanced to the specific site to be mapped in conjunction with the primary procedure (93620). Ventricular tachycardia is induced by programmed ventricular stimulation from the right and left ventricular apexes. The earliest activation site is determined and the diastolic pressure is recorded on the endocardial activation map during the ventricular tachycardia. Intracardiac electrograms with surface electrocardiograms are simultaneously displayed and recorded on a multichannel oscilloscopic photographic recorder.

Coding Tips

When medically necessary, report moderate (conscious) sedation provided by the performing physician with 99151-99153. When provided by another physician, report 99155-99157. Report 93613 in addition to 93620. Only one mapping procedure may be reported with a comprehensive electrophysiologic evaluation (93620) or intracardiac catheter ablation (93563). Three-dimensional mapping (93613) is the higher valued service and should be reported instead of 93609 when both are performed. Do not report 93613 with 93609 or 93654. Fluoroscopic guidance is included in electrophysiological procedures and should not be reported separately. For noninvasive arrhythmia localization and mapping, see 0745T.

ICD-10-CM Diagnostic Codes

This/these CPT code(s) are add-on code(s). See the primary procedure code that this code is performed with for your ICD-10-CM code selections. Diagnostic code(s) would be the same as the actual procedure performed.

AMA: **93613** 2021,Dec

Relative Value Units/Medicare Edits

Non-Facility RVU	Work	PE	MP	Total
93613	5.23	2.08	1.21	8.52
Facility RVU	**Work**	**PE**	**MP**	**Total**
93613	5.23	2.08	1.21	8.52

	FUD	Status	MUE	Modifiers				IOM Reference
93613	N/A	A	1(3)	N/A	N/A	N/A	80*	None

* with documentation

Terms To Know

dysrhythmia. Abnormality or disturbance in rhythm.

electrophysiologic studies. Electrical stimulation and monitoring to diagnose heart conduction abnormalities that predispose patients to bradyarrhythmias and to determine a patient's chance for developing ventricular and supraventricular tachyarrhythmias.

moderate sedation. Medically controlled state of depressed consciousness, with or without analgesia, while maintaining the patient's airway, protective reflexes, and ability to respond to stimulation or verbal commands.

ventricular tachycardia. Excessively rapid ventricular rhythm of the heart, usually more than 150 beats per minute, with an origin beat generated in the ventricle, commonly from atrioventricular dissociation.

93615-93616

93615 Esophageal recording of atrial electrogram with or without ventricular electrogram(s);

93616 with pacing

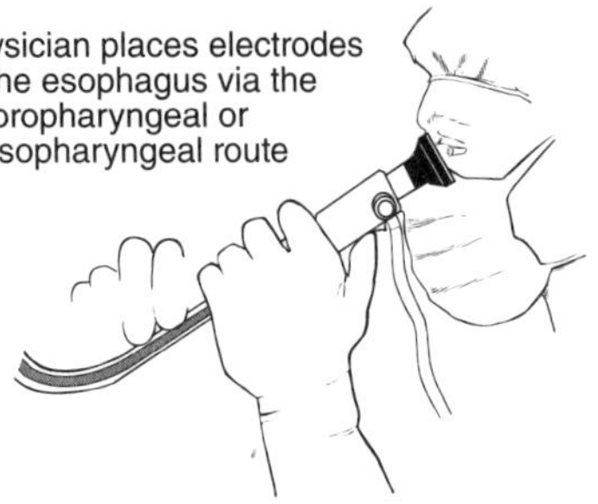

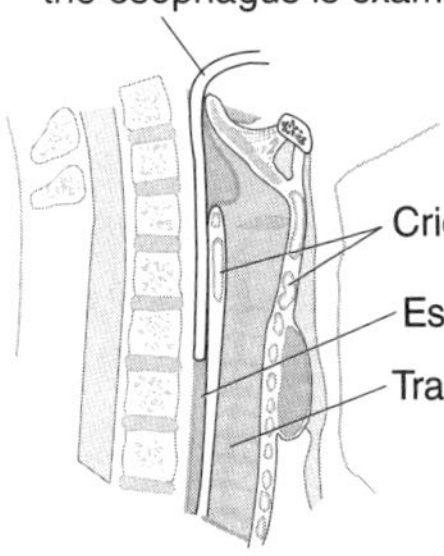

Explanation

The physician places electrodes into the esophagus via an oropharyngeal or nasopharyngeal route. The physician attaches the catheter to an electrical recording device to allow depiction of the esophageal electrograms obtained from electrodes on the catheter tip. The physician moves the catheter tip to the esophageal site that provides the optimal signal and obtains recordings. The physician compares the esophageal and surface electrograms to identify the mechanism of the arrhythmia. Report 93616 when the physician measures the heart's electrical function using a catheter placed into the patient's esophagus. The recording electrode at the end of the probe measures electrical activity of the atrium by pacing with or without recording activity of the ventricle.

Coding Tips

When medically necessary, report moderate (conscious) sedation provided by the performing physician with 99151-99153. When provided by another physician, report 99155-99157. As exempt from modifier 51, 93615 and 93616 have not been designated in CPT as add-on services/procedures. However, codes identified as exempt from modifier 51 are not subject to multiple procedure rules. No reimbursement reduction or modifier 51 is applied. Procedures 93615 and 93616 have both a technical and professional component. To report only the professional component, append modifier 26. To report only the technical component, append modifier TC. To report the complete procedure (i.e., both the professional and technical components), submit without a modifier. Fluoroscopic guidance is included in electrophysiological procedures and should not be reported separately.

ICD-10-CM Diagnostic Codes

I44.0	Atrioventricular block, first degree
I44.1	Atrioventricular block, second degree
I44.2	Atrioventricular block, complete
I44.39	Other atrioventricular block
I45.4	Nonspecific intraventricular block
I45.5	Other specified heart block
I45.6	Pre-excitation syndrome
I45.89	Other specified conduction disorders
I47.0	Re-entry ventricular arrhythmia
I47.11	Inappropriate sinus tachycardia, so stated
I47.21	Torsades de pointes
I47.29	Other ventricular tachycardia
I48.0	Paroxysmal atrial fibrillation
I48.11	Longstanding persistent atrial fibrillation
I48.19	Other persistent atrial fibrillation
I48.21	Permanent atrial fibrillation
I48.3	Typical atrial flutter
I48.4	Atypical atrial flutter
I49.01	Ventricular fibrillation
I49.02	Ventricular flutter

AMA: 93615 2021,Dec **93616** 2021,Dec

Relative Value Units/Medicare Edits

Non-Facility RVU	Work	PE	MP	Total
93615	0.0	0.0	0.0	0.0
93616	0.0	0.0	0.0	0.0
Facility RVU	**Work**	**PE**	**MP**	**Total**
93615	0.0	0.0	0.0	0.0
93616	0.0	0.0	0.0	0.0

	FUD	Status	MUE	Modifiers				IOM Reference
93615	0	C	1(3)	N/A	N/A	N/A	80*	None
93616	0	C	1(3)	N/A	N/A	N/A	80*	

* with documentation

Terms To Know

arrhythmias. Heart disorder of rhythm or rate, due to an electrical conduction system malfunction.

dysrhythmia. Abnormality or disturbance in rhythm.

Medicine

93618

93618 Induction of arrhythmia by electrical pacing

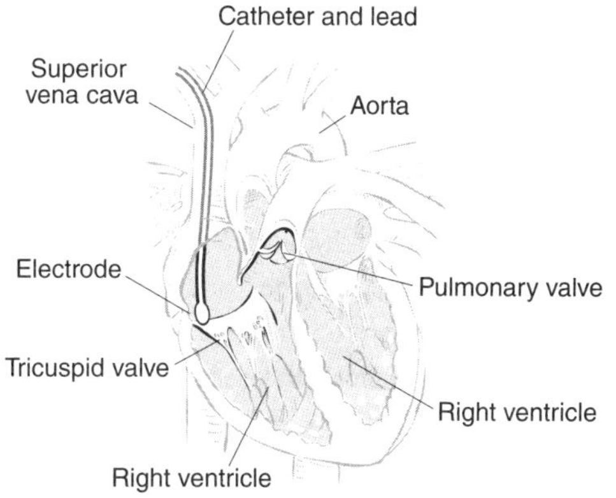

Arrhythmia is induced through electrical pacing. Usually the procedure is performed in conjunction with mapping of an area of the heart

Explanation

The physician places an appropriate arterial or venous sheath, usually femoral, to allow access to the chamber to be studied. The physician advances an electrical catheter through the sheath and into the appropriate chamber under fluoroscopic guidance. The physician attaches the catheter to an electrical pacing device to allow transmission of pacing impulses through the catheter to the heart chamber of interest. The physician stimulates the heart with rapid pacing or programmed electrical stimulation until the arrhythmia is induced.

Coding Tips

When medically necessary, report moderate (conscious) sedation provided by the performing physician with 99151-99153. When provided by another physician, report 99155-99157. As exempt from modifier 51, 93618 has not been designated in CPT as an add-on service/procedure. However, codes identified as exempt from modifier 51 are not subject to multiple procedure rules. No reimbursement reduction or modifier 51 is applied. Procedure 93618 has both a technical and professional component. To report only the professional component, append modifier 26. To report only the technical component, append modifier TC. To report the complete procedure (i.e., both the professional and technical components), submit without a modifier. Fluoroscopic guidance is included in electrophysiological procedures and should not be reported separately. Procedure 93618 reports induction of arrhythmia only. For comprehensive electrophysiologic evaluation, including induction of arrhythmia, see 93620–93622. Do not report 93618 with 93619, 93620–93622, 93653, 93654, or 93656. For intracardiac phonocardiogram, see 93799. Moderate sedation performed with 93618 is considered to be an integral part of the procedure and is not reported separately. However, anesthesia services (00100–01999) may be billed separately when performed by a physician (or other qualified provider) other than the physician performing the procedure.

ICD-10-CM Diagnostic Codes

I45.89	Other specified conduction disorders
I47.0	Re-entry ventricular arrhythmia
I47.11	Inappropriate sinus tachycardia, so stated
I47.21	Torsades de pointes
I47.29	Other ventricular tachycardia
I48.0	Paroxysmal atrial fibrillation
I48.11	Longstanding persistent atrial fibrillation
I48.19	Other persistent atrial fibrillation
I48.21	Permanent atrial fibrillation
I48.3	Typical atrial flutter
I48.4	Atypical atrial flutter
I49.01	Ventricular fibrillation
I49.02	Ventricular flutter
I49.1	Atrial premature depolarization
I49.2	Junctional premature depolarization
I49.3	Ventricular premature depolarization
I49.49	Other premature depolarization
I49.5	Sick sinus syndrome
I49.8	Other specified cardiac arrhythmias
R55	Syncope and collapse

AMA: **93618** 2021,Dec

Relative Value Units/Medicare Edits

Non-Facility RVU	Work	PE	MP	Total
93618	0.0	0.0	0.0	0.0
Facility RVU	**Work**	**PE**	**MP**	**Total**
93618	0.0	0.0	0.0	0.0

	FUD	Status	MUE	Modifiers				IOM Reference
93618	0	C	1(3)	N/A	N/A	N/A	80*	None

* with documentation

Terms To Know

arrhythmias. Heart disorder of rhythm or rate, due to an electrical conduction system malfunction.

fluoroscopy. Radiology technique that allows visual examination of part of the body or a function of an organ using a device that projects an x-ray image on a fluorescent screen.

93619

93619 Comprehensive electrophysiologic evaluation with right atrial pacing and recording, right ventricular pacing and recording, His bundle recording, including insertion and repositioning of multiple electrode catheters, without induction or attempted induction of arrhythmia

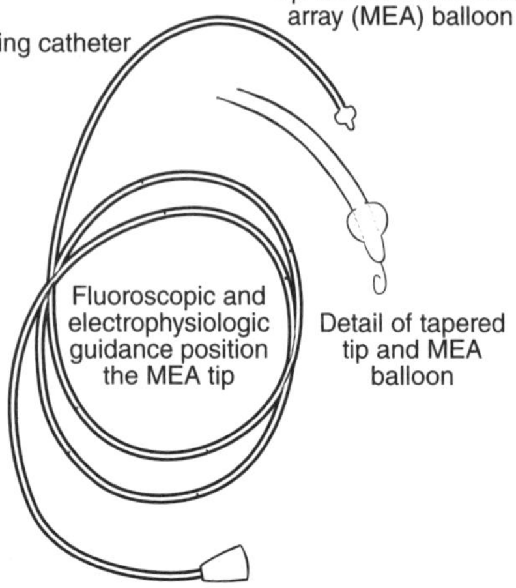

The right atrium and right ventricle are paced and recorded; the His bundle along the septum is recorded without any attempt to induce arrhythmia

Explanation

The physician places three venous sheaths, usually in one or both femoral veins, using standard techniques. The physician advances three electrical catheters through the venous sheaths and into the right heart under fluoroscopic guidance. The physician attaches the three catheters to an electrical recording device to allow depiction of the intracardiac electrograms obtained from electrodes on the catheter tips. The physician moves the tips of the three catheters to the right atrium, the bundle of His, and the right ventricle and obtains recordings.

Coding Tips

When medically necessary, report moderate (conscious) sedation provided by the performing physician with 99151-99153. When provided by another physician, report 99155-99157. Procedure 93619 has both a technical and professional component. To report only the professional component, append modifier 26. To report only the technical component, append modifier TC. To report the complete procedure (i.e., both the professional and technical components), submit without a modifier. Fluoroscopic guidance is included in electrophysiological procedures and should not be reported separately. Do not report 93619 with 93600, 93602, 93603, 93610, 93612, 93618, 93620–93622, or 93653–93657.

ICD-10-CM Diagnostic Codes

I44.0	Atrioventricular block, first degree
I44.1	Atrioventricular block, second degree
I44.2	Atrioventricular block, complete
I44.30	Unspecified atrioventricular block
I44.39	Other atrioventricular block
I44.4	Left anterior fascicular block
I44.5	Left posterior fascicular block
I44.69	Other fascicular block
I45.0	Right fascicular block
I45.19	Other right bundle-branch block
I45.2	Bifascicular block
I45.3	Trifascicular block
I45.4	Nonspecific intraventricular block
I45.5	Other specified heart block
I45.6	Pre-excitation syndrome
I45.89	Other specified conduction disorders
I47.0	Re-entry ventricular arrhythmia
I47.11	Inappropriate sinus tachycardia, so stated
I47.21	Torsades de pointes
I47.29	Other ventricular tachycardia
I48.0	Paroxysmal atrial fibrillation
I48.11	Longstanding persistent atrial fibrillation
I48.19	Other persistent atrial fibrillation
I48.21	Permanent atrial fibrillation
I48.3	Typical atrial flutter
I48.4	Atypical atrial flutter
I49.01	Ventricular fibrillation
I49.02	Ventricular flutter
I49.1	Atrial premature depolarization
I49.2	Junctional premature depolarization
I49.3	Ventricular premature depolarization
I49.49	Other premature depolarization
I49.5	Sick sinus syndrome
I49.8	Other specified cardiac arrhythmias
P29.81	Cardiac arrest of newborn N
R55	Syncope and collapse

AMA: **93619** 2023,May; 2021,Dec

Relative Value Units/Medicare Edits

Non-Facility RVU	Work	PE	MP	Total
93619	0.0	0.0	0.0	0.0
Facility RVU	**Work**	**PE**	**MP**	**Total**
93619	0.0	0.0	0.0	0.0

	FUD	Status	MUE	Modifiers				IOM Reference
93619	0	C	1(3)	51	N/A	N/A	80*	None

* with documentation

Medicine

93620

93620 Comprehensive electrophysiologic evaluation including insertion and repositioning of multiple electrode catheters with induction or attempted induction of arrhythmia; with right atrial pacing and recording, right ventricular pacing and recording, His bundle recording

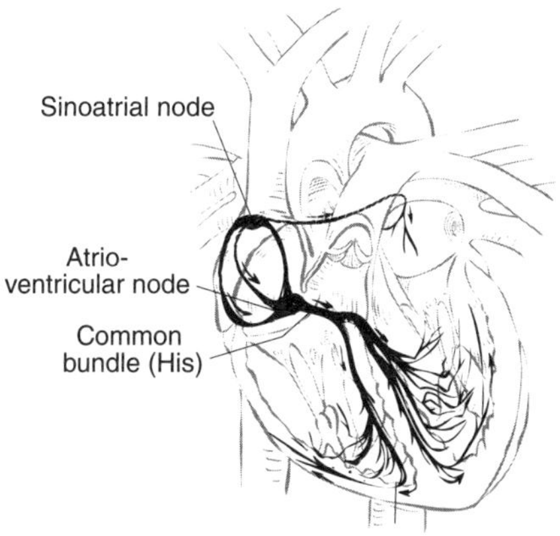

Conduction system of the heart

Explanation

The electrophysiologist places three venous sheaths, usually in one or both femoral veins, using standard techniques. Three electrical catheters are threaded through the venous sheaths and into the right heart under fluoroscopic guidance. The catheters are attached to an electrical recording device to allow depiction of the intracardiac electrograms obtained from electrodes on the catheter tips. The physician moves the tips of the catheters to the high right atrium, the bundle of His, and the right ventricle and obtains recordings. The physician then attaches the catheters to an electrical pacing device to allow transmission of pacing impulses through the catheters to the different heart chambers. The physician stimulates the heart with rapid pacing or programmed electrical stimulation in an attempt to induce an arrhythmia.

Coding Tips

When medically necessary, report moderate (conscious) sedation provided by the performing physician with 99151-99153. When provided by another physician, report 99155-99157. Procedure 93620 has both a technical and professional component. To report only the professional component, append modifier 26. To report only the technical component, append modifier TC. To report the complete procedure (i.e., both the professional and technical components), submit without a modifier. Fluoroscopic guidance is included in electrophysiological procedures and should not be reported separately. Do not report 93620 with 93600, 93602, 93603, 93610, 93612, 93618, 93619, or 93653–93657.

ICD-10-CM Diagnostic Codes

I44.0	Atrioventricular block, first degree
I44.1	Atrioventricular block, second degree
I44.2	Atrioventricular block, complete
I44.39	Other atrioventricular block
I44.4	Left anterior fascicular block
I44.5	Left posterior fascicular block
I44.69	Other fascicular block
I45.0	Right fascicular block
I45.19	Other right bundle-branch block
I45.2	Bifascicular block
I45.3	Trifascicular block
I45.4	Nonspecific intraventricular block
I45.5	Other specified heart block
I45.6	Pre-excitation syndrome
I45.89	Other specified conduction disorders
I46.2	Cardiac arrest due to underlying cardiac condition
I46.8	Cardiac arrest due to other underlying condition
I47.0	Re-entry ventricular arrhythmia
I47.11	Inappropriate sinus tachycardia, so stated
I47.21	Torsades de pointes
I47.29	Other ventricular tachycardia
I48.0	Paroxysmal atrial fibrillation
I48.11	Longstanding persistent atrial fibrillation
I48.21	Permanent atrial fibrillation
I48.3	Typical atrial flutter
I48.4	Atypical atrial flutter
I49.01	Ventricular fibrillation
I49.02	Ventricular flutter
I49.1	Atrial premature depolarization
I49.2	Junctional premature depolarization
I49.3	Ventricular premature depolarization
I49.49	Other premature depolarization
I49.5	Sick sinus syndrome
I49.8	Other specified cardiac arrhythmias
P29.81	Cardiac arrest of newborn N
R55	Syncope and collapse

AMA: 93620 2023,Oct; 2023,May; 2021,Dec

Relative Value Units/Medicare Edits

Non-Facility RVU	Work	PE	MP	Total
93620	0.0	0.0	0.0	0.0
Facility RVU	**Work**	**PE**	**MP**	**Total**
93620	0.0	0.0	0.0	0.0

	FUD	Status	MUE	Modifiers				IOM Reference
93620	0	C	1(3)	51	N/A	N/A	80*	None

* with documentation

Terms To Know

arrhythmias. Heart disorder of rhythm or rate, due to an electrical conduction system malfunction.

dysrhythmia. Abnormality or disturbance in rhythm.

fluoroscopy. Radiology technique that allows visual examination of part of the body or a function of an organ using a device that projects an x-ray image on a fluorescent screen.

Lown (-Ganong)-Levine syndrome. Electrocardiographic disorder indicated by a short P-R interval with normal duration of the QRS complex.

 ● New ▲ Revised + Add On ★ Telemedicine [Resequenced] ☑ Laterality

93621

\+ **93621** Comprehensive electrophysiologic evaluation including insertion and repositioning of multiple electrode catheters with induction or attempted induction of arrhythmia; with left atrial pacing and recording from coronary sinus or left atrium (List separately in addition to code for primary procedure)

Explanation

The physician places four central venous sheaths using standard techniques. Four electrical catheters are threaded through the venous sheaths and into the right heart under fluoroscopic guidance. The catheters are attached to an electrical recording device to allow depiction of the intracardiac electrograms obtained from electrodes on the catheter tips. The physician moves the tips of the catheters to the high right atrium, the bundle of His, the right ventricle, and through the coronary sinus to the left atrium and obtains recordings. The physician attaches the catheters to an electrical pacing device to allow transmission of pacing impulses through the catheters to the different heart chambers. The physician stimulates the heart with rapid pacing or programmed electrical stimulation in an attempt to induce an arrhythmia.

Coding Tips

When medically necessary, report moderate (conscious) sedation provided by the performing physician with 99151-99153. When provided by another physician, report 99155-99157. Report 93621 in addition to 93620. Do not report 93621 with 93656. Procedure 93621 has both a technical and professional component. To report only the professional component, append modifier 26. To report only the technical component, append modifier TC. To report the complete procedure (i.e., both the professional and technical components), submit without a modifier. Fluoroscopic guidance is included in electrophysiological procedures and should not be reported separately.

ICD-10-CM Diagnostic Codes

This/these CPT code(s) are add-on code(s). See the primary procedure code that this code is performed with for your ICD-10-CM code selections. Diagnostic code(s) would be the same as the actual procedure performed.

AMA: 93621 2023,May; 2021,Dec

Relative Value Units/Medicare Edits

Non-Facility RVU	Work	PE	MP	Total
93621	0.0	0.0	0.0	0.0
Facility RVU	**Work**	**PE**	**MP**	**Total**
93621	0.0	0.0	0.0	0.0

	FUD	Status	MUE	Modifiers				IOM Reference
93621	N/A	C	1(3)	N/A	N/A	N/A	80*	None

* with documentation

Terms To Know

arrhythmia. Irregular heartbeat.

electrophysiologic studies. Electrical stimulation and monitoring to diagnose heart conduction abnormalities that predispose patients to bradyarrhythmias and to determine a patient's chance for developing ventricular and supraventricular tachyarrhythmias.

93622

\+ **93622** Comprehensive electrophysiologic evaluation including insertion and repositioning of multiple electrode catheters with induction or attempted induction of arrhythmia; with left ventricular pacing and recording (List separately in addition to code for primary procedure)

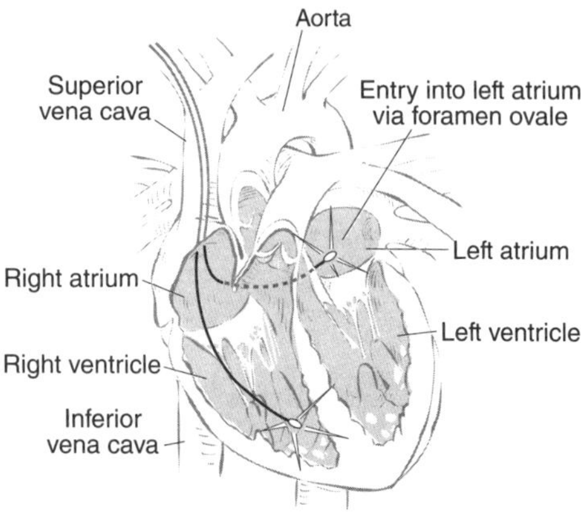

The left ventricle is paced and recorded, either remotely from the right side of the heart or intraventricularly

Explanation

The physician places three central venous sheaths and an arterial sheath using standard techniques. The physician advances four electrical catheters through these sheaths and into the heart under fluoroscopic guidance. The physician attaches the four catheters to an electrical recording device to allow depiction of the intracardiac electrograms obtained from electrodes on the catheter tips. The physician moves the tips of the four catheters to the right atrium, the bundle of His, the right ventricle, and the left ventricle and obtains recordings. The physician may attach the catheters to an electrical pacing device to allow transmission of pacing impulses through the catheters to the different heart chambers. The physician may stimulate the heart with rapid pacing or programmed electrical stimulation in an attempt to induce an arrhythmia.

Coding Tips

When medically necessary, report moderate (conscious) sedation provided by the performing physician with 99151-99153. When provided by another physician, report 99155-99157. Report 93622 in addition to 93620, 93653, or 93656. Do not report 93622 with 93654. Procedure 93622 has both a technical and professional component. To report only the professional component, append modifier 26. To report only the technical component, append modifier TC. To report the complete procedure (i.e., both the professional and technical components), submit without a modifier. Fluoroscopic guidance is included in electrophysiological procedures and should not be reported separately. For noninvasive arrhythmia localization and mapping, see 0745T.

ICD-10-CM Diagnostic Codes

This/these CPT code(s) are add-on code(s). See the primary procedure code that this code is performed with for your ICD-10-CM code selections. Diagnostic code(s) would be the same as the actual procedure performed.

AMA: 93622 2023,May; 2021,Dec

Relative Value Units/Medicare Edits

Non-Facility RVU	Work	PE	MP	Total
93622	0.0	0.0	0.0	0.0
Facility RVU	Work	PE	MP	Total
93622	0.0	0.0	0.0	0.0

	FUD	Status	MUE	Modifiers				IOM Reference
93622	N/A	C	1(3)	N/A	N/A	N/A	80*	None

* with documentation

Terms To Know

arrhythmias. Heart disorder of rhythm or rate, due to an electrical conduction system malfunction.

bundle of His. Bundle of modified cardiac fibers that begins at the atrioventricular node and passes through the right atrioventricular fibrous ring to the interventricular septum, where it divides into two branches. Bundle of His recordings are taken for intracardiac electrograms.

fluoroscopy. Radiology technique that allows visual examination of part of the body or a function of an organ using a device that projects an x-ray image on a fluorescent screen.

Lown (-Ganong)-Levine syndrome. Electrocardiographic disorder indicated by a short P-R interval with normal duration of the QRS complex.

moderate sedation. Medically controlled state of depressed consciousness, with or without analgesia, while maintaining the patient's airway, protective reflexes, and ability to respond to stimulation or verbal commands.

93623

\+ **93623** Programmed stimulation and pacing after intravenous drug infusion (List separately in addition to code for primary procedure)

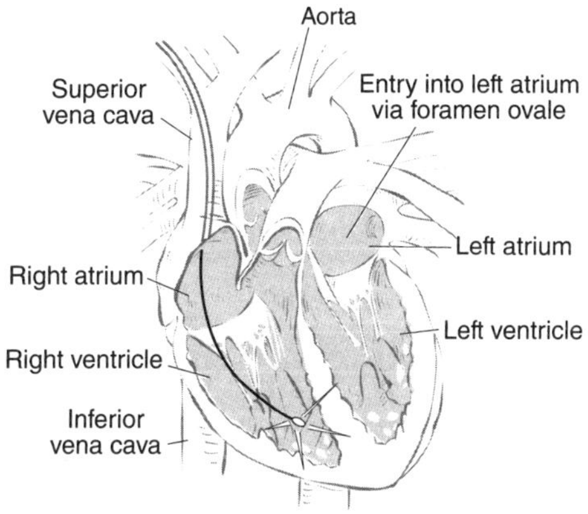

Stimulation and pacing is carried out as specified in previous codes, but an IV drug infusion occurs as a component of this procedure

Explanation

Following a comprehensive electrophysiological study with or without attempted or actual induction of an arrhythmia, before the electrode catheters are removed, an intravenous drug, such as isoproterenol, is infused. The physician attaches the catheter to an electrical pacing device to allow transmission of pacing impulses through the catheter to the heart chamber of interest. The heart is stimulated using rapid pacing or programmed electrical stimulation in an attempt to induce an arrhythmia. This code is reported in addition to the code for the primary electrophysiological procedure.

Coding Tips

Report 93623 in addition to 93610, 93612, 93619, 93620, 93653, 93654, or 93656. Procedure 93623 has both a technical and professional component. To report only the professional component, append modifier 26. To report only the technical component, append modifier TC. To report the complete procedure (i.e., both the professional and technical components), submit without a modifier. Only report 93623 once per day. Fluoroscopic guidance is included in electrophysiological procedures and should not be reported separately.

ICD-10-CM Diagnostic Codes

This/these CPT code(s) are add-on code(s). See the primary procedure code that this code is performed with for your ICD-10-CM code selections. Diagnostic code(s) would be the same as the actual procedure performed.

Relative Value Units/Medicare Edits

Non-Facility RVU	Work	PE	MP	Total
93623	0.0	0.0	0.0	0.0
Facility RVU	Work	PE	MP	Total
93623	0.0	0.0	0.0	0.0

	FUD	Status	MUE	Modifiers				IOM Reference
93623	N/A	C	1(3)	N/A	N/A	N/A	80*	None

* with documentation

93624

93624 Electrophysiologic follow-up study with pacing and recording to test effectiveness of therapy, including induction or attempted induction of arrhythmia

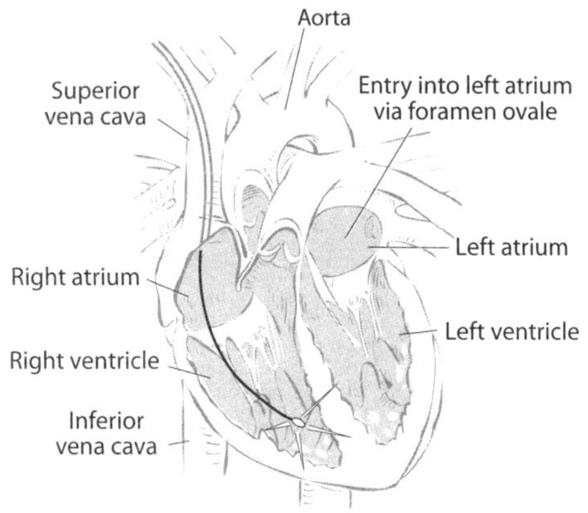

A follow-up EPS is performed with pacing and recording to test the effectiveness of therapy

Explanation

Following administration of therapy (antiarrhythmic drugs, surgery, ablation, etc.), the physician places an appropriate arterial or venous sheath, usually femoral, to allow access to the chamber to be studied. Under fluoroscopic guidance, the physician advances an electrical catheter through the sheath and into the appropriate chamber. An intravenous drug, such as isoproterenol, is infused. The physician attaches the catheter to an electrical pacing device to allow transmission of pacing impulses through the catheter to the heart chamber of interest. The physician stimulates the heart with rapid pacing or programmed electrical stimulation in an attempt to induce an arrhythmia.

Coding Tips

When medically necessary, report moderate (conscious) sedation provided by the performing physician with 99151-99153. When provided by another physician, report 99155-99157. Procedure 93624 has both a technical and professional component. To report only the professional component, append modifier 26. To report only the technical component, append modifier TC. To report the complete procedure (i.e., both the professional and technical components), submit without a modifier. Fluoroscopic guidance is included in electrophysiological procedures and should not be reported separately.

ICD-10-CM Diagnostic Codes

I44.0	Atrioventricular block, first degree
I44.1	Atrioventricular block, second degree
I44.2	Atrioventricular block, complete
I44.39	Other atrioventricular block
I44.4	Left anterior fascicular block
I44.5	Left posterior fascicular block
I44.69	Other fascicular block
I45.0	Right fascicular block
I45.19	Other right bundle-branch block
I45.2	Bifascicular block
I45.3	Trifascicular block
I45.4	Nonspecific intraventricular block
I45.5	Other specified heart block
I45.6	Pre-excitation syndrome
I45.89	Other specified conduction disorders
I46.2	Cardiac arrest due to underlying cardiac condition
I46.8	Cardiac arrest due to other underlying condition
I47.0	Re-entry ventricular arrhythmia
I47.11	Inappropriate sinus tachycardia, so stated
I47.21	Torsades de pointes
I47.29	Other ventricular tachycardia
I48.0	Paroxysmal atrial fibrillation
I48.11	Longstanding persistent atrial fibrillation
I48.19	Other persistent atrial fibrillation
I48.21	Permanent atrial fibrillation
I48.3	Typical atrial flutter
I48.4	Atypical atrial flutter
I49.01	Ventricular fibrillation
I49.02	Ventricular flutter
I49.1	Atrial premature depolarization
I49.2	Junctional premature depolarization
I49.3	Ventricular premature depolarization
I49.49	Other premature depolarization
I49.5	Sick sinus syndrome
I49.8	Other specified cardiac arrhythmias

Relative Value Units/Medicare Edits

Non-Facility RVU	Work	PE	MP	Total
93624	0.0	0.0	0.0	0.0
Facility RVU	**Work**	**PE**	**MP**	**Total**
93624	0.0	0.0	0.0	0.0

	FUD	Status	MUE	Modifiers				IOM Reference
93624	0	C	1(3)	51	N/A	N/A	80*	None

* with documentation

93631

93631 Intra-operative epicardial and endocardial pacing and mapping to localize the site of tachycardia or zone of slow conduction for surgical correction

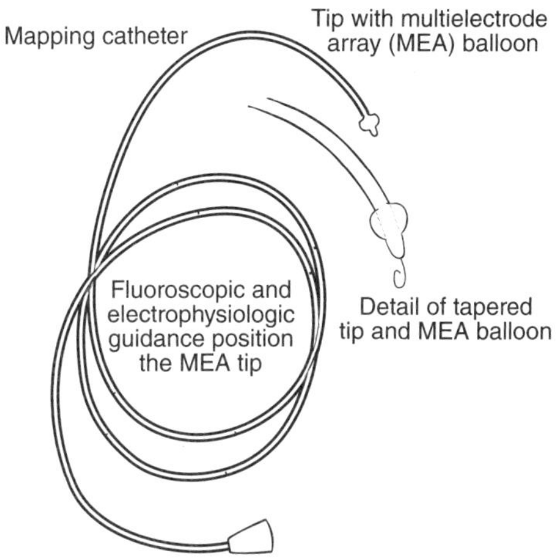

The physician places mapping and pacing catheters inside the heart prior to or during surgery using a standard transvenous approach. The tachycardia site or zone of slow conduction is localized so that it can be surgically corrected

Explanation

The purpose of this procedure is to localize the site of tachycardia during open-heart surgery to allow surgical correction of the tachycardia. The physician may place pacing or mapping catheters inside the heart prior to or during surgery using a standard transvenous approach. Additionally, the surgeon will place electrical probes on the outside (epicardium) of the heart in order to allow additional mapping. The physician attaches the catheters and probes to an electrical recording device to allow depiction of the electrograms obtained from electrodes on the catheter and probe tips. The surgeon's electrical probe can be moved around the outside of the heart to allow comparison of electrical activation times from different regions. The physician may attach the catheters to an electrical pacing device to allow transmission of pacing impulses through the catheters to the different heart chambers. The physician may stimulate the heart with rapid pacing or programmed electrical stimulation in an attempt to induce an arrhythmia.

Coding Tips

When an open heart ablation procedure is performed, the cardiothoracic surgeon typically performs the ablation component (33250–33261) and the electrophysiologist performs the pacing and mapping component (93631). Modifiers for multiple procedures, co-surgeons, and assistant surgeons are not reported with the two components because the individual codes describe the separate components that each physician performs. Procedure 93631 has both a technical and professional component. To report only the professional component, append modifier 26. To report only the technical component, append modifier TC. To report the complete procedure (i.e., both the professional and technical components), submit without a modifier.

ICD-10-CM Diagnostic Codes

I45.89	Other specified conduction disorders
I47.0	Re-entry ventricular arrhythmia
I47.11	Inappropriate sinus tachycardia, so stated
I47.21	Torsades de pointes
I47.29	Other ventricular tachycardia
I48.0	Paroxysmal atrial fibrillation
I48.11	Longstanding persistent atrial fibrillation
I48.19	Other persistent atrial fibrillation
I48.21	Permanent atrial fibrillation
I48.3	Typical atrial flutter
I48.4	Atypical atrial flutter
I49.01	Ventricular fibrillation
I49.02	Ventricular flutter
I49.1	Atrial premature depolarization
I49.2	Junctional premature depolarization
I49.3	Ventricular premature depolarization
I49.49	Other premature depolarization
I49.5	Sick sinus syndrome
I49.8	Other specified cardiac arrhythmias

Relative Value Units/Medicare Edits

Non-Facility RVU	Work	PE	MP	Total
93631	0.0	0.0	0.0	0.0
Facility RVU	**Work**	**PE**	**MP**	**Total**
93631	0.0	0.0	0.0	0.0

	FUD	Status	MUE	Modifiers				IOM Reference
93631	0	C	1(3)	N/A	N/A	N/A	80*	None

* with documentation

Terms To Know

arrhythmia. Irregular heartbeat.

supraventricular tachycardia. Rapid beating of the heart, usually pertains to more than 100 beats per minute and can be as high as 250 beats per minute. SVT is caused by abnormal electrical impulses originating at the AV node or above it in the atria (upper chambers) of the heart.

Medicine

93640-93641

93640 Electrophysiologic evaluation of single or dual chamber pacing cardioverter-defibrillator leads including defibrillation threshold evaluation (induction of arrhythmia, evaluation of sensing and pacing for arrhythmia termination) at time of initial implantation or replacement;

93641 with testing of single or dual chamber pacing cardioverter-defibrillator pulse generator

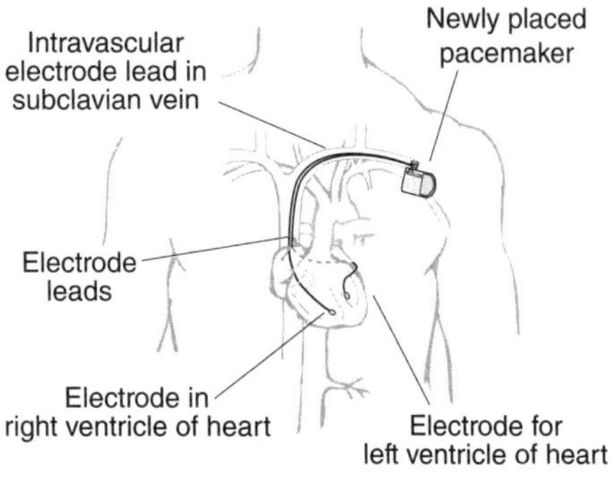

Testing is performed on cardioverter-defibrillator leads and pulse generator to ensure that they are functioning properly

Explanation

The purpose of this study is to ensure that the cardioverter-defibrillator (ICD) leads are positioned well and working properly, to guarantee proper function of this device in the future. Leads are typically placed in the heart via the subclavian vein, but occasionally defibrillation patches are placed on the epicardium or under the skin. To test the leads, the physician records cardiac electrical signals and paces the heart through the leads. The physician may test the leads using the actual ICD or by hooking the leads to an external device. The physician uses the leads to pace the heart into an arrhythmia, such as ventricular tachycardia or fibrillation. The ICD or external device detects the arrhythmia and shocks the heart through the ICD leads. The physician may perform this test with several different levels of shock to ensure that the ICD can reliably terminate the arrhythmia. In 93640, only the leads are tested. In 93641, both the leads and the cardioverter-defibrillator pulse generator are tested.

Coding Tips

When medically necessary, report moderate (conscious) sedation provided by the performing physician with 99151-99153. When provided by another physician, report 99155-99157. Codes 93640 and 93641 are reported in addition to the insertion codes at the time of implantation or replacement of the single or dual chamber pacing cardioverter-defibrillator electrode leads (93640) or pulse generator (93641). Induction of arrhythmia is included in 93640 and 93641. Do not report 93618 separately. Procedures 93640 and 93641 have both a technical and professional component. To report only the professional component, append modifier 26. To report only the technical component, append modifier TC. To report the complete procedure (i.e., both the professional and technical components), submit without a modifier. For subsequent or periodic electronic analysis and/or reprogramming of single or dual chamber pacing cardioverter-defibrillators, see 93282, 93283, 93289, 93292, 93295, and 93642.

ICD-10-CM Diagnostic Codes

I45.89	Other specified conduction disorders
I47.0	Re-entry ventricular arrhythmia
I47.11	Inappropriate sinus tachycardia, so stated
I47.21	Torsades de pointes
I47.29	Other ventricular tachycardia
I48.0	Paroxysmal atrial fibrillation
I48.11	Longstanding persistent atrial fibrillation
I48.19	Other persistent atrial fibrillation
I48.21	Permanent atrial fibrillation
I48.3	Typical atrial flutter
I48.4	Atypical atrial flutter
I49.01	Ventricular fibrillation
I49.02	Ventricular flutter
I49.1	Atrial premature depolarization
I49.2	Junctional premature depolarization
I49.3	Ventricular premature depolarization
I49.49	Other premature depolarization
I49.5	Sick sinus syndrome
I49.8	Other specified cardiac arrhythmias
T82.817A	Embolism due to cardiac prosthetic devices, implants and grafts, initial encounter
T82.827A	Fibrosis due to cardiac prosthetic devices, implants and grafts, initial encounter
T82.837A	Hemorrhage due to cardiac prosthetic devices, implants and grafts, initial encounter
T82.847A	Pain due to cardiac prosthetic devices, implants and grafts, initial encounter
T82.857A	Stenosis of other cardiac prosthetic devices, implants and grafts, initial encounter
T82.867A	Thrombosis due to cardiac prosthetic devices, implants and grafts, initial encounter
T82.897A	Other specified complication of cardiac prosthetic devices, implants and grafts, initial encounter
Z45.02	Encounter for adjustment and management of automatic implantable cardiac defibrillator
Z95.810	Presence of automatic (implantable) cardiac defibrillator

Relative Value Units/Medicare Edits

Non-Facility RVU	Work	PE	MP	Total
93640	0.0	0.0	0.0	0.0
93641	0.0	0.0	0.0	0.0
Facility RVU	**Work**	**PE**	**MP**	**Total**
93640	0.0	0.0	0.0	0.0
93641	0.0	0.0	0.0	0.0

	FUD	Status	MUE	Modifiers				IOM Reference
93640	0	C	1(3)	51	N/A	N/A	80*	None
93641	0	C	1(2)	51	N/A	N/A	80*	

* with documentation

93642

93642 Electrophysiologic evaluation of single or dual chamber transvenous pacing cardioverter-defibrillator (includes defibrillation threshold evaluation, induction of arrhythmia, evaluation of sensing and pacing for arrhythmia termination, and programming or reprogramming of sensing or therapeutic parameters)

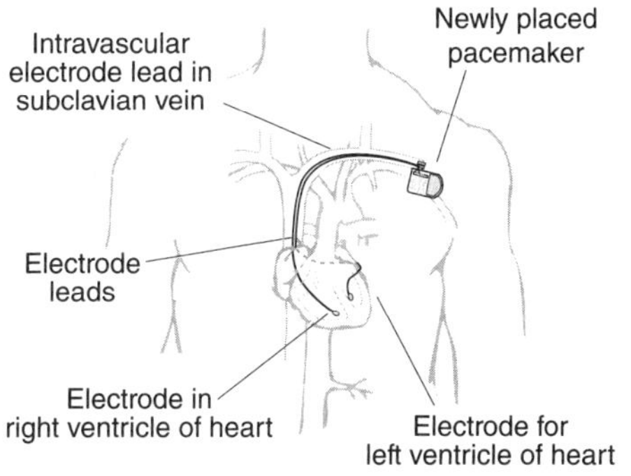

Testing is performed on cardioverter-defibrillator leads and pulse generator to ensure that they are functioning properly

Explanation

The purpose of this study is to ensure that the transvenous pacing cardioverter-defibrillator (ICD) and ICD leads are positioned well and working properly, to guarantee proper function of this device in the future. The physician records cardiac electrical signals from the leads and paces the heart through the leads to determine pacing threshold. The physician uses the ICD pulse generator to pace the heart into an arrhythmia, such as ventricular tachycardia or fibrillation. The ICD detects and terminates the arrhythmia using pacing or shocking the heart through the ICD lead. The physician may reprogram the ICD's treatment parameters to optimize the device function to best treat the patient's arrhythmia.

Coding Tips

When medically necessary, report moderate (conscious) sedation provided by the performing physician with 99151-99153. When provided by another physician, report 99155-99157. Code 93642 reports subsequent or periodic electronic analysis and/or reprogramming of a transvenous pacing cardioverter-defibrillator. When electrophysiologic evaluation of a pacing cardioverter-defibrillator is performed at the time of initial implantation or replacement, report 93640 or 93641 instead of 93642. Procedure 93642 has both a technical and professional component. To report only the professional component, append modifier 26. To report only the technical component, append modifier TC. To report the complete procedure (i.e., both the professional and technical components), submit without a modifier.

ICD-10-CM Diagnostic Codes

I45.89	Other specified conduction disorders
I47.0	Re-entry ventricular arrhythmia
I47.11	Inappropriate sinus tachycardia, so stated
I47.21	Torsades de pointes
I47.29	Other ventricular tachycardia
I48.0	Paroxysmal atrial fibrillation
I48.11	Longstanding persistent atrial fibrillation
I48.19	Other persistent atrial fibrillation
I48.21	Permanent atrial fibrillation
I48.3	Typical atrial flutter
I48.4	Atypical atrial flutter
I49.01	Ventricular fibrillation
I49.02	Ventricular flutter
I49.1	Atrial premature depolarization
I49.2	Junctional premature depolarization
I49.3	Ventricular premature depolarization
I49.49	Other premature depolarization
I49.5	Sick sinus syndrome
I49.8	Other specified cardiac arrhythmias
T82.817A	Embolism due to cardiac prosthetic devices, implants and grafts, initial encounter
T82.827A	Fibrosis due to cardiac prosthetic devices, implants and grafts, initial encounter
T82.837A	Hemorrhage due to cardiac prosthetic devices, implants and grafts, initial encounter
T82.847A	Pain due to cardiac prosthetic devices, implants and grafts, initial encounter
T82.857A	Stenosis of other cardiac prosthetic devices, implants and grafts, initial encounter
T82.867A	Thrombosis due to cardiac prosthetic devices, implants and grafts, initial encounter
T82.897A	Other specified complication of cardiac prosthetic devices, implants and grafts, initial encounter
Z45.02	Encounter for adjustment and management of automatic implantable cardiac defibrillator
Z95.810	Presence of automatic (implantable) cardiac defibrillator

AMA: **93642** 2021,Dec

Relative Value Units/Medicare Edits

Non-Facility RVU	Work	PE	MP	Total
93642	4.63	4.22	0.92	9.77
Facility RVU	**Work**	**PE**	**MP**	**Total**
93642	4.63	4.22	0.92	9.77

	FUD	Status	MUE	Modifiers				IOM Reference
93642	0	A	1(3)	51	N/A	N/A	80*	None

* with documentation

Terms To Know

arrhythmias. Heart disorder of rhythm or rate, due to an electrical conduction system malfunction.

cardioverter-defibrillator. Device that uses both low energy cardioversion or defibrillating shocks and antitachycardia pacing to treat ventricular tachycardia or ventricular fibrillation.

93644

93644 Electrophysiologic evaluation of subcutaneous implantable defibrillator (includes defibrillation threshold evaluation, induction of arrhythmia, evaluation of sensing for arrhythmia termination, and programming or reprogramming of sensing or therapeutic parameters)

Explanation

A study is performed to ensure that the subcutaneous implantable defibrillator system and leads are positioned well and working properly in order to guarantee proper function. The physician records cardiac electrical signals from the leads and paces the heart through the leads to determine pacing threshold. The physician uses the pulse generator to pace the heart into an arrhythmia, such as ventricular tachycardia or fibrillation. The system detects and terminates the arrhythmia using pacing or shocking the heart through the lead. The physician may reprogram the treatment parameters to optimize the device function to best treat the patient's arrhythmia.

Coding Tips

When medically necessary, report moderate (conscious) sedation provided by the performing physician with 99151-99153. When provided by another physician, report 99155-99157. For recurrent electrophysiologic evaluation of device, see 93260 and 93261. Do not report 93644 with 33270 during the same encounter for subcutaneous defibrillator insertion. For electrophysiologic evaluation of single or dual chamber implantable defibrillator leads including threshold evaluation at the time of implant or replacement, see 93640. For electrophysiologic evaluation of a single or dual chamber implantable defibrillator generator at the time of implant or replacement, see 93641. For recurrent analysis and/or reprogramming of single or dual chamber implantable defibrillators, see 93282, 93283, 93289, 93292, 93295, and 93642. For electrophysiologic evaluation of a single or dual chamber transvenous pacing cardioverter-defibrillator, see 93642.

ICD-10-CM Diagnostic Codes

I45.89	Other specified conduction disorders
I47.0	Re-entry ventricular arrhythmia
I47.11	Inappropriate sinus tachycardia, so stated
I47.21	Torsades de pointes
I47.29	Other ventricular tachycardia
I48.0	Paroxysmal atrial fibrillation
I48.11	Longstanding persistent atrial fibrillation
I48.19	Other persistent atrial fibrillation
I48.21	Permanent atrial fibrillation
I48.3	Typical atrial flutter
I48.4	Atypical atrial flutter
I49.01	Ventricular fibrillation
I49.02	Ventricular flutter
I49.1	Atrial premature depolarization
I49.2	Junctional premature depolarization
I49.3	Ventricular premature depolarization
I49.49	Other premature depolarization
I49.5	Sick sinus syndrome
I49.8	Other specified cardiac arrhythmias
T82.817A	Embolism due to cardiac prosthetic devices, implants and grafts, initial encounter
T82.827A	Fibrosis due to cardiac prosthetic devices, implants and grafts, initial encounter
T82.837A	Hemorrhage due to cardiac prosthetic devices, implants and grafts, initial encounter
T82.847A	Pain due to cardiac prosthetic devices, implants and grafts, initial encounter
T82.855A	Stenosis of coronary artery stent, initial encounter
T82.857A	Stenosis of other cardiac prosthetic devices, implants and grafts, initial encounter
T82.867A	Thrombosis due to cardiac prosthetic devices, implants and grafts, initial encounter
T82.897A	Other specified complication of cardiac prosthetic devices, implants and grafts, initial encounter
Z45.02	Encounter for adjustment and management of automatic implantable cardiac defibrillator
Z95.810	Presence of automatic (implantable) cardiac defibrillator

Relative Value Units/Medicare Edits

Non-Facility RVU	Work	PE	MP	Total
93644	3.04	2.55	0.1	5.69
Facility RVU	**Work**	**PE**	**MP**	**Total**
93644	3.04	2.55	0.1	5.69

	FUD	Status	MUE	Modifiers				IOM Reference
93644	0	A	1(3)	51	N/A	N/A	80*	None

* with documentation

Terms To Know

arrhythmia. Irregular heartbeat.

defibrillator system. System that includes a pulse generator and electrodes, implanted in the same manner as the pacemaker systems.

electrophysiologic studies. Electrical stimulation and monitoring to diagnose heart conduction abnormalities that predispose patients to bradyarrhythmias and to determine a patient's chance for developing ventricular and supraventricular tachyarrhythmias.

paroxysmal supraventricular tachycardia. Rapid heartbeat that starts above the ventricles and occurs sporadically.

supraventricular tachycardia. Rapid beating of the heart, usually pertains to more than 100 beats per minute and can be as high as 250 beats per minute. SVT is caused by abnormal electrical impulses originating at the AV node or above it in the atria (upper chambers) of the heart.

93650

93650 Intracardiac catheter ablation of atrioventricular node function, atrioventricular conduction for creation of complete heart block, with or without temporary pacemaker placement

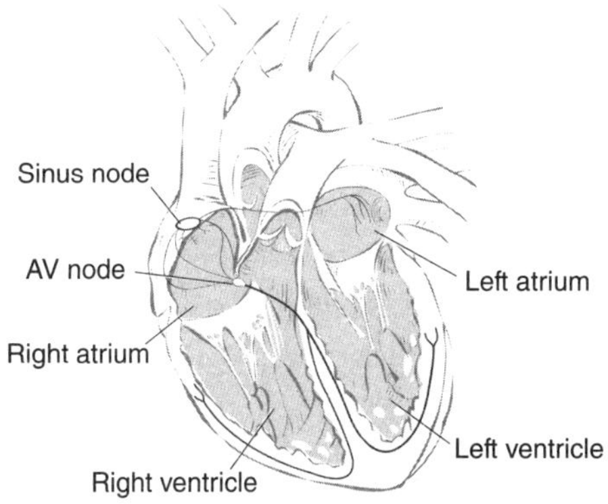

The atrioventricular (AV) node is ablated by intracardiac catheter. The elimination of AV function is usually to address atrial fibrillation. A temporary pacemaker may be placed as part of the procedure since the result is total stoppage of the heart's electromuscular function

Explanation

The purpose of this procedure is to create complete heart block, usually for control of the ventricular rate during atrial arrhythmias. The physician places a venous sheath, usually in a femoral vein, using standard techniques. The physician advances an electrical catheter through the venous sheath and into the right heart using fluoroscopic guidance. The physician attaches the catheter to an electrical recording device to allow depiction of the intracardiac electrograms obtained from electrodes on the catheter tip. The physician moves the catheter tip to the bundle of His, on the anteroseptal tricuspid annulus, and obtains recordings. Alternatively, the physician may obtain similar recordings by placing a catheter into the left ventricular outflow tract via the aorta. The physician maps the His bundle area and ablates the His bundle by sending cautery (radiofrequency) current through the catheter. The physician may also place a temporary pacing catheter in the right ventricle for this procedure.

Coding Tips

When medically necessary, report moderate (conscious) sedation provided by the performing physician with 99151-99153. When provided by another physician, report 99155-99157. Note that intracardiac catheter ablations are specific to the type of arrhythmia being treated. Code 93650 reports ablation of atrioventricular node function usually performed to control ventricular rate during atrial arrhythmias. For treatment of supraventricular tachycardia by intracardiac ablation, see 93653. For treatment of ventricular tachycardia by intracardiac ablation, see 93654. Fluoroscopic guidance is included in electrophysiological procedures and should not be reported separately.

ICD-10-CM Diagnostic Codes

I48.0	Paroxysmal atrial fibrillation
I48.11	Longstanding persistent atrial fibrillation
I48.19	Other persistent atrial fibrillation
I48.21	Permanent atrial fibrillation
I48.3	Typical atrial flutter
I48.4	Atypical atrial flutter
I48.91	Unspecified atrial fibrillation
I48.92	Unspecified atrial flutter
I49.1	Atrial premature depolarization

Relative Value Units/Medicare Edits

Non-Facility RVU	Work	PE	MP	Total
93650	10.24	4.44	2.32	17.0
Facility RVU	**Work**	**PE**	**MP**	**Total**
93650	10.24	4.44	2.32	17.0

	FUD	Status	MUE	Modifiers				IOM Reference
93650	0	A	1(2)	51	N/A	N/A	80*	None

* with documentation

Terms To Know

arrhythmias. Heart disorder of rhythm or rate, due to an electrical conduction system malfunction.

atrioventricular block. Condition in which there is a disturbance of electrical conduction, such as a delay, intermittence, or absence in the transmission of an impulse from the atria to the ventricles and categorized according to degree of severity.

cardiac arrest. Sudden, unexpected cessation of cardiac action, including absence of heart sounds and/or blood pressure.

cautery. Destruction or burning of tissue by means of a hot instrument, an electric current, or a caustic chemical, such as silver nitrate.

ventricular tachycardia. Excessively rapid ventricular rhythm of the heart, usually more than 150 beats per minute, with an origin beat generated in the ventricle, commonly from atrioventricular dissociation.

93653-93654

93653 Comprehensive electrophysiologic evaluation with insertion and repositioning of multiple electrode catheters, induction or attempted induction of an arrhythmia with right atrial pacing and recording and catheter ablation of arrhythmogenic focus, including intracardiac electrophysiologic 3-dimensional mapping, right ventricular pacing and recording, left atrial pacing and recording from coronary sinus or left atrium, and His bundle recording, when performed; with treatment of supraventricular tachycardia by ablation of fast or slow atrioventricular pathway, accessory atrioventricular connection, cavo-tricuspid isthmus or other single atrial focus or source of atrial re-entry

93654 with treatment of ventricular tachycardia or focus of ventricular ectopy including left ventricular pacing and recording, when performed

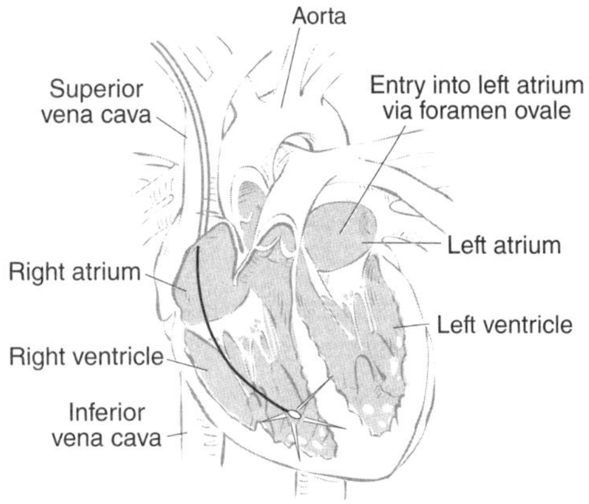

Electrophysiologic evaluation of right heart

Explanation

Catheter ablation is performed on cardiac tissue. In 93653, ablation is performed on dual atrioventricular nodal pathways, accessory atrioventricular connections, or other atrial foci causing supraventricular tachycardia (SVT). In 93654, ablation is performed on the cardiac tissue causing ventricular tachycardia or ectopy. For either procedure, the physician places three venous sheaths, usually in one or both femoral veins, using standard techniques. The physician advances three electrical catheters through the venous sheaths and into the right heart under fluoroscopic guidance. The three catheters are attached to an electrical recording device to allow depiction of the intracardiac electrograms obtained from electrodes on the catheter tips. The tips of the three catheters are moved to the right atrium, the bundle of His, left atrium and atrial pacing, and the right ventricle and recordings are obtained when clinically indicated. Selective destruction (ablation) of cardiac tissue to correct the SVT (93653) or the tachycardia or ectopy (93654) is based on the recordings. These codes include the use of three-dimensional mapping software when used.

Coding Tips

When medically necessary, report moderate (conscious) sedation provided by the performing physician with 99151-99153. When provided by another physician, report 99155-99157. Do not report 93653 with 93600–93603, 93610, 93612, 93613, 93618–93621, 93654, or 93656. Do not report 93654 with 93279–93284, 93286–93289, 93600–93603, 93609, 93610, 93612, 93613, 93618–93622, 93653, or 93656.

ICD-10-CM Diagnostic Codes

I44.39	Other atrioventricular block
I44.4	Left anterior fascicular block
I44.5	Left posterior fascicular block
I44.69	Other fascicular block
I45.0	Right fascicular block
I45.19	Other right bundle-branch block
I45.2	Bifascicular block
I45.3	Trifascicular block
I45.4	Nonspecific intraventricular block
I45.6	Pre-excitation syndrome
I45.89	Other specified conduction disorders
I46.2	Cardiac arrest due to underlying cardiac condition
I46.8	Cardiac arrest due to other underlying condition
I47.0	Re-entry ventricular arrhythmia
I47.11	Inappropriate sinus tachycardia, so stated
I47.21	Torsades de pointes
I47.29	Other ventricular tachycardia
I48.0	Paroxysmal atrial fibrillation
I48.11	Longstanding persistent atrial fibrillation
I48.19	Other persistent atrial fibrillation
I48.21	Permanent atrial fibrillation
I48.3	Typical atrial flutter
I48.4	Atypical atrial flutter
I49.01	Ventricular fibrillation
I49.02	Ventricular flutter
I49.2	Junctional premature depolarization
I49.8	Other specified cardiac arrhythmias

AMA: 93653 2024,Sep; 2023,Oct; 2021,Dec **93654** 2024,Sep; 2021,Dec

Relative Value Units/Medicare Edits

Non-Facility RVU	Work	PE	MP	Total
93653	15.0	6.0	3.42	24.42
93654	18.1	7.2	4.12	29.42
Facility RVU	**Work**	**PE**	**MP**	**Total**
93653	15.0	6.0	3.42	24.42
93654	18.1	7.2	4.12	29.42

	FUD	Status	MUE	Modifiers				IOM Reference
93653	0	A	1(3)	51	N/A	N/A	80*	None
93654	0	A	1(3)	51	N/A	N/A	80*	

* with documentation

93655

\+ **93655** Intracardiac catheter ablation of a discrete mechanism of arrhythmia which is distinct from the primary ablated mechanism, including repeat diagnostic maneuvers, to treat a spontaneous or induced arrhythmia (List separately in addition to code for primary procedure)

Explanation

After the initial treatment (ablation) for supraventricular or ventricular tachycardia, a postablation evaluation is performed. If there is a new (not previously diagnosed) or different mechanism causing the arrhythmia found on this evaluation, this is recorded and additional cardiac tissue is destroyed via the catheter to correct the newly discovered spontaneous or induced arrhythmia.

Coding Tips

When medically necessary, report moderate (conscious) sedation provided by the performing physician with 99151-99153. When provided by another physician, report 99155-99157. Report 93655 in addition to 93653, 93654, or 93656. This code is used when a separate, non-atrial fibrillation tachycardia has been separately diagnosed following pulmonary vein isolation.

ICD-10-CM Diagnostic Codes

This/these CPT code(s) are add-on code(s). See the primary procedure code that this code is performed with for your ICD-10-CM code selections. Diagnostic code(s) would be the same as the actual procedure performed.

AMA: **93655** 2021,Dec

Relative Value Units/Medicare Edits

Non-Facility RVU	Work	PE	MP	Total
93655	5.5	2.2	1.25	8.95
Facility RVU	**Work**	**PE**	**MP**	**Total**
93655	5.5	2.2	1.25	8.95

	FUD	Status	MUE	Modifiers				IOM Reference
93655	N/A	A	2(3)	N/A	N/A	N/A	80*	None

* with documentation

Terms To Know

ablation. Removal or destruction of a body part or tissue or its function. Ablation may be performed by surgical means, hormones, drugs, radiofrequency, heat, chemical application, or other methods.

supraventricular tachycardia. Rapid beating of the heart, usually pertains to more than 100 beats per minute and can be as high as 250 beats per minute. SVT is caused by abnormal electrical impulses originating at the AV node or above it in the atria (upper chambers) of the heart.

ventricular fibrillation. Cardiac arrhythmia in which ventricular myocardial fibers are rapidly and repetitively excited from a random or ectopic focus of electrical impulse, causing the muscle fibers to contract in an erratic manner without corresponding contraction of the ventricles. The condition requires immediate restoration of normal cardiac rhythm, often by electroshock through paddles placed on the chest.

93656-93657

▲ **93656** Comprehensive electrophysiologic evaluation with transseptal catheterizations, insertion and repositioning of multiple electrode catheters, induction or attempted induction of an arrhythmia including left or right atrial pacing/recording, and intracardiac catheter ablation of atrial fibrillation by pulmonary vein isolation, including intracardiac electrophysiologic 3-dimensional mapping, intracardiac echocardiography with imaging supervision and interpretation, right ventricular pacing/recording, and His bundle recording, when performed

\+ **93657** Additional linear or focal intracardiac catheter ablation of the left or right atrium for treatment of atrial fibrillation remaining after completion of pulmonary vein isolation (List separately in addition to code for primary procedure)

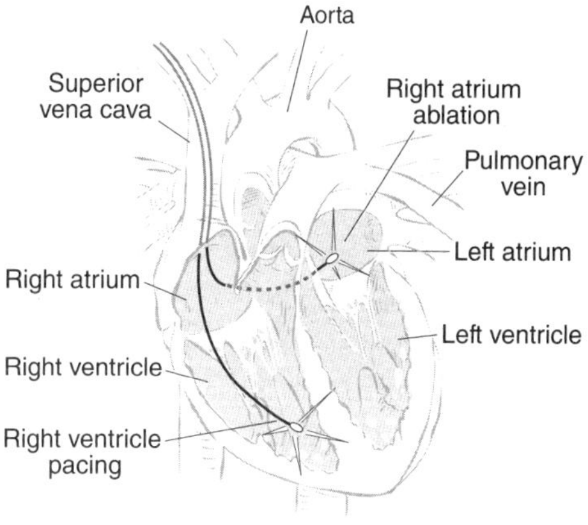

The left ventricle is paced and recorded and the pulmonary vein isolated

Explanation

During ablation by pulmonary vein isolation, also called pulmonary vein antrum isolation (PVAI), cardiac tissue responsible for the electrical irritability that causes atrial fibrillation is found at the opening of each of the four pulmonary veins that terminate in the left atrium. The physician places three venous sheaths, usually in one or both femoral veins, using standard techniques. Three electrical catheters are advanced through the venous sheaths into the right heart under fluoroscopic guidance and the septum is punctured for access to the left atrium. The physician attaches the three catheters to an electrical recording device to allow depiction of the intracardiac electrograms obtained from electrodes on the catheter tips. The tips of the three catheters are moved to the left atrium and selective destruction (ablation) of the cardiac tissue at the opening of the pulmonary veins is performed to correct the atrial fibrillation. The three catheters may also be maneuvered to the bundle of His and the right ventricle for pacing and to obtain recording. Report 93656 for the PVAI procedure. This code includes the use of three-dimensional mapping software when employed. Report 93657 when a postablation evaluation is performed after the initial PVAI and a new (not previously diagnosed) or different mechanism causing the atrial fibrillation is found and ablated.

Coding Tips

When medically necessary, report moderate (conscious) sedation provided by the performing physician with 99151-99153. When provided by another physician, report 99155-99157. Report 93657 in addition to 93656. These codes would not be reported if ablation to isolate the pulmonary veins is not performed. Do not report 93656 with 93279–93284, 93286–93289, 93462, 93600, 93602, 93603, 93610, 93612, 93613, 93618, 93619, 93620, 93621, 93653,

93654, or 93662. For treatment of SVT or ventricular tachycardia via intracardiac catheter ablation of arrhythmogenic focus, see 93653 and 93654.

ICD-10-CM Diagnostic Codes

I44.39	Other atrioventricular block
I44.4	Left anterior fascicular block
I44.5	Left posterior fascicular block
I44.69	Other fascicular block
I45.0	Right fascicular block
I45.19	Other right bundle-branch block
I45.2	Bifascicular block
I45.3	Trifascicular block
I45.4	Nonspecific intraventricular block
I45.6	Pre-excitation syndrome
I45.89	Other specified conduction disorders
I46.2	Cardiac arrest due to underlying cardiac condition
I46.8	Cardiac arrest due to other underlying condition
I47.0	Re-entry ventricular arrhythmia
I47.11	Inappropriate sinus tachycardia, so stated
I47.21	Torsades de pointes
I47.29	Other ventricular tachycardia
I48.0	Paroxysmal atrial fibrillation
I48.11	Longstanding persistent atrial fibrillation
I48.19	Other persistent atrial fibrillation
I48.21	Permanent atrial fibrillation
I48.3	Typical atrial flutter
I48.4	Atypical atrial flutter
I49.01	Ventricular fibrillation
I49.02	Ventricular flutter
I49.2	Junctional premature depolarization
I49.8	Other specified cardiac arrhythmias

AMA: 93656 2024,Sep; 2023,Oct; 2021,Dec; 2020,Nov; 2019,Sep **93657** 2020,Nov; 2019,Sep

Relative Value Units/Medicare Edits

Non-Facility RVU	Work	PE	MP	Total
93656	17.0	6.82	3.87	27.69
93657	5.5	2.21	1.25	8.96
Facility RVU	**Work**	**PE**	**MP**	**Total**
93656	17.0	6.82	3.87	27.69
93657	5.5	2.21	1.25	8.96

	FUD	Status	MUE	Modifiers				IOM Reference
93656	0	A	1(3)	51	N/A	N/A	80*	None
93657	N/A	A	2(3)	N/A	N/A	N/A	80*	

* with documentation

93662

\+ **93662** Intracardiac echocardiography during therapeutic/diagnostic intervention, including imaging supervision and interpretation (List separately in addition to code for primary procedure)

Explanation

During separately reportable electrophysiologic evaluation or intracardiac catheter ablation of arrhythmogenic focus, intracardiac echocardiography (ICE) is performed. ICE uses intravascular ultrasound imaging systems in the cardiac chambers providing direct endocardial visualization. A single rotating transducer that provides a 360-degree field of view in a plane transverse to the long axis of the catheter is introduced through a long vascular sheath. Access is typically via the femoral vein. The transducer is directed to various sites within the heart. During electrophysiologic evaluation, ICE is used to guide placement of mapping and stimulating catheters. During intracardiac ablation procedures, ICE allows for precise anatomic localization of the ablation catheter tip in relation to endocardial structures. Since the focus of some arrhythmias can be anatomically determined, it also allows the ablative procedure to be performed using anatomic landmarks.

Coding Tips

Report 93662 in addition to 33274, 33275, 33340, 33361–33366, 33418, 33477, 33741, 33745, 92986, 92987, 92990, 92997, 93451–93461, 93505, 93580–93583, 93590, 93591, 93593–93597, 93620, 93653, 93654, 0345T, 0483T, 0484T, and 0543T–0545T. Do not report 93662 with 92961, 0569T, 0570T, or 0613T. Electrophysiologic evaluation or intracardiac catheter ablation procedures are reported separately.

ICD-10-CM Diagnostic Codes

This/these CPT code(s) are add-on code(s). See the primary procedure code that this code is performed with for your ICD-10-CM code selections. Diagnostic code(s) would be the same as the actual procedure performed.

AMA: 93662 2022,Sep; 2022,Jul; 2021,Dec

Relative Value Units/Medicare Edits

Non-Facility RVU	Work	PE	MP	Total
93662	0.0	0.0	0.0	0.0
Facility RVU	**Work**	**PE**	**MP**	**Total**
93662	0.0	0.0	0.0	0.0

	FUD	Status	MUE	Modifiers				IOM Reference
93662	N/A	C	1(3)	N/A	N/A	N/A	80*	None

* with documentation

Terms To Know

catheterization. Use or insertion of a tubular device into a duct, blood vessel, hollow organ, or body cavity for injecting or withdrawing fluids for diagnostic or therapeutic purposes.

diagnostic procedures. Procedure performed on a patient to obtain information to assess the medical condition of the patient or to identify a disease and to determine the nature and severity of an illness or injury.

electrophysiologic studies. Electrical stimulation and monitoring to diagnose heart conduction abnormalities that predispose patients to bradyarrhythmias and to determine a patient's chance for developing ventricular and supraventricular tachyarrhythmias.

G0248-G0250

G0248 Demonstration, prior to initiation of home INR monitoring, for patient with either mechanical heart valve(s), chronic atrial fibrillation, or venous thromboembolism who meets Medicare coverage criteria, under the direction of a physician; includes: face-to-face demonstration of use and care of the INR monitor, obtaining at least one blood sample, provision of instructions for reporting home INR test results, and documentation of patient's ability to perform testing and report results

G0249 Provision of test materials and equipment for home INR monitoring of patient with either mechanical heart valve(s), chronic atrial fibrillation, or venous thromboembolism who meets Medicare coverage criteria; includes: provision of materials for use in the home and reporting of test results to physician; testing not occurring more frequently than once a week; testing materials, billing units of service include four tests

G0250 Physician review, interpretation, and patient management of home INR testing for patient with either mechanical heart valve(s), chronic atrial fibrillation, or venous thromboembolism who meets Medicare coverage criteria; testing not occurring more frequently than once a week; billing units of service include four tests

Explanation

Patients with a mechanical heart valve, chronic atrial fibrillation, or venous thromboembolism are at risk of developing intracardiac or intravascular thrombi and are frequently managed with long-term use of warfarin anticoagulation. Periodic monitoring is necessary to maintain a therapeutic effect of the anticoagulation treatment and reduce thromboembolic and hemorrhagic events. The use of the internationalized normalized ratio (INR) (rather than the prothrombin time) provides a result that is independent of the laboratory reagents used. The INR is the ratio of the patient's prothrombin time compared to the mean prothrombin time for a group of normal individuals. Patient self-testing and self-management through the use of a home INR monitor improve the time in therapeutic rate and hence clinical outcomes. Portable coagulometers that measure the prothrombin time and calculate the INR with the use of a drop of whole blood allow the patient to do self-testing.

Coding Tips

Medicare covers the use of home PT/INR monitoring when prescribed by a physician and when the patient has been anticoagulated for at least three months before using the home INR device, has undergone a face-to-face educational program on anticoagulation management, has demonstrated the correct use of the device prior to use in the home, continues to correctly use the device, and self-testing with the device does not occur more than once a week. Since G0250 is a professional service furnished by a physician, it is not payable under the outpatient prospective payment services (OPPS).

ICD-10-CM Diagnostic Codes

D68.51	Activated protein C resistance
D68.52	Prothrombin gene mutation
D68.59	Other primary thrombophilia
D68.61	Antiphospholipid syndrome
D68.62	Lupus anticoagulant syndrome
I26.01	Septic pulmonary embolism with acute cor pulmonale
I26.02	Saddle embolus of pulmonary artery with acute cor pulmonale
I26.09	Other pulmonary embolism with acute cor pulmonale
I26.90	Septic pulmonary embolism without acute cor pulmonale
I26.92	Saddle embolus of pulmonary artery without acute cor pulmonale
I26.93	Single subsegmental thrombotic pulmonary embolism without acute cor pulmonale
I26.94	Multiple subsegmental thrombotic pulmonary emboli without acute cor pulmonale
I48.0	Paroxysmal atrial fibrillation
I48.11	Longstanding persistent atrial fibrillation
I48.19	Other persistent atrial fibrillation
I48.21	Permanent atrial fibrillation
I80.01	Phlebitis and thrombophlebitis of superficial vessels of right lower extremity ☑
I80.02	Phlebitis and thrombophlebitis of superficial vessels of left lower extremity ☑
I80.03	Phlebitis and thrombophlebitis of superficial vessels of lower extremities, bilateral ☑
I80.11	Phlebitis and thrombophlebitis of right femoral vein ☑
I80.12	Phlebitis and thrombophlebitis of left femoral vein ☑
I80.13	Phlebitis and thrombophlebitis of femoral vein, bilateral ☑
I80.211	Phlebitis and thrombophlebitis of right iliac vein ☑
I80.212	Phlebitis and thrombophlebitis of left iliac vein ☑
I80.213	Phlebitis and thrombophlebitis of iliac vein, bilateral ☑
I80.221	Phlebitis and thrombophlebitis of right popliteal vein ☑
I80.222	Phlebitis and thrombophlebitis of left popliteal vein ☑
I80.223	Phlebitis and thrombophlebitis of popliteal vein, bilateral ☑
I80.231	Phlebitis and thrombophlebitis of right tibial vein ☑
I80.232	Phlebitis and thrombophlebitis of left tibial vein ☑
I80.233	Phlebitis and thrombophlebitis of tibial vein, bilateral ☑
I80.291	Phlebitis and thrombophlebitis of other deep vessels of right lower extremity ☑
I80.292	Phlebitis and thrombophlebitis of other deep vessels of left lower extremity ☑
I80.293	Phlebitis and thrombophlebitis of other deep vessels of lower extremity, bilateral ☑
I80.8	Phlebitis and thrombophlebitis of other sites
I82.0	Budd-Chiari syndrome
I82.1	Thrombophlebitis migrans
I82.220	Acute embolism and thrombosis of inferior vena cava
I82.221	Chronic embolism and thrombosis of inferior vena cava
T80.0XXA	Air embolism following infusion, transfusion and therapeutic injection, initial encounter
T82.817A	Embolism due to cardiac prosthetic devices, implants and grafts, initial encounter
T82.818A	Embolism due to vascular prosthetic devices, implants and grafts, initial encounter
Z95.2	Presence of prosthetic heart valve

Relative Value Units/Medicare Edits

Non-Facility RVU	Work	PE	MP	Total
G0248	0.0	2.96	0.04	3.0
G0249	0.0	1.96	0.01	1.97
G0250	0.18	0.07	0.01	0.26
Facility RVU	**Work**	**PE**	**MP**	**Total**
G0248	0.0	2.96	0.04	3.0
G0249	0.0	1.96	0.01	1.97
G0250	0.18	0.07	0.01	0.26

	FUD	Status	MUE	Modifiers				IOM Reference
G0248	N/A	R	1(2)	N/A	N/A	N/A	80*	None
G0249	N/A	R	3(3)	N/A	N/A	N/A	80*	
G0250	N/A	R	1(2)	N/A	N/A	N/A	80*	

* with documentation

Terms To Know

anticoagulant. Substance that reduces or eradicates the blood's ability to clot.

atrial fibrillation. Cardiac arrhythmia caused by small areas of muscle fibers becoming erratically and spontaneously activated through multiple circuits in uncoordinated phases of depolarization and repolarization.

embolism. Obstruction of a blood vessel resulting from a clot or foreign substance.

thrombosis. Condition arising from the presence or formation of blood clots within a blood vessel that may cause vascular obstruction and insufficient oxygenation.

G0278

G0278 Iliac and/or femoral artery angiography, nonselective, bilateral or ipsilateral to catheter insertion, performed at the same time as cardiac catheterization and/or coronary angiography, includes positioning or placement of the catheter in the distal aorta or ipsilateral femoral or iliac artery, injection of dye, production of permanent images, and radiologic supervision and interpretation (List separately in addition to primary procedure)

Explanation

An iliac artery is radiologically examined using contrast material at the same time as cardiac catheterization. The catheter that has been threaded over the guidewire from the access site is positioned nonselectively in the distal aorta or iliac artery. Contrast medium is injected and a series of permanent images are taken to visualize the vessels and evaluate any abnormalities. The catheter is removed and pressure applied to the site. Radiological supervision and interpretation is included. List this code separately in addition to the code for the main cardiac catheterization procedure.

Coding Tips

Report this procedure with cardiac catheterization codes 93451–93462. An examination of the iliac or femoral vessels is not ordinarily indicated during a cardiac catheterization. However, angiography and interventions on these vessels at the same time as the catheterization may be reported for conditions that would have required investigation and treatments whether or not a cardiac catheterization was performed. To be eligible for Medicare payment, the medical record must substantiate that these services were medically reasonable and necessary in accordance with accepted practice standards. Do not report G0278 if the iliac angiogram is performed only to determine the type of closure.

ICD-10-CM Diagnostic Codes

This/these CPT code(s) are add-on code(s). See the primary procedure code that this code is performed with for your ICD-10-CM code selections.

Relative Value Units/Medicare Edits

Non-Facility RVU	Work	PE	MP	Total
G0278	0.25	0.09	0.06	0.4
Facility RVU	**Work**	**PE**	**MP**	**Total**
G0278	0.25	0.09	0.06	0.4

	FUD	Status	MUE	Modifiers				IOM Reference
G0278	N/A	A	1(2)	N/A	N/A	N/A	80*	None

* with documentation

Terms To Know

angiography. Radiographic imaging of the arteries. Imaging may be performed to study the vasculature of any given organ, body system, or area of circulation such as the brain, heart, chest, kidneys, limbs, gastrointestinal tract, aorta, and pulmonary circulation to visualize the formation and the function of the blood vessels to detect problems such as a blockage or stricture. A catheter is inserted through an accessible blood vessel and the artery is injected with a radiopaque contrast material after which x-rays are taken.

G0403-G0405

G0403 Electrocardiogram, routine ECG with 12 leads; performed as a screening for the initial preventive physical examination with interpretation and report

G0404 Electrocardiogram, routine ECG with 12 leads; tracing only, without interpretation and report, performed as a screening for the initial preventive physical examination

G0405 Electrocardiogram, routine ECG with 12 leads; interpretation and report only, performed as a screening for the initial preventive physical examination

Explanation

Electrocardiogram (ECG) services are performed as a component of the initial preventive physical examination provided to a new beneficiary during the first 12 months of Medicare enrollment. Twelve electrodes are placed on a patient's chest to record electrical activity of the heart. A physician interprets the findings. Code G0403 includes interpretation and report of findings; G0404 includes a tracing only, without interpretation and report findings; and G0405 includes interpretation and report only.

Coding Tips

These codes are billable when it is a result of a referral from an initial preventive physical examination (IPPE).

ICD-10-CM Diagnostic Codes

Z13.6 Encounter for screening for cardiovascular disorders

Relative Value Units/Medicare Edits

Non-Facility RVU	Work	PE	MP	Total
G0403	0.17	0.24	0.02	0.43
G0404	0.0	0.18	0.01	0.19
G0405	0.17	0.06	0.01	0.24
Facility RVU	**Work**	**PE**	**MP**	**Total**
G0403	0.17	0.24	0.02	0.43
G0404	0.0	0.18	0.01	0.19
G0405	0.17	0.06	0.01	0.24

	FUD	Status	MUE	Modifiers				IOM Reference
G0403	N/A	A	1(2)	N/A	N/A	N/A	80*	None
G0404	N/A	A	1(2)	N/A	N/A	N/A	80*	
G0405	N/A	A	1(2)	N/A	N/A	N/A	80*	

* with documentation

HCPCS

G0023-G0024

G0023 Principal illness navigation services by certified or trained auxiliary personnel under the direction of a physician or other practitioner, including a patient navigator, 60 minutes per calendar month, in the following activities:

G0024 Principal illness navigation services, additional 30 minutes per calendar month (list separately in addition to G0023)

Explanation

Principal Illness Navigation (PIN) services are performed by certified or trained auxiliary personnel under the direction of a physician or other practitioner. PIN services are provided to Medicare patients with high-risk conditions who receive a patient-centered assessment to better identify their needs and connect them to clinical and support resources. High-risk conditions for which PIN services are provided include, but are not limited to, congestive heart failure (CHF), chronic kidney disease (CKD), dementia, cancer, HIV/AIDS, organ failure, substance use disorder (SUD), and mental health conditions. PIN services are provided during an initial visit and in subsequent visits to establish ongoing support and direction as the patient connects to disease-specific resources related to their high-risk condition. Examples of PIN services include establishing a comprehensive record of the patient's health history along with their cultural and linguistic identities, aligning care coordination, targeting illness-specific health education, providing health-care system navigation, building patient self-advocacy skills, and enabling access to services that address unmet social determinations of health (SDOH) needs. Report G0023 for the first 60 minutes of PIN services provided per calendar month. Report G0024 for each additional 30 minutes of PIN services provided per calendar month; list separately in addition to G0023.

Relative Value Units/Medicare Edits

Non-Facility RVU	Work	PE	MP	Total
G0023	1.0	1.35	0.07	2.42
G0024	0.7	0.76	0.05	1.51
Facility RVU	**Work**	**PE**	**MP**	**Total**
G0023	1.0	0.42	0.07	1.49
G0024	0.7	0.29	0.05	1.04

G0136

G0136 Administration of a standardized, evidence-based social determinants of health risk assessment tool, 5 to 15 minutes

Explanation

A physician or other qualified health care professional administers an assessment of an individual's social determinants of health (SDOH) or identified social risk factors that may influence the diagnosis and treatment of medical conditions. SDOH can limit the provider's ability to diagnose or treat a condition and the patient's ability to follow the prescribed treatment plan. This service is reported in addition to an E/M service or the annual wellness visit (AWV). This service may only be reported once every six months. This service is approved by Medicare as a telehealth service and may be performed by staff under incident-to guidelines.

Relative Value Units/Medicare Edits

Non-Facility RVU	Work	PE	MP	Total
G0136	0.18	0.38	0.01	0.57
Facility RVU	**Work**	**PE**	**MP**	**Total**
G0136	0.18	0.08	0.01	0.27

G0140, G0146

G0140 Principal illness navigation-peer support by certified or trained auxiliary personnel under the direction of a physician or other practitioner, including a certified peer specialist, 60 minutes per calendar month, in the following activities:

G0146 Principal illness navigation-peer support, additional 30 minutes per calendar month (list separately in addition to G0140)

Explanation

Principal Illness Navigation (PIN) services are performed with peer support (PIN-PS) from certified or trained auxiliary personnel under the direction of a physician or other practitioner, including a certified peer specialist. Peer support specialists may include individuals who have experience with the patient's shared high-risk illness. Principles of peer support specialists include empathy and shared personal experience, focus on individual patient strengths, and provision of support to patients as they work toward recovery and/or management of their illness within their plan of care. PIN services are provided to Medicare patients with high-risk conditions who receive a patient-centered assessment to better identify their needs and connect them to clinical and support resources. High-risk conditions for which PIN-PS services are given include behavioral health conditions that otherwise satisfy the definition of a high-risk condition(s). PIN-PS services are provided during an initial visit and in subsequent visits to establish ongoing support and direction as the patient connects to disease-specific resources related to their high-risk condition. Examples of PIN services include establishing a comprehensive record of the patient's health history along with their cultural and linguistic identities, aligning care coordination, targeting illness-specific health education, providing health-care system navigation, building patient self-advocacy skills, and enabling access to services that address unmet social determinations of health (SDOH) needs. Report G0140 for the first 60 minutes of PIN-PS services provided per calendar month. Report G0146 for each additional 30 minutes of PIN-PS services provided per calendar month; list separately in addition to G0140.

Relative Value Units/Medicare Edits

Non-Facility RVU	Work	PE	MP	Total
G0140	1.0	1.35	0.07	2.42
G0146	0.7	0.76	0.05	1.51
Facility RVU	**Work**	**PE**	**MP**	**Total**
G0140	1.0	0.42	0.07	1.49
G0146	0.7	0.29	0.05	1.04

G0288

G0288 Reconstruction, computed tomographic angiography of aorta for surgical planning for vascular surgery

Explanation

Report this code for the computer reconstruction of computerized tomography (CT) generated angiographic images of the aorta for the purpose of planning vascular surgery.

Relative Value Units/Medicare Edits

Non-Facility RVU	Work	PE	MP	Total
G0288	0.0	1.22	0.09	1.31
Facility RVU	**Work**	**PE**	**MP**	**Total**
G0288	0.0	1.22	0.09	1.31

G0316

G0316 Prolonged hospital inpatient or observation care evaluation and management service(s) beyond the total time for the primary service (when the primary service has been selected using time on the date of the primary service); each additional 15 minutes by the physician or qualified healthcare professional, with or without direct patient contact (list separately in addition to CPT codes 99223, 99233, and 99236 for hospital inpatient or observation care evaluation and management services). (Do not report G0316 on the same date of service as other prolonged services for evaluation and management codes 99358, 99359, 99418, 99415, 99416). (Do not report G0316 for any time unit less than 15 minutes)

Explanation

The physician or qualified health care professional provides prolonged hospital inpatient or observation care (including partial hospitalization) evaluation and management (E/M) services, with or without direct patient contact. Report G0316 as an add-on code to represent each additional 15 minutes of services provided beyond the greatest amount of allowed time of the highest-level primary E/M service. These primary services include initial or subsequent inpatient or observation care, as well as that for patients whose admission and discharge occur on the same day, and do not differentiate between new or established patients.

Relative Value Units/Medicare Edits

Non-Facility RVU	Work	PE	MP	Total
G0316	0.61	0.3	0.04	0.95
Facility RVU	**Work**	**PE**	**MP**	**Total**
G0316	0.61	0.25	0.04	0.9

G0317

G0317 Prolonged nursing facility evaluation and management service(s) beyond the total time for the primary service (when the primary service has been selected using time on the date of the primary service); each additional 15 minutes by the physician or qualified healthcare professional, with or without direct patient contact (list separately in addition to CPT codes 99306, 99310 for nursing facility evaluation and management services). (Do not report G0317 on the same date of service as other prolonged services for evaluation and management codes 99358, 99359, 99418). (Do not report G0317 for any time unit less than 15 minutes)

Explanation

The physician or qualified health care professional provides prolonged nursing facility evaluation and management (E/M) services, with or without direct patient contact. Report G0317 as an add-on code to represent each additional 15 minutes of services provided beyond the greatest amount of allowed time of the highest-level primary E/M service. These primary services include initial or subsequent nursing facility care that may be provided in nursing facilities and skilled nursing facilities, or for services in psychiatric residential treatment centers or intermediate care facilities for patients with intellectual disabilities. They do not differentiate between new or established patients.

Relative Value Units/Medicare Edits

Non-Facility RVU	Work	PE	MP	Total
G0317	0.61	0.3	0.04	0.95
Facility RVU	**Work**	**PE**	**MP**	**Total**
G0317	0.61	0.25	0.04	0.9

G0318

G0318 Prolonged home or residence evaluation and management service(s) beyond the total time for the primary service (when the primary service has been selected using time on the date of the primary service); each additional 15 minutes by the physician or qualified healthcare professional, with or without direct patient contact (list separately in addition to CPT codes 99345, 99350 for home or residence evaluation and management services). (Do not report G0318 on the same date of service as other prolonged services for evaluation and management codes 99358, 99359, 99417). (Do not report G0318 for any time unit less than 15 minutes)

Explanation

The physician or qualified health care professional provides prolonged evaluation and management (E/M) services, with or without direct patient contact, in a home or residence. Report G0318 as an add-on code to represent each additional 15 minutes of services provided beyond the greatest amount of allowed time of the highest-level primary E/M service. These primary services include the evaluation and management of a new or an established patient in a private residence or temporary lodging. Short-term accommodations such as a hotel, campground, hostel, or cruise ship are included, along with assisted living facility, group home, custodial care facility, or residential substance abuse treatment facility.

Relative Value Units/Medicare Edits

Non-Facility RVU	Work	PE	MP	Total
G0318	0.61	0.27	0.05	0.93
Facility RVU	**Work**	**PE**	**MP**	**Total**
G0318	0.61	0.23	0.05	0.89

G0422-G0423

G0422 Intensive cardiac rehabilitation; with or without continuous ECG monitoring with exercise, per session

G0423 Intensive cardiac rehabilitation; with or without continuous ECG monitoring; without exercise, per session

Explanation

Cardiac rehabilitation is a medically supervised program intended to help people with heart problems. The program includes training and education on the risk factors of heart disease, such as smoking, high blood pressure, and lack of exercise. Encouragement is given to adopt a healthy lifestyle by increasing physical activity, developing stress coping techniques, and adopting a healthy diet. The program may or may not include exercise and continuous ECG monitoring. Intensive cardiac rehabilitation (ICR) sessions are limited to 72 one-hour sessions, up to six sessions per day, over a period of up to 18 weeks.

Relative Value Units/Medicare Edits

Non-Facility RVU	Work	PE	MP	Total
G0422	1.92	1.81	0.12	3.85
G0423	1.92	1.81	0.12	3.85
Facility RVU	**Work**	**PE**	**MP**	**Total**
G0422	1.92	1.81	0.12	3.85
G0423	1.92	1.81	0.12	3.85

G0446

G0446 Annual, face-to-face intensive behavioral therapy for cardiovascular disease, individual, 15 minutes

Explanation

Annual intensive behavioral therapy for cardiovascular disease for risk reduction is reported with this code. Risk reduction includes encouraging aspirin therapy for the primary prevention of cardiovascular disease when the benefits outweigh the risks for men ages 45 to 70 years and women 55 to 79 years; screening for high blood pressure for patients 18 years and older; and intensive behavioral counseling to promote a healthy diet for adults with hyperlipidemia, hypertension, advancing age, and any other risk factors for cardiovascular and diet-related chronic disease. Behavioral counseling interventions should include the following Five A's approach that has been adopted by the United States Preventive Services Task Force (USPSTF): Assess: Ask about/assess behavioral health risk(s) and factors affecting choice of behavior and change goals/methods; Advise: Give clear, specific, and personalized behavior change advice, including information about personal health harms and benefits; Agree: Collaboratively select appropriate treatment goals and methods based on the patient's interest in and willingness to change the behavior; Assist: Using behavior change techniques (self-help and/or counseling), aid the patient in achieving agreed-upon goals by acquiring the skills, confidence, and social/environmental supports for behavior change, supplemented with adjunctive medical treatments when appropriate; Arrange: Schedule follow-up contacts (in person or by telephone) to provide ongoing assistance/support and to adjust the treatment plan as needed, including referral to more intensive or specialized treatment.

Relative Value Units/Medicare Edits

Non-Facility RVU	Work	PE	MP	Total
G0446	0.45	0.28	0.03	0.76
Facility RVU	**Work**	**PE**	**MP**	**Total**
G0446	0.45	0.2	0.03	0.68

G0447

G0447 Face-to-face behavioral counseling for obesity, 15 minutes

Explanation

Behavioral counseling for obesity is reported with this code. The United States Preventive Services Task Force (USPSTF) considers body mass index (BMI) a good indication of morbidity and mortality because of being overweight or obese. BMI is calculated using the following formula: BMI = (weight in pounds / (height in inches x height in inches)) x 703. Obese adults are considered those that have a BMI >=30 kg/m2. Behavioral counseling and behavior modification can be an effective combination to produce moderate, sustainable weight loss. The patients should have the following services: screening for obesity using BMI, assessment of food and nutritional intake, and counseling to include diet and exercise. Behavioral counseling interventions should include the following Five A's approach that has been developed by the United States Preventive Services Task Force (USPSTF): Assess: Ask about/assess behavioral health risk(s) and factors affecting choice of behavior and change goals/methods; Advise: Give clear, specific, and personalized behavior change advice, including information about personal health harms and benefits; Agree: Collaboratively select appropriate treatment goals and methods based on the patient's interest in and willingness to change the behavior; Assist: Using behavior change techniques (self-help and/or counseling), aid the patient in achieving agreed-upon goals by acquiring the skills, confidence, and social/environmental supports for behavior change, supplemented with adjunctive medical treatments when appropriate; Arrange: Schedule follow-up contacts (in person or by telephone) to provide ongoing assistance/support and to adjust the treatment plan as needed, including referral to more intensive or specialized treatment.

Relative Value Units/Medicare Edits

Non-Facility RVU	Work	PE	MP	Total
G0447	0.45	0.28	0.03	0.76
Facility RVU	**Work**	**PE**	**MP**	**Total**
G0447	0.45	0.19	0.03	0.67

G0563

● **G0563** Stereotactic body radiation therapy, treatment delivery, per fraction to 1 or more lesions, including image guidance and real-time positron emissions-based delivery adjustments to 1 or more lesions, entire course not to exceed 5 fractions

Explanation

Stereotactic body radiation therapy (SRBT) is a radiation therapy technique that uses special equipment to position a patient and precisely deliver a large radiation dose to a discrete tumor site while minimizing damage to healthy tissue. This code reports treatment delivery, including image guidance and real-time positron emissions-based delivery adjustments. This code is assigned for a course of SRBT per fraction, not to exceed five fractions, to one or more lesions.

Relative Value Units/Medicare Edits

Non-Facility RVU	Work	PE	MP	Total
G0563				
Facility RVU	**Work**	**PE**	**MP**	**Total**
G0563				

G9037

● **G9037** Interprofessional telephone/internet/electronic health record clinical question/request for specialty recommendations by a treating/requesting physician or other qualified health care professional for the care of the patient (i.e., not for professional education or scheduling) and may include subsequent follow up on the specialist's recommendations; 30 minutes

Explanation

Interprofessional telephone/internet/electronic health record consultation services (Making Care Primary [MCP] e-Consult [MEC]) are utilized when the attending qualified clinician requests the input of a physician or qualified clinician with specific knowledge of the condition. This specialist may assist in diagnosis or treatment of the patient without seeing the patient and often occurs when the situation is urgent and/or complex in nature. The patient may be a new or established patient with a new problem or exacerbation of a current problem in the eyes of the consultant. This code may not be reported for transfer of care or to schedule a face-to-face with the consultant. This discussion includes appropriate review of medical records, laboratory and radiology results, medication review/tolerance, and pathology results. The patient's medical record should contain an e-consult with an explanation as to the medical necessity of the request and the consultant response to the e-consult. Report G9037 when encounters of 30 minutes of the clinician's time is spent preparing for or communicating with the consultant. This code includes time spent by the provider describing the request in the e-consult, time interpreting the consultant's response, and the time spent discussing the findings with the patient. This consultation service is distinct clinical work from pre-visit planning for any subsequent E/M visits; if the e-consult findings are discussed in a subsequent visit, the discussion time should be counted in that E/M service. This code cannot be reported the same day as 99452 for the same MCP beneficiary by the same MCP clinician.

Relative Value Units/Medicare Edits

Non-Facility RVU	Work	PE	MP	Total
G9037	0.57	0.59	0.04	1.2
Facility RVU	**Work**	**PE**	**MP**	**Total**
G9037	0.57	0.59	0.04	1.2

G9157

G9157 Transesophageal Doppler used for cardiac monitoring

Explanation

Transesophageal Doppler is an ultrasound diagnostic procedure that uses low energy sound waves to provide noninvasive visualization. This code is specific to Medicare coverage of transesophageal Doppler monitoring of cardiac output for ventilated patients in the ICU and operative patients with a need for intraoperative fluid optimization. This service is only covered in a hospital setting or ambulatory surgical center and is included in the Inpatient Prospective Payment System payment.

Relative Value Units/Medicare Edits

Non-Facility RVU	Work	PE	MP	Total
G9157	2.2	0.4	0.18	2.78
Facility RVU	**Work**	**PE**	**MP**	**Total**
G9157	2.2	0.4	0.18	2.78

Q0035

Q0035 Cardiokymography

Explanation

Cardiokymography involves the use of a noninvasive device to record the anterior left ventricle segmental wall motion. The device typically consists of a 5 cm diameter capacitive plate transducer as part of a high-frequency, low-power oscillator with recording probe. Changes in wall motion affect the magnetic field and thus the oscillatory frequency, which is then recorded on a multichannel analog waveform polygraph. Medicare and most payers cover this type of test only as an adjunct to electrocardiographic stress testing to evaluate coronary artery disease and only when specific clinical indications are present. For male patients there must be atypical angina pectoris or nonischemic chest pain. For female patients, there must be angina, either typical or atypical.

Relative Value Units/Medicare Edits

Non-Facility RVU	Work	PE	MP	Total
Q0035	0.17	0.34	0.02	0.53
Facility RVU	**Work**	**PE**	**MP**	**Total**
Q0035	0.17	0.34	0.02	0.53

31611

31611 Construction of tracheoesophageal fistula and subsequent insertion of an alaryngeal speech prosthesis (eg, voice button, Blom-Singer prosthesis)

Explanation

The physician constructs a tracheal esophageal fistula for vocalization. The physician makes a horizontal neck incision and dissects the tissues between the tracheostoma and the esophagus. The esophagus is incised and a laryngeal speech prosthesis is inserted between the esophagus and the trachea, creating a fistula. The prosthesis, called a voice button or a Blom-Singer prosthesis, is a one-way valve enabling the patient to phonate. The physician closes the incision around the prosthesis.

Relative Value Units/Medicare Edits

Non-Facility RVU	Work	PE	MP	Total
31611	6.0	9.31	0.9	16.21
Facility RVU	**Work**	**PE**	**MP**	**Total**
31611	6.0	9.31	0.9	16.21

31613-31614

31613 Tracheostoma revision; simple, without flap rotation
31614 complex, with flap rotation

Explanation

The physician revises a tracheal stoma. The physician incises the stoma area and resects redundant scar tissue or a poorly healing wound. The skin is re-anastomosed and sewn to the stoma in sutured layers. Report 31613 for performance of a simple revision and 31614 if a complex procedure is performed with flap rotation.

Relative Value Units/Medicare Edits

Non-Facility RVU	Work	PE	MP	Total
31613	4.71	7.32	0.77	12.8
31614	8.63	11.53	1.32	21.48
Facility RVU	**Work**	**PE**	**MP**	**Total**
31613	4.71	7.32	0.77	12.8
31614	8.63	11.53	1.32	21.48

31622-31624

31622 Bronchoscopy, rigid or flexible, including fluoroscopic guidance, when performed; diagnostic, with cell washing, when performed (separate procedure)
31623 with brushing or protected brushings
31624 with bronchial alveolar lavage

Explanation

The physician views the airway using a flexible fiberoptic or rigid bronchoscope that is introduced under appropriate anesthesia through the nasal or oral cavity. The bronchoscope is inserted and advanced through the nasal or oral cavity, past the larynx to inspect the bronchus. In 31622, after diagnostic visualization of the bronchus, cell washings may be obtained through the bronchoscope. In 31623, sample lung tissue is obtained with brushings or protected brushing through the scope. In 31624, the bronchoscopy includes bronchial alveolar lavage, which allows lung tissue to be sampled by irrigating with saline followed by suctioning the fluid. The bronchoscope is removed. These codes include fluoroscopic guidance, when performed.

Relative Value Units/Medicare Edits

Non-Facility RVU	Work	PE	MP	Total
31622	2.53	4.64	0.31	7.48
31623	2.63	5.35	0.23	8.21
31624	2.63	4.77	0.24	7.64
Facility RVU	**Work**	**PE**	**MP**	**Total**
31622	2.53	1.06	0.31	3.9
31623	2.63	1.01	0.23	3.87
31624	2.63	1.05	0.24	3.92

31625

31625 Bronchoscopy, rigid or flexible, including fluoroscopic guidance, when performed; with bronchial or endobronchial biopsy(s), single or multiple sites

Explanation

The physician views the airway using a flexible fiberoptic or rigid bronchoscope that is introduced through the nasal or oral cavity. The airway is anesthetized. The bronchoscope is inserted and advanced through the nasal or oral cavity, past the larynx to inspect the bronchus, including fluoroscopic guidance, if used. After diagnostic visualization of the bronchus, a sample of bronchial or endobronchial tissue is removed for study. More than one site may be biopsied. Bleeding is assessed and controlled, and the bronchoscope is removed.

Relative Value Units/Medicare Edits

Non-Facility RVU	Work	PE	MP	Total
31625	3.11	7.02	0.3	10.43
Facility RVU	**Work**	**PE**	**MP**	**Total**
31625	3.11	1.17	0.3	4.58

31626

31626 Bronchoscopy, rigid or flexible, including fluoroscopic guidance, when performed; with placement of fiducial markers, single or multiple

Explanation

The physician views the airway using a flexible fiberoptic or rigid bronchoscope that is introduced through the nasal or oral cavity. The airway is anesthetized. The bronchoscope is inserted and advanced through the nasal or oral cavity, past the larynx to inspect the bronchus, including fluoroscopic guidance, if used. After diagnostic visualization of the bronchus, one or more fiducial markers are placed.

Relative Value Units/Medicare Edits

Non-Facility RVU	Work	PE	MP	Total
31626	3.91	19.07	0.46	23.44
Facility RVU	**Work**	**PE**	**MP**	**Total**
31626	3.91	1.41	0.46	5.78

31627

\+ **31627** Bronchoscopy, rigid or flexible, including fluoroscopic guidance, when performed; with computer-assisted, image-guided navigation (List separately in addition to code for primary procedure[s])

Explanation

The physician views the airway using a flexible fiberoptic or rigid bronchoscope that is introduced through the nasal or oral cavity. The airway is anesthetized. The bronchoscope is inserted and advanced through the nasal or oral cavity, past the larynx to inspect the bronchus, including fluoroscopic guidance, if used. This code reports the use of computer-assisted, image-guided navigation, and includes 3D reconstruction.

Relative Value Units/Medicare Edits

Non-Facility RVU	Work	PE	MP	Total
31627	2.0	29.6	0.21	31.81
Facility RVU	**Work**	**PE**	**MP**	**Total**
31627	2.0	0.61	0.21	2.82

31628-31629

31628 Bronchoscopy, rigid or flexible, including fluoroscopic guidance, when performed; with transbronchial lung biopsy(s), single lobe

31629 with transbronchial needle aspiration biopsy(s), trachea, main stem and/or lobar bronchus(i)

Explanation

The physician views the airway using a flexible fiberoptic or rigid bronchoscope that is introduced under appropriate anesthesia through the nasal or oral cavity. The bronchoscope is inserted and advanced through the nasal or oral cavity, past the larynx to inspect the bronchus, including fluoroscopic guidance, if used. After diagnostic visualization of the bronchus, the physician passes closed biopsy forceps (31628) through a channel in the bronchoscope and through the bronchial wall to obtain one or more lung tissue samples from a single lobe. Alternately, the physician passes a needle (31629) through a channel in the bronchoscope and through the bronchial wall to obtain one or more aspiration biopsies of the trachea, main stem, and/or lobar bronchi. Bleeding is assessed and controlled, and the bronchoscope is removed.

Relative Value Units/Medicare Edits

Non-Facility RVU	Work	PE	MP	Total
31628	3.55	7.25	0.31	11.11
31629	3.75	9.41	0.36	13.52
Facility RVU	**Work**	**PE**	**MP**	**Total**
31628	3.55	1.29	0.31	5.15
31629	3.75	1.36	0.36	5.47

31630-31631

31630 Bronchoscopy, rigid or flexible, including fluoroscopic guidance, when performed; with tracheal/bronchial dilation or closed reduction of fracture

31631 with placement of tracheal stent(s) (includes tracheal/bronchial dilation as required)

Explanation

The physician performs tracheal/bronchial dilation or closed fracture reduction using a flexible fiberoptic or rigid bronchoscope introduced through the nasal or oral cavity. The physician uses the views obtained through the bronchoscope to identify any narrowing or fracture of the trachea or bronchus. The physician introduces a wire through the narrowed or fractured part of the airway and removes the bronchoscope. A series of dilators or stents are passed over the wire to open the airway until sufficient dilation or closed reduction of the stricture or fracture is accomplished. This may be done with or without fluoroscopic guidance. In 31631, the physician places a tracheal stent or stents using a flexible fiberoptic or rigid bronchoscope introduced through the nasal or oral cavity, using local anesthesia of the patient's airway. The physician uses the views obtained through the bronchoscope to identify any narrowing or area of the trachea that requires stenting for support. The physician introduces a wire through the narrowed part of the trachea and removes the bronchoscope. If dilation is first required, a series of dilators are passed over the wire to open the airway until sufficient tracheal/bronchial dilation is accomplished. A stent is passed over the wire to the target area in the trachea and positioned in place to maintain an open airway.

Relative Value Units/Medicare Edits

Non-Facility RVU	Work	PE	MP	Total
31630	3.81	1.55	0.46	5.82
31631	4.36	1.75	0.52	6.63
Facility RVU	**Work**	**PE**	**MP**	**Total**
31630	3.81	1.55	0.46	5.82
31631	4.36	1.75	0.52	6.63

31632-31633

\+ **31632** Bronchoscopy, rigid or flexible, including fluoroscopic guidance, when performed; with transbronchial lung biopsy(s), each additional lobe (List separately in addition to code for primary procedure)

\+ **31633** with transbronchial needle aspiration biopsy(s), each additional lobe (List separately in addition to code for primary procedure)

Explanation

The physician views the airway using a flexible fiberoptic or rigid bronchoscope that is introduced under appropriate anesthesia through the nasal or oral cavity. The bronchoscope is inserted. It is advanced through the larynx to the bronchus. Fluoroscopy (x-ray) may be used to assist with navigation of the bronchoscope tip to the abnormal tissue to be biopsied. In 31632, the physician passes closed biopsy forceps through a channel in the bronchoscope, through the bronchial wall, and obtains tissue samples in one lobe. Report 31632 for each additional lobe in which this is done. In 31633, a needle is passed through a channel in the bronchoscope, into the trachea, main stem, and/or a lobe of the bronchus, and an aspiration biopsy is obtained. Report 31633 for each additional lobe in which this is done.

Relative Value Units/Medicare Edits

Non-Facility RVU	Work	PE	MP	Total
31632	1.03	0.81	0.09	1.93
31633	1.32	0.95	0.13	2.4
Facility RVU	**Work**	**PE**	**MP**	**Total**
31632	1.03	0.31	0.09	1.43
31633	1.32	0.39	0.13	1.84

31634

31634 Bronchoscopy, rigid or flexible, including fluoroscopic guidance, when performed; with balloon occlusion, with assessment of air leak, with administration of occlusive substance (eg, fibrin glue), if performed

Explanation

The physician treats a bronchopleural fistula (BPF) with bronchoscopic balloon occlusion. BPF is often a serious postoperative complication of thoracic surgery, although it can also occur as a complication in a diseased lung or a previously normal lung. The physician views the airway using a flexible fiberoptic or rigid bronchoscope that is introduced through the nasal or oral cavity. The airway is anesthetized. The bronchoscope is inserted. It is advanced through the larynx to the bronchus. Fluoroscopy (x-ray) may be used to assist with navigation of the bronchoscope tip to the area of the air leak, which is then assessed. A balloon catheter is placed at the site of the leak and inflated until the leak is occluded. Keeping the inflated catheter in this position, an appropriate sealant (e.g., fibrin) may be injected. Once effective sealing is verified, the catheter and bronchoscope are removed.

Relative Value Units/Medicare Edits

Non-Facility RVU	Work	PE	MP	Total
31634	3.75	39.7	0.37	43.82
Facility RVU	**Work**	**PE**	**MP**	**Total**
31634	3.75	1.39	0.37	5.51

31635

31635 Bronchoscopy, rigid or flexible, including fluoroscopic guidance, when performed; with removal of foreign body

Explanation

The physician views the airway using a flexible fiberoptic or rigid bronchoscope introduced through the nasal or oral cavity, using local anesthesia of the patient's airway. The physician uses the views obtained through the bronchoscope to locate the foreign body within the airway. The physician passes a snare, basket, or biopsy forceps through a channel in the bronchoscope to grasp the foreign body. The bronchoscope and foreign body are removed. This may be done with or without fluoroscopic guidance.

Relative Value Units/Medicare Edits

Non-Facility RVU	Work	PE	MP	Total
31635	3.42	4.97	0.38	8.77
Facility RVU	**Work**	**PE**	**MP**	**Total**
31635	3.42	1.35	0.38	5.15

31636-31638

31636 Bronchoscopy, rigid or flexible, including fluoroscopic guidance, when performed; with placement of bronchial stent(s) (includes tracheal/bronchial dilation as required), initial bronchus

\+ **31637** Bronchoscopy, rigid or flexible, including fluoroscopic guidance, when performed; each additional major bronchus stented (List separately in addition to code for primary procedure)

31638 with revision of tracheal or bronchial stent inserted at previous session (includes tracheal/bronchial dilation as required)

Explanation

A rigid or flexible bronchoscopy is performed, with or without fluoroscopic guidance, to place a bronchial stent. The type of stent used, as well as the level of patency vs. obstruction in the airway, will vary the placement technique. Initial assessment with the bronchoscope is done to determine the lesion's size and location. If fluoroscopy is used, the distal target position for stent placement is marked with a radiopaque object, such as a treated paperclip taped to the chest. If the airway is near completely occluded, a flexible tipped guidewire is placed through the bronchoscope, a balloon catheter is fed over the guidewire, and initial dilation is done. With the bronchoscope removed and the wire still in place, the stent, such as woven mesh or single wire stent with polyurethane covering, is passed over the guidewire by a stent catheter just past the obstruction. The stent is deployed by slowly sliding the plastic sheath covering back until it is snugly fitted. Report 31636 for the initial bronchial stent placement, 31637 for each additional major bronchus stented, and 31638 for the revision of a stent inserted in a previous session.

Relative Value Units/Medicare Edits

Non-Facility RVU	Work	PE	MP	Total
31636	4.3	1.58	0.46	6.34
31637	1.58	0.49	0.15	2.22
31638	4.88	1.82	0.5	7.2
Facility RVU	**Work**	**PE**	**MP**	**Total**
31636	4.3	1.58	0.46	6.34
31637	1.58	0.49	0.15	2.22
31638	4.88	1.82	0.5	7.2

31640-31641

31640 Bronchoscopy, rigid or flexible, including fluoroscopic guidance, when performed; with excision of tumor

31641 with destruction of tumor or relief of stenosis by any method other than excision (eg, laser therapy, cryotherapy)

Explanation

In 31640, the physician views the airway using a flexible fiberoptic or rigid bronchoscope introduced through the nasal or oral cavity, using local anesthesia of the patient's airway. The physician uses the views obtained through the bronchoscope to identify the tumor from within the airway. The physician may use fluoroscopy (x-ray) to assist with navigation of the bronchoscope tip to the abnormal tissue. The physician passes forceps through channels in the bronchoscope to grasp and excise the tumor. The bronchoscope is removed. This may be done with or without fluoroscopic guidance. In 31641, the physician views the airway using a bronchoscope introduced through the nasal or oral cavity, using local anesthesia of the patient's airway. The physician uses the views obtained through the bronchoscope to identify the tumor and/or area of stenosis from within the airway. Fluoroscopy (x-ray) may be used to assist with navigation of the bronchoscope tip to the abnormal tissue and is included when performed. The physician passes a laser or freezing (cryo) probe through a channel in the bronchoscope to destroy the tumor or any areas of stenosis. The bronchoscope is removed.

Relative Value Units/Medicare Edits

Non-Facility RVU	Work	PE	MP	Total
31640	4.93	1.81	0.5	7.24
31641	5.02	1.89	0.53	7.44
Facility RVU	**Work**	**PE**	**MP**	**Total**
31640	4.93	1.81	0.5	7.24
31641	5.02	1.89	0.53	7.44

31643

31643 Bronchoscopy, rigid or flexible, including fluoroscopic guidance, when performed; with placement of catheter(s) for intracavitary radioelement application

Explanation

The physician views the airway using a bronchoscope with a fiberoptic camera and operating device. The airway is anesthetized and the bronchoscope is introduced through the nasal or oral cavity and advanced through the bronchus. A catheter is inserted through the bronchoscope into a lung cavity and is placed at the site where, in a separately reportable procedure, intracavitary radioelements will be applied. This code includes the use of fluoroscopic guidance, when performed.

Relative Value Units/Medicare Edits

Non-Facility RVU	Work	PE	MP	Total
31643	3.49	1.2	0.27	4.96
Facility RVU	**Work**	**PE**	**MP**	**Total**
31643	3.49	1.2	0.27	4.96

31645-31646

31645 Bronchoscopy, rigid or flexible, including fluoroscopic guidance, when performed; with therapeutic aspiration of tracheobronchial tree, initial

31646 with therapeutic aspiration of tracheobronchial tree, subsequent

Explanation

The physician views the airway using a bronchoscope introduced under appropriate anesthesia through the nasal or oral cavity. The physician uses the views obtained through the bronchoscope to identify the closest approach to the fluid collection from within the airway. The physician may use fluoroscopy (x-ray) to assist with navigation of the bronchoscope tip to the fluid collection. The physician passes a catheter through a channel in the bronchoscope and aspirates the tracheobronchial tree. Alternately, the physician passes a needle through a channel in the bronchoscope into the fluid collection and aspirates fluid through the needle. The bronchoscope is removed. Report 31645 for the initial treatment only. Report 31646 for any subsequent aspiration procedures performed during the same hospital stay. These codes include the use of fluoroscopic guidance, when performed.

Relative Value Units/Medicare Edits

Non-Facility RVU	Work	PE	MP	Total
31645	2.88	5.04	0.29	8.21
31646	2.78	1.12	0.27	4.17
Facility RVU	**Work**	**PE**	**MP**	**Total**
31645	2.88	1.15	0.29	4.32
31646	2.78	1.12	0.27	4.17

31717

31717 Catheterization with bronchial brush biopsy

Explanation

The physician catheterizes the trachea to obtain a bronchial brush biopsy. The physician inserts a needle through the cricoid cartilage or the trachea. A catheter is passed over the needle and a brush is placed through the catheter to obtain bronchial tissue. A bronchoscope may be used to guide the brush. The brush is withdrawn through the catheter and both are removed. The incision may be closed with sutures.

Relative Value Units/Medicare Edits

Non-Facility RVU	Work	PE	MP	Total
31717	2.12	6.26	0.17	8.55
Facility RVU	**Work**	**PE**	**MP**	**Total**
31717	2.12	0.83	0.17	3.12

31720-31725

31720 Catheter aspiration (separate procedure); nasotracheal

31725 tracheobronchial with fiberscope, bedside

Explanation

The physician aspirates sputum from the lungs using a nasal tracheal catheter. The physician passes a suction catheter through the nose into the trachea. Saline may be used to liquify secretions. The secretions are removed with suction and the catheter is removed. Report 31725 if a tracheobronchial approach with fiberscope is used at bedside.

Relative Value Units/Medicare Edits

Non-Facility RVU	Work	PE	MP	Total
31720	1.06	0.29	0.08	1.43
31725	1.71	0.47	0.14	2.32
Facility RVU	**Work**	**PE**	**MP**	**Total**
31720	1.06	0.29	0.08	1.43
31725	1.71	0.47	0.14	2.32

31730

31730 Transtracheal (percutaneous) introduction of needle wire dilator/stent or indwelling tube for oxygen therapy

Explanation

The physician introduces a needle wire dilator/stent into the trachea to relieve a subglottic stenosis. The physician places a needle through the cricoid membrane or trachea. A wire is passed through the needle and the needle is removed. A series of dilators or stents are passed over the wire to open the trachea. When sufficient dilation is gained, a stent or indwelling tube for oxygen therapy is left in place to maintain patency.

Relative Value Units/Medicare Edits

Non-Facility RVU	Work	PE	MP	Total
31730	2.85	27.98	0.58	31.41
Facility RVU	**Work**	**PE**	**MP**	**Total**
31730	2.85	0.96	0.58	4.39

31770-31775

31770 Bronchoplasty; graft repair
31775 excision stenosis and anastomosis

Explanation

The physician repairs a bronchus. The physician makes a lateral thoracotomy incision to access the bronchus. An autograft or Silastic stent may be used to repair the bronchus in 31770. A chest tube is inserted and the wound is closed in sutured layers. Report 31775 if an excision stenosis and anastomosis are performed with this procedure.

Relative Value Units/Medicare Edits

Non-Facility RVU	Work	PE	MP	Total
31770	23.54	9.89	5.81	39.24
31775	24.59	10.68	6.08	41.35
Facility RVU	**Work**	**PE**	**MP**	**Total**
31770	23.54	9.89	5.81	39.24
31775	24.59	10.68	6.08	41.35

31781

31781 Excision tracheal stenosis and anastomosis; cervicothoracic

Explanation

The physician excises a tracheal stenosis and re-anastomoses the trachea. The physician makes a cervicothoracic incision to access the stenosis. The trachea is incised and the stenosis is resected. The proximal and distal portions of the trachea are brought together and closed with sutures. The wound is closed in sutured layers.

Relative Value Units/Medicare Edits

Non-Facility RVU	Work	PE	MP	Total
31781	24.85	14.61	3.62	43.08
Facility RVU	**Work**	**PE**	**MP**	**Total**
31781	24.85	14.61	3.62	43.08

31786

31786 Excision of tracheal tumor or carcinoma; thoracic

Explanation

The physician excises a tracheal tumor or carcinoma. The physician makes a thoracic approach to access the mass. The trachea is incised and the mass is resected. If necessary, the proximal and distal portions of the trachea are brought together and closed with sutures. The wound is sutured in layers.

Relative Value Units/Medicare Edits

Non-Facility RVU	Work	PE	MP	Total
31786	25.42	10.91	6.28	42.61
Facility RVU	**Work**	**PE**	**MP**	**Total**
31786	25.42	10.91	6.28	42.61

31805

31805 Suture of tracheal wound or injury; intrathoracic

Explanation

The physician closes a wound or injury of the intrathoracic trachea. The physician debrides the wound and closes the trachea with sutures. The tissues are sutured in layers.

Relative Value Units/Medicare Edits

Non-Facility RVU	Work	PE	MP	Total
31805	13.42	7.61	3.32	24.35
Facility RVU	**Work**	**PE**	**MP**	**Total**
31805	13.42	7.61	3.32	24.35

31820-31825

31820 Surgical closure tracheostomy or fistula; without plastic repair
31825 with plastic repair

Explanation

The physician closes a tracheostomy or fistula. The physician excises the scarred tissue forming the tracheostomy or fistula. If the trachea has healed, it is closed with sutures. The remaining tissues of the tracheostomy or fistula are pulled together and the wound is sutured in layers. Report 31820 if the tracheostomy or fistula is closed without plastic repair; report 31825 if the tracheostomy or fistula is closed with plastic repair of the skin made to hide the repair.

Relative Value Units/Medicare Edits

Non-Facility RVU	Work	PE	MP	Total
31820	4.64	8.09	0.72	13.45
31825	7.07	10.46	1.06	18.59
Facility RVU	**Work**	**PE**	**MP**	**Total**
31820	4.64	4.7	0.72	10.06
31825	7.07	6.57	1.06	14.7

36400

36400 Venipuncture, younger than age 3 years, necessitating the skill of a physician or other qualified health care professional, not to be used for routine venipuncture; femoral or jugular vein

Explanation

A needle is inserted through the skin to puncture the femoral or jugular vein of a child younger than age 3. The needle is inserted into the vein and used for the withdrawal of blood for diagnostic study or for the therapeutic infusion of intravenous medication. A soft flexible catheter may be placed for prolonged therapy. Once the procedure is complete, the needle or catheter is withdrawn and pressure is applied over the puncture site to control bleeding. Use this code for venipuncture when it necessitates the skill of a physician or other qualified health care professional. Do not use this code when routine venipuncture is performed.

Relative Value Units/Medicare Edits

Non-Facility RVU	Work	PE	MP	Total
36400	0.38	0.41	0.03	0.82
Facility RVU	**Work**	**PE**	**MP**	**Total**
36400	0.38	0.14	0.03	0.55

36405-36406

36405 Venipuncture, younger than age 3 years, necessitating the skill of a physician or other qualified health care professional, not to be used for routine venipuncture; scalp vein

36406 other vein

Explanation

A needle is inserted through the skin to puncture a vein of a child younger than age 3. In 36405, the scalp vein is punctured and in 36406, a vein other than the femoral, jugular, or scalp vein is used. The needle is inserted into the vein and used for the withdrawal of blood or for the therapeutic infusion of intravenous medication. A soft flexible catheter may be placed for prolonged therapy. Once the procedure is complete, the needle or catheter is withdrawn and pressure is applied over the puncture site to control bleeding. Use these codes when venipuncture necessitates the skill of a physician or other qualified health care professional. Do not use these codes when routine venipuncture is performed.

Relative Value Units/Medicare Edits

Non-Facility RVU	Work	PE	MP	Total
36405	0.31	0.39	0.02	0.72
36406	0.18	0.34	0.01	0.53
Facility RVU	**Work**	**PE**	**MP**	**Total**
36405	0.31	0.11	0.02	0.44
36406	0.18	0.07	0.01	0.26

36410

36410 Venipuncture, age 3 years or older, necessitating the skill of a physician or other qualified health care professional (separate procedure), for diagnostic or therapeutic purposes (not to be used for routine venipuncture)

Explanation

A needle is inserted through the skin to puncture a vein of a person 3 years of age or older. The needle is inserted into the vein and used for the withdrawal of blood for diagnostic study or for the therapeutic infusion of intravenous medication. A soft flexible catheter may be placed for prolonged therapy. Once the procedure is complete, the needle or catheter is withdrawn and pressure is applied over the puncture site to control bleeding. Use this code when the venipuncture necessitates the skills of a physician or other qualified health care professional. Do not use this code when routine venipuncture is performed.

Relative Value Units/Medicare Edits

Non-Facility RVU	Work	PE	MP	Total
36410	0.18	0.33	0.02	0.53
Facility RVU	**Work**	**PE**	**MP**	**Total**
36410	0.18	0.07	0.02	0.27

36415-36416

36415 Collection of venous blood by venipuncture

36416 Collection of capillary blood specimen (eg, finger, heel, ear stick)

Explanation

A needle is inserted into the skin over a vein to puncture the blood vessel and withdraw blood for venous collection in 36415. In 36416, a prick is made into the finger, heel, or ear and capillary blood that pools at the puncture site is collected in a pipette. In either case, the blood is used for diagnostic study and no catheter is placed.

36420-36425

36420 Venipuncture, cutdown; younger than age 1 year

36425 age 1 or over

Explanation

The physician makes an incision in the skin directly over the vessel and dissects the area surrounding the vein. A needle is passed into the vein for the withdrawal of blood or for the infusion of intravenous medication of a patient under 12 months of age (in 36420) or over 12 months of age (in 36425). A catheter may be left behind. Once the procedure is complete, the incision is repaired with a layered closure.

Relative Value Units/Medicare Edits

Non-Facility RVU	Work	PE	MP	Total
36420	1.01	0.18	0.22	1.41
36425	0.76	0.3	0.11	1.17
Facility RVU	**Work**	**PE**	**MP**	**Total**
36420	1.01	0.18	0.22	1.41
36425	0.76	0.3	0.11	1.17

36430

36430 Transfusion, blood or blood components

Explanation

The physician transfuses blood or blood components to a patient. The physician establishes venous access with a needle and catheter and transfuses the blood products.

Relative Value Units/Medicare Edits

Non-Facility RVU	Work	PE	MP	Total
36430	0.0	1.24	0.03	1.27
Facility RVU	**Work**	**PE**	**MP**	**Total**
36430	0.0	1.24	0.03	1.27

36440

36440 Push transfusion, blood, 2 years or younger

Explanation

The physician performs a push transfusion on a child 2 years old and under. The physician calculates the amount of blood to be transfused and slowly injects it into the patient using a needle or existing catheter.

Relative Value Units/Medicare Edits

Non-Facility RVU	Work	PE	MP	Total
36440	1.03	0.38	0.07	1.48
Facility RVU	**Work**	**PE**	**MP**	**Total**
36440	1.03	0.38	0.07	1.48

36481

36481 Percutaneous portal vein catheterization by any method

Explanation

The physician numbs the right lateral abdominal wall with local anesthetic. The physician places a large needle through the skin into the liver, maneuvering the needle through the liver into the intrahepatic portal vein, injecting contrast under fluoroscope for localization. The physician places a wire through the needle, retrograde into the portal vein. The physician removes the wire over the needle, and advances a catheter over the wire, through the skin and liver into the portal vein. The physician secures the catheter with suture. Alternative methods include placing a catheter via the internal jugular vein or using a transsplenic approach.

Relative Value Units/Medicare Edits

Non-Facility RVU	Work	PE	MP	Total
36481	6.73	43.29	0.74	50.76
Facility RVU	**Work**	**PE**	**MP**	**Total**
36481	6.73	2.0	0.74	9.47

36510

36510 Catheterization of umbilical vein for diagnosis or therapy, newborn

Explanation

The physician catheterizes the umbilical vein for diagnostic or therapeutic purposes. The physician cleanses the umbilical cord stump and locates the umbilical vein. A catheter is inserted in the vein for reasons including blood sampling or administering medication.

Relative Value Units/Medicare Edits

Non-Facility RVU	Work	PE	MP	Total
36510	1.09	1.41	0.08	2.58
Facility RVU	**Work**	**PE**	**MP**	**Total**
36510	1.09	0.4	0.08	1.57

36660

36660 Catheterization, umbilical artery, newborn, for diagnosis or therapy

Explanation

The physician catheterizes an umbilical artery in a newborn for diagnostic or therapeutic purposes. The physician prepares the umbilical artery and passes a catheter sheath inside the lumen for arterial access. The catheter is attached to a pressure line that maintains patency of the arterial lumen. The access is used for diagnostic or therapeutic purposes, allowing the drawing of blood for tests or instillation of medication.

Relative Value Units/Medicare Edits

Non-Facility RVU	Work	PE	MP	Total
36660	1.4	0.51	0.1	2.01
Facility RVU	**Work**	**PE**	**MP**	**Total**
36660	1.4	0.51	0.1	2.01

71045-71048

71045 Radiologic examination, chest; single view
71046 2 views
71047 3 views
71048 4 or more views

Explanation

In 71045, a single x-ray is taken of the patient's chest. Report 71046 for two views; 71047 for three views; and 71048 for four or more views.

Relative Value Units/Medicare Edits

Non-Facility RVU	Work	PE	MP	Total
71045	0.18	0.57	0.02	0.77
71046	0.22	0.77	0.02	1.01
71047	0.27	0.98	0.02	1.27
71048	0.31	1.04	0.02	1.37
Facility RVU	**Work**	**PE**	**MP**	**Total**
71045	0.18	0.57	0.02	0.77
71046	0.22	0.77	0.02	1.01
71047	0.27	0.98	0.02	1.27
71048	0.31	1.04	0.02	1.37

74018-74021

74018 Radiologic examination, abdomen; 1 view
74019 2 views
74021 3 or more views

Explanation

In 74018, a single x-ray is taken of the patient's abdomen. Because an abdominal x-ray usually precedes another diagnostic imaging procedure, it is not coded separately unless performed as a separately identifiable examination. Report 74019 for two views and 74021 for three or more views.

Relative Value Units/Medicare Edits

Non-Facility RVU	Work	PE	MP	Total
74018	0.18	0.71	0.02	0.91
74019	0.23	0.85	0.02	1.1
74021	0.27	1.0	0.02	1.29
Facility RVU	**Work**	**PE**	**MP**	**Total**
74018	0.18	0.71	0.02	0.91
74019	0.23	0.85	0.02	1.1
74021	0.27	1.0	0.02	1.29

75557-75559

75557 Cardiac magnetic resonance imaging for morphology and function without contrast material;

75559 with stress imaging

Explanation

Cardiac magnetic resonance imaging (MRI) is a radiation-free, noninvasive technique that produces high quality, detailed, three-dimensional imaging of complex congenital heart defects, as well as functional cardiac analysis. MRI uses the natural magnetic properties of the hydrogen atoms in our bodies that emit radiofrequency signals when exposed to radio waves within a strong electromagnetic field. These signals are processed and converted by the computer into high-resolution images. Patients with metallic or electronic implants or foreign bodies cannot be exposed to MRI. The patient must remain still while lying on a motorized table within the large, circular MRI tunnel. A sedative may be administered. Imaging is performed by obtaining tomographic cuts from the base to the apex and/or the interior to the posterior in order to interrogate the entire heart. Function studies may include observation of the atria and/or ventricles, qualitative and quantitative assessment of ventricular function, and obtaining numerical values for ejection fraction (EF) ventricular volumes, ventricular mass, and cardiac output. Code 75557 describes the observation of the cardiac function and morphology without administration of a contrast agent. Report 75559 if stress imaging is included. Following dobutamine injection, which mimics the effects of exercise on the heart and induces ischemia, the physician evaluates the left ventricular wall's ability to move during physical stress.

Relative Value Units/Medicare Edits

Non-Facility RVU	Work	PE	MP	Total
75557	2.35	6.11	0.12	8.58
75559	2.95	8.48	0.11	11.54
Facility RVU	**Work**	**PE**	**MP**	**Total**
75557	2.35	6.11	0.12	8.58
75559	2.95	8.48	0.11	11.54

75561-75565

75561 Cardiac magnetic resonance imaging for morphology and function without contrast material(s), followed by contrast material(s) and further sequences;

75563 with stress imaging

\+ **75565** Cardiac magnetic resonance imaging for velocity flow mapping (List separately in addition to code for primary procedure)

Explanation

Cardiac magnetic resonance imaging (MRI) is a radiation-free, noninvasive technique that produces high quality, detailed, three-dimensional imaging of complex congenital heart defects, as well as functional cardiac analysis. MRI uses the natural magnetic properties of the hydrogen atoms in our bodies that emit radiofrequency signals when exposed to radio waves within a strong electromagnetic field. These signals are processed and converted by the computer into high-resolution images. Patients with metallic or electronic implants or foreign bodies cannot be exposed to MRI. The patient must remain still while lying on a motorized table within the large, circular MRI tunnel. A sedative may be administered. Images are first obtained without contrast materials, followed by administration of contrast materials and further sequences. Imaging is performed by obtaining tomographic cuts from the base to the apex and/or the interior to the posterior in order to interrogate the entire heart. Function studies may include observation of the atria and/or ventricles, qualitative and quantitative assessment of ventricular function, and obtaining numerical values for ejection fraction (EF) ventricular volumes, ventricular mass, and cardiac output. Report 75561 for observation of cardiac function and morphology. Report 75563 if stress imaging is included. Following dobutamine injection, which mimics the effects of exercise on the heart and induces ischemia, the physician evaluates the left ventricular wall's ability to move during physical stress. If velocity flow mapping is performed, report 75565 in addition to the code for the primary procedure.

Relative Value Units/Medicare Edits

Non-Facility RVU	Work	PE	MP	Total
75561	2.6	8.47	0.14	11.21
75563	3.0	9.93	0.14	13.07
75565	0.25	1.14	0.01	1.4
Facility RVU	**Work**	**PE**	**MP**	**Total**
75561	2.6	8.47	0.14	11.21
75563	3.0	9.93	0.14	13.07
75565	0.25	1.14	0.01	1.4

75571

75571 Computed tomography, heart, without contrast material, with quantitative evaluation of coronary calcium

Explanation

Computed tomography directs multiple narrow beams of x-rays around the body structure being studied and uses computer imaging to produce thin, cross-sectional views of various layers (or slices) of the body. It is useful for the evaluation of calcium deposits on the coronary tree. Patients are required to remain motionless during the study. This code reports the CT of the heart and quantitative evaluation of calcium deposits in the coronary tree. High levels of calcium deposits in the heart triple a person's likelihood of suffering an adverse coronary event (e.g., myocardial infarct, cardiac arrest, etc.).

Relative Value Units/Medicare Edits

Non-Facility RVU	Work	PE	MP	Total
75571	0.58	2.44	0.05	3.07
Facility RVU	**Work**	**PE**	**MP**	**Total**
75571	0.58	2.44	0.05	3.07

75572-75574

75572 Computed tomography, heart, with contrast material, for evaluation of cardiac structure and morphology (including 3D image postprocessing, assessment of cardiac function, and evaluation of venous structures, if performed)

75573 Computed tomography, heart, with contrast material, for evaluation of cardiac structure and morphology in the setting of congenital heart disease (including 3D image postprocessing, assessment of left ventricular [LV] cardiac function, right ventricular [RV] structure and function and evaluation of vascular structures, if performed)

75574 Computed tomographic angiography, heart, coronary arteries and bypass grafts (when present), with contrast material, including 3D image postprocessing (including evaluation of cardiac structure and morphology, assessment of cardiac function, and evaluation of venous structures, if performed)

Explanation

The physician performs computed tomography (CT) of the heart utilizing contrast materials to evaluate cardiac structure and morphology. CT directs multiple, thin beams of x-rays at the body and uses computer imaging to produce thin, cross-sectional views of various layers of the body. It is useful in the evaluation of soft tissue. Because patients are required to be motionless during CT, this creates issues when producing CT images of the heart, which is continually moving rhythmically. In a cardiac gating technique, the patient is undergoing CT while attached to ECG leads. CT image acquisition is triggered by the ECG, allowing for coordination of imaging with periods of movement and rest within the heart. Code 75572 includes 3D image postprocessing, assessment of cardiac function, and evaluation of venous structures, if performed. Code 75573 reports CT of a heart with congenital anomalies, also performed utilizing contrast materials to evaluate cardiac structure and morphology. This code includes 3D image postprocessing, assessment of left ventricular (LV) cardiac function, right ventricular (RV) structure and function, and evaluation of vascular structures, if performed. Report 75574 for CT of the heart utilizing contrast materials in conjunction with computerized tomographic angiography (CTA) to evaluate the heart, coronary arteries, and any bypass grafts that are present. In addition to the CT imaging of the heart as described previously, a CTA of native and anomalous coronary arteries and coronary bypass grafts is obtained. CTA is a procedure used for imaging of vessels to detect aneurysms, blood clots, and other vascular irregularities. Contrast media is rapidly infused intravenously, at intervals, usually with an automatic injector. The patient's heart is scanned with thin section axial or spiral mode x-ray beams. Three-dimensional images are generated and postprocessing reconstruction is done at a workstation on the scanner. Vessel wall thickness and the venous anatomy of the heart are evaluated. This code also includes 3D image postprocessing (including evaluation of cardiac structure and morphology, assessment of cardiac function, and evaluation of venous structures, if performed).

Relative Value Units/Medicare Edits

Non-Facility RVU	Work	PE	MP	Total
75572	1.75	5.14	0.11	7.0
75573	2.55	6.63	0.16	9.34
75574	2.4	7.35	0.15	9.9
Facility RVU	**Work**	**PE**	**MP**	**Total**
75572	1.75	5.14	0.11	7.0
75573	2.55	6.63	0.16	9.34
75574	2.4	7.35	0.15	9.9

75580

75580 Noninvasive estimate of coronary fractional flow reserve (FFR) derived from augmentative software analysis of the data set from a coronary computed tomography angiography, with interpretation and report by a physician or other qualified health care professional

Explanation

A proprietary noninvasive fractional flow reserve (FFR) technology is used to assist a physician in evaluating the degree of coronary artery disease (CAD) that a patient has, including how a CAD blockage can affect blood flow to the heart with much greater accuracy based on combining anatomy (coronary CT angiogram) and physiology. This technology allows clinicians to personalize a patient's care plan and reduce the likelihood of needing more invasive procedures. The patient undergoes a coronary computed tomography (CT) angiogram. Data from this test is securely uploaded from the hospital's system to a cloud server. The FFR process creates a personalized, digital, three-dimensional representation of the patient's coronary arteries and employs robust algorithms to help determine and replicate coronary blood flow. The model can also determine any potential effect of blockages on coronary blood flow. Once the process is complete, the physician receives the patient's results through a secure web interface and selects the best treatment course for the patient. This artificial intelligence technology is considered augmentative, which means the machine analyzes and/or quantifies the data to produce clinically meaningful output, and a physician or other qualified health care professional provides an interpretation and report.

Relative Value Units/Medicare Edits

Non-Facility RVU	Work	PE	MP	Total
75580	0.75	26.28	0.09	27.12
Facility RVU	**Work**	**PE**	**MP**	**Total**
75580	0.75	26.28	0.09	27.12

75898

75898 Angiography through existing catheter for follow-up study for transcatheter therapy, embolization or infusion, other than for thrombolysis

Explanation

Angiography is performed during or following transcatheter infusion or embolization through the existing catheter to reassess the therapy's effectiveness. A radiopaque contrast medium is injected through the catheter and by fluoroscopic images recorded of the vessel, the radiologist interprets the status of the blood vessel and the effectiveness of treatment rendered.

75989

75989 Radiological guidance (ie, fluoroscopy, ultrasound, or computed tomography), for percutaneous drainage (eg, abscess, specimen collection), with placement of catheter, radiological supervision and interpretation

Explanation

Fluoroscopic, ultrasonic, or CT guidance may be used for percutaneous drainage of an abscess or to obtain a specimen and place a tube or catheter. Once the abscess is located, the skin is punctured with a needle to begin draining. A catheter may be advanced over a guidewire inserted through the needle and into the abscess cavity. The tract to the outside is dilated to facilitate placing a percutaneous drainage tube. The cavity is aspirated and the drainage tube placed at the lowest point to ensure complete drainage. The drainage tube is secured to suction drainage. This code reports the radiological supervision and interpretation only for this procedure.

Relative Value Units/Medicare Edits

Non-Facility RVU	Work	PE	MP	Total
75989	1.19	2.06	0.09	3.34
Facility RVU	**Work**	**PE**	**MP**	**Total**
75989	1.19	2.06	0.09	3.34

76120-76125

76120 Cineradiography/videoradiography, except where specifically included

\+ **76125** Cineradiography/videoradiography to complement routine examination (List separately in addition to code for primary procedure)

Explanation

Cineradiography uses high speed x-ray films to take a series of images of an organ or system in motion such as the vocal cords or heart. These images taken in exposure ranges of nanoseconds to milliseconds are like the individual frames of a motion picture. This allows the movement to be frozen and tracked very minutely to gather information about time-varying characteristics. Use 76120 when performed alone and not specifically included as part of the procedure. Use 76125 when cineradiography is performed in conjunction with a routine exam.

Relative Value Units/Medicare Edits

Non-Facility RVU	Work	PE	MP	Total
76120	0.38	3.12	0.04	3.54
76125	0.0	0.0	0.0	0.0
Facility RVU	**Work**	**PE**	**MP**	**Total**
76120	0.38	3.12	0.04	3.54
76125	0.0	0.0	0.0	0.0

76604

76604 Ultrasound, chest (includes mediastinum), real time with image documentation

Explanation

Diagnostic ultrasound is an imaging technique bouncing sound waves far above the level of human perception through interior body structures. The sound waves pass through different densities of tissue and reflect back to a receiving unit at varying speeds. The unit converts the waves to electrical pulses that are immediately displayed in picture form on screen. Real time scanning displays structure images and movement with time. This code reports ultrasound and real time for the chest, including the mediastinum.

Relative Value Units/Medicare Edits

Non-Facility RVU	Work	PE	MP	Total
76604	0.59	1.08	0.04	1.71
Facility RVU	**Work**	**PE**	**MP**	**Total**
76604	0.59	1.08	0.04	1.71

76700-76705

76700 Ultrasound, abdominal, real time with image documentation; complete

76705 limited (eg, single organ, quadrant, follow-up)

Explanation

Diagnostic ultrasound is an imaging technique bouncing sound waves far above the level of human perception through interior body structures. The sound waves pass through different densities of tissue and reflect back to a receiving unit at varying speeds. The unit converts the waves to electrical pulses that are immediately displayed in picture form on screen. Real time scanning displays structure images and movement with time. Report 76700 for ultrasound and real time of the entire abdomen and 76705 for a single quadrant or organ of the abdomen.

Relative Value Units/Medicare Edits

Non-Facility RVU	Work	PE	MP	Total
76700	0.81	2.62	0.06	3.49
76705	0.59	1.98	0.04	2.61
Facility RVU	**Work**	**PE**	**MP**	**Total**
76700	0.81	2.62	0.06	3.49
76705	0.59	1.98	0.04	2.61

76706

76706 Ultrasound, abdominal aorta, real time with image documentation, screening study for abdominal aortic aneurysm (AAA)

Explanation

Screening ultrasound of the abdominal aorta with real time image documentation is the imaging technique of bouncing sound waves far above the level of human perception through interior body structures. The sound waves pass through different densities of tissue and reflect back to a receiving unit at varying speeds. The unit converts the waves to electrical pulses that are immediately displayed in picture form on screen. Real time scanning gathers and displays structural images and movement with time. This procedure is used as a tool to evaluate for abdominal aortic aneurysms (AAA) by viewing how the flow of blood moves through the abdominal aorta, which shows defects within the artery typical for an AAA. The U.S. Preventive Services Task Force has suggested screening be performed on men ages 65 to 75 who are or have been smokers, as well as men age 60 and older with family history of AAA.

Relative Value Units/Medicare Edits

Non-Facility RVU	Work	PE	MP	Total
76706	0.55	2.61	0.04	3.2
Facility RVU	**Work**	**PE**	**MP**	**Total**
76706	0.55	2.61	0.04	3.2

76932

76932 Ultrasonic guidance for endomyocardial biopsy, imaging supervision and interpretation

Explanation

The physician takes a biopsy of muscle tissue from within the heart guided by ultrasound. Ultrasound is an imaging technique bouncing sound waves far above the level of human perception through interior body structures. The sound waves pass through different densities of tissue and reflect back to a receiving unit, which converts the waves to electrical pulses that are immediately displayed in picture form on screen. The physician threads a biopsy catheter to the heart through a central intravenous line often inserted into the femoral vein and takes tissue samples of the heart's septum. This code reports the imaging supervision and interpretation only for this procedure.

76937

\+ **76937** Ultrasound guidance for vascular access requiring ultrasound evaluation of potential access sites, documentation of selected vessel patency, concurrent realtime ultrasound visualization of vascular needle entry, with permanent recording and reporting (List separately in addition to code for primary procedure)

Explanation

This is an add-on code to report ultrasound guidance used in conjunction with procedures requiring vascular access. For example: a tunneled, centrally inserted CVAD is inserted without subcutaneous port or pump. The site over the access vein (e.g., subclavian, jugular) is injected with local anesthesia and punctured with a needle or accessed by cutdown approach. A guidewire is inserted. A subcutaneous tunnel is created using a blunt pair of forceps or sharp tunneling tools, over the clavicle from the anterior chest wall to the venotomy site, which is dilated to the right size. The catheter is passed through this tunnel over the guidewire and into the target vein. Report 76937 for the ultrasound guidance used for this procedure, including the evaluation of potential vascular access sites or the patency of selected vessels; guidance during needle entry and catheter manipulation; and verification of final catheter positioning. This code includes permanent recording and reporting.

Relative Value Units/Medicare Edits

Non-Facility RVU	Work	PE	MP	Total
76937	0.3	0.81	0.04	1.15
Facility RVU	**Work**	**PE**	**MP**	**Total**
76937	0.3	0.81	0.04	1.15

76978-76979

76978 Ultrasound, targeted dynamic microbubble sonographic contrast characterization (non-cardiac); initial lesion

\+ **76979** each additional lesion with separate injection (List separately in addition to code for primary procedure)

Explanation

Contrast-enhanced ultrasound (CEUS) imaging using microbubbles as an intravascular contrast agent has shown to be extremely effective in measuring blood flow in the heart and other organs; imaging blood perfusion in organs; describing and defining lesions, particularly focal liver lesions; and evaluating therapy responses. Microbubbles are approximately the same size as a red blood cell and are made up of a gas (e.g., perfluoro gas) enclosed with a phospholipid shell and have the ability to reflect ultrasound waves, enhance the reflections of the ultrasound waves, and create a unique image. There is a variety of microbubble contrast agents that vary based on the shell and gas core composition, as well as whether they are targeted or untargeted. Currently, all FDA-approved microbubbles are considered "untargeted," meaning they are used in clinics today; "targeted" microbubbles are in preclinical development. The microbubbles are administered using a small bolus or via continuous intravenous infusion into the circulation system and remain in the bloodstream for about five minutes. The technician directs the ultrasound waves to the area being evaluated; once the microbubbles pass into the ultrasound waves, the microbubbles produce a "fingerprint-like" harmonic reverberating sound within the ultrasound field vastly different from surrounding tissue that can be detected using microbubble-specific software. The system subsequently produces a contrast-enhanced real-time image. Microbubbles as a contrast agent are better tolerated over MR and CT agents, do not have as many side-effects and, when present, the side effects are typically less severe, and are not as toxic to the kidneys. Report 76978 for the initial lesion targeted and 76979 for each additional lesion with separate injection.

Relative Value Units/Medicare Edits

Non-Facility RVU	Work	PE	MP	Total
76978	1.62	4.93	0.1	6.65
76979	0.85	3.38	0.05	4.28
Facility RVU	**Work**	**PE**	**MP**	**Total**
76978	1.62	4.93	0.1	6.65
76979	0.85	3.38	0.05	4.28

76984

76984 Ultrasound, intraoperative thoracic aorta (eg, epiaortic), diagnostic

Explanation

Diagnostic epiaortic ultrasonography is used to evaluate the ascending aorta during a cardiac procedure and identify aspects of the procedure that may affect the intraoperative plan (e.g., change in bypass targets or cannulation strategy, identifying additional anomalies). It is often performed when other diagnostic modalities such as transesophageal echocardiography (TEE) or visual or manual inspection are not adequate. Ultrasound is an imaging technique that produces bouncing sound waves far above the level of human perception through interior body structures. The sound waves pass through different densities of tissue and reflect back to a receiving unit, which converts the waves to electrical pulses that are immediately displayed in picture form on a screen. A diagnostic epiaortic ultrasound examination may include the aortic arch, sinotubular junction, innominate artery origin, and the proximal, mid, and distal segments of the ascending aorta.

76987-76989

76987 Intraoperative epicardial cardiac ultrasound (ie, echocardiography) for congenital heart disease, diagnostic; including placement and manipulation of transducer, image acquisition, interpretation and report

76988 Intraoperative epicardial cardiac ultrasound (ie, echocardiography) for congenital heart disease, diagnostic; placement, manipulation of transducer, and image acquisition only

76989 Intraoperative epicardial cardiac ultrasound (ie, echocardiography) for congenital heart disease, diagnostic; interpretation and report only

Explanation

Diagnostic epicardial ultrasonography is used to evaluate cardiac structures for a patient with congenital heart disease during a cardiac procedure and identify aspects of the procedure that may affect the intraoperative plan (e.g., change in bypass targets or cannulation strategy, identifying additional anomalies). This type of cardiac ultrasound, or echocardiography, is often performed on pediatric or adult patients when a transesophageal echocardiography (TEE) is not feasible or is contraindicated. Ultrasound is an imaging technique that produces bouncing sound waves far above the level of human perception through interior body structures. The sound waves pass through different densities of tissue and reflect back to a receiving unit, which converts the waves to electrical pulses that are immediately displayed in picture form on a screen. An ultrasound probe is placed directly on the epicardial surface of the heart. The resulting two-dimensional image allows the provider to detect any residual or previously undetected cardiac defects in a patient with congenital heart disease. Report 76987 for placement and manipulation of the transducer, including obtaining images and interpretation and report; 76988 for placement and manipulation of the transducer and obtaining images only; and 76989 for interpretation and report only.

77001

+ **77001** Fluoroscopic guidance for central venous access device placement, replacement (catheter only or complete), or removal (includes fluoroscopic guidance for vascular access and catheter manipulation, any necessary contrast injections through access site or catheter with related venography radiologic supervision and interpretation, and radiographic documentation of final catheter position) (List separately in addition to code for primary procedure)

Explanation

This code reports the fluoroscopic guidance for placement, replacement, or removal of a central venous access device (CVAD) to be used in conjunction with the code for the procedure. For example, a tunneled, centrally inserted CVAD is inserted without subcutaneous port or pump. The site over the access vein (e.g., subclavian, jugular) is injected with local anesthesia and punctured with a needle or accessed by cutdown approach. A guidewire is inserted. A subcutaneous tunnel is created using a blunt pair of forceps or sharp tunneling tools over the clavicle from the anterior chest wall to the venotomy site, which is dilated to the right size. The catheter is passed through this tunnel over the guidewire and into the target vein. Fluoroscopy is used throughout the procedure to guide catheter placement and to check the positioning of the catheter tip. This code includes any contrast injections done through the access site or through the catheter with the necessary corresponding radiological supervision and interpretation of the venography, and the radiographic check of final catheter position.

Relative Value Units/Medicare Edits

Non-Facility RVU	Work	PE	MP	Total
77001	0.38	2.53	0.05	2.96
Facility RVU	**Work**	**PE**	**MP**	**Total**
77001	0.38	2.53	0.05	2.96

77002

+ **77002** Fluoroscopic guidance for needle placement (eg, biopsy, aspiration, injection, localization device) (List separately in addition to code for primary procedure)

Explanation

Fluoroscopic guidance produces x-ray images shown on a screen to assist in visualization of the anatomy, instrument insertion, and/or contrast. This code is specifically reported when utilized for needle biopsy or fine needle aspiration. A cutting biopsy or fine needle is inserted into the target area and the position reaffirmed by fluoroscopy. This is done for an internal mass or lesion that has been positively identified by other diagnostic imaging performed earlier.

Relative Value Units/Medicare Edits

Non-Facility RVU	Work	PE	MP	Total
77002	0.54	2.9	0.04	3.48
Facility RVU	**Work**	**PE**	**MP**	**Total**
77002	0.54	2.9	0.04	3.48

78414

78414 Determination of central c-v hemodynamics (non-imaging) (eg, ejection fraction with probe technique) with or without pharmacologic intervention or exercise, single or multiple determinations

Explanation

Measurement of central cardiovascular hemodynamics, such as left ventricular ejection fraction, is performed noninvasively using a scintillation probe. Using chest x-rays or echocardiography, the proper location for the probe is marked on the chest wall. An intravenous bolus of radiotracer and/or exercise may be introduced. The probe is applied and the variations in left ventricular volume changes are recorded and measured.

78428

78428 Cardiac shunt detection

Explanation

For detecting right to left cardiac shunts, radiolabeled macroaggregated albumin is used, which is trapped by the lungs and will be identified in the systemic circulation if a right to left shunt is present. For left to right shunts, the first pass technique is used. A bolus of radionuclide is injected and rapid image frames are acquired as it moves in the venous system through the chambers of the heart. Early recirculation detected would identify a left to right shunt.

Relative Value Units/Medicare Edits

Non-Facility RVU	Work	PE	MP	Total
78428	0.78	4.36	0.07	5.21
Facility RVU	**Work**	**PE**	**MP**	**Total**
78428	0.78	4.36	0.07	5.21

78445

78445 Non-cardiac vascular flow imaging (ie, angiography, venography)

Explanation

Nuclear imaging for non-cardiac vascular flow studies may be performed to test for arterial or venous peripheral vascular diseases or injuries, graft patency, and even catheter malfunctions. In radionuclide angiography, for example, red blood cells from the patient are tagged with radioactivity and injected intravenously. A scintillation camera positioned over the arterial area of interest detects the radioactivity in the blood and takes a series of dynamic images every 2 to 3 seconds immediately after injection, followed by static images. These are recorded on computer and/or film to be studied at different frame rates, times, and intensities. Normal flow is demonstrated as swift and unimpeded. Luminal narrowing or widening, blood flow obstructions and occlusions, and extraluminal accumulation of the radioactive cells can be visualized for diagnostic purposes.

Relative Value Units/Medicare Edits

Non-Facility RVU	Work	PE	MP	Total
78445	0.49	5.08	0.09	5.66
Facility RVU	**Work**	**PE**	**MP**	**Total**
78445	0.49	5.08	0.09	5.66

78451-78452

78451 Myocardial perfusion imaging, tomographic (SPECT) (including attenuation correction, qualitative or quantitative wall motion, ejection fraction by first pass or gated technique, additional quantification, when performed); single study, at rest or stress (exercise or pharmacologic)

78452 multiple studies, at rest and/or stress (exercise or pharmacologic) and/or redistribution and/or rest reinjection

Explanation

For tomographic myocardial perfusion imaging, the patient receives an intravenous injection of a radionuclide, usually thallium or technetium-99m, which localizes only in nonischemic tissue. SPECT (single photon emission computed tomographic) images of the heart are taken immediately to identify areas of perfusion vs. infarction. SPECT imaging differs from planar imaging by using a single or multiple-head camera that rotates around the patient to give three-dimensional tomographic imaging of the heart displayed in thin slices. In the nonstress version of the procedure, radionuclide is injected and images are taken without stress induction. In 78451, a single study is performed at rest or stress. If the test is to be done at a stress condition, it is induced with the standard treadmill exercise test or pharmacologically with the infusion of a vasodilator. In 78452, multiple studies are done at rest and/or stress with a second injection of radionuclide given again in the redistribution and/or resting phase just prior to resting images being taken. These codes also include attenuation correction (AC), which provides a more accurate diagnostic image for diagnosing defects or infarcted areas by raising the importance of radioactivity distribution counts arising from certain areas. For instance, counts from the anterior wall may be reduced or impeded by the presence of the breast. These codes also include qualitative or quantitative wall motion, ejection fraction (EF) by first pass or gated technique, and additional quantification, when performed.

Relative Value Units/Medicare Edits

Non-Facility RVU	Work	PE	MP	Total
78451	1.38	7.91	0.1	9.39
78452	1.62	11.23	0.14	12.99
Facility RVU	**Work**	**PE**	**MP**	**Total**
78451	1.38	7.91	0.1	9.39
78452	1.62	11.23	0.14	12.99

78453-78454

78453 Myocardial perfusion imaging, planar (including qualitative or quantitative wall motion, ejection fraction by first pass or gated technique, additional quantification, when performed); single study, at rest or stress (exercise or pharmacologic)

78454 multiple studies, at rest and/or stress (exercise or pharmacologic) and/or redistribution and/or rest reinjection

Explanation

For planar myocardial perfusion imaging, stress is induced with the standard treadmill exercise test or pharmacologically with the infusion of a vasodilator, if the test is to be done at stress conditions. The patient receives an intravenous injection of a radionuclide, usually thallium or technetium-99m, which localizes only in nonischemic tissue. Planar images of the heart are scanned immediately with a gamma camera that detects the radiation in the heart tissue to identify areas of infarction. In the nonstress version of the procedure, radionuclide is injected and images taken without stress induction. In 78453, a single study is performed at rest or stress. In 78454, multiple procedures are done at rest and/or at stress with a second injection of radionuclide given again in the redistribution or resting phase just prior to resting images being taken. For tests performed during pharmacological or exercise-induced stress, report the appropriate stress testing code. These codes also include qualitative or quantitative wall motion, ejection fraction (EF) by first pass or gated technique, and additional quantification, when performed.

Relative Value Units/Medicare Edits

Non-Facility RVU	Work	PE	MP	Total
78453	1.0	6.91	0.08	7.99
78454	1.34	10.46	0.14	11.94
Facility RVU	**Work**	**PE**	**MP**	**Total**
78453	1.0	6.91	0.08	7.99
78454	1.34	10.46	0.14	11.94

78456

78456 Acute venous thrombosis imaging, peptide

Explanation

Diagnostic nuclear imaging for acute venous thrombosis imaging uses radiolabeled peptides. Peptides are short-string proteins that attach to platelets, which are essential in blood clotting, and localize at sites where clots are present or beginning to form. Images from a scintillation, or gamma camera, are taken by detecting the gamma radiation from the radiotracer in the peptides attached to the blood component and these images can identify clots as soon as 10 minutes after the injection. Usually another set of images is done after 60 to 90 minutes following the injection as the image quality tends to improve with time after the injection. If a scan showed significantly increased uptake in any region of one leg compared to the other, or more intense uptake on delayed imaging, deep venous thrombosis is suspected.

Relative Value Units/Medicare Edits

Non-Facility RVU	Work	PE	MP	Total
78456	1.0	7.56	0.09	8.65
Facility RVU	**Work**	**PE**	**MP**	**Total**
78456	1.0	7.56	0.09	8.65

78457-78458

78457 Venous thrombosis imaging, venogram; unilateral

78458 bilateral

Explanation

A diagnostic nuclear venogram is done to identify the presence and location of thrombi (blood clots) within the venous system. An intravenous injection of a radiopharmaceutical into one or both extremities, most often the legs, is first performed. This is followed by rapid sequence imaging as the radiopharmaceutical passes through the venous system. Unilateral imaging for venous thrombosis is reported with 78457; bilateral imaging is reported with 78458. Bilateral studies may be performed even when only one leg is symptomatic for deep-vein thrombus as the normal extremity if used for comparison purposes.

Relative Value Units/Medicare Edits

Non-Facility RVU	Work	PE	MP	Total
78457	0.77	3.69	0.18	4.64
78458	0.9	4.79	0.09	5.78
Facility RVU	**Work**	**PE**	**MP**	**Total**
78457	0.77	3.69	0.18	4.64
78458	0.9	4.79	0.09	5.78

78459 [78429]

78459 Myocardial imaging, positron emission tomography (PET), metabolic evaluation study (including ventricular wall motion[s] and/or ejection fraction[s], when performed), single study;

78429 Myocardial imaging, positron emission tomography (PET), metabolic evaluation study (including ventricular wall motion[s] and/or ejection fraction[s], when performed), single study; with concurrently acquired computed tomography transmission scan

Explanation

In 78459, the cardiac muscle is imaged using data received from positron-emitting radionuclides administered to the patient by intravenous injection. The collision of the positrons emitted by the radionuclide with the negatively-charged electrons normally present in tissue is computer-synthesized to produce an image, usually in color. This image shows the presence or absence of ischemic or fibrotic cardiac tissue and allows evaluation of metabolic functioning of cardiac tissue. A test to determine the percentage of blood that is pumped out of a filled ventricle with each heartbeat, known as the ejection fraction, may also be undertaken at this time, as well as evaluation of ventricular wall motion. In 78429, a computed tomography (CT) scan is performed concurrently with the above-described PET study utilizing a combination PET/CT camera. Data sets obtained from the CT and PET are joined electronically by the scanner's computer system and can be viewed interactively by the clinician on a workstation, combining both excellent anatomic detail and physiologic information regarding metabolic activity.

78466-78469

78466 Myocardial imaging, infarct avid, planar; qualitative or quantitative
78468 with ejection fraction by first pass technique
78469 tomographic SPECT with or without quantification

Explanation

A radionuclide is injected intravenously that localizes in recently (under 72-hours) infarcted myocardial tissue. Multiple cardiac images are obtained between one and four hours after injection of the isotope. The location and extent of infarct can be determined by the presence of the radionuclide in the heart tissue. In 78468, first-pass technique is utilized. In first-pass technique, a bolus of Technetium-99m or other radionuclide is injected and visualized as it moves through the venous system into the right atrium, right ventricle, pulmonary artery, lungs, left atrium, left ventricle, and aorta. Several cardia cycles are generally observed. Ejection fraction measurements from both the right and left ventricle are calculated by determining the change in radioactivity over time. In 78469, SPECT images are obtained. SPECT images are tomographic reconstructions derived from a single- or multiple-head gamma camera that rotates around the patient. Tomographic imaging displays the heart in thin slices allowing better separation of myocardial and nonmyocardial structures. SPECT imaging is helpful in identifying small infarcts that are sometimes missed using planar imaging alone.

Relative Value Units/Medicare Edits

Non-Facility RVU	Work	PE	MP	Total
78466	0.69	4.25	0.06	5.0
78468	0.8	4.63	0.07	5.5
78469	0.92	5.17	0.07	6.16
Facility RVU	**Work**	**PE**	**MP**	**Total**
78466	0.69	4.25	0.06	5.0
78468	0.8	4.63	0.07	5.5
78469	0.92	5.17	0.07	6.16

78472-78473

78472 Cardiac blood pool imaging, gated equilibrium; planar, single study at rest or stress (exercise and/or pharmacologic), wall motion study plus ejection fraction, with or without additional quantitative processing
78473 multiple studies, wall motion study plus ejection fraction, at rest and stress (exercise and/or pharmacologic), with or without additional quantification

Explanation

Radionuclide, which will adhere to the patient's red blood cells, is injected intravenously for cardiac blood pool imaging. Multiple images of the heart, synchronized with the electrocardiographic RR interval (ECG gated), are taken several minutes later, after the radionuclide has spread through the blood pool. These images are computer synthesized and data is generated to produce a video display of cardiac wall motion, calculation of left ventricular ejection fractions, and images based on computer manipulation of the data received. In 78472, the procedure is performed as a single study at rest or stress, not both; in 78473, the procedure is performed at both rest and stress. For tests performed during pharmacological or exercise-induced stress, report the appropriate stress testing code also.

Relative Value Units/Medicare Edits

Non-Facility RVU	Work	PE	MP	Total
78472	0.98	5.25	0.08	6.31
78473	1.47	6.47	0.1	8.04
Facility RVU	**Work**	**PE**	**MP**	**Total**
78472	0.98	5.25	0.08	6.31
78473	1.47	6.47	0.1	8.04

78481-78483

78481 Cardiac blood pool imaging (planar), first pass technique; single study, at rest or with stress (exercise and/or pharmacologic), wall motion study plus ejection fraction, with or without quantification
78483 multiple studies, at rest and with stress (exercise and/or pharmacologic), wall motion study plus ejection fraction, with or without quantification

Explanation

A bolus of radionuclide is injected intravenously for cardiac blood pool imaging, first pass technique. As the radioisotope passes through the cardiac chambers, rapid sequence imaging and computer generation of data and images is done to produce a video display of cardiac wall motion, calculation of ventricular ejection fractions, and images based on computer manipulation of the data received. This technique provides information about the functional status of the heart at rest or in response to stress. In 78481, the procedure is performed as a single study at rest or stress, not both; in 78483, the procedure is performed at rest and stress. For tests performed during pharmacological or exercise-induced stress, report the appropriate stress testing code also.

Relative Value Units/Medicare Edits

Non-Facility RVU	Work	PE	MP	Total
78481	0.98	3.91	0.07	4.96
78483	1.47	5.1	0.09	6.66
Facility RVU	**Work**	**PE**	**MP**	**Total**
78481	0.98	3.91	0.07	4.96
78483	1.47	5.1	0.09	6.66

78491, 78492

78491 Myocardial imaging, positron emission tomography (PET), perfusion study (including ventricular wall motion[s] and/or ejection fraction[s], when performed); single study, at rest or stress (exercise or pharmacologic)
78492 multiple studies at rest and stress (exercise or pharmacologic)

Explanation

The cardiac muscle is imaged using data received from positron-emitting radionuclides administered to the patient by intravenous injection. The collision of the positrons emitted by the radionuclide with the negatively-charged electrons normally present in tissue is computer-synthesized to produce an image, usually in color, which shows the presence or absence of perfusion into normal or ischemic cardiac tissue. A determination of the percentage of blood that is pumped out of a filled ventricle with each heartbeat, known as the ejection fraction, may also be made at this time, as well as evaluation of ventricular wall motion. Report 78491 if the procedure is performed as a single study at rest or during exercise or pharmacologic-induced stress. Report 78492 for multiple studies at rest and during exercise or pharmacologic-induced stress.

[78430, 78431]

78430 Myocardial imaging, positron emission tomography (PET), perfusion study (including ventricular wall motion[s] and/or ejection fraction[s], when performed); single study, at rest or stress (exercise or pharmacologic), with concurrently acquired computed tomography transmission scan

78431 Myocardial imaging, positron emission tomography (PET), perfusion study (including ventricular wall motion[s] and/or ejection fraction[s], when performed); multiple studies at rest and stress (exercise or pharmacologic), with concurrently acquired computed tomography transmission scan

Explanation

The cardiac muscle is imaged using data received from positron-emitting radionuclides administered to the patient by intravenous injection. The collision of the positrons emitted by the radionuclide with the negatively-charged electrons normally present in tissue is computer-synthesized to produce an image, usually in color, which shows the presence or absence of perfusion into normal or ischemic cardiac tissue. A determination of the percentage of blood that is pumped out of a filled ventricle with each heartbeat, known as the ejection fraction, may also be made at this time, as well as evaluation of ventricular wall motion. A computed tomography (CT) scan is performed concurrently with the aforementioned PET study utilizing a combination PET/CT camera. Data sets obtained from the CT and PET are joined electronically by the scanner's computer system and can be viewed interactively by the clinician on a work station, combining both excellent anatomic detail and pertinent physiologic information. Report 78430 if the procedure is performed as a single study at rest or during exercise or pharmacologic-induced stress. Report 78431 for multiple studies at rest and during exercise or pharmacologic-induced stress.

[78432, 78433]

78432 Myocardial imaging, positron emission tomography (PET), combined perfusion with metabolic evaluation study (including ventricular wall motion[s] and/or ejection fraction[s], when performed), dual radiotracer (eg, myocardial viability);

78433 Myocardial imaging, positron emission tomography (PET), combined perfusion with metabolic evaluation study (including ventricular wall motion[s] and/or ejection fraction[s], when performed), dual radiotracer (eg, myocardial viability); with concurrently acquired computed tomography transmission scan

Explanation

In 78432, a myocardial viability study is undertaken using dual radiotracers such as rubidium-82 (to measure blood flow) and 18F-fluorodeoxyglucose or FDG (to measure whether heart muscle cells are alive) that are administered to the patient by intravenous injection. The collision of the positrons emitted by the radionuclide with the negatively-charged electrons normally present in tissue is computer-synthesized to produce an image, usually in color, which shows the presence or absence of ischemic or fibrotic cardiac tissue and allows evaluation of its metabolic functioning. It also reveals the presence or absence of perfusion into these tissues. A determination of the percentage of blood that is pumped out of a filled ventricle with each heartbeat, known as the ejection fraction, may also be made at this time, as well as evaluation of ventricular wall motion. The procedure is performed to assess myocardial viability. In 78433, a computed tomography (CT) scan is performed concurrently with the above-described PET study utilizing a combination PET/CT camera. Data sets obtained from the CT and PET are joined electronically by the scanner's computer system and can be viewed interactively by the clinician on a workstation, combining both excellent anatomic detail and pertinent physiologic information.

[78434]

\+ **78434** Absolute quantitation of myocardial blood flow (AQMBF), positron emission tomography (PET), rest and pharmacologic stress (List separately in addition to code for primary procedure)

Explanation

The physician performs absolute quantitation of myocardial blood flow during rest and pharmacologic stress using positron emission tomography (PET). Absolute quantitation of myocardial blood flow (MBF) by PET is an established method and superior tool in the detection, analysis, and management of epicardial and microvascular coronary artery disease (CAD) and provides clinicians the ability to measure, in a noninvasive manner, MBF in milliliters per minute, per gram of tissue. Positron emission tomography is a radionuclide imaging technique for noninvasive quantification of MBF. The process of evaluating myocardial perfusion is a key aspect in diagnosing and determining outcomes for cases of suspected or known CAD. Resting MBF is the total amount of blood flow received by the myocardium per minute, per gram of tissue and may be impacted by a myriad of factors including, but not limited to, the patient's age, gender, blood pressure, and heart rate. Normal values for MBF at rest range from 0.6 to 1.3 mL/min/g. Stress MBF, also referred to as hyperemic blood flow, describes the highest amount of blood flow that can be provided to the heart during the topmost period of vasodilation of the heart's vascular bed. Typically, to reach this maximum vasodilation, the patient receives vasodilators or inotropic agents via IV to simulate stress as well as a cold pressor test (CPT) and mental stress tests. Stress MBF may be impacted by a number of factors including, but not limited to, caffeine, increased microvascular tone and resistance, and coronary risk factors. Report 78434 in addition to the code for the primary procedure.

78494

78494 Cardiac blood pool imaging, gated equilibrium, SPECT, at rest, wall motion study plus ejection fraction, with or without quantitative processing

Explanation

Radionuclide, which will adhere to the patient's red blood cells, is injected intravenously for cardiac blood pool imaging, gated equilibrium. Multiple SPECT (single photon emission computed tomography) images of the heart, synchronized with the electrocardiographic RR interval (ECG gated), are taken several minutes later, after the radionuclide has spread through the blood pool. These SPECT images are taken by a rotating single or multiple-head camera for three-dimensional views of cross-sectional slices and provide better contrast in imaging and greater accuracy than planar scans. The SPECT images are computer synthesized and data is generated to produce a video display of cardiac wall motion, calculation of ventricular ejection fractions, and images based on computer manipulation of the data received.

Relative Value Units/Medicare Edits

Non-Facility RVU	Work	PE	MP	Total
78494	1.19	5.09	0.08	6.36
Facility RVU	**Work**	**PE**	**MP**	**Total**
78494	1.19	5.09	0.08	6.36

78496

\+ **78496** Cardiac blood pool imaging, gated equilibrium, single study, at rest, with right ventricular ejection fraction by first pass technique (List separately in addition to code for primary procedure)

Explanation

A bolus of radionuclide is injected intravenously for cardiac blood pool imaging with right ventricular ejection fraction by first pass technique. As the radioisotope in the venous system passes through the cardiac chambers, rapid sequence imaging, synchronized with the electrocardiographic RR interval (ECG gated), is done. This first pass technique provides information for right ventricular ejection fraction calculation not possible with static gated images which do not show right ventricular count in isolation. This test for functional status of the heart is done as a single study at rest in addition to the primary procedure.

Relative Value Units/Medicare Edits

Non-Facility RVU	Work	PE	MP	Total
78496	0.5	0.73	0.03	1.26
Facility RVU	**Work**	**PE**	**MP**	**Total**
78496	0.5	0.73	0.03	1.26

80051

80051 Electrolyte panel This panel must include the following: Carbon dioxide (bicarbonate) (82374) Chloride (82435) Potassium (84132) Sodium (84295)

Explanation

An electrolyte panel includes the following tests: carbon dioxide (82374), chloride (82435), potassium (84132), and sodium (84295). Blood specimen is obtained by venipuncture. See specific codes for additional information about the listed tests.

80061

80061 Lipid panel This panel must include the following: Cholesterol, serum, total (82465) Lipoprotein, direct measurement, high density cholesterol (HDL cholesterol) (83718) Triglycerides (84478)

Explanation

A lipid panel includes the following tests: total serum cholesterol (82465), high-density cholesterol (HDL cholesterol) by direct measurement (83718), and triglycerides (84478). Blood specimen is obtained by venipuncture. See specific codes for additional information about the listed tests.

80162-80163

80162 Digoxin; total
80163 free

Explanation

Digoxin is used principally to treat conditions surrounding congestive heart failure, such as arrhythmias, atrial fibrillation, and tachycardia. Test specimens may be drawn during peak and trough periods, which is shortly after administration and again just before the next administration when serum concentration is at its lowest. Method for total digoxin (80162) is high performance liquid chromatography (HPLC) or gas liquid chromatography (GLC) and is used to determine dosage. Free digoxin levels are useful in determining digoxin toxicity. A protein-free ultrafiltrate is prepared from the patient's serum, and the digoxin in the ultrafiltrate (free digoxin) is measured by fluorescence polarization immunoassay. Report 80162 for total serum levels and 80163 when free digoxin is assayed.

81000

81000 Urinalysis, by dip stick or tablet reagent for bilirubin, glucose, hemoglobin, ketones, leukocytes, nitrite, pH, protein, specific gravity, urobilinogen, any number of these constituents; non-automated, with microscopy

Explanation

This type of test may be ordered by the brand name product and the analytes tested. Although, screens are considered to show the presence of an analyte (qualitative), some newer products are semi-quantitative. Many are plastic strips that contain sites impregnated with chemicals that react with urine when the strip is dipped into a specimen. The result is a color change that is compared against a standardized chart. Most strips will test for numerous analytes, as well as for pH and specific gravity. Tablets work in a similar fashion. A drop of urine is placed on the tablet and a chemical reaction causes a color change that is compared to a standard chart. Usually, only a single analyte is under consideration, per tablet. Code 81000 involves a manual (nonautomated) test and includes a microscopic examination. Microscopy involves examination of the urine sediments or solids. The urine is first centrifuged in a graduated tube to concentrate the sediments. Samples (either wet or dry) are examined, usually under both high and low power, and abnormal constituents are noted. These may include a wide range of biological abnormalities, such as blood cells, casts, and bacteria, as well as chemical anomalies, such as crystals.

81001

81001 Urinalysis, by dip stick or tablet reagent for bilirubin, glucose, hemoglobin, ketones, leukocytes, nitrite, pH, protein, specific gravity, urobilinogen, any number of these constituents; automated, with microscopy

Explanation

This type of test may be ordered by the type of processor used and the analytes tested. The testing methodology is similar to the manual strips, except that the color change caused by the chemical reaction with urine is processed and read mechanically. The strip is exposed to the urine sample and is mechanically fed through a processor that reads the colors emitted by the reaction. The unit will be calibrated according to international standards and readings have a high degree of accuracy. The result may be displayed on a monitor, but is always printed or recorded in some form. Code 81001 also includes microscopy. Microscopy involves examination of the urine sediments or solids. The urine is first centrifuged in a graduated tube to concentrate the sediments. Samples (wet or dry) are examined, usually under both high and low power, and abnormal constituents are noted. These may include a wide range of biological abnormalities, such as blood cells, casts, and bacteria, as well as chemical anomalies, such as crystals.

81002

81002 Urinalysis, by dip stick or tablet reagent for bilirubin, glucose, hemoglobin, ketones, leukocytes, nitrite, pH, protein, specific gravity, urobilinogen, any number of these constituents; non-automated, without microscopy

Explanation

This type of test may be ordered by the brand name product and the analytes tested. Although usually considered screens to show the presence of an analyte (qualitative), some newer products are semi-quantitative. Many are plastic strips that contain sites impregnated with chemicals that react with urine when the strip is dipped into a specimen. The result is a color change that is compared against a standardized chart. Most strips will test for numerous analytes, as well as for pH and specific gravity. Tablets work in a similar fashion. A drop of urine is placed on the tablet and a chemical reaction causes a color change that is compared to a standard chart. Usually only a single analyte is under consideration per tablet, however. Code 81002 does not include a microscopic examination of the urine sample or its components.

81003

81003 Urinalysis, by dip stick or tablet reagent for bilirubin, glucose, hemoglobin, ketones, leukocytes, nitrite, pH, protein, specific gravity, urobilinogen, any number of these constituents; automated, without microscopy

Explanation

This type of test may be ordered by the type of processor used and the analytes tested. The testing methodology is similar to the manual strips, except that the color change caused by the chemical reaction with urine is processed and read mechanically. The strip is exposed to the urine sample and is fed through a processor that reads the colors emitted by the reaction. The unit will be calibrated according to international standards and readings have a high degree of accuracy. The result may be displayed on a monitor, but is always printed or recorded in some form. Code 81003 does not include a microscopic examination of the urine sample or its components.

82465

82465 Cholesterol, serum or whole blood, total

Explanation

Cholesterol level is a risk indicator for atherosclerosis and myocardial infarction. Blood specimen is obtained by venipuncture. Method is enzymatic. This test reports total cholesterol in serum or whole blood.

82550

82550 Creatine kinase (CK), (CPK); total

Explanation

This test may be requested as creatine kinase (CK) or creatine phosphokinase (CPK). Blood specimen is obtained by venipuncture. Method is enzymatic, kinetic, or spectrophotometry. This code reports total CK. Creatine kinase is an enzyme found in striated muscle and it is released following injury. Elevated CK levels are primarily associated with myocardial infarction, trauma and surgery, but CK levels may be elevated with a number of other conditions as well.

82552

82552 Creatine kinase (CK), (CPK); isoenzymes

Explanation

This test may be requested as creatine kinase (CK) isoenzymes or creatine phosphokinase (CPK) isoenzymes. Method is electrophoresis (EP), column ion-exchange chromatography. Creatine kinase consists of three isoenzymes, each of which is composed of two units, muscle (MM), brain (BB), or muscle and brain (MB). CK1 (BB) is found primarily in the brain and smooth muscle, CK2 (MB) in cardiac muscle, and CK3 (MM) in skeletal muscle. Because elevated CK levels are indicative of injury to the cells, quantifying the levels of each isoenzyme may assist in pinpointing the injured site.

82553

82553 Creatine kinase (CK), (CPK); MB fraction only

Explanation

This test may be requested as creatine kinase (CK) MB fraction, creatine phosphokinase (CPK) MB fraction, or CK2. Methods include immunochemical, fluorometric radial partition, microparticle enzyme immunoassay, immunoenzymetric, or chemiluminometric. Creatine kinase consists of three isoenzymes, which are each composed of two units, muscle (MM), brain (BB), or muscle and brain (MB). CK1 (BB) is found primarily in the brain and smooth muscle, CK2 (MB) in cardiac muscle, and CK3 (MM) in skeletal muscle. This code tests for the MB or CK2 fraction only.

82554

82554 Creatine kinase (CK), (CPK); isoforms

Explanation

This test may be requested as CK isoforms or CPK isoforms. Blood specimen is obtained by venipuncture. Methods include electrophoresis (EP), high performance liquid chromatography (HPLC), and isoelectric focusing (IEF). Creatine kinase consists of three isoenzymes, which are each composed of two units, muscle (MM), brain (BB), or muscle and brain (MB). CK1 (BB) is found primarily in the brain and smooth muscle, CK2 (MB) in cardiac muscle, and CK3 (MM) in skeletal muscle. These isoenzymes can be further subdivided into isoforms which are designated by the isoenzyme (MM, MB, BB) followed by a number (e.g., 1, 2, 3) Examples include CK-MB1, CK-MB2.

82800

82800 Gases, blood, pH only

Explanation

This test may be requested as blood pH. Blood pH is tested to identify acidemia or alkalemia. Arterial puncture is preferred, but venipuncture may also be performed. Method is glass pH electrode or potentiometry.

82803-82805

82803 Gases, blood, any combination of pH, pCO2, pO2, CO2, HCO3 (including calculated O2 saturation);

82805 with O2 saturation, by direct measurement, except pulse oximetry

Explanation

These tests may be requested as arterial blood gases (ABGs). Blood gases are usually requested to evaluate disturbances of acid-base balance, which may be caused by respiratory or metabolic disorders. Blood specimen is obtained by arterial puncture. Code 82803 reports any combination of pH, pCO2, pO2, CO2, and HCO3, including calculated O2 saturation. Code 82805 reports any combination of the same gases, but O2 saturation is performed by direct measurement. Method is selective electrode, potentiometry, or spectrophotometry (O2 saturation).

82810

82810 Gases, blood, O2 saturation only, by direct measurement, except pulse oximetry

Explanation

This test may be requested as O2. Oxygen saturation is the percent of the oxygen in the blood that combines with hemoglobin. Blood specimen is obtained by arterial puncture. Method is spectrophotometry.

82820

82820 Hemoglobin-oxygen affinity (pO2 for 50% hemoglobin saturation with oxygen)

Explanation

This test may be requested as oxygen, P50 or as pO2, P50. This test is performed to measure the affinity of hemoglobin for oxygen, which allows evaluation of oxygen delivery to body tissues. Blood specimen is obtained by arterial puncture. Method is spectrophotometry or potentiometry.

82948

82948 Glucose; blood, reagent strip

Explanation

This test is used to monitor disorders of carbohydrate metabolism. Blood specimen is obtained by finger stick. A drop of blood is placed on the reagent strip for a specified amount of time. When the prescribed amount of time has elapsed, the strip is blotted and the reagent strip is compared to a color chart. Method is reagent strip with visual comparison.

83036-83037

83036 Hemoglobin; glycosylated (A1C)

83037 Hemoglobin; glycosylated (A1C) by device cleared by FDA for home use

Explanation

These tests may also be known as HbA1C. A blood specimen is collected. Glycosylated hemoglobin levels reflect the average level of glucose in the blood over a three-month period. Methods may include high-performance liquid chromatography and ion exchange chromatography (83036) or FDA approved home monitoring device (83037).

83615

83615 Lactate dehydrogenase (LD), (LDH);

Explanation

This test may also be ordered as LD or LDH. The test is a measure of LD or LDH, which is found in many body tissues, particularly the heart, liver, red blood cells, and kidneys. Methods used are lactate to pyruvate or pyruvate to lactate. This test may be ordered for a wide variety of disorders, including renal diseases and congestive heart failure.

83625

83625 Lactate dehydrogenase (LD), (LDH); isoenzymes, separation and quantitation

Explanation

This test may be ordered as LDH isoenzymes or LD isoenzymes. Three serial blood specimens are collected at 6-8 hour intervals to detect changes in the LD isoenzymes. Shifts in the values of five clinically significant LD fractions monitored over time create diagnostic patterns that correlate with diseases such as myocardial infarction, renal infarction and hepatic congestion. This allows for the differential diagnosis of numerous conditions. Method is by electrophoresis or immunochemical methods, including immunoprecipitation. This test may be ordered for a wide variety of reasons, and results may point to numerous diagnoses.

83701

83701 Lipoprotein, blood; high resolution fractionation and quantitation of lipoproteins including lipoprotein subclasses when performed (eg, electrophoresis, ultracentrifugation)

Explanation

This test may be referred to as Type III fractionation. Type III hyperlipoproteinemia is an inherited disorder whereby both the cholesterol and triglycerides show high plasma concentrations. This particular test is usually performed following previous tests to further isolate abnormal beta-lipoproteins. The patient is told to fast. Blood is drawn by venipuncture. The test may be performed by various methods including ultracentrifugation or electrophoresis. Ultracentrifugation is more common and is considered the traditional standard for accuracy in high-density lipoproteins (HDL) subclass quantitation.

83718

83718 Lipoprotein, direct measurement; high density cholesterol (HDL cholesterol)

Explanation

This test may be requested as HDL, HDLC, or HDL cholesterol. Lipoproteins are compounds composed of lipids bound to proteins, which are transported through the blood. High-density lipoprotein (HDL) is frequently referred to as "good cholesterol," or "friendly lipid," as it is responsible for decreasing plaque deposits in blood vessels. High levels of HDL decrease the risk of premature coronary artery disease. This code reports direct measurement only, normally performed using an enzymatic or precipitation method.

83719

83719 Lipoprotein, direct measurement; VLDL cholesterol

Explanation

This test measures VLDL, the lipoprotein that carries triglycerides in the blood. The test is useful to determine a patient's risk of arteriosclerotic occlusive disease, as well as other cholesterol-related disorders. The method used is electrophoresis and may first involve ultracentrifugation.

83721

83721 Lipoprotein, direct measurement; LDL cholesterol

Explanation

This test may also be referred to as LDL-C. It measures the amount of low-density lipoprotein (LDL), also known as "bad cholesterol." The test is useful to determine the patient's risk of coronary heart disease (CHD), among other disorders. Method may be by precipitation procedure with results derived by the Friedewald formula.

83789

83789 Mass spectrometry and tandem mass spectrometry (eg, MS, MS/MS, MALDI, MS-TOF, QTOF), non-drug analyte(s) not elsewhere specified, qualitative or quantitative, each specimen

Explanation

This test identifies the presence of (qualitative), and measures the amount of (quantifies), specific analytes in protein. Specimen varies. Method is mass spectrometry (MS). The test is used for identifying the chemical makeup and structure of a substance. Tandem MS (MS/MS) is one type of MS using sequential analysis to provide structural information by establishing relationships between substances. Others include quadrupole/time-of-flight (Q/TOF) and matrix-assisted laser desorption/ionization (MALDI). This test assists in identifying the chemical makeup and structure of a substance, analyzing viruses, sequencing and analyzing peptides and proteins, and providing information on such life-threatening diseases as AIDS and various types of skin cancers as well as quantifies (measures) the amount of analyte in the specimen.

84132

84132 Potassium; serum, plasma or whole blood

Explanation

This test may be requested as K or K+. Potassium is the major electrolyte found in intracellular fluids. Potassium influences skeletal and cardiac muscle activity. Very small fluctuations outside the normal range may cause significant health risk, including muscle weakness and cardiac arrhythmias. Blood specimen is serum, plasma, or whole blood. Methods include atomic absorption spectrometry (AAS), ion-selective electrode (ISE), and flame emission spectroscopy (FES).

84450

84450 Transferase; aspartate amino (AST) (SGOT)

Explanation

This test is usually referred to as aspartate aminotransferase (AST) or as serum glutamic oxaloacetic transaminase (SGOT). AST is an enzyme found primarily in heart muscle and the liver. Serum levels are low unless there is cellular damage, at which time large amounts are released into circulation. AST levels are increased following acute myocardial infarction (MI). Liver disease may also cause elevated levels of AST. Blood specimen is serum or plasma. Method is spectrophotometry, kinetic assay, and enzymatic.

84478

84478 Triglycerides

Explanation

This test may be requested as trig. Triglycerides are blood lipids that are transported through the circulatory system by lipoproteins. Triglycerides contribute to atherosclerosis and other arterial diseases. Blood specimen is serum or plasma. Method is enzymatic or colorimetry.

84512

84512 Troponin, qualitative

Explanation

This may also be known as troponin regulatory complex. The specimen is plasma. Cardiac troponins are markers for myocardial muscle damage. Qualitative tests (positive/negative results) are primarily used to rule-in or rule-out myocardial infarction. Several bedside, point-of-care type assays are available. Methods are radioimmunoassay, enzyme-linked immunosorbent assay, and immunoenzymatic assay may also be seen.

85002

85002 Bleeding time

Explanation

This test may be ordered as a bleeding time or as an Ivy bleeding time. A small, superficial wound is nicked in the patient's forearm. Essentially, the amount of time it takes for the wound to stop bleeding is recorded at bedside. The Ivy bleeding time test is one standardized method. All methods are manual or point of care. A bleeding time is a rough measure of platelet (thrombocyte) function. The test is often performed on a preoperative patient.

85004

85004 Blood count; automated differential WBC count

Explanation

This test may be ordered as a blood count with automated differential. The specimen is whole blood. Method is automated cell counter. The blood count typically includes a measurement of normal cell constituents including white blood cells or leukocytes, red blood cells, and platelets. In addition, this test includes a differential count of the white blood cells or "diff" in which the following leukocytes are differentiated and counted automatically: neutrophils or granulocytes, lymphocytes, monocytes, eosinophils, and basophils.

85007-85008

85007 Blood count; blood smear, microscopic examination with manual differential WBC count

85008 blood smear, microscopic examination without manual differential WBC count

Explanation

These tests may be ordered as a manual blood smear examination, RBC smear, peripheral blood smear, or RBC morphology without differential parameters in 85008 and with manual WBC differential in 85007. The specimen is whole blood. The method is manual testing. A blood smear is prepared and microscopically examined for the presence of normal cell constituents, including white blood cells, red blood cells, and platelets. In 85008, the white blood cell and platelet or thrombocyte counts are estimated and red cell morphology is commented on if abnormal. In 85007, a manual differential of white blood cells is included in which the following leukocytes are differentiated: neutrophils or granulocytes, lymphocytes, monocytes, eosinophils, and basophils.

85009

85009 Blood count; manual differential WBC count, buffy coat

Explanation

This test may be ordered as a buffy coat differential or as a differential WBC count, buffy coat. Specimen is whole blood. Other collection types (e.g., finger stick or heel stick) do not yield the volume of blood required for this test. Method is manual testing. The whole blood is centrifuged to concentrate the white blood cells, and a manual WBC differential is performed in which the following leukocytes are differentiated: neutrophils or granulocytes, lymphocytes, monocytes, eosinophils, and basophils. This test is usually performed when the number of WBCs or leukocytes is abnormally low and the presence of abnormal white cells (e.g., blasts or cancer cells) is suspected clinically.

85013

85013 Blood count; spun microhematocrit

Explanation

This test may be ordered as a microhematocrit, a spun microhematocrit, or a "spun crit." The specimen (whole blood) is by finger stick or heel stick in infants. The sample is placed in a tube and into a microcentrifuge device. The vials can be read manually against a chart for the volume of packed red cells or a digital reader in the centrifuge device. A spun microhematocrit only reports the volume of packed red cells. It is typically performed at sites where limited testing is available, the patient is a very difficult blood draw, or on infants.

85014

85014 Blood count; hematocrit (Hct)

Explanation

This test may be ordered as a hematocrit, Hmt, or Hct. The specimen is whole blood. Method is automated cell counter. The hematocrit or volume of packed red cells (VPRC) in the blood sample is calculated by multiplying the red blood cell count or RBC times the mean corpuscular volume or MCV.

85018

85018 Blood count; hemoglobin (Hgb)

Explanation

This test may be ordered as hemoglobin, Hgb, or hemoglobin concentration. The specimen is whole blood. Method is usually automated cell counter but a manual method is seen in labs with a limited test menu and blood bank drawing stations. Hemoglobin is an index of the oxygen-carrying capacity of the blood.

85025-85027

85025 Blood count; complete (CBC), automated (Hgb, Hct, RBC, WBC and platelet count) and automated differential WBC count

85027 complete (CBC), automated (Hgb, Hct, RBC, WBC and platelet count)

Explanation

These tests may be ordered as a complete automated blood count (CBC). The specimen is whole blood. Method is automated cell counter. These codes include the measurement of erythrocytes (red blood cells or RBC), leukocytes (white blood cells or WBC), hemoglobin, hematocrit (volume of packed red blood cells or VPRC), platelet or thrombocyte count, and indices (mean corpuscular hemoglobin or MCH, mean corpuscular hemoglobin concentration or MCHC, mean corpuscular volume or MCV, and red cell distribution width or RDW). Code 85025 includes an automated differential of the white blood cells or "diff" in which the following leukocytes are differentiated: neutrophils or granulocytes, lymphocytes, monocytes, eosinophils, and basophils. Report 85027 if the complete CBC, or automated blood count, is done without the differential WBC count.

85032

85032 Blood count; manual cell count (erythrocyte, leukocyte, or platelet) each

Explanation

This code reports a manual cell count done for red blood cells (erythrocytes), white blood cells (leukocytes), or platelets (thrombocytes), each. The specimen is whole blood. The method is manual examination and counting.

85041

85041 Blood count; red blood cell (RBC), automated

Explanation

This test may be ordered as red blood cell count or RBC. The specimen is by whole blood. Method is automated cell counter.

85044

85044 Blood count; reticulocyte, manual

Explanation

This test may be ordered as a manual reticulocyte count or as a manual "retic." The specimen is whole blood. Method is manual. A blood smear is prepared and stained with a dye that highlights the reticulum in the immature red blood cells, or the reticulocytes. The reticulocytes reported as a percentage of total red blood cells.

85045

85045 Blood count; reticulocyte, automated

Explanation

This test may be ordered as an automated reticulocyte count, an "auto retic," or a reticulocyte by flow cytometry. The specimen is whole blood. Method is automated cell counter or flow cytometer. Reticulocytes are immature red blood cells that still contain mitochondria and ribosomes. The reticulocytes are reported as a percentage of total red blood cells.

85337

85337 Thrombomodulin

Explanation

This test may be ordered as a thrombomodulin assay. The specimen is plasma. The method is usually automated coagulation instrument but may be manual. Thrombomodulin is a protein involved in activation of the clot dissolution or lysis process.

85348

85348 Coagulation time; other methods

Explanation

This test may be ordered as a clotting time. The specimen is whole blood finger stick or, in infants, heel stick. Methods vary, as the formal description implies. Point-of-care testing often involves a hand held instrument that gives some measurement of whole blood clotting time.

85396

85396 Coagulation/fibrinolysis assay, whole blood (eg, viscoelastic clot assessment), including use of any pharmacologic additive(s), as indicated, including interpretation and written report, per day

Explanation

A coagulation/fibrinolysis assay is done on whole blood to assess the viscoelastic properties of blood as it clots. Information about the kinetics of clot formation and growth and the strength and stability of the formed clot provides a more global assessment about hemostatic function as a whole dynamic process. The interaction between fibrinogen, platelets, and the protein coagulation process are measured in viscoelastic assays as clotting happens, and followed through to clot lysis. This is invaluable in surgical circumstances for patients who have been treated with anticoagulants, or are suspected of thromboembolic disease.

Relative Value Units/Medicare Edits

Non-Facility RVU	Work	PE	MP	Total
85396	0.37	0.18	0.02	0.57
Facility RVU	**Work**	**PE**	**MP**	**Total**
85396	0.37	0.18	0.02	0.57

85576

85576 Platelet, aggregation (in vitro), each agent

Explanation

This test may be ordered as a platelet aggregation study, or as an in vitro platelet aggregation study. Specimen is plasma. The method may be platelet aggregometer. Platelet function is measured by observing the amount of platelet clumping that occurs when certain chemicals are added to a solution of platelets. The test is an in vitro enactment of the platelet aggregation that occurs naturally at the site of vascular injury. The test may be used to detect von Willebrand's disease or other inherited platelet-related disorders.

85610

85610 Prothrombin time;

Explanation

This test may be ordered as a prothrombin time (PT), a prothrombin, or as simply PT. The specimen is plasma. Method is one-stage using an automated device. The prothrombin time is prolonged when deficiencies of coagulation factors II, V, VII, or X are present. More commonly, this test monitors the effectiveness of the anticoagulant drug Coumadin or warfarin, prescribed to patients who have had blood clots or myocardial infarction.

85611

85611 Prothrombin time; substitution, plasma fractions, each

Explanation

This test may be ordered as a diluted prothrombin time (PT), a prothrombin 1:1, or as plasma diluted PT. The specimen is plasma. Addition or dilution with normal plasma differentiates between a clotting factor deficiency and a circulating anticoagulant. Prolonged prothrombin times due to a clotting factor deficiency will shorten to normal with the addition of normal plasma while a prolonged prothrombin time due to a circulating anticoagulant may increase with the addition of normal plasma.

85651

85651 Sedimentation rate, erythrocyte; non-automated

Explanation

This test may be ordered as an erythrocyte sedimentation rate (ESR), a Westergren sedimentation rate, Wintrobe sedimentation rate, or simply as a "sed rate." The specimen is whole blood. This test is a non-specific screening test for a number of diseases including anemia, disorders of protein production such as multiple myeloma, other conditions that alter the size and/or shape of red cells or erythrocytes, and to screen diseases that cause an increase or decrease in the amount of protein in the plasma. Further studies are often launched by ESR results. The method is manual. A variety of procedures have been used over time to study sedimentation rate. A common one performed manually is the Westergren tube.

85652

85652 Sedimentation rate, erythrocyte; automated

Explanation

This test may be ordered as a Zeta sedimentation rate or as a Zeta sed rate. Specimen is whole blood. Method is centrifugation; this is an automated test. This test is a non-specific screening test for a number of diseases including anemia, disorders of protein production such as multiple myeloma, and other conditions that alter the size and/or shape of red cells or erythrocytes. This test may also be used to screen diseases that cause an increase or decrease in the amount of protein in the plasma or liquid portion of the blood.

85730

85730 Thromboplastin time, partial (PTT); plasma or whole blood

Explanation

This test may be ordered as a partial thromboplastin time or PTT, or as an activated partial thromboplastin time or APTT. The specimen is plasma. The method is automated coagulation instrument. The partial thromboplastin time is prolonged when deficiencies of coagulation factors VIII, IX, XI, and XII are present. This test is used to monitor the effectiveness of the anticoagulant drug heparin, which is prescribed for patients who have had blood clots or heart attacks.

85732

85732 Thromboplastin time, partial (PTT); substitution, plasma fractions, each

Explanation

This test may be ordered as a diluted partial thromboplastin time, a PTT or APTT 1:1, or as a plasma diluted PTT or APTT. The specimen is plasma. The method is automated coagulation instrument. Addition of or dilution with normal plasma differentiates between a clotting factor deficiency and a circulating anticoagulant. Prolonged partial thromboplastin times due to a clotting factor deficiency will shorten to normal with the addition of normal plasma while a prolonged PTT due to a circulating anticoagulant may increase with the addition of normal plasma.

86147

86147 Cardiolipin (phospholipid) antibody, each Ig class

Explanation

This test may also be ordered as antiphospholipid antibody or anticardiolipin antibodies (ACA). The specimen is serum. Method is enzyme-linked immunoassay (ELISA). The test may be used to classify patients with recurrent venous or arterial thrombosis, thrombocytopenia (low platelet count), recurrent fetal loss, and acquired valvular heart disease, and systemic lupus erythematosus (SLE).

86590

86590 Streptokinase, antibody

Explanation

This test is commonly ordered as ASO. The specimen is serum. The test is useful for detection of antibody to an extracellular antigenic product of group A streptococci and commonly used to detect previous exposure to group A strep. The test may be performed by latex agglutination or enzyme-linked immunosorbent assay (ELISA).

86828-86829

86828 Antibody to human leukocyte antigens (HLA), solid phase assays (eg, microspheres or beads, ELISA, flow cytometry); qualitative assessment of the presence or absence of antibody(ies) to HLA Class I and Class II HLA antigens

86829 qualitative assessment of the presence or absence of antibody(ies) to HLA Class I or Class II HLA antigens

Explanation

These tests are commonly used to predict the histocompatibility between a patient and a donor to predict and prevent graft versus host disease (GVHD) or transplanted organ rejection. Human leukocyte antigens (HLA) are a group of genes found on chromosome 6. There are two types of HLA: class I and class II. The higher number of anti-HLA antibodies the higher the chance of a reaction to donor tissue. The specimen is blood. The method is enzyme-linked immunosorbent assay (ELISA) technique and the use of fluorescent beads with HLA molecules bound to their surface, which can be used in conventional flow cytometry or in conjunction with Luminex instrumentation. Report 86828 if the presence or absence of both HLA class I and II antibodies are assessed. Report 86829 when only one HLA class antibody is qualified.

87086-87088

87086 Culture, bacterial; quantitative colony count, urine

87088 with isolation and presumptive identification of each isolate, urine

Explanation

These codes report the performance of a urine bacterial culture with a calibrated inoculating device so that a colony count accurately correlates with the number of organisms in the urine. In 87088, isolation and presumptive identification of bacteria recovered from the sample is done by means of identifying colony morphology, subculturing organisms to selective media and the performance of a gram stain or other simple test to identify bacteria to the genus level. There are several automated systems that detect the presence of bacteria using colorimetric, radiometric, or spectrophotometric means. In 87086, quantified colony count numbers within the urine sample are measured.

87181

87181 Susceptibility studies, antimicrobial agent; agar dilution method, per agent (eg, antibiotic gradient strip)

Explanation

A susceptibility study is performed to determine the effectiveness of an antimicrobial agent against microorganisms. This test is performed to assist the treating provider in determining which drug will be the most effective for treatment of an infection. The methodology is agar dilution. Varying concentrations of an antimicrobial agent are introduced into agar, a culture medium used to grow microorganisms. This introduction is performed using an instrument such as an antibiotic gradient strip. The test result is expressed as the minimum inhibitory concentration (MIC), which is the lowest concentration of the antimicrobial agent needed to inhibit growth of an organism. This code is reported once per agent.

87271

87271 Infectious agent antigen detection by immunofluorescent technique; Cytomegalovirus, direct fluorescent antibody (DFA)

Explanation

A cytomegalovirus is detected by direct fluorescent antibody (DFA) staining technique. The presence of the infectious agent microorganism is detected indirectly when the fluorescent reaction of the dye is seen under a special microscope. The cytomegalovirus is isolated in cell culture for the test. Specimens include throat swabs, CSF, and blood samples. A cytomegalovirus is any virus in the Betaherpesvirinae subfamily.

90380-90381

90380 Respiratory syncytial virus, monoclonal antibody, seasonal dose; 0.5 mL dosage, for intramuscular use

90381 Respiratory syncytial virus, monoclonal antibody, seasonal dose; 1 mL dosage, for intramuscular use

Explanation

These codes report a monoclonal antibody injection prepared for seasonal respiratory syncytial virus (RSV). The monoclonal antibodies (IgG) target the RSV virus, inhibiting its replication and reducing the severity and occurrence of RSV infections. It is intended for intramuscular use in neonates and infants younger than 8 months of age who are in their first RSV season and certain at-risk infants and children 8 through 19 months of age before their second RSV season. Report 90380 for administration of the 0.5 mL dosage; 90381 for administration of the 1 mL dosage. These codes report the monoclonal antibody product only and should be reported with the appropriate administration code.

90471-90472

90471 Immunization administration (includes percutaneous, intradermal, subcutaneous, or intramuscular injections); 1 vaccine (single or combination vaccine/toxoid)

\+ **90472** each additional vaccine (single or combination vaccine/toxoid) (List separately in addition to code for primary procedure)

Explanation

A physician, nurse, or medical assistant administers an injectable (percutaneous, intradermal, subcutaneous, or intramuscular) immunization to the patient. It may be a single vaccine or a combination vaccine/toxoid in one immunization administration (e.g., diphtheria, pertussis, and tetanus toxoids are in a single DPT immunization). Report 90471 for one vaccine and 90472 for each additional vaccine (single or combination vaccine/toxoid).

Relative Value Units/Medicare Edits

Non-Facility RVU	Work	PE	MP	Total
90471	0.17	0.44	0.01	0.62
90472	0.15	0.28	0.01	0.44
Facility RVU	**Work**	**PE**	**MP**	**Total**
90471	0.17	0.44	0.01	0.62
90472	0.15	0.28	0.01	0.44

[90480]

90480 Immunization administration by intramuscular injection of severe acute respiratory syndrome coronavirus 2 (SARS-CoV-2) (coronavirus disease [COVID-19]) vaccine, single dose

Explanation

This code reports the immunization administration of a single dose vaccine against severe acute respiratory syndrome coronavirus 2, also known as SARS-CoV-2, coronavirus disease, or COVID-19. A vaccine produces active immunization by inducing the immune system to build its own antibodies against specific microorganisms/viruses. The body retains memory of the antibody production pattern for long-term protection. This code includes vaccine risk/benefit counseling, when performed, and can be reported for a patient of any age. This code reports the administration only and should be reported with the appropriate product code.

[91304]

91304 Severe acute respiratory syndrome coronavirus 2 (SARS-CoV-2) (coronavirus disease [COVID-19]) vaccine, recombinant spike protein nanoparticle, saponin-based adjuvant, 5 mcg/0.5 mL dosage, for intramuscular use

Explanation

This code reports a recombinant spike protein nanoparticle vaccine against severe acute respiratory syndrome coronavirus 2, also known as SARS-CoV-2, coronavirus disease, or COVID-19. A vaccine produces active immunization by inducing the immune system to build its own antibodies against specific microorganisms/viruses. The body retains memory of the antibody production pattern for long-term protection. This vaccine is intended for intramuscular use in patients ages 12 years and older. It contains a saponin-based adjuvant, a plant glycoside that is designed to enhance the effectiveness of the vaccine. This code is specific to the Novavax 5 mcg/0.5 mL dosage vaccine. This code reports the vaccine product only and should be reported with the appropriate administration code.

[91318]

91318 Severe acute respiratory syndrome coronavirus 2 (SARS-CoV-2) (coronavirus disease [COVID-19]) vaccine, mRNA-LNP, spike protein, 3 mcg/0.3 mL dosage, tris-sucrose formulation, for intramuscular use

Explanation

This code reports a spike protein vaccine against severe acute respiratory syndrome coronavirus 2, also known as SARS-CoV-2, coronavirus disease, or COVID-19. A vaccine produces active immunization by inducing the immune system to build its own antibodies against specific microorganisms/viruses. The body retains memory of the antibody production pattern for long-term protection. Based on messenger RNA (mRNA) that utilizes a lipid nanoparticle (LNP) as a delivery platform, this vaccine is intended for intramuscular use in patients ages 6 months through 4 years. This code is specific to the Pfizer-BioNTech 3 mcg/0.3 mL dosage vaccine that is based on a tris-sucrose buffer. This code reports the vaccine product only and should be reported with the appropriate administration code.

[91319]

91319 Severe acute respiratory syndrome coronavirus 2 (SARS-CoV-2) (coronavirus disease [COVID-19]) vaccine, mRNA-LNP, spike protein, 10 mcg/0.3 mL dosage, tris-sucrose formulation, for intramuscular use

Explanation

This code reports a spike protein vaccine against severe acute respiratory syndrome coronavirus 2, also known as SARS-CoV-2, coronavirus disease, or COVID-19. A vaccine produces active immunization by inducing the immune system to build its own antibodies against specific microorganisms/viruses. The body retains memory of the antibody production pattern for long-term protection. Based on messenger RNA (mRNA) that utilizes a lipid nanoparticle (LNP) as a delivery platform, this vaccine is intended for intramuscular use in patients ages 5 years through 11 years. This code is specific to the Pfizer-BioNTech 10 mcg/0.3 mL dosage vaccine that is based on a tris-sucrose buffer. This code reports the vaccine product only and should be reported with the appropriate administration code.

[91320]

91320 Severe acute respiratory syndrome coronavirus 2 (SARS-CoV-2) (coronavirus disease [COVID-19]) vaccine, mRNA-LNP, spike protein, 30 mcg/0.3 mL dosage, tris-sucrose formulation, for intramuscular use

Explanation

This code reports a spike protein vaccine against severe acute respiratory syndrome coronavirus 2, also known as SARS-CoV-2, coronavirus disease, or COVID-19. A vaccine produces active immunization by inducing the immune system to build its own antibodies against specific microorganisms/viruses. The body retains memory of the antibody production pattern for long-term protection. Based on messenger RNA (mRNA) that utilizes a lipid nanoparticle (LNP) as a delivery platform, this vaccine is intended for intramuscular use in patients ages 12 years and older. This code is specific to the Pfizer-BioNTech 30 mcg/0.3 mL dosage vaccine that is based on a tris-sucrose buffer. This code reports the vaccine product only and should be reported with the appropriate administration code.

[91321]

91321 Severe acute respiratory syndrome coronavirus 2 (SARS-CoV-2) (coronavirus disease [COVID-19]) vaccine, mRNA-LNP, 25 mcg/0.25 mL dosage, for intramuscular use

Explanation

This code reports a vaccine against severe acute respiratory syndrome coronavirus 2, also known as SARS-CoV-2, coronavirus disease, or COVID-19. A vaccine produces active immunization by inducing the immune system to build its own antibodies against specific microorganisms/viruses. The body retains memory of the antibody production pattern for long-term protection. Based on messenger RNA (mRNA) that utilizes a lipid nanoparticle (LNP) as a delivery platform, this vaccine is intended for intramuscular use in patients ages 6 months through 11 years. This code is specific to the Moderna 25 mcg/0.25 mL dosage vaccine. This code reports the vaccine product only and should be reported with the appropriate administration code.

[91322]

91322 Severe acute respiratory syndrome coronavirus 2 (SARS-CoV-2) (coronavirus disease [COVID-19]) vaccine, mRNA-LNP, 50 mcg/0.5 mL dosage, for intramuscular use

Explanation

This code reports a vaccine against severe acute respiratory syndrome coronavirus 2, also known as SARS-CoV-2, coronavirus disease, or COVID-19. A vaccine produces active immunization by inducing the immune system to build its own antibodies against specific microorganisms/viruses. The body retains memory of the antibody production pattern for long-term protection. Based on messenger RNA (mRNA) that utilizes a lipid nanoparticle (LNP) as a delivery platform, this vaccine is intended for intramuscular use in patients ages 12 years and older. This code is specific to the Moderna 50 mcg/0.5 mL dosage vaccine. This code reports the vaccine product only and should be reported with the appropriate administration code.

90657-90658

90657 Influenza virus vaccine, trivalent (IIV3), split virus, 0.25 mL dosage, for intramuscular use

90658 Influenza virus vaccine, trivalent (IIV3), split virus, 0.5 mL dosage, for intramuscular use

Explanation

These codes report the supply of the vaccine only. A vaccine produces active immunization by inducing the immune system to build its own antibodies against specific microorganisms/viruses. The body retains memory of the antibody production pattern for long-term protection. A split virus suspension of three (two influenza A and one influenza B) (IIV3) of the most prevalent strains of influenza is prepared for intramuscular use. Report 90657 for a 0.25 mL dose and 90658 for a 0.5 mL dose. The vaccine induces active immunity to the highly contagious infection of the respiratory tract caused by a myxovirus and transmitted by airborne droplet infection. Report these codes with the appropriate administration code.

[90674]

90674 Influenza virus vaccine, quadrivalent (ccIIV4), derived from cell cultures, subunit, preservative and antibiotic free, 0.5 mL dosage, for intramuscular use

Explanation

A vaccine produces active immunization by inducing the immune system to build its own antibodies against specific microorganisms/viruses. The body retains memory of the antibody production pattern for long-term protection. A suspension of the prevalent strain of influenza virus that has been derived from cell cultures is prepared for intramuscular use. Cell culture-derived vaccines are those in which the virus is grown in mammalian cells rather than egg-derived. The vaccine provides active immunity to the highly contagious infection of the respiratory tract caused by a myxovirus and transmitted by airborne droplet infection. This vaccine (ccIIV4) is preservative and antibiotic-free. This code reports a subunit in a .50 mL dose and should be reported with the appropriate administration code.

90678-90679

90678 Respiratory syncytial virus vaccine, preF, subunit, bivalent, for intramuscular use

90679 Respiratory syncytial virus vaccine, preF, recombinant, subunit, adjuvanted, for intramuscular use

Explanation

Code 90678 reports a nonadjuvanted vaccine for immunization against respiratory syncytial virus (RSV). A vaccine produces active immunization by inducing the immune system to build its own antibodies against specific microorganisms/viruses. The body retains memory of the antibody production pattern for long-term protection. This single-dose bivalent RSV prefusion (preF) vaccine, made up of two proteins selected to optimize protection against RSV A and B strains, is intended for intramuscular use in adults ages 60 years and older. In addition, it is approved for adults in their second or third trimester of pregnancy; antibodies to the RSV antigens are transferred placentally to provide passive immunization that protects infants from birth through 6 months of age. Report 90679 for a single-dose preF recombinant vaccine that includes an adjuvant to strengthen the immune response. The inclusion of an adjuvant enhances the vaccine's effectiveness, ensuring a robust and sustained immune reaction following administration. This vaccine, also intended for intramuscular use, is approved for individuals 60 years of age and older. These codes report the vaccine product only and should be reported with the appropriate administration code.

[90683]

90683 Respiratory syncytial virus vaccine, mRNA lipid nanoparticles, for intramuscular use

Explanation

This code reports a vaccine based on messenger RNA (mRNA) technology, enclosed within lipid nanoparticles (LNP), to combat respiratory syncytial virus (RSV), a common respiratory pathogen. A vaccine produces active immunization by inducing the immune system to build its own antibodies against specific microorganisms/viruses. The body retains memory of the antibody production pattern for long-term protection. This vaccine instructs the body's cells to produce prefusion F glycoprotein, which triggers antibodies to recognize and neutralize RSV. It is intended for intramuscular use in patients 60 years of age and older. This code reports the vaccine product only and should be reported with the appropriate administration code.

90732

90732 Pneumococcal polysaccharide vaccine, 23-valent (PPSV23), adult or immunosuppressed patient dosage, when administered to individuals 2 years or older, for subcutaneous or intramuscular use

Explanation

This code reports supply of a vaccine only. A vaccine produces active immunization by inducing the immune system to build its own antibodies against specific microorganisms/viruses. The body retains memory of these antibody production patterns for long-term protection. This code reports a pneumococcal polysaccharide vaccine, 23-valent (PPSV23), adult or immunosuppressed patient dosage, for subcutaneous or intramuscular administration to patients 2 years of age or older. Report this code with the appropriate administration code.

93000-93010

93000 Electrocardiogram, routine ECG with at least 12 leads; with interpretation and report

93005 tracing only, without interpretation and report

93010 interpretation and report only

Explanation

Multiple electrodes are placed on a patient's chest to record the electrical activity of the heart. A physician interprets the findings. Report 93000 for the combined technical and professional components of an ECG; 93005 for the technical component only; and 93010 for the professional component only.

Relative Value Units/Medicare Edits

Non-Facility RVU	Work	PE	MP	Total
93000	0.17	0.24	0.02	0.43
93005	0.0	0.18	0.01	0.19
93010	0.17	0.06	0.01	0.24
Facility RVU	**Work**	**PE**	**MP**	**Total**
93000	0.17	0.24	0.02	0.43
93005	0.0	0.18	0.01	0.19
93010	0.17	0.06	0.01	0.24

93015-93018

93015 Cardiovascular stress test using maximal or submaximal treadmill or bicycle exercise, continuous electrocardiographic monitoring, and/or pharmacological stress; with supervision, interpretation and report

93016 supervision only, without interpretation and report

93017 tracing only, without interpretation and report

93018 interpretation and report only

Explanation

A continuous recording of electrical activity of the heart is acquired by an assistant supervised by a qualified health care professional while the patient is exercising on a treadmill or bicycle and/or given medicines. The stress on the heart during the test is monitored. Code 93015 includes the test, supervision, and interpretation of the report; 93016 includes only the supervision of the test; 93017 includes performing the test only; and 93018 is reported for the interpretation of a previously performed test.

Relative Value Units/Medicare Edits

Non-Facility RVU	Work	PE	MP	Total
93015	0.75	1.37	0.04	2.16
93016	0.45	0.16	0.01	0.62
93017	0.0	1.11	0.02	1.13
93018	0.3	0.1	0.01	0.41
Facility RVU	**Work**	**PE**	**MP**	**Total**
93015	0.75	1.37	0.04	2.16
93016	0.45	0.16	0.01	0.62
93017	0.0	1.11	0.02	1.13
93018	0.3	0.1	0.01	0.41

93024

93024 Ergonovine provocation test

Explanation

The purpose of the study is to evaluate for coronary artery spasm. If ergonovine is not available, certain other ergot medications may be infused for the same purpose. Following baseline coronary angiography (coded elsewhere), the physician infuses gradually escalating doses of ergonovine into a peripheral vein, while monitoring for chest discomfort and electrocardiographic changes. Repeat angiography is performed during ergonovine infusion to assess the size of the coronary lumen. If the patient develops symptomatic coronary spasm, the physician may directly infuse vasodilating medications through the intracoronary catheter to relieve the problem.

Relative Value Units/Medicare Edits

Non-Facility RVU	Work	PE	MP	Total
93024	1.17	2.11	0.07	3.35
Facility RVU	**Work**	**PE**	**MP**	**Total**
93024	1.17	2.11	0.07	3.35

93025

93025 Microvolt T-wave alternans for assessment of ventricular arrhythmias

Explanation

T-Wave Alternans testing is an electrocardiographic method of measuring the alternating electrical amplitude from beat to beat on an electrocardiogram and is used as a method of evaluating ventricular arrhythmia risk. Microvolt T-wave alternans can be measured during exercise or pharmacologic stress, or during cardiac pacing, using a spectral analytic method with equipment that is able to detect as little as one microvolt of T-wave alternans. In electrode placement for a 12-lead ECG, the health care provider positions the leads on the wrists and ankles or shoulders and groins. Left leg electrodes are placed below the heart (but not on the chest), preferably below the umbilicus. The sensing electrodes look at the inferior surface of the heart, the left or lateral side of the heart, and at the right side of the heart.

Relative Value Units/Medicare Edits

Non-Facility RVU	Work	PE	MP	Total
93025	0.75	2.96	0.04	3.75
Facility RVU	**Work**	**PE**	**MP**	**Total**
93025	0.75	2.96	0.04	3.75

93040-93042

93040 Rhythm ECG, 1-3 leads; with interpretation and report
93041 tracing only without interpretation and report
93042 interpretation and report only

Explanation

An assistant records the electrical activity of the heart by placing one to three electrodes on a patient's chest in a predetermined pattern. Report 93040 when the physician interprets the report. Report 93041 when only the tracing is performed. Report 93042 when a physician interprets a previously acquired report.

Relative Value Units/Medicare Edits

Non-Facility RVU	Work	PE	MP	Total
93040	0.15	0.22	0.02	0.39
93041	0.0	0.18	0.01	0.19
93042	0.15	0.04	0.01	0.2
Facility RVU	**Work**	**PE**	**MP**	**Total**
93040	0.15	0.22	0.02	0.39
93041	0.0	0.18	0.01	0.19
93042	0.15	0.04	0.01	0.2

93050

93050 Arterial pressure waveform analysis for assessment of central arterial pressures, includes obtaining waveform(s), digitization and application of nonlinear mathematical transformations to determine central arterial pressures and augmentation index, with interpretation and report, upper extremity artery, non-invasive

Explanation

Blood pressure pulse wave analysis measures the blood pressure at the heart rather than in the arm as with traditional blood pressure cuffs, as well as providing information regarding the interaction of the heart and blood vessels. The brachial blood pressure is obtained to calibrate the radial pressure waveform. The pressure sensor wand (tonometer) is placed on the wrist where the strongest pulse is present. The pressure waveforms are transmitted and displayed on a data collection screen on a computer. After there is at least 10 seconds of data displayed, the data is captured. The data reflects average central aortic waveform, pressure measurements, and central parameters, as well as reference ranges. The augmentation index can be acquired by direct measurement or acquired pressure waveforms. This index is a percentage of pressure from systolic rise over pressure waves. The nonlinear mathematical transformation can be utilized to differentiate between active and rest blood pressure coinciding with the systolic and diastolic process. This code includes the digitization of the data, as well as the use of nonlinear mathematical transformation to determine pressure, augmentation index, and the provider interpretation and report.

Relative Value Units/Medicare Edits

Non-Facility RVU	Work	PE	MP	Total
93050	0.17	0.29	0.02	0.48
Facility RVU	**Work**	**PE**	**MP**	**Total**
93050	0.17	0.29	0.02	0.48

93224-93227

93224 External electrocardiographic recording up to 48 hours by continuous rhythm recording and storage; includes recording, scanning analysis with report, review and interpretation by a physician or other qualified health care professional
93225 recording (includes connection, recording, and disconnection)
93226 scanning analysis with report
93227 review and interpretation by a physician or other qualified health care professional

Explanation

The purpose of this study is to evaluate the patient's ambient heart rhythm during a full daily cycle. The physician or other qualified health care professional instructs the patient in the use of an external electrocardiographic (ECG) recorder, also known as a Holter monitor. A technician places ECG leads on the patient's chest, and the patient wears the recorder for up to 48 hours. During this time, there is continuous rhythm recording and storage. The patient returns the device, and the recorded heart rhythm is played back into digital format by a technician. The technician uses a scanning methodology to classify different ECG waveforms and to generate a report. The generated report describes the overall rhythm and significant arrhythmias. Code 93224 reports the recording, scanning analysis with report, provider review of the data, and the provision of a final interpretation in a report. Code 93225 reports the recording only, which includes connection, recording of data, and disconnection. Code 93226 reports only the scanning analysis with report. Code 93227 reports only the provider review and interpretation.

Relative Value Units/Medicare Edits

Non-Facility RVU	Work	PE	MP	Total
93224	0.39	1.74	0.03	2.16
93225	0.0	0.54	0.01	0.55
93226	0.0	1.06	0.01	1.07
93227	0.39	0.14	0.01	0.54
Facility RVU	**Work**	**PE**	**MP**	**Total**
93224	0.39	1.74	0.03	2.16
93225	0.0	0.54	0.01	0.55
93226	0.0	1.06	0.01	1.07
93227	0.39	0.14	0.01	0.54

[93241, 93242, 93243, 93244]

93241 External electrocardiographic recording for more than 48 hours up to 7 days by continuous rhythm recording and storage; includes recording, scanning analysis with report, review and interpretation
93242 External electrocardiographic recording for more than 48 hours up to 7 days by continuous rhythm recording and storage; recording (includes connection and initial recording)
93243 External electrocardiographic recording for more than 48 hours up to 7 days by continuous rhythm recording and storage; scanning analysis with report
93244 External electrocardiographic recording for more than 48 hours up to 7 days by continuous rhythm recording and storage; review and interpretation

Explanation

Long-term external electrocardiographic (ECG) recording is a diagnostic procedure that provides continuous rhythm recording of the patient's heart while the patient is engaged in the activities of daily living. The purpose of the study is to evaluate the patient's ambient heart rhythm during a full daily cycle. Rhythm disturbances and waveform abnormalities are detected; information is provided regarding the frequency of these disturbances. The physician or other qualified health care provider instructs the patient in the use of the external ECG recorder. A technician places ECG leads on the patient's chest, and the patient wears the recorder for 48 hours up to seven days. During this time there is continuous rhythm recording and storage. The patient returns the device and the recorded heart rhythm is converted into digital format by a technician. The technician uses a scanning methodology to classify different ECG waveforms and to generate a report. The generated report describes the overall rhythm and significant arrhythmias. Code 93241 reports the recording, scanning analysis with report, provider review of the data, and the provision of a final interpretation in a report. Code 93242 reports the recording only, which includes the connection and initial recording of data. Code 93243 reports only the scanning analysis with report. Code 93244 reports only the provider review and interpretation.

Relative Value Units/Medicare Edits

Non-Facility RVU	Work	PE	MP	Total
93241	0.5	7.21	0.04	7.75
93242	0.0	0.35	0.01	0.36
93243	0.0	6.7	0.01	6.71
93244	0.5	0.16	0.02	0.68
Facility RVU	**Work**	**PE**	**MP**	**Total**
93241	0.5	7.21	0.04	7.75
93242	0.0	0.35	0.01	0.36
93243	0.0	6.7	0.01	6.71
93244	0.5	0.16	0.02	0.68

[93245, 93246, 93247, 93248]

93245 External electrocardiographic recording for more than 7 days up to 15 days by continuous rhythm recording and storage; includes recording, scanning analysis with report, review and interpretation

93246 External electrocardiographic recording for more than 7 days up to 15 days by continuous rhythm recording and storage; recording (includes connection and initial recording)

93247 External electrocardiographic recording for more than 7 days up to 15 days by continuous rhythm recording and storage; scanning analysis with report

93248 External electrocardiographic recording for more than 7 days up to 15 days by continuous rhythm recording and storage; review and interpretation

Explanation

Long-term external electrocardiographic (ECG) recording is a diagnostic procedure that provides continuous rhythm recording of the patient's heart while the patient is engaged in the activities of daily living. The purpose of the study is to evaluate the patient's ambient heart rhythm during a full daily cycle. Rhythm disturbances and waveform abnormalities are detected; information is provided regarding the frequency of these disturbances. The physician or other qualified health care provider instructs the patient in the use of the external ECG recorder. A technician places ECG leads on the patient's chest, and the patient wears the recorder for more than seven days up to 15 days. During this time there is continuous rhythm recording and storage. The patient returns the device and the recorded heart rhythm is converted into digital format by a technician. The technician uses a scanning methodology to classify different ECG waveforms and to generate a report. The generated report describes the overall rhythm and significant arrhythmias. Code 93245 reports the recording, scanning analysis with report, provider review of the data, and the provision of a final interpretation in a report. Code 93246 reports the recording only, which includes the connection and initial recording of data. Code 93247 reports only the scanning analysis with report. Code 93248 reports only the provider review and interpretation.

Relative Value Units/Medicare Edits

Non-Facility RVU	Work	PE	MP	Total
93245	0.55	7.56	0.04	8.15
93246	0.0	0.35	0.01	0.36
93247	0.0	7.03	0.01	7.04
93248	0.55	0.18	0.02	0.75
Facility RVU	**Work**	**PE**	**MP**	**Total**
93245	0.55	7.56	0.04	8.15
93246	0.0	0.35	0.01	0.36
93247	0.0	7.03	0.01	7.04
93248	0.55	0.18	0.02	0.75

93228-93229

★93228 External mobile cardiovascular telemetry with electrocardiographic recording, concurrent computerized real time data analysis and greater than 24 hours of accessible ECG data storage (retrievable with query) with ECG triggered and patient selected events transmitted to a remote attended surveillance center for up to 30 days; review and interpretation with report by a physician or other qualified health care professional

★93229 technical support for connection and patient instructions for use, attended surveillance, analysis and transmission of daily and emergent data reports as prescribed by a physician or other qualified health care professional

Explanation

Mobile cardiovascular telemetry (MCT) uses external electrodes placed on the patient's body to continuously record electrocardiographic rhythm. Data segments are transmitted to a remote surveillance location by phone signal (cellular or landline); this is accomplished automatically and does not require patient intervention. Selected rhythm segments may be triggered for transmission automatically by rapid and slow heart rates or by the patient during a symptomatic episode. Data are analyzed continuously in real time. A remote technician responds to the alerts from the external device, reviewing the data and notifying the physician or other qualified health care professional depending on the stipulated criteria. Report 93228 for provider review and interpretation with report and 93229 for technical support, which includes connection, instructions to the patient for use, attended surveillance, analysis, and transmission of daily and emergent data reports per provider protocol. These codes may be reported only once per 30-day period.

Relative Value Units/Medicare Edits

Non-Facility RVU	Work	PE	MP	Total
93228	0.48	0.23	0.03	0.74
93229	0.0	24.33	0.09	24.42
Facility RVU	**Work**	**PE**	**MP**	**Total**
93228	0.48	0.23	0.03	0.74
93229	0.0	24.33	0.09	24.42

93268-93272

★93268 External patient and, when performed, auto activated electrocardiographic rhythm derived event recording with symptom-related memory loop with remote download capability up to 30 days, 24-hour attended monitoring; includes transmission, review and interpretation by a physician or other qualified health care professional

★93270 recording (includes connection, recording, and disconnection)

★93271 transmission and analysis

★93272 review and interpretation by a physician or other qualified health care professional

Explanation

The purpose of this study is to evaluate the patient's ambient heart rhythm during symptoms. The physician or other qualified health care professional instructs the patient in the use of an external rhythm monitor. A technician places ECG leads on the patient's chest, and the monitor uses a symptom-related memory loop mechanism with remote download capability up to 30 days to record the patient's rhythm. During symptoms, the patient activates the monitor by pressing a button. The resulting recording includes ECG activity prior to and during symptoms. The patient uses the device to transmit the recording over the telephone line, allowing a rhythm printout to be generated. The provider reviews and interprets this rhythm strip. Code 93268 reports transmission and provider review and interpretation. Code 93270 reports the recording only (including connection, recording, and disconnection). Code 93271 reports transmission download and analysis. Code 93272 reports only the provider review and interpretation.

Relative Value Units/Medicare Edits

Non-Facility RVU	Work	PE	MP	Total
93268	0.52	4.69	0.04	5.25
93270	0.0	0.24	0.01	0.25
93271	0.0	4.28	0.01	4.29
93272	0.52	0.17	0.02	0.71
Facility RVU	**Work**	**PE**	**MP**	**Total**
93268	0.52	4.69	0.04	5.25
93270	0.0	0.24	0.01	0.25
93271	0.0	4.28	0.01	4.29
93272	0.52	0.17	0.02	0.71

93278

93278 Signal-averaged electrocardiography (SAECG), with or without ECG

Explanation

Electrodes placed on a patient's chest record the heart's electrical activity. This technique uses signal-averaged electrocardiography (SAECG) and may include a standard electrocardiogram.

Relative Value Units/Medicare Edits

Non-Facility RVU	Work	PE	MP	Total
93278	0.25	0.68	0.02	0.95
Facility RVU	**Work**	**PE**	**MP**	**Total**
93278	0.25	0.68	0.02	0.95

[93264]

93264 Remote monitoring of a wireless pulmonary artery pressure sensor for up to 30 days, including at least weekly downloads of pulmonary artery pressure recordings, interpretation(s), trend analysis, and report(s) by a physician or other qualified health care professional

Explanation

A pulmonary pressure monitoring system, a device comprised of a battery-free sensor such as the CardioMEMS™, permits ongoing monitoring and measurement of a patient's heartrate as well as systolic, diastolic, and mean pressures in a patient diagnosed with non-rhythm related cardiac conditions (i.e., heart failure). Pulmonary arterial pressure (PAP) readings transmitted from an internally implanted sensor to a wireless electronic unit are subsequently transmitted to an internet-based file server or monitored by a surveillance technician with results sent to an online portal that can be accessed by the patient's treating health care provider. Through accurate monitoring of patients diagnosed with heart failure (HF) for exacerbations, it is possible to minimize the need for additional hospitalizations and the associated complications and allow for early pharmacological intervention.

Relative Value Units/Medicare Edits

Non-Facility RVU	Work	PE	MP	Total
93264	0.7	0.76	0.08	1.54
Facility RVU	**Work**	**PE**	**MP**	**Total**
93264	0.7	0.27	0.08	1.05

93279-93281

93279 Programming device evaluation (in person) with iterative adjustment of the implantable device to test the function of the device and select optimal permanent programmed values with analysis, review and report by a physician or other qualified health care professional; single lead pacemaker system or leadless pacemaker system in one cardiac chamber

93280 dual lead pacemaker system

93281 multiple lead pacemaker system

Explanation

A programming device evaluation is performed in person in order to test the device's function and select the most favorable permanent programmed values. Patients with previously implanted pacemakers require periodic programming device evaluations. This diagnostic procedure includes a face-to-face assessment of all device functions. Components that must be evaluated in order to assign a code from this range include the battery, leads, capture and sensing function, heart rhythm, and programmed parameters. Stored and measured data regarding these components are retrieved using an office, hospital, or emergency room instrument. This information is assessed to discern battery voltage, lead impedance, and settings for rhythm treatment and tachycardia detection, as well as to determine the pacemaker's current programming. If necessary, the sensing value and rate response, upper and lower heart rates, AV intervals, pacing voltage and pulse duration, and diagnostics are adjusted. These codes include physician or other qualified health care professional review, interpretation, and report, and are assigned per procedure. Report 93279 for evaluation of a single-lead pacemaker or leadless system (one in which there is pacing and sensing function in only one chamber of the heart). Report 93280 for evaluation of a dual-lead device (one with pacing and sensing function in only two chambers). Report 93281 for evaluation of a multiple-lead device (one with pacing and sensing function in three or more chambers).

Relative Value Units/Medicare Edits

Non-Facility RVU	Work	PE	MP	Total
93279	0.65	1.33	0.03	2.01
93280	0.77	1.55	0.03	2.35
93281	0.85	1.61	0.04	2.5
Facility RVU	**Work**	**PE**	**MP**	**Total**
93279	0.65	1.33	0.03	2.01
93280	0.77	1.55	0.03	2.35
93281	0.85	1.61	0.04	2.5

93282-93284

93282 Programming device evaluation (in person) with iterative adjustment of the implantable device to test the function of the device and select optimal permanent programmed values with analysis, review and report by a physician or other qualified health care professional; single lead transvenous implantable defibrillator system

93283 dual lead transvenous implantable defibrillator system

93284 multiple lead transvenous implantable defibrillator system

Explanation

A programming device evaluation is performed in person in order to test the device's function and select the most favorable permanent programmed values. Patients with transvenous implantable defibrillator systems require periodic programming device evaluations. This diagnostic procedure includes a face-to-face assessment of all device functions. Components that must be evaluated in order to assign a code from this range include the battery, leads, programmed parameters, presence or absence of therapy for ventricular tachyarrhythmias, and heart rhythm. Stored and measured data regarding these components are retrieved using an office, hospital, or emergency room instrument. This information is assessed to discern battery voltage, lead impedance, and settings for rhythm treatment and tachycardia detection, as well as to determine the defibrillator's current programming. If necessary, the sensing value and sensor rate response, upper and lower heart rates, AV intervals, pacing voltage and pulse duration, and diagnostics are adjusted. Ventricular tachycardia detection and therapies may also be altered. These codes include physician or other qualified health care professional review, interpretation, and report, and are assigned per procedure. Report 93282 for evaluation of a single-lead system (one in which there is pacing and sensing function in only one chamber of the heart). Report 93283 for evaluation of a dual-lead device (one with pacing and sensing function in only two chambers). Report 93284 for evaluation of a multiple-lead device (one with pacing and sensing function in three or more chambers).

Relative Value Units/Medicare Edits

Non-Facility RVU	Work	PE	MP	Total
93282	0.85	1.48	0.04	2.37
93283	1.15	1.71	0.05	2.91
93284	1.25	1.84	0.05	3.14
Facility RVU	**Work**	**PE**	**MP**	**Total**
93282	0.85	1.48	0.04	2.37
93283	1.15	1.71	0.05	2.91
93284	1.25	1.84	0.05	3.14

[93260]

93260 Programming device evaluation (in person) with iterative adjustment of the implantable device to test the function of the device and select optimal permanent programmed values with analysis, review and report by a physician or other qualified health care professional; implantable subcutaneous lead defibrillator system

Explanation

A programming device evaluation is performed in person in order to test the device's function and select the most favorable permanent programmed values. Patients with previously placed subcutaneous implantable defibrillator systems require periodic programming device evaluations. This diagnostic procedure includes a face-to-face assessment of all device functions, including analysis, review, and report by a physician or other qualified health care professional. Components that must be evaluated in order to assign a code from this range include the battery, leads, capture and sensing function, heart rhythm, and programmed parameters. Stored and measured data regarding these components are retrieved using an office, hospital, or emergency room instrument. This information is assessed to discern battery voltage, lead impedance, and settings, as well as to determine the system's current programming. If necessary, the parameters are reprogrammed.

Relative Value Units/Medicare Edits

Non-Facility RVU	Work	PE	MP	Total
93260	0.85	1.37	0.04	2.26
Facility RVU	**Work**	**PE**	**MP**	**Total**
93260	0.85	1.37	0.04	2.26

93285

93285 Programming device evaluation (in person) with iterative adjustment of the implantable device to test the function of the device and select optimal permanent programmed values with analysis, review and report by a physician or other qualified health care professional; subcutaneous cardiac rhythm monitor system

Explanation

A programming device evaluation is performed in person in order to test the device's function and select the most favorable permanent programmed values. Patients with previously placed subcutaneous cardiac rhythm monitor systems require periodic programming device evaluations. This diagnostic procedure includes a face-to-face assessment of all device functions. Components that must be evaluated include heartrate and rhythm during recorded episodes (patient-initiated and device algorithm detected events), as well as programmed parameters. Stored and measured data are retrieved using an office, hospital, or emergency room instrument. This information is assessed to discern current programming and to evaluate specific aspects of the device's function. If necessary, the bradycardia and tachycardia detection criteria are adjusted. This code includes physician or other qualified health care professional review, interpretation, and report, and is assigned per procedure.

Relative Value Units/Medicare Edits

Non-Facility RVU	Work	PE	MP	Total
93285	0.52	1.24	0.03	1.79
Facility RVU	**Work**	**PE**	**MP**	**Total**
93285	0.52	1.24	0.03	1.79

93286-93287

93286 Peri-procedural device evaluation (in person) and programming of device system parameters before or after a surgery, procedure, or test with analysis, review and report by a physician or other qualified health care professional; single, dual, or multiple lead pacemaker system, or leadless pacemaker system

93287 single, dual, or multiple lead implantable defibrillator system

Explanation

A programming device evaluation is performed in person in order to test the device's function and select the most favorable permanent programmed values. Patients with a previously implanted pacemaker or defibrillator systems may require adjustment of the device to patient-specific settings prior to a surgery, test, or procedure. The device system data is interrogated to evaluate the battery, leads, and sensors, as well as the stored patient and system measurements. If necessary, the device is programmed to settings appropriate for the surgery, test, or procedure. A postprocedure evaluation and programming may also be performed, with adjustments as required. Report 93286 for evaluation of a single-, dual-, or multiple-lead implantable pacemaker system or leadless pacemaker system. Report 93287 for evaluation of a single-, dual-, or multiple-lead implantable defibrillator system. Both codes include physician or other qualified health care professional analysis, review, and report.

Relative Value Units/Medicare Edits

Non-Facility RVU	Work	PE	MP	Total
93286	0.3	1.03	0.02	1.35
93287	0.45	1.09	0.02	1.56
Facility RVU	**Work**	**PE**	**MP**	**Total**
93286	0.3	1.03	0.02	1.35
93287	0.45	1.09	0.02	1.56

93288-93292 [93261]

93288 Interrogation device evaluation (in person) with analysis, review and report by a physician or other qualified health care professional, includes connection, recording and disconnection per patient encounter; single, dual, or multiple lead pacemaker system, or leadless pacemaker system

93289 single, dual, or multiple lead transvenous implantable defibrillator system, including analysis of heart rhythm derived data elements

93261 Interrogation device evaluation (in person) with analysis, review and report by a physician or other qualified health care professional, includes connection, recording and disconnection per patient encounter; implantable subcutaneous lead defibrillator system

93290 implantable cardiovascular physiologic monitor system, including analysis of 1 or more recorded physiologic cardiovascular data elements from all internal and external sensors

93291 subcutaneous cardiac rhythm monitor system, including heart rhythm derived data analysis

93292 wearable defibrillator system

Explanation

Patients with a previously implanted device, such as a cardiac pacemaker, implantable cardioverter-defibrillator (ICD), implantable cardiovascular monitor (ICM), or implantable loop recorder (ILR), require periodic interrogation device evaluations. This diagnostic procedure includes a face-to-face assessment of all device functions. Components that must be evaluated to assign 93288 include the battery, lead(s), capture and sensing function, heart rhythm, and programmed parameters of a single-, dual-, or multiple-lead pacemaker system. Code 93289 requires evaluation of the battery, lead(s), capture and sensing function, heart rhythm derived elements, presence or absence of therapy for ventricular tachyarrhythmias, and programmed parameters of a single-, dual-, or multiple-lead ICD system. Report 93261 for an interrogation device evaluation of an implantable subcutaneous lead defibrillation system. Code 93290 requires analysis of at least one recorded physiologic cardiovascular data element obtained from internal or external sensors and evaluation of programmed parameters of an ICM. Code 93291 requires evaluation of heart rate and rhythm during recorded episodes (from both patient-initiated and device algorithm detected events), as well as evaluation of programmed parameters of an ILR. Report 93292 for an interrogation device evaluation of a wearable defibrillation system. These codes include physician or other qualified health care professional analysis, review, and report. They also include connection, recording, and disconnection, and are assigned per procedure.

Relative Value Units/Medicare Edits

Non-Facility RVU	Work	PE	MP	Total
93261	0.74	1.31	0.03	2.08
93288	0.43	1.23	0.02	1.68
93289	0.75	1.36	0.04	2.15
93290	0.43	1.13	0.03	1.59
93291	0.37	1.07	0.02	1.46
93292	0.43	1.07	0.03	1.53
Facility RVU	**Work**	**PE**	**MP**	**Total**
93261	0.74	1.31	0.03	2.08
93288	0.43	1.23	0.02	1.68
93289	0.75	1.36	0.04	2.15
93290	0.43	1.13	0.03	1.59
93291	0.37	1.07	0.02	1.46
93292	0.43	1.07	0.03	1.53

93293

93293 Transtelephonic rhythm strip pacemaker evaluation(s) single, dual, or multiple lead pacemaker system, includes recording with and without magnet application with analysis, review and report(s) by a physician or other qualified health care professional, up to 90 days

Explanation

Patients with previously implanted pacemakers require periodic analysis of pacemaker function. A pacemaker may be implanted to control a patient's irregular heartbeat. This code applies to transtelephonic pacemaker monitoring, a form of evaluation in which the patient sends a rhythm strip over the telephone using a transmitter. This transmission is recorded by a receiving location using a receiver/recorder. The rhythm strip is recorded with and without a magnet being applied over the pacemaker and is assessed for heart rate and rhythm, as well as atrial and ventricular capture and sensing (if observed). The pacemaker's battery status is also determined. Code 93293 may be reported for a single, dual, or multiple lead pacemaker system, and includes physician or other qualified health care professional analysis, review, and report. This code should be reported only once per 90-day period.

Relative Value Units/Medicare Edits

Non-Facility RVU	Work	PE	MP	Total
93293	0.31	0.99	0.02	1.32
Facility RVU	**Work**	**PE**	**MP**	**Total**
93293	0.31	0.99	0.02	1.32

93294-93296

93294 Interrogation device evaluation(s) (remote), up to 90 days; single, dual, or multiple lead pacemaker system, or leadless pacemaker system with interim analysis, review(s) and report(s) by a physician or other qualified health care professional

93295 single, dual, or multiple lead implantable defibrillator system with interim analysis, review(s) and report(s) by a physician or other qualified health care professional

93296 single, dual, or multiple lead pacemaker system, leadless pacemaker system, or implantable defibrillator system, remote data acquisition(s), receipt of transmissions and technician review, technical support and distribution of results

Explanation

Patients with a previously implanted device, such as a cardiac pacemaker or implantable defibrillator, require periodic interrogation device evaluations. These codes report remote evaluations only and apply to single-, dual-, multiple-lead or leadless devices. Code 93294 reports the remote evaluation of a pacemaker system with interim physician or other qualified health care professional analysis, review, and report. Components that must be evaluated in order to assign this code include the battery, lead(s), capture and sensing function, heart rhythm, and programmed parameters. Code 93295 reports the remote evaluation of an implantable defibrillator system with interim physician or other qualified health care professional analysis, review, and report. Required evaluation components include the battery, lead(s), capture and sensing function, heart rhythm derived elements, presence or absence of therapy for ventricular tachyarrhythmias, and programmed parameters. Code 93296 reports the acquisition of remote data, transmission receipt and technician review, technical support, and result distribution and applies to pacemaker and defibrillator systems. Codes from this range may be reported only once per 90-day period.

Relative Value Units/Medicare Edits

Non-Facility RVU	Work	PE	MP	Total
93294	0.6	0.23	0.04	0.87
93295	0.74	0.29	0.05	1.08
93296	0.0	0.63	0.01	0.64
Facility RVU	**Work**	**PE**	**MP**	**Total**
93294	0.6	0.23	0.04	0.87
93295	0.74	0.29	0.05	1.08
93296	0.0	0.63	0.01	0.64

93297-93298

93297 Interrogation device evaluation(s), (remote) up to 30 days; implantable cardiovascular physiologic monitor system, including analysis of 1 or more recorded physiologic cardiovascular data elements from all internal and external sensors, analysis, review(s) and report(s) by a physician or other qualified health care professional

93298 subcutaneous cardiac rhythm monitor system, including analysis of recorded heart rhythm data, analysis, review(s) and report(s) by a physician or other qualified health care professional

Explanation

Patients with a previously implanted device, such as an implantable cardiovascular physiologic monitor (ICM) or subcutaneous cardiac rhythm monitor system, require periodic interrogation device evaluations. These codes report remote evaluations only and may be reported once per 30-day period. Report 93297 for the remote evaluation of an ICM, which includes the analysis of at least one recorded physiologic cardiovascular data element obtained from internal or external sensors. Physician or other qualified health care professional analysis, review, and report are also included. Report 93298 for the analysis of recorded heart rhythm data; this code also includes the provider's review and report.

Relative Value Units/Medicare Edits

Non-Facility RVU	Work	PE	MP	Total
93297	0.52	1.26	0.03	1.81
93298	0.52	2.49	0.04	3.05
Facility RVU	**Work**	**PE**	**MP**	**Total**
93297	0.52	1.26	0.03	1.81
93298	0.52	2.49	0.04	3.05

93303-93304

93303 Transthoracic echocardiography for congenital cardiac anomalies; complete

93304 follow-up or limited study

Explanation

Transducers are placed on the patient's chest to record an echocardiograph, which uses ultrasound to visualize the heart's function, blood flow, valves, and chambers. Report 93303 for a complete evaluation for congenital defects. Report 93304 for a follow-up or a limited evaluation for congenital defects.

Relative Value Units/Medicare Edits

Non-Facility RVU	Work	PE	MP	Total
93303	1.3	5.21	0.07	6.58
93304	0.75	3.86	0.05	4.66
Facility RVU	**Work**	**PE**	**MP**	**Total**
93303	1.3	5.21	0.07	6.58
93304	0.75	3.86	0.05	4.66

93306-93308

93306 Echocardiography, transthoracic, real-time with image documentation (2D), includes M-mode recording, when performed, complete, with spectral Doppler echocardiography, and with color flow Doppler echocardiography

93307 Echocardiography, transthoracic, real-time with image documentation (2D), includes M-mode recording, when performed, complete, without spectral or color Doppler echocardiography

93308 Echocardiography, transthoracic, real-time with image documentation (2D), includes M-mode recording, when performed, follow-up or limited study

Explanation

This is a noninvasive study that uses ultrasound to visualize the heart's function, blood flow, valves, and chambers. Two-dimensional echocardiography, also referred to as real-time imaging, is performed using multiple transducers or a rotating transducer, and these images are recorded on videotape. Computer reconstruction provides the two-dimensional image of specific planes of the heart. M-mode, when performed, provides additional detail of specific portions of the heart. A stationary ultrasound beam is directed at the area of the heart requiring additional study. Report 93306 for a complete evaluation that includes spectral and color flow Doppler, which provide information regarding intracardiac blood flow and hemodynamics. Report 93307 for a complete evaluation but without spectral or color flow Doppler. Report 93308 for a follow-up or limited study.

Relative Value Units/Medicare Edits

Non-Facility RVU	Work	PE	MP	Total
93306	1.46	4.35	0.08	5.89
93307	0.92	3.12	0.05	4.09
93308	0.53	2.39	0.04	2.96
Facility RVU	**Work**	**PE**	**MP**	**Total**
93306	1.46	4.35	0.08	5.89
93307	0.92	3.12	0.05	4.09
93308	0.53	2.39	0.04	2.96

93312-93314

93312 Echocardiography, transesophageal, real-time with image documentation (2D) (with or without M-mode recording); including probe placement, image acquisition, interpretation and report

93313 placement of transesophageal probe only

93314 image acquisition, interpretation and report only

Explanation

Transesophageal echocardiograph (TEE) is an invasive technique whereby the transducer is placed at the tip of an endoscope and introduced into the patient's esophagus to record a two-dimensional echocardiograph. This set of codes should be used for TEE used to diagnose cardiac sources of emboli, prosthetic heart valve malfunction, endocarditis, aortic dissection, cardiac tumors, and valvular heart disease excluding congenital heart disease. Code 93312 applies to a complete evaluation including probe placement, image acquisition, and the physician's interpretation. Report 93313 for probe placement only. Report 93314 for image acquisition, physician interpretation, and report only.

Relative Value Units/Medicare Edits

Non-Facility RVU	Work	PE	MP	Total
93312	2.3	4.65	0.11	7.06
93313	0.26	0.05	0.02	0.33
93314	1.85	4.73	0.19	6.77
Facility RVU	**Work**	**PE**	**MP**	**Total**
93312	2.3	4.65	0.11	7.06
93313	0.26	0.05	0.02	0.33
93314	1.85	4.73	0.19	6.77

93315-93317

93315 Transesophageal echocardiography for congenital cardiac anomalies; including probe placement, image acquisition, interpretation and report

93316 placement of transesophageal probe only

93317 image acquisition, interpretation and report only

Explanation

Transesophageal echocardiograph (TEE) is an invasive technique whereby the transducer is placed at the tip of an endoscope and introduced into the patient's esophagus to record a two-dimensional echocardiograph. This set of codes should be used for TEE used to diagnose cardiac sources of emboli, prosthetic heart valve malfunction, endocarditis, aortic dissection, cardiac tumors, and valvular heart disease excluding congenital heart disease. The set of codes is specific to evaluations for congenital defects. Code 93315 applies to a complete evaluation for congenital defects including probe placement, image acquisition, and the physician's interpretation. Report 93316 for probe placement only. Report 93317 for image acquisition, physician interpretation, and report only.

Relative Value Units/Medicare Edits

Non-Facility RVU	Work	PE	MP	Total
93315	0.0	0.0	0.0	0.0
93316	0.6	0.11	0.05	0.76
93317	0.0	0.0	0.0	0.0
Facility RVU	**Work**	**PE**	**MP**	**Total**
93315	0.0	0.0	0.0	0.0
93316	0.6	0.11	0.05	0.76
93317	0.0	0.0	0.0	0.0

[93319]

\+ **93319** 3D echocardiographic imaging and postprocessing during transesophageal echocardiography, or during transthoracic echocardiography for congenital cardiac anomalies, for the assessment of cardiac structure(s) (eg, cardiac chambers and valves, left atrial appendage, interatrial septum, interventricular septum) and function, when performed (List separately in addition to code for echocardiographic imaging)

Explanation

The physician performs 3D echocardiographic imaging/postprocessing during the same procedural episode as transesophageal or transthoracic echocardiography performed to evaluate congenital cardiac abnormalities. Cardiac structures are assessed and may include chambers and valves, interatrial or interventricular septum, or left atrial appendage. Cardiac function may also be assessed at this time.

Relative Value Units/Medicare Edits

Non-Facility RVU	Work	PE	MP	Total
93319	0.5	1.12	0.04	1.66
Facility RVU	**Work**	**PE**	**MP**	**Total**
93319	0.5	0.15	0.04	0.69

93318

93318 Echocardiography, transesophageal (TEE) for monitoring purposes, including probe placement, real time 2-dimensional image acquisition and interpretation leading to ongoing (continuous) assessment of (dynamically changing) cardiac pumping function and to therapeutic measures on an immediate time basis

Explanation

Transesophageal echocardiograph (TEE) is an invasive technique whereby the transducer is placed at the tip of an endoscope and introduced into the patient's esophagus to record a two-dimensional echocardiograph. TEE provides high-quality, real-time images of the beating heart and mediastinal structures. This code reports ongoing hemodynamic monitoring using TEE. TEE may be used to monitor critically ill patients in the intensive care unit as well as patients in certain operative settings. In both the intensive care unit and the operating room, it is used to monitor cardiac function including cardiac preload, contractility, and valve function in patients with acute hemodynamic decompensation. In addition, TEE may also be used to assess and monitor mediastinal, heart, lung, and aortic injury resulting from blunt chest trauma even in patients undergoing other life-saving procedures.

93320-93321

+ **93320** Doppler echocardiography, pulsed wave and/or continuous wave with spectral display (List separately in addition to codes for echocardiographic imaging); complete

+ **93321** follow-up or limited study (List separately in addition to codes for echocardiographic imaging)

Explanation

Transducers are placed on a patient's chest to record a Doppler echocardiograph, which uses ultrasound to visualize blood flow velocity, direction, and type of flow in different locations in the heart. Doppler studies can be displayed on a strip chart or video recorder. Report 93320 for a complete evaluation and 93321 for limited or follow-up studies.

Relative Value Units/Medicare Edits

Non-Facility RVU	Work	PE	MP	Total
93320	0.38	1.12	0.02	1.52
93321	0.15	0.59	0.01	0.75
Facility RVU	**Work**	**PE**	**MP**	**Total**
93320	0.38	1.12	0.02	1.52
93321	0.15	0.59	0.01	0.75

93325

+ **93325** Doppler echocardiography color flow velocity mapping (List separately in addition to codes for echocardiography)

Explanation

The technique for Doppler color flow velocity mapping is similar to that of other echocardiographs with transducers being placed on the patient's chest to record cardiac activity. Color Doppler is two-dimensional Doppler in which the signal is encoded with color to more clearly identify flow direction. List 93325 separately in addition to the code for echocardiography (76825, 76826, 76827, 76828, 93303, 93304, 93308, 93312, 93314, 93315, 93317, 93350, and 93351).

Relative Value Units/Medicare Edits

Non-Facility RVU	Work	PE	MP	Total
93325	0.07	0.63	0.0	0.7
Facility RVU	**Work**	**PE**	**MP**	**Total**
93325	0.07	0.63	0.0	0.7

93350-93352

93350 Echocardiography, transthoracic, real-time with image documentation (2D), includes M-mode recording, when performed, during rest and cardiovascular stress test using treadmill, bicycle exercise and/or pharmacologically induced stress, with interpretation and report;

93351 including performance of continuous electrocardiographic monitoring, with supervision by a physician or other qualified health care professional

+ **93352** Use of echocardiographic contrast agent during stress echocardiography (List separately in addition to code for primary procedure)

Explanation

Transducers are placed on a patient's chest to record a two-dimensional echocardiograph, which uses ultrasound to visualize the heart's function, blood flow, valves, and chambers. In 93350, the echocardiography is completed while the patient is at rest and exercising on a treadmill or stationary bicycle with or without medication and includes M-mode recording, when performed. Code 93351 also includes the performance of continuous electrocardiographic monitoring with supervision by the physician or other qualified health care professional. Code 93352 is assigned as an additional code to report the use of an echocardiographic contrast agent during the stress test and should not be reported more than once per stress echocardiogram. Supply of the contrast agent and/or the drugs used in pharmacologic stress are reported separately in addition to these procedure codes.

Relative Value Units/Medicare Edits

Non-Facility RVU	Work	PE	MP	Total
93350	1.46	4.03	0.07	5.56
93351	1.75	5.11	0.1	6.96
93352	0.19	0.83	0.02	1.04
Facility RVU	**Work**	**PE**	**MP**	**Total**
93350	1.46	4.03	0.07	5.56
93351	1.75	5.11	0.1	6.96
93352	0.19	0.83	0.02	1.04

[93356]

+ **93356** Myocardial strain imaging using speckle tracking-derived assessment of myocardial mechanics (List separately in addition to codes for echocardiography imaging)

Explanation

Myocardial strain imaging, also referred to as echocardiographic strain imaging or deformation (lengthening, shortening, or thickening) imaging, was initially utilized as a feature of Doppler imaging where velocity information is regenerated into strain rate. New technology, known as speckle tracking echocardiography (STE), utilizes image-processing algorithms to track areas of interest. Used in conjunction with two-dimensional or three-dimensional echocardiography for determining the multidirectional components of left ventricular (LV) deformation, these areas contain blocks of 20 to 40 pixels that contain constant patterns referred to as speckles. These markers or fingerprints are helpful in outlining irregularities by comprehensive assessment of regional myocardial function, specifically by discriminating between active and passive myocardial wall movement. Strain rate data assists in early detection of myocardial dysfunction and is beneficial in therapeutic decisions and follow-up of previous cardiac surgery. Report 93356 in addition to applicable codes for echocardiography imaging.

Relative Value Units/Medicare Edits

Non-Facility RVU	Work	PE	MP	Total
93356	0.24	0.85	0.02	1.11
Facility RVU	**Work**	**PE**	**MP**	**Total**
93356	0.24	0.08	0.02	0.34

93660

93660 Evaluation of cardiovascular function with tilt table evaluation, with continuous ECG monitoring and intermittent blood pressure monitoring, with or without pharmacological intervention

Explanation

The purpose of this procedure is to evaluate the patient's susceptibility to neurocardiogenic syncope. The physician secures the patient to the tilt table and attaches ECG leads to the chest. The physician also attaches an intermittent blood pressure monitor. The physician tilts the table, with the patient on it, and monitors the patient's symptoms, heart rhythm, and blood pressure. The physician may infuse medication, such as isoproterenol, through a standard intravenous catheter and repeat the tilt test.

Relative Value Units/Medicare Edits

Non-Facility RVU	Work	PE	MP	Total
93660	1.89	2.88	0.09	4.86
Facility RVU	Work	PE	MP	Total
93660	1.89	2.88	0.09	4.86

93668

93668 Peripheral arterial disease (PAD) rehabilitation, per session

Explanation

An exercise physiologist or nurse supervises rehabilitation exercises in a patient diagnosed with peripheral arterial disease (PAD). Rehabilitation for PAD is provided using either a motorized treadmill or a track. The patient is supervised during physical exercise sessions lasting between 45-60 minutes in order to achieve symptom-limited claudication. The supervising provider monitors the patient's claudication threshold and other cardiovascular limitations and adjusts the level of activity in order to reduce claudication symptoms and increase exercise tolerance.

Relative Value Units/Medicare Edits

Non-Facility RVU	Work	PE	MP	Total
93668	0.0	0.43	0.01	0.44
Facility RVU	Work	PE	MP	Total
93668	0.0	0.43	0.01	0.44

93701

93701 Bioimpedance-derived physiologic cardiovascular analysis

Explanation

Bioimpedance is a noninvasive, continuous measurement of blood flow, respiration, and other cardiopulmonary dynamics, using a patient's thorax as an impedance transducer. The health care provider attaches the patient to the bioimpedance system with solid-gel electrodes placed along the widest dimension of the thorax. The electrical bioimpedance measurement current is passed through the thorax in a direction parallel with the spine between a pair of electrodes placed on the upper neck and a pair of electrodes placed on the upper abdomen. On its way through the thorax, the measurement current seeks the shortest and the most conductive pathway. As a result, the majority of the thoracic electrical bioimpedance (TEB) measurement current flows through the thoracic aorta and superior and inferior vena. The measurement current produces a high-frequency voltage across the impedance of the thorax, sensed by two other pairs of electrodes placed at the beginning of the thorax and the end of the thorax. The sensing electrodes also detect the ECG signal. The heart rate is derived from the R-R intervals of the ECG signal.

Relative Value Units/Medicare Edits

Non-Facility RVU	Work	PE	MP	Total
93701	0.0	0.8	0.01	0.81
Facility RVU	Work	PE	MP	Total
93701	0.0	0.8	0.01	0.81

93702

93702 Bioimpedance spectroscopy (BIS), extracellular fluid analysis for lymphedema assessment(s)

Explanation

Bioimpedance spectroscopy (BIS) is an accurate, reproducible, and noninvasive method that detects alterations in extracellular fluid volume differences between the limbs using a device called an impedance plethysmograph. Skin electrodes are applied to the limb. A small alternating current is passed through the limb via these electrodes, and the impedance (opposition) to the current's flow is measured. This measurement is subsequently converted to fluid levels. Differences in extracellular fluid levels between the limbs can be an early indication of lymphedema (swelling from fluid buildup caused by inadequate functioning of the lymphatic system).

Relative Value Units/Medicare Edits

Non-Facility RVU	Work	PE	MP	Total
93702	0.0	3.65	0.02	3.67
Facility RVU	Work	PE	MP	Total
93702	0.0	3.65	0.02	3.67

93724

93724 Electronic analysis of antitachycardia pacemaker system (includes electrocardiographic recording, programming of device, induction and termination of tachycardia via implanted pacemaker, and interpretation of recordings)

Explanation

Patients with previously implanted pacemakers require periodic analysis of pacemaker function. This code applies to routine electronic analysis of pacemakers used to control irregularly fast heartbeats (antitachycardial) and includes electrocardiogram, programming, tests, and physician interpretation of the tests.

Relative Value Units/Medicare Edits

Non-Facility RVU	Work	PE	MP	Total
93724	4.88	3.24	0.16	8.28
Facility RVU	Work	PE	MP	Total
93724	4.88	3.24	0.16	8.28

93740

93740 Temperature gradient studies

Explanation

Temperature gradient studies assess heart or circulatory functions by contrasting temperatures of certain vessels via an intravenous catheter.

Relative Value Units/Medicare Edits

Non-Facility RVU	Work	PE	MP	Total
93740	0.16	0.06	0.01	0.23
Facility RVU	Work	PE	MP	Total
93740	0.16	0.06	0.01	0.23

93745

93745 Initial set-up and programming by a physician or other qualified health care professional of wearable cardioverter-defibrillator includes initial programming of system, establishing baseline electronic ECG, transmission of data to data repository, patient instruction in wearing system and patient reporting of problems or events

Explanation

The physician or other qualified health care professional performs initial set-up and programming of a wearable cardioverter-defibrillator. A wearable cardioverter-defibrillator is an external device that includes a monitor, electrodes, and an alarm contained in a vest-like garment that is worn 24 hours a day by

 ● New ▲ Revised + Add On ★ Telemedicine [Resequenced]

the patient. The wearable cardioverter-defibrillator is used to detect, monitor, and treat life-threatening tachycardia and fibrillation that can lead to sudden cardiac arrest and death. The wearable cardioverter-defibrillator works by restoring a normal rhythm using low frequency shocks (cardioversion) or by returning a fast, disordered rhythm to normal rhythm by means of high-energy shock(s) (defibrillation). This code reports the initial programming of the system by the provider that includes establishing a baseline ECG. The initial set-up also includes verifying data transmission to a data repository, patient instruction on wearing the device, and patient reporting of events or problems with the device.

93750

93750 Interrogation of ventricular assist device (VAD), in person, with physician or other qualified health care professional analysis of device parameters (eg, drivelines, alarms, power surges), review of device function (eg, flow and volume status, septum status, recovery), with programming, if performed, and report

Explanation

Patients with a previously implanted ventricular assist device (VAD) require periodic interrogation of the device. Code 93750 reports a diagnostic procedure that is performed in person and includes a face-to-face assessment of all device functions. Components that must be evaluated include device parameters (alarms, drivelines, and power surges) and a review of the device function (flow/volume status, septum status, and recovery). This code includes physician or other qualified health care professional analysis, review, and report. It also includes device programming, if performed.

Relative Value Units/Medicare Edits

Non-Facility RVU	Work	PE	MP	Total
93750	0.75	0.65	0.12	1.52
Facility RVU	**Work**	**PE**	**MP**	**Total**
93750	0.75	0.31	0.12	1.18

93770

93770 Determination of venous pressure

Explanation

Venous blood pressure is measured to assess heart and circulatory system functions. This code applies to the peripheral measurement.

Relative Value Units/Medicare Edits

Non-Facility RVU	Work	PE	MP	Total
93770	0.16	0.06	0.01	0.23
Facility RVU	**Work**	**PE**	**MP**	**Total**
93770	0.16	0.06	0.01	0.23

93784-93790

93784 Ambulatory blood pressure monitoring, utilizing report-generating software, automated, worn continuously for 24 hours or longer; including recording, scanning analysis, interpretation and report

93786 recording only

93788 scanning analysis with report

93790 review with interpretation and report

Explanation

A patient's ambient blood pressure is evaluated during a 24-hour period. A technician attaches the blood pressure monitor to the patient, who wears the monitor continuously for 24 hours. During this period, the device obtains blood pressure measurements and records them on automated report-generating software. Ambulatory blood pressure monitoring (ABPM) may be useful for patients with suspected masked or white coat hypertension. Report 93784 for the complete procedure, including interpretation and report. Report 93786 for the recording only. Report 93788 when a technician scans the data and generates a data summary. Report 93790 for review and interpretation of the data and a subsequent report of the findings.

Relative Value Units/Medicare Edits

Non-Facility RVU	Work	PE	MP	Total
93784	0.38	0.97	0.03	1.38
93786	0.0	0.67	0.01	0.68
93788	0.0	0.16	0.01	0.17
93790	0.38	0.14	0.01	0.53
Facility RVU	**Work**	**PE**	**MP**	**Total**
93784	0.38	0.97	0.03	1.38
93786	0.0	0.67	0.01	0.68
93788	0.0	0.16	0.01	0.17
93790	0.38	0.14	0.01	0.53

93792-93793

93792 Patient/caregiver training for initiation of home international normalized ratio (INR) monitoring under the direction of a physician or other qualified health care professional, face-to-face, including use and care of the INR monitor, obtaining blood sample, instructions for reporting home INR test results, and documentation of patient's/caregiver's ability to perform testing and report results

93793 Anticoagulant management for a patient taking warfarin, must include review and interpretation of a new home, office, or lab international normalized ratio (INR) test result, patient instructions, dosage adjustment (as needed), and scheduling of additional test(s), when performed

Explanation

Home and outpatient international normalized ratio (INR) monitoring is anticoagulant management of warfarin therapy, including ordering, review, and interpretation of new INR test results; patient instructions; and dosage adjustments, as appropriate. In 93792, face-to-face, clinician-directed training is started for the patient and/or caregiver for in-home INR monitoring to include proper use and care of the INR monitoring device, instructions for obtaining blood samples, and reporting INR test results. A documented determination as to the patient's and/or caregiver's ability to adequately perform testing and reporting is also required. Report 93793 for review and interpretation of a new home, office, or lab INR test result with instructions and dosage modifications, as necessary, as well as the scheduling of any additional tests, when performed.

Relative Value Units/Medicare Edits

Non-Facility RVU	Work	PE	MP	Total
93792	0.0	2.08	0.03	2.11
93793	0.18	0.15	0.01	0.34
Facility RVU	**Work**	**PE**	**MP**	**Total**
93792	0.0	2.08	0.03	2.11
93793	0.18	0.15	0.01	0.34

93797-93798

93797 Physician or other qualified health care professional services for outpatient cardiac rehabilitation; without continuous ECG monitoring (per session)

93798 with continuous ECG monitoring (per session)

Explanation

Patients with severe cardiac disease, particularly those who have had myocardial infarctions, surgery on the coronary vessels, and other occlusive coronary artery diseases, often require outpatient rehabilitation. A physician or other qualified health care professional supervises outpatient cardiac rehabilitation in areas of exercise, diet, and related modalities. Report 93798 when continuous electrocardiogram monitoring is provided.

Relative Value Units/Medicare Edits

Non-Facility RVU	Work	PE	MP	Total
93797	0.18	0.32	0.01	0.51
93798	0.28	0.47	0.02	0.77
Facility RVU	**Work**	**PE**	**MP**	**Total**
93797	0.18	0.07	0.01	0.26
93798	0.28	0.1	0.02	0.4

93880-93882

93880 Duplex scan of extracranial arteries; complete bilateral study
93882 unilateral or limited study

Explanation

The physician or an assistant performs a Duplex ultrasound scan, which is a combination of real-time and Doppler studies of the extracranial arteries in the head and neck to evaluate vascular blood flow in relation to blockage. Ultrasound uses high frequency sound waves to provide an image. Report 93880 when the procedure is performed on both sides of the head and neck. Report 93882 when a unilateral (one side of the head or neck) or limited study is performed.

Relative Value Units/Medicare Edits

Non-Facility RVU	Work	PE	MP	Total
93880	0.8	4.8	0.1	5.7
93882	0.5	3.16	0.08	3.74
Facility RVU	**Work**	**PE**	**MP**	**Total**
93880	0.8	4.8	0.1	5.7
93882	0.5	3.16	0.08	3.74

93886-93888

93886 Transcranial Doppler study of the intracranial arteries; complete study
93888 limited study

Explanation

The physician or an assistant performs a Doppler ultrasound scan of the intracranial arteries in the head and neck to evaluate vascular blood flow in relation to blockage. Code 93886 applies to a complete study of the intracranial arteries. Code 93888 applies to a limited study of the intracranial arteries.

Relative Value Units/Medicare Edits

Non-Facility RVU	Work	PE	MP	Total
93886	0.91	7.24	0.08	8.23
93888	0.5	4.24	0.05	4.79
Facility RVU	**Work**	**PE**	**MP**	**Total**
93886	0.91	7.24	0.08	8.23
93888	0.5	4.24	0.05	4.79

93892-93893

93892 Transcranial Doppler study of the intracranial arteries; emboli detection without intravenous microbubble injection
▲ **93893** venous-arterial shunt detection with intravenous microbubble injection

Explanation

The physician performs a transcranial Doppler (TCD) study of the intracranial arteries for emboli or venous-arterial shunt detection. TCD is a noninvasive ultrasound technology used to evaluate blood flow in the major intracranial arteries. In 93892, emboli detection without intravenous microbubble injection is performed. Intracranial circulating microemboli appear as high intensity transient signals in the TCD waveform. In 93893, venous-arterial shunt detection is performed with intravenous microbubble injection. A venous-arterial shunt is an abnormal connection between the venous and arterial systems. Gas-filled microbubbles are administered intravenously to increase the Doppler signal intensity from the blood for better visualization of the intracranial arteries.

Relative Value Units/Medicare Edits

Non-Facility RVU	Work	PE	MP	Total
93892	1.15	8.57	0.1	9.82
93893	1.15	10.82	0.12	12.09
Facility RVU	**Work**	**PE**	**MP**	**Total**
93892	1.15	8.57	0.1	9.82
93893	1.15	10.82	0.12	12.09

[93896, 93897, 93898]

+● **93896** Vasoreactivity study performed with transcranial Doppler study of intracranial arteries, complete (List separately in addition to code for primary procedure)
+● **93897** Emboli detection without intravenous microbubble injection performed with transcranial Doppler study of intracranial arteries, complete (List separately in addition to code for primary procedure)
+● **93898** Venous-arterial shunt detection with intravenous microbubble injection performed with transcranial Doppler study of intracranial arteries, complete (List separately in addition to code for primary procedure)

Explanation

The physician performs a vasoreactivity study, emboli detection without intravenous microbubble injection, or venous-arterial shunt detection with intravenous microbubble injection on the same day as a complete transcranial Doppler (TCD) study. TCD is a noninvasive ultrasound technology used to evaluate blood flow in the major intracranial arteries. In 93896, the physician performs a vasoreactivity study of the intracranial arteries to identify cerebrovascular disease. Vasoreactivity, also referred to as vasomotor reactivity, measures changes in blood flow velocity in response to a pharmacologic or other agent. TCD of the intracranial arteries is performed, and flow velocity is measured. A pharmacologic or other agent is administered, and TCD with flow velocity measurement is repeated. Changes in blood flow velocity in the intracranial arteries are compared and analyzed. In 93897, emboli detection without intravenous microbubble injection is performed. Intracranial circulating microemboli appear as high intensity transient signals in the TCD waveform. In 93898, venous-arterial shunt detection is performed with intravenous microbubble injection. A venous-arterial shunt is an abnormal connection between the venous and arterial systems. Gas-filled microbubbles are administered intravenously to increase the Doppler signal intensity from the blood for better visualization of the intracranial arteries. These are add-on codes and are reported in addition to the complete TCD study.

Relative Value Units/Medicare Edits

Non-Facility RVU	Work	PE	MP	Total
93896				
93897				
93898				
Facility RVU	**Work**	**PE**	**MP**	**Total**
93896				
93897				
93898				

93895

93895 Quantitative carotid intima media thickness and carotid atheroma evaluation, bilateral

Explanation

Carotid intima media thickness (IMT) study is a noninvasive assessment performed on the common carotid artery bilaterally. The measurements of the inner two artery layers, the intima and the media, are used as risk factor indicators for atherosclerosis and coronary heart disease. This test is performed by scanning with high-resolution B mode ultrasonography and using computer enhancement and analysis to determine the thickness of the intima and media of the carotid artery. The results evaluate for any thickening or signs of anatomical changes from early atherosclerotic disease.

93922-93923

93922 Limited bilateral noninvasive physiologic studies of upper or lower extremity arteries, (eg, for lower extremity: ankle/brachial indices at distal posterior tibial and anterior tibial/dorsalis pedis arteries plus bidirectional, Doppler waveform recording and analysis at 1-2 levels, or ankle/brachial indices at distal posterior tibial and anterior tibial/dorsalis pedis arteries plus volume plethysmography at 1-2 levels, or ankle/brachial indices at distal posterior tibial and anterior tibial/dorsalis pedis arteries with, transcutaneous oxygen tension measurement at 1-2 levels)

93923 Complete bilateral noninvasive physiologic studies of upper or lower extremity arteries, 3 or more levels (eg, for lower extremity: ankle/brachial indices at distal posterior tibial and anterior tibial/dorsalis pedis arteries plus segmental blood pressure measurements with bidirectional Doppler waveform recording and analysis, at 3 or more levels, or ankle/brachial indices at distal posterior tibial and anterior tibial/dorsalis pedis arteries plus segmental volume plethysmography at 3 or more levels, or ankle/brachial indices at distal posterior tibial and anterior tibial/dorsalis pedis arteries plus segmental transcutaneous oxygen tension measurements at 3 or more levels), or single level study with provocative functional maneuvers (eg, measurements with postural provocative tests, or measurements with reactive hyperemia)

Explanation

The physician or assistant physician evaluates the arteries of the arms or legs to check blood flow in relation to blockage. In one method, the physician places a transducer on each leg at a prescribed level and measures the change in blood-handling characteristics during constriction by pneumatic cuffs. The technique is similar to constriction and measuring of tension in the vascular system, but the medium may change. Report 93922 for ultrasound, plethysmography, and oxygen tension measurements in a bilateral evaluation limited to one or two levels. When a unilateral study of one to two levels is performed, report 93922 with modifier 52. This code is also applicable to a unilateral study when three or more levels are recorded or if provocative functional maneuvers are performed. Report 93923 for a complete bilateral study of three or more levels or a single-level study with provocative functional maneuvers.

Relative Value Units/Medicare Edits

Non-Facility RVU	Work	PE	MP	Total
93922	0.25	2.17	0.05	2.47
93923	0.45	3.37	0.09	3.91
Facility RVU	**Work**	**PE**	**MP**	**Total**
93922	0.25	2.17	0.05	2.47
93923	0.45	3.37	0.09	3.91

93924

93924 Noninvasive physiologic studies of lower extremity arteries, at rest and following treadmill stress testing, (ie, bidirectional Doppler waveform or volume plethysmography recording and analysis at rest with ankle/brachial indices immediately after and at timed intervals following performance of a standardized protocol on a motorized treadmill plus recording of time of onset of claudication or other symptoms, maximal walking time, and time to recovery) complete bilateral study

Explanation

The physician or assistant evaluates the arteries of the legs to check blood flow in relation to blockage. This code applies to ultrasound and oxygen tension measurements in a bilateral evaluation that occurs before and after a treadmill stress test.

Relative Value Units/Medicare Edits

Non-Facility RVU	Work	PE	MP	Total
93924	0.5	4.21	0.09	4.8
Facility RVU	**Work**	**PE**	**MP**	**Total**
93924	0.5	4.21	0.09	4.8

93925-93926

93925 Duplex scan of lower extremity arteries or arterial bypass grafts; complete bilateral study

93926 unilateral or limited study

Explanation

The physician or assistant evaluates the arteries of the legs bilaterally to check blood flow in relation to blockage by use of Duplex ultrasonography, which is a combination of real-time and Doppler studies. Code 93925 refers to a complete bilateral study. Code 93926 applies to studies of one leg or limited areas of both legs.

Relative Value Units/Medicare Edits

Non-Facility RVU	Work	PE	MP	Total
93925	0.8	6.3	0.11	7.21
93926	0.5	3.74	0.08	4.32
Facility RVU	**Work**	**PE**	**MP**	**Total**
93925	0.8	6.3	0.11	7.21
93926	0.5	3.74	0.08	4.32

93930-93931

93930 Duplex scan of upper extremity arteries or arterial bypass grafts; complete bilateral study

93931 unilateral or limited study

Explanation

A diagnostic study is performed on the upper extremity arteries or arterial bypass grafts. A duplex scan involves a two-dimensional ultrasonic scan, which provides a two-dimensional display of the structure. Code 93930 reports a procedure performed on both arms (complete bilateral study). Code 93931 applies to studies of one arm or limited areas of both arms.

Relative Value Units/Medicare Edits

Non-Facility RVU	Work	PE	MP	Total
93930	0.8	5.03	0.11	5.94
93931	0.5	3.14	0.07	3.71
Facility RVU	**Work**	**PE**	**MP**	**Total**
93930	0.8	5.03	0.11	5.94
93931	0.5	3.14	0.07	3.71

93970-93971

93970 Duplex scan of extremity veins including responses to compression and other maneuvers; complete bilateral study

93971 unilateral or limited study

Explanation

The physician or assistant performs a Duplex ultrasound scan, which is a combination of real-time and Doppler studies, of the veins in the arms or legs to evaluate vascular blood flow in relation to blockage. Code 93970 applies to complete responses to compression and other tests on both sides (complete bilateral study). Code 93971 applies to complete responses to compression and other tests and includes one side or limited areas of both sides.

Relative Value Units/Medicare Edits

Non-Facility RVU	Work	PE	MP	Total
93970	0.7	4.82	0.09	5.61
93971	0.45	3.07	0.05	3.57
Facility RVU	**Work**	**PE**	**MP**	**Total**
93970	0.7	4.82	0.09	5.61
93971	0.45	3.07	0.05	3.57

93975-93976

93975 Duplex scan of arterial inflow and venous outflow of abdominal, pelvic, scrotal contents and/or retroperitoneal organs; complete study

93976 limited study

Explanation

The physician or assistant performs a Duplex ultrasound scan, which is a combination of real-time and Doppler studies, of the arteries and veins in the abdominal, pelvic, or genitorectal areas to evaluate vascular blood flow in relation to blockage. Code 93975 applies to a complete bilateral evaluation. Code 93976 applies to a limited evaluation.

Relative Value Units/Medicare Edits

Non-Facility RVU	Work	PE	MP	Total
93975	1.16	6.64	0.13	7.93
93976	0.8	3.89	0.07	4.76
Facility RVU	**Work**	**PE**	**MP**	**Total**
93975	1.16	6.64	0.13	7.93
93976	0.8	3.89	0.07	4.76

93978-93979

93978 Duplex scan of aorta, inferior vena cava, iliac vasculature, or bypass grafts; complete study

93979 unilateral or limited study

Explanation

The physician or assistant performs a Duplex ultrasound scan, which is a combination of real-time and Doppler studies, of the arteries and veins in the aorta, inferior vena cava, or iliac areas to evaluate vascular blood flow in relation to blockage. Code 93978 applies to a complete bilateral evaluation. Code 93979 applies to one side or limited areas of both sides.

Relative Value Units/Medicare Edits

Non-Facility RVU	Work	PE	MP	Total
93978	0.8	4.48	0.13	5.41
93979	0.5	2.96	0.08	3.54
Facility RVU	**Work**	**PE**	**MP**	**Total**
93978	0.8	4.48	0.13	5.41
93979	0.5	2.96	0.08	3.54

93980-93981

93980 Duplex scan of arterial inflow and venous outflow of penile vessels; complete study

93981 follow-up or limited study

Explanation

The physician performs a Duplex ultrasound scan, producing real-time images integrating B-mode two-dimensional structure with Doppler mapping or imaging of motion with time, of the arteries and veins in the penis to evaluate vascular blood flow in and out of the penis in relation to blockages. Report 93980 for a complete evaluation and 93981 for a follow-up or a limited study.

Relative Value Units/Medicare Edits

Non-Facility RVU	Work	PE	MP	Total
93980	1.25	2.2	0.06	3.51
93981	0.44	1.64	0.04	2.12
Facility RVU	**Work**	**PE**	**MP**	**Total**
93980	1.25	2.2	0.06	3.51
93981	0.44	1.64	0.04	2.12

93985-93986

93985 Duplex scan of arterial inflow and venous outflow for preoperative vessel assessment prior to creation of hemodialysis access; complete bilateral study

93986 Duplex scan of arterial inflow and venous outflow for preoperative vessel assessment prior to creation of hemodialysis access; complete unilateral study

Explanation

The physician performs a Duplex ultrasound scan, producing real-time images integrating B-mode two-dimensional structure with Doppler mapping or imaging of motion with time for preoperative assessment of vascular blood flow prior to the creation of a hemodialysis access. This assessment includes the arterial inflow and venous outflow. Native arteriovenous fistula (AVF) is the preferred vascular access for hemodialysis patients, lasting longer and having fewer complications than grafts and central venous catheters. The use of the Doppler ultrasound (DUS) in preoperative vascular mapping enables identification of vessels that are most appropriate for fistula construction. Report 93985 for a complete bilateral study and 93986 for a complete unilateral study.

Relative Value Units/Medicare Edits

Non-Facility RVU	Work	PE	MP	Total
93985	0.8	6.47	0.16	7.43
93986	0.5	3.77	0.1	4.37
Facility RVU	**Work**	**PE**	**MP**	**Total**
93985	0.8	6.47	0.16	7.43
93986	0.5	3.77	0.1	4.37

93990

93990 Duplex scan of hemodialysis access (including arterial inflow, body of access and venous outflow)

Explanation

The physician performs a Duplex ultrasound scan, producing real-time images integrating B-mode two-dimensional structure with Doppler mapping or imaging of motion with time, of a hemodialysis access site, including the arterial inflow, body of the access site or device, and venous outflow, to evaluate vascular blood flow in relation to blockage.

Relative Value Units/Medicare Edits

Non-Facility RVU	Work	PE	MP	Total
93990	0.5	3.8	0.11	4.41
Facility RVU	**Work**	**PE**	**MP**	**Total**
93990	0.5	3.8	0.11	4.41

94002-94004

94002 Ventilation assist and management, initiation of pressure or volume preset ventilators for assisted or controlled breathing; hospital inpatient/observation, initial day

94003 Ventilation assist and management, initiation of pressure or volume preset ventilators for assisted or controlled breathing; hospital inpatient/observation, each subsequent day

94004 nursing facility, per day

Explanation

A mechanical ventilator is applied with a mask over the nose and mouth or through a tube placed into the trachea for patients requiring help breathing due to a lung disorder. Intermittent positive pressure breathing uses positive pressure during the inspiration phase of breathing. Code 94002 applies to ventilation assistance using adjustments in volume and pressure on the initial day of treatment in a hospital to an inpatient or observation patient and 94003 is reported for ventilation assistance to a hospital inpatient or observation patient provided on subsequent days. Ventilation assistance and management provided to a nursing facility patient is reported with 94004 on a per day basis.

Relative Value Units/Medicare Edits

Non-Facility RVU	Work	PE	MP	Total
94002	1.99	0.55	0.16	2.7
94003	1.37	0.42	0.11	1.9
94004	1.0	0.33	0.08	1.41
Facility RVU	**Work**	**PE**	**MP**	**Total**
94002	1.99	0.55	0.16	2.7
94003	1.37	0.42	0.11	1.9
94004	1.0	0.33	0.08	1.41

94150

94150 Vital capacity, total (separate procedure)

Explanation

This procedure measures the largest volume of air a patient can expire from his lungs. The patient amount of air inhaled and exhaled is measured and calculated with body size to determine the capacity of the lungs. This test is important for determining the threshold of capacity needed for vitality in patients with compromised respiration. For men, this is typically four to five liters; for women, this is normally three to four liters. It is normally performed as a part of a larger procedure and should only be billed separately when performed alone.

Relative Value Units/Medicare Edits

Non-Facility RVU	Work	PE	MP	Total
94150	0.07	0.67	0.02	0.76
Facility RVU	**Work**	**PE**	**MP**	**Total**
94150	0.07	0.67	0.02	0.76

94617 [94619]

94617 Exercise test for bronchospasm, including pre- and post-spirometry and pulse oximetry; with electrocardiographic recording(s)

94619 Exercise test for bronchospasm, including pre- and post-spirometry and pulse oximetry; without electrocardiographic recording(s)

Explanation

An exercise-induced bronchospasm (EIB) test is performed to diagnose EIB based on the difference in lung function postexercise rather than on symptoms. Bronchospasm, an occurrence that happens when the lungs shrink during exercise, makes it difficult to breathe. The clinician conducts a pre- and post-spirometry test that measures the amount of air a patient inhales and how much air is being exhaled. An EIB test typically involves rapidly increasing the intensity of the exercise, such as cycling or running, over a period of about two to four minutes duration in order to have the patient reach a high rate of breathing dry air via the use of a nasal clip. Exercise is continued until the patient's heartrate is 80 to 90 percent of the predicted maximum or once the patient's breathing reaches 68, 72, or 73 (17.5 to 21 times FEV1). The patient must maintain this level for an additional four to six minutes. Studies have shown that running helps reach these targets faster than any other type of exercise. Measurement of the patient's oxygen level is by pulse oximetry. An electrocardiography (ECG, EKG) is performed to monitor the heart in 94617. Report 94619 when the test is conducted without electrocardiographic recordings.

Relative Value Units/Medicare Edits

Non-Facility RVU	Work	PE	MP	Total
94617	0.7	1.93	0.04	2.67
94619	0.49	1.43	0.03	1.95
Facility RVU	**Work**	**PE**	**MP**	**Total**
94617	0.7	1.93	0.04	2.67
94619	0.49	1.43	0.03	1.95

94618-94621

94618 Pulmonary stress testing (eg, 6-minute walk test), including measurement of heart rate, oximetry, and oxygen titration, when performed

94621 Cardiopulmonary exercise testing, including measurements of minute ventilation, CO2 production, O2 uptake, and electrocardiographic recordings

Explanation

In 94618, a pulmonary exercise stress test is performed to determine how much air is moving in and out of the lungs during exercise and to establish where breathing problems are occurring, since they may be in the lungs, heart, or circulation. An exercise stress test is done with the patient riding a stationary bike (ergometer) or walking on a treadmill. Heartrate, breathing, and blood pressure are monitored before beginning the exercise. Basic ventilation studies are performed with a spirometer and recording device as the patient breathes through a mouthpiece and connecting tube while a nose clip prevents nasal breathing. Measurement of the patient's oxygen level by pulse oximetry is included, as well as oxygen titration and heartrate, when performed. In 94621, cardiopulmonary exercise testing is performed. Electrodes are placed on the upper body to monitor the heart. Throughout the process, blood samples may be taken to measure oxygen uptake and carbon dioxide waste products in the blood, as well as other tests including minute ventilation and an electrocardiogram (ECG, EKG).

Relative Value Units/Medicare Edits

Non-Facility RVU	Work	PE	MP	Total
94618	0.48	0.51	0.03	1.02
94621	1.42	3.11	0.11	4.64
Facility RVU	**Work**	**PE**	**MP**	**Total**
94618	0.48	0.51	0.03	1.02
94621	1.42	3.11	0.11	4.64

96160-96161

★**96160** Administration of patient-focused health risk assessment instrument (eg, health hazard appraisal) with scoring and documentation, per standardized instrument

★**96161** Administration of caregiver-focused health risk assessment instrument (eg, depression inventory) for the benefit of the patient, with scoring and documentation, per standardized instrument

Explanation

A provision in the Patient Protection and Affordable Care Act of 2010 (ACA) established a Medicare Wellness Visit, which included a Health Risk Assessment (HRA) and customized wellness or prevention plan. HRAs are typically completed by a patient or caregiver prior to the encounter with a physician or other qualified health care professional, but can involve the assistance of the clinician and/or staff members. The HRA tool is purposefully designed to be brief, straightforward, and easy to comprehend with questions such as patient demographic information, personal and/or family history, a self-assessment of how the patient interprets his/her health to be, risk factors, biometric measurements, and compliance. Completion of the HRA tool takes approximately 20 minutes and may be done via the internet or on a paper-based document. Assessments that emphasize a patient or caregiver focus may be referred to as HRA plus assessments and as such should be person centered and culturally appropriate in all areas, including, but not limited to, the assessment instrument, the administration process of the assessment, clinician communication with the patient regarding findings, as well as followup and monitoring. Additionally, the patient-focused HRA takes into consideration the importance of care support services over and above the health care system; for example, by family members, community support services, or even in the workplace setting where the individual receiving care is not deemed to be a "patient." An emphasis is also placed on cultural competency as means of limited health disparities through respect of the patient's beliefs and understanding the mental and physical ways a patient can experience illness and health and working together to establish a health plan. Another area of patient-focused care involves areas of importance to patients as consumers, such as convenience as well as increasing outcomes that matter to patients; for example, improved quality of life and function. Similarly, caregiver-focused assessment tools serve to identify areas of concern such as stress levels, depression, and the burdens placed on the caregiver. HRAs contribute to the goals of the government to drive health improvements, quality of life, and value for the health care delivery system in the United States. Report 96160 for administration of a patient-focused health risk assessment tool and 96161 for administration of a caregiver-focused assessment tool. Both codes include scoring and documentation of the assessment tool.

Relative Value Units/Medicare Edits

Non-Facility RVU	Work	PE	MP	Total
96160	0.0	0.09	0.0	0.09
96161	0.0	0.09	0.0	0.09
Facility RVU	**Work**	**PE**	**MP**	**Total**
96160	0.0	0.09	0.0	0.09
96161	0.0	0.09	0.0	0.09

96360-96361

96360 Intravenous infusion, hydration; initial, 31 minutes to 1 hour

\+ **96361** each additional hour (List separately in addition to code for primary procedure)

Explanation

A physician or an assistant under direct physician supervision infuses a hydration solution (prepackaged fluid and electrolytes) for 31 minutes to one hour through an intravenous catheter inserted by needle into a patient's vein or by infusion through an existing indwelling intravascular access catheter or port. Report 96361 for each additional hour beyond the first hour. Intravenous infusion for hydration lasting 30 minutes or less is not reported.

Relative Value Units/Medicare Edits

Non-Facility RVU	Work	PE	MP	Total
96360	0.17	0.79	0.01	0.97
96361	0.09	0.27	0.01	0.37
Facility RVU	**Work**	**PE**	**MP**	**Total**
96360	0.17	0.79	0.01	0.97
96361	0.09	0.27	0.01	0.37

96365-96368

96365 Intravenous infusion, for therapy, prophylaxis, or diagnosis (specify substance or drug); initial, up to 1 hour

\+ **96366** each additional hour (List separately in addition to code for primary procedure)

\+ **96367** additional sequential infusion of a new drug/substance, up to 1 hour (List separately in addition to code for primary procedure)

\+ **96368** concurrent infusion (List separately in addition to code for primary procedure)

Explanation

A physician or an assistant under direct physician supervision injects or infuses a therapeutic, prophylactic (preventive), or diagnostic medication other than chemotherapy or other highly complex drugs or biologic agents via intravenous route. Infusions are administered through an intravenous catheter inserted by needle into a patient's vein or by injection or infusion through an existing indwelling intravascular access catheter or port. Report 96365 for the initial hour and 96366 for each additional hour. Report 96367 for each additional sequential infusion of a different substance or drug, up to one hour, and 96368 for each concurrent infusion of substances other than chemotherapy or other highly complex drugs or biologic agents.

Relative Value Units/Medicare Edits

Non-Facility RVU	Work	PE	MP	Total
96365	0.21	1.63	0.04	1.88
96366	0.18	0.42	0.01	0.61
96367	0.19	0.65	0.01	0.85
96368	0.17	0.41	0.01	0.59
Facility RVU	**Work**	**PE**	**MP**	**Total**
96365	0.21	1.63	0.04	1.88
96366	0.18	0.42	0.01	0.61
96367	0.19	0.65	0.01	0.85
96368	0.17	0.41	0.01	0.59

96369-96371

96369 Subcutaneous infusion for therapy or prophylaxis (specify substance or drug); initial, up to 1 hour, including pump set-up and establishment of subcutaneous infusion site(s)

\+ **96370** each additional hour (List separately in addition to code for primary procedure)

\+ **96371** additional pump set-up with establishment of new subcutaneous infusion site(s) (List separately in addition to code for primary procedure)

Explanation

A physician or an assistant under direct physician supervision infuses a therapeutic or prophylactic (preventive) medication other than chemotherapy or other highly complex drug or biologic agent via a subcutaneous route. Indications for subcutaneous infusion may include coma, dysphagia, nausea/vomiting, intestinal obstruction, malabsorption, or extreme weakness. Infusions are administered through a needle inserted beneath the skin; common infusion sites include the upper arm, shoulder, abdomen, and thigh. Report 96369 for infusions lasting longer than 15 minutes and up to one hour. This code includes pump set-up and the establishment of subcutaneous infusion sites. Report 96370 for each additional hour and 96371 for an additional pump set-up with the establishment of new subcutaneous infusion sites. Codes 96369 and 96371 should be reported only once per encounter.

Relative Value Units/Medicare Edits

Non-Facility RVU	Work	PE	MP	Total
96369	0.21	4.0	0.03	4.24
96370	0.18	0.29	0.01	0.48
96371	0.0	1.8	0.01	1.81
Facility RVU	**Work**	**PE**	**MP**	**Total**
96369	0.21	4.0	0.03	4.24
96370	0.18	0.29	0.01	0.48
96371	0.0	1.8	0.01	1.81

96372-96376

96372 Therapeutic, prophylactic, or diagnostic injection (specify substance or drug); subcutaneous or intramuscular

96373 intra-arterial

96374 intravenous push, single or initial substance/drug

\+ **96375** each additional sequential intravenous push of a new substance/drug (List separately in addition to code for primary procedure)

\+ **96376** Therapeutic, prophylactic, or diagnostic injection (specify substance or drug); each additional sequential intravenous push of the same substance/drug provided in a facility (List separately in addition to code for primary procedure)

Explanation

The physician or an assistant under direct physician supervision administers a therapeutic, prophylactic, or diagnostic substance by subcutaneous or intramuscular injection (96372), intra-arterial injection (96373), or by push into an intravenous catheter or intravascular access device (96374 for a single or initial substance, 96375 for each additional sequential IV push of a new substance, and 96376 for each additional sequential IV push of the same substance after 30 minutes have elapsed). The push technique involves an infusion of 15 minutes or less, or one in which the physician or supervised assistant is continuously present to administer the injection and observe the patient. Code 96376 may be reported only by facilities.

Relative Value Units/Medicare Edits

Non-Facility RVU	Work	PE	MP	Total
96372	0.17	0.25	0.01	0.43
96373	0.17	0.38	0.01	0.56
96374	0.18	0.9	0.02	1.1
96375	0.1	0.35	0.01	0.46
96376	0.0	0.0	0.0	0.0
Facility RVU	**Work**	**PE**	**MP**	**Total**
96372	0.17	0.25	0.01	0.43
96373	0.17	0.38	0.01	0.56
96374	0.18	0.9	0.02	1.1
96375	0.1	0.35	0.01	0.46
96376	0.0	0.0	0.0	0.0

98980-98981

98980 Remote therapeutic monitoring treatment management services, physician or other qualified health care professional time in a calendar month requiring at least one interactive communication with the patient or caregiver during the calendar month; first 20 minutes

\+ **98981** Remote therapeutic monitoring treatment management services, physician or other qualified health care professional time in a calendar month requiring at least one interactive communication with the patient or caregiver during the calendar month; each additional 20 minutes (List separately in addition to code for primary procedure)

Explanation

The physician or other qualified health care professional (QHP) provides therapeutic monitoring treatment management services remotely to a patient under an individualized treatment plan. The results of remote therapeutic monitoring that has been ordered by a physician or QHP are used in this service, which requires at least one interactive communication with the patient or the patient's caregiver. Report 98980 for the first completed 20 minutes of time spent by the physician or QHP in a calendar month; this is reported once regardless of the number of monitoring modalities performed. Report 98981 for each additional 20 minutes.

Relative Value Units/Medicare Edits

Non-Facility RVU	Work	PE	MP	Total
98980	0.62	0.86	0.04	1.52
98981	0.61	0.55	0.04	1.2
Facility RVU	**Work**	**PE**	**MP**	**Total**
98980	0.62	0.25	0.04	0.91
98981	0.61	0.25	0.04	0.9

99026-99027

99026 Hospital mandated on call service; in-hospital, each hour
99027 out-of-hospital, each hour

Explanation

These codes report the time for hospital mandated on call service provided by the physician and do not include prolonged physician attendance time for standby services or the time spent performing other reportable procedures or services. Report 99026 for each hour of hospital mandated on call service spent in the hospital and 99027 for each hour of hospital mandated on call service spent outside the hospital.

99070, 99072

99070 Supplies and materials (except spectacles), provided by the physician or other qualified health care professional over and above those usually included with the office visit or other services rendered (list drugs, trays, supplies, or materials provided)
99072 Additional supplies, materials, and clinical staff time over and above those usually included in an office visit or other nonfacility service(s), when performed during a Public Health Emergency, as defined by law, due to respiratory-transmitted infectious disease

Explanation

Code 99070 is adjunct to basic services rendered. The physician or other qualified provider reports this code to indicate supplies and materials provided over and above those usually included with an office visit or services rendered. This code does not include eyeglasses; report the appropriate supply code if eyeglasses are provided. List drugs, trays, supplies, and other materials provided when using this code. Code 99072 reports additional supplies, materials, and clinical staff time necessary to perform safety protocols only during a public health emergency (PHE) due to respiratory-transmitted infectious disease. Examples include cleaning supplies, face shields and surgical masks, pre-visit screenings and instructions, and symptom checks upon patient's arrival to the office. Extra precautions, over and above those usually included in an office visit or other non-facility services, are taken to ensure the safety of patients and health care professionals during in-person interactions while allowing for the provision of evaluation, treatment, or procedural services. Use of this code does not depend on a specific patient diagnosis. It may be reported only once per in-person patient encounter per provider identification number.

99190-99192

99190 Assembly and operation of pump with oxygenator or heat exchanger (with or without ECG and/or pressure monitoring); each hour
99191 45 minutes
99192 30 minutes

Explanation

The health care provider assembles and operates a pump with an oxygenator or heat exchanger. Report 99190 to identify each hour; 99191 to report 45 minutes; and 99192 to report 30 minutes.

99195

99195 Phlebotomy, therapeutic (separate procedure)

Explanation

The health care provider draws blood from the patient to right dramatically imbalanced blood levels (i.e., hemoglobin, potassium salts). The procedure is similar to drawing blood from a donor, but a number of pints may be taken to reduce the imbalance. Blood removal is performed under a physician's direction.

Relative Value Units/Medicare Edits

Non-Facility RVU	Work	PE	MP	Total
99195	0.0	2.81	0.06	2.87
Facility RVU	**Work**	**PE**	**MP**	**Total**
99195	0.0	2.81	0.06	2.87

0234T-0238T

0234T Transluminal peripheral atherectomy, open or percutaneous, including radiological supervision and interpretation; renal artery
0235T visceral artery (except renal), each vessel
0236T abdominal aorta
0237T brachiocephalic trunk and branches, each vessel
0238T iliac artery, each vessel

Explanation

The physician treats a stenosed artery percutaneously or via open surgical incision to relieve a blockage. In the percutaneous approach, a needle punctures the skin at the access site and is followed by a guidewire and an introducer sheath to protect and enclose the opening. A series of catheters and guidewires are inserted until the stenosed area has been traversed. An atherectomy catheter is manipulated to the study area and activated to cut or drill a channel through the plaque lesion and reopen the artery. Contrast medium is injected to fluoroscopically visualize the degree of luminal opening. The process may be repeated with a larger diameter catheter if necessary. In the open surgical approach, the physician creates a femoral cutdown incision to expose one of the femoral arteries. The physician punctures the femoral artery with a large needle and passes a guidewire via the needle into the artery. The physician removes the needle while leaving the guidewire in place, enlarges the arterial opening slightly with a blade, and slides an introducer sheath over the guidewire into the arterial lumen. The physician slides a guidewire through the atherectomy catheter or device and inserts the guidewire/atherectomy catheter combination through the introducer sheath into the stenosed vessel. The atherectomy device is fluoroscopically positioned at the area of stenosis and then activated to remove the stenotic tissue. The physician rechecks the diameter of the lesion by angiography. Several passes with the atherectomy device may be required. The physician removes the atherectomy catheter, guidewire, and introducer sheath, closing the femoral arteriotomy with suture. Report 0234T when the blockage occurs in the renal artery; 0235T in a visceral artery; 0236T in the abdominal aorta; 0237T in the brachiocephalic trunk and branches; and 0238T in the iliac artery.

0266T-0271T

0266T Implantation or replacement of carotid sinus baroreflex activation device; total system (includes generator placement, unilateral or bilateral lead placement, intra-operative interrogation, programming, and repositioning, when performed)

0267T lead only, unilateral (includes intra-operative interrogation, programming, and repositioning, when performed)

0268T pulse generator only (includes intra-operative interrogation, programming, and repositioning, when performed)

0269T Revision or removal of carotid sinus baroreflex activation device; total system (includes generator placement, unilateral or bilateral lead placement, intra-operative interrogation, programming, and repositioning, when performed)

0270T lead only, unilateral (includes intra-operative interrogation, programming, and repositioning, when performed)

0271T pulse generator only (includes intra-operative interrogation, programming, and repositioning, when performed)

Explanation

A carotid sinus baroreflex activation system is implanted for the treatment of advanced heart failure and refractory hypertension. One proprietary stimulation device works by activating the body's baroreceptors (pressure sensors found within the walls of the carotid arteries that regulate heart rate and blood pressure). Consisting of an implantable pulse generator (IPG), a single 2 mm coated carotid sinus lead (electrode), and a wireless programmer system, the device prompts the body's natural reflexes to control blood pressure and the causal elements of heart failure progression. With the patient under general anesthesia, an incision is made on the left or right side of the neck and the soft tissues are dissected until the common carotid artery is located. The electrode, with a 7 mm silicone backer, is sutured to the carotid artery to activate the baroreceptors. An incision is made below the clavicle to form a pocket for the baroreflex activation generator. The wire attached to the electrode is tunneled beneath the skin to the generator pocket and connected to the IPG, which controls the baroreflex activation energy. The physician programs the IPG based on the patient's individual requirements. The IPG is secured within the surgically created pocket. The system is tested, and all incisions are closed routinely. Report 0266T for insertion or replacement of the entire carotid sinus baroreflex activation system (generator and lead); report 0267T for unilateral lead insertion or replacement; and report 0268T for insertion or replacement of the pulse generator only. Report 0269T for revision or removal of the entire carotid sinus baroreflex activation system (generator and lead); report 0270T for unilateral lead revision or removal; and report 0271T for revision or removal of the pulse generator only. These codes include intraoperative interrogation, programming, and repositioning.

0272T-0273T

0272T Interrogation device evaluation (in person), carotid sinus baroreflex activation system, including telemetric iterative communication with the implantable device to monitor device diagnostics and programmed therapy values, with interpretation and report (eg, battery status, lead impedance, pulse amplitude, pulse width, therapy frequency, pathway mode, burst mode, therapy start/stop times each day);

0273T with programming

Explanation

The purpose of these studies is to ensure that the carotid sinus baroreflex activation system is positioned well and working properly in order to guarantee proper function of the system in the future. A carotid sinus baroreflex activation system is implanted for refractory hypertension. The baroreflex sends signals to the brain to naturally regulate blood pressure. The insertion of this system allows the signals to be triggered artificially, causing the body to lower blood pressure. There are two components to a baroreflex activation system: a generator, which is positioned in a pocket below the clavicle, and electrodes (leads), one placed on each carotid sinus in the neck. The physician interrogates the device using the wireless programmer and collects and reports information including battery status, lead impedance, pulse amplitude and width, therapy frequency, pathway and burst modes, and therapy start and stop times. This interrogation must be performed in person. Report 0272T for the evaluation and 0273T if programming is performed in addition to the evaluation.

0331T-0332T

0331T Myocardial sympathetic innervation imaging, planar qualitative and quantitative assessment;

0332T Myocardial sympathetic innervation imaging, planar qualitative and quantitative assessment; with tomographic SPECT

Explanation

Myocardial sympathetic innervation imaging is performed to help assess cardiac nerve activity in patients with heart failure. Iodine meta-iodobenzylguanidine (MIBG) is injected intravenously. Planar images are taken at 15 minutes (early) and four hours (late) after injection to test the MIBG concentration levels in the myocardial sympathetic nerve endings. Qualitative and quantitative studies are performed using the average count per pixel and decrease in counts between early and late images. Report 0332T if single-photon emission computed tomography imaging is performed after the early and late planar images.

0338T-0339T

0338T Transcatheter renal sympathetic denervation, percutaneous approach including arterial puncture, selective catheter placement(s) renal artery(ies), fluoroscopy, contrast injection(s), intraprocedural roadmapping and radiological supervision and interpretation, including pressure gradient measurements, flush aortogram and diagnostic renal angiography when performed; unilateral

0339T bilateral

Explanation

A small incision is made over the femoral artery and a catheter with an electrode on the tip is inserted. Using fluoroscopic guidance, the catheter is maneuvered to the renal artery. The catheter is connected to a radiofrequency generator that delivers lower powered, precisely focused bursts of energy to disrupt the surrounding renal nerves and reduce the renal contribution to central blood pressure elevation. Report 0338T for a unilateral procedure and 0339T when performed bilaterally.

0342T

0342T Therapeutic apheresis with selective HDL delipidation and plasma reinfusion

Explanation

Therapeutic apheresis with selective high-density lipoprotein (HDL) delipidation and plasma reinfusion is a procedure in which plasma is removed from the body by apheresis, processed through a delipidation device, and returned to the patient. This technique may be employed to reduce atherosclerosis development in cardiovascular disease. Vascular access is established. A bag of the patient's blood is collected and the plasma is separated from the rest of the blood constituents. The red blood cells may be returned to the bloodstream. The plasma is treated, removing the cholesterol from HDL (good cholesterol), which results in what is known as pre-beta-HDL. This pre-beta-HDL infused plasma is considered delipidated plasma. The delipidated plasma is infused back into the patient once a week for seven weeks.

0345T

0345T Transcatheter mitral valve repair percutaneous approach via the coronary sinus

Explanation

A percutaneous mitral valve repair is performed. The right atrium of the heart is accessed using a catheter inserted in the internal jugular or subclavian vein. The coronary sinus is located and intubated with the compressed device within a sheath. An anchor, which resembles and functions much like a stent, on one end of the device is placed in the great cardiac vein and another is placed at the coronary sinus ostium and expanded, holding them in place. The anchors are connected by a bridge or wire. The bridge is made of dissolvable material that dissipates over time and pulls the anchors together, closing the mitral annulus. If the wire technique is used, the wire is pulled to bring the anchors closer together to shorten the mitral annulus before the anchors are expanded. Coronary compression may be assessed by angiogram and tension of the anchors adjusted. The sheath and catheter are removed and any wounds closed.

0408T-0411T

0408T Insertion or replacement of permanent cardiac contractility modulation system, including contractility evaluation when performed, and programming of sensing and therapeutic parameters; pulse generator with transvenous electrodes

0409T pulse generator only

0410T atrial electrode only

0411T ventricular electrode only

Explanation

Cardiac contractility modulation (CCM) is utilized to improve ventricular pump function and for patients who have normal QRS duration. The device consists of a programmable and rechargeable generator, powered by a lithium battery. The patient is given local anesthesia and the device is implanted within a pocket on the right side of the chest below the collarbone with an electrode fixed on the carotid sinus. One incision allows access to the cervical vagal nerve with another incision made for insertion of the right ventricular electrode. The vagal electrode is connected to the generator via subcutaneous tunnel. This unit includes three standard leads placed transvenously into the right side of the heart: one in the right atrium for sensing and two in the right ventricle for sensing and delivery of impulses. These impulses do not change the cardiac sequence (rhythm), but instead modify contractility by sending high-energy impulses to the myocardium during the refractory period. The unit allows the patient the ability to recharge the battery with an external charger that operates transcutaneously. This is required once a week and typically takes about 90 minutes. Programming and interrogation follows the same process as a pacemaker. Report 0408T for insertion or replacement of the entire system, including evaluation and programming when performed; 0409T for insertion or replacement of the pulse generator only; 0410T for insertion or replacement of the atrial electrode only; and 0411T for insertion or replacement of the ventricular electrode only.

0412T-0413T

0412T Removal of permanent cardiac contractility modulation system; pulse generator only

0413T transvenous electrode (atrial or ventricular)

Explanation

In 0412T, the physician removes a cardiac contractility modulation (CCM) system. The pocket is opened. The existing system is disconnected from the wire and removed. In 0413T, the electrodes are removed (atrial or ventricular). Previous insertion incisions may be reopened for removal of electrodes, which are disconnected from the generator as well as the vagal nerve, right atrium, and right ventricle.

0414T

0414T Removal and replacement of permanent cardiac contractility modulation system pulse generator only

Explanation

The physician removes and replaces a cardiac contractility modulation (CCM) system generator. The pocket is opened. The existing system is disconnected form the wire and removed. The electrodes remain in position and a new CCM system is inserted into the pocket. The electrodes are connected to the new system and tested. The pocket is closed.

0415T

0415T Repositioning of previously implanted cardiac contractility modulation transvenous electrode, (atrial or ventricular lead)

Explanation

The physician repositions a previously implanted cardiac contractility modulation transvenous electrode (atrial or ventricular lead). The physician gains access transvenously with imaging guidance and the electrode is repositioned. Depending on the extent of the work, the electrode may require reconnection to the generator, which would be tested for appropriate function. The incisions are closed.

0416T

0416T Relocation of skin pocket for implanted cardiac contractility modulation pulse generator

Explanation

The physician relocates a cardiac contractility modulation (CCM) system generator due to complications from the original generator placement. The pocket is opened and the generator is removed. A new pocket is formed within the subcutaneous tissue in close proximity of the existing electrodes. The electrodes are brought through a new subcutaneous tunnel into the new pocket. The old pocket is closed. The new or existing generator is inserted into the pocket and the electrodes are attached and tested. The pocket is closed.

0417T-0418T

0417T Programming device evaluation (in person) with iterative adjustment of the implantable device to test the function of the device and select optimal permanent programmed values with analysis, including review and report, implantable cardiac contractility modulation system

0418T Interrogation device evaluation (in person) with analysis, review and report, includes connection, recording and disconnection per patient encounter, implantable cardiac contractility modulation system

Explanation

A programming device evaluation (0417T) or interrogation (0418T) is performed in person in order to test the device's function and select the most favorable permanent programmed values. Patients with previously implanted cardiac contractility modulation (CCM) systems require periodic programming device evaluations. These diagnostic procedures include a face-to-face assessment of all device functions. Components that must be evaluated in order to assign a code from this range include the battery, leads, capture and sensing function, and programmed parameters. Stored and measured data regarding these components are retrieved using an office, hospital, or emergency room instrument. This information is assessed to discern battery voltage, lead impedance, and settings, as well as to determine the device's current programming. In 0417T, if necessary, the sensing value and rate response, upper and lower heart rates, impulses, and diagnostics are adjusted. These codes include physician or other qualified health care professional analysis, review, interpretation, and report, and are assigned per procedure. They also include connection, recording, and disconnection.

0439T

+ **0439T** Myocardial contrast perfusion echocardiography, at rest or with stress, for assessment of myocardial ischemia or viability (List separately in addition to code for primary procedure)

Explanation

Myocardial contrast perfusion echocardiography is used to examine myocardial microcirculation. Intravenous infusion of contrast containing microbubbles that exist primarily within the vascular space and maintain intravascular characteristics similar to red blood cells is utilized. Injection of contrast into the venous system may also be used since the microbubbles will continue circulating for approximately three to five minutes after injection. Low intensity ultrasound is necessary in order to avoid destroying the microbubbles. The perfusion is analyzed as the microbubbles are destroyed with a burst of high intensity ultrasound and the rate of restoration is evaluated as the microbubbles flow back into myocardial circulation. This evaluation can determine the velocity and peak myocardial signal intensity allowing for quantification of any changes. This imaging provides improved resolution that enables the physician to detect perfusion defects that may not be seen in lower resolution imaging.

0483T-0484T

0483T Transcatheter mitral valve implantation/replacement (TMVI) with prosthetic valve; percutaneous approach, including transseptal puncture, when performed

0484T transthoracic exposure (eg, thoracotomy, transapical)

Explanation

The physician performs transcatheter mitral valve implantation or replacement (TMVI). Mitral regurgitation (MR) is a condition that may be treated with transcatheter mitral valve implantation or replacement (TMVI/TMVR) in patients who are at high risk for open heart surgery. In 0483T, the procedure is performed via a percutaneous approach and includes a transseptal puncture, when performed. Under general anesthesia, the physician makes an incision over a lower extremity vessel, usually the femoral vein. A catheter with a specially designed prosthesis is maneuvered through the vessels to the heart under fluoroscopic imaging guidance. The catheter is threaded through the inferior vena cava to the right atrium where the interatrial wall or septum is punctured to access the left atrium. When the left atrium is accessed, the catheter is further advanced through the mitral valve and to the left ventricle. A stent-based prosthesis is implanted within the mitral annulus. In 0484T, under general anesthesia, the physician makes a left lateral mini-thoracotomy. The transapical puncture involves using a large bore needle to puncture the chest wall directly into the left ventricular cavity. A small incision is made between ribs (usually the fifth or sixth intercostal space) on the lower left side of the patient's chest to achieve direct access to the heart. A catheter is inserted following the guidewire to the mitral valve. A balloon is inflated to compress the native valve. The self-expanding prosthesis is introduced through the catheter, partially uncovered. Once in the left atrium, the catheter is deployed and secured using polyethylene tether fastened to an epicardial pad. Pledgeted sutures are placed. The tether tension is modified after the prosthesis has been deployed to ensure optimal placement of the device but also to limit movement of it within the annulus. No cardiopulmonary bypass or rapid ventricular pacing is required during the procedure. These procedures include vascular access, catheterization, balloon valvuloplasty, deploying the valve, repositioning the valve as needed, temporary pacemaker insertion for rapid pacing, and access site closure, when performed. Angiography, radiological supervision and interpretation, intraprocedural roadmapping to guide TMVI (e.g., contrast injections, fluoroscopy), left ventriculography (e.g., to assess mitral regurgitation for guidance of TMVI), and completion angiography are also included.

[0623T, 0624T, 0625T, 0626T]

0623T Automated quantification and characterization of coronary atherosclerotic plaque to assess severity of coronary disease, using data from coronary computed tomographic angiography; data preparation and transmission, computerized analysis of data, with review of computerized analysis output to reconcile discordant data, interpretation and report

0624T Automated quantification and characterization of coronary atherosclerotic plaque to assess severity of coronary disease, using data from coronary computed tomographic angiography; data preparation and transmission

0625T Automated quantification and characterization of coronary atherosclerotic plaque to assess severity of coronary disease, using data from coronary computed tomographic angiography; computerized analysis of data from coronary computed tomographic angiography

0626T Automated quantification and characterization of coronary atherosclerotic plaque to assess severity of coronary disease, using data from coronary computed tomographic angiography; review of computerized analysis output to reconcile discordant data, interpretation and report

Explanation

Using data from a coronary computed tomographic angiogram (CTA) that is reported separately, the severity of coronary artery disease is assessed by automated quantification/characterization of atherosclerotic plaque. This web-based service uses computerized algorithms to evaluate the degree and severity of disease; the computer-generated findings are then provided to the physician or other qualified healthcare professional in an interactive format for their final review and report. Report 0624T for data preparation and transmission only; 0625T for the computerized analysis only of data derived from the CTA; 0626T for review of the computerized analysis output to resolve conflicting data and subsequent interpretation and report; and 0623T if all components of the prior listed codes are included. These codes may be reported once per coronary CTA.

[0523T]

+ **0523T** Intraprocedural coronary fractional flow reserve (FFR) with 3D functional mapping of color-coded FFR values for the coronary tree, derived from coronary angiogram data, for real-time review and interpretation of possible atherosclerotic stenosis(es) intervention (List separately in addition to code for primary procedure)

Explanation

Noninvasive 3-dimensional (3-D) fractional flow reserve (FFR) enabled interpretation is performed during a coronary angiography procedure for possible atherosclerotic stenosis as an aid to the physician in making a determination for whether a percutaneous coronary intervention (PCI) is indicated and whether revascularization occurs in each angiography procedure performed. Medically recognized standards generally recommend that revascularization by percutaneous coronary intervention (PCI) is to be performed when the patient's stenosis of >50 percent is observed of the left main (LM) stem or proximal left anterior descending (LAD) coronary artery during angiography, the patient has one remaining patent vessel, or the patient suffers from two- or three-vessel disease with a left ventricular ejection fraction <40 percent. The Cathworks FFRangio™ System is a proprietary FFR platform that accurately conveys evidence-based multi-vessel physiologic measurements to enable the physician to confirm whether or not to proceed with intraprocedural PCI therapy.

0505T

0505T Endovenous femoral-popliteal arterial revascularization, with transcatheter placement of intravascular stent graft(s) and closure by any method, including percutaneous or open vascular access, ultrasound guidance for vascular access when performed, all catheterization(s) and intraprocedural roadmapping and imaging guidance necessary to complete the intervention, all associated radiological supervision and interpretation, when performed, with crossing of the occlusive lesion in an extraluminal fashion

Explanation

The physician bypasses an occlusion or stenosis in the femoral or femoropopliteal arterial segment of the leg by skirting the blocked area using the adjacent femoropopliteal vein as a pathway to place proprietary covered stents. In one method, the physician obtains access to the femoral artery opposite that of the affected limb (contralateral) and advances a guidewire over the aortic bifurcation to the occluded site in the affected femoral artery. A second access is obtained distally on this same side (ipsilateral) in the tibial vein. Proximal and distal anastomoses are created above and below the area of occlusion using a crossing device, a snare cage, and guidewires. Following balloon dilation of both proximal and distal anastomosis sites, stent grafts are inserted and deployed in an overlapping fashion from the popliteal artery into the femoral vein, and from the femoral vein into the femoral artery. Once dilated, the stents create an endograft bypass around the occlusion, utilizing the vein as a conduit. Final angiograms are obtained to verify patency and the incision sites are closed.

[0620T]

0620T Endovascular venous arterialization, tibial or peroneal vein, with transcatheter placement of intravascular stent graft(s) and closure by any method, including percutaneous or open vascular access, ultrasound guidance for vascular access when performed, all catheterization(s) and intraprocedural roadmapping and imaging guidance necessary to complete the intervention, all associated radiological supervision and interpretation, when performed

Explanation

The physician performs endovascular venous arterialization of the tibial or peroneal vein with transcatheter placement of one or more intravascular stent grafts in patients suffering from critical limb ischemia. In this chronic condition, there is lack of blood circulation to the foot due to blockages of the arteries in the leg. In one proprietary method, catheters are inserted under ultrasound guidance into the tibial vein at the level of the ankle and into the femoral artery at the level of the groin. Both catheters are advanced simultaneously toward each other; during this time, ultrasound waves are emitted by the arterial catheter toward the receiving venous catheter to assist the physician in determining the most optimal location for channel creation from the artery to the vein. An embedded needle within the arterial ultrasound catheter crosses over and is inserted into the vein, creating the connection between artery and vein. The physician inflates a small angioplasty balloon to allow for the passage of other devices. A valvulotome consisting of a small basket with minute incision hooks is introduced to cut through valves near the bottom of the foot in order to maximize the arterial flow to the vein into the foot. The severed valves are rendered incompetent, allowing oxygenated blood to flow forward and into the foot. Finally, several self-expanding covered metal stents are placed to act as permanent conduits for blood flow to the foot. Catheters are removed, incision sites are closed, and the patient observed. This code includes ultrasound guidance for vascular access, all intraprocedural roadmapping, catheterizations, and imaging guidance necessary to complete the procedure, and all associated radiological supervision and interpretation when performed.

0515T-0517T

0515T Insertion of wireless cardiac stimulator for left ventricular pacing, including device interrogation and programming, and imaging supervision and interpretation, when performed; complete system (includes electrode and generator [transmitter and battery])

0516T electrode only

0517T both components of pulse generator (battery and transmitter) only

Explanation

The physician inserts a wireless cardiac stimulator for left ventricular pacing. Wireless cardiac stimulator systems include a wireless endocardial left ventricular electrode that is typically implanted in the artery of the left ventricular wall. The electrode is wirelessly powered via ultrasound pulses originating from a transmitter implanted into one of two subcutaneous pockets created on the chest wall. The cardiac stimulator system also includes a pulse generator, which is comprised of two separate elements: a transmitter and a battery. The battery is housed in the other chest wall pocket. The battery and the electrode are connected via a subcutaneously tunneled cable. This system provides biventricular pacing by sensing right ventricular pacing output from a previously placed conventional device (i.e., pacemaker or defibrillator using uni- or biventricular leads) that subsequently transmits an ultrasound pulse to the wireless electrode inserted onto the left ventricle endocardium, resulting in a left ventricular pacing pulse emission. Patients who have both a wireless device and a conventional pacing device require separate programming and interrogation of each device. Report 0515T for insertion of the complete wireless cardiac stimulation system; 0516T for insertion of the electrode only; and 0517T for insertion of the pulse generator only, including both the battery and transmitter. All codes include programming and interrogation and all echocardiography and imaging, when performed.

0518T, 0519T-0520T [0861T]

0861T Removal of pulse generator for wireless cardiac stimulator for left ventricular pacing; both components (battery and transmitter)

0518T battery component only

0519T Removal and replacement of pulse generator for wireless cardiac stimulator for left ventricular pacing, including device interrogation and programming; both components (battery and transmitter)

0520T battery component only

Explanation

The physician removes a pulse generator battery and/or transmitter for a wireless cardiac stimulator for left ventricular pacing. Wireless cardiac stimulator systems include a wireless endocardial left ventricular electrode that is typically implanted in the artery of the left ventricular wall. The electrode is wirelessly powered via ultrasound pulses originating from a transmitter implanted into one of two subcutaneous pockets created on the chest wall. The cardiac stimulator system also includes a pulse generator, which is comprised of two separate elements: a transmitter and a battery. The battery is housed in the other chest wall pocket. The battery and the electrode are connected via a subcutaneously tunneled cable. This system provides biventricular pacing by sensing right ventricular pacing output from a previously placed conventional device (i.e., pacemaker or defibrillator using uni- or biventricular leads) that subsequently transmits an ultrasound pulse to the wireless electrode inserted onto the left ventricle endocardium, resulting in a left ventricular pacing pulse emission. Patients who have both a wireless device and a conventional pacing device require separate programming and interrogation of each device. Report 0861T for removal of the pulse generator, including both the battery and transmitter; 0518T for removal of the battery only; 0519T for removal with replacement of the pulse generator, including both battery and transmitter; and 0520T when only the battery component is removed and replaced. Codes 0519T and 0520T include device interrogation and programming.

[0862T, 0863T]

0862T Relocation of pulse generator for wireless cardiac stimulator for left ventricular pacing, including device interrogation and programming; battery component only

0863T Relocation of pulse generator for wireless cardiac stimulator for left ventricular pacing, including device interrogation and programming; transmitter component only

Explanation

The physician relocates a pulse generator for a wireless cardiac stimulator for left ventricular pacing. Wireless cardiac stimulator systems include a wireless endocardial left ventricular electrode that is typically implanted in the artery of the left ventricular wall. The electrode is wirelessly powered via ultrasound pulses originating from a transmitter implanted into one of two subcutaneous pockets created on the chest wall. The cardiac stimulator system also includes a pulse generator, which is comprised of two separate elements: a transmitter and a battery. The battery is housed in the other chest wall pocket. The battery and the electrode are connected via a subcutaneously tunneled cable. This system provides biventricular pacing by sensing right ventricular pacing output from a previously placed conventional device (i.e., pacemaker or defibrillator using uni- or biventricular leads) that subsequently transmits an ultrasound pulse to the wireless electrode inserted onto the left ventricle endocardium, resulting in a left ventricular pacing pulse emission. Patients who have both a wireless device and a conventional pacing device require separate programming and interrogation of each device. Report 0862T for relocation of the pulse generator battery only; 0863T for the transmitter only. These codes include device interrogation and programming.

0521T-0522T

0521T Interrogation device evaluation (in person) with analysis, review and report, includes connection, recording, and disconnection per patient encounter, wireless cardiac stimulator for left ventricular pacing

0522T Programming device evaluation (in person) with iterative adjustment of the implantable device to test the function of the device and select optimal permanent programmed values with analysis, including review and report, wireless cardiac stimulator for left ventricular pacing

Explanation

The physician or other qualified health care provider performs an in-person interrogation or programming device evaluation for a wireless cardiac stimulator for left ventricular pacing. Wireless cardiac stimulator systems include a wireless endocardial left ventricular electrode that is typically implanted in the artery of the left ventricular wall. The electrode is wirelessly powered via ultrasound pulses originating from a transmitter implanted into one of two subcutaneous pockets created on the chest wall. The cardiac stimulator system also includes a pulse generator, which is comprised of two separate elements: a transmitter and a battery. The battery is housed in the other chest wall pocket. The battery and the electrode are connected via a subcutaneously tunneled cable. This system provides biventricular pacing by sensing right ventricular pacing output from a previously placed conventional device (i.e., pacemaker or defibrillator using uni- or biventricular leads) that subsequently transmits an ultrasound pulse to the wireless electrode inserted onto the left ventricle endocardium, resulting in a left ventricular pacing pulse emission. Patients who have both a wireless device and a conventional pacing device require separate programming and interrogation of each device. Report 0521T for interrogation evaluation, including analysis, review, and report. This code includes connection, recording, and disconnection and is reported per patient encounter. Report 0522T for a programming device evaluation, including analysis, review, and report. This code includes adjustment of the device to test the function and select optimal programmed values.

0524T

0524T Endovenous catheter directed chemical ablation with balloon isolation of incompetent extremity vein, open or percutaneous, including all vascular access, catheter manipulation, diagnostic imaging, imaging guidance and monitoring

Explanation

Endovascular catheter-directed chemical ablation with balloon isolation (i.e., balloon sclerotherapy) describes treatment of varicose veins in an extremity by incorporating two familiar procedures: sclerotherapy and balloon catheterization as a minimally invasive and cost-effective treatment option. Traditional catheter-based endovenous sclerotherapy can often have negative effects to the overall body system resulting from the combination of air and the sclerosing agent. The physician uses a double lumen balloon catheter as a means of separating or isolating venous blood, allowing the physician to use the minimal amount of sclerosing agent needed while removing the excess amounts and subsequently limiting the potential for systemic risk. Vein occlusion occurs when the physician carefully retracts the expanded balloon containing the captured sclerotherapeutic agent in between.

0525T-0527T

0525T Insertion or replacement of intracardiac ischemia monitoring system, including testing of the lead and monitor, initial system programming, and imaging supervision and interpretation; complete system (electrode and implantable monitor)

0526T electrode only

0527T implantable monitor only

Explanation

An intracardiac ischemia monitoring system analyzes and records cardiac data to detect ischemic events. If an ischemic event is occurring, the device sends out auditory, visual, and vibrational alerts to the patient to seek medical care immediately. Access to the central caval veins is obtained through the subclavian vein or jugular vein. The vein is penetrated with a large needle and a guidewire is passed through. A fluoroscope is used to guide a standard pacemaker intracardiac lead to the right ventricular apex. A pocket for an implantable device (IMD) that analyzes and records the cardiac data is created and the lead is tested. The lead is connected to the IMD and the subcutaneous pocket is closed. Report 0525T for insertion or replacement of the complete system (electrode and implantable monitor). Report 0526T for insertion or replacement of the electrode only; report 0527T for implantable monitor only. All imaging, including supervision and interpretation, is included in these services.

0528T-0529T

0528T Programming device evaluation (in person) of intracardiac ischemia monitoring system with iterative adjustment of programmed values, with analysis, review, and report

0529T Interrogation device evaluation (in person) of intracardiac ischemia monitoring system with analysis, review, and report

Explanation

An intracardiac ischemia monitoring system analyzes and records cardiac data to detect ischemic events. If an ischemic event is occurring, the device sends out auditory, visual, and vibrational alerts to the patient to seek medical care immediately. In 0528T, a programming device evaluation is performed in person in order to test the functioning of the device and to select the most favorable permanent programming values. Patients with previously implanted monitoring systems require periodic programming device evaluations. This diagnostic procedure includes a face-to-face assessment of all device functions. Stored and measured data regarding these components are retrieved using an office, hospital, or emergency department instrument. This information is assessed in order to discern lead impedance and settings for detection, as well as to determine the system's current programming. If necessary, sensing values and diagnostics are adjusted. In 0529T, only an in-person device interrogation (extraction of data accumulated in a medical device) is performed, accessing the stored and measured data. Both of these codes include clinician analysis, review, and report.

0530T-0532T

0530T Removal of intracardiac ischemia monitoring system, including all imaging supervision and interpretation; complete system (electrode and implantable monitor)

0531T electrode only

0532T implantable monitor only

Explanation

An intracardiac ischemia monitoring system analyzes and records cardiac data to detect ischemic events. If an ischemic event is occurring, the device sends out auditory, visual, and vibrational alerts to the patient to seek medical care immediately. In 0530T, the subcutaneous pocket incision is reopened and the complete system (electrode and implantable monitor) is disconnected from the cardiac lead and removed. The lead is dissected from the scar tissue that has formed around it. Once the lead is completely freed, it is removed. Report 0531T for electrode removal only and 0532T when only the implantable monitor is removed.

0543T

0543T Transapical mitral valve repair, including transthoracic echocardiography, when performed, with placement of artificial chordae tendineae

Explanation

This procedure describes treatment for patients with mitral regurgitation, a progressive condition where the mitral valve does not close appropriately resulting in blood leaking back through the mitral valve. The surgeon performs a thoracotomy and places a proprietary system designed for use when the patient's native chordae tendineae (tough, tendinous type strands of the heart) become elongated or rupture from the disease process. The system contains expandable "jaws" that are used to hold the mitral valve leaflet or cusp and an average of three to four artificial chordae are inserted around the edge of the leaflet in order to rehang the prolapsed leaflet. Transesophageal echocardiography (TEE) is used as guidance to reduce the amount of blood leaking back into the mitral valve by varying the lengths of the artificial chordae. Once the appropriate level has been determined, the chordae are fastened to a small piece of absorbent material and attached to the outer layer of the heart wall.

0544T-0545T

0544T Transcatheter mitral valve annulus reconstruction, with implantation of adjustable annulus reconstruction device, percutaneous approach including transseptal puncture

0545T Transcatheter tricuspid valve annulus reconstruction with implantation of adjustable annulus reconstruction device, percutaneous approach

Explanation

The physician performs a transcatheter mitral valve annulus reconstruction with the implantation of an adjustable annulus reconstructive device. A proprietary system is used in these procedures, comprised of three components: the implant catheter (IC) itself, a guide catheter (GC), and a transseptal steerable sheath (TSS). The implant is made of a contraction wire with a covering made of a polyester fabric that is secured along the back annulus of the mitral valve by stainless steel anchors. Once fastened down, the implant is contracted under fluoroscopy and echocardiography imaging in order to reach the optimum constraint and amount of valvular regurgitation. The surgeon accesses the mitral valve using a percutaneous, catheter-delivered approach going through the femoral vein and the inferior vena cava. A transseptal puncture under transesophageal echocardiography (TEE) imaging is performed to identify the interatrial septum over the back middle mitral commissure, the area where the posterior leaflets or cusps are located. A transseptal steerable sheath (TSS) is introduced into the left atrium using a guidewire and the implant delivery system is advanced through the TSS and into the left atrium. It is positioned to line up with the top of the IC near the front lateral trigone using TEE guidance. Anchors are moved through the fabric of the implant and into the annular tissue to ensure the implant is securely fastened. Once secure, the tip of the IC continues to be moved along to each continuous point of anchoring on the commissure. When the last anchor is positioned in the trigone near the posterior medial commissure, the implant is disconnected from the IC with an average of 12 to 17 anchors required based on the length of the implant. Typically, this system and treatment is most often used for patients with functional mitral regurgitation (FMR) and more recently functional tricuspid regurgitation (FTR). Angiography, all radiological supervision and interpretation, intraprocedural road mapping, ventriculography required for device implantation, and adjustment are included. Report 0545T for reconstruction of the tricuspid valve annulus with an implanted adjustable annulus reconstruction device in a similar manner.

[0643T]

0643T Transcatheter left ventricular restoration device implantation including right and left heart catheterization and left ventriculography when performed, arterial approach

Explanation

Using a proprietary, transcatheter-based structural heart device, the cardiac surgeon, in conjunction with an interventional cardiologist, treats post-myocardial infarction scar tissue on the left ventricle in a beating-heart, minimally invasive procedure. Via a combined right internal jugular transvenous and left lateral mini-thoracotomy approach under fluoroscopic guidance, the physician implants titanium micro-anchor pairs intended to remodel the ventricle in order to reduce wall stress and improve blood flow. The internal (hinged) anchor is placed inside the right ventricle of the heart through the jugular vein, while the external (locking) anchor is placed on the outside of the left ventricle through the thoracoscope, which is inserted via a small incision between two ribs. The anchor pairs are connected by a tether. Once the anchors are in position, the physicians gently pull them toward each other, resulting in the anchor pairs excluding the scar tissue from the healthy tissue on the left ventricle. This isolates the nonfunctioning part of the heart muscle, allowing the remaining healthy tissue to work more effectively. An average of two to three anchor pairs are typically implanted. Left and right heart catheterization and left ventriculography, when performed, are included in this procedure.

0559T-0560T

0559T Anatomic model 3D-printed from image data set(s); first individually prepared and processed component of an anatomic structure

\+ **0560T** each additional individually prepared and processed component of an anatomic structure (List separately in addition to code for primary procedure)

Explanation

These codes describe the creation of three-dimensional (3D) printed models of individually prepared and processed elements of anatomic structures, such as bones, arteries, veins, nerves, ureters, muscles, tendons, ligaments, joints, visceral organs, and the brain. Models may be comprised of one or more distinct parts and incorporate various colors and materials. Uses of 3D-printed anatomic models are continuing to increase for a number of applications including, but not limited to, surgery planning, preparing and practicing for the procedure, training and education of health care professionals, and for patient education.

0561T-0562T

0561T Anatomic guide 3D-printed and designed from image data set(s); first anatomic guide

\+ **0562T** each additional anatomic guide (List separately in addition to code for primary procedure)

Explanation

Three-dimensional (3D) printed cutting or drilling guides are patient-specific surgery guides combining individualized imaging information that is used by the surgeon to navigate a procedure. Each guide is a sole, distinctive tool created to be an exact fit to the patient's natural anatomy customized to precisely match every intervention aspect, such as position and angles that mirror the actual surgery. The use of guides saves considerable time and resources; the predictability permitted by the guides allows for greater confidence in the operation room, which subsequently improves patient outcomes. In some cases, the surgery may require the use of a 3D-printed model and cutting or drilling guide for the same patient.

0569T-0570T

0569T Transcatheter tricuspid valve repair, percutaneous approach; initial prosthesis

\+ **0570T** each additional prosthesis during same session (List separately in addition to code for primary procedure)

Explanation

The physician performs a transcatheter tricuspid valve repair utilizing a percutaneous approach. Transcatheter devices currently in clinical testing include annuloplasty devices (suture, direct, or ring), coaptation devices, and heterotopic caval valve implantation. In one repair method, the surgeon accesses the tricuspid valve using a percutaneous, catheter-delivered approach through the left subclavian or axillary vein. An expandable, foam-filled balloon spacer is advanced through a sheath introducer and is stabilized by a rail that is anchored at the right ventricular apex. This device is intended to reduce the regurgitant orifice area by reducing malcoaptation of the tricuspid leaflets. Report 0569T for the initial prosthesis and 0570T for each additional prosthesis used during the same session.

[0646T]

0646T Transcatheter tricuspid valve implantation (TTVI)/replacement with prosthetic valve, percutaneous approach, including right heart catheterization, temporary pacemaker insertion, and selective right ventricular or right atrial angiography, when performed

Explanation

The physician implants or replaces the tricuspid valve with a prosthetic valve using a percutaneous, transcatheter approach; vascular access is typically gained via the jugular or femoral vein. Tricuspid regurgitation occurs when a diseased, damaged, or malfunctioning tricuspid valve fails to close properly, causing blood to flow backward from the right ventricle to the right atrium. Transcatheter tricuspid valve replacement or implantation (TTVR/TTVI) is most often performed on patients with symptomatic tricuspid regurgitation that are high risk or not eligible for traditional open chest surgery. One proprietary device is a bioprosthetic valve created from bovine tissue and polyester fabric. Set inside a flexible metal structure, it can be placed within the patient's own tricuspid valve. The physician gains access to the femoral vein. Under imaging guidance, a catheter with the prosthetic valve is maneuvered through the vessels to the point of placement in the tricuspid valve, where it is deployed. Code 0646T includes right heart catheterization, temporary pacemaker insertion, and selective right ventricular or right atrial angiography, if performed.

0571T-0574T, 0580T [0614T]

0571T Insertion or replacement of implantable cardioverter-defibrillator system with substernal electrode(s), including all imaging guidance and electrophysiological evaluation (includes defibrillation threshold evaluation, induction of arrhythmia, evaluation of sensing for arrhythmia termination, and programming or reprogramming of sensing or therapeutic parameters), when performed

0572T Insertion of substernal implantable defibrillator electrode

0573T Removal of substernal implantable defibrillator electrode

0574T Repositioning of previously implanted substernal implantable defibrillator-pacing electrode

0580T Removal of substernal implantable defibrillator pulse generator only

0614T Removal and replacement of substernal implantable defibrillator pulse generator

Explanation

The physician inserts an implantable cardioverter-defibrillator system that consists of a subcutaneous pulse generator and at least one substernal electrode. Under appropriate anesthesia, the physician creates a subcutaneous pocket over the lateral ribcage and places the generator. Without entering the pericardial cavity, the electrode is tunneled subcutaneously and placed into the substernal anterior mediastinum, where it performs defibrillation and antitachycardia pacing. This electrode does not perform chronic pacing. All imaging guidance is included, as is the electrophysiological evaluation, which includes evaluation of the defibrillation threshold, arrhythmia induction, evaluation of sensing for termination of arrhythmia, and programming/reprogramming of sensing or therapeutic parameters. Report 0571T for initial insertion of the entire system. Report 0571T along with 0573T and 0580T if the pulse generator and substernal electrodes are removed and subsequently replaced during the same operative episode. Report 0572T for insertion only of the electrode and 0573T for removal only. Report 0573T in conjunction with 0580T if both the pulse generator and electrodes are removed and not replaced. Report 0574T for repositioning of a previously implanted substernal electrode. Report 0580T for removal of the pulse generator only and 0614T if the pulse generator only is concurrently removed and replaced.

0575T-0576T

0575T Programming device evaluation (in person) of implantable cardioverter-defibrillator system with substernal electrode, with iterative adjustment of the implantable device to test the function of the device and select optimal permanent programmed values with analysis, review and report by a physician or other qualified health care professional

0576T Interrogation device evaluation (in person) of implantable cardioverter-defibrillator system with substernal electrode, with analysis, review and report by a physician or other qualified health care professional, includes connection, recording and disconnection per patient encounter

Explanation

A physician or other qualified health care provider performs device evaluations of an implantable cardioverter-defibrillator system with substernal electrode. In 0575T, a programming device evaluation is performed, consisting of repetitive adjustments of the device to test function and select optimal permanent programmed values. In 0576T, an interrogation device evaluation is performed, which includes connection, recording, and disconnection per patient encounter. These codes include analysis, review, and report.

0577T

0577T Electrophysiologic evaluation of implantable cardioverter-defibrillator system with substernal electrode (includes defibrillation threshold evaluation, induction of arrhythmia, evaluation of sensing for arrhythmia termination, and programming or reprogramming of sensing or therapeutic parameters)

Explanation

A physician or other qualified health care provider performs an electrophysiologic evaluation of an implantable cardioverter-defibrillator system with substernal electrode. This includes evaluation of defibrillation threshold, arrhythmia induction, evaluation of sensing for arrhythmia termination, and programming or reprogramming of sensing or therapeutic parameters.

0578T-0579T

0578T Interrogation device evaluation(s) (remote), up to 90 days, substernal lead implantable cardioverter-defibrillator system with interim analysis, review(s) and report(s) by a physician or other qualified health care professional

0579T Interrogation device evaluation(s) (remote), up to 90 days, substernal lead implantable cardioverter-defibrillator system, remote data acquisition(s), receipt of transmissions and technician review, technical support and distribution of results

Explanation

These codes report remote (up to 90 days) evaluations of a substernal lead implantable cardioverter-defibrillator system. In 0578T, a physician or other qualified health care professional provides interim analysis with review and report. In 0579T, included components are remote data acquisition, receipt of transmissions and technician review, technical support, and distribution of results. These codes may be reported once per 90 days.

0607T-0608T

0607T Remote monitoring of an external continuous pulmonary fluid monitoring system, including measurement of radiofrequency-derived pulmonary fluid levels, heart rate, respiration rate, activity, posture, and cardiovascular rhythm (eg, ECG data), transmitted to a remote 24-hour attended surveillance center; set-up and patient education on use of equipment

0608T analysis of data received and transmission of reports to the physician or other qualified health care professional

Explanation

This proprietary device uses a "chest patch" sensor and radiofrequency signals to provide continuous external mobile pulmonary fluid monitoring. The noninvasive system, which monitors heart and respiratory rates, lung fluid levels, activity, posture, and EKG data, consists of a chest patch made of copper-based sensors, a microprocessor unit, and a mobile application. Parameters are measured and multiple vital signs are derived from a single measurement at 40 samples per second, making this technology particularly useful for heart failure and hemodialysis patients. Report 0607T for initial set-up and patient education on the use of the equipment and 0608T for data analysis/report transmission to the physician or other qualified health care professional.

0613T

0613T Percutaneous transcatheter implantation of interatrial septal shunt device, including right and left heart catheterization, intracardiac echocardiography, and imaging guidance by the proceduralist, when performed

Explanation

The interatrial shunt device creates a shunt or "passage" connecting the two atria of the heart. This allows excess blood to flow between the chambers, regulating high pressure in the left atrium and stabilizing left ventricular function without overloading the right heart. The device is typically placed by an interventional cardiologist during a catheterization procedure; right and left heart catheterization, intracardiac echocardiography, and imaging guidance are included in this code when those services are performed in conjunction with the shunt implantation. The patient is placed under general anesthesia. Using a percutaneous approach, the procedure is performed through a transfemoral venous approach under fluoroscopic and transendoscopic echocardiographic (TEE) guidance. The physician places a catheter sheath into the femoral vein and advances the catheter over a guidewire, using fluoroscopic guidance, to the left atrium. The catheter is used to create a transseptal puncture in the intra-atrial septum. The catheter is then withdrawn, leaving the guidewire in place. The device is inserted through an introducer sheath and over the guidewire using a dedicated shunt delivery system designed to deploy the device at the target location across the atrial septum. The device remains in the opening in the septum, allowing blood to flow from the high pressure left side to the lower pressure right side. At the end of the procedure, the guidewire and deployment device are removed. Pressure is placed over the incision for 20 to 30 minutes to stem bleeding. The patient is observed for a period afterward.

0644T

0644T Transcatheter removal or debulking of intracardiac mass (eg, vegetations, thrombus) via suction (eg, vacuum, aspiration) device, percutaneous approach, with intraoperative reinfusion of aspirated blood, including imaging guidance, when performed

Explanation

The physician percutaneously removes or debulks intracardiac vegetations, frequently in the treatment of infective endocarditis, using a vacuum or aspiration suction device. Venous access is gained through the right internal jugular vein, the left femoral vein and artery, and the right femoral vein. Heparin is administered. Percutaneous insertion of a cannula into the left femoral vein is achieved to permit blood reinfusion. The right internal jugular vein is dilated using an inflow cannula, dilator, and guidewire. The apparatus is advanced under fluoroscopic guidance to the level of the right atrium; the dilator and guidewire are removed, and the cardiopulmonary bypass circuit is prepared. The proprietary suction system is inserted via the right jugular vein cannula, in this scenario, to the level of the tricuspid valve and the vegetation is aspirated under transesophageal echo guidance using suction in the form of venous extracorporeal bypass. The filtration system allows the aspirated blood to be filtered, removing vegetation. The blood is then reinfused through the left femoral vein. A final echocardiogram is performed to confirm that the infective vegetation has been completely aspirated. Heparin is partially reversed, and the physician removes all catheters and access cannulas. A variation of this procedure may also be used to remove intracardiac masses caused by thrombus.

0645T

0645T Transcatheter implantation of coronary sinus reduction device including vascular access and closure, right heart catheterization, venous angiography, coronary sinus angiography, imaging guidance, and supervision and interpretation, when performed

Explanation

The physician implants a coronary sinus reduction (CSR) device using a percutaneous, transcatheter approach in a patient suffering from chronic refractory angina. The device, which creates a focal narrowing and increases coronary venous pressure, consists of a stainless steel mesh pre-mounted on an hourglass-shaped balloon catheter. The physician accesses the right jugular vein percutaneously and advances a diagnostic catheter to the right atrium, where the central venous pressure is recorded. The coronary sinus is selectively engaged and contrast is injected to assess the vessel's anatomy. The physician exchanges a guiding catheter over the wire, positions it distally in the coronary sinus, and advances the reduction device to the targeted implantation site. The guiding catheter is then retracted, exposing the device and allowing the balloon to inflate and the CSR to expand. After the balloon catheter deflates, it is retrieved and a final angiogram is obtained to rule out any complications such as migration or perforation, to evaluate positioning, and to confirm the narrowing.

0650T

0650T Programming device evaluation (remote) of subcutaneous cardiac rhythm monitor system, with iterative adjustment of the implantable device to test the function of the device and select optimal permanently programmed values with analysis, review and report by a physician or other qualified health care professional

Explanation

Subcutaneous cardiac rhythm monitors provide uninterrupted, long-term cardiac monitoring for those whose symptoms occur too sporadically to be adequately detected by shorter-term external monitoring methods. Also known as insertable cardiac monitors or implantable loop recorders, these monitors are indicated for adults who exhibit symptoms (e.g., chest pain, dizziness, palpitations, shortness of breath, or syncope) that may indicate a cardiac arrhythmia. They are also indicated for those who are at risk of developing an abnormal heart rhythm. Report 0650T for remote programming of these devices. The physician or other qualified health care professional reviews automatically recorded as well as patient-activated rhythm episodes to assure that arrhythmias are identified accurately, and recording parameters are reviewed and adjusted. Stored and trended historical data are used for comparison to current data measurements and the device function is evaluated for signal strength. Battery life, total memory capacity, and recording capacity parameters are reviewed. Following a thorough examination of all device parameters, a decision is made regarding the adequacy; any changes needed to optimize performance are made and saved in the remote monitoring system.

0659T

0659T Transcatheter intracoronary infusion of supersaturated oxygen in conjunction with percutaneous coronary revascularization during acute myocardial infarction, including catheter placement, imaging guidance (eg, fluoroscopy), angiography, and radiologic supervision and interpretation

Explanation

The physician delivers supersaturated oxygen (SSO2) therapy to a patient suffering a left anterior descending (LAD) ST-elevation myocardial infarction (also known as a widowmaker because of the high mortality rate). Device components of the proprietary system include a console, cartridge, and SSO2 catheter. Immediately following primary percutaneous coronary intervention (PCI) with stenting that is performed within six hours of symptom onset, arterial blood drawn from the existing access site is combined with a highly oxygenated saline solution. The hyperoxemic blood is then delivered by the SSO2 infusion catheter using the femoral access site over a 60-minute period to the affected artery. The pO2 content of the superoxygenated infusion is seven to 10 times higher than that of normal arterial blood, which allows a high rate of oxygen diffusion into the ischemic tissue. Report this code in addition to 92941 for the percutaneous coronary revascularization procedure performed during the acute myocardial infarction.

0674T-0682T

0674T Laparoscopic insertion of new or replacement of permanent implantable synchronized diaphragmatic stimulation system for augmentation of cardiac function, including an implantable pulse generator and diaphragmatic lead(s)

0675T Laparoscopic insertion of new or replacement of diaphragmatic lead(s), permanent implantable synchronized diaphragmatic stimulation system for augmentation of cardiac function, including connection to an existing pulse generator; first lead

+ **0676T** Laparoscopic insertion of new or replacement of diaphragmatic lead(s), permanent implantable synchronized diaphragmatic stimulation system for augmentation of cardiac function, including connection to an existing pulse generator; each additional lead (List separately in addition to code for primary procedure)

0677T Laparoscopic repositioning of diaphragmatic lead(s), permanent implantable synchronized diaphragmatic stimulation system for augmentation of cardiac function, including connection to an existing pulse generator; first repositioned lead

+ **0678T** Laparoscopic repositioning of diaphragmatic lead(s), permanent implantable synchronized diaphragmatic stimulation system for augmentation of cardiac function, including connection to an existing pulse generator; each additional repositioned lead (List separately in addition to code for primary procedure)

0679T Laparoscopic removal of diaphragmatic lead(s), permanent implantable synchronized diaphragmatic stimulation system for augmentation of cardiac function

0680T Insertion or replacement of pulse generator only, permanent implantable synchronized diaphragmatic stimulation system for augmentation of cardiac function, with connection to existing lead(s)

0681T Relocation of pulse generator only, permanent implantable synchronized diaphragmatic stimulation system for augmentation of cardiac function, with connection to existing dual leads

0682T Removal of pulse generator only, permanent implantable synchronized diaphragmatic stimulation system for augmentation of cardiac function

Explanation

The physician inserts or replaces a synchronized diaphragmatic stimulation system for augmentation of cardiac function using a standard laparoscopic approach. The system consists of a pulse generator and two or more diaphragmatic leads (electrodes), which deliver synchronized diaphragmatic stimulation (SDS) pulses that cause the muscles of the diaphragm to contract. These contractions are gated to the cardiac cycle and increase intrathoracic pressure, improving both cardiac output and left ventricular function. Under appropriate anesthesia, the physician implants the electrodes in the muscle of the diaphragm using standard laparoscopic technique. The lead wires are tunneled under the skin to the chest area, where the physician has created a subcutaneous pocket for the pulse generator in the pectoral region. The electrodes are connected to the generator and tested prior to pocket closure. Report 0674T for insertion or replacement of the entire SDS system; 0675T for insertion or replacement of the first diaphragmatic lead with connection to an existing pulse generator and 0676T for each additional lead; 0677T for repositioning or relocation of the first diaphragmatic lead with connection to an existing pulse generator and 0678T for each additional lead; and 0679T for the removal of one or more diaphragmatic leads without replacement. Report 0680T for insertion or replacement of the subcutaneous pulse generator only, with connection to the existing leads; 0681T for relocation or repositioning of the pulse generator only, with connection to the existing leads; and 0682T for removal of the pulse generator only. All codes reporting insertion, replacement, or repositioning/relocation include both interrogation and programming by the implant physician when performed.

0683T-0685T

0683T Programming device evaluation (in-person) with iterative adjustment of the implantable device to test the function of the device and select optimal permanent programmed values with analysis, review and report by a physician or other qualified health care professional, permanent implantable synchronized diaphragmatic stimulation system for augmentation of cardiac function

0684T Peri-procedural device evaluation (in-person) and programming of device system parameters before or after a surgery, procedure, or test with analysis, review, and report by a physician or other qualified health care professional, permanent implantable synchronized diaphragmatic stimulation system for augmentation of cardiac function

0685T Interrogation device evaluation (in-person) with analysis, review and report by a physician or other qualified health care professional, including connection, recording and disconnection per patient encounter, permanent implantable synchronized diaphragmatic stimulation system for augmentation of cardiac function

Explanation

The physician performs an in-person device evaluation of an existing permanent implantable synchronized diaphragmatic stimulation system (SDS). In 0683T, a programming device evaluation is performed in order to test the device's function and select the most favorable permanent programmed values. This involves device adjustments made in a stepwise or iterative fashion. In 0684T, evaluation and programming of SDS parameters are performed prior to or following a surgery, procedure, or test. In 0685T, an interrogation device evaluation is performed that involves connecting, recording, and disconnecting the device; this is reported once per patient encounter. All codes include analysis, review, and report by the physician or other qualified health care professional.

0695T-0696T

0695T Body surface-activation mapping of pacemaker or pacing cardioverter-defibrillator lead(s) to optimize electrical synchrony, cardiac resynchronization therapy device, including connection, recording, disconnection, review, and report; at time of implant or replacement

0696T Body surface-activation mapping of pacemaker or pacing cardioverter-defibrillator lead(s) to optimize electrical synchrony, cardiac resynchronization therapy device, including connection, recording, disconnection, review, and report; at time of follow-up interrogation or programming device evaluation

Explanation

These codes report the electrophysiologic evaluation of pacemaker or pacing cardioverter-defibrillator leads using body surface mapping. Report 0695T when this procedure is performed with the insertion or replacement of pacing electrodes in the cardiac venous system for left ventricular pacing. Report 0696T when this procedure is performed at the time of follow-up interrogation or programming device evaluation.

0716T

0716T Cardiac acoustic waveform recording with automated analysis and generation of coronary artery disease risk score

Explanation

The health care provider determines coronary artery disease risk scores aided in part by acoustic waveform recordings. Using a computer-aided electronic auscultatory device, the acoustic signals of the heart are acquired, recorded, and analyzed by means of acoustic signal processing algorithms. Recordings from an acoustic sensor are analyzed by the computer to detect certain heart sounds, such as S1, S2, or suspected murmurs, and the results are displayed via a graphic user interface.

0744T

0744T Insertion of bioprosthetic valve, open, femoral vein, including duplex ultrasound imaging guidance, when performed, including autogenous or nonautogenous patch graft (eg, polyester, ePTFE, bovine pericardium), when performed

Explanation

The physician uses an open approach to make a 6- to 8-inch incision in the upper thigh to visualize the femoral vein. Clamps are applied to the proximal and distal sites of the target area on the femoral vein. The physician makes a 2 to 3 cm lengthwise incision to open the femoral vein, then inserts a proprietary bioprosthetic valve intended to reduce and eliminate venous reflux, a major cause of deep vein thrombosis (DVT) and chronic venous insufficiency (CVI), into the open femoral vein and sutures the stabilization ring of the valve frame to the wall of the femoral vein. Once the valve is secured in place, the physician sutures the femoral vein and removes the proximal and distal clamps, allowing blood flow to resume through the femoral vein. The patient may require general or regional anesthesia for the procedure. Autogenous or nonautogenous patch graft and duplex ultrasound imaging guidance are included when performed.

0745T-0747T

0745T Cardiac focal ablation utilizing radiation therapy for arrhythmia; noninvasive arrhythmia localization and mapping of arrhythmia site (nidus), derived from anatomical image data (eg, CT, MRI, or myocardial perfusion scan) and electrical data (eg, 12-lead ECG data), and identification of areas of avoidance

0746T Cardiac focal ablation utilizing radiation therapy for arrhythmia; conversion of arrhythmia localization and mapping of arrhythmia site (nidus) into a multidimensional radiation treatment plan

0747T Cardiac focal ablation utilizing radiation therapy for arrhythmia; delivery of radiation therapy, arrhythmia

Explanation

The physician administers noninvasive radiation therapy (RT) with a proprietary RT system to a target segment of the heart for the purpose of ablating, or scarring, cardiac tissue to correct an arrhythmia, such as ventricular tachycardia. In preparation, the cardiologist or cardiology team conducts testing and imaging (MRI, ECG, PET, or CT) to map precisely where the arrhythmia is originating in the heart. The provider uses this imaging and mapping information to plan and deliver targeted radiation treatment. Prior to radiation administration, the motion of the heart is measured when respiratory motion is a concern or when management of the movement may spare healthy tissue. The patient is brought to the radiation therapy lab and placed supine on the treatment table. The RT system is then used to direct radiation beams to the targeted cardiac site, often using the gray scale to refer to the amount of energy absorbed by the tissue. The patient receives "beam on" therapy for five to seven minutes. In one method, the provider targets the heart with a single dose of stereotactic body radiation therapy (SBRT), which is used commonly in cancer treatment and requires no general anesthesia. Report 0745T for the localization/mapping of the arrhythmia, 0746T for the conversion of this information into a multidimensional radiation treatment plan, and 0747T for the delivery of the radiation therapy directed at the arrhythmia.

0793T

0793T Percutaneous transcatheter thermal ablation of nerves innervating the pulmonary arteries, including right heart catheterization, pulmonary artery angiography, and all imaging guidance

Explanation

The physician performs transcatheter pulmonary artery (PA) thermal ablation of selective nerves that innervate the pulmonary arteries to reduce PA pressure in patients with pulmonary arterial hypertension (PAH). Right heart catheterization is conducted under fluoroscopic guidance to measure pulmonary artery hemodynamics. The physician advances a guide catheter through the sheath over a guidewire to the pulmonary artery, followed by a therapeutic radiofrequency catheter. Position is verified using fluoroscopy. Therapeutic radiofrequency energy is applied transmurally to nerve fibers in the main pulmonary artery trunk and its bifurcation, using thermal heat to cause denervation. The guide catheter and radiofrequency catheter may be repositioned to further deliver thermal denervation in the left and right pulmonary arteries. This code includes the right heart catheterization, angiography of the pulmonary artery, and all imaging guidance.

0795T-0797T

0795T Transcatheter insertion of permanent dual-chamber leadless pacemaker, including imaging guidance (eg, fluoroscopy, venous ultrasound, right atrial angiography, right ventriculography, femoral venography) and device evaluation (eg, interrogation or programming), when performed; complete system (ie, right atrial and right ventricular pacemaker components)

0796T right atrial pacemaker component (when an existing right ventricular single leadless pacemaker exists to create a dual-chamber leadless pacemaker system)

0797T right ventricular pacemaker component (when part of a dual-chamber leadless pacemaker system)

Explanation

The physician performs transcatheter insertion of a permanent dual-chamber leadless pacemaker. This system has two pacemakers: one implanted in the right atrium and the other in the right ventricle. Each has its own built-in battery and electrode. The femoral vein is entered using ultrasound guidance, followed by femoral venography for anatomy identification. A guidewire is advanced to the heart via the femoral vein, followed by dilation and upsizing of a femoral sheath. A leadless pacemaker introducer is inserted into the femoral vein, then the guidewire is removed. A delivery catheter is used to feed the leadless pacemaker system through the femoral vein to the inferior vena cava into the right atrium and through the tricuspid valve into the right ventricle via the introducer. Each pacemaker is anchored into the endocardium of its respective chamber with tines or a screw-in helix; a gentle tug conducted under fluoroscopy ensures pacemaker fixation to the chamber wall. The two pacemakers are positioned in accordance with the manufacturer for direct communication prior to release from the catheter. After validation of placement and stabilization of hemodynamics, the physician removes the delivery system and sheath, and sutures the access site closed. The pacemaker's software platform is used for data analysis and programming based on the patient's needs. These codes include imaging guidance and device evaluation, when performed. Report 0795T for insertion of a permanent dual-chamber leadless pacemaker complete system; 0796T for insertion of a right atrial pacemaker component when an existing right ventricular single leadless pacemaker exists to create a dual-chamber leadless pacemaker system; and 0797T for insertion of a right ventricular pacemaker component when it is part of a dual-chamber leadless pacemaker system.

0798T-0800T

0798T Transcatheter removal of permanent dual-chamber leadless pacemaker, including imaging guidance (eg, fluoroscopy, venous ultrasound, right atrial angiography, right ventriculography, femoral venography), when performed; complete system (ie, right atrial and right ventricular pacemaker components)

0799T Transcatheter removal of permanent dual-chamber leadless pacemaker, including imaging guidance (eg, fluoroscopy, venous ultrasound, right atrial angiography, right ventriculography, femoral venography), when performed; right atrial pacemaker component

0800T Transcatheter removal of permanent dual-chamber leadless pacemaker, including imaging guidance (eg, fluoroscopy, venous ultrasound, right atrial angiography, right ventriculography, femoral venography), when performed; right ventricular pacemaker component (when part of a dual-chamber leadless pacemaker system)

Explanation

The physician performs transcatheter removal of a permanent dual-chamber leadless pacemaker. For one proprietary system, the pacemaker device contains a docking button that facilitates retrieval. Other leadless pacemakers have tines, made specifically for placement positioning and removal. The femoral vein is entered using ultrasound guidance, followed by femoral venography for anatomy identification. A guidewire is advanced to the heart via the femoral vein, followed by dilation and upsizing of a femoral sheath. A pacemaker retrieval introducer is inserted into the femoral vein and the guidewire is removed. The physician inserts a retrieval catheter system that has a single-loop or multiple-loop snare. With continued imaging guidance, the retrieval catheter is advanced to the right atrium and/or right ventricle where the snare is looped around the pacemaker's tines or docking button. Once the pacemaker is securely snared, both the pacemaker and retrieval catheter system are pulled to the edge of a delivery cup, and then further pulled into the retrieval sheath. Both the pacemaker and retrieval system are extracted from the patient's body. The physician removes the delivery system and sheath and sutures the access site closed. Leadless pacemakers may also be removed in a similar snare fashion, but with a steerable sheath, also under fluoroscopic guidance. These codes include imaging guidance and device evaluation, when performed. Report 0798T for removal of a permanent dual-chamber leadless pacemaker complete system; 0799T for removal of a right atrial pacemaker component; and 0800T for removal of a right ventricular pacemaker component when it is part of a dual-chamber leadless pacemaker system.

0801T-0803T

0801T Transcatheter removal and replacement of permanent dual-chamber leadless pacemaker, including imaging guidance (eg, fluoroscopy, venous ultrasound, right atrial angiography, right ventriculography, femoral venography) and device evaluation (eg, interrogation or programming), when performed; dual-chamber system (ie, right atrial and right ventricular pacemaker components)

0802T Transcatheter removal and replacement of permanent dual-chamber leadless pacemaker, including imaging guidance (eg, fluoroscopy, venous ultrasound, right atrial angiography, right ventriculography, femoral venography) and device evaluation (eg, interrogation or programming), when performed; right atrial pacemaker component

0803T Transcatheter removal and replacement of permanent dual-chamber leadless pacemaker, including imaging guidance (eg, fluoroscopy, venous ultrasound, right atrial angiography, right ventriculography, femoral venography) and device evaluation (eg, interrogation or programming), when performed; right ventricular pacemaker component (when part of a dual-chamber leadless pacemaker system)

Explanation

The physician performs transcatheter removal and replacement of one or both components of a permanent dual-chamber leadless pacemaker. The physician removes the old pacemaker by a transcatheter approach through the femoral vein. Imaging guidance is used for insertion of a guidewire, followed by a retrieval catheter system or steerable sheath. The old pacemaker is snared by its tines or docking button and retrieved from the patient's body. A leadless pacemaker introducer is inserted into the femoral vein. A delivery catheter is used to feed the new leadless pacemaker system through the femoral vein to the inferior vena cava into the right atrium and through the tricuspid valve into the right ventricle via the introducer. The pacemaker is positioned in accordance with the manufacturer for direct communication prior to release from the catheter and anchored into the endocardium of its respective chamber. The physician removes the delivery system and sheath and sutures the access site closed. These codes include imaging guidance and device evaluation, when performed. Report 0801T for transcatheter removal and replacement of a permanent dual-chamber leadless pacemaker for an entire system including right atrial and right ventricular pacemaker components; 0802T for transcatheter removal and replacement of a right atrial pacemaker component; and 0803T for transcatheter removal and replacement of a right ventricular pacemaker component when it is part of a dual-chamber leadless pacemaker system.

0804T

0804T Programming device evaluation (in person) with iterative adjustment of implantable device to test the function of device and to select optimal permanent programmed values, with analysis, review, and report, by a physician or other qualified health care professional, leadless pacemaker system in dual cardiac chambers

Explanation

A programming device evaluation is performed in person to assess the dual-chamber leadless pacemaker's function and select the most favorable permanent programmed values. The device system data is interrogated to evaluate the battery and hardware, as well as the stored patient and system measurements. If necessary, the device is programmed to settings appropriate for a test or procedure. Postprocedure evaluation and programming may also be performed, with adjustments as required. This code includes physician or other qualified health care professional analysis, review, and report.

0805T-0806T

0805T Transcatheter superior and inferior vena cava prosthetic valve implantation (ie, caval valve implantation [CAVI]); percutaneous femoral vein approach

0806T open femoral vein approach

Explanation

Caval valve implantation (CAVI) is a type of transcatheter therapy composed of two self-expanding valves that are inserted and advanced percutaneously, then deployed into the inferior and superior vena cava to assist or replace the function of the tricuspid valve in patients with severe tricuspid regurgitation (TR) and heart failure. One proprietary system consists of two bioprosthetic self-expanding nitinol structures with bovine pericardium leaflets, one for the superior vena cava (SVC) and one for the inferior vena cava (IVC), both of which are pre-mounted on a valve delivery system. Sizing selection is based on premeasurements via CT scanning. For this system, three access sites are required: one through the right common femoral vein for system delivery and two through the left common femoral vein for a Swan-Ganz catheter at the right pulmonary artery and a pigtail that assists with control injections and SVC angiography. The physician places a guidewire via percutaneous femoral vein approach with fluoroscopic guidance and advances it to the SVC. A sheath is advanced to the site, after which the guidewire is removed. Fluoroscopy, transesophageal echocardiography, and ventriculography may be used to advance the valve delivery catheter to the vena cava and confirm positioning for deployment. The device's three hooks are released to ensure attachment. The delivery system is re-sheathed and removed from the patient. For deployment of the IVC portion, venography of the hepatic veins may be conducted for deployment reference. The IVC prosthesis is deployed and stabilized, and device hooks are released for further implantation and stabilization. The delivery system is re-sheathed and removed from the patient. Report 0805T if a percutaneous femoral vein approach is used; 0806T for an open femoral approach. These codes include vascular access, placement of access sheath, transseptal puncture, advancement of CAVI delivery system, and positioning and deployment of the device, when performed. Radiological supervision and interpretation and angiography performed for CAVI guidance are not reported separately.

0823T-0825T

0823T Transcatheter insertion of permanent single-chamber leadless pacemaker, right atrial, including imaging guidance (eg, fluoroscopy, venous ultrasound, right atrial angiography and/or right ventriculography, femoral venography, cavography) and device evaluation (eg, interrogation or programming), when performed

0824T Transcatheter removal of permanent single-chamber leadless pacemaker, right atrial, including imaging guidance (eg, fluoroscopy, venous ultrasound, right atrial angiography and/or right ventriculography, femoral venography, cavography), when performed

0825T Transcatheter removal and replacement of permanent single-chamber leadless pacemaker, right atrial, including imaging guidance (eg, fluoroscopy, venous ultrasound, right atrial angiography and/or right ventriculography, femoral venography, cavography) and device evaluation (eg, interrogation or programming), when performed

Explanation

The physician performs transcatheter insertion, removal, or replacement of a right atrial permanent single-chamber leadless pacemaker. This system includes a pulse generator, electrode, and built-in battery. After accessing the femoral vein, a guidewire is advanced to the heart, followed by dilation and upsizing of a femoral sheath. A leadless pacemaker introducer is inserted into the femoral vein, then the guidewire is removed. A delivery catheter is used to feed the leadless pacemaker system through the femoral vein to the inferior vena cava into the right atrium via the introducer. The pacemaker is anchored into the endocardium of the chamber with tines or a screw-in helix; a gentle tug conducted under fluoroscopy ensures pacemaker fixation to the chamber wall. The pacemaker is positioned in accordance with the manufacturer for direct communication prior to release from the catheter. After validation of placement and stabilization of hemodynamics, the physician removes the delivery system and sheath, and sutures the access site closed. The pacemaker's software platform is used for data analysis and programming based on the patient's needs. These codes include imaging guidance and device evaluation, when performed. Report 0823T for insertion of the pacemaker, 0824T for removal, and 0825T for removal and replacement.

0826T

0826T Programming device evaluation (in person) with iterative adjustment of the implantable device to test the function of the device and select optimal permanent programmed values with analysis, review and report by a physician or other qualified health care professional, leadless pacemaker system in single-cardiac chamber

Explanation

A programming device evaluation is performed in person for a single-chamber leadless pacemaker to test the device's function and select the most favorable permanent programmed values. Patients with previously implanted pacemakers require periodic programming device evaluations. This diagnostic procedure includes a face-to-face assessment of all device functions. Components that must be evaluated to assign this code include the battery, leads, capture and sensing function, heart rhythm, and programmed parameters. Stored and measured data regarding these components are retrieved using an office, hospital, or emergency room instrument. This information is assessed to discern battery voltage, lead impedance, and settings for rhythm treatment and tachycardia detection, as well as to determine the pacemaker's current programming. If necessary, the sensing value and rate response, upper and lower heart rates, AV intervals, pacing voltage and pulse duration, and diagnostics are adjusted. This code includes physician or other qualified health care professional review, interpretation, and report.

0876T

● **0876T** Duplex scan of hemodialysis fistula, computer-aided, limited (volume flow, diameter, and depth, including only body of fistula)

Explanation

The technician performs a limited, computer-aided Duplex ultrasound scan, producing real-time images integrating B-mode two-dimensional structure with Doppler mapping or imaging of motion with time, of a hemodialysis fistula. Using a proprietary, automated ultrasound device, data is collected to assess the volume flow rate, diameter, and depth of the body of the fistula to determine if the fistula has matured.

0893T

● **0893T** Noninvasive assessment of blood oxygenation, gas exchange efficiency, and cardiorespiratory status, with physician or other qualified health care professional interpretation and report

Explanation

A gas exchange monitor analyzes exhaled gas samples to determine a patient's cardiorespiratory status. A sensor, or pulse oximeter, is placed on the finger to measure oxygen levels in the blood. A clip is placed on the patient's nose, and the patient is instructed to breathe through a mouthpiece that collects samples of the patient's breath to measure O2 and CO2 gas levels from the lungs. A physician or other qualified health care professional interprets the results from the gas exchange monitor and prepares a written report.

0897T

● **0897T** Noninvasive augmentative arrhythmia analysis derived from quantitative computational cardiac arrhythmia simulations, based on selected intervals of interest from 12-lead electrocardiogram and uploaded clinical parameters, including uploading clinical parameters with interpretation and report

Explanation

The patient undergoes a 12-lead electrocardiogram (EKG). Utilizing a proprietary software program, the EKG and relevant clinical parameters are uploaded to a processing platform. Areas of interest are selected from the EKG recording, and maps are generated to identify focal and fibrillation arrhythmias, atrial and ventricular pacing, and beat-by-beat cardiac data in 2D and 3D. This artificial intelligence technology is considered augmentative, which means the machine analyzes and/or quantifies the data to produce clinically meaningful output, and a physician or other qualified health care professional provides an interpretation and report.

0899T-0900T

+● **0899T** Noninvasive determination of absolute quantitation of myocardial blood flow (AQMBF), derived from augmentative algorithmic analysis of the dataset acquired via contrast cardiac magnetic resonance (CMR), pharmacologic stress, with interpretation and report by a physician or other qualified health care professional (List separately in addition to code for primary procedure)

+● **0900T** Noninvasive estimate of absolute quantitation of myocardial blood flow (AQMBF), derived from assistive algorithmic analysis of the dataset acquired via contrast cardiac magnetic resonance (CMR), pharmacologic stress, with interpretation and report by a physician or other qualified health care professional (List separately in addition to code for primary procedure)

Explanation

The patient undergoes contrast cardiac magnetic resonance (CMR) imaging, a radiation-free, noninvasive technique that produces high quality, detailed, three-dimensional imaging of complex congenital heart defects, as well as functional cardiac analysis. Absolute quantitation of myocardial blood flow (MBF) is the volume of blood transiting through tissue at a certain rate, usually in milliliters per minute per gram of tissue (mL/min/g). The MBF measurement reflects coronary microcirculation and can be used to evaluate for coronary risk factors and myocardial disease. Stress MBF, also referred to as hyperemic blood flow, describes the highest amount of blood flow that can be provided to the heart during the topmost period of vasodilation of the heart's vascular bed. Typically, to reach this maximum vasodilation, the patient receives vasodilators or inotropic agents via IV to simulate stress. Utilizing a proprietary software program, the CMR images are uploaded to a processing platform for MBF calculations. Report 0899T for an absolute quantitation of myocardial blood flow determination from an augmentative algorithmic analysis from an artificial intelligence application, which means the machine analyzes and/or quantifies the data to produce clinically meaningful output. Report 0900T for an absolute quantitation of myocardial blood flow estimate from an assistive algorithmic analysis from an artificial intelligence application, which means the machine detects clinically relevant data but does not analyze it or make conclusions. These codes require an interpretation and report by the physician or other qualified health care professional and are reported in addition to the code for the primary procedure.

0902T

● **0902T** QTc interval derived by augmentative algorithmic analysis of input from an external, patient-activated mobile ECG device

Explanation

Proprietary technology is used to determine the corrected QT interval (QTc) using data from an external electrocardiogram (ECG) device. After selecting the appropriate options in the associated mobile application on a smartphone or tablet, the patient places both thumbs over two electrodes on the top of the ECG device. The electrode on the bottom of the device is held against the left knee or ankle. An ECG recording is captured in less than a minute, and the QT interval is measured. A QT interval represents the time between the start of the Q wave and the end of the T wave on an ECG. A prolonged QT interval can be an indication of a higher risk for ventricular arrythmias or a side effect from certain medications. QTc estimates the QT interval at a standard 60 beats per minute heart rate, allowing the physician to compare the QT intervals over time at different heart rates. This artificial intelligence technology is considered augmentative, which means the machine analyzes and/or quantifies the data to produce clinically meaningful output, and a physician or other qualified health care professional provides an interpretation and report.

0903T-0905T

- ● **0903T** Electrocardiogram, algorithmically generated 12-lead ECG from a reduced-lead ECG; with interpretation and report
- ● **0904T** tracing only
- ● **0905T** interpretation and report only

Explanation

A 12-lead electrocardiogram (ECG) is generated with reduced leads using artificial intelligence algorithms. The proprietary system consists of an ECG module and a single cable with five electrode connectors. After selecting the appropriate options in the associated mobile application on a smartphone or tablet, electrodes are placed on the chest and limbs by a qualified health care professional or trained personnel. The system provides simultaneous measurements of four channels (leads I, II, V2, V4) with calculations of the remaining limb leads (III, aVR, aVL, aVF). The remaining four precordial leads are synthesized using machine-learning algorithms. Report 0903T for the combined professional and technical components of an ECG, including the tracing and interpretation and report; 0904T for the tracing only; and 0905T for the interpretation and report only.

0913T-0914T

- ● **0913T** Percutaneous transcatheter therapeutic drug delivery by intracoronary drug-delivery balloon (eg, drug-coated, drug-eluting), including mechanical dilation by nondrug-delivery balloon angioplasty, endoluminal imaging using intravascular ultrasound (IVUS) or optical coherence tomography (OCT) when performed, imaging supervision, interpretation, and report, single major coronary artery or branch
- +● **0914T** Percutaneous transcatheter therapeutic drug delivery by intracoronary drug-delivery balloon (eg, drug-coated, drug-eluting) performed on a separate target lesion from the target lesion treated with balloon angioplasty, coronary stent placement or coronary atherectomy, including mechanical dilation by nondrug-delivery balloon angioplasty, endoluminal imaging using intravascular ultrasound (IVUS) or optical coherence tomography (OCT) when performed, imaging supervision, interpretation, and report, single major coronary artery or branch (List separately in addition to code for percutaneous coronary stent or atherectomy intervention)

Explanation

The physician places a catheter percutaneously (through the skin) for treatment of occlusive disease of the major coronary arteries or branches. An introducer sheath is placed in an artery, typically the femoral artery, using percutaneous puncture. The angiography catheter is advanced through the introducer sheath into the ascending aorta and directed, under fluoroscopic guidance, to the opening of the coronary artery. Following mechanical dilation with a non-drug balloon, a drug-coated balloon is advanced. The balloon's outer surface is coated with a therapeutic drug (paclitaxel) that is delivered directly to the stenosis site. Intravascular ultrasound (IVUS) or optical coherence tomography (OCT) endoluminal imaging may be used during the procedure. For IVUS, a catheter is placed over the guidewire. The ultrasound probe is used to obtain images from inside the vessel to assess area and extent of disease prior to interventional therapy, as well as adequacy of therapy after interventional therapy. The ultrasound probe provides a two-dimensional, cross-sectional view of the vessel or graft as the probe is advanced and withdrawn along the area of interest. When the ultrasound examination is complete, the catheter is removed. In OCT, light is utilized instead of sound to provide cross-sectional images in high resolution within the lumen. Report 0913T for percutaneous transcatheter drug delivery balloon intervention for a single major coronary artery or branch. Report add-on code 0914T in addition to the code for a percutaneous stent or atherectomy intervention when the balloon intervention is performed on a separate target lesion than the target lesion treated during balloon angioplasty, stent placement, or atherectomy. These codes include IVUS and OCT, when performed, and imaging supervision, interpretation, and report.

0915T-0918T

- ● **0915T** Insertion of permanent cardiac contractility modulation-defibrillation system component(s), including fluoroscopic guidance, and evaluation and programming of sensing and therapeutic parameters; pulse generator and dual transvenous electrodes/leads (pacing and defibrillation)
- ● **0916T** pulse generator only
- ● **0917T** single transvenous lead (pacing or defibrillation) only
- ● **0918T** dual transvenous leads (pacing and defibrillation) only

Explanation

Cardiac contractility modulation-defibrillation (CCM-D) is utilized to improve cardiac output in patients with moderate to severe heart failure. A defibrillator component is included that can provide shock therapy or pacing when an abnormal heart rhythm is detected. The device consists of a programmable and rechargeable generator powered by a lithium battery, a defibrillator lead, and pacemaker lead. Under local anesthesia, dissection is performed directly on top of the fascia in the left pectoral region of the chest to create a subcutaneous pocket. The defibrillator lead is placed in a mid-septum location, while the pacing lead is placed at least 2 cm away on the high septum. Once the leads are placed, they are tested and connected to the pulse generator that is placed in the previously prepared pocket. Sensing and therapeutic parameters are evaluated and programmed as appropriate. The subcutaneous pocket is closed with sutures. Report 0915T for insertion of the pulse generator with dual transvenous leads (pacing and defibrillation); 0916T for insertion of the pulse generator only; 0917T for insertion of a single transvenous lead (pacing or defibrillation) only; and 0918T for dual transvenous leads (pacing and defibrillation) only. These codes include imaging guidance, catheterization, and device evaluation and programming.

0919T-0922T

- ● **0919T** Removal of a permanent cardiac contractility modulation-defibrillation system component(s); pulse generator only
- ● **0920T** single transvenous pacing lead only
- ● **0921T** single transvenous defibrillation lead only
- ● **0922T** dual (pacing and defibrillation) transvenous leads only

Explanation

The physician removes a component of a cardiac contractility modulation-defibrillation (CCM-D) device. In 0919T, only the pulse generator is removed. Under local anesthesia, an incision is made into the previously created subcutaneous pocket. Leads are disconnected and capped. The generator is removed, and the incision is closed with sutures. Report 0920T when only the pacing lead is removed; 0921T when only the defibrillation lead is removed; and 0922T when both the pacing and defibrillation leads are removed.

0923T

- ● **0923T** Removal and replacement of permanent cardiac contractility modulation-defibrillation pulse generator only

Explanation

The physician removes and replaces a cardiac contractility modulation-defibrillation (CCM-D) pulse generator. Under local anesthesia, an incision is made into the previously created subcutaneous pocket. Leads are disconnected, and the generator is removed. A new pulse generator is inserted into the pocket. Existing leads are connected to the new generator and tested. The incision is closed with sutures.

0924T

- **0924T** Repositioning of previously implanted cardiac contractility modulation-defibrillation transvenous electrode(s)/lead(s), including fluoroscopic guidance and programming of sensing and therapeutic parameters

Explanation

The physician repositions one or more previously implanted cardiac contractility modulation-defibrillation (CCM-D) transvenous electrodes/leads due to displacement or abnormal function. An incision is made to access the lead. Fluoroscopy is used to identify the current placement of the lead and reposition it. The lead is secured in place and tested after connection to the pulse generator is verified. The incision is closed with sutures. This code includes fluoroscopic guidance and programming of the sensing and therapeutic parameters.

0925T

- **0925T** Relocation of skin pocket for implanted cardiac contractility modulation-defibrillation pulse generator

Explanation

The physician relocates the skin pocket for a cardiac contractility modulation-defibrillation (CCM-D) pulse generator due to complications or because the tissue in the area needs to be irradiated. Under local anesthesia, an incision is made into the previously created subcutaneous pocket. Leads are disconnected, and the generator is removed. If a hematoma or abscess is present, it is incised and drained, and this is not reported separately. The pocket is closed with sutures. In a new location, dissection is performed directly on top of the fascia to create a new subcutaneous pocket. The pulse generator is placed in the pocket. Existing leads are connected to the generator and tested. The incision is closed with sutures. This code includes all work associated with the original subcutaneous pocket and creation of a new pocket.

0926T

- **0926T** Programming device evaluation (in person) with iterative adjustment of the implantable device to test the function of the device and select optimal permanent programmed values with analysis, including review and report, implantable cardiac contractility modulation-defibrillation system

Explanation

A programming device evaluation is performed in person to test contractility modulation-defibrillation (CCM-D) device function and select the most favorable permanent programmed values. Patients with previously implanted CCM-D systems require periodic programming device evaluations. This diagnostic procedure includes a face-to-face assessment of all device functions, including sensing and therapeutic parameters. Current settings are analyzed, and the settings may be adjusted to maintain optimal function of the CCM-D device for the individual patient. This code includes the review and report.

0927T-0929T

- **0927T** Interrogation device evaluation (in person) with analysis, review, and report, including connection, recording, and disconnection, per patient encounter, implantable cardiac contractility modulation-defibrillation system
- **0928T** Interrogation device evaluation (remote), up to 90 days, cardiac contractility modulation-defibrillation system with interim analysis and report(s) by a physician or other qualified health care professional
- **0929T** Interrogation device evaluation (remote), up to 90 days, cardiac contractility modulation-defibrillation system, remote data acquisition(s), receipt of transmissions, technician review, technical support, and distribution of results

Explanation

An interrogation device evaluation is performed for an implantable contractility modulation-defibrillation (CCM-D) system. Interrogation may include testing of the function of the battery, lead(s), capture and sensing function, heart rhythm, and programmed parameters. In 0927T, interrogation is performed in person in a face-to-face assessment. This code includes the analysis, review, report, connection/disconnection, and recording. This code is reported once per patient encounter. In 0928T, a physician or other qualified health care professional provides interim analysis with report for remote device interrogation for a period of up to 90 days. In 0929T, included components are remote data acquisition, receipt of transmissions, technician review, technical support, and distribution of results for remote device interrogation for a period of up to 90 days.

0930T-0931T

- **0930T** Electrophysiologic evaluation of cardiac contractility modulation-defibrillator leads, including defibrillation-threshold evaluation (induction of arrhythmia, evaluation of sensing and therapy for arrhythmia termination), at time of initial implantation or replacement with testing of cardiac contractility modulation-defibrillator pulse generator
- **0931T** Electrophysiologic evaluation of cardiac contractility modulation-defibrillator leads, including defibrillation-threshold evaluation (induction of arrhythmia, evaluation of sensing and therapy for arrhythmia termination), separate from initial implantation or replacement with testing of cardiac contractility modulation-defibrillator pulse generator

Explanation

A physician or other qualified health care provider performs an electrophysiologic evaluation of contractility modulation-defibrillator (CCM-D) leads. This includes evaluation of a defibrillation threshold including arrhythmia induction with evaluation of sensing and therapy for arrhythmia termination. Report 0930T when the evaluation is performed at the time of the initial implantation or replacement with testing of the CCM-D pulse generator. Report 0931T when the evaluation is performed during a separate encounter from the initial implantation or replacement with testing of the pulse generator.

0932T

- **0932T** Noninvasive detection of heart failure derived from augmentative analysis of an echocardiogram that demonstrated preserved ejection fraction, with interpretation and report by a physician or other qualified health care professional

Explanation

Echocardiography image post processing is utilized to detect heart failure with preserved ejection fraction (HFpEF) in adult patients undergoing routine functional cardiovascular assessment using echocardiography. Utilized by an interpreting qualified health care professional (QHP) who determines that the echocardiogram demonstrates a preserved ejection fraction, the noninvasive proprietary device provides information that may be useful in the detection of heart failure. The device is an automated machine learning-based decision support system that takes input from Digital Imaging and Communications in Medicine (DICOM) files of 2D echocardiogram imaging data with an apical four-chamber view. The software employs an artificial intelligence (AI) model to produce an estimate of the absence or presence of HFpEF to the interpreting QHP. The QHP uses this data with other medical information to assist with the diagnosis of the patient. This code reports the interpretation and report of the data produced by the automated machine learning-based decision support system. The echocardiography is performed separately.

0933T

- **0933T** Transcatheter implantation of wireless left atrial pressure sensor for long-term left atrial pressure monitoring, including sensor calibration and deployment, right heart catheterization, transseptal puncture, imaging guidance, and radiological supervision and interpretation

Explanation

The physician implants a wireless atrial pressure sensor via right heart catheterization. The sensor allows for long-term, remote monitoring of left atrial pressure in patients with symptomatic heart failure. The physician gains access to the femoral vein. Under imaging guidance, a catheter is advanced from the femoral vein into the right atrium. The interatrial wall or septum is punctured, and the catheter is passed into the left atrium. Using a proprietary delivery system, the sensor is advanced to the interatrial septum and deployed. Calibration of the sensor is performed. This code includes all imaging guidance and radiological supervision and interpretation.

0934T

- **0934T** Remote monitoring of a wireless left atrial pressure sensor for up to 30 days, including data from daily uploads of left atrial pressure recordings, interpretation(s) and trend analysis, with adjustments to the diuretics plan, treatment paradigm thresholds, medications or lifestyle modifications, when performed, and report(s) by a physician or other qualified health care professional

Explanation

A wireless left atrial pressure sensor allows for long-term, remote monitoring of left atrial pressure (LAP) in patients with symptomatic heart failure. LAP readings are transmitted from a sensor that has been implanted in the interatrial septum. The sensory implant has no battery or leads; the patient wears a portable belt across the chest that powers the implant and transmits real-time LAP data to a cloud-based system. The patient can monitor the readings using a mobile application and adjust diuretics according to a prescribed treatment plan, or the provider can intervene with additional guidance. This code includes remote monitoring of the sensor for a 30-day period; do not report this code for monitoring if the duration is less than 16 days. Analysis of LAP trends with interpretation and report is performed by the physician or other qualified health care professional with any necessary adjustments to treatment paradigm thresholds, diuretics and other medications, or lifestyle recommendations.

0937T-0940T

- **0937T** External electrocardiographic recording for greater than 15 days up to 30 days by continuous rhythm recording and storage; including recording, scanning analysis with report, review and interpretation by a physician or other qualified health care professional
- **0938T** recording (including connection and initial recording)
- **0939T** scanning analysis with report
- **0940T** review and interpretation by a physician or other qualified health care professional

Explanation

Long-term external electrocardiographic (ECG) recording is a diagnostic procedure that provides continuous rhythm recording of the patient's heart while the patient is engaged in the activities of daily living. The purpose of the study is to evaluate the patient's ambient heart rhythm during a full daily cycle. Rhythm disturbances and waveform abnormalities are detected; information is provided regarding the frequency of these disturbances. The physician or other qualified health care provider instructs the patient in the use of the external ECG recorder. A technician places ECG leads on the patient's chest, and the patient wears the recorder for more than 15 days up to 30 days. During this time there is continuous rhythm recording and storage. The patient returns the device, and the recorded heart rhythm is converted into digital format by a technician. The technician uses a scanning methodology to classify different ECG waveforms and to generate a report. The generated report describes the overall rhythm and significant arrhythmias. Code 0937T reports the recording, scanning analysis with report, provider review of the data, and the provision of a final interpretation in a report. Code 0938T reports the recording only, which includes the connection and initial recording of data. Code 0939T reports only the scanning analysis with report. Code 0940T reports only the provider review and interpretation.

Correct Coding Initiative Update 30.3

❖Indicates Mutually Exclusive Edit

0234T 01924-01926, 0213T, 0216T, 0596T-0597T, 11000-11006, 11042-11047, 34713-34716, 34812, 34820, 34833-34834, 35201-35206, 35226-35236, 35256-35266, 35286, 36000, 36002-36005, 36400-36410, 36420-36430, 36440, 36500, 36591-36592, 36600-36640, 37184, 43752, 49000-49002, 51701-51703, 61645-61650, 62320-62327, 64400, 64405-64408, 64415-64435, 64445-64454, 64461, 64463, 64479, 64483, 64486-64490, 64493, 64505, 64510-64530, 69990, 75893, 76000, 76942, 76998, 77002, 93000-93010, 93040-93042, 93050, 93318, 93355, 94002, 94200, 94680-94690, 95812-95816, 95819, 95822, 95829, 95955, 96360, 96365, 96372, 96374-96377, 96523, 97597-97598, 97602, 99155, 99156, 99157, 99446-99449, 99451-99452, G0471

0235T 01924-01926, 0213T, 0216T, 0596T-0597T, 11000-11006, 11042-11047, 34713-34716, 34812, 34820, 34833-34834, 35201-35206, 35226-35236, 35256-35266, 35286, 36000, 36002-36005, 36400-36410, 36420-36430, 36440, 36500, 36591-36592, 36600-36640, 37184, 43752, 49000-49002, 51701-51703, 61645-61650, 62320-62327, 64400, 64405-64408, 64415-64435, 64445-64454, 64461, 64463, 64479, 64483, 64486-64490, 64493, 64505, 64510-64530, 69990, 75726, 75736, 75774, 75893, 76000, 76942, 76998, 77002, 93000-93010, 93040-93042, 93050, 93318, 93355, 94002, 94200, 94680-94690, 95812-95816, 95819, 95822, 95829, 95955, 96360, 96365, 96372, 96374-96377, 96523, 97597-97598, 97602, 99155, 99156, 99157, 99446-99449, 99451-99452, G0471

0236T 01924-01926, 0213T, 0216T, 0596T-0597T, 11000-11006, 11042-11047, 32551, 32556-32557, 34713-34716, 34812, 34820, 34833-34834, 35201-35206, 35226-35236, 35256-35266, 35286, 36000, 36002-36005, 36400-36410, 36420-36430, 36440, 36500, 36591-36592, 36600-36640, 37184, 43752, 49000-49002, 51701-51703, 61645-61650, 62320-62327, 64400, 64405-64408, 64415-64435, 64445-64454, 64461, 64463, 64479, 64483, 64486-64490, 64493, 64505, 64510-64530, 69990, 75600, 75605, 75625, 75630, 75635, 75893, 76000, 76942, 76998, 77002, 93000-93010, 93040-93042, 93050, 93318, 93355, 94002, 94200, 94680-94690, 95812-95816, 95819, 95822, 95829, 95955, 96360, 96365, 96372, 96374-96377, 96523, 97597-97598, 97602, 99155, 99156, 99157, 99446-99449, 99451-99452, G0471

0237T 01924-01926, 0213T, 0216T, 0596T-0597T, 11000-11006, 11042-11047, 34715-34716, 34834, 35201-35206, 35226-35236, 35256-35266, 35286, 36000, 36002-36005, 36400-36410, 36420-36430, 36440, 36500, 36591-36592, 36600-36640, 37184, 43752, 51701-51703, 61645-61650, 62320-62327, 64400, 64405-64408, 64415-64435, 64445-64454, 64461, 64463, 64479, 64483, 64486-64490, 64493, 64505, 64510-64530, 69990, 75605, 75710, 75716, 75893, 76000, 76942, 76998, 77002, 93000-93010, 93040-93042, 93050, 93318, 93355, 94002, 94200, 94680-94690, 95812-95816, 95819, 95822, 95829, 95955, 96360, 96365, 96372, 96374-96377, 96523, 97597-97598, 97602, 99155, 99156, 99157, 99446-99449, 99451-99452, G0471

0238T 01924, 0596T-0597T, 11000-11006, 11042-11047, 35201-35206, 35226-35236, 35256-35266, 35286, 36000, 36002-36005, 36400-36410, 36420-36430, 36440, 36500, 36591-36592, 36600-36640, 43752, 51701-51703, 61650, 62320-62327, 64400, 64405-64408, 64415-64435, 64445-64454, 64461, 64463, 64479, 64483, 64486-64490, 64493, 64505, 64510-64530, 69990, 75630, 75635, 75710, 75716, 75736, 75774, 75893, 76000, 76942, 76998, 77002, 93000-93010, 93040-93042, 93050, 93318, 93355, 94002, 94200, 94680-94690, 95812-95816, 95819, 95822, 95829, 95955, 96360, 96365, 96372, 96374-96377, 96523, 97597-97598, 97602, 99155, 99156, 99157, 99446-99449, 99451-99452, G0471

0266T 0213T, 0216T, 0267T, 0268T, 0269T, 0270T, 0271T, 0272T, 0273T, 0596T-0597T, 0708T-0709T, 11000-11006, 11042-11047, 36000, 36400-36410, 36420-36430, 36440, 36591-36592, 36600, 36640, 43752, 51701-51703, 61650, 62320-62327, 64400, 64405-64408, 64415-64435, 64445-64454, 64461, 64463, 64479, 64483, 64486-64490, 64493, 64505, 64510-64530, 69990, 93000-93010, 93040-93042, 93318, 93355, 94002, 94200, 94680-94690, 95812-95816, 95819, 95822, 95829, 95955, 96360, 96365, 96372, 96374-96377, 96523, 97597-97598, 97602, 99155, 99156, 99157, 99446-99449, 99451-99452, G0471

0267T 0213T, 0216T, 0270T, 0272T, 0273T, 0596T-0597T, 0708T-0709T, 11000-11006, 11042-11047, 36000, 36400-36410, 36420-36430, 36440, 36591-36592, 36600, 36640, 43752, 51701-51703, 61650, 62320-62327, 64400, 64405-64408, 64415-64435, 64445-64454, 64461, 64463, 64479, 64483, 64486-64490, 64493, 64505, 64510-64530, 69990, 93000-93010, 93040-93042, 93318, 93355, 94002, 94200, 94680-94690, 95812-95816, 95819, 95822, 95829, 95955, 96360, 96365, 96372, 96374-96377, 96523, 97597-97598, 97602, 99155, 99156, 99157, 99446-99449, 99451-99452, G0471

0268T 0213T, 0216T, 0270T, 0271T, 0272T, 0273T, 0596T-0597T, 0708T-0709T, 11000-11006, 11042-11047, 36000, 36400-36410, 36420-36430, 36440, 36591-36592, 36600, 36640, 43752, 51701-51703, 61650, 62320-62327, 64400, 64405-64408, 64415-64435, 64445-64454, 64461, 64463, 64479, 64483, 64486-64490, 64493, 64505, 64510-64530, 69990, 93000-93010, 93040-93042, 93318, 93355, 94002, 94200, 94680-94690, 95812-95816, 95819, 95822, 95829, 95955, 96360, 96365, 96372, 96374-96377, 96523, 97597-97598, 97602, 99155, 99156, 99157, 99446-99449, 99451-99452, G0471

0269T 0213T, 0216T, 0267T, 0268T, 0270T, 0271T, 0272T, 0273T, 0596T-0597T, 0708T-0709T, 11000-11006, 11042-11047, 36000, 36400-36410, 36420-36430, 36440, 36591-36592, 36600, 36640, 43752, 51701-51703, 61650, 62320-62327, 64400, 64405-64408, 64415-64435, 64445-64454, 64461, 64463, 64479, 64483, 64486-64490, 64493, 64505, 64510-64530, 69990, 93000-93010, 93040-93042, 93318, 93355, 94002, 94200, 94680-94690, 95812-95816, 95819, 95822, 95829, 95955, 96360, 96365, 96372, 96374-96377, 96523, 97597-97598, 97602, 99155, 99156, 99157, 99446-99449, 99451-99452, G0471

0270T 0213T, 0216T, 0272T, 0273T, 0596T-0597T, 0708T-0709T, 11000-11006, 11042-11047, 36000, 36400-36410, 36420-36430, 36440, 36591-36592, 36600, 36640, 43752, 51701-51703, 61650, 62320-62327, 64400, 64405-64408, 64415-64435, 64445-64454, 64461, 64463, 64479, 64483, 64486-64490, 64493, 64505, 64510-64530, 69990, 93000-93010, 93040-93042, 93318, 93355, 94002, 94200, 94680-94690, 95812-95816, 95819, 95822, 95829, 95955, 96360, 96365, 96372, 96374-96377, 96523, 97597-97598, 97602, 99155, 99156, 99157, 99446-99449, 99451-99452, G0471

0271T 0213T, 0216T, 0267T, 0270T, 0272T, 0273T, 0596T-0597T, 0708T-0709T, 11000-11006, 11042-11047, 36000, 36400-36410, 36420-36430, 36440, 36591-36592, 36600, 36640, 43752, 51701-51703, 61650, 62320-62327, 64400, 64405-64408, 64415-64435, 64445-64454, 64461, 64463, 64479, 64483, 64486-64490, 64493, 64505, 64510-64530, 69990, 93000-93010, 93040-93042, 93318, 93355, 94002, 94200, 94680-94690, 95812-95816, 95819, 95822, 95829, 95955, 96360, 96365, 96372, 96374-96377, 96523, 97597-97598, 97602, 99155, 99156, 99157, 99446-99449, 99451-99452, G0471

0272T 0213T, 0216T, 0596T-0597T, 0708T-0709T, 36000, 36400-36410, 36420-36430, 36440, 36591-36592, 36600, 36640, 43752, 51701-51703, 61650, 62320-62327, 64400, 64405-64408, 64415-64435, 64445-64454, 64461, 64463, 64479, 64483, 64486-64490, 64493, 64505, 64510-64530, 69990, 93000-93010, 93040-93042, 93318, 93355, 94002, 94200, 94680-94690, 95812-95816, 95819, 95822, 95829, 95955, 96360, 96365, 96372, 96374-96377, 96523, 99155, 99156, 99157, 99446-99449, 99451-99452, G0471

0273T 0213T, 0216T, 0272T, 0596T-0597T, 0708T-0709T, 36000, 36400-36410, 36420-36430, 36440, 36591-36592, 36600, 36640, 43752, 51701-51703, 61650, 62320-62327, 64400, 64405-64408, 64415-64435, 64445-64454, 64461, 64463, 64479, 64483, 64486-64490, 64493, 64505, 64510-64530, 69990, 93000-93010, 93040-93042, 93318, 93355, 94002, 94200, 94680-94690, 95812-95816, 95819, 95822, 95829, 95955, 96360, 96365, 96372, 96374-96377, 96523, 99155, 99156, 99157, 99446-99449, 99451-99452, G0471

0331T 0694T, 0708T-0709T, 36000, 36005, 36410, 36591-36592, 76000, 76376-76377, 96360, 96365, 96372, 96374-96377, 96523

0332T 0331T, 0694T, 0708T-0709T, 36000, 36005, 36410, 36591-36592, 76000, 76376-76377, 96360, 96365, 96372, 96374-96377, 96523

0338T 0213T, 0216T, 0596T-0597T, 0708T-0709T, 12001-12007, 12011-12057, 13100-13133, 13151-13153, 35201-35206, 35226-35236, 35256-35266, 35286, 36000, 36140, 36160-36200, 36245-36248, 36251-36254, 36400-36410, 36420-36430, 36440, 36591-36592, 36600, 36640, 43752, 51701-51703, 61650, 62320-62327, 64400, 64405-64408, 64415-64435, 64445-64454, 64461, 64463, 64479, 64483, 64486-64490, 64493, 64505, 64510-64530, 69990, 75625, 75630, 76000, 77002, 92012-92014, 93000-93010, 93040-93042, 93050, 93318, 93355, 94002, 94200, 94680-94690, 95812-95816, 95819, 95822, 95829, 95955, 96360, 96365, 96372, 96374-96377, 96523, 99155, 99156, 99157, 99211-99215, 99221-99223, 99231-99239, 99242-99245, 99252-99255, 99291-99292, 99304-99310, 99315-99316, 99347-99350, 99374-99375, 99377-99378, 99446-99449, 99451-99452, G0269, G0463, G0471

0339T 0213T, 0216T, 0338T, 0596T-0597T, 0708T-0709T, 12001-12007, 12011-12057, 13100-13133, 13151-13153, 35201-35206, 35226-35236, 35256-35266, 35286, 36000, 36140, 36160-36200, 36245-36248, 36251-36254, 36400-36410, 36420-36430, 36440, 36591-36592, 36600, 36640, 43752, 51701-51703, 61650, 62320-62327, 64400, 64405-64408, 64415-64435, 64445-64454, 64461, 64463, 64479, 64483, 64486-64490, 64493, 64505, 64510-64530, 69990, 75625, 75630, 76000, 77002, 92012-92014, 93000-93010, 93040-93042, 93050, 93318, 93355, 94002, 94200, 94680-94690, 95812-95816, 95819, 95822, 95829, 95955, 96360, 96365, 96372, 96374-96377, 96523, 99155, 99156, 99157, 99211-99215, 99221-99223, 99231-99239, 99242-99245, 99252-99255, 99291-99292, 99304-99310, 99315-99316, 99347-99350, 99374-99375, 99377-99378, 99446-99449, 99451-99452, G0269, G0463, G0471

0342T 0213T, 0216T, 0596T-0597T, 0708T-0709T, 12001-12007, 12011-12057, 13100-13133, 13151-13153, 36000, 36400-36410, 36420-36430, 36440, 36591-36592, 36600, 36640, 43752, 51701-51703, 61650, 62320-62327, 64400, 64405-64408, 64415-64435, 64445-64454, 64461, 64463, 64479, 64483, 64486-64490, 64493, 64505, 64510-64530, 69990, 92012-92014, 93000-93010, 93040-93042, 93318, 93355, 94002, 94200, 94680-94690, 95812-95816, 95819, 95822, 95829, 95955, 96360, 96365, 96372, 96374-96377, 96523, 99155, 99156, 99157, 99211-99215, 99221-99223, 99231-99239, 99242-99245, 99252-99255, 99291-99292, 99304-99310, 99315-99316, 99347-99350, 99374-99375, 99377-99378, G0463, G0471

0345T 01920, 01924, 01926, 0213T, 0216T, 0484T*, 0596T-0597T, 0632T, 0708T-0709T, 12001-12007, 12011-12057, 13100-13133, 13151-13153, 32554-32557, 33210-33211, 33310-33315, 33419, 35201-35207, 35211-35286, 36000, 36010, 36013-36100, 36140, 36160-36200, 36400-36410, 36420-36430, 36440, 36500, 36555-36556, 36568-36569, 36572-36573, 36591-36592, 36600-36640, 43752, 51701-51703, 61650, 62320-62327, 64400, 64405-64408, 64415-64435, 64445-64454, 64461, 64463, 64479, 64483, 64486-64490, 64493, 64505, 64510-64530, 69990, 75600, 75605, 75625, 75630, 75710, 75716, 75741, 75743, 75746, 75756, 75893, 76000, 76496, 76942, 76998, 77002, 78635, 92012-92014, 92961, 93000-93010, 93040-93042, 93050, 93306-93308, 93312-93318, 93320-93325, 93355, 93451-93462, 93503, 93563-93565, 93567, 93593-93598, 94002, 94200, 94680-94690, 95812-95816, 95819, 95822, 95829, 95955, 96360, 96365, 96372-96377, 96523, 99155, 99156, 99157, 99211-99215, 99221-99223, 99231-99239, 99242-99245, 99252-99255, 99291-99292, 99304-99310, 99315-99316, 99347-99350, 99374-99375, 99377-99378, 99446-99449, 99451-99452, G0269, G0463, G0471, G9157, J0670, J1644

0408T 00530, 00534, 0213T, 0216T, 0409T, 0410T, 0411T, 0414T, 0415T, 0416T, 0417T, 0418T, 0525T, 0526T, 0527T, 0528T, 0529T, 0575T-0576T, 0596T-0597T, 0632T, 0708T-0709T, 11000-11006, 11042-11047, 12001-12007, 12011-12057, 13100-13133, 13151-13153, 35201-35206, 35226-35236, 35256-35266, 35286, 36000, 36005-36013, 36140, 36400-36410, 36420-36430, 36440, 36555-36556, 36568-36569, 36572-36573, 36591-36592, 36600, 36640, 43752, 51701-51703, 61650, 62320-62327, 64400, 64405-64408, 64415-64435, 64445-64454, 64461, 64463, 64479, 64483, 64486-64490, 64493, 64505, 64510-64530, 69990, 76000, 76942, 76998, 77001-77002, 92012-92014, 92960-92961, 93000-93010, 93040-93042, 93260-93261, 93286-93287, 93318, 93355, 93452-93453, 93458-93461, 93595, 93600-93603, 93610-93612, 94002, 94200, 94680-94690, 95812-95816, 95819, 95822, 95829, 95955, 96360, 96365, 96372, 96374-96377, 96523, 97597-97598, 97602, 99155, 99156, 99157, 99211-99215, 99221-99223, 99231-99239, 99242-99245, 99252-99255, 99291-99292, 99304-99310, 99315-99316, 99347-99350, 99374-99375, 99377-99378, 99446-99449, 99451-99452, 99495-99496, G0463, G0471

0409T 00530, 00534, 0213T, 0216T, 0412T, 0416T, 0417T, 0418T, 0525T, 0526T, 0527T, 0528T, 0529T, 0530T, 0531T-0532T, 0575T-0576T, 0596T-0597T, 0708T-0709T, 11000-11006, 11042-11047, 12001-12007, 12011-12057, 13100-13133, 13151-13153, 33275, 36000, 36005, 36400-36410, 36420-36430, 36440, 36591-36592, 36600, 36640, 43752, 51701-51703, 61650, 62320-62327, 64400, 64405-64408, 64415-64435, 64445-64454, 64461, 64463, 64479, 64483, 64486-64490, 64493, 64505, 64510-64530, 69990, 76000, 76942, 76998, 77002, 92012-92014, 92960-92961, 93000-93010, 93040-93042, 93260-93261, 93286-93287, 93318, 93355, 93452-93453, 93458-93461, 93595, 93600-93603, 93610-93612, 94002, 94200, 94680-94690, 95812-95816, 95819, 95822, 95829, 95955, 96360, 96365, 96372, 96374-96377, 96523, 97597-97598, 97602, 99155, 99156, 99157, 99211-99215, 99221-99223, 99231-99239, 99242-99245, 99252-99255, 99291-99292, 99304-99310, 99315-99316, 99347-99350, 99374-99375, 99377-99378, 99446-99449, 99451-99452, 99495-99496, G0463, G0471

0410T 00530, 00534, 0213T, 0216T, 0409T, 0414T, 0415T, 0416T, 0417T, 0418T, 0525T, 0526T, 0527T, 0528T, 0529T, 0575T-0576T, 0596T-0597T, 0632T, 0708T-0709T, 11000-11006, 11042-11047, 12001-12007, 12011-12057, 13100-13133, 13151-13153, 35201-35206, 35226-35236, 35256-35266, 35286, 36000, 36005-36013, 36140, 36400-36410, 36420-36430, 36440, 36555-36556, 36568-36569, 36572-36573, 36591-36592, 36600, 36640, 43752, 51701-51703, 61650, 62320-62327, 64400, 64405-64408, 64415-64435, 64445-64454, 64461, 64463, 64479, 64483, 64486-64490, 64493, 64505, 64510-64530, 69990, 76000, 76942, 76998, 77001-77002, 92012-92014, 92960-92961, 93000-93010, 93040-93042, 93260-93261, 93286-93287, 93318, 93355, 93452-93453,

93458-93461, 93595, 93600-93603, 93610-93612, 94002, 94200, 94680-94690, 95812-95816, 95819, 95822, 95829, 95955, 96360, 96365, 96372, 96374-96377, 96523, 97597-97598, 97602, 99155, 99156, 99157, 99211-99215, 99221-99223, 99231-99239, 99242-99245, 99252-99255, 99291-99292, 99304-99310, 99315-99316, 99347-99350, 99374-99375, 99377-99378, 99446-99449, 99451-99452, 99495-99496, G0463, G0471

0411T 00530, 00534, 0213T, 0216T, 0409T, 0414T, 0415T, 0416T, 0417T, 0418T, 0525T, 0526T, 0527T, 0528T, 0529T, 0575T-0576T, 0596T-0597T, 0632T, 0708T-0709T, 11000-11006, 11042-11047, 12001-12007, 12011-12057, 13100-13133, 13151-13153, 35201-35206, 35226-35236, 35256-35266, 35286, 36000, 36005-36013, 36140, 36400-36410, 36420-36430, 36440, 36555-36556, 36568-36569, 36572-36573, 36591-36592, 36600, 36640, 43752, 51701-51703, 61650, 62320-62327, 64400, 64405-64408, 64415-64435, 64445-64454, 64461, 64463, 64479, 64483, 64486-64490, 64493, 64505, 64510-64530, 69990, 76000, 76942, 76998, 77001-77002, 92012-92014, 92960-92961, 93000-93010, 93040-93042, 93260-93261, 93286-93287, 93318, 93355, 93452-93453, 93458-93461, 93595, 93600-93603, 93610-93612, 94002, 94200, 94680-94690, 95812-95816, 95819, 95822, 95829, 95955, 96360, 96365, 96372, 96374-96377, 96523, 97597-97598, 97602, 99155, 99156, 99157, 99211-99215, 99221-99223, 99231-99239, 99242-99245, 99252-99255, 99291-99292, 99304-99310, 99315-99316, 99347-99350, 99374-99375, 99377-99378, 99446-99449, 99451-99452, 99495-99496, G0463, G0471

0412T 00530, 00534, 0213T, 0216T, 0415T, 0417T, 0418T, 0525T, 0526T, 0527T, 0528T, 0529T, 0575T-0576T, 0596T-0597T, 0708T-0709T, 11000-11006, 11042-11047, 12001-12007, 12011-12057, 13100-13133, 13151-13153, 36000, 36005, 36400-36410, 36420-36430, 36440, 36591-36592, 36600, 36640, 43752, 51701-51703, 61650, 62320-62327, 64400, 64405-64408, 64415-64435, 64445-64454, 64461, 64463, 64479, 64483, 64486-64490, 64493, 64505, 64510-64530, 69990, 76000, 76942, 76998, 77002, 92012-92014, 92960-92961, 93000-93010, 93040-93042, 93260-93261, 93318, 93355, 94002, 94200, 94680-94690, 95812-95816, 95819, 95822, 95829, 95955, 96360, 96365, 96372, 96374-96377, 96523, 97597-97598, 97602, 99155, 99156, 99157, 99211-99215, 99221-99223, 99231-99239, 99242-99245, 99252-99255, 99291-99292, 99304-99310, 99315-99316, 99347-99350, 99374-99375, 99377-99378, 99446-99449, 99451-99452, 99495-99496, G0463, G0471

0413T 00530, 00534, 0213T, 0216T, 0415T, 0416T, 0417T, 0418T, 0525T, 0526T, 0527T, 0528T, 0529T, 0575T-0576T, 0596T-0597T, 0632T, 0708T-0709T, 11000-11006, 11042-11047, 12001-12007, 12011-12057, 13100-13133, 13151-13153, 35201-35206, 35226-35236, 35256-35266, 35286, 36000, 36005-36013, 36140, 36400-36410, 36420-36430, 36440, 36555-36556, 36568-36569, 36572-36573, 36591-36592, 36600, 36640, 43752, 51701-51703, 61650, 62320-62327, 64400, 64405-64408, 64415-64435, 64445-64454, 64461, 64463, 64479, 64483, 64486-64490, 64493, 64505, 64510-64530, 69990, 76000, 76942, 76998, 77001-77002, 92012-92014, 92960-92961, 93000-93010, 93040-93042, 93260-93261, 93318, 93355, 94002, 94200, 94680-94690, 95812-95816, 95819, 95822, 95829, 95955, 96360, 96365, 96372, 96374-96377, 96523, 97597-97598, 97602, 99155, 99156, 99157, 99211-99215, 99221-99223, 99231-99239, 99242-99245, 99252-99255, 99291-99292, 99304-99310, 99315-99316, 99347-99350, 99374-99375, 99377-99378, 99446-99449, 99451-99452, 99495-99496, G0463, G0471

0414T 00530, 00534, 0213T, 0216T, 0409T, 0412T, 0415T, 0416T❖, 0417T, 0418T, 0525T, 0526T, 0527T, 0528T, 0529T, 0530T, 0531T-0532T, 0575T-0576T, 0596T-0597T, 0708T-0709T, 11000-11006, 11042-11047, 12001-12007, 12011-12057, 13100-13133, 13151-13153, 36000, 36005, 36400-36410, 36420-36430, 36440, 36591-36592, 36600, 36640, 43752, 51701-51703, 61650, 62320-62327, 64400, 64405-64408, 64415-64435, 64445-64454, 64461, 64463, 64479, 64483, 64486-64490, 64493, 64505, 64510-64530, 69990, 76000, 76942, 76998, 77002, 92012-92014, 93000-93010, 93040-93042, 93260-93261, 93286-93287, 93318, 93355, 93452-93453, 93458-93461, 93595, 93600-93603, 93610-93612, 94002, 94200, 94680-94690, 95812-95816, 95819, 95822, 95829, 95955, 96360, 96365, 96372, 96374-96377, 96523, 97597-97598, 97602, 99155, 99156, 99157, 99211-99215, 99221-99223, 99231-99239, 99242-99245, 99252-99255, 99291-99292, 99304-99310, 99315-99316, 99347-99350, 99374-99375, 99377-99378, 99446-99449, 99451-99452, 99495-99496, G0463, G0471

0415T 00530, 00540, 0213T, 0216T, 0416T, 0417T, 0418T, 0525T, 0526T, 0527T, 0528T, 0529T, 0575T-0576T, 0596T-0597T, 0632T, 0708T-0709T, 12001-12007, 12011-12057, 13100-13133, 13151-13153, 35201-35206, 35226-35236, 35256-35266, 35286, 36000, 36005-36013, 36140, 36400-36410, 36420-36430, 36440, 36555-36556, 36568-36569, 36572-36573, 36591-36592, 36600, 36640, 43752, 51701-51703, 61650, 62320-62327, 64400, 64405-64408, 64415-64435, 64445-64454, 64461, 64463, 64479, 64483, 64486-64490, 64493, 64505, 64510-64530, 69990, 76000, 76942, 76998, 77001-77002, 92012-92014, 92960-92961, 93000-93010, 93040-93042, 93260-93261, 93286-93287, 93318, 93355, 93452-93453, 93458-93461, 93595, 93600-93603, 93610-93612, 94002, 94200, 94680-94690, 95812-95816, 95819, 95822, 95829, 95955, 96360, 96365, 96372, 96374-96377, 96523, 99155, 99156, 99157, 99211-99215, 99221-99223, 99231-99239, 99242-99245, 99252-99255, 99291-99292, 99304-99310, 99315-99316, 99347-99350, 99374-99375, 99377-99378, 99446-99449, 99451-99452, 99495-99496, G0463, G0471

0416T 00530, 00534, 0213T, 0216T, 0412T❖, 0417T, 0418T, 0525T, 0526T, 0527T, 0528T, 0529T, 0575T-0576T, 0596T-0597T, 0708T-0709T, 10060-10061, 10140, 10180, 11000-11006, 11042-11047, 12001-12007, 12011-12057, 13100-13133, 13151-13153, 36000, 36005, 36400-36410, 36420-36430, 36440, 36591-36592, 36600, 36640, 43752, 51701-51703, 61650, 62320-62327, 64400, 64405-64408, 64415-64435, 64445-64454, 64461, 64463, 64479, 64483, 64486-64490, 64493, 64505, 64510-64530, 69990, 76000, 76942, 76998, 77002, 92012-92014, 92960-92961, 93000-93010, 93040-93042, 93260-93261, 93318, 93355, 94002, 94200, 94680-94690, 95812-95816, 95819, 95822, 95829, 95955, 96360, 96365, 96372, 96374-96377, 96523, 97597-97598, 97602, 99155, 99156, 99157, 99211-99215, 99221-99223, 99231-99239, 99242-99245, 99252-99255, 99291-99292, 99304-99310, 99315-99316, 99347-99350, 99374-99375, 99377-99378, 99446-99449, 99451-99452, 99495-99496, G0463, G0471

0417T 0418T, 36591-36592, 93000-93010, 93040-93042, 93224-93229, 93241-93248, 93268, 93270-93272, 96523, 99446-99449, 99451-99452

0418T 36591-36592, 93000-93010, 93040-93042, 93224-93229, 93241-93248, 93268, 93270-93272, 96523, 99446-99449, 99451-99452

0439T 36591-36592, 96523

0483T 01920, 01924, 01926, 0213T, 0216T, 0345T❖, 0596T-0597T, 0632T, 0708T-0709T, 12001-12007, 12011-12057, 13100-13133, 13151-13153, 32554-32557, 33210-33211, 33254-33256, 33310-33315, 33419, 35201-35207, 35211-35286, 36000, 36010-36100, 36140, 36160-36200, 36215-36217, 36245-36247, 36400-36410, 36420-36430, 36440, 36500, 36555-36556, 36568-36569, 36572-36573, 36591-36592, 36600-36640, 43752, 51701-51703, 62320-62327, 64400, 64405-64408, 64415-64435, 64445-64454, 64461-64463, 64479-64505, 64510-64530, 69990, 75600, 75605, 75625, 75630, 75710, 75716, 75741, 75743, 75746, 75756, 75893, 76000, 76496, 76942, 76998, 77002, 78635, 92012-92014, 92961, 93000-93010, 93040-93042, 93306-93308, 93312-93318, 93320-93325, 93355, 93451-93462, 93503, 93563-93565, 93567, 93590,

93592-93598, 94002, 94200, 94680-94690, 95812-95816, 95819, 95822, 95829, 95955, 96360-96368, 96372-96377, 96523, 99155, 99156, 99157, 99211-99215, 99221-99223, 99231-99239, 99242-99245, 99252-99255, 99291-99292, 99304-99310, 99315-99316, 99347-99350, 99374-99375, 99377-99378, 99446-99449, 99451-99452, G0269, G0463, G0471, G9157, J0670, J1644

0484T 01920, 01924, 01926, 0213T, 0216T, 0596T-0597T, 0632T, 0708T-0709T, 11000-11006, 11042-11047, 12001-12007, 12011-12057, 13100-13133, 13151-13153, 20680, 21750, 32100, 32551, 32554-32557, 33140, 33210-33211, 33254-33256, 33310-33315, 33419, 35201-35207, 35211-35286, 36000, 36010-36100, 36140, 36160-36200, 36215-36217, 36245-36247, 36400-36410, 36420-36430, 36440, 36500, 36555-36556, 36568-36569, 36572-36573, 36591-36592, 36600-36640, 39000-39010, 43752, 51701-51703, 62320-62327, 64400, 64405-64408, 64415-64435, 64445-64454, 64461-64463, 64479-64505, 64510-64530, 69990, 75600, 75605, 75625, 75630, 75710, 75716, 75741, 75743, 75746, 75756, 75893, 76000, 76496, 76942, 76998, 77002, 78635, 92012-92014, 92961, 93000-93010, 93040-93042, 93306-93308, 93312-93318, 93320-93325, 93355, 93451-93462, 93503, 93563-93565, 93567, 93590, 93592-93598, 94002, 94200, 94680-94690, 95812-95816, 95819, 95822, 95829, 95955, 96360-96368, 96372-96377, 96523, 97597-97598, 97602, 99155, 99156, 99157, 99211-99215, 99221-99223, 99231-99239, 99242-99245, 99252-99255, 99291-99292, 99304-99310, 99315-99316, 99347-99350, 99374-99375, 99377-99378, 99446-99449, 99451-99452, G0269, G0463, G0471, G9157, J0670, J1644

0505T 01924, 0596T-0597T, 0708T-0709T, 11000-11006, 11042-11047, 12001-12007, 12011-12057, 13100-13133, 13151-13153, 34713-34716, 34812-34820, 34833-34834, 35201-35206, 35226-35236, 35256-35266, 35286, 35302-35303, 36000, 36002-36012, 36140, 36160-36200, 36245-36247, 36400-36410, 36420-36430, 36440, 36500, 36591-36592, 36600-36640, 37186, 37224-37227, 37236-37239, 37246-37249, 43752, 51701-51703, 62320-62327, 64400, 64405-64408, 64415-64435, 64445-64454, 64461-64463, 64479-64505, 64510-64530, 69990, 75630, 75710, 75716, 75736, 75774, 75893, 76000, 76937, 76942, 76998, 77002, 92012-92014, 93000-93010, 93040-93042, 93050, 93318, 93355, 94002, 94200, 94680-94690, 95812-95816, 95819, 95822, 95829, 95955, 96360-96368, 96372, 96374-96377, 96523, 97597-97598, 97602, 99155, 99156, 99157, 99211-99215, 99221-99223, 99231-99239, 99242-99245, 99252-99255, 99291-99292, 99304-99310, 99315-99316, 99347-99350, 99374-99375, 99377-99378, 99446-99449, 99451-99452, 99495-99496, G0269, G0463, G0471, J0670, J1642, J1644

0515T 00530, 00534, 0213T, 0216T, 0516T, 0517T, 0518T, 0519T, 0520T, 0521T, 0522T, 0571T-0574T, 0575T-0576T, 0578T-0579T, 0580T, 0596T-0597T, 0614T, 0650T, 0708T-0709T, 0861T-0863T, 11000-11006, 11042-11047, 12001-12007, 12011-12057, 13100-13133, 13151-13153, 32100, 33206-33208, 33210-33218, 33220-33229, 33230-33231, 33233-33238, 33240-33241, 33243-33244, 33249, 33262-33264, 33270-33275, 35201-35207, 35211-35286, 36000, 36100, 36140, 36160-36200, 36215-36217, 36221, 36400-36410, 36420-36430, 36440, 36555-36556, 36568-36569, 36591-36592, 36600, 36640, 39010, 43752, 51701-51703, 62320-62327, 64400, 64405-64408, 64415-64435, 64445-64454, 64461-64463, 64479-64505, 64510-64530, 69990, 76000, 76380, 76937, 76942, 76998, 77001-77002, 77012, 77021, 92012-92014, 92960-92961, 93000-93010, 93040-93042, 93260-93261, 93279, 93280, 93281-93298, 93303-93304, 93306-93308, 93312-93318, 93320-93355, 93452-93453, 93458-93461, 93565, 93595-93597, 93600-93603, 93610-93612, 94002, 94200, 94680-94690, 95812-95816, 95819, 95822, 95829, 95955, 96360-96368, 96372, 96374-96377, 96523, 97597-97598, 97602, 99155, 99156, 99157, 99211-99215, 99221-99223, 99231-99239, 99242-99245, 99252-99255, 99291-99292, 99304-99310, 99315-99316, 99347-99350, 99374-99375, 99377-99378, 99446-99449, 99495-99496, G0448, G0463, G0471

0516T 00530, 00534, 0213T, 0216T, 0517T, 0518T, 0519T, 0520T, 0521T, 0522T, 0571T-0574T, 0575T-0576T, 0578T-0579T, 0580T, 0596T-0597T, 0650T, 0708T-0709T, 0861T, 11000-11006, 11042-11047, 12001-12007, 12011-12057, 13100-13133, 13151-13153, 33206-33207, 33210-33216, 33218, 33221-33229, 33230-33231, 33233-33238, 33240-33241, 33243-33244, 33249, 33270-33273, 33275, 35201-35207, 35211-35286, 36000, 36100, 36140, 36160-36200, 36215-36217, 36221, 36400-36410, 36420-36430, 36440, 36555-36556, 36568-36569, 36591-36592, 36600, 36640, 43752, 51701-51703, 62320-62327, 64400, 64405-64408, 64415-64435, 64445-64454, 64461-64463, 64479-64505, 64510-64530, 69990, 76000, 76380, 76937, 76942, 76998, 77001-77002, 77012, 77021, 92012-92014, 92960-92961, 93000-93010, 93040-93042, 93260-93261, 93279, 93280, 93281-93298, 93303-93304, 93306-93308, 93312-93318, 93320-93355, 93452-93453, 93458-93461, 93565, 93595-93597, 93600-93603, 93610-93612, 94002, 94200, 94680-94690, 95812-95816, 95819, 95822, 95829, 95955, 96360-96368, 96372, 96374-96377, 96523, 97597-97598, 97602, 99155, 99156, 99157, 99211-99215, 99221-99223, 99231-99239, 99242-99245, 99252-99255, 99291-99292, 99304-99310, 99315-99316, 99347-99350, 99374-99375, 99377-99378, 99446-99449, 99495-99496, G0448, G0463, G0471

0517T 00530, 00534, 0213T, 0216T, 0518T, 0519T, 0520T, 0521T, 0522T, 0571T-0574T, 0575T-0576T, 0578T-0579T, 0580T, 0596T-0597T, 0650T, 0708T-0709T, 0861T-0863T, 11000-11006, 11042-11047, 12001-12007, 12011-12057, 13100-13133, 13151-13153, 33206-33208, 33210-33218, 33220-33229, 33230-33231, 33233-33238, 33240-33241, 33243-33244, 33249, 33270-33275, 36000, 36005, 36400-36410, 36420-36430, 36440, 36591-36592, 36600, 36640, 43752, 51701-51703, 62320-62327, 64400, 64405-64408, 64415-64435, 64445-64454, 64461-64463, 64479-64505, 64510-64530, 69990, 76000, 76380, 76937, 76942, 76998, 77002, 77012, 77021, 92012-92014, 92960-92961, 93000-93010, 93040-93042, 93260-93261, 93279, 93280, 93281-93298, 93303-93304, 93306-93308, 93312-93318, 93320-93355, 93595-93597, 93600-93603, 93610-93612, 94002, 94200, 94680-94690, 95812-95816, 95819, 95822, 95829, 95955, 96360-96368, 96372, 96374-96377, 96523, 97597-97598, 97602, 99155, 99156, 99157, 99211-99215, 99221-99223, 99231-99239, 99242-99245, 99252-99255, 99291-99292, 99304-99310, 99315-99316, 99347-99350, 99374-99375, 99377-99378, 99446-99449, 99495-99496, G0463, G0471

0518T 00530, 00534, 0213T, 0216T, 0521T, 0522T, 0574T, 0575T-0576T, 0578T-0579T, 0596T-0597T, 0650T, 0708T-0709T, 0861T-0863T, 11000-11006, 11042-11047, 12001-12007, 12011-12057, 13100-13133, 13151-13153, 33210-33211, 33215, 36000, 36005, 36400-36410, 36420-36430, 36440, 36591-36592, 36600, 36640, 43752, 51701-51703, 62320-62327, 64400, 64405-64408, 64415-64435, 64445-64454, 64461-64463, 64479-64505, 64510-64530, 69990, 76000, 76380, 76937, 76942, 76998, 77002, 77012, 77021, 92012-92014, 92960-92961, 93000-93010, 93040-93042, 93260-93261, 93279, 93280, 93281-93298, 93303-93304, 93306-93308, 93312-93318, 93320-93355, 93595-93597, 94002, 94200, 94680-94690, 95812-95816, 95819, 95822, 95829, 95955, 96360-96368, 96372, 96374-96377, 96523, 97597-97598, 97602, 99155, 99156, 99157, 99211-99215, 99221-99223, 99231-99239, 99242-99245, 99252-99255, 99291-99292, 99304-99310, 99315-99316, 99347-99350, 99374-99375, 99377-99378, 99446-99449, 99495-99496, G0463, G0471

0519T 00530, 00534, 0213T, 0216T, 0518T, 0521T, 0522T, 0574T, 0575T-0576T, 0578T-0579T, 0580T, 0596T-0597T, 0650T, 0708T-0709T, 0861T-0863T, 11000-11006, 11042-11047, 12001-12007, 12011-12057, 13100-13133, 13151-13153, 33210-33211, 33215-33217, 33230-33231, 33240-33241,

36000, 36005, 36400-36410, 36420-36430, 36440, 36591-36592, 36600, 36640, 43752, 51701-51703, 62320-62327, 64400, 64405-64408, 64415-64435, 64445-64454, 64461-64463, 64479-64505, 64510-64530, 69990, 76000, 76380, 76937, 76942, 76998, 77002, 77012, 77021, 92012-92014, 93000-93010, 93040-93042, 93260-93261, 93279, 93280, 93281-93298, 93303-93304, 93306-93308, 93312-93318, 93320-93355, 93595-93597, 93600-93603, 93610-93612, 94002, 94200, 94680-94690, 95812-95816, 95819, 95822, 95829, 95955, 96360-96368, 96372, 96374-96377, 96523, 97597-97598, 97602, 99155, 99156, 99157, 99211-99215, 99221-99223, 99231-99239, 99242-99245, 99252-99255, 99291-99292, 99304-99310, 99315-99316, 99347-99350, 99374-99375, 99377-99378, 99446-99449, 99495-99496, G0463, G0471

0520T 00530, 00534, 0213T, 0216T, 0518T, 0519T, 0521T, 0522T, 0571T, 0574T, 0575T-0576T, 0578T-0579T, 0596T-0597T, 0614T, 0650T, 0708T-0709T, 0861T-0863T, 11000-11006, 11042-11047, 12001-12007, 12011-12057, 13100-13133, 13151-13153, 32100, 33210-33211, 33215-33217, 33223-33226, 33230-33231, 33240, 33262-33264, 35201-35207, 35211-35286, 36000, 36100, 36140, 36160-36200, 36215-36217, 36221, 36400-36410, 36420-36430, 36440, 36555-36556, 36568-36569, 36591-36592, 36600, 36640, 39010, 43752, 51701-51703, 62320-62327, 64400, 64405-64408, 64415-64435, 64445-64454, 64461-64463, 64479-64505, 64510-64530, 69990, 76000, 76380, 76937, 76942, 76998, 77001-77002, 77012, 77021, 92012-92014, 92960-92961, 93000-93010, 93040-93042, 93260-93261, 93279, 93280, 93281-93298, 93303-93304, 93306-93308, 93312-93318, 93320-93355, 93452-93453, 93458-93461, 93565, 93595-93597, 93600-93603, 93610-93612, 94002, 94200, 94680-94690, 95812-95816, 95819, 95822, 95829, 95955, 96360-96368, 96372, 96374-96377, 96523, 97597-97598, 97602, 99155, 99156, 99157, 99211-99215, 99221-99223, 99231-99239, 99242-99245, 99252-99255, 99291-99292, 99304-99310, 99315-99316, 99347-99350, 99374-99375, 99377-99378, 99446-99449, 99495-99496, G0448, G0463, G0471

0521T 0579T, 0861T, 0863T, 36591-36592, 93000-93010, 93040-93042, 93224-93229, 93241-93248, 93261, 93268, 93270-93272, 93279, 93280, 93286-93287, 93291, 93294, 93296-93298, 96523, 99446-99449

0522T 0521T, 0576T, 0650T, 0861T, 36591-36592, 93000-93010, 93040-93042, 93224-93229, 93241-93248, 93261, 93268, 93270-93272, 93285-93289, 93291, 93745, 96523, 99446-99449

0523T 0213T, 0216T, 0596T-0597T, 0694T, 0708T-0709T, 12001-12007, 12011-12057, 13100-13133, 13151-13153, 33210-33211, 36000, 36400-36410, 36420-36430, 36440, 36591-36592, 36600, 36640, 43752, 51701-51703, 62320-62327, 64400, 64405-64408, 64415-64435, 64445-64454, 64461-64463, 64479-64505, 64510-64530, 69990, 76376-76377, 92012-92014, 93000-93010, 93040-93042, 93318, 93355, 94002, 94200, 94680-94690, 95812-95816, 95819, 95822, 95829, 95955, 96360-96368, 96372, 96374-96377, 96523, 99155, 99156, 99157, 99211-99215, 99221-99223, 99231-99239, 99242-99245, 99252-99255, 99291-99292, 99304-99310, 99315-99316, 99347-99350, 99374-99375, 99377-99378, 99446-99449

0524T 0213T, 0216T, 0596T-0597T, 0708T-0709T, 12001-12007, 12011-12057, 13100-13133, 13151-13153, 29581, 35201-35207, 35211-35286, 36000, 36002-36012, 36400-36410, 36420-36430, 36440, 36474, 36476, 36479, 36591-36592, 36600, 36640, 37241, 43752, 51701-51703, 62320-62327, 64400, 64405-64408, 64415-64435, 64445-64454, 64461-64463, 64479-64505, 64510-64530, 69990, 75894, 76000, 76380, 76937, 76940, 76942, 76998, 77002, 77012-77013, 77021-77022, 92012-92014, 93000-93010, 93040-93042, 93318, 93355, 93970-93971, 93985-93986, 94002, 94200, 94680-94690, 95812-95816, 95819, 95822, 95829, 95955, 96360-96368, 96372, 96374-96377, 96523, 99155, 99156, 99157, 99211-99215, 99221-99223, 99231-99239, 99242-99245, 99252-99255, 99291-99292, 99304-99310, 99315-99316, 99347-99350, 99374-99375, 99377-99378, 99446-99449, 99495-99496, G0463, G0471, J0670

0525T 00530, 00534, 0213T, 0216T, 0417T, 0418T, 0526T, 0527T, 0528T, 0529T, 0575T, 0579T, 0596T-0597T, 0632T, 0650T, 0708T-0709T, 11000-11006, 11042-11047, 12001-12007, 12011-12057, 13100-13133, 13151-13153, 36000, 36005-36013, 36140, 36400-36410, 36420-36430, 36440, 36555-36556, 36568-36569, 36591-36592, 36600, 36640, 43752, 51701-51703, 61650, 62320-62327, 64400, 64405-64408, 64415-64435, 64445-64454, 64461, 64463, 64479, 64483, 64486-64490, 64493, 64505, 64510-64530, 69990, 76000, 76942, 76998, 77001-77002, 92960-92961, 93000-93010, 93040-93042, 93050, 93224-93229, 93241-93248, 93268, 93270-93272, 93279, 93285-93286, 93288, 93290-93293, 93296-93297, 93318, 93355, 93602, 94002, 94200, 94680-94690, 95812-95816, 95819, 95822, 95829, 95955, 96360, 96365, 96372, 96374-96377, 96523, 97597-97598, 97602, 99155, 99156, 99157, 99446-99449, G0471

0526T 00530, 00534, 0213T, 0216T, 0417T, 0418T, 0528T, 0529T, 0575T, 0579T, 0596T-0597T, 0632T, 0650T, 0708T-0709T, 11000-11006, 11042-11047, 12001-12007, 12011-12057, 13100-13133, 13151-13153, 36000, 36005-36013, 36140, 36400-36410, 36420-36430, 36440, 36555-36556, 36568-36569, 36591-36592, 36600, 36640, 43752, 51701-51703, 61650, 62320-62327, 64400, 64405-64408, 64415-64435, 64445-64454, 64461, 64463, 64479, 64483, 64486-64490, 64493, 64505, 64510-64530, 69990, 76000, 76942, 76998, 77001-77002, 92960-92961, 93000-93010, 93040-93042, 93224-93229, 93241-93248, 93268, 93270-93272, 93279, 93285-93286, 93288, 93290-93293, 93296-93297, 93318, 93355, 94002, 94200, 94680-94690, 95812-95816, 95819, 95822, 95829, 95955, 96360, 96365, 96372, 96374-96377, 96523, 97597-97598, 97602, 99155, 99156, 99157, 99446-99449, G0471

0527T 00530, 00534, 0213T, 0216T, 0417T, 0418T, 0526T, 0528T, 0529T, 0575T, 0579T, 0596T-0597T, 0650T, 0708T-0709T, 11000-11006, 11042-11047, 12001-12007, 12011-12057, 13100-13133, 13151-13153, 36000, 36005, 36400-36410, 36420-36430, 36440, 36591-36592, 36600, 36640, 43752, 51701-51703, 61650, 62320-62327, 64400, 64405-64408, 64415-64435, 64445-64454, 64461, 64463, 64479, 64483, 64486-64490, 64493, 64505, 64510-64530, 69990, 76000, 76942, 76998, 92960-92961, 93000-93010, 93040-93042, 93224-93229, 93241-93248, 93268, 93270-93272, 93279, 93285-93286, 93288, 93290-93293, 93296-93297, 93318, 93355, 94002, 94200, 94680-94690, 95812-95816, 95819, 95822, 95829, 95955, 96360, 96365, 96372, 96374-96377, 96523, 97597-97598, 97602, 99155, 99156, 99157, 99446-99449, G0471

0528T 0418T, 0529T, 0650T, 36591-36592, 93000-93010, 93040-93042, 93224-93229, 93241-93248, 93268, 93270-93272, 93285-93288, 93291, 96523, 99446-99449

0529T 0579T, 36591-36592, 93000-93010, 93286, 93296, 96523, 99446-99449

0530T 00530, 00534, 0213T, 0216T, 0415T, 0416T❖, 0417T, 0418T, 0528T, 0529T, 0575T-0576T, 0578T-0579T, 0596T-0597T, 0632T, 0650T, 0708T-0709T, 11000-11006, 11042-11047, 12001-12007, 12011-12057, 13100-13133, 13151-13153, 33210-33211, 33215, 36000, 36005-36013, 36140, 36400-36410, 36420-36430, 36440, 36555-36556, 36568-36569, 36591-36592, 36600, 36640, 43752, 51701-51703, 61650, 62320-62327, 64400, 64405-64408, 64415-64435, 64445-64454, 64461, 64463, 64479, 64483, 64486-64490, 64493, 64505, 64510-64530, 69990, 76000, 76942, 76998, 77001-77002, 92960-92961, 93000-93010, 93040-93042, 93260-93261, 93279, 93280, 93281-93298, 93318, 93355, 94002,

94200, 94680-94690, 95812-95816, 95819, 95822, 95829, 95955, 96360, 96365, 96372, 96374-96377, 96523, 97597-97598, 97602, 99155, 99156, 99157, 99446-99449, G0471

0531T 00530, 00534, 0213T, 0216T, 0415T, 0416T❖, 0417T, 0418T, 0528T, 0529T, 0575T-0576T, 0578T-0579T, 0596T-0597T, 0632T, 0650T, 0708T-0709T, 11000-11006, 11042-11047, 12001-12007, 12011-12057, 13100-13133, 13151-13153, 33210-33211, 33215, 36000, 36005-36013, 36140, 36400-36410, 36420-36430, 36440, 36555-36556, 36568-36569, 36591-36592, 36600, 36640, 43752, 51701-51703, 61650, 62320-62327, 64400, 64405-64408, 64415-64435, 64445-64454, 64461, 64463, 64479, 64483, 64486-64490, 64493, 64505, 64510-64530, 69990, 76000, 76942, 76998, 77001-77002, 92960-92961, 93000-93010, 93040-93042, 93260-93261, 93279, 93280, 93281-93298, 93318, 93355, 94002, 94200, 94680-94690, 95812-95816, 95819, 95822, 95829, 95955, 96360, 96365, 96372, 96374-96377, 96523, 97597-97598, 97602, 99155, 99156, 99157, 99446-99449, G0471

0532T 00530, 00534, 0213T, 0216T, 0415T, 0416T❖, 0417T, 0418T, 0528T, 0529T, 0575T-0576T, 0578T-0579T, 0596T-0597T, 0632T, 0650T, 0708T-0709T, 11000-11006, 11042-11047, 12001-12007, 12011-12057, 13100-13133, 13151-13153, 33210-33211, 33215, 36000, 36005-36013, 36140, 36400-36410, 36420-36430, 36440, 36555-36556, 36568-36569, 36591-36592, 36600, 36640, 43752, 51701-51703, 61650, 62320-62327, 64400, 64405-64408, 64415-64435, 64445-64454, 64461, 64463, 64479, 64483, 64486-64490, 64493, 64505, 64510-64530, 69990, 76000, 76942, 76998, 77001-77002, 92960-92961, 93000-93010, 93040-93042, 93260-93261, 93279, 93280, 93281-93298, 93318, 93355, 94002, 94200, 94680-94690, 95812-95816, 95819, 95822, 95829, 95955, 96360, 96365, 96372, 96374-96377, 96523, 97597-97598, 97602, 99155, 99156, 99157, 99446-99449, G0471

0543T 0213T, 0216T, 0345T❖, 0483T❖, 0484T❖, 0632T, 0643T❖, 11000-11006, 11042-11047, 12042-12047, 13131-13133, 20680, 21750, 32100, 32551, 32554-32557, 33140, 33210-33211, 33254-33256, 33310-33315, 33418-33419, 35207, 35221, 35236-35246, 35271-35276, 35820, 36010-36014, 36140, 36160-36200, 36215-36217, 36245-36247, 36591-36592, 39000-39010, 64450, 92960-92961, 92987, 93318, 93355, 93590, 93592, 96376, 96523, 97597-97598, 97602, 99304-99310, 99315-99316, 99347-99350, 99374-99375, 99377-99378, 99446-99449, 99451-99452, 99495-99496, G0463, G0471

0544T 01920, 01924, 01926, 0213T, 0216T, 0345T❖, 0483T❖, 0484T❖, 0632T, 0643T❖, 12042-12047, 13131-13133, 32554-32557, 33210-33211, 33254-33256, 33310-33315, 33418-33419, 35207, 35221, 35236-35256, 35281-35286, 36010, 36013-36100, 36140, 36160-36200, 36500, 36555-36556, 36568-36569, 36572-36573, 36591-36592, 36620-36625, 64450, 75600, 75605, 75625, 75630, 75710, 75716, 75741, 75743, 75746, 75756, 75893, 76496, 76942, 76998, 77002, 78635, 92961, 93306-93308, 93312-93318, 93320-93325, 93355, 93503, 93564-93565, 93567, 93590, 93592-93598, 96373, 96376, 96523, 99304-99310, 99315-99316, 99347-99350, 99374-99375, 99377-99378, 99446-99449, 99451-99452, G0269, G0463, G0471, G9157, J0670, J1644

0545T 0596T-0597T, 0632T, 0708T-0709T, 11000-11006, 11042-11047, 12021-12047, 13100-13133, 20680, 21750, 32100, 32551, 32554-32557, 33140, 33210-33211, 33254-33256, 33310-33315, 35201-35206, 35211-35216, 35226, 35251-35256, 35281-35286, 35820, 36000, 36400-36410, 36420-36430, 36440, 36591-36592, 36600, 36640, 39000-39010, 43752, 51701-51703, 62320-62327, 64400, 64405-64408, 64415-64435, 64445-64450, 64461-64463, 64479-64505, 64510-64530, 69990, 76000, 92960-92961, 93000-93010, 93040-93042, 93306-93308, 93312-93318, 93320-93325, 93355, 93451-93461, 93564, 93566, 93593-93598, 94002, 94200, 94680-94690, 95812-95816, 95819, 95822, 95829, 95955, 96360-96368, 96372, 96374-96377, 96523, 97597-97598, 97602, 99155, 99156, 99157, 99211-99215, 99221-99223, 99231-99239, 99242-99245, 99252-99255, 99291-99292, 99304-99310, 99315-99316, 99347-99350, 99374-99375, 99377-99378, 99446-99449, 99451-99452, 99495-99496, G0463, G0471

0559T 0694T, 76376-76377

0560T 0694T, 76376-76377

0561T 0694T, 76376-76377

0562T 0694T, 76376-76377

0569T 0213T, 0216T, 36430, 64450, 93318, 93593-93598, 93662, 96376

0570T 0213T, 0216T, 64450, 93318, 93593-93598, 93662, 96376

0571T 00530, 00534, 00540, 0213T, 0216T, 0521T, 0522T, 0525T, 0526T, 0527T, 0528T, 0529T, 0572T, 0575T-0577T, 0632T, 11000-11006, 11042-11047, 32100, 33202-33203, 33236-33238, 33243, 33250-33251, 33254-33259, 33261, 33265-33266, 35201-35206, 35226-35236, 35256-35266, 35286, 36005-36013, 36140, 36555-36556, 36568-36569, 36572-36573, 36591-36592, 39010, 64450, 76998, 77001, 92960-92961, 93318, 93355, 93600-93603, 93610-93612, 93640-93641, 96376, 96523, 97597-97598, 97602, 99446-99449, 99451-99452, 99495-99496, G0463, G0471

0572T 00530, 00540, 0213T, 0216T, 0521T, 0522T, 0575T-0577T, 11000-11006, 11042-11047, 33202-33203, 33236-33238, 33243, 33250-33251, 33254-33259, 33261, 33265-33266, 36591-36592, 64450, 76998, 92960-92961, 93318, 93355, 93600-93603, 93610-93612, 93640-93641, 96376, 96523, 97597-97598, 97602, 99446-99449, 99451-99452, G0471

0573T 00530, 00540, 0213T, 0216T, 0521T, 0522T, 0575T-0577T, 11000-11006, 11042-11047, 33202-33203, 33236-33238, 33243, 33250-33251, 33254-33259, 33261, 33265-33266, 36591-36592, 64450, 76998, 92960-92961, 93318, 93355, 93640-93641, 96376, 96523, 97597-97598, 97602, 99446-99449, 99451-99452, G0471

0574T 00530, 00540, 0213T, 0216T, 0521T, 0522T, 0525T, 0526T, 0527T, 0528T, 0529T, 0530T, 0531T-0532T, 0572T, 0575T-0577T, 0632T, 11000-11006, 11042-11047, 33202-33203, 33236-33238, 33243, 33250-33251, 33254-33259, 33261, 33265-33266, 35201-35206, 35226-35236, 35256-35266, 35286, 36005-36013, 36140, 36555-36556, 36568-36569, 36572-36573, 36591-36592, 64450, 75860, 76998, 77001, 92960-92961, 93318, 93355, 93600-93603, 93610-93612, 93640-93641, 96376, 96523, 97597-97598, 97602, 99446-99449, 99451-99452, 99495-99496, G0448❖, G0463, G0471

0575T 0418T, 0521T, 0529T, 0576T, 0580T, 0734T, 33202-33203, 33236-33238, 33243, 33250-33251, 33254-33259, 33261, 33265-33266, 36591-36592, 93000-93010, 93040-93042, 93224-93229, 93241-93248, 93640-93642, 93745, 96523, 98980, 99091, 99446-99449, 99451-99452, 99457

0576T 0417T, 0418T❖, 0525T, 0526T, 0527T, 0528T, 0734T, 33202-33203, 33236-33238, 33243, 33250-33251, 33254-33259, 33261, 33265-33266, 36591-36592, 93000-93010, 93040-93042, 93224-93229, 93241-93248, 93640-93641, 96523, 98980, 99091, 99446-99449, 99451-99452, 99457

0577T 00410, 00534-00537, 0213T, 0216T, 0521T❖, 0522T❖, 0580T, 0596T-0597T, 0632T, 0708T-0709T, 12001-12007, 12011-12057, 13100-13133, 13151-13153, 33202-33203, 33236-33238, 33243, 33250-33251, 33254-33259, 33261, 33265-33266, 36000, 36005-36013, 36140, 36400-36410, 36420-36430, 36440, 36555-36556, 36568-36569, 36572-36573, 36591-36592, 36600, 36640, 43752, 51701-51703, 62320-62327, 64400, 64405-64408, 64415-64435, 64445-64450, 64461-64463, 64479-64505, 64510-64530, 76942, 76998, 92012-92014, 92950, 92960-92961, 93000-93010, 93040-93042, 93050, 93318, 93355, 93451-93461, 93563, 93565-93568, 93593-93597, 93618, 93640-93641,

94002, 94200, 94680-94690, 95812-95816, 95819, 95822, 95829, 95955, 96360-96368, 96372, 96374-96377, 96523, 99155, 99156, 99157, 99211-99215, 99221-99223, 99231-99239, 99242-99245, 99252-99255, 99291-99292, 99304-99310, 99315-99316, 99347-99350, 99374-99375, 99377-99378, 99446-99449, 99451-99452, 99495-99496, G0463, G0471

0578T 0521T, 0525T, 0526T, 0527T, 0529T, 0576T, 0733T, 33202-33203, 33236-33238, 33243, 33250-33251, 33254-33259, 33261, 33265-33266, 36591-36592, 93000-93010, 93040-93042, 93224-93229, 93241-93248, 93640-93641, 96523, 98975-98977, 99453-99454

0579T 0576T, 0733T-0734T, 33202-33203, 33236-33238, 33243, 33250-33251, 33254-33259, 33261, 33265-33266, 36591-36592, 93000-93010, 93040-93042, 93224-93229, 93241-93248, 93640-93641, 96523, 98975-98977, 98980, 99091, 99453-99454, 99457

0580T 00530, 00534, 0213T, 0216T, 0521T, 0522T, 0525T, 0526T, 0527T, 0528T, 0529T, 0572T, 0576T, 11000-11006, 11042-11047, 33202-33203, 33236-33238, 33243, 33250-33251, 33254-33259, 33261, 33265-33266, 36005, 36591-36592, 64450, 76000, 76942, 76998, 77002, 92960-92961, 93318, 93355, 93640-93641, 96376, 96523, 97597-97598, 97602, 99446-99449, 99451-99452, 99495-99496, G0463, G0471

0607T No CCI edits apply to this code.

0608T No CCI edits apply to this code.

0613T 01926, 0213T, 0216T, 0708T-0709T, 11000-11006, 11042-11047, 12001-12007, 12011-12057, 13100-13133, 13151-13153, 33210-33211, 35201-35207, 35211-35286, 35702-35703, 36000, 36400-36410, 36420-36430, 36440, 36500, 36591-36592, 36600, 36640, 43752, 51701-51703, 62320-62327, 64400, 64405-64408, 64415-64435, 64445-64454, 64461-64463, 64479-64505, 64510-64530, 69990, 75893, 76000, 76937, 76942, 76998, 77002, 92012-92014, 92961, 93000-93010, 93040-93042, 93050, 93313-93314, 93318, 93355, 93451-93462, 93593-93598, 93662, 94002, 94200, 94680-94690, 95812-95816, 95819, 95822, 95829, 95955, 96360-96368, 96372-96377, 96523, 97597-97598, 97602, 99155, 99156, 99157, 99211-99215, 99221-99223, 99231-99239, 99242-99245, 99252-99255, 99291-99292, 99304-99310, 99315-99316, 99347-99350, 99374-99375, 99377-99378, 99446-99449, 99451-99452, 99495-99496, G0463, G0471

0614T 00530, 00534, 0213T, 0216T, 0521T, 0522T, 0525T, 0526T, 0527T, 0528T, 0529T, 0571T-0574T, 0575T-0579T, 0580T, 0650T, 0708T-0709T, 11000-11006, 11042-11047, 12001-12007, 12011-12057, 13100-13133, 13151-13153, 33210-33211, 33215-33217, 33230-33231, 33240-33241, 33262, 33270, 35201-35207, 35211-35286, 36000, 36005, 36400-36410, 36420-36430, 36440, 36591-36592, 36600, 36640, 43752, 51701-51703, 62320-62327, 64400, 64405-64408, 64415-64435, 64445-64454, 64461-64463, 64479-64505, 64510-64530, 69990, 76000, 76942, 76998, 92012-92014, 93000-93010, 93040-93042, 93260-93261, 93264, 93279, 93280, 93281-93298, 93318, 93355, 93600-93603, 93610-93612, 94002, 94200, 94680-94690, 95812-95816, 95819, 95822, 95829, 95955, 96360-96368, 96372, 96374-96377, 96523, 97597-97598, 97602, 99155, 99156, 99157, 99211-99215, 99221-99223, 99231-99239, 99242-99245, 99252-99255, 99291-99292, 99304-99310, 99315-99316, 99347-99350, 99374-99375, 99377-99378, 99446-99449, 99451-99452, 99495-99496, G0463, G0471

0620T 01924, 0213T, 0216T, 0708T-0709T, 11000-11006, 11042-11047, 12001-12007, 12011-12057, 13100-13133, 13151-13153, 35201-35207, 35211-35286, 36000, 36002-36012, 36140, 36160-36200, 36245-36247, 36400-36410, 36420-36430, 36440, 36500, 36591-36592, 36600-36640, 37228-37235, 37238-37239, 37246-37249, 43752, 51701-51703, 62320-62327, 64400, 64405-64408, 64415-64435, 64445-64454, 64461-64463, 64479-64505, 64510-64530, 69990, 75630, 75710, 75716, 75736, 75774, 75820, 75822, 75893, 76000, 76380, 76937, 76942, 76998, 77002, 77012, 77021, 92012-92014, 93000-93010, 93040-93042, 93050, 93318, 93355, 94002, 94200, 94680-94690, 95812-95816, 95819, 95822, 95829, 95955, 96360-96368, 96372, 96374-96377, 96523, 97597-97598, 97602, 99155, 99156, 99157, 99211-99215, 99221-99223, 99231-99239, 99242-99245, 99252-99255, 99291-99292, 99304-99310, 99315-99316, 99347-99350, 99374-99375, 99377-99378, 99446-99449, 99451-99452, 99495-99496, G0269, G0463, G0471, J0670, J1642, J1644

0623T 0624T-0626T, 0694T, 0711T, 36591-36592, 76376-76377, 96523

0624T 0694T, 36591-36592, 76376-76377, 96523

0625T 0694T, 36591-36592, 76376-76377, 96523

0626T 0694T, 36591-36592, 76376-76377, 96523

0643T 01920, 01924, 01926, 0213T, 0216T, 0345T❖, 0483T❖, 0596T-0597T, 0632T, 11000-11006, 11042-11047, 12001-12007, 12011-12057, 13100-13133, 13151-13153, 20680, 21750, 32100, 32551, 32554-32557, 33140, 33210-33211, 33254-33256, 33310-33315, 33419, 35201-35207, 35211-35286, 35820, 36000, 36010-36100, 36140, 36160-36200, 36215-36217, 36245-36247, 36400-36410, 36420-36430, 36440, 36500, 36555-36556, 36568-36569, 36572-36573, 36591-36592, 36600-36640, 39000-39010, 43752, 51701-51703, 62320-62327, 64400, 64405-64408, 64415-64435, 64445-64454, 64461-64463, 64479-64505, 64510-64530, 69990, 75600, 75605, 75625, 75630, 75710, 75716, 75741, 75743, 75746, 75756, 75893, 76000, 76496, 76942, 76998, 77002, 78635, 92012-92014, 92953-92971, 93000-93010, 93040-93042, 93306-93308, 93312-93318, 93320-93325, 93355, 93451-93464, 93503, 93563-93565, 93567, 93590, 93592-93597, 94002, 94200, 94680-94690, 95812-95816, 95819, 95822, 95829, 95955, 96360-96368, 96372-96377, 96523, 97597-97598, 97602, 99155, 99156, 99157, 99211-99215, 99221-99223, 99231-99239, 99242-99245, 99252-99255, 99291-99292, 99304-99310, 99315-99316, 99347-99350, 99374-99375, 99377-99378, 99446-99449, 99451-99452, 99495-99496, G0269, G0463, G0471, G9157, J0670, J1644

0644T 0213T, 0216T, 12001-12007, 12011-12057, 13100-13133, 13151-13153, 33210-33211, 33254-33256, 33310-33315, 33951-33956, 33965-33966, 33969, 33984-33986, 35820, 36000, 36010-36100, 36140, 36160-36200, 36215-36218, 36245-36248, 36400-36410, 36420-36430, 36440, 36600, 36640, 37187-37188, 43752, 51701-51703, 62320-62327, 64400, 64405-64408, 64415-64435, 64445-64450, 64461-64463, 64479-64505, 64510-64530, 69990, 76000, 76942, 76998, 77002, 92012-92014, 93000-93010, 93040-93042, 93306-93308, 93312-93318, 93320-93325, 93355, 93451-93462, 93563-93568, 93593-93598, 94002, 94200, 94680-94690, 95812-95816, 95819, 95822, 95829, 95955, 96360-96368, 96372, 96374-96377, 99155, 99156, 99157, 99211-99215, 99221-99223, 99231-99239, 99242-99245, 99252-99255, 99291-99292, 99315-99316, 99347-99350, 99374-99375, 99377-99378, G0269

0645T 01916, 01924-01926, 0213T, 0216T, 11000-11006, 11042-11047, 12001-12007, 12011-12057, 13100-13133, 13151-13153, 33210-33211, 33254-33256, 33310-33315, 35201-35206, 35211-35226, 35236-35246, 35261-35266, 35286, 35820, 36000, 36005-36013, 36400-36410, 36420-36430, 36440, 36500, 36591-36592, 36598-36600, 36640, 37246-37247, 37252-37253, 43752, 51701-51703, 62320-62327, 64400, 64405-64408, 64415-64435, 64445-64450, 64461-64463, 64479-64505, 64510-64530, 69990, 75825, 75827, 75860, 76000, 76937, 76942, 76998, 77001-77002, 92012-92014, 93000-93010, 93040-93042, 93306-93308, 93312-93318, 93320-93325, 93355, 93451-93462, 93563-93568, 93593-93598, 93662, 94002, 94200, 94680-94690, 95812-95816, 95819, 95822, 95829, 95955, 96360-96368, 96372,

96374-96377, 96523, 97597-97598, 97602, 99155, 99156, 99157, 99211-99215, 99221-99223, 99231-99239, 99242-99245, 99252-99255, 99291-99292, 99315-99316, 99347-99350, 99374-99375, 99377-99378, 99446-99449, 99451-99452, G0269

0646T 0213T, 0216T, 0545T❖, 0569T❖, 11000-11006, 11042-11047, 12001-12007, 12011-12057, 13100-13133, 13151-13153, 20680, 21750, 32100, 32551, 32554-32557, 33140, 33210-33211, 33254-33256, 33310-33315, 35201-35206, 35211-35216, 35226, 35251-35256, 35281-35286, 35820, 36000, 36400-36410, 36420-36430, 36440, 36591-36592, 36600, 36640, 39000-39010, 43752, 51701-51703, 62320-62327, 64400, 64405-64408, 64415-64435, 64445-64450, 64461-64463, 64479-64505, 64510-64530, 69990, 76000, 92012-92014, 92960-92961, 93000-93010, 93040-93042, 93306-93308, 93312-93318, 93320-93325, 93355, 93451-93461, 93503, 93564, 93566, 93593-93597, 93662, 94002, 94200, 94680-94690, 95812-95816, 95819, 95822, 95829, 95955, 96360-96368, 96372, 96374-96377, 96523, 97597-97598, 97602, 99155, 99156, 99157, 99211-99215, 99221-99223, 99231-99239, 99242-99245, 99252-99255, 99291-99292, 99304-99310, 99315-99316, 99347-99350, 99374-99375, 99377-99378, 99446-99449, 99451-99452, 99495-99496, G0463, G0471

0650T 0571T-0574T, 0575T-0579T, 0580T, 0734T, 36591-36592, 93224-93229, 93241-93248, 93260, 93268, 93270-93272, 93279, 93280, 93281-93282, 93284-93285, 93287-93288, 93291, 93298, 96523, 99091, 99446-99449, 99451-99452, 99457-99458, 99474

0659T 01924-01926, 0596T-0597T, 0632T, 11000-11006, 11042-11047, 33210, 34713-34714, 34812-34813, 35201-35206, 35226-35236, 35256-35266, 35286, 36140, 36160-36200, 36215-36217, 36245-36247, 36591-36592, 36620-36625, 37236, 37246-37247❖, 64451-64454, 75893, 76000, 77001-77002, 92961, 92975, 93050, 93224-93227❖, 93241-93248❖, 93355, 93454-93461, 93463, 93563-93564, 96373, 96523, 97597-97598, 97602, 99304-99310, 99446-99449, 99451-99452, 99495-99496, C9600❖, C9602❖, C9604❖, C9606❖, G0269, G0463, G0471

0674T 0213T, 0216T, 0596T-0597T, 0675T-0685T, 11000-11006, 11042-11047, 12001-12007, 12011-12057, 13100-13133, 13151-13153, 36000, 36400-36410, 36420-36430, 36440, 36591-36592, 36600, 36640, 43752, 44005, 47001, 49082-49084, 49320, 49400, 50715, 51701-51703, 57410, 62320-62327, 64400, 64405-64408, 64415-64435, 64445-64454, 64461-64463, 64479-64505, 64510-64530, 69990, 76000, 77001-77002, 92012-92014, 93000-93010, 93040-93042, 93318, 93355, 94002, 94200, 94680-94690, 95812-95816, 95819, 95822, 95829, 95955, 96360-96368, 96372, 96374-96377, 96523, 97597-97598, 97602, 99155, 99156, 99157, 99211-99215, 99221-99223, 99231-99239, 99242-99245, 99252-99255, 99291-99292, 99304-99310, 99315-99316, 99347-99350, 99374-99375, 99377-99378, 99446-99449, 99451-99452, 99495-99496, G0463, G0471

0675T 0213T, 0216T, 0596T-0597T, 0677T-0685T, 11000-11006, 11042-11047, 12001-12007, 12011-12057, 13100-13133, 13151-13153, 36000, 36400-36410, 36420-36430, 36440, 36591-36592, 36600, 36640, 43752, 44005, 47001, 49082-49084, 49320, 49400, 50715, 51701-51703, 57410, 62320-62327, 64400, 64405-64408, 64415-64435, 64445-64454, 64461-64463, 64479-64505, 64510-64530, 69990, 76000, 77001-77002, 92012-92014, 93000-93010, 93040-93042, 93318, 93355, 94002, 94200, 94680-94690, 95812-95816, 95819, 95822, 95829, 95955, 96360-96368, 96372, 96374-96377, 96523, 97597-97598, 97602, 99155, 99156, 99157, 99211-99215, 99221-99223, 99231-99239, 99242-99245, 99252-99255, 99291-99292, 99304-99310, 99315-99316, 99347-99350, 99374-99375, 99377-99378, 99446-99449, 99451-99452, 99495-99496, G0463, G0471

0676T 0213T, 0216T, 0596T-0597T, 0678T, 0683T-0685T, 11000-11006, 11042-11047, 12001-12007, 12011-12057, 13100-13133, 13151-13153, 36000, 36400-36410, 36420-36430, 36440, 36591-36592, 36600, 36640, 43752, 44005, 47001, 49082-49084, 49320, 49400, 50715, 51701-51703, 57410, 62320-62327, 64400, 64405-64408, 64415-64435, 64445-64454, 64461-64463, 64479-64505, 64510-64530, 69990, 76000, 77001-77002, 92012-92014, 93000-93010, 93040-93042, 93318, 93355, 94002, 94200, 94680-94690, 95812-95816, 95819, 95822, 95829, 95955, 96360-96368, 96372, 96374-96377, 96523, 97597-97598, 97602, 99155, 99156, 99157, 99211-99215, 99221-99223, 99231-99239, 99242-99245, 99252-99255, 99291-99292, 99304-99310, 99315-99316, 99347-99350, 99374-99375, 99377-99378, 99446-99449, 99451-99452, 99495-99496, G0463, G0471

0677T 0213T, 0216T, 0596T-0597T, 0676T, 0679T-0685T, 12001-12007, 12011-12057, 13100-13133, 13151-13153, 36000, 36400-36410, 36420-36430, 36440, 36591-36592, 36600, 36640, 43752, 44005, 47001, 49082-49084, 49320, 49400, 50715, 51701-51703, 57410, 62320-62327, 64400, 64405-64408, 64415-64435, 64445-64454, 64461-64463, 64479-64505, 64510-64530, 69990, 76000, 77001-77002, 92012-92014, 93000-93010, 93040-93042, 93318, 93355, 94002, 94200, 94680-94690, 95812-95816, 95819, 95822, 95829, 95955, 96360-96368, 96372, 96374-96377, 96523, 99155, 99156, 99157, 99211-99215, 99221-99223, 99231-99239, 99242-99245, 99252-99255, 99291-99292, 99304-99310, 99315-99316, 99347-99350, 99374-99375, 99377-99378, 99446-99449, 99451-99452, 99495-99496, G0463, G0471

0678T 0213T, 0216T, 0596T-0597T, 0683T-0685T, 12001-12007, 12011-12057, 13100-13133, 13151-13153, 36000, 36400-36410, 36420-36430, 36440, 36591-36592, 36600, 36640, 43752, 44005, 47001, 49082-49084, 49320, 49400, 50715, 51701-51703, 57410, 62320-62327, 64400, 64405-64408, 64415-64435, 64445-64454, 64461-64463, 64479-64505, 64510-64530, 69990, 76000, 77001-77002, 92012-92014, 93000-93010, 93040-93042, 93318, 93355, 94002, 94200, 94680-94690, 95812-95816, 95819, 95822, 95829, 95955, 96360-96368, 96372, 96374-96377, 96523, 99155, 99156, 99157, 99211-99215, 99221-99223, 99231-99239, 99242-99245, 99252-99255, 99291-99292, 99304-99310, 99315-99316, 99347-99350, 99374-99375, 99377-99378, 99446-99449, 99451-99452, 99495-99496, G0463, G0471

0679T 0213T, 0216T, 0596T-0597T, 0676T, 0678T, 0680T-0685T, 11000-11006, 11042-11047, 12001-12007, 12011-12057, 13100-13133, 13151-13153, 36000, 36400-36410, 36420-36430, 36440, 36591-36592, 36600, 36640, 43752, 44005, 47001, 49082-49084, 49320, 49400, 50715, 51701-51703, 57410, 62320-62327, 64400, 64405-64408, 64415-64435, 64445-64454, 64461-64463, 64479-64505, 64510-64530, 69990, 76000, 77001-77002, 92012-92014, 93000-93010, 93040-93042, 93318, 93355, 94002, 94200, 94680-94690, 95812-95816, 95819, 95822, 95829, 95955, 96360-96368, 96372, 96374-96377, 96523, 97597-97598, 97602, 99155, 99156, 99157, 99211-99215, 99221-99223, 99231-99239, 99242-99245, 99252-99255, 99291-99292, 99304-99310, 99315-99316, 99347-99350, 99374-99375, 99377-99378, 99446-99449, 99451-99452, 99495-99496, G0463, G0471

0680T 0213T, 0216T, 0676T, 0678T, 0681T-0685T, 11000-11006, 11042-11047, 12001-12007, 12011-12057, 13100-13133, 13151-13153, 36000, 36400-36410, 36420-36430, 36440, 36591-36592, 36600, 36640, 43752, 51701-51703, 62320-62327, 64400, 64405-64408, 64415-64435, 64445-64450, 64461-64463, 64479-64505, 64510-64530, 69990, 92012-92014, 93000-93010, 93040-93042, 93318, 94002, 94200, 94680-94690, 95812-95816, 95819, 95822, 95829, 95955, 96360-96368, 96372, 96374-96377, 96523, 97597-97598, 97602, 99155, 99156, 99157, 99211-99215, 99221-99223, 99231-99239, 99242-99245,

99252-99255, 99291-99292, 99315-99316, 99347-99350, 99374-99375, 99377-99378

0681T 0213T, 0216T, 0676T, 0678T, 0682T-0685T, 11000-11006, 11042-11047, 12001-12007, 12011-12057, 13100-13133, 13151-13153, 36000, 36400-36410, 36420-36430, 36440, 36591-36592, 36600, 36640, 43752, 51701-51703, 62320-62327, 64400, 64405-64408, 64415-64435, 64445-64450, 64461-64463, 64479-64505, 64510-64530, 69990, 92012-92014, 93000-93010, 93040-93042, 93318, 94002, 94200, 94680-94690, 95812-95816, 95819, 95822, 95829, 95955, 96360-96368, 96372, 96374-96377, 96523, 97597-97598, 97602, 99155, 99156, 99157, 99211-99215, 99221-99223, 99231-99239, 99242-99245, 99252-99255, 99291-99292, 99315-99316, 99347-99350, 99374-99375, 99377-99378

0682T 0213T, 0216T, 0676T, 0678T, 0683T-0685T, 11000-11006, 11042-11047, 12001-12007, 12011-12057, 13100-13133, 13151-13153, 36000, 36400-36410, 36420-36430, 36440, 36591-36592, 36600, 36640, 43752, 51701-51703, 62320-62327, 64400, 64405-64408, 64415-64435, 64445-64450, 64461-64463, 64479-64505, 64510-64530, 69990, 92012-92014, 93000-93010, 93040-93042, 93318, 94002, 94200, 94680-94690, 95812-95816, 95819, 95822, 95829, 95955, 96360-96368, 96372, 96374-96377, 96523, 97597-97598, 97602, 99155, 99156, 99157, 99211-99215, 99221-99223, 99231-99239, 99242-99245, 99252-99255, 99291-99292, 99315-99316, 99347-99350, 99374-99375, 99377-99378

0683T 0684T-0685T, 36591-36592, 96523

0684T 0685T, 36591-36592, 96523

0685T 36591-36592, 96523

0695T 00410, 00530, 00537, 00540, 0213T, 0216T, 0521T, 0522T, 0525T, 0526T, 0527T, 0528T, 0529T, 0530T, 0531T-0532T, 0571T-0574T, 0575T-0579T, 0580T, 0596T-0597T, 0614T, 0632T, 11000-11006, 11042-11047, 12001-12007, 12011-12057, 13100-13133, 13151-13153, 33202-33208, 33210-33218, 33220-33223, 33227-33229, 33230-33231, 33233-33238, 33240-33241, 33243-33244, 33249, 33250-33251, 33254-33259, 33261-33275, 35201-35206, 35226-35236, 35256-35266, 35286, 36000, 36005-36013, 36140, 36400-36410, 36420-36430, 36440, 36591-36592, 36600, 36640, 43752, 51701-51703, 62320-62327, 64400, 64405-64408, 64415-64435, 64445-64454, 64461-64463, 64479-64505, 64510-64530, 69990, 75860, 76000, 76942, 76998, 77001-77002, 92012-92014, 92950, 92960-92961, 93000-93010, 93040-93042, 93050, 93260-93261, 93264, 93279, 93280, 93281-93298, 93318, 93355, 93451-93461, 93563, 93565-93568, 93600-93603, 93610-93612, 94002, 94200, 94680-94690, 95812-95816, 95819, 95822, 95829, 95955, 96360-96368, 96372, 96374-96377, 96523, 97597-97598, 97602, 99155, 99156, 99157, 99211-99215, 99221-99223, 99231-99239, 99242-99245, 99252-99255, 99291-99292, 99304-99310, 99315-99316, 99347-99350, 99374-99375, 99377-99378, 99446-99449, 99451-99452, 99495-99496, G0463, G0471

0696T 00410, 00537, 0213T, 0216T, 0521T❖, 0522T❖, 0525T, 0526T, 0527T, 0528T❖, 0571T-0574T, 0575T-0579T, 0580T, 0596T-0597T, 0632T, 0734T, 12001-12007, 12011-12057, 13100-13133, 13151-13153, 33210-33211, 35201-35206, 35226-35236, 35256-35266, 35286, 36000, 36005-36013, 36140, 36400-36410, 36420-36430, 36440, 36600, 36640, 43752, 51701-51703, 62320-62327, 64400, 64405-64408, 64415-64435, 64445-64454, 64461-64463, 64479-64505, 64510-64530, 76000, 76942, 76998, 77001-77002, 92012-92014, 92950, 92960-92961, 93000-93010, 93040-93042, 93050, 93224-93229, 93241-93248, 93260-93261, 93264, 93268, 93270-93272, 93278-93279❖, 93280❖, 93282-93283, 93285, 93290-93298, 93318, 93355, 93451-93461, 93563, 93565-93568, 93610-93612, 94002, 94200, 94680-94690, 95812-95816, 95819, 95822, 95829, 95955, 96360-96368, 96372, 96374-96377, 99091, 99155, 99156, 99157, 99211-99215, 99221-99223, 99231-99239, 99242-99245, 99252-99255, 99291-99292, 99304-99310, 99315-99316, 99347-99350, 99374-99375, 99377-99378, 99446-99449, 99451-99452, 99457-99458, 99474, 99495-99496, G0463, G0471

0716T 0213T, 0216T, 12001-12007, 12011-12057, 13100-13133, 13151-13153, 36000, 36400-36410, 36420-36430, 36440, 36591-36592, 36600, 36640, 43752, 51701-51703, 62320-62327, 64400, 64405-64408, 64415-64435, 64445-64450, 64461-64463, 64479-64505, 64510-64530, 69990, 92012-92014, 93000-93010, 93040-93042, 93318, 94002, 94200, 94680-94690, 95812-95816, 95819, 95822, 95829, 95955, 96360-96368, 96372, 96374-96377, 96523, 99155, 99156, 99157, 99211-99215, 99221-99223, 99231-99239, 99242-99245, 99252-99255, 99291-99292, 99315-99316, 99347-99350, 99374-99375, 99377-99378

0744T 0213T, 0216T, 11000-11006, 11042-11047, 12001-12007, 12011-12057, 13100-13133, 13151-13153, 34501, 34510, 36000, 36400-36410, 36420-36430, 36440, 36591-36592, 36600, 36640, 43752, 51701-51703, 62320-62327, 64400, 64405-64408, 64415-64435, 64445-64450, 64461-64463, 64479-64505, 64510-64530, 69990, 76998, 92012-92014, 93000-93010, 93040-93042, 93318, 93971, 94002, 94200, 94680-94690, 95812-95816, 95819, 95822, 95829, 95955, 96360-96368, 96372, 96374-96377, 96523, 97597-97598, 97602, 99155, 99156, 99157, 99211-99215, 99221-99223, 99231-99239, 99242-99245, 99252-99255, 99291-99292, 99315-99316, 99347-99350, 99374-99375, 99377-99378

0745T 0213T, 0216T, 12001-12007, 12011-12057, 13100-13133, 13151-13153, 36000, 36400-36410, 36420-36430, 36440, 36591-36592, 36600, 36640, 43752, 51701-51703, 62320-62327, 64400, 64405-64408, 64415-64435, 64445-64450, 64461-64463, 64479-64505, 64510-64530, 69990, 92012-92014, 93000-93010, 93040-93042, 93318, 94002, 94200, 94680-94690, 95812-95816, 95819, 95822, 95829, 95955, 96360-96368, 96372, 96374-96377, 96523, 99155, 99156, 99157, 99211-99215, 99221-99223, 99231-99239, 99242-99245, 99252-99255, 99291-99292, 99315-99316, 99347-99350, 99374-99375, 99377-99378

0746T 0213T, 0216T, 12001-12007, 12011-12057, 13100-13133, 13151-13153, 36000, 36400-36410, 36420-36430, 36440, 36591-36592, 36600, 36640, 43752, 51701-51703, 62320-62327, 64400, 64405-64408, 64415-64435, 64445-64450, 64461-64463, 64479-64505, 64510-64530, 69990, 92012-92014, 93000-93010, 93040-93042, 93318, 94002, 94200, 94680-94690, 95812-95816, 95819, 95822, 95829, 95955, 96360-96368, 96372, 96374-96377, 96523, 99155, 99156, 99157, 99211-99215, 99221-99223, 99231-99239, 99242-99245, 99252-99255, 99291-99292, 99315-99316, 99347-99350, 99374-99375, 99377-99378

0747T 0213T, 0216T, 12001-12007, 12011-12057, 13100-13133, 13151-13153, 36000, 36400-36410, 36420-36430, 36440, 36591-36592, 36600, 36640, 43752, 51701-51703, 62320-62327, 64400, 64405-64408, 64415-64435, 64445-64450, 64461-64463, 64479-64505, 64510-64530, 69990, 92012-92014, 93000-93010, 93040-93042, 93318, 94002, 94200, 94680-94690, 95812-95816, 95819, 95822, 95829, 95955, 96360-96368, 96372, 96374-96377, 96523, 99155, 99156, 99157, 99211-99215, 99221-99223, 99231-99239, 99242-99245, 99252-99255, 99291-99292, 99315-99316, 99347-99350, 99374-99375, 99377-99378

0793T 35201-35207, 35211-35286, 36591-36592, 96523

0795T 0823T, 0825T, 11000, 11004-11006, 11042-11044, 35201-35207, 35211-35286, 36591-36592, 96523, 97597, 97602

0796T 0823T, 0825T, 11000, 11004-11006, 11042-11044, 35201-35207, 35211-35286, 36591-36592, 96523, 97597, 97602

0797T 0823T, 0825T, 11000, 11004-11006, 11042-11044, 35201-35207, 35211-35286, 36591-36592, 96523, 97597, 97602

0798T 11000, 11004-11006, 11042-11044, 35201-35207, 35211-35286, 36591-36592, 96523, 97597, 97602

0799T 0824T, 11000, 11004-11006, 11042-11044, 35201-35207, 35211-35286, 36591-36592, 96523, 97597, 97602

0800T 11000, 11004-11006, 11042-11044, 35201-35207, 35211-35286, 36591-36592, 96523, 97597, 97602

0801T 11000, 11004-11006, 11042-11044, 35201-35207, 35211-35286, 36591-36592, 96523, 97597, 97602

0802T 0823T, 0825T, 11000, 11004-11006, 11042-11044, 35201-35207, 35211-35286, 36591-36592, 96523, 97597, 97602

0803T 11000, 11004-11006, 11042-11044, 35201-35207, 35211-35286, 36591-36592, 96523, 97597, 97602

0804T 36591-36592, 96523

0805T 35201-35207, 35211-35286, 36591-36592, 96523

0806T 35201-35207, 35211-35286, 36591-36592, 96523

0823T 0826T, 11000, 11004-11006, 11042-11044, 35201-35207, 35211-35286, 36591-36592, 96523, 97597, 97602

0824T 0826T, 11000, 11004-11006, 11042-11044, 35201-35207, 35211-35286, 36591-36592, 96523, 97597, 97602

0825T 0826T, 11000, 11004-11006, 11042-11044, 33274, 35201-35207, 35211-35286, 36591-36592, 96523, 97597, 97602

0826T 36591-36592, 96523

0861T 11000, 11004-11006, 11042-11044, 35231-35286, 36591-36592, 96523, 97597, 97602

0862T 0521T, 0522T, 0861T, 11000, 11004-11006, 11042-11044, 35231-35286, 36591-36592, 96523, 97597, 97602

0863T 0522T, 0861T, 11000, 11004-11006, 11042-11044, 35231-35286, 36591-36592, 76000, 76998, 93303-93304, 93306-93308, 93312-93355, 93452-93453, 93458-93461, 93565, 93586, 93595-93597, 96523, 97597, 97602

0876T No CCI edits apply to this code.

0893T No CCI edits apply to this code.

0897T No CCI edits apply to this code.

0899T No CCI edits apply to this code.

0900T No CCI edits apply to this code.

0902T No CCI edits apply to this code.

0903T No CCI edits apply to this code.

0904T No CCI edits apply to this code.

0905T No CCI edits apply to this code.

0913T No CCI edits apply to this code.

0914T No CCI edits apply to this code.

0915T No CCI edits apply to this code.

0916T No CCI edits apply to this code.

0917T No CCI edits apply to this code.

0918T No CCI edits apply to this code.

0919T No CCI edits apply to this code.

0920T No CCI edits apply to this code.

0921T No CCI edits apply to this code.

0922T No CCI edits apply to this code.

0923T No CCI edits apply to this code.

0924T No CCI edits apply to this code.

0925T No CCI edits apply to this code.

0926T No CCI edits apply to this code.

0927T No CCI edits apply to this code.

0928T No CCI edits apply to this code.

0929T No CCI edits apply to this code.

0930T No CCI edits apply to this code.

0931T No CCI edits apply to this code.

0932T No CCI edits apply to this code.

0933T No CCI edits apply to this code.

0934T No CCI edits apply to this code.

0937T No CCI edits apply to this code.

0938T No CCI edits apply to this code.

0939T No CCI edits apply to this code.

0940T No CCI edits apply to this code.

20101 0213T, 0216T, 0596T-0597T, 11000, 11042-11044, 12001-12007, 12011-12057, 13100-13133, 13151-13152, 13160, 36000, 36400-36410, 36420-36430, 36440, 36591-36592, 36600, 36640, 43752, 51701-51703, 62320-62327, 64400, 64405-64408, 64415-64435, 64445-64454, 64461-64463, 64479-64505, 64510-64530, 69990, 92012-92014, 93000-93010, 93040-93042, 93318, 93355, 94002, 94200, 94680-94690, 95812-95816, 95819, 95822, 95829, 95955, 96360-96368, 96372, 96374-96377, 96523, 97597-97598, 97602-97608, 99155, 99156, 99157, 99211-99215, 99221-99223, 99231-99239, 99242-99245, 99252-99255, 99291-99292, 99304-99310, 99315-99316, 99347-99350, 99374-99375, 99377-99378, 99446-99449, 99451-99452, 99495-99496, G0168, G0463, G0471, J0670

20985 0213T, 0216T, 36000, 36410, 36591-36592, 61650, 62324-62327, 64415-64417, 64450, 64454, 64486-64490, 64493, 69990, 76000, 76380, 76942, 76998, 77001-77002, 77011-77012, 77021, 96360, 96365, 96372, 96374-96377, 96523

21501 0213T, 0216T, 0596T-0597T, 0708T-0709T, 10030, 10060, 10140, 10160, 12001-12007, 12011-12057, 13100-13133, 13151-13153, 20100-20101, 21555, 35800, 36000, 36400-36410, 36420-36430, 36440, 36591-36592, 36600, 36640, 43752, 49185, 49424, 51701-51703, 62320-62327, 64400, 64405-64408, 64415-64435, 64445-64454, 64461-64463, 64479-64505, 64510-64530, 69990, 92012-92014, 93000-93010, 93040-93042, 93318, 93355, 94002, 94200, 94680-94690, 95812-95816, 95819, 95822, 95829, 95955, 96360-96368, 96372, 96374-96377, 96523, 97597-97598, 97602-97608, 99155, 99156, 99157, 99211-99215, 99221-99223, 99231-99239, 99242-99245, 99252-99255, 99291-99292, 99304-99310, 99315-99316, 99347-99350, 99374-99375, 99377-99378, 99446-99449, 99451-99452, 99495-99496, G0463, G0471, J0670

21502 0213T, 0216T, 0596T-0597T, 0708T-0709T, 10030, 10060, 10140, 10160, 11000-11006, 11010-11011, 11042-11047, 12001-12007, 12011-12057, 13100-13133, 13151-13153, 20101, 20220, 21501, 36000, 36400-36410, 36420-36430, 36440, 36591-36592, 36600, 36640, 43752, 51701-51703, 62320-62327, 64400, 64405-64408, 64415-64435, 64445-64454, 64461-64463, 64479-64505, 64510-64530, 69990, 92012-92014, 93000-93010, 93040-93042, 93318, 93355, 94002, 94200, 94680-94690, 95812-95816, 95819, 95822, 95829, 95955, 96360-96368, 96372, 96374-96377, 96523, 97597-97598, 97602-97608, 99155, 99156, 99157, 99211-99215, 99221-99223, 99231-99239, 99242-99245, 99252-99255, 99291-99292, 99304-99310, 99315-99316, 99347-99350, 99374-99375, 99377-99378, 99446-99449, 99451-99452, 99495-99496, G0463, G0471

21510 00550, 0213T, 0216T, 0596T-0597T, 0707T-0709T, 0869T, 10030, 10060, 10140, 10160, 11010-11011, 12001-12007, 12011-12057, 13100-13133,

13151-13153, 20101, 20615, 36000, 36400-36410, 36420-36430, 36440, 36591-36592, 36600, 36640, 43752, 51701-51703, 62320-62327, 64400, 64405-64408, 64415-64435, 64445-64454, 64461-64463, 64479-64505, 64510-64530, 69990, 92012-92014, 93000-93010, 93040-93042, 93318, 93355, 94002, 94200, 94680-94690, 95812-95816, 95819, 95822, 95829, 95955, 96360-96368, 96372, 96374-96377, 96523, 97597-97598, 97602-97608, 99155, 99156, 99157, 99211-99215, 99221-99223, 99231-99239, 99242-99245, 99252-99255, 99291-99292, 99304-99310, 99315-99316, 99347-99350, 99374-99375, 99377-99378, 99446-99449, 99451-99452, 99495-99496, G0463, G0471

21550 0213T, 0216T, 0596T-0597T, 0708T-0709T, 10005, 10007, 10009, 10011, 10021, 10030, 10060, 10140, 10160, 12001-12007, 12011-12057, 13100-13133, 13151-13153, 20100, 36000, 36400-36410, 36420-36430, 36440, 36591-36592, 36600, 36640, 38500, 38531, 43752, 51701-51703, 62320-62327, 64400, 64405-64408, 64415-64435, 64445-64454, 64461-64463, 64479-64505, 64510-64530, 69990, 92012-92014, 93000-93010, 93040-93042, 93318, 93355, 94002, 94200, 94680-94690, 95812-95816, 95819, 95822, 95829, 95955, 96360-96368, 96372, 96374-96377, 96523, 99155, 99156, 99157, 99211-99215, 99221-99223, 99231-99239, 99242-99245, 99252-99255, 99291-99292, 99304-99310, 99315-99316, 99347-99350, 99374-99375, 99377-99378, 99446-99449, 99451-99452, 99495-99496, G0463, G0471, J0670

21552 0213T, 0216T, 0596T-0597T, 0708T-0709T, 10005, 10007, 10009, 10011, 10021, 10030, 10060, 10140, 10160, 11000-11006, 11010-11012❖, 11042-11047, 12001-12007, 12011-12057, 13100-13133, 13151-13153, 21501, 21550, 21555, 36000, 36400-36410, 36420-36430, 36440, 36591-36592, 36600, 36640, 38500-38520❖, 38531-38555❖, 38700❖, 38720❖, 38724❖, 43752, 51701-51703, 62320-62327, 64400, 64405-64408, 64415-64435, 64445-64454, 64461-64463, 64479-64505, 64510-64530, 69990, 92012-92014, 93000-93010, 93040-93042, 93318, 93355, 94002, 94200, 94680-94690, 95812-95816, 95819, 95822, 95829, 95955, 96360-96368, 96372, 96374-96377, 96523, 97597-97598, 97602, 99155, 99156, 99157, 99211-99215, 99221-99223, 99231-99239, 99242-99245, 99252-99255, 99291-99292, 99304-99310, 99315-99316, 99347-99350, 99374-99375, 99377-99378, 99446-99449, 99451-99452, 99495-99496, G0463, G0471

21554 0213T, 0216T, 0596T-0597T, 0708T-0709T, 10005, 10007, 10009, 10011, 10021, 10030, 10060, 10140, 10160, 11000-11006, 11010-11012❖, 11042-11047, 12001-12007, 12011-12057, 13100-13133, 13151-13153, 21501, 21550-21552, 21555-21556, 36000, 36400-36410, 36420-36430, 36440, 36591-36592, 36600, 36640, 38500-38520❖, 38531-38555❖, 38700❖, 38720❖, 38724❖, 43752, 51701-51703, 62320-62327, 64400, 64405-64408, 64415-64435, 64445-64454, 64461-64463, 64479-64505, 64510-64530, 69990, 92012-92014, 93000-93010, 93040-93042, 93318, 93355, 94002, 94200, 94680-94690, 95812-95816, 95819, 95822, 95829, 95955, 96360-96368, 96372, 96374-96377, 96523, 97597-97598, 97602, 99155, 99156, 99157, 99211-99215, 99221-99223, 99231-99239, 99242-99245, 99252-99255, 99291-99292, 99304-99310, 99315-99316, 99347-99350, 99374-99375, 99377-99378, 99446-99449, 99451-99452, 99495-99496, G0463, G0471

21555 0596T-0597T, 0708T-0709T, 10005, 10007, 10009, 10011, 10021, 10030, 10060, 10140, 10160, 11000-11006, 11010-11012❖, 11042-11047, 12001-12007, 12011-12057, 13100-13133, 13151-13153, 21550, 36000, 36400-36410, 36420-36430, 36440, 36591-36592, 36600, 36640, 38500-38520❖, 38531-38555❖, 38700❖, 38720❖, 38724❖, 43752, 51701-51703, 62320-62327, 64400, 64405-64408, 64415-64435, 64445-64454, 64461-64463, 64479-64505, 64510-64530, 69990, 92012-92014, 93000-93010, 93040-93042, 93318, 93355, 94002, 94200, 94680-94690, 95812-95816, 95819, 95822, 95829, 95955, 96360-96368, 96372, 96374-96377, 96523, 97597-97598, 97602, 99155, 99156, 99157, 99211-99215, 99221-99223, 99231-99239, 99242-99245, 99252-99255, 99291-99292, 99304-99310, 99315-99316, 99347-99350, 99374-99375, 99377-99378, 99446-99449, 99451-99452, 99495-99496, G0463, G0471, J0670

21556 0596T-0597T, 0708T-0709T, 10005, 10007, 10009, 10011, 10021, 10030, 10060, 10140, 10160, 11000-11006, 11010-11012❖, 11042-11047, 12001-12007, 12011-12057, 13100-13133, 13151-13153, 21501, 21550-21552, 21555, 36000, 36400-36410, 36420-36430, 36440, 36591-36592, 36600, 36640, 38500-38520❖, 38531-38555❖, 38700❖, 38720❖, 38724❖, 43752, 51701-51703, 62320-62327, 64400, 64405-64408, 64415-64435, 64445-64454, 64461-64463, 64479-64505, 64510-64530, 69990, 92012-92014, 93000-93010, 93040-93042, 93318, 93355, 94002, 94200, 94680-94690, 95812-95816, 95819, 95822, 95829, 95955, 96360-96368, 96372, 96374-96377, 96523, 97597-97598, 97602, 99155, 99156, 99157, 99211-99215, 99221-99223, 99231-99239, 99242-99245, 99252-99255, 99291-99292, 99304-99310, 99315-99316, 99347-99350, 99374-99375, 99377-99378, 99446-99449, 99451-99452, 99495-99496, G0463, G0471

21557 0213T, 0216T, 0596T-0597T, 0708T-0709T, 10005, 10007, 10009, 10011, 10021, 10030, 10060, 10140, 10160, 11000-11006, 11010-11012❖, 11042-11047, 12001-12007, 12011-12057, 13100-13133, 13151-13153, 21501, 21550-21556, 36000, 36400-36410, 36420-36430, 36440, 36591-36592, 36600, 36640, 38500-38520❖, 38531-38555❖, 38700❖, 38720❖, 38724❖, 43752, 51701-51703, 62320-62327, 64400, 64405-64408, 64415-64435, 64445-64454, 64461-64463, 64479-64505, 64510-64530, 69990, 92012-92014, 93000-93010, 93040-93042, 93318, 93355, 94002, 94200, 94680-94690, 95812-95816, 95819, 95822, 95829, 95955, 96360-96368, 96372, 96374-96377, 96523, 97597-97598, 97602, 99155, 99156, 99157, 99211-99215, 99221-99223, 99231-99239, 99242-99245, 99252-99255, 99291-99292, 99304-99310, 99315-99316, 99347-99350, 99374-99375, 99377-99378, 99446-99449, 99451-99452, 99495-99496, G0463, G0471

21558 0213T, 0216T, 0596T-0597T, 0708T-0709T, 10005, 10007, 10009, 10011, 10021, 10030, 10060, 10140, 10160, 11000-11006, 11010-11012❖, 11042-11047, 12001-12007, 12011-12057, 13100-13133, 13151-13153, 21501, 21550-21557, 36000, 36400-36410, 36420-36430, 36440, 36591-36592, 36600, 36640, 38500-38520❖, 38531-38555❖, 38700❖, 38720❖, 38724❖, 43752, 51701-51703, 62320-62327, 64400, 64405-64408, 64415-64435, 64445-64454, 64461-64463, 64479-64505, 64510-64530, 69990, 92012-92014, 93000-93010, 93040-93042, 93318, 93355, 94002, 94200, 94680-94690, 95812-95816, 95819, 95822, 95829, 95955, 96360-96368, 96372, 96374-96377, 96523, 97597-97598, 97602, 99155, 99156, 99157, 99211-99215, 99221-99223, 99231-99239, 99242-99245, 99252-99255, 99291-99292, 99304-99310, 99315-99316, 99347-99350, 99374-99375, 99377-99378, 99446-99449, 99451-99452, 99495-99496, G0463, G0471

21600 0213T, 0216T, 0596T-0597T, 0708T-0709T, 11000-11006, 11012❖, 11042-11047, 12001-12007, 12011-12057, 13100-13133, 13151-13153, 21610, 35820, 36000, 36400-36410, 36420-36430, 36440, 36591-36592, 36600, 36640, 43752, 49010, 51701-51703, 62320-62327, 64400, 64405-64408, 64415-64435, 64445-64454, 64461-64463, 64479-64505, 64510-64530, 69990, 92012-92014, 93000-93010, 93040-93042, 93318, 93355, 94002, 94200, 94680-94690, 95812-95816, 95819, 95822, 95829, 95955, 96360-96368, 96372, 96374-96377, 96523, 97597-97598, 97602, 99155, 99156, 99157, 99211-99215, 99221-99223, 99231-99239, 99242-99245, 99252-99255, 99291-99292, 99304-99310, 99315-99316, 99347-99350, 99374-99375, 99377-99378, 99446-99449, 99451-99452, 99495-99496, G0463, G0471

21601 00400, 0213T, 0216T, 0596T-0597T, 0708T-0709T, 10035, 11000-11001, 11042-11047, 12001-12007, 12020-12047, 13100-13133, 19081, 19083, 19085, 19100, 19120, 19281, 19283, 19285, 19287, 32556-32557, 36000, 36400-36410, 36420-36430, 36440, 36591-36592, 36600, 36640, 43752, 51701-51703, 62320-62327, 64400, 64405-64408, 64415-64435, 64445-64454, 64461-64463, 64479-64505, 64510-64530, 69990, 93000-93010, 93040-93042, 93318, 93355, 94002, 94200, 94680-94690, 95812-95816, 95819, 95822, 95829, 95955, 96360-96368, 96372, 96374-96377, 96523, 97597-97598, 97602, 99155, 99156, 99157, 99211-99215, 99221-99223, 99231-99239, 99242-99245, 99252-99255, 99291-99292, 99304-99310, 99315-99316, 99347-99350, 99374-99375, 99377-99378, 99446-99449, 99451-99452, 99495-99496, G0463, G0471

21602 00400, 0213T, 0216T, 0596T-0597T, 0708T-0709T, 10035, 11000-11001, 11042-11047, 12001-12007, 12020-12047, 13100-13133, 19081, 19083, 19085, 19100, 19120, 19281, 19283, 19285, 19287, 21601, 32556-32557, 36000, 36400-36410, 36420-36430, 36440, 36591-36592, 36600, 36640, 43752, 51701-51703, 62320-62327, 64400, 64405-64408, 64415-64435, 64445-64454, 64461-64463, 64479-64505, 64510-64530, 69990, 93000-93010, 93040-93042, 93318, 93355, 94002, 94200, 94680-94690, 95812-95816, 95819, 95822, 95829, 95955, 96360-96368, 96372, 96374-96377, 96523, 97597-97598, 97602, 99155, 99156, 99157, 99211-99215, 99221-99223, 99231-99239, 99242-99245, 99252-99255, 99291-99292, 99304-99310, 99315-99316, 99347-99350, 99374-99375, 99377-99378, 99446-99449, 99451-99452, 99495-99496, G0463, G0471

21603 00400, 0213T, 0216T, 0596T-0597T, 0708T-0709T, 10035, 11000-11001, 11042-11047, 12001-12007, 12020-12047, 13100-13133, 19081, 19083, 19085, 19100, 19120, 19281, 19283, 19285, 19287, 21601-21602, 32556-32557, 36000, 36400-36410, 36420-36430, 36440, 36591-36592, 36600, 36640, 43752, 51701-51703, 62320-62327, 64400, 64405-64408, 64415-64435, 64445-64454, 64461-64463, 64479-64505, 64510-64530, 69990, 93000-93010, 93040-93042, 93318, 93355, 94002, 94200, 94680-94690, 95812-95816, 95819, 95822, 95829, 95955, 96360-96368, 96372, 96374-96377, 96523, 97597-97598, 97602, 99155, 99156, 99157, 99211-99215, 99221-99223, 99231-99239, 99242-99245, 99252-99255, 99291-99292, 99304-99310, 99315-99316, 99347-99350, 99374-99375, 99377-99378, 99446-99449, 99451-99452, 99495-99496, G0463, G0471

21610 0213T, 0216T, 0596T-0597T, 0708T-0709T, 11000-11006, 11042-11047, 12001-12007, 12011-12057, 13100-13133, 13151-13153, 20101, 36000, 36400-36410, 36420-36430, 36440, 36591-36592, 36600, 36640, 37616, 43752, 51701-51703, 62320-62327, 64400, 64405-64408, 64415-64435, 64445-64454, 64461-64463, 64479-64505, 64510-64530, 69990, 92012-92014, 93000-93010, 93040-93042, 93318, 93355, 94002, 94200, 94680-94690, 95812-95816, 95819, 95822, 95829, 95955, 96360-96368, 96372, 96374-96377, 96523, 97597-97598, 97602, 99155, 99156, 99157, 99211-99215, 99221-99223, 99231-99239, 99242-99245, 99252-99255, 99291-99292, 99304-99310, 99315-99316, 99347-99350, 99374-99375, 99377-99378, 99446-99449, 99451-99452, 99495-99496, G0463, G0471

21615 0213T, 0216T, 0596T-0597T, 0708T-0709T, 11000-11006, 11042-11047, 12001-12007, 12011-12057, 13100-13133, 13151-13153, 20101, 21600, 21610, 36000, 36400-36410, 36420-36430, 36440, 36591-36592, 36600, 36640, 43752, 51701-51703, 62320-62327, 64400, 64405-64408, 64415-64435, 64445-64454, 64461-64463, 64479-64505, 64510-64530, 69990, 92012-92014, 93000-93010, 93040-93042, 93318, 93355, 94002, 94200, 94680-94690, 95812-95816, 95819, 95822, 95829, 95955, 96360-96368, 96372, 96374-96377, 96523, 97597-97598, 97602, 99155, 99156, 99157, 99211-99215, 99221-99223, 99231-99239, 99242-99245, 99252-99255, 99291-99292, 99304-99310, 99315-99316, 99347-99350, 99374-99375, 99377-99378, 99446-99449, 99451-99452, 99495-99496, G0463, G0471

21616 0213T, 0216T, 0596T-0597T, 0708T-0709T, 11000-11006, 11042-11047, 12001-12007, 12011-12057, 13100-13133, 13151-13153, 20101, 21600, 21610-21615, 36000, 36400-36410, 36420-36430, 36440, 36591-36592, 36600, 36640, 43752, 51701-51703, 62320-62327, 64400, 64405-64408, 64415-64435, 64445-64454, 64461-64463, 64479-64505, 64510-64530, 69990, 92012-92014, 93000-93010, 93040-93042, 93318, 93355, 94002, 94200, 94680-94690, 95812-95816, 95819, 95822, 95829, 95955, 96360-96368, 96372, 96374-96377, 96523, 97597-97598, 97602, 99155, 99156, 99157, 99211-99215, 99221-99223, 99231-99239, 99242-99245, 99252-99255, 99291-99292, 99304-99310, 99315-99316, 99347-99350, 99374-99375, 99377-99378, 99446-99449, 99451-99452, 99495-99496, G0463, G0471

21620 00550, 0213T, 0216T, 0596T-0597T, 0708T-0709T, 11000-11006, 11012❖, 11042-11047, 12001-12007, 12011-12057, 13100-13133, 13151-13153, 20101, 20220-20225, 20240-20245, 21750, 35820, 36000, 36400-36410, 36420-36430, 36440, 36591-36592, 36600, 36640, 43752, 51701-51703, 62320-62327, 64400, 64405-64408, 64415-64435, 64445-64454, 64461-64463, 64479-64505, 64510-64530, 69990, 92012-92014, 93000-93010, 93040-93042, 93318, 93355, 94002, 94200, 94680-94690, 95812-95816, 95819, 95822, 95829, 95955, 96360-96368, 96372, 96374-96377, 96523, 97597-97598, 97602, 99155, 99156, 99157, 99211-99215, 99221-99223, 99231-99239, 99242-99245, 99252-99255, 99291-99292, 99304-99310, 99315-99316, 99347-99350, 99374-99375, 99377-99378, 99446-99449, 99451-99452, 99495-99496, G0463, G0471

21627 00550, 0213T, 0216T, 0596T-0597T, 0708T-0709T, 11012❖, 12001-12007, 12011-12057, 13100-13133, 13151-13153, 20101, 20500, 20670-20680, 35820, 36000, 36400-36410, 36420-36430, 36440, 36591-36592, 36600, 36640, 43752, 51701-51703, 62320-62327, 64400, 64405-64408, 64415-64435, 64445-64454, 64461-64463, 64479-64505, 64510-64530, 69990, 92012-92014, 93000-93010, 93040-93042, 93318, 93355, 94002, 94200, 94680-94690, 95812-95816, 95819, 95822, 95829, 95955, 96360-96368, 96372, 96374-96377, 96523, 99155, 99156, 99157, 99211-99215, 99221-99223, 99231-99239, 99242-99245, 99252-99255, 99291-99292, 99304-99310, 99315-99316, 99347-99350, 99374-99375, 99377-99378, 99446-99449, 99451-99452, 99495-99496, G0463, G0471

21630 00550, 0213T, 0216T, 0596T-0597T, 0708T-0709T, 10030, 10060, 10140, 10160, 11000-11006, 11042-11047, 12001-12007, 12011-12057, 13100-13133, 13151-13153, 20101, 20650, 20670-20680, 21600, 21620-21627, 21750, 35820, 36000, 36400-36410, 36420-36430, 36440, 36591-36592, 36600, 36640, 43752, 51701-51703, 62320-62327, 64400, 64405-64408, 64415-64435, 64445-64454, 64461-64463, 64479-64505, 64510-64530, 69990, 92012-92014, 93000-93010, 93040-93042, 93318, 93355, 94002, 94200, 94680-94690, 95812-95816, 95819, 95822, 95829, 95955, 96360-96368, 96372, 96374-96377, 96523, 97597-97598, 97602, 99155, 99156, 99157, 99211-99215, 99221-99223, 99231-99239, 99242-99245, 99252-99255, 99291-99292, 99304-99310, 99315-99316, 99347-99350, 99374-99375, 99377-99378, 99446-99449, 99451-99452, 99495-99496, G0463, G0471

21700 0213T, 0216T, 0596T-0597T, 0708T-0709T, 11000-11006, 11012❖, 11042-11047, 12001-12007, 12011-12057, 13100-13133, 13151-13153, 36000, 36400-36410, 36420-36430, 36440, 36591-36592, 36600, 36640, 43752, 51701-51703, 62320-62327, 64400, 64405-64408, 64415-64435, 64445-64454, 64461-64463, 64479-64505, 64510-64530, 69990, 92012-92014, 93000-93010, 93040-93042, 93318, 93355, 94002, 94200, 94680-94690, 95812-95816, 95819, 95822, 95829, 95955, 96360-96368,

96372, 96374-96377, 96523, 97597-97598, 97602, 99155, 99156, 99157, 99211-99215, 99221-99223, 99231-99239, 99242-99245, 99252-99255, 99291-99292, 99304-99310, 99315-99316, 99347-99350, 99374-99375, 99377-99378, 99446-99449, 99451-99452, 99495-99496, G0463, G0471

21705 0213T, 0216T, 0596T-0597T, 0708T-0709T, 11000-11006, 11042-11047, 12001-12007, 12011-12057, 13100-13133, 13151-13153, 21700, 36000, 36400-36410, 36420-36430, 36440, 36591-36592, 36600, 36640, 43752, 51701-51703, 62320-62327, 64400, 64405-64408, 64415-64435, 64445-64454, 64461-64463, 64479-64505, 64510-64530, 69990, 92012-92014, 93000-93010, 93040-93042, 93318, 93355, 94002, 94200, 94680-94690, 95812-95816, 95819, 95822, 95829, 95955, 96360-96368, 96372, 96374-96377, 96523, 97597-97598, 97602, 99155, 99156, 99157, 99211-99215, 99221-99223, 99231-99239, 99242-99245, 99252-99255, 99291-99292, 99304-99310, 99315-99316, 99347-99350, 99374-99375, 99377-99378, 99446-99449, 99451-99452, 99495-99496, G0463, G0471

21740 0213T, 0216T, 0596T-0597T, 0708T-0709T, 12001-12007, 12011-12057, 13100-13133, 13151-13153, 21600, 21610, 21620, 21742-21743, 29000-29015, 29035-29058, 29200, 36000, 36400-36410, 36420-36430, 36440, 36591-36592, 36600, 36640, 43752, 51701-51703, 62320-62327, 64400, 64405-64408, 64415-64435, 64445-64454, 64461-64463, 64479-64505, 64510-64530, 69990, 92012-92014, 93000-93010, 93040-93042, 93318, 93355, 94002, 94200, 94680-94690, 95812-95816, 95819, 95822, 95829, 95955, 96360-96368, 96372, 96374-96377, 96523, 99155, 99156, 99157, 99211-99215, 99221-99223, 99231-99239, 99242-99245, 99252-99255, 99291-99292, 99304-99310, 99315-99316, 99347-99350, 99374-99375, 99377-99378, 99446-99449, 99451-99452, 99495-99496, G0463, G0471

21742 0213T, 0216T, 0596T-0597T, 0708T-0709T, 12001-12007, 12011-12057, 13100-13133, 13151-13153, 21610, 29000-29015, 29035-29058, 29200, 32601, 32604, 32606-32609, 36000, 36400-36410, 36420-36430, 36440, 36591-36592, 36600, 36640, 43752, 51701-51703, 62320-62327, 64400, 64405-64408, 64415-64435, 64445-64454, 64461-64463, 64479-64505, 64510-64530, 69990, 92012-92014, 93000-93010, 93040-93042, 93318, 93355, 94002, 94200, 94680-94690, 95812-95816, 95819, 95822, 95829, 95955, 96360-96368, 96372, 96374-96377, 96523, 99155, 99156, 99157, 99211-99215, 99221-99223, 99231-99239, 99242-99245, 99252-99255, 99291-99292, 99304-99310, 99315-99316, 99347-99350, 99374-99375, 99377-99378, 99446-99449, 99451-99452, 99495-99496, G0463, G0471

21743 0213T, 0216T, 0596T-0597T, 0708T-0709T, 12001-12007, 12011-12057, 13100-13133, 13151-13153, 21610, 21742✦, 29000-29015, 29035-29058, 29200, 32601, 32604, 32606-32609, 36000, 36400-36410, 36420-36430, 36440, 36591-36592, 36600, 36640, 43752, 51701-51703, 62320-62327, 64400, 64405-64408, 64415-64435, 64445-64454, 64461-64463, 64479-64505, 64510-64530, 69990, 92012-92014, 93000-93010, 93040-93042, 93318, 93355, 94002, 94200, 94680-94690, 95812-95816, 95819, 95822, 95829, 95955, 96360-96368, 96372, 96374-96377, 96523, 99155, 99156, 99157, 99211-99215, 99221-99223, 99231-99239, 99242-99245, 99252-99255, 99291-99292, 99304-99310, 99315-99316, 99347-99350, 99374-99375, 99377-99378, 99446-99449, 99451-99452, 99495-99496, G0463, G0471

21750 00550, 0213T, 0216T, 0596T-0597T, 0708T-0709T, 11000-11006, 11042-11047, 12001-12007, 12011-12057, 13100-13133, 13151-13153, 20650, 20670-20680, 21627, 35820, 36000, 36400-36410, 36420-36430, 36440, 36591-36592, 36600, 36640, 43752, 51701-51703, 62320-62327, 64400, 64405-64408, 64415-64435, 64445-64454, 64461-64463, 64479-64505, 64510-64530, 69990, 92012-92014, 93000-93010, 93040-93042, 93318, 93355, 94002, 94200, 94680-94690, 95812-95816, 95819, 95822, 95829, 95955, 96360-96368, 96372, 96374-96377, 96523, 97597-97598, 97602, 99155, 99156, 99157, 99211-99215, 99221-99223, 99231-99239, 99242-99245, 99252-99255, 99291-99292, 99304-99310, 99315-99316, 99347-99350, 99374-99375, 99377-99378, 99446-99449, 99451-99452, 99495-99496, G0463, G0471

21811 0213T, 0216T, 0594T-0597T, 0708T-0709T, 12001-12007, 12011-12057, 13100-13133, 13151-13153, 20650, 20690, 20692, 20696, 29200, 29700-29710, 32601, 36000, 36400-36410, 36420-36430, 36440, 36591-36592, 36600, 36640, 43752, 51701-51703, 62320-62327, 64400, 64405-64408, 64415-64435, 64445-64454, 64461-64463, 64479-64505, 64510-64530, 69990, 92012-92014, 93000-93010, 93040-93042, 93318, 93355, 94002, 94200, 94680-94690, 95812-95816, 95819, 95822, 95829, 95955, 96360-96368, 96372, 96374-96377, 96523, 97597-97598, 97602-97608, 99155, 99156, 99157, 99211-99215, 99221-99223, 99231-99239, 99242-99245, 99252-99255, 99291-99292, 99304-99310, 99315-99316, 99347-99350, 99374-99375, 99377-99378, 99446-99449, 99451-99452, 99495-99496, G0463, G0471

21812 0213T, 0216T, 0594T-0597T, 0708T-0709T, 12001-12007, 12011-12057, 13100-13133, 13151-13153, 20650, 20690, 20692, 20696, 21811, 29200, 29700-29710, 32601, 36000, 36400-36410, 36420-36430, 36440, 36591-36592, 36600, 36640, 43752, 51701-51703, 62320-62327, 64400, 64405-64408, 64415-64435, 64445-64454, 64461-64463, 64479-64505, 64510-64530, 69990, 92012-92014, 93000-93010, 93040-93042, 93318, 93355, 94002, 94200, 94680-94690, 95812-95816, 95819, 95822, 95829, 95955, 96360-96368, 96372, 96374-96377, 96523, 97597-97598, 97602-97608, 99155, 99156, 99157, 99211-99215, 99221-99223, 99231-99239, 99242-99245, 99252-99255, 99291-99292, 99304-99310, 99315-99316, 99347-99350, 99374-99375, 99377-99378, 99446-99449, 99451-99452, 99495-99496, G0463, G0471

21813 0213T, 0216T, 0594T-0597T, 0708T-0709T, 12001-12007, 12011-12057, 13100-13133, 13151-13153, 20650, 20690, 20692, 20696, 21811-21812, 29200, 29700-29710, 32601, 36000, 36400-36410, 36420-36430, 36440, 36591-36592, 36600, 36640, 43752, 51701-51703, 62320-62327, 64400, 64405-64408, 64415-64435, 64445-64454, 64461-64463, 64479-64505, 64510-64530, 69990, 92012-92014, 93000-93010, 93040-93042, 93318, 93355, 94002, 94200, 94680-94690, 95812-95816, 95819, 95822, 95829, 95955, 96360-96368, 96372, 96374-96377, 96523, 97597-97598, 97602-97608, 99155, 99156, 99157, 99211-99215, 99221-99223, 99231-99239, 99242-99245, 99252-99255, 99291-99292, 99304-99310, 99315-99316, 99347-99350, 99374-99375, 99377-99378, 99446-99449, 99451-99452, 99495-99496, G0463, G0471

21820 00550, 0213T, 0216T, 0596T-0597T, 0708T-0709T, 12001-12007, 12011-12057, 13100-13133, 13151-13153, 21750, 29200, 29700-29710, 36000, 36400-36410, 36420-36430, 36440, 36591-36592, 36600, 36640, 43752, 51701-51703, 62320-62327, 64400, 64405-64408, 64415-64435, 64445-64454, 64461-64463, 64479-64505, 64510-64530, 69990, 92012-92014, 93000-93010, 93040-93042, 93318, 93355, 94002, 94200, 94680-94690, 95812-95816, 95819, 95822, 95829, 95955, 96360-96368, 96372, 96374-96377, 96523, 97597-97598, 97602-97608, 99155, 99156, 99157, 99211-99215, 99221-99223, 99231-99239, 99242-99245, 99252-99255, 99291-99292, 99304-99310, 99315-99316, 99347-99350, 99374-99375, 99377-99378, 99446-99449, 99451-99452, 99495-99496, G0463, G0471

21825 00550, 0213T, 0216T, 0594T-0597T, 0708T-0709T, 12001-12007, 12011-12057, 13100-13133, 13151-13153, 20650, 20690, 20692, 20696-20697, 21750, 21820, 29200, 29700-29710, 36000, 36400-36410, 36420-36430, 36440, 36591-36592, 36600, 36640, 43752, 51701-51703, 62320-62327, 64400, 64405-64408, 64415-64435, 64445-64454,

64461-64463, 64479-64505, 64510-64530, 69990, 92012-92014, 93000-93010, 93040-93042, 93318, 93355, 94002, 94200, 94680-94690, 95812-95816, 95819, 95822, 95829, 95955, 96360-96368, 96372, 96374-96377, 96523, 97597-97598, 97602-97608, 99155, 99156, 99157, 99211-99215, 99221-99223, 99231-99239, 99242-99245, 99252-99255, 99291-99292, 99304-99310, 99315-99316, 99347-99350, 99374-99375, 99377-99378, 99446-99449, 99451-99452, 99495-99496, G0463, G0471

31500 00320, 00326, 0596T-0597T, 0708T-0709T, 12001-12007, 12011-12057, 13100-13133, 13151-13153, 31505, 31510-31531, 31536-31541, 31560-31578, 36000, 36400-36410, 36420-36430, 36440, 36591-36592, 36600, 36640, 43752, 51701-51703, 64461-64463, 64486-64495, 69990, 71045-71047, 92012-92014, 92502, 93000-93010, 93040-93042, 93318, 93355, 94002, 94200, 94680-94690, 95812-95816, 95819, 95822, 95829, 95955, 96360-96368, 96372, 96374-96377, 96523, 99155, 99156, 99157, 99211-99215, 99221-99223, 99231-99239, 99242-99245, 99252-99255, 99291-99292, 99304-99310, 99315-99316, 99347-99350, 99374-99375, 99377-99378, 99446-99449, 99451-99452, 99495-99496, G0463, G0471

31515 00326, 0213T, 0216T, 0596T-0597T, 0708T-0709T, 12001-12007, 12011-12057, 13100-13133, 13151-13153, 31505, 31575❖, 36000, 36400-36410, 36420-36430, 36440, 36591-36592, 36600, 36640, 43752, 51701-51703, 62320-62327, 64400, 64405-64408, 64415-64435, 64445-64454, 64461-64463, 64479-64505, 64510-64530, 69705-69706, 69990, 76000, 77001-77002, 92012-92014, 92502, 92511, 93000-93010, 93040-93042, 93318, 93355, 94002, 94200, 94680-94690, 95812-95816, 95819, 95822, 95829, 95955, 96360-96368, 96372, 96374-96377, 96523, 99155, 99156, 99157, 99211-99215, 99221-99223, 99231-99239, 99242-99245, 99252-99255, 99291-99292, 99304-99310, 99315-99316, 99347-99350, 99374-99375, 99377-99378, 99446-99449, 99451-99452, 99495-99496, G0463, G0471, J0670

31520 00320, 00326, 0213T, 0216T, 0596T-0597T, 0708T-0709T, 12001-12007, 12011-12057, 13100-13133, 13151-13153, 31505, 31575❖, 36000, 36400-36410, 36420-36430, 36440, 36591-36592, 36600, 36640, 43752, 51701-51703, 62320-62327, 64400, 64405-64408, 64415-64435, 64445-64454, 64461-64463, 64479-64505, 64510-64530, 69705-69706, 69990, 76000, 77001-77002, 92012-92014, 92502, 92511, 93000-93010, 93040-93042, 93318, 93355, 94002, 94200, 94680-94690, 95812-95816, 95819, 95822, 95829, 95955, 96360-96368, 96372, 96374-96377, 96523, 99155, 99156, 99157, 99211-99215, 99221-99223, 99231-99239, 99242-99245, 99252-99255, 99291-99292, 99304-99310, 99315-99316, 99347-99350, 99374-99375, 99377-99378, 99446-99449, 99451-99452, 99495-99496, G0463, G0471

31525 00320, 00326, 0213T, 0216T, 0596T-0597T, 0708T-0709T, 12001-12007, 12011-12057, 13100-13133, 13151-13153, 31505, 31575❖, 36000, 36400-36410, 36420-36430, 36440, 36591-36592, 36600, 36640, 42800, 42806, 43752, 51701-51703, 62320-62327, 64400, 64405-64408, 64415-64435, 64445-64454, 64461-64463, 64479-64505, 64510-64530, 69705-69706, 69990, 76000, 77001-77002, 92012-92014, 92502, 92511, 93000-93010, 93040-93042, 93318, 93355, 94002, 94200, 94680-94690, 95812-95816, 95819, 95822, 95829, 95955, 96360-96368, 96372, 96374-96377, 96523, 99155, 99156, 99157, 99211-99215, 99221-99223, 99231-99239, 99242-99245, 99252-99255, 99291-99292, 99304-99310, 99315-99316, 99347-99350, 99374-99375, 99377-99378, 99446-99449, 99451-99452, 99495-99496, G0463, G0471, J0670

31526 00320, 00326, 0213T, 0216T, 0596T-0597T, 0708T-0709T, 12001-12007, 12011-12057, 13100-13133, 13151-13153, 31505, 31575❖, 36000, 36400-36410, 36420-36430, 36440, 36591-36592, 36600, 36640, 43752, 51701-51703, 62320-62327, 64400, 64405-64408, 64415-64435, 64445-64454, 64461-64463, 64479-64505, 64510-64530, 69705-69706, 69990, 76000, 77001-77002, 92012-92014, 92502, 92511, 93000-93010, 93040-93042, 93318, 93355, 94002, 94200, 94680-94690, 95812-95816, 95819, 95822, 95829, 95955, 96360-96368, 96372, 96374-96377, 96523, 99155, 99156, 99157, 99211-99215, 99221-99223, 99231-99239, 99242-99245, 99252-99255, 99291-99292, 99304-99310, 99315-99316, 99347-99350, 99374-99375, 99377-99378, 99446-99449, 99451-99452, 99495-99496, G0463, G0471

31527 00326, 0213T, 0216T, 0596T-0597T, 0708T-0709T, 11000-11006, 11042-11047, 12001-12007, 12011-12057, 13100-13133, 13151-13153, 31505, 31525, 31575❖, 36000, 36400-36410, 36420-36430, 36440, 36591-36592, 36600, 36640, 43752, 51701-51703, 62320-62327, 64400, 64405-64408, 64415-64435, 64445-64454, 64461-64463, 64479-64505, 64510-64530, 69705-69706, 69990, 76000, 77001-77002, 92012-92014, 92502, 92511, 93000-93010, 93040-93042, 93318, 93355, 94002, 94200, 94680-94690, 95812-95816, 95819, 95822, 95829, 95955, 96360-96368, 96372, 96374-96377, 96523, 97597-97598, 97602, 99155, 99156, 99157, 99211-99215, 99221-99223, 99231-99239, 99242-99245, 99252-99255, 99291-99292, 99304-99310, 99315-99316, 99347-99350, 99374-99375, 99377-99378, 99446-99449, 99451-99452, 99495-99496, G0463, G0471

31528 00320, 00326, 0213T, 0216T, 0596T-0597T, 0708T-0709T, 12001-12007, 12011-12057, 13100-13133, 13151-13153, 31505, 31525, 31529❖, 31575❖, 36000, 36400-36410, 36420-36430, 36440, 36591-36592, 36600, 36640, 43752, 51701-51703, 62320-62327, 64400, 64405-64408, 64415-64435, 64445-64454, 64461-64463, 64479-64505, 64510-64530, 69705-69706, 69990, 76000, 77001-77002, 92012-92014, 92502, 92511, 93000-93010, 93040-93042, 93318, 93355, 94002, 94200, 94680-94690, 95812-95816, 95819, 95822, 95829, 95955, 96360-96368, 96372, 96374-96377, 96523, 99155, 99156, 99157, 99211-99215, 99221-99223, 99231-99239, 99242-99245, 99252-99255, 99291-99292, 99304-99310, 99315-99316, 99347-99350, 99374-99375, 99377-99378, 99446-99449, 99451-99452, 99495-99496, G0463, G0471

31529 00320, 00326, 0213T, 0216T, 0596T-0597T, 0708T-0709T, 12001-12007, 12011-12057, 13100-13133, 13151-13153, 31505, 31525, 31575❖, 36000, 36400-36410, 36420-36430, 36440, 36591-36592, 36600, 36640, 43752, 51701-51703, 62320-62327, 64400, 64405-64408, 64415-64435, 64445-64454, 64461-64463, 64479-64505, 64510-64530, 69705-69706, 69990, 76000, 77001-77002, 92012-92014, 92502, 92511, 93000-93010, 93040-93042, 93318, 93355, 94002, 94200, 94680-94690, 95812-95816, 95819, 95822, 95829, 95955, 96360-96368, 96372, 96374-96377, 96523, 99155, 99156, 99157, 99211-99215, 99221-99223, 99231-99239, 99242-99245, 99252-99255, 99291-99292, 99304-99310, 99315-99316, 99347-99350, 99374-99375, 99377-99378, 99446-99449, 99451-99452, 99495-99496, G0463, G0471

31592 00520, 0213T, 0216T, 0565T, 0596T-0597T, 0708T-0709T, 11000-11006, 11042-11047, 12001-12007, 12011-12057, 13100-13133, 13151-13153, 14040-14041, 14301, 15574, 15620, 15650, 15733, 15756, 15760-15769, 31600-31601, 31780-31781❖, 31800, 31820-31830, 36000, 36400-36410, 36420-36430, 36440, 36591-36592, 36600, 36640, 43752, 51701-51703, 62320-62327, 64400, 64405-64408, 64415-64435, 64445-64454, 64461-64463, 64479-64505, 64510-64530, 69990, 92012-92014, 92502, 93000-93010, 93040-93042, 93318, 93355, 94002, 94200, 94680-94690, 95812-95816, 95819, 95822, 95829, 95955, 96360-96368, 96372, 96374-96377, 96523, 97597-97598, 97602, 99155, 99156, 99157, 99211-99215, 99221-99223, 99231-99239, 99242-99245, 99252-99255, 99291-99292, 99304-99310, 99315-99316, 99347-99350, 99374-99375, 99377-99378, 99446-99449, 99451-99452, 99495-99496, G0463, G0471, J0670

31600 00320, 00326, 00520, 0213T, 0216T, 0596T-0597T, 0708T-0709T, 12001-12007, 12011-12057, 13100-13133, 13151-13153, 31502, 31603-31605, 31622, 31634, 31647, 36000, 36400-36410, 36420-36430, 36440, 36591-36592, 36600, 36640, 43752, 51701-51703, 62320-62327, 64400, 64405-64408, 64415-64435, 64445-64454, 64461-64463, 64479-64505, 64510-64530, 69990, 92012-92014, 92502, 93000-93010, 93040-93042, 93318, 93355, 94002, 94200, 94680-94690, 95812-95816, 95819, 95822, 95829, 95955, 96360-96368, 96372, 96374-96377, 96523, 99155, 99156, 99157, 99211-99215, 99221-99223, 99231-99239, 99242-99245, 99252-99255, 99291-99292, 99304-99310, 99315-99316, 99347-99350, 99374-99375, 99377-99378, 99446-99449, 99451-99452, 99495-99496, G0463, G0471

31601 00320, 00326, 00520, 0213T, 0216T, 0596T-0597T, 0708T-0709T, 12001-12007, 12011-12057, 13100-13133, 13151-13153, 31605, 36000, 36400-36410, 36420-36430, 36440, 36591-36592, 36600, 36640, 43752, 51701-51703, 62320-62327, 64400, 64405-64408, 64415-64435, 64445-64454, 64461-64463, 64479-64505, 64510-64530, 69990, 92012-92014, 92502, 93000-93010, 93040-93042, 93318, 93355, 94002, 94200, 94680-94690, 95812-95816, 95819, 95822, 95829, 95955, 96360-96368, 96372, 96374-96377, 96523, 99155, 99156, 99157, 99211-99215, 99221-99223, 99231-99239, 99242-99245, 99252-99255, 99291-99292, 99304-99310, 99315-99316, 99347-99350, 99374-99375, 99377-99378, 99446-99449, 99451-99452, 99495-99496, G0463, G0471

31603 00320, 00326, 00520, 0213T, 0216T, 0596T-0597T, 0708T-0709T, 12001-12007, 12011-12057, 13100-13133, 13151-13153, 31525-31526, 31575, 31610❖, 31613-31614❖, 36000, 36400-36410, 36420-36430, 36440, 36591-36592, 36600, 36640, 43752, 51701-51703, 62320-62327, 64400, 64405-64408, 64415-64435, 64445-64454, 64461-64463, 64479-64505, 64510-64530, 69990, 92012-92014, 92502, 93000-93010, 93040-93042, 93318, 93355, 94002, 94200, 94680-94690, 95812-95816, 95819, 95822, 95829, 95955, 96360-96368, 96372, 96374-96377, 96523, 99155, 99156, 99157, 99211-99215, 99221-99223, 99231-99239, 99242-99245, 99252-99255, 99291-99292, 99304-99310, 99315-99316, 99347-99350, 99374-99375, 99377-99378, 99446-99449, 99451-99452, 99495-99496, G0463, G0471

31605 00320, 00326, 00520, 0213T, 0216T, 0596T-0597T, 0708T-0709T, 12001-12007, 12011-12057, 13100-13133, 13151-13153, 31603❖, 31610❖, 31613-31614❖, 36000, 36400-36410, 36420-36430, 36440, 36591-36592, 36600, 36640, 43752, 51701-51703, 62320-62327, 64400, 64405-64408, 64415-64435, 64445-64454, 64461-64463, 64479-64505, 64510-64530, 69990, 92012-92014, 92502, 93000-93010, 93040-93042, 93318, 93355, 94002, 94200, 94680-94690, 95812-95816, 95819, 95822, 95829, 95955, 96360-96368, 96372, 96374-96377, 96523, 99155, 99156, 99157, 99211-99215, 99221-99223, 99231-99239, 99242-99245, 99252-99255, 99291-99292, 99304-99310, 99315-99316, 99347-99350, 99374-99375, 99377-99378, 99446-99449, 99451-99452, 99495-99496, G0463, G0471

31610 00320, 00326, 00520, 0213T, 0216T, 0596T-0597T, 0708T-0709T, 12001-12007, 12011-12057, 13100-13133, 13151-13153, 31600-31601, 36000, 36400-36410, 36420-36430, 36440, 36591-36592, 36600, 36640, 43752, 51701-51703, 62320-62327, 64400, 64405-64408, 64415-64435, 64445-64454, 64461-64463, 64479-64505, 64510-64530, 69990, 92012-92014, 92502, 93000-93010, 93040-93042, 93318, 93355, 94002, 94200, 94680-94690, 95812-95816, 95819, 95822, 95829, 95955, 96360-96368, 96372, 96374-96377, 96523, 99155, 99156, 99157, 99211-99215, 99221-99223, 99231-99239, 99242-99245, 99252-99255, 99291-99292, 99304-99310, 99315-99316, 99347-99350, 99374-99375, 99377-99378, 99446-99449, 99451-99452, 99495-99496, G0463, G0471

31611 00320, 00326, 00520, 0213T, 0216T, 0596T-0597T, 0708T-0709T, 11000-11006, 11042-11047, 12001-12007, 12011-12057, 13100-13133, 13151-13153, 31525-31526, 31575, 31600-31601, 31614❖, 36000, 36400-36410, 36420-36430, 36440, 36591-36592, 36600, 36640, 43752, 51701-51703, 62320-62327, 64400, 64405-64408, 64415-64435, 64445-64454, 64461-64463, 64479-64505, 64510-64530, 69990, 92012-92014, 92502, 93000-93010, 93040-93042, 93318, 93355, 94002, 94200, 94680-94690, 95812-95816, 95819, 95822, 95829, 95955, 96360-96368, 96372, 96374-96377, 96523, 97597-97598, 97602, 99155, 99156, 99157, 99211-99215, 99221-99223, 99231-99239, 99242-99245, 99252-99255, 99291-99292, 99304-99310, 99315-99316, 99347-99350, 99374-99375, 99377-99378, 99446-99449, 99451-99452, 99495-99496, G0463, G0471

31612 00320, 00326, 00520, 0213T, 0216T, 0596T-0597T, 0708T-0709T, 12001-12007, 12011-12057, 13100-13133, 13151-13153, 31525-31526, 31575, 31600-31605❖, 31610-31611❖, 31613-31614❖, 36000, 36400-36410, 36420-36430, 36440, 36591-36592, 36600, 36640, 43752, 51701-51703, 62320-62327, 64400, 64405-64408, 64415-64435, 64445-64454, 64461-64463, 64479-64505, 64510-64530, 69990, 89220, 92012-92014, 92502, 93000-93010, 93040-93042, 93318, 93355, 94002, 94200, 94680-94690, 95812-95816, 95819, 95822, 95829, 95955, 96360-96368, 96372, 96374-96377, 96523, 99155, 99156, 99157, 99211-99215, 99221-99223, 99231-99239, 99242-99245, 99252-99255, 99291-99292, 99304-99310, 99315-99316, 99347-99350, 99374-99375, 99377-99378, 99446-99449, 99451-99452, 99495-99496, G0463, G0471, J0670

31613 00320, 00326, 00520, 0213T, 0216T, 0596T-0597T, 0708T-0709T, 11000-11006, 11042-11047, 12001-12007, 12011-12057, 13100-13133, 13151-13153, 31525-31526, 31575, 31600-31601, 31610-31611❖, 36000, 36400-36410, 36420-36430, 36440, 36591-36592, 36600, 36640, 43752, 51701-51703, 62320-62327, 64400, 64405-64408, 64415-64435, 64445-64454, 64461-64463, 64479-64505, 64510-64530, 69990, 92012-92014, 92502, 93000-93010, 93040-93042, 93318, 93355, 94002, 94200, 94680-94690, 95812-95816, 95819, 95822, 95829, 95955, 96360-96368, 96372, 96374-96377, 96523, 97597-97598, 97602, 99155, 99156, 99157, 99211-99215, 99221-99223, 99231-99239, 99242-99245, 99252-99255, 99291-99292, 99304-99310, 99315-99316, 99347-99350, 99374-99375, 99377-99378, 99446-99449, 99451-99452, 99495-99496, G0463, G0471

31614 00320, 00326, 00520, 0213T, 0216T, 0596T-0597T, 0708T-0709T, 11000-11006, 11042-11047, 12001-12007, 12011-12057, 13100-13133, 13151-13153, 31515, 31525-31526, 31575, 31600-31601, 31610❖, 31613, 36000, 36400-36410, 36420-36430, 36440, 36591-36592, 36600, 36640, 43752, 51701-51703, 62320-62327, 64400, 64405-64408, 64415-64435, 64445-64454, 64461-64463, 64479-64505, 64510-64530, 69990, 92012-92014, 92502, 93000-93010, 93040-93042, 93318, 93355, 94002, 94200, 94680-94690, 95812-95816, 95819, 95822, 95829, 95955, 96360-96368, 96372, 96374-96377, 96523, 97597-97598, 97602, 99155, 99156, 99157, 99211-99215, 99221-99223, 99231-99239, 99242-99245, 99252-99255, 99291-99292, 99304-99310, 99315-99316, 99347-99350, 99374-99375, 99377-99378, 99446-99449, 99451-99452, 99495-99496, G0463, G0471

31615 00320, 00326, 00520, 0213T, 0216T, 0596T-0597T, 0708T-0709T, 0781T-0782T❖, 12001-12007, 12011-12057, 13100-13133, 13151-13153, 31525-31526, 31575, 31610❖, 31622-31625❖, 31628-31631❖, 31635❖, 31640-31648❖, 31651❖, 31660-31661❖, 31717❖, 31720-31725, 36000, 36400-36410, 36420-36430, 36440, 36591-36592, 36600, 36640, 43752, 51701-51703, 62320-62327, 64400, 64405-64408, 64415-64435, 64445-64454, 64461-64463, 64479-64505, 64510-64530, 69990, 76000, 77001-77002, 89220, 92012-92014, 93000-93010,

93040-93042, 93318, 93355, 94002, 94200, 94680-94690, 95812-95816, 95819, 95822, 95829, 95955, 96360-96368, 96372, 96374-96377, 96523, 99155, 99156, 99157, 99211-99215, 99221-99223, 99231-99239, 99242-99245, 99252-99255, 99291-99292, 99304-99310, 99315-99316, 99347-99350, 99374-99375, 99377-99378, 99446-99449, 99451-99452, 99495-99496, G0463, G0471, J0670

31622 00520, 0213T, 0216T, 0596T-0597T, 0708T-0709T, 12001-12007, 12011-12057, 13100-13133, 13151-13153, 31231, 31525, 31535, 31575, 31717, 31720-31725, 36000, 36400-36410, 36420-36430, 36440, 36591-36592, 36600, 36640, 43752, 51701-51703, 62320-62327, 64400, 64405-64408, 64415-64435, 64445-64454, 64461-64463, 64479-64505, 64510-64530, 69705-69706, 69990, 76000, 77001-77002, 89220, 92012-92014, 92511, 93000-93010, 93040-93042, 93318, 93355, 94002, 94200, 94680-94690, 95812-95816, 95819, 95822, 95829, 95955, 96360-96368, 96372, 96374-96377, 96523, 99155, 99156, 99157, 99211-99215, 99221-99223, 99231-99239, 99242-99245, 99252-99255, 99291-99292, 99304-99310, 99315-99316, 99347-99350, 99374-99375, 99377-99378, 99446-99449, 99451-99452, 99495-99496, G0463, G0471, J0670

31623 00520, 00528-00529, 0213T, 0216T, 0596T-0597T, 0708T-0709T, 12001-12007, 12011-12057, 13100-13133, 13151-13153, 31231, 31525-31526, 31535, 31575, 31622, 31634, 31647, 31717, 31720-31725, 36000, 36400-36410, 36420-36430, 36440, 36591-36592, 36600, 36640, 43752, 51701-51703, 62320-62327, 64400, 64405-64408, 64415-64435, 64445-64454, 64461-64463, 64479-64505, 64510-64530, 69705-69706, 69990, 76000, 77001-77002, 89220, 92012-92014, 92511, 93000-93010, 93040-93042, 93318, 93355, 94002, 94200, 94680-94690, 95812-95816, 95819, 95822, 95829, 95955, 96360-96368, 96372, 96374-96377, 96523, 99155, 99156, 99157, 99211-99215, 99221-99223, 99231-99239, 99242-99245, 99252-99255, 99291-99292, 99304-99310, 99315-99316, 99347-99350, 99374-99375, 99377-99378, 99446-99449, 99451-99452, 99495-99496, G0463, G0471, J0670

31624 00520, 00528-00529, 0213T, 0216T, 0596T-0597T, 0708T-0709T, 12001-12007, 12011-12057, 13100-13133, 13151-13153, 31231, 31525-31526, 31535, 31575, 31622, 31634, 31647, 31717, 31720-31725, 36000, 36400-36410, 36420-36430, 36440, 36591-36592, 36600, 36640, 43752, 51701-51703, 62320-62327, 64400, 64405-64408, 64415-64435, 64445-64454, 64461-64463, 64479-64505, 64510-64530, 69705-69706, 69990, 76000, 77001-77002, 89220, 92012-92014, 92511, 93000-93010, 93040-93042, 93318, 93355, 94002, 94200, 94680-94690, 95812-95816, 95819, 95822, 95829, 95955, 96360-96368, 96372, 96374-96377, 96523, 99155, 99156, 99157, 99211-99215, 99221-99223, 99231-99239, 99242-99245, 99252-99255, 99291-99292, 99304-99310, 99315-99316, 99347-99350, 99374-99375, 99377-99378, 99446-99449, 99451-99452, 99495-99496, G0463, G0471, J0670

31625 00520, 0213T, 0216T, 0596T-0597T, 0708T-0709T, 10005, 10007, 10009, 10011, 10021, 12001-12007, 12011-12057, 13100-13133, 13151-13153, 31231, 31525-31526, 31535, 31575, 31622, 31634, 31647, 31717, 31720-31725, 36000, 36400-36410, 36420-36430, 36440, 36591-36592, 36600, 36640, 43752, 51701-51703, 62320-62327, 64400, 64405-64408, 64415-64435, 64445-64454, 64461-64463, 64479-64505, 64510-64530, 69705-69706, 69990, 76000, 77001-77002, 89220, 92012-92014, 92511, 93000-93010, 93040-93042, 93318, 93355, 94002, 94200, 94680-94690, 95812-95816, 95819, 95822, 95829, 95955, 96360-96368, 96372, 96374-96377, 96523, 99155, 99156, 99157, 99211-99215, 99221-99223, 99231-99239, 99242-99245, 99252-99255, 99291-99292, 99304-99310, 99315-99316, 99347-99350, 99374-99375, 99377-99378, 99446-99449, 99451-99452, 99495-99496, G0463, G0471, J0670

31626 00520, 00528-00529, 0213T, 0216T, 0596T-0597T, 0708T-0709T, 10035-10036✦, 12001-12007, 12011-12057, 13100-13133, 13151-13153, 31231, 31525-31526, 31535, 31575, 31615✦, 31622, 31634, 31643✦, 31647, 31717, 31720-31725, 36000, 36400-36410, 36420-36430, 36440, 36591-36592, 36600, 36640, 43752, 51701-51703, 62320-62327, 64400, 64405-64408, 64415-64435, 64445-64454, 64461-64463, 64479-64505, 64510-64530, 69705-69706, 69990, 76000, 77001-77002, 89220, 92012-92014, 92511, 93000-93010, 93040-93042, 93318, 93355, 94002, 94200, 94680-94690, 95812-95816, 95819, 95822, 95829, 95955, 96360-96368, 96372, 96374-96377, 96523, 99155, 99156, 99157, 99211-99215, 99221-99223, 99231-99239, 99242-99245, 99252-99255, 99291-99292, 99304-99310, 99315-99316, 99347-99350, 99374-99375, 99377-99378, 99446-99449, 99451-99452, 99495-99496, G0463, G0471, J0670

31627 0213T, 0216T, 0596T-0597T, 0694T, 0708T-0709T, 36000, 36400-36410, 36420-36430, 36440, 36591-36592, 36600, 36640, 43752, 51701-51703, 61650, 62320-62327, 64400, 64405-64408, 64415-64435, 64445-64454, 64461, 64463, 64479, 64483, 64486-64490, 64493, 64505, 64510-64530, 69990, 76000, 76376-76377, 77001-77002, 93000-93010, 93040-93042, 93318, 93355, 94002, 94200, 94680-94690, 95812-95816, 95819, 95822, 95829, 95955, 96360, 96365, 96372, 96374-96377, 96523, 99155, 99156, 99157, G0471

31628 00520, 0213T, 0216T, 0596T-0597T, 0708T-0709T, 0782T, 10005, 10007, 10009, 10011, 10021, 12001-12007, 12011-12057, 13100-13133, 13151-13153, 31231, 31525-31526, 31535-31541, 31575, 31622, 31625, 31634, 31647, 31717, 31720-31725, 36000, 36400-36410, 36420-36430, 36440, 36591-36592, 36600, 36640, 43752, 51701-51703, 62320-62327, 64400, 64405-64408, 64415-64435, 64445-64454, 64461-64463, 64479-64505, 64510-64530, 69705-69706, 69990, 76000, 77001-77002, 89220, 92012-92014, 92511, 93000-93010, 93040-93042, 93318, 93355, 94002, 94200, 94680-94690, 95812-95816, 95819, 95822, 95829, 95955, 96360-96368, 96372, 96374-96377, 96523, 99155, 99156, 99157, 99211-99215, 99221-99223, 99231-99239, 99242-99245, 99252-99255, 99291-99292, 99304-99310, 99315-99316, 99347-99350, 99374-99375, 99377-99378, 99446-99449, 99451-99452, 99495-99496, G0463, G0471, J0670

31629 00520, 0213T, 0216T, 0596T-0597T, 0708T-0709T, 0782T, 10005, 10007, 10009, 10011, 10021, 12001-12007, 12011-12057, 13100-13133, 13151-13153, 31231, 31525-31526, 31535-31541, 31575, 31622, 31625, 31634, 31647, 31717, 31725, 36000, 36400-36410, 36420-36430, 36440, 36591-36592, 36600, 36640, 43752, 51701-51703, 62320-62327, 64400, 64405-64408, 64415-64435, 64445-64454, 64461-64463, 64479-64505, 64510-64530, 69705-69706, 69990, 76000, 77001-77002, 89220, 92012-92014, 92511, 93000-93010, 93040-93042, 93318, 93355, 94002, 94200, 94680-94690, 95812-95816, 95819, 95822, 95829, 95955, 96360-96368, 96372, 96374-96377, 96523, 99155, 99156, 99157, 99211-99215, 99221-99223, 99231-99239, 99242-99245, 99252-99255, 99291-99292, 99304-99310, 99315-99316, 99347-99350, 99374-99375, 99377-99378, 99446-99449, 99451-99452, 99495-99496, G0463, G0471, J0670

31630 00520, 0213T, 0216T, 0596T-0597T, 0708T-0709T, 12001-12007, 12011-12057, 13100-13133, 13151-13153, 31231, 31525-31526, 31535-31541, 31575, 31622, 31634, 31647, 31717, 31720-31725, 36000, 36400-36410, 36420-36430, 36440, 36591-36592, 36600, 36640, 43752, 51701-51703, 62320-62327, 64400, 64405-64408, 64415-64435, 64445-64454, 64461-64463, 64479-64505, 64510-64530, 69705-69706, 69990, 76000, 77001-77002, 89220, 92012-92014, 92511, 93000-93010, 93040-93042, 93318, 93355, 94002, 94200, 94680-94690, 95812-95816, 95819, 95822, 95829, 95955, 96360-96368, 96372, 96374-96377, 96523, 99155, 99156, 99157, 99211-99215, 99221-99223, 99231-99239,

99242-99245, 99252-99255, 99291-99292, 99304-99310, 99315-99316, 99347-99350, 99374-99375, 99377-99378, 99446-99449, 99451-99452, 99495-99496, G0463, G0471

31631 00520, 0213T, 0216T, 0596T-0597T, 0708T-0709T, 12001-12007, 12011-12057, 13100-13133, 13151-13153, 31231, 31525-31526, 31535-31541, 31575, 31622, 31630, 31634, 31647, 31717, 31720-31725, 36000, 36400-36410, 36420-36430, 36440, 36591-36592, 36600, 36640, 43752, 51701-51703, 62320-62327, 64400, 64405-64408, 64415-64435, 64445-64454, 64461-64463, 64479-64505, 64510-64530, 69705-69706, 69990, 76000, 77001-77002, 89220, 92012-92014, 92511, 93000-93010, 93040-93042, 93318, 93355, 94002, 94200, 94680-94690, 95812-95816, 95819, 95822, 95829, 95955, 96360-96368, 96372, 96374-96377, 96523, 99155, 99156, 99157, 99211-99215, 99221-99223, 99231-99239, 99242-99245, 99252-99255, 99291-99292, 99304-99310, 99315-99316, 99347-99350, 99374-99375, 99377-99378, 99446-99449, 99451-99452, 99495-99496, G0463, G0471

31632 10005, 10007, 10009, 10011, 10021, 36591-36592, 77001, 89220, 96523

31633 10005, 10007, 10009, 10011, 10021, 36591-36592, 77001, 89220, 96523

31634 00520, 0213T, 0216T, 0596T-0597T, 0708T-0709T, 12001-12007, 12011-12057, 13100-13133, 13151-13153, 31231, 31525-31526, 31535, 31575, 31615❖, 31622, 31717, 31720-31725, 36000, 36400-36410, 36420-36430, 36440, 36591-36592, 36600, 36640, 43752, 51701-51703, 62320-62327, 64400, 64405-64408, 64415-64435, 64445-64454, 64461-64463, 64479-64505, 64510-64530, 69705-69706, 69990, 76000, 77002, 89220, 92012-92014, 92511, 93000-93010, 93040-93042, 93318, 93355, 94002, 94200, 94680-94690, 95812-95816, 95819, 95822, 95829, 95955, 96360-96368, 96372, 96374-96377, 96523, 99155, 99156, 99157, 99211-99215, 99221-99223, 99231-99239, 99242-99245, 99252-99255, 99291-99292, 99304-99310, 99315-99316, 99347-99350, 99374-99375, 99377-99378, 99446-99449, 99451-99452, 99495-99496, G0463, G0471, J0670

31635 00520, 0213T, 0216T, 0596T-0597T, 0708T-0709T, 11000-11006, 11042-11047, 12001-12007, 12011-12057, 13100-13133, 13151-13153, 31231, 31525-31526, 31535-31541, 31575, 31622, 31634, 31647-31648❖, 31717, 31720-31725, 36000, 36400-36410, 36420-36430, 36440, 36591-36592, 36600, 36640, 43752, 51701-51703, 62320-62327, 64400, 64405-64408, 64415-64435, 64445-64454, 64461-64463, 64479-64505, 64510-64530, 69705-69706, 69990, 76000, 77001-77002, 89220, 92012-92014, 92511, 93000-93010, 93040-93042, 93318, 93355, 94002, 94200, 94680-94690, 95812-95816, 95819, 95822, 95829, 95955, 96360-96368, 96372, 96374-96377, 96523, 97597-97598, 97602, 99155, 99156, 99157, 99211-99215, 99221-99223, 99231-99239, 99242-99245, 99252-99255, 99291-99292, 99304-99310, 99315-99316, 99347-99350, 99374-99375, 99377-99378, 99446-99449, 99451-99452, 99495-99496, G0463, G0471

31636 00520, 0213T, 0216T, 0596T-0597T, 0708T-0709T, 12001-12007, 12011-12057, 13100-13133, 13151-13153, 31231, 31525-31526, 31535-31541, 31575, 31615❖, 31622, 31630, 31634, 31647, 31717, 31720-31725, 36000, 36400-36410, 36420-36430, 36440, 36591-36592, 36600, 36640, 43752, 51701-51703, 62320-62327, 64400, 64405-64408, 64415-64435, 64445-64454, 64461-64463, 64479-64505, 64510-64530, 69705-69706, 69990, 76000, 77001-77002, 92012-92014, 92511, 93000-93010, 93040-93042, 93318, 93355, 94002, 94200, 94680-94690, 95812-95816, 95819, 95822, 95829, 95955, 96360-96368, 96372, 96374-96377, 96523, 99155, 99156, 99157, 99211-99215, 99221-99223, 99231-99239, 99242-99245, 99252-99255, 99291-99292, 99304-99310, 99315-99316, 99347-99350, 99374-99375, 99377-99378, 99446-99449, 99451-99452, 99495-99496, G0463, G0471

31637 36591-36592, 77001, 96523

31638 00520, 0213T, 0216T, 0596T-0597T, 0708T-0709T, 0781T❖, 11000-11006, 11042-11047, 12001-12007, 12011-12057, 13100-13133, 13151-13153, 31231, 31525-31526, 31535-31541, 31575, 31615❖, 31622, 31630-31631❖, 31634, 31636❖, 31647, 31717, 31720-31725, 36000, 36400-36410, 36420-36430, 36440, 36591-36592, 36600, 36640, 43752, 51701-51703, 62320-62327, 64400, 64405-64408, 64415-64435, 64445-64454, 64461-64463, 64479-64505, 64510-64530, 69705-69706, 69990, 76000, 77001-77002, 92012-92014, 92511, 93000-93010, 93040-93042, 93318, 93355, 94002, 94200, 94680-94690, 95812-95816, 95819, 95822, 95829, 95955, 96360-96368, 96372, 96374-96377, 96523, 97597-97598, 97602, 99155, 99156, 99157, 99211-99215, 99221-99223, 99231-99239, 99242-99245, 99252-99255, 99291-99292, 99304-99310, 99315-99316, 99347-99350, 99374-99375, 99377-99378, 99446-99449, 99451-99452, 99495-99496, G0463, G0471

31640 00520, 0213T, 0216T, 0596T-0597T, 0708T-0709T, 0782T, 11000-11006, 11042-11047, 12001-12007, 12011-12057, 13100-13133, 13151-13153, 31231, 31525-31526, 31535-31541, 31575, 31622, 31625, 31634, 31647, 31660-31661❖, 31717, 31720-31725, 36000, 36400-36410, 36420-36430, 36440, 36591-36592, 36600, 36640, 43752, 51701-51703, 62320-62327, 64400, 64405-64408, 64415-64435, 64445-64454, 64461-64463, 64479-64505, 64510-64530, 69705-69706, 69990, 76000, 77001-77002, 89220, 92012-92014, 92511, 93000-93010, 93040-93042, 93318, 93355, 94002, 94200, 94680-94690, 95812-95816, 95819, 95822, 95829, 95955, 96360-96368, 96372, 96374-96377, 96523, 97597-97598, 97602, 99155, 99156, 99157, 99211-99215, 99221-99223, 99231-99239, 99242-99245, 99252-99255, 99291-99292, 99304-99310, 99315-99316, 99347-99350, 99374-99375, 99377-99378, 99446-99449, 99451-99452, 99495-99496, G0463, G0471

31641 00520, 0213T, 0216T, 0596T-0597T, 0708T-0709T, 0782T, 11000-11006, 11042-11047, 12001-12007, 12011-12057, 13100-13133, 13151-13153, 31231, 31525-31526, 31535-31541, 31575, 31622, 31625, 31634, 31640❖, 31647, 31651, 31717, 31720, 36000, 36400-36410, 36420-36430, 36440, 36591-36592, 36600, 36640, 43752, 51701-51703, 62320-62327, 64400, 64405-64408, 64415-64435, 64445-64454, 64461-64463, 64479-64505, 64510-64530, 69705-69706, 69990, 76000, 77001-77002, 89220, 92012-92014, 92511, 93000-93010, 93040-93042, 93318, 93355, 94002, 94200, 94680-94690, 95812-95816, 95819, 95822, 95829, 95955, 96360-96368, 96372, 96374-96377, 96523, 97597-97598, 97602, 99155, 99156, 99157, 99211-99215, 99221-99223, 99231-99239, 99242-99245, 99252-99255, 99291-99292, 99304-99310, 99315-99316, 99347-99350, 99374-99375, 99377-99378, 99446-99449, 99451-99452, 99495-99496, G0463, G0471

31643 00520, 00528-00529, 0213T, 0216T, 0596T-0597T, 0708T-0709T, 12001-12007, 12011-12057, 13100-13133, 13151-13153, 31231, 31525-31526, 31535, 31575, 31622, 31634, 31647, 31717, 31720-31725, 36000, 36400-36410, 36420-36430, 36440, 36591-36592, 36600, 36640, 43752, 51701-51703, 62320-62327, 64400, 64405-64408, 64415-64435, 64445-64454, 64461-64463, 64479-64505, 64510-64530, 69705-69706, 69990, 76000, 77001-77002, 89220, 92012-92014, 92511, 93000-93010, 93040-93042, 93318, 93355, 94002, 94200, 94680-94690, 95812-95816, 95819, 95822, 95829, 95955, 96360-96368, 96372, 96374-96377, 96523, 99155, 99156, 99157, 99211-99215, 99221-99223, 99231-99239, 99242-99245, 99252-99255, 99291-99292, 99304-99310, 99315-99316, 99347-99350, 99374-99375, 99377-99378, 99446-99449, 99451-99452, 99495-99496, G0463, G0471

31645 00520, 0213T, 0216T, 0596T-0597T, 0708T-0709T, 12001-12007, 12011-12057, 13100-13133, 13151-13153, 31231, 31525-31526, 31535, 31540, 31575, 31622, 31634, 31647, 31717, 31720-31725, 36000, 36400-36410, 36420-36430, 36440, 36591-36592, 36600, 36640, 43752, 51701-51703, 62320-62327, 64400, 64405-64408, 64415-64435, 64445-64454, 64461-64463, 64479-64505, 64510-64530, 69705-69706, 69990, 76000, 77001-77002, 89220, 92012-92014, 92511, 93000-93010, 93040-93042, 93318, 93355, 94002, 94200, 94680-94690, 95812-95816, 95819, 95822, 95829, 95955, 96360-96368, 96372, 96374-96377, 96523, 99155, 99156, 99157, 99211-99215, 99221-99223, 99231-99239, 99242-99245, 99252-99255, 99291-99292, 99304-99310, 99315-99316, 99347-99350, 99374-99375, 99377-99378, 99446-99449, 99451-99452, 99495-99496, G0463, G0471, J0670

31646 00520, 0213T, 0216T, 0596T-0597T, 0708T-0709T, 12001-12007, 12011-12057, 13100-13133, 13151-13153, 31231, 31525-31526, 31535-31541, 31575, 31622, 31634, 31645✦, 31647, 31717, 31720-31725, 36000, 36400-36410, 36420-36430, 36440, 36591-36592, 36600, 36640, 43752, 51701-51703, 62320-62327, 64400, 64405-64408, 64415-64435, 64445-64454, 64461-64463, 64479-64505, 64510-64530, 69705-69706, 69990, 76000, 77001-77002, 89220, 92012-92014, 92511, 93000-93010, 93040-93042, 93318, 93355, 94002, 94200, 94680-94690, 95812-95816, 95819, 95822, 95829, 95955, 96360-96368, 96372, 96374-96377, 96523, 99155, 99156, 99157, 99211-99215, 99221-99223, 99231-99239, 99242-99245, 99252-99255, 99291-99292, 99304-99310, 99315-99316, 99347-99350, 99374-99375, 99377-99378, 99446-99449, 99451-99452, 99495-99496, G0463, G0471, J0670

31717 00520, 0213T, 0216T, 0596T-0597T, 0708T-0709T, 10005, 10007, 10009, 10011, 10021, 12001-12007, 12011-12057, 13100-13133, 13151-13153, 36000, 36400-36410, 36420-36430, 36440, 36591-36592, 36600, 36640, 43752, 51701-51703, 62320-62327, 64400, 64405-64408, 64415-64435, 64445-64454, 64461-64463, 64479-64505, 64510-64530, 69990, 89220, 92012-92014, 93000-93010, 93040-93042, 93318, 93355, 94002, 94200, 94680-94690, 95812-95816, 95819, 95822, 95829, 95955, 96360-96368, 96372, 96374-96377, 96523, 99155, 99156, 99157, 99211-99215, 99221-99223, 99231-99239, 99242-99245, 99252-99255, 99291-99292, 99304-99310, 99315-99316, 99347-99350, 99374-99375, 99377-99378, 99446-99449, 99451-99452, 99495-99496, G0463, G0471, J0670

31720 00520, 0213T, 0216T, 0596T-0597T, 0708T-0709T, 12001-12007, 12011-12057, 13100-13133, 13151-13153, 36000, 36400-36410, 36420-36430, 36440, 36591-36592, 36600, 36640, 43752, 51701-51703, 62320-62327, 64400, 64405-64408, 64415-64435, 64445-64454, 64461-64463, 64479-64505, 64510-64530, 69990, 89220, 92012-92014, 93000-93010, 93040-93042, 93318, 93355, 94002, 94200, 94680-94690, 95812-95816, 95819, 95822, 95829, 95955, 96360-96368, 96372, 96374-96377, 96523, 99155, 99156, 99157, 99211-99215, 99221-99223, 99231-99239, 99242-99245, 99252-99255, 99291-99292, 99304-99310, 99315-99316, 99347-99350, 99374-99375, 99377-99378, 99446-99449, 99451-99452, 99495-99496, G0463, G0471

31725 00520, 0213T, 0216T, 0596T-0597T, 0708T-0709T, 12001-12007, 12011-12057, 13100-13133, 13151-13153, 36000, 36400-36410, 36420-36430, 36440, 36591-36592, 36600, 36640, 43752, 51701-51703, 62320-62327, 64400, 64405-64408, 64415-64435, 64445-64454, 64461-64463, 64479-64505, 64510-64530, 69990, 89220, 92012-92014, 93000-93010, 93040-93042, 93318, 93355, 94002, 94200, 94680-94690, 95812-95816, 95819, 95822, 95829, 95955, 96360-96368, 96372, 96374-96377, 96523, 99155, 99156, 99157, 99211-99215, 99221-99223, 99231-99239, 99242-99245, 99252-99255, 99291-99292, 99304-99310, 99315-99316, 99347-99350, 99374-99375, 99377-99378, 99446-99449, 99451-99452, 99495-99496, G0463, G0471

31730 00520, 0213T, 0216T, 0596T-0597T, 0708T-0709T, 12001-12007, 12011-12057, 13100-13133, 13151-13153, 36000, 36400-36410, 36420-36430, 36440, 36591-36592, 36600, 36640, 43752, 51701-51703, 62320-62327, 64400, 64405-64408, 64415-64435, 64445-64454, 64461-64463, 64479-64505, 64510-64530, 69990, 92012-92014, 92502, 93000-93010, 93040-93042, 93318, 93355, 94002, 94200, 94680-94690, 95812-95816, 95819, 95822, 95829, 95955, 96360-96368, 96372, 96374-96377, 96523, 99155, 99156, 99157, 99211-99215, 99221-99223, 99231-99239, 99242-99245, 99252-99255, 99291-99292, 99304-99310, 99315-99316, 99347-99350, 99374-99375, 99377-99378, 99446-99449, 99451-99452, 99495-99496, G0463, G0471, J0670

31760 00520, 0213T, 0216T, 0596T-0597T, 0708T-0709T, 11000-11006, 11042-11047, 12001-12007, 12011-12057, 13100-13133, 13151-13153, 31805, 36000, 36400-36410, 36420-36430, 36440, 36591-36592, 36600, 36640, 39000-39010, 43752, 51701-51703, 62320-62327, 64400, 64405-64408, 64415-64435, 64445-64454, 64461-64463, 64479-64505, 64510-64530, 69990, 92012-92014, 93000-93010, 93040-93042, 93318, 93355, 94002, 94200, 94680-94690, 95812-95816, 95819, 95822, 95829, 95955, 96360-96368, 96372, 96374-96377, 96523, 97597-97598, 97602, 99155, 99156, 99157, 99211-99215, 99221-99223, 99231-99239, 99242-99245, 99252-99255, 99291-99292, 99304-99310, 99315-99316, 99347-99350, 99374-99375, 99377-99378, 99446-99449, 99451-99452, 99495-99496, G0463, G0471

31770 00520, 0213T, 0216T, 0596T-0597T, 0708T-0709T, 11000-11006, 11042-11047, 12001-12007, 12011-12057, 13100-13133, 13151-13153, 31775✦, 32100, 36000, 36400-36410, 36420-36430, 36440, 36591-36592, 36600, 36640, 39000-39010, 43752, 51701-51703, 62320-62327, 64400, 64405-64408, 64415-64435, 64445-64454, 64461-64463, 64479-64505, 64510-64530, 69990, 92012-92014, 93000-93010, 93040-93042, 93318, 93355, 94002, 94200, 94680-94690, 95812-95816, 95819, 95822, 95829, 95955, 96360-96368, 96372, 96374-96377, 96523, 97597-97598, 97602, 99155, 99156, 99157, 99211-99215, 99221-99223, 99231-99239, 99242-99245, 99252-99255, 99291-99292, 99304-99310, 99315-99316, 99347-99350, 99374-99375, 99377-99378, 99446-99449, 99451-99452, 99495-99496, G0463, G0471

31775 00520, 0213T, 0216T, 0596T-0597T, 0708T-0709T, 11000-11006, 11042-11047, 12001-12007, 12011-12057, 13100-13133, 13151-13153, 32100, 36000, 36400-36410, 36420-36430, 36440, 36591-36592, 36600, 36640, 39000-39010, 43752, 51701-51703, 62320-62327, 64400, 64405-64408, 64415-64435, 64445-64454, 64461-64463, 64479-64505, 64510-64530, 69990, 92012-92014, 93000-93010, 93040-93042, 93318, 93355, 94002, 94200, 94680-94690, 95812-95816, 95819, 95822, 95829, 95955, 96360-96368, 96372, 96374-96377, 96523, 97597-97598, 97602, 99155, 99156, 99157, 99211-99215, 99221-99223, 99231-99239, 99242-99245, 99252-99255, 99291-99292, 99304-99310, 99315-99316, 99347-99350, 99374-99375, 99377-99378, 99446-99449, 99451-99452, 99495-99496, G0463, G0471

31781 00520, 0213T, 0216T, 0596T-0597T, 0708T-0709T, 11000-11006, 11042-11047, 12001-12007, 12011-12057, 13100-13133, 13151-13153, 32100, 36000, 36400-36410, 36420-36430, 36440, 36591-36592, 36600, 36640, 39000-39010, 43752, 51701-51703, 62320-62327, 64400, 64405-64408, 64415-64435, 64445-64454, 64461-64463, 64479-64505, 64510-64530, 69990, 92012-92014, 93000-93010, 93040-93042, 93318, 93355, 94002, 94200, 94680-94690, 95812-95816, 95819, 95822, 95829, 95955, 96360-96368, 96372, 96374-96377, 96523, 97597-97598, 97602, 99155, 99156, 99157, 99211-99215, 99221-99223, 99231-99239, 99242-99245, 99252-99255, 99291-99292, 99304-99310, 99315-99316, 99347-99350, 99374-99375, 99377-99378, 99446-99449, 99451-99452, 99495-99496, G0463, G0471

31786 00520, 0213T, 0216T, 0596T-0597T, 0708T-0709T, 11000-11006, 11042-11047, 12001-12007, 12011-12057, 13100-13133, 13151-13153, 31805, 32100, 33267, 36000, 36400-36410, 36420-36430, 36440, 36591-36592, 36600, 36640, 39000-39010, 43752, 51701-51703, 62320-62327, 64400, 64405-64408, 64415-64435, 64445-64454, 64461-64463, 64479-64505, 64510-64530, 69990, 92012-92014, 93000-93010, 93040-93042, 93318, 93355, 94002, 94200, 94680-94690, 95812-95816, 95819, 95822, 95829, 95955, 96360-96368, 96372, 96374-96377, 96523, 97597-97598, 97602, 99155, 99156, 99157, 99211-99215, 99221-99223, 99231-99239, 99242-99245, 99252-99255, 99291-99292, 99304-99310, 99315-99316, 99347-99350, 99374-99375, 99377-99378, 99446-99449, 99451-99452, 99495-99496, G0463, G0471

31805 00520, 0213T, 0216T, 0596T-0597T, 0708T-0709T, 12001-12007, 12011-12057, 13100-13133, 13151-13153, 32100, 36000, 36400-36410, 36420-36430, 36440, 36591-36592, 36600, 36640, 39000-39010, 43752, 51701-51703, 62320-62327, 64400, 64405-64408, 64415-64435, 64445-64454, 64461-64463, 64479-64505, 64510-64530, 69990, 92012-92014, 93000-93010, 93040-93042, 93318, 93355, 94002, 94200, 94680-94690, 95812-95816, 95819, 95822, 95829, 95955, 96360-96368, 96372, 96374-96377, 96523, 99155, 99156, 99157, 99211-99215, 99221-99223, 99231-99239, 99242-99245, 99252-99255, 99291-99292, 99304-99310, 99315-99316, 99347-99350, 99374-99375, 99377-99378, 99446-99449, 99451-99452, 99495-99496, G0463, G0471

31820 00520, 0213T, 0216T, 0596T-0597T, 0708T-0709T, 11000-11006, 11042-11047, 12001-12007, 12011-12057, 13100-13133, 13151-13153, 31830❖, 36000, 36400-36410, 36420-36430, 36440, 36591-36592, 36600, 36640, 43752, 51701-51703, 62320-62327, 64400, 64405-64408, 64415-64435, 64445-64454, 64461-64463, 64479-64505, 64510-64530, 69990, 92012-92014, 92502, 93000-93010, 93040-93042, 93318, 93355, 94002, 94200, 94680-94690, 95812-95816, 95819, 95822, 95829, 95955, 96360-96368, 96372, 96374-96377, 96523, 97597-97598, 97602, 99155, 99156, 99157, 99211-99215, 99221-99223, 99231-99239, 99242-99245, 99252-99255, 99291-99292, 99304-99310, 99315-99316, 99347-99350, 99374-99375, 99377-99378, 99446-99449, 99451-99452, 99495-99496, G0463, G0471, J0670

31825 00520, 0213T, 0216T, 0596T-0597T, 0708T-0709T, 11000-11006, 11042-11047, 12001-12007, 12011-12057, 13100-13133, 13151-13153, 31820, 36000, 36400-36410, 36420-36430, 36440, 36591-36592, 36600, 36640, 43752, 51701-51703, 62320-62327, 64400, 64405-64408, 64415-64435, 64445-64454, 64461-64463, 64479-64505, 64510-64530, 69990, 92012-92014, 92502, 93000-93010, 93040-93042, 93318, 93355, 94002, 94200, 94680-94690, 95812-95816, 95819, 95822, 95829, 95955, 96360-96368, 96372, 96374-96377, 96523, 97597-97598, 97602, 99155, 99156, 99157, 99211-99215, 99221-99223, 99231-99239, 99242-99245, 99252-99255, 99291-99292, 99304-99310, 99315-99316, 99347-99350, 99374-99375, 99377-99378, 99446-99449, 99451-99452, 99495-99496, G0463, G0471, J0670

32035 0213T, 0216T, 0596T-0597T, 0708T-0709T, 11000-11006, 11042-11047, 12001-12007, 12011-12057, 13100-13133, 13151-13153, 32036❖, 32096-32098, 32220-32225, 32551, 32556-32557, 32601, 32607-32609, 32900, 36000, 36400-36410, 36420-36430, 36440, 36591-36592, 36600, 36640, 43752, 51701-51703, 62320-62327, 64400, 64405-64408, 64415-64435, 64445-64454, 64461-64463, 64479-64505, 64510-64530, 69990, 92012-92014, 93000-93010, 93040-93042, 93318, 93355, 94002, 94200, 94680-94690, 95812-95816, 95819, 95822, 95829, 95955, 96360-96368, 96372, 96374-96377, 96523, 97597-97598, 97602, 99155, 99156, 99157, 99211-99215, 99221-99223, 99231-99239, 99242-99245, 99252-99255, 99291-99292, 99304-99310, 99315-99316, 99347-99350, 99374-99375, 99377-99378, 99446-99449, 99451-99452, 99495-99496, G0463, G0471

32036 0213T, 0216T, 0596T-0597T, 0708T-0709T, 12001-12007, 12011-12057, 13100-13133, 13151-13153, 32096-32098, 32220-32225, 32551, 32556-32557, 32601, 32607-32609, 36000, 36400-36410, 36420-36430, 36440, 36591-36592, 36600, 36640, 43752, 51701-51703, 62320-62327, 64400, 64405-64408, 64415-64435, 64445-64454, 64461-64463, 64479-64505, 64510-64530, 69990, 92012-92014, 93000-93010, 93040-93042, 93318, 93355, 94002, 94200, 94680-94690, 95812-95816, 95819, 95822, 95829, 95955, 96360-96368, 96372, 96374-96377, 96523, 99155, 99156, 99157, 99211-99215, 99221-99223, 99231-99239, 99242-99245, 99252-99255, 99291-99292, 99304-99310, 99315-99316, 99347-99350, 99374-99375, 99377-99378, 99446-99449, 99451-99452, 99495-99496, G0463, G0471

32096 0213T, 0216T, 0596T-0597T, 0708T-0709T, 10005, 10007, 10009, 10011, 10021, 11000-11006, 11042-11047, 12001-12007, 12011-12057, 13100-13133, 13151-13153, 20101, 21600, 31622, 31634, 31647, 32098-32100, 32220-32225, 32310, 32408❖, 32551, 32556-32601, 32607-32609, 36000, 36400-36410, 36420-36430, 36440, 36591-36592, 36600, 36640, 43752, 51701-51703, 62320-62327, 64400, 64405-64408, 64415-64435, 64445-64454, 64461-64463, 64479-64505, 64510-64530, 69990, 92012-92014, 93000-93010, 93040-93042, 93318, 93355, 94002, 94200, 94680-94690, 95812-95816, 95819, 95822, 95829, 95955, 96360-96368, 96372, 96374-96377, 96523, 97597-97598, 97602, 99155, 99156, 99157, 99211-99215, 99221-99223, 99231-99239, 99242-99245, 99252-99255, 99291-99292, 99304-99310, 99315-99316, 99347-99350, 99374-99375, 99377-99378, 99446-99449, 99451-99452, 99495-99496, G0463, G0471

32097 0213T, 0216T, 0596T-0597T, 0708T-0709T, 10005, 10007, 10009, 10011, 10021, 11000-11006, 11042-11047, 12001-12007, 12011-12057, 13100-13133, 13151-13153, 20101, 21600, 31622, 31634, 31647, 32096❖, 32098-32100, 32220-32225, 32310, 32408❖, 32551, 32556-32601, 32607-32609, 36000, 36400-36410, 36420-36430, 36440, 36591-36592, 36600, 36640, 43752, 51701-51703, 62320-62327, 64400, 64405-64408, 64415-64435, 64445-64454, 64461-64463, 64479-64505, 64510-64530, 69990, 92012-92014, 93000-93010, 93040-93042, 93318, 93355, 94002, 94200, 94680-94690, 95812-95816, 95819, 95822, 95829, 95955, 96360-96368, 96372, 96374-96377, 96523, 97597-97598, 97602, 99155, 99156, 99157, 99211-99215, 99221-99223, 99231-99239, 99242-99245, 99252-99255, 99291-99292, 99304-99310, 99315-99316, 99347-99350, 99374-99375, 99377-99378, 99446-99449, 99451-99452, 99495-99496, G0463, G0471

32098 0213T, 0216T, 0596T-0597T, 0708T-0709T, 10005, 10007, 10009, 10011, 10021, 11000-11006, 11042-11047, 12001-12007, 12011-12057, 13100-13133, 13151-13153, 20101, 21600, 31622, 31634, 31647, 32100, 32220-32225, 32310, 32400❖, 32408❖, 32551, 32556-32601, 32607-32609, 36000, 36400-36410, 36420-36430, 36440, 36591-36592, 36600, 36640, 43752, 51701-51703, 62320-62327, 64400, 64405-64408, 64415-64435, 64445-64454, 64461-64463, 64479-64505, 64510-64530, 69990, 92012-92014, 93000-93010, 93040-93042, 93318, 93355, 94002, 94200, 94680-94690, 95812-95816, 95819, 95822, 95829, 95955, 96360-96368, 96372, 96374-96377, 96523, 97597-97598, 97602, 99155, 99156, 99157, 99211-99215, 99221-99223, 99231-99239, 99242-99245, 99252-99255, 99291-99292, 99304-99310, 99315-99316, 99347-99350, 99374-99375, 99377-99378, 99446-99449, 99451-99452, 99495-99496, G0463, G0471

32100 0213T, 0216T, 0596T-0597T, 0708T-0709T, 11000-11006, 11042-11047, 12001-12007, 12011-12057, 13100-13133, 13151-13153, 20101, 21600-21603, 31622, 31634, 31647, 32200, 32215, 32225, 32310, 32551, 32556-32601, 32607-32609, 33025, 36000, 36400-36410, 36420-36430, 36440, 36591-36592, 36600, 36640, 43752, 51701-51703, 62320-62327, 64400, 64405-64408, 64415-64435, 64445-64454,

64461-64463, 64479-64505, 64510-64530, 69990, 92012-92014, 93000-93010, 93040-93042, 93318, 93355, 94002, 94200, 94680-94690, 95812-95816, 95819, 95822, 95829, 95955, 96360-96368, 96372, 96374-96377, 96523, 97597-97598, 97602, 99155, 99156, 99157, 99211-99215, 99221-99223, 99231-99239, 99242-99245, 99252-99255, 99291-99292, 99304-99310, 99315-99316, 99347-99350, 99374-99375, 99377-99378, 99446-99449, 99451-99452, 99495-99496, G0463, G0471

32110 0213T, 0216T, 0596T-0597T, 0708T-0709T, 11000-11006, 11042-11047, 12001-12007, 12011-12057, 13100-13133, 13151-13153, 20101, 31622, 31634, 31647, 32096-32100, 32200, 32220-32225, 32551, 32556-32601, 32607-32609, 33025, 33267, 36000, 36400-36410, 36420-36430, 36440, 36591-36592, 36600, 36640, 43752, 51701-51703, 62320-62327, 64400, 64405-64408, 64415-64435, 64445-64454, 64461-64463, 64479-64505, 64510-64530, 69990, 92012-92014, 93000-93010, 93040-93042, 93318, 93355, 94002, 94200, 94680-94690, 95812-95816, 95819, 95822, 95829, 95955, 96360-96368, 96372, 96374-96377, 96523, 97597-97598, 97602, 99155, 99156, 99157, 99211-99215, 99221-99223, 99231-99239, 99242-99245, 99252-99255, 99291-99292, 99304-99310, 99315-99316, 99347-99350, 99374-99375, 99377-99378, 99446-99449, 99451-99452, 99495-99496, G0463, G0471

32120 0213T, 0216T, 0596T-0597T, 0708T-0709T, 11000-11006, 11042-11047, 12001-12007, 12011-12057, 13100-13133, 13151-13153, 20101, 31622, 31634, 31647, 32096-32100, 32110❖, 32215-32225, 32551, 32556-32557, 32601, 32607-32609, 36000, 36400-36410, 36420-36430, 36440, 36591-36592, 36600, 36640, 43752, 51701-51703, 62320-62327, 64400, 64405-64408, 64415-64435, 64445-64454, 64461-64463, 64479-64505, 64510-64530, 69990, 92012-92014, 93000-93010, 93040-93042, 93318, 93355, 94002, 94200, 94680-94690, 95812-95816, 95819, 95822, 95829, 95955, 96360-96368, 96372, 96374-96377, 96523, 97597-97598, 97602, 99155, 99156, 99157, 99211-99215, 99221-99223, 99231-99239, 99242-99245, 99252-99255, 99291-99292, 99304-99310, 99315-99316, 99347-99350, 99374-99375, 99377-99378, 99446-99449, 99451-99452, 99495-99496, G0463, G0471

32124 0213T, 0216T, 0596T-0597T, 0708T-0709T, 11000-11006, 11042-11047, 12001-12007, 12011-12057, 13100-13133, 13151-13153, 20101, 31622, 31634, 31647, 32096-32100, 32200, 32215-32225, 32551, 32556-32601, 32607-32609, 32654, 32940❖, 36000, 36400-36410, 36420-36430, 36440, 36591-36592, 36600, 36640, 43752, 51701-51703, 62320-62327, 64400, 64405-64408, 64415-64435, 64445-64454, 64461-64463, 64479-64505, 64510-64530, 69990, 92012-92014, 93000-93010, 93040-93042, 93318, 93355, 94002, 94200, 94680-94690, 95812-95816, 95819, 95822, 95829, 95955, 96360-96368, 96372, 96374-96377, 96523, 97597-97598, 97602, 99155, 99156, 99157, 99211-99215, 99221-99223, 99231-99239, 99242-99245, 99252-99255, 99291-99292, 99304-99310, 99315-99316, 99347-99350, 99374-99375, 99377-99378,

32141 0213T, 0216T, 0596T-0597T, 0708T-0709T, 11000-11006, 11042-11047, 12001-12007, 12011-12057, 13100-13133, 13151-13153, 20101, 31622, 31634, 31647, 32096-32100, 32200, 32215-32225, 32551, 32556-32601, 32607-32609, 32654, 33267, 36000, 36400-36410, 36420-36430, 36440, 36591-36592, 36600, 36640, 43752, 51701-51703, 62320-62327, 64400, 64405-64408, 64415-64435, 64445-64454, 64461-64463, 64479-64505, 64510-64530, 69990, 92012-92014, 93000-93010, 93040-93042, 93318, 93355, 94002, 94200, 94680-94690, 95812-95816, 95819, 95822, 95829, 95955, 96360-96368, 96372, 96374-96377, 96523, 97597-97598, 97602, 99155, 99156, 99157, 99211-99215, 99221-99223, 99231-99239, 99242-99245, 99252-99255, 99291-99292, 99304-99310, 99315-99316, 99347-99350, 99374-99375, 99377-99378, 99446-99449, 99451-99452, 99495-99496, G0463, G0471

32150 0213T, 0216T, 0596T-0597T, 0708T-0709T, 11000-11006, 11042-11047, 12001-12007, 12011-12057, 13100-13133, 13151-13153, 20101, 31622, 31634, 31647, 32096-32100, 32200, 32215-32225, 32551, 32556-32601, 32607-32609, 32654, 36000, 36400-36410, 36420-36430, 36440, 36591-36592, 36600, 36640, 43752, 51701-51703, 62320-62327, 64400, 64405-64408, 64415-64435, 64445-64454, 64461-64463, 64479-64505, 64510-64530, 69990, 92012-92014, 93000-93010, 93040-93042, 93318, 93355, 94002, 94200, 94680-94690, 95812-95816, 95819, 95822, 95829, 95955, 96360-96368, 96372, 96374-96377, 96523, 97597-97598, 97602, 99155, 99156, 99157, 99211-99215, 99221-99223, 99231-99239, 99242-99245, 99252-99255, 99291-99292, 99304-99310, 99315-99316, 99347-99350, 99374-99375, 99377-99378, 99446-99449, 99451-99452, 99495-99496, G0463, G0471

32151 0213T, 0216T, 0596T-0597T, 0708T-0709T, 11000-11006, 11042-11047, 12001-12007, 12011-12057, 13100-13133, 13151-13153, 20101, 31622, 31634, 31647, 32096-32100, 32200, 32215-32225, 32551, 32556-32562, 32654, 36000, 36400-36410, 36420-36430, 36440, 36591-36592, 36600, 36640, 43752, 51701-51703, 62320-62327, 64400, 64405-64408, 64415-64435, 64445-64454, 64461-64463, 64479-64505, 64510-64530, 69990, 92012-92014, 93000-93010, 93040-93042, 93318, 93355, 94002, 94200, 94680-94690, 95812-95816, 95819, 95822, 95829, 95955, 96360-96368, 96372, 96374-96377, 96523, 97597-97598, 97602, 99155, 99156, 99157, 99211-99215, 99221-99223, 99231-99239, 99242-99245, 99252-99255, 99291-99292, 99304-99310, 99315-99316, 99347-99350, 99374-99375, 99377-99378, 99446-99449, 99451-99452, 99495-99496, G0463, G0471

32160 0213T, 0216T, 0596T-0597T, 0708T-0709T, 11000-11006, 11042-11047, 12001-12007, 12011-12057, 13100-13133, 13151-13153, 20101, 31622, 31634, 31647, 32096-32100, 32215-32225, 32551, 32556-32557, 32601, 32607-32609, 32654, 36000, 36400-36410, 36420-36430, 36440, 36591-36592, 36600, 36640, 43752, 51701-51703, 62320-62327, 64400, 64405-64408, 64415-64435, 64445-64454, 64461-64463, 64479-64505,

IMPORTANT

Note: The following URL and password will provide you with access to download and view the complete list of CCI edits:

https://www.optumcoding.com/productupdates

2025 password: **CAS25**

Please note that you should log in each quarter to ensure you receive the most current updates.

CPT Index

A

- **Abdomen, Abdominal**
  - Aorta
    - Aneurysm, 34813, 34830, 34841, 35081 [34718]
    - Thromboendarterectomy, 35331
  - Aortic Aneurysm, 34813, 34830, 34841, 35081 [34718]
  - Artery
    - Ligation, 37617
  - Bypass Graft, 35907
  - Exploration
    - for Postoperative Hemorrhage, Infection, or Thrombosis, 35840
  - Insertion
    - Venous Shunt, 49425
  - Intraperitoneal
    - Catheter Exit Site, 49436
    - Catheter Insertion, 49425, 49435
    - Shunt
      - Insertion, 49425
      - Ligation, 49428
      - Removal, 49429
      - Revision, 49426
  - Repair
    - Blood Vessel, 35221
      - with
        - Other Graft, 35281
        - Vein Graft, 35251
  - Revision
    - Venous Shunt, 49426
  - Ultrasound, 76700-76706
  - Wall
    - Reconstruction, 49905
  - X-ray, 74018
- **ABG**, 82803-82805
- **Ablation**
  - Atria, 33258
  - Endovenous, 0524T [36482]
  - Heart
    - Arrhythmogenic Focus, 33251, 33261, 93653
    - Atrioventricular Focus, 93650, 93654
    - Focal by Radiation Therapy, 0745T
    - Intracardiac Pacing and Mapping, 93631
      - Follow-up Study, 93624
      - Stimulation and Pacing, 93623
  - Lung
    - Tumor
      - Cryoablation, [32994]
      - Radiofrequency, 32998
  - Nerve
    - Percutaneous, 0793T
  - Pulmonary Tumor
    - Cryoablation, [32994]
    - Radiofrequency, 32998
  - Radiofrequency
    - Lung Tumor(s), 32998
  - Supraventricular Arrhythmogenic Focus, 33251
  - Vein
    - Endovenous, 0524T [36482]
  - Ventricular Arrhythmogenic Focus, 33261
- **Abscess**
  - Lung
    - Endoscopic, 31646
    - Open, 32200
  - Lymph Node, 38300-38305
  - Neck, 21502
  - Thoracostomy, 32551
  - Thorax, 21502
    - Bone Abscess, 21510
  - X-ray, 75989
- **Acidity/Alkalinity**
  - Blood Gasses, 82805
- **Acoustic**
  - Recording
    - Waveform, Cardiac, 0716T
- **Activated Partial Thromboplastin Time**, 85730-85732
- **Adhesion, Adhesions**
  - Lungs
    - Pneumolysis, 32124, 32940
- **Administration**
  - Health Risk Assessment, 96161
  - Immunization/Vaccination
    - Severe Acute Respiratory Syndrome Coronavirus (SARS-CoV-2 [COVID-19]), [90480]
  - Infusion/Injection
    - Therapeutic, Diagnostic, Prophylactic, 96365
  - Occlusive Substance During Bronchoscopy, 31634
  - Pharmacologic Agent w/Monitoring
    - with Monitoring, 93463
- **Advance Care Planning**, 99498
- **Advance Directives**, 99498
- **Advanced Life Support**
  - Physician Direction, 99288
- **AFBG**, 35539-35540, 35646
- **Aggregation**
  - Platelet, 85576
- **AICD (Pacing Cardioverter–Defibrillator)**, 33223, 93282, 93289, 93292, 93295, 0571T
  - Heart
    - Defibrillator, 93282, 93292, 93295 [33262]
    - Pacemaker, [33221, 33229]
- **Alcohol**
  - Abuse Screening and Intervention, 99409
- **Allograft Preparation**
  - Heart, 33933, 33944
  - Lung, 32856, 33933
- **Allograft**
  - Aortic Valve, 33406, 33413
  - Lung Transplant, 32850
- **ALS**, 99288
- **Aminotransferase**
  - Aspartate (SGOT), 84450
- **Analysis**
  - Cardiac Rhythm Monitor System, 93285, 93291, 93298, 0650T
  - Cardiac Stimulator, Wireless, 0521T
  - Cardiovascular Physiologic Monitoring System, 93290, 93297
  - Electronic
    - Antitachycardia Pacemaker, 93724
    - Cardioverter–Defibrillator
      - Data Analysis, 93289, 93296
      - Initial Evaluation, 93641
      - Substernal, Implantable, 0575T
    - Leads, 93641
    - Pacemaker, 93288, 93293
    - Wearable Cardiac Device, 93288
  - Implantable Defibrillator, 93287, 93289, 93296
  - Pacemaker, 93279, 93288, 93293
  - Physiologic Data, Remote, [99091, 99454, 99457]
- **Anastomosis**
  - Arteriovenous Fistula
    - Direct, 36821
    - Revision, 36832-36833
      - with Thrombectomy, 36833
      - without Thrombectomy, 36832
    - with Bypass Graft, 35686
    - with Graft, 36825-36830, 36832
    - with Thrombectomy, 36831
  - Artery
    - to Aorta, 33606
  - Broncho–Bronchial, 32486
  - Caval to Mesenteric, 37160
  - Cavopulmonary, 33622, 33768
  - Excision
    - Trachea, 31781
  - Portocaval, 37140
  - Pulmonary, 33606
  - Renoportal, 37145
  - Vein
    - Saphenopopliteal, 34530
- **Anatomic**
  - Guide, 3D Printed, 0562T
- **Anatomic** — *continued*
  - Model, 3D Printed, 0560T
- **Anesthesia**
  - Pleurectomy, 32320, 32656
- **Aneurysm Repair**
  - Aorta
    - Abdominal, 34813, 34830, 34841, 35081 [34718]
    - Thoracoabdominal, 33877
  - Axillary Artery, 35011-35013
  - Brachial Artery, 35011-35013
  - Carotid Artery, 35001-35002
  - Celiac Artery, 35121-35122
  - Femoral Artery, 35141-35142
  - Hepatic Artery, 35121-35122
  - Iliac Artery, 35132 [34717]
  - Innominate Artery, 35021-35022
  - Mesenteric Artery, 35121-35122
  - Popliteal Artery, 35151-35152
  - Radial Artery, 35045
  - Renal Artery, 35121-35122
  - Splenic Artery, 35111-35112
  - Subclavian Artery, 35001-35002, 35021-35022
  - Thoracic Aorta, 33889
  - Thoracoabdominal Aorta, 33877
  - Ulnar Artery, 35045
- **Aneurysm, Aorta, Abdominal**
  - Screening Study, 76706
- **Angiography**
  - Abdominal Aorta, [34717]
  - Aortography
    - Injection, 93567
  - Arteriovenous Shunt, 36901
  - Atrial, 93566
  - Bypass Graft, 93455, 93457, 93459
  - Carotid Artery, 36221
  - Cervico-Vertebral Arch, 36221
  - Congenital Heart, 93564
  - Coronary Artery, 93563
    - Coronary Calcium Evaluation, 75571
    - Flow Velocity Measurement During Angiography, 93571-93572
  - Dialysis Circuit, Diagnostic, 36901
    - with Balloon Angioplasty, 36902
    - with Mechanical Thrombectomy, 36904
    - with Stent Placement, 36903
  - Endovascular Repair, [34717]
  - Heart Vessels
    - Injection, 93563, 93566
  - Innominate Artery, 36223, 36225
  - Intracoronary Infusion
    - with Percutaneous Coronary Revascularization, 0659T
  - Intracranial Carotid, 36224
  - Left Heart
    - Injection, 93565
  - Lung
    - Injection Pulmonary Artery, 93569 [93573]
  - Non-cardiac Vascular Flow Imaging, 78445
  - Nuclear Medicine, 78445
  - Pulmonary Artery
    - Injection, 93569 [93573]
  - Right Heart
    - Injection, 93457, 93566
  - Shunt, Dialysis, 36901
  - Subclavian Artery, 36225
  - Transcatheter Therapy
    - Embolization, 75898
    - Infusion, 75898
  - Ventricular, 93566
  - Vertebral Artery, 36221, 36226, 36228
- **Angioplasty**
  - Aorta, 33897 [37247]
  - Axillary Artery, [37247]
  - Blood Vessel Patch, 35201
  - Brachiocephalic Artery, [37247]
  - Common Carotid Artery with Stent Placement, 37218
  - Coronary Artery
    - Percutaneous Transluminal, [92920]
- **Angioplasty** — *continued*
  - Coronary Artery — *continued*
    - Percutaneous Transluminal — *continued*
      - with Atherectomy, [92925, 92933]
      - with Stent, [92937]
  - Dialysis Circuit, 36903, 36905
  - Femoral Artery, 37224
  - for Revascularization
    - Coronary, [92938, 92941]
    - Coronary Bypass Graft(s), [92938, 92941]
    - Femoral, 37224
    - Iliac, 37220
    - Peroneal, 37228
    - Popliteal, 37224
    - Tibial, 37228
  - Iliac Artery, 37220
  - Innominate Artery with Stent Placement, 37217-37218
  - Peroneal Artery, 37228
  - Popliteal Artery, 37224
  - Pulmonary Artery
    - Percutaneous Transluminal, 92997-92998
  - Renal or Visceral Artery, [37247]
  - Subclavian Artery, [37247]
  - Tibioperoneal Artery, 37228
  - Transluminal
    - Aorta, 33897
    - Arterial, 36903, 36906
    - Coronary, [92920, 92925, 92928, 92934, 92938, 92941, 92943]
    - Dialysis Circuit, 36905
    - Percutaneous, 33897
    - Pulmonary, 92998
  - Vein Patch Graft, 35879, 35884
  - Venous, [37249]
  - Visceral Artery, [37247]
    - Endovascular, 34841
  - with Placement Intravascular Stent, 37217-37218, 37236
- **Angioscopy**
  - Noncoronary vessels, 35400
- **Antibody Identification**
  - Leukocyte Antibodies, 86828
  - Solid Phase Assay, 86828
- **Antibody**
  - Cardiolipin, 86147
  - Human Leukocyte Antigens (HLA), 86828
  - Streptokinase, 86590
- **Anticoagulant Management**, 93793
- **Antigen Detection**
  - Immunofluorescence
    - Cytomegalovirus, 87271
- **Antimicrobial/Antibiotic Sensitivity**
  - Agar Dilution Method, 87181
- **Antistreptokinase Titer**, 86590
- **Aorta**
  - Abdominal
    - Aneurysm, 34813, 34830, 34841, 35081 [34718]
      - Screening, 76706
    - Thromboendarterectomy, 35331
  - Anastomosis
    - to Pulmonary Artery, 33606
  - Angiogram
    - Injection, 93567
  - Angioplasty, 33897 [37246]
  - Ascending
    - Graft, 33864
  - Balloon
    - Insertion, 33967, 33970, 33973
    - Removal, 33968, 33971, 33974
  - Catheterization
    - Catheter, 36200
    - Intracatheter, 36160
    - Needle, 36160
  - Circulation Assist
    - Insertion, 33967, 33970, 33973
    - Removal, 33968, 33971, 33974
  - Coarctation, 33840, 33894

 [Resequenced]

Aorta — *continued*
  Conduit to Heart, 33404
  Excision
    Coarctation, 33840
  Graft, 33864-33866, 33875
  Hemiarch Graft, 33866
  Infrarenal
    Endovascular Repair, 34701, 34845 [34718]
  Insertion
    Balloon Device, 33967, 33970, 33973
    Catheter, 36200
    Graft, 33335, 33864-33866
    Intracatheter, 36160
    Needle, 36160
  Removal
    Balloon Assist Device, 33968, 33971, 33974
  Repair, 33321, 33802-33803
    Aneurysm
      Abdominal, 34813, 34830, 34841, 35081 [34718]
      Ascending, 33864
      Sinus of Valsalva, 33720
      Thoracoabdominal, 33877
      Transverse Arch, 33871
    Aortic Anomalies, 33800
    Aortic Arch, 33853
    Coarctation, 33840, 33894
    Graft, 33871
      Ascending, 33864
    Hypoplastic or Interrupted Aortic Arch
      with Cardiopulmonary Bypass, 33853
      without Cardiopulmonary Bypass, 33852
    Thoracic Aneurysm with Graft, 33871
      Endovascular, 33880
    Translocation Aortic Root, 33783
    Transposition of the Great Vessels, 33770
  Suspension, 33800
  Suture, 33321
  Thromboendarterectomy, 35331
  Ultrasound, 76706
  Valve
    Implantation, 33366
    Incision, 33415
    Repair, 33391
      Gusset Aortoplasty, 33417
      Left Ventricle, 33414
      Stenosis
        Idiopathic Hypertrophic, 33416
        Subvalvular, 33415
        Supravalvular, 33417
      Valvuloplasty
        Open
          Complex, 33391
          with Cardiopulmonary Bypass, 33390
    Replacement
      Open, [33440]
      Transcatheter, 33366
      with Allograft Valve, 33406
      with Aortic Annulus Enlargement, 33412
      with Cardiopulmonary Bypass, 33367, 33406-33410
      with Prosthesis, 33366, 33405
      with Stentless Tissue Valve, 33410
      with Translocation Pulmonary Valve, 33413
      with Transventricular Aortic Annulus Enlargement, [33440]
  Visceral
    Endovascular Repair, 34841
Aortic Stenosis
  Repair, 33415
    Nikaidoh Procedure, 33783
    Supravalvular, 33417
Aortography, 93567
Aortoiliac
  Embolectomy, 34151-34201

Aortoiliac — *continued*
  Thrombectomy, 34151-34201
Aortopexy, 33800
Aortoplasty
  Supravalvular Stenosis, 33417
Apheresis
  Therapeutic, 36511
    with Selective HDL Delipidation and Plasma Reinfusion, 0342T
Apical-Aortic Conduit, 33404
Apnea
  Central
    Neurostimulator System, [33276]
Application
  Pulmonary Artery Bands, 33620
Arm
  Lower
    Artery
      Ligation, 37618
    Bypass Graft, 35903
    Exploration
      Blood Vessel, 35860
    Repair
      Blood Vessel with Other Graft, 35266
      Blood Vessel with Vein Graft, 35236
  Upper
    Artery
      Ligation, 37618
    Bypass Graft, 35903
    Exploration
      Blood Vessel, 35860
    Repair
      Blood Vessel with Other Graft, 35266
      Blood Vessel with Vein Graft, 35236
Arrhythmias
  Induction, 93618
Arrhythmogenic Focus
  Heart
    Destruction, 33251, 33261, 93653
Arterial Pressure
  Non-invasive Waveform Analysis, 93050
Arterial Puncture, 36600
Arteriosus, Ductus
  Closure, Transcatheter, 93582
  Repair, 33820
Arteriosus, Truncus
  Repair, 33786
Arteriovenous Anastomosis, 36818
Arteriovenous Fistula
  Cannulization
    Vein, 36815
  Creation, 36830
    Percutaneous, [36837]
  Repair
    Abdomen, 35182
      Acquired or Traumatic, 35189
    Head, 35180
      Acquired or Traumatic, 35188
    Lower Extremity, 35184
      Acquired or Traumatic, 35190
    Neck, 35180
      Acquired or Traumatic, 35188
    Thorax, 35182
      Acquired or Traumatic, 35189
    Upper Extremity, 35184
      Acquired or Traumatic, 35190
  Revision
    Hemodialysis Graft or Fistula
      with Thrombectomy, 36833
      without Thrombectomy, 36832
  Thrombectomy
    Dialysis Circuit, 36904
Arteriovenous Malformation
  Iliac Artery
    Repair, [34718]
  Vascular Embolization, 37242
Arteriovenous Shunt
  Angiography, 36901
  Aorta to Pulmonary Artery, 33755-33762
  Blalock-Taussig, 33750
  Dialysis Circuit, 36901

Arteriovenous Shunt — *continued*
  Peritoneal-Venous
    Evaluation, 49427
    Insertion, 49425
    Ligation, 49428
    Removal, 49429
    Revision, 49426
  Potts-Smith Shunt, 33762
  Subclavian to Pulmonary Artery, 33750
  Thomas Shunt, 36835
  Waterson Shunt, 33755
Artery
  Abdomen
    Catheterization, 36245
    Ligation, 37617
  Aorta
    Aneurysm Screening Study, 76706
    Angioplasty, 33897 [37247]
  Aortobi-iliac
    Bypass Graft, 35538, 35638
  Aortobifemoral
    Bypass Graft, 35540
  Aortocarotid
    Bypass Graft, 35526, 35626
  Aortofemoral
    Bypass Graft, 35539
  Aortoiliac
    Bypass Graft, 35537, 35637
    Embolectomy, 34151-34201
    Thrombectomy, 34151-34201
  Aortoiliofemoral, 35363
  Aortoinnominate
    Bypass Graft, 35526, 35626
  Aortosubclavian
    Bypass Graft, 35526, 35626
  Arm
    Harvest of Artery for Coronary Artery Bypass Graft, 35600
    Transluminal, 0234T
  Atherectomy
    Brachiocephalic, 0237T
    Coronary, [92924]
    Femoral, 37225, 37227
    Iliac, 0238T
    Peroneal, 37229, 37231, 37233, 37235
    Popliteal, 37225, 37227
    Renal, 0234T
    Tibial, 37229, 37231, 37233, 37235
    Transluminal, 0234T [92924]
    Visceral, 0235T
  Axillary
    Aneurysm, 35011-35013
    Angioplasty, [37247]
    Bypass Graft, 35522, 35533, 35623, 35650-35654
    Embolectomy, 34101
    Exposure, 34716
    Thrombectomy, 34101
    Thromboendarterectomy, 35321
  Biopsy
    Transcatheter, 37200
  Brachial
    Aneurysm, 35011-35013
    Angiography, [34834]
    Bypass Graft, 35510, 35512, 35522, 35525
    Embolectomy, 34101
    Exposure, [34834]
    Thrombectomy, 34101
    Thromboendarterectomy, 35321
  Brachiocephalic
    Angioplasty, [37247]
    Atherectomy, 0237T
    Catheterization, 36215
  Bypass Graft
    with Composite Graft, 35682
      Autogenous
        Three or More Segments
          Two Locations, 35683
        Two Segments
          Two Locations, 35682
  Cannulization
    to Vein, 36818
  Carotid
    Aneurysm, 35001

Artery — *continued*
  Carotid — *continued*
    Baroflex Activation Device
      Implantation, 0266T
      Interrogation Evaluation, 0273T
      Removal, 0269T
      Replacement, 0266T
      Revision, 0269T
    Bypass Graft, 33891, 35510, 35526, 35606, 35626, 35642
    Catheterization, 36100, 36221, 36228
    Embolectomy, 34001
    Excision, 60605
    Exploration, 35701
    Ligation, 37600
    Reimplantation, 35691, 35695
    Stent Placement
      Transcatheter, 37218
      Transposition, 33889, 35691, 35695
    Thrombectomy, 34001
    Thromboendarterectomy, 35301, 35390
    Transposition, 33889, 35691, 35695
  Catheterization
    Abdominal, 36245
    Aorta, 36200
      Thoracic, Nonselective, 36221
      Translumbar, 36160
    AV Shunt, 36902
      with Stent Insertion, 36903
    Brachiocephalic Branch, 36215
    Carotid, 36100
      Common Carotid, Selective, 36222-36223
      External Carotid, Selective, 36227
      Internal Carotid, Selective, 36224
        Each Intracranial Branch, 36228
    Dialysis Circuit, 36902
    Extremity, 36140
    Innominate, Selective, 36223
    Lower Extremity, 36245
    Pelvic, 36245
    Pulmonary, 36013
    Renal, 36251
      Angioplasty, 36902, 36905, 36907 [37247]
    Thoracic Branch, 36215
    Vertebral, Selective
      Each Intracranial Branch, 36228
  Celiac
    Aneurysm, 35121-35122
    Bypass Graft, 35531, 35631
    Embolectomy, 34151
    Endoprosthesis, 34841
    Thrombectomy, 34151
    Thromboendarterectomy, 35341
  Chest
    Ligation, 37616
  Coronary
    Angiography, [92925, 92934]
    Atherectomy, [92925, 92934]
    Bypass
      Arterial, 33533
      Combined Arterial and Venous, 33517
      Venous, 33510
    Graft, 33505
    Ligation, 33502
    Repair, 33507
    Thrombectomy
      Percutaneous, [92973]
    Thrombolysis, [92975, 92977]
    Translocation, 33507
    Unroofing, 33507
  Extracranial
    Vascular Studies
      Duplex Scan, 93882
  Extremities
    Vascular Studies, 93924
      Bypass Grafts Extremities, 93925
  Extremity
    Bypass Graft Revision, 35883
    Catheterization, 36140, 36245

Artery — *continued*
Extremity — *continued*
Ligation, 37618
Femoral
Aneurysm, 35141-35142
Angioplasty, 37224
Atherectomy, 37225, 37227, 37229, 37231
Bypass Graft, 35521, 35533, 35540, 35558, 35566, 35621, 35646-35650, 35666, 35700
Bypass Graft Revision, 35884
Bypass In Situ, 35585
Embolectomy, 34201
Exploration, 35703
Exposure, 34714, 34813 [34812]
Thrombectomy, 34201
Thromboendarterectomy, 35302, 35372
Great Vessel Repair, 33770
Harvest
Endoscopic for Bypass Graft, 33509
Open for Bypass Graft, 35600
Hepatic
Aneurysm, 35121-35122
Iliac
Aneurysm, 35132
Angioplasty, 37220
Atherectomy, 0238T
Bypass Graft, 35537, 35563-35565, 35632, 35638, 35663-35665
Embolectomy, 34151-34201
Endoprosthesis, [34718]
Exposure, [34820, 34833]
Occlusion Device, 34808
Revascularization, 37220
Thrombectomy, 34151-34201
Thromboendarterectomy, 35351, 35361-35363
Iliоceliac
Bypass Graft, 35632
Iliofemoral
Bypass Graft, 35565, 35665
Thromboendarterectomy, 35355, 35363
Iliomesenteric
Bypass Graft, 35633
Iliorenal
Bypass Graft, 35634
Innominate
Aneurysm, 35021-35022
Catheterization, 36223, 36225
Embolectomy, 34001, 34101
Stent Placement
Transcatheter, 37217-37218
Thrombectomy, 34001, 34101
Thromboendarterectomy, 35311
Intracranial
Anastomosis, 33606
Leg
Catheterization, 36245
Mesenteric
Aneurysm, 35121-35122
Bypass Graft, 35331, 35631
Embolectomy, 34151
Endoprosthesis, 34841
Thrombectomy, 34151
Thromboendarterectomy, 35341
Neck
Ligation, 37615
Pelvic
Catheterization, 36245
Peripheral Arterial Rehabilitation, 93668
Peroneal
Angioplasty, 37228
Atherectomy, 37229, 37231, 37233, 37235
Bypass Graft, 35566, 35571, 35666-35671
Bypass In Situ, 35585-35587
Embolectomy, 34203
Thrombectomy, 34203
Thromboendarterectomy, 35306
Popliteal
Aneurysm, 35151-35152
Angioplasty, 37224

Artery — *continued*
Popliteal — *continued*
Atherectomy, 37225, 37227
Bypass Graft, 35556, 35571, 35583, 35623, 35656, 35671, 35700
Bypass In Situ, 35583, 35587
Embolectomy, 34203
Exploration, 35703
Thrombectomy, 34203
Thromboendarterectomy, 35303
Pulmonary
Anastomosis, 33606
Angioplasty, 92998
Banding, 33620, 33622, 33690
Embolectomy, 33910, 33916
Endarterectomy, 33916
Ligation, 33924
Pressure Sensor Insertion, 33289
Repair, 33690, 33926
Arborization Anomalies, 33926
Atresia, 33920
Stenosis, 33917
Radial
Aneurysm, 35045
Embolectomy, 34111
Thrombectomy, 34111
Rehabilitation, 93668
Reimplantation
Carotid, 35691, 35694-35695
Subclavian, 35693
Vertebral, 35693
Visceral, 35697
Renal
Aneurysm, 35121-35122
Angiography, 36251
Angioplasty, [37246]
Atherectomy, 0234T
Bypass Graft, 35536, 35560, 35631, 35636
Catheterization, 36251
Embolectomy, 34151
Endoprosthesis, 34841
Thrombectomy, 34151
Thromboendarterectomy, 35341
Repair
Angioplasty
Radiological Supervision, 36902, 36905
Direct, 35201
with Other Graft, 35261
with Vein Graft, 35231
Revision
Hemodialysis Graft or Fistula
Open without Revision, 36831
Revision
with Thrombectomy, 36833
without Thrombectomy, 36832
Splenic
Aneurysm, 35111-35112
Angioplasty, [37247]
Bypass Graft, 35536, 35636
Stent Insertion
Dialysis Segment, 36903, 36906, 36908
Subclavian
Aneurysm, 35002, 35022
Angioplasty, [37247]
Bypass Graft, 35506, 35512, 35526, 35606, 35626, 35645
Catheterization, 36225
Embolectomy, 34001
Exposure, 34716
Reimplantation, 35693
Thrombectomy, 34001
Thromboendarterectomy, 35301, 35311
Transposition, 33889, 35693
Superficial Femoral
Thromboendarterectomy, 35302
Temporal
Biopsy, 37609
Ligation, 37609
Thoracic
Catheterization, 33621, 36215
Thrombectomy, 37184

Artery — *continued*
Thrombectomy — *continued*
Dialysis Circuit, 36904
Hemodialysis Graft or Fistula, 36831
Other Than Hemodialysis Graft or Fistula, 35875 [37247]
Thrombolysis (Noncoronary), 37211, 37214
Tibial
Angioplasty, 37228
Atherectomy, 37229, 37231, 37233, 37235
Bypass Graft, 35566, 35571, 35623, 35666-35671
Bypass In Situ, 35585-35587
Embolectomy, 34203
Thrombectomy, 34203
Thromboendarterectomy, 35306
Tibial-Tibial
Bypass Graft, 35570
Tibial/Peroneal Trunk-Tibial
Bypass Graft, 35570
Tibioperoneal
Angioplasty, 37228
Atherectomy, 37229, 37231, 37233, 37235
Tibioperoneal Trunk Thromboendarterectomy, 35304
Transcatheter Therapy, 75898
with Angiography, 75898
Transposition
Carotid, 33889, 35691, 35694-35695
Subclavian, 33889, 35693
Vertebral, 35691-35693
Ulnar
Aneurysm, 35045
Bypass Graft, 35523
Embolectomy, 34111
Thrombectomy, 34111
Vascular Study
Extremities, 93922-93923
Vertebral
Aneurysm, 35005
Bypass Graft, 35508, 35515, 35642-35645
Catheterization, 36100
Reimplantation, 35693
Thromboendarterectomy, 35301
Transposition, 35693
Visceral
Angioplasty, [37247]
Atherectomy, 0235T
Reimplantation, 35697
ASAT, 84450
Aspartate Aminotransferase, 84450
Aspiration
Bronchi
Endoscopy, 31629, 31633, 31645-31646, 31725
Bronchus
Nasotracheal, 31720
Catheter
Nasotracheal, 31720
Tracheobronchial, 31725
Laryngoscopy
Direct, 31515
Lung, 32555
Pericardium, 33016
Pleural Cavity, 32555
Trachea, 31612
Nasotracheal, 31720
Puncture, 31612
Tracheobronchial, 31646, 31725
Transbronchial, 31629
Assessment
Cardiorespiratory, Noninvasive, 0893T
Health Risk
Caregiver-Focused, 96161
Patient-Focused, 96160
Online/Telephone
Consult Physician, 99446 [99452]
Physician, [99421]
Virtual Check-in, [98016]
Assisted
Circulation, 33946, 33967, 33970, 33973, 33976, 33979, 33991 [33995, 33997]

Assistive Analysis
Cardiac Magnetic Resonance
Absolute Quantitation Myocardial Blood Flow (AQMBF) Estimate, 0900T
AST, 84450
Atherectomy
Aorta, 0236T
Brachiocephalic, 0237T
Coronary, [92925, 92933]
Femoral, 37225, 37227
Iliac, 0238T
Peroneal, 37229, 37231, 37233, 37235
Popliteal, 37225, 37227, 37233, 37235
Renal, 0234T
Tibial, 37229, 37231, 37233, 37235
Tibioperoneal, 37229, 37231, 37233, 37235
Transluminal
Abdominal Aorta, 0236T
Brachiocephalic Trunk and Branches, 0237T
Coronary, [92924]
Iliac, 0238T
Renal, 0234T
Visceral, 0235T
Visceral, 0235T
ATP Creatine Phosphotransferase, 82550-82552
Atresia
Pulmonary Artery, 33920
Tetralogy of Fallot, 33697
Tricuspid, 33615
Atria
Ablation, 33254, 33266
Baffle Procedure, 33774
Blalock-Hanlon Operation, 33735
Cor Triatriatum Repair, 33732
Cuff Preparation, 32856
Electrogram, 93616
Endoscopy
Surgical, 33266
Left Atrial Appendage
Closure
with Implant, 33340
Exclusion
Open, [33267, 33268]
Thoracoscopic, [33269]
Membrane Resection, 33732
Rashkind Procedure, 33741
Reconstruction, 33254, 33266
Septectomy, 33735, 33741
Septostomy, 33735, 33741
Surgical, 33266
Thrombus, 33310
Atrial Electrogram
Esophageal Recording, 93615-93616
Attendance and Resuscitation Services
Newborn, 99464
Audio-only Visit, [98008-98015]
Audio-video Visit, [98000-98007]
Augmentation
Pulmonary Valve Outflow, 33478
Augmentative Analysis
Arrhythmia, 0897T
Cardiac Magnetic Resonance
Absolute Quantitation Myocardial Blood Flow (AQMBF) Determination, 0899T
Computed Tomography
Angiography
Coronary Fractional Flow Reserve (FFR), 75580
Echocardiogram
Heart Failure with Preserved Ejection Fraction, 0932T
QTc Interval, 0902T
Automated
Quantification/Characterization
Coronary Atherosclerotic Plaque, [0623T]
AV Fistula (Arteriovenous Fistula)
Cannulization
Vein, 36815
Repair
Abdomen, 35182
Acquired or Traumatic, 35189

AV Fistula (Arteriovenous Fistula) — *continued*
Repair — *continued*
Head, 35180
Acquired or Traumatic, 35188
Lower Extremity, 35184
Acquired or Traumatic, 35190
Neck, 35180
Acquired or Traumatic, 35188
Thorax, 35182
Acquired or Traumatic, 35189
Upper Extremity, 35184
Acquired or Traumatic, 35190
Revision
Hemodialysis Graft or Fistula
with Thrombectomy, 36833
without Thrombectomy, 36832
Thrombectomy
Dialysis Graft
without Revision, 36831
AV Shunt (Arteriovenous Shunt)
Dialysis Circuit, 36902
AVF, 36815

B

Babcock's Operation, 37700
Balloon Assisted Device
Aorta, 33967
Balloon, Cardiac Catheter, Insertion, 33967
Banding
Artery
Fistula, 37607
Pulmonary, 33690
Application, 33620
Removal, 33622
Baroreflex Activation Device
Implantation/Replacement, 0266T
Interrogation Evaluation, 0273T
Revision/Removal, 0269T
Bentall Procedure, 33863
Bicuspid Valve
Incision, 33420-33422
Repair, 33420
Replacement, 33430
Bilobectomy, 32482, 32670
Bioimpedance
Cardiovascular Analysis, 93701
Extracellular Fluid, 93702
Bioprosthetic Valve Insertion
Femoral, 0744T
Biopsy
Artery, 37200
Temporal, 37609
Bronchi
Catheterization, 31717
Endoscopic, 31627, 31632-31633
Brush
Bronchi, 31717
Heart, 93505
Lung
Bronchoscopy, 31625, 31629, 31633
Needle, 32400-32408
Thoracoscopy, 32601, 32608
Thoracotomy, 32097
Transbronchial, 31629, 31633
Lymph Nodes
Mediastinum, 39010, 39402
Mediastinum, 39402
Needle, 32408
Neck, 21550
Needle
Fluoroscopic Guidance, 77002
Lung, 32400-32408
Mediastinum, 32408
Pleura, 32400
Transbronchial, 31629, 31633
Pericardial Sac, 32604
Pericardium, 39010
Pleura, 32098, 32400, 32609
Needle, 32400
Thoracoscopy, 32609
Thoracotomy, 32098
Thorax, 21550
Transcatheter, 37200
Vein, 37200
Birthing Room
Attendance at Delivery, 99464
Resuscitation, 99465
Blalock-Taussig Procedure, 33750
Bleeding Time, 85002
Blom-Singer Prosthesis, 31611
Blood Pressure
Baroactivation Device, 0266T
Central Arterial Analysis, Non-invasive, 93050
Monitoring, 24 hour, [93898]
Venous, 93770
Blood Vessel(s)
Angioscopy
Noncoronary, 35400
Exploration
Abdomen, 35840
Carotid Artery, 35701
Chest, 35820
Extremity, 35860
Femoral Artery, 35703
Neck, 35800
Popliteal Artery, 35703
Great
Suture, 33321
Harvest
Endoscopic, 33509
Open
Lower Extremity Vein, 35572
Upper Extremity Artery, 35600
Upper Extremity Vein, 35500
Repair
Abdomen, 35221, 35251, 35281
with Composite Graft, 35682
with Other Graft, 35281
with Vein Graft, 35251
Aorta, 33321
Chest, 35211-35216
with Composite Graft, 35682
with Other Graft, 35271-35276
with Vein Graft, 35241-35246
Direct, 35201
Finger, 35207
Graft Defect, 35870
Great Vessels, 33321
Hand, 35207
Intra-abdominal, 35221, 35251, 35281
Intrathoracic, 35211-35216, 35241-35246, 35271-35276
Lower Extremity, 35226, 35256, 35286
with Composite Graft, 35682
with Other Graft, 35281
with Vein Graft, 35256
Neck, 35201
with Composite Graft, 35682
with Other Graft, 35261
with Vein Graft, 35231
Upper Extremity, 35206, 35236, 35266
with Composite Graft, 35682
with Other Graft, 35266
with Vein Graft, 35236
Shunt Creation
Direct, 36821
Thomas Shunt, 36835
with Bypass Graft, 35686
with Graft, 36825-36830
with Transposition, 36818
Shunt Revision
with Graft, 36832
Suture Repair, Great Vessels, 33321
Blood
Bleeding Time, 85002
Cell
Exchange, 36511
Sedimentation Rate
Automated, 85652
Manual, 85651
Cell Count
Blood Smear, 85007-85008
Complete Blood Count (CBC), 85025-85027
Differential WBC Count, 85004, 85009
Hematocrit, 85014
Hemoglobin, 85018
Blood — *continued*
Cell Count — *continued*
Hemogram
Manual, 85032
Microhematocrit, 85013
Red Blood Cells, 85032
White Blood Cell, 85032
Clot
Dissolve
Coronary Vessel, [92975, 92977]
Inhibitors, 85337
Removal
Artery, 34001, 37184
Catheter, 36593
Dialysis Graft, 36831, 36833
External Cannula, 36861
Graft, Arterial or Venous, 35876
Pericardial Sac, 32658
Pericardiotomy, 33020
Vascular Access Device, 36593
Vein, 34001, 37188
Vena Cava, 34401
Coagulation Factor
Inhibition Test, 85337
Partial Thromboplastin Time, 85732
Gases
CO2, 82803
HCO3, 82803
Hemoglobin-Oxygen Affinity, 82820
O2, 82805
O2 Saturation, 82805-82810
pCO2, 82803
pH, 82800-82803
pO2, 82803, 82820
Nuclear Medicine
Flow Imaging, 78445
Plasma
Exchange, 36516
Platelet
Aggregation, 85576
Count, 85008
Manual Count, 85032
Pool Imaging, 78472-78483, 78494-78496
Smear
Microscopic Examination, 85008
Test(s)
Panels
Electrolyte, 80051
Lipid Panel, 80061
Transfusion, 36430-36440
Push
Infant, 36440
Boarding Home Care, [99425, 99437, 99491]
BOH, 93600
Bone
Insertion
Needle, 36680
Brachial Plexus
Injection
Anesthetic or Steroid, 64415-64416
Brain
Angiography, 36100
Doppler Transcranial, [93896]
Breast
Excision
Tumors, 21601
Tumor
Excision
Chest Wall, 21601
with Ribs, 21601
Brock Operation, 33474
Bronchi
Allograft, 32856
Aspiration
Catheter, 31725
Endoscopic, 31629, 31633, 31646
Biopsy
Endoscopic, 31627, 31632-31633
Brushing
Protected Brushing, 31623
Catheterization
Insertion
with Intracavitary Radioelement, 31643
with Bronchial Brush Biopsy, 31717
Bronchi — *continued*
Endoscopy
Aspiration, 31645-31646
Biopsy, 31625, 31628-31629, 31632-31633
Destruction
Lesion, 31641
Tumor, 31641
Dilation, 31631, 31636
Excision
Lesion, 31640
Exploration, 31622
with Balloon Occlusion, 31634
Foreign Body Removal, 31635
Fracture, 31630
Lesion, 31640-31641
Stenosis, 31641
Tumor, 31640-31641
Exploration, 31622
Fracture
Endoscopy, 31630
Needle Biopsy, 31629, 31633
Reconstruction
Anastomosis, 31775, 32486
Graft Repair, 31770
Stenosis, 31775
Removal
Foreign Body, 31635
Repair
Fistula, 32815, 32906
Stenosis, 31641
Stenosis
Endoscopic Treatment, 31641
Stent
Placement, 31637
Revision, 31638
Testing
Bronchospasm Evaluation, 94617 [94619]
Pulmonary Stress Test, 94618
Tumor
Excision, 31640
Bronchial Alveolar Lavage, 31624
Bronchial Brush Biopsy
with Catheterization, 31717
Bronchial Brushings
Protected Brushing, 31623
Broncho-Bronchial Anastomosis, 32486
Bronchoalveolar Lavage, 31624
Bronchoplasty, 32501
Excision Stenosis and Anastomosis, 31775
Graft Repair, 31770
Reconstruction, Bronchi, 32501
Graft Repair, 31770
Stenosis, 31775
Bronchopulmonary Lavage, 31624
Bronchoscopy
Alveolar Lavage, 31624
Aspiration, 31629, 31633, 31646, 31725
Balloon Occlusion, 31634
Biopsy, 31627, 31632-31633
Brushing, Protected Brushing, 31623
Catheter Placement
Intracavity Radioelement, 31643
Computer-Assisted Image-Guided Navigation, 31627
Destruction
Lesion, 31641
Tumor, 31614
Diagnostic, 31623, 31643
Dilation, 31631, 31636
Exploration, 31622
Fiducial Marker Placement, 31626
Foreign Body Removal, 31635
Fracture, 31630
Needle Biopsy, 31629, 31633
Removal
Foreign Body, 31635
Tumor, 31640-31641
Stenosis, 31641
Stent Placement, 31631, 31637
Stent Revision, 31638
Tumor
Destruction, 31641
Excision, 31640
via Existing Tracheostomy, 31615

Bronchospasm Evaluation
- Exercise Test, 94617 [94619]

Brush Biopsy
- Bronchi, 31717

Bulla
- Lung
  - Excision–Plication, 32141
    - Endoscopic, 32655

Button
- Voice Prosthesis, 31611

Bypass Graft
- Aortobi-iliac, 35538, 35638
- Aortobifemoral, 35540, 35646
- Aortocarotid, 35526, 35626
- Aortoceliac, 35531, 35631
- Aortofemoral, 35539, 35647
- Aortoiliac, 35537, 35637
- Aortoinnominate, 35526, 35626
- Aortomesenteric, 35531, 35631
- Aortorenal, 35560, 35631
- Aortosubclavian, 35526, 35626
- Axillary Artery, 35522, 35533, 35623, 35650-35654
- Brachial Artery, 35510, 35512, 35523
- Brachial-Ulnar or -Radial, 35523
- Carotid Artery, 33891, 35510, 35601-35606, 35642
- Celiac Artery, 35341, 35632
- Coronary Artery
  - Arterial, 33533
  - Arterial-Venous, 33517, 33521, 33530
  - Venous Graft, 33510
- Excision
  - Abdomen, 35907
  - Extremity, 35903
  - Neck, 35901
  - Thorax, 35905
- Femoral Artery, 35521, 35533, 35539-35558, 35566, 35621, 35646-35647, 35654, 35666, 35700
- Harvest
  - Endoscopic
    - Artery, 33509
    - Vein, 33508
  - Open
    - Lower Extremity Vein, 35572
    - Upper Extremity Artery, 35600
    - Upper Extremity Vein, 35500
- Hepatorenal, 35535
- Iliac Artery, 35537-35538, 35563, 35637-35638, 35663
- Ilio-Celiac, 35632
- Ilio-Mesenteric, 35633
- Iliofemoral, 35565, 35665
- Ilioiliac, 35563, 35663
- Iliorenal, 35634
- Mesenteric Artery, 35531, 35631
- Peroneal Artery, 35566-35570, 35585-35587, 35666-35671
- Peroneal-Tibial Vein, 35570
- Placement
  - Vein Patch, 35685
- Popliteal Artery, 35556, 35571, 35583, 35623, 35656, 35671, 35700
- Renal Artery, 35536, 35560, 35631, 35636
- Reoperation, 35700
- Repair
  - Abdomen, 35907
  - Extremity, 35903
    - Lower Extremity
      - with Composite Graft, 35682
  - Neck, 35901
  - Thorax, 35905
- Revascularization
  - Extremity, 35903
  - Neck, 35901
  - Thorax, 35905
- Revision
  - Lower Extremity
    - Femoral Artery, 35884
    - with Angioplasty, 35879
    - with Vein Interposition, 35881
- Secondary Repair, 35870
- Splenic Artery, 35536, 35636

Bypass Graft — *continued*
- Subclavian Artery, 35506, 35512, 35526, 35606, 35626, 35645, 35694
- Thrombectomy, 35875-35876, 37184
  - Other Than Hemodialysis Graft or Fistula, 35876
- Tibial Artery, 35566, 35571, 35623, 35666-35671
- Tibial-Tibial Vein, 35570
- Vertebral Artery, 35508, 35515, 35642-35645
- with Composite Graft, 35682
  - Autogenous
    - Three or More Segments
      - Two Locations, 35683
    - Two Segments
      - Two Locations, 35682

Bypass In Situ
- Femoral Artery, 35585
- Peroneal Artery, 35585-35587
- Popliteal Artery, 35583, 35587
- Tibial Artery, 35585-35587
- Ventricular Restoration, 33548

Bypass
- Cardiopulmonary, 33510

C

CABG, 33505, 33510

Cannulation
- Arterial, 36620-36625
- Arteriovenous, 36810-36815
- Vein to Vein, 36800

Cannulization
- Arteriovenous (AV), 36810-36815, 36901
- Declotting, 36593, 36860-36861
- Dialysis Circuit, 36901
- ECMO
  - Insertion, 33951
  - Removal, [33965]
  - Repositioning, 33957
- External
  - Declotting, 36861
- Vein to Vein, 36800

Carbon Dioxide
- Blood or Urine, 82803

Cardiac Acoustic Waveform Recording, 0716T

Cardiac Catheterization
- Angiography
  - Bypass Graft(s), 93455, 93457, 93459, 93461
  - Congenital Heart, 93564
  - Coronary, 93563, 93571
  - Left Atrium, 93565
  - Left Ventricle, 93565
  - Pulmonary, 93569 [93573]
  - Right Atrium, 93566
  - Right Ventricle, 93566
- Combined Left and Right Heart, 93453, 93461
  - for Congenital Anomalies, 93597
  - with Ventriculography, 93453, 93461
- Flow Directed, 93503
- Flow Measurement, 93572
- for Biopsy, 93505
- for Congenital Anomalies
  - Left, 93595
  - Right, 93593
  - Right and Left, 93597
- for Dilution Studies, 93598
- for Measurement of O2 Cardiac Output, 93451
- for Opacification
  - Bypass Grafts, 93564
- for Stent Placement, 33621
- for Supravalvular Aortography, 93567
- Imaging, 93569 [93573]
- Injection, 93569 [93573]
- Insertion Swan-Ganz, 93503
- Left Heart
  - By Transseptal Puncture, 93462
  - for Congenital Anomalies, 93595
  - for Transapical Puncture, 93462
  - with Ventriculography, 93452, 93565
- Pacemaker, 33210
- Right Heart, 36013, 93451, 93457
  - for Congenital Anomalies, 93593

Cardiac Contractility Modulation System, 0408T, 0915T

Cardiac Event Recorder (wearable), [93247]

Cardiac Magnetic Resonance Imaging (CMRI)
- Absolute Quantitation Myocardial Blood Flow (AQMBF)
  - Assistive Analysis, 0900T
  - Augmentative Analysis, 0899T
- Morphology and Function, 75557-75563
- Stress Imaging, 75559, 75563
- Velocity Flow Mapping, 75565
- without Contrast, 75557

Cardiac Massage
- Thoracotomy, 32160

Cardiac Output Measurement
- by Indicator Dilution, 93598

Cardiac Rehabilitation, 93797-93798

Cardiac Rhythm Monitor System
- Analysis, 93285, 93291, 93298, 0650T
- Implantation, 33285
- Programming Device Evaluation, 0650T
- Removal, 33286

Cardiectomy
- Donor, 33930, 33940

Cardio Defibrillator (Implantable)
- Transvenous Device
  - Insertion
    - Electrode, 33217
    - Pulse Generator, 33240 [33231]
    - System, 33249
  - Interrogation Device Evaluation, 93289
    - Periprocedural, 93287
    - Remote, 93296
  - Relocation
    - Skin Pocket, 33223
  - Removal
    - Electrode, 33244
    - Pulse Generator, 33241 [33262]
  - Repair Electrode, 33218-33220
  - Reposition Electrode, 33215, 33226
- Wearable, 93745
  - Data Analysis, 93292

Cardioassist, 92970-92971

Cardiolipin Antibody, 86147

Cardiology
- Diagnostic
  - Atrial Electrogram
    - Esophageal Recording, 93615-93616
  - Bioimpedance Analysis, 93701
  - Cardiac Rhythm Monitor System
    - Data Analysis, 93291, 93298
    - Evaluation and Programming, 93285, 0650T
  - Electrophysiologic
    - Follow-up Study, 93624
    - with Myocardial Contrast Perfusion, 0439T
  - Endoluminal Imaging, [92979]
  - Ergonovine Provocation Test, 93024
  - Evaluation
    - Heart Device, 93640
  - Heart
    - Stimulation and Pacing, 93623
  - Implantable Defibrillator
    - Data Analysis, 93289, 93296
    - Evaluation of Programming, 93287, 93289, 93292, 93296, 93641
  - Implantable Monitor
    - Data Analysis, 93290, 93298
  - Intracardiac Pacing and Mapping, 93631
    - 3D Mapping, 93613, 93654
    - Follow-up Study, 93624
    - Stimulation and Pacing, 93623
  - Intracardiac Pacing and Recording
    - Arrhythmia Induction, 93618, 93624, 93641, 93653
    - Bundle of His, 93600, 93619, 93654, 93656
    - Intra–atrial, 93602, 93610, 93616, 93656
    - Left Ventricle, 93654

Cardiology — *continued*
- Diagnostic — *continued*
  - Intracardiac Pacing and Recording — *continued*
    - Right Ventricle, 93603, 93653, 93656
    - Tachycardia Sites, 93609
    - Ventricular, 93612
  - M Mode and Real Time, [93319]
  - Pacemaker Testing, 93642
    - Antitachycardia System, 93724
    - Data Analysis, 93288, 93293
    - Dual Chamber, 93280, 93288, 93293
    - Evaluation of Device Programming, 93279, 93286, 93288, 93290, 93293, 93296
    - Leads, 93641
    - Single Chamber, 93279, 93288, 93294
  - Perfusion Imaging, 78451 [78430]
  - Strain Imaging, [93356]
  - Stress Tests
    - Drug Induced, 93024
    - MUGA (Multiple Gated Acquisition), 78483
  - Temperature Gradient Studies, 93740
  - Tilt Table Evaluation, 93660
  - Venous Pressure Determination, 93784-93790
- Therapeutic
  - Ablation, 93650-93653
  - Cardioassist, 92970-92971
  - Cardiopulmonary Resuscitation, 92950
  - Cardioversion, 92960-92961
  - Endoluminal Imaging, [92979]
  - Implantable Defibrillator
    - Data Analysis, 93289, 93296
    - Evaluation of Device Programming, 93287, 93289, 93292, 93296
    - Initial Set-up and Programming, 93745
  - Pacing
    - Transcutaneous, Temporary, 92953
  - Rehabilitation, 93668, 93798
  - Thrombolysis
    - Coronary Vessel, [92977]
  - Thrombolysis, Coronary, [92977]
  - Valvuloplasty
    - Open, 33391
    - Percutaneous, 92986, 92990

Cardiopulmonary Bypass
- Aortic Valve Replacement, Transcatheter, 33367
- Lung Transplant with
  - Double, 32854
  - Single, 32852
- with Prosthetic Valve Repair, 33496

Cardiopulmonary Exercise Testing, 94621

Cardiopulmonary Resuscitation, 92950

Cardiotomy, 33310-33315

Cardiovascular Physiologic Monitor System
- Analysis, 93290, 93298

Cardioversion, 92960-92961

Care Management Services
- Advanced Care Planning, 99498
- Chronic Care Management, [99437, 99439, 99490, 99491]
  - Complex, 99487-99489
- Principal Care Management, [99424]
- Transitional Care, 99496

Care Plan Oversight Services
- Home Health Agency Care, 99374
- Home, Domiciliary, or Rest Home, [99425, 99437, 99491]
- Hospice, 99378
- Nursing Facility, 99380

Caregiver
- Focused Assessment, 96161

Carotid Artery
- Baroreflex Activation Device
  - Implantation/Replantation, 0266T

Carotid Artery — *continued*
Baroreflex Activation Device — *continued*
Interrogation Evaluation, 0273T
Revision/Removal, 0269T
Excision, 60605
Ligation, 37600
Stent, Transcatheter Placement, 37218
Carotid Body
Lesion
Carotid Artery, 60605
Excision, 60600
Carotid Sinus Baroreflex Activation Device
Implantation, 0266T
Interrogation Device Evaluation, 0272T-0273T
Removal, 0269T
Replacement, 0266T
Case Management Services
Team Conferences, 99366
Catheter
Aspiration
Nasotracheal, 31720
Tracheobronchial, 31725
Biopsy, Transcatheter, 37200
Blood Specimen Collection, 36592
Bronchus for Intracavitary Radioelement Application, 31643
Central Venous
Repair, 36575
Replacement, 36580-36581, 36584
Repositioning, 36597
Declotting, 36593, 36861
Drainage
Pleural, 32557
Embolectomy, 34001-34051, 34111-34203
Endovenous Ablation, 0524T
Flow Directed, 93503
Infusion
Brachial Plexus, 64416
Installation
Fibrinolysis, 32562
Pleurodesis, 32560
Intracatheter
Obstruction Clearance, 36596
Pericatheter
Obstruction Clearance, 36595
Placement
Bronchus
for Intracavitary Radioelement Placement, 31643
Stent, 33621
Wireless Physiologic Sensor, 34701
Removal
Central Venous, 36589
Foreign Body, 37197
Obstruction, 36596
Pleural Catheter, 32552
Repair
Central Venous, 36575
Replacement
Central Venous, 36581, 36584
Repositioning, 36597
Thrombectomy, 34001-34051, 34111-34451
Transcatheter Therapy, 36640-36660, 37211
Catheterization
Abdominal Artery, 36245
Aorta, 36160
Arterial
Aorta, 36200, 36221
Translumbar, 36160
Arteriovenous Shunt
Dialysis Circuit, 36901
Cutdown, 36625
Intracatheter/Needle, 36140
Percutaneous, 36620
Selective Placement, 36215, 36222
Superselective Placement, 36254
Arteriovenous Shunt
Dialysis Circuit, 36901
Brachiocephalic Artery, 36215
Bronchus
for Intracavitary Radioelement Application, 31643
with Bronchial Brush Biopsy, 31717

Catheterization — *continued*
Cardiac
Combined Left and Right Heart, 93453, 93461
for Congenital Anomalies, 93597
with Ventriculography, 93453, 93461
Flow Directed, 93503
Flow Measurement, 93572
for Angiography
Bypass Graft(s), 93455, 93457, 93459
Congenital Heart, 93564
Coronary, 93563
Left Atrial, 93565
Left Ventricular, 93565
Pulmonary, 93569 [93573]
Right Atrial, 93566
Right Ventricular, 93566
for Biopsy, 93505
for Congenital Anomalies
Left, 93595
Right, 93593
Right and Left, 93597
for Dilution Studies, 93598
for Measurement O2, Cardiac Output, 93451
for Opacification
Bypass Graft, 93564
for Stent Placement, 33621
for Supravalvular Aortography, 93567
Imaging, 93569 [93573]
Injection, 93569 [93573]
Insertion Swan-Ganz, 93503
Left Heart
by Transapical Puncture, 93462
by Transseptal Puncture through Intact Septum, 93462
for Congenital Anomalies, 93595
with Ventriculography, 93452, 93565
Pacemaker, 33210
Right Heart, 36013, 93451, 93457
for Congenital Anomalies, 93593
Carotid Artery, 36100, 36221, 36228
Central, 36555, 36561-36563, 36566, 36578-36580
Cerebral Artery, 36215
Dialysis Circuit, 36901
Extremity Artery, 36140
Innominate Artery, 36223, 36225
Interstitial Radioelement Application
Lung, 31643
Legs, 36245
Nasotracheal, 31720
Nasotracheobronchi, 31720
Newborn
Umbilical Vein, 36510
Pelvic Artery, 36245
Peripheral, 36584 [36572]
Placement
Arterial Coronary Conduit without Left Heart Catheterization, 93455
Coronary Artery without Left Heart Catheterization, 93455
Venous Coronary Bypass Graft without Left Heart Catheterization, 93455
Pleural Cavity, 32552
Portal Vein, 36481
Pulmonary Artery, 36013
Removal
Obstructive Material
Intracatheter, 36596
Pericatheter, 36595
Renal Artery, 36251
Subclavian Artery, 36225
Thoracic Artery, 36215
Tracheobronchi, 31725
Umbilical Artery, 36660
Umbilical Vein, 36510
Vena Cava, 36010
Venous
Central–Line, 36555, 36561-36563, 36566, 36578-36580
First Order, 36011

Catheterization — *continued*
Venous — *continued*
Intracatheter, 36000
Needle, 36000
Organ Blood, 36500
Peripheral, 36569, 36571, 36585 [36573]
Second Order, 36012
Umbilical Vein, 36510
Vertebral Artery, 36100, 36221, 36226, 36228
Wireless Pressure Sensor
Left Atrial, 0933T
Pulmonary, 33289
Caval Valve Implantation (CAVI), 0806T
CAVB, 93650
CAVI (Caval Valve Implantation), 0806T
Cell
Count
Bacterial Colony, 87086
Central Shunt, 33764
Central Sleep Apnea
Neurostimulator System, [33276]
Central Venous Catheter (CVC)
Insertion
Central, 36555, 36561-36563, 36566, 36578-36580
Non-tunneled, 36556
Peripheral, 36569, 36585 [36573]
with Port, 36571
Tunneled
with Port, 36561, 36566
with Pump, 36563
without Port or Pump, 36558, 36565
Removal, 36589
Repair, 36576
Replacement, 36580, 36584
Catheter Only, 36578
Repositioning, 36597
Central Venous Catheter Removal, 36589
Cerebral Vessel(s)
Thrombolysis, 37195
Chemical
Ablation, Endovenous, 0524T
Chemistry Tests
Organ or Disease Oriented Panel
Electrolyte, 80051
Lipid Panel, 80061
Chemotherapy or Highly Complex Agent/Drug
Arterial Catheterization, 36640
Intra–arterial
Catheterization, 36640
Infusion Pump Insertion, 36260
Pump Services
Intra–arterial
Insertion, 36260
Removal/Revision, 36262
Chest Wall
Reconstruction, 49904
Lung Tumor Resection, 32504
Trauma, 32820
Repair, 32905
Closure, 32810
Fistula, 32906
Lung Hernia, 32800
Resection, 32503
Tumor
Ablation, 32998 [32994]
Excision, 21601
Chest
Artery
Ligation, 37616
Cavity
Bypass Graft, 35905
Thoracoscopy
Exploration, 32601
Surgical, 32650
Therapeutic, 32654
Diagnostic Imaging
Ultrasound, 76604
Exploration
Blood Vessel, 35820
Penetrating Wound, 20101
Postoperative
Hemorrhage, 35820

Chest — *continued*
Exploration — *continued*
Postoperative — *continued*
Infection, 35820
Thrombosis, 35820
Funnel
Reconstructive Repair, 21742
with Thoracoscopy, 21743
Repair
Blood Vessel, 35211-35216
with Other Graft, 35271-35276
with Vein Graft, 35241-35246
Tube, 32551
Ultrasound, 76604
Wound Exploration
Penetrating, 20101
X-ray, 71047
Complete (four views) with Fluoroscopy, 71048
Partial (two views) with Fluoroscopy, 71046
Stereo, 71045
Chloride
Panels
Electrolyte, 80051
Cholesterol
Lipid Panel, 80061
Measurement
HDL, 83718
VLDL, 83719
Serum, 82465
Chromatography
Hemoglobin, 83036
Cimino Type Procedure, 36821
Circulation Assist
Aortic, 33967, 33970
Balloon Counterpulsation, 33967, 33970
Removal, 33971
Cardioassist Method
External, 92971
Internal, 92970
External, 33946
CK, 82550
Total, 82550
Clagett Procedure
Chest Wall, Repair, Closure, 32810
Closure
Atrial Appendage
with Implant, 33340
Atrial Septal Defect, 33641, 33647
Atrioventricular Valve, 33600
Cardiac Valve, 33600-33602
Fistula
Bronchi, 32815
Chest Wall, 32906
Patent Ductus Arteriosus, 93582
Semilunar Valve, 33602
Septal Defect, 33615
Ventricular, 33675, 33681, 93581
Sternotomy, 21750
Ventricular Septal Defect, 33675, 33681, 93581
Clot
Assay, 85396
Dissolve
Coronary Vessel, [92975, 92977]
Inhibitors, 85337
Removal
Artery, 34001, 37184
Catheter, 36593
Dialysis Graft, 36831, 36833
External Cannula, 36861
Graft, Arterial or Venous, 35876
Pericardial Sac, 32658
Pericardiotomy, 33020
Vascular Access Device, 36593
Vein, 34001, 37188
Vena Cava, 34001
Clotting
Factor
Inhibition Test, 85337
Partial Thromboplastin Time, 85732
Inhibitors, 85337
Test
Factor Inhibitor, 85337
Mixed Screen, 85611, 85732

Clotting — *continued*
Test — *continued*
Thrombomodulin, 85337
CMRI (Cardiac Magnetic Resonance Imaging)
Absolute Quantitation Myocardial Blood Flow (AQMBF)
Assistive Analysis, 0900T
Augmentative Analysis, 0899T
Stress Imaging, 75559, 75563
Velocity Flow Mapping, 75565
without Contrast, 75557
Coagulation
Factor III, 85730-85732
Coccidioidin Test
Streptokinase, Antibody, 86590
Collection and Processing
Radiological Guidance, 75989
Specimen
Capillary, 36416
Ear, 36416
Implantable Venous Access Device, 36591
Vein, 36415
Venous Access Device, 36591
Venous Blood, 36415, 36592
Venous Catheter, 36592
Washings
Bronchial, 31622
Commissurotomy
Right Ventricular, 33476, 33478
Complex Chronic Care Management Services, 99487-99489 [99437, 99439, 99490, 99491]
Composite Graft
Vein, 35682
Autogenous
Three or More Segments
Two Locations, 35683
Two Segments
Two Locations, 35682
Computed Tomographic Angiography
Heart, 75574
Computed Tomography (CT Scan)
Drainage, 75898
Heart, 75571
with Contrast
Cardiac Structure and Morphology, 75573
Heart, 75572
without Contrast
Heart, 75571
Computer
Analysis
Electrocardiographic Data, 93228
Assisted Navigation
Orthopedic Surgery, 20985
Conference
Medical
with Interdisciplinary Team, 99366
Congenital Heart Anomaly
Catheterization
Injection, 93564
Left Heart, 93595
Right and Left Heart, 93597
Right Heart, 93593
Closure
Interatrial Communication, 93580
Ventricular Septal Defect, 93581
Echocardiography
3D Imaging During Procedure, [93319]
Congenital Anomalies
Transesophageal, 93315
Transthoracic, 93304
Guidance for Intracardiac or Great Vessel Intervention, 93355
Treatment Ventricular Ectopy, 93654
Venography
Azygos/hemiazygos, [93585]
Coronary sinus, [93586]
Superior vena cava, [93584]
Venovenous collaterals, [93587]
Construction
Apical-Aortic Conduit, 33404
Arterial
Conduit, 33608, 33920
Construction — *continued*
Arterial — *continued*
Tunnel, 33505
Tracheoesophageal Fistula, 31611
Consultation
Inpatient/Observation, 99252
Interprofessional Online/Telephone, 99446 [99452]
Office/Outpatient, 99242
Contrast Material
Injection
Arteriovenous Dialysis Shunt
Dialysis Circuit, 36901
Central Venous Access Device, 36598
Peritoneal
Evaluation Venous Shunt, 49427
Renal Angiography, 36251
Coronary Artery
Angioplasty
with Atherectomy, [92934, 92938, 92941, 92943]
with Placement Stent, [92928, 92934, 92938, 92941, 92943]
Atherectomy, [92925]
Bypass Graft (CABG), 33505, 33510
Arterial, 33533
Arterial–Venous, 33517
Harvest
Upper Extremity Artery, 35600
Upper Extremity Vein, 35500
Reoperation, 33530
Venous, 33510
Ligation, 33502
Placement
Radiation Delivery Device, [92974]
Reconstruction, 33864
Repair, 33507
Revascularization, [92938, 92941, 92943]
Thrombectomy, [92973]
Thrombolysis, [92975, 92977]
Translocation, 33507
Unroofing, 33507
Ventricular Restoration, 33548
Coronary Atherosclerotic Plaque
Automated Quantification/Characterization, [0623T, 0624T, 0625T, 0626T]
Coronary Endarterectomy, 33572
Coronary Fractional Flow Reserve
Noninvasive, 75580 [0523T]
Coronary Lithotripsy
Transluminal, [92972]
Coronary Sinus Reduction Device, 0645T
Coronary
Thrombectomy
Percutaneous, [92973]
Costotransversectomy, 21610
COTD (Cardiac Output Thermodilution), 93598
Counseling and /or Risk Factor Reduction Intervention – Preventive Medicine, Individual Counseling
Behavior Change Interventions, 99406
Caregiver-focused, 96161
Patient-focused, 96160
Preventive Medicine, 99412
Counseling, Preventive
Group, 99411-99412
Individual, 99401
Counseling
Smoking and Tobacco Use Cessation, 99407
CPB, 32852, 32854, 33496, 33505, 33510, 33533
CPK
Isoenzymes, 82552
Isoforms, 82554
MB Fraction Only, 82553
Total, 82550
CPR (Cardiopulmonary Resuscitation), 92950
Creatine Kinase (Total), 82550
Creatine Phosphokinase
Blood, 82552
Total, 82550
Creatine, 82554
Creation
Arteriovenous
Fistula, 35686, 36825-36830
Percutaneous, [36837]
Catheter Exit Site, 49436
Creation — *continued*
Cavopulmonary Anastomosis, 33622
Complete Heart Block, 93650
Iliac Artery Conduit, [34833]
Pericardial Window, 32659, 33025
Shunt
Intracardiac, Transcatheter, 33745-33746
Speech Prosthesis, 31611
Cricothyroid Membrane
Incision, 31605
CRIT, 85013
Critical Care Services
Cardiopulmonary Resuscitation, 92950
Evaluation and Management, 99292, 99468
Neonatal
Initial, 99468
Subsequent, 99469
Pediatric
Initial, 99471, 99475
Subsequent, 99472, 99476
Cryofixation
for Transplantation, 32850, 33930, 33940
Cryopreservation
for Transplantation, 32850, 33930, 33940
Cryosurgery
Tumor
Lung, [32994]
Cryotherapy
Ablation
Lung Tumor, [32994]
Destruction
Bronchial Tumor, 31641
CT Scan
Angiography
Heart, 75574
Drainage, 75989
Heart
Evaluation
Angiography, 75574
Coronary Calcium, 75571
Structure and Morphology, 75573
Optical Coherence Tomography
Endoluminal, [92978, 92979]
CVAD (Central Venous Access Device)
Insertion
Central, 36555, 36561-36563, 36566, 36578-36580
Peripheral, 36569, 36571, 36585 [36573]
Removal, 36589
Repair, 36575
Replacement, 36580
Repositioning, 36597
CXR, 71047
Cyst
Excision
Mediastinum, 32662
Pericardial, 32661
Resection, 33050
Lung
Incision and Drainage, 32200
Removal, 32140
Mediastinal
Excision, 32662
Resection, 39200
Pericardial
Excision, 33050
Cytomegalovirus
Antigen Detection
Direct Fluorescence, 87271

D

Damus–Kaye–Stansel Procedure, 33606
David Procedure, 33864
Debridement
Sternum, 21627
Debulking Procedure
Intracardiac Mass, 0644T
Declotting
Artery, 34001, 37184
Catheter, 36593
Dialysis Graft, 36831, 36833
External Cannula, 36861
Graft, Arterial or Venous, 35876
Declotting — *continued*
Pericardial Sac, 32658
Pericardiotomy, 33020
Vascular Access Device, 36593
Vein, 34001, 37188
Vena Cava, 34401
Decompression
Trachea, 33800
Decortication
Lung, 32220-32225, 32320, 32652
Endoscopic, 32651-32652
Partial, 32225
Total, 32220
with Parietal Pleurectomy, 32320
Defibrillator/Defibrillator Pacemaker
Implantable
Data Analysis, 93289, 93296 [93260]
Evaluation, 93283, 93287, 93289, 93292, 93296, 93641 [33270, 93260]
Insertion, 33240 [33231, 33270]
Electrodes, 33217, 33224 [33271]
Interrogation, 93289, 93296 [93261]
Programming, 93287 [33270]
Removal, 33233, 33241 [33262]
Electrode, 33244 [33272]
Repair
Leads, Dual Chamber, 33220
Leads, Single Chamber, 33218
Replacement, 33249 [33262, 33264]
Repositioning
Electrodes, 33215, 33226 [33273]
Revise Pocket Chest, 33223
Wearable Device, 93292, 93745
Delorme Operation, 33031
Denervation
Sympathetic
Transcatheter Percutaneous, 0339T
Destruction
Arrhythmogenic Focus
Heart, 33250-33251, 33261
Device
Cerebral Embolic Protection, 33370
Coronary Sinus Reduction Device, 0645T
Drug Delivery
Transcatheter
Therapeutic, 0914T
Iliac Artery Occlusion Device
Insertion, 34808
Programming, 93644 [93260, 93261]
Venous Access
Collection of Blood Specimen, 36592
Implanted, 36591
Venous Catheter, 36592
Fluoroscopic Guidance, 77001
Insertion
Catheter, 36578
Central, 36560
Obstruction Clearance, 36595-36596
Peripheral, 36570-36571
Removal, 36590
Repair, 36576
Replacement, 36582-36583, 36585
Obstruction Clearance, 36596
Removal, 36590
Repair, 36576
Replacement, 36583, 36585
Catheter, 36578
Ventricular Assist, 33983 [33995, 33997]
Ventricular Restoration, [0643T]
Dialysis
Arteriovenous Fistula
Revision
without Thrombectomy, 36832
Thrombectomy, 36831
Arteriovenous Shunt, 36901
Revision
with Thrombectomy, 36833
Thrombectomy, 36831
Dialysis Circuit, 36901
Hemodialysis
Fistula
Duplex Scan, 0876T

Diaphragmatic Stimulation System
Evaluation/Interrogation, 0685T
Insertion or Replacement, 0674T
Pulse Generator Only, 0680T
Programming, 0683T
Removal, 0679T
Pulse Generator Only, 0682T
Repositioning, 0678T
Pulse Generator Only, 0681T
Differential Count
White Blood Cell Count, 85007, 85009
Digoxin
Assay, 80163
Blood or Urine, 80162
Dilation
Aortic Valve, 33391
Bronchi
Endoscopy, 31630, 31636
Larynx
Endoscopy, 31528-31529
Trachea
Endoscopic, 31630-31631, 31636
Discectomy
Lumbar, [0614T]
Discharge Services
Inpatient or Observation, 99239
Same Date Admit/Discharge, 99234
Dissection
Donor Organs
Heart, 33944
Heart/Lung, 33933
Lung, 32855
Infrarenal Aneurysm, 34830 [34718]
Mediastinal, 60522
Neurovascular, 32503
Division
Muscle
Neck
Scalenus Anticus, 21700-21705
Saphenous Vein, 37700-37735
Donor Procedures
Heart Excision, 33940
Heart–Lung Excision, 33930
Lung, 32850
Doppler Echocardiography, 93320
3D Imaging During Procedure for Congenital Anomalies, [93319]
Hemodialysis
Access, 93990
Prior to Access Creation, 93985
Fistula, 0876T
Intracardiac, 93662
Strain Imaging, [93356]
Transesophageal, 93318
Transthoracic, 93306
with Myocardial Contrast Perfusion, 0439T
Doppler Scan
Arterial Studies
Coronary Flow Reserve, 93572
Extracranial, 93882
Extremities, 93922
Intracranial, [93896]
Dor Procedure, 33548
Drainage
Abscess
Contrast Injection
with X-ray, 75989
Lung
Bronchoscopy, 31646
Open, 32200
Lymph Node, 38300-38305
Neck
Incision and Drainage, 21501-21502
Thoracostomy, 32551
Thorax
Incision and Drainage, 21501-21502
X-ray, 75989
Cyst
Lung, 32200
Empyema, 32036, 32810
Lymph Node, 38305
Mediastinum, 39010
Pericardial Sac, 32659
Pericardium, 33025
Drainage — *continued*
Pleura, 32557
Radiologic Guidance, 75989
Sinus Venosus, 33645
Via Tube Thoracostomy, 32551
Drug Assay
Digoxin, 80163
Drug Screen, 99409
Drug
Administration For
Cardiac Assessments, 93463
Infusion
Intravenous, 96365
Infusion, 96365
Ductus Arteriosus
Repair, 33820
Transcatheter Percutaneous Closure, 93582
Duplex Scan
Arterial Studies
Aorta, 93978-93979
Extracranial, 93880-93882
Lower Extremity, 93925-93926
Penile, 93980-93981
Upper Extremity, 93930-93931
Visceral, 93975
Hemodialysis
Access, 93990
Prior to Access Creation, 93985
Fistula, 0876T
Venous Studies
Extremity, 93970-93971
Penile, 93980-93981

E

Ear
Collection of Blood From, 36416
Ebstein Anomaly Repair, 33468
ECHO, 93306, 93314-93315, 93350 [93319, 93356]
Echocardiography
Augmentative Analysis
Heart Failure with Preserved Ejection Fraction, 0932T
Cardiac, 93320
Intracardiac, 93662
Strain Imaging, [93356]
Transesophageal, 93318
Transthoracic, 93306
with Myocardial Contrast Perfusion, 0439T
with Stress Test, [93356]
Doppler, 93350, 93662 [93319]
for Assessment of Myocardial Ischemia/Viability, 0439T
for Congenital Anomalies
3D Imaging During Procedure, [93319]
Transesophageal, 93315
Transthoracic, 93303-93304
Intracardiac, 93662
Intraoperative, 76987
M Mode and Real Time, 93306
Myocardial Contrast Perfusion, 0439T
Strain Imaging, [93356]
Stress Test, 93351
with Contrast, 93352
with Myocardial Contrast Perfusion, 0439T
Transesophageal, [93319]
for Congenital Anomalies, 93315
3D Imaging During Procedure, [93319]
for Guidance Intracardiac or Great Vessel Intervention, 93355
for Monitoring Purposes, 93318
Transthoracic, 93306 [93356]
for Congenital Anomalies, 93303-93304
3D Imaging During Procedure, [93319]
with Myocardial Contrast Perfusion, 0439T
with Stress Test, [93356]
Echography
Abdomen, 76705
Cardiac, 93306, 93321, 93662, 0439T [93356]
Echography — *continued*
Cardiac — *continued*
Guidance for Biopsy, 76932
Chest, 76604
Extracranial Arteries, 93880-93882
Heart, 93306, 93321, 93662, 0439T [93356]
Guidance for Biopsy, 76932
Intracranial Arteries, [93896]
ECLS (Extracorporeal Life Support Services)
Cannulization
Insertion, 33951
Removal, [33965]
Repositioning, 33957
Creation Graft Conduit, [33987]
Daily Management, 33949
Initiation, 33947
Left Heart Vent Insertion, [33988]
Left Heart Vent Removal, [33989]
ECMO (Extracorporeal Membrane Oxygenation)
Cannulization
Insertion, 33951
Removal, [33965]
Repositioning, 33957
Creation Graft Conduit, [33987]
Daily Management, 33949
Initiation, 33947
Left Heart Vent Insertion, [33988]
Left Heart Vent Removal, [33989]
ED, 99281
Electrical Stimulation
Cardiac, 93623
Induction of Arrhythmia, 93618
Electrocardiography (ECG, EKG)
12-Lead ECG, 93000
16 Days up to 30 Days, 0937T
24–hour Monitoring, [93247]
48 Hours up to 7 Days, [93241, 93242, 93243, 93244]
7 Days up to 15 Days, [93245, 93246, 93247, 93248]
Algorithmically Generated 12-Lead, 0903T
Augmentative
Arrhythmia Analysis, 0897T
Heart Failure Detection, 0932T
Evaluation, 93000, 93010
External Recording
48-Hours Duration, [93243]
Auto Activated, 93268
Interpretation, 93272 [93244, 93248]
Mobile
Greater Than 24 Hours, 93229
Patient Activated, 93268
Transmission and Evaluation, 93268, 93271
Up to 30 Days Download, 93268
Holter Monitors, 93224
Microvolt T-Wave Alternans, 93025
Mobile Telemetry, 93229
Monitoring
with Attended Surveillance
Cardiovascular Telemetry with Physician Review and Report, 93228
Technical Support, 93229
Recording, [93248]
Rhythm
1-3 Leads, 93040
Evaluation, 93042
Interpretation and Report Only, 93042
Microvolt T-Wave Alternans, 93025
Recording, [93242, 93246]
Review and Interpretation, [93244, 93248]
Scanning Analysis with Report, [93243, 93247]
Tracing and Evaluation, 93040
Tracing Only without Interpretation and Report, 93005, 93041
Routine; at Least 12 Leads, 93000
Interpretation and Report Only, 93010
Tracing Only, without Interpretation and Report, 93005
with Interpretation and Report, 93000
Signal Averaged, 93278
Symptom-Related Memory Loop, 93268
Electrocardiography (ECG, EKG) — *continued*
Tracing, 93005
Electrogram, Atrial
Esophageal Recording, 93615-93616
Electronic Analysis
Cardiac Rhythm Monitor System, 93285, 93291, 93298
Data Analysis, 93291, 93298
Evaluation of Programming, 93285, 93291, 93298, 0650T
Cardioverter–Defibrillator
Evaluation
in Person, 93289, 93640, 93642, 0576T
Remote, 93296, 0579T
with Reprogramming, 93287, 93642-93644, 0577T
without Reprogramming, 93289, 93292, 93295, 93641
Data Analysis, 93289
Defibrillator, 93282, 93289, 93292, 93295
Electrophoresis
High Resolution, 83701
Electrophysiology Procedure
Intracardiac, 93644
Eloesser Procedure, 32035-32036
Eloesser Thoracoplasty, 32905
Embolectomy
Aortoiliac Artery, 34151-34201
Axillary Artery, 34101
Brachial Artery, 34101
Carotid Artery, 34001
Celiac Artery, 34151
Femoral, 34201
Iliac, 34151-34201
Innominate Artery, 34001
Mesentery Artery, 34151
Peroneal Artery, 34203
Popliteal Artery, 34201-34203
Pulmonary Artery, 33910
Radial Artery, 34111
Renal Artery, 34151
Subclavian Artery, 34001
Tibial Artery, 34203
Ulnar Artery, 34111
Embolic Protection Device
Insertion
Cerebral, 33370
Embolization
Arterial (Not Hemorrhage or Tumor), 37242
Hemorrhage
Arterial, 37244
Venous, 37244
Infarction, 37243
Leiomyomata, 37243
Lymphatic Extravasation, 37244
Organ Ischemia, 37243
Tumors, 37243
Venous Malformations, 37241
Emergency Department Services, 99281
Physician Direction of Advanced Life Support, 99288
Empyema
Closure
Chest Wall, 32810
Empyemectomy, 32540
Enucleation, 32540
Thoracostomy, 32035-32036, 32551
Empyemectomy, 32540
EMS, 99288
Endarterectomy
Coronary Artery, 33572
Anomaly, 33507
Pulmonary, 33916
Endograft
Aorta, 34701
Iliac Artery, [34717]
Infrarenal Artery, 34701
Endoluminal Imaging, [92979]
Endomyocardial
Biopsy, 93505
Endoscopy
Atria, 33266
Bronchi
Aspiration, 31646

- **Endoscopy** — *continued*
  - Bronchi — *continued*
    - Biopsy, 31625, 31632-31633
    - Computer-Assisted Image Guidance, 31627
    - Destruction
      - Lesion, 31641
      - Tumor, 31641
    - Dilation, 31631, 31636
    - Excision Tumor, 31640
    - Exploration, 31622
    - Lavage, 31624
    - Lesion, 31641
      - Destruction, 31641
    - Needle Biopsy, 31629, 31633
    - Occlusion, 31634
    - Placement
      - Fiducial Marker, 31626
      - Radioelement Catheter, 31643
      - Stent, 31631, 31637
    - Removal
      - Foreign Body, 31635
    - Revision
      - Stent, 31638
    - Specimen Collection, 31624
    - Stenosis, 31641
    - Tracheobronchoscopy, 31615
    - Tumor
      - Destruction, 31641
    - Ultrasound
      - Destruction, 31641
      - Excision, 31640
  - Chest Cavity
    - Diagnostic, 32604
    - Exploration, 32601
    - Surgical, 32671
    - with Biopsy, 32607
  - Heart
    - Atria, 33266
  - Larynx
    - Aspiration, 31515
    - Diagnostic, 31525-31526
      - Newborn, 31520
    - Dilation, 31529
    - Direct
      - Diagnostic, 31520, 31526
    - Exploration, 31520
    - Insertion Obturator, 31527
  - Lung, Biopsy, 31628, 31632
  - Mediastinoscopy
    - Biopsy, 39402
    - Exploration, 39401
  - Trachea
    - Biopsy, 31629
    - Dilation, 31631, 31636
    - Stent Placement, 31631
    - via Tracheostomy, 31615
  - Vascular
    - Surgical, 33509, 37500
- **Endotracheal Tube**
  - Intubation, 31500
- **Endovascular**
  - Repair
    - Angiography, [34717]
    - Aorta
      - Abdominal Aneurysm
        - Endograft Placement, [34717]
        - with Open Exposure, 34716
      - Coarctation, 33894
      - Descending Thoracic, 33880
      - Open After Failed Endovascular Repair, 34830
      - Visceral
        - Fenestrated Endograft, 34841
        - Modular Endograft, 34845
        - Unibody Endograft, 34845
    - Endograft
      - Aorta, 34701
      - Iliac Artery, [34717]
      - Infrarenal Artery, 34701
    - Femoral Artery, 34713
    - Iliac Artery, 34702
    - Iliac Artery Bifurcation, [34717]
- **Endovascular** — *continued*
  - Repair — *continued*
    - Infrarenal Abdominal Aorta
      - with Endograft, 34701, 34845 [34718]
    - Lower Extremity, 37220
    - Physician Planning 90 Minutes, 34839
    - Vena Cava, 37191
    - Visceral Aorta
      - with Endograft, 34841
  - Therapy
    - Ablation
      - Vein, 36473
  - Venous Arterialization
    - Tibial or Peroneal Vein, [0620T]
- **Endovenous Catheter Ablation**, 36473, 0524T [36483]
- **Endovenous Femoral-Popliteal Revascularization**, 0505T
- **Enucleation**
  - Pleural, 32540
- **EPS**, 93644
- **ER**, 99281
- **Ergonovine Provocation Test**, 93024
- **Esophagomyotomy**, 32665
  - Heller Type, 32665
  - Thoracoscopic, 32665
- **Esophagus**
  - Repair
    - Heller Esophagomyotomy, 32665
- **ESR**, 85651-85652
- **Established Patient Services**
  - Audio-only Visit, [98012-98015]
  - Audio-video Visit, [98004-98007]
  - Consultations
    - Inpatient/Observation, 99252
    - Office/Outpatient, 99242
    - Online/Telephone, 99446 [99452]
  - Critical Care, 99292
  - Emergency Department Services, 99281
  - Inpatient or Observation, 99221, 99231
    - Consultations, 99252
    - Discharge Management, 99239
    - Same Date Admit/Discharge, 99234
  - Nursing Facility, 99304
  - Office/Outpatient Visit, 99211
  - Online E/M
    - Consultations, 99446 [99452]
    - Physician, [99421]
  - Preventive, 99391
  - Prolonged
    - Inpatient or Observation, [99418]
    - Outpatient, [99417]
  - Transitional Care Management, 99496
  - Virtual Check-in, [98016]
- **Evaluation and Management (E/M) Services**
  - Advance Care Planning, 99498
  - Advanced Life Support
    - Physician Direction, 99288
  - Alcohol and/or Substance Abuse, 99409
  - Audio-only Visit, [98008-98015]
  - Audio-video Visit, [98000-98007]
  - Care Management Services
    - Advanced Care Planning, 99498
    - Chronic Care Management, [99437, 99439, 99490, 99491]
      - Complex, 99489
    - Principal Care Management, [99424]
    - Transitional Care, 99496
  - Care Plan Oversight
    - Home Health Agency Care, 99374
    - Home, Domiciliary, or Rest Home Care, [99425, 99437, 99491]
    - Hospice, 99378
    - Nursing Facility, 99380
  - Consultations
    - Inpatient or Observation, 99252
    - Interprofessional Internet/Telephone Electronic Health, 99446 [99452]
    - Office or Outpatient, 99242
  - Critical Care, 99292
  - Discharge Management
    - Inpatient or Observation, 99239
      - Same Date Admit/Discharge, 99234
- **Evaluation and Management (E/M) Services** — *continued*
  - Emergency Department, 99281
  - Emergency Medical Service (EMS), Direction, 99288
  - Inpatient or Observation, 99221, 99231
    - Consultations, 99252
    - Discharge Management, 99239
      - Same Date Admit/Discharge, 99234
    - Neonate, 99469
    - Pediatric, 99472, 99476
    - Prolonged Services, [99418]
    - Same Date Admit/Discharge, 99234
  - Internet/Online/Telephone Communication
    - Consult Physician/QHP, 99446 [99452]
    - Physician/QHP, [99421]
  - Neonatal
    - Critical Care, 99469
  - Nursing Facility
    - Care Plan Oversight, 99380
    - Initial Care, 99304
    - Subsequent Care, 99307
  - Office/Outpatient, 99202
    - Consultations, 99242
    - Prolonged Services, [99417]
  - Pediatric
    - Critical Care, 99472, 99476
  - Preventive
    - Group Counseling, 99412
    - Individual Behavior Change Interventions, 99406
    - Individual Counseling, 99401
  - Prolonged, 99358 [99418]
  - Remote Physiologic Monitoring, [99091, 99454, 99474]
    - Treatment Management, [99458]
  - Smoking and Tobacco Cessation Counseling, 99407
  - Standby Services, 99360
  - Team Conference, 99366
  - Telemedicine, [98000-98016]
  - Transitional Care Management, 99496
  - Virtual Check-in, [98016]
- **Evaluation**
  - Electrophysiologic, 93654, 93656
  - Implantable Cardioverter-Defibrillator Device
    - Interrogation, 93289, 93292, 93295, 93641, 0576T, 0578T-0579T
    - Programming, 93287, 93642-93644, 0575T, 0577T [93260]
  - Interrogation Device Evaluation, 93289, 93292, 93295, 93641, 0576T, 0578T-0579T
  - Pacemaker, 93279, 93286, 93288, 93293, 93296, 93724
    - Leadless, 93279, 93286, 93288, 93294, 93296, 0804T, 0826T
- **EVAR (Endovascular Aortic Repair)**, [34717]
- **Exchange**
  - Blood Components, 36511
- **Excision**
  - Aorta
    - Coarctation, 33840
  - Atrial Septum, 33736
  - Bullae
    - Lung, 32141
      - Endoscopic, 32655
  - Bypass Graft, 35901
  - Carotid Artery, 60605
  - Chest Wall Tumor, 21601
  - Cyst
    - Lung, 32140
    - Mediastinum, 32662
    - Pericardial, 33050
      - Endoscopic, 32661
  - Embolectomy/Thrombectomy
    - Aortoiliac Artery, 34151-34201
    - Axillary Artery, 34101
    - Brachial Artery, 34101
    - Carotid Artery, 34001
    - Celiac Artery, 34151
    - Femoral Artery, 34201
    - Heart, 33315
    - Iliac Artery, 34151-34201
- **Excision** — *continued*
  - Embolectomy/Thrombectomy — *continued*
    - Innominate Artery, 34001
    - Mesentery Artery, 34151
    - Peroneal Artery, 34203
    - Popliteal Artery, 34203
    - Radial Artery, 34111
    - Renal Artery, 34151
    - Subclavian Artery, 34001
    - Tibial Artery, 34203
    - Ulnar Artery, 34111
  - Embolism
    - Pulmonary Artery, 33910
  - Empyema
    - Lung, 32540
    - Pleural, 32540
  - Heart
    - Donor, 33940
    - Lung
      - Donor, 33930
  - Lesion
    - Carotid Body, 60600-60605
  - Lung, 32442, 32488
    - Bronchus Resection, 32486
    - Bullae
      - Endoscopic, 32655
    - Completion, 32488
    - Emphysematous, 32491
    - Heart
      - Donor, 33930
    - Lobe, 32480-32482
    - Pneumonectomy, 32442
    - Segment, 32484
    - Total, 32442
    - Tumor
      - with Reconstruction, 32504
      - with Resection, 32503
    - Wedge Resection, 32505
      - Endoscopic, 32666
  - Lymph Nodes
    - Mediastinal, 38746
    - Paratracheal, 38746
    - Thoracic, 38746
  - Pericardium, 33030-33031
    - Endoscopic, 32659
  - Pleura, 32310-32320
    - Endoscopic, 32656
  - Ribs, 21603, 32900
  - Sternum, 21620, 21630
  - Thrombectomy
    - Axillary Vein, 34490
    - Bypass Graft, 35875-35876
    - Femoropopliteal Vein, 34401
    - Iliac Vein, 34401
    - Subclavian Vein, 34471-34490
    - Vena Cava, 34401
  - Thromboendarterectomy
    - Aorta, Abdominal, 35331
    - Aortoiliac, 35361
    - Aortoiliofemoral, 35363
    - Axillary Artery, 35321
    - Brachial Artery, 35321
    - Carotid Artery, 35301, 35390
    - Celiac Artery, 35341
    - Femoral Artery, 35302, 35371-35372
    - Iliac, 35361-35363
    - Iliac Artery, 35351
    - Iliofemoral Artery, 35355, 35363
    - Innominate Artery, 35311
    - Mesenteric Artery, 35341
    - Peroneal Artery, 35306
    - Popliteal Artery, 35303
    - Renal Artery, 35341
    - Subclavian Artery, 35301, 35311, 35331, 35390
    - Superficial Femoral Artery, 35302
    - Tibial Artery, 35306
    - Tibioperoneal Trunk, 35304
    - Vertebral Artery, 35301, 35390
  - Thymus Gland, 60521
  - Thyroid Gland
    - Total
      - Sternal Split
        - Transthoracic, 60270

- **Excision** — *continued*
  - Trachea
    - Stenosis, 31781
  - Tricuspid Valve, 33463
  - Tumor/Lesion
    - Bronchi, 31640
    - Carotid Body, 60605
    - Chest Wall, 21601
    - Heart, 33120-33130
    - Mediastinum, 32662, 39220
    - Neck, [21552]
    - Pericardium, 32661, 33050
    - Pulmonary, 32504
    - Thorax, [21552]
  - Vein
    - Varicose, 37765-37766
- **Exclusion**
  - Left Atrial Appendage
    - Open, [33268]
    - Thoracoscopic, [33269]
- **Exercise Stress Tests**, 93464
- **Exercise Test**
  - Bronchospasm, 94617 [94619]
  - Cardiopulmonary, 94621
- **Exploration**
  - Abdomen
    - Blood Vessel, 35840
  - Artery
    - Brachial, 35702
    - Carotid, 35701
    - Femoral, 35703
    - Lower Extremity, 35703
    - Popliteal, 35703
    - Subclavian, 35701
    - Upper Extremity, 35702
  - Blood Vessel
    - Abdomen, 35840
    - Chest, 35820
    - Extremity, 35860
    - Neck, 35800
  - Bronchi
    - Endoscopy, 31622
  - Bronchoscopy, 31622
  - Chest
    - Penetrating Wound, 20101
    - Thoracoscopy, 32601
    - Thoracotomy, 32100
  - Heart, 33310-33315
  - Larynx, 31520
  - Mediastinum, 39000-39010
- **Extracorporeal Circulation**
  - Cannulization
    - Insertion, 33951
    - Removal, [33965]
    - Repositioning, 33957
  - Daily Management, 33949
  - Initiation, 33947
- **Extracorporeal Immunoadsorption**, 36516
- **Extracorporeal Life Support Services (ECLS)**
  - Cannulization
    - Insertion, 33951
    - Removal, [33965]
    - Repositioning, 33957
  - Daily Management, 33949
  - Initiation, 33947
- **Extracorporeal Membrane Oxygenation (ECMO)**
  - Cannulization
    - Insertion, 33951
    - Removal, [33965]
    - Repositioning, 33957
  - Daily Management, 33949
  - Initiation, 33947
- **Extremity**
  - Lower
    - Harvest of Vein for Bypass Graft, 35500
    - Harvest of Vein for Vascular Reconstruction, 35572
    - Repair of Blood Vessel, 35286
    - Revision, 35879-35881
  - Testing
    - Vascular Diagnostics, 93924
  - Upper
    - Harvest of Artery for Coronary Artery Bypass Graft, 35600
- **Extremity** — *continued*
  - Upper — *continued*
    - Harvest of Vein for Bypass Graft, 35500
    - Repair of Blood Vessel, 35206

F

- **Factor**
  - Blood Coagulation
    - III, 85730-85732
- **Fenestration Procedure**
  - Tracheostomy, 31610
- **FFR (Fractional Flow Reserve)**, 75580 [0523T]
- **Fibrillation**
  - Atrial, 33254
- **Fibrin Deposit**
  - Removal, 32150
- **Fibrinolysis**
  - Assay, 85396
  - Pleural Cavity
    - Instillation of Agent, 32562
- **Fine Needle Aspiration**
  - Evaluation
    - Lung, 32408
    - Mediastinum, 32408
    - Pleura, 32400
- **Finger**
  - Collection of Blood, 36415-36416
  - Repair
    - Blood Vessel, 35207
- **Fistula**
  - Arteriovenous, 36831
    - Injection, 36901
    - Revision
      - with Thrombectomy, 36831
      - without Thrombectomy, 36832
    - Thrombectomy without revision, 36831
  - Autogenous Graft, 36825
  - Bronchi
    - Repair, 32815
  - Chest Wall
    - Repair, 32906
  - Hemodialysis
    - Duplex Scan, 0876T
  - Tracheoesophageal
    - Speech Prosthesis, 31611
- **Flap**
  - Free
    - Microvascular Transfer, 49906
    - Omental, 49906
  - Omentum
    - Free
      - with Microvascular Anastomosis, 49906
- **Flick Method Testing**, 93598
- **Fluoroscopy**
  - Chest
    - Bronchoscopy, 31634
    - Complete (Four views), 71048
    - Partial (Two views), 71046
  - Drain Abscess, 75989
  - Needle Biopsy, 77002
  - Venous Access Device, 36598, 77001
- **Fontan Procedure**, 33615-33617
- **Foreign Body**
  - Removal
    - Bronchi, 31635
    - Lung, 32151
    - Mediastinum, 39000-39010
    - Pericardium, 33020
      - Endoscopic, 32658
    - Pleura, 32150-32151
      - Endoscopic, 32653
- **Fractional Flow Reserve (FFR)**, 75580 [0523T]
- **Fracture Treatment**
  - Bronchi
    - Endoscopy, 31630
  - Rib
    - Open, 21811
  - Sternum
    - Closed, 21820
    - Open, 21825
  - Trachea
    - Endoscopic, 31630
- **Fusion**
  - Pleural Cavity, 32560

G

- **Gago Procedure**
  - Repair, Tricuspid Valve, 33463
- **GHb**, 83036
- **Glenn Procedure**, 33622, 33767
- **Globulin**
  - Immune, 90381
- **Glutamic Aspartic Transaminase**, 84450
- **Glycohemoglobin**, 83037
- **Graft**
  - Aorta, 33845, 33852, 33859, 33864-33871
  - Artery
    - Coronary, 33505
  - Cartilage
    - Rib to Face
      - Three or More Segments
        - Two Locations, 35682-35683
  - Composite, 35682
  - Hepatorenal, 35535
  - Peroneal-Tibial, 35570
  - Tibial-Tibial, 35570
  - Tibial/Peroneal Trunk-Tibial, 35570
  - Vein
    - Cross–over, 34520
- **Great Vessel(s)**
  - Shunt
    - Aorta to Pulmonary Artery
      - Ascending, 33755
      - Descending, 33762
    - Central, 33764
    - Subclavian to Pulmonary Artery, 33750
    - Vena Cava to Pulmonary Artery, 33766-33767
- **Greenfield Filter Insertion**, 37191
- **Guide**
  - 3D Printed, Anatomic, 0562T
- **Gunther Tulip Filter Insertion**, 37191

H

- **Hand**
  - Repair
    - Blood Vessel, 35207
- **Harvesting**
  - Endoscopic
    - Artery for Bypass Graft, 33509
    - Vein for Bypass Graft, 33508
  - Lower Extremity Vein for Vascular Reconstruction, 35572
  - Upper Extremity Artery
    - for Coronary Artery Bypass Graft, 35600
  - Upper Extremity Vein
    - for Bypass Graft, 35500
- **Hct**, 85013-85014
- **HDL (High Density Lipoprotein)**, 83718
- **Health Behavior**
  - Alcohol and/or Substance Abuse, 99409
  - Smoking and Tobacco Cessation, 99407
- **Health Risk Assessment Instrument**, 96161
- **Heart Biopsy**
  - Ultrasound, Radiologic Guidance, 76932
- **Heart Vessels**
  - Angiography, 93563
  - Angioplasty, [92920, 92928, 92938, 92941, 92943]
  - Injection, 93569 [93573]
  - Insertion
    - Graft, 33335
  - Thrombolysis, [92977]
  - Valvuloplasty
    - Percutaneous, 92987
- **Heart**
  - Ablation
    - Arrhythmogenic Focus
      - Open, 33257
    - Ventricular Septum
      - Transcatheter Alcohol Septal Ablation, 93583
  - Allograft Preparation, 33933, 33944
- **Heart** — *continued*
  - Angiography
    - Injection, 93569 [93573]
  - Aortic Arch
    - with Cardiopulmonary Bypass, 33853
    - without Cardiopulmonary Bypass, 33852
  - Aortic Valve
    - Implantation, 33366 [33440]
    - Repair
      - Left Ventricle, 33414
      - Transcatheter Closure, 93591
    - Replacement, [33440]
      - Transcatheter, 33366
      - with Cardiopulmonary Bypass, 33406-33410
  - Arrhythmogenic Focus
    - Destruction, 33250-33251, 33261
  - Biopsy, 93505
    - Radiologic Guidance, 76932
  - Blood Vessel
    - Repair, 33321
  - Cardiac Output Measurements
    - by Indicator Dilution, 93598
  - Cardiac Rehabilitation, 93797-93798
  - Cardiac Rhythm Monitor System
    - Insertion, 93291
    - Interrogation, 93298
    - Programming, 93285, 0650T
  - Cardioassist, 92970-92971
  - Cardiopulmonary Bypass
    - Lung Transplant, 32852, 32854
    - Replacement Ventricular Assist Device, 33983
  - Cardioverter–Defibrillator
    - Evaluation and Testing, 93640-93642, 0575T
  - Catheterization, 93451
    - Combined Left and Right Heart, 93597
    - Flow–Directed, 93503
    - Left Heart, 93595
    - Right Heart, 93593
  - Closure
    - Patent Ductus Arteriosus, 93582
    - Septal Defect, 33615
      - Ventricular, 33675, 33681, 33776, 33780, 93581
    - Valve
      - Atrioventricular, 33600
      - Semilunar, 33602
  - Commissurotomy, Right Ventricle, 33476, 33478
  - CT Scan, 75571
    - Angiography, 75574
  - Defibrillator
    - Removal, 33243-33244
      - Pulse Generator Only, 33241
    - Repair, 33218-33220
    - Replacement, Leads, 33216-33217, 33249
    - Wearable Device, 93745
  - Destruction
    - Arrhythmogenic Focus, 33250, 33261
  - Electrical Recording
    - 3D Mapping, 93613
    - Atria, 93602
    - Atrial Electrogram, Esophageal (or Transesophageal), 93615-93616
    - Bundle of His, 93600
    - Right Ventricle, 93603
    - Tachycardia Sites, 93609
  - Electroconversion, 92960-92961
  - Electrode
    - Insertion, 33202
  - Electrophysiologic Follow–up Study, 93624
  - Electrophysiology Procedures, 93644
  - Endoscopy
    - Atrial, 33266
  - Evaluation of Device, 93640
  - Excision
    - Donor, 33930, 33940
    - Tricuspid Valve, 33460, 33465
  - Exploration, 33310-33315
  - Fibrillation
    - Atrial, 33254, 33256

[Resequenced]

Heart — *continued*
Hemodynamic Monitoring
with Pharmacologic Agent, 93463
with Physiologic Exercise Study, 93464
Implantable Defibrillator
Data Analysis, 93289, 93296
Evaluation
In Person, 93287, 93289
Remote, 93296
Initial Setup and Programming, 93745
Insertion Electrodes, 33216-33217, 33224, 33249
Pulse Generator, 33240
Insertion, [33230]
Removal, 33241
Replacement, [33262]
System, 33249 [33270]
Reposition Electrodes, 33215, 33226
Implantation
Artificial Heart, Intracorporeal, 33927
Intracorporeal, 33979
Total Replacement Heart System, Intracorporeal, 33927
Ventricular Assist Device
Extracorporeal, 33976, 33981
Intracorporeal, 33979, 33983
Percutaneous, 33991 [33995]
Incision
Atrial, 33254, 33256
Exploration, 33310-33315
Injection
Radiologic, 93566
Insertion
Balloon Device, 33973
Defibrillator, 33213
Electrode, 33210-33211, 33215, 33224
Pacemaker, 33206, 33212-33213
Catheter, 33210
Pulse Generator, [33221]
Ventricular Assist Device
Extracorporeal, 33976, 33981
Intracorporeal, 33979, 33983
Percutaneous, 33991 [33995]
Intraoperative Pacing and Mapping, 93631
Ligation
Fistula, 37607
Magnetic Resonance Imaging (MRI), 75565
with Velocity Flow Mapping, 75565
without Contrast Material, 75557
Myocardial Contrast Perfusion, 0439T
Myocardial Strain Imaging, [93356]
Myocardial Sympathetic Innervation Imaging, 0332T
Myocardium
Imaging, Nuclear, 78466
Perfusion Study, 78451
Sympathetic Innervation Imaging, 0332T
Nuclear Medicine
Blood Flow Study, 78414
Blood Pool Imaging, 78472-78483, 78494-78496
Myocardial Imaging, 78466
Myocardial Perfusion, 78451, 0439T
Shunt Detection (Test), 78428
Open Chest Massage, 32160
Output, 93598
Pacemaker
Conversion, 33214
Evaluation
In Person, 93279, 93286, 93288
Remote, 93293, 93296
Insertion, 33206
Pulse Generator, 33212-33213
Leadless
Dual-Chamber
Evaluation/Programming, 0804T
Insertion, 0795T
Removal, 0798T
Replacement, 0801T
Right Atrial
Insertion, 0823T
Programming, 0826T
Removal, 0824T

Heart — *continued*
Pacemaker — *continued*
Leadless — *continued*
Right Atrial — *continued*
Replacement, 0825T
Ventricular
Insertion, [33274]
Removal, [33275]
Replacement, [33274]
Removal, [33229]
Replacement, 33206
Catheter, 33210
Upgrade, 33214
Pacing
Arrhythmia Induction, 93618
Atria, 93610
Transcutaneous
Temporary, 92953
Ventricular, 93612
Positron Emission Tomography (PET), 78459 [78429, 78434]
Perfusion Study, 78491 [78430]
Reconstruction
Atrial Septum, 33736
Vena Cava, 34502
Recording
Left Ventricle, 93622
Right Ventricle, 93603
Tachycardia Sites, 93609
Removal
Balloon Device, 33974
Electrode, 33238
Ventricular Assist Device, 33977-33978
Intracorporeal, 33980
Removal Single/Dual Chamber
Electrodes, 33243-33244
Pulse Generator, 33241
Repair, 33218-33220
Repair
Anomaly, 33615-33617
Aortic Valve, 93591
Atrial Septum, 33254, 33256, 33641, 33647, 93580
Internal Shunt Device, 0613T
Atrioventricular Canal, 33660-33665
Complete, 33670
Prosthetic Valve, 33670
Atrioventricular Valve, 33660-33665
Cor Triatriatum, 33732
Electrode, 33218
Fenestration, 93580
Prosthetic Valve, 33670
Infundibular, 33476, 33478
Mitral Valve, 33420, 93591
Myocardium, 33542
Outflow Tract, 33476, 33478
Patent Ductus Arteriosus, 93582
Postinfarction, 33542-33545
Prosthetic Valve Dysfunction, 33496
Sinus Venosus, 33645
Tetralogy of Fallot, 33697, 33924
Tricuspid Valve, 33464, 0570T
Ventricle, 33611-33612
Obstruction, 33619
Ventricular Septum, 33545, 33647, 33681, 33697, 93581
Wound, 33300-33305
Replacement
Artificial Heart, Intracorporeal, 33928
Electrode, 33210-33211, 33217
Mitral Valve, 33430
Total Replacement Heart System, Intracorporeal, 33928
Tricuspid Valve, 33465
Ventricular Assist Device, 33981
Repositioning
Electrode, 33215, 33217, 33226
Tricuspid Valve, 33468
Resuscitation, 92950
Septal Defect
Repair
Ablation, 93583
Atrial, 33641, 33660
Closure, 33615, 33647

Heart — *continued*
Septal Defect — *continued*
Repair — *continued*
Atrial — *continued*
Internal Shunt Device, 0613T
Nikaidoh Procedure, 33783
Closure
Atrial, 33615, 33647
Percutaneous Transcatheter, 93583
Ventricular, 33647, 33675, 93581
Obliteration
Aortopulmonary, 33814
Ventricular, 33697, 33783
Closure, 33647, 33675, 93581
Post-infarction Defect, 33545
Septectomy, 33736
Septostomy, 33736
Transcatheter, Congenital Anomaly, 33741
Stimulation and Pacing, 93623
Thrombectomy, 33315
Ventricular Assist Device, 33976
Intracorporeal, 33979
Transplantation, 33935, 33945
Allograft Preparation, 33933, 33944
Tumor
Excision, 33120-33130
Ultrasound
Myocardial Strain Imaging, [93356]
Radiologic Guidance, 76932
Ventriculomyectomy, 33416
Ventriculomyotomy, 33416
Wound
Repair, 33300-33305
Heller Procedure, 32665
Hemapheresis, 36511
Hematoma
Incision and Drainage
Neck, 21501-21502
Thorax, 21501-21502
Hemodialysis
Duplex Scan
Access, 93990
Prior to Access Creation, 93985
Fistula, 0876T
Hemoglobin
Analysis
O2 Affinity, 82820
Hemogram
Manual, 85014-85018, 85032
Hemorrhage
Chest Cavity
Endoscopic Control, 32654
Lung, 32110
Hemothorax
Thoracostomy, 32551
Hernia
Repair
Lung, 32800
Hicks–Pitney Test
Thromboplastin, Partial Time, 85730-85732
High Density Lipoprotein, 83718
HLA
Antibody Detection, 86828
Holter Monitor, 93224
Home/Residence Services
Anticoagulation Management, 93793
Hospital Services
Inpatient/Observation
Discharge Management, 99239
Initial Care, 99221
Newborn and/or Pediatric, 99465, 99469, 99472, 99476
Prolonged, [99418]
Same Day Admit/Discharge, 99234
Subsequent Care, 99231
Hydration, 96361

I

IA, 36140, 36260
IAB, 33973
IABP, 33973
IAC, 33973
II, Coagulation Factor, 85611
Immune Globulins
Administration, 96365, 96372
Respiratory Syncytial Virus (RSV), 90380
Immunoadsorption
Extracorporeal, 36516
Implant
Artificial Heart, Intracorporeal, 33927
Cardiac Rhythm Monitor, 33285
Carotid Sinus Baroreflex Activation Device, 0266T
Coronary Sinus Reduction Device, 0645T
Defibrillator System, 33240 [33271]
Interatrial Septal Shunt
Percutaneous, Transcatheter, 0613T
Reservoir Vascular Access Device
Declotting, 36593
Total Replacement Heart System, Intracorporeal, 33927
Tricuspid Valve Prosthetic, [0646T]
Ventricular Assist Device, 33976
Intracorporeal, 33979
Ventricular Restoration Device
Left, [0643T]
Incision and Drainage
Abscess
Lung, 32200
Lymph Node, 38300-38305
Neck, 21501-21502
Thorax, 21501-21502
Cyst
Lung, 32200
Hematoma
Neck, 21502
Thorax, 21502
Incision
Aortic Valve, 33391
for Stenosis, 33415
Atrial Septum, 33736
Brachial Artery
Exposure, [34834]
Cricothyroid Membrane, 31605
Exploration
Heart, 33315
Femoral Artery
Exposure, 34813 [34812]
Heart
Exploration, 33310-33315
Iliac Artery
Exposure, [34820, 34833]
Lung
Biopsy, 32097
Decortication, 32220-32225
Mitral Valve, 33420-33422
Pericardium, 33030-33031
with Clot Removal, 33020
with Foreign Body Removal, 33020
with Tube Insertion, 33017
Pleural Cavity
Empyema, 32035-32036
Pneumothorax, 32551
Pulmonary Valve, 33474
Thorax
Empyema, 32035-32036
Pneumothorax, 32551
Trachea
Emergency, 31603-31605
Planned, 31600
Younger Than Two Years, 31601
with Flaps, 31610
Incompetent Vein
Endovenous Ablation, [36483]
Injection, 36471 [36466]
Indicator Dilution Studies, 93598
Infectious Agent Detection
Antigen Detection
Immunofluorescence
Cytomegalovirus, 87271
Infusion
Cerebral
Intravenous for Thrombolysis, 37195
Hydration, 96361
Intra-arterial, 96373
Intraosseous, 36680

 [Resequenced]

Infusion — *continued*
Intravenous (IV), 96365
Hydration, 96361
Pump Services
Intra-arterial
Insertion, 36260
Removal/Revision, 36262
Intravenous
Insertion, 36563
Removal/Revision, 36576-36578, 36590
Subcutaneous, 96369
Transcatheter Therapy, 37211, 75898
Injection
Angiography
Heart Vessels, 93569 [93573]
Cardiac Catheterization, 93569 [93573]
Contrast
Central Venous Access Device, 36598
Extremity
Pseudoaneurysm, 36002
Hydration, 96361
Intra-arterial, 96373
Intramuscular, 96372
Intravenous (IV), 96365
Hydration, 96361
Left Heart
Radiologic, 93563
Right Heart
Injection of Radiologic Substance, 93566
Sclerosing Agent
Intravenous, 36471 [36466]
Spider Veins, 36468
Shunt
Peritoneal
Venous, 49427
Spider Veins
Telangiectasia, 36468
Subcutaneous (SC)
Infusion, 96369
Injection, 96372
Therapeutic
Extremity Pseudoaneurysm, 36002
Lung, 32960
Thoracic Cavity
Instillation, 32561
Thoracoscopic, 32650
Thrombolytic, 37184
Trachea
Puncture, 31612
Venography, 36005
Inpatient or Observation Services, 99221, 99231
Consultations, 99252
Discharge Management, 99239
Same Date Admit/Discharge, 99234
Neonate, 99469
Pediatric, 99472, 99476
Prolonged Services, [99418]
Same Date Admit/Discharge, 99234
INR Monitoring, 93793
INR Test Review, 93793
Insertion
Balloon
Intra–aortic, 33967, 33973
Cannula
Arteriovenous, 36810-36815
Vein to Vein, 36800
Catheter
Abdomen, 36584, 49435 [36573]
Abdominal Artery, 36245
Aorta, 36200
Brachiocephalic Artery, 36215
Bronchi, 31717
Bronchus
for Intracavitary Radioelement Application, 31643
Cardiac
Flow Directed, 93503
Flow Directed, 93503
Lower Extremity Artery, 36245
Nasotracheal, 31720
Pelvic Artery, 36245
Pleural Cavity, 32550
Portal Vein, 36481

Insertion — *continued*
Catheter — *continued*
Pulmonary Artery, 36013
Pressure Sensor, 33289
Renal Artery, 36251
Right Heart, 36013
Thoracic Artery, 36215
Tracheobronchial, 31725
Transthoracic, 33621
Vena Cava, 36010
Venous, 36011-36012, 36416, 36500-36510, 36555, 36569, 36584 [36573]
Defibrillator
Heart, 33212-33213, 0571T
Leads, 33216-33217
Pulse Generator Only, 33240
Electrode
Heart, 33202, 33211, 33215, 33224, 0572T [33271]
Endotracheal Tube
Emergency Intubation, 31500
Graft
Aorta, 33335, 33866
Heart Vessel, 33335
Iliac Artery
Occlusion Device, 34808
Implantable Defibrillator
Leads, 33217, 33224
Pulse Generator Only, [33230]
Infusion Pump
Intra-arterial, 36260
Intravenous, 36563
Intracatheter/Needle
Aorta, 36160
Arteriovenous Dialysis Circuit, 36901
Intraarterial, 36140
Intravenous, 36000
Venous, 36000
IVC Filter, 37191
Needle
Bone, 36680
Intraosseous, 36680
Needle Wire Dilator
Stent
Trachea, 31730
Transtracheal for Oxygen, 31720
Obturator/Larynx, 31527
Pacemaker, 33206, 33213 [33221]
Leadless, 0795T, 0823T [33274]
PICC Line, 36569, 36584 [36573]
Prosthesis
Button
Larynx (Voice), 31611
Obturator, Larynx, 31527
Speech Aid, 31611
Vascular
Bypass Graft, 35681
Endovascular
Abdominal Aorta, 34845
Aorta, 34701
Delayed Placement, 34711
Aortic Valve, 33366
Celiac Artery, 34841
Cerebral Embolic Protection Device, 33370
Enhanced Fixation Device, 34712
Femoral Artery Closure, 34713
Iliac Artery, [34717]
Delayed Placement, 34711
Occlusion Device, 34808
Ilio-iliac, 34708
Infrarenal Abdominal Aortic, 34701, 34709, 34711, 34845
Mesenteric Artery, 34841
Mitral Valve, 33419, 0345T
Physician Planning, 34839
Pulmonary Valve, 33477
Renal Artery, 34841

Insertion — *continued*
Prosthesis — *continued*
Vascular — *continued*
Endovascular — *continued*
Shunt
Ascending Aorta to Pulmonary Artery, 33755
Central, 33764
Descending Aorta to Pulmonary Artery, 33762
Intracardiac, Transcatheter, 33746
Subclavian to Pulmonary Artery, 33750
Superior Vena Cava to Pulmonary Artery, 33767
Second Superior Vena Cava, 33768
Thoracic Aorta, 33880
Visceral Aortic/Artery, 34841
Open
Aorta, 33851
Aortic Arch, 33853
Aortic Valve, 33405
Artery Exposure for Endovascular Prosthesis Delivery, 34714, 34716 [34820, 34834]
Atrioventricular Valve, 33670
Brachial Artery, [34834]
Femoral Vein, 0744T
Infrarenal Aortic, 34830
Mitral Valve, 33426
Pulmonary Valve, 33475
Valve Prosthesis Repair, 33496
Ventricular Patch, 33548
Pulse Generator
Heart, 33212-33213
Shunt, 36835
Abdomen
Vein, 49425
Venous, 49426
Interatrial Septal Shunt
Percutaneous, Transcatheter, 0613T
Tube
Trachea, 31730
Venous Access Device
Central, 36560
Peripheral, 36570-36571
Venous Shunt
Abdomen, 49425
Ventricular Assist Device
Extracorporeal, 33976, 33981
Intracorporeal, 33979, 33983
Percutaneous, 33991 [33995]
Wireless Cardiac Stimulator, [0861T]
Instillation
Agent for Pleurodesis, 32561
Intermediate Care Facility (ICF) Visits
Care Plan Oversight, 99380
Initial Care, 99304
Subsequent Care, 99307
International Normalized Ratio
Test Review, 93793
Internet/Online/Telephone Communication Service
Interprofessional Consult, 99446 [99452]
Physician, [99421]
Interprofessional Online/Telephone Consultation, 99446 [99452]
Interrogation
Cardiac Rhythm Monitor System, 93285, 93291, 93298, 0650T
Cardiac Stimulator, 0521T
Cardio-Defibrillator, 93289, 93292, 93295
Cardiovascular Physiologic Monitoring System, 93290, 93298

Interrogation — *continued*
Carotid Sinus Baroreflex Activation Device, 0273T
Pacemaker, 93288, 93294, 93296
Ventricular Assist Device, 93750
Interruption
Vein
Femoral, 37650
Iliac, 37660
Intra-aortic Balloon Pump Insertion, 33967
Intra-arterial Infusion/Injection, 96373
Pump, 36260
Intracardiac
Echocardiography, 93662
Ischemia Monitoring System
Insertion
Electrode Only, 0526T
Implantable Monitor Only, 0527T
Monitoring System, 0525T
Interrogation, 0529T
Programming, 0528T
Removal
Complete System, 0530T
Electrode Only, 0531T
Implantable Monitor Only, 0532T
Replacement, 0525T
Mass
Removal/Debulking, 0644T
Shunt
Transcatheter, 33745-33746
Intracardiac Ischemia Monitoring, 0525T
Intracoronary
Drug Delivery
Transcatheter Balloon, 0914T
Oxygen Infusion
with Percutaneous Coronary Revascularization, 0659T
Intramuscular (IM) Injection, 96372
Intraoperative
Coronary Fractional Flow Reserve (FFR), [0523T]
Ultrasound
Epicardial Cardiac, 76987
Thoracic Aorta, 76984
Intravascular Ultrasound
Intraoperative Noncoronary Vessel, 37253
Intravascular Vena Cava Filter (IVC), 37191
Insertion, 37191
Removal, 37193
Reposition, 37192
Intravenous (IV), 96361-96365
Introduction
Needle or Catheter
Aorta, 36160-36200
Arterial System
Brachiocephalic Branch, 36215
Lower Extremity, 36245
Pelvic Branch, 36245
AV Shunt
Dialysis Circuit, 36901
Carotid, 36100
Extremity Artery, 36140
Vertebral Artery, 36100
Intubation
Endotracheal Tube, 31500
IVC Filter
Insertion, 37191
Removal, 37193
Reposition, 37192
Ivy Bleeding Time, 85002

J

Jatene Procedure
Repair, Great Arteries, 33770

K

K+, 84132
Kinase Creatine
Blood, 82552
Konno Procedure, 33412

L

Lactic Dehydrogenase, 83615-83625

Laparoscopy
Diaphragmatic Stimulation System
Insertion or Replacement, 0674T
Removal, Lead(s), 0679T
Repositioning, 0678T
Laryngoplasty
Cricotracheal Resection, 31592
Laryngoscopy
Exploration, 31520
Newborn, 31520
Larynx
Aspiration
Endoscopy, 31515
Dilation
Endoscopic, 31528-31529
Endoscopy
Exploration, 31520
Exploration
Endoscopic, 31520
Insertion
Obturator, 31527
Laser Surgery
Bronchi, 31641
Incompetent Vein, 36479
Myocardium, 33141
Revascularization, 33141
Tumor
Bronchi, 31641
Lavage
Lung
Bronchial, 31624
Total, 32997
LD (Lactic Dehydrogenase), 83615
LDH, 83615-83625
LDL, 83721
Leg
Lower
Artery
Ligation, 37618
Bypass Graft, 35903
Exploration
Blood Vessel, 35860
Repair
Blood Vessel, 35226
with Other Graft, 35286
with Vein Graft, 35256
Upper
Artery
Ligation, 37618
Bypass Graft, 35903
Exploration
Blood Vessel, 35860
Repair
Blood Vessel
with Other Graft, 35286
with Vein Graft, 35256
Leiomyomata
Embolization, 37243
Lesion
Carotid Body
Excision, 60600-60605
Lymph Node
Incision and Drainage, 38300-38305
Leukapheresis, 36511
Leukocyte Count, 85032
LeVeen Shunt
Insertion, 49425
Revision, 49426
Ligation
Artery
Abdomen, 37617
Carotid, 37600
Chest, 37616
Coronary, 33502
Extremity, 37618
Fistula, 37607
Neck, 37615
Temporal, 37609
Inferior Vena Cava, 37619
Shunt
Aorta
Pulmonary, 33924
Peritoneal
Venous, 49428
Thoracic Duct
Thoracic Approach, 38381
Ligation — *continued*
Thyroid Vessels, 37615
Vein
Clusters, 37785
Femoral, 37650
Iliac, 37660
Jugular, Internal, 37565
Perforator, 37761
Saphenous, 37718, 37780
Vena Cava, 37619
Linton Procedure, 37760
Lipoprotein
LDL, 83701, 83721
Lithotripsy
Coronary
Transluminal, [92972]
Liver
Ultrasound Scan (LUSS), 76705
Lobectomy
Lung, 32482, 32663, 32670
Sleeve, 32486
Segmental, 32663
Sleeve, 32486
Long Term Care Facility Visits
Care Plan Oversight, 99380
Initial, 99304
Subsequent, 99307
Lung
Ablation, 32998 [32994]
Abscess
Incision and Drainage, 32200
Angiography
Injection, 93569 [93573]
Biopsy
Bronchoscopy, 31625, 31629, 31633
Needle, 32400-32408
Thoracoscopy, 32607
Thoracotomy, 32096
Bullae
Excision, 32141
Endoscopic, 32655
Cyst
Incision and Drainage, 32200
Removal, 32140
Decortication
Endoscopic, 32651-32652
Partial, 32225
Total, 32220
with Parietal Pleurectomy, 32320
Empyema
Excision, 32540
Excision
Bronchus Resection, 32486
Completion, 32488
Donor, 33930
Heart Lung, 33930
Lung, 32850
Emphysematous, 32491
Empyema, 32540
Lobe, 32480-32482
Segment, 32484
Total, 32442
Tumor, 32504
Wedge Resection, 32505
Endoscopic, 32666
Foreign Body
Removal, 32151
Hemorrhage, 32110
Injection
Radiologic, 93569 [93573]
Lavage
Bronchial, 31624
Total, 32997
Lysis
Adhesions, 32124
Needle Biopsy, 32408
Pneumolysis, 32940
Pneumothorax, 32960
Removal
Bilobectomy, 32482
Bronchoplasty, 32501
Completion Pneumonectomy, 32488
Extrapleural, 32445
Single Lobe, 32480
Single Segment, 32484
Sleeve Lobectomy, 32486
Lung — *continued*
Removal — *continued*
Sleeve Pneumonectomy, 32442
Total Pneumonectomy, 32442
Two Lobes, 32482
Volume Reduction, 32491
Wedge Resection, 32505
Repair
Hernia, 32800
Segmentectomy, 32484
Tear
Repair, 32110
Thoracotomy, 32110
Biopsy, 32096
Cardiac Massage, 32160
for Postoperative Complications, 32120
Removal
Bullae, 32141
Cyst, 32140
Intrapleural Foreign Body, 32150
Intrapulmonary Foreign Body, 32151
Repair, 32110
with Excision–Plication of Bullae, 32141
with Open Intrapleural Pneumonolysis, 32124
Transplantation, 32851, 33935
Allograft Preparation, 32856, 33933
Donor Pneumonectomy
Heart–Lung, 33930
Lung, 32850
Tumor
Removal, 32504
Volume Reduction
Emphysematous, 32491
LUSS (Liver Ultrasound Scan), 76705
LVRS, 32491
Lymph Node(s)
Abscess
Incision and Drainage, 38300-38305
Excision
Thoracic, 38746
Removal
Thoracic, 38746
Lymphadenectomy
Mediastinal, 32674
Thoracic, 38746
Lymphadenitis
Incision and Drainage, 38300-38305
Lysis
Adhesions
Lung, 32124

M

Mandated Services
Hospital, On Call, 99026-99027
Mass Spectrometry and Tandem Mass Spectrometry
Analyte(s), 83789
Massage
Cardiac, 32160
Mayo Operation
Varicose Vein Removal, 37718, 37780-37785
Maze Procedure, 33258, 33266
Mediastinoscopy
with Biopsy, 39402
Mediastinotomy
Cervical Approach, 39000
Transthoracic Approach, 39010
Mediastinum
Cyst
Excision, 32662, 39200
Endoscopy
Biopsy, 39402
Exploration, 39401
Exploration, 39000-39010
Incision and Drainage, 39000-39010
Lymphadenectomy, 32674
Needle Biopsy, 32408
Removal
Foreign Body, 39000-39010
Tumor
Excision, 32662, 39220
Medical Team Conference, 99366
Microvolt T-Wave Alternans, 93025
Mitral Valve
Implantation or Replacement
Percutaneous, 0483T
Transthoracic, 0484T
Incision, 33420-33422
Repair, 33420
Incision, 33420-33422
Transcatheter, 33419, 93590, 93592, 0345T
Replacement, 33430
Model
3D Printed, Anatomic, 0560T
Modulation System, Cardiac, 0408T, 0915T
Molecular
Oxygen Saturation, 82805
Monitoring
Ablation Therapy
Incompetent Vein, 36473, 36479, 0524T [36483]
Arterial Catheterization, 36620
Blood Pressure, 24 hour, 93784
Cardiac
Cardiovascular Physiologic System, 93290, 93297
Ischemia System
Insertion
Complete System, 0525T
Electrode Only, 0526T
Implantable Monitor Only, 0527T
Interrogation, 0529T
Programming, 0528T
Removal
Complete System, 0530T
Electrode Only, 0531T
Implantable Monitor Only, 0532T
Replacement, 0525T
Rhythm, 33286
Subcutaneous, 93285, 93291, 93298, 0650T
Contrast
Catheter, 93503
Electrocardiography
Auto-Activated, 93268
Mobile
More than 24 Hours, 93229
Patient Activated, 93268
Time
More than 48 Hours Up to 7 Days, [93241]
More than 7 Days Up to 15 Days, [93245]
Up to 30 Days, 93268
Up to 48 Hours, 93224
Transmission and Evaluation, 93268, 93271
Hemodynamic Pulmonary Artery Pressure, 33289 [93264]
INR, 93793
Physiologic Parameters
Remote, [99454]
Treatment Management Services, [99458]
Prolonged
Cognitive Care Assess/Plan, [99417]
Evaluation & Management
After/Before Direct Patient Care, 99358
Clinical Staff Care, [99416]
Home/Residence, [99417]
Inpatient/Observation, [99418]
Outpatient, [99417]
Pulmonary Fluid System, 0607T-0608T
Remote Services
Cardiac Systems
Cardiac Contractility Modulation, 0418T, 0926T
Cardiac Rhythm, Subcutaneous, 93285, 93291, 93298, 0650T
Cardiovascular Physiologic, 93290, 93297

Monitoring — *continued*
Remote Services — *continued*
Cardiac Systems — *continued*
Defibrillator, 93287, 93289, 93292, 93296, 93644, 0575T-0576T [93260, 93261]
Ischemia, 0529T
Left Atrial Pressure Sensor, 0934T
Pacemaker, 93279, 93286, 93288, 93293, 93296, 93724, 0804T, 0826T
Pulmonary Artery Pressure Sensor, [93264]
Synchronized Diaphragmatic Stimulation (SDS), 0683T
Physiologic Monitoring
Data Collection/Interpretation, [99091, 99474]
Education, [99454]
Treatment Management, [99458]
Treatment Management, 98981
Therapeutic, Remote
Treatment Management Services, 98981
Mosenthal Test, 81002
MRI (Magnetic Resonance Imaging)
Heart
Complete Study, 75565
Flow Mapping, 75565
MTWA (Microvolt T-Wave Alternans), 93025
MUGA (Multiple Gated Acquisition), 78453-78454, 78473, 78483
Muscle Division
Scalenus Anticus, 21700-21705
Musculoskeletal System
Computer Assisted Surgical Navigational Procedure, 20985
Mustard Procedure, 33774
MVR, 33430
Myocardial
Imaging, 78466-78469, 0332T [93356]
Perfusion Imaging, 78451, 0439T [78432]
Positron Emission Tomography (PET), 78459 [78430]
Repair
Postinfarction, 33542
Myocardium, 33141
Myofibroma
Embolization, 37243

N

Navigation
Computer Assisted, 20985
Neck Muscle
Division, Scalenus Anticus, 21700-21705
Neck
Artery
Ligation, 37615
Biopsy, 21550
Bypass Graft, 35901
Exploration
Blood Vessels, 35800
Incision and Drainage
Abscess, 21501-21502
Hematoma, 21501-21502
Repair
Blood Vessel, 35201
with Other Graft, 35261
with Vein Graft, 35231
Tumor, [21552]
Needle Biopsy
Bronchi, 31629, 31633
Fluoroscopic Guidance, 77002
Lung, 32400-32408
Mediastinum, 32408
Pleura, 32400
Transbronchial, 31629, 31633
Needle Wire
Introduction
Trachea, 31730
Neonatal Critical Care, 99469
Nerves
Ablation, 0793T
Neurostimulator
Phrenic Nerve
Device Evaluation, [93151]
Insertion, [33276]
Sensing Lead, [33277]
Interrogation
with Programming, [93152]
without Programming, [93153]
Removal Only
Complete System, [33278]
Pulse Generator Only, [33280]
Tranvenous Lead Only, [33279]
Replacement
Pulse Generator Only, [33287]
Tranvenous Lead Only, [33288]
Repositioning, [33281]
Therapy Activation, [93150]
New Patient Services
Audio-only Visit, [98008-98011]
Audio-video Visit, [98000-98003]
Consultations
Inpatient/Observation, 99252
Office/Outpatient, 99242
Online/Telephone, 99446 [99452]
Critical Care, 99292
Emergency Department, 99281
Inpatient/Observation, 99221, 99231
Consultations, 99252
Discharge Management, 99239
Same Day Admit/Discharge, 99234
Nursing Facility, 99304
Office/Outpatient Visit, 99202
Prolonged
Inpatient or Observation, [99418]
Outpatient, [99417]
Newborn Care
Attendance at Delivery, 99464
Critical Care, 99469
Laryngoscopy, 31520
Resuscitation, 99465
Standby for C-Section, 99360
Umbilical Artery Catheterization, 36660
Nikaidoh Procedure, 33783
Nitrate Reduction Test
Urinalysis, 81001
Non-invasive Arterial Pressure, 93050
Norwood Procedure, 33619, 33622
Nuclear Medicine, [78429]
Blood
Flow Imaging, Noncardiac, 78445
Diagnostic, [78429]
Heart, [78432]
Blood Flow, 78414 [78434]
Blood Pool Imaging, 78472-78483, 78494-78496
Myocardial Imaging, 78459-78466 [78429, 78434]
Myocardial Perfusion, 78451, 0439T [78432]
Shunt Detection, 78428
Vascular Flow, Noncardiac, 78445
Venous Thrombosis, 78456
Nucleic Medicine
Vein
Thrombosis Imaging, 78456
Nursing Facility Services
Care Plan Oversight, 99379-99380
Initial Care, 99304
Subsequent Care, 99307
Nuss Procedure
with Thoracoscopy, 21743
without Thoracoscopy, 21742

O

O2 Saturation, 82810
Observation/Inpatient Services
Discharge Management, 99239
Initial, 99221
Same Date Admit/Discharge, 99234
Subsequent, 99231
Obstruction Clearance
Venous Access Device, 36596
Obturator Prosthesis
Insertion
Larynx, 31527
Occlusive Disease of Artery, 35001, 35005, 35081, 35091, 35102, 35111, 35121, 35131, 35141, 35151
Office/Outpatient Services
Consultation, 99242
Established Patient, 99211
New Patient, 99202
Prolonged Service, [99418]
Omentum
Flap, 49904
Free
with Microvascular Anastomosis, 49906
One Stage Prothrombin Time, 85611
Online/Internet/Telephone Assessment/Management
Interprofessional Consult, 99446 [99452]
Physician, [99421]
Operation/Procedure
Babcock, 37700
Blalock-Hanlon, 33735
Blalock-Taussig, 33750
Brock, 33474
Damus-Kaye-Stansel, 33606
Dor, 33548
Fontan, 33617
Heller, 32665
Norwood, 33612, 33619
SVR, SAVER, 33548
Optical Coherence Tomography
Endoluminal Imaging Coronary Graft or Vessel, [92979]
Organ or Disease Oriented Panel
Electrolyte, 80051
Lipid Panel, 80061
Ostectomy
Rib, 21502, 21600, 21610, 21616
Sternum, 21620
Osteomyelitis
Incision
Thorax, 21510
Outpatient Visit, 99202
Output, Cardiac
by Indicator Dilution, 93598
Oxygen Saturation, 82810

P

Pacemaker, Heart
Conversion, 33214
Electronic Analysis
Antitachycardia System, 93724
Electrophysiologic Evaluation, 93641
Evaluation, 93279, 93286, 93288, 93293, 93296
Leadless, 0804T
Insertion, 33206
Electrode(s), 33202, 33211, 33217, 33224
Leadless, 0795T, 0823T
Pulse Generator, 33213, 33240
Interrogation, 93294, 93296
Leadless
Dual-Chamber
Evaluation/Programming, 0804T
Insertion, 0795T
Removal, 0798T
Replacement, 0801T
Right Atrial
Insertion, 0823T
Programming, 0826T
Removal, 0824T
Replacement, 0825T
Ventricular
Insertion, [33274]
Removal, [33275]
Replacement, [33274]
Programming, 93279
Leadless, 0804T, 0826T
Relocation
Skin Pocket, 33223
Removal, 33237
Electrodes, 33235, 33238, 33244
Leadless, 0798T, 0824T [33275]
with Replacement, 0801T, 0825T [33274]
Pacemaker, Heart — *continued*
Removal — *continued*
Pulse Generator
Implantable Defibrillator, 33241
Pacemaker, 33233
Repair
Electrode(s), 33220
Leads, 33220
Replacement, 33206
Catheter, 33210
Electrode(s), 33211
Leadless, 0801T, 0825T [33274]
Leads, 33211
Pulse Generator, 33213
Repositioning
Electrodes, 33215, 33226, 33249
Telephonic Analysis, 93293
Upgrade, 33214
Pain Management
Intravenous Therapy, 96360
Pancoast Tumor Resection, 32504
Partial Thromboplastin Time, 85732
Patent Ductus Arteriosus
Closure, 93582
Patient-focused Health Risk Assessment, 96160
Peak Flow Rate, 94150
Pectus Carinatum
Reconstructive Repair, 21742
with Thoracoscopy, 21743
Pectus Excavatum Repair
Reconstructive Repair, 21742
with Thoracoscopy, 21743
Pediatric Critical Care
Initial, 99471
Subsequent, 99472
Percutaneous
Ablation
Nerve, 0793T
Arteriovenous Fistula Creation, [36837]
Atherectomies, 37225, 37227, 37229, 37231, 37233, 37235, 0234T
Transcatheter
Interatrial Septal Shunt, 0613T
Transluminal Angioplasty
Aortic, 33897 [37247]
Brachiocephalic, [37247]
Coronary Artery, [92920]
with Atherectomy, [92925, 92933]
with Stent, [92937]
Femoral, Popliteal, 37224
Iliac, 37220
Pulmonary, 92997-92998
Renal, [37247]
Tibioperoneal, 37228
Vein, [37249]
Visceral, [37247]
Transluminal Coronary Lithotripsy, [92972]
Perfusion
Myocardial, 78451
Imaging, 78466, 0439T
Positron Emission Tomography (PET)
Myocardial Imaging, [78430]
Pericardial Cyst
Excision, 33050
Thoracoscopic, 32661
Pericardial Sac
Biopsy, 32604
Drainage, 32659
Pericardial Window
for Drainage, 33025
Thoracoscopic, 32659
Pericardiectomies, 33031
Endoscopic, 32659
Pericardiectomy
Complete, 33031
Subtotal, 33031
Pericardiocentesis, 33016
Pericardiostomy
Tube, 33017
Pericardiotomy
Removal
Clot/Foreign Body, 33020
via Thoracoscopy, 32658

[Resequenced]

Pericardium
Cyst
Excision, 32661, 33050
Excision, 32659, 33031
Incision, 33031
Removal
Clot, 33020
Foreign Body, 33020
with Tube, 33017
Incision and Drainage, 33025
Puncture Aspiration, 33016
Removal
Clot
Endoscopic, 32658
Foreign Body
Endoscopic, 32658
Tumor
Excision, 32661, 33050
Peripheral Artery Disease (PAD), 93668
Rehabilitation, 93668
Peritoneum
Ligation
Shunt, 49428
Removal
Shunt, 49429
Venous Shunt, 49427
Persistent Truncus Arteriosus
Repair, 33786
PET Scan
Heart, 78414
Absolute Quantitation, [78434]
Blood Pool Imaging, 78473-78483, 78494-78496
Myocardial Imaging, 78459-78466 [78429]
Myocardial Perfusion, 78451, 0439T [78431]
pH
Blood Gases, 82805
Pheresis, 36511
Phlebectasia
Ablation, 36473
Removal, 37718, 37765
with Tissue Excision, 37760
Phlebectomy
Stab, 37766
Phlebographies, 78445, 78458
Injection, 36005
Phleborrhaphy
Femoral, 37650
Iliac, 37660
Phlebotomy
Therapeutic, 99195
Phosphocreatine Phosphotransferase, ADP, 82552
Phosphokinase, Creatine, 82552
Phosphotransferase, ADP Phosphocreatine, 82552
Physical Examination
Office and/or Other Outpatient Services, 99202
Physician Services
Care Management
Chronic, [99437, 99439]
Complex, 99487-99489
Principal, [99424]
Transitional, 99496
Care Plan Oversight
Domiciliary Facility, [99425, 99437, 99491]
Home Health Agency Care, 99374
Home/Residence Care, [99425, 99437, 99491]
Hospice, 99377-99378
Nursing Facility, 99379-99380
Supervision, 99379
Case Management, 99366
Consultations
Interprofessional Online/Telephone, 99446 [99452]
Direction, Advanced Life Support, 99288
Online/Internet/Telephone, [99421]
Prolonged, [99418]
Standby, 99360
Team Conference, 99367
PICC Line Insertion, 36569, 36584 [36573]
Placement
Bronchial Stent, 31637
Catheter
Aneurysm Sac Pressure Sensor, 34701
Bronchus
for Intracavitary Radioelement Application, 31643
Pleural, 32550
Renal Artery, 36251
Catheter, Cardiac, 93503
Endovascular Prosthesis
Aorta, 33883, 34701
Fenestrated Endograft, 34841
Iliac Artery, [34717]
Fiducial Markers
Intrathoracic, 32553
Guidance Catheter
Abscess, 75989
Specimen, 75989
Interstitial Device
Intrathoracic, 32553
Intravascular Stent
Cervical Carotid Artery, 37216
Innominate Artery, 37218
Intrathoracic Common Carotid Artery, 37218
IVC Filter, 37191
Needle
Bone, 36680
Pressure Sensor, 34701
Radiation Delivery Device
Intracoronary Artery, [92974]
Pleural Cavity, 32553
Sensor, Wireless
Endovascular Repair, 34701
Tracheal Stent, 31631
Transcatheter Stent
Carotid Artery, 37218
Physiologic Sensor, 34701
Platelet
Aggregation, 85576
Blood, 85025
Count, 85032
Plethysmography
Extremities, 93922-93923
Pleura
Biopsy, 32098, 32400
Decortication, 32320
Empyema
Excision, 32540
Excision, 32310-32320
Endoscopic, 32656
Foreign Body
Removal, 32150-32151
Incision, 32320
Needle Biopsy, 32400
Removal
Foreign Body, 32150, 32653
Repair, 32215
Thoracotomy, 32096, 32100
Pleural Cavity
Catheterization, 32550
Fusion, 32560
Incision
Empyema, 32035-32036
Pneumothorax, 32551
Puncture and Drainage, 32554
Thoracostomy, 32035-32036
Pleural Scarification
for Repeat Pneumothorax, 32215
Pleurectomy
Parietal, 32310-32320
Endoscopic, 32656
Pleuritis, Purulent, 21502
Pleurodesis
Agent for Pleurodesis, 32560
Endoscopic, 32650
Plication
Bullae, 32141
Pneumolysis, 32940
Pneumonectomy, 32442, 32671
Completion, 32488
Donor, 32850, 33930
Sleeve, 32442
Pneumonolysis, 32940
Intrapleural, 32652
Pneumonolysis — *continued*
Open Intrapleural, 32124
Pneumonostomy, 32200
Pneumothorax
Agent for Pleurodesis, 32560
Pleural Scarification for Repeat, 32215
Therapeutic
Injection Intrapleural Air, 32960
Port-A-Cath
Insertion, [36572]
Removal, 36589
Replacement, 36575
Port
Peripheral
Insertion, [36573]
Removal, 36590
Replacement, 36578, 36585
Venous Access
Insertion, 36561, 36566
Removal, 36590
Repair, 36576
Replacement, 36578, 36583
Positron Emission Tomography (PET)
Heart, 78414
Absolute Quantitation, [78434]
Blood Pool Imaging, 78473-78483, 78494-78496
Myocardial Imaging, 78459-78466 [78429]
Myocardial Perfusion, 78451, 0439T [78431]
Potassium
Serum, 84132
Potts-Smith Procedure, 33762
Preparation
for Transplantation
Heart, 33933, 33944
Heart/Lung, 33933
Lung, 32856, 33933
Pressure Sensor, Aneurysm, 34701
Pressure, Blood
24-Hour Monitoring, 93784
Venous, 93770
Pressure, Venous, 93770
Preventive Medicine
Administration and Interpretation of Health Risk Assessment, 96161
Counseling and/or Risk Factor Reduction Intervention, 99407
Established Patient Exam, 99391
Intervention, 99407
Behavior Change, 99406
Group Counseling, 99412
Individual Counseling, 99401
Principal Care Management Services, [99424, 99425, 99426, 99427]
Programming
Cardiac Rhythm Monitor System, 93285, 0650T
Cardiac Stimulator, Wireless, 0522T
Defibrillator System, 93287
Pacemaker, 93279, 93286, 93724
Leadless, 93279, 93286, 0804T
Right Atrial, 0826T
Prolonged Services
Before or After Direct Patient Contact, 99358
Clinical Staff, Face-to-Face Time, [99416]
Office, [99416]
Physician Standby Services, 99360
with or without Direct Patient Contact, Other Than Office
Cognitive Care/Assessment, [99417]
Inpatient/Observation, [99418]
Outpatient, [99417]
Prosthesis
Button
Larynx (Voice), 31611
Obturator
Larynx, 31527
Speech Aid, 31611
Vascular
Bypass Graft, 35681
Endovascular
Abdominal Aorta, 34845
Aorta, 34701
Prosthesis — *continued*
Vascular — *continued*
Endovascular — *continued*
Aorta — *continued*
Delayed Placement, 34711
Aortic Valve, 33366
Celiac Artery, 34841
Cerebral Embolic Protection Device, 33370
Enhanced Fixation Device, 34712
Femoral Artery Closure, 34713
Iliac Artery, [34717]
Delayed Placement, 34711
Occlusion Device, 34808
Ilio-iliac, 34708
Infrarenal Abdominal Aortic, 34701, 34709, 34711, 34845
Mesenteric Artery, 34841
Mitral Valve, 33419, 0345T
Physician Planning, 34839
Pulmonary Valve, 33477
Renal Artery, 34841
Shunt
Ascending Aorta to Pulmonary Artery, 33755
Central, 33764
Descending Aorta to Pulmonary Artery, 33762
Intracardiac, Transcatheter, 33746
Subclavian to Pulmonary Artery, 33750
Superior Vena Cava to Pulmonary Artery, 33767
Second Superior Vena Cava, 33768
Thoracic Aorta, 33880
Valve Prosthesis Repair, 33496
Ventricular Patch, 33548
Visceral Aortic/Artery, 34841
Open
Aorta, 33851
Aortic Arch, 33853
Aortic Valve, 33405
Artery Exposure for Endovascular Prosthesis Delivery, 34713, 34714, 34716, 34813 [34820, 34834]
Atrioventricular Valve, 33670
Brachial Artery, [34834]
Femoral Vein, 0744T
Infrarenal Aortic, 34830
Mitral Valve, 33426
Pulmonary Valve, 33475
Valve Prosthesis Repair, 33496
Ventricular Patch, 33548
Protein C Activator, 85337
Protein
Urine
by Dipstick, 81001
Prothrombin
Time, 85610-85611
Prothrombinase
Partial Time, 85730-85732
Protime, 85611
PT, 85611
PTA, 36903, 36906, 37220, 92998 [37246]
PTCA
Artery, Aortic, [37247]
PTT, 85730-85732
Pulmonary
Artery
Angiography Injection, 93569 [93573]
Angioplasty, 92998
Banding, 33690
Catheterization, 36013
Embolism, 33910
Percutaneous Transluminal Angioplasty, 92998
Pressure Sensor
Insertion, 33289
Remote Monitoring, [93264]

[Resequenced]

Pulmonary — *continued*
Artery — *continued*
Reimplantation, 33788
Repair, 33690, 33920, 33926
Reimplantation, 33788
Shunt
from Aorta, 33755-33762
from Vena Cava, 33767
Subclavian, 33750
Systemic-to-Pulmonary Ligation/Takedown, 33924
Transection, 33922
Decortication, 32220-32225, 32320, 32652
Fluid Monitoring System, 0608T
Hemorrhage, 32110
Valve
Incision/Repair, 33474
Replacement, 33475
Vein
Repair
Complete, 33730
Partial, 33724
Stenosis, 33726
Pulmonology
Diagnostic
Hemoglobin Oxygen Affinity, 82820
Stress Test, 94618
Vital Capacity, 94150
Therapeutic
Ventilation Assist, 94002
Pulse Generator
Heart
Insertion/Replacement, 33212-33213
Pulse Rate Increased
Heart
Recording, 93609
Pump Services
Oxygenator/Heat Exchange, 99190
Puncture
Artery, 36600
Aspiration
Pericardium, 33016
Pleural Cavity, 32555
Tracheal, 31612
Chest
Aspiration, 32555
Drainage, 32557
Pericardium, 33016
Pleural Cavity
Aspiration, 32555
Drainage, 32557
Tracheal, 31612
Pyothorax
Incision and Drainage, 21501-21502

Q

QTc Interval
Augmentative Analysis, 0902T
Quantitative Carotid Atheroma Evaluation, 93895
Quantitative Carotid Intima Media Thickness Evaluation, 93895
Quick Test
Prothrombin Time, 85610-85611

R

Radial Arteries
Aneurysm, 35045
Embolectomy, 34111
Thrombectomy, 34111
Radiation Therapy
Cardiac Focal Ablation for Arrhythmia, 0745T
Radioelement Substance
Catheter Placement
Bronchus, 31643
Rapid Heart Rate
Heart
Recording, 93609
Raskind Procedure, 33736
Rastelli Procedure, 33786
RBC, 85007, 85014, 85041, 85652
Reconstruction
Abdominal Wall
Omental Flap, 49905

Reconstruction — *continued*
Apical–Aortic Conduit, 33404
Atrial, 33258
Endoscopic, 33266
Open, 33258
Bronchi
Graft Repair, 31770
Stenosis, 31775
with Lobectomy, 32501
with Segmentectomy, 32501
Cardiac Anomaly, 33622
Chest Wall
Omental Flap, 49905
Trauma, 32820
Conduit
Apical–Aortic, 33404
Heart
Atrial, 33258
Endoscopic, 33266
Open, 33258
Atrial Septum, 33736
Pulmonary Artery Shunt, 33924
Vena Cava, 34502
Mitral Valve Annulus, 0545T
Sternum, 21742
with Thoracoscopy, 21743
Trachea
Graft Repair, 31770
Intrathoracic, 31760
Tricuspid Valve Annulus, 0545T
Vena Cava, 34502
Red Blood Cell (RBC)
Count, 85032
Hematocrit, 85014
Morphology, 85007
Platelet Estimation, 85007
Sedimentation Rate
Automated, 85652
Manual, 85651
Reductase, Lactic Cytochrome, 83615-83625
Reduction
Fracture
Bronchi, Bronchus
Closed
Endoscopic Treatment, 31630
Rib
Open Treatment, 21811
Sternum
Open Treatment, 21825
Trachea, Tracheal
Closed
Endoscopic Treatment, 31630
Lung Volume, 32491
Rehabilitation
Artery
Occlusive Disease, 93668
Cardiac, 93797-93798
Rehydration, 96361
Reimplantation
Arteries
Aorta Prosthesis, 35697
Carotid, 35691, 35694-35695
Subclavian, 35693
Vertebral, 35691-35693
Visceral, 35697
Coronary Ostia, 33783
Pulmonary Artery, 33788
Relocation
Defibrillator Site
Chest, 33223
Pacemaker Site
Chest, 33222
Remote
Monitoring Services
Cardiac Systems
Cardiac Contractility Modulation, 0418T, 0926T
Cardiac Rhythm, Subcutaneous, 93285, 93291, 93298, 0650T
Cardiovascular Physiologic, 93290, 93297

Remote — *continued*
Monitoring Services — *continued*
Cardiac Systems — *continued*
Defibrillator, 93287, 93289, 93292, 93296, 93644, 0575T-0576T [93260, 93261]
Ischemia, 0529T
Left Atrial Pressure Sensor, 0934T
Pacemaker, 93279, 93286, 93292, 93296, 93724, 0804T, 0826T
Pulmonary Artery Pressure Sensor, [93264]
Synchronized Diaphragmatic Stimulation (SDS), 0683T
Physiologic Monitoring
Data Collection/Interpretation, [99091, 99474]
Education, [99454]
Treatment Management, [99458]
Treatment Management, 98981
Removal
Balloon
Intra–aortic, 33974
Balloon Assist Device
Intra–aortic, 33968, 33971
Blood Component
Apheresis, 36511
Cardiac Event Recorder, 33286
Carotid Sinus Baroreflex Activation Device, 0270T
Catheter
Central Venous, 36589
Pleural, 32552
Clot
Pericardium, 33020
Endoscopic, 32658
Defibrillator
Heart, 33244
Pulse Generator Only, 33241
via Thoracotomy, 33243
Subcutaneous Defibrillator Electrode Removal, [33272]
Subcutaneous Pulse Generator, 33241 [0614T, 33262]
Electrode
Heart, 33234, 0573T, 0580T
Embolus, Artery
Aortoiliac, 34201
Axillary, 34101
Brachial, 34101
Carotid, 34001
Celiac, 34151
Femoropopliteal, 34201
Iliac, 34151-34201
Innominate, 34001
Mesentery, 34151
Peroneal, 34203
Popliteal, 34203
Pulmonary, 33910
Radial, 34111
Renal, 34151
Subclavian, 34001
Tibial, 34203
Ulnar, 34111
Fibrin Deposit, 32150
Foreign Bodies
Bronchi, 31635
Lung, 31635, 32151
Mediastinum, 39000-39010
Pericardium, 33020
Endoscopic, 32658
Pleura, 32150-32151
Endoscopic, 32653
Implantable Defibrillator, 33241
Infusion Pump
Intra–arterial, 36262
Intravenous, 36590
Intra–aortic Balloon, 33974
Assist Device, 33968, 33971
Intracardiac Mass, 0644T
Intravascular Vena Cava (IVC) Filter, 37193
Lung
Apical Tumor, 32504
Bronchoplasty, 32501

Removal — *continued*
Lung — *continued*
Completion Pneumonectomy, 32488
Cyst, 32140
Emphysematous, 32491
Extrapleural, 32445
Pneumonectomy, 32442
Single Lobe, 32480
Single Segment, 32484
Sleeve Lobectomy, 32486
Sleeve Pneumonectomy, 32442
Two Lobes, 32482
Volume Reduction, 32491
Lymph Nodes
Thoracic, 38746
Mass, Intracardiac, 0644T
Pacemaker, [33229]
Leadless, 0798T, 0824T [33275]
Pulse Generator
Substernal Implantable Defibrillator, [0614T]
Shunt
Heart, 33924
Peritoneum, 49429
Vein
Clusters, 37785
Perforation, 37760
Saphenous, 37718, 37780
Secondary, 37785
Varicose, 37765-37766
Ventricular Assist Device, 33977-33978
Intracorporeal, 33980
Renal Arteries
Aneurysm, 35122
Angiography, 36251
Angioplasty, [37247]
Atherectomy, 0234T
Bypass Graft, 35536, 35560, 35632
Embolectomy, 34151
Thrombectomy, 34151
Thromboendarterectomy, 35341
Renal Dialysis
Duplex Scan
Access, 93990
Prior to Access Creation, 93985
Fistula, 0876T
Renal Disease Services
Arteriovenous Fistula
Revision, 36832-36833
Thrombectomy, 36831
Arteriovenous Shunt
Revision, 36832-36833
Thrombectomy, 36831
Reoperation
Carotid
Thromboendarterectomy, 35390
Coronary Artery Bypass
Valve Procedure, 33530
Distal Vessel Bypass, 35700
Repair
Abdomen
Hernia, 49435
Aneurysm
Aorta
Abdominal, 34701, 34830, 34841, 35081
Iliac Vessels, 35103, 37220 [34717]
Visceral Vessels, 35092
Infrarenal, 34701, 34830
Thoracic, 33883
Arteriovenous, 36832
Axillary-Brachial Artery, 35011-35013
Carotid Artery, 35002
Endovascular
Abdominal Aorta, [34718]
Iliac Artery, 35103, 37220 [34717]
Infrarenal Artery, 34701
Thoracic Aorta, 33880
Visceral Aorta, 34841
Femoral, 35142
Hepatic, Celiac, Renal, or Mesenteric Artery, 35122
Iliac Artery, 34701, 35132
Innominate, Subclavian Artery, 35022

[Resequenced]

Repair — *continued*
- Aneurysm — *continued*
  - Popliteal Artery, 35152
  - Radial or Ulnar Artery, 35045
  - Sinus of Valsalva, 33720
  - Subclavian Artery, 35002, 35022
  - Vertebral Artery, 35005
- Anomaly
  - Artery Arborization, 33926
  - Cardiac, 33608-33610, 33615-33617
  - Coronary Artery, 33507
  - Pulmonary Venous Return, 33730
- Aorta, 33321, 33802-33803
  - Coarctation, 33840, 33894
  - Graft, 33859, 33871
  - Thoracic
    - Endovascular, 33880, 33894
    - Prosthesis Placement, 33886
  - Visceral
    - Endovascular, 34841
- Aortic Arch
  - with Cardiopulmonary Bypass, 33853
  - without Cardiopulmonary Bypass, 33852
- Aortic Valve, 93591
  - Obstruction
    - Outflow Tract, 33414
  - Septal Hypertrophy, 33416
  - Stenosis, 33415
  - Valvuloplasty, 93591
- Arteriovenous Aneurysm, 36832
- Arteriovenous Fistula
  - Abdomen, 35182
    - Acquired or Traumatic, 35189
  - Extremities, 35184
    - Acquired or Traumatic, 35190
  - Head, 35180
    - Acquired or Traumatic, 35188
  - Neck, 35180
    - Acquired or Traumatic, 35188
  - Thorax, 35182
    - Acquired or Traumatic, 35189
- Artery
  - Angioplasty, 36903, 36905
    - Aorta, 33897 [37247]
    - Axillary, [37247]
    - Brachiocephalic, [37247]
  - Bypass Graft, 35570, 35633, 35697
  - Bypass In-Situ, 35583
  - Bypass Venous Graft, 33510, 35523
  - Coronary
    - Anomalous, 33507
  - Dialysis Circuit, 36903, 36905
  - Iliac, 35103, 37220 [34717]
  - Occlusive Disease, 35001, 35005, 35045-35081, 35091, 35102, 35111, 35121, 35131, 35141, 35151
  - Pulmonary, 33690, 33926
  - Renal, [37247]
  - Renal or Visceral, [37247]
  - Subclavian, [37247]
  - Thromboendarterectomy, 35304, 35390
  - Venous Graft, 33510, 35523
  - Visceral, [37247]
- Atria
  - Laparoscopic, 33266
  - Open, 33254
- Atrial Fibrillation, 33254, 33256
- Atrioventricular Canal, 33660
- Blood Vessel(s)
  - Abdomen, 35221, 35251, 35281
    - with Other Graft, 35281
    - with Vein Graft, 35251
  - Chest, 35211-35216
    - with Other Graft, 35271-35276
    - with Vein Graft, 35241-35246
  - Finger, 35207
  - Graft Defect, 35870
  - Hand, 35207
  - Intrathoracic, 35211-35216, 35241-35246, 35271-35276
  - Lower Extremity, 35226, 35256, 35286
    - with Other Graft, 35286
    - with Vein Graft, 35256

Repair — *continued*
- Blood Vessel(s) — *continued*
  - Neck, 35201, 35231, 35261
    - with Other Graft, 35261
    - with Vein Graft, 35231
  - Upper Extremity, 35206, 35236, 35266
    - with Other Graft, 35266
    - with Vein Graft, 35236
- Bronchi, 31770, 32501
  - Fistula, 32815
- Bypass Graft, 35901
  - Fistula, 35870
- Cannula, 36860-36861
- Central Venous Catheter, 36576
- Chest Wall, 32905
  - Closure, 32810
  - Fistula, 32906
  - Pectus Excavatum, 21740
- Cor Triatriatum or Supravalvular Mitral Ring, 33732
- Coronary Chamber Fistula, 33500-33501
- Defibrillator, Heart, 33218-33220
- Ductus Arteriosus, 33820
- Dysfunction
  - Prosthetic Valve, 33406
- Electrode, 33220
- Fistula
  - Coronary, 33501
  - Graft-Enteric Fistula, 35870
  - Sinus of Valsalva, 33702-33710
- Great Arteries, 33770
- Great Vessel, 33321
- Heart
  - Anomaly, 33600
  - Atria
    - Laparoscopic, 33266
    - Open, 33254
  - Atrioventricular Canal, 33660-33665
    - Complete, 33670
  - Atrioventricular Valve, 33660-33665
  - Blood Vessel, 33321
  - Cor Triatriatum, 33732
  - Fibrillation, 33254, 33256
  - Infundibular, 33476, 33478
  - Mitral Valve, 33420, 93590, 93592
  - Myocardium, 33542
  - Outflow Tract, 33476, 33478
  - Post-infarction, 33542-33545
  - Prosthetic Valve, 33670, 33852-33853
  - Prosthetic Valve Dysfunction, 33496
  - Pulmonary Artery Shunt, 33924
  - Pulmonary Valve, 33474
  - Septal Defect, 33545, 33608-33610, 33681, 33697
    - Atrial and Ventricular, 33647
    - Atrium, 33641
  - Sinus Venosus, 33645
  - Tetralogy of Fallot, 33692
  - Tricuspid Valve, 33465, 0570T
  - Ventricle, 33611-33612
    - Obstruction, 33619
  - Wound, 33300-33305
- Hernia
  - Lung, 32800
- Hypoplasia
  - Aortic Arch, 33619
- Iliac Artery, 35103, 37220 [34717]
- Lung
  - Hernia, 32800
  - Pneumolysis, 32940
  - Tear, 32110
- Mitral Valve, 33420, 93590, 93592, 0544T
- Neck Muscles
  - Scalenus Anticus, 21700-21705
- Obstruction
  - Ventricular Outflow, 33414, 33619
- Pacemaker
  - Heart
    - Electrode(s), 33218-33220
- Pectus Carinatum, 21742
  - with Thoracoscopy, 21743
- Pectus Excavatum, 21742
  - with Thoracoscopy, 21743
- Pectus Excavatum or Carinatum, 21740, 21743
- Pleura, 32215

Repair — *continued*
- Pulmonary Artery, 33917-33920, 33926
  - Reimplantation, 33788
- Pulmonary Valve, 33474
- Pulmonary Venous
  - Anomaly, 33724
  - Stenosis, 33726
- Scalenus Anticus, 21700-21705
- Septal Defect
  - Ablation, 93583
  - Atrial, 33641, 33660
    - Closure, 33615, 33647
    - Internal Shunt Device, 0613T
    - Nikaidoh Procedure, 33783
  - Closure
    - Atrial, 33615, 33647
    - Percutaneous Transcatheter, 93583
    - Ventricular, 33647, 33675, 93581
  - Obliteration
    - Aortopulmonary, 33814
  - Ventricular, 33697, 33783
    - Closure, 33647, 33675, 93581
    - Post-infarction Defect, 33545
- Septectomy, 33736
- Septostomy, 33736
  - Transcatheter, Congenital Anomaly, 33741
- Stenosis
  - Pulmonary, 33783
- Tear
  - Lung, 32110
- Tetralogy of Fallot, 33692-33697
- Trachea
  - Fistula
    - with Plastic Repair, 31825
    - without Plastic Repair, 31820
  - Stenosis, 31781
  - Stoma, 31613-31614
    - with Plastic Repair, 31825
    - without Plastic Repair, 31820
  - Wound
    - Intrathoracic, 31805
- Transposition
  - Great Arteries, 33771-33774
- Tricuspid Valve, 33463, 0545T, 0570T
- Truncus Arteriosus
  - Rastelli Type, 33786
- Vein
  - Angioplasty, [37249]
  - Femoral, 34501
  - Graft, 34520
  - Insertion Bioprosthetic Valve, 0744T
  - Pulmonary, 33730
  - Transposition, 34510
- Wound
  - Cardiac, 33300-33305

Repeat Surgeries
- Carotid
  - Thromboendarterectomy, 35390
- Coronary Artery Bypass
  - Valve Procedure, 33530
- Distal Vessel Bypass, 35700

Replacement
- Aortic Valve, [33440]
  - Transcatheter, 33366
  - with Translocation Pulmonary Valve, [33440]
- Artificial Heart
  - Intracorporeal, 33929
- Cardioverter–Defibrillator, 33249 [0614T, 33262]
- Carotid Sinus Baroreflex Activation Device, 0266T
- Electrode
  - Heart, 33210-33211, 33216-33217
- Heart
  - Defibrillator
    - Leads, 33249
- Mitral Valve, 33430
- Pacemaker, 33206 [33227]
  - Catheter, 33210
  - Electrode, 33210-33211, 33216-33217
  - Leadless, 0801T, 0825T [33274]
  - Pulse Generator, [33221, 33229]

Replacement — *continued*
- Pacing Cardioverter–Defibrillator
  - Leads, 33243-33244
  - Pulse Generator Only, 33241
- Pulmonary Valve, 33475
- Total Replacement Heart System
  - Intracorporeal, 33929
- Tricuspid Valve, 33465
  - Prosthetic Device, [0646T]
- Venous Access Device, 36582-36583, 36585
  - Catheter, 36578
- Venous Catheter
  - Central, 36580-36581, 36584
- Ventricular Assist Device, 33981

Repositioning
- Central Venous Catheter, Previously Placed, 36597
- Defibrillator, [33273]
- Electrode
  - Heart, 33215, 33226, 0574T
- Intravascular Vena Cava Filter, 37192
- Tricuspid Valve, 33468

Resection
- Aortic Valve Stenosis, 33415
- Bullae, 32141
- Chest Wall, 21601, 32900
- Cyst
  - Mediastinal, 39200
- Emphysematous Lung, 32672
- Lung, 32491, 32504, 32672
- Myocardium
  - Aneurysm, 33542
  - Septal Defect, 33545
- Pancoast Tumor, 32504
- Radical
  - Lymph Node(s)
    - Thoracic, 38746
  - Neck, 21558
  - Sternum, 21558
  - Thorax, 21558
- Ribs, 21601, 32900
- Thoracotomy Wedge, 32505
- Thymus, 32673
- Tumor
  - Lung, 32504
  - Mediastinal, 39220
  - Pericardial, 33050

Respiratory Syncytial Virus (RSV)
- Administration
  - Other, 90471-90472

Rest Home Visit
- Care Plan Oversight, [99425, 99437, 99491]

Restoration
- Ventricular, 33548
  - Device, [0643T]

Resuscitation
- Cardiac Massage via Thoracotomy, 32160
- Cardiopulmonary (CPR), 92950

Reticulocyte
- Count, 85045

Revascularization
- Distal Upper Extremity
  - with Interval Ligation, 36838
- Femoral, Popliteal Artery, 37224, 0505T
- Heart
  - Myocardial Resection, 33542
- Iliac Artery, 37220
- Interval Ligation
  - Distal Upper Extremity, 36838
- Peroneal, Tibial, 37228
- Popliteal, Femoral Artery, 37224
- Tibial, Peroneal Artery, 37228
- Transmyocardial, 33141
- with Intracoronary Infusion, 0659T

Revision
- Abdomen
  - Peritoneal-Venous Shunt, 49426
- Aorta, 33404
- Atrial, 33254
- Bronchial Stent, 31638
- Bronchus, 32501
- Bypass Graft
  - Vein Patch, 35685
- Carotid Sinus Baroreflex Activation Device, 0269T

Revision — *continued*
Infusion Pump
Intra-arterial, 36261
Intravenous, 36578, 36583
Lower Extremity Arterial Bypass, 35881
Venous Access Device, 36578, 36583, 36585
Ventricle
Ventriculomyectomy, 33416
Ventriculomyotomy, 33416
Rhythm Monitor, Cardiac, 33286
Rib
Excision, 21603, 32900
Fracture Treatment
Open, 21811
Resection, 21601, 32900
Right Atrioventricular Valve, 33464
Right Heart Cardiac Catheterization, 93457
for Congenital Anomalies, 93593
Risk Factor Reduction Intervention
Behavior Change Interventions, 99406
Group Counseling, 99412
Individual Counseling, 99401
Ross Procedure, 33413
Ross-Konno Procedure, [33440]

S

SAECG, 93278
Salivary Gland Virus
Antigen Detection
Direct Fluorescence, 87271
Sang–Park Procedure
Septectomy, Atrial, 33736-33741
SAST, 84450
SAVER (Surgical Anterior Ventricular Endocardial Restoration), 33548
Scalenotomy, 21705
Scalenus Anticus
Division, 21705
Scarification of Pleura
Agent for Pleurodesis, 32560
Endoscopic, 32650
Scarification
Pleural, 32215
Schede Procedure, 32906
Sclerotherapy
Venous, 36468
Screening
Abdominal Aortic Aneurysm (AAA), 76706
Drug
Alcohol and/or Substance Abuse, 99409
Scribner Cannulization, 36810
Second Look Surgery
Carotid Thromboendarterectomy, 35390
Coronary Artery Bypass, 33530
Distal Vessel Bypass, 35700
Valve Procedure, 33530
Sedimentation Rate
Blood Cell
Automated, 85652
Manual, 85651
Segmentectomy
Lung, 32484, 32669
Senning Procedure
Repair, Great Arteries, 33774
Senning Type, 33774
Sensor
Transcatheter Placement
Left Atrial Pressure, 0933T
Pulmonary, 33289
Septal Defect
Repair
Ablation, 93583
Atrial, 33641, 33660
Closure, 33615, 33647
Internal Shunt Device, 0613T
Nikaidoh Procedure, 33783
Closure
Atrial, 33615, 33647
Percutaneous Transcatheter, 93583
Ventricular, 33647, 33675, 93581
Obliteration
Aortopulmonary, 33814
Ventricular, 33697, 33783
Closure, 33647, 33675, 93581

Septal Defect — *continued*
Repair — *continued*
Ventricular — *continued*
Post-infarction Defect, 33545
Septectomy, 33736
Septostomy, 33736
Transcatheter, Congenital Anomaly, 33741
Septectomy
Atrial, 33736
Closed, 33735
Septostomy
Atrial, 33736-33741
Serum
CPK, 82550
SG, 93503
SGOT, 84450
Shunt(s)
Arteriovenous Shunt
Dialysis Circuit, 36901
Creation
Arteriovenous
Direct, 36821
Thomas Shunt, 36835
Transposition, 36818
with Bypass Graft, 35686
with Graft, 36830
Intracardiac, 33745-33746
Great Vessel
Aorta
Pulmonary, 33924
Aortic Pulmonary Artery
Ascending, 33755
Descending, 33762
Central, 33764
Subclavian–Pulmonary Artery, 33750
Vena Cava to Pulmonary Artery, 33768
Intra–atrial, 33736
Intracardiac, 33745-33746
LeVeen
Insertion, 49425
Ligation, 49428
Removal, 49429
Revision, 49426
Peritoneal
Venous
Injection, 49427
Ligation, 49428
Removal, 49429
Pulmonary Artery
from Aorta, 33762, 33924
from Vena Cava, 33767
Subclavian, 33750
Revision
Arteriovenous, 36832
Transcatheter Intracardiac (TIS), 33745-33746
Signal–Averaged Electrocardiography, 93278
Sinus Venosus
Repair, 33645
Six-Minute Walk Test, 94618
Skilled Nursing Facilities (SNFs)
Care Plan Oversight, 99380
Initial Care, 99304
Subsequent Care, 99307
Sleep Apnea
Central
Neurostimulator System, [33276, 33288]
Smoking and Tobacco Cessation, 99407
Special Services
Analysis
Remote Physiologic Data, [99091]
On Call, Hospital Mandated, 99026-99027
Prolonged Attendance, [99418]
Public Health Emergency (PHE)
Respiratory-Transmitted Infectious Disease, 99072
Pump Services, 99190
Remote Physiological Monitoring, [99091, 99454, 99457]
Supply of Materials, 99070, 99072
Specimen Collection
Venous Catheter, 36592

SPECT
Heart
Myocardial Imaging, 78459, 78466 [78431]
Myocardial Perfusion, 78451, 0439T [78431]
Spectrometry
Mass Analyte(s), 83789
Spectroscopy
Bioimpedance, 93702
Speech
Prosthesis
Creation, 31611
Insertion, 31611
Spring Water Cyst, 33050
Excision, 33050
via Thoracoscopy, 32661
Standby Services, Physician, 99360
Stenosis
Aortic
Repair, 33415
Supravalvular, 33417
Bronchi, 31641
Reconstruction, 31775
Excision
Trachea, 31781
Repair
Trachea, 31781
Tracheal, 31781
Stent
Intravascular, 37218, 37236, 0505T
Placement
Bronchoscopy, 31631, 31637
Transcatheter
Intravascular, 37218, 37236
Revision
Bronchoscopy, 31638
Tracheal
via Bronchoscopy, 31631
Revision, 31638
Stereotaxis
Computer-Assisted
Orthopedic Surgery, 20985
Sternal Fracture
Closed Treatment, 21820
Open Treatment, 21825
Sternotomy
Closure, 21750
Sternum
Debridement, 21627
Excision, 21620, 21630
Fracture Treatment
Closed, 21820
Open, 21825
Ostectomy, 21620
Radical Resection, 21630
Reconstruction, 21742, 21750
with Thoracoscopy, 21743
Stimulators, Cardiac, 33203 [0863T]
Streptokinase, Antibody, 86590
Stress Tests
Cardiovascular
Echocardiography, 93351
with Contrast, 93352
Multiple Gated Acquisition (MUGA), 78472-78473
Myocardial Perfusion Imaging, 78451, 0439T
Pulmonary, 94618
Subclavian Arteries
Aneurysm, 35002, 35022
Angioplasty, [37247]
Bypass Graft, 35506, 35512, 35526, 35606, 35626, 35645
Embolectomy, 34001
Thrombectomy, 34001
Thromboendarterectomy, 35301, 35311
Transposition, 33889
Subcutaneous Implantable Defibrillator Device
Electrophysiologic Evaluation, [33270]
Insertion, [33270]
Defibrillator Electrode, [33271]
Implantable Defibrillator System and Electrode, [33270]

Subcutaneous Implantable Defibrillator Device — *continued*
Insertion — *continued*
Pulse Generator with Existing Electrode, 33240
Interrogation Device Evaluation (In Person), [93261]
Programming Device Evaluation (In Person), [93260]
Removal
Electrode Only, [33272]
Pulse Generator Only, 33241
with Replacement, [33262]
Repositioning Electrode or Pulse Generator, [33273]
Subcutaneous
Infusion, 96369
Injection, 96372
Substance and/or Alcohol Abuse Screening and Intervention, 99409
Supervision
Home Health Agency Patient, 99374
Supply
Materials, 99070, 99072
Surgical
Collapse Therapy, Thoracoplasty, 32906
Revision
Cardiac Valve Procedure, 33530
Carotid Thromboendarterectomy, 35390
Coronary Artery Bypass, 33530
Distal Vessel Bypass, 35700
Ventricular Restoration, 33548
Suspension
Aorta, 33800
Suture
Aorta, 33320-33321
Great Vessel, 33321
Thoracic Duct
Thoracic Approach, 38381
Trachea
Fistula, 31825
with Plastic Repair, 31825
without Plastic Repair, 31820
Stoma, 31825
with Plastic Repair, 31825
without Plastic Repair, 31820
Wound
Intrathoracic, 31805
Vein
Femoral, 37650
Iliac, 37660
Vena Cava, 37619
SVR (Surgical Ventricular Restoration), 33548
Swan-Ganz Catheter Insertion, 93503
Sympathectomy
Renal, 0339T
Thoracic, 32664
with Rib Excision, 21616
Syrinx
Pulmonary Fluid Monitoring, 0607T-0608T
System, Body
Cardiovascular, [33276]
Mediastinum/Diaphragm, 39402
System
Cardiac Contractility Modulation, 0408T, 0915T
Diaphragmatic Stimulation
Evaluation/Interrogation, 0685T
Insertion or Replacement, 0674T
Pulse Generator Only, 0680T
Programming, 0683T
Removal, 0679T
Pulse Generator Only, 0682T
Repositioning, 0678T
Pulse Generator Only, 0681T
Neurostimulator
Central Sleep Apnea, [33276, 33288]
Pulmonary Fluid Monitoring, 0608T

T

Tachycardia
Heart
Recording, 93609
Takeuchi Procedure, 33505

[Resequenced]

TBNA (Transbronchial Needle Aspiration), 31629, 31633
TCD (Transcranial Doppler), [93896]
Technique
Pericardial Window, 33017
Technology-based Service
Virtual Check-in, [98016]
TEE, [93319]
Telangiectasia
Injection, 36468
Telemedicine, [98000-98016]
Telephone/Internet/Online Services
Consultation, 99446 [99452]
Pacemaker Analysis, 93293
Temperature Gradient Studies, 93740
Temporal Arteries
Biopsy, 37609
Ligation, 37609
TEP (Tracheoesophageal Puncture), 31611
Testing
Exercise
Bronchospasm, 94617 [94619]
Cardiopulmonary, 94621
Tetralogy of Fallot, 33697, 33924
Therapeutic
Apheresis, 36511
Thoracectomy, 32906
Thoracentesis, 32555
Thoracic
Anterior Ramus
Anesthetic or Steroid Injection, 64416
Arteries
Catheterization, 36215
Cavity
Bypass Graft Excision, 35905
Endoscopy
Exploration, 32601
Surgical, 32671
Duct
Ligation
Thoracic Approach, 38381
Suture
Thoracic Approach, 38381
Empyema
Incision and Drainage, 21502
Thoracoplasty, 32905
with Closure Bronchopleural Fistula, 32906
Thoracoscopy
Biopsy, 32607
Diagnostic, 32608
Surgical, 32671
Control Traumatic Hemorrhage, 32654
Creation Pericardial Window, 32659
Esophagomyotomy, 32665
Excision
Mediastinal Cyst, Tumor and/or Mass, 32662
Pericardial Cyst, Tumor and/or Mass, 32661
Lymphadenectomy, 32674
Parietal Pleurectomy, 32656
Partial Pulmonary Decortication, 32651
Pleurodesis, 32650
Removal
Clot, 32658
Foreign Body, 32653, 32658
Lung, 32671
Single Lobe, 32663
Single Lung Segment, 32669
Two Lobes, 32670
Resection
Thymus, 32673
Resection-Plication
Bullae, 32655
Emphysematous Lung, 32672
Sternum Reconstruction, 21743
Thoracic Sympathectomy, 32664
Total Pulmonary Decortication, 32652
Wedge Resection, 32666
Thoracostomy
Empyema, 32035-32036
Tube, 32551
Thoracotomy
Biopsy, 32096
Thoracotomy — *continued*
Cardiac Massage, 32160
Cyst Removal, 32140
Exploration, 32100
for Postoperative Complications, 32120
Hemorrhage, 32110
Lung Repair, 32110
Open Intrapleural Pneumolysis, 32124
Removal
Bullae, 32141
Cyst, 32140
Defibrillator, 33243
Electrodes, 33238
Foreign Body
Intrapleural, 32150
Intrapulmonary, 32151
Pacemaker, 33236-33237
Resection-Plication of Bullae, 32141
Transmyocardial Laser Revascularization, 33140-33141
Wedge Resection, 32505
Thorax
Biopsy, 21550
Incision
Empyema, 32035-32036
Pneumothorax, 32551
Incision and Drainage
Abscess, 21501-21502
Deep, 21510
Hematoma, 21501-21502
Tumor, [21552]
Thrombectomy
Aortoiliac Artery, 34151-34201
Arterial, Mechanical, 37185
Arteriovenous Fistula
Graft, 36904
Axillary Artery, 34101
Axillary Vein, 34490
Brachial Artery, 34101
Bypass Graft, 35875-35876
Noncoronary/Nonintracranial, 37184
Carotid Artery, 34001
Celiac Artery, 34151
Dialysis Circuit, 36904
Dialysis Graft
without Revision, 36831
Femoral, 34201
Femoropopliteal Vein, 34421-34451
Iliac Artery, 34151-34201
Iliac Vein, 34401
Innominate Artery, 34001
Mesenteric Artery, 34151
Percutaneous
Coronary Artery, [92973]
Noncoronary, Nonintracranial, 37184
Vein, 37188
Peroneal Artery, 34203
Popliteal Artery, 34203
Radial Artery, 34111
Renal Artery, 34151
Subclavian Artery, 34001
Subclavian Vein, 34471-34490
Tibial Artery, 34203
Ulnar Artery, 34111
Vena Cava, 34401
Venous, Mechanical, 37188
Thrombocyte (Platelet)
Aggregation, 85576
Count, 85008
Manual Count, 85032
Thromboendarterectomy
Aorta, Abdominal, 35331
Aortoiliofemoral Artery, 35363
Axillary Artery, 35321
Brachial Artery, 35321
Carotid Artery, 35301, 35390
Celiac Artery, 35341
Femoral Artery, 35302, 35372
Iliac Artery, 35351, 35361-35363
Iliofemoral Artery, 35355, 35363
Innominate Artery, 35311
Mesenteric Artery, 35341
Peroneal Artery, 35306
Popliteal Artery, 35303
Renal Artery, 35341
Subclavian Artery, 35301, 35311
Thromboendarterectomy — *continued*
Tibial Artery, 35306
Vertebral Artery, 35301
Thrombolysis
Cerebral
Intravenous Infusion, 37195
Coronary Vessels, [92977]
Cranial Vessels, 37195
Other Than Coronary or Intracranial, 37211
Thrombomodulin, 85337
Thromboplastin
Partial Time, 85730-85732
Thymectomy, 60521
Sternal Split
Transthoracic Approach, 60521-60522
Thymus Gland
Excision, 60521
Thyroid Gland
Excision
Total
Sternal Split
Transthoracic Approach, 60270
Thyroidectomy
Total
Sternal Split
Transthoracic Approach, 60270
Tibial
Arteries
Bypass Graft, 35570
Bypass In-Situ, 35587
Embolectomy, 34203
Thrombectomy, 34203
Thromboendarterectomy, 35306
TIS (Transcatheter Intracardiac Shunt), 33745-33746
Tissue Factor
Partial Time, 85732
TMR (Transmyocardial Revascularization), 33141
TMVI, 0484T
Tomographic SPECT
Myocardial Imaging, 78469
Tomography
Computed
Heart, 75571
Touroff Operation/Ligation, Artery, Neck, 37615
TR3SVR, 33548
Trachea
Aspiration, 31720
Catheter, 31720-31725
Dilation, 31631, 31636
Endoscopy
via Tracheostomy, 31615
Excision
Stenosis, 31781
Fistula
Repair, 31825
with Plastic Repair, 31825
without Plastic Repair, 31820
Fracture Treatment
Endoscopic, 31630
Incision
Emergency, 31603-31605
Planned, 31600-31601
with Flaps, 31610
Introduction
Needle Wire, 31730
Puncture
Aspiration and or Injection, 31612
Reconstruction
Graft Repair, 31770
Intrathoracic, 31760
Repair
Intrathoracic, 31760
Stoma, 31613-31614
Stenosis
Excision, 31781
Repair, 31781
Stoma
Repair, 31825
with Plastic Repair, 31825
without Plastic Repair, 31820
Trachea — *continued*
Tumor
Excision
Thoracic, 31786
Wound
Suture
Intrathoracic, 31805
Tracheal
Stent
Placement, 31631
Tube, 31500
Tracheobronchoscopy
via Tracheostomy, 31615
Tracheoesophageal Fistula
Speech Prosthesis, 31611
Tracheoplasty
Intrathoracic, 31760
Tracheoscopy, 31515
Tracheostoma
Revision, 31613-31614
Tracheostomy
Emergency, 31603-31605
Planned, 31600-31601
Surgical Closure
with Plastic Repair, 31825
without Plastic Repair, 31820
Tracheobronchoscopy Through, 31615
with Flaps, 31610
Transaminase
Glutamic Oxaloacetic, 84450
Transapical Mitral Valve Repair, 0543T
Transbronchial Needle Aspiration (TBNA), 31629, 31633
Transcatheter
Biopsy, 37200
Closure
Left Atrial Appendage, 33340
Percutaneous, Heart, 93582
Denervation
Renal Sympathetic, 0339T
Drug Delivery
Intracoronary Balloon, 0914T
Embolization
Vascular, 37241
Endovascular Venous Arterialization
Tibial or Peroneal Vein, [0620T]
Implantation and/or Replacement
Cerebral Embolic Protection Device, 33370
Coronary Sinus Reduction Device, 0645T
Interatrial Septal Shunt, 0613T
Left Atrial Pressure Sensor, 0933T
Mitral Valve
Percutaneous, 0483T
Transthoracic, 0484T
Tricuspid Valve, Prosthetic, [0646T]
Occlusion
Vascular, 37241
Placement
Intravascular Stent(s), 37218, 37236
Wireless Physiologic Sensor, 34701
Reconstruction
Mitral Valve Annulus, 0544T
Tricuspid Valve Annulus, 0545T
Removal
Foreign Body, 37197
Intracardiac Mass, 0644T
Restoration
Device
Left Ventricular, [0643T]
Shunt
Intracardiac, 33745-33746
Therapy
Infusion, 37211, 75898
Septal Reduction, 93583
Transcranial
Doppler Study (TCD), [93896]
Transection
Pulmonary Artery, 33922
Transesophageal
Echocardiography, [93319]
3D Imaging During Procedure for Congenital Anomalies, [93319]
Guidance for Intracardiac or Great Vessel Intervention, 93355

- **Transferase**
  - Aspartate Amino, 84450
  - Glutamic Oxaloacetic, 84450
- **Transfusion**
  - Blood, 36430
    - Push
      - Infant, 36440
- **Transitional Care Management**, 99496
- **Translocation**
  - Aortic Root, 33783
- **Transluminal**
  - Angioplasty
    - Arterial, 36903, 36906
    - Coronary, [92920]
    - Percutaneous, 33897
    - Radiological Supervision, [37247]
  - Atherectomies, 37227, 37229, 37231, 37233, 37235, 0234T [92925, 92934, 92938, 92941, 92943, 92973]
- **Transmyocardial Laser Revascularization**, 33140-33141
- **Transplantation**
  - Heart, 33945
    - Allograft Preparation, 33933, 33944
  - Heart–Lung, 33935
  - Lung
    - Allograft Preparation, 32856, 33933
    - Donor Pneumonectomy, 32850
    - Double with Cardiopulmonary Bypass, 32854
    - Double, without Cardiopulmonary Bypass, 32853
    - Single, with Cardiopulmonary Bypass, 32852
    - Single, without Cardiopulmonary Bypass, 32851
- **Transposition**
  - Arteries
    - Carotid, 33889, 35691, 35694-35695
    - Subclavian, 33889, 35693
    - Vertebral, 35691-35693
  - Great Arteries
    - Repair, 33770
  - Vein Valve, 34510
- **Transthoracic Echocardiography**, 0439T [93319, 93356]
  - 3D Imaging During Procedure for Congenital Anomalies, [93319]
- **Trendelenburg Operation**, 37785
- **Triacylglycerol**, 84478
- **Tricuspid Valve**
  - Excision, 33460
  - Repair, 33463, 0570T
  - Replace, 33465
    - Prosthetic Device, [0646T]
  - Repositioning, 33468
- **Triglycerides**, 84478
- **Troponin**
  - Qualitative, 84512
- **Truncus Arteriosus**
  - Repair, 33786
- **Truncus Brachiocephalicus**
  - Angioplasty, [37247]
  - Atherectomy, 0237T
  - Catheterization, 36215
- **Tube Placement**
  - Chest, 32551
- **Tubes**
  - Chest, 32551
  - Endotracheal, 31500
- **Tumor/Lesion**
  - Bronchi, 31641
  - Carotid Body, 60605
  - Chest Wall, 21601, 32998 [32994]
  - Heart, 33130
  - Lung, 32504, 32998 [32994]
  - Mediastinum, 32662, 39220
  - Neck, [21552]
  - Pericardium, 32661, 33050
  - Pleura, 32998 [32994]
  - Pulmonary, 32504, 32998 [32994]
  - Thorax, [21552]

U

- **UAC**, 36660
- **UCX (Urine Culture)**, 87088
- **Ulnar Arteries**
  - Aneurysm Repair, 35045
  - Embolectomy, 34111
  - Thrombectomy, 34111
- **Ultrasound**
  - Abdomen, 76700, 76706
  - Artery
    - Intracranial, [93896]
  - Chest, 76604
  - Drainage
    - Abscess, 75989
  - Guidance
    - Heart Biopsy, 76932
    - Pericardiocentesis, 33016
    - Vascular Access, 76937
  - Intraoperative
    - Epicardial Cardiac, 76987-76989
    - Thoracic Aorta, 76984
  - Intravascular
    - Intraoperative, 37253
  - Screening Study, Abdomen, 76706
- **Umbilical**
  - Vein Catheterization, 36510
- **Unlisted Services or Procedures**
  - Cineradiography, 76120-76125
  - Radiocinematographies, 76125
  - Videoradiography, 76125
- **Urinalysis**, 81001
  - Automated, 81001, 81003
  - Routine, 81002
  - without Microscopy, 81002
- **Urine**
  - Blood, 81001
  - Colony Count, 87086
  - Tests, 81001
- **Urothromboplastin**
  - Partial Time, 85732
- **UVC**, 36510

V

- **Vaccines**
  - Administration
    - Severe Acute Respiratory Syndrome Coronavirus (SARS-CoV-2 [COVID-19]), [90480]
  - Respiratory Syncytial Virus (RSV)
    - Monoclonal Antibody, 90380
      - Nonseasonal
        - Administration, 96372
      - Seasonal, 90381
    - Nonseasonal, 90679 [90683]
    - Seasonal, 90381
  - Severe Acute Respiratory Syndrome Coronavirus (SARS-CoV-2 [COVID-19]), [91304, 91318, 91319, 91320, 91321, 91322]
- **Valva Atrioventricularis Sinistra (Valva Mitralis)**
  - Incision, 33420-33422
  - Repair, 33420
    - Transcatheter, 33419
  - Replacement, 33430
- **Valve Stenosis, Aortic**
  - Repair, 33415
    - Supravalvular, 33417
- **Valve**
  - Aortic
    - Repair, Left Ventricle, 33414
    - Replacement, [33440]
  - Bicuspid
    - Incision, 33420-33422
    - Repair, 33420
      - Transcatheter, 33419
    - Replacement, 33430
  - Mitral
    - Incision, 33420-33422
    - Repair, 33420
      - Transcatheter, 33419
    - Replacement, 33430
  - Pulmonary
    - Incision, 33474
    - Repair, 33474
    - Replacement, 33475
  - Tricuspid
    - Excision, 33460
- **Valve** — *continued*
  - Tricuspid — *continued*
    - Implant
      - Prosthetic, [0646T]
    - Repair, 33463, 0570T
    - Replace, 33465
      - Prosthetic, [0646T]
    - Reposition, 33468
- **Valvectomy**
  - Tricuspid Valve, 33460
- **Valvotomy**
  - Mitral Valve, 33420-33422
  - Pulmonary Valve, 33474
  - Reoperation, 33530
- **Valvuloplasty**
  - Aortic Valve, 33391
  - Femoral Vein, 34501
  - Mitral Valve, 33425
  - Percutaneous Balloon
    - Aortic Valve, 92986
    - Mitral Valve, 92987
    - Pulmonary Valve, 92990
  - Prosthetic Valve, 33496
  - Reoperation, 33530
  - Tricuspid Valve, 33463, 0570T
- **Varicose Vein**
  - Ablation, 36473
  - Removal, 37718-37735, 37765
  - Secondary Varicosity, 37785
  - with Tissue Excision, 37735-37760
- **Vascular Procedure(s)**
  - Angioscopy
    - Noncoronary Vessels, 35400
  - Brachytherapy
    - Intracoronary Artery, [92974]
  - Endoluminal Imaging
    - Coronary Vessels, [92979]
  - Endoscopy
    - Surgical, 37500
  - Harvest
    - Lower Extremity Vein, 35572
  - Thrombolysis
    - Coronary Vessels, [92977]
    - Cranial Vessels, 37195
- **Vascular Rehabilitation**, 93668
- **Vascular Studies**
  - Angioscopy
    - Aorta, 93978-93979
    - Noncoronary Vessels, 35400
  - Arterial
    - Extracranial, 93882
    - Extremities, 93922
    - Intracranial, [93896]
    - Lower Extremity, 93922
    - Upper Extremity, 93930-93931
  - Blood Pressure Monitoring, 24 Hour, 93784
  - Hemodialysis Access, 93990
    - Prior to Access Creation, 93985
  - Hemodialysis Fistula, 0876T
  - Penile Vessels, 93980-93981
  - Temperature Gradient, 93740
  - Venous Studies
    - Extremities, 93971
    - Venous Pressure, 93770
  - Visceral Studies, 93975
- **Vascular Surgery**
  - Endoscopy, 37500
- **Vein**
  - Ablation
    - Endovenous, 36473
  - Anastomosis
    - Caval to Mesenteric, 37160
    - Portocaval, 37140
    - Renoportal, 37145
    - Saphenopopliteal, 34530
    - Vein, 34530
      - to Vein, 37140
  - Angioplasty
    - Transluminal, 36902, 36905, 36907 [37249]
  - Arm
    - Harvest of Vein for Bypass Graft, 35500
  - Axillary
    - Thrombectomy, 34490
- **Vein** — *continued*
  - Biopsy
    - Transcatheter, 37200
  - Cannulization
    - to Artery, 36810-36815
    - to Vein, 36800
  - Catheterization
    - Central Insertion, 36555, 36561-36563, 36566, 36578-36580
    - Organ Blood, 36500
    - Peripheral Insertion, 36569, 36571, 36585 [36573]
    - Removal, 36589
    - Repair, 36575
    - Replacement, 36578, 36584
    - Umbilical, 36510
  - Endoscopic Harvest
    - for Bypass Graft, 33508
  - External Cannula Declotting, 36860-36861
  - Extremity
    - Non–invasive Studies, 93971
  - Femoral
    - Repair, 34501
      - Insertion Bioprosthetic Valve, 0744T
  - Femoropopliteal
    - Thrombectomy, 34421-34451
  - Guidance
    - Fluoroscopic, 77001
    - Ultrasound, 76937
  - Heart
    - Venography, [93584]
  - Iliac
    - Thrombectomy, 34401-34451
  - Injection
    - Sclerosing Agent, 36468 [36466]
  - Insertion
    - IVC Filter, 37191
  - Interrupt
    - Femoral Vein, 37650
    - Iliac, 37660
    - Vena Cava, 37619
  - Leg
    - Harvest for Vascular Reconstruction, 35572
  - Ligation
    - Clusters, 37785
    - Jugular, 37565
    - Perforation, 37760
    - Saphenous, 37718, 37780
    - Secondary, 37785
  - Nuclear Medicine
    - Thrombosis Imaging, 78456
  - Portal
    - Catheterization, 36481
  - Pulmonary
    - Repair, 33730
  - Removal
    - Clusters, 37785
    - Saphenous, 37718, 37780
    - Varicose, 37765-37766
  - Repair
    - Angioplasty, [37249]
    - Graft, 34520
  - Stripping
    - Saphenous, 37718, 37780
  - Subclavian
    - Thrombectomy, 34471-34490
  - Thrombectomy
    - Other Than Hemodialysis Graft or Fistula, 35875-35876
  - Valve Transposition, 34510
  - Varicose
    - Ablation, 36473
    - Removal, 37718, 37765
    - Secondary Varicosity, 37785
    - with Tissue Excision, 37735-37760
  - Vena Cava
    - Thrombectomy, 34401
- **Vena Cava**
  - Catheterization, 36010
  - Interruption, 37619
  - Prosthetic Valve Implantation, 0806T
  - Reconstruction, 34502
- **Venesection**
  - Therapeutic, 99195

[Resequenced]

Venipuncture
Child/Adult
Cutdown, 36425
Percutaneous, 36410
Infant
Cutdown, 36420
Percutaneous, 36400
Routine, 36415
Venography
Heart, [93584, 93585, 93586, 93587, 93588]
Injection, 36005
Nuclear Medicine, 78445, 78457-78458
Venorrhaphy
Femoral, 37650
Iliac, 37660
Vena Cava, 37619
Venotomy
Therapeutic, 99195
Venous Access Device
Blood Collection, 36592
Declotting, 36593
Fluoroscopic Guidance, 77001
Insertion
Central, 36560
Peripheral, 36570-36571
Obstruction Clearance, 36595-36596
Removal, 36590
Repair, 36576
Replacement, 36582-36583, 36585
Catheter Only, 36578
Venous Blood Pressure, 93770
Venovenostomy
Saphenopopliteal, 34530
Ventilation Assist, 94002
Ventricular
Aneurysmectomy, 33542
Assist Device, 33983 [33995, 33997]
Ventricular — *continued*
Restoration Device, [0643T]
Ventriculomyectomy, 33416
Ventriculomyotomy, 33416
Vertebral
Arteries
Aneurysm, 35005
Bypass Graft, 35508, 35515, 35645
Catheterization, 36100
Thromboendarterectomy, 35301
Very Low Density Lipoprotein, 83719
Vessels Transposition, Great
Repair, 33770
Vicq D'Azyr Operation, 31600
Virtual Check-in, [98016]
Visceral Aorta Repair, 34841
Vital Capacity Measurement, 94150
VLDL, 83719
Voice Button
Speech Prosthesis, Creation, 31611
Volume
Reduction
Lung, 32491
Vulvectomy
Tricuspid Valve, 33463

W

Waterston Procedure, 33755
WBC, 85007, 85009, 85025
Wedge Resection
Chest, 32505, 32666
Well Child Care, 99391
Wellness Behavior
Alcohol and/or Substance Abuse, 99409
Smoking and Tobacco Cessation Counseling, 99407
Westergren Test
Sedimentation Rate, Blood Cell, 85651-85652
White Blood Cell
Count, 85032
Differential, 85004, 85009
Window, Pericardial, 33017
Wintrobe Test
Sedimentation Rate, Blood Cell, 85651-85652
Wireless
Cardiac Stimulator
For Left Ventricular Pacing
Insertion
Battery and Transmitter, 0517T
Complete System, 0515T
Electrode Only, 0516T
Interrogation, 0521T
Programming, 0522T
Relocation
Battery, [0862T]
Transmitter, [0863T]
Removal
Battery and Transmitter, [0861T]
Battery Only, 0518T
Removal with Replacement
Battery and Transmitter, 0519T
Battery Only, 0520T
Sensor
Left Atrial
Implantation, 0933T
Remote Monitoring, 0934T
Pulmonary, 33289
Remote Monitoring, [93264]
Wolff-Parkinson-White Procedure, 33250
Wound
Exploration
Penetrating
Chest, 20101
Suture
Trachea
Intrathoracic, 31805

X

X-ray
Abdomen, 74018
Chest
Complete (Four or More Views), 71048
Single View, 71045
Three Views, 71047
Two Views, 71046
with Contrast
Aorta, [34717]
Artery
Arteriovenous Shunt, 36901
Transcatheter Therapy, 75898
Angiogram, 75898
Central Venous Access Device, 36598
Iliac, [34717]

Y

Yacoub Procedure, 33864